Medical-Surgical Nursing
Concepts & Practice

Susan C. deWit, MSN, RN, CNS, PHN
Formerly, Instructor of Nursing
El Centro College
Dallas, Texas

Candice K. Kumagai, MSN, RN
Formerly, Instructor in Clinical Nursing
University of Texas at Austin
Austin, Texas

2nd Edition

ELSEVIER

ELSEVIER
SAUNDERS

3251 Riverport Lane
St. Louis, Missouri 63043
MEDICAL-SURGICAL NURSING: CONCEPTS & PRACTICE   ISBN: 978-1-4377-1707-5

Notices

Knowledge and best practice in this field are constantly changing. As new research and experience broaden our understanding, changes in research methods, professional practices, or medical treatment may become necessary.

Practitioners and researchers must always rely on their own experience and knowledge in evaluating and using any information, methods, compounds, or experiments described herein. In using such information or methods they should be mindful of their own safety and the safety of others, including parties for whom they have a professional responsibility.

With respect to any drug or pharmaceutical products identified, readers are advised to check the most current information provided (i) on procedures featured or (ii) by the manufacturer of each product to be administered, to verify the recommended dose or formula, the method and duration of administration, and contraindications. It is the responsibility of practitioners, relying on their own experience and knowledge of their patients, to make diagnoses, to determine dosages and the best treatment for each individual patient, and to take all appropriate safety precautions.

To the fullest extent of the law, neither the Publisher nor the authors, contributors, or editors, assume any liability for any injury and/or damage to persons or property as a matter of products liability, negligence or otherwise, or from any use or operation of any methods, products, instructions, or ideas contained in the material herein.

Previous edition copyrighted 2009

Library of Congress Cataloging-in-Publication Data
Medical-surgical nursing: concepts & practice / [edited by] Susan C. deWit, Candice Kumagai;
photographs by Jack Sanders. – 2nd ed.
    p.; cm.
  Includes bibliographical references and index.
  ISBN 978-1-4377-1707-5 (pbk. : alk. paper)
  I. DeWit, Susan C.   II. Kumagai, Candice K.
  [DNLM: 1. Perioperative Nursing. WY 161]

617′.0231–dc23   2011046197

Vice President: Loren Wilson
Executive Content Strategist: Teri Hines Burnham
Content Development Specialist: Tiffany Trautwein
Publishing Services Manager: Jeffrey Patterson
Senior Project Manager: Mary G. Stueck
Design Director: Karen Pauls
Marketing Manager: Kathleen Schlesinger

Printed in the United States of America

Last digit is the print number: 9 8 7 6 5 4 3

Selected Student Resources on Evolve

RESOURCES IN EVERY CHAPTER

Answer Guidelines for Critical Thinking Questions

Answers and Rationales for Review Questions for the NCLEX® Examination

Audio Glossary with pronunciations in English and Spanish

Bibliography and Suggested Readings

Body Spectrum A&P Coloring Book

Calculators

Helpful Phrases for Communicating in Spanish

Interactive Exercises and Activities

Interactive Review Questions for the NCLEX® Examination

Mathematics Review

Online Resources

SKILLS WITH SKILL PERFORMANCE CHECKLISTS

3-1	Starting the Primary Intravenous Infusion
3-2	Adding a New Solution to the Intravenous Infusion
3-3	Administering Intravenous Piggyback Medication
3-4	Adding Medication to an Intravenous Solution
3-5	Administering Medication via Saline or PRN Lock
3-6	Administering Medication with a Volume-Controlled Set
3-7	Administering an IV Bolus Medication (IV Push)
3-8	Discontinuing an Intravenous Infusion or PRN Lock
3-9	Administering Blood Products
14-1	Endotracheal and Tracheostomy Suctioning
14-2	Providing Tracheostomy Care
16-1	Phlebotomy and Obtaining Blood Samples with a Vacutainer System
29-1	Administering a Nasogastric/Duodenal Tube Feeding or Feeding via a PEG Tube
30-1	Steps for Changing an Ostomy Appliance
37-1	Combining Insulins
39-1	Assisting with a Pelvic Examination and Pap Test (Smear)

NURSING CARE PLANS

Chapter 19
Care of the Patient with a Venous Stasis Ulcer

Chapter 30
Care of the Patient with an Ostomy

Chapter 35
Care of the Patient with Renal Lithiasis

Chapter 46
Care of the Patient with Anxiety

Care of the Patient with Depression

Care of the Patient with Anorexia Nervosa

Chapter 49
Care of the Patient with Borderline Personality Disorder

PATIENT TEACHING

In addition to those in the textbook, the following Patient Teaching guidelines are available on Evolve.

Chapter 13
Guidelines for Effective Deep Breathing and Coughing

Chapter 15
How to Use a Metered-Dose Inhaler (MDI)

Oxygen Use in the Home

Self-Care Measures for Tuberculosis

Chapter 17
Precautions for the Patient with a Low Platelet Count (Thrombocytopenia)

Precautions for Preventing Infection for the Patient with a Low White Blood Cell Count

Chapter 22
Preparation for an EEG (Electroencephalogram)

Chapter 23
Care after Sustaining a Concussion

Chapter 26
Instilling Eye Drops

Chapter 29
Healing a Peptic Ulcer

Chapter 35
Hygiene Practices to Prevent Urinary Tract Infections

CLINICAL REFERENCES

Chapter 2
Admission Data Collection Form

Basic Care Worksheet

Interdisciplinary (Collaborative) Care Plan

Medication Reconciliation Form

Physical Assessment Form

Chapter 4
Consent for Surgery
Preoperative Checklist

Chapter 6
Health Promotion–*Healthy People 2020* Goals Related to
  Infectious Disease

Chapter 8
Health Promotion–*Healthy People 2020* Goals Related to
  Cancer

Chapter 9
Health Promotion–*Healthy People 2020* Goals Related to
  Rehabilitation
Katz Index of Independence in Activities of Daily
  Living
Minimum Data Set (MDS) 3.0
Rehabilitation Team Assessment Form
Team Conference Report
Team Kardex Form

Chapter 10
Immunization Schedule: 0 to 6 Years
Immunization Schedule: 7 to 18 Years
Immunization Schedule: Adult
Immunization Schedule: Catch-up, 4 Months to
  18 Years

Chapter 11
Health Promotion–*Healthy People 2020* Goals Related to
  HIV/AIDS

Chapter 15
Health Promotion–*Healthy People 2020* Goals Related to
  Lower Respiratory Disorders

Chapter 17
Health Promotion–*Healthy People 2020* Goals Related to Blood
  Disorders

Chapter 18
Health Promotion–*Healthy People 2020* Goals Related to
  Cardiovascular Health

Chapter 19
Health Promotion–*Healthy People 2020* Goals Related to
  Hypertension and Peripheral Vascular Disease

Chapter 20
Health Promotion–*Healthy People 2020* Objectives Related to
  Cardiovascular Disease

Chapter 21
Health Promotion–*Healthy People 2020* Goals Related to
  Cardiovascular Health
Health Promotion–*Healthy People 2020* Goals Related
  to Coronary Artery Disease and Myocardial
  Infarction

Chapter 22
Neurologic Assessment Flow Sheet

Chapter 24
Health Promotion–*Healthy People 2020* Goals Related to
  Stroke

Transient Ischemic Attack/Acute Ischemic Stroke
  Admission Form
Transient Ischemic Attack/Acute Ischemic Stroke Care Plan

Chapter 26
Health Promotion–*Healthy People 2020* Goals Related to
  Vision and Hearing

Chapter 27
Health Promotion–*Healthy People 2020* Goals Related to Eye
  and Ear Disorders

Chapter 33
Health Promotion–*Healthy People 2020* Goals Related to
  Arthritis and Osteoporosis

Chapter 35
Health Promotion–*Healthy People 2020* Goals Related to
  Chronic Kidney Disease

Chapter 38
Health Promotion–*Healthy People 2020* Goals Related to
  Diabetes and Hypoglycemia

Chapter 41
Health Promotion–*Healthy People 2020* Goals Related to
  Sexually Transmitted Infections

Chapter 43
PUSH Tool 3.0

Chapter 44
Health Promotion–*Healthy People 2020* Goals Related to
  Disaster and Bioterrorism

Chapter 46
Health Promotion–*Healthy People 2020* Goals Related to
  Anxiety, Mood, and Eating Disorders

Chapter 48
Health Promotion–*Healthy People 2020* Goals Related to
  Cognitive Disorders

Chapter 49
Health Promotion–*Healthy People 2020* Goals Related to
  Thought and Personality Disorders

ANIMATIONS

Chapter 10
Bacterial Replication
Virus and Surface Antigens

Chapter 15
Asthma
Hemothorax
Simple Pneumothorax and Tension Pneumothorax
Tuberculosis

Chapter 16
Differentiation of Blood Cells
Lymphocyte Function

Chapter 17
Hemophilia A
Sickle Cell Anemia
Thrombocytopenia

Chapter 18
Blood Clot Leading to Stroke
Chest Pain Radiating to Arm
Congestive Heart Failure
Function of Heart
Normal Cardiopulmonary Physiology
Normal Cardiopulmonary System
Pulmonary Embolus
Structure of the Heart
Vascular Tree: Heart, Aorta, Major Branches

Chapter 20
Atrial Fibrillation
Cardiac Arrest, Ventricular Fibrillation, External Heart
    Monitor
Ventricular Fibrillation

Chapter 21
Acute Coronary Syndrome (ACS), Acute Myocardial
    Infarction (AMI), Coronary Ischemia, Coronary Artery
    Disease
Coronary Artery Bypass Grafting (CABG)

Chapter 22
Brain Anatomy: Temporal Lobe, Brainstem, Cerebral
    Peduncle, Thalamus
Brain Lobes
Cranial Nerves

Chapter 23
Quadriplegia; Spinal Cord Injury
Spinal Cord Infarction
Spinal Cord Bleeding
Spine Structure

Chapter 24
Brain Abscess
Cerebellar Infarct; Stroke
Generalized Seizure
Meningitis
Subarachnoid Hemorrhage
TIA: Transient Ischemic Attack; CVA: Cerebrovascular
    Accident; Stroke; Brain Blood Clot

Chapter 25
Alzheimer's Disease
Guillain-Barré Syndrome
Parkinson's Disease

Chapter 26
Anatomy of Eye
Eye: Aqueous Humor, Vitreous Humor
Visual Pathway

Chapter 27
Retinal Detachment

Chapter 28
Abdominal Examination
Cirrhosis

Hepatobiliary Anatomy (Liver, Pancreas)
Passage of Food through Digestive Tract

Chapter 29
Bleeding Ulcer, Pathophysiology, Symptoms; Hematemesis
Perforated Duodenal Ulcer with Bleeding

Chapter 30
Appendicitis Symptoms
Diverticulitis
Inflamed Appendix, Appendicitis
Peritonitis, Ruptured Appendix

Chapter 33
Ankle Fracture
Dislocation of Bones (Hip, Knee, Shoulder, Elbow)
Hip Fracture, Femur Fracture, Femoral Fracture
Open Reduction Internal Fixation (ORIF) of Ankle

Chapter 34
Renal Anatomy and Function

Chapter 36
Adrenal Function

Chapter 39
Breast Cancer Spread; Metastasis
Chemotherapy
Radiation Therapy

Chapter 41
Pelvic Inflammatory Disease

Chapter 44
Anthrax

AUDIO CLIPS

Chapter 13
Bronchial Breath Sounds
Bronchovesicular Breath Sounds
High-Pitched Crackles
High-Pitched Wheeze
Low-Pitched Crackles
Low-Pitched Wheeze
Pericardial Friction Rub
Pleural Friction Rub
Stridor
Vesicular Breath Sounds

Chapter 18
Aortic Ejection Sound Related to S_1
Diastolic Murmur
Midsystolic Click Sound Related to S_1
Murmurs: Blowing, Harsh or Rough, and Rumble
Murmurs: High, Medium, and Low
Paradoxical Split Sound Related to S_2

Pulmonic Ejection Sound Related to S_1
S_1 at Various Locations
S_2 at Various Locations
Single S_1
Single S_2
Systolic Murmur
Fourth Heart Sound (S_4)
Fourth Heart Sound (S_4) with Bell Held Lightly then Applied Firmly
Third Heart Sound (S_3)
Wide Split Sound Related to S_2

VIDEO CLIPS

Chapter 13
Inspection and Palpation: Breathing and Respiratory Excursion, Anterior Chest
Inspection and Palpation: Respiration, Respiratory Excursion, and Tactile Fremitus
Posterior Chest
Palpation: Tactile Fremitus, Posterior Chest
Inspection and Percussion: Diaphragmatic Excursion
Percussion: Anterior Thorax

Chapter 18
Inspection and Palpation: Cardiac, Anterior Chest
Inspection and Palpation: Cardiac Auscultory Landmarks
Auscultation: Cardiac with Diaphragm
Auscultation: Cardiac with Bell
Auscultation: Cardiac with Diaphragm and Bell
Auscultation: Carotid Artery
Inspection and Palpation: Pulses, Lower Extremities

Chapter 22
Evaluation: Smell, Cranial Nerve I: Olfactory Nerve
Evaluation: Central Vision and Visual Acuity

Evaluation: Pupil Responses, Direct and Accomodation; Cranial Nerves III, IV, and VI: Oculomotor, Trochlear and Abducens Nerves
Evaluation: Light Touch; Face, Upper and Lower Extremities; Cranial Nerve V: Trigeminal Nerve
Inspection: Fine Motor Coordination, Upper Extremities
Inspection: Fine Motor Coordination, Lower Extremities

Chapter 26
Inspection and Palpation: External Ear
Inspection: Ear Canal
Inspection and Palpation: External Eye
Evaluation: Central Vision and Visual Acuity
Evaluation: Pupil Responses, Direct and Consensual
Inspection: Nose

Chapter 28
Auscultation: Abdomen, Bowel Sounds
Percussion: Abdomen
Percussion: Liver
Percussion: Spleen
Palpation: Abdomen Superficial and Deep

Chapter 32
Gait
Inspection: General Muscular Strength
Inspection and Palpation: Muscular Development

Chapter 39
Inspection: Female Breasts (Sitting)
Palpation: Female Breasts (Supine)
Inspection: External Genitalia
Inspection: Speculum Examination
Inspection and Palpation: Standing Position
Palpation: Inguinal Hernia Evaluation

*To my daughter and son-in-law, Kristen and Scott Webster,
who have given me a special grandson.*

*To all the students who will use this book to learn the art and science of nursing,
who one day may be taking care of me.*

*To my contributors, colleagues, and editors
who lend insight, support, and humor to the writing process.*

*To the memory of my aunt, "Bogie,"
who will always be in my heart.*

Susan C. deWit

*To my husband, Will,
who is always willing to stand by me,
no matter what hat I am wearing,
or how long I have been wearing it.*

*To my students,
who always make life fresh and interesting.*

Candice K. Kumagai

Contributors

Kim Cooper, MSN
Dean, School of Nursing
Ivy Tech Community College
Terre Haute, Indiana
Interactive Review Questions for the NCLEX®
  Examination
Interactive Exercises and Activities
Open-Book Quizzes
TEACH Lesson Plans
Test Bank

Carol Dallred, MSN, RNC, WHNP-BC
Advanced Practice Nurse
University of Texas
M.D. Anderson Cancer Center
Houston, Texas
Chapter 8   Care of Patients with Cancer
Chapter 9   Chronic Illness and Rehabilitation

Kelly Gosnell, RN, MSN
Associate Professor of Nursing
Ivy Tech Community College
Terre Haute, Indiana
Interactive Review Questions for the NCLEX®
  Examination
Interactive Exercises and Activities
Open-Book Quizzes
TEACH Lesson Plans
Test Bank

Signe S. Hill, BSN, RN, MA
Formerly, Instructor, Practical Nurse Program
Northeast Wisconsin Technical College
Green Bay, Wisconsin
Chapter 2   Critical Thinking and the Nursing Process

Helen Stephens Howlett, BSN, RN, MS
Formerly, Instructor, Practical Nurse Program
Northeast Wisconsin Technical College
Green Bay, Wisconsin
Chapter 1   Caring for Medical-Surgical Patients

Gloria Leifer, RN, MA, CNE
Professor, Obstetric and Pediatric Nursing
Riverside City College
Riverside, California
Chapter 39   Care of Women with Reproductive Disorders
Chapter 40   Care of Men with Reproductive Disorders
Chapter 41   Care of Patients with Sexually Transmitted
  Infections

Lauro Manalo, Jr., MSN, RN
Instructor, Associate Degree in Nursing Program
Allan Hancock College
Santa Maria, California
TEACH PowerPoint Slides with Audience Response System
  Questions

Trena L. Rich, RN, PHN, MSN, APRN, CIC
Director, Clinical Quality and Compliance
Patient Care Center
Western University of Health Sciences
Pomona, California
Chapter 6   Infection Prevention and Control
Chapter 10   The Immune and Lymphatic Systems
Chapter 11   Care of Patients with HIV/AIDS
Chapter 12   Care of Patients with Immune and Lymphatic
  Disorders

Reviewers

Kathy Lynn Burlingame, RN, MSN, CCRN, BSN, ADN
Academic Dean, Director of Nursing
Minnesota State Community and Technical College
Detroit Lakes, Minnesota

Dolores Cotton, RN, MSN
Practical Nursing Coordinator
Meridian Technology Center
Stillwater, Oklahoma

Gail E. Dunham RN, MSN
Professor of Nursing
Mid Michigan Community College
Harrison, Michigan

Ruth Ann Eckenstein, RN, MEd
Program Specialist
Oklahoma Department of Career and Technology
    Education
Stillwater, Oklahoma

Mary Gordon, MSN, CNS, PhD
Clinical Nurse Specialist
Children's Hospital of Houston
Houston, Texas

Nita Green, RN, MSN
Formerly, Nursing Program Director
Licensed Practical Nursing and Associate Degree
    Registered Nursing Programs
South Arkansas Community College
El Dorado, Arkansas

Janis Grimland
Interim Vocational Nursing Coordinator
Hill College
Hillsboro, Texas
Cleburne, Texas

Anna Allen Hamilton, RN, BSN, MS
Formerly, Instructor
McLennan Community College
Waco, Texas

Jeanne Hately, PhD, MSN, RN, PLNC
President
Professional Nurse Consultants, LLC
Aurora, Colorado

Phyllis Howard, RN, BSN
Program Coordinator, Practical Nursing Program
Ashland Community & Technical College
Ashland, Kentucky

Nina L. Hutchinson, MSN, RN
Assistant Professor
Chamberlain College of Nursing
St. Louis, Missouri

Rebecca A. Kelly, MSN, RN
Coordinator, Practical Nursing Program
Greater Altoona Career and Technology Center
Altoona, Pennsylvania

Jennifer A. Ponto, BSN, RN
Faculty, Vocational Nursing Program
South Plains College
Levelland, Texas

Beth Jackson-Rumbaoa, RN, BSN
Practical Nursing Coordinator
Boonslick Technical Education Center
Boonville, Missouri

Thomas M. Sadowski, BA, MA, GDipTESOL
Language Arts Department
Allan Hancock College
Santa Maria California

Russlyn A. St. John, RN, MSN
Professor, Practical Nursing
St. Charles Community College
Cottleville, Missouri

Anne P. Smith, MS, RD, LDN, CDE
Formerly, Senior Associate, Clinical Development
WellDoc, Inc.
Baltimore, Maryland

Holly Stromberg, RN, BSN, MSN, PHN, CCRN
Nursing Faculty, Allan Hancock College
Staff Nurse/Nurse Educator, Marian Medical Center
Santa Maria, California

Karen D. Winsor, RN, MSN, ACNS-BC
Clinical Nurse Specialist for Orthopedic Trauma
University Medical Center at Brackenridge
Austin, Texas

LPN Advisory Board

To the Instructor

ABOUT THE TEXT

Medical-Surgical Nursing: Concepts & Practice is written specifically for the LPN/LVN student who must be educated to work within a variety of settings, including hospitals, long-term care facilities, rehabilitation institutes, ambulatory clinics, physicians' offices, and home care agencies. All of the most common adult medical-surgical disorders are covered, but special attention is devoted to disorders most prevalent in our society. Special consideration is given to the elderly population, those with chronic illnesses, and others in long-term care settings.

This text builds on—but does not repeat—the concepts and skills presented in a fundamentals of nursing course. Many states are expanding LPN/LVN scope of practice, via certification, to include administration of intravenous (IV) fluids and medications, but others do not. Information on IV therapy is included within this text so that schools in states where such certification is possible will have the necessary educational materials.

With the expanding and changing role of the LPN/LVN there is an even greater need for **critical thinking** and the development of **clinical judgment.** These crucial skills are stressed throughout the clinical chapters (see p. xv) and again in the Study Guide. **Evidence-based practice** is designated with a special icon so students come to understand that the foundation of nursing care is in research. Although evidence-based practice research within the nursing community is still developing, medical evidence-based research—on which nurses often base patient teaching—is abundant. **Best practices** are highlighted throughout the narrative with an icon to emphasize cutting-edge information related to interventions.

The nursing process and its application to nursing care is an organizing principle throughout, and patients' needs are presented as the focus of nursing care. There is an emphasis on practical **assessment— including data collection**—to determine problems, monitor for the onset of complications, and evaluate the effectiveness of care. Data collection from the geriatric patient requires greater ability to elicit pertinent information from the patient and family, and the achievement of this skill is a major focus in this text. The text emphasizes the role of LPN/LVNs in data collection to assist the RN in choosing appropriate **nursing diagnoses** for each patient.

Planning holistic care must include consideration of the patient's cultural background and its impact on perception of health, illness, and health practices. **Implementation of nursing actions** is the heart of patient care and LPN/LVN practice. Nursing actions presented are specific, comprehensive, and organized by common care problems to decrease repetition of information within a chapter. This helps the student master concepts rather than memorize facts. Further interventions are discussed with each disorder as appropriate, and *safe practice* is emphasized throughout the text. Additional focal points are using **expected outcomes** and **evaluating** nursing care to ensure that those outcomes and goals have been met.

Patient teaching for health promotion and self-care is a basic function of the LPN/LVN. Each clinical chapter points out ways in which nurses can teach the public how to prevent many of the problems discussed. Self-care guidelines for the major disorders are presented, and relevant *Healthy People 2020* objectives have been identified and are incorporated on the Evolve website.

LPN/LVN nurse practice acts do not encompass **delegation** as a function. With a few exceptions, only RNs can delegate, although in many situations LPN/LVNs can assign tasks. Collaboration with other health care workers and the use of basic management skills to provide coordinated, cost-effective patient care is essential. In this text we particularly speak to the LPN/LVN management role in working with nursing assistants and assigning tasks appropriately.

PEDAGOGICAL FEATURES

Special pedagogical features throughout the text help you teach your students to understand the chapter content and apply it in practice:

- The text has been thoroughly updated with the new **NCLEX-PN Test Plan** in mind.
- Competencies identified through the **Quality and Safety Education for Nurses (QSEN) initiative**— and the associated knowledge, skills, and attitudes (KSAs)—have been integrated into the content and were a continual focus during the writing of this text and its ancillaries.
- The Joint Commission's **National Patient Safety Goals** are highlighted to help students integrate

safety measures and quality controls into their practice, and **Safety Alerts** remind students of specific safety concerns.

- The Joint Commission's **National Quality Core Measures** and the Institute for Healthcare Improvement's (IHI) **bundles** are described as additional measures for providing safe, effective, and quality care.
- The purpose of *Healthy People 2020* as a nationwide health improvement agenda is explained, and goals related to specific patient problems are available on the Evolve site for students. Other **Health Promotion** boxes throughout the text also emphasize the importance of health promotion, disease prevention, and reduction of health care costs.
- **Evidence-based practice** is designated with a special icon so that the student will see the thrust of nursing toward a foundation based in research.
- **Overview of Anatomy and Physiology** at the beginning of each system introduction chapter provides basic information for understanding the body system and its disorders. Normal physiologic changes associated with aging are presented for each body system.
- **The Nursing Process** provides a consistent framework for the disorders chapters.
- Separate **Theory** and **Clinical Practice objectives** highlight the chapter's main learning goals.
- **Concept Maps** found in disorders chapters are designed to help students visualize difficult material and to illustrate how a disorder's multiple symptoms, treatments, and side effects relate to each other.
- End-of-chapter **Review Questions for the NCLEX® Examination** include **multiple choice and alternate-format questions,** and an extensive set of Interactive Review questions for the NCLEX® Examination are located on the Evolve website for students.
- The easily understandable **writing style** is aimed at gaining and retaining student attention to reading assignments.
- The term "patient" is used rather than "client" because that is what is still used in hospitals. "Resident" is used for those in long-term care facilities.
- The use of "he" and "she" for patient, physician, and nurse varies from chapter to chapter to emphasize the diversity among these populations.
- An **English-as-a-Second Language (ESL) consultant** reviewed each chapter to make the text more user-friendly and understandable for the student with limited proficiency in English. A section in each chapter of the *Study Guide* has been designed to assist this student to more easily master the chapter content and to enhance English skills.
- **Bolded text** throughout the narrative emphasizes key concepts and practice.

ORGANIZATION OF THE TEXT

Unit I addresses medical-surgical nursing settings, nursing roles and issues, health care trends, assignment considerations, the nursing process, measures related to safe and effective care, and critical thinking. **Unit II** covers all the key medical-surgical nursing topics, including fluids and electrolytes, surgical patient care, infections, pain, cancer, palliative care, and a separate chapter on chronic illness, rehabilitation, and the interdisciplinary health care team. **Units III through XIV** cover all the body systems and their disorders, each unit beginning with a system overview, followed by specific disorders chapters. **Unit XV** addresses emergency and disaster management—including bioterrorism—as well as trauma and shock. **Unit XVI** is entirely devoted to mental health nursing and includes information on anxiety and mood disorders, eating disorders, cognitive disorders, thought and personality disorders, and substance abuse.

Content covering legal and ethical issues, nutrition considerations, care of the older adult, communication, cultural diversity, complementary and alternative therapies, patient teaching, home care, health promotion, and assignment and delegation have been integrated as appropriate rather than including individual chapters on these subjects (see pp. xv to xvi). End-of-life issues and palliative care are presented at the end of Chapter 8: *Care of Patients with Cancer.* **Chronic illness** and **rehabilitation care** are growing areas, and Chapter 9 addresses the differences in care approaches and nursing care for these individuals as well as the interaction of the interdisciplinary health care team. The care of patients with HIV/AIDs has been separated out in Chapter 11, and the chapters that cover cardiac content (18 through 21) have been rearranged and augmented.

LPN THREADS

The second edition of *Medical-Surgical Nursing: Concepts & Practice* shares some features and design elements with other Elsevier LPN/LVN textbooks. The purpose of these *LPN Threads* is to make it easier for students and instructors to use the variety of books required by the relatively brief and demanding LPN/LVN curriculum. The following features are included in the *LPN Threads*.

- A **reading level evaluation** is performed on every manuscript chapter during the book's development to increase the consistency among chapters and ensure the text is easy to understand.
- The **full-color design, cover, photos,** and **illustrations** are visually appealing and pedagogically useful.

- **Objectives** (numbered) begin each chapter and provide a framework for content and are especially important in providing the structure for the TEACH Lesson Plans for the textbook.
- **Key Terms** with phonetic pronunciations and page number references are listed at the beginning of each chapter. Key terms appear in color in the chapter and are defined briefly, with full definitions in the **Glossary.** The goal is to help the student reader with limited proficiency in English to develop a greater command of the pronunciation of scientific and nonscientific English terminology.
- A wide variety of **special features** relate to critical thinking, clinical practice, health promotion, safety, patient teaching, complementary and alternative therapies, communication, home health care, delegation and assignment, and more. Refer to the To the Student section of this introduction on pp. xv to xvi for descriptions.
- **Critical Thinking Questions** presented at the end of each chapter and with Nursing Care Plans give students opportunities to practice critical thinking and clinical decision-making skills with realistic patient scenarios. Answers are provided in the Student Resources section on the Evolve website.
- **Key Points** at the end of each chapter correlate to the objectives and serve as a useful chapter review.
- A full suite of **Instructor Resources** is available, including TEACH Lesson Plans and PowerPoint Slides, Test Bank, Image Collection, Open-Book Quizzes, and Answer Keys.
- In addition to consistent content, design, and support resources, these textbooks benefit from the advice and input of the **Elsevier LPN/LVN Advisory Board** (see p. xi)

TEACHING AND LEARNING PACKAGE

FOR THE INSTRUCTOR

The comprehensive and free Evolve Instructor Resources with TEACH Instructor Resource include the following:

- **Test Bank** with approximately 1400 multiple-choice and alternate-format questions with correct answer, rationale, textbook page reference, topic, step of the nursing process, objective, cognitive level, and NCLEX® category of client needs
- **TEACH Instructor Resource** with Lesson Plans and PowerPoint Slides with Audience Response System Questions that correlate each text and ancillary component
- **Image Collection** that contains all the illustrations and photographs in the textbook
- **Open-Book Quizzes** for each chapter that you can administer during class for pre- or post-lecture evaluation or as take-home assignments
- **Answer Keys** for Open-Book Quizzes and the Study Guide
- **Suggestions for Working with English as a Second Language (ESL) Students**

FOR THE STUDENT

The Evolve Student Resources include the following assets:
- **Animations** depicting anatomy, physiology, and pathophysiology
- **Answers and Rationales** for in-text Review Questions for the NCLEX® Examination
- **Answer Guidelines** for Critical Thinking Questions and Think Critically boxes
- **Audio Clips** of heart and lung sounds
- **Audio Glossary** with pronunciations in English and Spanish
- **Bibliography and Suggested Readings**
- **Body Spectrum A&P Coloring Book**
- **Bonus Content** including Skills, Skill Performance Checklists, Patient Teaching guidelines, Nursing Care Plans, and more
- **Calculators** for determining body mass index (BMI), body surface area, fluid deficit, Glasgow coma score, IV dosages, and conversion of units
- **Clinical Quick Companion,** a printable quick reference that includes essential information on assessments, lab values, procedures, selected disorders, and useful tools and guidelines
- **Clinical References,** including forms, checklists, tools, and relevant *Healthy People 2020* goals for specific patient problems
- **Fluids and Electrolytes Tutorial**
- **Helpful Phrases for Communicating in Spanish**
- **Interactive Exercises and Activities for each chapter**
- **Interactive Review Questions for the NCLEX® Examination**
- **Mathematics Review**
- **Online Resources**
- **Supplemental Image Collection**
- **Video clips** of patient assessment

The *Study Guide* (sold separately) is a valuable supplement to help students understand and apply the textbook content. Varied question and activity types provide students with learning tools for reinforcement and exploration of text material. Terminology, Short Answer, multiple choice and alternate-format Review Questions for the NCLEX® Examination, Critical Thinking Activities, and a special section called *Steps Toward Better Communication*—written by an ESL specialist—appear in most chapters. Other activity types include Completion, Identification, Review of Structure and Function, Priority Setting, and Application of Nursing Process. The Study Guide includes text page references for each question, and an Answer Key is provided for instructors on the Evolve website.

To the Student

READING AND REVIEW TOOLS

- **Objectives** introduce the chapter topics.
- **Key Terms** are listed with page number references, and difficult medical, nursing, or scientific terms are accompanied by simple phonetic pronunciations. Key terms are considered essential to understanding chapter content and are defined within the chapter. Key terms are in color the first time they appear in the narrative and are briefly defined in the text, with complete definitions in the Glossary.
- Each chapter ends with a *Get Ready for the NCLEX® Examination!* **section** that includes (1) **Key Points** that reiterate the chapter objectives and serve as a useful review of concepts; (2) a list of **Additional Resources** including the Study Guide, Evolve Resources, and Online Resources; (3) an extensive set of **Review Questions for the NCLEX® Examination** with answers located in Appendix D and Answers and Rationales on Evolve; and (4) **Critical Thinking Questions** with Answer Guidelines located on Evolve.
- **Reader References** in the back of the text cite evidence-based information and provide resources for enhancing knowledge. An expanded **Bibliography** and **Suggested Readings** are available on Evolve.

CHAPTER FEATURES

Assignment Considerations address situations in which the RN delegates tasks to the LPN/LVN or when the LPN/LVN assigns tasks to nurse assistants as allowed by each state's nurse practice act.

Think Critically boxes encourage students to synthesize information and apply concepts beyond the scope of the chapter.

Home Care Considerations focus on post-discharge adaptations of medical-surgical nursing care to the home environment.

Elder Care Points address the unique medical-surgical care issues that affect older adults and provide suggestions for assessment (data collection) and particular interventions for the long-term and home care patient.

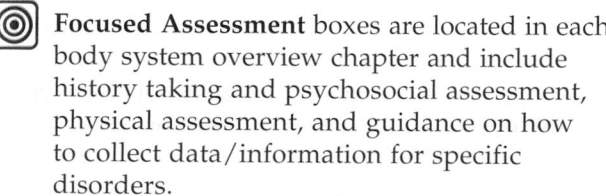

Focused Assessment boxes are located in each body system overview chapter and include history taking and psychosocial assessment, physical assessment, and guidance on how to collect data/information for specific disorders.

Clinical Cues provide guidance and advice related to the application of nursing care.

Nursing Care Plans, developed around specific case studies, include nursing diagnoses with an emphasis on patient goals and outcomes and questions to promote **critical thinking.**

Safety Alerts emphasize the importance of maintaining safety in patient care to protect patients, family, health care providers, and the public from accidents, spread of disease, and medication-related issues.

Health Promotion boxes emphasize healthy lifestyle choices, preventive behaviors, and screening tests.

Medication tables provide quick access to information about medications commonly used in medical-surgical nursing care.

Cultural Considerations explore select specific cultural preferences and how to address the needs of a culturally diverse patient and family.

Nutrition Considerations related to nursing care for specific disorders address the need for holistic care.

Patient Teaching boxes include step-by-step instructions and self-care guidelines.

Communication boxes provide guidance in therapeutic communication skills in realistic patient care situations.

Legal and Ethical Considerations present pertinent information about the legal issues and ethical dilemmas that may face the practicing nurse.

Complementary and Alternative Therapies boxes contain information on how nontraditional treatments for medical-surgical conditions may be used to complement traditional treatment.

Bonus Content, Clinical References, and other materials available on **Evolve** are referenced with icons in the margins where related text appears.

Animations depicting anatomy, physiology, and pathophysiology available on Evolve are referenced with icons in the margins where applicable.

Video clips of patient assessment available on Evolve are referenced with icons in the margins where applicable.

Evidence-Based Practice icons highlight current references to research in nursing and medical practice.

Best Practice icons highlight current information related to interventions.

Acknowledgments

We could not have managed to produce this text without the help of our chapter contributors—Helen Howlett, Signe Hill, Gloria Leifer, Trena Rich, and Carol Dallred. Our heart-felt gratitude goes to them. Thanks also go to the reviewers whose comments helped us to refine and clarify content as needed (see p. x).

Thanks to the following people for their hard work and dedication to prepare a great ancillary package with the textbook. The willingness of Larry Manalo to write and prepare the annotated PowerPoint Slides with Audience Response System Questions is greatly appreciated. He has done a commendable job. Kim Cooper and Kelly Gosnell updated and revised the Interactive Review Questions for the NCLEX® Examination; Interactive Exercises, Activities, and Critical Thinking Exercises; Open-Book Quizzes; TEACH Lesson Plans; and Test Bank, all of which are available on Evolve. Kim also wrote the lessons in the accompanying Virtual Clinical Excursions.

Thomas Sadowski did a phenomenal job with the ESL review and suggestions. He reviewed every chapter in the text and Study Guide, making suggestions on how to make information more understandable for the ESL students.

Thanks to Southwestern Washington Medical Center for allowing us to photograph within their facility. Their patients, staff, and administration are so willing to help with whatever they can for the education of nursing students. Jack Sanders is a talented, creative, professional photographer whose beautiful photos are seen throughout this book.

Thanks to Teri Hines-Burnham, Executive Content Strategist, and Tiffany Trautwein, Content Development Specialist, at Elsevier who have brought this project to fruition. Their dedication and friendship have kept the project on track. Mary Stueck, Senior Project Manager, makes the production process pleasurable. Her sense of humor always gets us through the tough parts and lightens the days. Mary is extremely good at her job. Christopher DeVito has done a fine job as copyeditor. The updated design of the book, which follows the Threads design of other Elsevier LPN/LVN texts, was provided by Karen Pauls. Danielle LeCompte, Marketing Manager has applied creative ideas to promote the book among students and instructors.

Teaching nursing has been one of the most exciting and gratifying phases of our lives. We hope this textbook and its ancillaries make your job as an instructor easier and class preparation more time-efficient. May your students find excitement and joy in learning and applying the information you impart in the clinical setting.

Susan C. deWit
Candice K. Kumagai

Contents

UNIT I Medical-Surgical Nursing Settings, Roles, and Issues

1 Caring for Medical-Surgical Patients, 1
Helen Stephens Howlett, BSN, RN, MS
Roles of Licensed Practical/Vocational
  Nurses, 1
    Uphold Clinical Standards, 2
    Provide Safe Patient Care, 2
    Teach Patients, 2
    Communicate Effectively, 2
    Work as a Collaborative Member of the
      Health Care Team, 2
    Advocate for the Patient, 3
Employment Opportunities, 3
Expanded Roles, 3
    Charge Nurse/Manager of Care, 3
Types of Health Care Financing, 4
    Health Insurance, 4
Goals for Health Care, 6
    Cost Containment, 6
    Health Promotion and *Healthy*
      People 2020, 6
    Holistic Care of Patients, 7

**2 Critical Thinking and the Nursing
Process, 14**
Signe S. Hill, BSN, RN, MA
Critical Thinking and Clinical
  Judgment, 14
    Factors that Influence Your Thinking and
      Nursing Care, 15
    Integrating Critical Thinking and the
      Nursing Process, 16
The Nursing Process, 16
    The Institute for Healthcare Improvement
      Bundles, 16
    The Joint Commission National Patient
      Safety Goals, 16
    The Joint Commission National Quality
      Core Measures, 17
Applying LPN/LVN Standards in Medical-
  Surgical Nursing, 17
    Assessment (Data Collection), 17
    Analysis and Nursing Diagnosis, 24
    Planning, 26
    Implementation, 26
    Evaluation, 27
Interdisciplinary (Collaborative)
  Care Plan, 27

UNIT II Medical-Surgical Patient Care Problems

**3 Fluids, Electrolytes, Acid-Base Balance, and
Intravenous Therapy, 30**
Distribution and Regulation of Body Fluids, 31
    Pathophysiology, 31
    Movement of Fluid and Electrolytes, 32
Fluid Imbalances, 33
    Pathophysiology, 33
    Deficient Fluid Volume, 34
    Excess Fluid Volume, 38
    Home Care, 40
Osmolality, 40
Electrolytes, 40
    Electrolyte Imbalances, 41
Acid-Base System, 45
    Physiology, 45
Acid-Base Imbalances, 47
    Pathophysiology, 47
    Arterial Blood Gas Analysis, 47
    Respiratory Acidosis, 48
    Metabolic Acidosis, 48
    Respiratory Alkalosis, 48
    Metabolic Alkalosis, 49
    Home Care, 50
Intravenous Fluid Therapy, 50
    Nursing Responsibilities in Administering
      IV Fluids, 51
    Calculating and Regulating the Rate
      of Flow, 53
    Nursing Management, 58
Community Care, 59

**4 Care of Preoperative and Intraoperative Surgical
Patients, 62**
Technological Advances in Surgery, 62
Autologous Blood for Transfusion, 64
Bloodless Surgery, 64
    Nursing Management, 64
Intraoperative Care, 74
The Surgical Team, 74
The Surgical Suite, 75
    The Surgical Holding Area, 75
    Roles of the Circulating Nurse and the Scrub
      Person, 75
Anesthesia, 75
    General Anesthesia, 76
    Regional Anesthesia, 76
    Procedural Sedation Anesthesia (Moderate
      Sedation), 76

Local Anesthesia, 76
Potential Intraoperative Complications, 77

5 Care of Postoperative Surgical Patients, 81
Immediate Postoperative Care, 81
Postanesthesia Care Unit, 81
Immediate Postoperative Care, 83
Nursing Management, 83
Discharge Planning, 94
Community Care, 97

6 Infection Prevention and Control, 100
Trena L. Rich, RN, PHN, MSN, APRN, CIC
The Infectious Process and Disease, 100
Factors that Influence Infectious
Disease, 101
Disease-Producing Pathogens, 101
The Body's Defense Against Infection, 103
Skin, 103
Normal Flora, 105
The Inflammatory Response, 105
The Immune Response, 108
Infection Prevention and Control, 108
Preventing and Controlling the Spread of
Infection, 108
Precaution Categories for Infection
Prevention and Control, 109
Health Care–Associated Infections, 111
The Cost of Health Care–Associated
Infections, 112
Nursing Interventions to Prevent Health
Care–Associated Infections, 114
Infection Surveillance and Reporting, 114
Medical Asepsis and Surgical
Asepsis, 115
Sepsis and Septic Shock, 115
Nursing Interventions for Patients with
Sepsis, 115
Nursing Management, 115
Community Care, 120
Home Care, 121
Long-Term Care, 121

7 Care of Patients with Pain, 124
Theories of Pain, 124
Classification of Pain, 125
Nociceptive Pain, 125
Neuropathic Pain, 126
Perception of Pain, 126
Acute versus Chronic Pain, 127
Acute Pain, 127
Chronic Pain, 128
Nursing Management, 128
Management of Pain, 134
Pharmacologic Approaches, 134
Nonpharmacologic Approaches, 138
Community Care, 140
Extended Care, 140
Home Care, 141

8 Care of Patients with Cancer, 144
Carol Dallred, MSN, RNC, WHNP, BC
The Impact of Cancer, 144
Physiology of Cancer, 145
Classification of Tumors, 146
Metastasis, 146
Causative Factors, 147
Chemical Carcinogens, 148
Promoters, 148
Chronic Irritation, 148
Physical Carcinogens, 148
Genetic Predisposition, 149
Contributing Factors, 149
Intrinsic Factors, 149
Stress, 150
Diet, 150
Measures to Prevent Cancer, 150
Diet and Nutrition, 150
Alcohol, 150
Environment, 150
Identifying High-Risk People, 151
Detection of Cancer, 151
Diagnostic Tests, 153
Laboratory Tests, 154
Nursing Management, 155
Common Therapies, Problems, and
Nursing Care, 158
Surgery, 158
Radiation Therapy, 159
Chemotherapy, 161
Hormone Therapy, 164
Immunotherapy Using Biologic Response
Modifiers, 165
Bone Marrow and Stem Cell
Transplantation, 165
Gene Therapy, 165
Evaluating the Effectiveness of Medical
Treatment, 166
Complementary and Integrative
Medicine, 166
Common Problems Related to Cancer or Cancer
Treatment, 166
Anorexia, Mucositis, and Weight
Loss, 166
Nausea, Vomiting, and Diarrhea, 167
Constipation, 167
Cystitis, 167
Immunosuppression, Bone Marrow
Suppression, and Infection, 168
Hyperuricemia, 169
Fatigue, 169
Alopecia, 169
Pain, 169
Patients with Metastatic Disease, 170
Fear and Ineffective Coping, 171
Oncologic Emergencies, 171

Care for the Dying Cancer Patient, 172
  Psychological Process of Death, 172
  Palliative Care, 172

9   **Chronic Illness and Rehabilitation, 177**
Carol Dallred, MSN, RNC, WHNP, BC
Chronic Illness, 177
  Preventing the Hazards of Immobility, 178
  Chronic Illness and Rehabilitation
    Care, 179
Rehabilitation, 187
  Rehabilitation Programs, 187
  The Rehabilitation Team, 188
  Nursing Management, 189
Home Care, 191
  The LPN/LVN in Home Care, 192
  The Family Caregiver, 192

UNIT III   Immune System

10   **The Immune and Lymphatic Systems, 195**
Trena L. Rich, RN, PHN, MSN, APRN, CIC
OVERVIEW OF ANATOMY AND
PHYSIOLOGY OF THE IMMUNE AND
LYMPHATIC SYSTEMS, 195
  What are the Organs and Structures of the
    Immune and Lymphatic Systems?, 195
  What are the Functions of the Immune and
    Lymphatic systems?, 196
  What Effects Does Aging have on the
    Immune and Lymphatic Systems?, 197
Protective Mechanisms of the Immune and
  Lymphatic Systems, 198
  Inflammatory Response, 198
  Immune Response, 198
Immune and Lymphatic System Disorders, 203
  Prevention of Immune and Lymphatic
    System Problems, 204
  Nursing Management, 205
Common Problems Related to the Immune and
  Lymphatic Systems, 209
  Fever, 209
  Nutrition, 212
  Immunosuppression, 212

11   **Care of Patients with HIV/AIDS, 215**
Trena L. Rich, RN, PHN, MSN, APRN, CIC
Disorders of Immune Deficiency, 215
  Human Immunodeficiency Virus (HIV) and
    Acquired Immunodeficiency Syndrome
    (AIDS), 215
  Nursing Management, 225

12   **Care of Patients with Immune and Lymphatic
     Disorders, 233**
Trena L. Rich, RN, PHN, MSN, APRN, CIC
IMMUNE DISORDERS, 233
Therapeutic Immunosuppression, 233

Diagnostic Tests and Treatment of Immune
  Deficiencies, 234
  Nursing Management, 235
Disorders of Inappropriate Immune
  Response, 236
  Allergy and Hypersensitivity, 236
  Nursing Management, 240
  Anaphylactic Reaction and Anaphylactic
    Shock, 241
Autoimmune Disorders, 243
  Systemic Lupus Erythematosus, 245
DISORDERS OF THE LYMPHATIC
SYSTEM, 249
Lymphoma, 249
  Hodgkin's Lymphoma, 249
  Non-Hodgkin's Lymphoma, 250
  Lymphedema, 253
  Fibromyalgia, 253

UNIT IV   Respiratory System

13   **The Respiratory System, 257**
OVERVIEW OF ANATOMY AND PHYSIOLOGY
OF THE RESPIRATORY SYSTEM, 257
  What Are the Functions of Each of the
    Structures of the Upper Respiratory
    System?, 257
  How Does the Epiglottis Protect the
    Airway?, 258
  How Is Speech Produced in the
    Larynx?, 258
  What Are the Functions of the Structures of
    the Lower Respiratory System?, 258
  How Is Oxygen Delivered to the Alveolar
    Membrane, Where It Can Diffuse into the
    Blood?, 258
  How Is the Lung Protected?, 258
  How Is Respiration Controlled?, 259
  How Do the Bones of the Thorax and the
    Respiratory Muscles Affect the
    Respiratory Process?, 259
  What Factors Can Affect the Exchange of
    Oxygen and Carbon Dioxide?, 259
  What Age-Related Changes Affect the
    Respiratory System?, 260
Causes of Respiratory Disorders, 260
Respiratory Disorders, 261
  Prevention, 261
  Nursing Management, 262
Common Respiratory Patient Care Problems, 271
  Ineffective Airway Clearance, 271
  Ineffective Breathing Patterns, 272
  Risk of Infection, 273
  Alterations in Nutrition and Hydration, 274
  Fatigue, 274

14 **Care of Patients with Disorders of the Upper Respiratory System, 277**
Disorders of the Nose and Sinuses, 277
    Upper Respiratory Infection (URI) (the Common Cold) and Rhinitis, 277
    Sinusitis, 279
    Epistaxis, 280
    Pharyngitis, 280
    Tonsillitis, 281
Obstruction and Trauma, 281
    Airway Obstruction and Respiratory Arrest, 281
    Obstructive Sleep Apnea, 282
    Nasal Fracture, 282
    Cancer of the Larynx, 283
Community Care, 289
    Home Care, 290
    Extended Care, 290

15 **Care of Patients with Disorders of the Lower Respiratory System, 293**
Respiratory Infectious Diseases, 293
    Acute Bronchitis, 293
    Influenza, 294
    Pneumonia, 295
    Empyema, 298
    Fungal Infections, 298
    Tuberculosis, 298
    Extrapulmonary Tuberculosis, 301
    Bronchiectasis, 301
    Occupational Lung Disorders, 302
    Interstitial Pulmonary Disease, 302
Restrictive Pulmonary Disorders, 302
    Pleurisy, 302
    Pleural Effusion, 302
Obstructive Pulmonary Disorders, 302
    Atelectasis, 303
    Chronic Obstructive Pulmonary Disease, 303
    Asthma, 305
    Lung Cancer, 310
Pulmonary Vascular Disorders, 311
    Pulmonary Embolism, 311
    Primary Pulmonary Hypertension, 312
    Lung Transplantation, 312
Chest Injuries, 312
    Pneumothorax and Hemothorax, 313
Lung Disorders, 314
    Pulmonary Edema, 314
    Adult (Acute) Respiratory Distress Syndrome, 314
    Respiratory Failure, 314
Common Therapeutic Measures, 315
    Intrathoracic Surgery, 315
    Medication Administration, 317
    Humidification, 320
    Pulmonary Hygiene, 321
    Oxygen Therapy, 323
    Mechanical Ventilation, 325
Community Care, 327

UNIT V   Hematologic System

16 **The Hematologic System, 331**
OVERVIEW OF ANATOMY AND PHYSIOLOGY OF THE HEMATOLOGIC SYSTEM, 331
    What Are the Functions of Blood?, 331
    What Are the Components of Blood?, 331
    What Are the Functions of the Plasma Proteins?, 331
    How Does the Body Produce Blood Cells?, 332
    What Are the Functions of the Red Blood Cells?, 332
    What Are the Functions of White Blood Cells?, 332
    What Are Platelets and What is Their Function?, 333
    How Does the Lymphatic System Interact with the Vascular System?, 334
    What Changes of the Hematologic System Occur with Aging?, 334
Causes of Hematologic Disorders, 334
Prevention of Hematologic Disorders, 335
Diagnostic Tests and Procedures, 336
    Nursing Management, 336
Common Problems Related to Disorders of the Hematologic System, 343
    Excessive Bleeding, 343
    Fatigue, 343
    Anorexia, 343
    Pain, 343
    Infection, 343
    Bone Marrow Failure, 344

17 **Care of Patients with Hematologic Disorders, 346**
Disorders of the Hematologic System, 346
    Anemia, 346
    Nursing Management, 349
    Aplastic Anemia, 352
    Sickle Cell Disease, 353
    Polycythemia Vera, 354
    Leukemia, 355
    Thrombocytopenia, 359
    Multiple Myeloma, 360
    Hemophilia, 361
    Disseminated Intravascular Coagulation, 362
Therapies Frequently Used in the Management of Hematologic Disorders, 362
    Transfusions, 362
    Leukapheresis, 364

Biologic Response Modifiers: Colony-
Stimulating Factor Therapy, 364
Bone Marrow and Stem Cell
Transplantation, 364
Oxygen Therapy, 366
Iron Therapy, 366
Vitamin B$_{12}$ Therapy, 367
Splenectomy, 367
Community Care, 367

UNIT VI   Cardiovascular System

18 The Cardiovascular System, 371
OVERVIEW OF ANATOMY AND PHYSIOLOGY
OF THE CARDIOVASCULAR SYSTEM, 371
What Are the Structures of the Heart and
Their Functions?, 371
What Causes the Heart to Contract and
Pump Blood?, 372
What Is the Cardiac Cycle?, 373
What Is the Ejection Fraction?, 373
How Does the Vascular System Function to
Carry Blood Throughout the Body?, 373
What Is the Blood Pressure and What
Affects It?, 374
What Changes Occur in the Cardiovascular
System with Aging?, 375
Cardiovascular Disease, 375
Women and Heart Disease, 375
Causes of Cardiovascular Disorders, 375
Prevention of Cardiovascular
Disease, 376
Diagnostic Tests and Procedures, 377
Nursing Management, 384
Common Problems of Patients with
Cardiovascular Disorders, 393
Fatigue and Dyspnea, 393
Fluid Overload (Edema), 393
Pain, 394
Altered Tissue Perfusion, 394
Impaired Tissue Integrity, 395

19 Care of Patients with Hypertension and
Peripheral Vascular Disease, 398
Hypertension, 398
Nursing Management, 404
Arteriosclerosis and Atherosclerosis, 406
Peripheral Vascular Disease, 406
Peripheral Arterial Disease (Arterial
Insufficiency), 407
Nursing Management, 409
Aneurysm, 411
Nursing Management, 412
Carotid Occlusion, 413
Buerger's Disease (Thromboangiitis
Obliterans), 413
Nursing Management, 413
Raynaud's Disease and Raynaud's
Phenomenon, 413

Venous Disorders, 414
Venous Thrombosis, 414
Superficial Thrombophlebitis, 415
Deep Vein Thrombosis, 415
Nursing Management, 416
Varicose Veins, 416
Chronic Venous Insufficiency, 420
Venous Stasis Ulcers, 421
Nursing Management, 422
Community Care, 423

20 Care of Patients with Cardiac Disorders, 426
Disorders of the Heart, 426
Heart Failure, 426
Nursing Management, 431
Cardiac Conduction Disorders
(Dysrhythmias), 435
Inflammatory and Infectious Diseases of
the Heart, 442
Infective Endocarditis, 442
Pericarditis, 443
Cardiomyopathy, 444
Cardiac Valve Disorders, 444
Mitral Stenosis, 445
Mitral Regurgitation (Insufficiency), 445
Aortic Stenosis, 445
Aortic Regurgitation (Insufficiency), 445
Treatment of Valve Disorders, 445
Cardiac Trauma, 446
Common Therapies and Their Nursing
Implications, 447
Oxygen Therapy, 447
Pharmacologic Agents, 447
Dietary Control, 447
Community Care, 448

21 Care of Patients with Coronary Artery Disease
and Cardiac Surgery, 451
Coronary Artery Disease, 451
Angina Pectoris, 453
Acute Coronary Syndrome and Myocardial
Infarction, 455
Cardiogenic Shock, 461
Surgical and Nonsurgical Treatment Options, 464
Percutaneous Transluminal Coronary
Angioplasty, 464
Transmyocardial Laser Revascularization, 464
Cardiac Surgery, 464
Community Care, 469

UNIT VII   Neurologic System

22 The Neurologic System, 472
OVERVIEW OF ANATOMY AND PHYSIOLOGY
OF THE NEUROLOGIC SYSTEM, 472
How Is the Nervous System Organized?,
472
How Does the Peripheral Nervous System
Interact with the Central Nervous System?,
474

How Is the Central Nervous System Protected?, 475
How Do Nerves Conduct Impulses?, 475
What Are the Special Characteristics of the Nervous System?, 477
What Changes Occur in the Nervous System with Aging?, 478
Causative Factors Involved in Neurologic Disorders, 478
Prevention of Neurologic Disorders, 478
Evaluation of Neurologic Status, 479
Cranial Nerves, 479
Coordination and Balance, 479
Neuromuscular Function Testing, 479
Reflexes, 479
Nursing Management, 485
Common Neurologic Patient Care Problems, 492
Ineffective Breathing Pattern, 492
Impaired Mobility, 492
Self-Care Deficit, 492
Dysphagia, 493
Incontinence, 493
Pain, 495
Confusion, 495
Aphasia, 495
Sexual Dysfunction, 496
Psychosocial Concerns, 497
Ineffective Family Coping, 497

23 Care of Patients with Head and Spinal Cord Injuries, 500
Head Injuries, 500
Increased Intracranial Pressure, 506
Nursing Management, 508
Injuries of the Spine and Spinal Cord, 509
Nursing Management, 515
Back Pain and Ruptured Intervertebral Disk ("Slipped Disk"), 517

24 Care of Patients with Disorders of the Brain, 523
Seizure Disorders and Epilepsy, 523
Nursing Management, 526
Transient Ischemic Attack, 527
Cerebrovascular Accident (Stroke, Brain Attack), 528
Nursing Management, 534
Brain Tumor, 539
Infectious and Inflammatory Disorders of the Nervous System, 541
Bacterial Meningitis, 541
Viral Meningitis, 543
Nursing Management, 543
Encephalitis, 544
Brain Abscess, 544
Headaches, 545
Migraine Headaches, 545
Cluster Headaches, 546
Tension Headaches, 546
Cranial Nerve Disorders, 546

Trigeminal Neuralgia (Tic Douloureux), 546
Nursing Management, 547
Bell's Palsy, 548

25 Care of Patients with Peripheral Nerve and Degenerative Neurologic Disorders, 551
Parkinson's Disease, 551
Nursing Management, 554
Multiple Sclerosis, 557
Nursing Management, 559
Alzheimer's Disease, 559
Amyotrophic Lateral Sclerosis, 559
Guillain-Barré Syndrome, 560
Nursing Management, 561
Poliomyelitis and Postpolio Syndrome, 562
Huntington's Disease, 562
Myasthenia Gravis, 562
Nursing Management, 563
Community Care, 565

UNIT VIII Sensory System

26 The Sensory System: Eye and Ear, 568
OVERVIEW OF ANATOMY AND PHYSIOLOGY OF THE EYE, 568
What Are the Structures of the Eye?, 568
What Are the Functions of the Eye Structures?, 569
What Changes Occur in the Eye with Aging?, 570
The Eye, 571
Eye Disorders, 571
Basic Eye Care, 571
Prevention of Eye Injury, 572
Prevention of Visual Loss, 572
Diagnostic Tests and Examinations, 573
Nursing Management, 573
Community Care, 579
OVERVIEW OF ANATOMY AND PHYSIOLOGY OF THE EAR, 579
What Are the Structures of the Ear?, 579
What Are the Functions of the Ear Structures?, 580
What Changes Occur in the Ear with Aging?, 580
The Ear, 581
Hearing Loss, 581
Nursing Management, 585
Common Problems of Patients with Ear Disorders, 588
Rehabilitation for Hearing Loss, 590
Community Care, 591

27 Care of Patients with Disorders of the Eyes and Ears, 594
Common Disorders of the Eye, 594
Errors of Refraction, 594
Uveitis, 595
Corneal Disorders, 595

Eye Trauma, 597
Cataract, 598
Glaucoma, 600
Open-Angle Glaucoma, 602
Narrow-Angle (Angle-Closure)
    Glaucoma, 605
Retinal Detachment, 605
Retinopathy, 608
Macular Degeneration, 608
Nursing Care of the Patient Having Eye
    Surgery, 610
    Preoperative Care, 610
    Postoperative Care, 611
Community Care, 611
    Resources for the Vision Impaired, 611
Common Disorders of the Ear, 612
    External Otitis, 612
    Impacted Cerumen and Foreign
        Bodies, 612
    Otitis Media, 612
    Labyrinthitis, 613
    Ménière's Disease (Ménière's Syndrome),
        613
    Acoustic Neuroma, 614
    Otosclerosis and Hearing Loss, 614
Nursing Care of the Patient Having Ear
    Surgery, 615
    Preoperative Care, 615
    Postoperative Care, 617
Community Care, 617

UNIT IX   Gastrointestinal System

28 The Gastrointestinal System, 620
    OVERVIEW OF ANATOMY AND PHYSIOLOGY
    OF THE GASTROINTESTINAL SYSTEM, 620
        What Are the Organs and Structures of the
            Gastrointestinal System?, 620
        What Are the Functions of the
            Gastrointestinal System?, 620
        What Effects Does Aging Have on the
            Gastrointestinal System?, 621
        What Are the Structures and Locations of the
            Accessory Organs?, 621
        What Are the Functions of the Gallbladder,
            Liver, and Pancreas?, 622
        How Does Aging Affect the Accessory
            Organs of Digestion?, 623
    The Gastrointestinal System, 623
        Gastrointestinal System Disorders, 623
        Nursing Management, 631
        Common Problems Related to the
            Gastrointestinal System, 633
29 Care of Patients with Disorders of the Upper
    Gastrointestinal System, 640
    Eating Disorders, 640
        Anorexia Nervosa, 640
        Bulimia Nervosa, 640
        Obesity, 640
        Nursing Management, 642
    Upper Gastrointestinal Disorders, 643
        Stomatitis, 643
        Dysphagia, 643
        Cancer of the Oral Cavity, 644
        Cancer of the Esophagus, 645
        Hiatal Hernia (Diaphragmatic Hernia), 645
        Gastroesophageal Reflux Disease, 646
        Gastroenteritis, 649
        Gastritis, 649
        Nursing Management, 652
        Peptic Ulcer, 650
        Gastric Cancer, 657
    Common Therapies for Disorders of the
        Gastrointestinal System, 658
        Gastrointestinal Decompression, 658
        Enteral Nutrition, 658
        Total Parenteral Nutrition, 660
30 Care of Patients with Disorders of the Lower
    Gastrointestinal System, 663
    Disorders of the Abdomen and Bowel, 663
        Abdominal and Inguinal Hernia, 663
        Irritable Bowel Syndrome, 664
        Diarrhea or Constipation, 665
        Diverticula, 665
        Intestinal Obstruction, 668
        Bowel Ischemia, 670
        Inflammatory Bowel Disease, 670
        Nursing Management, 672
        Appendicitis, 672
        Peritonitis, 673
        Malabsorption, 673
        Cancer of the Colon, 674
    Ostomy Surgery and Care, 679
        Colostomy, 679
        Ileostomy, 680
        Preoperative Nursing Care, 681
        Nursing Management, 681
    Anorectal Disorders, 685
        Hemorrhoids, 685
        Pilonidal Sinus (Pilonidal Cyst), 686
        Anorectal Abscess and Fistula, 686
    Community Care, 687
31 Care of Patients with Disorders of the
    Gallbladder, Liver, and Pancreas, 690
    Disorders of the Gallbladder, 690
        Cholelithiasis and Cholecystitis, 690
    Disorders of the Liver, 694
        Hepatitis, 694
        Nursing Management, 698
        Cirrhosis, 701
        Nursing Management, 703
        Liver Transplantation, 707
        Cancer of the Liver, 708
    Disorders of the Pancreas, 708

Acute Pancreatitis, 708
Chronic Pancreatitis, 710
Cancer of the Pancreas, 710
Community Care, 713

UNIT X   Musculoskeletal System

32 **The Musculoskeletal System, 716**
OVERVIEW OF ANATOMY AND PHYSIOLOGY
OF THE MUSCULOSKELETAL SYSTEM, 716
What Are the Structures of the
Musculoskeletal System?, 716
What Are the Functions of the Bones?, 717
What Are the Functions of the Muscles?, 718
What Changes Occur in the Musculoskeletal
System with Aging?, 718
Musculoskeletal Disorders, 718
Causes, 718
Prevention, 719
Nursing Management, 723

33 **Care of Patients with Musculoskeletal and
Connective Tissue Disorders, 734**
Connective Tissue Disorders, 734
Sprain, 734
Strain, 735
Dislocation, 735
Rotator Cuff Tear, 735
Anterior Cruciate Ligament Injury, 735
Meniscal Injury, 736
Achilles Tendon Rupture, 736
Bursitis, 736
Bunion (Hallux Valgus), 736
Carpal Tunnel Syndrome, 736
Fractures, 736
Nursing Management, 742
Inflammatory Disorders of the Musculoskeletal
System, 745
Lyme Disease, 745
Osteoarthritis, 745
Rheumatoid Arthritis, 746
Nursing Management, 750
Gout, 755
Osteoporosis, 755
Nursing Management, 757
Paget's Disease, 757
Bone Tumors, 757
Amputation, 758
Community Care, 760

UNIT XI   Urinary System

34 **The Urinary System, 764**
OVERVIEW OF ANATOMY AND PHYSIOLOGY
OF THE UROLOGIC SYSTEM, 764
What Are the Structures of the Urologic
System and How Do They Interrelate?, 764
What Are the Functions of the
Kidneys?, 765

What Are the Functions of the Ureters,
Bladder, and Urethra?, 765
What Changes Occur with Aging?, 766
The Urologic System, 766
Disorders of the Urologic System, 766
Nursing Management, 768
Common Urologic Problems, 777
Urinary Incontinence, 777
Urinary Retention, 782

35 **Care of Patients with Disorders of the Urinary
System, 785**
Inflammatory Disorders of the Urinary Tract, 785
Cystitis, 785
Urethritis, 788
Pyelonephritis, 788
Acute Glomerulonephritis, 789
Chronic Glomerulonephritis, 789
Nephrotic Syndrome, 790
Obstructions of the Urinary Tract, 790
Hydronephrosis, 790
Renal Stenosis, 791
Renal Stones, 791
Urologic System Trauma, 794
Trauma to Kidneys and Ureters, 794
Trauma to the Bladder, 794
Urologic System Cancers, 795
Cancer of the Bladder, 795
Cancer of the Kidney, 798
Renal Failure, 798
Acute Renal Failure, 798
Nursing Management, 801
Chronic Renal Failure, 801
Nursing Management, 808
Community Care, 811

UNIT XII   Endocrine System

36 **The Endocrine System, 818**
OVERVIEW OF ANATOMY AND PHYSIOLOGY
OF THE ENDOCRINE SYSTEM, 818
What Are the Organs and Structures of the
Endocrine System?, 818
What Are the Functions of the Endocrine
System?, 819
What Are the Effects of the Pituitary
Hormones?, 819
What Are the Effects of the Thyroid
Hormones?, 819
What Are the Functions of the Parathyroid
Glands?, 821
What Are the Functions of the Hormones
Secreted by the Adrenal Glands?, 821
What Is the Hormonal Function of the
Pancreas?, 821
What Are the Effects of Aging on the
Endocrine System?, 822
The Endocrine System, 822
Endocrine System Disorders, 823

Nursing Management, 829
Community Care, 831

37 Care of Patients with Pituitary, Thyroid, Parathyroid, and Adrenal Disorders, 833
Disorders of the Pituitary Gland, 833
  Pituitary Tumors, 833
  Hypofunction of the Pituitary Gland, 835
  Diabetes Insipidus, 835
  Syndrome of Inappropriate Antidiuretic Hormone, 837
Disorders of the Thyroid Gland, 838
  Goiter, 838
  Hyperthyroidism, 839
  Thyroidectomy, 840
  Hypothyroidism, 844
  Myxedema Coma, 845
  Thyroiditis, 845
  Thyroid Cancer, 845
Disorders of the Parathyroid Glands, 845
  Hypoparathyroidism, 845
  Hyperparathyroidism (von Recklinghausen's Disease), 846
Disorders of the Adrenal Glands, 847
  Pheochromocytoma, 847
  Adrenocortical Insufficiency (Addison's Disease), 847
  Acute Adrenal Insufficiency or Adrenal Crisis, 848
  Excess Adrenocortical Hormone (Cushing Syndrome), 852
Community Care, 853

38 Care of Patients with Diabetes and Hypoglycemia, 856
Diabetes Mellitus and Hypoglycemia, 856
  Diabetes Mellitus, 856
  Nursing Management, 867
  Hypoglycemia, 876
Community Care, 877

UNIT XIII   Reproductive System

39 Care of Women with Reproductive Disorders, 880
Gloria Leifer, RN, MA, CNE
OVERVIEW OF ANATOMY AND PHYSIOLOGY OF THE FEMALE REPRODUCTIVE SYSTEM, 881
  What Are the Primary External Structures of the Female Reproductive System?, 881
  What Are the Primary Internal Structures of the Female Reproductive System?, 881
  What Are the Accessory Organs of the Female Reproductive System?, 882
  What Are the Phases of the Female Reproductive Cycle during the Childbearing Years?, 882
  When Does Sexual Development Occur in the Fetus?, 882
  What Changes Take Place as Girls Mature into Women and Become Capable of Reproduction?, 882
  What Changes Take Place as a Woman Enters Menopause?, 882
  What Changes Occur with Aging?, 882
The Female Reproductive System, 883
  Menstruation, 883
  Normal Breasts, 883
  Contraception and Fertility, 883
  Menopause, 890
  Health Promotion and Disease Prevention, 892
Nursing Management, 894
Disorders of the Female Reproductive System, 902
  Menstrual Dysfunctions, 902
  Pelvic Relaxation Syndrome, 903
  Polycystic Ovarian Syndrome, 904
  Dysfunctional Uterine Bleeding, 904
  Abnormal Uterine Bleeding, 904
  Leiomyoma, 905
  Endometriosis, 906
  Inflammations of the Lower Genital Tract, 906
  Toxic Shock Syndrome, 906
  Cancer of the Reproductive Tract, 907
Disorders of the Breast, 908
  Benign Disorders of the Breast, 908
  Breast Cancer, 909
Home Care, 915
Community Care, 915

40 Care of Men with Reproductive Disorders, 918
Gloria Leifer, RN, MA, CNE
OVERVIEW OF ANATOMY AND PHYSIOLOGY OF THE MALE REPRODUCTIVE SYSTEM, 918
  What Are the Structures of the Male Reproductive System?, 918
  What Are the Functions of the Organs of the Male Reproductive System?, 919
  How Is Sperm Production Controlled?, 919
  What Changes Occur with Aging?, 920
The Male Reproductive System, 920
  Fertility, 920
  Contraception, 920
  Nursing Management, 921
Disorders of the Male Reproductive System, 923
  Erectile Dysfunction, 923
  Ejaculation Disorders, 924
  Infertility, 924
  Hydrocele, 925
  Varicocele, 926
  Testicular Torsion, 926
  Priapism, 926
  Peyronie's Disease, 927
  Benign Prostatic Hyperplasia, 927
  Inflammations and Infections of the Male Reproductive Tract, 932
  Cancer of the Male Reproductive Tract, 933
Community Care, 935

41 **Care of Patients with Sexually Transmitted Infections, 938**
Gloria Leifer, RN, MA, CNE
Common Infections of the Female Reproductive Tract, 939
Pelvic Inflammatory Disease, 939
Candidiasis, 939
Bacterial Vaginosis, 939
Risk Factors for Transmission of Sexually Transmitted Infections, 939
Prevention of Human Papillomavirus, 940
Lesions of Sexually Transmitted Infections, 940
Reporting Sexually Transmitted Infections, 940
Transmission of Sexually Transmitted Infections, 940
Common Diagnostic Tests, 941
Nursing Management, 941
Community Care, 950

UNIT XIV   Integumentary System

42 **The Integumentary System, 952**
OVERVIEW OF ANATOMY AND PHYSIOLOGY OF THE INTEGUMENTARY SYSTEM, 952
What Is the Structure of the Skin, Hair, and Nails?, 952
What Are the Functions of the Skin and Its Structures?, 953
What Changes Occur in the Skin and Its Structures with Aging?, 953
The Integumentary System, 954
Disorders of the Integumentary System, 954
Integrity of Skin, 956
Nursing Management, 958

43 **Care of Patients with Integumentary Disorders and Burns, 966**
Inflammatory Infections, 966
Dermatitis, 966
Acne, 967
Psoriasis, 969
Stevens-Johnson Syndrome, 969
Bacterial Infections, 970
Viral Infections, 970
Herpes Simplex, 970
Herpes Zoster, 971
Fungal Infections, 972
Tinea Pedis, 973
Parasitic Infections, 973
Pediculosis and Scabies, 973
Noninfectious Disorders of Skin, 974
Skin Cancer, 974
Pressure Ulcers, 977
Burns, 981
Nursing Management, 989
Community Care, 994

UNIT XV   Emergency and Disaster Management

44 **Care of Patients During Disasters, Bioterrorism Attacks, and Pandemic Infections, 997**
Disaster Preparedness and Response, 997
Community Preparedness, 999
Hospital Preparedness, 1000
Psychological Responses to Disaster, 1001
Triage, 1001
Preparing for Chemical, Nuclear, or Biologic Disasters, 1006
Chemical Disaster, 1006
Nuclear Disaster, 1009
Biologic Disaster, 1010
Pandemic Influenza Infection, 1015

45 **Care of Patients with Trauma or Shock, 1019**
Prevention of Accidents, 1019
Home Safety, 1019
Highway Safety, 1019
Water Safety, 1019
First Aid and Good Samaritan Laws, 1020
Emergency Care, 1021
Triage: Initial Survey, 1022
Airway and Respiration, 1022
Control of Bleeding, 1023
Neck and Spine Injuries, 1024
Chest Trauma, 1024
Abdominal Trauma, 1025
Multiple Trauma, 1026
Metabolic Emergencies, 1026
Insulin Reaction or Severe Hypoglycemia, 1026
Other Metabolic Emergencies, 1026
Injuries Caused by Extreme Heat and Cold, 1026
Heatstroke, 1026
Hypothermia, 1027
Frostbite, 1027
Poisoning, 1028
Accidental Poisoning, 1028
Food Poisoning, 1029
Inhaled Poisons, 1030
Bites and Stings, 1030
Human Bites, 1030
Animal Bites, 1030
Snakebite, 1030
Insect Bites and Stings, 1031
Electric Shock and Burns, 1031
Chemical Burns, 1032
Choking Emergencies, 1032
Cardiopulmonary Resuscitation, 1032
Shock, 1033
Signs and Symptoms, 1033
Hypovolemic Shock, 1033
Cardiogenic Shock, 1035
Obstructive Shock, 1036

Maldistribution of Fluids (Distributive Shock), 1036
Anaphylactic Shock, 1036
Neurogenic Shock, 1037
Sepsis and Septic Shock, 1037
Systemic Inflammatory Response Syndrome, 1038
Nursing Management, 1039
Psychological and Social Emergencies, 1040
The Combative Patient, 1040
Domestic Violence and Abuse, 1041

UNIT XVI   Mental Health Nursing of the Adult

46 Care of Patients with Anxiety, Mood, and Eating Disorders, 1045
Anxiety and Anxiety Disorders, 1045
Generalized Anxiety Disorder, 1046
Phobic Disorder, 1047
Obsessive-Compulsive Disorder, 1047
Post-Traumatic Stress Disorder, 1047
Nursing Management, 1048
Mood Disorders, 1051
Bipolar Disorder, 1051
Nursing Management, 1052
Major Depressive Disorder, 1055
Nursing Management, 1057
Suicidal Patients, 1059
Nursing Management, 1059
Eating Disorders, 1060
Anorexia Nervosa, 1060
Bulimia Nervosa, 1060
Treatment of Eating Disorders, 1061
Nursing Management, 1061
Community Care, 1062

47 Care of Patients with Substance Abuse Disorders, 1065
Substance and Alcohol Abuse, 1065
Signs and Symptoms, 1066
Effects of Substance Abuse on Family and Friends, 1067
Disorders Associated with Substance Abuse, 1068
Alcohol Abuse, 1068
Symptoms of Intoxication and Withdrawal, 1068
Abuse of Other Central Nervous System Depressants, 1071
Abuse of Opiates, 1073
Abuse of Stimulants, 1074
Abuse of Nicotine, 1075
Abuse of Cannabis, 1075
Abuse of Hallucinogens and Inhalants, 1076
Nursing Management, 1076
Community Care, 1081

48 Care of Patients with Cognitive Disorders, 1085
Overview of Cognitive Disorders, 1085
Delirium, 1085
Substance-Induced Delirium, 1086
Dementia, 1086
Alzheimer's Disease, 1087
Nursing Management, 1088
Vascular Dementia, 1093
AIDS Dementia Complex, 1093
Nursing Management, 1093
Community Care, 1099

49 Care of Patients with Thought and Personality Disorders, 1102
Overview of Thought Disorders, 1102
Neurotransmitters, 1102
Schizophrenia, 1103
Nursing Management, 1108
Overview of Personality Disorders, 1113
Borderline Personality Disorder, 1114
Nursing Management, 1114
Community Care, 1116

Appendices

Appendix A   **Most Common Laboratory Test Values, 1119**

Appendix B   **Standard Precautions, 1128**

Appendix C   **Standard Steps for All Nursing Procedures, 1130**

Appendix D   **Answers to Review Questions for the NCLEX® Examination, 1132**

Appendix E   **Standards of Practice and Educational Competencies of Graduates of Practical/Vocational Nursing Programs, 1134**

Appendix F   **NFLPN Nursing Practice Standards for the Licensed Practical/Vocational Nurse, 1137**

Appendix G   **American Hospital Association: The Patient Care Partnership— Understanding Expectations, Rights, and Responsibilities, 1140**

Reader References, 1142
Illustration Credits, 1159
Glossary, 1163
Index, 1185
NANDA-I–Approved Nursing Diagnoses, Inside back cover

Caring for Medical-Surgical Patients

Objectives

1. Describe each of the roles of the licensed practical/vocational nurse (LPN/LVN).
2. Identify 10 sites of employment for LPN/LVNs in medical-surgical nursing.
3. Explain the difference between a health maintenance organization (HMO) and a preferred provider organization (PPO).
4. Differentiate between Medicare and Medicaid in the areas of eligibility and services provided.
5. Describe how hospitals are reimbursed under the diagnosis-related group (DRG) system of Medicare, including care excluded from reimbursement.
6. Discuss four factors that contribute to rising health care costs.
7. Explain how *Healthy People 2020*—as a health promotion and prevention of illness strategy—could decrease health care costs.
8. Define and explain the importance of holistic care.
9. Explain how the nurse-patient relationship is established.
10. Discuss how psychological, social, cultural, and spiritual needs are incorporated in the LPN/LVN's plan of care.
11. Identify the relationship of unmet needs to withdrawn, dependent, hostile, and manipulative behavior.

Key Terms

acuity (ă-KŪ-ĭ-tē, p. 3)
advocate (ĂD-vō-kăt, p. 3)
biomedicine (BĪ-ō-MĔD-ĭ-sĭn, p. 10)
capitation (kă-pĭ-TĀ-shŭn, p. 4)
co-insurance (kō-ĭn-SHŪ-rĕnz, p. 4)
complementary and alternative medicine (CAM) (KŎM-plĕ-MĔN-tĕ-rē ănd ăl-TŬR-nă-tĭv MĔD-ĭ-sĭn, p. 10)
copayment (kō-PĀY-mĕnt, p. 4)
cost containment (kŏst kŏn-TĀN-mĕnt, p. 6)
deductible (dē-DŬK-tĭ-bŭl, p. 4)
delegation (DĔL-ĭ-GĀ-shŭn, p. 3)
dependent (dĕ-PĔN-dĕnt, p. 9)
diagnosis-related groups (DRGs) (dī-ăg-NŌ-sĭs rē-LĀ-tĕd grūpz, p. 5)
empathy (ĔM-pă-thē, p. 7)
fee-for-service (fē fŏr SĔR-vĭs, p. 4)
health maintenance organizations (HMOs) (hĕlth MĀN-tĕ-nĕnz ŏr-gă-nĭ-ZĀ-shŭnz, p. 5)

Healthy People 2020 (HĔLTH-ē PĒ-pl, p. 6)
holistic care (hō-LĬS-tĭk kār, p. 7)
managed care (MĂN-ăjd kār, p. 5)
Medicaid (mĕd-ĭ-KĀD, p. 6)
Medicare (mĕd-ĭ-KĀR, p. 5)
nonjudgmental (NŎN-jŭj-MĔN-tăl, p. 9)
nurse practice act (NPA) (nŭrz PRĂK-tĭs ăct, p. 1)
preferred provider organizations (PPOs) (prĕ-FŬRD prō-vī-dĕr ŏr-gă-nĭ-ZĀ-shŭnz, p. 5)
prospective payment system (PPS) (prŏs-PĔK-tĭv pā-mĕnt sĭs-tĕm, p. 5)
provider (prō-VĪ-dĕr, p. 4)
retrospective payment system (rĕt-rōs-PĔK-tĭv pā-mĕnt sĭs-tĕm, p. 5)
stereotypes (STĔR-ē-ō-tīps, p. 10)
unlicensed assistive personnel (UAP) (un-LĪ-sĕnst ă-SĬS-tĭv pĕr-sŏ-NĔL, p. 3)

Medical-surgical nursing involves care for adult patients with medical and/or surgical conditions that affect single or multiple body systems. Medical patients have diseases that require a variety of treatments, including medication and diet therapy. Surgical patients require operative procedures to treat diseases and/or trauma. Patients can have a single diagnosis of a medical or surgical condition or a combination of medical and surgical diagnoses.

ROLES OF LICENSED PRACTICAL/VOCATIONAL NURSES

Each state's **nurse practice act (NPA)** defines the role and scope of practice of licensed practical/vocational nurses (LPN/LVNs). Administrative rules and regulations and interpretations of the state's board of nursing provide more *specific* details and clarification. Some NPAs list specifically what LPN/LVNs can do, but the wording allows for changes in the roles of the LPN/LVN. This eliminates the need for state legislators to reopen the nurse practice act and revise it each time a change is required to accommodate evolving nursing roles. It is your responsibility to be aware of the law of the state in which you are employed. The LPN/LVN cares for patients within the scope of the state's NPA, and upholds clinical standards, provides safe patient care, serves as a patient advocate, teaches patients, and communicates effectively—all while functioning as a collaborative member of the health care team.

 Think Critically

Nurse practice acts vary considerably from state to state. Where can you obtain a copy of your state's NPA?

UPHOLD CLINICAL STANDARDS

Check your institution for guidelines and policies. The facility might restrict the LPN/LVN's role to less than the NPA allows, but **no employer can give nurses permission to do what their license says they cannot do.**

The National Association for Practical Nurse Education and Service, Inc. (NAPNES) and the National Federation of Licensed Practical Nurses, Inc. (NFLPN) are practical/vocational nursing organizations that provide standards to guide the role of the LPN/LVN (see Appendices E and F on Evolve and the Online Resources at the end of this chapter). These standards of practice—which echo the values and priorities of the profession and provide guidelines for safe and competent nursing care—may be used as a basis of prosecution or defense in a court of law.

PROVIDE SAFE PATIENT CARE

In the hospital acute care setting, the LPN/LVN may be engaged in total care for assigned patients, under the supervision of a registered nurse (RN). Total care duties involve being responsible for meeting patients' basic needs, with the goal of making patients as independent as possible to preserve their ability to care for themselves. LPN/LVNs cannot assume the role of the professional (registered) nurse, but they do participate in the nursing process by assisting the RN to assess (gather data on) patients and to plan and evaluate patient care. The LPN/LVN assists with personal hygiene, performs ordered treatments, initiates nursing interventions, and administers drugs. In other situations, the LPN/LVN might be used as a medication and treatment nurse for all patients on a team. If asked to do a procedure or treatment that was not taught in the educational program but is allowed by the NPA (e.g., monitoring blood transfusions), LPN/LVNs can obtain further training and have their new proficiency recorded in their personnel file.

TEACH PATIENTS

An important aspect of nursing care is to teach patients and families to care for themselves or loved ones to prevent complications, restore health, and prevent further illness. LPN/LVNs also teach basic hygiene and nutrition in the context of health promotion. Examples of teaching include reinforcing what the registered nurse or physician advises regarding scheduled diagnostic tests, upcoming surgery, how to treat a wound, or how to change a dressing. Other teaching activities concern how to take prescribed medication, what side effects to report, and the self-care activities and lifestyle changes required to promote rehabilitation and independence. LPN/LVNs contribute to the discharge plan by reinforcing discharge instructions and providing information to patients about community resources and self-help groups.

 Think Critically

Recall a time when you *reinforced* patient teaching, and rank your teaching effectiveness on a scale of 1 to 10. How would you improve your performance in another patient teaching situation? Do the same for other patient situations in which you *initiated* health teaching.

COMMUNICATE EFFECTIVELY

Therapeutic communication from the medical professional helps the patient develop trust in the quality of care and decreases anxiety about the medical situation. Therapeutic communication is also used when communicating with staff, especially when making requests. Call staff by name, to ensure their attention, and explain the purpose of the communication. Present requirements of a request and give a time line for completion. Obtain feedback that the request was understood, and provide appreciation for cooperation. Loudspeaker noise from paging systems is annoying to patients. Some agencies try to cut down on noise with wireless communication devices that clip on clothing and allow staff to contact each other, other departments, and physicians.

LPN/LVNs give objective and thorough end-of-shift reports and maintain objective documentation about the care given and the status of patients. Nursing documentation is used to receive approval for length of stay, and reimbursement of facility charges from insuring agencies.

WORK AS A COLLABORATIVE MEMBER OF THE HEALTH CARE TEAM

LPN/LVNs work with other members of the health care team (e.g., physician, RN, physical therapist, respiratory therapist, dietitian, pastoral care team, pharmacy personnel, and unlicensed assistive personnel [UAP]) to provide the patient with an integrated, comprehensive plan of care.

Think Critically

What is your role as a member of the team when in the clinical area? List three examples. To whom on staff do you communicate the care you give? To whom do you go with questions? What is your instructor's role?

ADVOCATE FOR THE PATIENT

Facility and unit routine can lead to an impersonal health care system that loses its focus on patients' rights. The American Hospital Association (AHA) has published *The Patient Care Partnership: Understanding Expectations, Rights and Responsibilities* (2003) (Appendix G). LPN/LVNs advocate for patients by standing up for patients' rights and ensuring that their needs are met.

 Clinical Cues

If a patient declines A.M. care (bath, brushing teeth, etc.), you can postpone it for a while, as your work schedule allows. You should fit it in before your shift is over. Leaving care to be done on the next shift burdens the oncoming staff, and is not considered acceptable practice. Listen to the patient's reasons for not wanting care. If it appears that care really is being refused for that complete day, talk with the staff nurse or charge nurse about it. The patient has the right to refuse care. Most often, if the benefits of care are explained, you can gain the patient's cooperation. Conferring with more experienced team members can help a new nurse determine when routine can be altered in the patient's best interests.

Advocating for a patient could be as simple as making arrangements for special food or meals at times other than those within the facility routine, or it may entail informing the physician of a patient concern.

 Think Critically

If you have had the opportunity to advocate for a patient, briefly describe what happened and how you felt about the effectiveness of your action.

EMPLOYMENT OPPORTUNITIES

Hospital employment involves very ill patients with complex needs (high acuity patients) and a fast-paced environment. Employment opportunities vary considerably geographically. The majority of graduate practical/vocational nurses are employed in long-term care, and many nursing jobs continue to move to community-based settings. Other sites of employment are listed in Box 1-1.

Think Critically

What are the current medical-surgical opportunities for employment where you live? List two agencies you may contact for this information.

Box 1-1 Various Sites of Employment for LPN/LVNs

AREAS WITHIN THE HOSPITAL
- Outpatient surgery
- Intermediate care unit (step-down unit)
- Intravenous (IV) therapy team*
- Emergency department

ADDITIONAL SITES FOR EMPLOYMENT OPPORTUNITIES
- Long-term care facility (nursing home)
- Ambulatory care
- Rehabilitation services (extended care, postacute care, subacute care)
- Hospice care
- Adult group homes
- Assisted living facilities
- Homes for developmentally disabled
- Home health care
- Ambulatory clinics
- Medical offices
- Hospice care agency
- Military service
- Dialysis center
- Jails and prisons

*Requires postgraduate education and certification.

EXPANDED ROLES

CHARGE NURSE/MANAGER OF CARE

The most common site of employment for the LPN/LVN is the nursing home or long-term care unit. In this setting, LPN/LVNs frequently assume the role of charge nurse. Many NPAs specifically state that the LPN/LVN charge nurse functions in a nursing home under the general supervision of an RN, who is either on site or is available by phone.

 Think Critically

What (if any) restriction(s) does your state's NPA place on the charge nurse position?

Delegation and Assignment

To *delegate* is to transfer authority and to assign is to distribute work. In the LPN/LVN context, delegation involves transferring to qualified unlicensed assistive personnel (UAP) the authority to perform a selected nursing task or activity in a selected patient situation that is within the job description of the LPN/LVN. Assignment involves assigning nursing tasks or activities within the job description of the UAP to a particular individual (National Council of State Boards of Nursing [NCSBN], 2005).

Delegation. Not all states allow LPN/LVNs to delegate nursing tasks or activities, and state NPAs vary greatly concerning protocol for delegation (Box 1-2). Check your state's NPA to determine whether you

Comparison of Assigning and Delegating by the LPN/LVN Charge Nurse

Ask yourself the following questions:

1. Are tasks/activities in nursing assistant's job description?
   When assigning: Yes.
   When delegating: No. The tasks/activities delegated are in the job description of the LPN/LVN. Specific tasks/activities are not listed. Delegated tasks/activities depend on the nurse practice act and patient situation.
2. May nursing assistant refuse nursing task/activity?
   When assigning: No, unless staff person thinks he or she is unqualified for the task/activity assignment.
   When delegating: Yes. In addition, the nursing assistant must voluntarily accept the task/activity.
3. What accountability is held for nursing task/activity?
   When assigning: The nursing assistant is accountable for completing the task/activity and in a safe manner.
   When delegating: The LPN/LVN is accountable for delegating the right task/activity to the right person.

Adapted from Hill, S., & Howlett, H. (2009). *Success in Practical/Vocational Nursing: From Student to Leader* (6th ed.). Philadelphia: Saunders, p. 288.

may delegate as an LPN/LVN charge nurse in your state. If your state gives you permission to delegate as an LPN/LVN, check if your place of employment gives permission for delegation in the facility's written policies. Delegation is a *voluntary* function. You do not *have* to delegate simply because the NPA and the facility allow it.

Your nursing program might include class material on delegation. However, a position paper from the NCSBN (the group that develops your licensing examination) states that delegation is a complex skill that new graduates are not prepared to carry out. The skill for delegation must be developed in the clinical area after graduation, usually by working with an experienced licensed nurse who serves as a role model and who provides advice and support on delegation (NCSBN, 2005).

During the LPN/LVN program, students learn the activities and procedures they will perform when licensed, and the reasons for performing them. Each patient situation determines which task/activity can be delegated; there is no specific list of tasks that can be delegated. Because a patient's condition can change so rapidly, judgment must be developed with experience as to what and when it is wise to delegate.

The NCSBN's position paper, *Delegation: Concepts and Decision-Making Process* (1995), provides a decision-making process to be used by licensed persons in clinical settings as a guide for delegation of nursing duties. The NCSBN identifies "Five Rights" to include when delegating:

1. *Right Task*—a task that can legally be delegated for a specific patient.
2. *Right Circumstances*—the patient is stable, independent nursing judgment is not required for the task, and resources to perform task are available.
3. *Right Person*—the person asked to perform the task is competent and qualified to do so.
4. *Right Direction/Communication*—objective and specific explanation of what should be done and when, what to report to the delegating nurse and when to make the report.
5. *Right Supervision*—the delegating nurse needs to monitor the performance of the task, to intervene when needed, to evaluate the results of the task, and to provide feedback to the unlicensed person.

Assignment. With heavy LPN/LVN workloads, many tasks may need to be assigned to nursing assistants or other UAP. Such tasks must be within the job description of the person to whom they are being assigned. The LPN/LVN should always consider the advisability of assigning the task; consider carefully another person's ability to carry out the task; and provide information about how the assigned task should be done, what should be recorded or reported, and to whom it should be reported.

TYPES OF HEALTH CARE FINANCING

HEALTH INSURANCE

Health insurance, like any type of insurance, spreads risk among the whole group of insureds. The young and the healthy generally do not claim as much as the elderly for health care, and (if the fee structure is equivalent for all) the young and healthy subsidize (support) the sick and older persons covered by the insurance provider.

The cost of health care services today generally makes payment directly by the patient (private pay) impossible. The traditional method of financing health care services, fee-for-service, involves direct reimbursement by an insurance company to a provider (a licensed health care person such as a physician, dentist, or nurse practitioner) whose health care services are covered by a health insurance plan. To improve their profit, insurance providers charge a deductible (the yearly amount an insured person must spend out-of-pocket for health care services *before* the insurance provider will begin to pay for services), a copayment (the amount an insured person must pay at the time of an office visit, prescription, or hospital service), and co-insurance (once a deductible is met, the percentage of the total bill paid by the insured person). The insurance company subtracts the amount the patient has paid from the total bill, and then pays the remainder.

Capitation, an alternative for fee-for-service payment, involves a set monthly fee charged by the provider of health care services for each member of the insurance group for a specific set of health care services. If services cost more than the monthly fee, the provider absorbs the cost of those services. At the end of the year, if any money is left over from the unused portions of monthly fees, the health care provider keeps this remainder as a profit.

Group Health Insurance

Group health insurance is a private insurance method of pooling individual contributions with the goal of protecting group members from financial disaster because of health care bills. When insured under a group health plan, an individual is said to have third-party coverage (a middleman), which pays a percentage of the individual's health care bills while the individual pays the balance. Employers offer most group health insurance in the United States (e.g., BlueCross BlueShield).

Managed Care. Managed care is a type of group health insurance developed to provide quality health care with cost and care utilization controls. This is accomplished by paying physicians to care for groups of patients for a set fee, and by limiting services. Medical necessity and the appropriateness of health care services are monitored by a utilization review system. Types of managed care systems include health maintenance organizations (HMOs) and preferred provider organizations (PPOs).

Government-Sponsored Health Insurance

Medicare. Medicare is a federal public insurance program that helps to partially finance health care for all persons over age 65 years (and their spouses), who have at least a 10-year (40 quarters) record in Medicare-covered employment, and who are citizens or permanent residents of the United States. Coverage is also given to persons under age 65 who are victims of end-stage renal disease or are permanently and totally disabled. Those eligible because of age or disability are entitled, by law, to the benefits of Medicare programs. In November 2003, Congress passed the Medicare Prescription Drug, Improvement, and Modernization Act, which is the largest expansion of Medicare since it began in 1965 (Box 1-3).

Before 1983, hospitals submitted a bill to the government for the total charges they incurred for Medicare patients and were reimbursed for the billed amount. Payment was based on actual costs and was called a retrospective payment system. The federal government was the first group to try to stop the skyrocketing cost of health care. In 1983, the Health Care Financing Administration (now the Centers for Medicare and Medicaid Services [CMS]) adopted a system called diagnosis-related groups (DRGs) or illness groups. This system pays hospitals a flat rate for Medicare services, and hospitals now know in advance how much they will be reimbursed by this prospective payment system (PPS).

Box 1-3   Basic Components of Medicare

MEDICARE PART A
- Is available without cost to those eligible for the program.
- Helps pay for inpatient hospital care, including drugs, supplies, laboratory tests, radiology, and intensive care unit.
- Covers 20 days after hospitalization for skilled nursing facility care for rehabilitation services, home health care services under certain conditions, and hospice care.
- Does not pay for nursing home custodial services (e.g., patients only needing help with activities of daily living, feeding), private rooms, telephones, or televisions provided by hospitals or skilled nursing facilities.

MEDICARE PART B
- Is similar to a major medical insurance plan and is funded by monthly premiums.
- Persons who elect to have this coverage pay a monthly premium based on income.
- Requires a deductible and pays 80% of most covered charges. The remaining 20% of charges are the responsibility of the patient.
- Helps pay for medically necessary physicians' services; outpatient hospital services (including emergency department visits); ambulance transportation; diagnostic tests, including laboratory services and mammography and Pap smear screenings; and physical therapy, occupational therapy, and speech therapy in a hospital outpatient department or Medicare-certified rehabilitation agency.
- Does not pay for most prescription drugs, routine physicals, services not related to treatment of illness or injury, dental care, dentures, cosmetic surgery, routine foot care, hearing aids, eye examinations, or glasses.

MEDICARE PART C
- Refers to Medicare Advantage plans, such as HMOs or regional PPOs.
- Provides Part A, B, and D benefits to persons who elect this type of coverage instead of the original fee-for-service program.

MEDICARE PART D
- Refers to the outpatient prescription drug benefit.
- Is available to all Medicare enrollees in the original fee-for-service program for an additional monthly fee.

Under the DRG system, the fee the government will pay for hospitalization depends on the DRG category (illness). Hospitals receive a flat fee for each patient's DRG category, *regardless of length of stay in the hospital;* thus hospitals have an incentive to treat patients and discharge them as quickly as possible. If the hospital keeps the patient longer than the government's fee will cover, and the patient cannot be reclassified in the DRG system, the hospital must absorb the difference in costs. However, if the acute care facility can treat the patient for less than the guaranteed reimbursement amount, *the facility can keep the difference in payment as profit.* Because Medicare patients, as all patients, are discharged sooner from hospitals than they were in the past, extended care units or skilled care facilities and home care are frequently used to continue convalescence. With the goal of improving quality of care and saving millions of taxpayer dollars each year, Medicare no longer covers specific preventable conditions of hospitalized patients (Box 1-4).

? Think Critically

Should Medicare pay for new, expensive, technological procedures that are developed to treat common medical problems of the elderly? Should cost-effectiveness enter the picture for treating Medicare patients? Explain the reasoning behind your answer.

Medicaid. The Medicaid program, which is funded jointly by the federal and state governments, provides medical assistance for eligible families and individuals with low incomes and few resources. The federal government establishes broad national guidelines for the program. Each state establishes its own program services and requirements, including eligibility. Proportionally, Medicaid is the second largest item in state budgets (Box 1-5).

GOALS FOR HEALTH CARE

The United States spends more on health care than any other country, yet approximately 47 million persons in the United States are uninsured. The increase in the elderly population taxes the Medicare system, because chronic illness incidence requires more frequent health care. The impending retirement of "baby

Box 1-4 Health Care–Associated Conditions Not Paid for by Medicare/Medicaid

- Foreign object left in the patient after surgery
- Air embolism
- Blood incompatibility
- Stage III and IV pressure ulcers
- Falls and trauma (fractures, dislocations, intracranial injuries, crushing injuries, burns, electrical shocks)
- Poor glycemic control (diabetic ketoacidosis, nonketotic hyperosmolar coma, hypoglycemic coma, secondary diabetes with ketoacidosis, secondary diabetes with hyperosmolarity)
- Catheter-related urinary tract infection
- Vascular catheter-associated infection
- Surgical site infection following coronary artery bypass graft, particularly mediastinitis (infection in the chest); following bariatric surgery, gastroenterostomy, laparoscopic gastric restrictive surgery, or orthopedic procedures
- Deep vein thrombosis or pulmonary embolism following total knee replacement or hip replacement.

Data from *www.cms.hhs.gov/apps/media/press/release.asp?Counter=3041.* Retrieved 29 October 2010.

Box 1-5 The Medicaid Program

- Medicaid is the second largest item in state budgets and covers over 39 million low-income children and parents, many in working families.
- Medicaid is the largest source of health insurance for children in the United States. The State Children's Health Insurance Program (SCHIP) supplements Medicaid by providing coverage for low-income children who are not covered by health insurance and do not qualify for Medicaid.
- Medicaid is the primary source of health and long-term care coverage for low-income individuals with disabilities or chronic illnesses and those who need mental health services and substance abuse treatment.
- Medicaid covers services that Medicare does not cover for low-income Medicare beneficiaries, including long-term care and vision and dental care. Medicare beneficiaries who are also enrolled in Medicaid are known as "dual eligibles."

boomers" (persons born in the period immediately following World War II) will tax the Medicare system even more. As strains on government support for health care increase, Medicare and Medicaid reimbursements to providers continue to decline.

Many persons are unable to afford health insurance premiums and some covered by a health insurance plan are unable to pay the plan's deductibles and copayments. Some retirees who received health insurance as part of their retirement benefits have had these benefits reduced or eliminated. Advances in technology make noninvasive diagnosis of some diseases possible, and technology helps treat these diseases with fewer complications and side effects, but these technologies are very expensive. The continually increasing costs of medications means that some patients cannot afford prescribed drugs.

COST CONTAINMENT

The driving force today in all health care facilities is cost containment (holding costs to within fixed limits, while remaining competitive in the health care marketplace). Health care agencies are interested in improving their agency's "bottom line" with business principles that reduce waste and inefficiency. Consumers would like the cost of health care to be reduced while high-quality care and service are maintained. Service, quality, and cost control are attributes of health care that need to be understood and considered in all clinical situations, and the LPN/LVN has the opportunity to identify wasteful practices and inefficient routines in the work setting (Box 1-6).

HEALTH PROMOTION AND *HEALTHY PEOPLE 2020*

Healthy People 2020 is a health promotion and disease prevention agenda by the U.S. Department of Health and Human Services to improve the health of all

| Box 1-6 | LPN/LVN Role in Containing Health Care Costs in the Work Setting |

1. Follow facility policy for charging patients for all supplies used in their care.
2. Follow facility policy for documenting patient care for reimbursement.
3. Organize patient care for effective and efficient use of time. If some aspect of care needs to be "redone," it would have been better and more time-efficient to do it right the first time.
4. Decrease patient length of stay by implementing nursing care to help prevent complications.
5. Meet the patient's needs, not your needs.

From Hill, S., & Howlett, H. (2009). *Success in Practical/Vocational Nursing: From Student to Leader* (6th ed.). Philadelphia: Saunders, p. 325.

people in the United States. It includes a set of health objectives based on the best available scientific knowledge. *Healthy People 2020* has the potential to affect the health of all U.S. citizens and reduce health care costs, but individuals, groups, and organizations must work together to incorporate *Healthy People 2020* into current programs, special events, publications, and meetings. Every LPN/LVN has the responsibility to educate patients about healthy lifestyles and assist the health of their communities through educational health promotion. Nurses can also model healthier lifestyles for their patients by not smoking, maintaining healthy eating habits, and exercising to manage weight.

Health Promotion

Healthy People 2020 Overarching Goals

- Attain high-quality, longer lives free of preventable disease and disability, and full of opportunities for progress.
- Achieve health equity, eliminate disparities, and improve the health of all groups.
- Create social and physical environments that promote good health for all.
- Promote quality of life, healthy development, and healthy behaviors across all life stages.

HOLISTIC CARE OF PATIENTS

Holistic care involves being aware of and attending to the physiologic, psychological, social, cultural, and spiritual needs of patients. Data for many of these needs can be collected, and interventions carried out, while administering care and treatments. Assisting with bathing, feeding, ambulating, and other physical care provides an opportunity to find out about dimensions of the patient's life beyond his or her physical problems. Use time with the patient constructively.

 Focused Assessment

Data Collection for Holistic Assessment

PHYSICAL ASSESSMENT
- List and prioritize assessments/data to be collected for specific medical and/or surgical diagnoses and treatments for the patient.

PSYCHOLOGICAL ASSESSMENT
- What is your greatest concern about this hospitalization?
- Is there anyone you do not want to visit you while in the hospital?
- Who are the significant persons in your life?
- Who is your source of support, for help with problems?
- Do you have any fears that may get in the way of diagnosis and treatment? Closed spaces, darkness, needles, etc.?
- Do you experience problems with eating? Too much? Too little? If so, how much of a weight gain or loss have you had in the past 2 months?
- Do you smoke? How much every day?
- Do you drink alcohol? What and how often?
- What do you do to relieve stressful feelings?
- Do you experience feeling hopeless or very sad? How often and what triggers the feeling?
- Is there anyone in your life who abuses you? Verbally? Physically? If so, describe how.
- Are you sexually active? If yes, are you satisfied with your sex life?

SOCIAL ASSESSMENT
- With whom do you live? How will your admission affect those with whom you live?
- Do you have a personal relationship with someone? If so, are you satisfied with this relationship?
- Do you have children? If so, who will care for your children while you are in the hospital?
- Are you employed? If so, how will your illness/accident/hospitalization affect your job? Do you have sick leave at work?
- Do you have health insurance?
- Who are the persons in your life who can be of help at this time?
- Will you be able to manage at home with bathing, meals, cleaning, laundry, errands, and obtaining your medications and/or needed equipment for your treatments?
- Are there any physical impediments (stairs, tub but no shower, etc.) that will make it difficult at home?

CULTURAL ASSESSMENT
- What are your beliefs or practices for staying well?
- What foods do you have in your diet that help you stay well?
- What foods in your diet help you recover when you are sick?
- Do you use complementary and alternative medicine (CAM)?
- If you use CAM, did you inform your physician of CAM use, including herbals?

SPIRITUAL ASSESSMENT
- How do you cope with problems or difficult situations?
- Do you believe in the power of prayer?
- Do you meditate or read spiritual materials?
- What are your beliefs about a higher power?
- If you have a relationship to a higher power, do you have a religious affiliation? If so, do you want a representative of your religious affiliation notified of your admission?
- Do you have any religious items that you wear on your person?

Meeting Psychological Needs

Use of Empathy. An important part of the nurse-patient relationship is the nurse's ability to display empathy. No one can know or feel what another experiences. Empathy involves accurately perceiving the patient's feelings and understanding their meanings, even though the nurse cannot experience the emotional impact of these feelings as the patient does.

No one can know or feel what another experiences, but empathy displays appreciation for what the other person is feeling.

The empathetic nurse conveys the interpretation of the patient's feelings back to the patient, for validation of their accuracy. In this way, the patient's feelings are valued and accepted as legitimate responses. An example of an empathetic statement by the nurse is, "You seem upset about your surgery tomorrow." In contrast, sympathy involves entering into feelings with patients and is displayed by sorrow and concern. An example of a sympathetic statement by the nurse is, "You poor thing. I had that surgery."

Patients judge their health care experiences by the nature of the help they receive. Scores on patient satisfaction surveys drop when care is impersonal.

Promote a Therapeutic Nurse-Patient Relationship.
The focus of the nurse-patient relationship is on the patient's problems and needs. The relationship is therapeutic, because it provides the patient with the help needed for healing or for a return to wellness. In comparison, a social relationship is not goal-directed, exists primarily for pleasure, and meets the needs of each person in the relationship. LPN/LVNs need to maintain boundaries when working with patients. Avoid using patient contact to meet personal needs (e.g., the need to be liked, for friendship, or for approval). LPN/LVNs need to develop awareness of their own personal needs, and to realize that those needs are appropriately met outside their professional roles, within their personal lives.

The nurse-patient relationship ends when the patient is discharged. Avoid the temptation to continue the relationship on a social basis, which means not allowing the exchange of addresses, phone/cell numbers, or e-mail addresses. It is not beneficial to patients to stay in contact with their nurses after discharge. Sometimes patients want to present nurses with gifts at the time of discharge. Check facility policy regarding this practice.

Establish trust. To develop a therapeutic relationship, trust needs to be established between patient and nurse. In today's health care system, time with patients is limited and each patient contact must be fully utilized. Knock before entering the room, give your name, identify yourself as a nursing student or LPN/LVN, and give the reason for your visit. Call patients by name and preferred title, explain how long you will be on duty, advise when meals arrive and when to expect physicians to visit, and so on. Explain what care will be given on the shift and when it will be offered.

Many older patients are not accustomed to the informality of having strangers address them by their given (first) name. Clarify how the patient would like to be addressed. Put the patient at ease with a pleasant, unhurried approach. Other behaviors to establish trust follow.

Use therapeutic communication skills. Communicate at the level of the patient's understanding. Active listening helps the patient express needs and feelings. Ask patients what they think and actively listen to their answers, as well as to their concerns and fears. Avoid judging the message or the patient. Avoid forming a response while the patient is speaking. Rephrase the message when the patient is finished, to verify that you understand the message. Make sure the patient's and your verbal and nonverbal communication are congruent. Answer all the patient's questions, when possible. Admit when you do not know the answer to a question, and find out and deliver the answer as soon as possible. The focus needs to be the physical and mental well-being of patients and the development of trust. Thank the patient for cooperation and attention. Avoid gossip, arguments, and complaints within patients' range of hearing. Patients may think that because staff cannot get along with each other, they cannot focus on the patients' needs.

Maintain patients' self-esteem. A major problem for patients of any age is the loss of self-esteem. In a health care setting, patients sometimes may be viewed as problems. Patients are sometimes dealt with as an illness (diagnosis) or as a behavior, instead of as a person who happens to have a particular illness or behavior. How often have you heard a patient referred to as "the hip fracture in 205" or "the depressed woman in 305"? Nurses and physicians are especially guilty of this demeaning practice. Some patients are talked down to, coddled, or treated as though they have no strengths. Identify the strengths of patients and find a way to support those strengths and thereby sustain patients' self-esteem.

> ### ? Think Critically
>
> If you have experienced an illness or injury or have a chronic illness, have you ever been treated in a demeaning way? How did it make you feel? How would you have liked to have been treated?

Display competence. A skilled and competent nurse builds a patient's confidence, which decreases a patient's anxiety. Focus on the patient and explain what procedures entail and what to expect before starting treatments. Patients expect nurses to be competent when performing treatments and have necessary equipment at hand before beginning a procedure. Leave the patient's environment clean and orderly after procedures.

Ensure pain control. Many nursing actions help to decrease patient stress, but pain control is an especially important action. Anticipate patients' pain control needs before they are expressed—for example, before painful procedures are administered, and before ambulating after surgery or a long illness. Assess the need for further pain medication before the next dose is due and determine whether the medication is effective. If pain medicine is not doing its job, speak to the physician and get the order changed. Give a back rub along with pain medication, when appropriate, for added relief.

Display compassion. Displaying compassion is considered "low-tech nursing," because no degree, advanced training, or increase in unit budget is required to display kindness and patience to patients. Treat patients with common courtesy, and see them as unique individuals worthy of respect. All health care workers need to be aware of the rights of the patient (see Appendix G). A good starting point is to view the patient as someone's spouse, relative, friend, or parent.

Use therapeutic touch. Touch can be reassuring, calming, and encouraging to patients. In this era of threats of sexual harassment, some nurses may be afraid to touch patients. Ask if touch is OK or touch an arm or a hand and be aware of the patient's reaction, to see if this gesture is acceptable. Be aware of cultural taboos about being touched.

Elder Care Points

- Please treat me with respect. Avoid treating me as if I have a mental impairment until you clarify by looking on my chart that I do have one. Avoid shouting at me until you clarify that I have a hearing deficit. Regardless, speak in a normal volume, with a medium to low pitch, and enunciate clearly.
- Be patient with me. It might take me longer to get out of bed, to walk to the bathroom, or to answer your repeated questions. If you need to give me information, give it to me slowly, and ask for feedback to see if I understood. It would help if you gave me printed information to read.
- If my family or friends are with me and you want information about me, ask me and let me speak for myself. Also, I want to be included in decision making and planning for my care. Ask me if I would mind being hugged or touched before you do so. If I don't mind, avoid patting me on the head like a child; that is demeaning. Be patient when I talk too much. I may be lonely. Treat me in a way you would want your mother, grandmother, or grandfather treated, or treat me as you would want to be treated if you were in my situation.

Patients Who Display Difficult Behaviors. A patient who is physically ill is also affected emotionally by the illness or injury. It is not unusual for patients to display behavior that is not their usual manner. Patients' emotional needs and the resulting behaviors are usually temporary and related to the stresses of illness. Occasionally, patient behavior is related to underlying disorders that will benefit from a psychiatric consultation or treatment (see Chapters 46 through 49). Even patients whose primary illness is a physical rather than psychological disorder can sometimes express emotional discomfort through **dependent,** withdrawn, hostile, or manipulative behavior. They may behave in ways that are confusing and are uncomfortable for the nurse who is not prepared to intervene effectively.

It is easier to deal with patients' behaviors if you understand that their responses to a particular situation are the best they are capable of offering at that particular time. The task of the nurse is to recognize that patients'

behavior results from the demands being placed on them at the moment. Appropriate nursing responses require kindness, understanding, and sometimes firmness. People may become childlike and fearful when they are ill or act as if they are unaffected by their illness. Patients appreciate having someone available to guide them through their ordeal in a therapeutic manner.

Think Critically

When you were assigned to a patient who had a manipulative pattern of behavior, did the patient remind you of someone you know personally? Ask yourself, did you "hang that person's face" on this patient, and respond to the patient accordingly? What was the result?

Meeting Social Needs

Inability to assume personal responsibilities can be a source of worry for patients and may interfere with a positive outcome after illness or surgery. Some patients are caring for aging parents, are grandparents who play an active, daily role in caring for grandchildren, or are a single parent with young children. If a patient lives alone, pet care may be a concern. When employed, patients might have used all their sick leave, may not have health insurance, or may carry a high insurance deductible. Patients enrolled in an educational program might be concerned about having to drop a course or leave a program because of time lost to hospitalization, diagnostic tests, or restrictions such as not being able to drive.

Think Critically

What impact would your admission today for an emergency appendectomy have on your life? How could you resolve your concerns? Who could help you in this situation?

Meeting Cultural Needs

Health care must accommodate patients of many cultural backgrounds. Patients may think and behave differently because of social class, religion, ethnic background, minority group status, marital status, or sexual preference. Avoid making judgments about people who are culturally different. Nurses should be open-minded and **nonjudgmental,** taking differences at face value, accepting people as they are, and giving high-quality care.

Think Critically

Can you give examples of judgmental behaviors you observed in staff members during your clinical rotation?

The philosophy of individual worth is the belief in the uniqueness and value of each human being. Nurses need to realize that individuals have the right to live according to personal beliefs and values *as long as those beliefs and values do not interfere with the rights of others and are within the law.*

Nursing students sometimes think that somewhere there is a recipe book that will tell them how to care for people who are different from themselves. Applying information to all individuals in a group can lead to assumptions, which are called **stereotypes.** A stereotype is a generic simplification used to describe all members of a group, without exception. Stereotyping provides an expectation that all individuals in a group will act in a particular way in a given situation, simply because these individuals are members of a cultural group. Stereotypes ignore individual differences that each person in every cultural group possesses. Members of any culture may have modified the degree to which they observe the values and practices of their culture. Information about cultural groups can help explain—but cannot predict—individual behavior.

🌐 Cultural Considerations

Cultural Preferences

- People from the Philippines may be shy and feel awkward in unfamiliar surroundings. They may give little direct eye contact. A family member should be allowed at the bedside at all times. The patient may be reluctant to venture out of the room to ambulate.
- Many Cambodians believe that the soul resides in the head and it is inappropriate to touch their heads without permission. Ask before touching the head when changing head dressings or applying eyedrops.
- Hmong from Southeast Asia prefer their own relatives as interpreters and may not trust a hospital-employed interpreter. The interpreter should be of the same sex as the patient, as neither Hmong men nor women may discuss or admit to intimate problems to an interpreter of the opposite sex.

When disease strikes, people may blame pathogens (germs), spirits, or an imbalance in the body. Some cultural groups have folk medicine rituals or special procedures to address maladies (e.g., rubbing the skin with the edge of a coin to release the toxins causing illness). Some groups have special persons who are charged with curing disease (physician, herbalist, shaman, or curandero). Some groups believe that special foods, or food combinations ("cold" foods for "hot" illness), or herbs (echinacea, feverfew) can prevent or cure illnesses. Others see no relationship between the diet and health. Some patients consider the prevention of illness as an attempt to control the future; they may wonder about the necessity to see a health care provider for preventive care (e.g., immunizations). Different beliefs of patients need to be respected.

Biomedicine. **Biomedicine** is the dominant health system in the United States and focuses on symptoms. The goal of biomedicine is to find the cause of disease and to eliminate or correct the problem. However, many Americans use methods that focus on the whole body—and not exclusively on symptoms—when treating disease.

Complementary and Alternative Medicine. **Complementary** (used in conjunction with biomedical treatments) **and alternative** (substituted for biomedical medicine) **medicine (CAM)** focus on assisting the body's own healing powers and restoring body balance. The National Center for Complementary and Alternative Medicine (NCCAM) of the National Institutes of Health researches and evaluates the effectiveness and safety of CAM therapies. Natural medicines often have not undergone scientific studies to determine correct doses, side effects, or risk of interactions with other medicines or foods. Patients need to be reminded that all herbals and supplements need to be included when they are asked for a list of drugs taken.

Meeting Spiritual Needs

Spirituality is an essential part of being human. A person's spirit may be thought to incorporate the beliefs and values that provide strength and hope, awareness of self (including inner strengths), and understanding of life's meaning and purpose. Patients have a spiritual self with spiritual needs, and patients may use spiritual practices to meet those needs. Examples of personal spiritual practices may include gardening, reading inspirational books, listening to music, meditating, praying, communing with nature, practicing breathing techniques, volunteering, expressing gratitude, and counting blessings.

Spirituality and *religion* are related terms, but they do not have the same meaning. Religion attempts to formalize and ritualize spiritual beliefs. Some patients fulfill spiritual needs by belonging to a religious denomination. The different rituals and practices of a religion can bring the security of the past into a crisis situation. Concrete symbols, such as books, pictures, icons, herb packets, beads, statues, jewelry, and other objects, can affirm patients' connection with their belief in a higher power. The value of patients' rituals and religious practices is determined by their faith, and is not subject to scientific evidence. Spirituality, on the other hand, does not necessarily include religion and its formal practice.

Crisis situations frequently surface in acute health care situations. Patients' beliefs and values can profoundly affect their response to these crises, attitude toward treatment, and rate of recovery. The need for spiritual care for patients and families may be intensified by hospitalization, pain experiences, chronic or incurable disease, terminal illness, or the death of a loved one (Box 1-7).

The pastoral care team allies with nurses in providing spiritual care for patients, but pastoral care workers do not relieve nurses of their responsibility to provide spiritual care. Follow agency policy for arranging visits of patients' clergy or spiritual advisors, when such visits are desired. Agency policies vary, and pastoral care policies are being tested nationwide.

Box 1-7   Spiritual Care Interventions

- Ask open-ended questions—ones that cannot be answered by "yes" or "no."
- Actively listen to the patient. Sit beside the patient. Make eye contact, if culturally appropriate.
- Be nonjudgmental of patients and their responses.
- Avoid giving advice or a lecture to the patient.
- Avoid being a proselytizer (a person who tries to convert another person to his or her own religion).
- Be aware of nonverbal messages from the patient.
- Understand the feelings of the patient but avoid adopting those feelings.
- Expect to learn from patients.

- Stay with the patient after the patient has received an unfavorable diagnosis.
- When patients request help with prayer, offer to pray with them if you are comfortable doing so.
- When the patient requests help with specific readings, offer to read to the patient.
- Assist the patient to participate in desired spiritual/religious rituals.
- Protect the patient's spiritual/religious articles. Do not remove them if they are being worn, unless required by emergency.

Adapted from Hill, S., & Howlett, H. (2009). *Success in Practical/Vocational Nursing: From Student to Leader* (6th ed.). Philadelphia: Saunders, p. 208.

Get Ready for the NCLEX® Examination!

Key Points

- Medical-surgical nursing is a vast nursing specialty that involves care for adult patients with medical and/or surgical conditions that affect one or more body systems.
- The most common site of employment for the LPN/LVN as charge nurse is the nursing home/long-term care facility.
- Qualities and skills needed by LPN/LVNs for medical-surgical nursing include upholding clinical practice standards, providing safe patient care, teaching patients, communicating effectively, working as a collaborative member of the health care team, and advocating for the patient.
- Each state's nurse practice act (NPA) defines what the LPN/LVN can and cannot do in practice, including delegating from the position of charge nurse.
- Assignment involves allocating tasks to unlicensed personnel—when those tasks are within their job descriptions, and once the patient has been declared stable.
- Delegation involves designating duties to unlicensed personnel that are in the job description of the LPN/LVN, are within the boundaries of the nurse practice act, and are advisable considering the patient situation.
- The fee-for-service method of financing health care services has been challenged by the capitation method of financing those services.
- Medicare and Medicaid are examples of government-sponsored health insurance in the United States.
- To help curb rising health care costs, the federal government adopted a payment system called diagnosis-related groups (DRGs) as part of Medicare.
- To help curb costs and increase the quality of care, Medicare will not reimburse for some conditions unless those conditions exist at the time of admission.
- The driving force in health care facilities is cost containment. LPN/LVNs play a role in containing health care costs in the work setting.
- Holistic care includes being aware of the physical, psychological, social, cultural, and spiritual needs of patients.
- The nurse-patient relationship is therapeutic and goal-directed, and ends when the patient is discharged.
- Trust is established with patients by using therapeutic communication skills, maintaining the patient's self-esteem, displaying competence in providing care, and displaying compassion for patients.
- The patient with a physical illness is also affected emotionally and may display dependent, hostile, or manipulative behaviors.

Additional Learning Resources

SG Go to your Study Guide for additional learning activities to help you master this chapter content.

evolve Go to your Evolve website (http://evolve.elsevier.com/deWit/medsurg) for the following FREE learning resources:
- Animations, audio, and video
- Answers and rationales for questions and activities
- Concept Map Creator
- Glossary with pronunciations in English and Spanish
- Interactive Review Questions and Exercises and more!

 Online Resources
- *Healthy People 2020,* www.healthypeople.gov
- National Council of State Boards of Nursing (NCSBN), www.ncsbn.org/Joint_statement.pdf
- National Federation of Licensed Practical Nurses (NFLPN), www.nflpn.org/practice-standards4web.pdf

Review Questions for the NCLEX® Examination

1. On initial assessment, the patient is found to be quite interested in asking questions about the nurse, evades personal questions, and is often silent while making no eye contact. These characteristics are more likely to be found in which behaviors?

   1. Withdrawn
   2. Manipulative
   3. Dependent
   4. Hostile

2. Which statement made by a patient strongly indicates dependent behavior?

   1. "I can do this by myself. I do not need help."
   2. "I will try to do this and will ask for help if needed."
   3. "Would you help me if I am not able to do it myself?"
   4. "I'm tired and I'd rather you help me dress."

3. A patient must decide between HMO or PPO health care plans that her employer offers. Which statement best describes coverage of the HMO plan?

   1. "All heath care bills are covered except yearly mammograms, annual physical exams, and routine colonoscopies."
   2. "Patients can only see physicians hired by the HMO whenever a visit or treatment is required—no exceptions."
   3. "I will have to pay a fixed monthly fee and a co-payment for each doctor's visit regardless of treatment needed."
   4. "I will have to pay charges as I leave the doctor's office and send the bills to the HMO for reimbursement."

4. Which condition is not paid for by Medicare if it develops after hospitalization?

   1. Hypokalemia
   2. Heart attack
   3. Hip fracture
   4. Meningitis

5. If the nurse is caring for a patient with an indwelling urinary catheter, which task can be delegated to the nursing assistant?

   1. Providing perineal care each morning and evening
   2. Collecting a urine specimen for laboratory testing
   3. Irrigating the catheter to ensure patency
   4. Instilling antibiotics for a urinary infection

6. In caring for patients with pressure ulcers, which task would be most appropriate to delegate to the nursing assistant?

   1. Providing assistance in making dietary choices, including fluids
   2. Participating in determining the appropriate type of wound care
   3. Repositioning the patient every 2 hours
   4. Describing condition of the wound and any drainage

7. The nurse finds a confused patient with a history of falls attempting to get out of bed. To maintain the patient's self-esteem and safety, the nurse's intervention should be to:

   1. apply physical restraints to keep the patient in bed.
   2. administer sedatives per doctor's order.
   3. install a bed alarm to notify staff.
   4. discover what the patient is searching for.

8. After providing discharge instructions to a patient following knee replacement, which statement by the patient indicates a need for further teaching?

   1. "I will wash my hands before changing my dressing."
   2. "I will be on strict bed rest to allow my knee to heal."
   3. "I will take analgesics before the pain gets worse."
   4. "I will be able to eat and drink as usual."

9. What should the nurse do before delegating a specific task? (Select all that apply.)

   1. Know the scope of practice.
   2. Be aware of the staff person's competency and experience.
   3. Seek approval from the facility administration.
   4. Determine stability of the patient's condition.
   5. Provide adequate explanation and oversight of the task.

10. The patients states, "I'm worried about this procedure." Which statement(s) would be therapeutic? (Select all that apply.)

    1. "You poor thing. I had a similar surgery."
    2. "You seem upset regarding your procedure."
    3. "Can you tell me what you mean by that?"
    4. "You will be fine. Your doctor is the best."
    5. "I will hold your hand during the entire procedure."

Critical Thinking Questions

Scenario A
During your clinical rotations, your instructors will schedule a clinical evaluation. Thinking about your clinical experience to date, consider the following.

1. What are your strong areas within the roles of the LPN/LVN? Give example corresponding behaviors for each role.

2. What are the roles of the LPN/LVN and corresponding behaviors for areas where you feel you need improvement?

3. What behaviors are necessary to improve the above roles during the rest of the medical-surgical rotation?

Scenario B
The U.S. federal government is faced with budget problems resulting in large deficits and the need to reduce spending. Congress suggests reducing spending by cuts in the Medicare and Medicaid programs. The congressional representative for your district asks for your opinion and your rationale in answer to each of the following questions.

1. Should Medicare pay the cost of coronary bypass surgery for an active 85-year-old person?

2. Should Medicaid pay for care in an extended-care facility for an 88-year-old person who has suffered a stroke and is long-term comatose?

3. Should Medicare or Medicaid pay for lifestyle prescription drugs (e.g., Viagra) for men eligible for these programs?

Scenario C
Bill Boyd, age 72, was surprised at the aloofness of the admission clerk as she "entered" him into the electronic system for a total knee replacement, his first hospital experience. Two personnel who assisted him to his assigned room called him "Bill." Neither introduced themselves or indicated the role they played in his admission. While wearing a patient gown with the opening down the front and waiting for a nurse to interview him, people kept coming into his room without knocking. One asked his wife if he drank coffee or tea with his meals. That night, the sound of TVs, the click and beep of machines, and staff talking in the halls prevented him from getting a good night's sleep before surgery.

1. List the things that went wrong with Mr. Boyd's admission-day experience.

2. Describe how you would have made admission day a better experience.

3. Explain the reasons for the things you chose to do differently.

Scenario D
Mario Villanuevo, a Mexican American, has a fracture of the right femur and is in balanced suspension traction. Neurovascular assessments are indicated every shift. The LPN/LVN documents that Mario moves the toes of his right foot on command and can feel the nurse touch different aspects of each toe. The pulse in the dorsalis pedis artery of the right foot is palpable and the foot is warm to touch. The LPN/LVN is unable to note any color changes because of the patient's dark skin tone.

1. How can the LPN/LVN student assess color of any patient who has dark skin tone?

2. What should the LPN/LVN student do if there is a question about finding the dorsalis pedis pulse?

3. If sensation is diminished, what should the LPN/LVN student do?

Critical Thinking and the Nursing Process

Objectives

Theory

1. Explain what critical thinking is in your own words.
2. Describe how critical thinking affects clinical judgment.
3. Discuss why nurses in all programs must learn to think critically.
4. Clarify your role in nursing process according to your state's nurse practice act.
5. Explain three fundamental beliefs about human life as the basis for nursing process.
6. Identify the source for LPN/LVN standards for nursing practice.

Clinical Practice

1. Explain how factors that influence critical thinking are experienced by you during patient care.
2. Provide a clinical example of how nursing process is used in the care of medical-surgical patients.

3. Provide an example of each of the following techniques of physical examination: inspection and observation, olfaction, auscultation, and percussion.
4. Prepare a list for beginning-of-shift assessment for a specific patient.
5. Write an example of a patient goal that is realistic, measurable, and time-referenced.
6. Differentiate between nursing orders and medical orders.
7. Explain the value of identifying the patient's actual problems that lead to nursing diagnoses.
8. Provide a clinical example of a bundle used to reduce the incidence of a deadly infection.
9. Explain the purpose of National Patient Safety Goals.
10. Explain how core measures relate to clinical care.

Key Terms

auscultation (ăw-skŭl-TĀ-shŭn, p. 20)
bundles (p. 16)
congruent (kŏn-GRŪ-ĕnt, p. 20)
Core Measures (p. 17)
critical thinking (p. 14)
data collection (DĀ-tă, p. 15)
evaluation (ĭh-văl-ū-Ā-shŭn, p. 15)
expected outcomes (p. 26)
goals (p. 26)
implementation (ĭm-plĭ-mĕn-TĀ-shŭn, p. 15)
inspection (p. 20)
interdisciplinary (collaborative) care plans (kŏ-LĂB-ĕr-ă-tĭv plănz, p. 27)
National Patient Safety Goals (NPSGs) (p. 16)

North American Nursing Diagnosis Association International (NANDA-I) (p. 24)
nursing diagnosis (p. 24)
nursing interventions (p. 26)
nursing process (p. 16)
objective data (ŏb-JĔK-tĭv DĀ-tă, p. 17)
observation (p. 20)
olfaction (ōl-FĂK-shŭn, p. 20)
palpation (păl-PĀ-shŭn, p. 20)
percussion (pĕr-KŬ-shŭn, p. 20)
planning (p. 15)
priority setting (p. 24)
subjective data (sŭb-JĔK-tĭv DĀ-tă, p. 17)

Critical thinking is a method for solving problems. In nursing practice, critical thinking incorporates the scientific method and always asks, "Is there a better way?" Developing critical thinking skills is a lifelong process and, as you practice the knowledge you are gaining, you become more skilled at thinking critically and applying new knowledge to patient care.

CRITICAL THINKING AND CLINICAL JUDGMENT

Critical thinking applied to clinical judgment in practical/vocational nursing can be described as:
• Purposeful, informed, and outcome focused (results oriented), requiring careful identification of patient problems, issues, and risks, and makes accurate

decisions about what is happening, what needs to be done, and what the priorities are for patient care.
- Driven by patient, family, and community health care needs.
- Based on principles of nursing process (Box 2-1) and the scientific method.
- Using both logic and intuition and is based on knowledge, skills, and the professional experience of the LPN/LVN.
- Guided by standards and ethical codes of the following organizations:
  - National Association of Practical Nurse Education and Service, Inc. (NAPNES) *Standards of Practice for Licensed Practical/Vocational Nurses* (see Appendix E) and *Code of Ethics*
  - National Federation of Licensed Practical Nurses, Inc. (NFLPN) *Nursing Practice Standards for the Licensed Practical/Vocational Nurse* (see Appendix F) and *The Code for Licensed Practical/Vocational Nurses*
- Calling for strategies that make the most of human potential (e.g., using individual strengths), and compensating for problems created by human nature (e.g., overcoming the powerful influence of personal beliefs, values, and prejudices).
- Meaning constantly reevaluating, self-correcting, and striving to improve (e.g., practicing skills, learning new skills, attending classes and workshops, and reading nursing journals) (Alfaro-Lefevre, 2009; Hill & Howlett, 2009).

Critical thinking involves expanding one's thinking beyond the obvious. The critical thinker (1) is willing to consider other ideas, (2) recognizes that there may be more than one way to do the right thing, and (3) realizes that there may not be a perfect solution. Judgments are based on facts (knowledge)—not on assumptions—and these facts are synthesized and applied to a patient situation. A critical thinker recognizes the patient's primary problems and makes decisions about how to prioritize the problems and how to deal with deviations from normal health status.

Box 2-1   **Four Phases of the Nursing Process for LPN/LVNs**

Data Collection: Assist the RN by a systematic gathering and review of information about the patient and communicating it to appropriate members of the health care team.
Planning: Assist the RN in the development of expected outcomes and interventions for a patient's plan of care.
Implementation: Provide planned nursing care to accomplish expected outcomes.
Evaluation: Compare actual outcomes of nursing care to expected outcomes and assist with updating the nursing care plan.

? Think Critically

Can you list three examples in which you might use critical thinking in the classroom?

Critical thinking is at its best when the brain is purposefully engaged. For example, while listening to a report at the beginning of the shift, pay attention to what the nurse is saying and think about how you will apply the information you have gained. Observe the critical thinking activities that take place among the nurses during the report as they collaborate in solving a patient-related problem. Observe the same elements later in the shift as nurses make decisions about patient care issues, about when to notify the physician, and the like. Consider the following when receiving report:
- Do I understand what is being said?
- What will I be expected to do?
- What are the priorities of nursing care?
- What areas need further clarification?
- What procedures will require instructor supervision?

Examine your thinking and the thinking of others, and apply the knowledge to patient care. Critical thinking is based on science and scientific principles and includes:
- Collecting data in an organized way
- Verifying data in an organized way
- Looking for gaps in information
- Analyzing the data

With the patient's needs in mind, apply critical thinking when developing a care plan. As a student and as a nurse, you must access, understand, recall, and use information as the basis for critical thinking in the clinical arena. Much of what you learn as a student involves exposure to sources of information, and how to access these sources quickly. Of course, some information must be committed to memory, and the more you use learned information, the easier it is to remember. As you practice putting information into your own words when planning patient care, you are reinforcing your comprehension of the information. Critical thinking allows the nurse to apply learned knowledge and principles to different patient care situations.

FACTORS THAT INFLUENCE YOUR THINKING AND NURSING CARE

Attitude

A major factor in learning to apply critical thinking is attitude. The critical thinker is humble and recognizes that he does not have all the answers; he also recognizes that his perceptions may be clouded by personal values and beliefs. The critical thinker makes an effort to consider evidence that is presented objectively.

Box 2-2	Actual Examples of Student Charting (How *Not* to Chart)

- Vaginal packing out. Dr. Heffle in.
- Dr. Jones in. Had large formed brown stool.
- On the second day the knee was better, and on the third day it disappeared.
- She is numb from the toes down.
- Patient was alert and nonresponsive.

Communication Skills

The critical thinker communicates effectively both orally and in writing. The critical thinker reflects on thoughts before speaking and presents information in a clear, concise manner. When documenting, the critical thinker clearly conveys to other health team members what was planned, the patient's reaction to any care offered or provided, and whether expected outcomes were met (Box 2-2).

? Think Critically

Recall the first time you gave a report on a patient. What was the general feedback you received? Has feedback changed with the most recent report you gave, and if so, in what way?

It is helpful to identify a nurse who is skilled at thinking critically and who can communicate clearly both verbally and through charting. This person, who might be an instructor or a nurse who works on the medical-surgical unit, can serve as a mentor to you as you learn to apply critical thinking and knowledge. The most effective mentor will be one who coaches by asking questions, rather than someone who merely provides answers.

INTEGRATING CRITICAL THINKING AND THE NURSING PROCESS

The NCSBN integrated critical thinking and the nursing process into all aspects of the practical/vocational licensing examination (NCLEX-PN®) in 2002. The NCSBN also clearly defined the LPN/LVN role in the nursing process.

? Think Critically

What does your state's nurse practice act (NPA) indicate about the role of the LPN/LVN? What questions do you have regarding clarification of the NPA?

If in doubt about the role of the LPN/LVN in the nursing process, direct your questions to your state's board of nursing. It is important to have studied the NPA of the state in which you work. According to NCSBN research, all U.S. states and territories identify a scope of practice for either LPNs or LVNs. However, the scope of practice allowed varies widely. Although

most LPN/LVN scopes of practice stipulate a directed role under the supervision of an RN, many scopes of practice differ in the areas of care planning, assessment, intravenous therapy, teaching, and delegation (Spector, 2005).

THE NURSING PROCESS

Nursing process is the language of nursing. It is an orderly way to assess a patient's response to current health status and to plan, implement, and evaluate the patient's response to nursing care. It is a way to communicate to all nursing personnel what is to be done and who is to do it, during all shifts. Nursing process provides a way to make changes in patient care if progress is not being made. The nursing process builds on a patient's strengths and creates a partnership between nurse and patient whenever possible. The goal of the nursing process is to alleviate, minimize, or prevent real or potential health problems.

THE INSTITUTE FOR HEALTHCARE IMPROVEMENT BUNDLES

The Institute for Healthcare Improvement (IHI) (2009) developed the concept of **bundles,** a collection of evidence-based (tested) interventions that—when delivered as a group—have been shown to offer reliable care to a patient undergoing high-risk treatment. Bundles usually consist of three to five interventions. Unlike checklists that may be the responsibility of a number of staff members (e.g., discharge checklist), a bundle is "owned" by particular staff members. The entire bundle is completed with no exception, within a specific time and in a specific space. An example is a Central Line Bundle, which consists of a set of five steps to help prevent catheter-related bloodstream infections—deadly infections that can be introduced through an intravenous (IV) line in a patient's vein. The steps are simple, commonsense tasks including using proper hygiene and sterile contact barriers, properly cleaning the patient's skin, finding the best possible vein for the IV line, checking every day for infection, and removing or changing the line only when needed (IHI, 2009).

THE JOINT COMMISSION NATIONAL PATIENT SAFETY GOALS

The purpose of The Joint Commission (TJC) **National Patient Safety Goals (NPSGs)** is to increase patient safety by preventing *sentinel events* (adverse events leading to complications and/or death). The NPSGs are reviewed yearly by TJC and a Sentinel Event Advisory Committee recommends possible goals to the TJC for decision. Each goal includes elements of performance (EPs)—formerly known as implementation expectations (IPs)—which include evidence-based methods to achieve the goals. Hospitals providing

Box 2-3	2011 Critical Access Hospital National Patient Safety Goals

The purpose of the National Patient Safety Goals is to improve patient safety. The goals focus on problems in health care safety and how to solve them.

Identify Patients Correctly

NPSG.01.01.01   Use at least two ways to identify patients (e.g., patient's name *and* date of birth) to make sure that each patient gets the correct medicine and treatment.

NPSG.01.03.01   Make sure that the correct patient gets the correct blood when giving a blood transfusion.

Improve Staff Communication

NPSG.02.03.01   Get important test results to the right staff person on time.

Use Medicines Safely

NPSG.03.04.01   Before a procedure, label medicines that are not labeled (e.g., medicines in syringes, cups and basins). Do this in the area where medicines and supplies are set up.

NPSG.03.05.01   Take extra care with patients who take medicines to thin their blood.

Prevent Infection

NPSG.07.01.01   Use the hand hygiene guidelines from the Centers for Disease Control and Prevention or the World Health Organization. Set goals for improving hand hygiene. Use the goals to improve hand hygiene.

NPSG.07.03.01   Use proven guidelines to prevent infections that are difficult to treat.

NPSG.07.04.01   Use proven guidelines to prevent infection of the blood from central lines.

NPSG.07.05.01   Use proven guidelines to prevent infection after surgery.

Check Patient Medicines

NPSG.08.01.01   Find out what medicines each patient is taking. Make sure that it is permissible for the patient to take any new medicines with their current medicines.

NPSG.08.02.01   Give a list of the patient's medicines to their next caregiver. Give the list to the patient's regular physician before the patient is discharged.

NPSG.08.03.01   Give a list of the patient's medicines to the patient and their family before the patient is discharged. Explain the list.

NPSG.08.04.01   Some patients may get medicine in small amounts or for a short time. Make sure that it is permissible for those patients to take those medicines with their current medicines.

Prevent Mistakes in Surgery

UP.01.01.01   Make sure that the correct surgery is done on the correct patient and at the correct place on the patient's body.

UP.01.02.01   Mark the correct place on the patient's body where the surgery is to be performed.

UP.01.03.01   Pause before the surgery to make sure that a mistake is not being made.

Data from the Joint Commission (TJC). (2010). *National Patient Safety Goals.* Retrieved from www.jointcommission.org/standards_information/npsgs.aspx.

care, treatment, and services relevant to these goals are expected to implement these elements of performance. Box 2-3 lists 2010 TJC NPSGs with a single definition (The Joint Commission, 2010).

THE JOINT COMMISSION NATIONAL QUALITY CORE MEASURES

The *Specifications Manual for Joint Commission National Quality Core Measures* includes sets of evidence-based, scientifically researched standards of care shown to improve clinical outcomes (TJC, 2010). **Core Measures** are used to treat the majority of patients who come to a hospital for a condition or illness that frequently develops complications (Box 2-4).

APPLYING LPN/LVN STANDARDS IN MEDICAL-SURGICAL NURSING

The five basic steps of the nursing process are (1) assessment (data collection), (2) nursing diagnosis, (3) planning, (4) implementation, and (5) evaluation. The LPN/LVN assists the RN with steps 1, 3, 4, and 5. The RN is responsible for formulating the nursing

diagnoses in step 2 from the assessment data obtained from all sources.

ASSESSMENT (DATA COLLECTION)

The purpose of data collection is to have a relevant database from which patient problems and potential problems may be identified. Data collection provides the basis for developing a problem list, from which nursing diagnoses will be developed.

Box 2-4	Core Measures with Selected Evidence-Based Interventions

Acute myocardial infarction (AMI): Receive aspirin at arrival.

Heart Failure (HF): Receive adult smoking cessation counseling.

Pneumonia (PN): Antibiotic administered within 6 hours of arrival.

Surgical care improvement: Recommended antibiotic to be given 1 hour preoperatively.

Data from the Joint Commission (TJC). (2010). *Core Measure Sets.* Retrieved from www.jointcommission.org/core_measure_set.

The LPN/LVN acts in a more independent role when participating in data collection (assessment) and during the implementation phase of the nursing process. LPN/LVNs systematically gather and review data about the patient and communicate their findings to appropriate members of the health care team. A complete database includes a thorough health history, physical assessment, psychosocial assessment, and cultural and spiritual assessments. Most health care facilities use a standardized form to follow in the admission database, so that data collection is as complete as possible. Both subjective data (data that the patient gives that cannot be seen or felt by another, such as pain) and objective data (data that can be verified by sight, smell, touch, or sound) are included.

If there is an immediate life-threatening problem, determine immediately what action must be taken and if additional expertise is needed to deal with the problem. Once the patient's physical condition is stabilized, a formal care plan can be developed (Nursing Care Plan 2-1).

★ Nursing Care Plan 2-1   Care of the Patient with Imbalanced Nutrition

Scenario

Mark Nielson, age 82, was admitted because of continued loss of weight and weakness. He is a frail-looking man who walks slowly and with hesitation. The patient has experienced loss of appetite, loss of weight, and loss of energy since his right lung lobectomy 3 years ago.

Problem/Nursing Diagnosis

Eats only 5% of each meal/Imbalanced nutrition, less than body requirements, related to loss of appetite and weakness

Supporting Assessment Data

Objective: Height 5'9", weight 128 lb, loss of 35 lb

Goals/Expected Outcomes	Nursing Interventions	Selected Rationale	Evaluation
Patient will eat 1500 calories of soft diet and drink 2000 mL of liquids each 24-hr period.	Six small meals at 8 A.M., 10 A.M., noon, 2 P.M., 4 P.M., and 6 P.M.	Small, attractively arranged soft diet of favorite foods will entice patient to eat without feeling too full.	By day 2, patient will be able to consume 1000 calories in a 24-hr period.
	Assist patient to chair using minimal assistance.	Sitting up encourages proper digestion.	Sitting up for all meals.
	Encourage self-feeding. Assist only if needed. Assess preferred diet.	Encourages independence. Patients eat more when presented with food they prefer.	Feeding self. Prefers chicken, mashed potatoes, gravy, creamed peas, and lemon pie.
	Set up tray for easy reach.	Preserves strength and helps patient overcome weakness.	Trays set up. Continue plan.
By day 4, patient will be able to remove lids and cut most of meat.	Open packages and milk carton. Remove lids. Cut meat.		
By day 2 will drink 1000 mL during 24-hr period.	Offer 240 mL of liquids at 6 A.M., 9 A.M., 11 A.M., 3 P.M., 5 P.M., 7 P.M., and 9 P.M. Vary choices. Likes apple juice, orange juice, ice cream, water, gelatin. Likes lemon-line soft drink at lunch and dinner. Enjoys tea at breakfast and 3 P.M. Record time, amount, and liquids taken.	A variety of favorite liquids in small amounts, alternating between meals, will be easier to consume.	Intake: 500 mL this shift.
Patient will verbalize increased energy and spend more time awake during the day.	Collect data on amount of hours patient is awake and the length and number of naps.	Provides objective data as a baseline.	Patient states that he feels more energetic and will decrease the length of morning and afternoon nap times to ½ hr each.

Critical Thinking Questions

1. What practical methods can the nurse use to entice the patient to eat, without actually feeding him?
2. What are measures that the nurse can use to encourage activity, without tiring the patient excessively?

Focused Assessment

Abbreviated General Patient Interview Guide

SOCIAL ASSESSMENT
- Are you married?
- Who lives with you?
- What kind of work do you do?
- Are you a member of a church or belong to any organizations?
- Do you have health insurance?
- How are things at home, if you are not there, because you are here in the hospital?
- Are there any medical problems that are common in your family?
- Have you had previous surgeries or serious injuries?
- In your life now, who is helpful to you?
- What prescription drugs do you take? What over-the-counter medicines?
- Do you smoke? How much?
- Do you drink alcohol? How often do you drink and how much?
- Are you allergic to any drugs? Foods? Other substances?
- What do you like to eat? Describe yesterday's meals and snacks.

PHYSICAL ASSESSMENT
- Why were you admitted here?
- What health problems do you have?
- Do you routinely see doctors? If so, for what?

REVIEW OF SYSTEMS (Ask questions regarding the following)

Head and Neck
Frequent headaches; dizziness, ringing of the ears, hearing problems; visual problems, glaucoma, cataracts, glasses or contact lenses; surgery of the brain, eyes, or ears; frequent colds; nasal allergies; sinus infections; frequent sore throats; hoarseness; trouble swallowing; swollen glands; mouth sores; date of last dental examination; history of thyroid problems; use of a hearing aid; difficulty sleeping; napping

Chest
Male and female: Cough, sputum production; asthma, wheezing, frequent bronchitis; history of pneumonia; tuberculosis, exposure to tuberculosis; exposure to occupational respiratory hazards; palpitations, chest pain; shortness of breath; history of heart problems, murmurs, hypertension; anemia; surgery
Female: Frequency of breast examinations; date of last mammogram; nipple discharge; breast lumps

Abdomen (Gastrointestinal Tract)
Indigestion; pain; nausea; vomiting; excessive thirst or hunger; frequency of bowel movements; change in bowel movements; rectal bleeding; black or tarry stools; constipation; diarrhea; excessive gas; hemorrhoids; history of gallbladder or liver problems

Genitourinary (Inquire with Cultural Sensitivity)
Male and female: Problems with urination; up at night to urinate; dribbling of urine; history of urinary tract infection; stones
Female: Sexual activity; sexual problems; menstrual cycle and any problems; last menstrual period; bleeding between periods or after menopause; vaginal discharge; date of last Pap smear; history of sexually transmitted infections or vaginal disorders
Male: Sexual activity; genital problems; penile discharge; history of sexually transmitted infections; sexual problems

Extremities and Musculoskeletal System
Joint pain or stiffness; back problems; muscle pain; limited range of motion; vascular problems in legs or arms; easy bruising; skin lesions; history of phlebitis; thrombophlebitis; gout, arthritis, fractures, injury

PSYCHOLOGICAL ASSESSMENT
- Are you experiencing anxiety? Depression?
- Do you have unusual memory problems?
- Do you have difficulty thinking?
- Are you ever confused?

Sources of Information
Review of Admission Forms. The admission form generally accompanies a patient to the unit. The Focused Assessment box at left covers questions for basic information such as the patient's name, reason for admission, and other important information. If the patient has been hospitalized in the past, previous records may be included. The physician's history and medical examination, if available, will provide the patient's physical and mental status. The medical diagnosis will guide the nurse in collecting assessment data and in identifying patient problems. Check to see if results of preliminary laboratory work, radiographs, or other test results are included. If available, read the current information before entering the patient's room; knowing current information will enhance your critical thinking and observation skills during your initial patient contact (and will keep you from repeating obvious questions).

 Think Critically

How many sources can you identify that would provide information for a nursing database on a patient who has been admitted to a long-term care facility?

Interview. Ask patients what they think is their major problem or "chief complaint." Other questions concern the present level of pain, when the last bowel movement occurred, problems with urination or appetite, difficulty sleeping, and whether patients have any additional concerns or complaints. The patient is the primary source of current information and knows more about the problem than anyone else.

If for some reason the patient is incapacitated, secondary sources of information are useful (e.g., spouse, significant other, relative, friend, or patient advocate). The secondary source can also help verify information that was provided by the patient. Box 2-5 provides suggestions for interviewing. The remainder of the admission form is filled out by the nurse and includes the status of advance directives, assessments for fall risk, pain level, pressure ulcer risk, nutrition requirements, and ability to perform activities of daily living. Psychosocial, cultural, and spiritual assessment data are gathered as well.

Elder Care Points

Plan extra time for an interview with a patient who is elderly. The elderly person who is ill may think and speak more slowly than expected, and often has a longer health history to relate than does a younger person.

After obtaining a list of current medications from the patient, a medication reconciliation form to identify and prevent *polypharmacy* (multiple drugs prescribed

Box 2-5 | Interview Suggestions

- Introduce yourself to the patient by name and as an LPN/LVN student.
- Be respectful.
- A patient is entitled to be addressed by his surname. Do so, unless the patient asks you to address him differently.
- Pull up a chair so that the patient can see you at his eye level and can hear you clearly.
- Speak slowly and clearly.
- Ask your questions without dropping your voice at the end of the sentence. Be alert to any hearing difficulty the patient may have.
- Give time for the patient to respond.
- Attempt to resolve incongruence between body language and responses.
- Ask for clarification if you are unsure what the patient means by a particular statement or response.
- Summarize for the patient what you think you heard during the interview.
- Ask the patient for any corrections or additions.

for the same condition by different physicians) is filled out. Medication reconciliation also reduces the risk of medication order errors and adverse interactions between drugs. Patient allergies and medications—prescription, over-the-counter, and herbal preparations and supplements—are included on the form, which is reviewed by both the physician and the pharmacist. Patients need to know that the information gathered will be recorded and used in planning their care.

Physical Assessment. Physical data collection usually begins with measuring the patient's blood pressure, pulse, respiration, temperature, weight, and height. *Accuracy is essential.* Data collection correlates current readings with the baseline data, with trends of past readings, with the patient's current clinical status, and with any medical care that has been provided. Such data yield significant information about the patient's condition and response to medication and other treatments. Complete assessments are performed daily.

Inspection and Observation. Inspection (looking) and observation (looking and noting) are important aspects of nursing assessment. Use your eyes to pick up clues about the patient's physical and mental condition. Note the patient's facial expression, posture, grimaces, movements, and whether answers are congruent (match the feeling tone of what is said). Inspect the hair, skin, nails, and oral mucous membranes for data about hydration and dental hygiene. Observe the patient's state of personal care. Is the hair combed, and are the nails clean and reasonably trimmed? Is there anything in the room that gives evidence of support systems, family, or friends?

Olfaction. Olfaction (smelling) can provide data about a patient's personal hygiene, as well as clues to possible illness. The sweet, fruity odor of acetone can be indicative of diabetic acidosis. The smell of newly mown clover can be present with hepatic coma. The smell of alcohol indicates the patient has been drinking. Sometimes patients with acute alcoholism may smell like aftershave, mouthwash, vanilla, Sterno, or other substances containing a high percentage of alcohol. Foul or metallic mouth odors usually indicate poor oral hygiene or periodontal disease. Odor from the nose may be indicative of chronic sinusitis with postnasal drip or an obstruction in the nasal passages.

Patients who have anemia, an endocrine problem, or a central nervous system abnormality may be trying to cover up unpleasant body odor with bath powder or heavy perfume. An unpleasant genital odor may indicate an infection, poor hygiene, or insufficient fluid intake (commonly found in female patients in long-term care facilities). Without additional attention, body areas that are unattended may become reddened, irritated, and sometimes infected.

Palpation. Palpate (touch) the patient's skin to learn if it feels healthy or if it is coarse, dry, swollen, cold, or clammy. Dryness may be related to dehydration and swelling may indicate edema (fluid in the tissues). If you depress the skin with your fingers and your touch leaves pitting (indentation) on the skin, edema is present. Measure and record the depth of pitting and the length of time the tissue remains indented. Palpation of the skin can provide additional information. Cold extremities may indicate poor circulation. Hot tissue may be the result of localized inflammation, and you will want to examine the area more carefully. Use your fingertips, not your thumb, to palpate the pulses. Use the flat of the hand to palpate the abdomen to determine whether it is soft or hard or if there are any tender areas. Palpate the breasts for abnormal growths. Premenopausal women may have masses in their breasts, making it difficult to determine which lumps are significant (this is a good time to ask assistance from your instructor, the staff RN, or the clinical nurse specialist).

Auscultation. Auscultation (listening) is an important skill in gathering data. Listen to the sounds of the patient's breathing—with a stethoscope and without a stethoscope. You may hear wheezing from constricted bronchi or stridor caused by a partial airway obstruction. Listening to the quality of a patient's cough will determine whether it is dry or moist. With the stethoscope, the sounds are amplified and you can auscultate normal, abnormal, or adventitious breath sounds (Figure 2-1). Listen to the apical pulse at the apex of the heart and on the abdomen for bowel sounds, listening carefully in each quadrant (Figure 2-2).

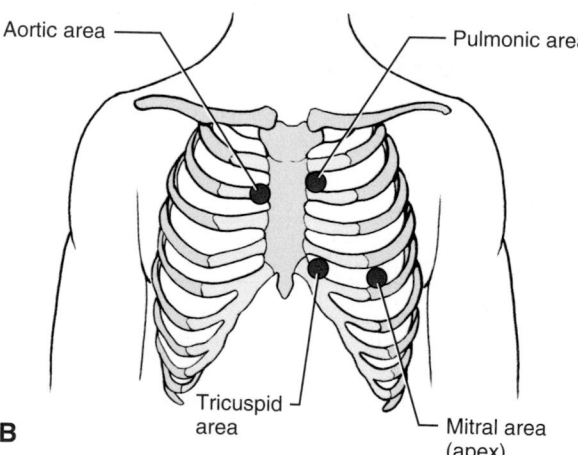

FIGURE 2-1   A, Place the stethoscope on the bare skin at these locations to hear the lung sounds. **B,** Place the stethoscope at the apex of the heart to listen to the apical pulse.

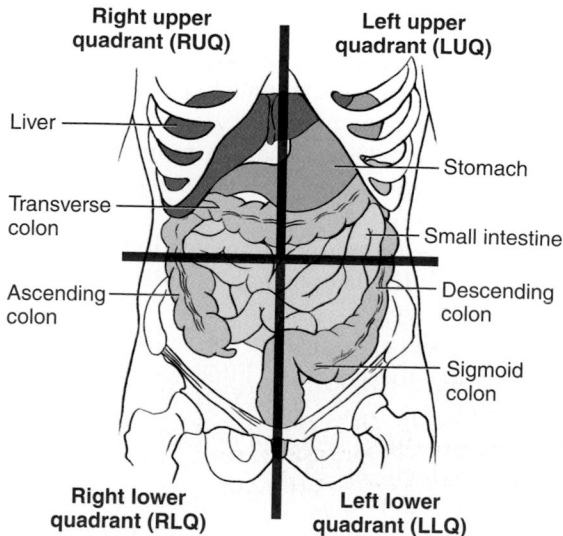

FIGURE 2-2 Listen for bowel sounds in all four quadrants of the abdomen.

Focused Assessment

Beginning-of-Shift Assessment

PHYSICAL REVIEW*

- Assess the patient's level of consciousness (LOC), including the patient's ability to respond quickly and appropriately and orientation to person, place, and time. Refer to the Glasgow Coma Scale in Chapter 22 for patients with neurologic problems.
- Check the patient's ability to think by asking questions within the client's capacity to think (mentate) (e.g., who is the President?).
- Observe skin color and texture and degree of moisture.
- Note the appearance of the eyes.
- Measure the vital signs (temperature, pulse, respiration, and blood pressure). Note rhythm and strength of the pulse, rhythm and depth of respiration, and respiratory effort.
- Ask the patient to describe any pain. Determine the location, severity, quality, and precipitating and alleviating factors.
- Auscultate the chest using the stethoscope. Listen for breath sounds, noting normal, abnormal, and adventitious breath sounds. Listen at the apex of the heart, checking for regularity of rhythm. Auscultate the apical pulse for 60 seconds to count the rate and note the rhythm of the heartbeat. It is difficult for the new nurse to pick up extra heart sounds, but you can determine if there is an increase or decrease in the heart rate.
- Assess the skin turgor (elasticity) by gently lifting the skin on the upper chest with your thumb and forefinger and observing the speed with which it snaps back when you let go.
- Observe the contour of the abdomen (e.g., flat, round, distended).
- When the patient is in a supine position or low Fowler's position, auscultate bowel sounds in all four quadrants.
- Gently palpate the abdomen with the palm side of the fingers, noting whether the abdomen is soft or firm. Also ask the patient whether he experiences any pain or discomfort, indicating areas of tenderness. Inquire about appetite and weight changes.
- Assess the patient's bowel and bladder status. Note the time of patient's last bowel movement (from the chart or by asking the patient) and whether or not flatus is being passed. Review the intake and output (I&O) for the past 24 hours. Observe and palpate the pubic area to assess bladder distention, especially if there is a discrepancy between the current and previous I&O. If the patient has an indwelling catheter, observe the characteristics of the urine in the drainage tube and the rate of drainage.
- Ask the patient to move each extremity. Observe the ability to actively move the joints through the range of motion and the coordination of the movements. If the patient is unable to actively move any joints, assist the patient with passive motion and note the degree of flexibility. Ask the patient to move extremities against resistance, to determine extremity strength. The nurse can also determine the patient's level of cooperation and ability to follow directions during the exercises.
- Compare the peripheral pulses bilaterally.
- Note the presence of any edema.

TUBES AND EQUIPMENT STATUS

- *Intravenous catheter:* Condition of site; fluid in progress, rate, additives; time next fluid is to be hung
- *Nasogastric tube:* Suction setting; amount and character of drainage; patency of tube; security of tube
- *Urinary catheter:* Character and quantity of drainage; tubing not positioned underneath patient
- *Dressings:* Location; drains in place; wound suction devices; amount and character of wound drainage
- *Pulse oximeter:* Intact probe; readings
- *Patient-controlled analgesia pump:* Properly functioning; correct medication infusing; amount of solution remaining
- *Traction:* Correct weight; body alignment; weights hanging free
- *Equipment:* Applied properly; functioning as ordered

*The physical review may include a head-to-toe assessment based on the patient's needs.

Percussion. Physicians, nurse practitioners, and physician assistants use percussion much more. By using a light, quick tapping on different surfaces of the body, they are able to tell the size, location, and density of different organs, especially in the chest, abdomen, and kidney areas. Percussion of the abdomen will reveal areas of excessive gas in the bowel.

Practical Daily Focused Assessment (Data Collection)

A full assessment (data collection) is completed on each assigned patient at admission, and then a daily *focused assessment* is directed to areas in which the patient is experiencing health problems. Focused assessment augments the admission assessment of the patient and is based on the identified problems, data from report, and medical diagnoses and treatment. Many hospitals have standardized forms for collecting head-to-toe data on the patient. Information from reviewing the patient's chart and care plan is used to identify areas in which focused assessment data should be collected. Ask for a demonstration of an appropriate head-to-toe assessment.

Chart Review

The face sheet of the chart provides demographic data such as address, marital status, insurance coverage, age, date of birth, occupation, significant others, and emergency contact information. The physician's history, physical examination, progress notes, and results of diagnostic tests give an overview of the patient's total health status and provide a summary of current health problems and progress toward resolving them. Allergy information should be identified as part of the admission information and displayed prominently on the front of the chart and at other locations as required by the facility's policies and procedures. The current physician's orders provide a clue as to the plan for that day (tests or treatments).

The medication profile sheets or medication administration record (MAR) lists the routine and as-needed (PRN) medications and provides documentation of medication administration. Consultation sheets or nursing documentation includes narrative notes and flow sheets that describe care provided to the patient and the patient's response to that care. Reviewing the nursing documentation provides a comprehensive picture of the patient's needs and will assist in preparing for beginning patient care.

Other clinicians such as the dietitian, respiratory therapist, and social worker contribute documentation to the patient's chart. Information provided by these clinicians completes the comprehensive picture of the patient. You must keep all information you gather private.

 Elder Care Points

You walk into your patient's room and find that Mr. Nethers, age 72, has been restrained because he pulled out his oxygen tube, IV line, and urinary catheter earlier in the morning. He has also attempted to get out of bed several times. Yesterday he was alert and had a lucid conversation with you. Mr. Nethers had surgery yesterday after you left the unit to go to class and you see in the documentation that he has been receiving codeine for pain. You recall when you looked up medications that codeine could have a severe behavioral side effect, especially for an older patient. You inform the medication nurse and request that she discuss the information with the physician before giving additional doses.

 Legal and Ethical Considerations

Protected Health Information

Any protected health information from a patient's chart must be carefully guarded to avoid violating the confidentiality component of the Health Insurance Portability and Accountability Act (HIPAA). Information that is retained by a student for educational purposes must be devoid of identifying information. Student preparation paperwork that contains protected health information must be destroyed according to the policies and procedures of the facility.

Prioritizing

After obtaining patient information, preparation for care entails planning and prioritization. Prioritizing care is the most important step in planning competent, timely patient care. Prioritizing of care includes when to give medications, measure vital signs, monitor blood glucose, change dressings, check IVs, and so on. Prioritizing also includes identifying which tasks are urgent, and which tasks can wait.

Nursing students often have only one patient assigned to them for clinical care. On graduation, it is rare to have an assignment of a single patient. The norm is four to six patients. During low staffing, expect the number of assigned patients to increase. Once you receive your assignments:

- Review the patient's chart, computer printout, or Kardex (whichever system is used for patient information).
- Look up required drug information for each routine and PRN drug listed, including IV solutions and additives.
- List focused assessments you will make, and data you will collect, both at intervals and before you go off duty.
- List procedures that will be performed and a list of equipment for each.
- Attend report and make additional notes, and question what you do not understand.

- Make rounds on all your assigned patients (unless a bedside report was given). Seeing the patient alerts you to changes that need immediate attention.

Your notes and lists are excellent organization tools for reporting vital signs, medications given, and treatments performed. Your care plan is necessary for evaluating patient progress toward goals and outcomes and can identify issues not yet addressed on the chart problem list.

 Think Critically

How will you use the patients' care plans to effectively receive and give report? What are the items to which you will pay greatest attention, or that you will emphasize?

Diagnostic Tests

Review laboratory and test data to identify general concerns and to confirm assessment findings. Most often, the diagnostic data help chart the patient's progress.

White Blood Cell Count. When the patient has an infection, an increased number of white blood cells (WBCs) are sent from the bone marrow to attack bacteria or viruses causing infection. An increased number of WBCs may occur with mild infections, appendicitis, pregnancy, leukemia, hemorrhage, and other conditions. Strenuous exercise, emotional distress, and anxiety can also cause an increase in WBCs. A low WBC count makes it harder for a patient to fight off infections and is also seen with illnesses such as mumps, lupus, cirrhosis of the liver, and cancer. In addition, radiation therapy and certain types of drug therapy tend to lower the WBC count. When looking up medications before giving them to the patient, notice if reduction in WBCs is a potential side effect. It is not prudent for a staff member with a cold or other infection to work with a patient who has a low WBC count. If you must care for such a patient, isolation barrier precautions should be maintained (gown, mask, gloves, etc.). If you are sick or infected, check with your supervisor before beginning to provide care.

Red Blood Cell Count. Red blood cells (RBCs) contain hemoglobin and carry oxygen and carbon dioxide in the blood. The RBC count determines if the number of RBCs in your body is low (anemia) or high (polycythemia). Common causes of an abnormal RBC count are iron deficiency anemia due to chronic blood loss (e.g., menstruation, small amounts of bleeding due to colon cancer), acute blood loss (e.g., acute bleeding, ulcer, trauma), hereditary disorders (e.g., sickle cell anemia), or improper diet. Polycythemia from low

oxygen in the blood or an unknown cause is relatively uncommon. Compare the laboratory value of the RBC count to information about the underlying disorder. Note any difference in vital signs that correlates with a high or a low RBC count.

Hemoglobin. Low hemoglobin (Hb) levels often indicate anemia; usually the patient with low Hb levels will also have a low RBC count and a low hematocrit (Hct). Signs and symptoms of anemia (paleness, shortness of breath, fatigue) will start to show when the Hb is too low. Women tend to normally have lower RBC counts and Hb levels than men. Be sure to check all three values (RBC count, Hb, and Hct) when scanning a lab report; correlate the RBC, Hb, and Hct counts with your observations of the patient.

Hematocrit. Hematocrit measures how much of the patient's blood is made up of RBCs. The hematocrit measurement (Hct) is useful in identifying anemia, the presence of liver disease, and RBC production in the bone marrow. Hematocrit increases during dehydration and, along with Hb, increases in polycythemia. If the patient has polycythemia, there is a risk of a stroke or myocardial infarction from a clot. Watch for signs of these problems.

Platelet Count. Platelets help stop bleeding after injury or surgery. The platelet count may change with bleeding disorders, heart disease, diabetes, inflammatory disease, and anemia. If your patient has bruising or is prone to bruising, a platelet count may be ordered. Be aware that patients may have brought in their own over-the-counter medications (such as aspirin) and herbal products (such as ginkgo biloba) that may affect the platelet count.

Glucose. High blood glucose after fasting for 12 hours suggests diabetes; additional tests will confirm the diagnosis. If the patient does have diabetes, you will be involved in coaching the patient to self-test glucose levels with a blood glucose meter. For some patients, the glucose level readings determine the amount of insulin they receive after each reading. The glucose level must be checked as ordered, and the correct amount of insulin must be given, on time. Once again, you will be able to track patient progress toward stabilizing the illness. A slightly elevated glucose is sometimes related to stress.

A low glucose level occurs with hypoglycemia. The patient will experience symptoms such as weakness, nausea, sweating, and confusion. A high-protein snack such as cheese may sustain the low-glucose patient longer than sweets, which raise the blood glucose level quickly, but for only a short period of time.

Hemoglobin A₁C. A hemoglobin A_{1C} (Hb A_{1C}) test provides an average blood glucose level for the past 2 to 3 months. It is considered the "gold standard" in determining if interventions for diabetes are working.

Thyroid-Stimulating Hormone. Thyroid-stimulating hormone (TSH) testing is the most sensitive way to identify both hypothyroidism and hyperthyroidism. TSH increases in primary hypothyroidism and decreases in hyperthyroidism. Check to see if the TSH is within normal limits.

Other Resources

Student nurses have more time to collect data than staff nurses have. As a student, take advantage of this added time. Course textbooks are the primary resource and other texts, journal articles, and the Internet can provide a wealth of information. Handheld devices with downloaded electronic books (e.g., medical-surgical, drug, and lab texts) provide instant access to clinical resources. Since there is no control over information placed on the Internet, resources should be evaluated carefully. Your instructor, pharmacists, dietitians, social workers, occupational therapists, physical therapists, physicians, and other specialists can provide valuable information about specific aspects of the patient. Work to gain a comprehensive picture of the patient's situation.

ANALYSIS AND NURSING DIAGNOSIS

The LPN/LVN reports data collection findings to the RN and assists in verifying, categorizing, and grouping the collected data in a logical order. The LPN/LVN also assists in analyzing the data to determine significant relationships among data, patient needs, and problems. A *prioritized* list of patient problems is developed. The focus is on actual and potential patient problems that can be addressed with independent nursing interventions. From the analysis, the RN chooses nursing diagnoses from the current **North American Nursing Diagnosis Association International (NANDA-I)** list (see inside back cover). The nursing diagnoses are general statements or stems labeling patient problems. The stem is then linked with the etiology (cause) and evidence (signs and symptoms) of the problem, making the nursing diagnosis statement specific to the patient.

Nursing care is based on the *priority* of patient problems. High-priority problems are dealt with first and lower priority problems are dealt with as time permits. The nursing diagnoses are based on all of the available patient data, including—but not limited to—the nursing assessment (subjective and objective) data, diagnostic test data, and the medical diagnosis. Placing a nursing diagnosis in the care plan means that the nurse is accepting accountability for accuracy of the statement. Permitting a problem to continue without

designating a nursing diagnosis can lead to patient harm (Alfaro-Lefevre, 2009).

 Think Critically

What is important in choosing the correct nursing diagnosis for a care plan? How would you determine that a nursing diagnosis on a facility care plan is appropriate for the patient?

It is important for a nurse to differentiate between a **nursing diagnosis** and a medical diagnosis. The physician is concerned with health problems that can be treated with surgery, medications, and other forms of therapy provided or prescribed by the physician. Nursing diagnoses identify the patient's response to an illness or a health condition. Nursing practice addresses physical, psychological, social, cultural, and spiritual comfort and well-being; the prevention of complications; and patient education. Nursing care focuses on preventing, minimizing, and alleviating specific health problems. Although the physician is responsible for managing medical problems, the nurse often uses clues from the medical diagnosis to identify patient problems and to develop accurate nursing diagnoses.

NANDA-I–approved stems are chosen by the RN, based on an analysis of available data. These approved stems label the patient problems that can be independently treated using nursing interventions. Other components of a nursing diagnosis make statements specific to the patient's situation, and direct the planning and implementation phases of the nursing process. A complete nursing diagnosis includes the problem (NANDA-I stem), the etiology (related causes of the problem), and the signs and symptoms (evidence of the problem).

The etiology component describes the known or suspected cause or causes of a problem (e.g., a patient's ineffective breathing patterns could be related to etiologies of reduced lung capacity, anxiety, or pain). The signs and symptoms of the problem describe the subjective and objective evidence of the problem (i.e., the diagnosis is supported [evidenced] by the assessment data). To follow our example, a patient's ineffective breathing pattern might be evidenced by a statement of shortness of breath, or by the nurse's observation of dyspnea (difficulty breathing), changes in respiratory rate or rhythm, or decreased oxygen saturation levels. The RN, after considering all of the available data relevant to the patient's respiratory function, might develop the following diagnosis statement: *Ineffective breathing related to abdominal incision pain as evidenced by shallow respirations and low pulse oximeter readings (89% to 92%).*

Actual problems are problems that the patient currently exhibits, and documentation should include all three components of the diagnosis statement (problem,

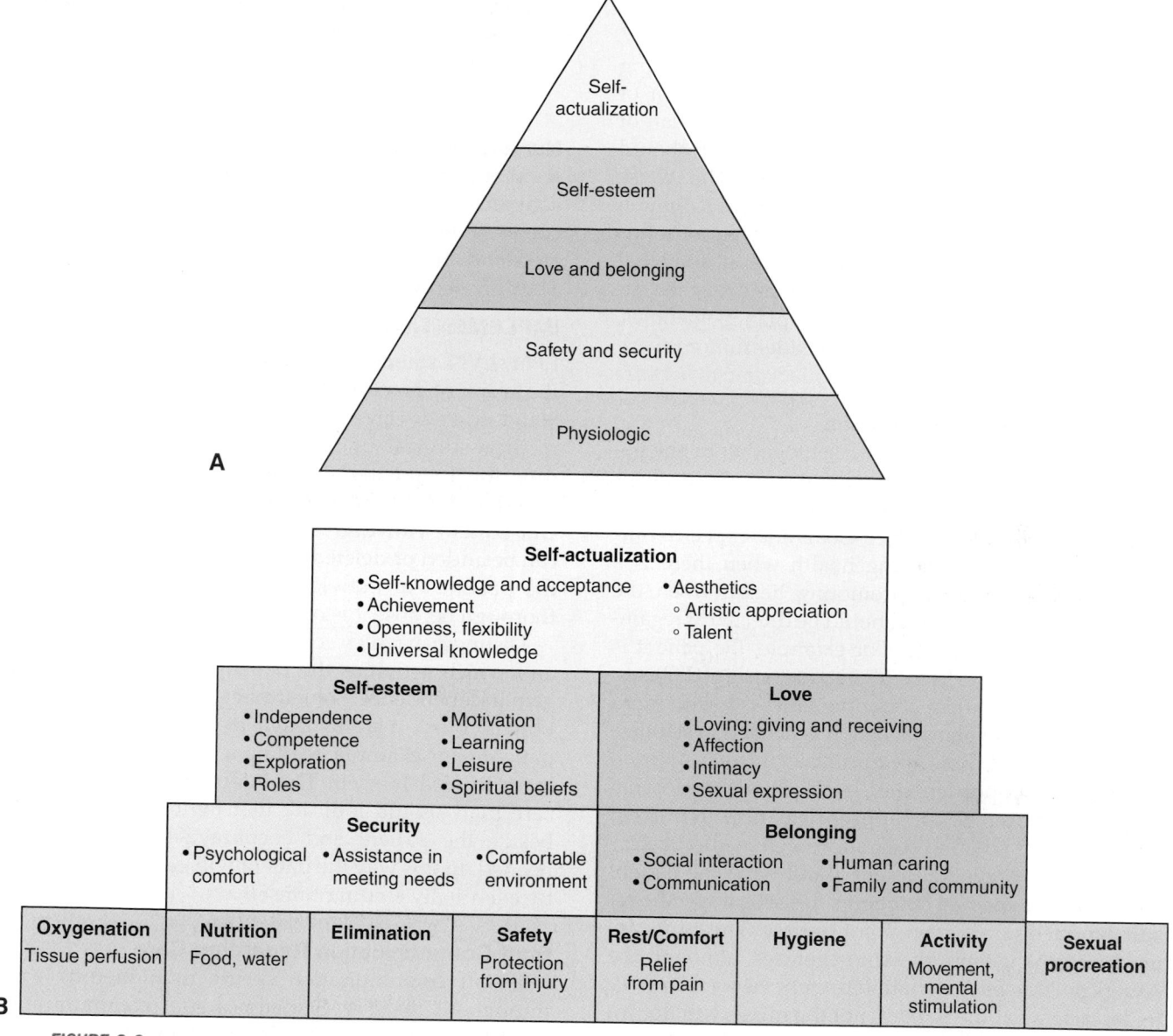

A,

B,

FIGURE 2-3 A, Maslow's hierarchy of needs. **B,** Evolving hierarchy of needs adapted by nursing to help determine priorities of care.

etiology, signs and symptoms). Sometimes the patient does not currently exhibit evidence of potential problems, but the data demonstrate that a problem could occur—these situations describe potential problems. Potential problem statements begin with the phrase "risk for" and include the NANDA-I stem and the etiology. An example of a potential problem is: *Risk for fluid volume deficit related to vomiting and diarrhea*. In this example, the patient is not currently showing signs of dehydration, but is at risk because of the fluid loss associated with vomiting and diarrhea. By identifying potential problems, the nurse is alerted to take preventive measures, rather than wait for a problem to materialize before taking action. The LPN/LVN is expected to be familiar with the NANDA-I list of nursing diagnoses.

Setting Priorities of Care

Priority setting is a method of handling problems and tasks according to the importance (priority) of the patient's problems. Maslow's hierarchy of needs is one way to prioritize nursing care (Figure 2-3). The lowest level of needs—those needed to sustain life, such as an airway and breathing—must be attended to immediately, even before a formal care plan is developed. All problems might not be included in the initial plan. Nursing diagnoses are listed on the care plan in order of priority. As problems are dealt with successfully, they are modified or discontinued. Other problems are added to the plan as they arise. Priority setting is a skill that must be developed in order to work efficiently and safely. While prioritizing it should become apparent if there is a need to assign some tasks to others.

PLANNING

LPN/LVN standards of care indicate that the LPN/LVN will use the nursing process in planning nursing care, and will assist the RN in the identification of health goals and interventions for a patient's plan of care. For a care plan to be effective, the patient should be involved in determining priorities. The nurse should collect data to determine the patient's opinion and knowledge of the situation and the need for information. Data regarding desired information, and what the patient is willing and able to do to improve the situation, are also gathered for the care plan. Sometimes, something that the nurse might consider minor is very important to the patient.

Goals and Expected Outcomes

All goals or expected outcomes, set together by the patient and the nurse, must be patient-centered, realistically achievable, measurable, and include a time frame within which they will be met. Goals and expected outcomes relate to (1) restoring health when there is a health problem and (2) promoting health when the patient's resources can and should be directed at regaining or maintaining health. For example, the patient is eager to learn how to live with the diagnosis of diabetes. You instruct the patient about the illness, how to monitor the glucose level, what action is needed to stabilize the glucose level, how to administer insulin, how to maintain a supportive diet, what kinds and what frequency of exercise are appropriate, how to prevent infections, and when to seek additional medical help.

Goals state a general intent about what the patient will achieve. Expected outcomes describe a specific result expected at a certain point in time. The terms are used interchangeably in some agencies, although the American Nurses Association prefers the term *outcome* to describe what the patient, not the nurse, will do. An outcome is written as *"The patient will..."*. Patient input is important in order to establish motivation to accomplish the outcome. Outcome statements are derived from the signs and symptoms included in the nursing diagnosis statement. The nurse, in conjunction with the patient, transforms the "evidenced by" component of the problem into an achievable, positive outcome statement.

The word "patient" is used as the subject of the statement. The outcome statements are written with a subject, an action verb, conditions or modifiers, and the criterion (standard) for desired performance. Expected outcomes should include:

- Patient activity that can be observed, or patient knowledge that can be assessed. Consider how "the patient will select *[action verb—can be measured or observed]* low-sodium foods from a list" provides a better indicator of knowledge than "the patient will understand *[passive verb]* a low-sodium diet."

- Description of how the patient's behavior will be measured, including the accuracy and quality of performance, and the time frame within which the objective is to be met.

Nursing Interventions

Nursing interventions are nursing actions and patient activities chosen to achieve the goals and expected outcomes. Independent nursing interventions can be initiated and implemented without a physician's order. They are written on the nursing care plan.

IMPLEMENTATION

LPN/LVN standards require providing care within the scope of practice to accomplish established goals. Standardized care plans are frequently found on medical-surgical units and include generic nursing care for frequently encountered patient problems. The standardized plan is not individualized for a specific patient. However, problems and/or interventions can be added or deleted if they are not appropriate for the patient. An individualized plan of care is more thorough because it is developed for a specific patient.

Distinguish which activities the nurse is to carry out, and which activities the patient must learn to do to gain independence. Sometimes when a nurse is exceptionally busy, it seems faster to do an activity for the patient—for example, feeding a patient who needs to learn to feed himself. The interventions listed in the care plan should indicate that the caregiver is to sit beside the patient and encourage him verbally, as needed. In this way the patient will gain independence by eventually feeding himself.

Staff Communication Regarding Care

Interstaff communication occurs in numerous ways throughout the day. Sometimes staff communication must be immediate in order to communicate urgent and relevant data that were discovered during an assessment of the patient. Urgent data are usually communicated verbally and may require immediate action.

Charting occurs on nurses' notes, treatment flow sheets, MARs, and activity flow sheets. Nurses also might chart on common charting forms with other health care providers. Many health care facilities are moving to electronic documentation and records management. An electronic health record (EHR) is a computerized comprehensive record of a patient's history and care across all facilities and admissions (deWit, 2009). For the sake of security, health care providers use passwords to obtain information from the record, or to record new information.

Think critically about what needs to be documented and be succinct in recording the information. Follow agency policy for the method of documentation to be used (e.g., problem-oriented record, focus charting, or charting by exception).

Report is conducted at the change of shifts according to facility protocol to ensure continuity of care for the patients. On some medical-surgical units, all the staff members listen to report on all of the patients, the advantage of which is that all of the nurses and nursing assistants are aware of the needs of every patient. Other units use an individualized report system in which the assigned nurse receives report on assigned patients only. Walking rounds are another method for change-of-shift report in which nurses go to patients' rooms and the departing nurse and patient describe what happened during the previous shift. They discuss what the departing nurse and patient see as priorities for the next shift. It is more time-consuming than other methods, but walking rounds provide a sense of partnering for the patient, and the arriving nurse has an opportunity to see and hear the patient before beginning care. It is especially helpful and saves time if the arriving nurse has the Kardex sheet or computer care plan in hand during report.

EVALUATION

The LPN/LVN standards require comparison of *actual* outcomes of patient care to the *expected* outcomes. This comparison is known as *evaluation*. Evaluation begins as soon as a nursing plan is implemented. To make the comparisons needed for evaluation, collect data with every patient contact, think critically about how the patient is progressing, and determine if there is a way to improve care. Daily evaluation is part of the natural flow of nursing process, regardless of the time frame established for patient outcomes. The collected and documented data demonstrate a patient's progress toward meeting the expected outcomes. If the data show a lack of progress toward meeting the expected outcomes via planned interventions, the interventions should be reviewed and revised.

INTERDISCIPLINARY (COLLABORATIVE) CARE PLAN

Interdisciplinary (collaborative) care plans require input from all health team members involved in patient care. The collaborative care plan is developed using the interdisciplinary focus of each professional (e.g., nurse, social worker, occupational therapist, recreational therapist). A separate care plan for each profession is considered repetitious. The focus of interdisciplinary planning is on patient problems rather than on nursing diagnosis, making the language used in the plan common to all professions. Interdisciplinary care plans have the following characteristics:

- The patient's medical diagnosis is used, rather than a nursing diagnosis.
- Observations (data collected) are shared among all providers involved in the care of the patient.
- A problem list is developed and prioritized. The patient's statement of problem(s) that led to admission is considered. **Priority is given to lifesaving/physiologic needs.**
- A shared care plan is created, identifying specific and shared responsibilities for all professions represented.
- The plan is discussed with the patient (when possible) or patient advocate. The team plays a supportive role during implementation of the plan.
- Documentation of progress is usually on a common form or computer record to allow easy access for all team members involved with the patient.
- Evaluation is ongoing, with periodic in-depth evaluation by the team during agreed-on dates. Interventions are deleted, added, and changed as needed.

Get Ready for the NCLEX® Examination!

Key Points

- Critical thinking generates new ideas and judges the worth of those ideas. Critical thinking prompts the LPN/LVN to ask what could be improved and what measures would prevent further harm to the patient.
- Clinical judgment is a proactive reasoning skill that uses critical thinking in the clinical area to determine the appropriate actions to take in specific situations.
- Factors that influence critical thinking and the decisions about nursing care include our culture, personal motivation, attitude, and verbal and written communication ability.
- Nursing process is an advanced problem-solving method used to collect and analyze data in order to plan, implement, and evaluate patient care in an orderly way. It is the language of nursing, and provides a method for nurses to communicate with regard to patient care.
- Goals and expected outcomes are patient centered and describe what the patient will achieve.
- Receiving a patient assignment and preparing a preliminary care plan before beginning patient care is considered safe practice for student nurses, as the NPAs in all states mandate student nurses to function equivalent to an LPN/LVN.
- Techniques of physical examination used by the LPN/LVN include inspection and observation, olfaction, palpation, percussion, and auscultation.

- Nurses need to be aware of common laboratory and other diagnostic tests and their relationship to common illness. Laboratory and diagnostic tests also provide a way to track the effectiveness of treatments and the emergence of side effects of select medications.
- Interdisciplinary (collaborative) care plans are used in health facilities where it is more convenient for all professions involved to have their plan of care interwoven with others. Medical diagnosis, rather than nursing diagnosis, is used here because of the number of disciplines involved.
- Staff communication takes place both verbally and by charting. Urgent communication is done verbally, and as soon as possible.
- A "bundle" is a collection of evidence-based interventions that—when delivered as a group—have been shown to improve patient outcomes.
- TJC National Patient Safety Goals focus on making patients safer by developing ways to prevent adverse incidents leading to serious complications or death.
- Core measures are evidence-based, scientifically researched standards of care used to treat the majority of patients who come to the hospital for specific conditions.

Additional Learning Resources

SG Go to your Study Guide for additional learning activities to help you master this chapter content.

evolve Go to your Evolve website (http://evolve.elsevier.com/deWit/medsurg) for the following FREE learning resources:
- Animations, audio, and video
- Answers and rationales for questions and activities
- Concept Map Creator
- Glossary with pronunciations in English and Spanish
- Interactive Review Questions and Exercises and more!

 Online Resources
- Critical thinking, http://hsc.unm.edu/consg/critical
- Critical thinking, www.criticalthinking.org/resources/HE/ctandnursing.cfm
- Nursing care plans, www.medi-smart.com/carepl.htm
- Nurse Together, www.nursetogether.com

Review Questions for the NCLEX® Examination

1. When caring for an elderly woman who developed a 5-cm pressure ulcer on her sacrum because of being immobilized and incontinent, an appropriate expected outcome would be that the:
   1. patient will be able to ambulate to the bathroom with minimal assistance.
   2. nurse will provide turning and repositioning schedules for the staff.
   3. patient will verbalize importance of using pressure-reducing devices and of frequent repositioning during her stay.
   4. family will be able to provide protein-rich foods during the hospital stay.

2. While dangling her feet at the bedside, a patient suddenly complains of "faintness and dizziness." An immediate nursing action would be to:
   1. check vital signs.
   2. assist the patient back to a supine position.
   3. open the airway.
   4. provide reassurance that everything is OK.

3. A nursing diagnosis addressing risk for falls would be most appropriate for which type of patient?
   1. An immobilized patient
   2. A patient with rashes
   3. A patient on antihypertensive medications
   4. A patient having elective surgery

4. Which patient statement indicates the need for further teaching regarding the use of an incentive spirometer?
   1. "I will inhale as deeply as possible each time I use the spirometer."
   2. "I need to slightly tilt the incentive spirometer to reduce effort."
   3. "To monitor progress, I will record the top volume achieved."
   4. "I may have trouble sealing the mouthpiece due to mouth dryness."

5. The nurse is collecting data from an elderly patient with a history of fractures hospitalized for elective gallbladder surgery. Along with general assessment, the nurse should include:
   1. determining orientation to person, place, and time.
   2. auscultating for a heart murmur.
   3. checking pulse oximetry.
   4. testing passive and active range of motion.

6. During report the word "bundle" is used in regard to a newly admitted patient. What is a "bundle"?
   1. A take-off on the old term "bundling" used to warm a person.
   2. A current name for a checklist of duties to be performed before discharge.
   3. A collection of evidenced-based interventions performed to decrease risk.
   4. A set of steps used with high-risk patients before discharge.

7. National Patient Safety Goals are formulated to:
   1. identify specific problem areas in patient safety and health care and possible solutions to these problems.
   2. measure or evaluate the outcomes of medical care and develop standards for improving care.
   3. meet the challenge of preparing future nurses so that they will have the skills and knowledge to decrease risks to the safety of the patient.
   4. ensure adequate nursing assessment of patients as they enter hospitals, in order to improve outcomes of care.

8. Assessing a patient's sleep patterns should include which aspect(s)? *(Select all that apply.)*
   1. Family history of sleep disorders
   2. Rituals associated with sleep
   3. Feelings of restfulness
   4. Diet choices
   5. Urinary habits

9. Which nursing action(s) should be implemented when addressing the needs of an elderly patient with the nursing diagnosis of *Imbalanced nutrition: less than body requirements related to poor dental condition? (Select all that apply.)*
   1. Encourage fluid intake if not contraindicated by the medical condition.
   2. Inspect oral cavity and condition of mucous membranes and teeth.
   3. Assist with swallowing.
   4. Initiate speech therapy and dietitian consult.
   5. Monitor daily caloric intake and weekly weights.

10. While obtaining the health history, the nurse finds that the patient is on long-term anticoagulant therapy. Which patient statement(s) would strongly correlate with excessive anticoagulant therapy? *(Select all that apply.)*
    1. "I have noticed some blood streaking in my bowel movements."
    2. "I have been embarrassed by frequent, uncontrollable gassiness."
    3. "My urine has been cloudy with occasional clots."
    4. "I readily bruise whenever I bump into anything."
    5. "I notice some blood when I floss my teeth."

Critical Thinking Questions

Scenario A
Review Critical Thinking and Clinical Judgment on pages 14–16. Consider how the critical thinking points discussed have helped you learn clinical judgment.

1. Describe an example from personal experience explaining how you used critical thinking and clinical judgment in a situation involving a patient, a patient's family member, or a friend.

2. Is there more you could have done, or could it have been done in a better way?

3. Did your action prevent harm to the person?

Scenario B
Mr. Nash is 68 years old and describes himself as a tough guy. He is currently on bed rest with his right leg in traction. He fell from his roof while adjusting the satellite dish. His main theme is, "What do I have to do to get out of here?" Although grumpy, Mr. Nash's positive attribute is that he will do whatever will get him released from the hospital. "I've got to smell my own air and I want my nightly martini!" A nursing diagnosis in his chart is *Impaired physical mobility related to right leg in traction.*

1. Write an example of a patient-centered expected outcome for Mr. Nash that is realistic, time referenced, and measurable.

2. Plan nursing interventions to meet the expected outcome you have written.

Scenario C
Since no jobs are currently available in the medical-surgical unit at the local hospital, you have applied at the mental health facility. You know that your medical-surgical observation skills will be useful in data collection (assessment). The mental health facility uses interdisciplinary care plans.

1. Explain the major differences in a nursing process–focused plan and an interdisciplinary plan.

2. What is the responsibility of each medical specialist for developing and carrying out the interdisciplinary plan?

Scenario D
You are assigned to a mixed medical-surgical nursing unit for your student assignment. You have arrived ½ hour early (at 6:30 A.M.) to begin preparation for patient care on the medical-surgical unit at the local hospital. Your assignment involves the following four patients:

Patient 1: Scheduled for abdominal surgery at 8 A.M.; arrives during report and says she was held up in traffic.
Patient 2: Newly diagnosed patient with diabetes, requiring blood glucose readings before each meal with a sliding scale diabetic teaching.
Patient 3: Total knee replacement 2 days ago who is scheduled for physical therapy (PT) at 10 A.M.
Patient 4: Has pneumonia, admitted during the night, oxygen at 4 L/min via nasal cannula, has an oxygen saturation monitor.

1. Which tasks are priorities?

2. How soon before surgery should the preoperative preparation start?

3. What time is glucose monitoring performed, and does the patient receive insulin based on the glucose reading?

4. When are IVs assessed?

5. What is required for preparation for PT?

6. Which patients need a full assessment?

7. Does Patient 3 have a dressing change and if so, when?

chapter

3

Fluids, Electrolytes, Acid-Base Balance, and Intravenous Therapy

http://evolve.elsevier.com/deWit/medsurg

Objectives

Theory

1. Recall the various functions fluid performs in the body.
2. Identify the body's mechanisms for fluid regulation.
3. Review three ways in which body fluids are continually being distributed among the body's fluid compartments.
4. Distinguish the signs and symptoms of various electrolyte imbalances.
5. Discuss why the elderly have more problems with fluid and electrolyte imbalances.
6. Recognize the disorders that cause specific fluid and electrolyte imbalances.
7. Compare the major causes of acid-base imbalances.
8. State interventions to correct an acid-base imbalance.
9. Discuss the steps in managing an intravenous infusion.
10. Describe the measures used to prevent the complications of intravenous therapy.

11. Identify intravenous fluids that are isotonic.
12. Discuss the principles of intravenous therapy.

Clinical Practice

1. Assess patients for signs of dehydration.
2. Correctly assess for and identify edema and signs of overhydration.
3. Apply knowledge of normal laboratory values in order to recognize electrolyte imbalances.
4. Carry out interventions to correct an electrolyte imbalance.
5. Determine if a patient has an acid-base imbalance.
6. Carry out measures to prevent the complications of intravenous therapy.
7. Compare interventions for the care of a patient receiving total parenteral nutrition with one undergoing intravenous therapy.

Key Terms

acidosis (ăh-sĭ-DŌ-sĭs, p. 41)
active transport (ĂK-tĭv, p. 33)
aldosterone (p. 32)
alkalosis (ăl-kă-LŌ-sĭs, p. 44)
anions (ĂN-ī-ŏnz, p. 40)
antidiuretic hormone (ADH) (ăn-tĭ-dī-ū-RĔT-ĭk HŎR-mōn, p. 31)
ascites (ăh-SĪ-tēz, p. 41)
atrial natriuretic peptide (ANP) (p. 32)
carpopedal spasm (spăzm, p. 44)
cations (KĂT-ī-ŏnz, p. 40)
dehydration (dē-hī-DRĀ-shŭn, p. 34)
diffusion (dĭ-FŪ-zhŭn, p. 32)
edema (ĕh-DĒ-mă, p. 39)
electrolytes (ĕh-LĔK-trō-līts, p. 40)
extracellular (ĕks-tră-SĔL-ū-lăr, p. 31)
filtration (fĭl-TRĀ-shŭn, p. 33)
hydrostatic pressure (hī-drō-STĂ-tĭk PRĔ-shŭr, p. 33)
hypercalcemia (hī-pĕr-kăl-SĒ-mē-ăh, p. 45)
hyperchloremia (hī-pĕr-klŏr-Ē-mē-ăh, p. 45)
hyperkalemia (hī-pĕr-kă-LĒ-mē-ăh, p. 44)
hypermagnesemia (hī-pĕr-măg-nĕ-SĒ-mē-ăh, p. 45)
hypernatremia (hī-pĕr-nă-TRĒ-mē-ăh, p. 41)
hyperphosphatemia (hī-pĕr-fŏs-fă-TĒ-mē-ăh, p. 45)
hypertonic (hī-pĕr-TŎN-ĭk, pp. 33, 51)

hyperventilation (hī-pĕr-vĕn-tĭ-LĀ-shŭn, p. 48)
hypervolemia (hī-pĕr-vō-LĒ-mē-ăh, p. 39)
hypocalcemia (hī-pō-kăl-SĒ-mē-ăh, p. 44)
hypochloremia (hī-pō-klŏr-Ē-mē-ăh, p. 45)
hypodermoclysis (hī-pō-dĕrm-ōk-LĪ-sĭs, p. 56)
hypokalemia (hī-pō-kă-LĒ-mē-ăh, p. 44)
hypomagnesemia (hī-pō-măg-nĕ-SĒ-mē-ăh, p. 45)
hyponatremia (hī-pō-nă-TRĒ-mē-ăh, p. 40)
hypophosphatemia (hī-pō-fŏs-făw-TĒ-mē-ăh, p. 45)
hypotonic (hī-pō-TŎN-ĭk, pp. 33, 51)
hypovolemia (hī-pō-vō-LĒ-mē-ăh, p. 39)
hypoxemia (hī-pŏk-SĒ-mē-ăh, p. 48)
insensible (p. 34)
interstitial (ĭn-tĕr-STĬSH-ăl, p. 32)
intracellular (ĭn-tră-SĔL-ū-lăr, p. 31)
intravascular (ĭn-tră-VĂS-cū-lăr, p. 32)
ions (ī-ŏnz, p. 32)
isotonic (ī-sō-TŎN-ĭk, pp. 33, 50)
ketoacidosis (kē-tō-ă-sĭ-DŌ-sĭs, p. 48)
osmolality (ŏz-mō-LĂ-lĭ-tē, p. 40)
osmosis (ŏz-MŌ-sĭs, p. 32)
stridor (STRĪ-dŏr, p. 49)
tetany (TĔT-ă-nē, p. 44)
transcellular (trăns-SĒ-lū-lăr, p. 32)
turgor (TŬR-gŏr, p. 34)

Over half of the human body's weight is water. Throughout life there is a gradual decline in the amount of body water. An infant's body is approximately 77% water, and an elderly person's body is about 45% water. **The elderly and the very young are more likely to experience severe consequences with even minor changes in their fluid balance.** Fatty tissue does not contain as much water as other tissues; thus the greater the amount of fat in the body, the less the percentage of body water. Maintaining a healthy weight is important to regulating the body's percentage of water. Keeping body fluids within a normal range is necessary because for every cell of every organ, life processes take place within fluid. The nutrients needed for life, reproduction, and the normal functioning of a cell must be dissolved or suspended in water. Moreover, the largest part of each cell is fluid. For all of the cell's life processes to take place, there must be a continuous exchange of water, glucose, oxygen, nutrients, electrolytes, and waste products. The four main functions of water in the body are to:

1. Be a vehicle for the transportation of substances to and from the cells.
2. Aid heat regulation by providing perspiration, which evaporates and cools the body.
3. Assist in maintenance of hydrogen (H^+) balance in the body.
4. Serve as a medium for the enzymatic action of digestion.

Table 3-1 shows sources of water and avenues of a body's water loss.

DISTRIBUTION AND REGULATION OF BODY FLUIDS

PATHOPHYSIOLOGY

Body fluids are continually in motion, moving in and out of the blood and lymph vessels, through the spaces surrounding the cells, and through the bodies of the cells themselves. Fluid within the cell is considered to be in one compartment (intracellular) and fluid outside the cell in another (extracellular) (Figure 3-1). The three types of extracellular fluid (ECF) and body fluid distribution are shown in Box 3-1. Excretion of the body's fluid is mainly achieved via the kidney. Control of fluid balance is managed by:

- *Osmoreceptors* in the hypothalamus sense the internal environment and promote the intake of fluid (thirst mechanism) when needed.
- Antidiuretic hormone (ADH) released by the posterior pituitary controls how much fluid leaves the

Table 3-1   Sources of Water and Avenues of Water Loss

SOURCES	24 HOURS (AVERAGE INTAKE)	AVENUE OF LOSS	AMOUNT OF LOSS (AVERAGE OUTPUT)
Oral fluids	1500 mL	Urine	1500 mL
Food	800 mL	Perspiration	400 mL
Metabolism	200 mL	Feces	200 mL
		Expired air	400 mL
Total	**2500 mL**		**2500 mL**

Adapted from deWit, S.C. (2009) *Fundamental Concepts and Skills for Nursing* (3rd ed.). Philadelphia: Saunders, p. 436.

FIGURE 3-1 Factors that influence body fluid distribution.

Box 3-1 Body Fluid Distribution

EXTRACELLULAR FLUID (outside of cells)
- Approximately ⅓ of total body water.
- Transports water, nutrients, oxygen, waste, etc., to and from the cells.
- Regulated by renal, metabolic, and neurologic factors.
- High in sodium (Na^+) content.

Intravascular Fluid
- Fluid within the blood vessels.
- Consists of plasma and fluid within blood cells.
- Contains large amounts of protein and electrolytes.

Interstitial Fluid
- Fluid in the spaces surrounding the cells.
- High in sodium (Na^+) content.

Transcellular Fluid
- Includes aqueous humor, saliva, cerebrospinal, pleural, peritoneal, synovial, and pericardial fluids, gastrointestinal secretions, and fluid in urinary system and lymphatics.

INTRACELLULAR FLUID (within cells)
- About ⅔ of total body fluid. Fluid contained within the cell walls. Most cell walls are permeable to water. High in potassium (K^+) content.

Modified from deWit, S.C. (2009). *Fundamental Concepts and Skills for Nursing* (3rd ed.). Philadelphia: Saunders, p. 437.

body in the urine and causes reabsorption of water from the kidney tubules.

- **Aldosterone** and **atrial natriuretic peptide (ANP)** regulate the reabsorption of water and sodium ions from the kidney tubules.
- Baroreceptors in the carotid sinus and aortic arch detect pressure changes indicating an increase or decrease in blood volume and stimulate the sympathetic or parasympathetic nervous system to return the pressure to normal.

Pain, nausea, and stress can also cause the release of ADH by the pituitary. When the ECF volume is low, or when sodium concentration is elevated, the adrenal cortex releases aldosterone, which causes reabsorption of sodium from the renal tubules. The *renin-angiotensin-aldosterone system* regulates the release of aldosterone. Renin is released when there is decreased blood flow to the kidney. Baroreceptors in the atrium of the heart detect fluid overload and stimulate the myocardium to release atrial natriuretic peptide. Atrial natriuretic peptide helps protect the body from fluid overload.

To be normally distributed within the body, water and the substances suspended or dissolved in water must move from compartment to compartment. As blood flows through the capillaries, fluid and solutes can move into the interstitial spaces, where nutrients and wastes can be exchanged by the cells of the body. Several processes accomplish the movement of fluids, electrolytes, nutrients, and waste products back and forth across the cell membranes (Figure 3-2).

MOVEMENT OF FLUID AND ELECTROLYTES

Passive Transport

Diffusion. Diffusion is the process by which substances move back and forth across the membrane until they are evenly distributed throughout the available space. As the plasma moves along a capillary, large amounts of fluid filter through pores in the capillary walls. The fluid moves into and out of the capillaries by filtering through the permeable capillary wall or cell membrane walls. There is a capillary hydrostatic pressure inside the capillary that pushes against the membrane of the capillary. **When the solution on one side of the membrane is more concentrated than the solution on the other side of the membrane, the particles in the more concentrated solution travel through the membrane to the less concentrated side in an attempt to equalize the concentration of the two solutions.** Diffusion is possible because of *kinetic* motion, which diffuses the molecules in the intracellular fluid (ICF) and the plasma. The molecules literally bounce off one another, mixing and stirring the body fluids.

Diffusion is a spontaneous mixing and moving that allows the exchange of molecules, ions (electrically charged particles), cellular nutrients, wastes, and other substances dissolved or suspended in body water. The direction of water flow depends on which side of the membrane has the greatest concentration of solutes. Substances will move from a high to a low concentration until the concentration on both sides of the membrane is equal. This is called *movement down a concentration gradient.* **Glucose, oxygen, carbon dioxide, water, and other small ions and molecules move by diffusion, which is a process of equalization.**

Diffusion may occur by movement along an electrical gradient as well. The attraction between particles of opposite charge and the repellent action between particles of like charge comprise an electrical gradient. Many intracellular proteins have a negative charge that tends to attract the positively charged sodium and potassium ions from the ECF.

Osmosis. Osmosis is the movement of pure solvent (liquid) across a membrane. **Water moves by osmosis.** When there are differences in concentration of fluids in the various compartments, osmotic pressure (what holds fluid in the vascular space) will move water from the area of lesser concentration of solutes to the area of greater concentration until the solutions in the compartments are of equal concentration. The process takes place via a *semipermeable membrane*—a membrane that allows some substances to pass through but prevents the passage of other substances. **Fluid moves between the interstitial and intracellular and the interstitial and intravascular compartments by osmosis.**

When living cells are surrounded by a solution that has the same concentration of particles, the water

FIGURE 3-2 Movement of water and electrolytes between compartments.

concentration of the ICF and the ECF will be equal. Such a solution is termed isotonic (of equal solute concentration). If cells are surrounded by a solution that has a greater concentration of solute than the cells, the water in the cells will move to the more concentrated solution and the cells will dehydrate and shrink. The solution is hypertonic (of greater concentration) in relation to the cells. If the cells are surrounded by a solution that has less solute than the cells, the solution is hypotonic (of less concentration) in relation to the cells. The particles within the cells exert osmotic pressure and draw water inward through the semipermeable membrane. The cells swell from the extra fluid (overhydrate). These concepts are important to the administration of intravenous fluids (see discussion later in this chapter). Solutions are classified as isotonic, hypertonic, or hypotonic according to their concentration of electrolytes and other solutes.

Think Critically

Can you describe to a classmate the difference between osmosis and diffusion?

Filtration. Filtration is the movement of water and solutes through a semipermeable membrane due to a pushing force on one side of the membrane. The pumping action of the heart creates hydrostatic pressure (pressure exerted by fluid) within the capillaries. Hydrostatic pressure causes fluid to press outward on the vessel. Water and electrolytes move through the capillary wall to the interstitial fluid. Filtration occurs in the kidney, where waste substances and excess water are eliminated.

Active Transport

In contrast to diffusion, osmosis, and filtration, active transport requires cellular energy, which can move molecules into cells regardless of their electrical charge or the concentrations already in the cell. Active transport **may move substances from an area of lower concentration to an area of higher concentration.** The energy source for the process is adenosine triphosphate (ATP). ATP is produced during the complex metabolic processes in the body's cells. Enzyme reactions metabolize carbon chains of sugars, fatty acids, and amino acids, yielding carbon dioxide, water, and high-energy phosphate bonds. **Amino acids, glucose, iron, hydrogen, sodium, potassium, and calcium are moved through the cell membrane by active transport.** The "sodium pump" is the mechanism by which sodium and potassium are moved into or out of the cell via active transport.

FLUID IMBALANCES

PATHOPHYSIOLOGY

Healthy people maintain fluid balance by drinking sufficient fluids and eating a balanced diet each day. Solid foods contain up to 85% water, and water is also produced in the body as a by-product of metabolism. **The healthy kidney balances the amount of substances entering and leaving the blood, helping to maintain normal concentrations of fluid and electrolytes.** Illness affects fluid balance in many ways. The patient may be unable to ingest food or liquids, there may be a problem with absorption from the intestinal tract, or there may be a kidney impairment that affects excretion or reabsorption of water and electrolytes. Any disease that affects circulation (e.g., heart failure) will ultimately affect the distribution and composition of body fluids. Extra fluid is lost when the metabolic rate is accelerated, such as occurs in fever, thyroid crisis, burns, severe trauma, and states of extreme stress. Perspiration can account for a fluid loss of up to 2 L/hr in an adult. For every degree of fever on the Celsius scale, an insensible (unaware of) water loss of 10% may occur. Perspiration and water lost in respiration are insensible losses. When the weather is hot and dry, water loss from the body is greater. Patients on mechanical ventilators, those with rapid respirations, and those with severe diarrhea or excessive amounts of fistula drainage also lose greater quantities of water. **Any seriously ill patient is at risk for a fluid and electrolyte imbalance.**

A fluid imbalance exists when there is an excess (too much) or a deficit (too little) of water in the body. When this occurs, there will be an accompanying imbalance in the substances dissolved in body water. When considering sodium imbalances, **it is important to remember that water follows sodium in the body, through osmosis.** The sodium concentration causes an osmotic pull, and water will go to where the sodium concentration is highest.

[?] Think Critically

Can you give an example of active transport taking place within the body?

DEFICIENT FLUID VOLUME

Those at risk for deficient fluid volume are patients who are unable to take in sufficient quantities of fluid because of impaired swallowing, extreme weakness, disorientation or coma, or the unavailability of water, and patients who lose excessive amounts of fluid through prolonged vomiting, diarrhea, hemorrhage, diaphoresis (sweating), excessive wound drainage, or diuretic therapy.

When a fluid deficit occurs, water moves from the cells into the interstitial and intravascular spaces. This movement of water out of the cells causes dehydration of the cells. Dehydration is treated by administering fluid orally or intravenously. For patients who will be unable to take in fluids or food on their own for an extended period, a feeding tube must be placed or total parenteral nutrition (TPN) started (see Chapter 30). Signs and symptoms of dehydration are presented in Box 3-2. **Turgor** (degree of elasticity) is checked by gently pinching up the skin over the abdomen, forearm, sternum, forehead, clavicle, or thigh (Figure 3-3). In a person with normal fluid balance, the pinched skin will immediately fall back to normal when released. If a

---

Box 3-2   Signs and Symptoms of Dehydration and Overhydration

SIGNS AND SYMPTOMS OF DEHYDRATION
- Thirst
- Poor skin turgor
- Weight loss
- Weakness
- Complaints of dizziness
- Postural hypotension
- Decreased urine production
- Dark, concentrated urine
- Dry, cracked lips and tongue
- Dry mucous membranes
- Sunken, soft eyeballs
- Thick saliva
- Dry, scaly skin
- Flat neck veins when lying down
- Rapid, weak, thready pulse
- Elevated temperature ≥100.6° F (38.1° C)
- Increased hematocrit
- High urine specific gravity with low volume

SIGNS AND SYMPTOMS OF OVERHYDRATION
- Weight gain
- Slow, bounding pulse
- Elevated blood pressure
- Firm subcutaneous tissues
- Possibly edema
- Possibly crackles in lungs on auscultation
- Lethargy, possibly seizures
- Possibly visible neck veins when lying down
- Decreased serum sodium
- Decreased hematocrit from hemodilution
- Low urine specific gravity with high volume

FIGURE 3-3 Testing tissue turgor.

fluid deficit is present, the skin may remain elevated or tented for several seconds. However, since pinching the skin to measure fluid deficit also measures skin elasticity, this test is not a valid indicator of fluid status in the elderly—whose skin is often inelastic and routinely tents when pinched. In the infant, dehydration is evident by sunken fontanels.

Clinical Cues

The most accurate measure of fluid gain or loss for any age group is weight change. A weight gain or loss of 2.2 lb (1 kg) in 24 hours indicates a gain or loss of 1 L of fluid.

 Elder Care Points

Fluid volume deficit is a common problem in the elderly. There is an age-related decline in total body water and a decrease in thirst sensation and taste that causes elderly people to become dehydrated more easily. If urinary incontinence problems are present, the person becomes reluctant to drink extra fluids. Thirst is a late sign of dehydration in the elderly.

Many elderly people rely on laxatives and enemas to clear the bowel. This practice can cause fluid volume deficit along with sodium and potassium loss. **Fluid volume deficit contributes to constipation and orthostatic hypotension with related dizziness and falls, and makes the person more susceptible to infection.**

A furrowed, dry tongue that is not the result of drug therapy indicates a fluid deficit. If the person has fever, this adds to the fluid loss. Because of the fluid and accompanying electrolyte losses, the person may become confused. Offering the patient small amounts of liquid and electrolyte solution frequently—if fluid can be kept down—helps prevent additional problems.

 Clinical Cues

Measure the blood pressure and pulse in the lying, sitting, and standing positions. If there is a systolic blood pressure drop of 20 mm Hg accompanied by a pulse rate increase of 10 beats per minute (bpm) at 1 minute after the position change, fluid volume deficit is suggested. This is termed *orthostatic* or *postural hypotension*.

Nursing Management. Provide an adequate fluid intake for those who are unable to do this for themselves. Include the patient's preferences for liquids on the plan of care. The patient should receive fruit juices, bouillon, and any other nutritious liquid tolerated (Nursing Care Plan 3-1).

A frequent cause of excessive fluid loss is abnormally rapid excretion of intestinal fluids, such as that which occurs from vomiting and diarrhea.

 Assignment Considerations

Increasing Fluid Intake

If a nursing assistant or unlicensed assistive personnel (UAP) is available to assist, *assign* the task of increasing fluid intake to that person. Work out a timed plan to help the patient with regular, periodic intake of fluids by mouth. Ask that the patient drink 4 oz of fluid every hour. Advise of any safety precautions regarding difficulty swallowing or need for assistance.

 Think Critically

Why is it important to the body's function to administer fluid and electrolytes during a fever?

Nausea and Vomiting

Nausea is a feeling of discomfort or an unpleasant sensation vaguely felt in the epigastrium and abdomen. It is a symptom of illness and is often accompanied by a tendency to vomit. Nausea is experienced when nerve endings in the stomach and other parts of the body are irritated. Irritated nerve endings in the stomach send messages to the part of the brain that controls the vomiting reflex; however, nerve cells in other parts of the body can trigger the same response. Pain can trigger the nausea-vomiting mechanism. Nausea and vomiting are an automatic response of the involuntary autonomic nervous system to unpleasant stimuli.

 Complementary and Alternative Therapies

Preventing Nausea

Sea bands (acupressure wristbands) are very helpful to many people who suffer from nausea and vomiting. They are available at most drugstores. Ginger tea is another alternative therapy that has proven helpful, as are small pieces of ginger candy.

Nausea and vomiting may occur from gastrointestinal irritation from foods, viruses, radiation of the mucosa, and some drugs and other chemicals. Certain types of anesthetics may trigger nausea, as may pregnancy.

 Safety Alert

Prolonged Vomiting

Prolonged vomiting can lead to sodium and potassium deficits and metabolic alkalosis, due to the loss of electrolytes and stomach acids.

The patient may complain of nausea or feeling "sick to my stomach," of queasiness, abdominal pain, epigastric discomfort or burning, and vomiting. The patient may also exhibit pallor; mild diaphoresis; cold, clammy skin; excessive salivation; and the patient may attempt to remain quiet and motionless. **If vomiting occurs, the vomitus should be observed for odor, color, contents (e.g., undigested food), and amount.** Noting and recording vomiting patterns, conditions that trigger vomiting, and quality of nausea as described by the patient can be helpful in planning treatment.

Medical treatment for nausea consists of administering one of the antiemetic drugs (Table 3-2). Antihistamines, sedatives and hypnotics, anticholinergics, phenothiazines, and other drugs are used to control nausea and vomiting. The patient is given nothing

⭐ Nursing Care Plan 3-1   Care of the Patient with Deficient Fluid Volume

Scenario
A 78-year-old woman is admitted to the hospital after 3 days of vomiting and diarrhea. She is confused, disoriented, dehydrated, and very weak.

Problem/Nursing Diagnosis
Vomiting and diarrhea/Deficient fluid volume related to fluid loss and inability to take in sufficient fluids.

Supporting Assessment Data
Subjective: Hx of vomiting and diarrhea for 3 days; unable to keep anything in stomach. Had eaten food at a church picnic on a hot day.

Objective: Furrowed tongue, tenting of skin on sternum, thick saliva, and dry mucous membranes; 3-lb weight loss from normal. Urine sp. gr. 1.030; scant urine; temp. 101.4° F (40° C).

Goals/Expected Outcomes	Nursing Interventions	Selected Rationale	Evaluation*
Diarrhea and vomiting will stop within 24 hours.	Medicate with antiemetic as ordered.	Antiemetic should stop vomiting.	IM injection of Vistaril given Z-track as ordered. Has not vomited in last hour.
Patient will be able to eat normally before discharge.	Initiate IV therapy as ordered.	IV therapy will replenish fluids and electrolytes in the body.	IV fluids infusing. Site clean, dry without redness.
Fluid balance will be reestablished within 72 hours.	Monitor IV site and fluid every hour.		
	Initiate I&O recording.	I&O record provides data to determine degree of fluid imbalance.	Two liquid stools. Continue plan.
	Keep patient clean and dry. Reduce odors in room to decrease nausea.	Odors contribute to nausea.	No odor in room.
	Provide assistance to bathroom as needed.	Assistance helps prevent falls in weak patients.	Assistance provided × 4.
	Protect perianal skin with ointment as ordered.	A barrier cream or ointment will protect the perianal skin from excoriation from diarrhea.	Perianal skin slightly reddened.
	When vomiting stops, administer medication for diarrhea as ordered.	Medication will slow or stop the diarrhea.	Took Lomotil tab with a sip of Gatorade.
	When able to take PO fluids, offer sips of electrolyte solution, and progress to a clear liquid diet.	Small sips of fluid are easier to keep in the stomach. Electrolyte solution replenishes low electrolytes.	Taking sips of Gatorade.
	Offer mouth care after vomiting and at least q 2 hr.	Mouth care promotes comfort and reduces nausea.	Mouth care provided.
	Monitor mucous membrane status and skin turgor.	Provides data about rehydration status.	Mucous membranes more moist.
	Weigh daily. Monitor electrolyte values.	Provides data about electrolyte imbalances.	Laboratory results not back yet. Continue plan.

Critical Thinking Questions
1. What would be other concerns that should be addressed in her care plan?
2. What do you think is the cause of her confusion and disorientation?

Key: *Hx*, history; *I&O*, intake and output; *IM*, intramuscular; *IV*, intravenous; *PO*, oral; *sp. gr.*, specific gravity; *temp.*, temperature.
*Evaluation data must be documented in the medical record.

Table 3-2   Drugs Commonly Prescribed for Vomiting and Diarrhea

CLASSIFICATION	ACTION	NURSING IMPLICATIONS	PATIENT TEACHING
Antiemetics			
Hydroxyzine (Vistaril, Atarax) Promethazine (Phenergan)	Antihistamine-antiemetic used to stop nausea and vomiting. Depresses the central nervous system (CNS).	Give by Z-track injection. Never give IV or subcutaneously. Monitor vital signs. Check compatibility before mixing with other drugs. Monitor for dizziness and hypotension. Observe for urinary retention.	Avoid concurrent alcohol ingestion or other CNS depressants. Avoid activities that require alertness. Raise patient slowly to prevent dizziness. Avoid prolonged sunlight.
Prochlorperazine maleate (Compazine)	Blocks chemoreceptor trigger zone, which in turn acts on vomiting center. Stops nausea and vomiting.	Monitor vital signs and for respiratory depression, especially in elderly. Check compatibilities before mixing with other drugs. Watch for seizures, muscle stiffness, and untoward reactions.	Avoid hazardous activities; avoid alcohol and other CNS depressants. Advise urine may be pink to reddish brown. Avoid the sun or use sunscreen and protective clothing. Report bleeding, rash, bruising, blurred vision, or clay-colored stools.
Ondansetron (Zofran)	Blocks serotonin peripherally, centrally, and in the small intestine.	Monitor for extrapyramidal signs (shuffling gait, tremors, grimacing, rigidity). Observe for rash or bronchospasm.	Report diarrhea, constipation, rash, change in respiration, or discomfort at IV insertion site.
Metoclopramide	Decreases reflux, stimulates stomach emptying, and raises threshold of chemoreceptor trigger zone.	Monitor for extrapyramidal symptoms with IV administration. Assess for rash. Monitor renal function, blood pressure, and heart rate.	Report involuntary eye, facial, or limb movements. Avoid alcohol.
Antidiarrheals			
Diphenoxylate atropine (Lomotil)	Slows intestinal motility. Slows or stops diarrhea.	Assess bowel pattern and monitor for constipation. Discontinue if not effective after 2 days of treatment.	Do not use alcohol or CNS depressants. Do not exceed the prescribed dosage. May be habit forming. Avoid hazardous activities.
Loperamide HCl (Imodium)	Works on intestinal muscles to decrease peristalsis; reduces volume and increases stool bulk. Slows or stops diarrhea.	Monitor stools and for electrolyte imbalances. Monitor for dehydration. Discontinue if not effective after 2 days of treatment.	Drowsiness may occur; do not operate machinery. Do not take other over-the-counter preparations.
Kaolin-pectin (Kaopectate)	Decreases gastric motility and water content of stool; acts as absorbent and demulcent.	Monitor bowel pattern. Monitor for dehydration and electrolyte imbalances.	Do not exceed recommended dosage. Shake suspension well. Take other medications 2 hr before or after administration.
Bismuth salts (Pepto-Bismol)	Inhibits prostaglandin synthesis responsible for gastrointestinal hypermotility; stimulates absorption of fluid and electrolytes. Prevents or stops diarrhea.	Monitor bowel pattern. Do not give to children under age 3.	Shake liquid before using. The tongue may darken and stools may turn black. Do not take other salicylates along with this medication. Stop taking if diarrhea has not stopped in 2 days.
Camphorated opium tincture (paregoric)	Opiate that acts to decrease intestinal motility.	Controlled substance. Addictive with long-term use. Monitor bowel function. May cause nausea and vomiting.	Do not exceed prescribed dosage. Causes CNS depression; do not operate machinery.

by mouth (kept NPO) until vomiting has stopped; afterward, the patient is started back on clear liquids, progressing slowly to a regular diet. Sips of carbonated drinks are usually tolerated well, at first.

Nursing Management. **Have the patient lie down and turn his head to one side, or have the patient sit and lower his head between the legs so that vomitus is not aspirated into the respiratory tract.** Hold an emesis basin close to the side of the face. Use a cool, damp washcloth to wipe the patient's face and the back of the neck. Have the patient breathe through the mouth. Provide mouth care after the episode. Sucking on ice chips helps reduce nausea in some patients. A quiet, cool, odor-free environment helps calm nausea. If nausea and vomiting persist, observe for dehydration.

 Elder Care Points

Older patients must be rehydrated cautiously. Any patient who has a cardiac problem is at risk for fluid overload from intravenous (IV) infusions. If a liter of fluid infuses too fast, it can cause the patient to go into heart failure. **If an IV infusion falls behind, do not make up for lost time by infusing fluid at a rate faster than ordered.**

Diarrhea

Diarrhea is defined as the rapid movement of fecal matter through the intestine. During diarrhea, patients absorb nutrients poorly and lose water and electrolytes. These electrolytic substances—especially the potassium needed by the body to prevent alkalosis—are lost in large amounts by patients with diarrhea.

Major diarrhea is related to local irritation of the intestinal mucosa, especially irritation caused by infectious agents, such as *Salmonella*, *Clostridium difficile*, and *Escherichia coli*; by gastrointestinal flu; and by chemicals. Chronic and prolonged diarrhea is typical of such disorders as ulcerative colitis, irritable bowel syndrome, allergies, lactose intolerance, and nontropical sprue. Obstruction to the flow of intestinal contents, such as from a tumor or a fecal impaction, also can produce diarrhea. Considerable potassium and sodium are lost during diarrhea.

To rest the intestines and stomach of a patient with acute diarrhea, limit the intake of foods. Once oral feedings are allowed, begin clear liquids and progress to bland liquids and then solid foods of increased calories and high-protein, high-carbohydrate content. Give rehydrating solutions containing glucose and electrolytes first. *Avoid iced fluids, carbonated drinks, whole milk, roughage, raw fruits, and highly seasoned foods.*

Medications prescribed for diarrhea depend on the cause of the disorder and the length of time the condition has been present (see Table 3-2). Mild cases usually respond well to kaolin and bismuth preparations (e.g., Kaopectate), which coat the intestinal tract and make the stools more firm. Bismuth subsalicylate (e.g., Pepto-Bismol) is the recommended treatment for "traveler's diarrhea"; given in advance of travel, bismuth subsalicylate may prevent this type of diarrhea. Diarrhea caused by infections may be treated with drugs that are specific for the causative organism. Depending on the organism responsible, it is sometimes advisable to allow the toxins to be eliminated naturally from the body, and so drugs may not be given initially. Diarrhea is characterized by frequent watery bowel movements, abdominal cramping, and general weakness. Diarrheic watery stools often contain mucus and are blood streaked. It is the consistency rather than the number of stools per day that is the hallmark of diarrhea. In some cases the number can be as high as 15 to 20 liquid stools. If the condition is chronic, the patient can suffer from dehydration, malnutrition, and anemia. Bowel sounds are likely to be gurgling and tinkling sounds that come in waves and are hyperactive. Note and record the number of stools during the shift and the characteristics of each stool and any associated pain.

 Think Critically

If a patient has food poisoning and suffers from vomiting and diarrhea, what type of fluid and electrolyte imbalance may the patient suffer?

Nursing Management. Nursing measures for diarrhea aim to provide physical and mental rest, to prevent unnecessary loss of water and nutrients, protect the rectal mucosa, and eventually replace lost fluids. Diarrhea can be associated with nervous tension and anxiety. The patient often is embarrassed by the condition and inconvenienced by frequent trips to the bathroom or the need to request a bedpan. This emotional stress only serves to make the condition worse. Help break the vicious cycle by maintaining a calm and dignified manner, accepting and understanding the patient's behavior, and providing privacy and a restful environment for the patient.

 Think Critically

How would you assess the patient with diarrhea for signs of dehydration?

EXCESS FLUID VOLUME

An excessive amount of *body water* usually occurs first in the extracellular compartment because this is where water enters and leaves the body. When people become ill, they may receive more water than they excrete, which can happen if they receive IV fluid too quickly, are given tap water enemas, or are persuaded to drink more fluids than they can eliminate. If these events happen, the patient will suffer a fluid volume excess. When any of these conditions is present, the patient is likely to suffer from *water intoxication.*

Impaired elimination, such as occurs in renal failure, is a major cause of fluid volume excess (see Box 3-2). An objective measure of water excess and circulatory overload is the hematocrit. The hematocrit measures the percentage of red blood cells in a volume of whole blood. When fluid volume excess occurs, hypervolemia (excessive blood volume) may also occur. Hypervolemia elevates blood pressure.

Clinical Cues

Normal hematocrit values range from 35 to 54 mL of red blood cells per 100 mL of whole blood, depending on age and sex. If there is an excess of water, the proportion of red blood cells to milliliters of blood will be lower, and the hematocrit will be below the normal values because of dilution by the water.

Urine concentration provides another clue to the fluid status. Urine concentration is commonly measured by specific gravity and compared with the specific gravity of distilled water, which is 1.000. Urine contains urea, electrolytes, and other substances, so its specific gravity will exceed 1.000 and ranges between 1.003 and 1.030. The average range is 1.010 to 1.025.

Edema

Edema is associated with the retention of water, sodium, and chloride and defined as an accumulation of freely moving interstitial fluid (fluid surrounding cells). Look for puffy eyelids and swollen hands. Edema also can occur in body cavities, as in the peritoneal cavity (ascites) and the cranial cavity. The accumulation of body fluids can affect almost all of the tissue spaces (*generalized edema*). Alternatively, fluid accumulation can affect a limited area (*localized edema*). Generalized edema occurs when the body's mechanisms for eliminating excess sodium fail. Edema becomes life threatening when accumulated fluids overload the circulatory system, as in congestive heart failure, and when fluids accumulate in the lungs, as in pulmonary edema.

Four general causes of edema are (1) a loss of plasma proteins, (2) obstruction of lymphatic circulation, (3) an increase in capillary permeability, and (4) an increase in capillary hydrostatic pressure.

Increased hydrostatic pressure causes pulmonary edema. A loss of plasma proteins decreases osmotic pressure in the vascular system causing fluid to leak from the vessels, leading to edema. A tumor or infection can damage a lymph node, or lymph nodes may be removed during cancer surgery. When lymph nodes are removed during mastectomy surgery, lymph may accumulate in the tissues resulting in *lymphedema.*

When an inflammatory response or infection occurs, histamine and other chemical mediators are released from the cells involved in the tissue injury. These chemicals cause increased capillary permeability, and more fluid moves into the interstitial spaces. Proteins leak into the interstitial spaces also, decreasing the osmotic pressure in the capillaries. Protein in the interstitial spaces holds fluid there rather than moving that fluid back into the capillaries. When fluid shifts from the vascular space (from the plasma) to the interstitial space, dehydration and hypovolemia (too little blood volume) can occur. The occurrence of the shift of fluid is termed *third spacing* and may occur with extensive trauma, burns, peritonitis, intestinal obstruction, nephrosis, sepsis, or cirrhosis of the liver in which there is an increase in capillary hydrostatic pressure or increased capillary membrane permeability.

? Think Critically

What characteristics would you expect to find in a urine specimen from a patient who is dehydrated? How would it differ from a urine specimen from a patient who has a fluid volume excess?

Localized edema often occurs with inflammation. Localized edema usually is nonpitting, does not come and go, and is characterized by tight, shiny skin that is stretched over a hard and red area. Causes of localized edema include trauma, allergies, burns, obstruction of lymph flow, and liver failure.

Dependent edema is noted in the feet, ankles, and lower legs, or in the sacral region of patients confined to bed or chair. Dependent edema is an effect of gravity and therefore can be somewhat relieved by elevating the affected body part 18 inches (or above heart level, when possible) and by repositioning the patient frequently. Pitting edema is common in patients with dependent edema. The name is derived from the fact that a pit or depression can be created by pressing a fingertip against the swollen tissue. **To check for pitting edema, press your thumb into the patient's skin at a bony prominence, such as the tibia or malleolus, and hold for 5 seconds.** If the depression, or "pit," remains for a while after the pressure is released, the patient has pitting edema. Assessing the severity and progress of pitting edema in the feet and ankles (pedal edema) can be done more accurately by rating the findings and comparing assessments from one shift to another (Figure 3-4).

The scale used for rating pedal edema is:

1+   Mild pitting—slight indentation with no swelling of the leg
2+   Moderate pitting—indentation subsides quickly
3+   Deep pitting—indentation remains for a short time; leg looks swollen
4+   Very deep pitting—indentation lasts a long time and leg is very swollen

FIGURE 3-4 Measuring pedal edema.

Treatment. Treatment of a fluid imbalance involves correcting the underlying cause and assisting the body to rebalance fluid content. For conditions of edema, fluid may be restricted or diuretic drugs may be administered to facilitate excretion of the excess fluid. A diuretic is a drug that prompts the kidneys to increase the excretion of fluid. Bed rest may be ordered to facilitate fluid excretion as the kidneys function best when the body is supine.

The patient is placed on a low-sodium diet. Elastic stockings or sequential compression devices are ordered for foot and leg edema. Intake and output recording is requested.

[?] Think Critically

Can you describe the assessments you would make to determine whether your 68-year-old patient is experiencing edema?

HOME CARE

For the patient with a fluid deficit, it is important to teach the patient and family how to measure fluid intake and output, and how to keep a log of the amounts. The patient should be encouraged to take small amounts of liquid every hour while awake. If the patient has been vomiting, it is better to let carbonated beverages go flat before drinking them, to decrease stomach distention.

If an elderly patient has been vomiting considerably for several hours or has had constant diarrhea without fluid intake, a visit to the emergency department is in order so that IV fluids can be given to prevent serious dehydration.

When the patient has a fluid excess, the patient should be weighed daily and a chart kept. The patient and family should be taught how to assess edema and to record findings. If edema is worsening or weight is rising, the physician should be notified.

OSMOLALITY

Nonelectrolyte solutes include protein, urea, glucose, creatinine, and bilirubin. Along with the electrolytes, these solutes contribute to the osmolality (concentration of the solution determined by the number of solutes in it) of the body fluid. Osmolality controls water movement and the body fluid distribution in the intracellular and

extracellular compartments. Potassium maintains the osmolality of the ICF. Sodium controls the osmolality of the ECF. Normal osmolality of body fluids is 280 to 294 milliosmoles per kilogram (mOsm/kg).

[?] Think Critically

Why should you watch for signs of fluid imbalance in any patient who has a serious infection or who has suffered considerable physical trauma?

ELECTROLYTES

Some molecules, when placed in solution, undergo a separation of their atoms into electrically charged ions. These molecules are called electrolytes because their atomic particles are capable of conducting an electrical current. The molecules of electrolytes break up into atomic particles that are either negatively charged (anions) or positively charged (cations). For example, when sodium chloride (table salt) is dissolved in body water, its molecules separate into sodium ions, which are positively charged (Na^+), and chloride ions, which are negatively charged (Cl^-).

Because electrolytes are electrically charged, they are chemically active. **This chemical activity allows for the creation of an electrical impulse across the cell membrane, making possible the transmission of nerve impulses, contraction of muscles, and excretion of hormones and other substances from glandular cells.** Thus electrolytes are essential to the normal functioning of the body.

ELECTROLYTE IMBALANCES

Electrolytes have many functions in the body. In order to determine if there is an electrolyte imbalance, you must know the normal range for each electrolyte (Table 3-3). Many disorders can cause a shift in electrolytes, and an imbalance—with too much or too little of an electrolyte circulating in the bloodstream or inside the cells of the body.

Sodium Imbalances

Hyponatremia. Hyponatremia, a deficit of sodium in the blood (Na^+ less than 135 mEq/L), is the most common electrolyte imbalance. Hyponatremia can occur from either a sodium loss or an excess of water. Decreased

Table 3-3 Normal Ranges and Functions of Major Electrolytes

ELECTROLYTE	NORMAL RANGE	SI UNITS	FUNCTION
Sodium (Na^+)	135–145 mEq/L	135–145 mmol/L	**Major cation of the extracellular fluid.** Major role in regulation of water balance. Regulates extracellular fluid volume through somatic pressure. **Water follows sodium concentration in the body.** Essential to the transmission of nerve impulses and helps maintain neuromuscular irritability. Important in controlling contractility of the heart. Helps maintain acid-base balance. Aids in maintenance of electroneutrality.
Potassium (K^+)	3.5–5.0 mEq/L	3.5–5.0 mmol/L	**Major intracellular cation.** Important to nerve transmission and muscle contraction. Helps maintain normal heart rhythm. Helps maintain plasma acid-base balance.
Calcium (Ca^{2+})	8.4–10.6 mg/dL	2.10–2.65 mmol/L	Involved in formation of bone and teeth. Necessary for blood coagulation. Essential for normal nerve and muscle activity.
Magnesium (Mg^{2+})	1.3–2.1 mg/dL	0.65–1.05 mmol/L	Necessary for building bones and teeth. Necessary for nerve transmission and is involved in muscle contraction. Plays an important role in many metabolic reactions, where it acts as a cofactor to cellular enzymes.
Phosphate (PO_4^-)	3.0–4.5 mg/dL	1.0–1.5 mmol/L	Necessary for formation of adenosine triphosphate (ATP). Cofactor in carbohydrate, protein, and lipid metabolism. Activates B-complex vitamins.
Chloride (Cl^-)	96–106 mEq/L	96–106 mmol/L	Helps maintain acid-base balance. Important to formation of hydrochloric acid for secretion to the stomach. Aids in maintaining plasma electroneutrality.
Bicarbonate (HCO_3^-)	22–26 mEq/L	23–29 mmol/L	A buffer that neutralizes excess acids in the body. Helps regulate acid-base balance.

From deWit, S.C. (2009). *Fundamental Concepts and Skills for Nursing* (3rd ed.). Philadelphia: Saunders, p. 437.

secretion of aldosterone results in sodium loss. Congestive heart failure, liver disease with ascites (abnormal accumulation of fluid within the peritoneal cavity), and chronic renal failure result in excessive water retention—without concurrent sodium retention—and this results in hypervolemia combined with hyponatremia. Decreased osmotic pressure in the extracellular compartment may cause a fluid shift into the cells. A decrease in blood pressure may occur. The average intake of sodium is 4 to 5 g/day. If there is a problem with water balance, sodium may be restricted in the diet. The consequence of hyponatremia is impaired nerve conduction. Table 3-4 presents the signs and symptoms, risk factors, and nursing interventions for hyponatremia.

Hypernatremia. Hypernatremia occurs when the sodium level rises above 145 mEq/L. Water loss from fever, respiratory infection, or watery diarrhea is the usual cause. The body tries to correct the situation by conserving water through reabsorption in the renal tubules. Another cause of hypernatremia is the excessive administration of sodium bicarbonate for the treatment of acidosis (excess acid or depletion of alkaline

substances in the blood and body tissues). Good tissue turgor and firm subcutaneous tissues occur during hypernatremia. Hypernatremia causes an osmotic shift of fluid from the cells to the interstitial spaces, causing a cellular dehydration and interruption of normal cell processes. **Sodium intake is restricted for the patient with hypernatremia** (see Table 3-4).

Nutrition Considerations

Foods High in Sodium*

Buttermilk	Ham
Canned meats or fish	Hot dogs
Canned soups	Olives
Canned vegetables	Pickles
Casserole and pasta mixes	Prepared mustard
Catsup	Preserved meats
Cheese (all kinds)	Processed foods
Delicatessen meats	Salted nuts
Dried fruits	Salted popcorn
Dried soup mixes	Salted snack foods
Foods containing monosodium glutamate (MSG)	Softened water
	Soy sauce
Frozen vegetables with sauces	Tomato or vegetable
Gravy mixes	juice

*Check all packaged food labels for sodium content.

Table 3-4   Electrolyte Imbalances and Nursing Interventions

SERUM VALUE	SIGNS AND SYMPTOMS	CAUSES/RISK FACTORS	NURSING INTERVENTIONS
Sodium—Normal Range: 135–145 mEq/L			
Hyponatremia <135 mEq/L	Central nervous system and neuromuscular changes resulting from failure of swollen cells to transmit electrical impulses Fatigue, lethargy, headache, mental confusion, altered level of consciousness, anxiety, coma, anorexia, nausea, vomiting, muscle cramps, seizures, decreased sensation and decreased blood pressure (BP)	Inadequate sodium intake, as in patients on low-sodium diets Excessive intake or retention of water (kidney failure and heart failure) Loss of bile, which is rich in sodium as a result of fistulas, drainage, gastrointestinal surgery, nausea and vomiting, and suction Loss of sodium through burn wounds Administration of intravenous (IV) fluids that do not contain electrolytes	Restrict water intake as ordered for patients with congestive heart failure, kidney failure, and inadequate antidiuretic hormone production. Liberalize diet of patient on low-sodium diet. Closely monitor patient receiving IV solutions to correct hyponatremia. Replace water loss with fluids containing sodium.
Hypernatremia >145 mEq/L	Dry mucous membranes, taut skin turgor, intense thirst, flushed skin, oliguria, and possibly elevated temperature Weakness, lethargy, irritability, twitching, seizures, coma, intracranial bleeding	High-sodium diet, inadequate water intake as in comatose, mentally confused, or debilitated patient Excessive sweating, diarrhea, failure of kidney to reabsorb water from urine Administration of high-protein, hyperosmotic tube feedings and osmotic diuretics	Encourage increased fluid intake. Measure intake and output (I&O). Give water between tube feedings. Restrict sodium intake. Monitor temperature.
Potassium—Normal Range: 3.5–5.0 mEq/L			
Hypokalemia <3.5 mEq/L	Abdominal pain, paralytic ileus, gaseous distention of intestines Cardiac dysrhythmias, muscle weakness, decreased reflexes, paralysis, urinary retention, increased urinary pH, lethargy, confusion, electrocardiogram (ECG) changes	Inadequate intake of potassium-rich foods Loss of potassium in urine when kidneys do not reabsorb the mineral Loss of potassium from intestinal tract as a result of diarrhea or vomiting, drainage from fistulas, overuse of gastric suction Improper use of diuretics	Instruct patients (especially those taking diuretics) about foods high in potassium content; encourage intake. Observe closely for signs of digitalis toxicity in patients taking this drug. Teach patients to watch for signs of hypokalemia. Administer potassium chloride supplement as ordered. Monitor I&O and cardiac rhythm.
Hyperkalemia >5.0 mEq/L	Muscle weakness, fatigue, hypotension, nausea, paresthesias, paralysis, cardiac dysrhythmias, ECG changes	Kidney failure, decreased kidney function Intestinal obstruction that prevents elimination or potassium in the feces Addison's disease, digitalis toxicity, uncontrolled diabetes mellitus, insulin deficit, crushing injuries, and burns Overuse of potassium-containing salt substitute, or overuse of potassium-sparing diuretic	Decrease intake of foods high in potassium. Increase fluid intake to enhance urinary excretion of potassium; provide adequate carbohydrate intake to prevent use of body proteins for energy. Carefully administer proper dose of insulin to diabetic patients. Instruct patient in proper use of salt substitutes containing potassium.

Adapted from deWit, S.C. (2009). *Fundamental Concepts and Skills for Nursing* (3rd ed.). Philadelphia: Saunders, pp. 443–444.

Table 3-4	Electrolyte Imbalances and Nursing Interventions—cont'd		
SERUM VALUE	**SIGNS AND SYMPTOMS**	**CAUSES/RISK FACTORS**	**NURSING INTERVENTIONS**
Calcium—Normal Range: 8.4–10.6 mg/dL			
Hypocalcemia <8.4 mg/dL	Paresthesias, abdominal cramps, weak pulse, decreased BP, seizures, muscle spasms, tetany, hand spasm, positive Chvostek's sign, positive Trousseau's sign, cardiac dysrhythmia, wheezing, dyspnea, difficulty swallowing, colic, cardiac failure, excessive blood transfusions	Metastatic cancer, inadequate dietary intake of calcium and vitamin D. Impaired absorption of calcium from intestinal tract, as in diarrhea, sprue, overuse of laxatives and enemas containing phosphates (phosphorus tends to be more readily absorbed from the intestinal tract than calcium and suppresses calcium retention in the body). The parathyroid regulates calcium and phosphorus levels. Hyposecretion of parathyroid hormone can result in hypocalcemia	Encourage adults to consume sufficient calcium from cheese, broccoli, shrimp, and other dietary sources. Have 10% calcium gluconate solution at bedside of patient having thyroidectomy in case of surgical damage to the parathyroid glands. Give all oral medicines containing calcium 30 min before meals to facilitate absorption.
Hypercalcemia >10.6 mg/dL	Anorexia, nausea, abdominal pain, constipation, muscle weakness, oliguria, confusion. Renal calculi, pathologic fractures, dysrhythmias, cardiac arrest	Excess intake of calcium, as in patient taking antacids indiscriminately. Excess intake of vitamin D. Conditions that cause movement of calcium out of bones and into extracellular fluid (e.g., bone tumor, multiple fractures). Tumors of the lung, stomach, and kidney, and multiple myeloma. Immobility and osteoporosis	Administer diuretics as prescribed to increase urinary output and calcium excretion. Monitor I&O; encourage high fluid intake (3000–4000 mL/day).
Magnesium—Normal Range: 1.3–2.1 mEq/L			
Hypomagnesemia <1.3 mEq/L	Insomnia, hyperactive reflexes, leg and foot cramps, twitching, tremors. Seizures, cardiac dysrhythmias, positive Chvostek's sign, positive Trousseau's sign, vertigo, hypocalcemia, and hypokalemia	Chronic malnutrition, chronic diarrhea. Bowel resection with ileostomy or colostomy. Chronic alcoholism. Thiazide diuretic use. Prolonged gastric suction. Acute pancreatitis. Biliary or intestinal fistula. Osmotic diuretic therapy. Diabetic ketoacidosis	Diet counseling to help patients at risk increase their level of magnesium (e.g., milk and cereals). Monitor IV infusions of magnesium closely. Monitor I&O.
Hypermagnesemia >2.1 mEq/L	Hypotension, sweating and flushing, nausea and vomiting. Muscle weakness, paralysis, respiratory depression. Cardiac dysrhythmias	Overuse of antacids and cathartics containing magnesium. Aspiration of sea water, as in near-drowning. Chronic kidney failure	Teach patients to avoid abuse of laxatives and antacids; instruct patients with renal problems to avoid over-the-counter drugs that contain magnesium. Encourage fluid intake to increase urinary excretion of magnesium if not contraindicated. Monitor I&O. Administer diuretics as ordered.

Continued

Table 3-4	Electrolyte Imbalances and Nursing Interventions—cont'd		
SERUM VALUE	**SIGNS AND SYMPTOMS**	**CAUSES/RISK FACTORS**	**NURSING INTERVENTIONS**
Phosphate—Normal Range: 3.0–4.5 mg/dL			
Hypophosphatemia	Confusion, seizures, numbness, weakness, possible coma Chronic state may cause rickets and osteomalacia	Vitamin D deficiency or hyperparathyroidism Use of aluminum-containing antacids	Assess for vitamin D deficiency, hyperparathyroidism, or overuse of aluminum-containing antacids.
Hyperphosphatemia	Anorexia, nausea, vomiting	Renal insufficiency	Assess for restlessness, confusion, chest pain, and cyanosis. Monitor respirations. Check all electrolyte levels.

Potassium Imbalances

Hypokalemia. Hypokalemia occurs when the potassium level falls below 3.5 mEq/L and may occur from a variety of causes. Hypokalemia can cause serious problems. See Table 3-4 for risk factors, signs and symptoms, and interventions for hypokalemia.

It is important to teach patients taking diuretics that are not potassium sparing to increase potassium in the diet, take potassium supplements as prescribed, and watch for signs of hypokalemia.

Severe hypokalemia (K+ less than 2.5 mEq/L) may cause cardiac arrest. Extra potassium must be given to help correct an imbalance.

Nutrition Considerations

Common Foods High in Potassium

Apricots	Orange juice
Avocado	Orange (1 med)
Baked potato with skin (small)	Pinto beans (½ cup)
Banana (1 med)	Prune juice (½ cup)
Cantaloupe (¼ med)	Prunes
Dates, chopped	Raisins, seedless
Figs	Spinach
Honeydew melon (¼ med)	Tomatoes
Mango	Winter squash

! Safety Alert

IV Potassium

Urine output must be at least 30 mL/hr before intravenous potassium is administered. Intravenous potassium must always be diluted before administration and is never given as a "push" (rapid, undiluted) injection.

Hyperkalemia. Hyperkalemia occurs when the serum potassium level rises above 5.0 mEq/L. The mechanical disruption of cell membranes causes a shift of potassium from the ICF to the ECF. This shift happens when extensive tissue damage occurs from burns or crush injuries. **Hyperkalemia can cause life-threatening cardiac dysrhythmia.**

Calcium Imbalances

Hypocalcemia. Hypocalcemia occurs when the calcium level drops below 8.4 mg/dL. Hypocalcemia occurs from disorders in which there is a shift of calcium into the bone. Removal or injury of the parathyroid glands during thyroidectomy causes parathyroid hormone deficiency and consequent hypocalcemia. Conditions causing alkalosis (excess of alkaline or decrease of acid substances in the blood and body fluids) may cause hypocalcemia. Hypocalcemia in renal failure results from retention of phosphate ions, which causes a loss of calcium ions. In addition, during renal failure, vitamin D is not activated, causing the loss of absorption of calcium from the intestinal tract.

- Calcium ions are needed for a variety of metabolic processes and enzyme reactions, including for blood clotting. Calcium deficit upsets the stability of nerve membranes, causing abnormalities in nerve conduction, and muscle contractions. Carpopedal spasm (also called Trousseau's sign), hyperactive reflexes, Chvostek's sign, and tetany (skeletal muscle spasm in which the muscles are in sustained contraction and causing spasm) may occur. Laryngospasm may occur if deficit is severe (see Table 3-4).
- Check for Trousseau's and Chvostek's signs when calcium or magnesium deficit is a possibility. To test for Trousseau's sign, place a blood pressure cuff on the arm and inflate above systolic pressure and hold for 3 minutes; if a spasm of the hand occurs, the reaction is positive (Figure 3-5). Chvostek's sign is assessed by tapping the facial nerve about an inch in front of the earlobe. A unilateral twitching of the face is a positive response (Figure 3-6). Test deep tendon reflexes by tapping a partially stretched muscle tendon with a percussion hammer. The extent of the reflex is scored from 0 to 4+, with 0 representing no response, 2+ a normal response, and 4+ a hyperactive response.

FIGURE 3-5 Palmar flexion (carpopedal spasm) indicating positive Trousseau's sign in hypocalcemia.

FIGURE 3-6 Facial muscle response indicating positive Chvostek's sign in hypocalcemia.

Hypercalcemia. Hypercalcemia occurs when the serum calcium level is above 10.6 mg/dL. This can occur during periods of lengthy immobilization, when calcium is mobilized from the bone, or when an excess of calcium or vitamin D is taken into the body. See Table 3-4 for signs and symptoms, risk factors, and interventions. Administer diuretics to increase calcium excretion, and encourage high fluid intake.

Magnesium Imbalances

Hypomagnesemia. Hypomagnesemia occurs when the serum level drops below 1.3 mEq/L and usually is present when hypokalemia and hypocalcemia occur. Magnesium is important in deoxyribonucleic acid (DNA) and protein synthesis, and in many enzyme reactions. Magnesium imbalances are rare, but can be caused by a variety of factors (see Table 3-4).

Hypermagnesemia. Hypermagnesemia is present when there is a serum level above 2.1 mEq/L. It can occur in the presence of renal failure or from overuse of magnesium-containing antacids and cathartics and is rare.

Anion Imbalances

Because of electroneutrality, imbalances of chloride, phosphate, and bicarbonate accompany cation imbalances. Hypochloremia (a level below 95 mEq/L) is associated with hyponatremia. Hypochloremia can also occur with severe vomiting and is seen as a compensatory decrease in acid-base disorders. Hyperchloremia (a level above 103 mEq/L) occurs along with hypernatremia and a form of metabolic acidosis. Hypophosphatemia occurs when the level falls below 3.0 mg/dL. Hypophosphatemia may result from use of aluminum-containing antacids that bind phosphate, vitamin D deficiency, or hyperparathyroidism. Hyperphosphatemia (a level above 4.5 mg/dL) commonly occurs in renal failure. See Table 3-4 for signs and symptoms of phosphate imbalance.

ACID-BASE SYSTEM

PHYSIOLOGY

It is crucial to maintain acid-base balance because cell enzymes function within a very narrow pH range. To understand the concept of acid-base balance and how it is maintained in the body fluids, you should be familiar with some basic facts about biochemistry and the terms commonly used in discussions of hydrogen ion concentration (Box 3-3).

Box 3-3 | **Some Chemistry Facts Related to Acid-Base Balance**

- An *acid* is defined as a substance capable of giving up a hydrogen ion during chemical exchange.
- A *base* is a substance capable of accepting a hydrogen ion.
- Acids react with bases to form water and a salt.
- **A reaction of an acid and a base to form water and a salt is a *neutralization* reaction because *both the acid and the base are neutralized.***
- Acids react with carbonates and bicarbonates to form carbon dioxide gas.
- The term *pH* refers to the concentration of hydrogen (H) in a solution. The "p" represents a *negative* logarithm, which is an inverse proportion. This means that **the higher the concentration of hydrogen ions in a solution, the lower the pH.** A higher pH indicates the opposite, that is, a lower concentration of hydrogen ions.
- A chemically neutral solution has a pH of 7.0.
- **The pH of the body's fluids is normally somewhat alkaline (between 7.35 and 7.45).**
- A pH below 7.25 or above 7.55 is considered life threatening.
- A pH above 7.8 *(alkalosis)* or a pH below 6.8 *(acidosis)* usually is fatal.
- A blood pH of 7.4 indicates a ratio of 1 part carbonic acid to 20 parts bicarbonate (base).
- Acidosis is the result of either a loss of base or an accumulation of acid.

Nutrients in the blood diffuse into the cells, where various metabolic processes take place. Metabolic wastes, including acids, from those cellular processes diffuse back from the cells to the blood. There are three mechanisms that control or try to rebalance pH:

- Buffer pairs circulating in the blood respond to pH changes quickly. The bicarbonate–carbonic acid buffer system is responsible for more than half of the buffering. Three other buffer systems in the body include the phosphate, hemoglobin, and protein systems.
- The respiratory system alters breathing rate and depth. Because carbon dioxide dissolves in the blood and combines with water to form carbonic acid, retaining or blowing off carbon dioxide helps retain or eliminate acids from the body.
- The kidneys change the excretion rate of acids and the production and absorption of bicarbonate ion. The kidneys are slow to compensate, but are the most effective compensating mechanism (Figure 3-7).

The bicarbonate–carbonic acid buffer system links an acid (carbon dioxide) with water and a base (bicarbonate ion). A buffer is a substance that increases the amount of acid or alkali in the solution to produce a unit change in pH. The balance of the bicarbonate ions and carbonic acid ions is controlled by the respiratory system and by the kidneys. The carbon dioxide produced by cell metabolism diffuses into the blood. There carbon dioxide reacts with water and forms carbonic acid. The carbonic acid dissociates (separates) to form hydrogen ions and bicarbonate ions, as needed. The process can be reversed in the lungs, freeing up carbon dioxide so it can be expired along with water, thereby reducing the total acid in the body.

Enzymes in the kidney promote the formation of hydrogen ions, which are excreted in the urine while the bicarbonate ions are returned to the blood. The kidneys, through the influence of aldosterone, can exchange hydrogen ions for sodium ions. Acids can be removed in the kidney by combining them with ammonia and other basic chemicals. Urine pH can vary from 4.5 to 8.0 as kidney compensation occurs.

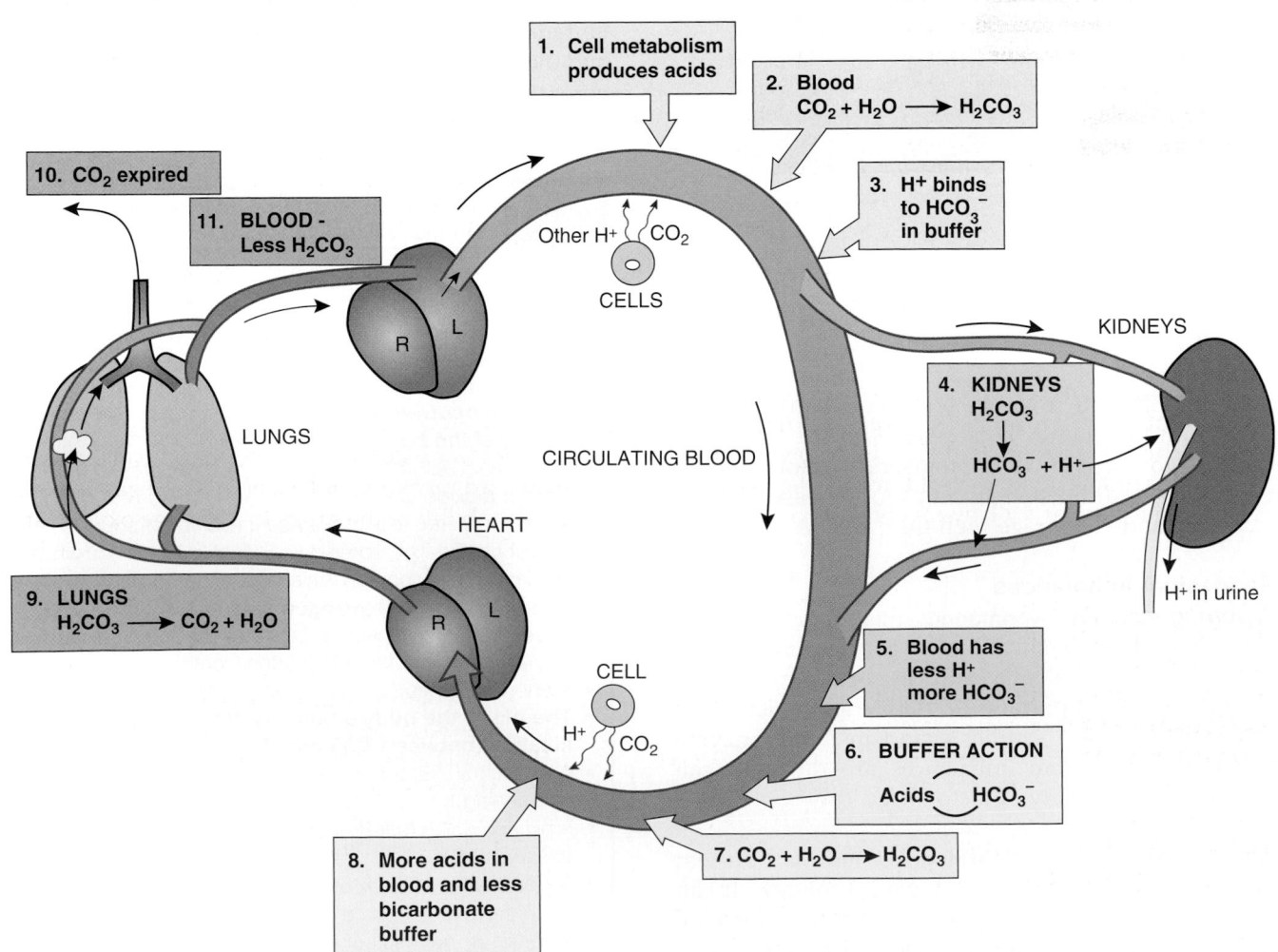

FIGURE 3-7 Regulation of acid-base balance by chemical buffers, respiratory system, and renal system.

ACID-BASE IMBALANCES

PATHOPHYSIOLOGY

Most of the body's metabolic activities produce carbon dioxide gas, which moves from the tissues into the blood, where it combines with water to form carbonic acid ($CO_2 + H_2O = H_2CO_3$). The body deals with this constant manufacture of acid in a number of ways so that the correct ratio of carbonic acid to bicarbonate can be maintained and an alkaline environment provided for normal cellular activities. If the ratio is not maintained, the acid-base balance is upset. The pH will either fall below the normal range and acidosis will occur, or pH will rise above normal range and alkalosis will be present. As long as the ratio of carbonic acid to bicarbonate is maintained at 1:20, the pH remains within normal limits. In a respiratory imbalance, the lungs retain or "blow off" (excrete) carbon dioxide (CO_2). In *hypoventilation,* the lungs do not eliminate enough CO_2, and CO_2 remains in the body, unites with water, and forms carbonic acid. The opposite is *hyperventilation,* in which too much CO_2 may be blown off.

The kidneys are the principal organs of control in maintaining a normal pH during metabolic activities because they either reabsorb or excrete bicarbonate. If they eliminate too much bicarbonate, acidosis will develop. Conversely, if they fail to eliminate enough bicarbonate and allow it to be reabsorbed into the bloodstream, alkalosis will develop.

In the presence of respiratory acidosis, the kidneys will retain and manufacture more bicarbonate than normal so that it is available to neutralize the excess acid. However, this is a slow process that takes from a few hours to several days. In the presence of respiratory alkalosis, the kidneys will increase their excretion of bicarbonate. **In response to metabolic acidosis, the patient will involuntarily hyperventilate to remove carbon dioxide so that CO_2 is not available to produce carbonic acid.** Should metabolic alkalosis develop, the patient will hypoventilate to retain the supply of carbon dioxide.

The foregoing information on acid-base balance, hydrogen ion concentration, and the carbon dioxide–bicarbonate ratio does not represent an in-depth explanation. Many complex chemical activities are involved in maintaining an internal environment that must be slightly alkaline for normal body function.

Because acidosis and alkalosis are common to a great variety of medical and surgical conditions of illness, the chapters on specific illnesses will frequently refer to problems of acid-base imbalance.

The four types of acid-base imbalances are shown in Table 3-5. To determine if an acid-base imbalance exists, the pH, $Paco_2$, and HCO_3^- are measured by arterial blood gas analysis. Imbalances may be acute or chronic. **An initial change in carbon dioxide is nearly always due to a respiratory disorder. Metabolic disorders show an initial change in bicarbonate ions.** Three control mechanisms continually work together to maintain acid-base balance: the respiratory system, the kidneys, and the bicarbonate buffer system. When an imbalance occurs, the lungs and kidneys try to *compensate* by working to bring the pH back toward normal limits.

ARTERIAL BLOOD GAS ANALYSIS

Studies of the percentages of gases (oxygen and carbon dioxide) in the blood and the hydrogen ion concentration (pH) are useful in assessing the status of both respiratory and metabolic acid-base imbalances. Blood gas studies are valuable indicators of a patient's progress toward recovery, or lack of it. Blood gas analyses reflect the ability of the lungs to exchange oxygen and carbon dioxide, the effectiveness of the kidneys in balancing retention and elimination of bicarbonate, and the effectiveness of the heart as a pump. The results of analyses of arterial blood gases (ABGs) are reported as follows:

- Pao_2—partial pressure (P) exerted by oxygen (O_2) in the arterial blood (a). **Normal value is 80 to 100 mm Hg; indicates the amount of oxygen carried in the blood.**
- $Paco_2$—partial pressure of carbon dioxide in the arterial blood. **Normal value is 35 to 45 mm Hg; indicates the amount of carbon dioxide in the blood.**
- pH—an expression of the extent to which the blood is alkaline or acid. **Normal value is 7.35 to 7.45.**

Table 3-5	The Four Acid-Base Imbalances	
IMBALANCE	**CAUSES**	**BLOOD GAS VALUES**
Respiratory acidosis	Slow, shallow respirations Respiratory congestion/ obstruction	pH <7.35 $Paco_2$ >45 mm Hg
Metabolic acidosis	Shock (poor circulation) Diabetic ketoacidosis Renal failure Diarrhea	pH <7.35 HCO_3^- <22 mEq/L
Respiratory alkalosis	Hyperventilation	pH >7.45 $Paco_2$ <35 mm Hg
Metabolic alkalosis	Vomiting Excessive antacid intake Hypokalemia	pH >7.45 HCO_3^- >26 mEq/L

From deWit, S.C. (2009). *Fundamental Concepts and Skills for Nursing* (3rd ed.). Philadelphia: Saunders, p. 447.

- SaO_2 (also abbreviated O_2 Sat.)—percentage of available hemoglobin that is saturated (Sa) with oxygen, that is, the ratio of the amount of oxygen that is combined with hemoglobin to the total amount of oxygen the hemoglobin can carry. **Normal value is 94% to 100%.**
- HCO_3^-—the level of plasma bicarbonate; an indicator of the metabolic acid-base status. **Normal value is 22 to 26 mEq/L.**
- Base excess or deficit—indicates the amount of blood buffer present. Alkalosis is present when this value is abnormally high. Abnormally low values indicate acidosis. Alkalosis is measured in "+" or "−" values.

RESPIRATORY ACIDOSIS

An increase in carbon dioxide levels occurs in a variety of disorders. It is seen in:

- Acute problems such as airway obstruction, pneumonia, asthma, chest injuries, or pulmonary edema
- Chronic obstructive pulmonary disease (COPD), such as emphysema
- With opiate use that depresses the respiratory rate

 Think Critically

What could you do to help prevent respiratory acidosis in a home care patient who has pneumonia?

A patient with COPD is most likely to develop acute acidosis when an infection of the respiratory tract further impairs breathing capacity and the removal of carbon dioxide. Signs and symptoms of respiratory acidosis include complaints of increasing difficulty in breathing, a history of respiratory obstruction (acute or chronic), dyspnea, weakness, dizziness, restlessness, sleepiness, and change in mental alertness.

The treatment for respiratory acidosis is establishment or maintenance of an airway. A tracheostomy or the insertion of an endotracheal tube may be necessary. Oxygen administration may be needed, and the assistance of a mechanical ventilator may be required. Conservative treatment is by postural drainage, deep-breathing exercises, bronchodilators, and antibiotics if indicated. Care must be taken when administering certain drugs that depress the respiratory center including narcotics, hypnotics, and tranquilizers.

The patient must be watched closely for respiratory and cardiac arrest. Should either occur, it will be necessary to maintain respiration and circulation artificially through cardiopulmonary resuscitation.

 Clinical Cues

In patients with COPD, the respiratory drive mechanism is altered, and oxygen can act as a respiratory depressant. Oxygen should be administered with great care to these patients (no more than 2 to 3 L/min) because it can cause respiratory arrest.

If a patient's history is unknown, oxygen is begun at a rate of 2 to 3 L/min until it is determined that a higher flow rate can be tolerated.

METABOLIC ACIDOSIS

An excessive loss of bicarbonate ions or an increased production or retention of hydrogen ions leads to metabolic acidosis. The main causes of metabolic acidosis are:

- Excessive loss of bicarbonate ions from diarrhea
- Renal failure
- Diabetic ketoacidosis
- Hyperkalemia

In diabetes mellitus, insulin insufficiency leads to excessive burning of fats, and the end product is fatty acids. When more energy than usual is expended, as in athletic competition, lactic acid builds up in the body as oxygenation of tissue falls. In kidney disease there is decreased excretion of acids and decreased production of bicarbonate. The increased buildup of acids causes metabolic acidosis.

The symptoms of metabolic acidosis include weakness, lethargy, headache, and confusion (Concept Map 3-1). If the acidosis is not relieved, these symptoms progress to stupor, unconsciousness, coma, and death. The breath of the patient may have a fruity odor owing to the presence of ketone bodies (ketoacidosis). Vomiting and diarrhea may occur and aggravate the metabolic imbalance because of the loss of fluids and electrolytes, which are essential to restoring the acid-base balance. When compensatory mechanisms are working to correct metabolic acidosis, the patient may have deep, rapid breathing (Kussmaul's respirations) and may secrete urine with a low pH.

Treatment of metabolic acidosis is aimed at the underlying cause. Insulin is administered if the patient is in diabetic ketoacidosis. Dialysis may be necessary to correct the problem in the patient with kidney failure. **Immediate treatment of severe metabolic acidosis requires administration of IV bicarbonate or lactate.**

RESPIRATORY ALKALOSIS

Alkalosis occurs less frequently than acidosis. Hyperventilation (a rapid respiratory rate) results in respiratory alkalosis. Hyperventilation is usually caused by:

- Anxiety
- High fever
- An overdose of aspirin

Patients hyperventilate for a variety of reasons, including hypoxemia (insufficient oxygen, which triggers an automatic increase in respiration), reactions to certain drugs, pain, and panic. The overzealous use of mechanical ventilation also can cause hyperventilation, when too much CO_2 is blown off. Head injuries may also lead to hyperventilation.

CONCEPT MAP 3-1 Causes, signs, and symptoms of metabolic acidosis.

Symptoms of respiratory alkalosis include deep, rapid breathing, tingling of the fingers, pallor around the mouth, dizziness, and spasms of the muscles of the hands.

Treatment for hyperventilation addresses the underlying disorder. The person may breathe through a re-breather mask temporarily, mixing the excessively exhaled carbon dioxide with oxygen so that carbon dioxide is reinhaled. If the underlying cause of respiratory alkalosis is panic, treatment is aimed at preventing further hyperventilation and helping the patient reestablish a normal level of carbon dioxide in the blood. Sedatives may be given to calm the patient. To aid in the retention of carbon dioxide, the patient may be instructed to hold the breath, or to breathe into a paper sack and re-breathe the carbon dioxide just exhaled. This recycling of carbon dioxide can eventually restore normal carbonic acid levels in the blood.

METABOLIC ALKALOSIS

Metabolic alkalosis follows a loss of hydrochloric acid from the stomach. Causes include:

- Vomiting
- Extensive gastrointestinal suction
- Hypokalemia
- Excessive use of antacids with bicarbonate

Hypokalemia causes this disorder because the kidney then retains K^+ while excreting H^+.

Other causes include drainage from intestinal fistula; diuresis resulting from potent diuretics that increase potassium loss in the urine; and steroid therapy, which causes retention of sodium and chloride and loss of potassium and hydrogen.

Symptoms of metabolic alkalosis include such neurologic signs as **irritability, disorientation, lethargy, muscle twitching, tingling and numbness of the fingers, and convulsions;** and respiratory manifestations such as **slow, shallow respirations, decreased chest movements, and cyanosis.** In addition, there may be symptoms of potassium and calcium depletion. If the alkalosis progresses, tetany will occur and seizures and coma will result. Tetany is characterized by severe muscle cramps, carpopedal spasms, laryngeal spasms, and stridor (shrill, harsh sound on inspiration).

Treatment is directed at correcting the underlying cause and attempting to restore the body fluids to a less alkaline state. Fluids and electrolytes are replaced orally and parenterally as needed. Emergency measures include the administration of an acidifying

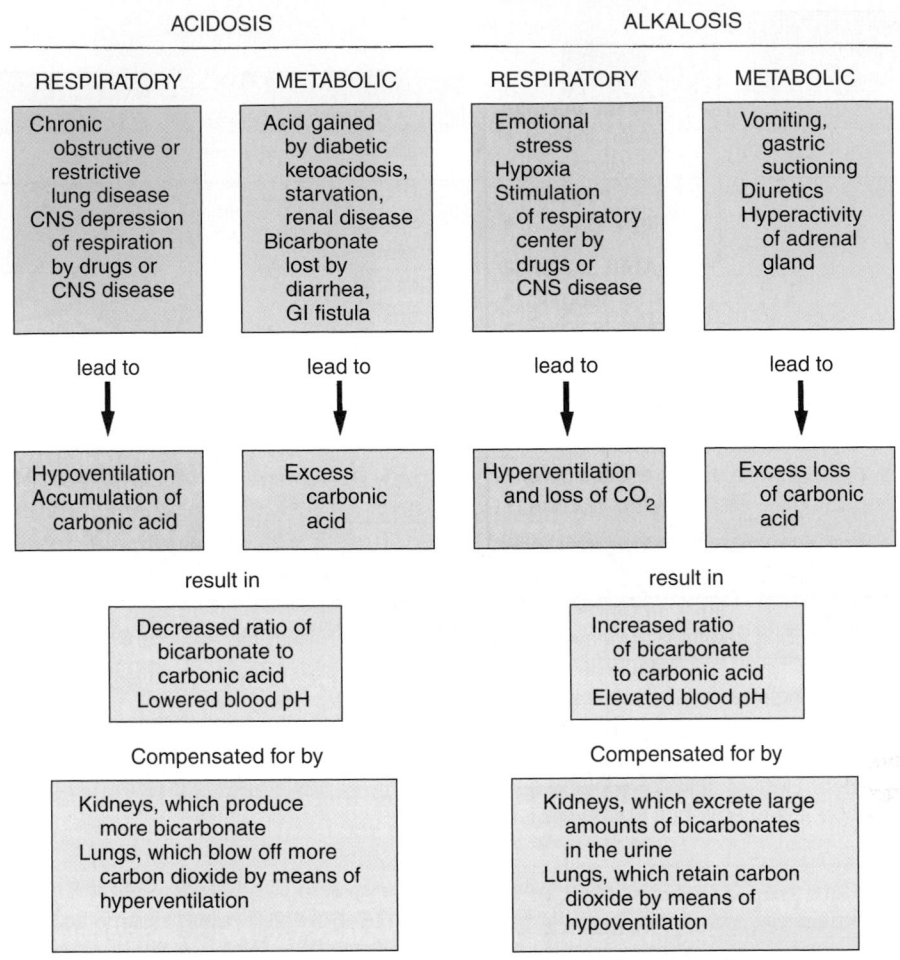

FIGURE 3-8 Comparison of causes, physiologic effects, and compensatory mechanisms for acidosis and alkalosis.

solution, such as ammonium chloride. Figure 3-8 compares the causes, physiologic effects, and compensatory mechanisms for acidosis and alkalosis.

? Think Critically

Can you identify the type of imbalance that might result from (1) rapid respiratory rate, (2) out-of-control diabetes, (3) renal failure, and (4) eating antacids for a nervous stomach?

HOME CARE

For the home care patient, teach about the requirements for fluid intake or restriction. Monitor adherence to sodium restriction by periodically checking the patient's food intake. Obtain feedback, to be certain the patient understands the instructions. Collaborate with the patient on the plan of care, in order to obtain patient compliance.

When acid-base imbalance occurs, control of the underlying disorder is a priority. Blood gases are monitored, and oxygen and electrolytes are administered as needed. Nursing measures to improve pulmonary function are instituted as appropriate.

? Think Critically

What measures could assist the patient who is in metabolic acidosis to achieve acid-base balance once more?

INTRAVENOUS FLUID THERAPY

Administering fluids through the veins is the most common means by which water, electrolytes, nutrients, and some drugs may be given when oral intake is not possible or must be supplemented. Intravenous therapy is often used when a fluid deficit is present or when there are electrolyte imbalances. Intravenous fluids may also be used to help reestablish acid-base balance. Medications are administered in an IV solution when rapid action is required. Total parenteral nutrition (TPN) is used for administering nutrients to patients with gastrointestinal problems who cannot take in nutrients in any other way.

Some terms related to the concentration of an IV fluid and its effect on cells are:

• **Isotonic**—a solution that has the same osmotic pressure as ICF. Body cells can be bathed in an isotonic solution without net flow of water across the cell membrane.

- Hypotonic—a solution that has a lower osmotic pressure (is less concentrated) than that of body fluids. Cells bathed in a hypotonic solution will swell as water passes from the less concentrated solution across the cell membrane and into the cell. *Note: Sterile distilled water is hypotonic and is never added to an IV solution.*
- Hypertonic—a solution that has a higher osmotic pressure than that of body fluids. Cells bathed in a hypertonic solution will shrink as water passes out of the cell into the fluid surrounding it.

An example of an isotonic solution is 0.9% normal saline. Hypotonic solutions are those with less than 5% glucose or with anions less than 150 mEq/L. Fluids commonly used in IV therapy are presented in Table 3-6.

Blood-related fluids that are given IV include whole blood, packed cells from which the plasma has been removed leaving only the red blood cells, and plasma. Whole blood is sometimes given to replace blood that has been lost through hemorrhage. Packed cells may be administered to patients with anemia or some other blood disorder, or to patients who cannot tolerate a large volume of fluid very well, such as those with renal disease or heart failure. Plasma is given to increase blood volume (as in shock), to provide protein, and to treat disorders of coagulation.

In the treatment of shock, *plasma expanders* are administered to increase the volume of plasma. Examples of plasma expanders are low-molecular-weight dextran, albumin, Hespan, and Plasmanate. Blood disorders and blood product administration are further presented in Chapter 17.

NURSING RESPONSIBILITIES IN ADMINISTERING IV FLUIDS

Responsibility for the safe and effective administration of IV fluids rests with every member of the nursing staff.

 Legal and Ethical Considerations

IV Therapy Guidelines

Check your state's nurse practice act to determine what aspects of IV therapy, if any, your state will allow the LPN/LVN to perform. With the continuation of the nursing shortage, a few states have expanded their LPN/LVN practice act to allow licensed LPN/LVNs to perform a variety of IV therapy functions. Other states are considering expanding their practice acts accordingly.

As with any therapeutic measure, IV therapy is not without its hazards to the patient. Many complications can be avoided through careful handling of equipment and meticulous monitoring of the patient's reaction to the fluids being administered.

 Safety Alert

IV Line Connection Safety

When connecting an IV solution or disconnecting a line, always trace the line to where it connects to the patient to make certain that it is an IV line and connects to an IV device. Many mistakes have been made by connecting an IV fluid to the wrong device.

The four goals of nursing care for a patient receiving an IV infusion are to (1) prevent infection, (2) minimize physical injury to the veins and surrounding tissues, (3) administer the correct fluid at the prescribed time and at a safe rate of flow, and (4) observe the patient's reaction to the fluid and medications being administered (Box 3-4).

All equipment and fluids used for IV therapy must be sterile and safe for administration. *Before any plastic bag or bottle of solution is added to an IV set, it must be checked for leaks and possible contamination.*

 Safety Alert

IV Solution Safety

A plastic bag of solution may be squeezed to check for leaks. Any solution that is discolored or has small particles, a white cloud, or film in it should not be used. If there is no vacuum in a bottle when it is opened, the solution may be contaminated. Gently invert the bag or bottle and hold it up to the light so you can see if there are any particles floating in it.

When a new bottle of fluid or additional medication is added to an IV infusion already in progress, strict surgical asepsis must be observed as there is a danger of introducing bacteria into the patient's blood system. Because of the danger of incompatibility, it is essential to check each drug and each solution to be certain they can be mixed. **Always wash your hands just before handling IV fluids and equipment. The port on the IV tubing into which the administration set of a piggyback medication is to be attached must be carefully and thoroughly wiped with a fresh alcohol swab before the tubing is attached to the container.**

There should be a clear occlusive (airtight) dressing over the IV insertion site. The edges of the dressing should adhere to the skin on all sides. Tubing should be secured so that accidental pulling on the tubing will not affect the IV cannula. Dressings are changed according to agency protocol, but usually are changed at least every 72 hours. If a dressing becomes loose, it should be removed and a new dressing applied (Box 3-5). Label tubing and dressing with the date.

The site of venipuncture should be watched closely for signs of inflammation. Redness, swelling, and heat

Table 3-6   Commonly Prescribed IV Solutions

SOLUTION	TONICITY	mOsm/kg	GLUCOSE (g/L)	INDICATIONS AND CONSIDERATIONS
Dextrose in Water				
5%	Isotonic	278	50	Provides free water necessary for renal excretion of solutes. Used to replace water losses and treat hypernatremia. Provides 170 calories/L. Does not provide any electrolytes.
10%	Hypertonic	556	100	Provides free water only, no electrolytes. Provides 340 calories/L.
Saline				
0.45%	Hypotonic	154	0	Provides free water in addition to Na^+ and Cl^-. Used to replace hypotonic fluid losses. Used as maintenance solution, although it does not replace daily losses of other electrolytes. Provides no calories.
0.9%	Isotonic	308	0	Used to expand intravascular volume and replace extracellular fluid losses. Only solution that may be administered with blood products. Contains Na^+ and Cl^- in excess of plasma levels. Does not provide free water, calories, other electrolytes. May cause intravascular overload or hyperchloremic acidosis.
3.0%	Hypertonic	1026	0	Used to treat symptomatic hyponatremia. Must be administered slowly and with extreme caution because it may cause dangerous intravascular volume overload and pulmonary edema.
Dextrose in Saline				
5% in 0.225%	Isotonic	355	50	Provides Na^+, Cl^-, and free water. Used to replace hypotonic losses and treat hypernatremia. Provides 170 calories/L.
5% in 0.45%	Hypertonic	432	50	Same as 0.45% NaCl except provides 170 calories/L.
5% in 0.9%	Hypertonic	586	50	Same as 0.45% NaCl except provides 170 calories/L.
Multiple Electrolyte Solutions				
Ringer's solution	Isotonic	309	0	Similar in composition to plasma except that it has excess Cl^-, no Mg^{2+}, and no HCO_3^-. Does not provide free water or calories. Used to expand the intravascular volume and replace extracellular fluid losses.
Lactated Ringer's (Hartmann's) solution	Isotonic	274	0	Similar in composition to normal plasma except does not contain Mg^{2+}. Used to treat losses from burns and lower gastrointestinal tract. May be used to treat mild metabolic acidosis but should not be used to treat lactic acidosis. Does not provide free water or calories.

Modified from Lewis, S.M., Heitkemper, M.M., Dirksen, S.R., et al. (2011). *Medical-Surgical Nursing: Assessment and Management of Clinical Problems* (8th ed.). St. Louis: Mosby.

in the area should be reported, as they are possible signs of phlebitis. Chills and an elevation of body temperature may indicate a bacterial infection. Table 3-7 presents the complications of IV therapy.

When an IV is discontinued, the tubing is clamped, all tape is removed, and the needle or catheter is gently, but quickly, withdrawn using *Standard Precautions* (see Appendix B). A dry, sterile gauze is held on the site with enough pressure to control the leakage of

blood and avoid the formation of a hematoma. If possible, raising the patient's limb for a minute or two to drain blood from the site of insertion will help prevent leakage of blood from the punctured vein.

A safety goal of The Joint Commission requires that at least two patient identifiers (neither being the patient's room number) must be used whenever IV fluid is administered. The nurse should check the patient's armband with the medication administration

Box 3-4   The Five Rights Applied to IV Therapy

Be sure you have:
1. The right solution with or without additives as ordered; the correct solution to follow what has been infusing
2. The right dose (amount) of solution and additive as ordered
3. The right route (peripheral IV, peripherally inserted central catheter [PICC], central line, port)
4. The right time (to infuse)
5. The right patient as identified with two identifiers

Additionally:
- Teach the patient the reason for administration of the fluid and/or drug and signs and symptoms of problems to report to you.
- Check for drug and latex allergies.
- Be aware of potential interactions with IV medications or irrigating solutions.
- Maintain sterility of all solutions, tubing, and connections.

Box 3-5   IV Therapy Guidelines

- **Keep IV fluid sterile.** Make sure that everything coming in contact with the solution is sterile, including the inside surface of the cannula hub, and all connecting points between the bag and drip chamber and between the tubing and the needle.
- **Protect the cannula site from contamination to avoid possible infection.** An airtight, transparent dressing is used over the cannula site.
- **Keep tubing free of air.** Clear tubing of air before connecting to the cannula. Do not allow the current bag to run dry before changing to the next one.
- **Hang fluids at the correct height.** Fluids flow through the tubing by the force of gravity. If there is negative pressure in the IV line, blood will flow back into the tubing. Keep the bag of fluid sufficiently above the level of the cannula site to maintain flow, but avoid having it too high because this significantly increases the effect of gravity.
- **Carefully regulate the rate of flow.** If the IV is behind schedule, do not open up the clamp and run in a large amount of fluid at one time to catch up. Rather, recalculate either (1) the span of time for the infusion or (2) the rate of drops per minute for the fluid to run at the ordered rate.
- **Track intake and output when a patient is receiving IV fluids or blood.** Keep accurate intake and output records and compare intake with output over 24 hours.
- **The solution to run in first should be hung the highest.** When a second bag is attached piggyback to a primary IV line, lower the primary bag without clamping the tubing so it will begin to flow when the piggyback has run in. Attach the piggyback beneath the roller clamp on the primary tubing.
- **Assess the site frequently for signs of complications.** Infiltration, swelling at the IV site, irritation of the vein, formation of a clot stopping the flow, or systemic reaction should be identified quickly. Signs of infiltration are pain or discomfort at the site caused by dislodgement of the needle or puncture of the vein. Vital signs should be taken several times a day to detect early signs of infection or adverse reaction.

Go to Evolve for step-by-step Skills related to IV therapy.

record for the correct name and the correct agency identification number, and then ask the patient to state his name.

Safety Alert

Five Rights for IV Therapy

The IV administration of fluids requires the same safety precautions as any other medication. Follow the Five Rights and the additional rules for drug administration (see Box 3-4). The label must be read and compared to the order or the medication administration record (MAR) three times to ensure that the correct solution is being given to the correct patient. The patient's ID band must be checked each time a solution is administered. Use two patient identifiers before administration.

CALCULATING AND REGULATING THE RATE OF FLOW

Rate of flow is an important factor in safe and effective IV therapy. Intravenous setups should be checked once every hour, to be certain that the fluid is running correctly and that there are no problems. When possible, use an IV pump that is set for the specific rate of flow to administer IV fluids. IV pumps, although not infallible, keep IV fluids flowing at the desired rate and act as safeguards, should a problem arise. **Even when an IV pump is used, you must check to see that it is delivering the solution accurately, as prescribed.** Principles that affect the rate of flow for IVs *not* administered by a pump are as follows:
- The higher the container is placed above the level of the patient's heart, the faster the rate of flow.
- The fuller the container, the faster the rate of flow.
- The more viscous (thicker) the fluid, the slower the flow; for example, packed red cells will flow more slowly than 5% dextrose in water.

- The larger the diameter of the needle and tubing, the faster the flow.
- The higher the pressure within the vein, the slower the flow. As an infusion progresses and the veins become fuller, the IV solution may drip more slowly.
- Fluid will pass through a straight tube faster than through one that is coiled or hanging below the level of the cannula.

There usually is a chart available to determine the number of drops that should be given per minute to administer a given amount of fluid in a specified time. The IV tubing package will contain information about the number of drops the set will deliver per milliliter. If a chart is not available, calculate the number of drops per minute to be infused. To check the rate of flow, you

Table 3-7 Complications of IV Therapy and Nursing Interventions

COMPLICATION	SIGNS AND SYMPTOMS	NURSING INTERVENTIONS
Local		
Infiltration	Arm swollen, tender, cool to touch; IV catheter may or may not have blood return	Remove IV catheter and restart IV in the other extremity.
Extravasation	Pain at insertion site, tender and cool to touch, IV flow slows, edema, burning, pale, fluid leaking around catheter Tissue sloughing may occur in 1–4 wk	Stop infusion immediately. Remove the IV catheter and restart in the other extremity. If drug is involved, aspirate from short cannula. Administer antidote if available. Apply cold compresses if not contraindicated. Photograph site. Monitor site for 24 hr. Provide written instructions for patient and family.
Phlebitis	Vein hard with skin red, swollen, tender, warm Blood return present IV infusion may or may not be sluggish	Remove IV catheter, document; apply warm, moist pack to the IV site. Restart IV in other extremity. Monitor frequently.
Thrombophlebitis	Site red, tender, warm IV infusion sluggish	Never irrigate the IV catheter; remove the IV catheter, notify the physician, restart IV in opposite extremity. Apply cool compresses initially, followed by warm compresses.
IV site skin infection	Site hot, red, painful but not hard or swollen IV infusion sluggish	Remove IV catheter, restart in opposite extremity, change entire administration system. Clean site with alcohol. Apply warm compresses. May send tip of catheter for culture.
Venous spasm	Slowing of infusion rate Cramping or pain at or above the insertion site Numbness in the area Inability to withdraw peripherally inserted central catheter (PICC) or mid-line catheter	Slow infusion rate and apply warm compresses. Do not apply tension to catheter or forcibly remove it. Encourage consumption of warm liquids. Keep extremity covered and dry.
Nerve damage	Tingling, "pins and needles" feeling, or numbness at or below the catheter insertion site	Immediately stop the cannula insertion if patient complains of severe pain. If sensations do not go away once the catheter is secured, remove the catheter.
Catheter embolus	Decrease in blood pressure (BP); pain along vein; weak, rapid pulse; cyanosis of nail beds; loss of consciousness	Remove IV catheter and inspect, place a tourniquet high on limb of IV site, notify physician, obtain x-ray, prepare for surgery to remove pieces.
Systemic		
Infection	Fever, chills, general malaise	Change the infusion system, notify the physician, obtain cultures as ordered.
Speed shock	Light-headedness or dizziness, flushed face, irregular pulse, decreased BP, loss of consciousness, cardiac arrest	Stop the infusion, notify the physician, monitor vital signs frequently. Run dextrose 5% in water at a keep-vein-open rate.
Circulatory overload	Shortness of breath, tachypnea, increased BP, moist cough, crackles, puffiness around eyes and dependent edema	Elevate head of the bed, keep patient warm, assess for edema, slow the infusion rate; notify the physician. Administer oxygen and diuretic as ordered.

must know how many drops should pass through the drip chamber in *1 minute.*

Once the number of drops per minute has been set and the IV infusion is flowing, the IV setup must be checked at 30- to 60-minute intervals to be sure that it continues to flow at the prescribed rate. As explained in the list of principles that affect the rate of flow, any number of factors can speed up or slow down the infusion.

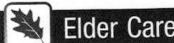 **Elder Care Points**

Elderly people and those with either renal or cardiac conditions cannot tolerate rapid administration of fluids. Check an infusing IV for these patients every 30 minutes.

If the IV slows down and has not been checked and readjusted for some time, **no attempt should be made to "catch up"** by speeding up the rate of flow beyond

Table 3-8   Troubleshooting IV Flow

CHECK	RATIONALE
Height of infusion container	Patient may have changed position. The container should be at least 36 inches above the heart.
System vent	Air vent may be absent or occluded, which will prevent the flow.
Position of tubing	Tubing may be kinked, obstructing flow. Tubing may be hanging below the bed, interfering with the gravity flow.
Position of the extremity where the site is located	Flexion of the extremity may have compressed the vein, slowing the flow.
Any possible obstruction to flow	A protective device on the limb may be too tight. Tape may be compressing the circumference of the extremity.
When filter was changed	Filter may be occluded.
Position of the cannula within the vessel	Cannula may be lying against the vessel wall, obstructing flow. Slightly turning the cannula to reposition the tip may cure the problem.
If other measures have not opened the line, attempt to aspirate blood from the cannula	A small clot may be obstructing the cannula. Aspiration may withdraw the clot.

that ordered. This can lead to circulatory overload and a volume excess that may produce pulmonary edema in susceptible people. Table 3-8 presents points to check when an IV solution will not run at the prescribed rate.

Clinical Cues

Whenever the patient who has an IV infusing is up out of bed, recheck the drop rate once back in bed. The fluid drop rate often changes when the patient is up and moving around.

Think Critically

How would you calculate the rate of flow for an order for "1000 mL of D₅W (dextrose 5% in water) over 8 hours" using a drip set that delivers 15 gtt/mL? How would the rate differ if the drip set delivers 20 drops (gtt)/mL? How would you calculate the flow rate for an order for "250 mL NS (normal saline) at 50 mL/hour" using a microdrip set (60 gtt/mL)?

Intravenous Intake

The total amount of IV fluid infused during the shift is calculated at the end of the shift. For example, say the beginning count is 350 mL (in the container at the beginning of the shift) and the 350 mL is infused during the shift; then (during the same shift) a new solution of 1000 mL is added and some additional infusion takes place—we calculate as follows:

	Count	Infused
Count at beginning of shift	350 mL	
New solution added at 11:30	1000 mL	350 mL
Count left at end of shift	525 mL	475 mL
Total amount of IV intake for shift		825 mL

Safety Alert

No Margin for Error

Intravenous therapy may become such a commonplace procedure to nurses that they are tempted to be complacent about it. However, it should never be thought of as a routine procedure that requires little attention. Any fluid or medication that enters a vein has an immediate effect. There is no margin for error in its administration.

Flushing PRN Locks or Central IV Lines

Flushing the catheter or line prevents contact and reactions between the fluid that was last infused and incompatible drugs. Flushing the catheter or line maintains patency of the lumen. Either normal saline alone or normal saline followed by a heparin solution is used.

Before using a PRN (as-needed) lock, flush the catheter according to agency policy to determine patency (openness) of the lumen and to flush out any heparinized solution. The procedure will depend on the type of valved catheter or positive fluid-displacement needleless device in place. When flushing the catheter, apply slow, gentle pressure to the syringe plunger. **If you feel any resistance, stop the procedure immediately.** Proceeding may force a clot into the venous circulation that will become an embolus that could cause severe damage to the patient. Aspirate for a brisk blood return from the catheter lumen, and then flush the blood from the catheter with the flush solution. Three to 10 mL of normal saline is used depending on the length of the catheter that is in place.

Safety Alert

Flushing IV Catheters

Do not use more than 30 mL of bacteriostatic normal saline within a 24-hour period to flush the catheter. Always use single-dose vials or syringes of solution for flushing. *Do not use a multiple-dose vial for this purpose as it may be contaminated and could cause infection.*

PRN locks and catheters should be flushed immediately following use or whenever an IV piggyback medication infusion is completed. Delay in disconnecting the intermittent infusion administration set and flushing the lock could allow blood backflow into the catheter lumen, because the infusion pressure drops lower than the venous pressure when the infusion is complete. In such a case, a clot can form, occluding the lumen. **Be aware of when an intermittent infusion should be completed, and at the appropriate time be at the bedside prepared to remove the piggyback infusion set and to flush the PRN lock.**

Clinical Cues

When heparinized saline is required to keep the lumen of a catheter patent, use a volume of the solution that is equal to twice the volume of the catheter lumen with the extension set or connectors added on. This will usually be between 5 and 10 mL; check your facility's policy.

Providing Central Line Care

If a gauze dressing is in place, provide site care every 24 to 48 hours per agency protocol. Transparent dressings require site care every 3 to 7 days. Every central line dressing should be examined once each shift, and the dressing should be changed if it is soiled. Central line dressing change and site care are sterile procedures. The Centers for Disease Control and Prevention (CDC) sets guidelines for prevention of catheter-related infections (CDC, 2002). The old dressing is removed using gloves. A Central Line Bundle has been developed by the Institute for Healthcare Improvement (IHI) to prevent infection from central lines. It has five components: optimal site selection, chlorhexidine skin antisepsis, hand hygiene, maximal barrier precautions, and daily review of whether the line is still necessary with prompt removal if it is not needed (IHI, 2010).

Blood Drawing. Drawing blood from a central line is not recommended unless venipuncture is not advisable. If a blood draw is performed, use strict aseptic technique. It is preferable to use needleless connectors and vacuum tubes for the procedure, rather than a needle and syringe or vacuum tube with needle.

Subcutaneous Infusion. Subcutaneous infusion is often used in home care or during hospice palliative care. Subcutaneous therapy is useful when the patient cannot tolerate oral medications, when injections are too painful, or when vascular access is too difficult to obtain. Pain management is the primary use, although several other types of drugs are infused in this manner.

Hypodermoclysis (the slow infusion of isotonic fluid into subcutaneous tissue) may be used for small volumes of fluid. Generally, the front and sides of the thighs, the hips, the area under the clavicle, and the upper abdomen are usual sites for hypodermoclysis. A butterfly needle or a special subcutaneous infusion device is used to provide access for the hypodermoclysis fluid.

Epidural Infusion. Epidural infusion is used to administer medication for pain control or for anesthesia (see Chapter 7).

Partial or Total Parenteral Nutrition. Many patients with fluid and electrolyte imbalances are nutritionally depleted. Partial parenteral nutrition (PPN) is given when a patient cannot maintain an adequate nutritional status with oral intake. PPN is given through a large peripheral vein in the arm. If sufficient nutrition cannot be delivered by oral intake and PPN, or by enteral feedings, TPN is begun. Figure 3-9 shows placement of a peripherally inserted central catheter and of a central venous catheter.

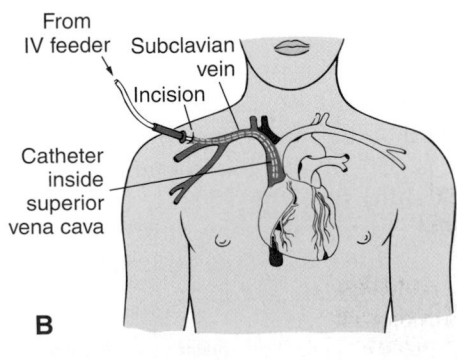

FIGURE 3-9 A, Placement of a peripherally inserted central catheter (PICC) through the antecubital fossa. **B,** Placement of a central venous catheter inserted into the subclavian vein.

TPN solution is made up of a nitrogen (protein) source, hypertonic dextrose, and supplementary vitamins and minerals. The solution is hypertonic and contains 1 calorie/mL or 1000 calories/L. Some solutions also contain lipids. Because of its degree of concentration, TPN solution must be infused through a central vein, usually the subclavian, where the high rate of blood flow quickly dilutes it. The Hickman, Broviac, and Groshong catheters are the most frequently used central line catheters, and they can be used for long-term therapy. TPN solution is administered with a pump or an infusion controller device so that the flow rate is constant.

! Safety Alert

Total Parenteral Nutrition (TPN) Safety Precaution

The flow rate for TPN solution is never changed to "catch up" on the amount of fluid that should have been infused if the flow has slowed for some reason. The hypertonic solution can draw fluid into the vascular system, causing fluid overload.

TPN solutions and catheters must be handled with strict asepsis, as the solution is an ideal medium for bacterial growth. Infection is a major complication of TPN. The TPN solution is mixed in the pharmacy under sterile conditions. There are many complications of TPN in addition to infection, including glucose intolerance, electrolyte imbalance, phlebitis, allergic reaction, and fluid overload. The port through which TPN is administered should not be used for any other solution. When beginning TPN, start the flow rate slowly at about 60 to 80 mL/hr, then gradually increase in increments of 25 mL/hr, until reaching the maintenance rate. This allows the body to adjust to the glucose load. During TPN carefully monitor the patient. Perform blood glucose determinations frequently during the stabilization period, which is usually the first week. If the patient's body has difficulty with glucose tolerance, insulin may be ordered and added to the TPN solution. At the end of therapy, taper down the flow rate for 1 to 2 hours before stopping the fluid, to allow the body to adjust.

PPN is used for patients in whom central venous access is not possible, or who need IV nutritional support for only 7 to 10 days. A solution of less concentration is given to these patients because the solution does not flow into a vessel with a large blood flow, which would dilute it. Box 3-6 summarizes the principles for administering TPN.

Free-flow protection must be used on all general-use and patient-controlled analgesia infusion pumps. Alarms should be tested regularly and are to be activated with appropriate settings, and be sufficiently audible at all times when an infusion pump is in use. Although important for any IV infusion, an alarm system is vitally important when TPN is being administered.

Box 3-6   Principles for Administration of TPN

- Placement of a central venous catheter must be verified by x-ray before beginning the infusion of the TPN solution.
- Use an infusion pump to administer TPN solution; start infusion slowly at first and increase to desired rate over a 24-hour period.
- If solution is administered cyclically (e.g., at night only), taper to the desired flow over 1 to 2 hours and taper flow down to 1 to 2 hours before completion.
- Check the amount actually infusing every 30 to 60 minutes; do not rely solely on the pump functioning accurately.
- Before administering other solutions or drugs through another lumen of the central line, check compatibility with the TPN solution.
- Monitor continuously for signs of complications such as glucose intolerance, infection, fluid volume excess, phlebitis, and sepsis.
- Record the intake and output accurately.
- Never speed up the solution flow rate beyond that ordered, even if it falls behind for some reason.

Focused Assessment

Data Collection for Problems of Fluid, Electrolyte, and Acid-Base Imbalance

Assess the following areas:
CURRENT ILLNESS
Head
- Alertness, orientation, dizziness, signs of confusion, irritability, restlessness
- Appearance of eyes and eyelids
- Condition of oral mucous membranes, tongue, thickness of saliva

Skin and Extremities
- Color, moisture, temperature, areas of discoloration
- Turgor
- Tightness of rings
- Evidence and degree of edema
- Strength of handgrip
- Cramping of muscles
- Reflexes
- Chvostek's sign
- Trousseau's sign

Laboratory and Diagnostic Tests
- Hematocrit changes
- Urine amount, color, odor, and specific gravity
- Electrolyte values
- Blood gas values
- Electrocardiogram T-wave changes

Vital Signs
- Blood pressure changes
- Pulse rate, rhythm, and character
- Temperature
- Respirations
- Change in weight

Lungs
- Breath sounds (any crackles?)

INTAKE AND OUTPUT
KNOWN DISEASE CONDITIONS
MEDICATIONS

❖ NURSING MANAGEMENT

■ Assessment (Data Collection)

First, assess the patient for *risk* of fluid, electrolyte, or acid-base imbalance, then assess for actual signs and symptoms of fluid, electrolyte, and acid-base imbalance. Question the patient about subjective signs and symptoms.

Elder Care Points

Remember that checking for tenting is not an accurate way to assess dehydration in the elderly because their skin loses elasticity with aging and will tent with normal hydration. It is better to check for dry mucous membranes, concentrated urine, and other signs and symptoms in these patients.

■ Nursing Diagnosis

Analyze the assessment data, identify problem areas, and choose nursing diagnoses. Common nursing diagnoses for patients with fluid, electrolyte, or acid-base imbalances are:

- Deficient fluid volume
- Excess fluid volume
- Risk for imbalanced fluid volume
- Ineffective tissue perfusion
- Decreased cardiac output
- Impaired gas exchange
- Ineffective breathing pattern
- Risk for injury related to IV fluid administration

Other nursing diagnoses may be appropriate as a result of the fluid, electrolyte, or acid-base imbalance—or may be related to the cause of the imbalance, for example, diarrhea.

■ Planning

The goal is to restore the patient's fluid, electrolyte, or acid-base balance. Write the individual, expected outcomes. Expected outcomes might be that the:

- Patient will exhibit normal skin turgor
- Patient's weight will stabilize at normal baseline
- Intake and output will be balanced
- Blood gases will return to normal
- Breath sounds will be clear to auscultation
- There will be no evidence of edema
- Electrolyte values will be within normal limits
- Patient will not experience complications of IV therapy

See Nursing Care Plan 3-1 for examples of expected outcomes with nursing interventions.

■ Implementation

When patients are unable to take in sufficient fluids on their own, work with the physician to provide adequate fluid and electrolytes. If patients can swallow and retain fluid, assist patients to frequently take small amounts of fluid. Establish a plan for assisting with both hot and cold liquid consumption. With conscientious care, the need for IV feeding can be avoided. It is helpful to assess what the patient prefers. In addition to water, offer the patient fruit juices, bouillon, Popsicles, soft drinks, or gelatin.

? Think Critically

What type of fluid and electrolyte imbalance is the patient who has intestinal flu and is suffering from both vomiting and diarrhea likely to have?

The patient with a fluid volume excess may have an order for fluid restriction. This means that the patient may take in only a certain amount of fluid over a 24-hour period. Work out a schedule of fluid intake so that liquids are spaced evenly and the patient does not receive all the allotted liquids in a short time. A typical schedule would be day, 600 mL; evening, 400 mL; night, 200 mL. If not prohibited, sugarless hard candies and chewing gum can help relieve thirst. Frequent oral care is essential.

Diuretics are often prescribed, particularly when there is a potential for congestive heart failure or pulmonary edema. For patients at such risk, daily weight and electrolyte status must be monitored, along with intake and output.

Assignment Considerations

Obtaining a Daily Weight

When assigning the daily weighing of patients to a nursing assistant or unlicensed assistive personnel (UAP), remind the person that weight should be measured before breakfast, with the patient in essentially the same amount of clothing as at the last measurement, and after voiding. The same scale should be used each day. This provides more reliable data for comparison. Any gain of 2 lb or more over 2 days should be reported to you immediately.

Skin care is particularly important in preventing a breakdown over an edematous area. The stretched skin is extremely fragile, has a decreased blood supply, and is no longer flexible. Keep bed linens dry and smooth and turn the patient frequently to relieve pressure over bony prominences. **Be very gentle in repositioning and turning the patient; to avoid friction on the skin, use a turning sheet. A break in edematous skin can quickly form a pressure ulcer.**

When acid-base imbalance occurs, institute control of the underlying disorder. Monitor blood gases, and administer oxygen and electrolytes as needed. Apply nursing measures to improve pulmonary function, as appropriate.

Think Critically

Your patient has a Pao$_2$ of 94, pH of 7.32, Paco$_2$ of 48, and HCO$_3^-$ of 26. What type of acid-base imbalance does he have?

▪ Evaluation

Every 24 hours, perform evaluations to see if nursing interventions are assisting the patient to meet expected outcomes. If the patient is not progressing toward achievement of the outcomes, problem-solve and think critically to determine why, then alter the plan of care appropriately. When a specific outcome is met, discontinue that portion of the plan.

COMMUNITY CARE

Nurses in long-term care facilities deal every day with the problems of delicate fluid balance in their elderly patients. These patients often are taking multiple drugs that can affect their fluid and electrolyte status. Diuretics in particular can upset fluid and electrolyte status. It is especially important that the long-term care and home care nurse be vigilant for the signs of hypokalemia (see Table 3-4). Potassium imbalances are particularly dangerous for the heart patient. Hypokalemia alters the way digitalis is metabolized in the body, and predisposes the patient to digitalis toxicity. Signs of digitalis toxicity are fatigue, anorexia, headache, blurred vision, yellow-green halos around lights, nausea, diarrhea, and cardiac dysrhythmias.

Clinical Cues

Any patient in a long-term care facility or at home who is taking digitalis and is experiencing nausea, vomiting, diarrhea, or fluid and electrolyte alterations should be questioned daily about symptoms of hypokalemia and digitalis toxicity.

Dehydration and hyponatremia from infection account for many of the hospital admissions of patients from long-term care facilities and home situations. It takes a caring, skillful nurse to see that long-term and home care patients take in enough fluids without interfering with their nutritional intake.

The home care nurse must collaborate with the infusion company nurse when the patient is receiving IV fluids at home or is on TPN. Clear instructions must be given to the patient and family regarding the IV therapy. The elderly patient who has a fluid volume excess from congestive heart failure may already have a diminished appetite. In this instance, restricting sodium in the diet may do more harm than good. The nurse, along with the physician, must make individual judgments about the patient's priority needs.

Patient Teaching

Home Care IV Therapy

Call the nurse when:
- Swelling, redness, or pain occurs at the IV site or along the vessel.
- The solution will not flow even after you have checked that the clamps are open.
- The solution leaks at the catheter site and you have checked to see that the tubing is firmly attached to the catheter.
- The patient's temperature rises above 100° F (38° C).

Telephone number _____

Get Ready for the NCLEX® Examination!

Key Points

- Fluid balance is essential because the life processes of every cell take place within fluid.
- The infant and the elderly are at greatest risk for fluid imbalance.
- Water has four main functions in the body.
- Body fluids are distributed in intracellular compartments and extracellular compartments.
- Control of fluid balance is managed by hormones and by the thirst mechanism.
- Fluids and solutes move within the body by diffusion, filtration, osmosis, and active transport.
- Tonicity refers to the amount of solutes in relation to the amount of fluid.
- Filtration occurs through a semipermeable membrane.
- Hydrostatic pressure causes filtration of fluid out of the intravascular system into the interstitial spaces.
- Water diffuses by osmosis.
- Diffusion moves water from the interstitial spaces into the cells.
- The kidney is a major factor in the regulation of fluid and electrolyte balance in the body.
- Fluid volume deficit may occur due to fluid losses or because of lack of fluid intake (see Table 3-1).
- A fluid deficit causes dehydration.

- Checking skin turgor is one way to assess for dehydration.
- Check the tongue and mucous membranes of the elderly to assess for dehydration.
- Weight change is the most accurate measure of fluid gain or loss.
- Fluid deficit is a common problem in the elderly.
- Electrolytes need to be replaced along with fluid when there has been a fluid deficit.
- Prolonged vomiting leads to sodium and potassium deficits and metabolic alkalosis.
- Position the vomiting patient so that aspiration of vomitus does not occur.
- Rehydrate the elderly dehydrated patient cautiously so that overhydration does not occur.
- Medications can be administered to help stop vomiting and diarrhea (see Table 3-2).
- Fluid volume excess leads to hypervolemia, edema, and possibly to pulmonary edema.
- Assessment will reveal elevated blood pressure and a full, bounding pulse.
- Edema may be localized or general; pitting edema may occur.
- Loss of plasma proteins may cause edema.
- When fluid shifts from the intravascular space to the interstitial spaces, hypovolemia may occur.
- With fluid excess, sensorium may be clouded.
- Edema may be treated with diuretic medications, a low-sodium diet, and elastic stockings or sequential compression devices.
- Electrolytes are responsible for the transmission of nerve impulses, contraction of muscles, and excretion of hormones (see Table 3-4).
- Urine output must be at least 30 mL/hr before IV potassium is given.
- Intravenous potassium is always diluted and never given as a bolus injection.
- Acid-base imbalances upset the normal function of the body's systems.
- The kidneys are the principal organ in controlling a normal pH; the lungs also assist.
- Too much carbonic acid in the body causes acidosis; too much bicarbonate in the body causes alkalosis.
- Changes in carbon dioxide are usually respiratory; changes in bicarbonate are usually metabolic.
- Diabetic ketoacidosis causes metabolic acidosis and can be life threatening.
- Arterial blood gases are analyzed to determine if there is an acid-base imbalance and to see what type of imbalance is present.
- Each acid-base imbalance has its own signs and symptoms and probable treatments.
- Every ill patient should be assessed for a fluid, electrolyte, and acid-base imbalance.
- Intravenous therapy can provide the patient with fluid, electrolytes, and nutrients.
- Intravenous fluids are isotonic, hypotonic, or hypertonic (see Table 3-6).

- Intravenous therapy must be administered in a strict aseptic manner.
- The "Five Rights" should be used when administering any IV fluid or drug (see Box 3-4).
- Monitoring for complications of IV therapy is a top priority (see Table 3-7).
- Rate of IV flow must be monitored closely; never rely solely on an IV pump.
- The elderly can become fluid overloaded very quickly.
- Subcutaneous infusion is mostly used for pain control.
- Total parenteral nutrition is used when a patient cannot obtain adequate nutrition by other means.

Additional Learning Resources

SG Go to your Study Guide for additional learning activities to help you master this chapter content.

 Go to your Evolve website (http://evolve.elsevier.com/deWit/medsurg) for the following FREE learning resources:
- Animations, audio, and video
- Answers and rationales for questions and activities
- Concept Map Creator
- Glossary with pronunciations in English and Spanish
- Interactive Review Questions and Exercises and more!

Online Resources
- Acid-base tutorials, http://fitsweb.uchc.edu/student/selectives/TimurGraham/Stepwise_approach.html; www.acid-base.com/
- Acid-base physiology, www.anaesthesiamcq.com/AcidBaseBook/ABindex.php; www.rapidlearningcenter.com/biology/anatomy-physiology/22-Fluid-Electrolyte-and-Acid-Base-Balance.html

Review Questions for the NCLEX® Examination

1. A patient who has congestive heart failure has a fluid excess with a weight gain of 1.5 pounds since yesterday and edematous ankles. Which physician's order has the highest priority?
   1. Maintain accurate intake and output.
   2. Monitor skin for signs of breakdown.
   3. Administer furosemide 20 mg PO once daily.
   4. Obtain daily weight.

2. The nurse is gathering data regarding the patient's risk for fluid volume deficit. Which factor puts the patient at immediate risk?
   1. Liver failure
   2. Viral gastroenteritis
   3. Lymph node dissection
   4. Protein-calorie malnutrition

3. The nurse appropriately elicits a sign of hypocalcemia by:
   1. tapping the face about 1 inch from the ear.
   2. palpating a partially stretched tendon.
   3. inspecting facial symmetry.
   4. applying pressure on the radial pulse.

4. At the beginning of the shift, there is 410 mL of fluid in the IV bag. A piggyback medication containing 150 mL is hung at 12:00 noon to run over 30 minutes. You hang a new bag of 1000 mL at 1:00 P.M. to run at 125 mL/hr. At the end of shift there is 250 mL left in the bag. The count for the total amount of fluid infused during your shift ending at 7:00 P.M. is:
   1. 1260 mL.
   2. 1285 mL.
   3. 1560 mL.
   4. 1310 mL.

5. In planning care for a patient with congestive heart failure, the nurse chooses the nursing diagnosis *Excess fluid volume related to inadequate cardiac output.* The nursing diagnosis would most likely be supported by which sign or symptom?
   1. Temperature of 101.5° F (38.6° C)
   2. Hematocrit 35%
   3. Fine crackles in the lung sounds
   4. Clear, yellow urine

6. Which would be the most accurate measurement in monitoring effective fluid resuscitation in a patient with severe dehydration?
   1. Weight
   2. Urine output
   3. Respirations
   4. Serum sodium

7. The nurse responds to a patient complaining of pain, burning, and wetness over the peripheral intravenous site. On assessment, the nurse finds that the intravenous insertion site is tender and cool to touch. These are signs and symptoms of:
   1. phlebitis.
   2. infiltration.
   3. infection.
   4. venous spasm.

8. What should the nurse monitor or measure when a patient is receiving a diuretic regularly? (*Select all that apply.*)
   1. Skin turgor and integrity
   2. Daily weight
   3. Electrolyte status
   4. Mentation
   5. Intake and output

9. Which patient(s) can be considered at high risk for fluid and electrolyte imbalance? (*Select all that apply.*)
   1. A 45-year-old woman with thyroid crisis
   2. A 35-year-old trauma victim on ventilator
   3. A 60-year-old woman with temperature of 99.6° F (37° C)
   4. A 70-year-old man on anticoagulant therapy
   5. A 30-year-old woman complaining of persistent diarrhea

10. An elderly man is admitted for severe disorientation, confusion, and general weakness. His spouse reports that the patient is not able to tolerate any food or fluids and has had several episodes of vomiting and diarrhea. Which imbalance(s) is the patient most likely experiencing? (*Select all that apply.*)
    1. Hypokalemia
    2. Metabolic acidosis
    3. Hyponatremia
    4. Respiratory alkalosis
    5. Hypochloremia

Critical Thinking Questions

Scenario A
Mrs. Thompson, age 64, is admitted to the hospital for congestive heart failure. She is very edematous. She is slightly confused on admission, and although she is not on absolute bed rest, she tells you she is too weak to get out of bed.

1. What type of diet would you expect the physician to order for Mrs. Thompson? Why?
2. Why are daily weights ordered for Mrs. Thompson? Why are those data important?
3. Mrs. Thompson is on fluid restrictions. How would you schedule her fluid intake?

Scenario B
Mr. Mendez, age 76, is admitted with dehydration and diarrhea. He is confused and listless.

1. What parameters would you assess to see if his fluid balance is improving?
2. What electrolyte imbalances would you expect to find?
3. Why would you need to keep a close eye on Mr. Mendez's IV that is ordered?
4. What acid-base imbalance is he likely to be experiencing?
5. What assessment data would tell you that Mr. Mendez's plan of care is working to rebalance his fluid and electrolytes?

Objectives

Theory

1. Discuss the advantages of current technological advances in surgery.
2. Identify the types of patients most at risk for surgical complications, and state why each patient is at risk.
3. Explain the preparation of patients physically, emotionally, and psychosocially for surgical procedures.
4. Plan and implement patient and family teaching to prevent postoperative complications.
5. Analyze the differences in the various types of anesthesia and list the advantages and disadvantages to the surgeon and the patient.

6. Compare the roles of the scrub nurse and the circulating nurse.

Clinical Practice

1. Perform a thorough nursing assessment for a preoperative patient.
2. Teach the patient postoperative exercises during the preoperative period.
3. Prepare a patient for surgery using a preoperative checklist.
4. Administer preoperative medications.
5. Document preoperative care and assessment data.
6. Observe during a patient's surgery.

Key Terms

anesthesia (ăn-ĕs-THĒ-zē-ă, p. 75)
atelectasis (ă-tĕ-LĔK-tā-sĭs, p. 67)
autologous (ăw-TŎL-ŏ-gŭs, p. 64)
capnography (kăp-NŎG-ră-fē, p. 76)
dehiscence (dē-HĬS-ĕntz, p. 67)
palliative (p. 63)

perioperative (pĕr-ē-ŎP-ĕr-ă-tĭv, p. 64)
pneumonia (nū-MŌ-nē-ă, p. 67)
prosthesis (prŏs-THĒ-sĭs, p. 65)
robotics (rō-bŏ-tĭks, p. 62)
stasis (STĀ-sĭs, p. 71)
thrombophlebitis (thrŏm-bō-flĕ-BĪ-tĭs, p. 71)

Surgery is performed for a variety of reasons (Table 4-1). For the patient, any type of surgery is a serious event. Knowing terminology specific to surgical procedures helps envision the procedure so that you may better prepare patients for surgery and care for them afterward (Box 4-1).

In a hospital or surgery center, surgery may be performed as a same-day or outpatient procedure, or as an inpatient procedure. Minor surgery is often performed in a physician's office. For any surgery, preparation is usually begun before admission. The patient undergoes diagnostic tests and is taught postoperative care during the days just before the scheduled surgery. The ability to deliver and reinforce teaching for postoperative and home care is crucial to the well-being and quick recovery of patients.

TECHNOLOGICAL ADVANCES IN SURGERY

Recently, laparoscopic and endoscopic procedures have replaced many "open" surgeries (in which a large incision is necessary). Minimally invasive laparoscopic surgery (done through small openings in the abdomen) can be performed more quickly. This results in less trauma to tissue, less inflammatory response and therefore less pain, and a faster recovery. For example, laparoscopic cholecystectomy for gallbladder removal has reduced a patient's recovery time from 6 weeks to approximately 1 week.

Endoscopic surgery (in which instruments are used to visualize interior structures of the body), operating microscopes, and lasers are commonplace in the surgical suite.

Robots have entered the operating room. Medical **robotics** (design of computerized, mechanical instruments) provides a key to less invasive, less traumatic surgeries. A medical robot is operated from a nearby computer while the surgeon views magnified three-dimensional images of the surgical field on the computer's screen. The robot's tiny camera has multiple lenses that allow magnification up to 12 times that of normal vision. There are assistants and a second surgeon next to the patient, but the primary surgeon at the computer uses the robot to perform the surgery.

Table 4-1	Selected Categories of Surgical Procedures	
CATEGORY	**DESCRIPTION**	**CONDITION OR SURGICAL PROCEDURE**
Reasons for Surgery		
Diagnostic	Performed to determine the origin and cause of a disorder or the cell type for cancer	Breast biopsy Exploratory laparotomy Arthroscopy
Curative	Performed to resolve a health problem by repairing or removing the cause	Laparoscopic cholecystectomy Mastectomy Hysterectomy
Restorative	Performed to improve a patient's functional ability	Total knee replacement Finger reimplantation
Palliative	Performed to relieve symptoms of a disease process, but does not cure	Colostomy Nerve root resection Tumor debulking Ileostomy
Cosmetic	Performed primarily to alter or enhance personal appearance	Liposuction Revision of scars Rhinoplasty Blepharoplasty
Urgency of Surgery		
Elective	Planned for correction of a nonacute problem	Cataract removal Hernia repair Hemorrhoidectomy Total joint replacement
Urgent	Requires prompt intervention; may be life threatening if treatment is delayed more than 24-48 hr	Intestinal obstruction Bladder obstruction Kidney or ureteral stones Bone fracture Eye injury Acute cholecystitis
Emergent	Requires immediate intervention because of life-threatening consequences	Gunshot or stab wound Severe bleeding Abdominal aortic aneurysm Compound fracture Appendectomy
Degree of Risk of Surgery		
Minor	Procedure without significant risk; often done with local anesthesia	Incision and drainage (I&D) Implantation of a venous access device (VAD) Muscle biopsy
Major	Procedure of greater risk, usually longer and more extensive than a minor procedure	Mitral valve replacement Pancreas transplant Lymph node dissection
Extent of Surgery		
Simple	Only the most overtly affected areas are involved in the surgery	Simple/partial mastectomy
Radical	Extensive surgery beyond the area obviously involved; is directed at finding a root cause	Radical prostatectomy Radical hysterectomy

From Ignatavicius, D.D., & Workman, M.L. (2010). *Medical-Surgical Nursing: Critical Thinking for Collaborative Care* (6th ed.). Philadelphia: Saunders, pp. 243–244.

Remote-controlled instruments are inserted through small incisions. A big advantage of using the robot is that it has "rock-steady" hands, providing precision that is beyond human dexterity. Because only small incisions are needed, the patient has less pain postoperatively and requires less time to heal. With robotic surgical techniques, the patient experiences less scarring (because incisions are smaller), and the small surgical wounds heal faster. Surgeries can be transmitted by way of videoconferencing to

| Box **4-1** | Terminology Used for Surgical Procedures |

Suffixes are often attached to a stem word to describe a surgical procedure. For example, *appendectomy* means cutting out the appendix.

- **-ectomy:** Cutting out or off (colectomy: cutting out a part of the colon)
- **-lysis:** Removal or destruction of (neurolysis: freeing a nerve from adhesions)
- **-oma:** Tumor (excision of a fibroma: removal of a connective tissue tumor)
- **-ostomy:** To furnish with an outlet (colostomy: creating an outlet for the colon from the body)
- **-otomy:** Cutting into (thoracotomy: cutting into the chest cavity)
- **-plasty:** Revision, molding, or repair of tissue (mammoplasty: revision of the breast)
- **-pexy:** Fixation, anchoring in place (orchiopexy: fixation of an undescended testicle in the scrotum)

locations around the world to enhance skill levels of surgeons everywhere.

AUTOLOGOUS BLOOD FOR TRANSFUSION

Since the mid-1980s, patients undergoing elective surgery have had the option of banking their own blood before surgery, in case a transfusion is needed. The patient's blood is withdrawn at the blood bank several weeks before the surgery, prepared, and stored. The blood is prepared for autologous (related to self) transfusion. Cell savers are used to collect and salvage blood during and after surgery, so the patient's own blood can be reinfused if the patient needs it. Access to autologous procedures has greatly decreased the anxiety of patients who fear infection with a blood-borne virus, such as human immunodeficiency virus or hepatitis B or C.

BLOODLESS SURGERY

Many patients opt for bloodless surgery to avoid completely the risk inherent in a blood transfusion. Bloodless surgery uses a combination of techniques to minimize blood loss and maximize blood volume and function. Epoetin alfa (Epogen, Procrit) may be given before surgery to stimulate red blood cell production, and hemostatic agents may be given before or during surgery to promote clotting (ADAM, 2009). During surgery, the surgeon may request induced hypotension or hypothermia to decrease oxygen demand.

Another bloodless surgical technique is hemodilution, in which several units of the patient's blood are removed and replaced with crystalloids or colloids to expand vascular volume. Hemodilution decreases blood viscosity, improves oxygen transport, and—if bleeding occurs during surgery—minimizes the loss of red blood cells.

 Cultural Considerations

Jehovah's Witness Patients and Blood Transfusions

Followers of Jehovah's Witness will not accept a blood transfusion from another person because of their religious beliefs. They believe that there are eternal consequences from receiving blood not their own. In the past, this precluded them from having certain major surgeries. Now bloodless surgery is one option for them.

❖ NURSING MANAGEMENT

Perioperative nursing refers to care of the patient before, during, and after surgery. The nurse plays a key role during the perioperative period.

■ Assessment (Data Collection)

Before surgery, the patient should be in the best possible physical condition. In emergencies, of course, physical condition cannot be controlled, but planned surgery may be postponed until the patient is physically able to withstand the stress of anesthesia and major surgery. To determine the patient's readiness for surgery, a thorough health assessment is conducted and risk factors are considered. In addition to the admission assessment data that are gathered when the patient is first admitted (see Chapter 1), the perioperative nurse gathers data specific to the surgical procedure and postoperative course. Thorough assessment facilitates planning of care during and after surgery.

 Elder Care Points

Patients over age 75 have surgical complication rates three times higher than those of younger adults. The elderly patient is less able to adjust and compensate for the stress of surgery, as physiologic reserves (cardiac, respiratory, renal) have already declined with age. The elderly patient is more likely to have impaired renal, hepatic, respiratory, and cardiac functions, and is susceptible to chronic diseases that cause vulnerability to fluid and electrolyte imbalances during and after surgery.

When assessing the presurgical patient, any significant deviations from normal range should be brought to the attention of the surgeon. For example, an elevated temperature might indicate an infection that would need to be brought under control before surgery. Knowing the patient's usual blood pressure reading is necessary for comparison after surgery, when postoperative shock is a concern. Height and weight are measured and charted before surgery so the anesthesiologist can accurately calculate anesthetic dosages. Allergies must be identified and noted on the front of the patient's chart and on an allergy bracelet worn on the patient's arm.

Focused Assessment

Preoperative Data Collection

HEALTH HISTORY AND PSYCHOSOCIAL ASSESSMENT
- Have you previously had surgery? What was your experience?
- What is the reason for this surgery?
- How do you feel about having this surgery?
- What do you know about this surgery and the before and after care?
- What are your expectations of this surgery?
- Have you or any family members ever experienced any problems with surgery or anesthesia?
- Will this surgery create any problems in your usual roles or relationships?
- Do you have any chronic illnesses?
- Have you gained or lost considerable weight recently?
- Do you have any allergies to medications, iodine, shellfish, adhesive tape, or latex?
- What medications, over-the-counter preparations, vitamins, herbs, and supplements do you take?
- Do you smoke? How much and for how many years?
- What is your usual use of alcohol?
- When was your last bowel movement?
- Do you have any problems with urination?
- Do you currently have an upper respiratory infection?
- Do you have any musculoskeletal problems that need to be addressed during positioning for surgery?
- Do you have health insurance?
- What people will be able to help you during your recovery?
- Will you be able to cope with inconveniences during your recovery without additional help?
- How do you usually cope with pain?
- Are there any particular concerns or fears that you have regarding the surgery now?

CULTURAL ASSESSMENT
- What is your primary language?
- Do you have any cultural or spiritual practices that you would like to observe during this period of surgery and recovery?
- What are your cultural customs regarding privacy, blood transfusions, and disposal of body parts?

SPIRITUAL ASSESSMENT
- Do you have spiritual or religious beliefs?
- Do you wish to talk with or see your spiritual or religious advisor?
- Is there any conflict between your value or belief system and this planned surgery?

PHYSICAL ASSESSMENT
- Measure height and weight.
- Measure vital signs.
- Auscultate the lungs and heart.
- Listen for bowel sounds.
- Check pulses and compare bilaterally.
- Gather basic neurologic data: level of consciousness, orientation to time, place, and person; ability to think, answer questions, and follow instructions.
- Assess skin status, integrity, moisture, and temperature.
- Assess for recent tattoos, piercings, and body jewelry.
- Assess for limitations in joint range of motion.
- Assess for muscle weakness.
- Assess for loose teeth, dentures, bridges, contact lenses, hearing aid, and other prostheses.

LABORATORY AND DIAGNOSTIC TEST DATA
- Verify that test results are in the chart.
- Note any abnormal findings.

 Safety Alert

Latex Allergy

The patient who is allergic to latex is at high risk of exposure during surgery when unconscious and unable to monitor the environment. The perioperative nurse must be constantly vigilant to keep anything with latex on it out of the patient's environment. Even rubber stoppers on medication bottles or IV containers can be a problem. The operating room must be prepared to be "latex free." A "latex-free" crash cart is kept at hand in case of emergency.

 Think Critically

Why would a localized infection be a contraindication for surgery in some instances?

It is particularly important to know if a patient is taking a corticosteroid, which can delay wound healing, alter fluid and electrolyte balance, and affect several metabolic functions in the body—factors that increase surgical risk. Patients should be questioned about medicines and eyedrops that may contain a corticosteroid. Corticosteroids should be tapered slowly before surgery, but never stopped abruptly. Vitamin E, aspirin and other nonsteroidal anti-inflammatory drugs (NSAIDs), and anticoagulants have a continuing effect on blood clotting for several days; these supplements and medicines are usually discontinued 7 to 14 days before surgery.

 Complementary and Alternative Therapies

Herbals and Supplements

Most anesthesiologists will ask patients to discontinue taking herbal supplements 2 to 3 weeks before surgery, as many herbal supplements interact with anesthetic agents or interfere with blood clotting. If doing without a supplement is not possible, the herbal supplement container should be brought to the anesthesiologist. Black cohosh, St. John's wort, feverfew, goldenseal, valerian, ginger, and ginkgo biloba all can have adverse effects either on clotting mechanisms or by interactions with other medications and anesthetics and should be stopped 2 to 3 weeks before surgery. It is best to stop all herbals before surgery. After surgery, the patient should ask the health care provider when each herb can be restarted.

Nutritional status and body weight are significant factors in healing and repair of the surgical site. Obesity presents problems related to such routine procedures as venipuncture and intubation for general anesthesia, and obesity causes prolonged uptake of anesthetic drugs.

The operating room personnel are notified if the patient is hard of hearing, is essentially blind when glasses are not in place, or has a **prosthesis** (artificial body part).

The news that surgery is needed usually comes as an emotional shock to patients and their families. Surgery causes changes in the routine of their lives that could result in personal and financial burdens on patients and their families. Surgery will alter the lives of some patients permanently, and possibly may leave them physically impaired. Others might expect to be greatly helped by the surgical procedure. In any event, there will be fears and misgivings about the prospect of undergoing anesthesia and surgery.

 Cultural Considerations

Financial Burden

Many Chinese do not purchase health insurance, and any hospitalization or major surgery may bring considerable financial hardship to the family.

 Cultural Considerations

Beliefs Regarding Surgery

Cultural beliefs and values regarding surgery must be taken into consideration. If the patient does not speak the same language as the surgical team, an interpreter should be enlisted to assist with communication. If a female patient's culture has strict rules for female attire, she needs assurance of sufficient privacy and protection of modesty to allay any fears she might have. Such issues and interventions must be conveyed to the surgical team. If there are certain cultural taboos regarding an aspect of the surgery, the surgical team needs to know them and plan a way to achieve a good outcome without violating such taboos. It is especially important to know whether the patient will accept a blood transfusion.

 Elder Care Points

Older patients who are experiencing serious depression are at high risk for complications of surgery because their motivation for recovery often is very low.

Determine whether the patient will have adequate help at home when discharged from the hospital. Many older people live alone, and although self-sufficient before surgery, may have difficulty preparing meals, bathing, or performing wound care while recovering from surgery.

Some people are concerned about whether they will "wake up" or survive the anesthesia and surgical procedure. Some patients have a strong spiritual belief that helps them cope independently with sickness, suffering, and death. Others may need help in finding the spiritual support they need. Still others do not want to discuss this particular facet of their lives. Allow time with clergy or a spiritual advisor before the surgical procedure, per the patient's desire.

Laboratory and Diagnostic Test Data

Box 4-2 lists the tests most frequently required before surgery. A chest radiograph is usually obtained, and an electrocardiogram is ordered for many patients

---

Box 4-2	Commonly Ordered Preoperative Laboratory Tests

- Complete blood count (CBC)
- Urinalysis (UA)
- Blood glucose*
- Electrolytes
- Prothrombin time (PT)
- Partial thromboplastin time (PTT)
- Blood type and crossmatch
- Liver function tests (AST, ALT, bilirubin)*
- Renal function tests (BUN, creatinine)*
- Beta-human chorionic gonadotropin†

Key: *ALT*, alanine aminotransferase; *AST*, aspartate aminotransferase; *BUN*, blood urea nitrogen.
*May be ordered as part of a metabolic panel or sequential multiple assay (SMA)-6 or SMA-12.
†To check for pregnancy in women of childbearing age.

over 40 years of age. If the patient has lung disease, pulmonary function tests may be ordered. If the laboratory reports indicate any abnormal values, surgery may be postponed. Most surgeons prefer to delay surgery if a patient's hemoglobin level is below 10 g/dL.

 Think Critically

Why would anemia make a patient a poor surgical candidate?

Surgery puts a strain on the cardiovascular, renal, and respiratory systems. Liver function is important because the liver is involved in synthesizing clotting factors, producing albumin, and metabolizing and detoxifying drugs. Although requesting preoperative diagnostic tests is the responsibility of the physician, you will need to explain to the patient why these tests have been ordered.

Surgical Risk Factors

Carefully assess the patient before surgery for risk of complications (Table 4-2). Infants and the elderly are at higher risk for complications of surgery due to either immature body systems or a decline in function of various body systems. Maintaining core body temperature is one concern when caring for these patients. Research has shown that quitting smoking and alcohol intake 3 to 8 weeks before surgery will reduce the incidence of serious postoperative complications (Tonnesen et al., 2009).

 Think Critically

What points would you make when explaining to a patient how smoking is harmful to the surgery patient?

Learning Needs

There is general information to be provided to the surgical patient about what will happen immediately before, during, and after surgery, as well as specific

Table 4-2 Surgical Risk Factors

FACTOR	KEY POINTS
Diabetes mellitus and other chronic diseases	Stress of surgery may cause swings in blood glucose levels that are difficult to control. Patient may receive intravenous insulin during and after surgery. Wound healing tends to be delayed in the diabetic patient, making the risk of **dehiscence** (wound separation) greater. There is a higher incidence of infection in surgical wounds in diabetic patients. Liver and kidney disease make it more difficult to metabolize and eliminate anesthesia and waste products.
Advanced age with inactivity	Healing is slower in elderly patients. The risk of disuse syndrome, hypostatic **pneumonia** (inflammation and consolidation in the lungs), and thrombus formation is higher in an inactive elderly person.
Very young person	Infants have difficulty with temperature control and in maintaining normal circulatory blood volume; they are at risk of dehydration.
Malnutrition	Inadequate nutritional stores lead to poor wound healing and skin breakdown.
Dehydration	Reduced circulating volume reduces kidney perfusion and predisposes the patient to a reduced urine output and thrombus formation. Dehydration also alters electrolyte values. The dehydrated patient is more at risk for problems with pressure areas during surgery.
Obesity	The extremely heavy patient does not breathe as deeply and is at risk of hypostatic pneumonia. Excessive fatty tissue also is a factor in poor wound healing.
Cardiovascular problems	Patients with hypertension, left ventricular hypertrophy, cardiac dysrhythmias, or history of congestive heart failure are at a higher risk for myocardial infarction from the stresses of surgery and anesthesia.
Peripheral vascular disease	Poor circulation in the extremities predisposes the patient to possible thrombus formation and pressure sores on the lower legs and feet. Anti-embolism stockings or devices are generally prescribed for use during and after surgery.
Liver disease	Interferes with normal blood clotting; liver cannot properly detoxify anesthetics and other drugs.
Respiratory disease	Inhaled anesthetics may irritate the respiratory mucosa, creating more secretions. With immobility there is greater probability of accumulated secretions and inflammation of the lungs and bronchial tree. Impaired oxygen–carbon dioxide exchange may cause acid-base imbalance.
Substance abuse or alcohol dependence	May alter reaction to anesthetic agents. Alcohol dependence may cause withdrawal symptoms if the use of alcohol is discontinued abruptly.
Smoking	Causes increased lung secretions from anesthesia and predisposes the patient to **atelectasis** (collapsed alveoli) and pneumonia, postoperatively. Smokers are more prone to thrombus formation.
Regular use of certain drugs	Aspirin, nonsteroidal anti-inflammatory drugs, and anticoagulants make the patient more prone to excessive bleeding. Corticosteroids reduce the body's response to infection and delay the healing process.
Excessive fear	Stimulates the sympathetic nervous system and causes the release of hormones, causing swings in the body's chemistry and vital signs. Increased muscle tension makes surgery more difficult. Physical manifestations of fear can interfere with achieving the desired state of anesthesia.

Adapted from deWit, S.C. (2009). *Fundamental Concepts and Skills for Nursing* (3rd ed.). Philadelphia: Saunders, p. 749.

preventive measures to be learned (see Implementation on pp. 70–75). If members of the family or supportive friends are expected to assist the patient during the postoperative period, they need to be instructed during teaching sessions.

Patient Teaching

General Preoperative Teaching

All surgical patients should receive information related to:
- **Preoperative procedures:** Enemas, skin preparation, care of belongings, restriction of food and liquid intake, and administration of bedtime sedatives and preoperative medication; time to come to the hospital

- **Technical information:** Anticipated surgical procedure; location of incisions; dressings, tubes, drains, catheters, or other equipment that is expected
- **Day of surgery:** Time surgery is scheduled, time to arrive at hospital or time patient is to leave her room, probable length of procedure, effects of preoperative medications, where family will wait, when and where family can see the patient after surgery, pain control, and postoperative routine
- **Postanesthesia care unit (PACU):** General environment (noise, lights, equipment), frequent taking of vital signs, pulse oximetry, and administration of oxygen
- **Surgical intensive care unit (SICU)** (if patient is to go there from PACU): Location of the unit, expected length of stay, and visiting privileges

■ Nursing Diagnosis

Based on the assessment, nursing diagnoses in the preoperative stage include both actual and potential problems. Examples of common preoperative nursing diagnoses are:

- Anxiety related to the surgical experience and outcome
- Fear related to risk for death, effects of impending surgery, or loss of control due to anesthesia
- Grieving related to impending loss of a body function or body part
- Deficient knowledge related to preoperative and postoperative routines
- Insomnia related to stress or unfamiliar environment
- Ineffective coping related to lack of problem-solving skills or adequate support
- Ineffective role performance related to inability to perform job duties or to care for children during hospitalization

Each diagnosis is supported by data obtained during the nursing assessment.

■ Planning

Specific expected outcomes will be written for each nursing diagnosis (Nursing Care Plan 4-1). However, there are general *nursing goals* for all preoperative patients. The expectation is that the patient will be:

- Prepared for surgery physically and emotionally
- Able to demonstrate deep breathing, coughing, and leg exercises
- Able to verbalize understanding of the procedure and the expectations for the postoperative period
- Able to maintain fluid and electrolyte balance throughout the perioperative period

When preoperative patients are assigned, you must plan your work for the shift carefully to have the patients ready for surgery without neglecting the needs of other assigned patients.

 Clinical Cues

At the beginning of the shift, check to see that any ordered preoperative medications are on hand. Check the surgery schedule and estimate the time needed to prepare the patient for surgery. If preoperative medications are ordered, calculate the dosages of preoperative medications ahead of time so that you will be prepared to quickly draw them up when the call comes from the operating room (OR) nurse to "preop" the patient.

■ Implementation

Preoperatively, your time is divided between preparing the patient for surgery and teaching the patient about what will happen and how to hasten recovery.

The same-day surgery patient receives teaching from the physician's office nurse or from a surgical intake nurse. Teaching sessions may be scheduled when the patient comes for diagnostic testing. Sending written instructions home with the patient reinforces what has been taught. Before entering the hospital for surgery, the patient should be given a phone number to call for answers to questions that may arise. Protocol may differ from one facility to another.

 Elder Care Points

It is particularly important to reinforce instruction and information given to the elderly patient. The anxiety of surgery, unfamiliar surroundings, diminished hearing and vision, and forgetfulness make learning more difficult and may decrease retention of information. Seek specific feedback periodically of points that are important for the patient to remember. Treat all patients with respect and dignity.

Consent for Surgery

Before the surgeon can perform an operation, written permission signed by either the patient, guardian, or whoever holds power of attorney must be obtained. This written consent protects the surgeon against claims of unauthorized surgery and provides the patient an opportunity to exercise the right of *informed consent.* In most hospitals, the "consent" is a printed form that the patient signs before surgery. The correct surgical procedure is written into the "consent." The surgeon explains the procedure, risks, and benefits; the nurse only witnesses the patient's signature. The patient must be mentally competent and give consent freely and without coercion. The consent form is attached to the patient's chart and is sent to the OR with the patient. **The nurse must always check that a consent form has been signed before giving the preoperative medication.**

 Legal and Ethical Considerations

Giving Surgical Consent

Mrs. Jones, age 66, was slightly confused due to dehydration when she was brought to the hospital. She has signed a surgical consent for a hip replacement, but her daughter feels she was confused when she signed the form and questions its validity. What would you do? How would the surgeon verify that Mrs. Jones was not confused when she signed the form?

 Clinical Cues

Patients have the right to change their minds and revoke consent up until the time of surgery. If a patient tells you the surgery is not wanted, delay preoperative preparations and explore the issue with the patient. If it appears the consent for surgery really is being revoked, notify the charge nurse and the surgeon.

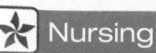

Scenario

A married 38-year-old woman, the mother of two children ages 16 and 14, is scheduled for a simple mastectomy as treatment for a localized malignant tumor that was detected by self-examination of her breasts.

Problem/Nursing Diagnosis

Cancer diagnosis/Fear related to cancer, disfigurement, and possible death.

Supporting Assessment Data

Subjective: Grandmother died of breast cancer.
Objective: Malignant tumor by biopsy, crying at intervals; states is worried about husband's reaction to the loss of the breast.

Goals/Expected Outcomes	Nursing Interventions	Selected Rationale	Evaluation
Patient will discuss fears openly by day 2.	Establish rapport and trust.	Establishing trust helps patient express fears and concerns.	Spent time with patient answering questions.
Patient will look at incisional area before discharge.	Encourage her to discuss fears with nurse and family.	Expressing fears decreases anxiety.	
Patient will identify spiritual support before discharge.	Encourage her to think of cancer as a challenge.	A positive perspective empowers the patient.	
Patient will talk about having cancer by postoperative day 2.	Help her to identify specific fears and deal with each one separately.	Decreases the fear of the unknown. Dispelling fear and anxiety makes learning easier.	Stated is afraid of chemotherapy. Is now using the word "cancer" when discussing her surgery. Discussed ways to meet the challenges of chemotherapy.
	Teach relaxation exercises to decrease anxiety.	Relaxation exercises help decrease anxiety.	Expressed willingness to learn a relaxation exercise. Tried relaxation exercises twice.
Patient will join support group for cancer patients after discharge.	Advise of community resources available to her.		Expressed appreciation for information about a support group.
Patient will utilize community resources after discharge.			

Problem/Nursing Diagnosis

Simple mastectomy scheduled/Knowledge deficit about preoperative routine and postoperative care.

Supporting Assessment Data

Subjective: States, "I've never had surgery before. What will I need to do?"
Objective: Puzzled expression on face.

Goals/Expected Outcomes	Nursing Interventions	Selected Rationale	Evaluation
Patient will verbalize understanding of preoperative procedures and requirements before surgery.	Do preoperative teaching for patient and family: routine procedures, NPO status, expected tubes and drains, equipment to expect in room, probable length of surgery, where family will wait, pain relief measures, handling of arm on operative side, coughing, deep breathing and leg exercises, ambulation, diet, daily postoperative routine.	Knowledge reduces fear of the unknown and anxiety.	Performed return demonstrations and verbalized understanding of routine and procedures.
Family will express understanding of what will happen preoperatively, where they will stay during surgery, and what to expect after surgery by end of teaching session			Family verbalized understanding of what to expect.
	Call pastor or chaplain if patient desires a visit.	Clergy can be a positive support in time of stress.	A pastoral visit is scheduled for this afternoon.
	Provide private time for patient and husband and patient and family.	Private time is necessary for serious discussions.	Will have private talk with husband and one with daughters later today. Continue plan.

Critical Thinking Questions

1. How would you specifically assess this patient's learning needs?
2. How could you assess for any cultural factors that would affect her learning or your teaching?

Think Critically

Why should the consent be signed before giving any preoperative medication? What happens if a patient has been given the preoperative medication and then it is discovered that the surgical consent form has not been signed?

Food and Fluids

Food and fluids will often be restricted for 8 hours before surgery, and the patient is placed on NPO (*nil per os*, which means "nothing by mouth") status. A light meal such as toast and clear fluids may be allowed up to 6 hours before surgery. Clear liquids such as black coffee, tea, apple juice, or carbonated beverages may be consumed up to 3 hours before surgery in elective cases (Maltby, 2000). Often the surgeon or anesthesiologist will allow an oral blood pressure medication, heart medication, or anticonvulsant to be taken with a sip of water the morning of surgery. Always check the physician's order before giving anything by mouth in the immediate preoperative period. The purpose of oral restriction is to prevent nausea, vomiting, and aspiration. **Confirm with the patient that the NPO order has been heeded.** Insulin may or may not be given; check the orders.

Clinical Cues

If a patient has not remained NPO for the prescribed period, surgery may be canceled.

Elimination

If the patient is having abdominal or colon surgery, enemas may be ordered to clear the bowel. Sometimes oral GoLYTELY solution is used. The patient may be placed on a special soft or liquid diet for the 3 days before surgery in order to decrease the content of the bowel.

When completing the preoperative checklist, ask the patient to empty the bladder (unless a catheter is in place). If the bladder is not empty, relaxation induced by medications and anesthesia causes the urge to urinate. The bladder should be emptied before any sedating medication is given.

Tubes and Equipment

If a nasogastric tube will be inserted during surgery for postoperative use, explain its purpose, its care, and what it will feel like to the patient. Give an estimate of how long the tube will remain in the stomach. The tube is usually removed when bowel sounds return and nausea has passed. If surgery has occurred in the stomach or intestinal tract, the tube may remain longer. Explain the function of other tubes such as drains, an intravenous (IV) line, oxygen delivery and monitoring devices, a chest tube, and a urinary catheter, as well as their care and probable duration of use.

Rest and Sedation

It is desirable for the patient to be as well rested as possible before surgery so the body is not compromised in meeting the stresses of anesthesia and surgical procedure. A sedative may be ordered for the patient the night before surgery, but the inpatient often must ask for it. Check on the patient frequently during the night. If the patient awakens and is restless, sit and listen and try to dispel fears, offer a soothing back rub, or give backup sedation as ordered. The patient scheduled for same-day surgery should take the sedative at home and retire early the night before because it may be necessary to arise early to enter the hospital.

Pain Control

Many surgeons order a patient-controlled analgesia (PCA) pump for their patients postoperatively. If a PCA pump is ordered, patients should receive instruction before surgery about the pump and how to operate it. If patients will be receiving injections for pain control, explain that this type of medication is ordered on an as-needed basis every 3 to 4 hours, and that patients must ask for it. Oral pain medication is usually ordered for every 4 to 6 hours as needed. Explain that asking for the pain medication before the pain becomes severe makes it easier to control the pain level. Teach the patient about the pain scale that is used at the facility.

Skin Preparation

The night or morning before surgery, the patient may be asked to shower with a special antibacterial cleanser to remove as many microorganisms from the skin as possible. On the morning of the surgery, hair may be removed from the operative site—this is done either in the surgical holding area or in the OR. As a Core Measure for reducing surgical site infection, use hair clippers only for hair removal before surgery (The Joint Commission [TJC], 2010). Explain to the patient the hair removal area to be prepared, the hair removal process, and the timing for hair removal. Nail polish is removed so that the pulse oximeter can function correctly when attached to the finger. Makeup is removed; note the presence of permanent makeup on the preoperative checklist. Ask about contact lenses and have them removed as well.

Elder Care Points

The elderly patient should be taught needed information in short segments, to prevent confusion and increase the patient's comprehension. Written reminders of key instructions should be given to the patient.

Preoperative Teaching

Teaching the patient correct breathing, coughing, turning, and leg exercises is a high priority during the preoperative period. It is helpful to have a relative or close friend present for these teaching sessions so this

FIGURE 4-1 Teaching foot and leg exercises.

person can later give coaching and encouragement to the patient. Instruct the patient about what to expect before, during, and after surgery. Help the same-day surgery patient devise a schedule for doing the necessary exercises.

Venous return is often hampered during the surgical procedure, due to the position assumed on the operating table and pooling of blood in the lower extremities. The stasis (slowing of flow) of blood places the patient at risk for thrombophlebitis (blood clot and inflammation of a vessel). Specific leg exercises help to prevent this complication (Figure 4-1). Explain the importance of doing the exercises, show the patient how to do each one, and ask for a return demonstration. One way to remind patients to do the exercises is to have them exercise whenever a commercial comes on, if they watch TV. The exercises should be done after surgery at least 5 to 10 times every hour while awake, until the patient is up and moving about normally.

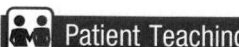 **Patient Teaching**

Postoperative Foot and Leg Exercises

- Flex and extend the right foot, moving the toes upward and downward, four or five times.
- Repeat with the left foot.
- Trace circles to the right with the right foot five times; repeat with circles to the left.
- Trace circles to the right with the left foot five times; repeat with circles to the left.
- Bend the right leg at the knee, sliding the foot back toward the buttocks as far as possible; raise the bent leg off the bed, extend the leg, and dorsiflex the foot; extend the foot and lower the leg to the bed.
- Bend the left leg at the knee, sliding the foot back toward the buttocks as far as possible; raise the bent leg off the bed, extend the leg, and dorsiflex the foot; extend the foot and lower the leg to the bed.
- Tighten the buttocks muscles for a count of 10 and release to exercise the quadriceps muscles.
- Repeat each exercise four more times.

FIGURE 4-2 Teaching deep breathing and coughing while splinting the incision.

Deep Breathing and Coughing. For deep breathing and coughing, it is preferable for the patient to sit up, with the back away from the mattress or chair. This allows for full lung expansion and clearing of excretions. The surgical chest or abdominal incision should be splinted with a pillow (Figure 4-2).

Clinical Cues

A small, firm "coughing pillow" can be made by folding a bath towel or a light blanket and securing it inside a pillow case with the ends tucked inside over the towel or blanket.

The surgeon may order use of an incentive spirometer. Instruct the patient in its use and supervise until the patient has mastered the technique.

 Patient Teaching

Lung Exercises

DEEP BREATHING
- Sit up away from the mattress.
- Take a deep breath in through the nose, hold for a few seconds, and slowly exhale.
- Repeat four more times.
- Perform every 2 hours during the day and when awakened at night for vital signs.

FORCED EXHALATION COUGHING
- Sit up away from the mattress.
- Splint the abdominal or chest incision and:
  - Take a deep breath through the nose and cough as you exhale with the mouth open, but covered with a tissue.
  - If you cannot move secretions with your cough, use a forced exhalation cough.
  - Take a deep breath through the nose and forcibly quickly exhale, producing a "huff" cough.
  - Repeat the process using three short "huffs" as you exhale to bring the secretions to the mouth, where they can be expectorated. Repeat until no secretions are audible in lungs, resting in between attempts.
  - Perform every 2 hours during the day and when awakened at night for vital signs.

USING AN INCENTIVE SPIROMETER

- Sit up away from the mattress.
- Insert the mouthpiece, covering it completely with the lips.
- Take a slow deep breath and hold it for at least 3 seconds.
- Exhale slowly, keeping the lips puckered.
- Breathe normally for a few breaths.
- Try to increase the inspired volume by at least 100 mL with each breath on the spirometer.
- Once maximal volume is achieved, attempt to inspire this volume 10 times, resting a few breaths in between each attempt.
- Clean the mouthpiece of the spirometer when finished.
- During the first 3 postoperative days, try to do this every hour.

Turning. Show the patient how to turn in bed by flexing the legs to relax the abdominal muscles, placing a pillow between the legs, grabbing on to the side of the bed, and slowly turning to the side. This maneuver is also used for getting up out of bed. A trapeze bar for orthopedic patients is very helpful for turning and repositioning.

Family Instructions. Advise the family to come to the hospital 1 to 1½ hours before surgery. The family should be told about the usual routines, where to wait, the approximate time before the patient may be expected to return, and what to anticipate in the way of tubes, equipment, and patient appearance after surgery. This knowledge keeps the family from thinking the patient has "taken a turn for the worse" when they see the extra equipment for suction, oxygen, or IV therapy in use after surgery. A warning about the occasional delays in starting surgery can keep the family from becoming excessively anxious if the patient is not back at the expected time.

Immediate Preoperative Care

The patient is usually dressed in a clean hospital gown, without underwear, for the operating room. Hair is covered with a surgical paper cap. Long hair should be fixed so that it can tangle only minimally and all hairpins and barrettes must be removed. Ask about body piercings and the presence of piercing jewelry, including the tongue and genital areas. Explain why *all* jewelry must be removed for safety due to electrocautery used during surgery and the danger of an electrical burn from conduction of electricity through metal.

Jewelry, along with money and credit cards, is given to a family member or relative to keep, or is secured in a valuables envelope and placed in a safe, according to facility policy. If a wedding band is to be worn to surgery, tape the ring to the finger without restricting circulation. Dentures are removed, placed in a labeled cup, and kept in a designated place, according to hospital policy. Sometimes the anesthesiologist will order the dentures left in place to facilitate the administration of anesthesia by mask. If a hearing aid is left in place, a very visible note should be placed on the front of the chart cover and placement of the hearing aid should be noted on the preoperative checklist sheet.

Verify that the identification bracelet matches the chart, to avoid any error or mix-up of patients in the operating room. Verify that the procedure site indicated on the surgical consent form is the same as what the patient states. The procedure site will be verified and marked on the patient before transport to surgery or in the preoperative holding area if not done previously.

Clinical Cues

Attend to all items on the preoperative checklist that can be handled ahead of time (Figure 4-3). This prevents hurrying, which can increase mistakes, and prevents delaying administration of any preoperative medication while the list is completed.

Most preoperative medications are given by the anesthesiologist. A medication to inhibit gastric acid secretion may be administered intravenously. Check that the surgical consent is signed and start any ordered medications on time. You may need to send an IV piggyback antibiotic to the OR with the patient. Often no medication is given before the patient is in the surgical area.

Safety Alert

Preventing Falls

If the patient has received a sedative preoperatively, remember to put up the side rails of the bed per facility protocol and lower the bed. Remind the patient not to get up without assistance. These are important patient safety measures after administering sedatives.

Preoperative medications may be given to:
- Reduce anxiety and promote a restful state
- Decrease secretion of mucus and other body fluids
- Counteract nausea and reduce emesis
- Enhance the effects of the anesthetic

Assist in transferring the patient to the stretcher when the transport person comes to take the patient to surgery. Compare the patient's identification bracelet name and numbers with the transport request sheet for accuracy. Check the chart to make certain that everything ordered has been done and complete final documentation.

 ### Cultural Considerations

Differences in Drug Metabolism

Asians, and particularly the Chinese, metabolize psychotropic drugs differently than other ethnic groups. Valium causes greater sedation with normal doses. Atropine is also metabolized differently and can greatly accelerate the heart rate. Asian patients should be monitored closely when receiving these drugs.

PREOP/PREPROCEDURE CHECKLIST/REPORT FORM			PATIENT LABEL

Date	Time		

Surgery/procedure		YES	
Correct patient ID band on		☐	

	On chart	☐
	Dictated	☐

History and Physical
H&P 24 hours to 30 days: update with "No Pertinent Change in History & Physical" stamp
H&P 31-180 days: H&P update form #2396
OB H&P Update for Surgery/Procedures form #2543

	YES	N/A
Initiate Anesthesia Preop order 101.S09. As appropriate initiate OB Anesthesia Order 144.P11	☐	
Include at least one page of patient ID stickers	☐	
Procedural consent: Signed/On Chart	☐	
Procedural site verified with patient/guardian	☐	N/A
Procedural site marked when laterality (including internal laterality), multiple structures (fingers, toes, lesions) or multiple levels (spine). Specify site: _____	☐	☐
Preop antibiotic given	☐	☐
Interpreter if needed	☐	☐
HBOC transfer report on chart (when applicable)	☐	☐
Acuscan MAR-LOS custom report on chart (when applicable)	☐	☐

OB   ☐ The Department of Social and Health Services consent for sterilization completed and on chart dated ≥ than 30 days prior to procedure (*unless meets exception criteria, listed in Standards of Care Notebook)
☐ Notify anesthesia provider

Diagnostic   ☐ Labs on chart   ☐ X-rays with patient (when appropriate)   ☐ When applicable Glucose: _____ /time _____
☐ Type and screen   ☐ ECG (when applicable)   Blood units available: # _____

Medications/IV   ☐ MAR on chart   ☐ IV/Saline lock in place   ☐ If TPN running, start second peripheral IV site

Belongings	Labeled	With Patient/Family	To OR
Contacts			
Glasses			
Hearing aids R L Both			
Dentures ☐ Upper ☐ Lower ☐ Partial			

Prep   ☐ Personal clothing removed   ☐ Prep completed
☐ Snap gown   ☐ Voided, time: _____   ☐ Foley
☐ Jewelry/body piercings: _____   ☐ None ☐ Taped ☐ Family   ☐ Patient registration safe
☐ Preop teaching done   Last oral/fluid intake: _____   Time: _____

Unit based or bedside procedures: FINAL VERIFICATION
☐ Correct patient   ☐ Correct side/site   ☐ Correct position
☐ Correct procedure   ☐ Correct equipment/trays

REPORT USING SBAR: Provide an opportunity to ask and answer questions. Include significant history/special needs.

2067 4/06

INITIALS/OR SIGNATURE IF SIGNATURE PAGE NOT USED

FIGURE 4-3 Preoperative checklist.

Elder Care Points

Because of decreasing liver and kidney function that occurs with age, elderly patients, especially those over 75, will need reduced dosages of preoperative narcotics and sedatives. Observe for signs of toxicity.

 Think Critically

How would you handle a situation in which a patient scheduled for an abdominal procedure has put back on underwear or jewelry after you finished doing the preoperative checklist?

Preparation of the Patient Unit

While patients are in surgery, prepare the room for their return. Make the bed with fresh linen; include a drawsheet between the shoulder and the knee area that can be used as a lift sheet to reposition the patient. For abdominal or perineal surgery, place an underpad at the hip area to catch excess drainage. Fan-fold the top covers to the far side of the bed or to the bottom of the bed. Raise the bed to the height of the stretcher that will return the patient, and arrange furniture so that the stretcher can be pulled up alongside the bed. Place the IV pole at the head of the bed.

Gather an emesis basin, tissues, frequent vital signs sheet or postoperative record, intake and output sheet, small towel and washcloth, and pen and place them on the bedside table or console (Figure 4-4). Connect oxygen and suction equipment if their need is anticipated. A thermometer, sphygmomanometer, pulse oximeter, and stethoscope should be close at hand on the patient's return to the unit. If a PCA pump, sequential pneumatic compression devices, or a passive range-of-motion machine will be needed, see that they are obtained and ready.

FIGURE 4-4 Room prepared for surgical patient's return.

Evaluation

Evaluation is accomplished by determining if the nursing goals have been met. If the patient is properly prepared for surgery, kept NPO, reasonably calm, and knowledgeable about the procedure and what is expected, the general goals have been met. If the preoperative medications were not given on time or the patient was not ready for transport at the appointed time, review your steps to see where improvement can occur. Data are gathered to determine if expected outcomes written for individual nursing diagnoses are being met (see Nursing Care Plan 4-1).

INTRAOPERATIVE CARE

In the surgical holding room, the circulating nurse will verify the patient's identification, verify that all preoperative orders have been accomplished, and verify that all relevant documents and diagnostic studies are available. The anesthesia care provider will start an IV line if one is not already in place. The surgical site will be verified and marked by the surgeon or a member of the operating team, and a Universal Protocol to prevent wrong site surgery is followed (TJC, 2009). When the OR is ready, the patient is transferred to the operating table. Patient identification is verified again by the circulating nurse.

 Safety Alert

Time-Out

Before surgery begins while all members of the team are present, a "time-out" occurs during which a final verification of the correct patient, procedure, site, and implants (if applicable) is performed. Any questions or concerns must be resolved before the procedure begins.

The patient is positioned with padding to prevent injury to nerves and to minimize pressure over bony prominences. Serious injury and pressure ulcers can develop from improper positioning or lack of padding for a surgical procedure (see Chapter 43). Safety straps are secured to safeguard the patient.

THE SURGICAL TEAM

The surgical team consists of the surgeon, surgical assistants, anesthesia care provider, circulating nurse, and scrub person. The surgeon is the head of the surgical team and may be a physician, an oral surgeon, or a podiatrist. The *first* surgical assistant is another physician, a surgical resident, or a specially trained and authorized RN. Other assistants may be RNs or LPN/LVNs. The surgeon, surgical assistants, and scrub nurse are sterile members, perform a surgical scrub or rub, and wear sterile gowns and gloves. They work within the sterile field.

THE SURGICAL SUITE

Operating rooms (ORs) are removed from other areas of the hospital and access is restricted to OR personnel and surgical patients. The OR is maintained as a positive pressure environment to reduce the entrance of microbes that might cause infection. The surgical suite is divided into three distinct areas to help keep the ORs as microbe free as possible. The unrestricted zone is essentially the control desk area. Street clothes may be permitted here. Semi-restricted zones include the hallways and outer regions of the ORs. The circulating nurse and anesthesia care providers work in these areas. Clean scrub clothes and caps are required. The restricted zone is the area surrounding the operating table and instrument trays and table. Personnel wear scrub clothes, sterile gowns, caps, shoe covers, masks, and sterile gloves within this area. Asepsis is the responsibility of all surgical personnel.

The temperature in the OR is kept at 66° to 70° F (18.9° to 21.1° C) to discourage microbial growth and to keep the surgical team comfortable under the bright lights and in the layers of surgical clothing. Cabinets, instrument tables, instrument trays, and disposal buckets are usually made of stainless steel that can be easily cleaned and disinfected. The restricted area is scrubbed down with disinfectant after each procedure. The entire room is kept scrupulously clean.

THE SURGICAL HOLDING AREA

The patient is transported to the holding area in the surgical suite. The holding area nurse greets the patient, reviews the medical record and the preoperative checklist, and verifies that the operative consent is signed, that a risk assessment is documented, and that the surgical site is marked as required. The nurse offers emotional support and answers any questions. The anesthesiologist may greet the patient, start an IV line if one has not been established, administer preoperative medications, and prepare the patient for anesthesia.

ROLES OF THE CIRCULATING NURSE AND THE SCRUB PERSON

A surgical technician or a specially trained nurse (LPN/LVN or RN) may be the scrub person. This person functions within the sterile area of the operating room (Box 4-3, Figure 4-5). **Sterile technique is maintained at all times. Any break in sterile technique should be immediately pointed out by the circulating nurse or any member of the OR team and remedied.**

The circulating nurse is responsible, along with the anesthesia care provider, for maintaining the safety and dignity of the patient and bringing needed items to the operating team, as well as many other duties (Box 4-4). The circulating nurse is the communication link between the OR and those outside the surgical suite.

Box 4-3	Major Functions of the Scrub Person

- Gathers all equipment for the procedure.
- Prepares all sterile supplies and instruments using sterile technique.
- Gowns and gloves surgeons on entry into operating room.
- Assists with sterile draping of the patient.
- Maintains sterility within the sterile field during surgery.
- Hands instruments and supplies to the operating team during surgery, anticipating what is needed.
- Maintains a neat instrument table.
- Labels and handles surgical specimens correctly.
- Maintains an accurate count of sponges, sharps, and instruments on the sterile field; verifies counts with the circulating nurse before and after surgery.
- Monitors for breaks in sterile technique and points them out.
- Cleans up after the surgery is over.

FIGURE 4-5 Scrub nurse setting up the instrument table in the operating room.

ANESTHESIA

Anesthesia (the loss of sensory perception) has been in use for surgical procedures since the 1840s. Newer anesthetics and techniques make anesthesia safer than ever, but **there is still a risk any time a patient is anesthetized.** The goals of anesthesia administration are to (1) prevent pain; (2) achieve adequate muscle relaxation; and (3) calm fear, ease anxiety, and induce forgetfulness of an unpleasant experience. Anesthetics are administered in a number of ways to achieve these goals (Table 4-3). Patients are classified according to their age, physical condition, and risk status and are assigned a risk potential. The choice of anesthesia depends on the type of surgical procedure to be performed and the risk potential. The anesthetic to be used is chosen by the anesthesia care provider, although it is discussed with the patient. The anesthesia care provider may be an anesthesiologist, another physician, or a certified registered nurse anesthetist (CRNA) who is supervised by an anesthesiologist.

| Box 4-4 | Major Functions of the Circulating Nurse |

- Coordinates care, oversees the environment, and cares for the patient in the operating room.
- Greets patient and performs patient assessment.
- Verifies that consent is signed and accurate and that surgical site is correctly marked.
- Checks medical record and preoperative forms for completeness.
- Sets up the operating room; adjusts lights, stools, and discard buckets; and ensures supplies and diagnostic support are available.
- Gathers and checks all equipment that is anticipated to be used, ensuring its safe function.
- Opens sterile supplies for scrub nurse.
- Provides needed padding and warming or cooling devices for the operating table.
- Assists with ties of surgical team's gowns.
- Assists with the transfer of the patient to the operating table and positions the patient.
- Places electrocautery ground pad under patient if electrocautery is to be used.
- Assists the anesthesia induction provider.
- May prep the patient's skin before sterile draping occurs.
- May insert a Foley catheter.
- Handles labeling and disposition of specimens.
- Coordinates activities with radiology and pathology departments.
- Monitors urine and blood loss during surgery and reports findings to the surgeon.
- Supplies, monitors, and documents the infusion of ordered fluids.
- Observes for breaks in sterile technique and announces them to the team.
- Monitors traffic and noise within the operating room.
- Communicates information on the surgery's progress to family during long procedures.
- Documents care, events, interventions, drugs, fluids, and findings.
- Assists with final count of sponges and sharps with the scrub person.
- Helps transfer patient to gurney and accompanies patient to recovery area, providing report of the surgery and patient condition to the recovery nurse.

GENERAL ANESTHESIA

General anesthesia is induced by the administration of an inhalant gas or by medication introduced intravenously. During general anesthesia, the patient is in a deep sleep state with muscle relaxation and is not aware of the surroundings. An endotracheal tube or nasal endotracheal catheter may be placed to maintain the airway. Placement of a laryngeal mask is another option. There are three stages of general anesthesia:

1. Induction—unconsciousness is induced
2. Maintenance—period during which the surgical procedure is performed
3. Emergence—surgery is completed and the patient is prepared to return to consciousness; neuromuscular blocking agents are reversed

 Elder Care Points

Obtaining an accurate height and weight of the elderly patient is very important for calculation of anesthetic agents and medication dosages. Kidney function is declining in the elderly person, and drugs are not eliminated from the body as quickly. Reduced dosages are often needed.

REGIONAL ANESTHESIA

Regional anesthesia is accomplished by administering a nerve block. It is often more economical than general anesthesia. Regional anesthesia may be accomplished by injecting the spinal, epidural, caudal, or peripheral nerve area. The block anesthetizes the local area or the area distal to the block. Spinal or epidural blocks are frequently used for high-risk patients undergoing pelvic or lower extremity surgery; epidural blocks are widely used in obstetric procedures.

PROCEDURAL SEDATION ANESTHESIA (MODERATE SEDATION)

A local anesthetic agent or regional anesthesia to numb the area plus IV sedation is used to provide systemic analgesia and sedation during a surgical procedure. The combination can be used for any procedure that can be done with local or regional anesthesia and is being used more and more frequently. The patient is monitored closely for blood pressure changes, oxygen saturation levels, and heart activity. Recently carbon dioxide levels have begun to be monitored by **capnography** (measurement of inhaled and exhaled carbon dioxide). Capnography provides a tracing that is a graphic representation of exhaled CO_2. The Microstream machine allows CO_2 monitoring without intubation with a nasal cannula–like device.

 Complementary and Alternative Therapies

Music's Effects

Music that the patient likes is known to have a calming effect on the preoperative patient. Research studying the use of music delivered by earphones to the patient during surgery is showing that music may reduce the amount of anesthesia and analgesia needed (Evans, 2007). The patient appears to become more relaxed and less anxious. Before and after surgery, listening to a blank CD through earphones appears to lower anxiety and pain, probably because the earphones decrease outside sensory stimulation.

LOCAL ANESTHESIA

Local anesthesia is used for minor procedures such as superficial tissue biopsies, surface cyst excision, insertion of a pacemaker, and insertion of vascular access devices. The patient who has had local anesthesia is transferred directly to the nursing unit and does not need care in the postanesthesia care unit (PACU, also called the postanesthesia recovery room [PAR or PARR] or postanesthesia recovery unit [PARU]) (see Chapter 5).

Table 4-3   Types of Anesthesia

TYPE	USE	ADVANTAGE
General		
Inhalation	Extensive surgery where it is desirable for patient to be unconscious with relaxed muscles.	Well controlled with assisted ventilation; few side effects.
Intravenous	Shorter surgery; rapid induction.	Little postoperative nausea or vomiting.
Regional		
Spinal	Surgery in lower half of body; for patients unable to undergo general anesthesia.	Patient can be conscious; does not require fasting. No nausea or vomiting from anesthesia.
Epidural	For gynecologic procedures and childbirth.	No diet restrictions postoperatively.
Nerve block	Foot surgery and some orthopedic surgeries.	Patient is conscious and can cooperate with instructions.
Local	Minor surgical procedures.	Can produce good pain control for many hours postoperatively; patient may remain conscious. Numbs an area for a short period of time.
Procedural/Conscious Sedation		
	Surgery of short duration where unconsciousness is undesirable.	Reversal is rapid, patient is unaware but can breathe without assistance. Little if any nausea or vomiting. Amnesia of surgery.
Other		
Hypnosis	Surgery in patients who are unable to have general anesthesia and where regional anesthesia is inappropriate.	No drug side effects.
Cryothermia	Surgery where patient cannot tolerate other anesthesia such as in life-threatening trauma.	Provides decrease in pain.

Go to Evolve for a table listing the types of anesthetic agents and their uses, advantages, and disadvantages.

POTENTIAL INTRAOPERATIVE COMPLICATIONS

Potential intraoperative complications of surgery include:

- Infection
- Fluid volume excess or deficit
- Hypothermia
- Malignant hyperthermia
- Injury related to positioning

No one with an active infection should be in the operating room. Surgical asepsis is practiced with great care to prevent contamination of the surgical site. Counts of sponges, needles, and instruments are performed to verify that no equipment has been left in a wound where it might cause a postoperative infection or complication.

Many associations and agencies have banded together to promote a program to decrease surgical infections and complications. Core Measures and National Patient Safety Goals include proper hair removal, timely antibiotic administration, blood glucose control, prevention of thromboembolic events, and prevention of adverse cardiac events (Bratzler, 2009; Griffin, 2005).

IV fluids are carefully regulated by the anesthesia care provider and the surgeon. The cool atmosphere, cool IV fluids, inhalation of cool anesthetic gases, and exposure of body surfaces will lower a patient's normal temperature. Body temperature is monitored during surgery to ensure that it does not become dangerously low. Sometimes hypothermia is desirable for certain lengthy procedures to decrease metabolic needs of the body. However, if the patient's temperature drops too low, warmed IV fluids may be administered, or a body warming device may be used. Hypothermia can adversely affect cardiac function and may make the body more susceptible to infection. Keeping the body at a normal temperature has been found to decrease postoperative wound infection and is especially important during colon surgery (Melling et al., 2002). Prophylactic antibiotics work best when given in the OR (Agency for Healthcare Research and Quality, 2007).

Malignant hyperthermia is an inherited disorder. In patients with malignant hyperthermia, muscle metabolism and heat production increase rapidly and uncontrollably in response to the stress of surgery and some anesthetic agents. Fever, tachycardia, cyanosis, tachypnea, muscle rigidity, diaphoresis, hypotension, and irregular heart rate develop. If not treated quickly, cardiac arrest can occur. The circulating nurse monitors the patient's temperature along with the anesthesia care provider. If the temperature begins to rise rapidly, anesthesia is discontinued and the surgical team takes measures to correct the physiologic problems.

During a surgical procedure the patient is placed in one position for an extended period of time. Such positioning places the patient at risk for injury, such as problems of immobility and pressure damage to the skin and underlying tissue. A variety of materials are used for padding pressure areas and stabilizing the patient's body. The circulating nurse must understand the risk factors for each surgical position and must pad joints and pressure areas accordingly. Joint problems and pressure ulcers can develop days after surgery from damage that occurred during the surgical procedure.

Get Ready for the NCLEX® Examination!

Key Points

- Surgical procedures vary in reason, urgency, degree of risk, and extent (see Table 4-1).
- The use of lasers, fiberoptic endoscopes with high-resolution video cameras, operating microscopes, and robotic technology has revolutionized surgery.
- Autologous transfusion or bloodless surgery techniques are reducing problems that can be caused by blood transfusions from outside donors.
- A thorough assessment is performed by the nurse, and any risk factors for surgery are identified (see Focused Assessment on p. 65).
- The elderly patient is at much greater risk from surgery and anesthesia than a younger adult.
- Cultural factors and preferences should always be assessed and considered.
- An appropriate individual nursing care plan is formulated for the preoperative period.
- The surgeon must obtain informed consent from the patient before surgery is performed.
- Preoperative procedures are performed in a timely manner.
- The method to be used for postoperative pain control is explained and discussed with the patient.
- Preoperative teaching of exercises to be performed postoperatively is very important; the patient is taught turning, leg, deep breathing, and coughing exercises.
- Immediate preoperative care includes checking to see that all jewelry and metal objects have been removed from the patient.
- A signed surgical consent form is checked before preoperative medication is administered.
- Once preoperative sedation (if ordered) is administered, the patient is cautioned to stay in bed to prevent falls.
- The patient's identity and the correct surgical site are carefully checked and marked before the patient is transported to surgery.
- After the patient leaves for surgery, the patient's room is prepared for postoperative care.
- A Universal Protocol is followed to prevent wrong-site surgery.
- Several measures are instituted to prevent surgical site infection and other complications.
- The operating room is kept as microbe free as possible.
- Surgical asepsis is the responsibility of the entire operating room staff.
- A "time-out" occurs just before the start of the surgical procedure to recheck the patient's identity, the surgical procedure to be performed, and the site of the surgery.
- The scrub person and the circulating nurse, along with the surgeon and anesthesiologist or CRNA, provide care for the patient while in the operating room.
- The circulating nurse and the scrub person have distinctly different roles.
- Anesthesia is used to prevent pain, to achieve adequate muscle relaxation, and to calm fear, allay anxiety, and induce amnesia of an unpleasant experience.
- Inhalant gases and intravenous medications are used to induce general anesthesia, and the patient progresses through stages of induction to total anesthesia.
- Regional anesthesia, procedural (moderate) sedation, or local anesthesia is used for many surgical procedures.
- There is a risk of several complications during the intraoperative period.
- Patients are positioned carefully and pressure points and joints are padded to prevent injury.
- The circulating nurse, anesthesia care provider, and surgeon observe for symptoms of complications, and measures are taken immediately to avert a problem.

Additional Learning Resources

SG Go to your Study Guide for additional learning activities to help you master this chapter content.

 Go to your Evolve website (http://evolve.elsevier.com/deWit/medsurg) for the following FREE learning resources:
- Animations, audio, and video
- Answers and rationales for questions and activities
- Concept Map Creator
- Glossary with pronunciations in English and Spanish
- Interactive Review Questions and Exercises and more!

🖱 Online Resources
- Surgery information, www.yoursurgery.com
- TJC performance measurement, www.jointcommission.org/PerformanceMeasurement.aspx
- Health on the Net Foundation, www.hon.ch/HONselect/Selection/E04.html

Review Questions for the NCLEX® Examination

1. The nurse reinforces the importance of turning, coughing, and deep breathing to a preoperative patient. Which patient statement indicates a need for further instruction?
   1. "I could place a pillow to brace my abdominal incision to reduce pain with coughing."

2. "I would lie still in bed to reduce the risk of injuring my surgical wound."
3. "Coughing would help reduce pneumonia."
4. "Immediately getting out of bed speeds up recuperation."

2. After same-day surgery, the patient is ready to go home when:

1. there is an adult there to drive the patient home.
2. the patient is alert, ambulatory, and able to empty the bladder.
3. pain is controlled with oral analgesia.
4. nausea has passed and the patient is taking fluids.

3. While reviewing the clinical history of a preoperative patient, which patient information warrants immediate notification of the physician?

1. Temperature 101.5° F (38.6° C)
2. Serum sodium 135 mg/dL
3. Bronchovesicular breath sounds
4. Blood pressure 135/80 mm Hg

4. While transferring from the preoperative area to the surgical suite, the patient asks, "Am I going to make it?" An appropriate response by a nurse would be:

1. "Everything will be all right."
2. "Didn't your physician discuss the possible adverse outcomes of the procedure?"
3. "You seem anxious. Tell me more about how you are feeling."
4. "Your physician has performed the procedure several times."

5. During a preoperative teaching session, the patient asks the nurse, "What is general anesthesia?" An accurate explanation would be that it:

1. is provision of a nerve block.
2. is administration of inhalant gas to produce unconsciousness.
3. results in local anesthesia.
4. results in mild sedation and systemic analgesia.

6. During major surgery, the patient is considered at risk for:

1. injury related to placement in one position for extended period of time.
2. altered nutrition: less than body requirements related to prolonged fasting.
3. hypervolemia from irrigating fluids used in surgery.
4. hypertension related to continuous infusion of fluids.

7. When teaching a patient using an incentive spirometer, the nurse determines that the patient's technique is correct if the patient is:

1. exhaling forcibly after holding the breath for 30 seconds.
2. using the spirometer for 5 breaths every hour.

3. taking slow, deep breaths and holding each for at least 3 seconds.
4. exhaling forcibly into the spirometer.

8. Regarding informed consent for a surgical procedure, the nurse is responsible for which aspect(s)? (Select all that apply.)

1. Verifying that the consent has been signed and witnessed before sending the patient to surgery
2. Explaining the risks and benefits of the procedure
3. Determining the mental capacity of the patient
4. Administering any preoperative medications after verification that the consent has been signed
5. Answering general questions regarding postoperative care

9. Which nursing intervention(s) would be considered critical in preoperative preparation of the patient? (Select all that apply.)

1. No solid food intake for at least 6 hours.
2. Allow clear liquids up to 2 hours before major procedures.
3. Ensure timely administration of insulin injections at all times.
4. Withhold all cardiac medications, antihypertensives, and anticonvulsants.
5. Confirm patient compliance with the nothing by mouth (NPO) status.

10. In discussing options for fluid resuscitation during major surgery, the physician indicated availability of bloodless surgery. Bloodless surgery may include which intervention(s)? (Select all that apply.)

1. Administration of Epogen
2. Administration of volume expanders
3. Induction of hypothermia
4. Banking blood before surgery
5. Autologous transfusion

Critical Thinking Questions

Scenario A

Your patient is scheduled for abdominal surgery this morning. You are assigned two other patients to care for as well. One of these patients is stable and will be going home. The other patient is going for a computed tomography (CT) scan at 9:30 A.M.

1. Describe in detail how you would plan your morning care for these three patients.

2. Your surgical patient shares with you that she is having second thoughts about having this surgery. How would you handle the situation?

3. You notice that the patient scheduled for surgery is wearing panties under her gown as she returns from emptying her bladder. You had told her to remove them earlier. How would you handle this situation?

Scenario B

On your first day on the surgical unit, you are assigned a patient who is scheduled for surgery at 10:00 A.M. The following preoperative medications are ordered: Lotensin 10 mg PO with sip of water and cefazolin 250 mg IV 1 hour before incision.

1. What would you check in the patient's chart as part of her preoperative preparation?

2. What steps would you take to complete the preoperative checklist and charting for this patient? When would you start the preoperative preparation?

3. When would you give the dose of Lotensin? How would you handle the dose of cefazolin?

Scenario C

The patient is scheduled for right hip surgery. You have been asked to have her sign the surgical consent form as her surgeon forgot to have her do it when he saw her last evening.

1. What should you do before asking the patient to sign the consent form?

2. She asks when and how she will be "prepped for surgery." What would you tell her?

3. She inquires as to when she will be able to see her family after surgery. What would you tell her?

Care of Postoperative Surgical Patients

Objectives

Theory

1. Describe the care of the patient in the postanesthesia care unit (PACU).
2. Identify points the PACU nurse should cover in report to the floor nurse.
3. Formulate a plan of care for a postoperative patient returning from the PACU.
4. Determine assessment factors for each potential postoperative complication.
5. Prepare the surgical patient for discharge.

Clinical Practice

1. Identify how to promote adequate ventilation of the lungs during recovery from anesthesia in the PACU.

2. Prepare to perform an immediate postoperative assessment when a patient returns to the nursing unit.
3. Apply interventions to prevent postoperative complications.
4. Assess for postoperative pain and provide comfort measures and pain relief.
5. Promote early ambulation and return to independence in activities of daily living.
6. Perform discharge teaching necessary for postoperative home self-care.

Key Terms

anaphylaxis (ă-nă-fă-LĂK-sĭs, p. 93)
atelectasis (ă-tĕ-LĔK-tă-sĭs, p. 84)
dehiscence (dĕ-HĬS-ĕntz, p. 91)
embolus (ĔM-bō-lŭs, p. 88)
evisceration (ē-vĭs-ĕr-Ā-shŭn, p. 91)
hematoma (hē-mă-TŌ-mă, p. 89)
malignant hyperthermia (MH) (hī-pĕr-THĔR-mē-ă, p. 93)

paralytic ileus (păr-ă-LĬT-ĭk ĬL-ē-ŭs, p. 87)
pneumonia (nū-MŌ-nē-ă, p. 86)
purulence (PŪ-rū-lĕns, p. 89)
seroma (sĕ-RŌ-mă, p. 89)
thrombophlebitis (thrŏm-bō-flĕ-BĪ-tĭs, p. 85)
thrombosis (thrŏm-BŌ-sĭs, p. 85)

IMMEDIATE POSTOPERATIVE CARE

POSTANESTHESIA CARE UNIT

When surgery with general anesthesia is completed, the patient is usually transferred to the postanesthesia care unit (PACU) adjacent to the surgical suites (Figure 5-1). Patients who have had spinal anesthesia for a major procedure go to the PACU also. Very critically ill patients, such as those recovering from open heart surgery, are often taken directly to the intensive care unit for anesthesia recovery. Surgical patients who had procedural sedation or a local or regional anesthetic are usually recovered in the ambulatory surgery area. The PACU nurse receives a verbal report from the anesthesia care provider about the procedure, blood loss, anesthesia administered, fluids infused, medications administered, and any problems encountered.

The patient is immediately attached to the cardiac and pulse oximeter monitors, and oxygen is usually administered if the patient had general anesthesia. Oxygen helps eliminate the anesthetic gases and helps

meet the increased metabolic demand for oxygen caused by surgery. Any respiratory problems are immediately addressed, as maintenance of airway and adequate ventilation takes priority. An oral airway may be in place because the anesthesia medications often cause the tongue to occlude the airway. Alternatively, the airway can be opened by moving the jaw forward (Figure 5-2). Suction is on and readily available to clear secretions. If needed, mechanical ventilation is provided. Warm blankets are placed over the patient, vital signs are assessed and compared with baseline readings, and a full neurologic assessment is performed. Neurologic assessment includes level of consciousness, orientation, sensory and motor status, and size, equality, and reactivity of the pupils. The patient may be asleep, drowsy but arousable, or awake.

Determine intake and output to assess function of the urinary system. Closely monitor urinary output. Check all intravenous (IV) lines for patency, verify the correct solutions along with the correct drip rate, and inspect

FIGURE 5-1 Nurse cares for patient in postanesthesia recovery unit.

FIGURE 5-2 Jaw-thrust maneuver to open the airway. The fingers are placed behind the angle of the jaw, lifting the jaw forward. As the jaw moves, the tongue comes forward, opening the airway.

Box 5-1	**Postanesthesia Care Unit Report to Nursing Unit Nurse**

GENERAL INFORMATION
- Patient name, age
- Diagnosis
- Allergies
- Stability level

SURGICAL DATA
- Surgeon's name
- Surgical procedure performed
- Length of surgery time
- Unexpected surgical events
- Vital sign trends during surgery
- Anesthetic administered
- Medications administered during surgery and recovery
- Amount of blood loss and replacement

POSTANESTHESIA CARE COURSE
- Vital signs and oxygen saturation
- Urine output
- Intravenous solutions and blood products administered, with amounts
- Tubes, drains, and equipment in use
- Results of any intraoperative laboratory or diagnostic tests (note whether patient/family has been told pathology results)
- Pain status and time of last dose of analgesia
- Any problems encountered

? **Think Critically**

What is the number one priority of care for the patient in the PACU?

wound drains and evacuation devices for proper function. Assess dressings for unexpected drainage.

Surgical recovery can take from 2 to 6 hours. Because patients are coming out of anesthesia through various stages and are unstable, keep the environment as quiet as possible. Briefly communicate with the staff in hushed tones. The patient may wake up confused and may need reorientation and reassurance that the surgery is over, that he is in the recovery room, and that his family member or relative has been notified. Once the patient is awake, family members are sometimes allowed to visit for a few minutes so that they are assured that their loved one is all right and recovering.

Assessments are performed at least every 15 minutes or according to the status of the patient. Assessment for complications of the particular surgery and anesthesia are ongoing. The patient remains in the PACU until the vital signs are stable and the patient is awake and able to respond to stimuli. A form of the Aldrete scoring system may be used to determine readiness for transfer. Activity, respiration, circulation, consciousness, skin color, and oxygen saturation are each given a score. The patient with a score of 9 or

10 is ready for transfer to the nursing unit. Report is given to the staff nurse (Box 5-1).

For many procedures the patient may be transferred from the operating room (OR) directly back to the same-day surgery unit. Monitor the patient's respirations, circulation, vital signs, neurologic status, fluid balance, wound drainage and dressings, and comfort level. When the vital signs are stable, the patient is allowed to sit up and then is ambulated. If discharge criteria are met, the patient may be discharged when able to ambulate unassisted and empty the bladder. Recovery time in the same-day surgery unit usually takes 1 to 3 hours. Discharge teaching is begun before the surgery and continues once the patient is again alert. Written instructions are always sent home with the patient. If the patient has undergone sedation, another adult driver must provide transportation home after same-day surgery. Advise surgery patients who have received anesthesia or procedural sedation not to resume normal activities or make important decisions for at least 24 hours after surgery. The phone number of the surgeon and signs and symptoms to report are written on the postoperative instruction sheet.

How would you assess a patient to determine whether or not the gag (swallowing) reflex has returned sufficiently after being sedated to allow him to have a few ice chips?

IMMEDIATE POSTOPERATIVE CARE

❖ NURSING MANAGEMENT

■ Assessment (Data Collection)

After the patient is transferred from recovery, check identity, settle the patient in bed, and perform an initial postoperative assessment. **Airway, breathing, and circulation are always the top priorities.** This provides a baseline against which frequent postoperative assessment data can be compared to prevent or quickly detect signs of complications. Vital signs are taken more frequently if they are unstable; this is a nursing judgment.

 Focused Assessment

Postoperative Assessment

AREA	ASSESSMENT	SCHEDULE
Airway	Lung sounds, depth and quality of air movement; respiratory rate Oxygen saturation Oxygen delivery at rate ordered and patent system	Auscultate lungs initially; respiratory rate q 15 min until fully aroused from anesthesia; then assess quality of respirations with vital signs assessment Note per vital signs schedule and whenever in room Check oxygen delivery system with initial assessment and each shift
Circulation	Auscultate heart; check peripheral pulses and sensation, especially distal to surgical site; assess skin color	Initially, q 4 hr × 2, then with vital signs; if surgery was on an extremity, assess each time vital signs are measured
Mental status	Level of consciousness and orientation	Initially and then with full vital signs
Vital signs	Temperature Blood pressure, pulse, and respirations	Check initially; then q 8 hr once stable Check q 15 min × 1 hr; q 30 min × 4; q 1 hr × 4; q 4 hr × 24–48 hr; or per agency protocol
Fluid status and hydration	Intravenous infusion site and flow rate Intake and output Skin turgor; oral membranes	Check initially and when in room Check each shift Check initially and each shift
Surgical site	Check for bleeding; mark drainage on dressing; assess wound drainage in containers	Initially and q 1 hr × 4; then with vital signs
Gastrointestinal	Auscultate bowel sounds; assess abdomen Check nasogastric drainage color, character, amount	Initially, then q 8 hr Check drainage whenever in room
Tubes	Check for patency and function of each	Initially; then with vital signs and after turning
Kidney function	Assess urine output from Foley catheter; must void within 8 hr if no Foley in place	Initially and q 1 hr × 4; then if >30 mL/hr, q 4 hr
Pain	Use a pain scale and observation of nonverbal behaviors	Initially and with vital signs; assess at least q 3 hr
Skin	Pressure areas over bony prominences	Initially and q 2 hr
Safety	All equipment is intact and safely functioning	Initially and each shift

Assignment Considerations

Postoperative Vital Signs

Because postoperative patients need close vigilance in the early postoperative period, it is best not to assign the taking of frequent vital signs to unlicensed assistive personnel (UAP) for the first couple of hours. Other parameters besides the measurement of vital signs need to be checked on a frequent schedule. After the first couple of hours, the task of vital sign measurement can be assigned to a UAP proficient in obtaining accurate measurements. Remind the UAP of exactly what to report: temperature elevation above 99.8° F (37.1° C), blood pressure alteration of a specific amount down or up from the baseline, tachycardia, and respiratory rate increase above or below normal range.

Monitoring for signs of the various surgical complications that may occur is a major nursing responsibility. **The first 72 hours after surgery require frequent observations to detect signs of postoperative complications.**

■ Nursing Diagnosis

Nursing diagnoses commonly used for postoperative patients who have undergone general anesthesia are:

- Impaired gas exchange related to the effect of anesthesia on the lungs

- Ineffective breathing pattern related to analgesia and pain
- Impaired skin integrity related to surgical incision
- Risk for infection related to surgical wound
- Risk for injury related to sedation, decreased level of consciousness, or excessive blood loss
- Acute pain related to disruption of tissue
- Ineffective airway clearance related to inability to breathe deeply and cough without discomfort
- Deficient fluid volume related to fluid loss and nothing by mouth (NPO) status
- Risk for constipation related to opioid analgesics, decreased mobility, and decreased peristalsis
- Self-care deficit, bathing/hygiene related to decreased mobility, use of tubes, and presence of dressings
- Ineffective tissue perfusion related to surgery, anesthesia, and positioning in the OR
- Ineffective coping related to loss of body part or change in body image
- Impaired urinary elimination related to effects of anesthesia or presence of catheter

For patients who have undergone spinal anesthesia, include all of the above diagnoses plus:

- Impaired physical mobility related to effects of spinal anesthesia
- Risk for injury related to decreased sensation and movement in lower extremities

■ Planning

The expected outcomes depend on the individual specific nursing diagnoses. General *nursing* goals are:

- Maintain patent airway and adequate respiratory exchange.
- Maintain adequate tissue perfusion.
- Promote normal physiologic body function.
- Prevent injury.
- Promote comfort and rest.
- Promote wound healing.
- Promote psychological adjustment to lifestyle or body image changes.
- Prevent postoperative complications.

When planning your work for the shift, allow time for frequent postoperative assessments. Careful planning is essential so that proper care for the early postoperative patient does not override the needs of other patients.

■ Implementation

Maintain Ventilation

The postoperative patient is at risk for respiratory problems from the effects of anesthesia on the lungs, being in one position for the duration of surgery, and limited mobility in the immediate postoperative period. **Maintaining a patent airway is a priority measure.** Unless contraindicated, the patient must be positioned on the side or with the head turned to the side to prevent aspiration until fully recovered, alert, and with the gag reflex intact. Monitor oxygen saturation closely, and administer oxygen as ordered.

 Elder Care Points

Providing adequate pain control for older patients has been shown to prevent respiratory complications because—with pain controlled—patients will breathe more deeply and are able to follow instructions for respiratory care (Shea et al., 2002).

Some degree of atelectasis (collapse of alveoli in the lungs) exists after anesthesia. A mild hypoxia is usually present for about 48 hours after surgery. A large percentage of all patients who have had either abdominal or thoracic surgery suffer from increasing atelectasis and pneumonitis. **If any area of the lung remains atelectatic for more than 72 hours, hypostatic pneumonia from retained secretions is likely to occur.**

Hypostatic pneumonia results when lack of movement or of position change causes stasis of secretions, which become a breeding ground for bacteria. Auscultate the lungs carefully for abnormal sounds indicating retained secretions, assess the rate and depth of breathing, and encourage the patient to deep breathe and cough every 2 hours. Coughing to remove secretions may be contraindicated for patients who have had a hernia repair or eye, ear, brain, jaw, or plastic surgery. Check the physician's orders. If the patient cannot cough effectively, instruct to "huff" cough (see Patient Teaching, Lung Exercises on pp. 71-72).

Be certain the patient turns every 2 hours, which changes the distribution of gas and blood flow in the lungs and helps move secretions. Early ambulation is ordered to promote ventilation. **Signs of complications for procedures other than thoracic surgery are complaints of shortness of breath, pain on inspiration, and extreme fatigue (which is related to hypoxemia).**

The use of an incentive spirometer is especially helpful to prevent atelectasis and hypoventilation (see Chapter 4). It should be used every hour while the patient is awake for the first 24 hours following surgery, and every 2 hours thereafter. The elderly patient may need extra coaching to master the spirometer technique.

 Elder Care Points

The risk of hypoventilation is greater in the elderly because lung expansion may be hampered by calcification of costal cartilage and weakened respiratory muscles.

A pulse oximeter may be used to determine blood oxygenation. Monitor oxygen readings periodically and report oxygen saturation (SaO_2) readings below 95%.

Maintain Circulation and Tissue Perfusion

When considerable blood is lost during surgery, a blood transfusion may be ordered. Autologous blood may be transfused if the patient donated blood several weeks before surgery or if the patient's blood was collected as it was lost during surgery. This blood is filtered and returned to the patient.

If surgery involves an extremity (arm, leg, foot, or hand) or if a procedure has been done to the pelvic area, the distal or peripheral pulse is checked during each full assessment. Swelling at the surgical site can compress vessels and decrease blood flow distal to the surgical site. The skin distal to the surgical site should be warm to the touch, and there should be brisk capillary refill in the fingers or toes. Color, movement, and sensation of the fingers and toes should be checked to detect nerve compression from swelling and edema.

Blood pressure and pulse should be compared with preoperative values to determine if there are significant changes. An increase in pulse may indicate that internal bleeding is occurring, but it can also signify incomplete pain control. Blood pressure falling below the patient's normal baseline level may indicate major bleeding.

Core Measures (The Joint Commission [TJC], 2008) require antithrombosis therapy after many surgeries. The use of antiembolic (elastic) stockings increases venous return from the legs and helps prevent stasis of blood in the lower extremities. The stockings should be checked frequently to ensure that they fit smoothly. They may be removed for 20 minutes per shift for bathing, to allow air circulation to the skin, and/or full skin inspection (Winslow & Brosz, 2008).

If the patient is at considerable risk of venous **thrombosis** (blood clot), the surgeon may order pneumatic sequential compression devices (SCDs) to be applied to the legs. SCDs alternately compress and release, squeezing the legs and propelling blood along the vessels (Figure 5-3). Orders for ambulation are written as soon as the patient is able to be up and walking.

FIGURE 5-3 Sequential compression devices in place to prevent thrombus formation.

 Clinical Cues

Compression stockings should be applied at least 2 hours preoperatively and worn until the patient is fully ambulatory. Problems occur if the stockings are not fitted correctly, particularly with thigh-high stockings.

Low-molecular-weight subcutaneous heparin injections may be ordered as a general precaution and for any patient who has a history of **thrombophlebitis** (clot and inflammation in a blood vessel). Patients undergoing hip surgery also receive heparin. Thrombophlebitis may not occur until after the fifth day of bed rest, when stasis has allowed a clot to form and irritate the vein. Question the patient about pain or tenderness in the legs. If the patient complains of leg pain, gently assess the skin for increased warmth, and notify the physician.

 Safety Alert

Preventing Embolus

Never massage the patient's legs, which might dislodge a blood clot and cause an embolus that could lodge in the lungs, heart, or brain, causing a pulmonary embolus, myocardial infarction, or stroke.

 Think Critically

The initial vital sign readings for your patient on return from surgery were blood pressure (BP) 138/86, pulse 76, respirations 14, temperature 97.7° F (36.5° C). An hour later they were BP 126/74, pulse 80, respirations 14, temperature 98.0° F (36.7° C). What action, if any, should you take?

Prevent Injury

Safety is a primary concern until the patient is fully recovered from anesthesia. Always leave the bed in the low position after administering care. Remind the patient to call for assistance as needed and be certain the call bell is within reach. Core Measures (The Joint Commission, 2011) require the use of interventions to prevent falls. Remember that you are the patient's advocate while the patient is still recovering from surgery and anesthesia or is under the influence of narcotic analgesia. Be certain that all appropriate safety measures are listed on the patient's care plan.

Reassure the patient who has had spinal anesthesia that it is normal for the legs to feel numb and heavy, and that feeling will soon return to normal. Maintain a flat position with only a pillow until feeling returns. Sense of position in space will return to the legs first, followed by sensation to deep pressure, voluntary movement, and finally feeling of superficial pain and temperature. A feeling of "pins and needles" in the legs is common. The patient is susceptible to hypotension until all effects of the spinal anesthesia are gone. Lying flat for 6 to 8 hours may decrease the chance of post–spinal anesthesia headache. If a headache develops, staying flat in bed reduces the pain. Keep IV fluid running as ordered. **Encourage the patient to drink a lot of fluids, including those containing caffeine.** The patient can turn the head to the side and sip from a straw while someone else holds the container. Fluids and caffeine raise the vascular pressure at the spinal puncture site and help to seal the hole.

 Think Critically

How would care for the patient who has had spinal anesthesia differ from care for the patient who has had general anesthesia?

Many surgical procedures last several hours, which means that the patient has been lying motionless, in a fixed position, on a hard table for a considerable time. Check pressure points related to the position that the patient was in during surgery and provide padding and appropriate positioning for areas that are painful (see Chapter 43).

 Think Critically

Your postoperative patient was placed in a right side-lying position during surgery. Which specific places should you check for signs of pressure problems? How would you position the patient who is complaining of pain in the right hip, as well as pain in the left flank where the surgery occurred?

 Elder Care Points

Because skin is fragile and there is less subcutaneous tissue in an elderly person, check bony prominences carefully for signs of breakdown. Joint strains can occur from the positioning necessary for certain types of surgery; perform position changes slowly and gently.

Prevent Infection

Use aseptic technique when caring for the postoperative patient. Good hand hygiene is the primary means of preventing infection. Dressing changes are performed with strict sterile technique while the patient is in the hospital; the patient may use clean technique at home. Encouraging fluid intake in order to flush the bladder will help prevent a bladder infection for the patient who was catheterized or has an indwelling catheter. Turning, coughing, deep breathing, and ambulation will assist in preventing pneumonia (inflammation and accumulation of exudate in the lung) from retained secretions and lack of movement. Aseptically handling drains and aseptically emptying wound drainage devices prevents the entry of microorganisms.

Core Measures (TJC, 2008) state that if the patient is receiving a prophylactic antibiotic, it must be discontinued within 24 hours after surgery. Assess the surgical wound area each shift and assess for signs of infection (e.g., local pain, increased tenderness, warmth, redness, or drainage of purulent material). Monitor the blood count for increasing leukocytes (white blood cells [WBCs]) and the body temperature for unexpected increase.

Maintain Fluid Balance and Elimination

Urine output is closely monitored after surgery. If the patient has an indwelling catheter, observe the urine in the bag every hour in the early postoperative period. Report urine flow less than 30 mL/hr to the charge nurse. Check the catheter to ensure that it is not kinked and that the connecting tubing is not lying beneath the patient. The patient without a catheter in place must void within 4 to 8 hours depending on the type of surgery undergone. If the patient is unable to empty the bladder spontaneously, obtain an order for catheterization. **If flow is less than 60 mL over a 2-hour period, the surgeon must be notified.**

 Assignment Considerations

Urinary Output

When a UAP is assigned to turn the patient every 2 hours, remind the UAP to check that the tubing of any indwelling catheter is not under the patient or crimped. If the UAP is assigned the task of emptying the Foley catheter bag at the end of the shift, ask that you be notified if there is less than 30 mL of urine per hour for the shift in the output. Verify that the UAP knows to maintain sterility of the urinary catheter system and to wipe the spout with an alcohol sponge after emptying the urine bag.

Patients usually return from surgery with an IV infusion running. Depending on the type of surgery, IV fluids may be continued for a few days or may be discontinued after the fluid has infused. Check orders to see that the correct solution is running. **No potassium additive should be given until the urine flow is at least 30 mL/hr.** Potassium may cause hyperkalemia if kidney function is not adequate. Assess the IV site for patency, flow rate, and complications each hour. Document all IV fluids administered as intake on the intake and output record.

As soon as the patient is conscious and the gag reflex has returned, offer a few ice chips or sips of water, unless there is an order to maintain NPO status. Document all oral intake, as well as IV fluids administered. At the end of each shift, calculate and document the difference between the intake and output. Because fluids were lost during surgery, the body will initially retain fluid. Postoperatively, the output will slowly increase until it is more than the intake; after 2 to 3 days, fluids should again be balanced.

Clinical Cues

A cup of ice equals ½ cup of water.

Anesthesia may cause nausea, and vomiting. Keep the emesis basin close by, and position the patient on the side to prevent aspiration. Check the orders to determine on which side the patient can be positioned. The surgeon usually writes an order for medication in the event of excessive nausea or vomiting. **To prevent stress on the incision and sutures, it is best to medicate the patient before actual vomiting occurs.**

Apply a cool cloth to the forehead and back of the neck, rinse the mouth, rid the room of odors, and provide a quiet environment to help reduce nausea. After emesis, mouth care should be provided. If vomiting is uncontrolled with medication, a nasogastric (NG) tube, which suctions stomach contents and prevents fluid and electrolyte loss, may need to be inserted.

Surgeons often place an NG tube after abdominal procedures because handling of the gastrointestinal tract and general anesthesia cause peristalsis to halt, which means that secretions will not flow through the system properly. The NG tube removes gathering secretions. When an NG tube is in place, check that the tube is positioned and functioning properly and that the suction is set according to orders. Assess the amount of drainage produced every 1 to 2 hours. If the drainage turns dark brown and grainy, it should be checked for blood using a special reagent. Report the presence of blood to the surgeon.

 Elder Care Points

Fluid and electrolyte shifts may cause confusion in the elderly patient after surgery. Skin and vessels in the elderly are more fragile, so the IV site must be assessed frequently for signs of infiltration. Adjustment to fluid shifts is more difficult, and the elderly patient is very prone to postural hypotension when changing to a standing position. Be sure to provide adequate support.

Promote Gastrointestinal Function

A healthy surgical patient may be kept on nothing but IV fluids for several days without developing a serious nutritional problem. If extensive tissue repair is required for healing, supplemental nutrition by enteral or parenteral feeding may be started (see Chapters 3 and 29 for details of enteral and total parenteral nutrition). A patient who is kept on IV fluids only will lose some weight as there are insufficient calories in the IV fluids to meet total daily requirements. A liter of 5% dextrose in water contains only 200 calories.

Eating after surgery with general anesthesia is not allowed until bowel sounds have returned, due to the risk of developing paralytic ileus (failure of forward movement of bowel contents).

 Clinical Cues

When permitted by the surgeon, chewing sugarless gum can speed bowel recovery after surgery. Gum chewing has also been shown to be effective for recovery from paralytic ileus (Barclay, 2006).

At least once per shift, listen for bowel sounds in all four quadrants. Once they are heard, the surgeon usually orders clear liquids, followed by full liquids, then a regular diet if the preceding diets have been tolerated. The patient may be allowed to eat right away after spinal anesthesia.

Discomfort from abdominal distention and considerable flatus may occur after general anesthesia because peristalsis ceases. Taking only small amounts of liquid or food at a time, drinking only tepid liquids, and refraining from drinking with a straw helps keep flatus to a minimum, and ambulating helps move and evacuate gas. If permitted, the patient can try resting in a slight Trendelenburg's position, with the legs and rectum higher than the stomach, which may assist in evacuation of flatus.

Once the patient is eating again, a bowel movement should occur within 2 to 3 days. If this does not occur, an order for a suppository or laxative may be needed to stimulate a bowel movement. Patients receiving narcotic analgesics may become constipated and require stool softeners or laxatives to produce normal bowel movements.

? **Think Critically**

Name four specific interventions to prevent constipation in a postoperative patient who is receiving narcotic analgesics for pain.

Promote Comfort

Pain and discomfort interfere with rest and inhibit the processes of healing and repair. Although analgesic drugs are almost always prescribed for the postoperative patient, comfort measures also should be used. Nonsteroidal anti-inflammatory drugs (NSAIDs) and non-narcotic analgesics work on both the peripheral and the central nervous systems to control pain and may be used to augment opioids. Opioids tend to depress respirations and the cough reflex and therefore may contribute to the development of pulmonary problems. Opioids also can increase the possibility of nausea and vomiting. Using other drugs in combination with opioids helps to control pain with the fewest side effects.

Pain must be reduced so that the patient will rest, turn, cough, and deep breathe frequently, and medication should be given consistently for the first 24 to 48 hours postoperatively. **Assess pain level and effectiveness of analgesia using a pain scale at least every**

3 hours. Remind the patient to request medication before the pain becomes severe.

If the patient complains of pain on transfer to the unit, refer to the notes from the recovery unit nurse. Note any medications administered both preoperatively and postoperatively. **When droperidol plus fentanyl (Innovar) is given preoperatively, narcotic pain medication should be reduced by half for 8 hours postoperatively to prevent serious respiratory depression.** If respirations are within normal limits and there is no contraindication to doing so, medicate the patient promptly with the ordered analgesic. If it is too soon to give more analgesia, reposition the patient, be sure the bladder is not distended and causing discomfort, check that the patient is warm enough, and use other comfort measures to relieve the pain, such as distraction and imagery. Note when analgesia is due and have it ready to administer at the appointed time.

Teach relaxation techniques that can help decrease the patient's discomfort (see Chapter 7). Pain medication may be administered by subcutaneous or intramuscular injection, intravenously, epidurally, or by intermittent administration of local anesthetic into the pleural space via an intrapleural catheter. Two methods commonly used for pain control are the epidural catheter and the patient-controlled analgesia pump. Pain, methods of pain control, and pain medications and their administration are discussed in greater detail in Chapter 7.

Operating rooms are kept very cool so that the staff members working under the bright lights do not become overheated and growth of organisms is inhibited. The patient's temperature in this environment often decreases, especially during prolonged abdominal surgery in which the peritoneal cavity has been open for a long period. Warming during surgery is recommended, and the Core Measures specifically state the importance of warming the patient undergoing colon surgery (TJC, 2008). Postoperatively, the patient may feel cold and should be kept warm with extra blankets or warmed bath blankets applied under the top covers. Placing socks on the patient's feet may help. Some anesthetic agents may cause tremors as they are metabolized. If uncontrollable shivering occurs, contact the physician for medication orders.

Dressings on extremities should be checked to be certain that they are not so tight that circulation is impaired. Check the pulse, skin temperature, sensation, and movement distal to the surgical site to evaluate circulation (neurovascular assessment). You should be able to slip your little finger between a dressing and the extremity.

Occasionally, continuous hiccoughs occur after surgery, making the patient quite uncomfortable. Having the patient breathe into a paper bag will often relieve the hiccoughs, and sedatives and tranquilizers are sometimes prescribed to promote relaxation and reduce irritation of the phrenic nerve. Severe, persistent cases of hiccoughs may require surgical interruption of impulses along the nerve pathways to remove the cause of the spasms of the diaphragm.

Complementary and Alternative Therapies

Stopping Hiccoughs

An alternative treatment for hiccoughs is to massage the earlobes. Massage activates the acupressure points, interrupting the hiccough reflex. Other commonly used remedies include:

- Fill a glass with at least 4 oz of water. Lean over a sink and drink the water from the back side of the glass. Drink continuously until the glass is empty.
- Stick a finger in each ear, and hold your breath.
- Drink from a glass that someone else is holding for you.
- Breathe into a paper bag deeply 20 times.
- Place a teaspoon of sugar or peanut butter on the tongue and let it slowly dissolve; the hiccoughs will be gone when the sugar or peanut butter has dissolved.

Promote Rest and Activity

The patient needs to sleep after surgery. Keep the room quiet and group nursing activities to prevent waking the patient more than necessary. At least every 2 hours, the patient must do leg exercises and change position. Orders for ambulation may begin within several hours after surgery. Raise the head of the bed first and let the body adjust to the position change. Then sit the patient on the side of the bed, allowing the legs to dangle over the side with the feet on the floor. After a few minutes, slowly assist the patient to stand. Assist the patient to walk around the room, or for at least a few steps. Use a gait belt and have someone assist you if the patient is very weak. Pain medication can be timed to decrease pain during ambulation if it does not make the patient too groggy.

Emphasize that exercise is vital to prevent circulatory problems and offer praise for all efforts. Keeping blood from pooling in the extremities helps prevent thrombus formation and embolus (a thrombus or clot that travels and lodges elsewhere in the body). Continue to ambulate, in the hospital or at home, on a set schedule until the patient is able to do so independently. In many hospitals, physical therapy orders will be written and the physical therapist will be responsible for ambulating the patient and overseeing range-of-motion exercises.

If the patient is on strict bed rest, range-of-motion exercises must be performed at least four times a day. The patient may do active range of motion on most joints, but passive range of motion on joints the patient is unable to exercise must be done unless physical therapy visits have been ordered. Family members also may help with these exercises.

Promote Wound Healing

Surgical incisions most often heal by primary, or first, intention (Table 5-1). Adequate rest, sufficient blood supply, and proper nutrition all promote wound healing. Rest decreases the metabolic rate and allows nutrients to be used for healing rather than activity. *Proteins* provide the amino acids that are the building blocks of tissue and are vital to the healing process. Blood transports amino acids and other elements needed for rebuilding tissue and is essential to healing. Good circulation ensures that blood reaches the wound. *Vitamin C* is necessary for collagen production, the formation of capillaries that bring blood to the healing tissues, and for resistance to infection. The minerals *zinc, copper,* and *iron* also assist in the formation of collagen.

🍎 Nutrition Considerations

Foods High in Vitamin C and Protein

FOODS HIGH IN VITAMIN C	FOODS HIGH IN PROTEIN
Citrus fruits and juices	Meats: chicken, beef, pork, lamb*
Strawberries	Cottage cheese
Cantaloupe	Milk*
Tomatoes	Cheese
Bell peppers	Peanut butter
Cabbage	Beans
Turnip or collard greens	Eggs
Broccoli	Ice cream
Mangos	Grain products: breads, pasta
Peaches	Tofu; soy products
Pineapple	
Potatoes	

*Meats and milk products contain the highest amounts of protein.

Table 5-1   Phases of Primary Intention Wound Healing*

PHASE	ACTIVITY
Phase I	
Acute inflammatory reaction (3–4 days)	Process of hemostasis. Constriction of blood vessels, platelet aggregation and the formation of fibrin, and epithelial cell migration. Phagocytosis occurs. Scab forms.
Phase II	
Proliferation and granulation (3rd or 4th day to 2–3 wk)	Macrophages clear debris, fibroblasts synthesize collagen, capillary networks are built, granulation tissue is formed. Closure by contracture begins.
Phase III	
Scar maturation and contracture (3–6 wk)	Remodeling with collagen lysis and synthesis; scar tissue thins and becomes paler, but stronger.

*A surgical incision most often heals by primary intention. Many accidental wounds and some infected wounds heal by secondary or tertiary intention.

⚡ Elder Care Points

- The elderly person often has chronic diseases that interfere with oxygenation, transport of nutrients to the cells, and removal of waste from the cells.
- Vitamin and mineral deficiencies are common in the elderly, contributing to poor wound healing.
- Regeneration of tissue takes more time in the elderly, partially because of the slower metabolic rate that occurs with age.

Factors Interfering with Wound Healing. Mechanical injury from friction, pressure, or abrasion—such as can occur when tape is removed—disrupts the healing tissue and prolongs wound healing. Physical injury destroys granulation tissue, which is the framework on which new cells grow and mature to form a covering for the wound. Handle all wounds gently and shield them from injury. When dressings are removed from a wound, take care not to dislodge granulation tissue. **Smoking decreases the amount of hemoglobin available to carry oxygen to the healing tissues and prolongs healing time.**

The presence of pathogenic organisms in a wound prolongs the inflammatory process and delays healing. Anti-infective drugs are sometimes given postoperatively to prevent wound infection, and should be administered as ordered to maintain appropriate blood levels of the drugs. Corticosteroids taken for a chronic condition will slow the healing process because they suppress the immune and inflammatory response. **Excessive stress, apprehension, and emotional disturbances seem to make the body more vulnerable to invasion by foreign organisms by depressing the immune system.** When under excessive stress, the body also is less able to mobilize the elements and cells that promote healing.

Interventions for Wound Care. The surgical wound should be inspected during dressing changes, or at least once a day. Assessment includes observing the incision line for signs of excessive swelling, formation of a hematoma (blood-filled swelling), seroma (serum-filled swelling), redness, and tearing of the skin or other signs of separation of the edges of skin that have been sutured together. Normally, a surgical wound is sealed within hours and little drainage is expected. Report and document evidence of bleeding, purulence (pus), or any other sign that the wound is not healing properly. Document the appearance of any drainage. Drainage may be serous (clear or very light yellow), serosanguineous (reddish yellow), or sanguineous (blood red). Documentation should include whether sutures or staples are intact and the wound edges are well approximated.

The best way to prevent hospital-acquired infection of a surgical wound is always to wash your hands before doing wound care or touching the patient, to use aseptic technique and Standard Precautions for dressing changes, and to change the dressings as ordered. Additional factors that may slow wound healing in a postoperative patient include vomiting, abdominal distention, and strenuous respiratory efforts, such as coughing and forcefully exhaling breaths of air without proper splinting of the incision. The wound should be properly splinted for coughing to prevent dehiscence of the incision (see Figure 4-2).

Dressings. Surgical dressings should be checked each time vital signs are taken for the first 24 hours after surgery, every 4 hours during the next 24 hours, and then at least every 8 hours as long as the surgical wound is covered with a dressing. If a wound is not expected to drain, but drainage is evident, the surgeon should be notified. If drainage is outlined and the time and date noted, the nurse can tell if the wound is draining more than it should over a period of hours. The surgeon usually does the first dressing change. If the dressing becomes saturated before this, it should be reinforced by placing more dressing material over the area. If it is within the orders, remove outer dressings—leaving those in direct contact with the wound—and secure new outer dressings in place. When there is excessive drainage, the dressing probably will require reinforcing every 4 hours. Changing the dressing more often than once a shift is not recommended because of the dangers of introducing infectious agents, of traumatizing the wound, and of interfering with tissue regeneration.

Each time the dressing is changed, the amount and characteristics of drainage on the dressing should be noted and documented. If the wound is infected, the odor of the drainage can give a clue as to the kind of organism causing the infection. A musty odor is characteristic of aerobic organisms. An acrid (sharp, stinging) or putrid (foul) odor is characteristic of anaerobes. Anaerobic infections are frequently seen in colorectal and vaginal surgery. An infected wound should be cultured to see what organism is causing the infection.

Drains. Drains are used to (1) prevent accumulation of fluids or air at the operative site; (2) protect suture lines; and (3) remove specific fluids, such as bile, cerebrospinal fluid, or drainage from an abscess. Drains not attached to a suction device are attached to a drainage bag or have dressings placed to catch the fluid. An example of a drain is the *Penrose*, which is inserted into the abdominal cavity or any other area where an abscess, fistula, or other condition requires drainage (Figure 5-4). A T-tube drain may be placed in the common bile duct after surgery on the gallbladder or liver.

Some drains are connected to an apparatus that creates continuous suction to facilitate removal of fluid and gas. If a drain is kinked, the accumulated fluid and gas can cause pain, create dead air space

FIGURE 5-4 Wound drain and suction devices. **A,** Penrose drain. **B,** T-tube drain. **C,** Hemovac drainage system. **D,** Jackson-Pratt drain and reservoir.

(which delays healing), damage the healing tissue at the suture lines, and delay healing by compressing surrounding capillaries and cutting off oxygen supply to the cells.

One kind of drain system is the closed-wound suction device (e.g., Hemovac). The drainage catheter is connected to a spring-loaded drum and is collapsed at least once a shift to create the desired suction, which pulls fluid into a collection area of the device.

Jackson-Pratt suction devices are about the size of the bulb on a blood pressure cuff and have a valve on top. The valve is opened to allow removal of fluid and to collapse the bulb; the valve is then closed to create negative pressure, which provides the suction. As drainage accumulates in the bulb, it is emptied and recompressed (Figure 5-5). This procedure should be done to Jackson-Pratt suction devices at least once per shift.

Removing Sutures and Staples. When an order is written to remove sutures or staples, check the order, gather the proper equipment, inform the patient about the procedure, correctly identify the patient, wash hands, don gloves, and inspect the incision carefully. For a long incision or an incision over a joint, remove every other suture or staple first (Figure 5-6). If the edges of the incision do not pull apart, remove the rest of the sutures or staples. Often *Steri-Strips* (small, reinforced strips of adhesive) are applied to hold the incision together until healing is complete.

Prevent Postoperative Complications

Table 5-2 summarizes the major postoperative complications and the nursing interventions to prevent them. Some complications are immediately life threatening.

FIGURE 5-5 Reactivating surgical wound suction devices by compressing the suction device after emptying the reservoir. **A,** Hemovac. **B,** Jackson-Pratt.

FIGURE 5-6 Surgical staples are removed with a special implement.

Wound Infection. Infection of a wound can occur in any surgical procedure, but it is more common in wounds caused by accidental injury and in wounds that were already infected at the time of surgery. A prophylactic antibiotic may be ordered to prevent the occurrence of postoperative wound infection. **If an infection is going to develop, it usually becomes apparent 2 to 7 days postoperatively.** Most patients will already be at home when postoperative infection becomes evident.

> ### Clinical Cues
>
> *Subjective* complaints that may indicate infection include fatigue, loss of appetite, headache, nausea, or general malaise or pain. *Objective* signs may include pain, redness, swelling and induration in the area, purulent drainage, fever, increased pulse rate, elevated WBC count, and swollen lymph nodes in adjacent areas.

If an infection occurs, cultures are obtained and appropriate antibiotics are given for a specific length of time. Wound irrigations may be ordered for an open, infected wound. Sterile normal saline is the most common solution for this purpose. The wound may be packed with dressings moistened with the sterile saline solution.

A noninfected wound should not be cleaned or irrigated with anything but sterile normal saline; other substances irritate the tissue and slow healing. Transmission-based isolation precautions or contact precautions are instituted when a wound is infected (see Chapter 6). Gowns and gloves are worn when performing dressing changes or when irrigating infected wounds. If splattering is likely, protective eyewear and masks are also worn. Soiled dressings and supplies are bagged in plastic barrier bags to be deposited in a biohazard trash receptacle. **Dressings from an infected wound should never be placed in the patient's room trash container.**

Dehiscence and Evisceration. When caring for a patient who has undergone abdominal surgery, you must be alert for possible disruption or separation of some or all the layers of the surgical wound. This is called dehiscence. If the wound completely separates and the contents of the abdominal cavity (viscera) protrude through the incision, the condition is called evisceration (Figure 5-7).

> ### Clinical Cues
>
> Dehiscence can occur at any time during the postoperative period, but it most commonly occurs between the 5th and 12th postoperative days—when the patient is feeling stronger and more active, but healing is not complete, or when infection has occurred. When checking an abdominal surgical wound, be particularly aware of any drainage on the dressing. There is often a noticeable increase in the amount of serosanguineous drainage on the dressing before the separation of the wound layers becomes apparent. Subjectively, the patient may not notice any symptoms until there is a feeling of "giving way" in the wound.

Wound separation or disruption usually is brought on by a sudden strain or stress on the suture lines (e.g., when the patient sneezes, coughs, or has an episode of retching and vomiting). **Patients most at risk for dehiscence and evisceration are those who are diabetic, obese, malnourished, or dehydrated; have a malignancy; have experienced multiple traumas to the abdomen; or have an infected wound.** Abdominal distention and broken sutures are other factors in

Table 5-2   Postoperative Complications

PROBLEM	SIGNS AND SYMPTOMS	PREVENTIVE INTERVENTIONS
Atelectasis	Decreased breath sounds over areas not aerating; dyspnea	Deep breathing and coughing; use of incentive spirometer; early ambulation; teach to cough properly.
Pneumonia: hypostatic, aspiration, or bacterial	Fever, malaise, increased sputum, purulent sputum, cough, flushed skin, dyspnea, pain on inspiration; abnormal breath sounds, crackles, rhonchi	Deep breathing, coughing, and frequent turning; early ambulation; incentive spirometer use; range-of-motion exercises if unable to ambulate; medication if bacterial.
Paralytic (adynamic) ileus	No bowel sounds 24–36 hr after surgery or fewer than 5 sounds/min	Monitor bowel sounds; encourage early ambulation; nothing by mouth as ordered. Do not feed until bowel sounds return.
Thrombophlebitis	Pain or warmth in calf of leg, swollen leg, warm area to touch on leg; possible temperature elevation	Encourage leg exercises; keep the patient well hydrated; encourage ambulation; use anti-embolic stockings or devices.
Urinary retention	Distended bladder; inability to void spontaneously	Palpate bladder; encourage voiding, catheterize if unable to void within 8 hr per order; medicate to increase urinary sphincter tone as ordered.
Urinary tract infection	Dysuria, frequency, foul-smelling urine	Force fluids when allowed; encourage frequent voiding; keep catheter clean and patent; use aseptic technique to empty drainage bag.
Wound infection	Redness, swelling, pain, warmth, drainage, fever, increased leukocytes, rapid pulse and respirations (fever 72 hr after surgery indicates infection in some system or in the wound)	Assess wound characteristics and drainage. Monitor white blood cell count and temperature. Use aseptic technique for wound care; encourage adequate nutrition and fluids; encourage activity.
Pulmonary embolus	Shortness of breath, anxiety, chest pain, rapid pulse and respirations, cyanosis, cough, bloody sputum	Anti-embolism stockings, adequate fluid intake, frequent turning or ambulation, preventive anticoagulant if ordered; leg exercises.
Hemorrhage and shock	Evidence of copious bleeding; decreased blood pressure, elevated pulse, cold clammy skin, decreased urinary output	Give blood or volume expander; stop bleeding. Place in shock position with feet and legs elevated and head flat; administer ordered medications to raise blood pressure; administer oxygen; frequent vital signs measurement.
Wound dehiscence or evisceration	Discharge of serosanguineous drainage from wound and sensation that "something gave"; separation of wound edges with intestines visible through abdominal incision	Teach to splint properly for coughing. Place patient supine; cover wound with sterile saline-soaked gauze or towels; return to operating room for repair; monitor for shock.
Fluid imbalance	Signs of overhydration: crackles in lungs, edema, weight gain Signs of dehydration: weight loss, diminished pulse, dry mucous membranes, decreased tissue turgor	Control intravenous flow rate. Monitor intake and output; correct imbalances. Output will be less than intake for first 72 hr after surgery with general anesthesia. Auscultate lungs each shift. Monitor weight; check for edema.
Malignant hyperthermia	High temperature, cardiac dysrhythmias, muscle rigidity, hypotension, tachypnea, and dark cola-colored urine	Genetic predisposition; can only monitor and treat symptoms; apply cooling blanket and ice packs. Give dantrolene as ordered.

Adapted from deWit, S.C. (2009). *Fundamental Concepts and Skills for Nursing* (3rd ed.). Philadelphia: Saunders, p. 772.

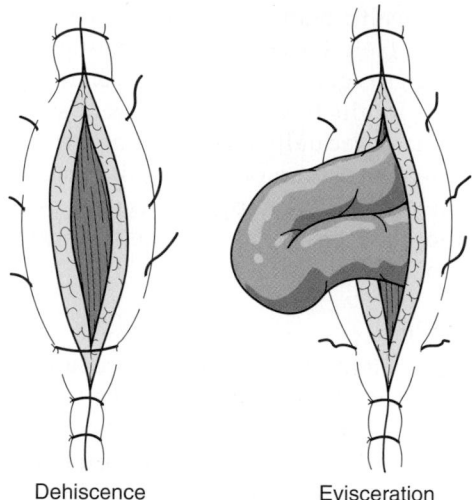

Dehiscence   Evisceration

FIGURE 5-7 Complications of wound healing: dehiscence and evisceration.

wound disruption. Wound dehiscence and evisceration create an emergency that requires immediate surgery and are very serious complications. After dehiscence and evisceration occur and before reparative surgery, the patient should lie supine with the knees flexed. The wound should be covered with a sterile towel or sterile dressings moistened with sterile normal saline.

 Home Care Considerations

In Case of Dehiscence or Evisceration

If dehiscence or evisceration occurs at home, moisten sterile gauze with sterile water (or fresh water if sterile is unavailable) and place over the exposed bowel to keep the bowel membrane moist. Immediately notify the home care agency or the physician, call someone to help, and have the patient lie supine with the moistened dressings in place.

 Think Critically

Identify seven assessment findings that together would indicate a wound infection.

Hemorrhage and Shock. The two most common complications of anesthesia and surgery are shock and infection. Shock, which can quickly develop into a life-threatening emergency, presents the most immediate danger to the patient. Shock disrupts normal physiologic function and can result from (1) failure of the heart to function as a pump (*cardiogenic shock*), as in cardiac arrest (see Chapter 21); (2) a low volume of blood (*hypovolemic shock*), as in hemorrhage; (3) collapse of the blood vessels as a result of faulty nervous system regulation (*neurogenic shock*) (see Chapter 23); (4) anaphylaxis (severe, allergic reaction), as in hypersensitivity to a drug or other allergen (see Chapter 12); and (5) sepsis, occurring when toxins

from bacteria relax and dilate blood vessels, resulting in a drop in blood pressure (see Chapters 6 and 45).

In the immediate postoperative period, the patient is most likely to suffer from cardiogenic, hypovolemic, or neurogenic shock. However, any of the five kinds of shock are possible after anesthesia and surgery. The symptoms of shock depend to some degree on the cause of circulatory failure.

 Clinical Cues

Early signs of impending hypovolemic shock from hemorrhage are thirst, restlessness, tachycardia, and tachypnea. Changes in the vital signs may be the only warning sign of neurogenic and cardiogenic shock.

As shock progresses, blood pressure begins to drop and pulse rate increases. Pulse may be bounding at first but becomes thready and indistinct as circulatory collapse occurs. Skin becomes cold and clammy, and pallor becomes evident. There may be air hunger with cyanosis of the lips and nail beds as a result of tissue hypoxia. As shock deepens, blood pressure continues to fall, and the patient loses consciousness, eventually becoming comatose. Untreated shock is fatal.

Both general and local anesthesia can bring about circulatory collapse. If there is evidence of shock, the patient should be placed in the supine position with the lower extremities elevated to add blood volume to the vital organs. **Patients in cardiogenic shock are placed in Fowler's position to lower the diaphragm and increase oxygenation as long as they do not become too hypotensive.** Pain contributes to the progression of shock; however, administering large doses of narcotics can decrease blood pressure further. Sometimes patients who develop shock also develop disseminated intravascular coagulation, a life-threatening disorder evidenced by bleeding from many sites (see Chapter 45).

Intravenous fluids and medications are important to prevent and treat shock. Supplemental oxygen is usually given to combat tissue hypoxia and cardiac response. See Chapter 45 for specific treatments for shock.

Malignant Hyperthermia. Malignant hyperthermia (MH) is a life-threatening complication of general anesthetic agents, including halothane, isoflurane, enflurane, and succinylcholine. MH occurs from a biochemical reaction in genetically predisposed persons. Signs of MH include high temperature, cardiac dysrhythmia, rigidity of the jaw or other muscles, hypotension, tachypnea, and dark cola-colored urine. A late sign of MH is an extremely high temperature of up to 111.2° F (44° C). Notify the anesthesiologist and surgeon immediately if any of these signs occurs. If it is not treated swiftly and effectively, MH is fatal. Dantrolene sodium (Dantrium) is infused rapidly to treat MH. The patient is immediately placed on a hypothermia blanket, ice bags are applied to the armpits and groin to cool the core of the body, and iced saline IV solutions and cold-solution enemas may be administered (Hommertzheim & Steinke, 2006).

Promote Psychological Adjustment

When surgery alters physical appearance, the patient may not only be concerned about the ability to perform self-care postoperatively but also have considerable changes in body image, particularly if there is extensive scarring. If part of an extremity, an organ, or part of a breast has been surgically removed, the necessary psychological adjustment is considerable and takes a lot of time.

 Communication

Recovering from Abdominal Surgery

Mrs. Wilson is a 74-year-old recovering from abdominal surgery. Although her body language tells her nurse she is experiencing pain, she has denied any need for pain medication since she administered her patient-controlled analgesia dose 3 hours before.

Nurse: "Mrs. Wilson, I would like to see you able to cough more vigorously, move about in bed more, and walk around more frequently. I think that if you would use your pain pump more often, you would be more comfortable doing your exercises and coughing."

Mrs. Wilson: "I'm not that uncomfortable, and those medications always cause problems for me."

Nurse: "Problems?"

Mrs. Wilson: "Yes, I get really constipated."

Nurse: "The doctor has a stool softener ordered for you to help prevent constipation, and by increasing fluids, we should be able to control that. Do you have other problems with the pain medication?"

Mrs. Wilson: "Yes, it makes me light-headed and unsteady on my feet."

Nurse: "If the pain medication makes you light-headed, we can switch you to a different medication, and one of us will stay with you when you are out of bed to see that you do not fall."

Mrs. Wilson: "I'm very afraid of falling, breaking a hip, and adding to my troubles."

Nurse: "By taking the medication and being more comfortable, you'll feel more like doing your exercises. That's how you can help prevent postoperative complications such as pneumonia or blood clots."

Mrs. Wilson: "I certainly don't want pneumonia or a blood clot!"

Nurse: "Moving about more will also increase circulation and help your wound to heal faster."

Mrs. Wilson: "O.K., I'll take the pain medication if it will help me prevent complications."

Assess the patient for signs of ineffective coping, including withdrawn, depressed behavior; less attention to grooming than before; and poor communication efforts. If these signs occur, work with the patient to identify areas of concern and collaborate

with other health team members to develop a plan of assistance. Help the patient by encouraging discussion of feelings regarding what has been removed and the effect it might have on the patient's life. Be an active listener; gradually focus the patient on the positives in life rather than on the loss incurred. It helps to refer the patient to a support group of people who have undergone a similar experience and are also learning to cope.

■ Evaluation

Evaluative statements regarding previously stated goals and expected outcomes might be:

- Lungs clear to auscultation; respirations 18
- Pulse 82, BP 136/86, peripheral pulses present
- Pain controlled for 4 hours with analgesia; states pain medication controls pain for about 4 hours
- Incision clean, dry, and without redness
- Patient expresses gladness that periods of pain and malaise will be gone
- No signs of thrombophlebitis or infection

Each nursing care plan is evaluated on whether the individual specific outcomes have been met. Further examples of evaluation are in Nursing Care Plan 5-1.

DISCHARGE PLANNING

With same-day surgery and early release from the hospital after inpatient surgery, it is vital that discharge planning be started at admission or several days before the surgery. Assess needs for home care. Will the patient need assistance with bathing, meals, or dressing changes? It may be necessary to arrange home health care with an aide to assist with bathing, and with a nurse to assess the patient's condition and provide wound care. Equipment, such as oxygen, suction, or an IV pump, may need to be ordered before discharge so that the transition to home goes smoothly.

 Cultural Considerations

Performing Wound Care

Although not overly modest, traditional Chinese people may hesitate in touching their own bodies, so it is important to assess who will perform wound care and change dressings at home. A home health nurse may need to be accessed, or teaching of another family member may be important.

Family or relatives must be included in discharge planning and teaching. Often it is a family member who will do the dressing changes, monitor for side effects of medication, alert the physician to signs of complications, and provide general support to the patient during recovery.

★ Nursing Care Plan 5-1   Care of the Patient Who Has Had a Simple Mastectomy

Scenario

A married 38-year-old woman and the mother of two children ages 16 and 14 underwent a simple mastectomy with sentinel node biopsy as treatment for a 4.5-cm malignant tumor.

Problem/Nursing Diagnosis

*Surgical incision/*Impaired skin integrity related to surgical wound.

Supporting Assessment Data

Objective: Right mastectomy; dressing on right chest.

Goals/Expected Outcomes	Nursing Interventions	Selected Rationale	Evaluation
Wound will be free of signs of infection at discharge.	Keep Jackson-Pratt suction functioning properly.	Suction is needed to pull drainage from operative site.	No signs of infection. Incision clean, dry, and without reddening.
Wound will heal completely within 6 weeks.	Note character and amount of drainage; document. Reinforce dressing as needed.	Helps detect excessive bleeding.	Draining small amounts of serosanguineous fluid. No need for dressing reinforcement.
	Assess for excessive bleeding q hr for 4 hr, then q 2 hr for first 24 hr.		Small amount of serosanguineous drainage in Jackson-Pratt.
	Assess pulses in arm q 2 hr to detect excessive swelling in arm.	Swelling in arm can cause nerve damage.	Minimal swelling in arm; pulses are 2+.
	Monitor temperature and white blood cell (WBC) count.	Temperature and WBC count trends will show if infection is developing.	No increase in temperature or WBC count.
	Assess wound for signs of infection with each dressing change. Change dressing q 8–24 hr as needed.	Sterile dressing helps prevent infection.	Wound clean and dry without signs of infection. Surgeon changed dressing this afternoon. Continue plan.

Problem/Nursing Diagnosis

*Surgery/*Pain related to surgical incision.

Supporting Assessment Data

Subjective: Complains of incisional pain and discomfort.
Objective: Right mastectomy; rates pain at 4 on pain scale.

Goals/Expected Outcomes	Nursing Interventions	Selected Rationale	Evaluation
Pain will be controlled by analgesia as noted by patient.	Instruct on use of patient-controlled analgesia (PCA).	Knowledge is needed to use PCA effectively.	Using PCA appropriately.
	Assess pain level q 3–4 hr.	Assessing pain level will demonstrate whether pain is adequately controlled.	Pain level consistently below 4.
	Provide comfort measures.	Comfort measures increase effect of analgesia.	Straightened bed; brought warmed blanket.
Pain is controlled by oral analgesia by discharge.	Administer analgesics as ordered.		Continue plan.

Problem/Nursing Diagnosis

*Anesthesia/*Potential for impaired gas exchange related to inhalation anesthesia.

Supporting Assessment Data

Objective: Had general anesthesia. Restricted mobility.
Subjective: "I don't like using the incentive spirometer. Do I have to cough? It hurts."

Continued

✦ Nursing Care Plan 5-1   Care of the Patient Who Has Had a Simple Mastectomy—cont'd

Goals/Expected Outcomes	Nursing Interventions	Selected Rationale	Evaluation
Patient will not have atelectasis by end of postoperative day 2.	Have patient use incentive spirometer q hr while awake.	Incentive spirometer use opens alveoli, decreasing atelectasis.	Using incentive spirometer; barely diminished breath sounds in lung bases.
	Have patient cough q 2 hr.	Coughing clears secretions from lung irritation due to anesthesia.	Coughed secretions are clear.
Lung sounds will be clear at discharge.	Auscultate lungs q 8 hr.	Auscultation determines status of breath sounds.	Lungs clear.
	Encourage ambulation. Monitor temperature, respirations, and oxygen saturation.		Ambulated × 2. Continue plan.

Problem/Nursing Diagnosis
Loss of breast/Risk for grieving related to loss of body part and perception of femininity.

Supporting Assessment Data
Objective: Right mastectomy.
Subjective: Expresses concern about husband's reaction to surgery.

Goals/Expected Outcomes	Nursing Interventions	Selected Rationale	Evaluation
Patient will verbalize feelings of self-worth and confidence.	Have patient list her strengths and positive attributes.	Focusing on strengths can help counter feelings of loss.	Is patient verbalizing feelings of confidence and self-worth? Not yet.
Patient will discuss sadness over loss of breast.	Encourage sharing of sad feelings and fears with husband.	Talking openly with husband may provide reassurance.	Expressed sadness over breast loss to husband.
	Talk with husband privately about his feelings.	Involvement will show her he still cares for her.	Husband reluctant to speak about the surgery or his feelings so far.
	Involve husband in patient's care.		
	Encourage daughters to discuss their feelings and fears with patient.		Daughters have not been in yet today.
	Encourage independence in patient.	Independence increases self-confidence.	Brushed her teeth. Continue plan.

Critical Thinking Questions
1. You auscultate the patient's lungs the evening after surgery, and sounds are diminished in the bases. What do you think it means?
2. What would you do if the radial pulse in the arm on the same side as the breast surgery becomes weaker and harder to detect?

When the patient is discharged, review specific instructions regarding care at home, including care of the incision or wound, diet requirements, activity level allowed, medications, and signs and symptoms of complications to report to the health care provider. Make certain the patient understands when to see the physician for follow-up. Send home sufficient supplies of items needed for dressing changes, and tell the patient and family where more items can be obtained. Make every attempt to ensure that the patient does not go home with unanswered questions.

Patient Teaching

Discharge Instructions for Same-Day Surgery Patient

DIET
- Type of diet and importance of proper nutrition for healing
- Dietary restrictions, if any
- Avoiding alcohol for first 24 hr after anesthesia
- Special dietary recommendations
- Recommended fluid intake

ACTIVITY
- Recommended exercise and frequency
- Instructions for special equipment: crutches, walker, cane, splint, etc.
- Schedule for deep breathing, coughing, and leg exercises; how long to continue these activities; remember to splint the incision when coughing and getting out of bed
- Recommended rest periods
- Activity restrictions (i.e., driving, intercourse, and lifting)
- Application, use, and care of anti-embolism stockings

WOUND CARE
- Hand hygiene
- Dressing changes and frequency
- Cleansing of wound; irrigations
- Drainage observations
- Signs to report
- Use of heat or cold packs
- Supplies and where to obtain them

TEMPERATURE MONITORING
- Record time and temperature
- Report temperature >100° F (38° C)

BATHING
- Type of bath
- Frequency

MEDICATIONS
- Analgesics
- Antibiotics
- Sedatives
- Vitamin supplements
- Other medications

PRECAUTIONS RELATED TO ANESTHESIA OR SIDE EFFECTS OF MEDICATION
- Caution regarding using machinery
- Caution regarding making decisions for 24 hr
- Drug interactions
- Potential for constipation
- Potential for urinary retention

SIGNS AND SYMPTOMS TO REPORT
- Elevated temperature
- Increasing malaise
- Severe pain or swelling
- Bleeding through bandage
- Decreased sensation below surgical site
- Severe nausea and vomiting

OTHER
- Scheduled follow-up appointment with the physician
- Expectation for return to usual activities
- Expectation for return to feeling normal

Think Critically

An elderly patient who has had a hip replacement and who has chronic lung disease is being discharged home to the care of a 78-year-old spouse. Which health care professionals would you collaborate with to plan appropriate continuing care for the patient?

COMMUNITY CARE

The patient may be given follow-up care at an outpatient clinic, physician's office, subacute care unit, rehabilitation unit, extended-care unit, or at the patient's home. The nurse case manager will coordinate the care of the whole team, collaborating with the social worker, physical therapist, respiratory therapist, nurse's aide, dietitian, pharmacist, physician, and other health care professionals. The nurse assesses the patient's condition and progress, performs treatments and procedures such as wound care, and reinforces teaching about the signs and symptoms of complications. The quality of nursing care delivered postoperatively often is the factor that prevents complications and rehospitalization.

Some physicians discharge patients who are ambulatory and normally self-sufficient, thinking that patients themselves can do complicated wound care. Most patients need assistance with anything more than a simple dressing change, which is particularly true if the patient lives alone. The nurse must verify that the patient can adequately perform self-care and collaborate with the patient, physician, social worker, and community agencies to secure the assistance the patient needs.

Home Care Considerations

General Points for Home Care for Postsurgical Patients

- The patient must know about each medication to be taken and when to take it.
- The diet, any restrictions, and guidelines for fluid intake are discussed.
- Alcohol must be avoided for 24 hr after surgery.
- Any restrictions on activity are listed; instructions for use of any special equipment such as crutches, splint, walker, and so forth are presented.
- Patients should not drive or make important decisions for 24 hr after anesthesia.
- The patient knows what type of bath is permitted.
- Cleansing and dressing of the wound are discussed, along with where to obtain supplies.
- Signs and symptoms to report to the surgeon are listed— temperature above 100° F (38° C), increasing malaise, severe pain or swelling, bleeding through the bandage, decreased sensation below the surgical site, or severe nausea and vomiting.
- Instructions for when to schedule a follow-up appointment with the physician.
- Written instructions should be sent home with the patient for all essential points of care and consultation.

Get Ready for the NCLEX® Examination!

Key Points

- Nurses in the recovery unit monitor patients very closely until they are fully aroused from anesthesia.
- Maintaining a patent airway is the highest priority.
- The nurse is vigilant for signs of complications and performs frequent assessments during the postoperative period.
- Nursing interventions are aimed at providing pain control, comfort, and fluid balance; protecting the patient from injury; maintaining vital functions; and preventing infection.
- The nurse tries to prevent or intervene in the many potential complications from surgery.
- Discharge planning begins at admission and covers all areas of basic needs, wound care, and activity restrictions.
- Written instructions regarding all aspects of postoperative care should be sent home with the patient.

Additional Learning Resources

SG Go to your Study Guide for additional learning activities to help you master this chapter content.

evolve Go to your Evolve website (http://evolve.elsevier.com/deWit/medsurg) for the following FREE learning resources:
- Animations, audio, and video
- Answers and rationales for questions and activities
- Concept Map Creator
- Glossary with pronunciations in English and Spanish
- Interactive Review Questions and Exercises and more!

 Online Resources
- Postoperative care, www.surgeryencyclopedia.com/Pa-St/Postoperative-Care.html

Review Questions for the NCLEX® Examination

1. A 32-year-old woman who has undergone bilateral radical mastectomy is withdrawn and quiet. She is afebrile with no apparent complaints of pain. Her dressings are dry and intact. Pulses are full on both upper extremities. Considering the data, the most appropriate nursing diagnosis at this time for this patient would be:
   1. Acute pain related to surgical incision.
   2. Risk for infection related to surgery.
   3. Disturbed body image related to loss of body parts.
   4. Impaired communication related to unknown causes.

2. In planning care for an elderly patient who had open reduction and internal fixation of the right femur, the nurse formulates the following nursing diagnoses: *Risk for infection related to surgical incision* and *compromised immunity associated with advanced age.* An appropriate expected outcome would be that the:
   1. nurse will monitor changes in temperature and laboratory values during the shift.

   2. patient will state some signs and symptoms of wound infection before discharge.
   3. nurse will teach aseptic techniques to the patient before discharge.
   4. patient will not develop a wound infection before discharge.

3. Which statement indicates a need for further teaching regarding the use of a patient-controlled analgesia (PCA) pump?
   1. "I control my pain medication by pressing the button."
   2. "To a certain extent, I control the amount of pain medication I can have."
   3. "I need to tell the nurse if the pain is not controlled well."
   4. "I need to call the nurse when I need pain medication."

4. To promote wound healing, the postoperative patient is instructed to eat foods high in protein. Which food choice warrants further patient teaching?
   1. Caesar salad with French bread and milk
   2. Tuna sandwich, carrot strips, and watermelon chunks
   3. Broccoli cheese soup, crackers, and an orange
   4. Broiled chicken breast, steamed broccoli, and mashed potatoes

5. After a series of instructions and demonstrations in preparation for home discharge, the postoperative patient is allowed to administer his own subcutaneous enoxaparin (Lovenox). Which patient action is an incorrect technique for the injection?
   1. Wiping the injection site with alcohol
   2. Aspirating blood before injecting the heparin
   3. Retaining the air bubble in the prefilled syringe
   4. Applying light pressure to the site with gauze after administration

6. On arrival from the postanesthesia care unit, the patient complains of severe thirst. The nurse finds that the patient is increasingly restless, tachypneic, and tachycardic. Considering the findings, what would the nurse likely suspect?
   1. Hypovolemia
   2. Cardiogenic shock
   3. Normal response to anesthesia
   4. Pain medication overdose

7. The patient is prescribed anti-embolism stockings. The patient asks, "Why do I need these stockings?" The best nursing response would be:
   1. "Your physician ordered these stockings."
   2. "These help prevent formation of clots in the legs."
   3. "These massage your legs to make you feel better."
   4. "You sound upset. Do these stockings bother you?"

8. The nurse performing an initial assessment of a postoperative patient notes the following: temperature 104.9° F (40.5° C), blood pressure 90/60, pulse 58, respirations 30, rigidity of the jaw muscles, and dark urine. The priority nursing action would be to:
   1. instruct the patient to relax and take deep breaths.
   2. notify the physician immediately.
   3. administer pain medications.
   4. give a tepid sponge bath.

9. While caring for the postoperative patient, the nurse must reinforce which measure(s) to reduce the incidence of complications? *(Select all that apply.)*
   1. Use the incentive spirometer every hour while awake.
   2. Ambulate the designated distance six times a day.
   3. After deep breathing, cough effectively every 4 hours.
   4. Turn or change position at least every 2 hours.
   5. Assess for pain and provide prompt relief.

10. What nursing action(s) would be appropriate when caring for a postoperative patient with a Jackson-Pratt wound drain? *(Select all that apply.)*
    1. Assess the wound drain for patency.
    2. Measure amount of drainage.
    3. Compress the bulb to reestablish pressure.
    4. Rinse the bulb after emptying with sterile water.
    5. Notify the physician when there is no drainage.

Critical Thinking Questions

Scenario A
Ms. Simpson just had a colon resection for a tumor, and you are assisting with her care in the PACU. She is waking up, but is still groggy and her breathing is somewhat shallow. She has a large dressing on the left side of the abdomen.

1. What would you do to improve her respiratory status?
2. Describe the method used to ensure an open airway.

Scenario B
You are assigned to care for a 37-year-old man who just had a same-day surgical repair of a ventral hernia with spinal anesthesia.

1. How does the care of this patient differ from that of a patient who had inhalation or general anesthesia?
2. If this patient has difficulty voiding after surgery, how could you assist him?
3. If he develops a spinal headache, what measures could be taken to decrease his discomfort?

Scenario C
Mrs. Stinson is a 78-year-old who underwent an abdominal hysterectomy and exploration for cancer of the uterus. She returned to the nursing unit from surgery 1 hour ago and has an IV infusion running into the right forearm. Her blood pressure has gradually fallen from 138/88 to 102/62. She is restless, complains of thirst, and is anxious.

1. What assessments would you make?
2. What actions would you take? In what order would you perform these actions?

Scenario D
Mr. Porter is a 66-year-old with a history of asthma and frequent respiratory infections. He is recovering from chest surgery.

1. What are his increased risks from hypostatic pneumonia?
2. What nursing actions would you implement to help prevent this complication?
3. What signs and symptoms would indicate that he might have hypostatic pneumonia?

Objectives

Theory

1. Analyze the factors that increase the risk of infection.
2. Discuss how the body uses its natural defensive mechanisms to protect against infection.
3. Explain how fever plays a role in the prevention of infection.
4. Describe the classic signs of infection.
5. Analyze situations that require the use of expanded precautions.
6. List the types of personal protective equipment and analyze situations for when they should be used.

7. Describe factors that make the elderly more susceptible to infections.
8. Analyze factors that may impair the process of healing and repair of damaged tissue.

Clinical Practice

1. Care for a patient whose condition requires extended precautions.
2. From a day's patient assignment, determine the factors present for each patient that are risk factors for infection.

Key Terms

acquired (ăk-KWĪ-ĕrd, p. 104)
agent (Ā-gĕnt, p. 100)
communicable (kŏ-MŪ-nĭ-kă-bŭl, p. 100)
disease (dĭ-ZĒZ, p. 100)
Expanded Precautions (prĕ-KĂW-shŭns, p. 109)
exudate (ĔKS-ū-dāt, p. 105)
hand hygiene (HĪ-gēn, p. 108)
health care–associated infection (HAI) (ĭn-FĔK-shŭn, p. 111)
host (hōst, p. 100)
immunity (ĭ-MŪ-nĭ-tē, p. 104)
infection (ĭn-FĔK-shŭn, p. 100)
inflammation (ĭn-flă-MĀ-shŭn, p. 105)
innate (p. 104)

macrophages (MĂK-rō-făj-ĕz, p. 105)
multidrug-resistant organism (MDRO) (MŬL-tĭ-drŭg rē-zĭs-tĕnt ŌR-găn-ĭz-ĕm, p. 116)
normal flora (NŌR-măl FLŌR-ă, p. 100)
pathogen (PĂTH-ō-gĕn, p. 101)
personal protective equipment (PPE) (PĔR-sŭn-ŭl prō-TĔK-shŭn ē-KWĬP-mĕnt, p. 109)
phagocytosis (făg-ō-sī-TŌ-sĭs, pp. 102, 105)
sepsis (SĔP-sĭs, p. 115)
shedding (shĕd-ĭng, p. 100)
Standard Precautions (STĂN-dĕrd prĕ-KĂW-shŭnz, p. 109)
susceptible (sŭs-SĔP-tĭ-bŭl, p. 100)
vectors (VĔK-tĕrz, p. 108)

THE INFECTIOUS PROCESS AND DISEASE

Normal flora (microorganisms that normally exist in the body and provide natural immunity against certain infections) are most often found on or in body systems that have some form of contact with the outside environment (Table 6-1). Normal flora prevents the most harmful microorganisms from colonizing the body. Understanding how the body defends itself against infection, and how to prevent further exposure to *pathogenic* (disease-producing) microorganisms, is crucial in order to provide safe and effective nursing care.

An infection is the presence and growth of pathogenic microorganisms, in a susceptible (lacking resistance) host, to the extent that tissue damage occurs. Infection can be communicable (can be passed from one person to another directly, through touch, or indirectly, by using a contaminated glass) and noncommunicable.

Disease is one possible outcome of an infection. Once an infection has occurred, the person is considered communicable until the organism is no longer shedding (to lose by natural process) from the body. This period of communicability varies by the type of pathogen involved and the host's ability to fight off the infecting agent (any substance capable of producing an effect, whether physical, chemical, or biologic). Bacteria, for example, after entering the body, must find a way to attach to a host (an organism in which another, usually parasitic organism, is nourished and harbored) cell in order to multiply. Once the organisms have found a place to multiply, they can then spread through the body via the circulatory or lymphatic system. **The development of an infection is dependent on the interrelationship among the host, the agent, and the environment.**

Table 6-1	Normal Flora of the Body*
SITE	**NORMAL FLORA**
Eye	Corynebacterium species Neisseria species Staphylococcus aureus Staphylococcus epidermidis Streptococcus species
Upper respiratory tract (nose, mouth, throat)	Corynebacterium species Enterobacter species Haemophilus species Klebsiella species Lactobacillus species Neisseria species Staphylococcus species Streptococcus viridans Various types of anaerobes
Skin	Corynebacterium species Staphylococcus aureus Staphylococcus epidermidis Streptococcus species Yeasts such as Candida and Pityrosporum
Small bowel and colon	Bacteroides species Clostridium perfringens Enterobacter species (i.e., coliform) Escherichia coli Streptococcus faecalis
Vagina	Corynebacterium species Klebsiella species Lactobacillus species Proteus species Pseudomonas species Staphylococcus species Streptococcus species

Adapted from deWit, S.C. (2009). *Fundamental Concepts and Skills for Nursing* (3rd ed.). Philadelphia: Elsevier Saunders.

*The central nervous system, lower respiratory tract, and upper and lower urinary tracts are normally sterile. This table lists only those organisms most commonly found in the various body systems. They can also cause illness or infection if they are able to invade another system within the body.

FACTORS THAT INFLUENCE INFECTIOUS DISEASE

Many factors concerning the host determine the type of response the body will have to an invading pathogen. *Risk* of exposure is influenced by the lifestyle, occupation, and socioeconomic status of the host. The underlying disease state, as well as the immunologic and nutritional status of the host, influences the *degree* of resistance or susceptibility the body will have to the pathogen. Environmental factors can also increase the likelihood of developing an infection (Figure 6-1). Other factors that influence infection or disease are listed in Box 6-1.

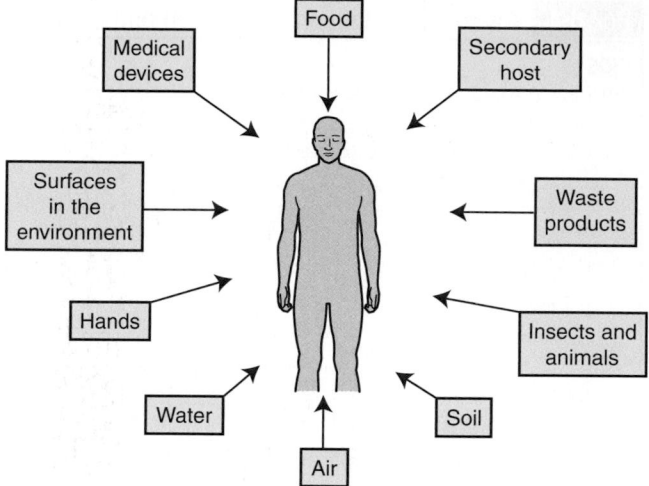

FIGURE 6-1 The environment and the spread of infection.

DISEASE-PRODUCING PATHOGENS

Any microorganism capable of producing disease is known as a pathogen. Once pathogens have entered the body, many are able to adapt to their new environment, enhancing survival and increasing their likelihood of causing illness or disease. Pathogens can be transmitted from one person to another through one of three routes: *airborne, contact,* or *droplet.* Hand hygiene is the number one way to prevent the spread or transmission of pathogenic microorganisms. Following respiratory etiquette by covering your cough/sneeze and performing hand hygiene afterward is another method to use in preventing the spread of infection.

Categories of Microorganisms

Nine categories of microorganisms are known to cause infection in humans: bacteria, viruses, protozoa, Rickettsia, chlamydia, fungi, mycoplasmas, helminths, and prions.

Bacteria. Bacteria are classified into three major categories, according to their shape, gram-staining properties, and requirements for oxygen. Round or spherical bacteria are referred to as *cocci,* rod-shaped bacteria are referred to as *bacilli,* and spiral or corkscrew-shaped bacteria are called *spirochetes.* Some bacteria grow in chains (streptococci), some grow in pairs (diplococci), and some grow in clusters (staphylococci).

Bacteria that require oxygen to live and reproduce are *aerobic;* those that cannot tolerate the presence of oxygen are *anaerobic.* When bacteria enter the body, they trigger the immune system to produce *antibodies* (proteins that fight and destroy antigens). Some bacteria produce poisonous substances called *endotoxins* (toxins that are found within the bacteria and are released when the cell breaks apart); others produce *exotoxins* (excreted by both gram-negative and gram-positive bacteria).

Factors that Influence Infection and Disease

HOST
Intrinsic (genetic predisposition [born with it])
    Age, sex, race
    Chronic diseases (e.g., diabetes mellitus)
Extrinsic (environmental):
    Personal behaviors (e.g., drugs, alcohol, hygiene, sexual
        practices)
    Occupation
    Socioeconomic status

AGENT
Dosage and duration of exposure to the infecting agent(s)
Biologic—bacterial, fungal, viral, protozoal microbes can be
    involved
Chemical—organic and inorganic, pesticides,
    pharmaceuticals
Physical—ionizing radiation, cold, heat, electricity, noise

ENVIRONMENT*
Coexisting chronic disease (e.g., hypertension, diabetes
    mellitus)
Living environment overcrowded (e.g., dormitory or prison
    setting)
Travel to country with endemic diseases such as
    tuberculosis or HIV/AIDS
Vectors (e.g., mosquitoes, flies, ticks, fleas)

Data from Mandell, G.L., Bennett, J.E., & Dolin, R. (Eds.). (2010). *Mandell, Douglas, and Bennett's Principles and Practice of Infectious Disease* (7th ed.). Philadelphia: Elsevier Saunders; Arias, K.M. (2010). *Quick Reference to Outbreak Investigation Prevention and Control in Health Care Settings, Critical Issues in Patient Safety* (2nd ed.). Boston: Jones & Bartlett; Brachman, P.S., & Evans, A.S. (2009). *Bacterial Infections of Humans: Epidemiology and Control* (4th ed.). New York: Springer.
HIV/AIDS, human immunodeficiency virus/acquired immunodeficiency syndrome.
*Environment includes not only the body, but also where one lives and works.

Different bacteria thrive under different environmental conditions. Some form *spores* (a protective covering over the original cell) to protect themselves against destruction from heat, cold, lack of water, toxic chemicals, and radiation. Examples of spore-forming infectious diseases are anthrax and botulism. Other bacteria thrive best in water, such as *Pseudomonas* species or *Legionella.* The bacterium that causes tuberculosis can survive for years in many environments. Some bacteria, such as *Staphylococcus aureus,* can survive in very high temperatures.

Different methods can be used to prevent infection and its spread. A physiologic response can stimulate the immune system to produce a fever and the body's immune response is triggered to destroy the invading pathogenic microorganism through phagocytosis (ingestion and digestion of bacteria). Another method is to clean, sterilize, or boil inanimate objects, such as a glass or surgical instruments, to prevent the spread of infection if the items are used by or on a patient. The correct antimicrobial agent must be given and completed as prescribed, otherwise the patient is at increased risk for developing infection with a multidrug-resistant organism.

Viruses. Viruses are not cells. They do not have cell walls and do not reproduce like other microbes. They cannot be treated with antibiotics or antifungals. They are composed of either deoxyribonucleic acid (DNA) or ribonucleic acid (RNA); have an outside coating made of protein; and are dependent on the cell they have invaded in order to survive and reproduce. Some viruses use the cytoplasm from the cell they have attacked to develop an "envelope" that makes it harder for the body's immune system to destroy them. Viruses have the ability to keep changing their protein markers, called *antigens,* making it difficult for the virus to be neutralized or killed by white blood cells (WBCs). Once viruses have established themselves in the body, they can trigger an immune response that is harmful to the cells. They can also damage cells by preventing protein synthesis from occurring. New viral elements can be released into the circulation either by the virus breaking down the wall of the cell it has invaded and releasing itself or from small offshoots that have burst, thereby infecting other cells.

Viruses are classified as one of three types: (1) latent—because they can reside in the body for years without producing symptoms and then suddenly cause an acute flare-up of symptoms (e.g., herpes simplex); (2) *oncogenic* (cancer causing)—because they have the ability to alter the cell walls to the point where the cells become malignant; and (3) active—where the virus enters the body, invades a number of cells, and infects the body (e.g., influenza and severe acute respiratory syndrome, which are discussed in Chapter 15).

Viruses, as well as bacteria, vary in their resistance to destruction by chemical disinfectants, but most are easily inactivated or destroyed by heat. However, some of the hepatitis viruses must be boiled as long as 30 minutes before they can be considered nonpathogenic. It is important to note that antibiotics do not help in a viral infection but antiviral agents, such as acyclovir, can help prevent a more virulent viral infection from occurring if taken at the first signs of illness.

Protozoa. Protozoa are one-celled parasitic organisms that have the ability to move. There are four main types, named by their method of travel within their environment. They are called either amebas, ciliates, flagellates, or sporozoa. These microorganisms are typically found in water and soil. Many protozoa species have the ability to lie dormant. Although thousands of species exist, only a few are pathogenic to humans. To cause disease, some protozoans have to be ingested whereas others are introduced into the body through the bite of a vector, such as a mosquito.

Rickettsia and Chlamydia. Rickettsia are small, round or rod-shaped bacteria that are often transmitted by the bites of body lice, ticks, and fleas. *Chlamydia* is also a bacterium, and is typically transmitted via close contact, especially sexual. Both are dependent on a living host.

Fungi. Fungi are very small, primitive organisms that grow on living plants, animals, and other decaying organic material. They thrive in warm, moist environments. Fungal infections in humans are called *mycoses* and are classified into three main types: (1) cutaneous mycoses, which grow in the outer layer of the skin; (2) subcutaneous mycoses, which involve the deeper layers of the skin, subcutaneous tissues, and sometimes bone; and (3) systemic or deep mycoses involving internal organs.

Fungal infections are difficult to eradicate once they have invaded a host, because fungi tend to form spores that are resistant to ordinary antimicrobial agents. Antifungal agents can be given topically or systemically, but can be toxic to the liver and the nervous system; therefore the course of treatment must be carried out cautiously and over a long period.

Fungal infections commonly found in immune-competent hosts include coccidioidomycosis (caused by *Coccidioides immitis*), histoplasmosis (caused by *Histoplasma capsulatum*), and blastomycosis (caused by *Blastomyces dermatitidis*). They are all systemic mycoses caused by inhalation of airborne spores. Once in the lung, the spores take root and then can spread to any part of the body. However, it is important to note that the majority of fungal infections are self-limited and do not cause clinical disease.

Opportunistic fungal infections (infections that occur in a person with a depressed immune system) are more typically found in patients who have some form of immune compromise and typically include species from *Candida, Cryptococcus* (can infect any organ in the body, including the brain and the meninges), and *Aspergillus* (found in soil, dust, and decomposing organic material).

Mycoplasmas. Mycoplasmas, once thought to be a virus, are very small organisms that do not have a cell wall. They are more like an extracellular parasite because they attach themselves to epithelial cells that line the body cavities and outer surfaces, such as the skin. They tend to be slow growing. For example, *Mycoplasma pneumoniae* can take up to 3 weeks to incubate before signs or symptoms begin to appear.

Other Infectious Agents

Helminths. Helminths are worms (either round, flat, or hook-like) and flukes. All are parasitic and are typically spread via the fecal-oral route. Pinworms are most commonly found in children and cause significant itching in the perianal area due to the eggs being laid outside the rectum. Flatworms, such as a tapeworm, can grow up to 50 feet long and live in the intestines. Hookworm and fluke infestations can easily penetrate the skin, are found in the blood, and invade organs such as the liver and lungs. Flatworms and flukes can cause significant weight loss and debilitation.

Prions. Although quite rare (one case per 1 million persons), prions are usually spread through eating meat, especially brain tissue that has been infected, or in even rarer cases, through corneal transplantation from a donor who had a prion infection (Centers for Disease Control and Prevention, 2010). Prions are extremely resistant to the typical methods used for killing most viruses, bacteria, and fungi. These organisms require a type of special cleaning and sterilization that can be especially hard on surgical instruments.

THE BODY'S DEFENSE AGAINST INFECTION

The four primary lines of defense the body has against infection are (1) the skin, (2) normal flora, (3) the inflammatory response, and (4) the immune response.

 Think Critically

In the work environment, where do you think you are most likely to come in contact with pathogens that might cause infection? What precautions can you take to prevent or lessen your risk of exposure?

SKIN

Mechanical and Chemical Barriers to Infection

Mechanical Barriers. Mechanical barriers are intact skin and mucous membranes. They are the primary defense the body has against invading microorganisms and infection. Skin, being the largest organ of the body, serves as a first line of defense against harmful agents in the environment. It functions as a protective covering for the more delicate and vulnerable underlying tissues and organs.

The portals of exit and entry provide the means by which pathogens move in and out of the body. For example, pathogens most frequently exit or enter the body where the skin and mucous membranes meet, such as through the mouth, nose, and gastrointestinal or genitourinary tracts, as well as through a cut in the skin.

Chemical Barriers. Chemical barriers assist the skin and mucous membranes in fighting off invasive organisms by the secretion of tears, saliva, and mucus. Lactic and fatty acids, which inhibit the growth of bacteria, are excreted via sweat and the sebaceous glands. Secretions from the mucous membranes lining the respiratory, gastrointestinal, and reproductive tracts contain an abundance of a bactericidal enzyme called *lysozyme.* This same enzyme is found in tears and saliva. Stomach acid and digestive enzymes kill off most swallowed microorganisms. Mucus produced by the respiratory tract helps capture a variety of inhaled particles. *Cilia* (tiny hairs), which line the respiratory tract, trap organisms and debris and then propel them up and out of the body with a wavelike action.

 Think Critically

What effect might medications such as Nexium and Prilosec (proton pump inhibitors), which reduce stomach acid, have on a person's general health? How will this affect a patient's ability to fight off pathogenic microorganisms that may be swallowed?

Protective and Defensive Mechanisms Against Infection

Our bodies have two forms of **immunity** (the body's ability to be unaffected by a particular disease or condition) against infections. They are **innate** (born with/natural) and **acquired** (develops throughout life) (Box 6-2). See Chapter 10 for more detail. When the body's defense mechanisms are stressed or exhausted, it is more susceptible to infection. Heredity, the degree of natural resistance, and one's own immune status are the greatest determinants of infection, but personal habits and behaviors are also factors to consider. General health, state of nutrition, hormone balance,

| Box 6-2 | Innate and Acquired Immunity |

INNATE IMMUNITY
- The body senses the presence of pathogenic microorganisms
- Genetic predisposition to respond to invasion in a specific way
- Responds rapidly to invasion of pathogenic microorganisms
- Elements consist of antibodies, phagocytes, natural killer cells, and mast cells

ACQUIRED IMMUNITY
- Cellular and humoral immunity are activated through T-cell and B-cell receptors
- Genetic rearrangement occurs throughout life
- Develops slowly once the body has been initially invaded
- Provides the body with protection with each subsequent exposure to the same pathogens
- Is the basic component for immunity induced via vaccination
- Elements consist of antibodies and cytotoxic and helper T cells

Adapted from Munford, R.S. (2010). Sepsis. In G.L. Mandell, J.E. Bennett, & R. Dolin (Eds.). *Mandell, Douglas, and Bennett's principles and Practice of Infectious Disease* (7th ed.). Philadelphia: Elsevier Saunders, pp. 906-926.

immune status, and the presence of a chronic disease, such as diabetes mellitus, may influence the degree of susceptibility a person may have to infection.

Fever. Fever is one of the primary mechanisms the body has to prevent infection from an invading microorganism. Once the immune system has determined that an invasion is trying to occur, it signals the hypothalamus in the brain to raise the body temperature. In an effort to fight off the infection, the body increases the heart rate and respiratory rate due to the increased metabolic and oxygen demand at the cellular level. Shivering occurs to increase the core body temperature, but the surrounding environment feels cooler than the new core body temperature, and the patient may complain of "freezing to death." It is at this point in the inflammatory response that fever is noticeably increased. In an attempt to decrease the body's temperature via evaporation, *diaphoresis* (sweating) occurs, and it is not unusual for the patient to not want to be covered by a blanket or sheet. This increased heat in the body creates a hostile environment to the microorganisms, and a person whose immune system is intact is able to destroy them more efficiently. Once the threat of infection is no longer present, the immune system again signals the hypothalamus and the body is able to start cooling down on its own.

 Think Critically

A patient asks you to explain what causes a person to have a temperature. Would the age of the patient be a factor you should consider in your teaching?

Nutrition. Poor nutrition predisposes a person to developing an infection because the body may not have sufficient protein stores to generate enough antibodies to help fight off an infection. The very young and the elderly have a less efficient immune system, and that is why it is important to ensure that these age groups have received the appropriate vaccinations and immunizations. Excessive stress is another factor that influences a person's immune status. Stress can increase blood cortisol levels, which will decrease the anti-inflammatory response of the body.

Elder Care Points

Many elderly do not eat sufficient protein because of monetary concerns or because of physical limitations that interfere with their ability to prepare a proper meal. Referral to a home delivery meal program may help to increase dietary intake of protein and other essential nutrients to help fight off infection.

Antigens. An antigen is a form of protein found on the outside of cells that has the ability to identify it as "self" (native) or "non-self" (foreign). Antigens can stimulate the immune response to wipe out microorganisms.

Table 6-2	Types of Antibodies
ANTIBODY	**DESCRIPTION**
IgM	Appears first if the body is exposed to an antigen. Will bind to antigen and work to clear the pathogen from the body.
IgG	Most abundant immunoglobulin found in the body. Crosses the placental barrier, reaching the developing fetus. Provides passive immunity until the fetus's own immune system can defend itself.
IgA	Found in tears, mucus, saliva, gastric fluid, colostrum, and sweat. Prevents pathogens from attaching to or penetrating epithelial cells, such as the skin.
IgE	Binds to mast cells and basophils and releases histamine and heparin. Stimulates a hypersensitive reaction, as seen in bronchial asthma or systemic anaphylaxis.
IgD	Works together with IgM. One function is to stimulate certain cells in the immune system; however, its overall role in the immune response is still unclear.

Antibodies. Antibodies, also known as immunoglobulins (Ig), are one part of acquired immunity. They have many functions, such as neutralizing toxins and killing invading pathogens. There are five types of antibodies: IgM, IgG, IgA, IgE, and IgD (Table 6-2). IgE has the ability to bind to mast cells and basophils and to release histamine and heparin. This in turn stimulates a hypersensitive reaction, as seen in bronchial asthma or systemic anaphylaxis.

Bone Marrow. The bone marrow is a major component in the body's defense system. Bone marrow plays an important role in the manufacturing of blood products that help the body defend itself against infection. These products are called *leukocytes, neutrophils, macrophages,* and *lymphocytes.*

Leukocytosis. Leukocytosis is an increased number of *leukocytes* (white blood cells), usually seen at the beginning of an infection when the person's immune system has not been overly stressed. Leukocytosis is seen more often with bacterial than viral infections. When infection does occur, the bone marrow is stimulated to produce and release more leukocytes to help the body fight infection.

Phagocytosis. The process of phagocytosis is a form of innate immunity. This is the body's first line of defense at the cellular level. Within the first few hours of the onset of the inflammatory process, the monocytes swell up (becoming macrophages) and migrate to the site of inflammation. Neutrophils, which are a type of leukocyte, are also released and have the ability to kill both aerobic and anaerobic organisms. After the macrophages and neutrophils engulf and destroy bacteria and other foreign matter, they die, producing an exudate (discharge) that is composed of tissue, fluid, dead cells, and their by-products. This exudate, usually yellow or green in color, is commonly known as *pus* and is a sign of infection.

Macrophages. Macrophages are *monocytes* (large leukocytes) that have left the bloodstream and have migrated into the tissues. They ingest and destroy pathogens and clear away the cellular debris and dead neutrophils in the latter stages of an infection. Macrophages cleanse the lymphatic fluid as it passes through the lymph nodes and perform a similar action on the blood as it passes through the liver and spleen.

Liver Cells. As part of the innate immune system, about 50% of all macrophage cells can be found in the liver's Kupffer cells. These macrophages act either to prevent invasion by pathogens mechanically or to neutralize the pathogen chemically (through the pH of body secretions). Macrophages also destroy bacteria that have found their way into the blood circulation through the liver's portal system. The body's defense mechanisms against pathogens are summarized in Table 6-3.

NORMAL FLORA

The flora that is normally present on the skin and in the mucous membranes, gastrointestinal tract, and vagina coexists with the body and controls the growth of harmful pathogens. When the amount of the normal flora is diminished, other pathogens may cause infection. When the body's immune system is suppressed for whatever reason, normal flora may grow out of control and cause infection. For example, *Candida albicans* causes a yeast infection (thrush) that frequently occurs after treatment with antibiotics, because the normal flora has been destroyed, allowing the *Candida* to flourish. Table 6-4 shows changes in the natural defense mechanisms that occur with age and cause the elderly to become more susceptible to infection.

THE INFLAMMATORY RESPONSE

Inflammation is an immediate, localized, protective response of the body to any kind of injury or damage to its cells or tissues. It is considered to be the second line

Table 6-3 The Body's Mechanism of Defense Against Infection

MECHANISM	FACTORS INVOLVED IN PROTECTION
Innate (natural) immunity	Determined by age, ethnicity, and genetics. Greater resistance to disease.
Antibody-mediated (humoral) immune response, (antigen-antibody; B lymphocytes)	Antibodies are produced against invading pathogens and inactivate or destroy them.
Cell-mediated immune response (T lymphocytes)	Sensitized T cells kill or inactivate antigens by chemical release or secretion of substances that destroy the antigen.
Inflammation	Cells damaged by pathogens release enzymes, and leukocytes are attracted to the area; the damaged area is "walled off" and phagocytosis disposes of the microorganisms and dead tissue.
Phagocytosis by white blood cells	Leukocytes, neutrophils, and macrophages (large monocytes) engulf, ingest, kill, and dispose of invading microorganisms.
Fever	May not always have fever with an infection, such as seen with immunocompromised or debilitated patients or in patients who have been on long-term corticosteroid therapy. Causes surface blood vessels to constrict, which leads to shivering in order to hold heat in the body (to kill the invading organisms). Increases metabolic rate, so can be problematic for patients with cardiorespiratory problems due to increased workload on the heart/circulatory system. Fever stops once the anti-inflammatory agents have helped to restore homeostasis.
Normal flora	Present on skin and in mucous membranes of oral cavity, gastrointestinal tract, and vagina. Helps prevent excessive growth of pathogens.
Intact skin	Skin is the first defense; slightly acid pH and normal flora present unfavorable environment for colonization of pathogens.
Mucous membranes	Mucous membranes, with their mucociliary action, provide mechanical protection against invasion of pathogens. Mucous secretions contain enzymes that inhibit many microorganisms. Respiratory system clears about 90% of introduced pathogens.
Gastrointestinal tract	Peristaltic action empties the gastrointestinal tract of pathogenic organisms. Acid pH of stomach secretions, bile, pancreatic enzymes, and mucus protects against invasion by harmful pathogens.
Genitourinary tract	Flushing of urine through the system washes out microorganisms. The acid pH of urine helps maintain a sterile environment in the system.

Table 6-4 Changes in Natural Defense Mechanisms that Occur with Age

CHANGE	CONSEQUENCE
Decreased skin turgor and greater skin friability	Skin is more susceptible to friction damage and tearing.
Decreased elasticity and atherosclerosis of peripheral vessels	Decreased blood flow to extremities produces slower wound healing.
Calcification of heart valves	Provides a location for bacteria to attach and cause endocarditis.
Stiffness of thorax from arthritis or aging changes, weakened respiratory muscles, decreased ciliary action from smoking or exposure to air pollution	Decreased ability to maintain good oxygenation leads to less respiratory reserve; greater tendency to retain secretions as cilia cannot move foreign substances and secretions as easily; cough reflex and effort are diminished.
Gastrointestinal tract motility is decreased as muscles weaken; acid production is decreased	Insufficient acid to inhibit growth of pathogens; decreased motility allows organisms to remain in gastrointestinal tract and multiply.
Prostate changes, bladder prolapse, and urethral strictures	Bladder is not completely emptied at each voiding, which allows for stagnation; provides medium for growth of pathogens.
Immune response decreases as bone marrow does not produce new blood cells as rapidly	Mobilization of body defenses to fight infection and heal wounds is slower.

Entry of bacteria or foreign particle

Tissue damage

Release of chemical mediators (complement, histamine, etc.)

Neutrophils and macrophages attracted to area (chemotaxis)

Increased capillary permeability (swelling → pain)

Vasodilation increases blood flow (redness and warmth)

Chronic inflammation with continued tissue damage

Increased number of phagocytes in area

Offending agents phagocytized

No bacteria remain   Some bacteria remain

Tissue repair

FIGURE 6-2 Steps in the inflammation process.

of defense to infection at the cellular level (Figure 6-2). Three basic purposes of the inflammatory response are to (1) neutralize and destroy harmful agents, (2) limit their spread to other tissues by walling off the organisms, and (3) prepare the damaged tissues for repair.

Inflammatory Changes

Changes that are part of the inflammatory response can occur locally, at the site of injury, and systemically. These changes involve (1) the cells of the damaged tissues and adjacent connective tissues; (2) the blood vessels in and near the site of injury; (3) the blood cells, particularly the leukocytes; (4) the macrophages

and phagocyte activity; (5) the immune system; and (6) the hormonal system. An inadequate inflammatory response, may cause active, systemic infection.

⬗ Clinical Cues

The five local signs and symptoms of inflammation are heat, redness, swelling, pain, and limitation or loss of function.

Signs and Symptoms of Inflammation

Local Reactions. Redness and *heat* are caused by the increased blood flow to the affected area. *Swelling* is the result of the increased permeability of the capillaries and the leakage of fluid from the blood into the tissue spaces around the cells. Blockage of lymphatic drainage from the site also contributes to the local swelling. *Pain,* caused by the chemicals released by the defensive cells and the accumulation of fluid in the area, irritates the nerve endings.

Systemic Reactions. Systemic reactions to inflammation are familiar to any of us who have had the flu or some other kind of generalized infection. Headache, *myalgia* (muscle aches), fever, diaphoresis, chills, *anorexia* (loss of appetite), and *malaise* (weakness) are some of the more common signs/symptoms a person may experience with a systemic infection. (Note: An inflammatory response can occur in the absence of an infection, such as rheumatoid arthritis or a histamine response due to an insect bite.)

Nursing care for patients who have a systemic infection includes providing for a balanced fluid intake and output, pain relief, and temperature control. Measures ensuring adequate nutrition and rest are employed. If there is an inadequate inflammatory response to a systemic infection, bacterial infections may spread elsewhere in the body and delay tissue repair and wound healing.

Chemical Release and Vascular Changes

The complement system is a group of proteins that lie dormant in the body until they have been activated through an encounter with a foreign substance. The activation of these proteins enhances phagocytosis and the inflammatory process. If viral invasion has occurred, the chemical *interferon* is released in order to protect the cells against further viral invasion. As soon as damage occurs, the blood vessels in the injured area briefly constrict and, as histamine and serotonin are released, they dilate so that more blood is brought to the damaged cells. The walls of the capillaries become more *permeable* (i.e., their pores enlarge) so that water, proteins, and defensive cells can seep into the fluid surrounding the damaged cells. One of the classic outward signs of inflammation is leakage of fluid into the spaces around the cells, producing a localized swelling or *edema.* This results in a "walling off" of the area and delays the spread of pathogens, toxins, and other harmful agents to the rest of the body.

THE IMMUNE RESPONSE

The third line of defense is the immune response, which attempts to defend and protect the body through a series of complex chemical and mechanical activities. These activities involve (1) the detection of entry by foreign agents as soon as they gain access to the body's cells; (2) immediate recognition of the agents as foreign or alien; and (3) the ability to distinguish one kind of foreign agent from another and to "remember" that particular agent if it appears again years later. The specific antibodies and antitoxins produced by the immune response are transported by the circulatory system to the tissue spaces that are surrounding the site of inflammation. They attack the foreign cells and neutralize the toxins those cells produce. The immune response is discussed more fully in Chapter 10.

Hormonal Response

Some hormones, such as cortisone, have an *anti-inflammatory* action that limits inflammation to the locally damaged tissues. Other hormones, such as aldosterone, are *proinflammatory*, which means that they stimulate the body's protective inflammatory response. Thus the hormones have a regulatory effect on the inflammatory process so that the response is well balanced and provides maximum benefit. Other hormones, such as those excreted by the adrenal glands, can interfere with healing, and in some cases of severe inflammation, the physician may prescribe an anti-inflammatory drug to relieve these symptoms.

The Chain of Infection

For an infectious disease to be spread from one person to another, certain conditions must be met. As seen in the links of a chain, infection occurs through a cyclical interrelated process (Figure 6-3). Prevention or control of infection is aimed at interrupting the chain of infection. This can include the performance of hand hygiene or the wearing of gloves to protect the hands or a cover gown to protect one's clothing.

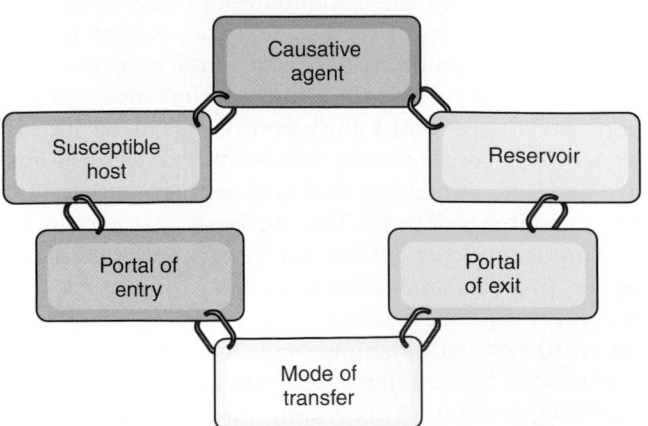

FIGURE 6-3 The cyclical process of infection. Each link of the infection cycle must be present and in the proper sequence to produce disease.

| Box **6-3** | Human Reservoirs |

CARRIER
Person has the actual infection but does not show any obvious signs or symptoms; typically does not take precautions to prevent the spread of infection and can transmit it to others

COLONIZED
Can transmit the pathogenic organisms by either direct or indirect contact with objects or within own environment

INFECTIOUS (SYMPTOMATIC)
Has obvious signs and symptoms of infection; less likely to spread infection as precautions are usually taken

The mechanism of transmission of a pathogenic agent within the environment or to another person is by either direct or indirect contact. **Vectors** such as mosquitoes, fleas, ticks, and flies can transmit pathogens through their bites or stings. (Refer to Chapter 15 for information on West Nile virus and avian flu, which are spread via a vector [mosquitoes or birds].)

The three most important aspects in the infection chain are the interaction of the *agent*, the *host*, and the *mode of transmission*.

A reservoir is any place a pathogen is normally found (Box 6-3). The reservoir can be *animate* (living) such as people, animals, and insects, or it can be *inanimate* (nonliving), as found in soil, in water, and on surfaces of objects such as a cup or bed rails. The body can be a reservoir because pathogenic organisms can grow and multiply *(colonize)* on the skin or inside the body without causing a specific immune response or an infection. Infectious agents can also be found in body excretions or secretions such as saliva, sputum, urine, feces, and wound drainage. Individuals who have become colonized with a specific pathogen, such as methicillin-resistant *Staphylococcus aureus* (MRSA) or vancomycin-resistant *enterococci* (VRE), can be asymptomatic carriers *(reservoirs)* and unknowingly spread the infection to others because they are not aware that they have been exposed and are now colonized with an organism that is known to be multidrug resistant. One of the *Healthy People 2020* objectives is to reduce the incidence of MRSA. In the home or community, contaminated or improperly cooked food, stagnant water, or sewage can also be a source of infection.

INFECTION PREVENTION AND CONTROL

PREVENTING AND CONTROLLING THE SPREAD OF INFECTION

Hand Hygiene

Hand hygiene is the primary intervention any health care provider can use to control the spread of infection. Hand hygiene can be performed with soap and water, if hands are visibly soiled, or an alcohol-based hand sanitizing solution for routine decontamination. It is important to note that hand hygiene must be performed *regardless* of whether gloves were worn while providing care to a patient. Artificial fingernails or extenders are not recommended for those health care providers who have direct patient contact because pathogens can be found beneath the nails.

Clinical Cues

Remove any rings or other forms of jewelry before washing hands with soap and water. Hand hygiene should be done with an approved soap under running water, using friction, for at least 15 to 30 seconds. Ensure that the areas in between fingers and the dorsal and palmar aspects of both hands are thoroughly rubbed.

PRECAUTION CATEGORIES FOR INFECTION PREVENTION AND CONTROL

Standard Precautions

Standard Precautions were mandated by the Centers for Disease Control and Prevention (CDC) in the 1980s (Box 6-4 and see Appendix B). These precautions are designed to prevent the transmission of microorganisms

Box 6-4 Standard Precautions

1. Use barrier precautions, such as gloves, gown, face mask, and protective eyewear, to prevent exposure of skin or mucous membranes to a patient's blood, body fluid, or other potentially infectious materials while providing care or assisting with a procedure with your patient.
   a. Change gloves between contact with one body part and another (e.g., respiratory and urinary).
   b. Perform hand hygiene immediately after removing gloves.
   c. Discard used gloves in the appropriate waste container; do not wash or reuse them.
2. Prevent injury by needle stick or cut from sharp instruments.
   a. Be cautious and attentive any time you are handling a needle or sharp instrument.
   b. Do not recap a used needle by hand; scoop the cap onto the needle on a flat surface or deploy the safety device attached to the needle.
   c. Immediately dispose of a used needle or other sharp instrument in the puncture-resistant container provided for that purpose in the room.
   d. Replace puncture-resistant containers when they are three-quarters full and as needed; do not attempt to push needles into a container that is too full.
3. Prevent possible self-contamination or exposure through broken skin.
   a. If you have open lesions or weeping dermatitis, do not give direct patient care or handle patient care equipment until the condition has resolved.
4. Prevent possible self-contamination during cardiopulmonary resuscitation.
   a. Use disposable mouthpiece or resuscitation bag for emergency mouth-to-mouth breathing.
   b. Wear the appropriate personal protective equipment (PPE) whenever possible.

from one patient to another, as well as to protect the health care worker from unnecessary exposure to infection. Standard Precautions are to be used on all patients because their potential for being colonized, or actually infectious, is not always known. Barrier precautions, such as gloves or isolation techniques that include the proper handling and disposal of secretions, excretions, and exudates, can prevent the transmission of pathogens from one person, or object, to another.

Expanded Precautions

Expanded Precautions incorporate Standard Precaution techniques with additional protective actions specific to the organism and location involved. These safety measures are to be implemented for patients with a suspected or confirmed infection or who are known to be colonized with a highly transmissible organism. These additional precautions are known as category-specific precautions and include the following: Airborne Infection Isolation, Contact Isolation, and Droplet Isolation. Health care facilities have information cards that are usually placed on the door to the patient's room to ensure that all who enter the room are made aware of the safety precautions and the personal protective equipment (PPE) that must be used before entry. Depending on the microorganism involved, the nurse verifies which types of Expanded Precautions are to be used. If unsure as to what types are needed, the nurse should contact the hospital infection control professional for guidance. The effectiveness of Standard Precautions and Expanded Precautions depends on rigorous compliance with the infection prevention and control precautions. See Table 6-5 for more information regarding category-specific isolation methods.

Think Critically

What type of Expanded Precautions would be necessary for a patient who is admitted with complications of varicella? What PPE would you need in order to assist this patient with activities of daily living?

Personal Protective Equipment

Personal protective equipment (PPE) is the use of some type of barrier to protect a person from exposure to blood-borne pathogens, body fluids, or other potentially infectious materials. These barriers include, but are not limited to, gloves, cover gowns, face masks, eye protections, and respirator masks. By law, health care facilities are required to provide PPE at no expense to the staff (Occupational Safety and Health Administration Bloodborne Pathogens Standards, 1910.132). If you suspect you have a latex allergy, contact your Occupational/Employee Health Services department so that a more detailed assessment can be made. If it is determined that a latex allergy does exist,

Table 6-5 Category-Specific Isolation Precautions (Expanded Precautions)

PRIVATE ROOM*	MASKS	GOWNS	GLOVES	COMMON DISEASES PLACED INTO ISOLATION CATEGORY
Airborne Infection Isolation				
Always; door to room must be kept closed at all times	Must wear a fit-tested NIOSH-approved N-95 respirator	No, unless draining wounds	No, unless draining wounds	Pulmonary or laryngeal tuberculosis, or draining tuberculous skin lesions; smallpox, viral hemorrhagic fever, Severe Acute Respiratory Syndrome (SARS); measles; varicella, disseminated zoster
Contact Precautions				
Preferred; cohorting of patients with same type of infection is acceptable	Situation dependent	Always; if patients are cohorted, staff must perform hand hygiene and change PPE *between* patients	Always; if patients are cohorted, staff must perform hand hygiene and change PPE *between* patients	Open or draining wounds, history of MRSA, VRE, ESBL positive; diarrhea; MDRO infections
Droplet Precautions				
Preferred; cohorting of patients with same type of infection is acceptable	Wear a surgical mask when entering room; patient should wear mask during transport and observe cough etiquette	Not usually	When helping with cough-inducing procedures or discarding of used tissues	Pneumonia, influenza, rubella, pertussis, streptococcal pharyngitis, meningitis caused by *Neisseria meningitidis* or *Haemophilus influenzae* type B

ESBL, extended spectrum beta lactamase; *MDRO,* multidrug-resistant organism; *MRSA,* methicillin-resistant *Staphylococcus aureus; NIOSH,* National Institute of Occupational Safety and Health; *PPE,* personal protective equipment; *VRE,* vancomycin-resistant enterococci.
*In most cases, patients infected with the same organism may share a room. For any patient in Expanded Precaution isolation, limit the time the patient is out of the room; notify receiving unit or department that the patient is in isolation so that appropriate measures can be taken before the arrival of the patient.

your facility is required to provide you with the appropriate PPE. Figure 6-4 shows methods for donning and removing PPE.

 Clinical Cues

Remember, when you are using PPE you cannot retrieve common items from your uniform pocket (e.g., pen, alcohol pad, or stethoscope). You must plan ahead and obtain a small stock of supplies and equipment that will remain in the patient's room.

Protective Environment

Patients with hematopoietic stem cell transplantation require highly specialized forms of expanded isolation techniques. Nurses and all staff who provide care to the transplant recipient receive detailed education and training on the appropriate care. Interventions include special airflow and filtration rooms with positive air pressure, smooth surfaces to aid in disinfection, and minimizing the length of time the patient is outside of the protective environment. Staff must be free from signs/symptoms of illness. For additional information, refer to the facility's policy and procedure manuals or the CDC's website, www.cdc.gov, for further guidance.

Respiratory Hygiene and Cough Etiquette

Two methods of preventing droplets from spreading to others are teaching people to cover the mouth when sneezing or coughing and turning one's head away to prevent coughing into the face of another (Figure 6-5). In addition, educating patients and families to dispose of soiled tissues in waste containers and to perform hand hygiene after contact with actual or potentially contaminated items is important. To prevent the transmission of pathogenic microorganisms to a patient, instruct the patient to avoid contact with others who may have an infection.

Transmission of an infectious organism can be interrupted at the portal of entry by using only clean or sterile items when caring for patients. Use of effective hand hygiene techniques by health care workers, visitors, and patients is key in the prevention of infection. Immunization and measures to boost immunity through proper nutrition and a healthy lifestyle also increase a person's resistance to infection. One of the *Healthy People 2020* objectives is to increase the proportion of adults who are immunized for influenza and pneumococcal disease. Table 6-6 on p. 113 lists factors that can make a host more susceptible to pathogens.

DONNING AND REMOVING PPE
Donning Personal Protective Equipment (PPE)
The type of PPE will vary based on the level of precautions required, such as Standard and Contact, Droplet, or Airborne Isolation Precautions.

Gown
- Fully cover torso from neck to knees, arms to end of wrist, and wrap around the back
- Fasten in back at neck and waist

Mask or respirator
- Secure ties or elastic band at middle of head and neck
- Fit flexible band to nose bridge
- Fit snug to face and below chin
- Fit-check respirator

Goggles or face shield
- Put over face and eyes and adjust to fit

Gloves
- Extend to cover wrist of isolation gown

SAFE WORK PRACTICES
- Keep hands away from face
- Limit surfaces touched
- Change gown and gloves when torn or heavily contaminated
- Perform hand hygiene

A

FIGURE 6-4 A, Donning personal protective equipment (PPE).

Continued

? Think Critically

What you would do if, while taking a blood pressure reading, you have a patient who sneezes or coughs and does not cover her nose or mouth? How would you respond? What type of education would benefit the patient? What additional precautions would you need to institute once the patient has left the examination room?

HEALTH CARE–ASSOCIATED INFECTIONS

A **health care–associated infection (HAI),** formerly known as a *nosocomial* infection, occurs when a patient is cared for in any kind of health care setting and acquires an infection. There are specific criteria for the infection to be classified as an HAI, such as length of time in the facility before the onset or appearance of the infection. Because health services are provided in a wide variety of locations, such as acute care facilities, outpatient surgery or dialysis centers, homes, and mobile clinics, it is sometimes difficult to determine just where the patient may have become infected.

Although inanimate objects such as needles, contaminated surgical instruments, and linens are major sources of infection in these settings, every patient is directly and indirectly in contact with large numbers of health care workers, each of whom could be the source of infection. That is why it is important to ensure that appropriate precautions, such as hand hygiene and Expanded Precaution techniques, are followed at all times. Table 6-7 presents HAI risk factors.

Removing Personal Protective Equipment (PPE)
Remove PPE at doorway before leaving patient room, or in anteroom; remove respirator outside of room.

Gloves
- Outside of gloves are contaminated!
- Grasp outside of glove with opposite gloved hand; peel off
- Hold removed glove in gloved hand
- Slide fingers of ungloved hand under remaining glove at wrist

Goggles or face shield
- Outside of goggles or face shield is contaminated!
- To remove, handle by "clean" head band or ear pieces
- Place in designated receptacle for reprocessing or in waste container

Gown
- Gown front and sleeves are contaminated!
- Unfasten neck, undo the waist ties
- Remove gown using a peeling motion; pull gown from each shoulder toward the same hand
- Gown will turn inside out
- Hold removed gown away from body, roll into a bundle, and discard into waste or linen receptacle

Mask or respirator
- Front of mask/respirator is contaminated—DO NOT TOUCH!
- Grasp bottom then top ties/elastics and remove
- Discard in waste container

Hand hygiene
- Perform immediately after removing all PPE!

B

FIGURE 6-4, cont'd **B,** Removing personal protective equipment (PPE).

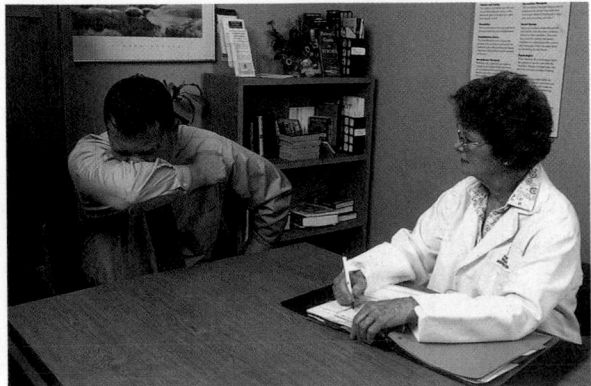

FIGURE 6-5 Covering your cough to help prevent the spread of infection.

THE COST OF HEALTH CARE–ASSOCIATED INFECTIONS

Human suffering, prolonged hospital stays, and time lost from work are some of the concerns with an HAI. Another cost is the increased expense of health care delivery. For example, the cost of treating a catheter-related bloodstream infection is estimated to be between $3700 and $29,000 (Institute for Healthcare Improvement, 2011). Because of the escalating cost of HAIs, Congress is working with multiple agencies to help design a more appropriate method of tracking and reporting HAIs so that there will be uniformity across the country and, hopefully, less confusion. Many states have already enacted mandatory reporting of HAIs to their state health departments.

Table 6-6 **Risk Factors for Increased Susceptibility to Infection**

RISK FACTOR	CONSEQUENCE
Altered defense mechanisms	Body damage from trauma, breaks in the skin or mucous membranes; fractures.
Below normal leukocyte (white blood cell) count	Bone marrow suppression from chemotherapy or toxic agents; genetic or acquired agranulocytosis, such as what is seen with chemotherapy drugs.
Age	Elderly patients and the very young are more susceptible to infection, probably because of declining or immature immune function.
Excessive stress or fatigue	These states seem to interfere with the body's normal defense mechanisms.
Malnutrition	Poor nutrition interferes with cell growth and replacement, which contributes to decreased immune function.
Alcoholism	Inhibits the immune system.
Preexisting chronic illnesses, such as diabetes mellitus, adrenal insufficiency, renal failure, or liver disease; serious illness such as pneumonia, peritonitis, etc.	These disease states upset the normal homeostatic balance within the body, impairing the normal defense mechanisms. Serious illness taxes the immune system, causing greater susceptibility to other pathogens.
Immunosuppressive treatment, chemotherapy, or corticosteroid treatment	Depresses the immune system or harms the bone marrow, decreasing the number of leukocytes. Corticosteroids depress the inflammatory response, inhibiting one of the body's defense mechanisms.
Invasive equipment or indwelling tubes	Fracture pins, endotracheal or tracheostomy tubes, intravenous cannulas, feeding tubes, and urinary catheters provide a potential route of entry for pathogens.
Smoking or inhalation of toxic chemicals	Inhibits ciliary action of the respiratory tract. Toxic chemicals may damage bone marrow, inhibiting the production of leukocytes.
Intravenous drug abuse	Allows introduction of microorganisms into the bloodstream from contaminated needles or from lack of aseptic technique.
Unsafe sexual practices (not knowing history or health status of sexual partner, not using condoms)	Allows entry of pathogenic organisms through the genital mucosal tissue.
Unsafe handling of needles and sharps	Potential for breaks in the skin through which pathogens may enter.

Adapted from Ignatavicius, D.D., & Workman, M.L. (2010). *Medical-Surgical Nursing: Critical Thinking for Collaborative Care* (6th ed.). Philadelphia: Elsevier Saunders.

Table 6-7 **Risk Factors for Health Care–Associated Infections**

RISK	SOURCE OR CAUSE
Impaired host defenses	Invasive tubes (i.e., endotracheal, nasogastric, enteral feeding) Position of the patient (i.e., supine vs. head of bed >30 degrees) Impaired or altered mental status; sedation Malnutrition, malignancy; immunosuppression
Introduction of microorganisms	Bacterial colonization Gastric pH neutralized due to H_2-receptor-blocking agents Lack of oral hygiene Acute vs. chronic sinusitis Invasive procedures; open wounds Contaminated respiratory equipment
Overgrowth of virulent organisms	Prolonged or inappropriate antibiotic use Iatrogenic (inadequate hand hygiene); multidrug-resistant organism infection Central venous lines (i.e., subclavian, femoral, peripherally inserted central catheter) Comorbid illness (e.g., diabetes mellitus, peripheral vascular disease) Frequent hospitalizations or exposure to invasive therapies Prolonged hospital stays

Adapted from Flanders, A.S., Collard, H.R., & Saint, S. (2006). Nosocomial pneumonia: State of the science. *American Journal of Infection Control, 34*, 84-93.

NURSING INTERVENTIONS TO PREVENT HEALTH CARE–ASSOCIATED INFECTIONS

Hand hygiene is the key to breaking the chain of infection; however, for it to be effective, you need to know what to use. For example, if the patient has an *S. aureus* infection, the health care worker can use (1) soap and water or (2) an alcohol-based hand sanitizer to cleanse the hands. However, if the patient has a *Clostridium difficile* or *Candida albicans* infection, the health care worker must use only soap and water to cleanse the hands. The alcohol in alcohol-based sanitizers only makes the spores for these organisms "sticky"; it does not kill them. In addition, if a patient with *C. difficile* is discharged, the housekeeping staff needs to know that the patient had this type of infection so that the appropriate cleaning agents will be used. The primary way to prevent infection is careful attention to hand hygiene before and after any direct patient contact, before and after any invasive or sterile procedure, after contact with infectious materials (e.g., wound drainage, feces, urine, or sputum), and before contact with immunocompromised patients. Reducing catheter-related infections is one of the 2011 National Patient Safety Goals and a *Healthy People 2020* objective. Interventions for this important goal include hand hygiene, use of a standardized kit for dressing changes, and chlorhexidine-based antiseptic for skin preparation.

Clinical Cue

In accordance with National Patient Safety Goals (The Joint Commission [TJC], 2010), compliance with guidelines for hand hygiene is one of the primary issues for reducing HAIs. Make a point of washing your hands in view of the patient and the family; this builds their confidence in you as a caregiver and demonstrates your attention to preventing infection.

Soiled or contaminated items should not be placed on the floor or remain in an uncovered trash container in the patient's room. Disposing of infectious materials, such as tissues, used dressings, soiled linens, and contaminated equipment, in covered, moisture-resistant biohazard containers helps contain the organism, as well as odors. Protecting patients from others with respiratory infections and from visitors with other communicable diseases is also appropriate. Table 6-8 reviews the major sites of HAIs, the infectious agents most often responsible, and some of the interventions nurses may take to prevent or control the spread of infection.

Along with preventive interventions and appropriate treatments, the nurse must continuously assess the patient to identify early signs of infection or its spread. It is also helpful to review and document each patient's immunization status against such infections as tetanus, pertussis, influenza, hepatitis B, pneumococcal pneumonia, and varicella.

INFECTION SURVEILLANCE AND REPORTING

Surveillance demands that nurses be alert for signs or symptoms of infection in patients under their care. For example, the nurse should routinely assess the patient for unexpected elevation of temperature; malaise; cough; loss of appetite; foul-smelling urine; new-onset diarrhea; and wounds that are red, swollen, painful, or have a foul-smelling discharge. It is important to note the color of the purulent drainage as it is helpful in identifying the kind of organism that may be causing an infection (e.g., *S. aureus* produces a golden discharge and *Pseudomonas aeruginosa* has bluish green discharge).

The nurse should pay particular attention to those patients who are more susceptible to infection. These patients include those who (1) are weakened by severe illness or injury; (2) have drainage tubes or catheters, intravenous cannulas, or other invasive devices for monitoring or treatment; (3) are very young or very

Table 6-8 Preventing and Controlling Health Care–Associated Infections

MOST COMMON SITES	NURSING INTERVENTIONS
Urinary tract	Catheterize only when absolutely necessary. Observe sterile technique when catheterizing. Keep drainage system for indwelling catheter closed, off the floor, and below bladder level at all times to avoid urine reflux. Empty urine drainage bag into clean container, without contaminating spout. Wipe spout with alcohol pad before securing it. Remove indwelling catheter as soon as possible to decrease risk of infection.
Surgical wounds	Administer prophylactic antimicrobials as ordered. Change soiled dressing and linens promptly. Dispose of them in the correct container. Ensure that patient has adequate nutrition and sufficient fluid intake.
Respiratory tract	Encourage the patient to cough, deep breathe, and move. Perform suctioning, tracheostomy care, and other procedures under aseptic technique. Protect patient from others with colds or other signs of infection.
Bloodstream (bacteremia)	Maintain meticulous aseptic technique in the administration of intravenous (IV) fluids. Follow recommended procedure for daily care of insertion site (including the dressing) and IV tubing and catheters. Assess site for increased redness, pain, or infiltration. Remove and insert new IV set per facility policy, and when indicated.

old; (4) have had recent surgery; or (5) are immuno-compromised. When an infection is suspected, the nurse reports this to the patient's health care provider. In certain situations, Expanded Precautions may need to be instituted even before culture results are available. If there is a question as to what type of Expanded Precautions to initiate, the nurse should contact the facility's infection control department.

MEDICAL ASEPSIS AND SURGICAL ASEPSIS

Medical Asepsis

Medical asepsis (the goal is to reduce microorganisms) includes hand hygiene, separation or isolation of the patient, use of appropriate precautions for the handling and disposing of contaminated articles, and other techniques devised to contain and destroy infectious agents, such as cleansing and disinfection.

Surgical Asepsis

Surgical asepsis (the goal is to completely eliminate microorganisms) involves the sterilizing of instruments, skin, linens, and other articles that will be used to perform surgery or other types of sterile procedures. This is because a surgical procedure typically requires that the first line of defense (i.e., the skin) be compromised in some way. Surgical asepsis must also be used when placing an intravenous catheter into a vein, when inserting a Foley catheter into the urinary bladder, during the placement of internal monitoring devices, or during other invasive procedures such as a cardiac angiogram. Hand hygiene for surgical asepsis is more vigorous and must be done according to the facility's policy and procedure. In a surgically aseptic environment, surgical gowns, face masks, and sterile gloves are necessary and must be put on and removed in a specific way. Procedures being performed at the bedside that require surgical asepsis, such as a central line placement, require that all persons in the room wear a face mask and head cover. The person performing the procedure must also wear sterile gloves and a sterile cover gown. The patient must be covered with sterile drapes, and only sterile equipment and supplies are to be used. The door to the room must be closed throughout the procedure (CDC, 2002).

SEPSIS AND SEPTIC SHOCK

If a patient's HAI or community-acquired infection is not adequately treated, the pathogen may enter the bloodstream, causing a bacteremia and sepsis with a systemic inflammatory response syndrome (SIRS). When microorganisms enter the bloodstream, they are carried throughout the body and may invade any tissue or body system. Symptoms of sepsis include, but are not limited to, tachycardia, increased cardiac output, *tachypnea* (rapid breathing), fever, and an elevated WBC count. An altered level of consciousness may also

occur. Sepsis is most commonly associated with bacterial invasion from gram-negative bacteria, such as *Pseudomonas aeruginosa, Escherichia coli,* and *Klebsiella pneumoniae,* or gram-positive bacteria such as *Staphylococcus aureus* and *Streptococcus pneumoniae.* The toxins secreted into the blood from these pathogens react with the blood vessels and cell membranes, stimulating a massive inflammatory and immune response. Increased capillary permeability with loss of fluid from the vascular space, cellular injury, and greatly increased cellular metabolic rates can result in septic shock. Refer to Chapter 45 for further information on SIRS and septic shock.

NURSING INTERVENTIONS FOR PATIENTS WITH SEPSIS

Patients who are at risk for sepsis must be identified and then closely monitored for changes from the baseline assessment, such as a change in mental status; the development of warm, dry, flushed skin; peripheral edema; a full, bounding pulse; normal to high blood pressure; and decreased urine output. The temperature may be normal or elevated, depending on the organism or organisms that are causing the sepsis. Pneumonia and postsurgical wound infections are two conditions that can lead to sepsis if not correctly treated, and some patients, often the elderly, experience *hypothermia* (below normal temperature) when septic.

Sepsis is diagnosed from the clinical presentation of the patient and the results of laboratory tests, such as elevated leukocyte count, decreased platelets, and serial blood cultures that may be positive for invading organisms. Antimicrobial sensitivities are done on these pathogens to determine which drugs would be most appropriate to treat the infection. Ensuring that the correct antimicrobial agents are prescribed in a timely manner decreases the risk of the patient developing a multidrug-resistant infection and eliminates the pathogens as quickly as possible.

Clinical Cues

If sepsis is discovered early, the chance of a full recovery is good. Septic shock can progress to the stage of tissue damage from microthrombus formation and disseminated intravascular coagulation (DIC), and the prognosis is poor and death may soon occur. Closely monitoring the patient who has an infection for signs of sepsis and reporting any such signs to the physician are extremely important.

❖ NURSING MANAGEMENT

■ Assessment (Data Collection)

Detecting infection in a patient requires a thorough nursing assessment. Subjective data can be obtained by asking the patient to describe symptoms and time of onset. Questions should also include whether the patient is or has had any of the following: pain, headache, stiff neck, fever, or chills. The interview is based on the patient's complaints, for example, if the patient states that it hurts to go to the bathroom, ask if there is also urgency or burning when trying to empty the bladder. With some signs and symptoms, it may be appropriate to ask if patients have traveled outside the country recently (i.e., amebic dysentery), or if they have been bitten by any insects before onset of symptoms (i.e., West Nile virus), or if they have a compromised immune system, either from disease or from drug exposure (i.e., chemotherapy agents). (Refer to Chapter 15 for more information on West Nile virus.)

 Clinical Cues

Subjective complaints that may indicate infection include fatigue, loss of appetite, headache, nausea, general malaise, and pain.

Objective data often point to the specific body system affected by the infection, but may also include systemic signs such as fever, increased pulse, or increased respiratory rate. Data collection includes assessing vital signs; auscultating the lungs to check for abnormal breath sounds; inspecting the skin for lesions or rashes; and checking the urine for cloudiness, discoloration, abnormal odor, and increased specific gravity. Bowel sounds are auscultated in all four quadrants, and then the abdomen is gently palpated for signs of tenderness. In addition, look for signs of local infection such as redness, swelling, or pain or tenderness on palpation or movement, heat in the affected area, and possibly loss of function of the affected body part.

Elder Care Points

Many elderly people, especially those over age 80, have a normally low body temperature. Because of decreased inflammatory and immune response, there may be very little rise in temperature in the presence of infection. Small increases in temperature in these patients may be quite significant. Signs of inflammation may not be present or may be less than what is typically seen in a younger person. A decrease in mental alertness, increased fatigue, or sudden onset of confusion, irritability, or apathy may be clues that an infection is present.

Diagnostic Tests

Laboratory data that may indicate infection include an elevated WBC count, changes in the distribution and number of the various types of leukocytes, an elevated erythrocyte sedimentation rate (ESR), and microbiology cultures that test positive for microorganisms.

Bacteriologic tests are done by culturing blood, body fluids, or waste products such as feces. Cultures are grown from specimens collected. When obtaining a culture, the nurse must be careful to (1) use aseptic technique, where indicated and with sterile equipment; (2) only collect fresh material from the suspected site, avoiding contamination by microbes from nearby tissues and fluids; and (3) use the appropriate container for the sample, making sure the container is correctly labeled and tightly covered to avoid spilling and contamination during transport to the laboratory.

Sensitivity tests are done in conjunction with microbiology cultures to determine which antimicrobials can most effectively destroy or inhibit the multiplication and growth of the specific infecting microbe. Once this has been determined, the drug that is most likely to kill the invading microorganism needs to be started as soon as possible. Inadequate dosages or delays in administration can lead to a genetic mutation of the pathogen involved or the development of a **multidrug-resistant organism (MDRO)**.

With some infectious diseases, intradermal skin tests are done to determine the presence of certain active or inactive diseases, such as tuberculosis, coccidioidomycosis, and candidiasis. Radiography (x-rays), computed tomography (CT), or magnetic resonance imaging (MRI) may be used to detect changes in the tissues or organs and to locate abscesses anywhere within the body.

■ Nursing Diagnosis

The specific type of infection and the problem it presents determine the correct nursing diagnosis. For example, if the patient has a urinary tract infection, the more specific nursing diagnosis would be *Alteration in urinary elimination*. In some cases, collaboration with other health team members helps establish the correct nursing diagnosis. Appropriate nursing diagnoses for patients with infection always include *Risk for infection* and *Risk for injury*. Any patient entering the hospital for surgery or an invasive procedure is at risk for an HAI. Therefore *Risk for infection* should be listed as a nursing diagnosis on the patient's care plan. The nursing diagnosis of *Deficient knowledge related to lack of knowledge about the disease, prevention of infection, or self-care* should always be considered (Nursing Care Plan 6-1).

■ Planning

The planning phase of the nursing process should take into account the physical strength of the patient and the need for rest. Every effort should be made to maintain the integrity of the skin and mucous membranes so that they continue to serve as effective barriers to infectious agents. Good skin care, oral hygiene, and personal cleanliness are essential. The psychological impact of Expanded Precautions must be addressed as some patients may feel "dirty" or that people are avoiding them because they have an infectious disease.

Scenario

Patient is a 28-year-old man who has been diagnosed with a lower abdominal wound infection that is culture positive for methicillin-resistant *Staphylococcus aureus* (MRSA). He is going to be discharged in 2 days.

Problem/Nursing Diagnosis

Wound infection/Impaired skin integrity related to infected abdominal wound.

Supporting Assessment Data

Objective: Drainage from abdominal wound is culture positive for MRSA, a multidrug-resistant organism (MDRO).

Goals/Expected Outcomes	Nursing Interventions	Selected Rationale	Evaluation
Infection will be controlled and not spread.	Place in Contact Precautions and explain purpose and requirement to patient and visitors.	To prevent the spread of infection to other patients and staff.	No evidence of spread of infection.
	Assist patient with bath to ensure skin has been cleaned.	Enables the nurse to do a thorough skin assessment.	Bathed.
	Change wound dressing as ordered and as needed.	Ensures that the wound is assessed at least daily and nurse can track progression of wound treatment.	Dressing changed, less drainage and redness.
	Monitor vital signs, complete blood count, microbiology cultures.	Indicates progress in resolving the infection.	Vital signs stable. WBC normalizing. Outcomes met.

Problem/Nursing Diagnosis

Has never cared for a wound/Deficit knowledge related to proper wound care at home.

Supporting Assessment Data

Subjective: States, "I don't know how to change the dressing."

Goals/Expected Outcomes	Nursing Interventions	Selected Rationale	Evaluation
Before discharge, the patient and family member will be able to: • Demonstrate proper hand hygiene techniques.	Demonstrate proper hand hygiene technique and observe patient and family member perform this task.	Providing opportunities for education and training throughout the hospital stay increases the knowledge base the patient or the caregiver can build on.	Patient verbalizes reasons for Contact Precautions; patient and family member demonstrate proper hand hygiene, wound cleansing, and dressing change techniques using medical asepsis; patient and family member verbalize signs and symptoms to report to physician and states that he understands how to take medication and why he must finish the prescription.
• State reasons for using Contact Precautions for dressing change. • Demonstrate dressing change, maintaining medical asepsis before discharge.	Demonstrate dressing change and wound cleansing procedure; obtain return demonstration from patient and family member before discharge.	Providing hands-on training increases the understanding of wound healing and need for appropriate wound care.	
• List signs and symptoms that should be reported to physician.	Instruct patient and family to watch for elevated temperature, increased redness, swelling, pain, or purulent discharge from wound, and to report any such findings to the physician.	Knowing what to look for and report decreases the risk of adverse outcomes.	
• State why it is important to complete the course of antibiotic therapy exactly as directed.	Explain importance of taking medication exactly as prescribed and of finishing entire prescription.	Taking antimicrobials as prescribed decreases the risk of the patient developing an MDRO infection.	Outcomes being met.

Critical Thinking Questions

1. What other nursing methods could you implement that would promote healing?
2. How would you recommend the patient's linens be laundered at home?

Cultural beliefs about infection and recovery should also be considered.

The nursing goals for recovery from infection include measures to help the patient:

- Use the body's own defensive and healing processes
- Obtain adequate rest, nutrition, and hydration
- Be as free from physical discomfort as possible
- Be free of as much mental anxiety or depression as possible
- Ensure that sufficient oxygen and blood are supplied to the infected tissues

Cultural Considerations

Hot and Cold Foods

Some Asian cultures believe that a balance of hot and cold foods should be eaten when a fever or infection is present. They believe that cold foods, such as watermelon or white radish soup, will help the body fight off the infection and retain its balance. Many Hispanic cultures believe that "hot" and "cold" forces are thrown out of balance when illness strikes. They may prefer cold foods such as dairy products, honey, or fresh vegetables when they are suffering from infection.

■ Implementation

Providing a quiet environment with uninterrupted rest periods is important in the recovery process. Relieving the discomforts of fever and muscle aches is accomplished by tepid sponge baths, ice bags, antipyretics, and massage. Warm compresses and the application of heat, as appropriate, can also promote healing. Mild physical exercise promotes circulation and helps some patients to relax. It can also increase blood circulation to an infected area. This ultimately will help to remove the metabolic wastes that were produced from the body.

Provide patient and family teaching regarding the infection, including the following:

- The purposes of diagnostic tests, treatments, and special precautions
- Why the family must help maintain medical asepsis to prevent the spread of infection to themselves and others

Administering Antimicrobial Agents

Administer the antimicrobial drugs on time to maintain effective blood levels. In addition, monitor the patient for drug side effects and evaluate the progress of the patient to determine whether the drug is effective in eradicating the infection. General nursing actions for the administration of an antimicrobial medication are shown in Table 6-9.

Before administering the prescribed drug, be familiar with the different antimicrobial agent classifications: antibacterial, antiviral, antifungal, and anthelmintic (Table 6-10).

 Complementary and Alternative Therapies

Prolonged antibiotic use can destroy the normal gastrointestinal flora and cause antibiotic-associated diarrhea. Probiotics are available in yogurt or in tablet, capsule, or powder form and may help to restore natural flora. Side effects include mild abdominal discomfort and flatulence. The patient should be encouraged to consult the health care provider before using probiotics.

Koivula, M. (2010). Intro to Probiotic Therapy. *Advance for Nurses.* http://nursing.advanceweb.com/Regional-Articles/Features/Intro-to-Probiotic-Therapy-4.aspx.

There are two primary categories of antibacterial agents: narrow spectrum and broad spectrum. Both kinds inhibit replication and growth of bacterial organisms. The most common side effects are nausea, vomiting, and diarrhea. The narrow-spectrum agents primarily work on a select type of microorganism such as a gram-positive organism that is susceptible to penicillin. A broad-spectrum antibiotic can attack a larger group of organisms. However, these agents can also cause superinfections because they wind up killing off many of the "good bacteria" in the body. A narrow-spectrum antibiotic is the preferred choice for treatment over a broad-spectrum agent because it primarily goes after the pathogenic organism and also reduces the risk of developing an MDRO infection.

Antiviral agents interfere with DNA or RNA synthesis required for the virus to duplicate itself. The most common side effects are headache, nausea, vomiting, anorexia, and diarrhea; more severe side effects include acute renal failure, encephalopathy, and bleeding disorders.

Antifungal agents increase permeability of the cell membrane by binding with certain components, leading to decreased nutrients to the cell. The most common side effects are headache, fever, chills, nausea, vomiting, and anorexia; more severe side effects include acute kidney and/or liver failure, and hemorrhagic gastroenteritis.

Anthelmintic agents cause paralysis of the invading parasite, and common side effects include dizziness, headache, fever, nausea, vomiting, anorexia, diarrhea, and rash.

Supporting Coping Mechanisms

Stress seems to make the body more vulnerable to invasion by foreign organisms by depressing the immune system. When under excessive stress, the body also is less able to mobilize the elements and cells that promote healing. The nurse should realize that the attitude shown toward a patient and the ways in which the nurse strives to meet the patient's needs could reduce stress and promote healing in ways that are not yet completely understood.

If the illness is lengthy, concerns about work and home responsibilities may cause anxiety or increase

Table 6-9   General Nursing Implications for the Administration of Antimicrobial Drugs

NURSING IMPLICATIONS	RATIONALE
Before Giving the Antimicrobial Drug	
• Check all drugs patient is receiving for drug interactions with the antimicrobial prescribed.	To prevent toxicity or lack of absorption
• Know the reason why the patient is to receive an antimicrobial drug (question the health care provider if the drug does not seem appropriate for the patient).	To help prevent drug administration errors
• Check that dosage of an antimicrobial drug is appropriate for the patient who may have decreased kidney or liver function.	To ensure drug levels do not build up to a toxic level
• Verify allergies with the patient before administering an antimicrobial drug.	To prevent allergic reaction or adverse outcomes
• Ensure cultures have been obtained before administering the antimicrobial agent. If culture and sensitivity results are available, verify that the drug that was ordered is one to which the organism is sensitive. If it is not, clarify the order with the health care provider.	To ensure medication being given is appropriate for the microorganism involved
• Check precautions for administration of the antimicrobial drug, especially when the patient is pregnant or lactating.	To prevent harm to the developing fetus or infant
When Giving an Antimicrobial Drug	
• Follow the "Five Rights" of medication administration.	To prevent errors and injury to the patient
• Give each dose of an antimicrobial drug as close to the scheduled time as possible.	To maintain a consistent blood level of the drug
• Check to see if serum drug levels have been ordered. Ensure that they are drawn as specified by the physician.	To ensure drug dosage is effective and to ensure toxicity will not occur
Monitor for Possible Side/Adverse Effects	
• The most common general side effects are gastrointestinal upset, anorexia, nausea, diarrhea, rash, and photosensitivity.	Knowing what the side effects are aids the nurse in effectively teaching the patient about what to observe for and report to the physician
• Monitor patient for signs of allergic reaction, such as rash, hives, itching, drug fever, swelling of the mucous membranes, difficulty breathing, or anaphylaxis.	To ensure appropriate interventions are instituted quickly and to prevent more severe outcomes up to, and including, death
• Check for signs of superinfection in patients taking high doses of an antimicrobial drug for an extended period of time (e.g., oral thrush, vaginal itching or discharge, diarrhea).	To ensure appropriate countermeasures can be instituted in a timely manner
Teach the Patient	
• Take the medication with a full glass of water.	To aid with absorption
• Take all of an antimicrobial drug prescription, regardless of whether the patient feels better and has no obvious signs or symptoms of infection.	To prevent the development of multidrug-resistant microorganisms
• Take the medication in relationship to meals. (Different drugs vary in this respect; some need to be taken with food and some should be taken on an empty stomach.)	For best absorption of the drug with minimal gastrointestinal side effects
• Discontinue the drug and notify the health care provider if an allergic reaction occurs.	To ensure treatment is instituted quickly and to prevent more severe outcomes up to, and including, death. May require an alternate type of antibiotic to be prescribed
• Use a sunblock and protective clothing when sun exposure is unavoidable when taking an antimicrobial agent that is known to cause photosensitivity.	To decrease the risk of sunburn
• Unless contraindicated, increase fluid intake to 2500–3000 mL/day, especially when taking a sulfa-type drug.	To prevent crystallization in the kidneys and promote drug excretion

Table 6-10   Antimicrobial Drug Classifications*

Antibacterial Agents

Narrow Spectrum
Gram-positive cocci and gram-positive bacilli
Penicillins G and V
Vancomycin
Erythromycin
Clindamycin
Gram-negative aerobes
Aminoglycosides: gentamicin, tobramycin, neomycin, and azithromycin
Cephalosporins:
   First generation (e.g., cefazolin [Ancef], cephalexin [Keflex])
   Second generation (e.g., cefaclor [Ceclor], cefotetan [Cefotan], cefuroxime [Zinacef])
Mycobacterium tuberculosis
Ethambutol
Isoniazid
Pyrazinamide
Rifampin

Broad Spectrum
Gram-positive cocci and gram-negative bacilli
Broad-spectrum penicillins (e.g., ampicillin)
Cephalosporins:
   Third generation (e.g., cefepime [Maxipime], cefixime [Suprax], cefotaxime [Claforan], ceftriaxone [Rocephin])
Tetracyclines (e.g., doxycycline, minocycline)
Carbapenems (e.g., imipenem and meropenem)
Sulfonamides (e.g., sulfasalazine, sulfisoxazole)

Antiviral Agents

Acyclovir
Amantadine
Azidothymidine
Saquinavir

Antifungal Agents

Amphotericin B
Ketoconazole
Itraconazole

Anthelmintic Agents

Pyrantel

Data from Lehne, R.A. (2010). *Pharmacology for Nursing Care* (7th ed.). Philadelphia: Elsevier Saunders; and Skidmore-Roth, L. (2011). *Mosby's Nursing Drug Reference* (24th ed.). Philadelphia: Elsevier Mosby.
*As with any other drug, it is important for the nurse to know what the drug is and what it is being given for, and to provide close nursing observation, especially if the patient has never received the drug in the past. Teaching the patient signs and symptoms to report is also an important part of providing safe and effective nursing care.

the patient's stress levels. Therefore collaboration with the social worker or case manager for solutions to such problems may be needed.

Patient Teaching for Preventing and Controlling Infection

Appropriate teaching is essential so that the patient and the patient's family will understand why specific precautions are necessary. Before beginning teaching, the nurse needs to find out how much the patient or family knows about the patient's condition and the problems that may arise. Nurses have an obligation to teach patients how to care for themselves and how to avoid infection through good personal hygiene.

 Patient Teaching

How to Prevent and Control Infection

Teach the patient and family:
- The ways in which the infection is transmitted
- How to perform proper hand hygiene
- Correct techniques for wound care
- The approved method for disinfecting or sanitizing equipment, supplies, and linens
- The correct method for proper handling and disposal of contaminated articles
- Any specific precautions for the type of infection the patient has

The patient taking antimicrobial medications at home must be taught how to take them, to take all the medication as prescribed, and not to discontinue taking any antimicrobial medication, even if symptoms are gone. Explain to the patient and the family that stopping before the full amount of medication has been taken can lead to a second outbreak of the infection and possibly a return to the hospital.

▪ Evaluation

Evaluation of the success of interventions includes data indicating:
- Temperature, pulse, and respirations are within normal range
- WBC count and ESR are within normal limits and cultures are negative (see Chapter 10 for more information on diagnostic tests and normal laboratory values).
- Ability to rest comfortably
- Absence of or decrease in severity of pain and discomfort
- Fluid and nutritional needs are being met

COMMUNITY CARE

As more nurses work in community settings, opportunities to educate the public about preventing the spread of infection become even more important. Controlling the spread of infectious diseases within the community is accomplished in conjunction with public health officials. Their major goals, and those of nurses who work with them, are to (1) promote sanitary standards in communities, (2) identify persons who are highly susceptible to infection and reduce their chances of developing an infectious disease, and (3) provide immunization programs to protect people against certain infectious diseases.

HOME CARE

The home care nurse must educate the patient and family members to help prevent infection. All people living in the home should be instructed to wash their hands as soon as they return home from being out in a public place. Microorganisms are picked up on the hands from a variety of items, such as shopping cart handles, elevator buttons, door handles, and telephone receivers. The incidence of colds and flu might be decreased if, during the heavy respiratory illness season, people who are at increased risk for infection would stay away from crowded stores and theaters where pathogens are likely to be airborne.

The home care nurse must teach the techniques of medical asepsis to patients and family members to prevent cross-infection from one person to another or the spread of infection in the patient. Hand hygiene is stressed, and family members are taught not to share personal items, especially toothbrushes or razors that might be contaminated by blood. Dishes and eating utensils are washed with soap and water or in the dishwasher. The patient's soiled linens, clothing, and towels should be washed as soon as possible or stored in sealed plastic bags until washed. Surfaces contaminated with traces of blood, urine, feces, or vomitus should be sanitized using a clean cloth, soap, and hot water, and then recleaned with a 1:10 solution of chlorine bleach and hot water. Within the home, the patient and family are taught to contain infectious wastes such as dressings and soiled tissues in a sealed, impermeable plastic bag. The bags can then be disposed of in the garbage cans outside of the home.

🏃 Health Promotion

What You Can Do to Prevent Infections at Home

1. Wash your hands often.
   - **When:** Before eating; before, during, and after handling/preparing food; before dressing a wound, giving medicine, or inserting contact lenses; after contact with body fluids or blood; after changing a diaper; after using the bathroom; after handling animals, their toys, leashes, or waste; after handling anything contaminated, such as trash, drainage, soil, etc.
   - **How:** Wet hands and apply soap, briskly rub hands together for 20 seconds, rinse thoroughly with warm water, and dry with a clean towel.
2. Routinely clean surfaces.
   - **In kitchen:** Clean counters, cutting boards, and all other surfaces before, during, and after preparing food, especially meat and poultry. Use hot, soapy water and scrub cutting boards well. Avoid wooden cutting boards, because they tend to hold more bacteria.
   - **In bathroom:** Clean and disinfect all surfaces routinely.
3. Handle and prepare food safely.
   - **Clean:** Clean hands and work surfaces often.
   - **Separate:** Do not cross-contaminate one food with another; use separate cutting boards for meat and fresh produce and keep food separate in the refrigerator.
   - **Cook:** Cook foods to proper temperatures; use a food thermometer. Find recommended food cooking temperatures at *www.fightbac.org/heatitup.cfm* or *www.isitdoneyet.gov*.
   - **Chill:** Refrigerate foods promptly. Do not thaw frozen foods on the countertop.
4. Get immunized.
   - Make sure you and your loved ones get the necessary shots suggested by your health care provider at the proper time, and maintain immunization records for the family. Ask your physician about special programs that provide free shots for your child.
5. Use antibiotics appropriately.
   - Take antibiotics exactly as prescribed by your health care provider. Antibiotics do not work against viruses such as colds or flu.
6. Be careful with pets.
   - Follow the immunization schedule for your pets as recommended by the vet.
   - Clean litter boxes daily.
   - Make sure your child does not put any object or hands in the mouth after touching animals.
   - Wash hands thoroughly after contact with animals, especially after visiting farms, petting zoos, and fairs.
   - Use flea and tick prevention treatment on cats and dogs.
7. Avoid contact with wild animals.
   - Do not leave food around and keep garbage cans sealed around your home.
   - Clear brush, grass, and debris around your home.
   - Seal any entrance holes to animal dens, if any are found inside or outside of your home.
   - Use insect repellent to prevent ticks.

Maintaining a healthy lifestyle that promotes an intact immune system increases a person's resistance to infection. Obtaining adequate sleep, eating properly, and exercising regularly all contribute to increased resistance to illness or infection. Adopting effective stress reduction techniques and using them regularly can also be beneficial.

LONG-TERM CARE

The elderly in long-term care facilities often have chronic illnesses that add to their susceptibility. Many elderly have low-grade infections of the urinary, respiratory, or gastrointestinal tract that can be easily passed on to others if hand hygiene is not consistently practiced. Provide assistance to residents to wash their hands before meals and after toileting, after being in community rooms such as the dining room or social activities lounge, and any time their hands become soiled. Cleaning incontinent patients promptly and maintaining skin integrity is an essential nursing function. Also, to help decrease the odors caused by incontinence, it is important to secure soiled linens in plastic linens bags before removal from the patient's room.

Get Ready for the NCLEX® Examination!

Key Points

- Normal flora is needed to help prevent harmful microorganisms from colonizing or infecting the body.
- An infection is the presence and growth of pathogenic microorganisms, in a susceptible host, to the extent that tissue damage occurs.
- The relationship between the host, the agent, and the environment is what determines whether an infection will or will not occur.
- A pathogen is any organism that, if allowed to grow, can cause infection or disease.
- There are multiple types of antimicrobial drugs that can be used to fight infection: antibiotics for bacterial infections, antivirals for viral infections, and antifungals for fungal infections.
- The body has mechanical barriers, such as the skin and mucous membranes, and chemical barriers, such as tears or saliva, that help fight against infection.
- Fever is one of the primary immune responses to fighting off invading microorganisms.
- Hand hygiene is the number one way to prevent the spread of infection.
- There are three types of Expanded Precautions: Airborne, Contact, and Droplet. Each requires different personal protective equipment and isolation protocols.
- Using respiratory hygiene and cough etiquette helps to prevent the spread of infection.
- Blood or other body fluid specimens for culture must be collected before the start of any antimicrobial agent.
- Assess how much the patient already knows about preventing the spread of infection and teach about hand hygiene, the correct use of antimicrobial agents, cleaning of wounds, and keeping the home environment clean.
- The nurse must model scrupulous hand hygiene compliance for patients and family members.

Additional Learning Resources

SG Go to your Study Guide for additional learning activities to help you master this chapter content.

evolve Go to your Evolve website (http://evolve.elsevier.com/deWit/medsurg) for the following FREE learning resources:
- Animations, audio, and video
- Answers and rationales for questions and activities
- Concept Map Creator
- Glossary with pronunciations in English and Spanish
- Interactive Review Questions and Exercises and more!

Online Resources
- Health care–associated infections, www.cdc.gov/hai
- Infection control, www.guideline.gov/content.aspx?id=15722&search=infection+control

Review Questions for the NCLEX® Examination

1. The nurse is admitting a patient with an infected abdominal wound. Wound cultures are positive for methicillin-resistant *Staphylococcus aureus*. Appropriate nursing care for this patient includes:
    1. monitoring temperature and white blood cell count.
    2. placing the patient on strict intake and output.
    3. instituting respiratory precautions.
    4. encouraging ambulation along the hallways.

2. During an assessment, the nurse notes fever, fatigue, general weakness, cold and clammy skin, nausea, vomiting, and diarrhea. What is an appropriate nursing diagnosis?
    1. Pain
    2. Deficient fluid volume
    3. Deficient knowledge
    4. Ineffective coping

3. Which patient instruction is most critical to a patient being discharged on antibiotic therapy?
    1. Wash your hands.
    2. Monitor urine color.
    3. Reduce stress.
    4. Take all the antibiotics as prescribed.

4. The nurse is observing a nursing student who must perform a dressing change for a patient. The nurse would intervene if the student:
    1. washes hands with soap under running water, using friction, for 20 seconds.
    2. removes rings and jewelry before washing hands with soap and water.
    3. washes hands before donning clean gloves to remove the old dressing.
    4. prepares supplies, dons sterile gloves, and removes the old dressing.

5. When determining the most appropriate antibiotic for an infection, the physician is likely to rely on:
    1. elevated white blood cells.
    2. culture and sensitivity.
    3. erythrocyte sedimentation rate.
    4. fever.

6. The nurse assumes the care of a patient with active pulmonary tuberculosis. Before entering the patient's room, what is an appropriate nursing action?
    1. Keep the door open to maintain continuous airflow.
    2. Wear a properly fit-tested N-95 mask.
    3. Don sterile gloves.
    4. Observe strict Standard Precautions.

7. The need for protective isolation and the parameters are being explained to the patient. She wails, "How can I hug my children when I am locked up in this room?" A likely nursing diagnosis would be:
   1. Pain.
   2. Altered nutrition.
   3. Deficient knowledge.
   4. Social isolation.

8. Which intervention would the nurse implement for a patient with active pulmonary tuberculosis who has social isolation related to imposed airborne precautions?
   1. Limit the number of visitors to immediate family.
   2. Suggest alternative means of contact such as e-mail and phone calls.
   3. Arrange for a nursing assistant to sit with the patient.
   4. Reinforce rationale for airborne precautions.

9. The nurse is caring for an elderly patient and notes a change in mental status. The skin is flushed, warm, and dry. There is a full, bounding pulse and a decreased urine output. What is the priority action?
   1. Alert the rapid response team for suspected sepsis.
   2. Call the physician to obtain an order for blood cultures.
   3. Take a full set of vital signs and compare them to the baseline.
   4. Check the patient's history to determine risk for sepsis.

10. Cross-infection among members of the household who take care of a relative with a severe infection can be prevented by which behavior(s)? *(Select all that apply.)*
    1. Share personal items.
    2. Practice hand hygiene.
    3. Use bleach to clean surfaces.
    4. Seal used dressings in impermeable bags.
    5. Wash soiled linens weekly.

Critical Thinking Questions

Scenario A
Mrs. Compton, age 44, is admitted to the hospital for a hysterectomy. During the admission assessment procedure, you notice a large, draining abscess in her axillary region. She also has a temperature of 100° F (37.7° C), and she tells you that she has not felt well for the past few days.

1. What would be your course of action following this assessment?

Scenario B
Mr. Lopez, age 18, has been admitted to the orthopedic unit following an automobile accident. He has sustained an open fracture of the femur and has been placed in traction.

1. What would be some expected signs and symptoms of inflammation that he might experience?

2. What specific problems might his care present for the nurse?

Scenario C
Mrs. Kay is an elderly woman, who comes to the clinic for treatment of an abrasion on her arm that she sustained "while picking up my cat." She is alert, oriented, and very cheerful and talkative. You notice that she is slightly underweight and that her clothes are not very clean.

1. What additional assessment might you make about the wound and the injury because she mentioned the cat?

2. What changes related to aging are likely to affect Mrs. Kay's natural defense mechanisms to fight infection?

3. Based on the scenario, identify issues that will affect wound healing and self-care for Mrs. Kay.

4. Explain why older adults may have a normal or even subnormal temperature in the presence of infection.

Care of Patients with Pain

Objectives

Theory

1. Demonstrate an understanding of the current view of pain as a specific entity requiring appropriate intervention.
2. Review the gate control theory of pain and its relationship to nursing care.
3. Compare nociceptive and neuropathic pain and the nursing care for each.
4. Explain how pain perception is affected by personal situations and cultural backgrounds.
5. Describe the false perceptions that underlie many current ideas about pain and pain management and assist patients to achieve a clearer, more factual understanding.

6. List the different pharmacologic approaches to pain management with examples of each.
7. Analyze the major differences between acute and chronic pain and their management.

Clinical Practice

1. Effectively use the nursing process for pain management.
2. Use appropriate pain evaluation tools for a variety of patients.
3. Recognize common side effects of analgesics and describe techniques for addressing them.
4. Employ nonpharmacologic approaches to pain management with a variety of patients.

Key Terms

acute pain (ă-KŪT pān, p. 127)
adjuvant (ĂJ-ŭ-vănt, p. 126)
buccal mucosa (BŪK-ăl MŪ-cō-să, p. 136)
chronic pain (KRŎN-ĭk pān, p. 127)
endorphins (ĕn-DŎR-fĭnz, p. 125)
epidural (Ĕ-pĭ-DŪ-rŭl, p. 136)
intractable pain (ĭn-TRĂC-tă-bŭl pān, p. 136)
modulation (p. 126)
neuropathic pain (nū-rō-PĂTH-ĭk pān, p. 126)

nociceptive pain (nō-sē-SĔP-tĭv pān, p. 125)
pain threshold (pān, p. 127)
pain tolerance (pān TŎL-ŭr-ŭns, p. 127)
perception (pĕr-CĔP-shŭn, p. 126)
phantom pain (FĂN-tŏm pān, p. 126)
placebos (plă-SĒ-bōz, p. 134)
referred pain (rĭ-FŬRD pān, p. 130)
transduction (trănz-DŬK-shŭn, p. 126)
transmission (trăns-MĬ-shŭn, p. 126)

THEORIES OF PAIN

Current thinking views pain not as just a symptom, but as a specific problem that needs to be treated. *Pain* is defined as a neurologic response to unpleasant stimuli. Pain receptors are abundantly distributed throughout the skin and in many deeper structures of the body. Receptors for pain do not become dulled with repeated stimulation and, under some conditions, repeated stimulation results in an increase in the acuteness of the pain sensation.

Pain results from the release of various chemicals from damaged cells, but the actual mechanism of pain is still poorly understood. It may be helpful to think of pain as being controlled by a "gate" in the central nervous system (Figure 7-1). When the gate is open, the pain sensation is allowed through. When the gate is closed, the pain sensation is blocked. The *gate control theory* recognizes that stimuli other than pain pass through the same gate. When a large volume of non-painful stimuli are competing for the gate, pain impulses may be blocked. A high volume of pain, however, may override other stimuli and pass through the gate, causing the individual to perceive the pain.

Aspects of this theory relate to nursing practice in several ways:

- Two types of nerve fibers—small-diameter and large-diameter—carry pain stimuli.
- Activity in the small-diameter nerve fibers seems to open the gate, and activity in the large-diameter nerve fibers seems to close it.
- Massage and vibration produce activity in the large-diameter nerve fibers.
- High levels of sensory input create brainstem impulses that seem to close the gate. Distraction in the form of activity or social interaction produces these brainstem impulses.

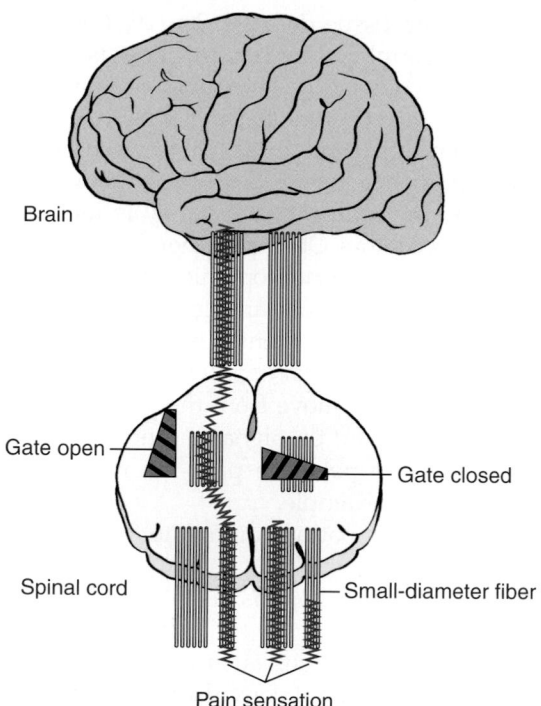

FIGURE 7-1 The gate control theory of pain.

- An increase in anxiety seems to open the gate, and a decrease in anxiety seems to close it. The fear that pain will not be controlled may actually increase pain intensity, and knowing that pain can be or is being controlled may reduce pain.

Another way of looking at pain and its management is the idea of "pieces of pain." The more intense the pain, the greater the number of pieces, and therefore a greater number of pieces of analgesia will be required to control pain. This idea states that inadequate analgesia results in leftover "pieces" of pain, and total relief or control has not been achieved.

The human body produces substances called **endorphins** (endogenous morphine) that attach to pain receptors and block pain sensation. Much is still unknown about endorphins and how they work, but their properties appear to modify and inhibit unpleasant stimuli, reduce anxiety, and relieve pain. Endorphins also may produce feelings of euphoria and well-being. For example, the "runner's high" may occur because endorphins are released after physical exercise.

CLASSIFICATION OF PAIN

There are two pathophysiologic classifications of pain: *nociceptive* and *neuropathic*.

NOCICEPTIVE PAIN

Nociceptive pain is associated with pain stimuli from either *somatic* (body tissue) or *visceral* (organs) structures. Somatic nociceptive pain arises from injury to tissue where pain receptors called nociceptors are located. These nociceptors may be found in skin, connective tissue, bones, joints, or muscles. Trauma, burns, or surgery may cause injuries triggering somatic nociceptive pain. Visceral nociceptive pain arises from pathophysiology in visceral organs such as the organs of the gastrointestinal tract. Pathologic conditions triggering visceral nociceptive pain include tumors and obstructions of the organs (Table 7-1).

Table 7-1   Physiologic Sources of Pain

PHYSIOLOGIC STRUCTURE	CHARACTERISTICS OF PAIN	SOURCES OF ACUTE POSTOPERATIVE PAIN	SOURCES OF CHRONIC PAIN SYNDROMES
Nociceptive Pain			
Somatic Pain			
Cutaneous or superficial: skin and subcutaneous tissues Deep somatic: bone, muscle, blood vessels, connective tissues	Sharp, burning, dull, aching, cramping	Incisional pain, pain at insertion sites of tubes and drains, wound complications, orthopedic procedures, skeletal muscle tissue	Bony metastases, osteoarthritis and rheumatoid arthritis, low back pain, peripheral vascular diseases
Visceral Pain			
Organs and the linings of the body cavities	Poorly localized Diffuse, deep cramping or splitting, sharp, stabbing	Chest tubes, abdominal tubes and drains, bladder distention or spasms, intestinal distention	Pancreatitis, liver metastases, colitis, appendicitis
Neuropathic Pain			
Nerve fibers, spinal cord, and central nervous system	Poorly localized Shooting, burning, fiery, shock-like, sharp, painful numbness	Phantom limb pain, postmastectomy pain, nerve compression	HIV-related pain, diabetic neuropathy, postherpetic neuralgia, chemotherapy-induced neuropathies, cancer-related nerve injury, radiculopathies

Adapted from Ignatavicius, D.D., & Workman, M.L. (2010). *Medical-Surgical Nursing: Critical Thinking for Collaborative Care* (6th ed.). Philadelphia: Elsevier Saunders, p. 38.

Four phases of pain are associated with nociceptive pain (Figure 7-2) (Lewis et al., 2011):

1. **Transduction** begins when tissue damage causes the release of substances that stimulate the nociceptors and initiate the sensation of pain.
2. **Transmission** involves movement of the pain sensation to the spinal cord.
3. **Perception** occurs when impulses reach the brain and the pain is recognized.
4. **Modulation** occurs when neurons in the brain send signals back down the spinal cord by release of neurotransmitters.

Aspects of nociceptive pain relate to nursing practice in several ways:

- Treatment of nociceptive pain may be directed toward one or all of the four phases.
- Nonsteroidal anti-inflammatory drugs (NSAIDs) work by blocking the production of the substances that trigger the nociceptors in the transduction phase.
- Opioids interfere with the transmission phase.
- Nonpharmacologic treatments, such as distraction and guided imagery, may be effective during the perception phase.
- Drugs that block neurotransmitter uptake work in the modulation stage.

NEUROPATHIC PAIN

Neuropathic pain is associated with a dysfunction of the nervous system that involves an abnormality in the processing of sensations. These dysfunctions in the nervous system are often associated with medical conditions rather than with tissue damage. The dysfunction may occur in the peripheral or central nervous system. In peripheral nervous system neuropathic pain, it is believed that pain receptors become sensitive to stimuli and send pain signals more easily. Nerve endings grow additional branches that send stronger pain signals to the brain. As the branches grow, they influence touch and warmth receptors. Other peripheral nervous system conditions may cause neuropathic pain. Neuropathic pain may be the result of damage to nerve roots such as compression or entrapment. Another dysfunction of the central nervous system occurs when the pain signal that would normally move from the periphery toward the brain reverses and the signal is sent in the opposite direction. **Phantom pain,** the pain felt in a limb after amputation, is an example.

Aspects of neuropathic pain relate to nursing practice in several ways:

- Analgesics and opioids usually do not relieve neuropathic pain.
- **Adjuvant** medications such as NSAIDs, tricyclic antidepressants, anticonvulsants, and corticosteroids relieve neuropathic pain.

PERCEPTION OF PAIN

Pain is a subjective experience. Only the patient knows the location of the pain, its degree of intensity, and which treatment regimen works and how long it is effective. Reactions to pain can vary widely from person to person and in the same individual under different circumstances.

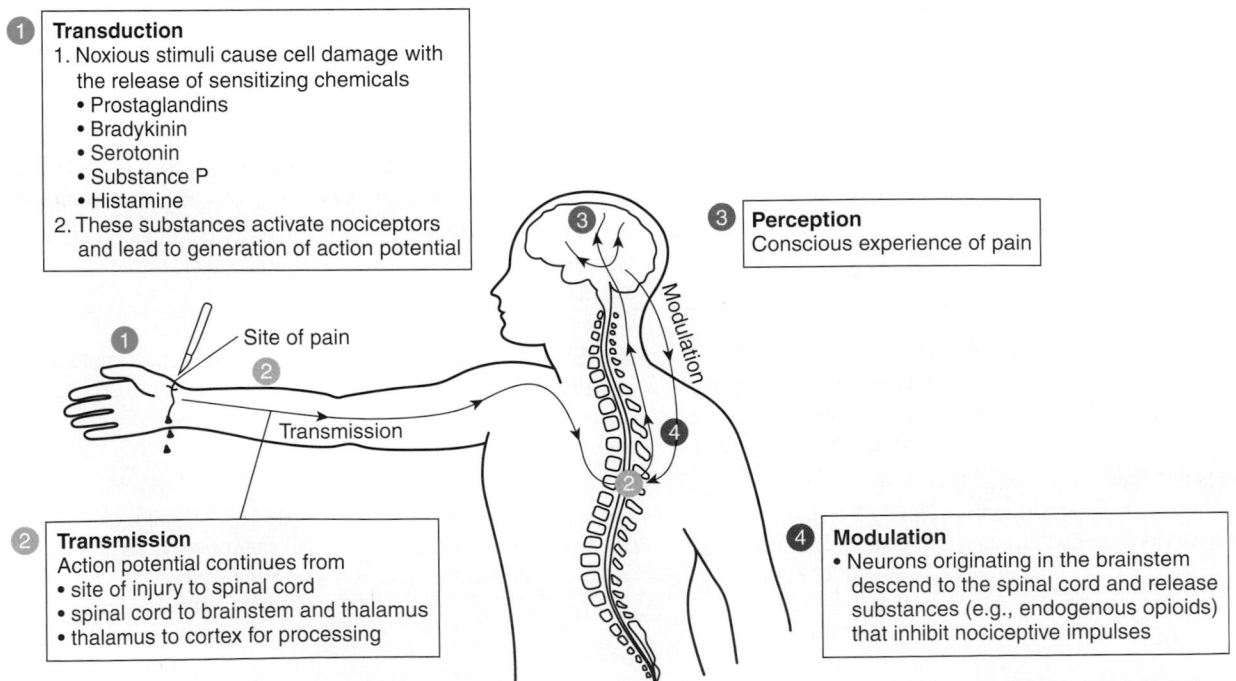

Transduction
1. Noxious stimuli cause cell damage with the release of sensitizing chemicals
   - Prostaglandins
   - Bradykinin
   - Serotonin
   - Substance P
   - Histamine
2. These substances activate nociceptors and lead to generation of action potential

Perception
Conscious experience of pain

Site of pain

Transmission

Modulation

Transmission
Action potential continues from
- site of injury to spinal cord
- spinal cord to brainstem and thalamus
- thalamus to cortex for processing

Modulation
- Neurons originating in the brainstem descend to the spinal cord and release substances (e.g., endogenous opioids) that inhibit nociceptive impulses

FIGURE 7-2 Nociceptive pain originates when tissue is injured. *1,* Transduction. *2,* Transmission. *3,* Perception. *4,* Modulation.

Pain threshold is the point at which pain is perceived. Relaxation and distraction strategies can alter the perception of pain. Pain tolerance is the length of time or the intensity of pain a person will endure before outwardly responding to it. Tolerance varies among people and is influenced by culture, pain experience, expectations, and role behaviors. People with acute pain (of recent onset, lasting less than 6 months) may have physiologic symptoms such as increased pulse and respiratory rates, increased blood pressure, diaphoresis, and increased muscle tension. They may also experience nausea and vomiting. People with chronic pain (lasting months or years) may have learned adaptive methods that allow them to have some control over their pain. Symptoms associated with chronic pain include irritability, depression, withdrawal, and insomnia. Coping with any pain takes a lot of energy, and patients who are debilitated are less able to withstand pain than are strong, robust people. Fatigue caused by pain can lead to an increase in pain perception.

Clinical Cue

Patients who have a substance abuse problem are not to be denied pain medication when they experience acute pain. Patients who are being treated for long-term chronic pain often require higher doses of pain medication after surgery or trauma.

Pain can cause a variety of physiologic responses, including increased respiratory rate, pulse, or blood pressure; muscle tension; sweating; flushing or pallor; and frowning or grimacing. Although the presence of any of these factors may indicate pain, their absence does not prove the absence of pain.

A person's cultural background influences feelings about pain. In much of Western culture it is considered valuable to have a high pain tolerance, particularly among men. Other cultures promote the idea that to endure pain is natural, or honorable. A nurse whose cultural background approves the "stiff upper lip"

approach to handling pain may see the patient who outwardly expresses pain as weak or manipulative. By contrast, those patients whose cultural upbringing causes them to hide and deny pain may suffer needlessly unless the nurse can intervene and help them to understand that analgesia will aid the healing process by encouraging movement and decreasing fatigue. Learning to accept without judgment the various ways of coping with and expressing pain is a very necessary process for nurses.

Elder Care Points

The idea that pain perception diminishes with age is false. In fact, perception of pain may actually increase with age, as the individual becomes frail, has more than one chronic ailment, and has fewer resources for tolerating pain.

ACUTE VERSUS CHRONIC PAIN

ACUTE PAIN

Patients with acute pain frequently experience fear and anxiety, which can take many forms. They may fear that something is seriously wrong, that they will never get relief from the pain, or that they will become addicted to the pain medication. The anxiety and fear of these patients frequently are alleviated by first providing adequate analgesia to relieve the pain and then educating them about their pain and the methods that can be used to control pain safely. Including patients in planning care reassures patients that health care professionals believe them and want to help.

Rely on the patient's report of pain and intervene to promote comfort. Table 7-2 compares acute and chronic pain. Some nurses hesitate to administer pain medication to patients with a history of drug abuse. Such patients may experience acute pain, for example, following surgery. The postoperative period is not the time to withhold pain medication from any patient. Concept Map 7-1 shows the various types and causes of pain.

Table 7-2 Acute versus Chronic Pain

	ACUTE	CHRONIC
Duration	Hours to days.	Months to years.
Prognosis for relief	Good; may resolve spontaneously or in response to analgesic therapy.	Poor unless complicating factors removed; spontaneous relief unusual.
Cause	Relatively easy to identify.	Sometimes cause is known, but diagnosis may be complex or undetermined.
Psychosocial effects	Usually transient or none. May temporarily disrupt normal activities or routine.	Can affect ability to earn a living, enjoy social activities, maintain self-esteem.
Effect of therapy	Medication usually beneficial, surgery often helpful.	Medications may be helpful, but patient may become dependent. Multiple medication regimen may be used. Surgery may help, but also may worsen the problem.

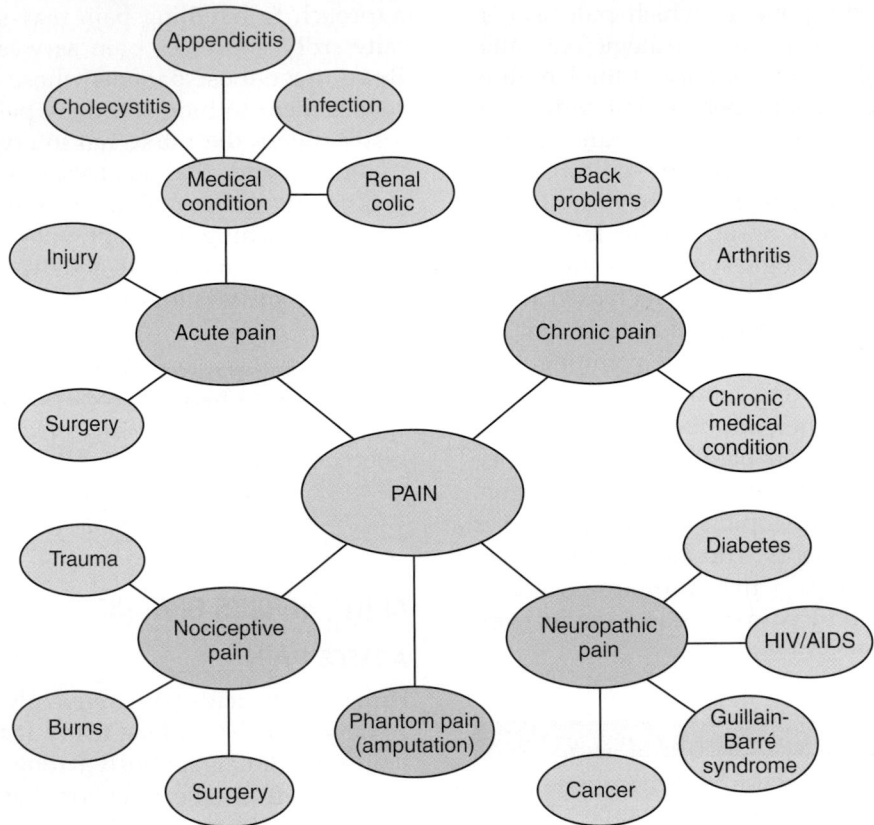

CONCEPT MAP 7-1 The various types and causes of pain.

CHRONIC PAIN

Chronic pain is commonly associated with depression. People who hurt most or all of the time frequently resign themselves to the idea that they can never again live a normal life. Research and the work of several outstanding pain centers and nurse and physician specialists now offer new pain relief techniques for sufferers of chronic pain. Many people whose lives were previously dictated by their pain now experience good control and have returned to normal, productive lives.

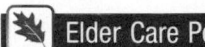 Elder Care Points

Between 50% and 70% of the elderly in the community have chronic pain. The most common conditions causing the pain are joint problems from osteoarthritis, degenerative disk disease from osteoporosis, low back pain, and pain from previous fracture sites. If their chronic pain is adequately controlled, quality of life is improved.

❖ NURSING MANAGEMENT
■ Assessment (Data Collection)

Because no technology can accurately and objectively measure pain, you must use a combination of evaluation methods, including observation and rating scales.

Observation

Appearance. The patient's face may look tense, drawn, or pale. There may be a grimace or even a look of fear.

Behavior. A normally verbal patient may become quiet or withdrawn. One who is normally pleasant may become irritable, demanding, or argumentative. The individual may protect or "cradle" the painful area with the hands or arms. Tears, refusal of food or drink, or any behavior that is out of the ordinary for the individual may be an indication of pain.

Activity Level. A person in pain often reduces activity to a minimum. Staying in bed, creeping slowly from place to place, stooping over during ambulation, and stopping frequently to rest or lean against a support can all indicate pain.

Verbalization. Many individuals in pain may verbalize their discomfort, but it is not always easy to interpret the degree of pain from what is said. Limited vocabulary, lack of experience in verbalizing abstract concepts, fear of disbelief or disapproval, cultural stoicism, and fear of becoming addicted to the analgesic all can impair the person's ability to communicate the degree of pain.

Physiologic Clues. Physiologic clues to pain include rapid, shallow, or guarded respirations, pallor, diaphoresis, increased pulse, elevated blood pressure, dilated pupils, and tenseness of the skeletal muscles. However, remember that problems other than pain can also cause these physiologic clues to occur. All physiologic changes must be fully assessed to determine the cause.

 Elder Care Points

Older patients may not report pain for a variety of reasons, and their pain is often undertreated. They may think pain is an expected part of aging. They may deny pain because it means they are getting older. They may not report pain because they feel they cannot afford the cost of tests or treatments. Elderly people often will say they have "soreness" or "discomfort" rather than pain. Assess further if such comments are made.

 Focused Assessment

The Patient with Pain

Ask the following questions while assessing a patient with pain:

LOCATION
- Where is your pain?
- Can you point to the pain?

CHARACTERISTICS
- Can you describe your pain?
- What words would you use to describe the pain? (Aching, burning, gnawing, sharp, stabbing, shooting, etc.)
- Is the pain constant or does it come and go?

QUANTITY
- How strong or intense is your pain?
- How strong is your pain on this scale?

PATTERN
- How long have you had this pain?
- Did the pain begin during activity, before eating, after eating?
- Did the pain start suddenly?
- Has the pain increased over time?

ASSOCIATED FACTORS
- Have you had other symptoms such as nausea and vomiting, shortness of breath, rapid heart rate, sweating?
- What does your family usually do when there is pain?
- Do you have any chronic problems that cause pain?

ALLEVIATING FACTORS
- What have you tried to relieve the pain? (Medication, certain position, application of heat or cold, distraction, etc.)
- Did it work?

AGGRAVATING FACTORS
- What, if anything, makes the pain increase?

Pain Rating Scales

Several rating scales have been developed for use in pain evaluation. **When using a pain rating scale, it is important that the nursing staff use it consistently and that the patient fully understands how to use it.** The type of scale being used and any pertinent information about how the patient uses the scale must be included in the patient care plan.

Numbered Scale. Numbered scales ask the patient to rate the degree of pain as a number from 0 to 5 or 0 to 10, with 0 indicating no pain and the highest number indicating the greatest amount of pain imaginable. The numbers in between show graduated levels of pain. The scale may be simply verbal, or it may actually be drawn on a piece of paper so the person can mark or point to the degree of pain. Number scales can be used very effectively with people who have a good understanding of the numerical concept and who like a strictly logical approach. They are not appropriate for young children, anyone who has difficulty with numbers, or anyone who is confused or disoriented.

Visual Scale. Some visual scales use photographs or simple drawings of faces with expressions showing a pain-free state (happy and smiling) that progress through a series of faces showing increased discomfort. The final picture shows a face either crying or with an intense grimace (Figure 7-3).

Color Scale. A color scale allows the patient to select colors that represent varying degrees of pain. Colored pieces of paper or plastic (e.g., poker chips), crayons, or markers can be used. The patient selects a color that represents no pain, a color that represents severe pain, and then one, two, or three other colors for pain levels in between. This scale is often used with children, but very young children cannot understand more than three or four possible choices.

Pieces of Pain Scale. This scale uses five poker chips or other identical, plain objects that represent "pieces" of pain. The patient indicates the degree of pain by selecting the number of chips that equals the intensity of pain being experienced.

Behavioral Pain (FLACC) Scale. This scale is used with patients who are cognitively impaired or cannot speak. The nurse assesses the patient's behavior in categories such as facial expression, limb movement,

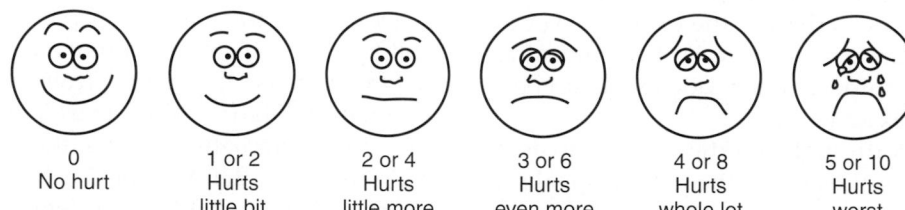

FIGURE 7-3 Wong-Baker FACES pain rating scale. For coding purposes, numbers 0, 2, 4, 6, 8, and 10 can be substituted for 0-5 system to accommodate a 0-10 system.

Face	**0** No particular expression or smile	**1** Occasional grimace or frown, withdrawn, disinterested	**2** Frequent to constant frown, clenched jaw, quivering chin
Legs	**0** Normal position or relaxed	**1** Uneasy, restless, tense	**2** Kicking, or legs drawn up
Activity	**0** Lying quietly, normal position, moves easily	**1** Squirming, shifting back and forth, tense	**2** Arched, rigid, or jerking
Cry	**0** No cry (awake or asleep)	**1** Moans or whimpers, occasional complaint	**2** Cries steadily, screams or sobs, frequent complaints
Consolability	**0** Content, relaxed	**1** Reassured by occasional touching, hugging, or talking to; distractible	**2** Difficult to console or comfort

FIGURE 7-4 FLACC scale for pain assessment used for cognitively impaired persons.

and activity level (Figure 7-4). A score from 0 to 2 is obtained for each category, and the category scores are added together to arrive at a pain score total of 0 to 10. It is useful when assessing the pain of confused or nonverbal adults, infants, and young children.

Elder Care Points

A more accurate assessment of pain in the elderly is obtained when several types of pain scales are used, such as a number scale, a visual scale, and a behavioral scale.

? Think Critically

Can you explain the difference between acute and chronic pain to someone?

Data Collection Difficulties

Much of the data gathered when assessing a patient's pain comes from conversation with the patient, which presents a variety of problems. The first problem is language itself. Concepts of the true meaning of words in a common language may vary greatly from person to person. It is important to discuss the common words used to describe pain and to agree on their meaning (Table 7-3). It also is important that documentation include the patient's exact words.

The need to work through an interpreter or to deal with language difficulties when the patient speaks a foreign language compounds the problem of communicating pain. Whenever possible, the nurse should use a medical professional (rather than a family member)

Table 7-3 **Common Terms to Help Patients Describe Pain**

Degree of pain (from least to most severe)	Absent, minimal, mild, moderate, fairly severe, severe, very or extremely severe, excruciating
Quality of pain	Crushing, tingling, itching, throbbing, pulsating, twisting, pulling, burning, searing, stabbing, tearing, biting, blinding, nauseating, debilitating
Frequency of pain	Constant, intermittent, occasional, related to something specific (e.g., only when coughs)

with a good knowledge of both languages as an interpreter. Most hospitals have a list of approved interpreters to assist in these situations. Patients may hide personal, embarrassing, or painful information if the interpreter is a family member or personal friend.

Describing the location of pain can be made difficult by the problem of **referred pain** (pain felt in a different part of the body from where it actually originates) (Figure 7-5). Heart pain may be felt in the jaw or radiating down the arm. Gastric pain may center in the area of the heart rather than the stomach. **There also is a tendency not to believe an individual's statement of pain if there is no outward appearance of pain.** For example, a patient watching

Cultural Considerations

Cultural Beliefs Affecting Pain Perception and Treatment

Various groups from different cultures may have beliefs about pain that differ from yours. Do recall, however, that just because a person is linked to a particular cultural group, it doesn't mean that he participates in the cultural practices of that group. Proper assessment of beliefs is very important.

Pain Expression and Meaning	Preferences and Action
WHITE (EUROPEAN; CAUCASIAN)	
Men display strong stoicism. Narcotic use brings fear of addiction for many. May dismiss the effects of pain and continue to work and carry out usual activities. May decrease use of pain medication quickly.	Prefer to use non-narcotic medications. Many prefer to use relaxation and distraction techniques rather than medication, or just to "tough it out."
HISPANIC	
Mexican Americans often feel that pain is "God's will" and are stoical. Pain may be seen as a consequence of immoral behavior. For some males, expressing pain shows weakness and may cause lack of respect. Other Hispanic groups tend to be expressive of pain and discomfort and may moan, groan, or cry, and such expression is seen as acceptable.	Many feel that injectable medication is better treatment for pain than a pill. Prayer, heat, and herbs may be used to treat pain.
BLACK (AFRICAN AMERICAN, AFRICAN NATIVE)	
Pain is often seen as a sign of sickness. May express pain openly, but this varies. Pain may be seen as something to just be endured.	Laying-on of hands and prayer are thought to help relieve pain. May rely on spiritual or religious belief to help endure pain.
ASIAN	
Varies among subgroups, but generally tend to be stoical. Bearing pain may be seen as a matter of family honor. May describe pain obliquely in terms of body symptoms. Some Filipinos view pain as a part of life and to endure it as honorable. Elders may fear addiction to pain medication.	May prefer oral or intravenous pain medication; injections may be seen as too invasive of privacy. May use applications of moist heat. Family may request pain medication for the patient.
AMERICAN INDIAN (NATIVE AMERICAN)	
Many believe that pain is something to be endured and will not ask for pain medication. Pain is often described in general body terms such as "I don't feel good." May not be aware that they can ask for medication for pain.	Many use traditional medicine men and rely on herbal preparations. May tell family or visitors about the pain rather than tell the health care provider.
ARAB	
View pain as something to be controlled and expect prompt treatment. May describe pain in terms of hot and cold. May express pain more openly to family than to health care providers.	Usually prefer injectable medication rather than pills.

an exciting football game with a friend may enjoy the game even if his surgical incision is quite painful. The lack of a grimace or of physiologic changes indicative of pain may be viewed as an absence of pain, when in fact the patient is using distraction as a way of coping with the presence of pain. People may fall asleep even though pain is severe, particularly if uncontrolled pain has left them in a state of exhaustion.

 Think Critically

Which pain scale would you use for a 24-year-old patient? Why? Which one would you use for a patient who is cognitively impaired? Why?

■ Nursing Diagnosis

The nursing diagnosis for pain frequently is "Pain related to" a cause. An example would be *Pain related to a fractured pelvis and fractured left femur.*

■ Planning

The overall goal is *relief* of pain. If that is impossible to achieve, the goal is *control* of pain. Plan the goals of nursing care by indicating actions that will promote the comfort of the patient during treatment and recovery. Planning should be a team effort that includes the patient, and both pharmacologic and nonpharmacologic interventions should be considered. Physician input comes as written orders and progress notes and may also be available through direct discussion. Include input from pharmacists, therapists, and other health care professionals in pain management. As recovery progresses, update the nursing care plan. The type of medication, method of delivery, and comfort measures will change as the patient's needs change. Planning must address all areas that affect the patient's pain management needs, including family situation, cultural influences, financial constraints, and whether pain is acute or chronic in nature (Nursing Care Plan 7-1).

■ Implementation

Reassess all patients for pain at the beginning of each hospital shift, clinic appointment, or home visit and revise interventions based on the findings. Appropriate interventions include providing an analgesic as ordered, using nonpharmacologic measures such as repositioning or massage (adjunctive measures), and reporting to the physician when measures are not

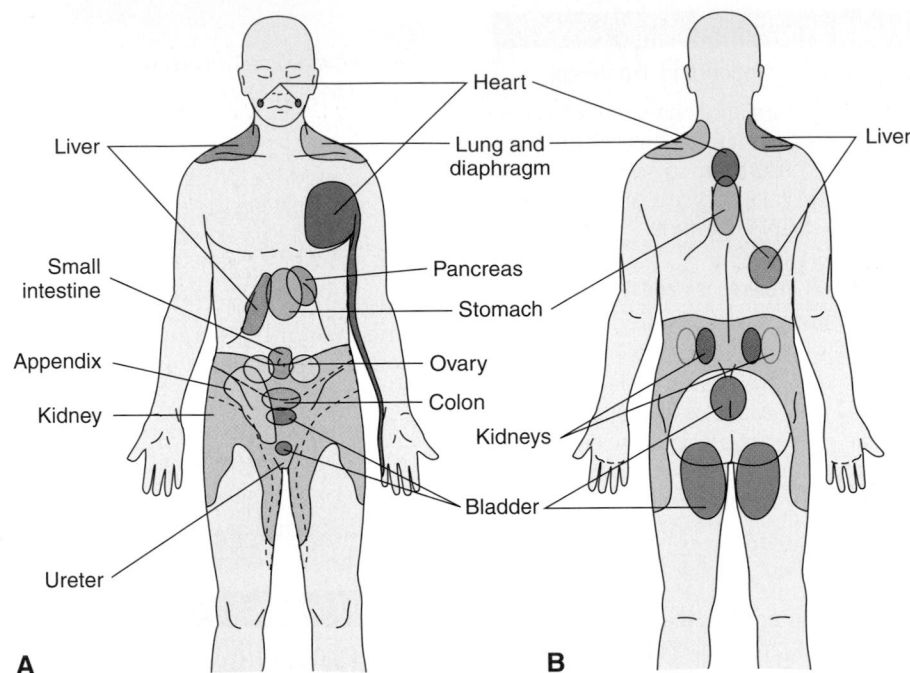

FIGURE 7-5 Usual sites of referred pain. **A,** Front. **B,** Back.

effective or have unwanted side effects. Implementation also includes teaching the patient and family how to monitor effects of treatment and report side effects. False perceptions of pain may need to be addressed (Table 7-4).

Preventing complications from medications is an important aspect of implementation. Specific actions include:

- Prominent documentation of any known drug allergies.
- Accurate recording of pertinent information obtained during the initial assessment phase, such as current medications, previous experience with pain, analgesics, and adjuncts to pain relief.
- Patient and family teaching regarding dose, frequency, and the need to first consult with the physician or nurse before taking any other medications to avoid dangerous interactions.
- Appropriate monitoring of effects of any medications given and prompt notification of the physician should medications fail to relieve pain or should problems occur.
- Accurate and complete documentation of any adverse reactions to treatment and communication of that information to other health care providers, to the patient, and to appropriate family members.

■ Evaluation

Ask the patient about the effectiveness of the pain control measures. How quickly did relief occur? How long did it last? To what degree was the pain controlled? Were there any unpleasant side effects? Whenever possible, use patient verbalization as the primary evaluation tool. For evaluation, use a pain assessment tool with the patient before the pain is treated and again after treatment to compare the patient's response.

If the patient is unable to verbalize, evaluate the objective signs. For instance, an aphasic stroke patient might thrash, moan, and look fearful when in pain, and evaluation of effective analgesia might include, "Mr. Jones lying quietly, free of facial tension, watching the activity around him. He did not moan when repositioned one hour after analgesic given."

🔹 Clinical Cues

Evaluation of the effectiveness of the pain control medication used should be based on the route of administration. Medications given by mouth may take 30 to 45 minutes to be effective. Injections are effective within 30 to 45 minutes. Intravenous medications are effective within 5 to 15 minutes.

■ Documentation

All measures to control pain must be accurately documented:

- Initial pain assessment (location, intensity, duration of the pain, and the method used to assess [e.g., pain scale, patient verbalization]; document aggravating and alleviating factors)
- Measures taken (e.g., analgesic medication, adjunctive measures)
- Evaluation of effectiveness of measures
- Physician notification of problems or concerns and physician response, if applicable
- Related patient or family education provided

★ Nursing Care Plan 7-1   Care of the Patient with Pain

Scenario

Mr. Osbourne, an 82-year-old patient with a history of cerebrovascular accident, has been admitted via the emergency department after a fall and left hip fracture. A total hip replacement was performed this morning. Orders include morphine sulfate via patient-controlled analgesia (PCA), which has just been started. Mr. Osbourne has complained of pain at 8 on a 0-to-10 scale. His blood pressure and pulse are slightly elevated, but his temperature and respirations are normal. He has been restless and moaning. You implement the following portion of his plan of care.

Problem/Nursing Diagnosis

Pain and muscle aching in left hip and leg/Pain related to surgical incision and replacement of hip.

Supporting Assessment Data

Subjective: Grimaces and moans when moves in bed; moves very cautiously; states muscles feel sore.
Objective: Incision at left hip; hip replacement on 5/17.

Goals/Expected Outcomes	Nursing Interventions	Selected Rationale	Evaluation
Patient will report pain at 0 to 3 on a 0-to-10 scale within 2 hr.	Teach to use the PCA pump.	Knowledge of how to use the pump allows the patient to use it correctly.	Using pump correctly, but without good relief.
	Encourage relaxation techniques, provide diversionary activities such as television and electronic games.	Relaxation and diversion are known to lessen pain by focusing the mind elsewhere.	Taught relaxation exercise. Does not wish to watch TV at present. Will use electronic poker game.
	Encourage use of the PCA before ambulation, exercise, or repositioning.	Medicating before activity reduces pain from the activity.	Medicated before physical therapy visit.
	Position in good body alignment.	When the body is in correct alignment, joints hurt less.	Repositioned in correct alignment with abduction pillow q 2 hr.
	Apply cold packs to reduce swelling over large bruise on lower thigh.	Cold reduces swelling by vasoconstriction and also dulls the perception of pain.	Cold pack over thigh for 20 min q hr × 8 hr.
	Observe frequently for pain relief and side effects of medication.	If pain is inadequately relieved, other measures to relieve it can be employed. Knowing if side effects are occurring allows measures to be taken to alleviate or prevent them.	No side effects noted other than drowsiness. Pain at 3.
	Keep abduction wedge in place.	Keeping leg abducted prevents dislocation of the hip and reduces pain.	Wedge in place when in bed.

Critical Thinking Questions

1. If the PCA pump medication is not controlling the pain adequately, what would you do?
2. Considering the age of the patient and the type of surgery, which possible side effects of the analgesia would be of greatest concern? What interventions would you use to try to counter the side effects and prevent problems?

 Patient Teaching

Managing Pain

Take medication before pain is severe; take medication regularly until pain is well controlled before lengthening time between doses. Use distraction, imagery, or relaxation exercises to augment the effect of pain medication.

Example of pain documentation. States pain level following physical therapy at 7 on a 0-to-10 scale.

Morphine sulfate 10 mg IM in the rt. deltoid. 45 minutes after injection, states pain level is now 2 to 3. Pulse 72, respirations 16, moving freely in bed. Discussed pain relief needs; suggested that he request pain medication before next therapy session.

 Think Critically

What do you think is the most difficult aspect of evaluating someone's pain?

Table 7-4 False Perceptions of Pain

FALSE PERCEPTION	FACT
If pain is really present, there must be a demonstrable cause.	**Pain can be present even though no cause can be found.** Although damage to the cells does lead to the release of chemicals that stimulate the pain receptors, in many cases pain may be present although no cellular abnormality can be found. The patient with a migraine headache may or may not suffer less than one with a brain tumor. We cannot say that just because the brain tumor can be shown on a brain scan and the headache cannot, the person with the brain tumor has greater pain than the person with the migraine headache.
The person who has a low tolerance for pain has no self-control and probably is emotionally immature or childish.	**Pain tolerance is a physiologic response to pain that is made more complex by psychosocial factors—many of which can be beyond the control of the patient.** Tolerance for pain is defined as that duration or intensity of pain the person is *willing* to endure without seeking relief. **Pain tolerance varies greatly from one individual to another and varies in the same person from time to time.** Nurses often place a high value on a patient's ability to feel pain without complaining or asking for relief. Those who value a high pain tolerance usually impose their own values on their patients by ignoring or belittling patient reports of pain. The person who should decide how willing he ought to be to tolerate pain is the one who is suffering pain.
The neonate is too neurologically immature to perceive or remember pain, so analgesia is unnecessary in this age group.	***Neonates do perceive and maintain memory of pain.*** They cry and pull away from procedures such as heelstick blood tests. Male infants cry and struggle when they are circumcised. Neonates with medical conditions that require repeated blood tests begin to cry and pull away as soon as someone grasps the foot as if to perform a blood test, indicating a memory of pain from previous heelsticks. Analgesia for neonates is appropriate during procedures or situations that would be known to cause pain in more mature patients.
Elderly patients have a decreased ability to perceive pain, and pain medicines are dangerous for them because of their age.	***Ability to express pain may be impaired by decreased cognitive function, but acute pain is still perceived.*** Age combined with physical impairments such as decreased kidney or liver function may reduce tolerance for various medications, but with appropriate dosage and monitoring, geriatric patients can have good pain management without severe side effects. Untreated pain will interfere with sleep, nutrition, healing, and general well-being.
Reactions to acute pain and chronic pain are the same.	**In general, acute pain is more often associated with anxiety and chronic pain with depression.** Emotional reactions such as anxiety and depression do not cause pain, but they can intensify pain. The management of acute and chronic pain is not the same, as discussed in the chapter text.
Addiction to pain-relieving drugs is always a hazard, and for the sake of the patient, nurses often must withhold a drug even though the patient asks for it.	**A very small percentage of patients (probably less than 1% and no more than 3%) become addicted to drugs administered for the purpose of relieving acute pain.** In spite of an abundance of evidence to the contrary, this mistaken belief about the dangers of addiction persists, causing needless suffering among patients who are denied adequate pain relief.
Placebos (substances prescribed that contain no medication, such as sterile saline or sugar pills) are very useful in assessing whether a patient actually has pain.	**There is no basis for believing that a patient who finds relief from pain after receiving a placebo has been pretending to have pain or that the reported pain has been "all in his mind."** The question of how placebos affect people and why they have a positive response in some and not in others is still poorly understood. However, there has been sufficient study of the subject to show that actual pain is sometimes well relieved by placebos.

MANAGEMENT OF PAIN

Effective pain management is not just a matter of giving the right medicine at the right time. It is a combination of pharmacologic and nonpharmacologic approaches that together give the individual the greatest possible degree of comfort for the longest possible time. The World Health Organization has made recommendations for a stepped approach to pharmacologic pain control (Figure 7-6).

 Home Care Considerations

Maintain Medication Record

Jot down the time pain medication is taken at home. It is easy to forget just when a medication has been taken. Writing down the time when medication was taken helps prevent overdosage and toxicity.

PHARMACOLOGIC APPROACHES

Analgesics and Routes of Administration

Table 7-5 lists common analgesics by category and action.

FIGURE 7-6 The analgesic ladder proposed by the World Health Organization.

Table 7-5   Analgesic Medications by Type, Primary Action, and Nursing Implications

TYPE OF DRUG AND PRIMARY ACTION	PRIMARY ACTION	EXAMPLES	NURSING IMPLICATIONS
Non-narcotic analgesics, including nonsteroidal anti-inflammatory drugs (NSAIDs)	Block pain at the peripheral nervous system level	Over-the-counter aspirin, acetaminophen, ibuprofen,* ketoprofen,* naproxen* Prescription naproxen, indomethacin, ibuprofen, ketoprofen	May be present in combination drugs. Various possible side effects of which to be aware.† Educate patients not to use in combination with over-the-counter dosage of same medication.
Narcotics (opioids)	Block pain at the central nervous system level	Morphine, meperidine, hydromorphone, codeine, fentanyl	Constipation common, can be severe. Can cause respiratory depression; antidote is naloxone (Narcan).
Medications with nonanalgesic primary actions used as adjuncts to pain control	Various mechanisms of action	Antidepressants: amitriptyline, imipramine, trazodone hydrochloride Anticonvulsants: phenytoin, carbamazepine, gabapentin, pregabalin Stimulants: caffeine, dextroamphetamine Muscle relaxants: carisoprodol, baclofen Chemotherapeutic agents: methotrexate	Varied due to different mechanisms of action. Always be aware of side effects and possible adverse reactions. May cause grogginess.

*Nonprescription dose.
†Note: Combination drugs are often used. These may combine two forms of analgesic (e.g., acetaminophen and codeine) or an analgesic with another type of medication, such as an antihistamine. It is important to be aware of what ingredients are contained in combination drugs to avoid administering excessive amounts of one of the components.

Oral Analgesics. An oral analgesic is any substance taken by mouth for the control of pain. Oral analgesics include over-the-counter (OTC) medications such as acetaminophen (Tylenol), aspirin, and ibuprofen (Advil, Motrin), and prescription medications such as codeine and morphine. Oral analgesics are available in extended-release forms that can provide 12 to 24 hours of pain relief (Aleve). Mexiletine (Mexitil) is currently used off-label (non–Food and Drug Administration [non-FDA] approved use) for the neuropathic pain of diabetes.

Safety Alert
Preventing Acetaminophen Overdose

When administering acetaminophen, check all other medications and OTC drugs the patient is receiving when administering doses of acetaminophen. Many OTC drugs combine acetaminophen with other drugs. Toxicity may occur if more than the total recommended safe dosage is ingested.

Intramuscular Analgesics. Intramuscular (IM) analgesics are substances injected into muscular tissue to control pain.

Subcutaneous Analgesics. Subcutaneous analgesics are medications injected or infused into *subcutaneous* (fatty tissue just beneath the skin) tissue to control pain.

Topical Analgesics. Topical analgesics are medications placed in a specific area on the skin and absorbed via the vascular system. Topical anesthetics such as EMLA (a mixture of lidocaine and prilocaine) are used to treat pain from minor procedures such as venipunctures. Capsaicin (Zostrix) (made from a substance in peppers) is used topically for joint and other pain.

Transdermal Patches. Transdermal patches placed on the skin rely on vascular uptake of pain medication. These patches can provide relief from systemic pain and are commonly used with patients who have chronic pain. Transdermal patches containing lidocaine may be used for local pain.

Safety Alert
Pain Patch

Fentanyl patches used for severe pain can cause death from overdose. Signs of overdose are difficulty breathing, shallow breathing, extreme sleepiness, and inability to think, talk, or walk normally. Faintness, dizziness, and confusion are other signs.

Clinical Cues

Always remove the old transdermal patch before applying a new one; cleanse the skin where the old patch has been. The patch must be removed before the patient undergoes an MRI to prevent a burn from the foil in the patch.

Buccal Swabs. Buccal swabs contain medication that is absorbed through the buccal mucosa (mucous membrane lining the inside of the mouth) and provides rapid relief from pain. Buccal swabs are commonly used with hospice patients.

Intravenous Analgesics. Intravenous (IV) analgesics are substances injected or infused over a prescribed time directly into the vascular system.

Patient-Controlled Analgesia. Patient-controlled analgesia (PCA) is an infusion device controlled by the patient that injects the prescribed dose of analgesia. The PCA machine is programmed so that the patient can decide when a dose is given, but cannot exceed the maximum dose or minimum time interval ordered by the physician. PCA analgesia is usually given IV, but may also be administered subcutaneously. Make certain that free-flow protection is in use on the PCA pump so that overdosage is not possible. Morphine and Dilaudid are most commonly used for PCA.

Epidural Analgesic. An epidural analgesic such as morphine is medication infused directly into the epidural space near the base of the spine using a programmable pump. An anesthesiologist inserts the infusion catheter. Patients receiving epidural analgesia need to be monitored for possible delayed respiratory suppression or apnea, bradycardia, hypotension, urinary retention, nausea and vomiting, and allergic reactions such as itching or hives. Report adverse symptoms to the anesthesiologist immediately, and observe the insertion site for signs of infection, localized allergic reaction, and leaking.

Peripheral Nerve Catheter. A peripheral nerve catheter is used to deliver local anesthetic to the sheath of a nerve. These catheters are typically used postoperatively for patients who have had total joint replacement.

Nonanalgesic Medications Used for Pain Control
Antidepressants. A number of antidepressant medications are effective in controlling some specific types of pain, such as nerve root pain. They may be given alone or in combination with other analgesic medications.

Chemotherapeutic Agents and Other Immunosuppressants. Occasionally drugs such as methotrexate (Rheumatrex) are used for intractable pain in rheumatoid conditions.

Anticonvulsants. Newer anticonvulsants, such as gabapentin (Neurontin), have been approved for treatment of neuropathic pain. Pregabalin (Lyrica) has been approved for the pain of fibromyalgia.

Muscle Relaxants. Muscle relaxants, such as baclofen, are often used adjunctively to ease spasm in patients with back pain, multiple sclerosis, and other neurologic and muscular disorders.

Invasive Treatments. Invasive treatments—such as sympathectomies, rhizotomies, and cordotomies, which sever the nerve conducting the pain—are now uncommon. Advances in pain management, including surgically implanted medication pumps and nerve stimulators, have made these invasive treatments unnecessary in most cases. A dorsal column stimulator may be implanted for pain after failed back surgery and for other pain syndromes. An epidural injection may be used to ease sciatic nerve pain. The medication dosage given directly to the spinal cord (intrathecal) is about 1/10 of the oral dose, so patients suffer no central nervous system side effects. They can work and drive while being relieved of severe pain.

Special Considerations in Pain Management
Pharmacologic analgesics, including OTC drugs, may be administered to patients in a health care facility only under a physician's order to prevent unwanted interactions with other prescribed medications. For example, aspirin, commonly taken for occasional headache and arthritis pain, is a powerful anticoagulant. Aspirin can lead to dangerous complications for someone with a bleeding disorder or who is taking another anticoagulant medication. Acetaminophen in high doses is toxic to the liver, and may be contraindicated in patients with a liver disorder. Alerting patients that OTC drugs can have serious interactions with their prescribed drugs is an important part of patient education.

 Elder Care Points

The very elderly frequently have reduced tolerance for medications. Smaller doses of analgesics may give effective relief without causing overwhelming sedation or disorientation. Elderly patients on analgesics must be monitored carefully, and the route of administration is a serious consideration. Intramuscular injections are not recommended for the elderly because diminished muscle and fatty tissue may affect the bioavailability of drugs.

Nurses' Responsibilities
In addition to following the "Five Rights" (right patient, right drug, right dose, right route, right time), the nurse has a variety of responsibilities when giving analgesic medications (Box 7-1).

Side Effects and Complications of Pain Medications
Probably the most common—and one of the most distressing—side effect of pain medication is constipation. Analgesics such as morphine, meperidine, and codeine slow peristalsis. Fecal material becomes

Box 7-1 Nursing Responsibilities When Administering Analgesics

1. Document drug, dose, route (including location of injection site for IM or subcutaneous injections), and reason for drug administration.
2. Monitor the effectiveness of pain relief after 15 to 30 minutes and at 1- to 2-hour intervals. Document the degree and duration of pain relief in the patient record.
3. If the analgesic is ineffective, determine whether a stronger analgesic is available to the patient and administer per physician order. If no other analgesic is available, notify the physician that the medication is not effective. Also notify the physician if the medication is initially effective but the duration of effect is too short to maintain patient comfort until the next dose may be given.
4. If the analgesic results in unwanted side effects (e.g., depressed vital signs, vomiting, or altered level of consciousness), monitor the patient closely and notify the physician before administering another analgesic dose.

compacted and dry because of the extended time of passage through the intestines. Patients receiving these medications for any length of time should be monitored carefully for regular, normal bowel movements. **Oral fluids must be increased if possible.** Stool softeners and fiber-based laxatives, such as psyllium (Metamucil), can be helpful if approved by the physician. Miralax also has proven very effective for opioid-induced constipation.

 Elder Care Points

Help prevent constipation in the elderly patient receiving a narcotic analgesic by encouraging the increased intake of fluids and fiber, administering an ordered stool softener, and monitoring for bloating, discomfort, and lack of daily bowel movement.

Some side effects, such as drowsiness and euphoria, generally only last for the first few days and then spontaneously disappear. Allergic reactions, such as itching and hives, must be reported immediately. Discontinue the medication and obtain an alternative order. The patient may need an antihistamine such as diphenhydramine (Benadryl) for relief of itching. Narcotic analgesics can depress the respiratory system to the point of apnea (no respiration). Should this occur, resuscitation must begin immediately. In the hospital setting, provide respiratory support and call the code team. In the home, physician's office, or clinic, provide respiratory support and call 911. The standard treatment for respiratory suppression from narcotics is naloxone (Narcan), an effective narcotic antagonist that can be given IM or IV.

The most feared side effect to analgesia—that of addiction to narcotics—in reality almost never occurs when pain medications are taken for real pain. **Patients** in pain have a right to expect that effective analgesia will be available to them. Dependence does occur with long-term use of many of the narcotic analgesics and they should not be stopped abruptly. When pain can be controlled with non-narcotic medications, the patient is tapered off of the narcotic analgesic.

 Legal and Ethical Considerations

Narcotic Pain Control at the End of Life

Patients and their families often worry that treating the terminally ill with sufficient pain medication to control pain may hasten death. However, no scientific evidence has proven that this can happen when opioids are used to control pain. Health care providers have a moral obligation to adequately treat pain even at the very end of life, and opioids must be administered for the purpose of relieving pain and not to purposefully hasten death (Lewis et al., 2011).

Elder Care Points

Some drugs are considered especially risky to administer to elderly patients. Tramadol (Ultram) and meperidine (Demerol) lower the seizure threshold and should be used cautiously (Titler et al., 2003).

NONPHARMACOLOGIC APPROACHES

A variety of methods exist for relieving pain without or in addition to medications. Using adjuncts can increase the effectiveness of pain medication and may decrease the frequency at which it is needed.

Sleep

Adequate sleep and rest are major factors in healing. **Rest increases pain tolerance and improves response to analgesia.** Allow adequate time between treatments for naps, and plan care to keep sleep interruptions to a minimum. For instance, take vital signs when the patient is awake to use the bathroom or requests pain medication. It is important to remember that exhaustion will cause a patient to sleep, even while experiencing severe pain, but such sleep is not as therapeutic. Appropriate analgesia combined with adequate rest promotes healing.

Heat

Gentle heat is very soothing for many types of pain. Gentle heat promotes vasodilation of the area, which promotes increased blood supply and movement of nutrients to the affected area. Sources include warm compresses, warm blankets, water-filled heating devices, Hydrocollator pads, whirlpools, tub baths, heat lamps, and chemical self-heating packs. Compresses and packs are usually left in place for 15 to

20 minutes, although gentle heat sources such as water-filled heating devices may be used over longer periods. Always check the temperature before applying heat, and monitor the patient closely for tolerance. To prevent injury to the skin, never apply a warm compress directly to the surface of the skin. The very young and the very old are particularly sensitive to heat. Anyone with an altered level of consciousness or loss of normal sensation may not realize something is too hot, and those with loss of movement may not be able to move away from the heat source when necessary.

 Elder Care Points

The skin of the elderly is thin and burns more easily. Stroke patients and those with diabetic neuropathy frequently have areas of lost or diminished sensation, and patients with senile dementia may not recognize that something is too hot. Even the alert and oriented elderly person frequently falls asleep and may be burned. Monitor any heat application very carefully. Do not apply heat to any areas where nerve damage or decreased sensation has occurred.

Menthol. When applied to the skin, menthol causes warming, which may have an analgesic effect. Mentholated products are usually massaged into the skin, giving the individual the benefit of both massage and warmth. They are available OTC but require a physician's order in a hospital or clinic setting. Do not use menthol with external heating devices to avoid overheating the skin surface. Caution the patient to wash hands well after applying to avoid contact of the menthol with the eyes or mucous membranes.

Cold

Cold is particularly helpful in reducing swelling through vasoconstriction. It also can be effective in relieving muscle spasms and some types of joint pain. Ice massage of sore muscles can be done by freezing water in a paper cup, then tearing away the edge of the cup to expose the ice, leaving the base of the cup as a handle. Some individuals are very sensitive to cold. If cold applications cause shivering, tensing of the muscles, or an increase in pain or spasm, discontinue their use.

 Clinical Cues

The effectiveness of cold is maximized in 15 to 20 minutes. Remove the source after that time.

Distraction

Any activity that takes a person's attention away from pain is termed a *distraction.* This includes watching TV, talking with friends, using a computer, or playing a game. People have an innate ability to distract themselves from their surroundings or situation. Health care workers may mistakenly interpret patients' ability to distract themselves as proof that there is no pain. Distracting activities can take the patient's mind off of pain momentarily, but distractions do not stop pain. Distraction can be helpful in bridging the time gap between giving an analgesic and the onset of pain relief.

Relaxation

Relaxation also is called "tension release" and involves the conscious relaxation of muscle groups. Tension release is frequently done as a progression, beginning at the feet and moving up the body, ending with the neck and facial muscles. Initially, the nurse can guide the patient verbally, slowly directing the attention to the next muscle group to be relaxed. After one or two sessions, many patients can effectively provide their own relaxation sequence.

Guided Imagery

Guided imagery involves assisting patients to form mental images of a pleasant environment where they are comfortable and happy. For some, the experience is visual; in their minds they "see" a beautiful place. For others, it is a process of achieving a feeling of comfort and peace. Either is highly effective in giving the patient a brief mental break from pain. These methods often are used during painful procedures, such as bone marrow extraction.

Meditation

Meditation involves the use of a focus point, which may be a sound, a repeated phrase (sometimes called a *mantra*), the sound of the breath as it moves in and out of the body, or a visual image. The visual image may be a picture or object that the patient gazes at, or it may be an imagined image (a candle's flame, a leaf moving with breeze, beach waves).

Hypnosis

Hypnosis, or therapeutic suggestion, should be done by a trained practitioner. It involves the use of focusing and relaxation to induce a trance-like state during which a patient receives suggestions that may be helpful after returning to a normal level of consciousness. Although people under hypnosis cannot be induced to do things they would ordinarily feel were wrong, this inducement remains a common fear. Reassurance may help, but hypnosis should be used only if the subject is comfortable with the idea and is open to its use.

Biofeedback

Biofeedback involves the use of a machine that uses electrodes attached to the skin to measure the degree of muscular tension. The machine has colored lights that change (usually red to yellow to green) and an audible tone that changes in pitch from higher to lower as the patient relaxes. The patient receives visual and auditory confirmation of self-induced relaxation. This technique is particularly effective with people who are highly competitive because it rewards success and allows them to "win" the game.

Music

Music used alone can be highly effective in bringing about relaxation and can be used as a focal point for meditation or to enhance other distracting activities. Nature sounds, including the ocean, running streams, breezes, rain, and birds singing, also can induce relaxation. Headphones allow the patient to be immersed in sound without disturbing others. Headphones with music can be used during loud or long diagnostic procedures such as magnetic resonance imaging (MRI).

Binders

Binders are helpful for strains, sprains, and wounds or surgical incisions that are packed. They support the tissues during movement, such as ambulation or coughing, which reduces the pain.

Massage

Once a mainstay of nursing comfort measures, massage (cutaneous stimulation) is again increasing in popularity. The use of long, firm strokes; short, soft, circular strokes; and occasionally gentle pounding with the sides of the hands stimulates circulation, relaxes muscles, and increases the general sense of well-being. When the painful area has inflammation, or consists of a wound or an incision, massaging another area of the body with gentle but firm pressure helps the patient direct attention away from the pain. Always be guided by the patient's sense of comfort. Use only the degree of pressure that is pleasant and relaxing.

Simple massage can be done by a family member with just a little instruction, giving them an opportunity to assist in the care in a positive and loving way. Massage should not be used on any area that has been reddened by pressure. This tissue is already compromised and massage can cause further damage through *shearing*, the traumatic pulling of tissue layers away from one another.

Acupuncture and Acupressure

Acupuncture originated centuries ago in China and involves the use of tiny needles inserted into the skin at specific points along lines called *meridians*, a concept similar to that of nerve pathways. In recent years it has gained favor in the United States as a pain control measure. Research has shown that acupuncture helps relieve back and headache pain (Doheny, 2010; Yuan et al., 2008). Acupressure involves the use of external finger pressure at the meridian points to achieve similar effects. Both acupuncture and acupressure require extensive training for proper use and should only be done by someone fully trained in these procedures.

Complementary and Alternative Therapies

Pain Relief

Complementary and alternative therapies are used more for pain relief than for anything else. Therapies used include relaxation, meditation, biofeedback, yoga, hypnosis, imagery, chiropractic, acupuncture, acupressure, massage, aromatherapy, and herbal preparations and supplements. Research from the National Institutes of Health has proven that acupuncture is effective for many patients for various pain problems.

Transcutaneous Electrical Nerve Stimulation

Transcutaneous electrical nerve stimulation (TENS) utilizes a small electrical stimulator attached to the skin with electrodes placed around the area of pain. A low current running between the electrodes acts to block pain sensation. The degree of stimulation can be controlled by the patient using dials on the stimulator. The application of TENS requires specific training and must be ordered by a physician (Figure 7-7). Some patients find TENS unpleasant rather than helpful. In such cases, the physician should be notified and an alternative method of pain control selected.

Spinal Cord Stimulator

The spinal cord stimulator is implanted in the epidural space adjacent to nerves that innervate the affected body area. This device is used for patients with chronic pain who have not responded to medications or other methods of pain management.

? **Think Critically**

What types of nonpharmacologic methods would you use for the patient who is complaining of muscle pain in the shoulder after an auto accident?

FIGURE 7-7 Instructing the patient on how to use a TENS unit.

COMMUNITY CARE

Community care for pain can take place in a variety of settings, with varying levels of training among direct caregivers. Nurses may need to work with the social worker before discharge to put in place all the necessary measures to control pain for the patient going home. Nurses in the community should help educate people about the complementary and alternative resources available to treat chronic pain.

EXTENDED CARE

Extended-care facilities may provide rehabilitative services, long-term care services, or both. Each type of care may include specific pain management needs. Patients undergoing rehabilitation often have acute pain related to therapy, particularly in the early phases. It is important that therapy be scheduled to allow for adequate rest and recovery time. It also is important that analgesic medication be given on a schedule that provides the patient with the greatest pain relief during therapy sessions. This assists the patient to cooperate with therapy, which in turn encourages a more rapid recovery. In planning, always include the patient, who knows best which medication and time schedule provides the most effective pain relief.

Long-term care facilities—also called nursing homes, skilled nursing facilities, transitional care units, and board and care homes—often have patients who live there for the last weeks, months, or even years of their lives. In such settings, the term *resident* is used, rather than *patient*. Residents may have pain following a fall, after dental work, or during a period of illness, and they may have chronic pain from arthritis, degenerative disorders, or cancer. Residents may be mentally alert and oriented, or be alert and confused, or have a decreased level of consciousness. However, each of these individuals can perceive pain and should be given appropriate analgesics when pain exists.

The nurse can be of great assistance to the physician in ordering analgesia by providing accurate information about the type of pain, the frequency, the intensity, and precipitating factors. For instance, a resident with degenerative arthritis and chronic joint pain may benefit from a routine oral analgesic such as acetaminophen (Tylenol) or ibuprofen (Motrin). Those with more severe chronic problems, such as cancer, may benefit from routine time-released medications such as MS Contin (oral morphine sulfate in a time-released tablet). As pain increases, more narcotic may be needed to gain relief, but remember that the very elderly or debilitated may be more drug sensitive. Monitor all medications carefully and work with the physician to ensure that the resident's pain is being appropriately addressed. Ideally, the resident is comfortable, alert, and able to participate in activities of choice. Nurses in the long-term care setting must make pain assessment and management a priority.

HOME CARE

The number of individuals receiving skilled and professional nursing care at home is increasing rapidly. Early discharge from the hospital is growing primarily to control escalating medical costs and because people generally are more comfortable and heal more rapidly in their home environment. Patients frequently go home from the hospital with peripheral or central IV lines providing analgesia. The nurse provides patient and family education on pain management in the home setting, which includes verbal and written instructions about the medication and any equipment used to dispense it. Telephone numbers that give the patient and family access to 24-hour assistance should be prominently displayed.

Just as in an inpatient setting, home care patients must be evaluated for the continued safety and effectiveness of the analgesic medication. The nurse must contact the physician any time the medication orders need to be adjusted. Adjuncts to pain management, such as simple massage, relaxation techniques, and the use of pillows, warmth, repositioning, or soft music, are readily taught to patients and families for use in the home care setting.

PCA medications sometimes are given subcutaneously rather than intravenously, particularly for those patients with poor peripheral venous access who are not candidates for a central line. A tiny needle is placed in the subcutaneous tissue on the abdomen and taped in place. Sites are changed at regular intervals to maintain good absorption of the medication and avoid damage to the tissues. The increased use of central IV catheters and ports and the availability of oral timed-release analgesics are making subcutaneous PCA devices much less common.

Current guidelines for home care by agencies such as Medicare require that case management be done by a licensed professional. This usually is a registered nurse, although the registered physical therapist may fill this role for patients whose only acute need is continued restorative therapy. The role of the LPN/LVN is that of direct patient care under the guidance of the case manager. The LPN/LVN may monitor an ongoing infusion and discontinue the infusion as needed, but must report any difficulties immediately to the case manager for intervention. Some states offer IV therapy certification for LPN/LVNs, which allows them to infuse medications.

The nurse must always be alert to an increase in pain due to changes in the disease process. The physician needs to be notified of the change so that appropriate measures, including adjusting or changing the medications, can take place.

Get Ready for the NCLEX® Examination!

Key Points

- Only the patient knows where the pain is and its degree of intensity.
- Pain is a neurologic response to unpleasant stimuli.
- The gate control theory states that when the gate is open, pain sensation is allowed through; when the gate is closed, pain is blocked.
- The patient should be asked to use an appropriate pain scale.
- Endorphins can block pain sensation.
- The two pathophysiologic classifications of pain are nociceptive and neuropathic.
- Nociceptive pain derives from stimulation of somatic or visceral structures.
- There are four phases of nociceptive pain: transduction, transmission, perception, and modulation.
- Neuropathic pain is from dysfunction of the nervous system.
- Neuropathic pain is relieved with NSAIDs, tricyclic antidepressants, anticonvulsants, and corticosteroids.
- Pain tolerance varies from one individual to another.
- Pain threshold is the point at which pain is perceived.
- Cultural factors and beliefs affect each person's perception of pain.
- Pain assessment/data collection includes the areas of appearance, behavior, activity level, verbalization, and physiologic clues.
- An interpreter may be required to gather correct data about a non–English-speaking patient's pain.
- Goals of care are (1) relief of pain and (2) control of pain.
- Pharmacologic and nonpharmacologic methods are used to treat pain.
- False perceptions about pain may affect care (see Table 7-4).
- Evaluating the effectiveness of measures used to relieve pain is a primary nursing responsibility.
- Always follow the "Five Rights" when administering pain medication.
- It is important to know all about the commonly used analgesics (see Table 7-5).
- Constipation is a common side effect of narcotic analgesia, and preventive measures should be used.
- Adequate sleep assists in controlling pain.
- Hypnosis and biofeedback have been proven to be effective for many people for a variety of types of pain.
- Chronic pain is common among the elderly in long-term care facilities.

Additional Learning Resources

SG Go to your Study Guide for additional learning activities to help you master this chapter content.

 evolve Go to your Evolve website (http://evolve.elsevier.com/deWit/medsurg) for the following FREE learning resources:

- Animations, audio, and video
- Answers and rationales for questions and activities
- Concept Map Creator
- Glossary with pronunciations in English and Spanish
- Interactive Review Questions and Exercises and more!

Online Resources

- American Chronic Pain Association, www.theacpa.org/default.aspx
- Pain assessment and management resources: http://ltctoolkit.rnao.ca/resources/pain; www.vachss.com/help_text/pain.html; www.stoppain.org; www.webmd.com/pain-management/default.htm

Review Questions for the NCLEX® Examination

1. An appropriate expected outcome for a patient with *Acute pain related to recent surgical procedure* would be:
   1. the patient will demonstrate use of patient-controlled analgesia pump.
   2. the nurse will assess for adequate pain relief.
   3. the incision will heal without infection.
   4. pain will be adequately controlled with a PCA pump.

2. The long-term care nurse is caring for an elderly male patient who appears to be withdrawn and quiet. He grimaces whenever he is touched. The *most* appropriate nursing action would be to:
   1. administer pain medication.
   2. assess for underlying causes of the patient's behavior.
   3. reposition him and check again in 2 hours.
   4. notify the physician.

3. A 25-year-old patient complains of moderate pain at his incision site. The nurse administers morphine sulfate intramuscularly. The most appropriate nursing action after the injection would be to:
   1. evaluate the effectiveness of the pain medication in 2 hours.
   2. encourage him to close his eyes and rest.
   3. suggest he play solitaire or watch something interesting on TV.
   4. administer ordered ibuprofen orally.

4. Before administering an opioid analgesic, it is *most* important to:
   1. check the blood pressure.
   2. provide other comfort measures first.
   3. assess for possible constipation.
   4. assess rate and depth of respirations.

5. A patient with chronic pain asks, "What is a TENS unit?" What is the best nursing response?
   1. "It is an implant in the epidural space adjacent to nerves that innervate the affected body area."
   2. "It provides a small electrical stimulus to the skin around the area of pain."
   3. "It involves the use of external finger pressure at the meridian points."
   4. "It supports the tissues during movement."

6. A patient who has osteoarthritis is experiencing right knee pain daily. This type of pain usually has the best result if treated by:
   1. oxycodone.
   2. ibuprofen.
   3. Lyrica.
   4. prednisone.

7. The nurse reinforces the need for safe administration of gentle heat to the nursing assistant. Which action by a nursing assistant indicates the need for further instruction?
   1. Applying a cold pack directly to the painful site
   2. Encouraging relaxation techniques to decrease pain
   3. Repositioning the patient for comfort
   4. Checking on the patient in 20 minutes after the heat application

8. After administering ketorolac (Toradol) 30 mg intramuscularly to a 30-year-old male patient, an immediate nursing action would be to:
   1. recap the needle.
   2. massage the area.
   3. check for pain relief in 45 minutes.
   4. encourage an activity that will provide distraction.

9. The nurse is assigned to care for a patient with an epidural for analgesia. Which sign or symptom related to this treatment would require immediate physician notification?
   1. Blood pressure 80/60 mm Hg
   2. Temperature 99.5° F (37.5° C)
   3. Respirations 12/min
   4. Urinary output less than 30 mL/hr

10. In determining the patient's perception of pain, which question(s) would be useful in assessing pain? *(Select all that apply.)*
    1. "Where are you hurting?"
    2. "What pain control measures have worked in the past?"
    3. "How would you describe your pain?"
    4. "What were you doing before the onset of the pain?"
    5. "Are you sleeping adequately?"

Critical Thinking Questions

Scenario A

Ann Jefferson, a 43-year-old woman, has suffered shoulder pain from an old healed fracture for several years. When the pain is too severe to be controlled with acetaminophen, her physician recommends that she use the oral narcotic analgesic he prescribed. However, Ann does not want to continue taking drugs that she "might become addicted to."

1. How would you respond to Ann's statement regarding her fear of addiction to the pain medication?

2. What other measures could you suggest for management of Ann's pain?

Scenario B

Fred Hickson, an African American construction worker, had a bowel resection 3 days ago. He is determined to get back to work quickly and is very cooperative about ambulation.

He refuses pain medication, stating, "I don't need it." You note that he stops frequently to lean against the wall, walks stooped over, and grimaces when no one is looking.

1. Why might Fred be refusing pain medication?

2. What information might you share regarding pain control and getting well after major surgery?

3. What suggestions might you make to Fred regarding his comfort?

Scenario C

Jim Tolliver, age 32, sprained his left ankle playing football with his friends this morning. He consults his neighbor (who is a nurse) about what to do as it is hurting a lot.

1. What should his nurse neighbor do first?

2. What should be suggested to Jim as to home treatment?

3. What precautions should the neighbor take regarding further treatment?

Objectives

Theory

1. Identify characteristics of neoplastic (abnormal tissue) growth.
2. Identify at least five factors that may contribute to the development of a malignancy.
3. State at least four practices that can contribute to prevention and early detection of cancers.
4. Include the recommendations of the American Cancer Society for routine checkups and detection of cancers into patient education.
5. Explain the advantages and disadvantages of the various treatments available for cancer.
6. Illustrate the major problems for a patient who is coping with side effects of radiation or chemotherapy for cancer, and state the appropriate nursing interventions.

7. Distinguish the stages of the grieving process experienced by the dying cancer patient.

Clinical Practice

1. Devise a general plan of nursing care for the patient receiving chemotherapy.
2. Formulate a teaching plan for the patient who has bone marrow suppression from cancer treatment.
3. Institute nursing interventions to help the patient cope with the common problems of cancer and its treatment.
4. Use appropriate nursing interventions to help patients and families deal with the psychosocial effects of cancer and its treatment.
5. Employ nursing interventions to help the cancer patient cope with death and dying.

Key Terms

benign (bĕ-NĪN, p. 145)
biopsy (BĪ-ŏp-sē, p. 153)
carcinogens (kăr-SĬN-ō-jĕnz, p. 147)
carcinoma (kăr-sĭ-NŌ-mă, p. 146)
cytology (sī-TŎL-ō-jē, p. 151)
cytotoxic (sī-tŏ-TŎK-sĭk, p. 162)
deoxyribonucleic acid (DNA) (dē-ŏx-ē-rī-bō-nū-KLĀ-ĭc ĂS-ĭd, p. 145)
encapsulated (ĕn-KĂP-sū-lāt-ĕd, p. 145)
hematoma (hē-mă-TŌ-mă, p. 146)
incidence (ĬN-sĕ-dĕns, p. 144)
leukemia (lū-kĒ-mē-ă, p. 146)
lymphoma (lĭm-FŌ-mă, p. 146)
malignant (mă-LĬG-nănt, p. 145)

melanoma (mĕl-ă-NŌ-mă, p. 146)
metastasis (mĕ-TĂS-tă-sĭs, p. 146)
mutation (mū-TĀ-shŭn, p. 147)
neoplasm (NĒ-ō-plăzm, p. 145)
occult blood (ŏ-KŬLT blŭd, p. 151)
oncogenes (ŎNGK-ō-jĕnz, p. 147)
palliative care (PĂL-ē-ă-tĭv, p. 172)
prognosis (prŏg-NŌ-sĭs, p. 146)
promoters (prō-MŌ-tĕrz, p. 148)
sarcoma (săr-kŌ-mă, p. 146)
TNM staging (p. 146)
transformation (trănz-fĕr-MĀ-shŭn, p. 149)
tumor markers (TŪ-mŏr, p. 154)
vesicants (VĔ-si-kĕnts, p. 163)

THE IMPACT OF CANCER

Cancer is a group of diseases that characteristically grow in an uncontrolled manner with the spread of abnormal cells. In many instances, however, the growth can be controlled by specific treatment. In the early 1900s, there was little hope for survival once cancer was detected. This year, 4 of 10 people who are diagnosed with cancer will be alive in 5 years.

Excluding skin cancer, about 1,529,560 new cases of invasive cancer will be diagnosed in 2010 (American Cancer Society [ACS], 2010). It is estimated that an

additional 1 million people in 2010 will be told that they have squamous cell skin cancer. The current rate of cancer is about the same as that of 1977, indicating little advance in the rate of cancer occurrence. The incidence of lung cancer in men declined during 2010 and the incidence in women stabilized. However, the incidence of breast cancer has increased over the past three decades and is mostly attributed to improved detection.

Death rates for many other major cancers have stabilized or declined since the 1930s. However, cancer still accounts for one in four deaths in the United States

Leading sites of new cancer cases and deaths – 2010 estimates

Estimated new cases*		Estimated deaths	
Male	**Female**	**Male**	**Female**
Prostate 217,730 (28%)	Breast 207,090 (28%)	Lung & bronchus 86,220 (29%)	Lung & bronchus 71,080 (26%)
Lung & bronchus 116,750 (15%)	Lung & bronchus 105,770 (14%)	Prostate 32,050 (11%)	Breast 39,840 (15%)
Colon & rectum 72,090 (9%)	Colon & rectum 70,480 (10%)	Colon & rectum 26,580 (9%)	Colon & rectum 24,790 (9%)
Urinary bladder 52,760 (7%)	Uterine corpus 43,470 (6%)	Pancreas 18,770 (6%)	Pancreas 18,030 (7%)
Melanoma of the skin 38,870 (5%)	Thyroid 33,930 (5%)	Liver & intrahepatic bile duct 12,720 (4%)	Ovary 13,850 (5%)
Non-Hodgkin lymphoma 35,380 (4%)	Non-Hodgkin lymphoma 30,160 (4%)	Leukemia 12,660 (4%)	Non-Hodgkin lymphoma 9,500 (4%)
Kidney & renal pelvis 35,370 (4%)	Melanoma of the skin 29,260 (4%)	Esophagus 11,650 (4%)	Leukemia 9,180 (3%)
Oral cavity & pharynx 25,420 (3%)	Kidney & renal pelvis 22,870 (3%)	Non-Hodgkin lymphoma 10,710 (4%)	Uterine corpus 7,950 (3%)
Leukemia 24,690 (3%)	Ovary 21,880 (3%)	Urinary bladder 10,410 (3%)	Liver & intrahepatic bile duct 6,190 (2%)
Pancreas 21,370 (3%)	Pancreas 21,770 (3%)	Kidney & renal pelvis 8,210 (3%)	Brain & other nervous system 5,720 (2%)
All sites 789,620 (100%)	All sites 739,940 (100%)	All sites 299,200 (100%)	All sites 270,290 (100%)

* Excludes basal and squamous cell skin cancers and in situ carcinoma except urinary bladder.

©2010, American Cancer Society, Inc., Surveillance and Health Policy Research

FIGURE 8-1 Leading sites of new cancer cases and deaths.

today. About 569,490 people will die from cancer in 2010 (1500 people per day). On the other hand, there are 11.1 million living Americans who have a history of cancer, and 68% of them were diagnosed over 5 years ago. **That means that 66% of cancer patients are surviving.** Because of earlier detection and improvements in treatment methods, patients who are diagnosed today may have much higher survival rates. More people can survive cancer if it is treated in its earliest stages. In fact, the American Cancer Society (ACS) estimates that if all the cancers that are detectable early *were diagnosed in localized stages,* the 5-year survival rate would be 95%. Figure 8-1 shows the leading sites of new cancer cases and deaths.

PHYSIOLOGY OF CANCER

The human body is continuously producing new cells to replace those cells that are worn out, and to repair damage done to cells by illness and injury. An abnormal replication of cells results in a neoplasm (new growth of tissue, or tumor), which is not beneficial. The word benign indicates a neoplasm that is usually harmless. Benign growths are almost always encapsulated (surrounded by a fibrous capsule). The capsule prevents the release of cells and restricts their spread to other parts of the body. Benign growths can, however, create problems if they press against and interfere with the normal structure and function of nearby organs.

The cells of malignant (uncontrolled growth that can lead to death) growths are quite different from normal cells. Cells that exhibit malignant growth are known as cancer. Cancerous growth changes a cell's deoxyribonucleic acid (DNA) makeup and function, and also the DNA structure and function of cells that are replicated; hence, cancer cells do not look like or behave like normal cells (Figure 8-2). DNA is the material that contains the genetic makeup of all future generations of a cell.

The nucleus of a malignant (cancer) cell is large and irregular. As the cancer cell divides and duplicates, it fails to follow the rules that regulate the reproduction of normal cells. Malignant cells do not seem to "know" when to stop multiplying. The offspring of cancerous cells *proliferate* (multiply) in great numbers, and they grow more and more disorganized, often forming tumorous masses. Some cancerous cells take on new characteristics, so that they do not resemble the cells of the original tissue. The malignant cells invade neighboring tissues and travel to other parts of the body. There they establish another colony of malignant cells. Their demand for nutrients depletes the supply of

FIGURE 8-2 Normal and malignant skeletal muscle cells. **A,** Normal skeletal muscle cells. Note that cells are well differentiated and similar in appearance. **B,** Malignant tumor cells in skeletal muscle (rhabdomyosarcoma).

nourishment available for normal cells. This spread of tumor cells is called metastasis (movement of cancer cells from the original cancer site to other areas of the body). **Not all malignant cells metastasize, but the great majority of malignant cells do.**

 Think Critically

Can you compare and contrast the aspects of a benign and a malignant tumor?

CLASSIFICATION OF TUMORS

Tumors are often classified according to the organs or tissues from which they first began to grow; alternatively, tumors are classified according to the substances of which they are formed. The suffix *-oma* means tumor; this suffix is used in the names of various kinds of growths or swellings. Remember that *-oma* simply means tumor; the suffix *-oma* can designate any swelling, including a swelling in which there is a collection of fluids, as well as a swelling containing malignant cells. For example, hematoma (another word for bruise) is a combination of *hema-*, meaning blood, and *-oma*, meaning a swelling or collection of fluid or cells.

The prefixes used in classifying neoplasms indicate the kind of tissue in which they originate. For example, a tumor arising from fatty (lipoid) tissue is called a *lipoma*. A *fibroma* is a tumor composed of fibrous tissue. A *leiomyofibroma* contains both smooth-muscle tissue and fibrous connective tissue. Lipomas, fibromas,

and leiomyomas are the most frequently occurring types of benign growths.

Malignant growths are divided into four main types. A sarcoma arises from mesenchymal tissues (bone, muscles, and other connective tissues). A carcinoma originates in epithelial tissues (skin and mucous membranes). These kinds of cancers make up the majority of cancers of the stomach, uterus, lungs, skin, and tongue. Leukemia and lymphoma are cancers of the blood-forming system. Malignancy of the pigment cells of the skin is called melanoma.

These are the main groups of cancers. More accurate naming can be done by adding modifying prefixes. For example, *osteosarcomas* arise from bone (*osteo-*), and *adenocarcinomas* arise from glandular (*adeno-*) structures.

METASTASIS

The word *metastasis* means the movement of cells from one part of the body to another. **Metastasis refers to the moving of these malignant cells to another site.** Malignant cells can metastasize by traveling in the blood and body fluids, in much the same way as do bacterial cells. It also is possible for free malignant cells to be directly transplanted from one organ to another during surgery when gloves and instruments that have these cells on them serve as vehicles for their transportation. Another way in which malignant cells can "contaminate" normal tissues and organs is by entering a body cavity and coming in contact with a healthy organ. For example, malignant cells may break off from a diseased organ, enter the abdominal cavity, and attach themselves to an ovary or the *mesentery* (tissues that connect the internal organs to the abdominal cavity wall) (Figure 8-3).

The prognosis (prediction of survival) for a patient with a malignancy depends on how much the malignant cells have attacked body tissues. A localized growth is one that remains at the original site *(in situ)* and has not yet released its cells, even though the growth may have invaded underlying tissues. At this stage the disease is much more easily destroyed.

A *regional* malignancy is one in which cells from the original malignancy have spread to the body area around the tumor, such as to nearby lymph nodes. The spread has been limited by the body's protective mechanisms. These cells may continue to grow and multiply, and if the regional cancer is not successfully treated, malignant cells will eventually break away and spread throughout the body. This creates an *advanced* cancer that is often fatal.

One system that identifies cancers by how much the malignancy has spread is the TNM staging system. The three basic parts of the system are *T* for primary tumor, *N* for regional nodes, and *M* for metastasis. The number written beside each letter indicates how much the malignancy has spread and attacked other tissues. For example, T1, N0, M0 means that the tumor is small

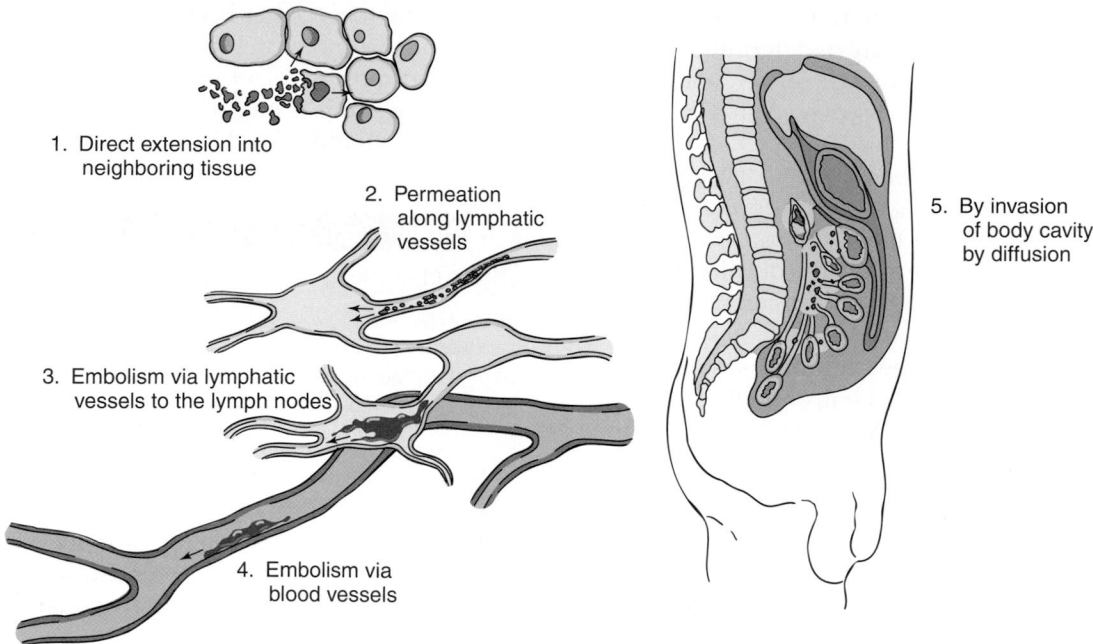

1. Direct extension into neighboring tissue

2. Permeation along lymphatic vessels

3. Embolism via lymphatic vessels to the lymph nodes

4. Embolism via blood vessels

5. By invasion of body cavity by diffusion

FIGURE 8-3 Modes of dissemination of cancer.

and localized (no involvement of regional lymph nodes and no metastasis). A label of T1, N2, M1 indicates a small (T1) tumor with moderate regional involvement (N2) that has metastasized to one distant site or organ (M1).

CAUSATIVE FACTORS

All cancer results from defects in the DNA of genes. These defects either are inherited or are caused by mutation (a permanent change in the DNA sequence of a gene) during a person's lifetime from exposure to chemicals or radiation. Several cancer-causing genes (oncogenes) are discovered each year. Oncogenes are mistakes in the instructions inside a cell's DNA genetic code, whereby newly created cells are no longer normal. The defective gene tells the new cells to multiply at a higher rate. Also, the defective coding prevents newly created defective cells from dying and being reabsorbed. This results in a tumor, or mass.

Tumor suppressor genes are healthy, normal genes that control the growth of cells in the body. Each person's body has a different ability to withstand the effects of cancer-causing substances (carcinogens), to mount a healthy immune response, and to repair damaged DNA. It is hoped that discoveries in molecular biology will allow individual risk profiles to be drawn that could be used to counsel people to avoid certain occupational and environmental exposures or to develop protective therapies.

In the external environment, many harmful agents exist that are known to be carcinogenic, and others are strongly suspected. **Among these harmful agents are certain chemicals, sources of radiation, and viruses** (Table 8-1). There are also some internal factors

Table **8-1**	Common Carcinogenic Substances
SUBSTANCE	**TYPE OF CANCER**
Asbestos	Lung, peritoneal, pericardial
Benzene	Acute myelocytic leukemia
Tobacco	Lung, mouth, pharynx, larynx, esophagus, pancreas, bladder, kidney
Alcoholic beverages	Mouth, pharynx, larynx, esophagus, liver
Ionizing radiation	Leukemia, tumors of most organs
Sunlight (ultraviolet rays)	Skin
Diethylstilbestrol (prenatally)	Vagina
Estrogens, synthetic	Endometrial
Androgens, synthetic	Liver
Vinyl chloride	Liver
Aromatic amines	Bladder
Arsenic (inorganic)	Lung, skin
Chromium	Lung
Nickel dust	Lung, nasal sinuses
Chronic hepatitis B or C infection	Liver
Human T-cell lymphotropic virus type 1 (HTLV-1)	Adult T-cell leukemia and lymphoma
Human papillomavirus (HPV)	Cervix, mouth and throat
Phenacetin	Renal pelvis, bladder
Alkylating agents (used for chemotherapy)	Acute myelocytic leukemia
Cyclosporine (used to prevent transplant rejection)	Non-Hodgkin's lymphoma

that affect an individual's ability to cope with malignant cells. Hormones play an undetermined role in the development and progress of cancer, and several inherited genes have been discovered that increase a person's chance of getting certain types of cancer. In some families there is a tendency to develop cancer in particular organs. This is shown in certain high-risk groups, described later in this chapter.

Another factor that enters into the development of a malignancy is age. Although cancer can strike at any age, older people are more susceptible. *Immunocompetence,* or the capability of one's immune system to deal with foreign cells—bacterial, viral, or malignant—is an important factor in the development of cancers; immunocompetence decreases with aging.

CHEMICAL CARCINOGENS

More than 200 years ago (1775), Sir Percival Pott linked the occurrence of cancer to a substance in the environment when he observed that cancer of the scrotum was common among the chimney sweeps of London. He attributed this high incidence of cancer to repeated accumulations of soot on the skin of these young men, whose occupation required continuous contact with the coal soot in the chimneys they cleaned. Since that time, almost 500 different chemical carcinogens have been identified.

> **? Think Critically**
>
> Can you identify three chemicals used in your home or your garden that are carcinogenic? How can you reduce your exposure to them and decrease the risk of cancer?

Many of the cancer-producing substances in the environment are related to occupations that involve repeated exposure to certain substances that are handled or inhaled. **Petrofluorocarbons (polychlorinated biphenyls or PCBs) and some pesticides (e.g., DDT) are known carcinogens.** These and other such chemicals decrease immunocompetence. For example, cancer of the skin often is related to the handling of pitch, asphalt, crude paraffin, and petroleum products. Lung cancer is linked to irritating substances in the air, such as tobacco smoke, asbestos, and chemical wastes from industry and automobiles. Cancer of the bladder is associated with certain substances in aniline dyes, which are present in the environment of workers in that industry. Vinyl chloride, nickel, arsenic, and chromate are linked to cancers in workers in industries that use those chemicals. Benzene, an ingredient in older unleaded gasoline, is linked to leukemia. These are but a few of the chemical agents that can contribute to the development of cancer in humans.

Chewing tobacco has been directly related to cancer of the tongue and structures of the mouth and throat. **Cigarette smoking is a known direct cause of cancer of the lung and is thought to be linked to esophageal, pancreatic, bladder, and kidney cancers.**

> **🏃 Health Promotion**
>
> **Effects of Smoking**
>
> Encourage those who smoke to quit. Ninety percent of lung cancers in men and 79% in women are related to smoking. Use of tobacco in conjunction with the intake of alcohol is related to several other types of cancer.

Immunosuppressive drugs used to suppress organ transplant rejection are a cause of non-Hodgkin's lymphoma. Synthetic estrogens are linked to a higher incidence of endometrial cancer. Many cancer drugs affect the immune system and can predispose to other types of cancer.

PROMOTERS

Promoters are substances that are not carcinogenic when found alone, but when they are in a person's body with a known carcinogen, cancer occurs faster. Alcohol is such a substance. When nicotine is present, cancers occur at a faster rate in those who are heavy consumers of alcohol than in those who use nicotine but do not drink alcohol. It is thought that about 90% of all head and neck cancers are tobacco plus alcohol related.

CHRONIC IRRITATION

In one of the earliest theories about the causes of cancer, a skin cancer was attributed to long-term chronic irritation of the skin and mucous membranes. Although this condition may be a *contributing cause* of cancer, chronic irritation alone usually does not lead to malignancy. There must be other factors present, particularly a mole on the skin and/or exposure to a chemical carcinogen or ultraviolet rays, in order for the skin cancer process to begin.

Research on chemicals that may have this same type of influence is ongoing. Most likely the second substance involved, although not directly carcinogenic, has a harmful effect on the immune system, making the person more susceptible to malignant cell growth.

PHYSICAL CARCINOGENS

Radiation

Radiation may originate from x-ray machines and radioactive elements or from the ultraviolet rays of the sun. These rays are capable of penetrating certain body tissues and causing the development of malignant cells in the affected area. The relationship of intense and prolonged exposure to these rays and the production of cancer cells was first discovered when it was noted that there was a high incidence of cancer, particularly leukemia, among people who pioneered studies of x-rays, or worked with radium or uranium. Later it was found that survivors of atomic blasts at Hiroshima and Nagasaki at the end of World War II suffered an unusually high incidence of leukemia.

There is continued concern about the danger that excessive radiation in the environment presents, especially the long-term effects that are not immediately apparent but may eventually prove to be related to malignancy. In addition to leukemia, cancers of the skin, bone marrow, breast, lung, and thyroid are believed to be closely linked to exposure to radiation.

The ultraviolet rays of the sun can produce skin cancer. The deterioration of the Earth's ozone layer is causing more ultraviolet rays to reach the earth than in the past, which compounds the problem. The susceptibility of the individual also is a factor: people with fair complexions have less protective pigment and therefore are more likely to develop skin cancer from ultraviolet radiation than are people with darker skin.

Radon Gas

People who live in areas that have more radon emission from the earth have a higher incidence of malignancy in the population than people in areas that are low in radon.

Viruses

In recent years, extensive research has been directed toward establishing a link between viruses and malignancy. Experiments involving animals have demonstrated that a number of cancers can be produced in animals by injecting them with a filtrate from virus-infected malignant growths. **The hepatitis B virus is carcinogenic for liver cancer.** The Epstein-Barr virus causes Burkitt's lymphoma. Cases of adult T-cell leukemia and lymphoma are caused by human T-cell lymphotropic virus. Several types of the human papillomavirus (HPV) cause cervical carcinoma and are related to throat and mouth cancer in nonsmokers. These viruses are known as *oncoviruses* because of their ability to cause cancer.

After the transformation (change into something else) of a normal cell into a precancerous state, the malignant cell requires many conditions favorable to its multiplication and growth into a cancerous tumor. **Viruses are capable of introducing new genetic material into a normal cell and transforming it into a malignant one.** Furthermore, cell reproduction can be altered when viruses interact with carcinogens. Viruses such as the human immunodeficiency virus (HIV) can damage the immune system and decrease immunocompetence, causing the body to become more susceptible to the growth of abnormal cells. Such damage also reduces the body's ability to fight off cancer-causing viruses, such as HPV. Some cancers—such as Kaposi sarcoma—are only seen in HIV-infected or severely immunocompromised patients (see Chapter 11 for more information).

GENETIC PREDISPOSITION

All cancers are caused by genes that malfunction and cause the overgrowth of cells. Research is revealing that there is a genetic predisposition to various types of cancer. It has been known for many years that breast cancer is more likely to occur in women who have a close female relative who developed breast cancer before age 50. Gene markers have been found for colon cancer, breast cancer, prostate cancer, pancreatic cancer, and leukemia. However, only 5% to 10% of cancers are related to a directly inherited gene. The remaining cancers are caused by genes that are damaged (mutated) throughout the lifetime, and are not inherited. Some people are more susceptible to these mutations.

 Cultural Considerations

Race Factors

Some populations are at a higher risk for certain types of cancer. For example, of the four types of melanoma, African Americans are most susceptible to the acral lentiginous type whereas whites are least susceptible to it. Lentigo maligna melanoma is found most often in Hawaii.

With the completion of the Human Genome Project, scientists are working to identify the genes that are related to specific cancers (National Cancer Institute, 2011). Currently, research is focused on finding genetic markers—or oncogenes—for other forms of cancer. Such markers, or the proteins they produce, could identify high-risk individuals who then might undergo more vigorous, regular diagnostic testing to detect any malignancy in the very earliest stages. Since several cancers have precursor lesions (such as adenomatous polyps in the colon) such early discovery would greatly increase survival rates.

CONTRIBUTING FACTORS

INTRINSIC FACTORS

Age, sex, and race are considered "predisposing factors" for certain types of cancers. Predisposition simply means that, statistically, certain types of cancer strike particular age, sex, or racial groups more frequently than others. For example, prostate cancer is far more common in black males than in white males. The incidence of cervical cancer is higher in black women than in white women. Breast cancer is more prevalent in white women than in Asian women. As for age factors, approximately 76% of cancers occur in people age 55 and older.

STRESS

Another factor that seems to play a role in the development of cancer is stress. Considerable stress over long periods has an adverse effect on the immune system; stress can make the immune system less effective in ridding the body of invading organisms and stress decreases the body's ability to destroy abnormal cells. Stress is one more factor that may tip the scales in favor of the growth of malignant cells. When one partner of a long-term relationship dies, the stress of the loss and adjustment to life without the partner seems to increase the likelihood of cancer in the surviving partner.

DIET

Most experts agree that approximately 30% of cancers could be reduced through proper nutrition and exercise. There is strong evidence that healthy diet and normal body weight are crucial in the control of cancer. Cancers of the breast, colon, rectum, endometrium, esophagus, uppermost abdomen, gallbladder, pancreas, liver, and kidney are all linked to excess weight and obesity. Although there is no universal agreement about the role of fiber in the prevention of malignancy, high-fiber foods such as fruits, vegetables, and cereals are recommended as a wholesome substitute for fatty foods.

MEASURES TO PREVENT CANCER

The nurse can be instrumental in educating the public about ways to prevent cancer. Each nurse should teach patients the following measures at every opportunity.

DIET AND NUTRITION

Encourage maintenance of normal weight. Obesity is considered a risk factor in many cancers. It also makes early detection of many cancers difficult. One study noted that men and women who were overweight by 40% or more have a 33% and 35% greater risk, respectively, for developing cancer than do persons with normal weight.

Nitrite and nitrate food additives are also known to be cancer *stimulators* (encouraging cancer). However, research has indicated that if foods containing nitrites are eaten in combination with foods containing vitamin C (ascorbic acid), the formation of nitrosamines is blocked. This means, for example, that if orange juice is consumed along with a meal containing bacon, there is less chance of carcinogenic nitrosamines damaging the body. In this instance, the vitamin C is a cancer *inhibitor* (discouraging cancer).

 Think Critically

If you saw that a package of meat contained nitrates, what other chemical would you expect to find in the package?

 Nutrition Considerations

Minimizing the Risk for Cancer

- Eat a varied diet and balance caloric intake with exercise to maintain a healthy weight.
- Limit red meat and processed meat intake. Eat fatty fish twice a week to increase omega-3 intake. Limit other fat intake, particularly saturated and *trans* fats. Substitute olive oil for cooking and salad dressings where possible.
- Eat five or more servings of a variety of vegetables and fruits each day. Include cruciferous vegetables, containing beta-carotene, tomatoes, onions and garlic, citrus fruits, and red and blue fruits and vegetables (cabbage, broccoli, Brussels sprouts, kohlrabi, cauliflower, carrots, yellow squash, sweet potatoes, red grapes, berries, and red cherries).
- Choose whole-grain foods over processed (refined) grains; include beans, whole-grain cereals, flaxseed, breads, and pastas to increase fiber intake daily.
- Keep alcohol consumption moderate: no more than two drinks or two glasses of wine or beer per day (one drink for women). No alcohol is best.
- Avoid smoked, salt-cured, nitrite-cured, and charred (blackened) foods.

From American Cancer Society: ACS guidelines on nutrition and physical activity for cancer prevention. Available at www.cancer.org/Healthy/EatHealthyGetActive.

These recommendations are from a report by a special committee on nutrition and cancer and are based on studies conducted for more than 20 years by the ACS's research program. Although no direct cause-and-effect relationship between diet and cancer has been demonstrated, there is ample evidence that avoidance of obesity and modification of the diet can help prevent some types of cancers.

 Think Critically

Can you identify three specific changes you could make in your personal diet that might decrease your cancer risk? What would you add to the diet, or what would you stop eating?

ALCOHOL

Moderation in the drinking of alcohol is recommended, because alcohol consumption alone has been shown to increase risk for several cancers. Excessive alcohol consumption also can lead to liver damage, and possibly to liver cancer.

ENVIRONMENT

Because groundwater is so often contaminated with chemicals that have leached into it from fertilizers, pesticides, and industrial wastes, it is wise to know the chemical makeup of the local water supply. If the geographic area is highly contaminated, filtered or bottled water might help prevent further damage to immunocompetence, and thereby decrease the incidence of cancer.

 Patient Teaching

Avoiding and Limiting Exposure to Carcinogens

- Knowing which substances used in the household, yard, and areas of recreation and at the place of work are carcinogenic and using protective measures against them can decrease exposure.
- The use of protective clothing, gloves, and mask as appropriate when spraying pesticides or chemicals or using chemical cleaners or strippers greatly decreases exposure.
- Being certain the area is well ventilated when using chemical cleaners indoors is protective.
- Thoroughly washing the hands and any exposed skin after using compounds containing carcinogenic chemicals provides protection.
- Using an appropriate sunscreen and protective clothing when outdoors, avoiding sunburns, and avoiding tanning salons and sunlamps greatly decreases the incidence of skin cancer.
- Australians have the highest rate of skin cancer in the world and have developed a message that is a good way to instruct your patients: **slip, slap, slop, strap—slip** on protective clothing, **slap** on a hat, **slop** on some sunscreen, and **strap** on sunglasses.
- Avoiding swimming and water sports in contaminated waters and avoiding eating fish from waters that have chemical contamination limit exposure.
- Washing or rinsing fruits and vegetables before preparing them for eating or cooking decreases exposure to agricultural pesticides.

IDENTIFYING HIGH-RISK PEOPLE

Studies of individuals who have developed cancer—their medical history, lifestyle, and family history—have shown that some people are more likely to develop certain kinds of cancer. Table 8-2 shows information on high-risk groups published by the ACS in order to develop an awareness of the need for frequent and thorough examinations to detect cancer early in those who are susceptible to developing a malignancy.

DETECTION OF CANCER

Cancer is a group of diseases. It can strike any organ of the body, affect different organs with different functions, and therefore can present an untold number of symptoms as it progresses. To be able to identify the symptoms of cancer in its earliest stages, it is important to be aware of its warning signals. The purpose of screening large segments of a population is to identify as many people with cancer as possible.

 Health Promotion

Warning Signs of Cancer

- Unusual bleeding or discharge
- A sore that does not heal
- A change in bowel or bladder habits
- A lump in the breast or other part of the body
- A nagging, persistent cough
- An obvious change in a mole
- Difficulty in swallowing

Elder Care Points

Elderly patients are at increasingly higher risk for developing cancer; their immune system is not as efficient as that of a younger person. Many of the cancer screening programs are suggested to begin at age 40 or 50.

In addition to the medical history and thorough physical examination that are essential components of any health status evaluation, the health care professional also conducts certain tests to determine whether a malignancy is present. Recommendations of the ACS for routine checkups and early detection of cancer are shown in Box 8-1.

One widely used technique to detect cancer is to examine cells under a microscope to determine whether they are malignant or premalignant. This technique is called **cytology,** and the most widely used cytology test is the Papanicolaou (Pap) smear to detect cervical cancer. A *cytologic examination* can be done by obtaining a sample of secretions containing cells that have been released from adjacent tissue. The technique involves either scraping or brushing a sample of cells from the area or collecting body secretions that contain cells. These secretions may be cervical discharges, sputum, gastric washings, pleural fluid, or urinary washings. The specimen is placed on a slide or put in a liquid medium and sent to a laboratory, where a specially trained technologist or pathologist examines the cells microscopically. If "suspicious" cells are found, the patient is referred to a health care professional for more extensive diagnostic tests. Another screening technique, used for colorectal cancer, is the simple test for **occult blood** (hidden blood) in the stool. This can be obtained through a fecal occult blood test (FOBT) or a newer test called the fecal immunochemical test (FIT). The person simply collects one or more stool specimens (depending on the particular test being used), applies a thin smear on the container provided, and returns the specimens to the health center, clinic, or clinical laboratory. **Occult blood in the stool is not always an indication of cancer of the bowel or rectum.** Other conditions also can produce this symptom.

Table 8-2 Major Risk Factors for Cancer

TYPE OF CANCER	RISK FACTORS	SIGNS
Lung	• Heavy smoker over age 50 • Smoked a pack a day for 20 years • Started smoking at age 15 or before • Exposure to environmental smoke • Exposure to asbestos, arsenic, certain chemicals in the workplace • Radiation or radon exposure • History of tuberculosis	Persistent cough, blood in the sputum, chest pain, recurring pneumonia or bronchitis
Breast	• History of breast cancer • History of some forms of breast biopsy • Close relatives with history of breast cancer • Early menarche; late menopause • Never had children; first child after age 30 • Lengthy exposure to cyclic estrogen • Higher educational and socioeconomic status • Consumption of alcohol	Lump in breast, nipple discharge, thickening, dimpling, nipple retraction, pain or tenderness of the nipple
Colon-rectum	• History of rectal polyps • Rectal polyps run in family • History of inflammatory bowel disease	Blood in stool; alteration in bowel pattern (e.g., constipation alternating with diarrhea)
Uterine-cervical	• Frequent sex in early teens or with many partners • History of HPV • Low socioeconomic status • Poor care during or following pregnancy • Smoking or history of smoking • Exposure to in-utero DES	Unusual bleeding or discharge
Uterine-endometrial	• Estrogen therapy • Tamoxifen therapy • Late menopause (after age 55) • History of infertility or failure to ovulate • Diabetes, high blood pressure, gallbladder disease, and obesity • Pelvic irradiation	Unusual bleeding or discharge
Skin	• Excessive exposure to sun or tanning booth • Fair complexion • Work with coal tar, pitch, or creosote	Change in the size, color, or appearance of a mole or spot on the skin; scaliness, oozing, bleeding or change in appearance of a bump or nodule; spread of pigmentation beyond the border; change in sensation of any skin lesion
Oral	• Heavy smoker and drinker • Use of smokeless tobacco • Poor oral hygiene • HPV	White patch in the mouth or on the tongue; nodules
Ovary	• History of ovarian cancer among close relatives • History of breast cancer • History of never having children	None until well advanced
Prostate	• Over age 65 • Black ancestry • History of family incidence of prostate cancer	Difficulty urinating; hesitancy, blood in the urine; need to urinate frequently; pain in lower back, pelvis, or upper thighs
Stomach	• History of stomach cancer among close relatives • Diet heavy in smoked, pickled, or salted foods • Some link with blood group A	Nonspecific; indigestion, feeling of fullness or pressure; pain and weight loss are late signs
Pancreas	• Smoking or other recreational drugs	No signs
Bladder	• Smoking	Painless blood in the urine; need for frequent urination
Leukemia	• Down syndrome • Exposure to excessive radiation • Exposure to benzene (unleaded gas) • HTLV-1 infection • Philadelphia chromosome	Frequent infections, easy bruising, fatigue, weight loss, nosebleeds, paleness

DES, diethylstilbestrol; *HPV,* human papillomavirus; *HTLV-1,* human T-cell lymphotropic virus type 1.

Box 8-1 **Routine Measures Recommended by the American Cancer Society for the Early Detection of Cancer**

BREAST
- Self-awareness of the condition of the women's own breasts, or monthly self-examination of breasts for lumps, nodules, or changes in contour; check by physician every 3 years until age 40, then every year.
- Appropriate screening age and intervals for mammograms is controversial. Beginning at age 40, a yearly mammogram is recommended by the American Cancer Society (ACS) and other major cancer institutions. The U.S. Preventive Services Task Force (USPSTF) recommends mammogram screening every 1-2 years beginning at age 50 (ACS, 2009).

COLON-RECTUM
At age 50, begin screening with one of the following:
- Yearly fecal occult blood test (FOBT) or fecal immunochemical test (FIT).*
- Flexible sigmoidoscopy every 5 years.*
- Both FOBT/FIT and flexible sigmoidoscopy (better than either alone)
- Double-contrast barium enema every 5 years.
- Colonoscopy every 10 years.

CERVIX AND UTERUS
- Pelvic examination every year.
- Yearly Pap test (or every 2 years if liquid based) beginning by age 21.
- Beginning at age 30, after three consecutive normal Pap tests or after a normal Pap test and a negative HPV test, the test may be performed every 2 to 3 years at the discretion of the physician. Women at high risk for cervical cancer should continue with annual Pap tests.
- Beginning at age 70, low-risk women with three normal Pap tests in a row, no abnormal Pap test in the last 10 years, and a negative HPV test may discontinue screening.
- Endometrial screening is not recommended. However, those at high risk for endometrial cancer should have an endometrial tissue biopsy taken yearly beginning at age 35 at the discretion of their primary care clinician.

TESTICLES AND PROSTATE
- At age 14, begin performing testicular self-examination (TSE) once a month.
- Beginning at age 40, baseline digital rectal examination (DRE); prostate-specific antigen (PSA) test should be

performed at age 50 on all men who have at least a 10-year life expectancy. If the PSA is <1 ng/mL, screening should continue at 5-year intervals. If the PSA is >1 ng/mL, or the patient is African American or has increased risk from family history, continue with annual screening. For a complete algorithm of appropriate prostate screening, consult the National Comprehensive Cancer Network (NCCN) Practice Guidelines (NCCN, 2009).

SKIN
- Self-examination of skin by all adults once a month to detect new lesions and monitor appearance of moles.
- Consultation with a dermatologist if pale, wax-like, pearly nodules, or red, scaly, sharply outlined patches are found.
- Melanoma may manifest as a mole that is asymmetrical one half to the other, or may have an irregular border, pigmentation that is not uniform throughout the mole, or a diameter greater than 6 mm. A dermatologist should be consulted if any of these changes are found.

ORAL
- Regular dental examinations.
- Consult physician or dentist if a white patch remains in mouth for more than a week, or a nodule is felt on the gums, tongue, or mucous membranes.
- Inspect the sides and bottom of the tongue every few months.

HIGH-RISK EXCEPTIONS
Each person is encouraged to confer with a physician and determine whether these recommendations are adequate in light of his or her personal history and risk factors. More frequent and thorough examinations are recommended for:
- Women with personal family histories of breast cancer.
- Women who began having sexual intercourse at an early age or those with many partners.
- Women who have a history of obesity, infertility, failure of ovulation, abnormal uterine bleeding, or estrogen therapy.
- Men at high risk for prostate cancer should begin testing at age 40.
- Men and women who have a personal family history of cancer of the rectum, familial polyposis, Gardner's syndrome, ulcerative colitis, or a history of polyps, and those with a family incidence of melanoma.

*These tests should be combined.

Research continues on identifying proteins produced by mutated DNA that might be used to diagnose various types of cancer. These tests may soon be available for those at high risk for bladder, cervical, lung, breast, colon, and prostate cancer. If these tests prove reliable, they may well be incorporated into a normal part of routine medical care.

Other procedures used to identify lesions that are possibly malignant include radiologic studies, endoscopy, sonography, magnetic resonance imaging, computed tomography, clinical laboratory testing of enzymes and other substances in the blood, and studies specific to the system in which the cancer is

suspected. Tests for viruses are now being done to identify increased risk for some cancers. For example, a test for the presence of high-risk types of HPV is available to identify women at risk for cervical cancer.

DIAGNOSTIC TESTS

Biopsy

Biopsy of a tumor and examination of the cells obtained are the most certain techniques for establishing a diagnosis of malignancy in most neoplasms. Malignancies involving blood cells, such as in leukemia, are diagnosed by examining these cells. A biopsy is the removal of living cells for the purpose of examining them under a microscope. The cells may be removed by surgical *excision* (cutting out) of a small part of a tumor, by the *aspiration* (suction) of cells through a needle introduced into the growth, or by brush biopsy. If the tumor is small, the entire growth may be removed. The specimen obtained is examined under the microscope by a pathologist.

If the sample is taken in the operating room and the surgeon is waiting for the results to determine the extent of surgery needed to remove all the malignant cells, the tissues may be frozen for quick examination. This technique is called *preparing a frozen section.*

New procedures, such as fine-needle aspiration (FNA) and *percutaneous* (through the skin) large-core breast biopsy, are used for diagnosing breast cancer without the disfigurement of traditional surgical breast biopsy. Breast biopsy is combined with imaging techniques such as ultrasound to verify correct placement of the biopsy needle. Then FNA is combined with computer analysis of the samples obtained.

Radiologic Studies

Mammography is a radiologic examination of the breast that is useful in diagnosing malignant growths, and x-ray films are particularly helpful in diagnosing bone and hollow organ tumors. Mortality rates can be cut by 31% when routine mammography screening is performed (Tabar et al., 2003). The respiratory, digestive, and urinary tracts can be visualized on a radiograph if a *radiopaque* (not penetrated by the x rays) substance is used. The substance passes through the hollow organ and, since it is radiopaque, the inner structure of the organ is clearly demonstrated on the radiograph.

Another radiologic technique involves the use of a radioactive substance (*radionuclide* or *isotope)* that is given to the patient before the x-ray filming. The isotope is a "tumor-seeking" chemical that searches for the tumor and may or may not concentrate around it. A special scanning apparatus moves back and forth over the subject's body; as the scanner moves, it records information about the concentration of the isotope in the area being examined. If the substance is concentrated in the tumor, the growth shows up as a "hot spot" on the screen of the scanning apparatus. If the tumor does not accept the isotope, the normal tissue around the tumor concentrates the isotope, and the tumor shows up as a "cold spot." This technique is commonly used in the investigation of thyroid tumors.

A commonly used radiologic scanning technique is *computed tomography (CT) scanning.* This method is noninvasive and involves relatively small amounts of radiation exposure for the subject. The term *noninvasive* means that no surgical procedures are needed to reveal the size, shape, contour, and density of an organ. The procedure requires minimal preparation.

In CT scanning, the x-ray source moves past the subject in one direction while the film moves in another. In this way, three-dimensional cross sections, or "slices," of tissue can be obtained. The scanner rotates an entire 180 degree (half circle) around the area being examined, filming as it rotates 1 degree at a time. Information received by the scanner is relayed to a computer, which presents an image of the tissues one slice at a time. The "picture" presented by the computer is an interpretation of the varying densities of tissues, fluids, and bones. Tumors, as well as other abnormal structures within the body tissues, can be seen in this way.

Another imaging technique is called *magnetic resonance imaging* (MRI). As in CT scanning, MRI produces views of "slices" of tissue. MRI can sometimes "see" tumors and abnormalities that other techniques miss. It is currently used as a breast screening tool—in addition to mammography—for patients at high risk for breast cancer because of family history. MRI can also be used in real time to monitor cancer treatments. Patients with pacemakers, certain metal fragments, clips, or shrapnel in the body cannot use MRI because the powerful magnets used in this technique can bend and twist metal and can damage the body.

Endoscopy

An endoscope is an instrument used for direct visualization of internal body parts. It is designed so that it can be inserted and passed along the interior of hollow organs and cavities.

Types of endoscopes include the colonoscope for the colon, the bronchoscope for the trachea and bronchi, the laparoscope for the contents of the abdominal or pelvic cavity, and the cystoscope for inside the bladder. During an endoscopy, a sample of cells may be taken from a suspicious area so they can be examined more precisely under a microscope (biopsy).

LABORATORY TESTS

Although no one blood test can establish a definite diagnosis of cancer, certain tests are used to ascertain specific information. A complete blood count is helpful in diagnosing leukemia. The presence of a high level of prostate-specific antigen (PSA) may indicate prostate cancer. Current recommendations include offering a baseline PSA test for men over age 50, to be repeated at various intervals depending on the patient's risk factors (Box 8-2).

Specialized tests for tumor markers have been developed. These tests detect biochemical substances synthesized and released into the bloodstream by tumor cells. However, these are not 100% accurate for diagnosing tumors because many of these substances also are produced by normal or embryonic cells and are also found in benign conditions. **Therefore tumor markers are mainly used to confirm a diagnosis, the response to therapy, or to detect a relapse.** CA-125 is

Box 8-2	Prostate-Specific Antigen (PSA) Test

- No sexual activity for 24 to 48 hours before the test
- Avoid test until after urinary tract infection is cleared
- Do not perform test after recent urinary tract surgery
- Collect blood sample before digital examination
- Prostatic acid phosphatase (PAP) is collected to confirm an elevated PSA
- Phosphatase gives information about extent of disease
- Alkaline phosphatase often elevated with bone cancer and liver metastasis

Box 8-3	Common Nursing Diagnoses Used for Patients with Cancer

- *Imbalanced nutrition (less than body requirements)* related to increased metabolic demand and nausea, vomiting, diarrhea, or mucositis
- *Risk for infection* related to bone marrow depression from therapy
- *Pain, acute or chronic,* related to effects of tumor on body structures or cancer therapy
- *Impaired skin integrity* related to surgical or radiation therapy
- *Disturbed body image* related to weight loss or hair loss
- *Risk for injury* to patient, staff, and visitors related to exposure to a radioactive implant
- *Impaired physical mobility* related to restricted activity secondary to a radioactive implant
- *Diarrhea* related to effects of cancer treatment
- *Constipation* related to effects of chemotherapy
- *Impaired urinary elimination* related to radiation therapy or secondary to effects of chemotherapy
- *Activity intolerance* related to fatigue
- *Deficient knowledge* related to drugs and side effects
- *Self-care deficit* (bathing/hygiene, dressing/grooming, feeding, toileting) related to weakness and fatigue
- *Fear* related to the possibility of dying
- *Ineffective individual coping* related to denial of significance of cancer
- *Compromised family coping* related to inability to function as a result of anxiety over patient's prognosis

used to detect the presence of ovarian cancer or its recurrence after therapy. Carcinoembryonic antigen (CEA) and CA 19-9 are tests used to detect the recurrence of gastrointestinal, pancreatic, and liver cancer after initial treatment, and CA 27-29 is used most frequently to follow the progress in breast cancer treatment and later to check for recurrence.

❖ NURSING MANAGEMENT

■ Assessment (Data Collection)

The first step is to find out whether the patient has been informed of the diagnosis and what is known about the illness and treatment. Some patients may suspect they have cancer but do not want to discuss it. Even those who have been informed may choose not to talk about it or ask any questions about their treatment. The fact that a patient cannot discuss her illness or seek help in dealing with the problems it presents may indicate how frightened she is and how much she needs help and understanding. The nurse must assess how the disease is affecting the patient's body and life, in order to plan comprehensive care.

A thorough assessment of the system where the cancer is located and a good general physical assessment provide a baseline on which changes in physical function caused by the cancer can be evaluated. A psychosocial assessment of the patient and family or significant others provides data that indicate psychosocial needs, and resources for support and care.

Finally, the nurse should determine how to assist the patient to make the most of the personal resources and abilities that the patient currently possesses. This could mean helping with adjustment to the emotional impact of only recently learning the diagnosis of cancer, or it could require helping the patient to deal with the pain and discomfort of advanced malignancy and to prepare for a peaceful death.

■ Nursing Diagnosis

Patients with cancer, depending on the stage of the disease, can have a great number of problems; a large number of nursing diagnoses may be appropriate. Specific diagnoses are chosen for the body systems and functions in which the disease or tumor is causing

disruption of homeostasis. Common general nursing diagnoses associated with a diagnosis of cancer can be found in Box 8-3.

■ Planning

Specific expected outcomes are written for each nursing diagnosis chosen, as appropriate for the patient (Nursing Care Plan 8-1). Planning is a collaborative process that includes the patient, the family, the physician, the oncologist, the nurse manager, the social worker, and other specialists on the health care team. The home care nurse, the infusion therapy company nurse, and the pharmacist often are involved in care, and should be included in the planning process. The nurse manager usually is the one who consults with the others of the team and coordinates the plan of care.

■ Implementation

See Nursing Care Plan 8-1 and the following sections for specific interventions.

■ Evaluation

Evaluation is based on determining whether the expected outcomes specified for the patient are being met or have been met. Constant assessment for signs of complications, side effects of therapy, nutritional

⭐ Nursing Care Plan 8-1   Care of the Patient with Cancer

Scenario
Mr. Pole is receiving chemotherapy for leukemia. This is his third round of weekly intravenous treatments. His platelet count is down to 185,000; he has had difficulty eating as a result of mucositis and anorexia. He states that he is mildly nauseated most of the time. He is 15 lb underweight.

Problem/Nursing Diagnosis
Undergoing chemotherapy/Risk for infection related to bone marrow suppression.

Supporting Assessment Data
Objective: Receiving chemotherapy drugs that suppress bone marrow.

Goals/Expected Outcomes	Nursing Interventions	Selected Rationale	Evaluation
Patient will remain free of infection.	Monitor WBCs (more susceptible to infection when <3000 and granulocyte count is <2000).	Neutropenia is a sign of immunosuppression.	WBCs 3200.
	Assess for signs of infection every shift.	Elevated temperature may indicate infection.	Temp. 98.8° F (37.1° C); no signs of infection.
	Teach good hygiene, mouth care, hand hygiene before meals and after using bathroom.	Hand hygiene prevents spread of infection.	Patient washing hands appropriately and using good hygiene.
	Use protective isolation techniques if needed.	If neutrophil count <500, initiate protective isolation.	Isolation not yet initiated.
	Encourage good nutrition and hydration.	Good nutrition and hydration minimizes irritation.	Taking sufficient food and fluid; continue plan.
	Give Neupogen as ordered.	Neupogen raises the WBC and neutrophil count.	Neupogen 300 mcg subcutaneously given 1 time/day.

Problem/Nursing Diagnosis
Receiving chemotherapy/Risk for injury related to impaired blood clotting ability.

Supporting Assessment Data
Objective: Receiving chemotherapy (chemotherapy treatment lowers platelets and extends bleeding time).

Goals/Expected Outcomes	Nursing Interventions	Selected Rationale	Evaluation
Patient will remain free from hemorrhage.	Monitor blood count; assess for bleeding of gums or bruising and bleeding into joints q shift.	Blood count plays an important role in blood clotting and bleeding.	WBCs 3200; platelet count 180,000.
	Observe for signs of bleeding: hematuria, melena, etc.		No signs of bleeding.
	Refrain from needle sticks as much as possible.		
	Give stool softener as ordered to prevent straining at stool and bleeding.	Hard stools can initiate bleeding in the rectum.	Stool soft; continue plan. Stool softener administered.
	Avoid rectal bleeding. Do not take temperature rectally.		Oral temp: 98.8° F (37.1° C).
	Brush teeth with very soft brush or tooth sponge. Do not floss.	Avoid bleeding gums.	Appropriate dental hygiene.

Problem/Nursing Diagnosis

Nauseated with no appetite/Alteration of nutrition (less than body requirements), related to nausea, vomiting, and mucositis.

Supporting Assessment Data

Subjective: "I feel nauseated."
Objective: Chemotherapy administration.

Goals/Expected Outcomes	**Nursing Interventions**	**Selected Rationale**	**Evaluation**
Patient will verbalize relief from nausea. Patient will be able to eat with minimal discomfort.	Keep room odor free; give mouth care before meals. Give ordered antiemetic before and during chemotherapy.	Odors may aggravate nausea. Antiemetics help prevent chemotherapy-induced nausea and vomiting (N&V).	Antiemetic 45 min before meals.
Patient will maintain present weight.	Assess mouth and mucous membranes q shift. Give meticulous mouth care q 2 hr. Use distraction, meditation, relaxation techniques. Give small, frequent feedings. Encourage added calories in meals and food supplements between meals.	Sore mouth may reduce food intake. N&V may be reduced with behavioral interventions. Experts recommend these dietary interventions.	Mucous membranes reddened, but intact. Mouth care: 7, 9, 11, 1, and 3 o'clock. Has not vomited this shift. Enriched shake taken between meals.

Problem/Nursing Diagnosis

Balding from chemotherapy/Body image disturbance related to alopecia and weight loss.

Supporting Assessment Data

Subjective: "I look awful; I don't want any visitors to see me."
Objective: Loss of considerable amount of hair from head.

Goals/Expected Outcomes	**Nursing Interventions**	**Selected Rationale**	**Evaluation**
Patient will adjust to new body image within 3 wk as evidenced by verbalization.	Encourage him to maintain sense of humor. Use caps, head bandana, and eyebrow pencil as needed. Assure him that hair will eventually grow back. Encourage verbalization of feelings; focus on strengths. Establish and maintain trusting relationship. Assess spiritual needs; help patient achieve spiritual consolation. Encourage him to obtain clothing that fits.	Humor is a positive coping strategy. Hair covering may reduce negative body image. Verbalization is a positive coping technique.	Has not yet lost hair; checking on purchase of wig; family is bringing head scarves. Talking more about feelings regarding weight loss and appearance. Continue plan.

Continued

⭐ **Nursing Care Plan 8-1**   **Care of the Patient with Cancer—cont'd**

Problem/Nursing Diagnosis
Expressing fear of dying/Fear related to diagnosis of cancer.

Supporting Assessment Data
Subjective: "Do you really think the treatment will cure my cancer? I'm afraid that I'll go through all this and it will just come back in a few months."

Goals/Expected Outcomes	Nursing Interventions	Selected Rationale	Evaluation
Patient will verbalize fears and develop coping mechanisms to decrease fear.	Encourage verbalization and identification of specific fears.	Verbalizing fears makes them easier to face.	Is verbalizing fears; encouraged to do same with family.
	Help him to explore ways to cope with fears.	Knowing what to expect helps people plan.	Used to meditate; encouraged to do so.
	Assess spiritual needs; contact minister or other as patient desires.	Patients have their own beliefs about death.	Began teaching imagery techniques.
	Offer support by active listening, offering hope in some form, and be there for patient.	Active listening provides comfort and strength.	Continue plan.
	Encourage expression of fears to significant others.	When significant others are aware of the patient's fears, they have a better understanding of behavior.	

Critical Thinking Questions
1. What is another nursing diagnosis that may apply to a patient who is receiving chemotherapy?
2. Why should the nurse be concerned about infection in a patient who is receiving chemotherapy?

---

status, and pain status is necessary. The nursing care plan must be changed when the interventions initially chosen are not effective in meeting the desired outcomes. Collaboration with the patient and the other members of the health care team is important to the success of care plan changes.

COMMON THERAPIES, PROBLEMS, AND NURSING CARE

There are three traditional modes of therapy for malignancies: surgery, radiation, and chemotherapy. Hormone manipulation, immunotherapy with biologic response modifiers, and bone marrow or stem cell transplantation are treatments combined with traditional therapies.

Each of the modes of treatment may be used singly or in combination with one or more of the other methods available. For example, chemotherapy may be used as an adjuvant (assisting treatment) after surgical removal of a tumor. The methods of treatment are chosen after consideration of many factors and are prescribed with the best interests of the patient in mind.

SURGERY

Surgery may be performed:
- To obtain a biopsy specimen.
- As prophylaxis (preventive treatment), such as in the removal of the ovaries of a woman whose mother had ovarian cancer.
- To determine the effectiveness of therapy by looking to see whether the initial tumor is reduced in size.
- For palliation (offering relief), as in *debulking* (removing as much as possible) a tumor to prevent pressure on adjacent structures or obstruction of vessels or the gastrointestinal tract.
- As an attempt at cure.

Reconstructive surgery also is associated with cancer treatment. The woman who has lost a breast to mastectomy may have the breast reconstructed. Other extremely mutilating forms of cancer surgery require reconstructive procedures after the initial procedure. Flap grafts in a patient who underwent radical neck surgery for cancer of the throat are an example.

Surgical removal of a malignant growth is the oldest method of treatment. It works very well for tumors that are easily accessible. Adjacent tissues that may contain malignant cells also are excised. Regional lymph nodes often harbor malignant cells, and these can then travel to distant parts of the body and establish a new cancer site, if not removed. Newer surgical procedures and techniques have significantly reduced the need for extensive surgical removal of adjacent tissues and structures. Radical mastectomy, for example, involves removal of the entire breast along with underlying pectoral muscle tissues and lymph nodes under the arm on the affected side. This procedure has been replaced almost completely by a modified radical mastectomy, or lumpectomy and sentinel node biopsy, combined with radiation and/or chemotherapy, which is far less traumatic and mutilating. If there is no evidence of metastasis, some patients are good candidates for simple removal of the tumor *(lumpectomy)*. The use of radiation and/or chemotherapy during, after, and sometimes before surgery has decreased the need for extensive removal of adjacent tissues and is associated with decreased recurrence.

RADIATION THERAPY

The source for radiation therapy is either a linear accelerator or a radioactive element or substance. The purpose of radiation is to destroy malignant cells (which are more sensitive to radiation than are normal cells) without permanent damage to adjacent body tissues.

Ionizing radiation can have both an immediate and a delayed effect on malignant cells. Ionizing radiation can damage the cell membrane immediately, causing *lysis* (bursting) or decomposition of the cell, or it can cause a break in both strands of the DNA in the cell's nucleus. **When a cell is damaged in this way, it will not die until it attempts to divide and replicate itself. The rate at which a particular kind of cell undergoes mitosis determines whether the effects of radiation will occur in a matter of days, months, or years.** This explains the delayed effects and side effects of radiation that might not be evident at the time of treatment but appear later. Normal cells have a greater ability to repair the DNA damage than do malignant cells. Some tissues are more sensitive to radiation than others, and this is taken into account when the physicist-physician calculates the dose of radiation needed to eradicate the tumor. The other factors considered are the sensitivity of the tumor to radiation, its location, and its size. Once calculated, the dose is *fractionalized,* meaning it is divided over many days, to deliver the optimum dosage with the least amount of effects to normal tissues. The course of radiation is spread over a period of days to weeks. The *rad,* or *radiation absorbed dose,* is the unit used for measuring dosages of radiation.

Teletherapy and brachytherapy are the two types of radiation delivery used to treat cancer. Teletherapy is *external*— the source of radiation is outside the patient.

Brachytherapy is *internal*—the source of radiation is a radioactive element or substance that has been implanted or injected into the body, to provide low doses in focused areas.

Because of improvements in tumor localization, beam direction, megavoltage machines, planning and prescribing the field to be irradiated, and determining the precise dosage needed, radiation therapy is far more beneficial and less harmful than it was when it was first pioneered. With the *linear accelerator* and its partner, the *cyclotron,* the damage to normal tissue can be minimized by keeping the dosage or degree of penetration accurate and by aiming the rays from several different angles. The latter technique increases the concentration of the rays in the area of the tumor with a minimum of damage to overlying tissues. Cobalt-60 machines deliver gamma rays and these machines are today much more efficient and precise than they were in the early years of radiation therapy.

External Radiation Therapy

The linear accelerator used for external radiation therapy produces extremely high-energy x-ray and electron beam irradiation that bombards the malignant cells and destroys them. Because malignant cells divide at an abnormally high rate, they are more susceptible to destruction than normal cells.

Modern radiation therapy has decreased the side effects of radiation therapy considerably. Since DNA is the critical target for radiation damage, the increased knowledge about DNA gained from the Human Genome Project has also helped streamline radiation therapy. The use of *stereotactic* (exact positioning in space) surgery is effective for small brain tumors (Figure 8-4). Many cancer research institutions have lead-lined surgical suites where intraoperative radiation therapy may be delivered directly to the affected area after tumor removal and before the incision is

FIGURE 8-4 Cyberknife used to deliver radiation to a small brain tumor. It is particularly useful for recurrence of tumor.

closed. Depending on the dosage (rads) given, the patient may not need to receive further radiation. This method has proven beneficial for cancers of the head and neck, abdomen, pelvis, and extremities and for patients with operable pancreatic cancer.

Nursing Care of Patients Undergoing External Beam Radiation Therapy.
Nursing care goals related to cancer radiation therapy include (1) helping the patient and family cope with the diagnosis of cancer and treatment with radiation therapy; and (2) teaching the patient and family how to recognize and manage the expected side effects of radiation.

Helping patients cope with radiation therapy. A lack of knowledge about the side effects of radiation and of how to cope with them can greatly add to the anxiety and stress that the patient feels. It is not unusual for a layperson to have some misconceptions about how radiation works, whether a patient can present a hazard to others while undergoing treatment, when the patient will begin to experience its effects, and how long it will be before the patient begins to recover from them.

Before the first treatment, the patient is told what therapeutic effects are anticipated, what it is like to have a treatment, and what is expected of her during the course of therapy. Because the patient will probably be treated on an outpatient basis, she should be encouraged to keep her scheduled appointments and notify the clinic if cancellation is necessary. Assurance that the source of radiation is in the machine only and that it is not possible to "contaminate" others with radioactivity should be provided. Someone should accompany the patient for initial treatments—preferably a family member or a close and trusted friend—who can provide emotional support. It is essential that time be set aside for the nurse to establish a trusting relationship with the patient, to prompt and answer any questions about therapy, and to provide an avenue for communication throughout the course of treatment.

Patient Teaching

Skin Care During Radiation Treatment

- Shower or wash the area once a day using warm water and mild soap; use the hand to wash the affected area rather than a washcloth. Dry with a soft, clean towel; pat, don't rub.
- Limit cold and sun exposure and when outdoors use a sunscreen with a sun protection factor (SPF) of at least 15.
- Do not use lotion, salve, or alcohol on the affected area unless prescribed by the radiologist.
- Do not remove any of the markings for radiation treatment.
- Wear loose, 100% cotton clothing over the irradiated area.
- Do not shave the area, or use an electric razor without the radiologist's permission.

Skin care during radiation therapy. With the advanced methods and computerized delivery of radiation, there is much less trauma to the skin from radiation

therapy than in previous years. The patient must understand that should skin damage occur, it is usually only temporary. In preparation for radiation therapy, the physician will outline the area to be exposed to radiation by marking it with indelible ink. The exposed area will need special care. Most clinics and hospitals have written procedures and precautions to be used to avoid unnecessary trauma to the exposed areas of skin.

Although skin damage is rare now, the degree of reaction of the skin to radiation is individual and should be assessed daily, either by the patient or by some knowledgeable person.

Think Critically

Can you list the points to be covered for care of the skin when teaching the patient who is to undergo external radiation therapy?

Teaching the patient and family how to recognize and help manage expected side effects is particularly important when the patient is not hospitalized. She will feel more in control if she is able to participate in assessing her condition and planning and implementing her care at home. It is unfair to expect either the patient or her family to remember everything they are told about her care. Therefore it is essential that they have some written information to refer to once they leave the clinic. They also should be encouraged to write down any questions they might have before the next visit, and to note any points on which they feel they need more information.

Internal Radiation Therapy

Radiation from *radioactive elements* has the same ionizing effect as that from linear accelerators; differing only in the source of radiation. Internal radiation therapy involves introducing a radioactive element into the body and may be administered in different ways: (1) it can be placed in a *sealed* container and inserted into a body cavity at the tumor site or placed directly into the tumor; or (2) it may be administered in an *unsealed* form and taken orally or injected by syringe.

To be effective, the radiation source must come into direct contact with the tumor tissue for a specified time. Most implants emit a lower level of radiation while in constant contact with the tumor cells. **Because the radiation source is within the patient, radiation is emitted for a period and can be a hazard to others. Nurses caring for patients receiving internal radiation must take extra precautions** (Box 8-4).

As soon as an element becomes radioactive, it begins to lose its characteristic of radioactivity. The rate at which it becomes less radioactive is called its *half-life*, which is the amount of time it takes for half of its

Box 8-4	**Precautionary Measures When a Patient Is Receiving Internal Radiation Therapy from a Sealed Source**

- Place the patient in a private room.
- Place a sign on the patient's door indicating that the patient is receiving internal radiation therapy.
- Observe principles of time and distance. Limit time spent in the room. Work as quickly and as efficiently as possible. Avoid standing near the part of the patient's body where the radioactive element is located; stand at the shoulders or the feet depending where the implant is located.
- Check all linens, bedpans, and emesis basins routinely to see if the sealed source has been accidentally lost from the tissue.
- If a sealed source is dislodged, but has not fallen out of the patient's body, notify the x-ray department at once. If the source has fallen out, *do not pick it up with your bare hands.* Use forceps and place it in a lead container.
- Most patients are placed on bed rest and instructed to remain in certain positions so that emanations from the element will reach the correct area.
- Visitors should spend limited time in the room.
- No children or pregnant women should visit.

Box 8-5	**Precautions When Caring for the Patient Receiving Internal Radiation from an Unsealed Source**

- Observe the principles of time, distance, and shielding for radiation protection.
- Wear gloves when handling bedpans, bed linens, and patient's clothes.
- Dispose of urine, feces, and vomitus according to policy.
- Handle dressings with forceps and dispose of them according to policy.
- Follow hospital procedure for disposal of patient's bed linens and clothing.

radioactivity to dissipate. The half-life of radium is about 1600 years, whereas the half-life of iodine is only about 8 days. **It is important that the nurse caring for a patient receiving sealed or unsealed sources of radiation know the element used, its half-life, and the ways in which it might be eliminated from the body.** Cesium is a radioactive element frequently used to treat malignancies of the mouth, tongue, vagina, and uterine cervix.

Some isotopes are given orally and others are administered into a body cavity. The isotopes are unsealed sources of radiation. If radioactivity is a hazard, it is a problem only for the duration of the half-life of the isotope. The substance is eliminated through body secretions such as sweat, sputum, vomit, urine, or feces. Examples of unsealed sources include iodine-131, which is in a solution and is swallowed by the patient; and phosphorus-32 and gold-198, which are administered by injection. Radioactive iodine is useful in the treatment of thyroid malignancies because that gland readily takes up iodine. Thus the radioactive element is delivered to the site of the tumor, where it can be more effective. The major hazard from radioactive iodine is in the patient's urine, but iodine is also excreted in the feces and sweat; therefore special precautions must be taken according to hospital policy (Box 8-5).

Principles of Radiation Protection

In general, the amount of radiation a nurse might receive while caring for a patient being treated with internal radioactive elements depends on three factors: (1) the distance between the nurse and the patient;

(2) the amount of time spent in actual proximity to the patient; and (3) the degree of shielding provided.

Distance is an important factor in reducing exposure to radiation. Doubling one's distance from a radioactive element reduces the exposure to one fourth, and tripling the distance reduces it to one ninth (Figure 8-5). Time spent near the source of radiation can be controlled by the nurse who plans his nursing care carefully, so that he can spend less time with the patient without sacrificing the quality of care given. The total time spent with a radioactive patient should be less than 30 minutes per 8-hour shift.

Shielding from radiation exposure must take into account the type of rays being emitted. The denser the shielding material, the less the possibility of penetration by the rays, and the better the protection. A lead shield that is 1-cm thick offers the same amount of protection as 5 cm of concrete or 30 cm of wood. Lead aprons give protection from diagnostic x rays, but do not provide adequate shielding from the *gamma rays* emitted by radium, cesium-137, and cobalt-60. Anyone in proximity to—or in contact with—a source of radiation should wear a radiation dosimeter badge (Figure 8-6). This badge measures the radiation dose that the individual has received through exposure to the source.

Hospitals where sealed sources of radiation are implanted into the body tissues to treat malignancies usually have written policies and procedures to guide personnel who are responsible for patient care. After the physician removes the source, the patient is no longer in need of special precautionary care. Special observations are necessary, however, in the event a systemic reaction develops. Table 8-3 lists the most common side effects of radiation therapy. For appropriate nursing care of problems related to radiation therapy, see the section on common problems related to cancer or cancer therapy.

CHEMOTHERAPY

The oncologist has a wide variety of drugs from which to choose when planning a course of treatment for a patient with cancer. He may choose to give a particular drug alone, or in combination with other drugs.

FIGURE 8-5 Time, distance, and shielding in radiation exposure. The nurse nearest the source of radioactivity (the patient) is more exposed; at 2 feet, exposure is more than of 15 times that of exposure at 8 feet. *mGy*, milligray.

FIGURE 8-6 Radiation dosimeter badge worn by personnel who might be exposed to radiation.

Chemotherapy may be used with other forms of therapy; for example, therapy may follow surgery and may occur before, during, or after radiation treatments, or with immunotherapy.

Among the drugs used to treat malignancies are the *antineoplastic* agents (Table 8-4). **The overall effect of antineoplastic drugs is to decrease the number of malignant cells in a generalized malignancy (such as leukemia) or to reduce the size of a localized tumor and thereby lessen the severity of symptoms.** Antineoplastic drugs are cytotoxic (poisonous to cells), and their damaging effects are not limited to malignant cells. However, normal cells do not reproduce in exactly the same way as malignant cells, and so normal cells are able to repair themselves more rapidly and effectively. Steroids often are used in combination with antineoplastic drugs for cancer treatment.

Drug combinations are used to treat certain types of cancers because different drugs are effective at different times in the growth and replication cycle of the tumor cell. This method offers the best chance of killing the most malignant cells. Chemotherapy is the preferred treatment for various kinds of leukemias,

Table 8-3	Common Side Effects of Radiation Therapy
TYPE AND AREA	**EFFECT**
External Radiation	
Head and neck	• Irritation of oral mucous membranes with oral pain and risk of infection • Loss of taste • Irritation of the pharynx and esophagus with nausea and indigestion • Increased intracranial pressure
Chest	• Inflammation of lung tissue with increased susceptibility to infection
Abdomen	• Nausea, vomiting, diarrhea, anorexia
Pelvis	• Diarrhea • Cystitis • Sexual dysfunction • Urethral and rectal stenosis
General side effects	• *Skin:* Change in texture and/or color; moist desquamation (rare); alopecia • *Blood:* Bone marrow depression with leukopenia, anemia, and thrombocytopenia • Depressed immune function • Fatigue
Internal Radiation	
General effects	• Elevated temperature • *Cervical implant:* Urinary frequency, diarrhea, nausea, vomiting, anorexia • *Head and neck implant:* Mucositis, oral pain and risk of infection, anorexia

some lymphomas, multiple myeloma, and many types of tumors resulting from metastasis.

Techniques of administration of antineoplastic agents include intra-arterial, intraperitoneal, intraventricular, and *intrathecal* (within a space of the spine), as

Table 8-4   Common Antineoplastic Drug Classes, Actions, and Major Side Effects

CLASSIFICATION AND EXAMPLES	ACTION	MAJOR SIDE EFFECTS*
Alkylating Agents		
Cyclophosphamide, doxorubicin, mechlorethamine, ifosfamide, melphalan, chlorambucil, busulfan, streptozocin, carmustin, lomustine, dacarbazine, temozolomide, thiotepa, altretamine, platinum (cisplatin, carboplatin, oxaliplatin)	Attach "alkyl groups" or organic side chains to the proteins in the cell, poisoning it; inhibit cell division	Bone marrow depression, nephrotoxicity with some Nausea, vomiting, diarrhea, dermatitis; hyperpigmentation Platinum: Hearing loss
Antimetabolites		
Methotrexate, 6-mercaptopurine, 6-thioguanine, 5-fluorouracil, capecitabine, gemcitabine, cytarabine, fludarabine, pemetrexed	Interfere with a specific cell phase, thereby preventing replication Some inhibit enzymes that make essential cellular constituents; others attach to DNA, interfering with replication	Bone marrow depression, stomatitis, intestinal ulceration, nausea, vomiting, diarrhea
Antitumor Antibiotics		
Bleomycin, dactinomycin, doxorubicin, epirubicin, idarubicin, daunorubicin, plicamycin, mitomycin-C, mitoxantrone	Injure cells by direct interaction with DNA, causing distortion Interfere with DNA or RNA synthesis	Bone marrow depression, some cause cardiotoxicity; stomatitis, alopecia Bleomycin causes pneumonitis and pulmonary fibrosis
Mitotic Inhibitors		
Vincristine, vinblastine, vinorelbine, etoposide	Interfere with mitosis Act during M phase of cell cycle to prevent cell division	Vincristine: Peripheral neuropathy, constipation Vinblastine: Bone marrow depression
Miscellaneous Agents		
Altretamine, asparaginase, etoposide, hydroxyurea, procarbazine, mitotane, teniposide, paclitaxel, imatinib mesylate, epirubicin, docetaxel, cladribine, rituximab, interleukin-2, interferon alpha	These drugs work in a variety of ways; consult information for each drug	Bone marrow depression is the major side effect of all except asparaginase and mitotane Asparaginase: Pancreatic dysfunction Mitotane: Central nervous system depression Paclitaxel: Peripheral neuropathy
Hormone-Related Agents		
Anti-estrogens (fulvestrant, tamoxifen, toremifene), aromatase inhibitors (anastrozole, exemestane, letrozole), progestins (egestrol acetate), estrogens, anti-androgens	Lowers circulating hormone levels to prevent hormone-related tumors	Hot flushes; deep venous thrombosis; cancer

*Each drug has specific side effects. Consult information regarding each individual drug before administration.

well as intravenous infusion. Cancers of the liver, ovary, and brain have sometimes shown better remission with intraventricular or intraperitoneal infusion treatment. An advance in chemotherapy has been the use of lower doses of multiple drugs to treat various types of malignancies. Because side effects are lessened when lower doses of a drug are used, several drugs can be used in combination to hit all phases of the cell cycle, destroying more malignant cells.

Often a central line or implanted injection port is used to administer chemotherapy drugs that are to be given over several weeks or months (Figure 8-7). The nurse cares for the central line and its insertion site according to hospital policy, using strict aseptic technique.

Many antineoplastic drugs are vesicants (chemicals causing tissue damage on direct contact) that can cause severe local injury if they escape from the vein into which they are administered. Administration should be only into veins that have good blood flow. If *extravasation* (escape from the vein into the tissue) occurs, the infusion is stopped immediately. The type of treatment required depends on the drug and amount that extravasated. **Should extravasation occur, consult the pharmacist, the policy and procedures manual, and the physician.**

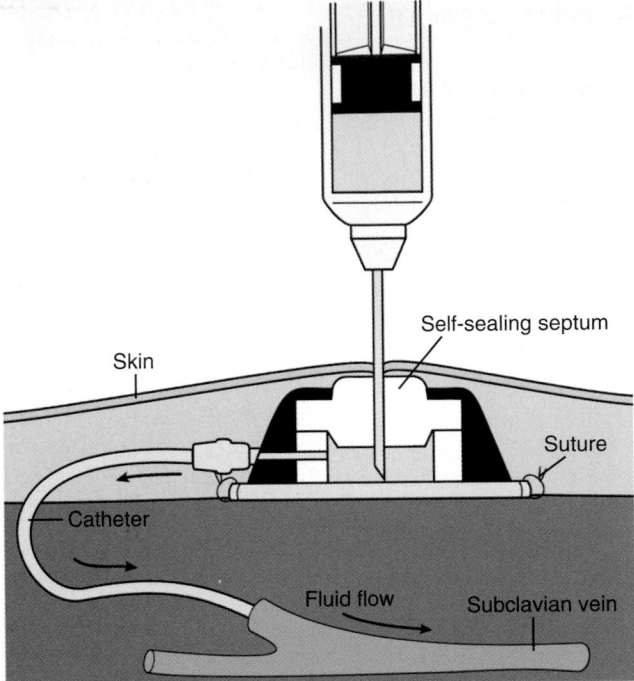

FIGURE 8-7 Implanted infusion port for administration of chemotherapy drugs or continuous morphine drip.

Table 8-5	Assessment for Toxic Effects of Chemotherapy*
SIDE EFFECT	**INTERVENTION**
Bone marrow suppression	Monitor red and white blood cell count and differential count for numbers of neutrophils and granulocytes; check platelet count.
Cardiotoxicity	Monitor for signs of congestive heart failure, such as pulmonary crackles, shortness of breath, tachycardia, weight gain, and peripheral edema. Monitor ECG.
Neurotoxicity	Monitor for weakness, paresthesias, sensory loss (particularly in feet), and decreased reflexes. Constipation and urinary hesitancy are other signs.
Pulmonary toxicity	Evidenced by pulmonary infiltrates and pulmonary fibrosis on x-ray. Monitor respiratory status closely; auscultate for decreased breath sounds and for crackles.
Hepatotoxicity	Monitor liver function tests: AST, ALT, bilirubin.
Nephrotoxicity	Monitor kidney function tests: creatinine and blood urea nitrogen; monitor urine output.
Ototoxicity	Monitor for tinnitus or hearing loss.

ALT, alanine aminotransferase; *AST,* aspartate aminotransferase; *ECG,* electrocardiogram.
*Many antineoplastic drugs are toxic to various organs of the body. Whenever a specific drug has one of these toxicities, include the specific assessment parameters for that toxicity in your regular assessment.

Some antineoplastic drugs have toxic effects that must be monitored. Table 8-5 presents the assessments necessary to detect various types of organ toxicity. One drug, dexrazoxane (Zinecard), appears to be heart-protective for patients receiving the cardiotoxic drug doxorubicin (Adriamycin). If a drug is toxic to the reproductive system, the patient should make a decision about banking sperm or eggs before beginning chemotherapy.

Nursing Care of Patients Receiving Chemotherapy

Nursing management of the patient receiving chemotherapy requires special knowledge and skills beyond those of basic nursing. The oncology nurse is a specialist who is able to give comprehensive nursing care because of years of study and experience. A full discussion of care of the patient receiving chemotherapy is therefore beyond the scope of this text. There are, however, some general principles that can be helpful to the nurse who encounters a patient receiving a course of chemotherapy for cancer, or a patient who is experiencing some of the toxic side effects of antineoplastic drugs.

Not all antineoplastic drugs produce every toxic side effect, and the oncologist plans therapy so that destruction of malignant cells is maximized and toxicity is minimized. **The toxicity associated with chemotherapy is most evident in the cells of the body that have a short life span and therefore must continuously reproduce to provide the body with the normal cells it needs. These types of cells include the blood cells, hair follicles, and epithelial cells of the mucous membranes lining the digestive tract. Most chemotherapeutics are excreted in the body fluids, so precautions should be taken. Remember, most of these drugs are *teratogenic* (can cause birth defects), so they should be avoided during pregnancy.**

Some of the side effects of chemotherapy are similar to the expected effects of radiation (see Table 8-4). Although the causes of the problems are different, assessment of the patient and symptomatic relief measures are the same. See Nursing Care Plan 8-1 for nursing interventions for selected problems in a patient receiving chemotherapy for cancer.

HORMONE THERAPY

Hormone therapy is used as an adjunct to other types of cancer therapy. It can slow tumor growth or prevent cancer recurrence. When a hormone is added to the body, the balance of naturally produced hormones changes. **Giving large amounts of one hormone prevents the uptake of other hormones. So if the tumor growth is aided by one type of hormone, giving**

another type prevents the uptake of the growth-promoting hormone and slows the progress of the tumor. Tamoxifen and aromatase inhibitors such as letrozole (Femara), used against certain types of breast cancer, are examples of hormone therapy. They have been shown to be chemopreventive for women with high risk factors and for recurrence for certain types of breast cancer (National Cancer Institute, 2010).

Side effects of hormone therapy depend on the type of hormone used. Androgens and anti–estrogen receptor drugs produce masculinizing effects, such as facial and chest hair. Menses may stop and breast tissue will shrink. These drugs cause fluid retention in women. Acne is another side effect of the androgens. Hypercalcemia and liver dysfunction can occur with prolonged therapy. In men taking estrogens or progestins to combat prostate cancer, there is a feminizing effect with decreased facial hair, a redistribution of body fat, breast development (*gynecomastia*), smoothing of the facial skin, and the risk of thrombus formation. Over time, some testicular and penile atrophy may occur, and it may become more difficult to attain and maintain an erection.

IMMUNOTHERAPY USING BIOLOGIC RESPONSE MODIFIERS

Biologic response modifiers (BRMs) are agents that manipulate the immune system in the hope of controlling or curing a malignancy with little or no toxic effect on normal cells. These agents either stimulate or suppress immune activity. The BRMs include interferons, interleukins, colony-stimulating factors, monoclonal antibodies, vaccines, gene therapy, and nonspecific immunomodulating agents. They essentially make the immune system function better. BRMs stimulate the immune system to recognize cancer cells and to institute action to destroy them. Some BRMs, such as colony-stimulating factor (CSF), work by enhancing a quicker recovery of the bone marrow after radiation or chemotherapy. CSF stimulates bone marrow to function more quickly. Neumega (interleukin-2) is a drug that stimulates thrombocyte (platelet) production. This drug is used to decrease the bleeding tendencies induced by chemotherapy, and could help create new chemotherapy protocols that are more effective against cancer cells.

Two types of BRMs are used to fight cancer: interleukins and interferons. **Interleukins help the immune system cells recognize and destroy abnormal cells. Interferons slow cell division in cancer cells, stimulate natural killer cells, delay the appearance of oncogenes, and assist cancerous cells to revert to more normal cells.** Both interleukins and interferons are manufactured using *recombinant* (artificial DNA sequence) DNA technology. Interleukin-2 is used for patients with melanoma, renal cell carcinoma, and

lymphoma. Interferons are used effectively against leukemia, melanoma, multiple myeloma, carcinoid tumors, and renal carcinoma. Both interleukins and interferons are very expensive to manufacture.

A second group of BRMs includes monoclonal antibodies (MoAbs) and tumor necrosis factor, both of which have direct antitumor effects. Genetic engineering techniques can produce the monoclonal antibodies, and thus this form of therapy holds much promise for the future. Rituximab (Rituxan) and trastuzumab (Herceptin) are examples of MoAbs that have been approved by the U.S. Food and Drug Administration. Rituxan is used in the treatment of non-Hodgkin's lymphoma, and Herceptin is used for the treatment of metastatic breast cancer in patients who produce an excess amount of a protein called HER-2.

The third group of BRMs contains agents that have varying functions. This group includes cancer vaccines, which may stimulate the immune system to attack the cancer cells (therapeutic) or stimulate the production of antibodies against a cancer-causing virus (prophylactic). Also included are nonspecific immunomodulating agents that may stimulate the immune system and either restore depressed immune function or increase immune inflammatory responses.

BONE MARROW AND STEM CELL TRANSPLANTATION

Bone marrow transplantation (BMT) is mainly used to correct the severe bone marrow damage caused by chemotherapy or radiation. Sometimes whole-body irradiation is used to treat a hematopoietic cancer such as leukemia or Hodgkin's disease. Irradiation of this sort totally incapacitates the body's bone marrow, and the patient would die if blood cells could not again be manufactured. Stem cells may be transplanted to overcome the devastating effects of chemotherapy or total body irradiation before bone marrow transplant. BMT and stem cell treatment are discussed in Chapter 17.

GENE THERAPY

As research reveals the genes thought to be responsible for various types of cancers, the possibility of gene splicing or replacement becomes a reality. Genetic engineering is still in its infancy, but scientists are hard at work hoping to make it a reality for cancer patients. The genes *BRCA1* and *BRCA2* are implicated in about half of the cases of inherited breast and ovarian cancer. Research has shown that when healthy *BRCA1* genes are injected into mice that have faulty *BRCA1* genes, tumor growth is slowed. This has proven true for other genes implicated in other types of cancer. Some day gene therapy may be the major treatment for cancer.

EVALUATING THE EFFECTIVENESS OF MEDICAL TREATMENT

The oncologist conducts an ongoing evaluation of each patient's status to determine how effective the prescribed treatment has been and to plan for a future course of therapy should it be needed. It is particularly important to know whether there has been a reduction in the size of the tumor and an abatement of the patient's symptoms. This is the purpose of "second-look surgery."

One test for monitoring the effectiveness of treatment is a measurement of CEA levels. This antigen is a glycoprotein that is produced during fetal life but is not normally present after birth. Its production may resume again, however, and CEA levels can be increased by some kinds of liver disease, heavy cigarette smoking, and especially by gastrointestinal and colorectal cancers. Because of the many and diverse conditions that can elevate CEA levels, the test cannot be used to diagnose cancer. However, it can be used as a tumor marker to evaluate the effectiveness of treatment, because CEA levels usually fall to within the normal range about 1 month after successful treatment of cancer. Other tumor markers, such as PSA for prostate cancer and CA-125 for ovarian cancer, are used to track the success of treatment and recurrence in those cancers.

COMPLEMENTARY AND INTEGRATIVE MEDICINE

Normally, the treatments and therapies already listed should be employed as the primary cancer treatment, but many patients choose to supplement their care with complementary therapeutic approaches, also known as complementary and integrative medicine (CIM). There are many of these approaches, but the most common are alternative medical systems, such as traditional Chinese medicine (including acupuncture), Ayurveda, homeopathy, and naturopathy; mind-body interventions, which include meditation, hypnosis, dance, music, and art therapy; biologically based treatments, such as herbal and plant therapies, nutrition, and biologic pharmacology; manipulative and body-based methods, which include chiropractic and osteopathic manipulation and massage therapy; and energy therapies, including biofield therapies such as Qi gong, Reiki, and Therapeutic Touch (Anderson, 2009).

In CIM, the therapies are used in addition to—but not as a replacement for—traditional Western (allopathic) medicine. When patients choose to use these approaches, the health care professional and the patient work together to find the therapies best suited to the patient's needs. It is important to form a partnership to promote the patient's health and well-being. The nurse also needs to understand the requirements for care of the patient undergoing these approaches, in order to be supportive and to help achieve the highest level of health possible.

COMMON PROBLEMS RELATED TO CANCER OR CANCER TREATMENT

The problems that occur in the cancer patient are complex, and depend on both the location and type of cancer and the therapy used to treat it. A discussion of the most common problems and the related nursing care is presented here.

ANOREXIA, MUCOSITIS, AND WEIGHT LOSS

Many cancer patients experience an alteration in taste. Often the first thing noticed is that red meat does not taste good. The taste of sweets also is altered. *Anorexia* (loss of appetite) often is associated with changes in taste and with inflammation of the mouth and tongue, which can cause the patient great difficulty in eating and drinking. The loss of appetite can quickly lead to deficiencies of protein and calories. **The patient with anorexia can experience a significant weight loss (2 or more pounds per week) and may suffer from severe malnutrition.** A synthetic substance derived from the female hormone progesterone, megestrol (Megace), has proven to work well to stimulate the appetite. A thorough routine for mouth care to minimize damage and anorexia should be started several days before the beginning of chemotherapy or radiation therapy to the head and neck. Radiation to the head or neck will produce some inflammatory changes in the mouth and often also in the pharynx and esophagus. Measures to combat this expected reaction include frequent oral intake of liquids that are not irritating chemically, the use of artificial saliva, and frequent and consistent mouth care.

Patients are encouraged to drink water as often as possible to help alleviate the discomfort of dryness of the mouth and tongue. However, drinking water will not completely resolve the problem. Artificial saliva combats mouth dryness in a different way and helps keep the mucous membranes soft and moist. It also helps to buffer the acidity in the mouth and thus to reduce irritation of the oral mucosa. Artificial saliva is available as a spray (Salivart) and a gel (Biotene oralbalance) and can be used by the patient as often as desired. If artificial saliva cannot be found at a local pharmacy, it can be obtained online from most of the online drugstores.

The patient undergoing chemotherapy may experience *mucositis* (irritation and inflammation of the mucosa) in the mouth. A major goal of mouth care (other than protection of the mucosa) is preservation of the teeth and prevention of gum infections. To accomplish this, the patient should be encouraged to accept as much responsibility as possible for frequent and consistent oral hygiene. She probably will need to be taught how to brush her teeth using a soft brush or tooth sponges (toothettes) and to employ gentle strokes. She also should be taught how to irrigate her mouth to remove debris and counteract acidity. The solutions most often used for this irrigation are normal saline, mild solutions of peroxide (1:5 ratio), or a bicarbonate of soda and salt solution (¼ to ½ tsp of baking soda and ⅛ to ¼ tsp salt in an 8-oz glass of water). Fluid intake must be increased to 3000 mL/day. Because of the risk of infection, toothbrushes should be rinsed with a bleach solution or hydrogen peroxide and then rinsed with water before reuse. Running toothbrushes through the dishwasher is another option for disinfection.

Relief of the mouth pain of mucositis or *stomatitis* (inflammation of the mouth) is provided by special topical compounds (such as Xylocaine Viscous) that are "swished and spit." Such compounds contain a topical anesthetic and an anti-inflammatory agent. **The patient is instructed *not* to swallow this solution.** The patient should avoid spicy foods, alcohol, and tobacco while undergoing treatment. The metabolic demand of malignant growth, the anorexia, and the mucositis that makes eating difficult all contribute to weight loss. Weight loss also can occur in cancer patients because of disturbances in their metabolism whereby the body metabolizes its own proteins for energy instead of using the carbohydrates available in the diet or in body fat. The body has to work hard to repair normal cells after cancer treatment. Initially, the patient's current weight should be noted and recorded and compared with her ideal weight. Her protein intake should be increased to compensate for the fact that cancer patients often metabolize their own tissues for energy, even though glucose may be readily available in the blood. Small, frequent feedings, attention to preferences for foods, and a pleasant and restful environment during meals are often helpful. Supplemental feedings to provide additional protein and calories can help avoid excessive weight loss and protein deficiency. Supplements taste better if they are served in glass or plastic rather than out of a metal container. The ACS has patient pamphlets available on ways to increase nutritional intake.

NAUSEA, VOMITING, AND DIARRHEA

Radiation therapy of the abdomen or lower back often produces nausea, vomiting, and diarrhea starting 7 to 10 days after the beginning of treatment. Various antineoplastic drugs also can produce these side effects. Antiemetic regimens should be chosen based on the potential of the chemotherapy regimen to cause nausea. Dose and timing vary for the antiemetic agents, but the regimen (consisting of several different drugs) is usually started 30 minutes to an hour before doses of chemotherapy and continued 1 to 2 days afterward. Antiemetics are used for nausea and vomiting resulting from radiation therapy as well. A class of antiemetics commonly used, serotonin antagonists, acts

on the chemoreceptor trigger zone for vomiting and has proven very beneficial to the chemotherapy patient. These drugs are working for previously resistant chemotherapy-induced nausea and vomiting.

Eating before treatment seems to decrease nausea. Eating toast or crackers before arising or engaging in activity during periods of nausea may decrease vomiting. Liquids, liquid supplements, or easily digested foods are given at 3- to 4-hour intervals in small amounts. Foods and liquids should be high in protein and calories, bland, lukewarm, and to the patient's taste. Meals should be eaten slowly and food chewed thoroughly. Carbonated drinks and tea are tolerated better than other liquids, but should be taken 1 hour before or after meals, not with meals. It is best not to lie down for at least 2 hours after a meal. Caffeine and rich or fatty foods should be avoided. The patient's environment should be free of bothersome smells, sights, or sounds. If food odor is nauseating, consider serving cold meals. Chewing gum or sucking on hard or sour candy, candied ginger, or ice helps reduce nausea in some patients. Nursing care involves providing comfort measures and mouth care. If nausea strikes, breathing slowly and deeply through the mouth may prevent vomiting. The patient is monitored for dehydration and electrolyte imbalances when excessive vomiting occurs.

Diarrhea may occur from radiation to the abdomen, lower back, or pelvis. Many of the chemotherapy drugs cause diarrhea because they affect the cells of the intestinal mucosa, causing inflammation. Treatment involves avoiding high-fiber foods that encourage rapid evacuation from the bowel and adding low-fiber foods such as bananas and cheese to the diet. Cleansing the rectal area and applying petroleum jelly, A&D ointment, or Desitin cream helps decrease discomfort and protects the skin from breakdown. The physician may prescribe a medication to decrease the number and frequency of bowel movements. The nurse must monitor the patient for signs of dehydration and electrolyte imbalance.

CONSTIPATION

Certain antineoplastic drugs, such as vincristine, vinblastine, and paclitaxel, cause constipation. Increasing fluids (as allowed), adding fiber to the diet, administering stool softeners and fiber laxatives, exercise, and monitoring vigilantly for the beginning signs of constipation are the usual measures taken. Suppositories or enemas may be necessary.

CYSTITIS

Cytoxan and ifosfamide may cause cystitis. The nurse monitors for hesitancy, urgency, and pain during urination. The urine is checked for cloudiness and signs of *hematuria* (blood in the urine). Fluids are increased to 2 to 3 L/day. The patient is encouraged to empty the bladder frequently. The antineoplastic drug is administered in the morning and/or early afternoon so that most of it can be flushed from the bladder before bedtime, so that the patient sleeps through the night.

IMMUNOSUPPRESSION, BONE MARROW SUPPRESSION, AND INFECTION

Suppression of the bone marrow is the major reason why doses of chemotherapy must be limited. When the marrow is suppressed (that is, its cell production is slowed) few new erythrocytes, leukocytes, or platelets are produced. This reduction decreases oxygen-carrying power and the patient experiences hypoxia and fatigue. Decreased platelets bring an increased risk of bleeding. A low leukocyte count means lower immune function and lower ability to fight infection.

All antineoplastic drugs cause some degree of bone marrow suppression, but some can cause severe suppression. The amount of suppression is dose related. Severe suppression is a life-threatening side effect for the patient. The suppression usually is temporary, and improvement in bone marrow function occurs within weeks to months of completed therapy. The white blood cell (WBC) count is monitored for a count of less than 3000/mm^3, indicating neutropenia. Filrastim or sargramostim is given to raise the neutrophil count and the WBC count. Often, administration of these agents is started before the WBC count drops too low.

The anemia resulting from antineoplastic therapy places an increased workload on the heart and lungs, as these organs attempt to oxygenate the body adequately. When the platelet count reaches a low of 50,000/mm^3, any small injury can lead to an episode of prolonged bleeding. At 20,000/mm^3, spontaneous bleeding that is difficult to control may occur. Therefore, at a count of 100,000/mm^3, the next dose of chemotherapy is withheld. If the count is less than 50,000/mm^3, bleeding precautions are observed (no invasive procedures), and if the count is less than 10,000 to 15,000/mm^3, the patient is transfused.

The increased danger of infection is an indication to the nurse to become very attentive to good, frequent, and thorough hand hygiene and to maintain strict asepsis in all aspects of patient care. If the neutrophil count is below 500 mm^3, follow the policy and procedures for protective isolation to prevent infection.

Patients with thrombocytopenia can take measures to help lower the risk of bleeding. An infusion of platelets may be administered if the count falls to 20,000/mm^3. The patient must be handled gently. Using a lift sheet helps in turning and repositioning the patient. Needle sticks for injections, laboratory specimens, and intravenous line starts are kept to a minimum. The smallest gauge needle possible for the

Patient Teaching

Cancer Treatment and Infection Prevention

- Wash your hands well with an antimicrobial soap or alcohol-based hand rub:
  - Before eating.
  - After using the toilet.
  - After blowing your nose.
  - After handling items many people have handled, such as railings, money, shopping carts, library books, newspapers, and pieces of mail.
  - After touching a pet.
  - After spending time out in public.
- Do not share personal care items (razor, toothbrush, toothpaste, washcloth, towels, deodorant, hand lotion, lipstick, etc.).
- Clean toothbrush by running it through the dishwasher or soaking it in a bleach or hydrogen peroxide solution.
- Stay away from people with respiratory or other infections.
- Bathe daily if possible; use an antimicrobial soap.
- Examine the mouth daily for sores or white patches; perform mouth care frequently.
- Examine the skin, especially the feet, for signs of broken areas daily.
- Wash dishes, utensils, and items used in cooking in hot sudsy water or run them through a dishwasher.
- Drink only fresh, bottled water.
- Do not reuse drinking cups or glasses without washing them.
- Keep lips moist with lip ice or petroleum jelly to avoid cracking.
- Stay out of crowded places.
- Eat only canned or cooked foods.
- If leukocyte count is extremely low, maintain a low-bacteria diet by avoiding salads, raw fruits and vegetables, undercooked meat, pepper, or paprika.
- Do not handle garden flowers, plants, or earth.
- Do not clean out cat litter boxes or bird cages.
- Have someone change water in flower arrangements if such are allowed.
- Monitor temperature daily.
- Be careful not to nick or scratch the skin.
- Report the following signs of infection to the physician immediately:
  - Temperature over 100° F (38° C).
  - Persistent cough.
  - Colored or foul-smelling drainage from wound or nose.
  - Presence of a boil or abscess.
  - Cloudy, foul-smelling urine or burning on urination.

task should be used. Pressure is applied to the site for 5 to 10 minutes or until bleeding stops. All urine and stool should be tested for the presence of blood. Abdominal girth is measured daily to check for internal bleeding. Ice is applied to any area that is bumped or injured.

The diet is modified to avoid irritating foods. Stool softeners are given to keep the stool soft and to prevent the Valsalva maneuver that occurs with constipation. No rectal suppositories or enemas are given, and rectal temperatures are contraindicated.

Patient Teaching

Prevent Bleeding and Bruising in the Patient with a Low Platelet Count

- Use a soft toothbrush and brush lightly; do not floss.
- Use only an electric razor or depilatory for shaving.
- Avoid constipation by increasing fluid and roughage in the diet; take a stool softener if needed.
- Caution health care workers not to use a tourniquet to obtain blood specimens.
- Tell health care workers what normal blood pressure is so that cuff is not pumped up excessively.
- Avoid nonprescription drugs that inhibit platelet function: aspirin, ibuprofen (Motrin, Advil), Alka-Seltzer. Check for salicylates that inhibit platelet function in all analgesic and cold medicines.
- Move around carefully to avoid bumping into things; avoid contact sports or any sport where falling is a risk.
- If a bump or injury occurs, apply ice to area for 1 hour.
- Avoid tight, constricting clothing or shoes.
- Do not wear jewelry with sharp edges.
- Use ample lubrication for intercourse; avoid anal intercourse.
- Avoid blowing the nose or picking at it; if you must blow, blow gently without occluding either nostril.

Immunosuppression may be treated with colony-stimulating factors (CSFs), such as granulocyte-macrophage colony-stimulating factor (GM-CSF), granulocyte colony-stimulating factor (G-CSF), or in limited cases epoetin (EPO), to increase leukocytes, granulocytes, and erythrocytes. Granulocyte-stimulating factors are questionable for patients with a cancer of the blood-forming organs, such as leukemia (unless whole-body irradiation has occurred) as there is a possibility that more abnormal cells will be produced. Granulocyte-stimulating factors are used after total body irradiation for Hodgkin's disease, acute lymphocytic lymphoma, and non-Hodgkin's lymphoma. They are given after the BMT has been completed.

? Think Critically

You came to work with a slightly scratchy throat and a drippy nose this morning. The charge nurse has assigned you to a cancer patient who has bone marrow suppression. What would you do in this situation?

HYPERURICEMIA

The antimetabolite drugs cause an increase in uric acid in the blood as cancer cells are destroyed. A high fluid intake helps prevent problems of *hyperuricemia* (high uric acid in the blood) that occurs. Allopurinol may be prescribed to decrease the incidence of gout caused by the hyperuricemia; it is started at the beginning of therapy in an effort to prevent the problem.

FATIGUE

The fatigue occurring from immunosuppression treatment itself requires an adjustment of lifestyle. Physically, the patient may feel tired and without energy. She may find that she is impatient and irritable and she may withdraw from her social environment. This decrease in activity may lead to a decline in function that is irreversible.

The nurse must instruct the patient about how to manage her fatigue. Fatigue management includes avoiding unnecessary bed rest, maintaining a good balance between energy and activity, minimizing emotional distress, maintaining activities of daily living, using energy-saving devices, and prioritizing activities. Maintaining a good nutritional status with high protein intake will help keep up energy levels. Supplemental feedings between meals often are necessary to ensure adequate calorie intake. Fluids should be increased to 3 L/day on day 3 of chemotherapy, unless contraindicated, to help flush the waste materials of killed cancer cells from the body and to decrease the toxicities of the antineoplastic drugs. Explain that fatigue is a normal result of cancer treatment, and that fatigue may continue for 2 to 3 months after completion of therapy. Light exercise such as walking tends to increase energy level (Kornmehl, 2007).

ALOPECIA

Hair loss (*alopecia*) resulting from chemotherapy is temporary. Occasionally, radiation therapy to the head causes permanent hair loss. Although some techniques—such as using ice caps or a tourniquet around the scalp during the administration of chemotherapy—have been somewhat effective, they are not recommended by oncologists. The reduction of circulation of the drug to the area may prevent the killing of cancer cells that are harbored in the blood or lymph vessels in the scalp and head.

Hair begins regrowth about a month after chemotherapy ends. The patient must be told that the new hair may be different in texture and color from the original hair. Before hair loss occurs, the patient should choose a wig or head cover to wear until the hair is regrown. Some offices of the ACS have wigs available for loan that have been donated by former patients. In today's times, it is popular to "sport" the baldness that results from treatment. Singer Melissa Etheridge made her first stage appearance after cancer treatment without any wig or cap. Whatever your patient decides, help her understand that society supports her as a unique individual.

PAIN

For many cancer patients, pain is a daily reality. Pain reduces appetite, limits activity, and interferes with sleep. Most cancer pain (90%) can be relieved or at least controlled by a combination of measures. Often, however, the pain of cancer is undertreated. Chapter 7 discusses all the modalities to control the patient's pain. Acupuncture has been validated as being useful to help control cancer pain (Paley et al., 2011).

Table 8-6 Common Drugs Effective for Cancer Pain

DRUG	BRAND NAME	DURATION (hr)	DOSAGE (mg)	SIDE EFFECTS
Common Oral Pain Relievers: Mild to Moderate Intensity				
Acetaminophen	Tylenol	3–4	650	Hepatic
Aspirin	Many brands	3–5	550	GI
Codeine	Many brands	3–5	32	CNS, GI
Hydrocodone combination	Vicodin	3–4	5	CNS, GI
Ibuprofen	Motrin, Advil	3–5	400	GI
Ketoprofen	Orudis	5–7	50	GI
Naproxen	Naprosyn	2–8	250	GI
Oxycodone	Roxicodone	3–6	5	CNS, GI
Piroxicam	Feldene	24	20	GI
Propoxyphene	Darvon	4–6	65	CNS

DRUG	BRAND NAME	DURATION (hr)	PARENTERAL DOSE (mg)	ORAL DOSE (mg)
Common Opioid Pain Relievers: Moderate to Severe Intensity				
Morphine	Generic	4–5	10	30
Controlled-release morphine	MS Contin	6–12	—	30
Hydromorphone	Dilaudid	3–4	1.5	4
Methadone	Dolophine	5–6	10	20
Fentanyl	Duragesic	1–2	0.1	0.025
Oxycodone	Roxicodone	3–6	—	5
Controlled-release oxycodone	OxyContin	12	—	10
Codeine	Generic	2–4	120	200

CNS, central nervous system; *GI*, gastrointestinal.

Table 8-6 lists current oral and intravenous medications proven effective against cancer pain. By putting aside worries about addiction to opiates, believing the patient's reports of pain and what relieves it, and concentrating on humane treatment of cancer patients, the nurse can be the instrument for helping the patient achieve a pain-free or pain-controlled existence. Adjunctive medications used along with analgesics to help control cancer pain may include steroids, antidepressants, and antiseizure drugs. In combination with analgesics, one or more of these drugs can be very effective.

Nonpharmacologic Interventions
Nonpharmacologic interventions are combined with oral, topical, and parenteral analgesia to achieve relief or good control of pain. Pain must be (1) assessed and documented regularly; (2) discussed openly with family, and the reports of pain must be believed and understood; (3) addressed with options that are appropriate for the setting and for family; and (4) treated with interventions in a timely fashion. **The main factor in pain treatment is to continue to seek a combination of interventions or different treatments until the pain is under control.** Pain should be reassessed 15 to 30 minutes after

parenteral drug administration and 1 hour after oral drugs are given. Medication doses should be scheduled regularly and around the clock to maintain a therapeutic drug level to prevent pain recurrence. The pain medication employed should be known to be effective for cancer pain. Pain control or relief greatly increases the quality of life for the cancer patient.

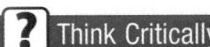 Think Critically

The pain control regimen for an assigned cancer patient is not working well. Can you write a role-play situation that would show your classmates how you would interact with the physician to obtain better pain control for your patient?

PATIENTS WITH METASTATIC DISEASE

A percentage of cancer patients experience metastasis. Table 8-7 shows the most common locations for metastasis for major cancers. Treatment options are usually the same as for primary cancer. Nursing care becomes more complex as more body systems are affected. All nurses caring for cancer patients should be aware of the possibility of metastasis and be alert for signs that might indicate it has occurred. To rule out metastasis,

Table 8-7	Common Sites of Metastasis for Different Cancer Types

CANCER TYPE	SITES OF METASTASIS
Breast cancer	Bone* Lung* Liver Brain
Lung cancer	Brain* Bone Liver Lymph nodes Pancreas
Colorectal cancer	Liver* Lymph nodes Adjacent structures
Prostate cancer	Bone (especially spine and legs)* Pelvic nodes
Melanoma	Gastrointestinal tract Lymph nodes Lung Brain
Primary brain cancer	Central nervous system

*Most common site of metastasis for the specific malignant neoplasm.
From Ignatavicius, D.D., & Workman, M.L. (2010). *Medical-Surgical Nursing: Critical Thinking for Collaborative Care* (6th ed.). Philadelphia: Elsevier Saunders, p. 405.

the patient is periodically assessed by the physician and bone scans are performed to detect metastasis to locations in the skeleton.

FEAR AND INEFFECTIVE COPING

The patient newly diagnosed with cancer faces enormous stress. **Knowledge about the disease, treatment options, and what will be experienced during each type of treatment greatly decreases fear in patients and families.** Knowing what to expect allows people to plan and feel confident that they will have some control over their experience. An assessment of the patient's and family's usual coping techniques is important in formulating the overall plan of care.

When a patient has been diagnosed with cancer, pay attention to the patient's partner. Give the partner enough knowledge to decrease anxiety, and the patient will be calmer. Be honest about the adverse effects of chemotherapy, immunotherapy, radiation therapy, and other treatments, but take a positive approach. Indicating that many patients feel a little nauseated with chemotherapy, but that there is medication that controls nausea very well, is better than telling the patient that there will not be any problems with the chemotherapy.

The nurse must consider psychosocial and spiritual care when working with the cancer patient, as the disease will affect every aspect of life in some way. The nurse's job is to be supportive, to assist the patient to use strengths in planning and fighting

the disease, and to coordinate family strengths in order to support the patient to continue with daily life.

Speak with the patient and partner about sexual concerns. Intimacy is to be encouraged. Unless the patient is recovering from surgery, has pathologic fractures, or is severely immunosuppressed, sexual intercourse should not be a serious problem. If sexual function has been altered by surgery or treatment, help the patient find other means of sexual expression and gratification.

Referral to a social worker may be needed to coordinate resources for treatment and care assistance. Care of the cancer patient is a collaborative process that involves many members of the health care team. Family, friends, individuals, and community groups are among the sources of support and encouragement that the cancer patient might need for self-care and to attain some level of independence and peace of mind.

Local chapters of the ACS and American Lung Association have a wide variety of services available to professionals and laypersons interested in caring for the cancer patient. These include an annotated bibliography of public, patient, and professional information and education materials, pamphlets and booklets, and audiovisual programs. To obtain materials from the ACS, one can write to or call the nearest ACS division. There are more than 3000 local ACS unit offices in the United States and Puerto Rico.

Learning as much as possible about the particular kind of cancer advises the patient of available options. Knowledge of the latest and most effective treatments should be gained before making a decision about treatment. Contacting the National Cancer Institute for the latest information is wise.

Throughout treatment, the patient should be actively seeking information. The patient must trust the physician and the hospital or treatment facility. Trust is not developed on the basis of someone else's recommendation alone. Encourage the patient to maintain a sense of humor and to look for a little pleasure and enjoyment in life on a daily basis to counteract the hours consumed by treatment.

ONCOLOGIC EMERGENCIES

An oncologic emergency can occur when a tumor grows so large it is compromising function of adjacent structures or when metabolic processes or normal coagulation processes are disrupted. There are six major oncologic emergencies:

1. *Tumor lysis syndrome:* rapid release of byproducts from cell destruction from cancer therapy; first sign is an elevated potassium level and this may cause renal failure, cardiac dysrhythmias, or asystole.
2. *Hypercalcemia:* calcium level rises above 11 mg/dL due to bone deterioration and release of secretion of parathyroid hormone by a tumor.

3. *Disseminated intravascular coagulation (DIC):* due to abnormal activation of clot formation, resulting in excessive consumption of platelets and blood coagulation factors.
4. *Pericardial effusion and cardiac tamponade:* invasion of cancer cells into the pericardial sac causing fluid secretion into the sac.
5. *Spinal cord compression:* related to metastatic tumor and bone collapse, causing impingement of the spinal cord.
6. *Superior vena cava syndrome:* occurs in lung cancer when affected lymph nodes block circulation in the vena cava.

When these emergencies occur, immediate action is taken to prevent severe injury or death.

CARE FOR THE DYING CANCER PATIENT

PSYCHOLOGICAL PROCESS OF DEATH

Though many more cancer patients are being cured, cancer is still the second leading cause of death in the United States. Sometimes cancer cannot be eliminated. In 2010, it is anticipated that 569,490 Americans will die from cancer. That amounts to 1500 patients who die from cancer every day. Oncology nurses need to understand the grief process and the process of death and dying and they need to apply knowledge about these processes compassionately when caring for cancer patients.

Grieving

Elisabeth Kübler-Ross introduced the world to the stages of grief and dying when her landmark book, *On Death and Dying,* was published in 1969. Kübler-Ross suggested that people go through several predictable junctures as they learn to adapt to the processes of loss or impending death. Not everyone goes through all the stages, nor do people go through stages in any set order. These five stages may apply to the grieving process when a body function or part is lost (such as a lost breast from cancer), a loved one dies, or one's own death is approaching (Box 8-6).

Fear

The patient feels and expresses many powerful emotions as she grieves the loss of her life. Almost all dying patients face varying levels of fear (Box 8-7). Caregivers are almost never successful in directly making

Box 8-6   Kübler-Ross' Stages of Dying

Denial (This can't happen to me!)
Anger (Why *me*?)
Bargaining (Yes me, *but*...)
Depression (It *is* me, I give up...)
Acceptance (I'm ready...)

Box 8-7   Common Fears of the Dying Patient

Almost all dying patients face varying levels of fear which may include fear of:
- The unknown
- Abandonment and loneliness
- Loss of relationships
- Loss of experiences in the future
- Dependency and loss of independence
- Pain

patients less afraid of death through talk. The nurse is most helpful to the patient in just "being there" for the patient and expressing caring. A nurse who is compassionate and soothing provides comfort and strength for the patient. In the same way, when a patient displays behavior that is upsetting to the family, the nurse can explain to the family that patients go through these stages and the behavior is not because the family has done something wrong. These are times that both the patient and family are in great need, and nursing support can be profoundly comforting.

When nurses care for dying patients regularly, they cannot help but reflect on their own mortality. It is important to review one's beliefs about death and dying and reaffirm those beliefs. In this way, it is possible to support patients who may have their own beliefs about the mysteries of death. Table 8-8 provides some common spiritual beliefs and practices.

Take a periodic inventory of your ability to provide care without "burnout." If you come to the point where you can only provide care in a detached and distant manner, you can no longer be supportive, compassionate, and understanding. When a nurse experiences the emotional distance that accompanies "burnout," it is time to take a break or to move on and let others provide care for the dying patient.

PALLIATIVE CARE

Patients are living longer with cancer than they have in the past. Extended time means steps must be taken to maintain as high a quality of life as possible for the dying cancer patient.

Palliative care, also called *comfort care,* is directed at meeting the needs of the dying patient by providing comfort while maintaining a high quality of life. Nurses who care for the dying patient have a unique opportunity to become an intimate part of the patient's life. The dying patient can be supported physically and emotionally, while the nurse maintains a professional role.

Whether assisting the patient in the hospital or at home, certain comfort measures are required. Palliative care requires a specialized body of knowledge and skill that can be difficult to obtain, and also to maintain, if the nurse is not routinely applying the skills. Clinical issues across the settings involve the following.

Table 8-8 Spiritual Beliefs and Practices Regarding Death

EXISTENCE OF DEITY	END-OF-LIFE (EOL) RITUALS	AFTERLIFE?	SPECIAL BELIEFS SURROUNDING EOL
Christianity			
Roman Catholic			
One triune deity: Father, Son, and Holy Spirit	Last Rites ("Anointing of the Sick")	Soul goes to purgatory, followed by eternity in heaven or hell	Catholics may be cremated, but the cremains must be interred, not scattered or kept
Protestant			
One triune deity: Father, Son, and Holy Spirit	No special rituals Minister may perform extreme unction	Consequences of actions on Earth dictate whether soul goes to heaven or hell and it happens immediately after death	Beliefs vary among sects; in general, cremation and autopsies are allowed
Judaism			
One God	*Halakhot* (contains accepted Jewish laws and customs of death and mourning)	Immortality of the soul; belief in afterlife among the Orthodox	Euthanasia, suicide, and assisted suicide are strictly forbidden The body is never left alone until burial Autopsy is discouraged The body must not be cremated
Buddhism			
No	Rituals to ensure that the consciousness leaves the body	Progression of the soul	Sick patients must not know they are dying
Hinduism			
Multitudes of gods and goddesses—being of ultimate oneness	*Antyesti samskara* (death rites) The Hindu dies at home, if possible Family member chants a mantra at moment of death	Progression of the soul—cycles of rebirth	*Mahaprasthana* (a vision of a tunnel of light) Death is a blissful time Avoidance of excessive drugs Body is cremated; only men go to cremation site
Islam			
One God (Allah), powerful but unknowable	Family members or an Imam (clergy) read Koran and offer prayers	Another world after death	Dying person should face Mecca before and after death
American Indian/Alaska Native			
Common concept is dual divinity: creator and mythical individual	May have Christian or Aboriginal traditions May smoke ceremonial pipe	In general, no precise belief May believe in reincarnation, or progression to another world	Traditional natives object to incorporation of their religious beliefs into other spiritual paths or into commercial affairs
African American			
Most believe in one deity	Important to incorporate prayer in coping with illness	Depends on actual religion, but most believe in an afterlife	More likely to request life-sustaining therapies Spiritual beliefs incorporated into treatment Physician is God's instrument

Anticipatory Guidance

The nurse can prepare the family and patient by anticipating the death to come: giving them guidance about physical changes, symptoms, and complications that may arise. This may also aid the patient and family in deciding about possible hospice care. There are two stages of dying: *pre-active,* which may take weeks or months; and *active,* which lasts only a few days (King & Klawitter, 2007). In the pre-active phase, patients know they are dying and exhibit this knowledge by withdrawing from social activities and attempting to put their affairs in order. Patients in this phase often report seeing loved ones who have already died. Patients in the pre-active phase become restless, have slow wound healing, and begin to have dependent edema (swelling in extremities, or even the entire body). When patients enter the active phase of dying (the final 2 to 3 days) they exhibit specific signs in breathing patterns and other body functions which indicate that death is imminent. Following are some active dying symptoms and associated nursing activities.

Terminal Hydration

A dying patient gradually reduces fluid intake. Dehydration can also increase due to the disease process. Also, a dry mouth and a feeling of thirst may be induced by the drugs being administered. The nurse must help educate the patient and family as to both the benefits and burdens of hydration. Many times, the course is for patients to choose what to take, and also to be allowed to refuse further nourishment. This is termed *patient-endorsed intake.*

End-Stage Symptom Management

Many expected symptoms are related to metabolic changes at the end of life. The last few days of patient life have been studied extensively. Recognize these latter symptoms and either alleviate them or help explain them to the patient and family. Since comfort is the goal of palliative care, administering only oral medications is the preferred choice. However, this may not be possible as death draws near, and it is also the goal to allow a pain-free death. In some cases it may be possible to administer transdermal and/or rectal pain medications.

Pain. Transdermal fentanyl has helped eliminate the burden of pain at the end of life. Sometimes this regimen is supplemented with rescue doses of morphine. Whatever the regimen, studies have shown that pain relief, either total or at least enough to make the pain tolerable, is possible 75% to 97% of the time.

Dyspnea. When patients are near death, they often subjectively feel as if they cannot get enough air. It is difficult to determine what causes this feeling, but several measures can be taken. The patient can be placed in Fowler's position, activities reduced, and air temperature adjusted, and medications such as bronchodilators can be given. Morphine may be given to ease breathing. It is important for the nurse to remember that this feeling can be very frightening for both the patient and family members, and aggressive treatment to lessen discomfort is important.

Death Rattle. Noisy ventilation is heard when patients can no longer clear their throats of normal secretions. Family members are often alarmed and are afraid the patient will choke to death. In these cases, scopolamine or atropine, drugs that are known to reduce secretions, may be used to quiet the patient and bring breathing back to normal.

Delirium. Dying patients may experience hallucinations and/or altered mental status. Nurses must first search for causes such as pain, positional discomfort, or bladder distention and address those physical problems. Next, the nurse should discuss the delirium with the patient's family and encourage the family to talk to the patient in quiet tones while remaining calm.

Nursing Resources

The palliative care nurse is an important element for the patient's and family's comfort during this transition. In September 2004, a certification examination for LPN/LVNs was launched by the National Board for Certification of Hospice and Palliative Nurses (NBCHPN). Detailed information is available by calling 1-888-519-9901 or visiting the NBCHPN website (see Online Resources below).

Get Ready for the NCLEX® Examination!

Key Points

- Cancer cells begin growing as a result of a change in normal body cells, probably a mutation in their DNA.
- Malignant cells can spread to other areas of the body.
- Tumors are classified according to the organs or tissues from which they first begin.
- All cancer results from defects in the DNA of genes.
- Harmful agents that are carcinogenic exist in the environment.
- Some people may have a genetic predisposition to some types of cancer.
- Age, sex, and race are considered predisposing factors for certain types of cancers.
- Changing certain lifestyle characteristics, such as quitting smoking, maintaining normal weight, reducing alcohol usage, avoiding and limiting exposure to carcinogens, and eating a varied diet, can lower the risk of cancer.
- Cytology, biopsy, radiologic studies, and laboratory tests are common methods used to diagnose cancer.
- Tumor markers detect biochemical substances synthesized and released into the bloodstream by tumor cells and are used mainly to confirm a diagnosis or response to a cancer therapy.
- Treatment modes of therapy for malignancies may include surgery, radiation, chemotherapy, hormone therapy, immunotherapy, and gene therapy.
- Nurses must protect themselves from overexposure to radiation.

- One of the most important areas of the patient's body to protect from radiation is the skin.
- Antineoplastic chemotherapy drugs are effective at different times in the growth and replication phases of the tumor cell cycle.
- Many antineoplastic drugs can cause tissue damage on direct contact, so the nurse must take care to protect patients from extravasation and administer the drugs into veins that have good blood flow.
- Biologic response modifiers manipulate the immune system to stimulate or suppress activity. These drugs assist the body in destroying cancer cells with minimal effect on normal tissue.
- Bone marrow and stem cell transplantation are used to correct damage caused by chemotherapy or radiation.
- Nausea, vomiting, diarrhea, and constipation are frequent complaints of cancer patients and require vigilant care.
- Cancer treatment may suppress the patient's bone marrow and the patient may develop thrombocytopenia, requiring therapy to be ceased for a period of time.
- The main factor in pain treatment is to continue to seek a combination of interventions or different treatments until the pain is under control.
- Many cancer patients and their families go through the five steps of grief that are recognized in patients experiencing loss.
- Palliative care is providing comfort for the dying patient and maintaining a high quality of life throughout the death process.

Additional Learning Resources

SG Go to your Study Guide for additional learning activities to help you master this chapter content.

*e*volve Go to your Evolve website (http://evolve.elsevier.com/deWit/medsurg) for the following FREE learning resources:
- Animations, audio, and video
- Answers and rationales for questions and activities
- Concept Map Creator
- Glossary with pronunciations in English and Spanish
- Interactive Review Questions and Exercises and more!

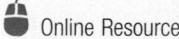
Online Resources
- American Cancer Society, www.cancer.org/docroot/home/index.asp
- Association of Cancer Online Resources, www.acor.org/index.html
- Complementary/integrative cancer therapy, www.mdanderson.org/education-and-research/resources-for-professionals/clinical-tools-and-resources/cimer/resources-and-links/index.html
- National Board for Certification of Hospice and Palliative Nurses, www.nbchpn.org
- National Cancer Institute, www.cancer.gov
- National Coalition for Cancer Survivorship, www.canceradvocacy.org
- OncoLink, www.oncolink.upenn.edu
- Online cancer resources, www.cancerindex.org/clinks6.htm

Review Questions for the NCLEX® Examination

1. There are two phases of dying: pre-active and active. A difference between the pre-active and active phases is:
   1. the pre-active phase lasts longer.
   2. patients in the active phase develop dependent edema.
   3. patients in the active phase report seeing relatives who have already died.
   4. patients in the pre-active phase begin developing Cheyne-Stokes breathing.

2. The nurse reinforces patient instructions regarding neutropenic precautions. Important topics should include the following except:
   1. pregnancy.
   2. diet restrictions.
   3. hand hygiene.
   4. social isolation.

3. A patient who recently had chemotherapy for lung cancer complains of uncontrollable nausea and vomiting with accompanying loss of appetite. An appropriate nursing diagnosis would be:
   1. *Ineffective coping.*
   2. *Deficient knowledge.*
   3. *Anticipatory grieving.*
   4. *Imbalanced nutrition: less than body requirements.*

4. The family members attending to the needs of a dying patient express distress regarding the noisy breathing. An important nursing action would be to:
   1. increase pain medications.
   2. administer atropine.
   3. reassure family members.
   4. consult a priest or a minister.

5. The patient is scheduled for bone marrow biopsy to confirm the diagnosis of leukemia. As the nurse reinforces physician instructions regarding the procedure, an appropriate nursing statement regarding bone marrow biopsy would be:
   1. "It is performed in the operating room."
   2. "It is a painless procedure."
   3. "It introduces a needle to aspirate tissue samples."
   4. "It requires a surgical incision."

6. Pain is not unique to cancer but is a common occurrence in cancer patients. An important point to keep in mind when employing pain control efforts is to:
   1. always try one type of intervention at a time and give it a chance to work before switching to a different intervention.
   2. seek a combination of interventions to offer the best pain control.
   3. try to avoid narcotics in order to protect the patient from drug addiction.
   4. refer the patient for psychological counseling if pain becomes an issue.

7. Before chemotherapy, a female patient expresses concerns regarding hair loss. She says that her partner would no longer love her because she will not be as attractive. An appropriate nursing diagnosis would be:
   1. *Disturbed body image* related to anticipated loss of hair.
   2. *Ineffective coping* due to perceived loss of relationship.
   3. *Powerlessness* related to chemotherapy.
   4. *Risk for impaired skin integrity* related to hair loss.

8. A patient had chemotherapy for non-Hodgkin's lymphoma 2 weeks ago. Based on the understanding of the effects of chemotherapy, the nurse would anticipate which clinical finding?
   1. Temperature 101.5° F (38.6° C)
   2. Elevated white blood cell count
   3. Easy bruising
   4. Change in hair color

9. A terminally ill female patient reminiscing about the "good old days" becomes increasingly confused. She talks of seeing relatives who have died. Which nursing intervention(s) would be appropriate? *(Select all that apply.)*
   1. Discuss the patient's behaviors with the family.
   2. Force oral fluids.
   3. Encourage the family to talk to the patient in quiet tones.
   4. Promote a calm environment.
   5. Apply physical restraints.

10. A 40-year-old woman is scheduled for external radiation therapy for breast cancer. To help the patient cope with her illness and the effects of radiation therapy, what should the nurse help her to focus on? *(Select all that apply.)*
    1. Complying with scheduled radiation therapies
    2. Taking precautions on exposing other family members
    3. Protecting the skin by applying lotion
    4. Wearing snug-fitting clothing
    5. Understanding the therapeutic effects and side effects of the treatment

Critical Thinking Activities

Scenario A
An acquaintance tells you that she has had a mole on her back for several years and it appears to be getting larger and darker. She states she is worried about the fact that it is getting bigger, but says that she is scared to go to the physician. She does not have health insurance and is worried about paying for the visit.

1. What is your obligation as a nurse in encouraging this person to see a physician at once?

2. What suggestions could you make about obtaining a medical opinion without incurring a lot of expense?

Scenario B
Ms. Allen went to her physician for a regular physical checkup and was told that she had malignant cells in the cervical secretions obtained from her Pap test. She had a biopsy of the cervix, and this, too, proved to contain malignant cells. She was admitted to the hospital, cesium was implanted in the cervix, and Ms. Allen was kept in bed in a private room during the treatment.

1. If you were assigned to give A.M. care to this patient, what special precautions would you take to protect yourself from excessive radiation?

2. What would be some signs and symptoms that you would watch for to determine whether Ms. Allen is having either a local or a systemic reaction to radiation?

Scenario C
Mary is a 19-year-old college student receiving chemotherapy for Hodgkin's disease.

1. Identify psychosocial problems you would expect Mary to have, and state the measures you would suggest to help her deal with them.

Scenario D
Alisha is a 40-year-old mother undergoing radiation therapy for ductal carcinoma of the breast. She has heard that acupuncture might help for the xerostomia (dry mouth) that she is experiencing. She has tried mouthwashes and various toothpastes, but still has the problem and her breath is interfering with her social life. She asks you for your opinion regarding acupuncture.

1. What should you tell Alisha about acupuncture and alternative approaches to this problem?

2. If you do not agree with complementary or integrative medicine, what is your obligation as a nurse to do in this situation?

Chronic Illness and Rehabilitation

Objectives

Theory

1. Define relevant nursing issues for patients with chronic illness.
2. Distinguish patients at risk for problems associated with immobility.
3. Describe the effect of immobility on each of the major systems of the body.
4. Explain the general goals for the resident in a long-term care facility and how to meet those goals.
5. Compare the role of the LPN/LVN in a long-term care facility of that in the hospital setting.
6. Describe the types of rehabilitation programs that might be found in a large city.
7. Apply the goals of rehabilitation.

8. Identify the members of the rehabilitation team and the collaborative care–giving process and state the role of each.
9. Explain the differences in philosophy and required attitude between the home care setting and the hospital.

Clinical Practice

1. Choose specific interventions to assist the patient with a chronic illness who is home-bound and has issues of loneliness.
2. When in a long-term care facility, discuss with the charge nurse the measures that are used for safety and fall prevention in that facility.
3. Observe a rehabilitation team conference to see how a collaborative care plan is created or updated.
4. From assessment data, identify areas of psychosocial need for a home care patient and family.

Key Terms

disability (dĭs-ă-BĬL-ĕ-tē, p. 177)
handicap (HĂN-dē-kăp, p. 177)
hemiparesis (hĕm-ē-pă-RĒ-sĭs, p. 187)
impairment (ĭm-PĂR-mĕnt, p. 177)

orthostatic hypotension (ōr-thō-STĀT-ĭk hī-pō-TĔN-shŭn, p. 183)
rehabilitation (rē-hă-bĭl-ĭ-TĀ-shŭn, p. 187)
sundowning (SŬN-doun-ĭng, p. 186)

Patients with chronic illnesses and disabilities are cared for in long-term care facilities, rehabilitation institutes, at home, at outpatient clinics, at rehabilitation agencies, and in physicians' offices. When working with patients who have a chronic illness, or who are disabled, nurses need to be skilled in providing care and comfort, promoting coping skills and adaptive living capabilities, promoting self-care for independent living, and fostering quality of life.

CHRONIC ILLNESS

Chronic illness affects millions of people. Diabetes, hypertension, heart disease, cancer, neurologic disorders (such as multiple sclerosis and stroke), asthma, arthritis, back disorders, and musculoskeletal deformities (such as those from arthritis and osteoporosis) all require continuous care. Although many people with a chronic illness can lead an active and productive life, about 46 million people in the United States have chronic illnesses or disabilities that interfere with normal function. People, and particularly the

elderly, may have more than one chronic illness, which makes treatment and care very complicated. Many health insurance companies have a case management department that oversees services for those with chronic illnesses. The terms *impairment, disability,* and *handicap* are encountered with patients who have a chronic illness. Impairment refers to dysfunction of a specific organ or body system. Disability indicates a difficulty in performing certain tasks because of impairment, and having a handicap means that there is a physical or mental defect or characteristic that prevents or restricts a person from participating in a normal life or limits the capacity to work; a handicap is usually related to a disability.

When chronic illness causes the loss of function, usual roles may be changed. The person may no longer be able to be the primary breadwinner, or hold whatever positions in the workforce or community that formerly were held. Changes in the person's role affect the family as well. Daily patterns are altered to accommodate treatments and therapy and to cope with the problems of disability. Sorrow is felt for all that has been lost. The patient may wonder, why did this happen to me? Spiritual distress may be experienced as the person is faced with the limitations of the illness or disability that has occurred. Holistic care that addresses spiritual and psychosocial needs as well as physical needs is essential.

Patients with a chronic illness often feel powerless, especially during the phases of diagnosis and early treatment. Patients realize that the chronic illness will dictate much of their course in life now, and that they have less control over what is happening to their body. Support of usual coping techniques—and teaching new ways to cope—help the patient effectively deal with the illness and the changes in life patterns it brings. Nurses can be instrumental in instilling hope for a good quality of life, despite the illness.

PREVENTING THE HAZARDS OF IMMOBILITY

Patients are immobilized to varying degrees and for different amounts of time. The multiple trauma patient may be on bed rest for several weeks. The patient with advanced multiple sclerosis may be able to move around only with a wheelchair. The patient who experiences great difficulty breathing from advanced lung disease or heart disease may have very little energy and does not move around much for that reason. Patients with spinal cord injury or brain damage from a stroke may be immobile for the rest of their lives. Patients who have pain or who have arthritic joints that cause pain with movement also tend to be less mobile. Patients who have any disorder requiring bed rest are at risk. All of these patients are subject to the problems of immobility.

Evaluate each patient situation and determine whether the patient is at risk for problems related to immobility. **Even if the patient is going to be immobile for only a few days, measures should be taken to prevent secondary problems.** Patients with disorders causing immobility should be assessed for the degree of risk for the various problems of immobility, and interventions to prevent them should be initiated (Box 9-1). **Early effects of immobility include a decrease in muscle strength, generalized weakness, easy fatigue, joint stiffness, decreased coordination, abdominal distention, and various metabolic changes detectable by laboratory test.** Table 9-1 presents the more severe problems with measures for prevention when lack of activity occurs for more than a few days.

The prevention of problems related to immobility begins the moment a patient first becomes ill or injured. Preventive actions must continue as long as the patient needs health care. The systems of the body work together as a whole and lack of activity affects more than one system. The effects vary depending on the general health of the individual, his age, the degree of immobility, and the length of time of inactivity or bed rest. Lack of mobility may begin a cycle that

Box **9-1**	Disorders that May Cause Immobility

- Multiple sclerosis
- Stroke
- Spinal cord injury
- Lower extremity amputation
- Head injury
- Multiple trauma
- Fractures of the knee, leg, ankle, hip, pelvis, or spine
- Neuromuscular disorders: muscular dystrophy, amyotrophic lateral sclerosis, poliomyelitis, cerebral palsy, myasthenia gravis, etc.
- Congenital deformities
- Burns
- Advanced metastatic cancer
- Advanced stages of chronic disorders such as Parkinson's disease, Alzheimer's disease, or Huntington's chorea
- Severe rheumatoid arthritis, osteoarthritis, and other forms of arthritis

leads to an ever-increasing loss of independence for the patient. As he becomes less able to move, the patient becomes more dependent, and as he becomes more dependent, he is less able to care for himself—which in turn leads to even more adverse effects from immobility. It is the nurse's responsibility to avoid the beginning of such a cycle by helping the patient maintain normal functioning of each body system to the highest degree possible (see Nursing Care Plan 9-1 on pp. 180–182).

 Elder Care Points

Although a lot of elderly people are active in their daily lives, many do not engage in daily exercise activity. When immobilized, these patients quickly lose what strength and flexibility they had, as muscle fibers atrophy quickly. It is much more difficult for these patients to regain mobility.

Assess the patient daily, looking closely at each body system in which a problem related to immobility might occur. Know the signs and symptoms of each type of problem and understand how to intervene to decrease or prevent it. The pathophysiology of the problems of immobility, including the signs and symptoms, medical treatment, and nursing care for each problem, is discussed in the relevant chapters of this text.

 Elder Care Points

Because of the changes in the various body systems that normally occur with aging, the elderly patient is at greatly increased risk for problems of immobility. Monitor closely for pressure sores, as well as hypostatic pneumonia, constipation, urinary problems, and inadequate nutritional intake due to anorexia. Attention to range-of-motion exercises is very important and often neglected.

Table 9-1	Prevention of the Common Hazards of Immobility
COMPLICATION	**PREVENTION**
Musculoskeletal	
Contractures	Range-of-motion exercises
Footdrop	Foot support while in bed, range-of-motion exercises, high-top tennis shoes
Osteoporosis	Range-of-motion exercises, ambulation if possible (walking)
Susceptibility to fractures	Weight-bearing exercises
Muscular atrophy	Passive or active range-of-motion exercises
Gastrointestinal	
Constipation	Increased activity level Increased fluid intake, fiber
Cardiovascular	
Decreased cardiac output	Range-of-motion exercises
Increased venous stasis	Exercise, support hose, or anti-embolism stockings
Thrombus formation	Exercise, support hose, or anti-embolism stockings
Embolism	Avoidance of leg massage, low-molecular-weight heparin
Neurologic	
Disorientation	Sleep-wake schedule in accord with light-dark pattern Reorientation (to person, place, and time) Control of sensory stimulation Avoidance of sudden position changes, tilt table
Renal/Urinary	
Calculi	Decreased dietary calcium level Increased fluid intake Maintenance of acidic urine
Infection	Increase fluids Use intermittent catheterization instead of indwelling if possible
Respiratory	
Pneumonia	Frequent repositioning in wheelchair or bed Respiratory exercises

CHRONIC ILLNESS AND REHABILITATION CARE

A chronic illness may develop following an acute illness or an accident. Some patients are transferred to a transitional unit or long-term care facility for a period of weeks for recovery after the most acute phase of illness or injury has passed. Many elderly, who have several chronic problems and deficits in self-care, enter long-term care facilities for the remainder of their lives. Other patients may enter a rehabilitation facility for an extended time. Some patients are discharged home to continue with rehabilitation services as an outpatient.

Long-Term Care

In the long-term care facility, an RN usually is the director of nurses. The RN supervisor manages the care for the entire facility on a 24-hour basis and delegates tasks to the LPN/LVN. An LPN/LVN often is the charge nurse, and certified nursing assistants (CNAs), patient care assistants, or restorative aides provide much of the basic direct care to the residents. An occupational therapist, physical therapist, speech pathologist, respiratory therapist, activity therapist, or other professional provides services as needed. A physician or advanced practice nurse supervises each resident's care program. Although the RN ultimately is responsible for the nursing care plan of each resident, the LPN/LVN charge nurse often is the person who admits the resident and initiates the plan of care. If the LPN/LVN initiates a plan of care, collaboration with the RN is necessary to ensure that the plan is appropriate and complete. The LPN/LVN performs treatments and wound care, regularly assists with gathering assessment data from the residents, organizes the shift's workload, administers medications, documents assessment findings and care given, assists with updating the nursing care plans, and assigns care tasks to patient care assistants. The LPN/LVN oversees care for a group of residents for a shift. The LPN/LVN assigns tasks to the patient care assistants. Those tasks may include assistance with toileting,

Text continued on p. 183

Nursing Care Plan 9-1 Care of an Immobilized Resident

Scenario
Carl Sanders is an 83-year-old man with weakness and debilitation and who has several chronic diseases. He has been transferred to the long-term care facility following a hospitalization for pneumonia.

Problem/Nursing Diagnosis
Cannot walk, turn, or reposition self/Impaired physical mobility related to weakness, debility, illness, and age.

Supporting Assessment Data
Objective: Needs assistance to turn, reposition in the bed, or walk.

Goals/Expected Outcomes	Nursing Interventions	Selected Rationale	Evaluation
Resident will maintain present joint mobility. Resident will perform active ROM of arms by discharge.	Perform ROM on joints tid. Assist to turn and reposition q 2 hr. Place in high Fowler's position for meals; assist to chair for lunch.	Regular ROM prevents frozen joints. Repositioning helps prevent pressure ulcers and hypostatic pneumonia.	Active ROM done twice this shift. Repositioned q 2 hr. Up in chair for meals. Breath sounds clear right; slightly diminished in left base.

Problem/Nursing Diagnosis
Break in skin with redness on left hip/Impaired skin integrity related to immobility and pressure over left trochanter.

Supporting Assessment Data
Subjective: "I can't move very much."
Objective: Too weak to reposition self; Stage I pressure ulcer over left trochanter.

Goals/Expected Outcomes	Nursing Interventions	Selected Rationale	Evaluation
Resident will have no evidence of more pressure damage to skin. Stage I pressure ulcer will heal within 3 wk.	Turn at least 2 q hr and more frequently if possible. Use supports for positioning and cushioning for relief of pressure. Keep reddened area clean, with clear film dressing in place; inspect q shift. Inspect all pressure points q 4 hr. Use turning sheet to turn patient.	Relieves pressure on dependent areas. Prevents pressure ulcers and keeps body in good anatomical alignment. Cleanliness prevents infection. Clear film dressing seals in moisture while allowing inspection. Identifies skin problems. Helps prevent shearing injuries from sliding resident on sheet.	Position adjusted q 1 hr. On pressure relief mattress; pressure relief cushion in chair. Clear dressing in place; reddening decreasing. Pressure points inspected q 4 hr. No new reddened areas. Turning sheet used for turning.

Problem/Nursing Diagnosis
Little stool passed/Constipation related to immobility.

Supporting Assessment Data
Subjective: "I feel constipated."
Objective: Only small amount of hard, dry stool passed once in last 4 days.

Goals/Expected Outcomes	Nursing Interventions	Selected Rationale	Evaluation
Resident will have normal bowel pattern by discharge.	Administer oil retention enema as ordered followed by suppository; monitor results. Assist to bedside commode after breakfast every day. Provide privacy. Give stool softener daily as ordered.	Oil will soften stool. Suppository stimulates bowel movement. Sitting on commode and privacy promote ease of bowel movement. Keeps stool soft.	Oil retention given; held for 20 min. Had large BM; suppository not needed. Assisted to commode after enema. Privacy provided. Received stool softener.

Goals/Expected Outcomes	Nursing Interventions	Selected Rationale	Evaluation
Resident will have normal pattern by discharge—cont'd	Increase fluids to 8 oz every hour while awake.	Keeps stool soft.	Took in at least 6 oz of fluid each hour; continue plan.
	Increase fiber in diet.	Adds bulk, helping to prevent constipation.	Ate a bran muffin at breakfast.
	Offer warm prune juice each morning.	Stimulates bowel and softens stool.	Warm prune juice taken before enema.

Problem/Nursing Diagnosis

Unable to walk/Risk for injury related to possible falls.

Supporting Assessment Data

Objective: Unable to walk without falling, gets confused after dark and tries to get out of bed.

Goals/Expected Outcomes	Nursing Interventions	Selected Rationale	Evaluation
Resident will not sustain fall in hospital.	Place call light and personal items within reach. Answer call light promptly.	Helps prevent him from trying to get out of bed without assistance.	Call bell and personal items on bed and bedside table within reach.
	Place an alarm device on the bed.	Alerts staff to attempt to get out of bed without assistance.	Bed alarm in place and functioning.
	Frequently reinforce instructions not to get up without assistance.		Reinforced not to get up without assistance q 2 hr.
	Assist to bedside commode and back to bed.	Prevents falling.	Assisted to bedside commode after enema.
	Keep low light on in room at night to decrease confusion.	Light helps maintain orientation to room.	Placed instruction on Computer Care Plan.
	Check on resident frequently; anticipate needs.	Anticipating needs helps keep resident from arising without assistance.	Checked on resident every hour during this shift.

Problem/Nursing Diagnosis

Recovering from pneumonia/Impaired mobility related to weakness and debility.

Supporting Assessment Data

Subjective: "I've really been sick; I'm so weak."
Objective: Lungs just cleared of secretions; breathes shallowly.

Goals/Expected Outcomes	Nursing Interventions	Selected Rationale	Evaluation
Resident will perform breathing exercises q 2 hr while awake.	Assist to sitting position for deep-breathing exercises, use of spirometer, and coughing q 2 hr.	Lungs can expand better when thoracic cage is not against the mattress.	Assisted to sit up and perform deep breathing and coughing. Used spirometer q 2 hr.
Lung fields will remain clear.	Encourage adequate fluid intake.	Keeps secretions more liquid and easier to expectorate.	Taking more fluid per hour (6 oz).
	Encourage to take deeper breaths during each commercial break when watching TV.	Aerates lower alveoli.	Encouraged to remember to take deep breaths during commercials on TV.
	Auscultate lungs each shift.	Detects changes in lungs.	Lungs clear right; slightly diminished sounds at left base.
	Turn q 2 hr.	Helps prevent hypostatic pneumonia.	Turned q 2 hr while in bed.

Continued

Problem/Nursing Diagnosis

Immobile for many days/Risk for ineffective tissue perfusion related to venous stasis.

Supporting Assessment Data

Subjective: "I've been mostly in bed for over a week."
Objective: Has been inactive and in bed most of the time for the past 10 days. History of previous thrombophlebitis in right leg.

Goals/Expected Outcomes	Nursing Interventions	Selected Rationale	Evaluation
Resident will not have evidence of thrombophlebitis or deep venous thrombosis.	Encourage active ROM of legs, feet, and ankles q 2 hr while awake.	Muscle movement compresses blood vessels, propelling blood to the heart.	Performing active ROM of legs, feet, and ankles after breathing exercises q 2 hr.
	Keep TED hose smoothly in place except for 30 min while bathing.	Elastic hose place pressure on vessels, encouraging venous return to the heart.	TEDs reapplied after bath.
	Encourage extra fluid intake.	Fluid prevents dehydration and hemoconcentration.	Offered fluid each time care provided.
	Assess for Homans' sign once per shift.	Homans' sign may indicate a thrombus (clot).	No positive Homans' sign.
	Visually inspect legs for reddening or swelling.	Reddening, swelling, or pain may indicate a thrombus or thrombophlebitis.	No reddening or swelling of legs and ankles.

Problem/Nursing Diagnosis

Immobile for 10 days/Risk for infection of the urinary tract related to immobility.

Supporting Assessment Data

Subjective: "I've had several bladder infections in the past."
Objective: Urine is concentrated and slightly cloudy.

Goals/Expected Outcomes	Nursing Interventions	Selected Rationale	Evaluation
Resident will not develop a urinary tract infection.	Increase fluid intake to at least 3000 mL/day.	Promotes more urine flow.	Is increasing fluid intake this shift.
	Encourage fluid intake hourly until 2 hr before bedtime.		Offering fluids each time care is given (q 1-2 hr).
	Assess for bladder distention q 4 hr.	Helps determine if bladder is being emptied sufficiently.	No bladder distention; voiding sufficient quantities.
	Observe characteristics of urine for signs of infection.	Cloudy, foul-smelling urine may indicate infection.	Urine is yellow, clear, and without foul odor.
	Measure intake and output.	Helps evaluate fluid intake.	Intake 1800 mL this shift. Output 1465 mL this shift.

Problem/Nursing Diagnosis

In bed in room most of time; roommate not able to communicate/Risk for loneliness related to lack of social interaction.

Supporting Assessment Data

Subjective: "I'm really sick of being in bed."
Objective: Roommate is aphasic and cannot communicate verbally.

Goals/Expected Outcomes	Nursing Interventions	Selected Rationale	Evaluation
Resident will maintain social contact.	Bring phone to resident and assist to call family members and friends.	Phone calls maintain contact with family and friends.	Phoned wife this morning. Says will call friend later this evening.
	Ask volunteers to play cards with him.	Playing cards with another provides social interaction.	Requested volunteer to play cards for late afternoon.
	Visit his room frequently.	Stopping in room provides social contact.	In room q 1 hr.
	Set up a schedule with family members for visits.	Spread out visits to help dispel loneliness.	Wife is trying to set up visiting schedule.

Critical Thinking Questions

1. What other psychosocial problems might this resident have?
2. Once he is stronger and able to walk with assistance, what measures could you take to help prevent him from falling?
3. What type of activities will help him to restore muscle strength?

bathing, feeding, ambulation, or range-of-motion (ROM) exercises; care of the resident unit; and transfer of residents from bed to chair. Patient care assistants are the core caregivers of the long-term care facility. The skillful LPN/LVN will establish rapport, harmony, and respect among the work team by valuing these workers, appreciating their contributions, and listening to their concerns.

 ## Assignment Considerations

Appropriate Assignments

When assigning tasks to unlicensed assistants (certified nursing assistants, patient care assistants, restorative aides), you must know that the person has shown competence at performing the task. Competencies of assistive personnel should be documented in their personnel files. Evaluation of task competence must be done at least annually. Give specific directions about what you want the person to do, how it is to be done, and what needs to be reported to you. You are responsible for the care of any resident or patient assigned to you. Do not assign unlicensed personnel to perform tasks for unstable patients.

When planning care for residents in a long-term care facility, the LPN/LVN must keep in mind that the overall goals of care for the facility are to provide a safe environment, assist the resident to maintain or attain as much function as possible, promote individual independence, and **allow the resident to maintain or achieve as much autonomy as possible.**

Safety. Providing a safe environment for a group of residents, many of whom may not be totally mentally competent, while allowing autonomy and independence is a great challenge. Two of the greatest safety concerns are to keep confused residents within the boundaries of the facility and to prevent falls. Those with physical disabilities need extra measures to ensure safety. National Patient Safety Goals (The Joint Commission [TJC], 2011) have been developed specifically for long-term care and rehabilitation facilities (Box 9-2). Meeting resident safety and independence needs without resorting to chemical or physical restraints requires caring, commitment, and ingenuity on the part of the nurse.

Fall Prevention. The first step in the prevention of falls is to recognize which residents are at greatest risk (Box 9-3). All residents are assessed for the risk of a fall on admission and whenever their condition changes (Box 9-4). The next step to prevent a fall is to recognize hazards in the environment that could precipitate a fall (Box 9-5).

Restorative programs focus on muscle strengthening and balance. Residents who are at risk for orthostatic hypotension (blood pressure that falls with position change from supine to sitting or standing) are taught ways to decrease the risk of falling. Be alert to the fact

---

Box 9-2	TJC National Patient Safety Goals

The 2010 National Patient Safety Goals that specifically pertain to long-term care and rehabilitation facilities include:

- **Identify residents correctly.** Use at least two ways to identify residents. For example, use the resident's name and date of birth. This is done to make sure that each resident gets the correct medicine and treatment.
- **Use medicines safely.** Take extra care with residents who take medicines to thin their blood.
- **Prevent infection.** Use the hand cleaning guidelines from the Centers for Disease Control and Prevention or the World Health Organization. Use proven guidelines to prevent infection of the blood from central lines.
- **Check resident medicines.** Find out what medicines each resident is taking. Make sure that it is OK for the resident to take any new medicines with their current medicines.
- **Prevent residents from falling.** Find out which residents are most likely to fall. For example, is the resident taking any medicines that might make him weak, dizzy, or sleepy? Take action to prevent falls for these residents.
- **Prevent bed sores.** Find out which residents are most likely to have bedsores. Take action to prevent bedsores in these patients. From time to time, recheck residents for bedsores.

From The Joint Commission. National Patient Safety Goals (2010): *Long Term Care.* The Joint Commission. (Retrieved from www.jointcommission.org/GeneralPublic/NPSG/10_npsgs.htm)

that a resident who was previously ambulating safely may be weakened if he has been recently sick with fever, urinary tract infection, flu, a cold, vomiting, or diarrhea. The resident who is receiving diuretic therapy must be assessed frequently for fluid and electrolyte imbalance that could cause weakness, dizziness, or confusion. Residents on diuretic therapy must receive prompt assistance for toileting when assistance is requested. The resident who needs narcotic therapy for pain or sedatives to sleep must be safeguarded. Instruct the resident to ring for assistance

---

Box 9-3	Problems and Disorders that Increase the Risk of Falls

- Musculoskeletal disorders that impair normal ambulation or balance
- Neurologic problems such as peripheral neuropathy affecting the feet
- Balance or gait problems resulting from stroke or inner ear problems
- Postural hypotension or dizziness caused by medications
- Impaired vision
- Impaired hearing
- Extreme weakness
- Oxygen deficit that may cause dizziness and loss of balance
- A history of previous falls

Box 9-4 **Fall Risk Assessment**

Place a check mark in front of the items that apply to the patient.

GENERAL INFORMATION
___ Age over 70
___ History of falls*
___ Confusion at times
___ Confused most of the time*
___ Impaired memory or judgment
___ Unable to follow directions*
___ Needs assistance with elimination
___ Visual impairment
___ Feels physically weak*

MEDICATIONS
___ Central nervous system suppressants (narcotic, sedative, tranquilizer, hypnotic, antidepressant, psychotropic, anticonvulsant)
___ Medication that causes orthostatic hypotension (antihypertensive, diuretic)*
___ Medication that may cause diarrhea (cathartic)
___ Medication that may alter blood glucose levels (insulin, hypoglycemics)

GAIT AND BALANCE
___ Poor balance when standing*
___ Balance problems when walking*
___ Swaying, lurching, or slapping gait*
___ Unstable when making turns*
___ Needs assistive device (walker, cane, holds on to furniture)*

*A check mark on any starred item indicates a risk for falls. A combination of four or more of the unstarred items indicates a risk for falls.
From deWit, S.C. (2009). *Fundamental Concepts and Skills for Nursing* (3rd ed.). Philadelphia: Elsevier Saunders, p. 325.

Box 9-5 **Interventions to Help Prevent Falls**

- Keep pathways free of objects.
- Remove loose rugs or secure with a nonslip pad.
- Place shoes and slippers underneath the bed or chair rather than in the pathway.
- Provide lighting without glare or deep shadows.
- Provide adequate night lighting for the pathway from the bed to the bathroom.
- Wipe up spilled liquids immediately.
- Keep wheels locked on all equipment when stationary.
- Place belongings within easy reach to prevent leaning from the bed or chair.
- Check to see that the call bell is within reach before leaving the room.
- Promptly answer call light to prevent the resident's arising without assistance.
- Encourage the use of supportive, sturdy footwear with nonslip soles for ambulation.
- Floor covering should not be slippery or highly patterned, and should be easily navigated when ambulating in common footwear or with assistive devices.
- Encourage residents to crouch down rather than bending over to pick up something, and to sit to dry the feet and pull on underwear and pants.
- Place grab bars by the toilet, in the bath or shower, along each set of stairs, and in the hallways.
- Provide chairs that are the proper height and depth to prevent "falling" into the chair or leaning far forward to arise from the chair.

---

should the need to arise from the bed or chair occur. The bed should be kept in the low position.

 Safety Alert

Medication Assessment

Assess all medications a resident is taking to determine the risk of medication-induced postural hypotension or dizziness. Medications that cause dizziness are a frequent contributor to falls. Over-the-counter medications should be considered, as well as prescription medications.

 Think Critically

Can you describe how you would determine just how at risk a new resident is for falls? Can you identify points that should be included in the assessment of a high risk for a fall?

Use of Security Devices and Alternative Measures.

When a resident frequently forgets instructions to call for assistance, repeatedly attempts to get up and falls, or interferes with medical treatment by pulling out ordered tubes or scratching at wounds, the use of security devices may be necessary. However, these devices should only be used when all else has failed. Research has provided strong evidence that restraints increase rather than decrease the risk for injury (Hollins & Stubbs, 2011). Chemical restraints are tranquilizers or sedatives that calm a resident and alter behavior. Physical and chemical restraint use is restricted by law and is applied only as a last resort for safety when a resident is a proven threat to self or others.

⚖ **Legal and Ethical Considerations**

Considering Restraints

Patient deaths have occurred due to improperly applied restraints. Laws require that they be used only as a last resort for safety after all other measures have been tried—such as sitters, family at the bedside, alarms, or distractions—and these other measures have failed. Documentation must be thorough, indicating specific alternative measures that have been tried and that the measures have failed. Document the time the restraint is applied, the condition of the patient at that time, interim assessments, the time the restraint is removed, and the condition of the patient at the time when the restraint is removed.

The purpose of such statutes is to ensure that restraints are used to protect residents, not to hinder their movements for the staff's convenience. Alternative measures are always tried first (Box 9-6). When a

Chronic Illness and Rehabilitation   **CHAPTER 9**   **185**

Box **9-6**	Measures Helpful to Prevent the Need for Security Devices

- Explore what may be upsetting the resident and causing agitation.
- Place the restless or high-risk resident in a room or location close to the nurses' station where he can be checked frequently and attempts to get up will be most likely observed.
- Reorient the acutely confused resident as frequently as possible.
- Use validation to reaffirm feelings and concerns of the resident with dementia.
- Provide distraction activities that keep the resident busy; give the person a "job" to do.
- If the resident is agitated, turn off the television and provide soft, soothing music.
- Provide familiar and cherished items that the resident can handle.
- Ask a family member to stay with the resident.
- Use a bed or chair alarm to alert nursing staff that the resident is attempting to get out of bed or chair unassisted.
- Remain with the unsteady, agitated, or confused resident when he is up and about.
- Leave another person in charge of your residents when leaving the unit for a meal break or other reason; specifically mention which residents need to be visually checked frequently.
- If a resident needs to get up at night frequently to urinate and does not call for assistance, restrict fluid intake after 6 P.M. if appropriate.
- Provide social and diversional activities to a resident confined to a wheelchair or bed so that boredom does not cause the person to try to get up and seek activity.
- Move the mattress onto a low platform or the floor so that it is easier for the resident to get in and out of bed without the risk of a fall.

Box **9-7**	Principles Related to the Use of Security and Safety Devices

- The use of safety or security devices must help the resident or be needed for the continuation of medical therapy.
- All devices that limit movement or immobilize must be ordered by a physician.
- Use the least amount of immobilization needed for the situation. For example, use mitts rather than wrist restraints if the resident cannot otherwise be prevented from pulling out tubes or lines.
- Apply the device snugly but not so tightly as to interfere with blood circulation or nerve function.
- If a security device is applied, check on the resident at least every 30 minutes. Assess for breathing, circulation, and possible nerve or skin impairment.
- An immobilization device must be removed and the resident's position changed at least every 2 hours. Active or passive exercises are performed for immobilized joints and muscles.
- Reassess need for the security measure every 4 to 8 hours.
- Meet needs for food, fluids, and toileting and assess these needs every 2 hours.
- Assess pain/comfort level and provide interventions as necessary.
- Document alternative measures taken and their success or failure. Document all pertinent data related to assessments when security devices are in place, when they were applied, and when removed.
- The physician should be notified as soon as the security device is deemed no longer necessary.

or repositioned every 2 hours. Thorough assessment of skin and circulation is done at that time. The restraint should be removed immediately after the risk has been lessened.

Managing Confusion and Disorientation. For the resident with mild confusion and disorientation, various techniques and measures are used to help maintain orientation. Reality orientation involves both the environment and the people who interact with the resident and should be an ongoing process. The environment is structured so that the resident has concrete and continual reminders of the year, day, and time of day. Environmental aids include a readable, up-to-date calendar, a clock, and the daily newspaper or local television or radio news (Figure 9-1).

Consistency in mealtimes, scheduled activities, treatments, and daily personal care routine also can be helpful. Limit the number of choices to be made during these activities. A time schedule for activities and events within the facility is posted in large type where the resident can refer to it frequently. Decorations for the next upcoming holiday give clues as to the current season of the year. Try to assign caregivers who are familiar to the resident, avoid placing the

security device is used, the least restrictive device is chosen. A variety of techniques help provide a restraint-free, yet safe, environment. The techniques depend on the type of population present in a facility. **All security devices must only be used as a last resort and must be ordered by a physician.** If a qualified, licensed nurse determines the need for a chemical or physical security device in an emergency, the need is specifically documented when the security device is applied. A physician's order for the security device must be written within 24 to 48 hours. Box 9-7 presents the principles related to the use of security and safety devices.

The resident who is immobilized with a security device must be checked visually at least every 30 minutes to ensure that the resident's body is in good alignment and that there are no problems. These checks must be documented. Whenever you are in the patient's room, check skin color for circulation in the affected body parts. Residents must be turned

<h1></h1>

FIGURE 9-1 Promoting reality orientation in the long-term care environment.

resident in unfamiliar situations, and limit visitors to one or two people at a time.

A positive and helpful approach is to respond continuously to the resident's confusion with honest and real information. Assess the possibility of a physical cause for the confusion, such as urinary tract infection, constipation, dehydration, or suboptimal pain control.

Nocturnal confusion (sundowning) occurs often among some elderly residents. Sensory deficits, such as impaired sight and hearing, add to the resident's confusion and anxiety at night when the environment becomes different because of darkness. A night-light that gives illumination without shining in the resident's eyes or causing frightening shadows can be used. Keep the call bell within reach and visit the resident frequently to calm and reassure. Moving the resident closer to the nurses' station, touching, and other signs of caring are all ways to intervene to minimize nocturnal confusion. A bed alarm that alerts staff when the resident attempts to get out of bed is helpful. Door alarms that announce when the resident has left his room, or designated area, may be used in place of security devices and prevent patients from wandering in unsafe areas. Keeping the resident active during the day and encouraging physical exercise helps promote sleep at night. **Listening to the resident to try to determine any possible cause of unrest or fear can often help solve the problem.**

Promoting Independence. The move to a long-term care facility is a major upheaval for the resident, particularly when it is for the remainder of the person's lifetime. Specific goals should be set with the resident to encourage independence in activities of daily living (ADLs) and in recreational activity. Perhaps a resident can pursue a former hobby, such as knitting or playing the piano, if such activities are available. Adaptive devices and a consultation with the dietitian may provide all the assistance that is necessary for self-feeding once again. Other adaptive devices can make daily living considerably easier (Table 9-2). **To promote a resident's independence, staff members should refrain from doing tasks that the resident is capable of doing himself.** For the resident who has had a stroke or suffers from debilitating arthritis or other musculoskeletal problem, use of adaptive devices can assist in the promotion of independence, provide some autonomy, and help to maintain function (Figure 9-2).

Table 9-2 Uses of Common Assistive-Adaptive Devices

DEVICE	USE
Buttonhook	Threaded through the buttonhole to enable patients with weak finger mobility to button shirts. Alternative uses include serving as a pencil holder.
Sock puller	Assists in putting on socks and compression stockings. Is placed in sock; then pulling on the strings pulls up the sock.
Extended shoe horn	Assists in putting on shoes for patients with decreased mobility. Alternative uses include turning light switches off or on while the patient is in a wheelchair.
Plate guard	Applied to a plate to assist patients with weak hand and arm mobility to feed themselves.
Gel pad	Placed under a plate or a glass to prevent dishes from slipping and moving. Alternative uses include placement under bathing and grooming items to prevent their movement.
Foam buildups	Applied to eating utensils to assist patients with weak hands to grasp and help feed themselves. Alternative uses include the application to pens and pencils to assist with writing, or over a buttonhook to assist with grasping the device.
Hook and loop fastener (Velcro) straps	Applied to utensils, a buttonhook, or a pencil to slip over the hand and provide a method of stabilizing the device when the patient's handgrasp is weak.
Long-handled reacher	Assists in obtaining items located on high shelves or at ground level for patients who are not able to change positions easily.
Elastic shoelaces or Velcro shoe closure	Prevents the need for tying shoes.

Adapted from Ignatavicius, D.D., & Workman, M.L. (2010). *Medical-Surgical Nursing: Critical Thinking for Collaborative Care* (6th ed.). Philadelphia: Elsevier Saunders, p. 103.

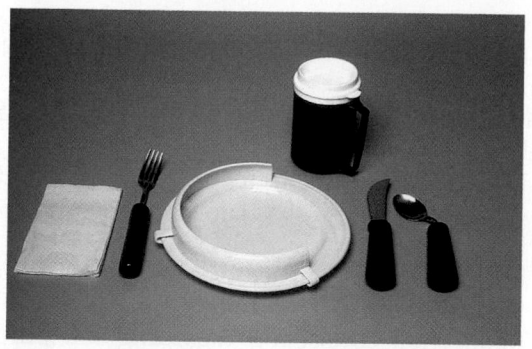

FIGURE 9-2 Adaptive devices to promote independence in eating.

Clinical Cues

Activity theory states that people will be happiest in direct proportion to how much activity they are able to maintain as they grow older. Continuity theory proposes that participation in activities and relationships that have been maintained over a long period of time contributes to a sense of well-being and allows a sense of integrity and continuity with the past. Finding out what activities have significant meaning for the resident, and seeing how those might be continued by making adaptations so that enjoyment in the activities is possible, can greatly enhance the quality of the resident's life.

? Think Critically

Can you think of three ways to foster independence in the new resident who is still quite weak, has suffered a stroke, and has right-sided **hemiparesis** (weakness)? He is right-handed.

Maintaining Function. Once a functional assessment has been completed, specific goals should be written to maintain the highest level of function possible for the resident. If the resident is ambulatory, exercise should be planned and encouraged on a daily basis. If the resident is not ambulatory, ROM exercises should be performed several times a day. Measures to promote continued bowel and bladder continence are essential. Assessing patterns of elimination and providing assistance for toileting as needed is a basic part of promoting continued function and protecting the resident's dignity. If the resident has been temporarily incontinent because of illness or surgery, a bowel or bladder retraining program is appropriate. Chapters 30 and 35 discuss such programs.

Mental stimulation is essential to maintaining a high level of cognitive functioning. Although resident preference and values should be considered in group television viewing areas, the staff should consider planning segments of time to turn on informational programs that are interesting. Scientific shows, travel shows, public television specials, and similar programs can stimulate thinking and encourage the sharing of thoughts on a variety of subjects. Assisting residents to work crossword puzzles is another way to help them keep an active mind. When a resident cannot write or read because of poor vision, group work on a puzzle is an option. Card games promote mental stimulation as well as social interaction. Group activities such as bingo, group singing, holiday celebrations, and entertainment acts provide socialization and stimulation. Continuing interest in lifelong activities is a factor in successful aging for many.

Documentation. Documentation in a long-term care facility is somewhat different from documentation in the hospital or in home care. For long-term care documentation, an admission assessment and an extensive 38-page Minimum Data Set (MDS) form that is required by the federal government are filled out. Bowel and bladder training assessment forms and training program forms, weekly pressure ulcer reports, and 24-hour intake and output records are some of the other documentation forms used in the long-term care facility.

REHABILITATION

Rehabilitation is the process whereby a disabled person is helped to achieve optimal function. A primary goal of rehabilitation is to minimize the deficit from the condition and maximize the abilities that are intact. It involves measures to achieve the highest possible levels of physical, emotional, psychological, and social function and well-being. Vocational rehabilitation is job retraining for the disabled under the Americans with Disabilities Act (ADA) to provide a means of contributing to self-support. Rehabilitation is concerned with achieving a better quality of life. The majority of patients who require rehabilitation services are disabled as a result of a chronic illness. Others have become disabled from trauma incurred during an accident. Several of the objectives for *Healthy People 2020* are rehabilitation oriented.

Each year about 8000 spinal cord injuries occur in the United States, and one out of four of the more than 2 million people who suffer head injuries annually have residual deficits. Another objective of *Healthy People 2020* is to reduce the incidence of secondary disabilities associated with injuries of the head and spinal cord. As the population ages, more people suffer heart attacks and strokes, which often leaves them with residual deficits. The need for rehabilitation services will continue to grow rapidly.

REHABILITATION PROGRAMS

Rehabilitation services are offered in freestanding rehabilitation hospitals, rehabilitation units in general hospitals, and skilled nursing home units where the patients stay for a few weeks.

Patients who have had a hip replacement often are placed in a skilled nursing facility for rehabilitation before returning home. Many communities have a hospital with an outpatient rehabilitation program for patients with cardiac and respiratory problems. Rehabilitation services are scarce in rural areas, and patients who have suffered neurologic injury or loss of musculoskeletal function due to amputation, trauma, or disease often have to go to a rehabilitation center miles away from home. Programs within large cities are often available for vision or hearing rehabilitation. YMCAs often have rehabilitation programs with water exercise for patients with severe arthritis. Most burn centers have comprehensive rehabilitation programs available for the burn patient. Rehabilitation programs have a philosophy that is based on three beliefs:

1. Each person is unique, whole within himself, and interdependent with his own environment.
2. Independence can be achieved within the limits of disability when the person is a full participant in managing his own life.
3. The goal is to enable patients to mobilize their own resources, choose goals, and attain them through their own efforts.

Rehabilitation involves a team effort directed at holistic care and involves a variety of disciplines.

 Elder Care Points

An elderly patient who has suffered a major loss of body function may not be initially receptive to rehabilitation efforts. It takes a skillful nurse to help motivate the patient to want to improve his functional ability. Sometimes introducing the patient to someone close to his own age who has been through a similar illness and has managed to regain some functions is the best "medicine." Gentle encouragement with praise for small efforts and accomplishments is better than trying to force the patient to perform exercises or practice tasks.

A respiratory rehabilitation program teaches self-care techniques to the patient that will help him attain a better quality of life. There are generally three components to a respiratory rehabilitation program:

1. Breathing exercises
2. Paced walking exercise
3. Correct use of inhaled medications

Patients are enrolled in the program for a number of weeks and interact with other patients who have the same problems. A nurse or respiratory therapist teaches the various breathing techniques, paced walking, and use of inhalers. The nurse conducts motivational group activities to increase the desire to participate in an exercise program and to display the benefits of following the program. Teaching how to avoid respiratory infections is reinforced. The nurse or respiratory therapist is available to encourage the patient and, while exercising, to evaluate the patient's progress in using the techniques taught. Vital signs are monitored periodically to determine the effect of exercise on cardiac and respiratory function. Some rehabilitation centers provide respiratory services that wean the patient from the ventilator and then work with him to improve respiratory function and functional capacity for ADLs.

Cardiac rehabilitation programs are usually outpatient based and consist of:

- Monitored exercise to increase strength and endurance and build collateral circulation to the heart
- Diet counseling and education to lower cholesterol, triglycerides, and body fat
- Medication counseling regarding the purpose, administration, and side effects of the prescribed medications
- Vital sign monitoring to determine the effect of exercise on the cardiovascular system
- Group sessions on stress reduction techniques
- Support group sessions for those experiencing depression or anxiety after surgery or a myocardial infarction

Such cardiac rehabilitation programs usually have a physician, nurses, physical therapist, dietitian, and psychologist or social worker on staff.

Rehabilitation after knee surgery and other musculoskeletal injuries is often performed on an outpatient basis. Either the physical therapist goes to the home or the patient travels to the physical therapy facility. Supervised exercise is performed to increase ROM, decrease pain, strengthen muscles, promote ambulation, and improve balance.

Patients with neurologic damage from a spinal cord or head injury may need to spend several months in a rehabilitation facility. Because of insurance limitations, inpatient treatment is not always possible. Rehabilitation efforts then need to be continued at home.

THE REHABILITATION TEAM

The nurse who works with rehabilitation patients must be flexible and creative and recognize that the patient is the "captain" of the rehabilitation team. The nurse's function is to assist the patient to achieve an optimal state of wellness as *defined by the patient*. It is very important that the nurses be nonjudgmental and not impose their own values and attitudes on the patient.

The rehabilitation nurse must be able to work collaboratively with other health team members. Besides the physician, occupational, physical, speech, cognitive, and recreational therapists, vocational counselors, and social workers are part of the team. The nurse assists in seeing to it that the patient correctly performs exercises and activities as instructed by such therapists and reinforces their teaching. A collaborative or interdisciplinary care plan is followed so that each member of the team is aware of what treatment and education the patient is receiving. Both short- and long-term goals are set. This provides for continuity of interdisciplinary care, recognizing the critical importance of each discipline in promoting positive outcomes for

FIGURE 9-3 The rehabilitation team conferring about the patient's care.

the patient. Team conferences are scheduled regularly for members to collaborate on the patient's care and evaluate rehabilitation progress (Figure 9-3).

The patient and family both undergo considerable stress during the rehabilitation period. Caregivers should assist both patient and family in developing positive coping techniques. A good sense of humor, gentle, firm people skills, patience, and the ability to provide solid encouragement are good tools for working with rehabilitation patients.

The philosophy of rehabilitation nursing is based on the recognition of the patient's need for independence. Learn to judge when the patient should be allowed to struggle to do something on his own, and learn to recognize when the patient's frustration is reaching a level at which assistance is needed.

Roles of the LPN/LVN in Rehabilitation

There are often two levels of LPN/LVNs employed in rehabilitation facilities. One is the licensed LPN/LVN I and the other is the licensed LPN/LVN II with intravenous therapy and Functional Independence Measure (FIM) certification. The LPN/LVN I does not infuse intravenous therapy, but does all other nursing activities except for assessments. The LPN/LVN II performs the same functions as the LPN/LVN I plus the tasks involved with intravenous infusions. At least a year of medical-surgical experience is required for employment as a nurse in a rehabilitation facility. The LPN/LVN initiates and participates in updating the team plan of care in collaboration with the RN to meet the patient's needs. The LPN/LVN assists with patient and family education by supporting the outlined teaching plan and reinforcing teaching. Any barriers to patient/caregiver readiness to learn are reported by the LPN/LVN to the supervisor. Recommendations are made by the nurses to team members on how to facilitate patient/caregiver learning. Learning outcomes are evaluated and documented. The LPN/LVN is an active participant and facilitator of both structured and nonstructured learning experiences. Leadership functions of the LPN/LVN are to supervise the patient

care assistants, the certified nursing assistants, and the nursing rehabilitation technicians. The LPN/LVN acts as a preceptor for unlicensed personnel as needed and appropriate. As a member of the team, the LPN/LVN carries out all normal patient care nursing duties, and provides input and feedback to the team. When assigned to do so, the LPN/LVN carries out quality improvement activities.

❖ NURSING MANAGEMENT

■ Assessment (Data Collection)

After obtaining a thorough history, a physical and psychosocial assessment are performed for each patient to establish a baseline; to determine physical limitations, ability to perform ADLs, and amount of assistance needed; and to identify present psychosocial difficulties.

A skin risk assessment and fall risk assessment are performed (see Chapter 43 for the pressure ulcer risk assessment tool). Patients covered by Medicare will have data filled in on the section of the MDS pertinent to rehabilitation. The patient's home environment is examined before discharge to determine whether physical features of the home, such as stairs, narrow doorways, or access to bathroom facilities, will present a problem. Questions about the neighborhood, such as the location of shopping centers and types of transportation available, are asked. Inquiries about who does the grocery shopping, cooking, errands, and housework for the patient are made.

The patient's usual daily schedule and habits of everyday living are examined, including sleeping, waking, eating, elimination patterns, hygiene, grooming, sexual activity, working, and leisure activities. A *functional assessment* of how the patient's disability has affected his former usual patterns (Box 9-8) focuses on the patient's present ability to perform ADLs, such as toileting, bathing, dressing, grooming, and ambulating, as well as his ability to use the telephone, shop, prepare food, and perform housekeeping chores. Various assessment tools are used to determine the patient's ability to function. A common one, the Katz Index of Independence in Activities of Daily Living, helps evaluate how much assistance the patient needs for various activities.

Box 9-8	Functional Independence Measure Scoring Categories

- Self-care
- Sphincter control
- Transfers
- Locomotion
- Communication
- Social cognition

A score of 0 or 1 is given in each category. Totaled scores indicate independent (6-7), modified dependence (3-5), or complete dependence (1-2).

Focused Assessment

For the Rehabilitation Patient

After reviewing the patient's history, the following data are collected by asking pertinent questions for each body system of function.

CARDIOVASCULAR
- Fatigue
- Chest pain
- Arrhythmia
- Fear of cardiac event

RESPIRATORY
- Activity tolerance
- Shortness of breath
- Fear of not being able to breathe

GASTROINTESTINAL/NUTRITION
- Dysphagia
- Anorexia, nausea, vomiting
- Eating pattern; amount of oral intake
- Weight loss or gain
- Bowel status; change in stool
- Serum albumin levels

URINARY
- Urinary pattern
- Fluid intake
- Retention
- Self-catheterization status
- Urinalysis and/or culture

NEUROLOGIC
- Motor function
- Sensation
- Cognitive abilities
- Assistive devices

MUSCULOSKELETAL
- Muscle strength
- Range of motion
- Endurance
- Fall risk assessment
- Assistive devices
- Safety measures

INTEGUMENTARY
- Skin condition
- Skin risk of breakdown
- Presence of lesions
- Measures to decrease risk of breakdown

DEGREE OF INDEPENDENCE
- Functional Independence Measure (FIM) scores per certified personnel assessment
- Ability for ADLs (Katz assessment, see p. 191)

PSYCHOSOCIAL
- Alteration in roles
- Financial concerns
- Support people
- Self-concept status
- Coping mechanisms
- Sexual concerns
- Employment/educational concerns
- Family strain
- Home environment alterations needed

MEDICATIONS
- Scheduled medications
- PRN (as-needed) medications

SAFETY
- All equipment in use checked for safety
- Risk assessments for falls and skin
- Prostheses applied correctly
- Adaptive equipment obtained

The Baird Body Image Assessment Tool is often used to perform a psychosocial assessment, which includes evaluating self-esteem and body image. Use of defense mechanisms, level of anxiety, and usual coping techniques are explored. To ascertain the patient's response to loss, ask the patient to describe feelings related to the loss of a body part or body function. The patient's support systems and the family's coping abilities also are determined. As rehabilitation progresses, the nurse performs a vocational assessment so that the vocational counselor can assist the patient in finding appropriate training, education, or employment after discharge from the rehabilitation program.

Patients with life-changing illness or injury, those who have suffered major loss of body function or former roles, and those who have lost most of their independence and social contacts may suffer from anger and depression. Assessing mental outlook is an ongoing nursing function. Should several signs of severe depression become evident, consult with the physician. The patient must be kept safe. Determining suicide potential in the depressed patient is important. Chapter 49 discusses assessment and intervention for depression and suicidal thought.

Sexual concerns should be addressed during the rehabilitation period. Help the patient identify problems and concerns and work to assist in finding means for sexual expression and gratification. If you are not comfortable or knowledgeable in this role, an appropriate referral to a psychologist or sex therapist should be made.

 Think Critically

Can you explain the difference between a physical assessment and a functional assessment?

■ Nursing Diagnosis

Nursing diagnoses appropriate for the patient undergoing rehabilitation are listed in Box 9-9. Individual nursing diagnoses are chosen based on the data collected.

■ Planning

An interdisciplinary plan of care is devised for each rehabilitation patient. Often there will be five or more health professionals involved. Periodic care conferences are essential for the members of the health care team to evaluate the progress of the patient, to share perceptions and ideas, and to revise the plan of care if it is not helping the patient to meet established expected outcomes. Depending on the situation, care conferences may occur once every 1 or 2 weeks or once a month. Both long-term and short-term goals will be set. Expected outcomes are written for each nursing diagnosis.

Box 9-9	Nursing Diagnoses Common for Patients in Rehabilitation

- *Impaired physical mobility* related to neuromuscular impairment, sensory-perceptual impairment, and/or pain
- *Self-care deficit (specify deficits)* related to perceptual or cognitive impairment and/or neuromuscular impairment
- *Risk for impaired skin integrity* related to alteration in sensation, mobility, or nutritional status
- *Risk for injury* related to musculoskeletal weakness or perceptual or cognitive impairment
- *Impaired urinary elimination* related to neurologic dysfunction or trauma or disease affecting spinal nerves
- *Constipation* related to neurologic impairment or immobility
- *Ineffective coping* related to added stressors or situational crisis
- *Compromised family coping* related to situational crisis and/or added stressors
- *Impaired home maintenance* related to neuromuscular impairment or perceptual or cognitive impairment
- *Deficient knowledge* related to self-care and techniques for rehabilitation
- *Disturbed body image* related to loss of normal function or traumatic injury and/or scarring
- *Sexual dysfunction* related to neuromuscular impairment, pain, or impaired mobility

■ Implementation and Evaluation

Interventions are carried out in a manner that encourages the patient to do as much for himself as possible. Praise is given for even small accomplishments or attempts at self-care. When working with the patient, observe for undue fatigue. Pace activities according to the patient's fatigue level. Physical and occupational therapists work closely with rehabilitation patients to help them adapt so that patients can perform ADLs (Figure 9-4). Speech therapists, activity therapists, and others will be involved in the implementation of the care plan. The patient will be kept very busy during rehabilitation.

Discharge planning is implemented from the time the patient enters rehabilitation. The family and patient will need resources within the community. Evaluation is performed by gathering data that show whether the goals and expected outcomes have been met.

HOME CARE

The majority of care in the community setting is given by home health and hospice agencies. Home health care is the preferred and most cost-effective method of health care delivery. Recent innovations in medical equipment have allowed more complex, high-technology care to be given at home. For the patient there are many benefits, both physically and psychologically. **The goal of home care is to keep the patient as well and independent as possible and enable him to stay at home.** The LPN/LVN must have 1 year's experience working in an acute care facility before being hired for home care in most states.

For home care, the RN acts as case manager and coordinates the care of all of the health care providers involved in the patient's care. The RN is responsible for the plan of care and for seeing that care is delivered in an uninterrupted manner. This nurse must act as a liaison with the other care providers to see to it that all efforts effectively complement one another. The LPN/LVN may perform treatments, perform appropriate delegated duties of the RN, or be employed to provide care in the home on a daily shift basis.

Home care nursing can prevent a patient's expensive readmission to a hospital or the entry into a long-term care facility. Home health care is family centered, and the family members are also responsible for the ongoing care of the patient. The nurse visits to intervene and see that the patient is provided comfort, that complications are prevented and health is improved, and to assist with rehabilitation (Figure 9-5).

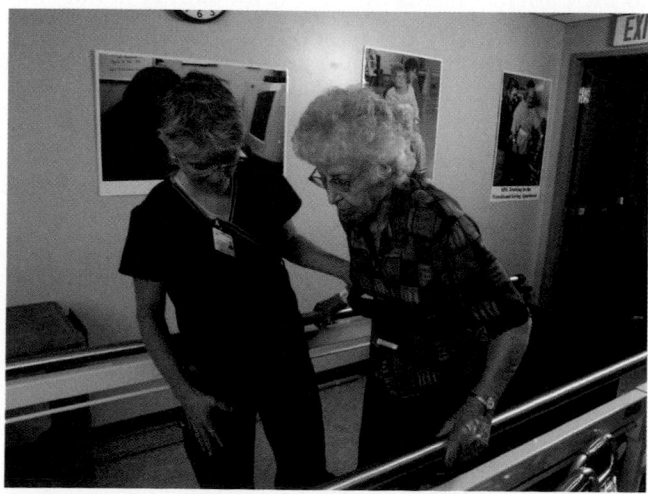

FIGURE 9-4 Physical therapist working with a patient on ambulation and muscle strengthening.

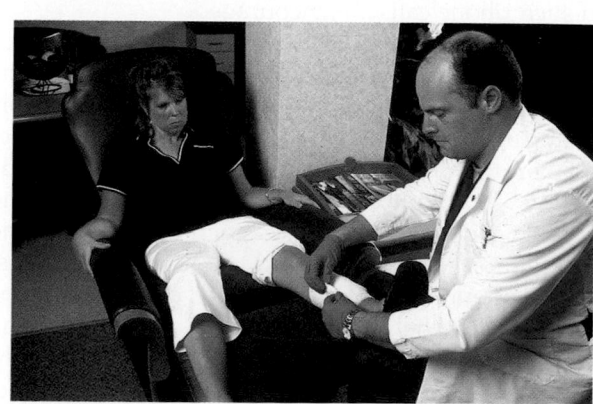

FIGURE 9-5 Home health nurse changing a dressing.

Because home health care is family centered, **the philosophy of the nurse must have a different focus. In the home care setting, the patient and family are in charge. The nurse is a guest in the home, and acts as a consultant, coordinator of care, provider of skilled care, teacher, and advocate.**

In home care, the patient and family are seeking the nurse's services and must be treated as valued customers. You must learn to be nonjudgmental of the patient, the family, and the living arrangements. Together, the nurse and patient and family set goals for care, and then establish boundaries of the nurse's role. Should the living situation not be ideal, furnishings and equipment lacking, or the home dirty, establish trust with the patient and family before trying to accomplish major changes. Be sensitive to the patient and family's cultural values, financial resources, and specific ways of doing things and try not to impose your own views. Work together with the patient and family to improve home safety, and share knowledge of available resources. **A home care nurse must be very flexible and creative in teaching patients and families ways to accomplish care of the patient while abiding by the principles of asepsis and safety.**

A large percentage of the home care nurse's time with the patient is spent evaluating physical and psychosocial status, signs of complications, side effects of medications, and effects of therapy. Both the safety of the home and the quality of nutritional and basic care are evaluated. The nurse is with the patient and is able to gather considerable useful data for the physician. Considerable time is spent consulting with physicians by phone, updating them on the patient's condition, seeking new orders, and collaborating about care needs. Each visit to the patient includes a physical assessment of the identified problems and of nutritional, home safety, elimination, skin, and psychosocial status. All findings are documented. The nurse also documents data indicating that home health nursing care is still needed. Between visits, the nurse may contact the patient or family to check on various aspects of care or to see whether there are any concerns. The patient and family may contact the agency or the nurse at any time, and such phone calls are encouraged.

Other functions of the home health nurse include performing wound care and dressing changes, organizing medications for scheduled administration, monitoring blood sugar levels, drawing blood samples for laboratory testing, giving injections or teaching injection technique, monitoring pain control, and monitoring enteral feedings. Teaching self-care and rehabilitation techniques and monitoring progress and compliance with treatment are primary nursing functions that help control health care costs and keep the patient from needing hospitalization. The home care nurse needs to be a strong advocate for the patient's needs and treatment.

The home care nurse provides considerable psychosocial care for the patient and family. Sometimes, the nurse is the only visitor the patient has. In this instance, the nurse becomes a sort of friend, providing social interaction as well as needed health care. The nurse must become knowledgeable about negotiating the complex medical care system and obtaining supplies, medications, or services when the patient does not have money for them. A full knowledge of the community's resources available to the patient is essential. Most home health agencies have lists of resources available. The medical social worker who has a liaison with the agency also can be of help. Whereas the hospital nurse stays out of financial concerns (except for referrals to the social worker) the home care nurse must try to help the patient find remedies to financial problems so that stress will be reduced and energies can be directed at healing and techniques of self-care.

> ### ? Think Critically
>
> Can you explain how you would go about trying to obtain a shower chair for a patient who cannot afford to buy or rent one?

THE LPN/LVN IN HOME CARE

Generally the LPN/LVN working in home care is under the supervision of the RN case manager. The LPN/LVN may be providing "private-duty" services for an unconscious patient who needs skilled care such as tracheal suctioning or tube feedings, performing home visits to change dressings or monitor blood sugar levels, or possibly acting as an in-agency supervisor by coordinating home health aide visits and supervising their work. The role of the LPN/LVN in home care is growing. The family provides assistance with personal care, and a home health aide may visit a few times a week to bathe the patient and shampoo hair. Homemaking is provided by family members, or by a homemaker aide. "Sitters" may be hired to attend to the patient's needs at night if the family is not able to provide this service.

Nursing care plans are formulated, considering 24-hour needs, in collaboration with the patient, the family or relatives, and all other health care providers. Case conferences are conducted regularly, even if they are done by the case manager on the telephone with the others involved in the patient's care. Medicare requires a case conference every 60 days when more than one discipline is involved in the patient's care.

THE FAMILY CAREGIVER

When a patient has considerable disability and cannot function independently, a family member often becomes the main caregiver. Depending on the degree of dependence of the patient, the caregiver may have an overwhelming task in caring for the patient, maintaining the house, obtaining food and supplies,

◎ Focused Assessment

Assessing Caregiver Stress

- What help do you have in caring for your spouse/relative?
- Are there more family members who might help out?
- What are your cultural values related to caregiving?
- Is your sleep often disturbed because you have to meet your spouse/relative's needs?
- Do you feel strained with all your family and caregiving responsibilities?
- Have you been feeling edgy or irritable lately?
- Are you feeling overwhelmed?
- Do you feel you cannot leave your relative alone?
- Have you been having crying spells?
- Are you having difficulty making decisions?
- Do you find you have trouble keeping your mind on what you are doing?
- Are you having frequent headaches, backaches, or muscle or stomach pain?
- Do you have any social contact?

cooking, and coordinating therapy or physician appointments. The caregiver's usual life is disrupted and social contacts are limited due to time constraints and fatigue. The nurse must assess the caregiver's stress levels regularly.

Some home care agencies have an assessment tool for this purpose. When caregiver stress is high, calling the agency social worker for a consultation can provide either more help for the caregiver, or a respite program that might provide the caregiver a few days of needed rest and relaxation. A respite program provides room, meals, and care for a patient while the caregiver is relieved of all responsibility.

Get Ready for the NCLEX® Examination!

Key Points

- Chronic illness interferes with normal function for about 43 million people in the United States.
- Hazards of immobility are numerous and can occur within just a few days for the immobile patient.
- It is a nursing responsibility to prevent hazards of immobility.
- The elderly are especially prone to develop problems of immobility.
- The LPN/LVN often works as a charge nurse in a long-term care facility.
- The LPN/LVN supervises the nursing assistants in the long-term care facility.
- Safety of residents is a primary goal in the long-term care facility.
- Much attention is directed to preventing resident falls.
- Security devices are only used to protect the resident, or others, and only as a last resort.
- Frequent assessment is essential when a security device is applied to a resident.
- Techniques to minimize confusion and disorientation are used consistently.
- Keeping the resident active during the day helps decrease nocturnal confusion.
- A goal of long-term care is to promote as much independence as possible for the resident.
- Long-term care facilities must help residents to maintain or regain function.
- Rehabilitation helps a disabled person to achieve optimal function.
- There are rehabilitation programs for patients with respiratory, heart, and musculoskeletal problems.
- Rehabilitation is a team effort of the patient and many health professionals.
- The nurse assists with determination of rehabilitation needs.
- Rehabilitation is carried out with a collaborative plan of care.

- Home care agencies provide continuing care in the community.
- LPN/LVNs are supervised by the physician or RN in the home care environment.
- In the home care setting, the patient and family are in charge; the nurse is a guest in the home.
- Home care nurses must be flexible and creative in order to accomplish needed care of the patient in the home.

Additional Learning Resources

SG Go to your Study Guide for additional learning activities to help you master this chapter content.

evolve Go to your Evolve website (http://evolve.elsevier.com/deWit/medsurg) for the following FREE learning resources:
- Animations, audio, and video
- Answers and rationales for questions and activities
- Concept Map Creator
- Glossary with pronunciations in English and Spanish
- Interactive Review Questions and Exercises and more!

 Online Resources
- National Council on Disability, www.ncd.gov
- National Rehabilitation Information Center, www.naric.com

Review Questions for the NCLEX® Examination

1. A 78-year-old woman is admitted with sudden onset of confusion and disorientation during the early evenings. Her family indicates that she is generally alert and oriented during the day. The nurse would likely recommend:
   1. keeping soft lighting without shadows on during the evening.
   2. promoting activity and physical exercise during the day.
   3. encouraging napping during the day.
   4. medicating with sleeping pills.

2. The nurse is assessing a patient's spouse for caregiver distress. Which question would be appropriate?
   1. "How long have you been married?"
   2. "What television shows do you watch?"
   3. "Are there any available resources to help you take care of your spouse?"
   4. "How is your fatigue level?"

3. A 56-year-old man is admitted for shoulder surgery. On transfer to the medical-surgical unit, the patient complains of pain when he raises his arm. The dressing is dry and intact. Vital signs are 120/60, HR 55, RR 12, and temperature 99° F (37° C). An appropriate nursing diagnosis would be:
   1. *Self-care deficit.*
   2. *Ineffective coping.*
   3. *Risk for infection.*
   4. *Impaired physical mobility.*

4. The nurse gives discharge instructions to an 80-year-old Asian woman who had open heart surgery. After detailing the importance of increasing activity, the patient smiles and nods her head. The nurse understands that the patient:
   1. understood the instructions.
   2. acknowledged the efforts of the nurse.
   3. demonstrated enthusiasm with increasing activity.
   4. may not understand the instructions.

5. During a home visit, the nurse finds scatter rugs all over the house, the kitchen sink full of dirty dishes, the toilet has a strong odor, and the pantry and refrigerator have several outdated food items. The 76-year-old patient is coherent with occasional forgetfulness, disheveled with stained clothing, and generally ungroomed. An appropriate nursing diagnosis would be:
   1. *Decisional conflict.*
   2. *Powerlessness.*
   3. *Self-care deficit.*
   4. *Imbalanced nutrition: less than body requirements.*

6. The nurse reinforces the use of an incentive spirometer to a patient with blunt chest injury. Understanding of nursing instructions is clear when the patient:
   1. exhales normally.
   2. takes rapid, shallow breaths.
   3. seals the mouthpiece during exhalation.
   4. tilts the incentive spirometer.

7. The nurse provides discharge instructions regarding home safety to a 78-year-old woman. Which patient statement indicates a need for further teaching?
   1. "Scatter rugs would be useful in decreasing glare from shiny floors."
   2. "My favorite slippers can be stored underneath my bed."
   3. "I need to have a handyman install grab bars in the bathroom."
   4. "I need to be really careful when picking up something."

8. The nurse admits a 70-year-old woman who is hard of hearing and has bilateral cataracts. The patient is taking antihypertensive medications. A priority nursing diagnosis would be:
   1. *Risk for falls.*
   2. *Impaired verbal communication.*
   3. *Deficient knowledge.*
   4. *Activity intolerance.*

9. After failure of less restrictive measures, the nurse decides to apply physical restraints to a confused elderly man. Which measure(s) must the nurse include to ensure safe use of physical restraints? *(Select all that apply.)*
   1. Promptly attend to the toileting needs of the patient.
   2. Reevaluate use of the restraints every shift.
   3. Ensure adequate nutrition and hydration.
   4. Administer scheduled doses of sedative-hypnotics.
   5. Provide frequent range-of-motion exercises.

10. The nurse suspects early complications of immobility in a 45-year-old patient admitted for multiple stab wounds to the chest. What sign would the nurse most likely find? *(Select all that apply.)*
    1. Increased muscle strength
    2. Generalized weakness
    3. Moist breath sounds
    4. Limited range of motion
    5. Pain with repositioning

Critical Thinking Activities

Scenario A

Mr. Porter has been discharged home and transferred to a home health nursing agency for continued care after suffering a stroke that has left him with left-sided hemiplegia and dysphagia. His wife will be taking care of him, but she has severe arthritis and cannot perform many needed tasks. You are assigned to provide "private-duty" care to him as he must have tube feedings.

1. What assessments would you make each day?

2. How would you collaborate with the case manager and the physical therapist?

3. How would you plan care for rehabilitation?

4. What would you teach Mr. Porter's wife about taking care of the equipment for his tube feeding?

Scenario B

Mrs. Robbins is a new resident in the long-term care facility in which you work. She is mentally alert, but needs assistance with bathing, dressing, and toileting because of arthritis and weakness and fatigue from heart failure. She can use a walker to ambulate short distances, but does not like to do so.

1. How would you promote independence and autonomy for this resident?

2. How can you promote maintenance of function for her?

3. How would you promote socialization for Mrs. Robbins?

The Immune and Lymphatic Systems

chapter

10

Objectives

Theory

1. Describe the body's innate (natural) immune response.
2. Compare and contrast the characteristics of innate and acquired immunity.
3. Describe the role of the lymphatic system in the immune response.
4. Identify the various ways in which immunity to disease occurs.
5. Analyze the factors that interfere with normal immune response.
6. Explain the role of immunizations in relation to immunity.

7. Compare and contrast the responsibilities of different members of the health care team in preventing infection in immunocompromised patients.

Clinical Practice

1. Identify assessments that indicate immune system function.
2. Describe precautions to be taken for patients with an impaired immune system.
3. Evaluate your patient's risk for infection during a clinical experience.

Key Terms

acquired immunity (ă-KWĪRD ĭ-MŪ-nĭ-tē, p. 202)
antibodies (ĂN-tĭ-bŏ-dēz, p. 197)
antigens (ĂN-tĭ-jĕnz, p. 198)
antigen-antibody response (ĂN-tĭ-jĕn ĂN-tĭ-bŏ-dē rē-SPŎNS, p. 201)
antitoxin (ĂN-tĭ-tŏk-sĭn, p. 200)
autoimmune disease (ăw-tō-ĭ-MŪN dĭ-ZĒZ, p. 199)
autoimmunity (ăw-tō-ĭ-MŪN-ĭ-tē, p. 202)
cell-mediated immunity (sĕl MĒ-dē-ā-tĕd ĭ-MŪ-nĭ-tē, p. 201)
complement system of proteins (PRŌ-tēnz, p. 202)
cytokines (SĪ-tō-kĭnz, p. 200)
homeostasis (hō-mē-ō-STĀ-sĭs, p. 198)

humoral immunity (HŪ-mŏr-ăl ĭ-MŪ-nĭ-tē, p. 200)
hyperpyrexia (hī-pĕr-pī-RĔX-ē-ă, p. 211)
iatrogenic (ī-ăt-rō-JĔN-ĭk, p. 203)
immune deficiency (ĭ-MŪN dĭ-FĬSH-ĭn-sē, p. 199)
immunization (ĭm-ū-nĭ-ZĀ-shŭn, p. 204)
immunoglobulins (ĭm-ū-nō-GLŎB-ū-lĭnz, p. 200)
immunoscintigraphy (ĭm-ū-nō-sĭn-TĬG-ră-fē, p. 206)
innate immunity (ĭ-NĀT ĭ-MŪ-nĭ-tē, p. 202)
lysis (LĪ-sĭs, p.200)
neutropenia (nū-trō-PĒ-nē-ă, p. 212)
passive immunity (PĂ-sĭv ĭ-MŪ-nĭ-tē, p. 202)
stromal cells (STRŌ-măl sĕlz, p. 199)
toxin (TŎK-sĕn, p. 200)

OVERVIEW OF ANATOMY AND PHYSIOLOGY OF THE IMMUNE AND LYMPHATIC SYSTEMS

WHAT ARE THE ORGANS AND STRUCTURES OF THE IMMUNE AND LYMPHATIC SYSTEMS?

- Bone marrow produces a type of stem cell that is able to produce all types of blood cells (white blood cells [WBCs], red blood cells [RBCs], and platelets), which then *differentiate* (acquire individual characteristics) into the cells of the hematologic and immune systems (Figure 10-1). B lymphocytes are produced and mature in the bone marrow and play a significant role in the humoral immune response.

- The thymus gland, located behind the sternum (breastbone), is the place where T lymphocytes mature and are released into the bloodstream.
- Lymph nodes and vessels circulate fluid called *lymph*. It contains nutrients such as proteins, glucose, monocytes, and lymphocytes. Lymph nodes (Figure 10-2) are also where most lymphocytes are initially exposed to foreign antigens such as bacteria, fungi, and viruses.
- The lymph vessels are located near the blood vessels and capillaries. The lymph system removes what is left over after the plasma has delivered nutrients to the cells.

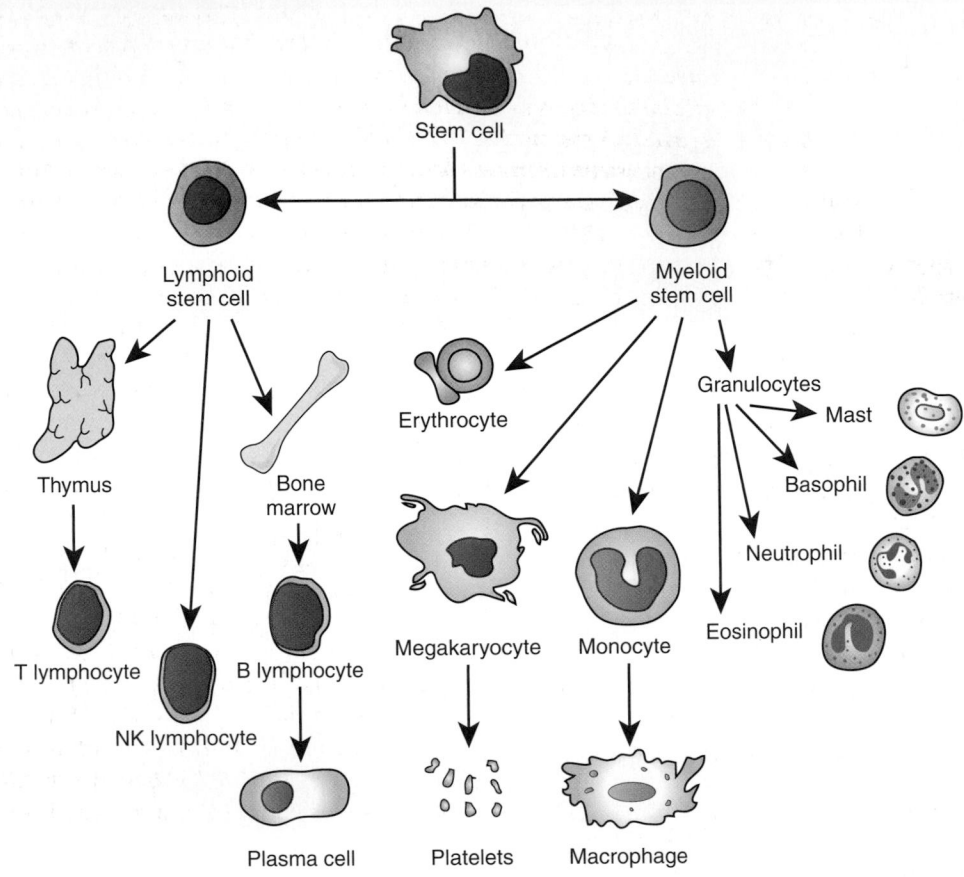

FIGURE 10-1 Maturation of blood cells.

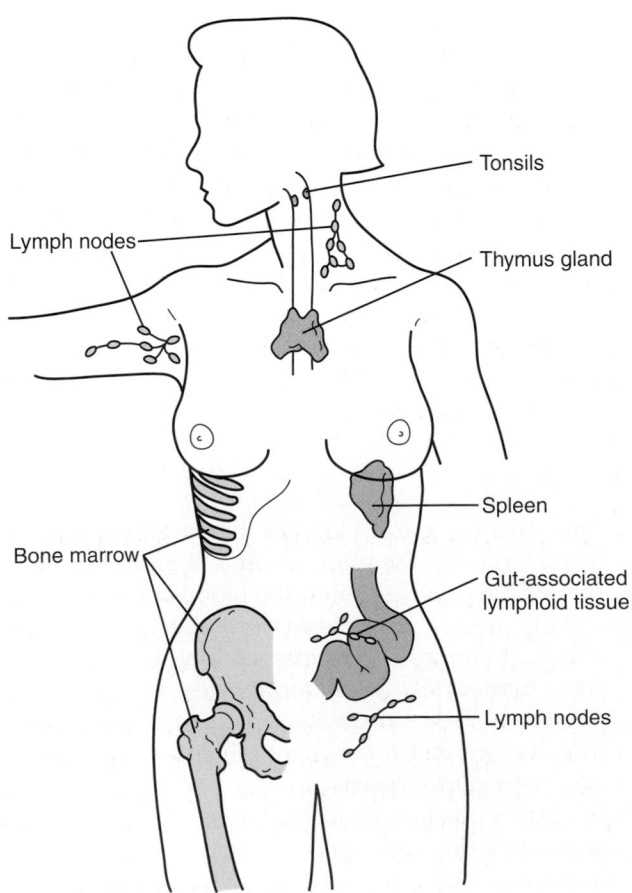

FIGURE 10-2 Organs of the immune system.

- The lymph fluid drains into large veins, blending with the plasma circulating in the bloodstream.
- Tonsils and adenoids are lymph tissues that guard the airway from inhaled microbes.
- The spleen filters blood, which allows lymphocytes to come into contact with any circulating organism, thus activating the appropriate lymphocyte response. It also filters out damaged or old RBCs, recycling the hemoglobin in the production of bilirubin.
- Peyer's patches are lymphoid tissue typically found in the ileum portion of the small bowel. These patches help defend against ingested pathogens.

WHAT ARE THE FUNCTIONS OF THE IMMUNE AND LYMPHATIC SYSTEMS?

- The immune and lymphatic systems work together to guard the body against pathogens and to eliminate them if they manage to pass through external barriers.
- The neutrophils and macrophages of the hematologic system assist the immune system by phagocytosis when an antigen is encountered.
- Chemical mediators, plasma cells, and B and T lymphocytes play active roles in the immune response (Table 10-1).
- Both humoral and cellular immunity are carried out by the lymphocytic cells, a specialized type of WBC that originates in the bone marrow.

Table 10-1   Major Components of the Immune System and Their Functions

COMPONENT	FUNCTION
Antigen	Foreign substance or component of cell that stimulates immune response
Antibody	Specific protein produced in humoral response to bind with antigen
Autoantibody	Antibodies against "self" antigen; attacks body's own tissues
Bone marrow	Source of stem cells, leukocytes, and maturation of B lymphocytes
Thymus	Gland located in the mediastinum, large in children, decreasing size in adults; site of maturation and proliferation of lymphocytes
Lymphatic tissue	Contains many lymphocytes; filters body fluids, removes foreign matter, immune response
Cells	
Neutrophils	White blood cells: for phagocytosis; nonspecific defense; active in inflammatory process
Basophils	White blood cells: bind immunoglobulin E; release histamine in anaphylaxis
Eosinophils	White blood cells: participate in allergic responses
Monocytes	White blood cells: migrate from the blood into tissues to become macrophages
Macrophages	Phagocytosis; process and present antigens to lymphocytes for the immune response
Mast cells	Release chemical mediators such as histamine in connective tissue
B lymphocytes	Humoral immunity–activating cell becomes an antibody-producing plasma cell or a B memory cell
Plasma cells	Develop from B lymphocytes and secrete specific antibodies
T lymphocytes	White blood cells: cell-mediated immunity
Cytotoxic or killer T cells	Destroy antigens, cancer cells, virus-infected cells
Memory T cells	Remember antigens and quickly stimulate immune response on reexposure
Helper T cells	Activate B and T cells; control or limit specific immune response
Natural killer (NK) lymphocytes	Destroy foreign cells, virus-infected cells
Chemical Mediators	
Complement	Group of inactive proteins in the circulation that when activated stimulate the release of other chemical mediators, promoting inflammation, chemotaxis, and phagocytosis
Histamine	Released from mast cells and basophils, particularly in allergic reactions; causes vasodilation and increased vascular permeability or edema, also contraction of bronchiolar smooth muscle, and pruritus
Kinins (e.g., bradykinin)	Cause vasodilation, increased permeability (edema) and pain
Prostaglandins	Group of lipids with varying effects; some cause inflammation, vasodilation, increased permeability, and pain
Leukotrienes	Group of lipids, derived from mast cells and basophils, that cause contraction of bronchiolar smooth muscle and have a role in development of inflammation
Cytokines (messengers)	Includes lymphokines, monokines, interferons, and interleukins; produced by macrophages and activated lymphocytes; stimulate activation and proliferation of B and T cells (communication between cells); involved in inflammation, fever, and leukocytosis
Chemotactic factors	Attract phagocytes to area of inflammation

From Dyer, R., & Gould, B.E. (2010). *Pathophysiology for the Health Professions* (4th ed.). Philadelphia: Elsevier Saunders, p. 37.

- T lymphocytes, which provide cell-mediated immunity, pass through the thymus and migrate to the lymph tissues throughout the body.
- B lymphocytes migrate to lymphoid tissue, where they wait in readiness to form either sensitized lymphocytes or antibodies (immunoglobulins that identify and neutralize foreign objects).
- The lymph system, in addition to facilitating the work of lymphocytes, also drains tissue fluid and puts it back into the circulation.
- Innate (natural) immunity is nonspecific immunity that is in humans when they are born, making them not susceptible to diseases of other species.
- Immunity can be acquired actively or passively.

WHAT EFFECTS DOES AGING HAVE ON THE IMMUNE AND LYMPHATIC SYSTEMS?

- Neonates are susceptible to infection due to an immature immune system.
- The thymus gland is largest during childhood and adolescence. After adolescence it begins to shrink in size and its production of T lymphocytes decreases.

- Aging causes skin to become thin, less elastic, and more prone to injury. The skin is the first barrier encountered by pathogens.
- Decreased ciliary action in the respiratory system and gastrointestinal tract results in decreased removal of potentially harmful organisms.
- The presence of chronic diseases can decrease the immune response.

PROTECTIVE MECHANISMS OF THE IMMUNE AND LYMPHATIC SYSTEMS

The immune and lymphatic systems work together to defend against threats from multiple sources inside and outside of the body. Except for the central nervous system, some portion of the lymphatic system is found in every part of the body. The sensory nervous system interacts with the lymphatic system by helping to alert the body to outside physical threats by relaying chemical signals back to the brain. Internally, the blood and lymphatic systems are constantly protecting against microscopic threats to homeostasis (tendency to maintain internal stability and balance). The hematologic system interacts in the production of specialized white blood cells that help fight infection and rid the body of foreign invaders. The primary job of the immune system is to protect the body from agents that can cause disease. A review of the structure and functions of the immune and lymphatic systems is necessary to understand immune responses.

The human body has multiple protective mechanisms. The first line of defense begins with the skin, tears, earwax, mucous membranes, and urinary tract. They all provide external barriers to prevent foreign substances and microorganisms from entering the body. Natural (innate) immunity is present in the body even before exposure to any unknown antigen occurs. What this means is that the body has the ability to recognize certain microorganisms as harmful, even without prior encounters. This recognition allows the body to immediately lodge a defense because the tissue damage created by the invading microorganisms releases certain chemicals within the body. These chemical triggers, such as histamine, lead to the activation of the inflammatory response, which then causes the blood and lymphatic systems to deliver certain types of WBCs, lymphocytes, proteins, and other nutrients to the affected area.

INFLAMMATORY RESPONSE

Trauma, pathogenic microorganisms, chemicals, or heat may cause injury to tissues inside and outside of the body. The first step in the body's defense mechanisms against this invasion is inflammation or the inflammatory response (see coverage of the inflammatory response in Chapter 6). If the injury is close to the external surface of the body, there will likely be obvious redness and swelling, and the area may also be warm and tender to the touch. These findings are due to select cells, proteins, and chemicals being sent to the affected area. The delivery of these substances increases blood flow to the site by dilating blood and lymphatic vessels upstream of the injury, resulting in warmth and redness. The same substances also affect downstream vessels, causing vasoconstriction and swelling. If the effects of swelling are not quickly controlled, the edema can compress nerve endings surrounding the area of injury, leading to a pain reaction.

The inflammatory response alone may be adequate in killing the invading organism by creating a hostile environment (see Figure 6-2). Protective proteins that are activated in the inflammatory response include the *complement system* of proteins. Several of these protein enzymes, when sequentially activated, form a "membrane attack complex" (MAC) that embeds itself into the cell membrane of the attacking microbe. This activation occurs when there is exposure of complement-binding sites on antibodies after they attach to antigens. This binding causes a break in the cell wall allowing for ions, such as salt, to enter the cell. The salt is followed by water, which causes swelling and bursting of the microbe.

The same WBCs, lymphocytes, proteins, and chemicals respond to internal tissue injury. The results are not as readily visible, but are detectable if appropriate assessments are conducted. The mechanisms of the inflammatory response combine with the immune response to eliminate foreign invaders (Figure 10-3).

IMMUNE RESPONSE

The immune response is a remarkable series of complex chemical and mechanical activities that take place in the body. These activities involve (1) constant surveillance to detect the entry of foreign agents (antigens) as soon as they gain access to the body's cells; (2) immediate recognition of the agents as "non-self" (i.e., foreign or alien); and (3) the ability to distinguish one kind of foreign agent from another and to remember that particular agent if it appears in the body again at a later time. The lymphatic system, thymus, spleen, lymph nodes, bone marrow, and Peyer's patches in the small intestine play a major role in the immune response (see Figure 10-2). As previously mentioned, many different cells, proteins, and chemicals assist in the body's defense against invading agents.

The immune response is usually triggered by the body's identification of something as foreign or "non-self." This recognition is essential for the body to respond to a foreign threat in an appropriate manner and to not react to tissues or cells that are typically recognized as "self." When an inappropriate

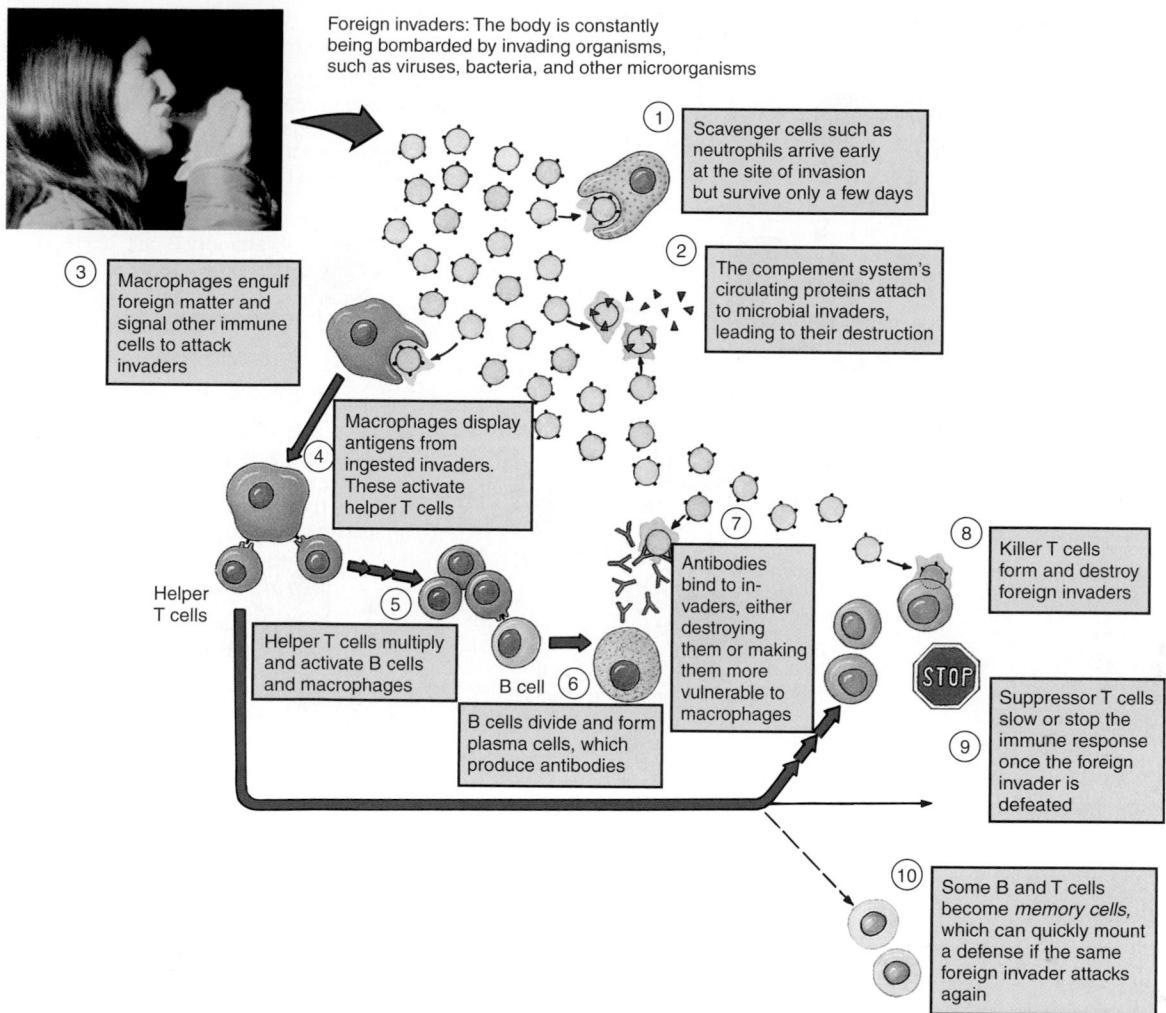

FIGURE 10-3 Action of the immune response against foreign invaders.

response happens, one of two types of disorders occurs. If there is a lack of appropriate response, an **immune deficiency** is present. The second type of disorder occurs when the body produces an immune response to a "self" cell or tissue, causing an **autoimmune disease.** It is important to recognize that while injury can activate a response by the immune system, massive trauma or chronic illness can inhibit the ability of this vitally important system to respond effectively.

Types of Immunity

Once a particular kind of foreign substance has been detected and identified, the body responds in two general ways. **It immediately produces a protein (called an *antibody*) that is specifically designed to do battle with the *antigen.* The immediate response is called a *humoral response. Humoral* refers to any fluid or semi-fluid. There is also a delayed response that involves the use of sensitized lymphocytes to attack whole cells, such as those of bacteria, viruses, and malignant (cancer) cells. This second kind of response is called a *cellular* or *cell-mediated* response.

The cells that mediate the response are the T lymphocytes. Examples of antigens include bacteria, viruses, fungi, and other infectious microorganisms, as well as the toxins they produce as they invade the body. Nonliving matter such as pollen, dust, and chemicals can also be antigens. For some people, certain foods are perceived by the body as antigens and result in an adverse reaction, such as anaphylaxis, when the particular food is eaten.

T cells and B cells interact with each other in complex ways. Helper T cells must interact with B cells before the B cells can become plasma or memory cells. The suppressor T cells regulate the amount of antibody that B cells produce. Both T cells and B cells are necessary for a normal immune response to occur. Acquired and inherited disorders can inhibit T- and B-cell activity.

Primary Humoral Response. Lymphocytic B cells are involved in humoral immunity and the production of antibodies. They arise from stem cells in the bone marrow and undergo a maturation process that involves bone marrow **stromal cells** (cells that contribute to the

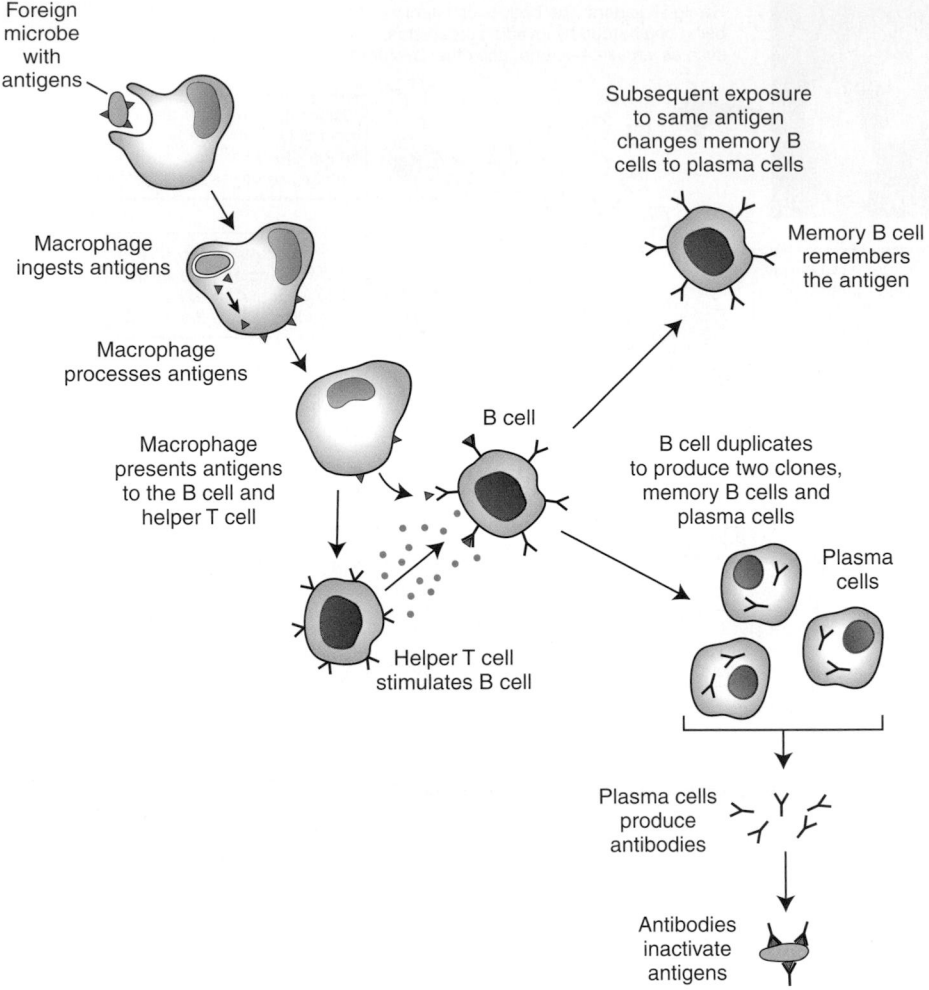

FIGURE 10-4 Humoral (antibody-mediated) immunity.

development of multiple tissues and blood cells) and their **cytokines** (messenger hormones). When mature, the B cells migrate to the lymph nodes. When stimulated by an antigen, a B cell becomes a plasma cell that secretes antibody molecules into the bloodstream. B cells secrete immunoglobulins called antibodies in response to the specific antigen they encounter. This is antibody-mediated or **humoral immunity** (Figure 10-4). Some of the antigen-stimulated B cells become memory cells. This mechanism is the basis for acquired immunity. The memory cells reactivate the plasma cells to produce large quantities of the specific type of antibody needed to fight the particular type of antigen, when the same antigen enters the body a second time. It is an immediate and potent response, and antibodies continue to be produced for many months.

When the body is exposed to a harmful substance, the immune system produces antibodies, which are a type of protein synthesized by plasma cells. These antibodies are also called **immunoglobulins.** There are five classes of immunoglobulins (Ig): IgA, IgD, IgE, IgG, and IgM. Each immunoglobulin is able to attach to the kind of antigen for which it is made (Table 10-2).

The antibody's ability to form a bond with its antigen is important to the destruction of the antigen, but it can sometimes result in damage to the body's own cells. Antibodies are found in the serum of blood and in other body fluids and tissues, including tears, saliva, breast milk, spinal fluid, interstitial fluid, lymph nodes, the spleen, and urine. An antibody can either destroy or inactivate its particular antigen by (1) mechanically harming it, (2) activating a complement system, or (3) causing the release of chemicals that affect the environment of the antigen.

Through a process called **lysis** the antibody prepares the antigen for ingestion by damaging the outer membrane of the antigen's cell. The damaged cell then ruptures, making its contents accessible for digestion by phagocytes.

If the antigen is a **toxin** (poison) produced by a bacterial or viral cell, the antibody produced to fight it is called an **antitoxin.** This antitoxin is capable of neutralizing the poisonous chemical of the antigen by covering the antigenic agent. An antitoxin is therefore a specific type of antibody that acts through the process of *neutralization.*

Table 10-2		Immunoglobulins and Their Functions	
CLASS	**PERCENT OF TOTAL***	**LOCATION**	**FUNCTION**
IgG	75–85	Blood plasma	Major antibody in primary and secondary immune responses; activates complement system; inactivates antigen; neutralizes toxins; crosses placenta to provide immunity for newborn; responsible for Rh reactions
IgA	5–15	Tears, saliva, mucus, breast milk, GI, pulmonary, prostatic and vaginal fluids	Protects mucous membranes on body surfaces; provides immunity for newborn; prevents antigens on food from being absorbed
IgM	5–10	Attached to B cells; released into plasma during immune response	First Ig to respond to microbial invasion; activates complement systems; causes antigens to clump together; responsible for transfusion reactions in the ABO blood typing system
IgD	0.2	Attached to B cells	Receptor sites for antigens on B cells; binding with antigen results in B-cell activation
IgE	0.5	Produced by plasma cells in mucous membranes and tonsils	Binds to mast cells and basophils, causing release of histamine; responsible for allergic reactions; helps fight off parasitic invasion

From Applegate, E. (2010). *The Anatomy and Physiology Learning System* (4th ed.). Philadelphia: Elsevier Saunders.
*Immunoglobulins.

When a bacterium or other antigen enters the body, it may encounter a B lymphocyte that is specific for that bacterium or antigen. The B lymphocyte becomes a plasma cell that secretes IgM (antibody), which attacks the bacterium or antigen. After the particular bacterium or antigen is encountered for the first time, it takes 4 to 8 days for the B lymphocyte to produce immunoglobulins that can attack. If the same bacterium or antigen enters the body again several months or even years later, the immunoglobulin response by the memory cells is much quicker so that the invading cells are attacked much sooner, typically 1 to 2 days after a reexposure. The major function of the humoral antigen-antibody response is to provide protection against acute, rapidly developing bacterial and viral diseases. The antigen-antibody response is also involved in allergic and transfusion reactions.

Secondary Cellular Response. **The second type of immunologic response of the body involves various interactions with antigens by T lymphocytes.** Unlike the humoral response, which takes place in the plasma, the cellular response involves whole cells called *sensitized lymphocytes* and occurs out in the tissues. They are said to be *sensitized* because they have been made sensitive to a specific antigen after their first contact with it. Subsequent exposure to the antigen to which they are sensitive triggers a host of chemical and mechanical activities, all designed to either destroy or inactivate the offending antigen.

Those lymphocytes destined to provide cellular immunity pass through the thymus and migrate to the lymph tissues throughout the body. These are called the *T lymphocytes* (the "T" is for thymus) and they are further divided into helper T cells, memory T cells, suppressor T cells, and sensitized T cells (killer cells). T cells provide defense against viral infections. Viruses are difficult to destroy because they inject themselves into host cells and reproduce themselves. T cells respond to foreign or abnormal molecules on the surface of cells. Host cells containing virus have small fragments of the virus slightly protruding from the cell membrane. T cells identify the virus fragment as foreign and kill the host cell. T cells and macrophages produce a variety of substances called *lymphokines* that help destroy antigens. Killer T cells attach themselves to cells bearing antigen and secrete toxic substances that kill the antigen-bearing cells. This cell-to-cell contact response is called **cell-mediated immunity** or cellular immunity (Figure 10-5).

The T lymphocytes mediate (indirectly accomplish) the cellular response. When an antigen is complex (e.g., a bacterium or another type of living cell), T lymphocytes that are specifically reactive with the particular antigen mediate the cellular response in several ways. These specific T lymphocytes enter the circulating fluids of the body from the lymphoid tissues, migrate widely, and react anywhere in the body where they encounter the particular antigen. Destruction of the antigen may occur by release of chemicals into the membrane of the target cell, by secretion of lymphokines such as interleukin-2 or T-cell growth factor, or by other processes. This direct contact by the T lymphocytes with an antigen is called *killer activity*, and such lymphocytes are named *killer T cells.* Cellular immune response is often termed *delayed hypersensitivity.* The larger the amount of antigen present, the greater the response of sensitized T lymphocytes.

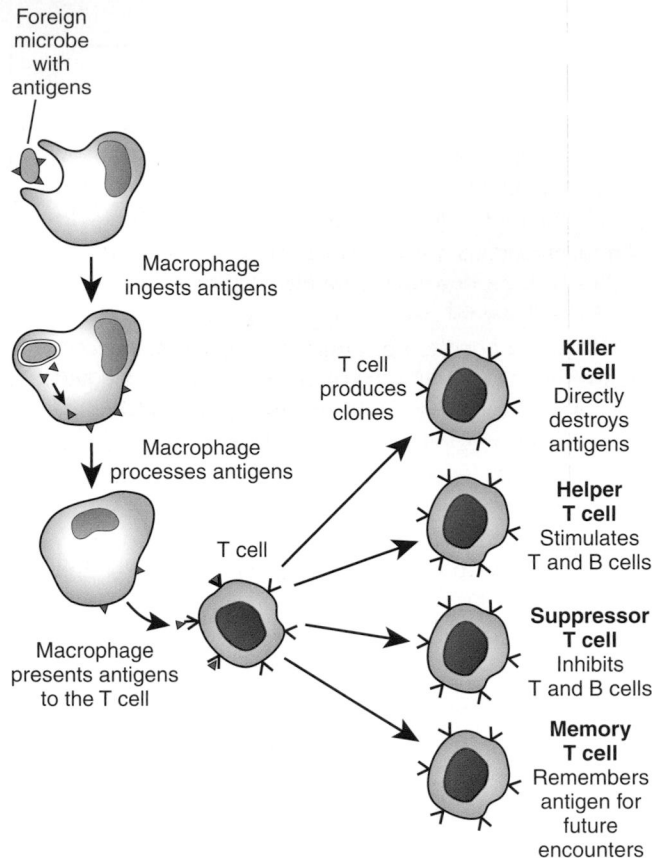

Foreign microbe with antigens

Macrophage ingests antigens

Macrophage processes antigens

T cell

Macrophage presents antigens to the T cell

T cell produces clones

Killer T cell
Directly destroys antigens

Helper T cell
Stimulates T and B cells

Suppressor T cell
Inhibits T and B cells

Memory T cell
Remembers antigen for future encounters

FIGURE 10-5 Cell-mediated immunity.

The **complement system of proteins** is a series of proteins produced in the liver that work with antibodies to destroy antigens. The complement system directly kills microbes by attaching to the cell wall and allowing salt and water into the cell, causing it to burst. It also assists in the inflammatory and immune response. The proteins of this system "complement" or assist the immune system.

The T lymphocytes perform immune surveillance for the body by detecting cells that enter the host and have foreign antigens on their surface. T lymphocytes are also defensive cells that patrol the blood and tissues. Sensitized T lymphocytes are the cause of allergic reactions. T cells are responsible for the inflammatory response present in people with a variety of autoimmune diseases. **Autoimmunity** means that there is a defective cellular immune response and antibodies are produced against normal parts of a person's body. These T lymphocytes, along with migrating macrophages, are responsible for rejecting transplanted organs as well. This is why transplanted tissue must have surface antigens that are very similar to those of the host (transplant recipient) tissue to be accepted by the host body.

Immunity Against Disease

There are two major types of immunity to specific disease: innate (natural) immunity and acquired (adaptive) immunity. **Innate immunity** is present at birth. **Acquired immunity** occurs by actively producing antibodies when the body has been invaded by pathogens, or by receiving an immunization that causes antibodies to a specific pathogen to form.

Innate (Natural) Immunity. Unique innate, or inborn, features of human cells make a person naturally immune to certain diseases. Humans are immune to some diseases simply by being human and are not susceptible to the same diseases as animals of other species. Some immunity is related to race, gender, or a particular inherited genetic makeup. Genetic factors present at birth may *predispose* individuals to immune disorders (Figure 10-6).

Acquired Immunity. In acquired immunity, a person can either actively produce her own antibodies or passively receive antibodies produced by another person or animal (**passive immunity**). *Passive natural immunity* is the type that is transmitted from mother to baby. The mother passes antibodies to the fetus in utero or after birth through breast milk. When the fetus is in utero, it passively receives some natural immunity when antibodies from the mother's bloodstream pass through the placenta and mix with the blood of the fetus. Those maternal antibodies are then present in the infant's blood at birth. More immunity can be passed to the infant through breast milk. Breast-feeding is the best way to protect the newborn from infectious disease. Depressed immune function in the mother can limit the benefits typically received from breast milk to her baby.

Administration of human immune globulin to boost the immune system is an example of *passive artificial immunity*. Human immune globulin, formerly called gamma globulin, contains antibodies against not just

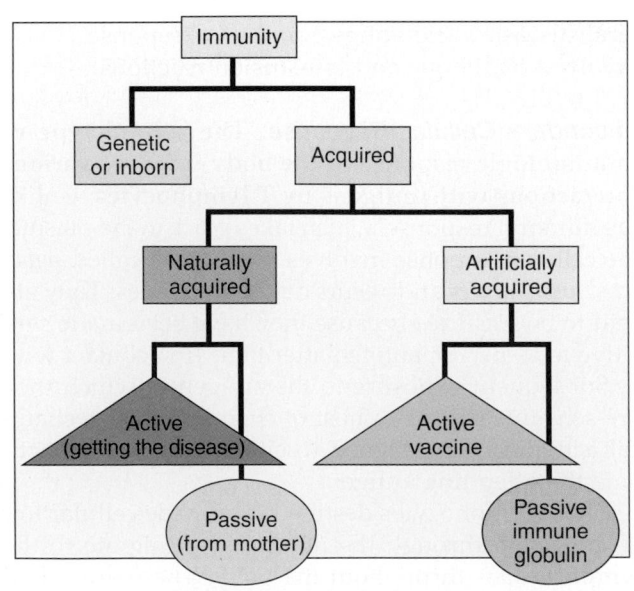

Immunity

Genetic or inborn

Acquired

Naturally acquired

Artificially acquired

Active (getting the disease)

Active vaccine

Passive (from mother)

Passive immune globulin

FIGURE 10-6 Types of immunity.

one, but many infectious diseases. It is developed from donated blood plasma and purified to prevent the spread of additional disease. This type of immune globulin is used when a susceptible person is exposed to or contracts a communicable disease such as hepatitis A, rubella, and varicella to help lessen the effects of the disease.

The blood serum from a horse contains ready-made antibodies and antitoxins against tetanus when the horse has been prepared with increasingly strong injections of that antigen. Antivenins that contain antibodies against snake venoms and the poisons produced by the black widow spider are also available. Injections that provide passive immunity should be given as early as possible in the disease as they only protect against further tissue damage. It is important to note that immune globulins, regardless of the source, cannot reverse damage already done.

Passive immunity is usually time limited as the antibodies provided only last for a specific period.

 Think Critically

What type of immunity is provided by a "flu shot"? How does an injection of human immune globulin protect a world traveler from hepatitis A?

Active naturally acquired immunity occurs when a person contracts and survives a disease. Once survival from a particular disease has occurred, the person is considered immune and should not fear contracting that particular disease again.

Active artificially acquired immunity occurs by vaccination or immunization. To provide active immunity to diseases by artificial means, the actual pathogenic microorganisms are grown and cultured in the laboratory. They are divided into single doses under rigid controls and made into vaccines. These specially treated microorganisms are weakened (attenuated) or killed so that they will stimulate the production of antibodies, but will not cause the disease itself. Vaccines from cowpox, tetanus, polio, influenza, measles, mumps, chickenpox, and hepatitis A and B viruses are examples of immunizing agents used to produce an active immunity in humans.

This method of stimulating the production of immunizing substances in the body is successful in situations in which there is time to wait for the person to build up her own defenses. This immunity does not last indefinitely. The body must be reminded of the need to produce more antibodies. To achieve this, a booster dose of an immunizing agent is given to jog the memory of the specific B cells and cause them to actively produce more antibodies. This is one reason why a yearly influenza vaccine is recommended and a booster for tetanus is recommended every 10 years.

IMMUNE AND LYMPHATIC SYSTEM DISORDERS

With all of the complexity of the human immune response, there are multiple natural areas of dysfunction that occur. One of the more commonly encountered reasons for alteration in immune function not caused by pathogenic factors is **iatrogenic**—a condition caused by medical treatment. Current therapies for asthma, inflammatory disorders, autoimmune disorders, and organ transplantation are all aimed at suppressing or attenuating the body's natural immune response. Although this effect is helpful in addressing the primary disorder, it also makes the patient more vulnerable to infection or other autoimmune diseases. Many over-the-counter medications have anti-inflammatory effects and are used to decrease pain caused by inflammation. The inflammation is the initiation of the immune process. Suppression of this response can hinder the body's ability to fight infection or disease.

 Elder Care Points

The older patient is at risk for problems with immunity due to decreased immune function. The older patient is more likely to have chronic illness and decreased nutritional intake. For those in long-term care facilities, living in close proximity to others makes transmission of communicable diseases easier if the appropriate Standard Precautions are not taken (see Chapter 6 and Appendix B).

Consumption of alcohol can alter the body's ability to launch an immune response. There are both long- and short-term effects of alcohol on the immune system. Two drinks can impair the ability of the B lymphocytes to produce antibodies and can affect T-cell activity. Long-term alcohol use leads to alteration in liver function and impaired nutrition, also altering immune function. Many other drugs, including cocaine, marijuana, and methamphetamines, also compromise the immune system.

Autoimmune disorders are caused by a malfunction of the body's immune system. When the body does not recognize tissues as "self," an autoimmune disorder occurs and the defense mechanisms are launched against the body's own tissues. The trigger for this dysfunction is largely unknown. Some conditions are thought to be initiated by a systemic infectious process and others by inherited factors.

 Health Promotion

Maintaining a Healthy Immune System

A healthy immune system is a function of a healthy body. Eating right and getting enough rest and exercise are all important in maintaining resistance to infection and disease. Frequently skipping meals, eating unhealthy meals, sleeping too little, or not exercising weakens the immune system and makes people more susceptible to pathogens.

Treat any patient with chronic substance abuse as immuno-compromised until proven otherwise.

PREVENTION OF IMMUNE AND LYMPHATIC SYSTEM PROBLEMS

Immunization

Before immunization and inoculation became commonplace, the only way an individual could acquire immunity was to contract the disease and survive. Today, immunity from immunizations is usually achieved by administering the vaccine in divided doses over weeks or months. This sets in motion the more powerful, longer lasting secondary immune responses. For example, infants are given immunizations at intervals during infancy and then periodically throughout early adolescence. To stimulate continued immunity, adults should have immunizations against tetanus and diphtheria every 10 years. The Centers for Disease Control and Prevention (CDC) also recommends that adults receive a one-time vaccine referred to as Tdap, which helps fight against tetanus, diphtheria, and pertussis. Patients should also be encouraged to discuss, with their health care providers, whether they should receive a hepatitis B vaccine booster.

Nursing Implications. The nurse plays a major role in providing education regarding the importance of immunizations. Vaccine-preventable diseases cause disabilities and deaths every year. Nurses can have significant influence by encouraging the public to participate in immunization programs recommended by public health officials and by helping to identify people in need of immunization. *Healthy People 2020* Goal 14 is to reduce or eliminate cases of vaccine-preventable diseases.

An important aspect of health teaching is to improve the general public's awareness of the importance of immunization as a means of avoiding certain diseases and their consequences. Despite the availability of vaccines against poliomyelitis, measles, rubella, mumps, and other potentially dangerous diseases, there still are many children who have not been adequately immunized. This is particularly true in areas populated by people who do not have easy access to the health care system. Nurses have a responsibility to inform the public on the purpose and importance of immunization in terms the layperson can understand. Figure 10-7 shows the secondary response and longer lasting immunity provided by a second injection of an antigen.

Legal and Ethical Considerations

Immunizations

Immunizations are a proven way to decrease illness for individuals and the spread of diseases in communities. Some religious and cultural practices forbid immunizations. How can the needs of society be balanced with the rights of individuals?

Parents should be told why immunization is important for their children and be warned of the dangers faced by children who are not adequately immunized. The nurse must present this information in such a way that the parents do not feel threatened or badgered. Older adults and others who are particularly susceptible to influenza and pneumococcal pneumonia should also be immunized according to the recommendations of public health officials. Health care workers should be immunized annually for influenza so they do not transmit the disease to susceptible patient populations. The CDC has recommended immunization schedules for all ages, including those who have never been vaccinated.

Circumstances that require the modifying or postponing of immunization include fevers, immune deficiency disease, immunosuppressive therapy, and administration of human immune globulin,

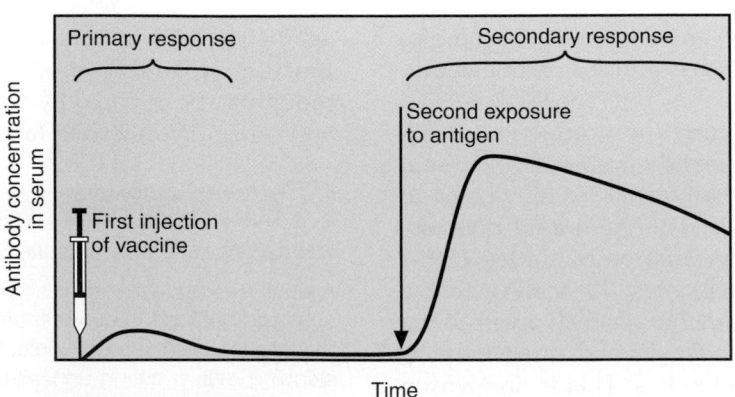

FIGURE 10-7 Comparison of primary and secondary immune response.

plasma, or whole blood transfusion 6 to 8 weeks before the immunization. Select immunizations are also contraindicated immediately before and during pregnancy and when a person is taking certain drugs; however, the influenza vaccine is not one of them. Brochures accompanying these drugs will state whether they prohibit the administration of an immunizing agent. The vaccine for tuberculosis (TB), bacille Calmette-Guérin (BCG), is not routinely used in the United States because of the low incidence of TB. In countries where TB is more prevalent, BCG is given; therefore individuals who have received vaccine will have a positive TB skin test for a number of years.

Whenever an immunizing agent is to be administered, precautions must be taken to ensure, as much as possible, that the patient is not hypersensitive to the components of the agent. Religious orientation is also important to consider as some vaccine products are made using pork or bovine serum and are strictly forbidden by their religious tenets. Many times chicken embryos, horse serum, and other substances are used to make the vaccine or immune serum. These substances can produce a serious allergic reaction in people who are hypersensitive to them. Immunizing agents that are most often associated with anaphylaxis, a potentially fatal reaction, include tetanus antitoxin, botulism antitoxin, diphtheria antitoxin, rabies antitoxin, and antilymphocyte globulin.

It is imperative that a history of allergies in the patient and her family be obtained before administering an immunizing agent. It also should be determined whether the patient has an immune deficiency disease of any kind that would prevent a normal immune response to the immunizing agent. If a patient does have a history of allergies or an immune deficiency, the health care provider should be made aware of this fact before the immunizing agent is given. If the patient has had an allergic reaction to the specific agent she is supposed to receive, the drug must not be given.

There are times when a skin sensitivity test is indicated before any serum is administered to a patient. Skin testing for sensitivity should not be confused with skin testing for diagnostic purposes. Testing for sensitivity is done to determine whether a minute amount of the immunizing agent will produce a local reaction. If it does, chances are the patient will have a severe reaction if the agent is given systemically. Botulism antitoxin is an example of a treatment that mandates a "scratch test" be performed before its administration.

In spite of these precautions, it is possible that a patient will suffer from hypersensitivity to an immunizing agent. To avoid serious problems, the nurse should always be prepared to act quickly and effectively in such an emergency. In all patient care areas where immunizing agents are administered, emergency equipment should be readily available. As an extra precaution to ensure prompt treatment of a hypersensitivity reaction if one occurs, it is advisable for people receiving immunizing agents to remain in the clinic or office for 15 to 20 minutes after an injection is given. This practice is in accordance with the National Patient Safety Goal of recognizing and quickly responding to changes in a patient's condition.

In addition to enhancing the immune system by administering immunizations, the nurse should instruct the patient in other measures for maintaining a healthy immune system. Keeping the body healthy is the best way to preserve immune function. Not smoking, staying physically active, getting adequate rest, and eating a balanced diet are all measures that should be encouraged.

 Complementary and Alternative Therapies
Garlic Assists Immune Action

Garlic has been used for centuries to increase resistance to the common cold and other infections. It has a variety of actions, including antilipidemic, antitriglyceride, antiplatelet, antioxidant, cancer preventive, and antimicrobial. It inhibits the growth of both gram-positive and gram-negative organisms and is effective against certain fungi, viruses, and helminths. Because garlic interacts with many drugs, the health care provider should be consulted before administration. It should not be used by pregnant women as it may induce labor. Patients on anticoagulants need to know that it may extend the action.

❖ NURSING MANAGEMENT
▪ Assessment (Data Collection)

If the immune system is functioning normally, there will be an absence of physical signs and symptoms. It is when the system is activated and doing its job or is unable to mount an active defense that detectable physical signs and symptoms may become evident.

Since the function of the immune system is to guard the body against microbial invasion, it is important to assess for signs and symptoms of infection. These include fever, redness, swelling, and exudate from open skin areas. Patients who have a known infection but do not exhibit obvious signs and symptoms of infection should be evaluated for an immune deficiency. Another indicator of a depressed or inadequate immune response is recurrent infections or infections of common organisms to which individuals with normal immune systems are not susceptible. A thorough history should be gathered.

Focused Assessment

Data Collection for the Lymphatic and Immune Systems

- What immunizations have you had? When were you last immunized for tetanus, diphtheria, and influenza?
- Have you had a recent infection or a recurrence of infection?
- Do you have any allergies?
- Do you have any chronic illnesses such as diabetes, rheumatoid arthritis, inflammatory bowel disease, Crohn's disease, lung disease, renal disease, or acquired immunodeficiency syndrome?
- Have you ever had cancer? Radiation therapy? Chemotherapy?
- Have you recently had surgery or a blood transfusion?
- Do you get sick frequently?
- Have you traveled out of the country?
- What do you usually eat in a day?
- Has your weight changed lately?
- Do you smoke, drink, or use illicit drugs?
- Have you been exposed to industrial/agricultural chemicals?
- Have you been exposed to industrial radiation?
- Are you on any medications?
- Do you take any supplements or herbal preparations?
- Do you see a physician regularly?
- Are you under excessive stress at home or in your job?
- Are you sexually active? Are you monogamous? (Try to determine sexual orientation.)

Previously diagnosed diseases affecting the immune system, immunizations, medications (including herbal supplements), allergies, and nutritional status are important areas to explore. The patient should also be questioned about any recent surgeries, blood transfusions, and diagnoses of chronic illnesses. Habits and lifestyle questions are also important to include in the data collection. Since important diseases affecting the immune system can be transmitted through the exchange of blood and body fluids, asking about the use of illicit drugs and sexual history are very important. Information regarding smoking history and exposure to environmental and industrial radiation or pollutants should also be obtained.

Physical Assessment

The skin is a major defense against access to the body by microorganisms. It is important to do a thorough assessment of the skin to identify any potential entryways for organisms. Remember to assess those areas where catheters, tubes, and other medical devices may penetrate the skin barrier. The skin may show excessive immune reaction, as in an allergic response resulting in hives or other skin eruptions.

Clinical Cues

Latex allergy can be another cause of redness at tube sites if the tube or the occlusive dressing contains latex.

When the immune response is activated, lymph nodes may become swollen and tender and can be evaluated by palpation. Nodes in the neck, axillae, and groin areas are those most commonly examined because they are closer to the skin surface. Data obtained from a head-to-toe physical assessment provide important information regarding immune and lymphatic system function.

Focused Assessment

Physical Assessment of the Lymphatic and Immune Systems

- Take vital signs, noting if there is an increase in temperature or pulse rate.
- Measure height and weight.
- Inspect the skin for color, turgor, texture, and presence of lesions.
- Assess extremities for edema.
- Inspect ears, eyes, nose, and throat for drainage, redness, or exudate.
- Palpate lymph nodes in the neck to identify enlargement or tenderness.
- Auscultate lung fields and assess work of breathing.
- Analyze laboratory results such as complete blood count (CBC), C-reactive protein, and antibody screening tests.

Diagnostic Tests, Procedures, and Nursing Implications

Skin Testing. *Skin testing* is one of the most commonly used techniques to measure immunity and to identify people who may have a dormant infectious disease. These tests include the *Schick test* to determine susceptibility to diphtheria and the *tuberculin skin test* (Mantoux test) to identify those who might need treatment for TB. The Mantoux test and other tests for TB are covered in Chapter 15.

Several types of skin testing may also be done to identify allergens that are causing allergic symptoms in an individual. A scratch test (also called a prick or puncture test) may be done by dropping extracts of allergens into scratches made on the skin. Intradermal injection of allergens is used to detect allergies to insect venom or penicillin. Patches containing allergens that might cause contact dermatitis are placed in direct contact with the skin. Inflammation and itching identify those allergens that provoke the immune system.

Laboratory Tests. Laboratory tests on blood and serum also give important information regarding the status of the immune system. A CBC gives information regarding the number of circulating WBCs. The differential indicates what percentage of the total WBC count is accounted for by the different cells. An increased white count indicates that the immune system has been activated (Table 10-3). If a specific disease or condition is suspected, blood testing can determine if antibodies to that disease or condition are present.

Imaging Studies. Immunoscintigraphy is a nuclear medicine imaging procedure in which antibodies labeled with radioactive isotope are injected into the

Table 10-3 Diagnostic Tests for Disorders of the Immune and Lymphatic Systems*

TEST AND NORMAL RANGE	PURPOSE	DESCRIPTION	NURSING IMPLICATIONS
Complete Blood Count (CBC)			
	Determine whether abnormalities are present in the numbers of blood cells or types of blood cells; assess the amount of hemoglobin present Useful to diagnose anemia	Fill a lavender-top tube containing EDTA with a venous sample of blood. Use a site where there is little chance of dilution from intravenous solution. Mix the blood and the EDTA by gently rotating the tube.	Warn the patient that a "stick" is about to occur, but that the pain will be short lived. Apply pressure directly to the puncture site after withdrawing the needle; at the antecubital space, do **not** have the patient flex the arm as this tends to cause a hematoma.
Erythrocytes			
Hemoglobin: females: 12.0-16.0 g/dL; males: 13.0-18.0 g/dL Red blood cell count: females: 4.2-5.4 million/mm³; males: 4.6-6.2 million/mm³ Hematocrit: females: 37%-47%; males: 40%-54%			
Leukocytes			
White blood cell (WBC) count: 4500-11,000/mm³			
Differential Count			
Granulocytes 　Neutrophils: 54%-62% of WBCs 　Eosinophils: 1%-3% of WBCs 　Basophils: 0%-1% of WBCs Agranulocytes 　Lymphocytes: 25%-33% of WBCs 　Monocytes: 3%-7% of WBCs Thrombocytes (platelets): 150,000-400,000/mm³ of blood Mean corpuscular hemoglobin (Hgb) (MCH): 26-34 pg/cell Mean corpuscular Hgb concentration (MCHC): 32-36 mg/dL Mean corpuscular volume (MCV): 80-96 μm³			
Lymphangiogram			
Normal-size vessels and nodes without filling defects	Detect abnormalities in the lymphatic system, especially cancer	Dye is injected intradermally between the first three toes of each foot while the patient is supine. Local anesthesia is injected, and an incision is made in the dorsum of the foot to inject iodine contrast material directly into a lymphatic vessel over a 1½-hr period. X-rays are taken of the abdomen, pelvis, and upper body.	Repeat films are taken in 24 hr. Obtain written consent. Assess for allergy to iodine or shellfish. Explain procedure. Postprocedure, elevate legs for 24 hr to decrease swelling. Assess for signs of infection and oil embolism q 4 hr × 24 hr.
Spleen Sonogram			
Proper size, shape, and position	Detect structural abnormalities of the spleen	An ultrasound wand is moved over the abdomen in the area of the spleen with the patient supine on the examining table.	Explain that the test typically takes about 30 min.

*Diagnostic tests for human immunodeficiency virus are presented in Chapter 11. Bone marrow aspiration is covered in Chapter 16.

Continued

Table 10-3 Diagnostic Tests for Disorders of the Immune and Lymphatic Systems—cont'd

TEST AND NORMAL RANGE	PURPOSE	DESCRIPTION	NURSING IMPLICATIONS
Spleen Scan			
Looks at the distribution of radioactive erythrocytes throughout the spleen	Detect anatomical changes in the spleen; determine invasion of Hodgkin's or metastatic disease Usually done in conjunction with a liver scan	A radioactive nuclide colloid is injected intravenously. After about 20 min, a minimum of three views are obtained. Radiation exposure is about 0.5 rad (equal to about 1 yr of natural radiation exposure to the body). Schedule scan before tests using barium.	Explain that a substance will be injected and, after about 20 min, scanning begins. Radiation exposure is minimal. The test takes about 60 min.
Immunoglobulins, Serum			
IgG: 564-1765 mg/dL IgA: 85-385 mg/dL IgM: 53-375 mg/dL IgD: 0-14 mg/dL IgE: 0 <100 IU/mL	Used to detect and monitor quantities of antibodies circulating in the blood Useful for monitoring hypersensitivity diseases, immune deficiencies, autoimmune diseases, and chronic infections	Serum is placed on a slide containing agar gel and an electrical current is passed through the gel. The immunoglobulins are separated out and electrophoresed according to the quantity and difference in electrical charge.	No fasting or special preparation is required. Requires drawing 7-10 mL of blood.
Complement Assays			
Total serum complement (CH_{50}): 40-1000 units/mL C3 (mature T cells): 1200-1500 mcg/mL C4 (helper T cells): 350-600 mcg/mL	Used to monitor immune disorders; genetic complement deficiencies; treatment response	In the presence of antibody/ antigen complexes, the complement system is overly activated, and the complement components are "consumed" or used up.	No fasting or special preparation is required. Requires drawing 7-10 mL of blood.
C-reactive protein (CRP) <8 mcg/mL	Detect the presence of an inflammatory process	CRP is initiated by antigen-immune complexes, bacteria, fungi, and trauma. It interacts with the complement system.	Explain that fasting may be required for 4-12 hr. Water is permitted. Requires drawing a blood sample. Cigarette smoking can cause increased levels. Alcohol consumption can decrease levels. Estrogens and progesterones may cause increased levels. Statins, fibrins, and niacin may cause decreased levels.
Lymph Node Biopsy			
Negative for abnormal cells or infectious agents	Detect changes in tissue; identify autoimmune disease or detect the spread of malignancy	Tissue is obtained by needle aspiration, excision, or needle punch using aseptic technique.	Fasting may be required. Sedation and/or local anesthesia will be administered. Biopsied material is placed in formaldehyde. Label and transport to the laboratory immediately. A dry sterile dressing is applied to the biopsy site. Instruct the patient to watch for signs of infection: increasing pain, redness, swelling, purulent drainage, or fever >101° F (38.3° C).

Table 10-3	Diagnostic Tests for Disorders of the Immune and Lymphatic Systems—cont'd		
TEST AND NORMAL RANGE	**PURPOSE**	**DESCRIPTION**	**NURSING IMPLICATIONS**
Culture			
	Determine organism responsible for infection	A sample of exudate, fluid, or tissue is taken from the suspected infected area.	The procedures for collecting bacterial, viral, and fungal samples are different. Consult agency protocol. Gather the correct culture tubes and culture media. Label all containers before collecting the specimen(s). Transport the specimen(s) to the laboratory immediately.

bloodstream. The isotope emits gamma rays that can be detected by the imaging equipment. Computers construct a picture of sites in the body where the antibody accumulates. The primary use of this technique is for identification of neoplasms, as well as in locating and confirming areas of infection, such as in osteomyelitis. Current research is investigating techniques for "tagging" other cellular components of the immune system with radioactive substances that can then be visualized with nuclear medicine equipment.

Computed tomography (CT), magnetic resonance imaging (MRI), and positron emission tomography (PET) can all be used to evaluate the thymus gland and other tissue structures of the immune system.

▪ Nursing Diagnosis

Nursing diagnoses commonly encountered for patients with immune and lymphatic disorders are numerous (Table 10-4).

▪ Planning

Planning is based on the particular problems identified for the individual patient (see Table 10-4). General nursing goals include:
- Protect from infection
- Improve health status
- Maintain a high degree of wellness to promote optimal immune function

▪ Implementation

Nursing interventions include all methods for prevention of spread of infection. Meticulous adherence to Standard Precautions, including appropriate hand hygiene, is essential. Additional protection from infection may include implementation of protective isolation. Promotion of balanced, adequate nutrition is essential in maintaining or regaining optimal immune function.

 Assignment Considerations

Instructing Certified Nursing Assistants (CNAs) and Unlicensed Assistive Personnel (UAP)

When assigning patients or tasks to CNAs or UAP, remember to share that a patient is immunocompromised (very susceptible to infection) and that it is important to be extra diligent about complying with hand hygiene and transmission-based isolation protocols. Ask them to help restrict the presence of people who have an infection in the patient's room. Remind them that it is important that the patient obtain sufficient rest and not be continually disturbed. Ask the CNA/UAP to report any new skin lesion, irritation, or redness that is noticed during bathing or repositioning. State that you want to know if the urine has a foul odor. Remember at the end of the shift to thank the person for the help provided.

Psychosocial care to decrease fear, help deal with lifestyle or role changes, and reduce stress is important in caring for the whole person. Patient teaching regarding the disorder, treatment, signs of complications, and self-care is an effective way to reduce stress and fear. Nursing care for specific disorders of the immune and lymphatic system is presented in Chapter 12.

▪ Evaluation

Determination of whether expected outcomes are being met includes assessing for signs and symptoms of immune function. This includes gathering physical data, as well as monitoring laboratory and diagnostic study results for improvement. Temperature and other vital signs are also good indicators of immune function. General well-being and side effects of medications should also be monitored in evaluating the effectiveness of nursing and medical interventions.

COMMON PROBLEMS RELATED TO THE IMMUNE AND LYMPHATIC SYSTEMS

FEVER

A rise in body temperature typically signals a normal immune system response to infection. The rise in temperature is only one component for fighting off the

Table 10-4	Common Nursing Diagnoses and Interventions for Patients with Alteration in Immune and Lymphatic Function	
NURSING DIAGNOSIS	**GOALS/EXPECTED OUTCOMES**	**NURSING INTERVENTIONS**
Excessive Immune Response		
Risk for ineffective breathing pattern related to excessive immune response	Patient will maintain a patent airway and adequate oxygenation	Maintain patent airway. Assess respiratory function q 2–4 hr. Provide supplemental oxygen as needed and ordered.
Risk for hyperthermia secondary to inflammatory response	Patient will maintain core temperature within normal range	Monitor temperature. Administer antipyretics as indicated. Initiate cooling measures if indicated. Monitor intake and output. Encourage fluid intake.
Risk for impaired skin integrity secondary to allergens	Patient's skin will be intact and without redness or rash or hives	Assess for rash or hives. Administer topical and systemic medications as ordered. Keep skin clean and dry, use lotions for lubrication. Refrain from bathing in hot water. Suggest use of ice to decrease itching. Keep nails short to reduce risk of injury from scratching. Provide distraction activities to shift focus from itching.
Anxiety related to threatened health status	Patient will assist with lessening symptoms through various techniques Patient's anxiety will decrease by discharge	Assess level of anxiety. If patient is having respiratory difficulty, stay with the patient. Explain to the patient what is being done to help her and what she can do to lessen the symptoms. Teach relaxation exercises.
Deficient Immune Response		
Infection, either actual or risk for, secondary to decreased resistance	Patient will remain free of infection or, if infection occurs, it will be promptly identified and treated	Maintain infection control standards to prevent health care–associated infections. Assess for signs and symptoms of infection. Aggressively treat infection if it occurs. Instruct patient in techniques to prevent acquisition of infection.
Risk for impaired social interaction resulting in social isolation	Patient will participate in social activities within ability	Encourage interaction using technology to maintain relationships and prevent infections. Provide positive reinforcement when the patient participates socially. Provide education regarding modes of transmission so that social interactions can be safely undertaken.
Risk for imbalanced body temperature secondary to illness	Maintain body temperature within normal range	Monitor core body temperature. Maintain a comfortable ambient temperature. Restore/maintain temperature within patient's normal range.
Risk for imbalanced nutrition: less than body requirements secondary to loss of appetite	Maintain stable weight	Assess presence and degree of nausea or loss of appetite. Assist patient to make a dietary plan including favorite foods. Consult with dietitian and health care team. Offer frequent small meals. Promote an odor-free, relaxing atmosphere for meals.
Deficient knowledge regarding disease process and prevention of infection transmission	Patient and family will verbalize understanding of disease process, treatment, and necessary precautions	Assess readiness to learn. Provide information in multiple formats: verbal, visual media, written. Teach necessary precautions to prevent infection. Provide positive reinforcement. Use team and group teaching as appropriate. Provide access to other information sources. Refer to community agencies and support groups.

Table 10-4	Common Nursing Diagnoses and Interventions for Patients with Alteration in Immune and Lymphatic Function—cont'd	
NURSING DIAGNOSIS	**GOALS/EXPECTED OUTCOMES**	**NURSING INTERVENTIONS**
Lymph System Disorders		
Acute pain related to disease process	Patient's pain will be reduced and kept within range acceptable to patient	Teach patient use of pain scale for reporting of pain. Accept patient's report of pain. Monitor vital signs. Provide comfort measures. Instruct and encourage relaxation, imagery, and diversional activities. Administer analgesics as needed to maintain acceptable comfort level. Encourage adequate rest periods. Work with patient and family to identify effective strategies for pain management.
Imbalanced nutrition: less than body requirements secondary to disease process	Patient will maintain present or ideal body weight	Determine ability to chew and swallow. Identify patient food preferences. Offer frequent small meals. Weigh daily. Promote relaxing meal environment. Provide oral care before and after meals.
Powerlessness related to disease process	Patient will become actively involved in care and will make choices related to care	Assess patient's knowledge and perception of condition. Identify patient support systems. Listen to patient's expressions of feelings. Show concern for patient as an individual. Treat patient's decisions with respect. Encourage realistic goal setting. Provide opportunities for the patient to control as many events as restrictions allow.
Body image disturbance related to lymphedema	Patient will verbalize understanding of body changes	Teach patient and family about pathophysiology of lymphedema. Institute measures to reduce lymphedema: elevation of extremity and use of pressure sleeve as ordered. Teach measures to prevent lymphedema recurrence. Support patient decision making. Refer to appropriate support groups.

invaders by promoting a hostile environment. There is a significant amount of evidence-based research that shows how fever is helpful to the immune system. However, there is continued controversy about when to treat an elevation in body temperature. *Hyperthermia* or fever related to infections can cause discomfort, and excessive fever can lead to complications such as seizures. Decreasing body temperature by physical or pharmaceutical means promotes comfort for the individual but may decrease the effectiveness of the body's efforts to eliminate pathogenic microorganisms. Excessive fever (hyperpyrexia) is usually treated with antipyretics and cooling measures.

Nursing Management

Cooling measures can be as simple as removing excess coverings or as complex as using mechanical cooling blankets and cooled intravenous fluids. Usual nursing measures for decreasing body temperature include sponging with tepid water. Cold water is contraindicated because rapid cooling can induce shivering, which can drive the temperature back up.

 Clinical Cues

Sometimes body temperature can be lowered by placing ice bags in the axillae and groin area. Be sure to insulate the packs with a cloth before placing them on the body. These areas have good blood circulation and can help with cooling the core body temperature.

The ideal treatment for fever is to address the cause. Appropriate antimicrobial therapy can reduce fever by fighting the infection. Allergic inflammatory responses can be treated with corticosteroids. Anti-inflammatory medications such as aspirin, ibuprofen, or naproxen may also be administered to lower the temperature.

NUTRITION

Anorexia (decreased desire for food) often accompanies fever, infection, and use of antimicrobial agents. Adequate amounts of fluid, calories, vitamins, and protein are essential in maintaining the immune system and rebuilding tissues affected by infection. Increased body temperature causes an increased metabolic rate. This increase in cellular metabolism uses more oxygen and water than under normal circumstances. Respiratory and heart rates increase with the core body temperature; therefore if a high temperature is not brought under control and fluids replenished, the body ceases to function at an optimum level and could lead to shock or even death.

Nursing Management

Offering favorite fluids and foods in small portions can sometimes tempt the appetite. When febrile, individuals often prefer cold or frozen items. Easily digested food items are usually more tempting such as soup, ices, pops, and clear (nonpulp) juices.

IMMUNOSUPPRESSION

Many patients can be immunosuppressed either from the disease process or from medical treatment. This makes the person highly susceptible to common microorganisms. Patients who have to take daily corticosteroids for any reason, such as those with chronic asthma, post–organ transplantation patients, or patients who are receiving chemotherapy, are immunosuppressed. Individuals with diabetes mellitus may also have a depressed immune system.

Nursing Management

Hospital settings are known for having a high concentration of pathogens simply because of the variety of patient illnesses. In the hospital environment, **it is critical that all standard infection prevention and control protocols be implemented and followed by everyone without fail.** Patients with neutropenia (less than normal amount of WBCs) may need additional precautions. Transmission-based isolation precautions refer to procedures that may be implemented to protect immunosuppressed patients from exposure to infectious microorganisms. In some cases, the precautions may also include restrictions on fresh fruits, vegetables, and flowers. Visitors who may have an infectious disorder may also be restricted from walking in the halls or going into populated areas such as a gift shop or cafeteria. Regardless of what is implemented, the principle is the same—preventing the transmission of potentially infective microorganisms to other patients, regardless of their immune status. These measures may include specially constructed rooms with positive airflow, monitoring of water purity, and monitoring of air vents for the presence of pathogenic microorganisms. The degree to which these measures are implemented is determined by the degree of immunosuppression. Any patient who is ill and hospitalized has an immune system under stress. Health care staff meticulously adhering to Standard Precautions and, if needed, transmission-based precautions will help protect patients. Chapter 17 presents more on the care of a neutropenic patient.

 Think Critically

What devices, tools, equipment, or other objects are routinely carried from patient to patient without disinfection? Where do they fit in the chain of infection? What can you, as a health care provider, do about reducing transmission of microorganisms?

Get Ready for the NCLEX® Examination!

Key Points

- The immune and lymphatic systems protect the body against microscopic threats to homeostasis.
- The inflammatory response is the first step in the immune response.
- Antibodies are proteins that fight antigens.
- B and T lymphocytes are major forces in fighting infection.
- The body produces a humoral (immediate) and cellular (delayed) response to antigens.
- Chronic consumption of alcohol can alter the body's ability to launch an immune response.
- Active artificially acquired immunity occurs by vaccination or immunization.

- Immunizations introduce pathogens to the body in a controlled way, allowing the body to produce antibodies to prevent future illness.
- The nurse plays a major role in providing patient education regarding the importance of immunizations to public health.
- Decreased immune response puts the patient at risk for infection.
- Measures such as hand hygiene and strict adherence to Standard Precautions should always be implemented, regardless of immune status, to prevent health care–associated infections.
- Good nutrition and healthy lifestyle choices are important for a healthy immune system.
- Immunosuppression can be caused by treatment for conditions such as asthma and cancer.

Additional Learning Resources

SG Go to your Study Guide for additional learning activities to help you master this chapter content.

 Go to your Evolve website (http://evolve.elsevier.com/deWit/medsurg) for the following FREE learning resources:
- Animations, audio, and video
- Answers and rationales for questions and activities
- Concept Map Creator
- Glossary with pronunciations in English and Spanish
- Interactive Review Questions and Exercises and more!

Online Resources
- Centers for Disease Control and Prevention, www.cdc.gov

Review Questions for the NCLEX® Examination

1. The administration of weak or attenuated microorganisms to stimulate the production of antibodies without causing a full-blown disease is referred to as:
   1. active naturally acquired immunity.
   2. active artificially acquired immunity.
   3. passive natural immunity.
   4. passive artificial immunity.

2. The nurse demonstrates understanding of passive natural immunity when he makes which statement?
   1. "Breastfeeding is the best way to enhance the infant's immunity."
   2. "Timely vaccination could easily provide protection from hepatitis."
   3. "The skin provides passive natural immunity for warding off diseases."
   4. "Administration of human immune globulins boosts the immunity."

3. Before administering antibodies against tetanus, which patient statement would indicate a need for further nursing assessment?
   1. "I have reactions to horse serum."
   2. "I cannot have any seafood."
   3. "I have lactose intolerance."
   4. "I do not like eggs."

4. During a health promotion outreach for older adults, the nurse discusses the physiologic changes in aging that increase susceptibility to infection. Which statement is true?
   1. "With advanced age, the skin becomes tough and leathery."
   2. "Decreased cilia in the lung provide a more hospitable environment to harmful organisms."
   3. "Decreased normal flora in the intestines causes the harboring of pathogens."
   4. "Repeated infections build up immune responses."

5. The patient is newly diagnosed with an autoimmune thyroid disease. When the nurse discusses the patient's questions and concerns, the patient asks, "What did the physician mean by autoimmune disease?" What is the most appropriate response?
   1. "The body's immune defenses fail to respond to the pathogenic agents."
   2. "Immune defenses are attacking the normal body cells."
   3. "There is a break in the body's defenses."
   4. "The physician was able to identify the underlying cause of the disorder."

6. The nurse assesses the condition of a sacral pressure ulcer on an immobilized patient. Which sign or symptom indicates the presence of infection?
   1. Warm to touch
   2. Pink wound surface
   3. Wound culture <10,000 colonies
   4. Purulent drainage

7. While caring for an immunocompromised patient, which action by a nursing assistant indicates a need for instruction and supervision by a licensed nurse?
   1. Reporting changes in the physical characteristics of the urine
   2. Allowing all family members in the patient's room at all times
   3. Meticulous hand hygiene before entering the patient's room
   4. Turning the patient while bathing the patient

8. During the data collection process, the patient indicates, "I take garlic pills to reduce my risk for cancer." What is an appropriate nursing response?
   1. "How much and how often do you take your garlic pills?"
   2. "Have you been screened for cancer?"
   3. "What other herbal medications are you taking?"
   4. "You sound worried. Could you talk more about it?"

9. The patient needs to have blood drawn for C-reactive protein. What is an important preprocedure instruction?
   1. Hormone replacement therapy can increase the level of C-reactive protein.
   2. Cigarette smoking is never advised, but will not affect the level of C-reactive protein.
   3. Your morning dose of niacin and simvastatin will not affect the outcomes of the test.
   4. The procedure requires a 4- to 12-hour fast with no water intake.

10. Before receiving antivenin, the patient asks, "How does the antivenin work?" Which statement demonstrates that the nurse has knowledge of the medication?
    1. "The antivenin provides a lifelong protection from any snake bite."
    2. "The antivenin must be given as early as possible to afford immediate reversal of the subsequent effects of the venom."
    3. "The antivenin reverses the effects of the poisonous snake bite."
    4. "The antivenin cannot be given to patients who are allergic to eggs."

Critical Thinking Activities

Scenario A
Mr. Green, an 80-year-old farmer, is admitted with pneumonia. His vital signs are: temperature 103° F (39.4° C) (oral), blood pressure 136/78 mm Hg, heart rate 100 bpm, respirations 28 breaths/min, and no complaint of pain.

1. What assessment data indicate that the immune system is active?

2. Describe how the body is reacting to the lung infection. Which type of immunity will help fight the infection?

3. List appropriate nursing interventions for Mr. Green.

Scenario B
Mrs. Hope brings her newborn into the pediatrician's office. She is seeking information.

1. Mrs. Hope asks when she should bring her baby in for immunizations. What will you tell her?

2. Explain how immunizations help protect the body.

3. Discuss what information should be given so that Mrs. Hope could identify if her baby has had a reaction to an immunization.

Care of Patients with HIV/AIDS

Objectives

Theory

1. Summarize the modes of transmission for HIV.
2. List the tests used to diagnose HIV and to monitor the immune status of an HIV-positive patient.
3. Identify the signs and symptoms of AIDS.
4. Analyze conditions where opportunistic infections (viral, bacterial, fungal, parasitic) are likely to occur.
5. List the primary categories of highly active antiretroviral therapy (HAART) and common side effects of each.
6. Identify the nursing diagnoses needed for a patient with AIDS.
7. Explain wasting syndrome and nursing interventions.

Clinical Practice

1. Perform nursing interventions needed for opportunistic infections.
2. Implement a teaching plan for a patient being started on HAART.
3. Review a nursing care plan for an HIV/AIDS patient hospitalized with a low CD4 count.
4. During a clinical rotation, review the facility's policy for exposure to blood or body fluids from an HIV-positive patient.

Key Terms

acquired immunodeficiency syndrome (AIDS) (ă-KWĪRD ĭm-ū-nō-dĕ-FĬSH-ĕn-sē SĬN-drōm, p. 217)
anasarca (p. 226)
dermatomes (p. 221)
disseminated (p. 223)
human immunodeficiency virus (HIV) (ĭm-ū-nō-dĕ-FĬSH-ĕn-sē VĪ-rŭs, p. 217)
immune deficiency (ĭ-MŪN dĕ-FĬSH-ĕn-sē, p. 215)
immunocompetence (p. 215)

opportunistic infections (OIs) (ŏp-pŏr-tū-NĬS-tĭk ĭn-FĔK-shŭnz, p. 217)
prodrome (p. 221)
protease inhibitors (PIs) (prō-tē-ās ĭn-hĬb-ĭ-tŏrz, p. 222)
replicate (RĔP-lĭ-kāt, p. 217)
retrovirus (rĕ-trō-VĪ-rŭs, p. 217)
reverse transcriptase (rē-VĔRS trănz-SCRĬP-tās, p. 217)
sentinel infections (SĔN-tĭ-nĕl ĭn-FĔK-shŭnz, p. 219)
suppression (sū-PRĔ-shŭn, p. 217)
wasting syndrome (p. 229)

Immunocompetence occurs when a threat to the immune system stimulates certain physiologic responses (i.e., the vascular system, initiation of chemical responses, and the release of white blood cells) to protect the body against invasion from microorganisms or toxins.

Abnormal responses of the immune system are typically the result of an infection, medical therapy, or exposure to select toxins. An immune deficiency can occur when there is insufficient production of antibodies, immune cells, or both.

Acquired immune deficiency can result from human immunodeficiency virus (HIV) infection or administration of chemotherapy for cancer can temporarily reduce the ability of the bone marrow to produce white blood cells (WBCs).

DISORDERS OF IMMUNE DEFICIENCY

HUMAN IMMUNODEFICIENCY VIRUS (HIV) AND ACQUIRED IMMUNODEFICIENCY SYNDROME (AIDS)

In the early years, HIV was a fatal disease and treatment involved comfort measures and hospice care. Today, there is still no cure for HIV/AIDS, but there are approximately 16 approved HIV medications, and the prognosis for HIV has dramatically improved with early diagnosis. HIV is now considered a chronic controllable disease which requires adherence to prescribed medications, routine appointments, and recommended HIV tests (Figure 11-1, on the following page).

① HIV virus: HIV genetic material encoated by a protein shell. GP120 proteins are able to attach to CD4 receptors on the surface of the host's CD4+ T cells.

GP120 proteins

HIV genetic material

Enzymes used during life cycle

② HIV attaches to the surface of host's CD4+ lymphocyte.

STOP Nucleoside reverse transcriptase inhibitors integrate into the new viral DNA and block its building process.

STOP Protease inhibitors prevent the assembly and release of the new HIV virions.

Host's CD4+ lymphocyte

⑤ The new HIV DNA enters the host cell and becomes integrated with the host DNA (using the enzyme integrase). The host cell begins to make new virus particles called virions.

CD4+ cell nucleus

STOP Investigational drugs that inhibit entry include attachment inhibitors and coreceptor binding inhibitors.

⑥ The enzyme protease cuts the long virion chains into new HIV virus particles.

STOP Fusion inhibitors prevent HIV from entering healthy T cells.

④ To replicate, HIV RNA must be made into double-stranded DNA. The enzyme reverse transcriptase is needed for this step.

⑦ The new virus particles "bud" out from the host cell and begin the process again in other CD4+ lymphocytes. The host cell dies.

③ The virus cell membrane fuses with the host cell's membrane, allowing the HIV particle to release its RNA and enzymes into the host cell.

STOP Nonnucleoside reverse transcriptase inhibitors bind to reverse transcriptase and prevent HIV RNA from converting to DNA.

FIGURE 11-1 The steps in the life cycle of HIV with correlation to medications.

Pathophysiology

Human immunodeficiency virus (HIV)/acquired immunodeficiency syndrome (AIDS) is the most serious of the immune deficiency disorders. A person with AIDS also has HIV; however, a person with HIV does not necessarily have AIDS. Current research shows that those who are HIV positive will usually not develop AIDS if compliant with effective HIV treatment.

HIV is a retrovirus that integrates itself into the genetic material of the host cell, changing the proviral DNA and encoding structural, regulatory, and accessory proteins within the cell. A **retrovirus** differs from other viruses because of an enzyme called **reverse transcriptase,** which helps the virus reproduce in the host cell. HIV primarily attaches to the CD4 cell wall receptors found on lymphocytes and some monocytes. The virus must go through several stages (Table 11-1) before it can effectively infect a host cell. Once infected with HIV, the host cell and the ability of the cell-mediated immune response is seriously impaired. Once the infection occurs in the CD4 lymphocytes and produces HIV, the CD4 cell itself dies.

The most recent revision of the definitions of AIDS and HIV infection by the Centers for Disease Control and Prevention (CDC) was done in 1993. (See Evolve for the classification system for HIV.) **Suppression** or inhibition of the immune response as a result of HIV infection is the cause of AIDS. HIV-1 is the most common cause of HIV infection in the United States, Europe, and Asia. HIV-2 is widespread in western Africa. Research shows that HIV-2 spreads at a lower rate, has a lower plasma viral load, takes longer to incubate, and persons with this strain have

a lesser risk of developing full-blown AIDS (American Academy of HIV Medicine, 2007).

HIV-1 and HIV-2 are both *retroviruses* and have only ribonucleic acid (RNA) as their genetic material. When they **replicate** (reproduce), their genetic material is placed in the deoxyribonucleic acid (DNA) of the host cell. The resulting new DNA continues the process of replication, and produces as many as 50 million to 2 billion viral particles a day. These viral particles are released from the host cell into the circulatory system, where they infect other cells, such as macrophages and lymphoid tissue.

The T cells that have the protein CD4 on their surface are known as CD4 positive (CD4+) and as T helper cells. Normally CD4+ T cells activate B cells, natural killer cells, and phagocytes. These cells participate in both cellular and humoral immunity. The infected person becomes more prone to **opportunistic infections (OIs),** including normal flora found in the body (see Chapter 6). The diagnosis of AIDS is usually made in an HIV-infected patient with a CD4 T-lymphocyte count less than 200 cells/μL or with a specific OI being diagnosed.

Transmission

Research has shown that HIV cannot be transmitted by casual contact, routine nursing care (which includes following Standard Precautions), or by household contact. The *only* mode of transmission is by exposure to HIV-infected blood, body fluids, or tissue (Box 11-1). Any break in skin or mucous membranes is an entry portal for HIV. The highest risks for becoming infected with HIV are: having unprotected sex (oral, vaginal, or anal) or sharing needles and syringes with an HIV-infected person and maternal-fetal exposure.

A CDC report in 2009 stated that as of 2007, there were 42,495 newly confirmed cases of HIV in the United States (CDC, 2009a). The largest proportion of new cases (53%) was found in men having sex with other men (known as MSM). The increased numbers

Table 11-1 The Life Cycle of HIV

STAGE	ACTION
Entry	Virus binds to envelope protein to CD4 molecule causing virus to fuse to host cell. Fusion releases RNA and HIV-1 proteins into the target cell cytoplasm.
Reverse transcription	RNA is transcribed into double-stranded DNA through the encoded protein. This phase is very error prone and can lead to mutations.
Integration	The new DNA inserts into the host gene.
Viral mRNA and protein expression	Viral protein production is activated and T cells are modified by HIV-1 protease.
Assembly and budding	Virus then attaches to host plasma membrane and new virions are produced.

mRNA, memory RNA (ribonucleic acid).

Box 11-1 Additional Modes of Human Immunodeficiency Virus (HIV) Exposure

- Percutaneous exposure through an open-bore needle stick with an HIV-contaminated needle
- Not using a latex condom or dental dam during sexual intercourse or activity
- Maternal transmission, referred to as vertical transmission, to an infant through vaginal delivery or breast milk
- Receiving a transfusion of HIV-infected blood or blood products
- Receiving an organ transplant from an HIV-positive person

of heterosexual cases may be from a bisexual MSM engaging in unprotected sex with a female partner. The second highest rate (32%) of HIV-positive cases is found in the heterosexual population, especially among those involved in the high-risk behaviors (CDC, 2009a).

An unsafe practice that is a known method of HIV transmission is to be the receptive partner in anal or vaginal intercourse without using some form of barrier precaution such as a latex condom. Participating in unprotected anal intercourse with an HIV-positive partner will increase the risk of exposure via the microscopic tears that can occur in the lining of the anus (a lining that is thinner than the vaginal walls).

🏃 Health Promotion

Safe Sexual Practices

Barrier protection must be practiced with every sexual encounter, in order to prevent transmission of HIV or other infectious diseases. Latex condoms are more impermeable than other types of condoms. Polyurethane and deproteinized latex condoms are available for those allergic to latex. Condoms should not be stored in wallets, glove compartments, or hot or sunny areas, because the temperature will degrade the integrity of the condom material. Lambskin condoms help prevent pregnancy but may allow the virus to seep through; therefore they do not prevent transmission of HIV. Spermicides may help in preventing pregnancy, but they may cause tissue irritation and thereby increase the risk of injury to the mucous membranes. The only guaranteed way to prevent sexual transmission is through abstinence.

Another unsafe practice is orogenital (fellatio or cunnilingus) or oroanal (rimming) stimulation without a barrier (dental dam). Contact with any body fluids, such as semen or vaginal secretions and blood, must absolutely be avoided when the partner has HIV.

There is no reason for HIV-infected individuals to completely discontinue sexual activity. Touch and various forms of intimacy are important parts of any relationship. However, there is a need to reduce the risk of transmitting the virus to others and to prevent exposure to other sexually transmitted infections, as additional infection is more difficult to treat when the immune system is compromised by HIV.

Tattoos and Body Piercings. To date, there have been no documented cases of HIV transmission from tattoos and body piercings. However, there have been a significant number of confirmed cases of hepatitis B transmission from these activities and HIV and hepatitis B are transmitted in the same manner. There is a risk if needles and instruments for tattooing are not properly disinfected and sterilized between uses and if leftover ink is used. For tattoos and piercings, it is important to use licensed businesses which follow blood-borne

pathogen procedures and other safety measures (Lehman et al., 2010).

Blood Products. For more than 25 years, all blood, blood products, and prospective organ donors have been screened for blood-borne pathogens such as hepatitis and HIV. According to the CDC, the current risk of contracting HIV from receiving a blood transfusion, blood products, or a donated organ or tissue is extremely small, even in populations with a high incidence of HIV infection.

Vaccine Development

The International AIDS Vaccine Initiative, which includes a network of professional researchers and physicians in more than 23 countries, seeks effective treatments for AIDS and an effective HIV vaccine. HIV mutates rapidly and to date, almost 2 million mutations have been found among slightly fewer than 56,000 individuals infected with HIV (CDC, 2010). Mutations are found in newly infected as well as chronically infected individuals. People who take antiretroviral medications and have unprotected sex, or who share needles and syringes among intravenous drug users increase the risk of spreading the drug-resistant strains of HIV. Developing a vaccine is extremely challenging and currently, the primary emphasis is on preventing the spread of HIV.

Prevention Through Education

Providing basic understandable information helps to dispel the myths and fears associated with becoming infected with HIV. A nurse can contribute to prevention, in accordance with the *Healthy People 2020* objectives to reduce the incidence of HIV/AIDS, by obtaining accurate facts related to HIV and by educating others—patients, colleagues, and the community—about their individual roles in helping to prevent the spread of this virus. Nurses must also assess for risk behaviors and implement individualized education.

🌐 Cultural Considerations

HIV and Minorities in the United States

HIV reporting in the United States indicates that more than 74% of new HIV infections occur among minorities, specifically, African Americans and Hispanics (CDC, 2009b). Factors that may increase HIV/AIDS among minority groups include:

- Lack of culturally sensitive and high-quality information about HIV risk and prevention
- Socioeconomic status and limited access to health care
- Health beliefs concerning sexual practices, roles of women, the value of children, and HIV treatment
- The high cost of highly active antiretroviral therapy (HAART)

Data from www.cdc.gov/hiv/topics/surveillance/resources/slides/race-ethnicity/index.htm.

Signs and Symptoms

Some people infected with HIV have no symptoms for many years. A person's preexisting health status influences the length of time needed for the humoral (antibody-mediated) and cellular (cell-mediated) immune responses to lodge a defense against HIV. Some newly infected individuals have no symptoms; other individuals may have flulike symptoms, which may be accompanied by maculopapular rash and lymphadenopathy. However, the HIV test may be negative at this phase of the disease.

As the immune system begins to fail, symptoms of **sentinel infections** (opportunistic infections that indicate immunosuppression) appear, such as oral thrush, recurrent vaginal yeast infections, or skin disorders. HIV has variable clinical presentations and latent periods without obvious symptoms. Often, the initial signs and symptoms of HIV infection are similar to flu: fever, fatigue, diarrhea, and loss of appetite. These symptoms may be ignored and the infected person typically does not seek health care until more obvious signs or symptoms begin to appear, such as skin rashes, night sweats, swollen lymph glands, and significant unintended weight loss. Symptoms may disappear and then recur and take longer to resolve. Additional illnesses (recurrent yeast infections or pneumonias, memory or movement problems) may prompt the person to seek treatment.

Diagnosis

Testing is available through a physician, local public health clinic, community agency, or by home test kit (Box 11-2). Home Access HIV-1 Test System is the only self-test kit that is approved by the Food and Drug Administration (FDA). The patient can anonymously purchase the kit, collect the required specimen, and send it to a specified lab and receive coded results through the mail. Other testing products on the market are not approved by the FDA because of their questionable methods or results; therefore patients must be advised about products.

Clinical laboratories and some physician offices have rapid HIV tests that can be performed with oral fluids and in some cases with urine. HIV tests search for antibodies to the virus. After exposure to HIV, there may be a delay before antibodies appear in the blood. A negative HIV test after initial exposure is not considered final; a second test, using a different test method than the first test, must be conducted 1 to 3 months later. The most common test used in a clinical laboratory setting is the enzyme-linked immunosorbent assay (ELISA). Most HIV experts recommend that a confirmatory ELISA test be performed for any positive rapid HIV test. A positive HIV ELISA test is usually confirmed by performing a Western blot (WB) HIV gene sequence test. The HIV Western blot test can be negative, positive, or indeterminate.

Box 11-2   HIV Tests

ENZYME-LINKED IMMUNOSORBENT ASSAY (ELISA), A TYPE OF ENZYME IMMUNOASSAY (EIA)
- Normal value: Negative.
- HIV-antibody screening test (positives must be confirmed with a Western blot).
- Antibody assays do not detect HIV antibody in the earliest stages of the infection. (HIV antibody may be detected normally from 2 weeks to 6 months after the acute infection.)
- False-positive ELISA may be seen in the presence of maternal antibodies.
- Sensitivity: 98%.

WESTERN BLOT (WB)
- Normal value: Negative.
- HIV-antibody test used to confirm a positive ELISA.
- False-positive WB may be seen in the presence of maternal antibodies.

POLYMERASE CHAIN REACTION (PCR)
- Normal value: Negative.
- A qualitative measurement of cell-associated proviral DNA.
- Sensitivity: 100%.

IMMUNOFLUORESCENT ANTIBODY ASSAY (IFA)
- Normal value: Negative.
- Sensitivity: 99.8%.

CD4 CELL COUNT
- Normal value: 500 to 1500 cells/μL.
- Values below 200 cells/μL prompt treatment.

A negative Western blot test means that the positive ELISA test was a false positive. A positive HIV Western blot confirms the true positive nature of the ELISA positive test. An indeterminate test means that this test cannot be adequately read and is not an early positive test. The patient may also have other tests for concurrent hepatitis or sexually transmitted infections.

It is recommended that any sexually active adult between ages 15 and 65 be offered HIV testing at the time of a complete physical examination (CDC, 2006). The age group included is a point of controversy. It is estimated that 25% of HIV-infected patients are unaware of their HIV infection and thus may be unintentionally infecting others (Box 11-3). The CDC has previously recommended HIV testing in pregnant women. If the patient elects to "opt out" of HIV testing, a note is made in the clinical record that the patient has declined HIV testing. It is now not necessary to get a specific request for HIV testing or perform pretest and post-test HIV counseling; however, it is important for the nurse to be familiar with state or local HIV testing requirements. The results of HIV antibody tests are confidential patient information.

Box 11-3 Centers for Disease Control and Prevention Recommendations for HIV Testing

- HIV screening is recommended for patients in all health care settings after the patient is notified that testing will be performed unless the patient declines (opt-out screening).
- Persons at high risk for HIV infection should be screened for HIV at least annually.
- Separate written consent for HIV testing should not be required; general consent for medical care should be considered sufficient to encompass consent for HIV testing.
- Prevention counseling should not be required with HIV diagnostic testing or as part of HIV screening programs in health care settings.

Adapted from Anish, P., Mahajan, A.P., Stemple, L., et al. (2009). Consistency of state statutes with the Centers for Disease Control and Prevention HIV testing

Management of HIV Infection

When an individual is confirmed to have HIV, a comprehensive history and physical examination for health status should be conducted, including additional baseline laboratory and diagnostic studies (Table 11-2). A CD4 lymphocyte count should be performed to establish the stage of HIV infection and to assist in determining when to initiate antiretroviral therapy (ART) and prophylaxis for OIs.

Choice of optimal therapy is based on clinical data and individual factors, such as past health status,

medication history, quality-of-life issues, and patient expectations of therapy. The World Health Organization (WHO) has established standard criteria for staging HIV infection (Box 11-4). Genotyping or phenotyping blood tests to detect a drug-resistant strain of HIV are strongly recommended before starting drug therapy. Certain viral subtypes have a higher likelihood of developing drug resistance than others, and may require closer monitoring. Table 11-3 presents the current classes of antiretroviral medications with select nursing implications and side effects. Typically a three-drug regimen that often includes two nucleoside reverse transcriptase inhibitors (NRTIs) and one nonnucleoside reverse transcriptase inhibitors (NNRTI) will be prescribed. Occasionally, a protease inhibitor (PI) will be prescribed.

The most effective current treatment is highly active antiretroviral therapy (HAART), a combination of available drugs recommended for HIV. This therapy is also effective against other conditions common to HIV/AIDS. OIs are treated with drugs specific to their cause, and sometimes antimicrobials are given to prevent infection. As the disease progresses, many patients with HIV/AIDS and/or chronic conditions become too ill to work. It is estimated that drug therapy and laboratory testing for HIV/AIDS combined costs at least $25,000 a year per patient and well over $600,000 if a patient lives with HIV/AIDS for 20 years or more.

Table 11-2 Additional Laboratory and Diagnostic Studies for Patients Newly Diagnosed with HIV*

LABORATORY/DIAGNOSTIC STUDY	PURPOSE
HIV antibody confirmatory study	Confirm diagnosis of HIV
CD4 count (reported as cells/µL)	Identify what stage of HIV infection patient may be in; can be used to determine when to start prophylactic therapy for OIs; should be obtained every few months to assess immune and/or therapeutic response and evaluate need for starting antiretroviral therapy (ART)
Quantitative plasma HIV-RNA level (viral load, reported as copies/mL)	Assess degree of clinical progression; help determine need for starting ART and if it needs adjustment
Drug resistance test (genotype: mutations, phenotype: viral replication)	Determine which ART will be most effective; prevent further development of drug-resistant strain of HIV
Complete blood cell (CBC) count	Assess for anemia, leukopenia, and thrombocytopenia; certain ARTs may be less effective if any of these are present
Comprehensive chemistry panel (includes electrolytes, BUN/creatinine, liver enzymes, cholesterol/triglycerides, glucose)	Determine baseline kidney and liver function, as well as lipid profile; results can be used to determine potential for complications with proposed ART
Sexually transmitted infections	Establish if treatment is needed
Toxoplasma gondii IgG	Detects prior exposure; if positive in the newly diagnosed HIV positive, patient is at increased risk of developing CNS difficulties when CD level is <100 µL
Hepatitis A, B, C	Determines if prior exposure to hepatitis and also indicates need for vaccination against hepatitis A and B

Adapted from American Academy of HIV Medicine: *AAHIVM Fundamentals of HIV Medicine for the HIV Specialist.* (2007). Chicago: The Academy.
BUN, blood urea nitrogen; CNS, central nervous system; IgG, immunoglobulin G; OIs, opportunistic infections.
*Additional testing may also include tuberculosis; Pap smear for women, and PSA level and prostate examination for men; CMV and eye examination along with routine health maintenance examinations based on age of patient.

Box 11-4 — World Health Organization Classification System for HIV Infection and Staging

CLINICAL STAGE I
- Asymptomatic infection
- Persistent generalized lymphadenopathy
- Acute retroviral infection
- *Performance scale 1:* Asymptomatic, normal activity

CLINICAL STAGE II
- Moderate unintentional weight loss <10% of body weight
- Minor mucocutaneous manifestations (e.g., dermatitis, prurigo, fungal nail infections, angular cheilitis)
- Herpes zoster within previous 5 years
- Recurrent upper respiratory tract infections
- *Performance scale 2:* Symptoms, but nearly fully ambulatory

CLINICAL STAGE III
- Severe unintentional weight loss >10% body weight
- Chronic diarrhea >1 month
- Prolonged fever >1 month (constant or intermittent)
- Oral candidiasis
- Oral hairy leukoplakia
- Pulmonary tuberculosis within the previous year
- Severe bacterial infections
- Vulvovaginal candidiasis
- *Performance scale 3:* In bed more than normal but <50% of normal daytime during the previous month

CLINICAL STAGE IV
- HIV wasting syndrome
- *Pneumocystis jiroveci* (formerly *carinii*) pneumonia
- Toxoplasmosis of the brain
- Cryptosporidiosis with diarrhea >1 month
- Isosporiasis with diarrhea >1 month
- Cryptococcosis, extrapulmonary
- Cytomegalovirus disease of an organ other than liver, spleen, or lymph node
- Herpes simplex virus infection, mucocutaneous
- Progressive multifocal leukoencephalopathy
- Any disseminated endemic mycosis (e.g., histoplasmosis)
- Candidiasis of the esophagus, trachea, bronchi, or lung
- Atypical mycobacteriosis, disseminated
- Nontyphoid *Salmonella* septicemia
- Extrapulmonary tuberculosis
- Lymphoma
- Kaposi sarcoma
- HIV encephalopathy
- *Performance scale 4:* In bed >50% of normal daytime during previous month

From AETC National Resource Center. (2009). HIV Classification: CDC and WHO Staging Systems. Retrieved from www.aidsetc.org/aidsetc?page=cm-105_disease#b-4.

Think Critically
How would you go about helping a patient who has AIDS find a way to afford the medications needed to control the disease?

Complementary and Alternative Therapies
Use of Alternative Therapies by Patients with HIV

Relaxation, meditation, Reiki, and imagery can help decrease stress. Acupressure and acupuncture may help control pain. There is controversy regarding using herbal and other substances to boost the immune system because some can interfere with HAART. The primary health care provider should be consulted.

Complications
Opportunistic Infections. *Opportunistic infections* (OIs) are defined as diseases caused by microorganisms commonly present in the environment or the body, that only cause disease when there is a weakening or suppression of the immune system.

Viral Infections. HIV/AIDS patients can have problems with herpes simplex virus types 1 and 2 (HSV-1 and HSV-2), cytomegalovirus (CMV), and varicella-zoster virus (VZV), commonly referred to as shingles. In HIV-infected individuals, a herpesvirus usually manifests as outbreaks in the oral, genital, and perirectal areas. Patients experience a **prodrome** (early symptoms) of itching and tingling 24 to 48 hours before the actual outbreak of vesicles. Most herpesviruses cause the formation of vesicles that contain clear liquid. This fluid is highly infectious and great care must be taken not to infect other areas of the body, especially the eyes. A herpes eye infection should be promptly treated as it can cause scarring on the cornea and affect vision. Chronic ulcerative lesions may form after the vesicles rupture. Symptoms of fever, pain, bleeding, lymph node enlargement, headache, myalgia, and malaise may occur if the infection becomes systemic.

Herpes Simplex Virus Type 1 and Type 2. HSV-1 and HSV-2 can be transmitted sexually. HSV-1 usually occurs in the nose, mouth, pharynx, and esophagus. HSV-2 generally appears in the genital, perineal, and perirectal areas, more commonly referred to as genital herpes. Because of cross-infection, HSV-2 may be cultured from the usual HSV-1 sites, and vice versa. It is important to note that HSV-1 and HSV-2 can occur in immunocompetent persons.

Varicella-zoster virus (VZV). After infection with chickenpox, the virus becomes dormant in the base of nerve pathways. Stress can reactivate the virus and vesicles will form along one or more **dermatomes** (nerve tracts). The symptoms of shingles are itching and tingling along the affected nerve accompanied by burning and shooting pain, headache, and low-grade fever. As the fluid-filled vesicles rupture, the virus can infect other areas of the body. Cross-infection can be prevented by using good hand hygiene practices and, if hospitalized, by following transmission-based isolation precautions.

Table 11-3   **Classifications of Antiretroviral Medications for HIV/AIDS Therapy***

CLASSIFICATION	ACTIVITY	NURSING IMPLICATIONS AND SIDE EFFECTS*
Nucleoside reverse transcriptase inhibitors (NRTIs)	Block conversion from RNA to DNA thus preventing HIV genetic material from entering host cells	Monitor hepatic and renal function, CBC. Assess for signs of abdominal pain, nausea, vomiting, dizziness, neuropathy, difficulty in vision, hearing, touch, and balance. If sore throat, fatigue, shortness of breath, or flulike symptoms occur, drug class may need to be modified or discontinued completely.
Nucleotide reverse transcriptase inhibitor	Prevents the virus from altering healthy CD4 cells	Monitor renal function. Assess for abdominal bloating.
Nonnucleoside reverse transcriptase inhibitors (NNRTIs)	Act by binding to and disabling reverse transcriptase, a protein that is needed for replication of HIV	Monitor hepatic function, and if on anticoagulants, coagulation levels. Monitor for headaches, dysphoria, dizziness, insomnia, and nightmares. Diarrhea occurs in some patients. Contraindicated in pregnancy.
Protease inhibitors (PIs)	Work at the last stage of the viral reproduction cycle by preventing the virus from maturing and cause the release of immature viruses, which are then unable to infect other host cells	Monitor serum lipid levels, glucose, bilirubin levels. Higher incidence of nephrolithiasis. Most must be given with food and adequate hydration is required.
Others: Coreceptor antagonist Fusion inhibitors Integrase inhibitor Multiple-class inhibitors	Block virus from binding, fusing, and entering into CD4 cells	Usually given to patients with higher risk of drug resistance. Assess for headaches, nausea, vomiting, skin rash. Must rotate injection sites because of local irritation.

Adapted from Romanelli, F., & Matheny, S. (2009). HIV Infection: The role of primary care. *Am Fam Physician 80*(9), 946–952.
For the most current recommendations, go to the National Institutes of Health website: www.aidsinfo.nih.gov/guidelines.
*Refer to current drug reference materials for drugs prescribed and review side effects and patient teaching recommendations.

! Safety Alert

Varicella (Chickenpox) Transmission

Any nurse who has never had varicella (chickenpox) or has not been successfully immunized against it, should not be assigned to care for a patient with herpes zoster. Pregnant nurses should not care for any patient with herpes lesions as the virus may harm the fetus.

VZV in the immunosuppressed can last for weeks rather than days. For some, the presence of VZV is the first indication of undiagnosed HIV. Recurrent VZV infections may occur because of immune suppression and may signal the onset of other OIs.

Complications of VZV infection include scarring and postherpetic neuralgia that manifests as prolonged pain at the site. Varicella pneumonia and varicella encephalitis can also occur.

The drug of choice is oral acyclovir (Zovirax); intravenous acyclovir is given for severe cases. The treatment for acyclovir-resistant strains is usually with foscarnet (Foscavir). Foscarnet must be given through a central venous access catheter. It is also nephrotoxic; therefore preinfusion and postinfusion hydration with normal saline may be given and monitoring of creatinine and blood urea nitrogen is necessary.

? Think Critically

If you saw a lesion on the thigh of a female patient and were not certain if it was a herpes lesion, what would you do?

Cytomegalovirus. Cytomegalovirus (CMV) is transmitted by contact with body fluids. In households and child care centers, CMV is spread through hand-to-mouth contact with infected body fluids. CMV can also be passed to a fetus in utero, or to a newborn during the birth process, during breast-feeding or during a blood transfusion. Organ transplant recipients are at increased risk because of immunosuppressant drugs. A CD4 count less than 50 cells/µL increases the risk of acquiring CMV. The two most common sites of infection are the retina (may cause blindness) and the gastrointestinal (GI) tract (causing abdominal cramps, diarrhea, weight loss, and anorexia).

The first sign of CMV in the eye is loss of peripheral vision. Treatment for CMV retinitis must be started early and continued to preserve vision. The antiviral drugs will slow (but not cure) CMV retinitis and include ganciclovir (Cytovene), foscarnet, and cidofovir (Vistide). Ganciclovir can be delivered via an intravitreal implant, which is placed by a surgeon in the posterior segment of the eye to deliver the drug directly to the site of infection.

CMV infection in the GI tract manifests as painful swallowing related to ulceration of the esophagus and colitis symptoms which include fever, diarrhea and abdominal pain. Pulmonary infections caused by CMV typically produce severe shortness of breath, dyspnea on exertion, and nonproductive cough. CNS symptoms from CMV may be memory loss, muscle weakness, paralysis, lethargy, headache, numbness in the extremities, and personality changes.

Cidofovir is given via a central venous catheter. To minimize the potential for nephrotoxicity, probenecid and intravenous normal saline should be administered with each dose of cidofovir. The patient should increase oral fluid intake and any fluid loss (e.g., vomiting or diarrhea) must be replaced to prevent kidney damage.

Hepatitis. HIV-positive patients who also have hepatitis B need antiretroviral medications. Co-infection makes each disease more difficult to treat. Infection with hepatitis C is common in HIV-positive individuals because the mode of transmission for both viruses is similar. Many of the medications used for treatment of HIV can be hepatotoxic; thus careful monitoring and drug dosing is necessary. See Chapter 31 for information related to hepatitis.

Bacterial infections

Mycobacterium tuberculosis. HIV infection promotes the progression of latent tuberculosis (TB) infection to active disease and it can also cause a relapse in previously treated patients. *Mycobacterium tuberculosis* (MTb) may manifest as a pulmonary infection, but in approximately 50% of people infected with HIV, MTb is found in sites such as the central nervous system (CNS), skin, bone, GI tract, liver, and spleen. (See Chapter 15 for additional information on pulmonary tuberculosis.)

Mycobacterium avium complex (MAC). MAC infections are primarily caused by *M. avium intracellulare*. The respiratory system and GI tract are usually affected; however, the bone marrow and the circulatory system may also be affected. Symptoms may include fevers, night sweats, weight loss, lymphadenopathy, malaise, and organ disease. MAC becomes a threat when the CD4 count is below 100 cells/μL. Physicians will initiate prophylaxis for MAC and order serial blood and sputum cultures to determine if disseminated (widespread) disease is present. Culture results can take up to 4 to 6 weeks. The viral amplification test can be used to differentiate between MTb and MAC, because the treatment and infection control are markedly different for the two diseases.

Fungal infections

Cryptococcosis. Cryptococcosis, caused by *Cryptococcus neoformans*, is the fourth most common OI for those with HIV/AIDS. This fungus is found in pigeon droppings and in the soil. In individuals with a low CD4 count, generally about 100 cells/μL, cryptococcosis may manifest as fungal meningitis or disseminated disease.

Typical sites of cryptococcosis infection are the lungs (which is the usual entry point) and the CNS. Cryptococcosis also may appear in the bone, prostate, and skin. Symptoms are any—or all—of the following: fever, headache, visual changes, nausea, vomiting, nuchal rigidity, confusion, and altered mental status. Neurologic changes and seizures may also occur.

Treatment for disseminated cryptococcosis is generally with an IV antifungal drug, such as amphotericin B. This drug is nephrotoxic and should be discontinued at the first signs of toxicity. Common side effects with amphotericin B include fever and shakes *(rigors)*. The primary care provider may premedicate the patient before the infusion with antipyretics, antiemetics, antihistamines or meperidine (Demerol). Initially the patient receives daily treatments of amphotericin B. Treatments may be reduced to 3 to 5 days a week to decrease renal toxicity. The amphotericin B medication is best given via a central venous access device.

Fluconazole (Diflucan) is an antifungal that may be given orally or IV, and is used for long-term management of cryptococcosis. The oral form of fluconazole does not cause the renal toxicity and the depletion of potassium, magnesium, and phosphate that commonly occurs with amphotericin B.

Histoplasmosis. The causative agent for histoplasmosis is *Histoplasma capsulatum*. Histoplasmosis is endemic (commonly found) in the Ohio, Missouri, and Mississippi river valleys. The organism is typically found in bat and bird droppings and once dry, it easily becomes aerosolized and the fungal spores can be inhaled. Generally histoplasmosis manifests as a pulmonary infection, but may become disseminated and can also involve the skin. The most common clinical findings include fever, hepatomegaly, splenomegaly, and generalized lymphadenopathy. Symptoms may also include dyspnea, weight loss, and cough. Initial therapy is similar to that for *Cryptococcus* infection.

Coccidioidomycosis. This disease is commonly caused by *Coccidioides immitis*, and is also sometimes referred to as "Cocci" or "valley fever." It is considered endemic in the southwestern United States and California. The fungus is found primarily in the soil; rain after a long period of drought causes the release of the fungal spores into the air. This infection is not transmitted from person to person. Healthy people may have minimal symptoms and require no treatment. However, in the immunocompromised person, severe pulmonary infection or death may occur. Initial symptoms begin as a flulike illness and some may develop a cutaneous rash. Hemoptysis or empyema can occur in more diffuse pulmonary infection. Diagnosis includes chest radiograph, computed tomography (CT) scan, and microbiologic cultures of body fluids, including sputum. Tissue biopsies may also be performed. Treatment consists of antifungal agents such as oral fluconazole or, in more severe cases, IV amphotericin B. If the patient survives the initial infection, oral antifungal agents become a lifetime therapy.

Candidiasis. *Candida albicans* can affect the skin, mucous membranes in the mouth, vagina, GI, or urinary tract. In HIV-infected individuals, oral infections usually manifest as white patches on the surface of the tongue and buccal mucosa. When involving the pharynx, esophagus, and hard palate, symptoms of sore throat and altered taste sensation are present. This condition is commonly referred to as *thrush* and is one of the defining symptoms for AIDS. Esophageal candidiasis can cause difficulty or pain when swallowing. Nystatin (Mycostatin) swish and swallow is the treatment for oral and esophageal thrush. Repeated outbreaks of vaginal candidiasis (yeast infection) may be the initial symptom of HIV infection in women. Fluconazole orally or vaginally is the most common treatment for recurrent *Candida* infections.

Pneumocystis jiroveci (formerly *carinii*). *Pneumocystis jiroveci* pneumonia (PCP) is also called *pneumocystosis*. The causative agent was originally thought to be a protozoan *(Pneumocystis carinii)*, but more research resulted in its reclassification as a fungus *(Pneumocystis jiroveci)* in 2002 (Stringer et al., 2002). The organism is present in the environment and is usually inhaled during childhood (Ponce et al., 2010). When the CD4 count is 200 cells/μL or less, *P. jiroveci* becomes activated. The symptoms may be a nonproductive cough, shortness of breath, dyspnea on exertion, chest discomfort, fever, malaise, night sweats, and weight loss. *P. jiroveci* may also infect other sites such as the CNS, eyes, GI tract, and lymph nodes.

Trimethoprim-sulfamethoxazole (Bactrim, Septra) is recommended for first-line therapy. However, more than 25% of patients taking this sulfa-based drug develop an allergy. In this situation, dapsone or aerosolized pentamidine can be used for treatment and as a prophylaxis. PCP also is seen after chemotherapy for cancer and in organ transplant patients because of therapeutic immune suppression to prevent organ rejection.

Parasitic infections

Toxoplasmosis. Toxoplasmosis (toxo) is caused by a *protozoan* (a unicellular organism) called *Toxoplasma gondii.* The organism is found in wild game, lamb, and venison. Cats—both wild and domestic—can be infected with toxo by eating infected prey such as birds or mice, or by ingesting contaminated meat or soil that passes into their feces. Within 24 hours the oocysts (toxo eggs) in the feces become spores, which can remain in the environment for more than a year. In the individual with a normal immune system, an infection can cause flulike symptoms or may cause a severe inflammatory response. If the toxo survives, cysts can form in the brain, muscles, and heart. In immunosuppression, the cysts break down and infect the patient's body.

🏃 Health Promotion

Preventing Toxoplasmosis

Toxoplasma gondii, the organism that causes toxoplasmosis, is found in poorly cooked meats, particularly pork, venison, and mutton. Immunosuppressed or pregnant individuals should not empty cat litter boxes or eat undercooked meat. Children's sand boxes and dirt play areas may contain cat feces. Gardeners routinely come in contact with soil that could be contaminated. *Toxoplasma* is transmitted by the individual swallowing the organism. Thorough hand hygiene using soap and water after contact with contaminated items can help prevent the spread of the organism.

The clinical manifestations may be nonspecific and include fever, headache, nausea and vomiting, and malaise. Usually CNS symptoms predominate, such as problems with motor skills and speech. Altered mental status, confusion, lethargy, cognitive impairment, and coma may also occur. A head CT scan is the usual diagnostic test for toxoplasmosis. Treatment includes pyrimethamine and sulfadiazine for as long as 6 weeks. Folinic acid should also be given to prevent hematologic side effects. Lifelong suppressive therapy consists of the same medications in smaller doses.

Cryptosporidiosis. Cryptosporidiosis is caused by a microscopic parasite, *Cryptosporidium parvum. Cryptosporidium*—an intestinal protozoan—manifests in HIV-infected individuals with severe, large-volume, foul-smelling, watery diarrhea. As the result of significant fluid losses, severe abdominal cramping, and malaise, an electrolyte imbalance (especially of sodium, potassium, and chloride) can occur. Cryptosporidiosis can also cause weight loss, dehydration, malabsorption, malnutrition, skin breakdown, and debilitation. The diarrhea may last anywhere from 4 to 20 days.

Cryptosporidium is easily spread by contaminated food or water or by direct contact with an infected person or animal. People with healthy immune systems can be infected, but the symptoms are usually self-limiting. Individuals with AIDS can become severely ill. There are no pharmacologic therapies that will eliminate the parasite. Most therapies are aimed at symptom control and replacement of lost fluid and electrolytes.

FIGURE 11-2 Kaposi sarcoma.

Neoplasms

Kaposi sarcoma. Kaposi sarcoma (KS) is one of the most frequent causes of malignancy in HIV-positive persons, and is more common in HIV-infected men than women (American Cancer Society, 2009). KS is caused by the human herpesvirus type 8. KS does not usually cause death.

KS appears as discolored areas on the skin, but can also form inside the mouth, lungs, and intestines (Figure 11-2). The skin discoloration may range from pink to red or purple. The lesions tend to darken over time. In people with olive or black skin, the lesions may appear dark brown or black. The discoloration is caused by the formation of many tiny blood vessels and cancer cells under the skin.

HAART can halt or even eliminate the progression of skin lesions in some individuals. Skin lesions can concurrently be treated with liquid nitrogen, surgically removed, or injected with anticancer drugs. Low-dose radiation therapy is used for small skin lesions. Larger doses are required for internal organs and lymph node involvement. Radiation treatment can reduce the size of tumors near lymph nodes; this improves lymph flow and decreases lymphedema (see Chapters 12 and 39). If KS has spread into internal organs and HAART treatment is insufficient, doxorubicin (Doxil), daunorubicin (DaunoXome), or paclitaxel (Taxol) may be added.

Lymphomas. Lymphomas are tumors of the tissues and cells of the lymphatic system. Non-Hodgkin's lymphoma (NHL) is the most common lymphoma in people with HIV/AIDS. Most cases of NHL are large B-cell lymphomas and have an approximate 2-year mortality rate. HAART therapy appears to slow its progression; however, death is the outcome in a large percentage of cases (Highleyman, 2009). See Chapter 12 for additional information on lymphomas.

Neurologic Complications.

HIV encephalopathy and AIDS dementia may occur at any point in the disease process. In some individuals it may be the only symptom. The neurologic signs and symptoms displayed could arise from the progression of the virus or they could be a result of opportunistic infections, tumors, or drug-related complications. The symptoms have a very subtle beginning and are difficult to differentiate from depression, Parkinson's disease, and Alzheimer's disease.

Treatment with HAART appears to be the most effective intervention by targeting the primary cause of the problem. Nursing interventions focus on preventing the individual from doing harm to self or to others and ensuring that daily needs are being met.

❖ NURSING MANAGEMENT

▪ Assessment (Data Collection)

The assessment should include a review of signs and symptoms, functional level (ability to perform activities of daily living [ADLs]), safety, self-care abilities, support systems, financial status, risk behaviors, living environment, and understanding of disease process, transmission, and therapeutic regimen. The assessment of the functional level is an ongoing assessment. One tool that is useful is the Karnofsky Performance Scale (Table 11-4).

History and Physical Assessment

The history should include a general assessment of the patient's past and present status. Previous history of HIV testing, such as blood donations or military service, might be important for the timing of HIV infection. Current prescription medications and treatments should be documented, to include whether the patient is on any experimental, herbal, immune complex boosting agents and other complementary and alternative therapies. If the patient has been HIV

Table 11-4	Karnofsky Performance Scale	
DESCRIPTION		**PERCENT (%)**
Normal; no complaints; no evidence of disease		100
Able to carry on normal activity; minor signs and symptoms of disease		90
Normal activity with effort; some signs and symptoms of disease		80
Cares for self; unable to carry on normal activity or do work		70
Requires occasional assistance, but is able to care for most personal needs		60
Requires considerable assistance and frequent medical care		50
Disabled; requires special care and assistance		40
Severely disabled; hospitalization indicated although death not imminent		30
Very sick; hospitalization necessary, requires active support treatment		20
Moribund; fatal processes progressing rapidly		10
Dead		0

Adapted from AETC. (2006). *Clinical Manual for Management of the HIV-infected Adult.* New Jersey, AETC National Resource Center, p. 10-1.

positive for some time, it is important to obtain a history of OIs. Ask if there is any history of respiratory illnesses that increase risk for current problems, such as bacterial or opportunistic pneumonia, chronic obstructive pulmonary disease, or asthma. Assess for smoking history. Determine if the patient has been tested for tuberculosis—if so, when, and what were the results? The neurologic history should include questions about pain or numbness in the extremities and changes in mental status (since HIV/AIDS can cause serious neurologic changes as the disease progresses). A sexual history is needed to ascertain risky behaviors such as multiple sexual partners and possible exposure to other sexually transmitted infections. Assessing for a history of substance use is also important to determine the risk of transmission. Discussing notification of sexual or needle-sharing partners is essential.

A complete head-to-toe physical evaluation should be performed. During the physical examination, particular attention should be given to eye and mouth condition, neurologic status, skin and lymph nodes, and any signs of OIs.

Focused Assessment

Data Collection for the HIV-Positive Patient

First gather a general health history, then:
- Obtain height, weight; note any loss from usual weight.
- Obtain vital signs. Assess for hypotension, orthostatic hypotension, and fever.
- Assess neurologic function, cognition, and neurovascular status.
- Determine level of consciousness, orientation to time and place, cognition, and concentration ability.
- Assess for visual changes.
- Determine if there has been a change in eating pattern.
- Evaluate ability to swallow.
- Determine presence of nausea, vomiting, or diarrhea. If diarrhea is present, note the volume and quantity and duration.
- Assess for dehydration and electrolyte imbalances (see Chapter 3).
- Auscultate the heart.
- Assess quality of respirations; auscultate breath sounds.
- Determine character of the cough and sputum if cough is present.
- Assess condition of skin and mucous membranes.
- Assess for peripheral and periorbital edema and lymphedema.
- Identify any psychosocial issues that may complicate or enhance care.

Changes in nutritional status could be caused by nausea, vomiting, or diarrhea related to the HAART regimen. Assess for signs of dehydration which can lead to potassium depletion, hyponatremia, and hypokalemia. Assess for pale mucous membranes and dry, flaky skin. If the patient has advanced AIDS, observe the patient for anasarca (generalized massive edema) in the trunk, extremities, and around the eyes. This occurs as a result of severe depletion of albumin caused by inadequate nutritional intake. The HIV/AIDS patient may experience changes in motor and sensory function, such as gait changes, imbalance, and changes in vision (particularly in peripheral visual fields). Clinical and situational depression related to the HIV/AIDS diagnosis—and other behavioral changes—may also be noted.

Psychosocial History. The psychosocial assessment should include a history of interpersonal relationships, educational level, and career information. It is important to determine if the patient has told his family of his HIV status. Examples of questions to ask include: Have you experienced multiple losses? What is your living situation? Do you live with someone who is helpful? Are you involved in any community organizations, such as a church, mosque, temple, or synagogue? Referrals (such as community-based AIDS organizations) are needed if the patient does not have a support network.

? Think Critically

A diagnosis of HIV affects a person's self-concept. How could you help a patient to voice his feelings about the diagnosis and find an effective means to cope with the disease?

■ Nursing Diagnosis

Table 11-5 identifies common nursing diagnoses, expected outcomes, and interventions that may be associated with systemic, psychosocial, or specific body system responses to HIV/AIDS.

■ Planning

An HIV-positive patient can have significant issues relating to financing, employment, housing, mental health, substance abuse, or other medical problems. HIV care is usually performed in an outpatient clinical setting and the health care team may include the patient, nurses, physicians, the dietitian, the pharmacist, the discharge planner, and the primary caregiver at home. Information related to the patient's social and economic status is critical for the team to develop and implement a successful treatment plan. The patient's ability to participate in the delivery of the plan of care must be periodically reassessed. If the patient is allowed to have a role in decisions and adjustments to the treatment plan, it increases the likelihood of compliance. The major nursing goals are listed in Box 11-5.

■ Implementation

In accordance with National Patient Safety Goals, Standard Precautions must be consistently used when caring for all patients (see Chapter 6 and Appendix B). For prevention of secondary infections, hand hygiene is critical for health care providers, the patient, and the family. Role modeling and teaching about the importance of hand hygiene happens during routine care. The nurse must also teach about decreasing infection risk in the home setting.

Table 11-5 Nursing Diagnoses and Interventions for the Patient with HIV/AIDS

NURSING DIAGNOSIS	EXPECTED OUTCOMES	NURSING INTERVENTIONS
Risk for infection as evidenced by elevated body temperature and depressed immune function	Patient will exhibit no signs of infection; normal temperature	Monitor body temperature daily. Monitor for outward signs of infections and for symptoms of opportunistic infection. Assess for signs of dehydration and altered mental status.
Impaired gas exchange as evidenced by excessive lung secretions and use of respiratory accessory muscles for breathing	Patient's oxygenation will improve to within baseline levels within 3 wk of beginning treatment	Encourage deep breathing and coughing as indicated. Conserve strength and oxygen by assisting with activities of daily living. Position patient to allow for maximum chest expansion. Monitor breathing patterns and breath sounds q 4 hr. Provide supplemental oxygen as ordered. Monitor blood gases as ordered. Suction airway PRN as ordered.
Impaired skin integrity as evidenced by multiple areas of skin abrasion and state of dehydration	No further areas of skin breakdown will occur Areas of abrasion will heal within 2 wk	Assess skin status q 4 hr; assess for areas of excoriation, lesions, rashes, and discoloration. Report changes from baseline findings. Change linens as needed if diaphoresis or incontinence is present to keep skin clean and dry. Use elbow and heel protectors and special mattress if patient is bedridden. Encourage adequate fluid intake per physical status. Monitor intake and output. Assess for signs of dehydration or fluid overload/edema q 4 hr.
Imbalanced nutrition: less than body requirements	Patient will not experience further weight loss	Assess patient's ability to take in food, chew, and swallow. Monitor weight twice a week. Record input and output. Administer antiemetics as ordered. Assess the availability of food within living situation. Assess ability of caregiver to meet patient's nutritional needs. Administer dietary supplements if required.
Pain related to pressure on nerves from Kaposi sarcoma and discomfort from peripheral neuropathy	Pain will be controlled within tolerable levels within 4 days	Assess pain level and patient's methods to relieve it. Relieve causes of pain by correcting underlying condition if possible. Administer pain medications as ordered; assess amount of relief provided by medication; if relief is not adequate, consult with physician for more effective protocol for pain relief; explore use of NSAIDs and antidepressant medications for pain relief in conjunction with other analgesics. Implement adjunctive therapies to assist with pain relief: massage, cold or hot applications, repositioning, distraction, meditation, imagery. Teach relaxation techniques.
Activity intolerance	Level of activity intolerance will improve within 1 mo	Encourage periods of rest alternated with periods of activity; plan activities according to usual stamina levels; change schedule of activities as degree of fatigue indicates need; assist with activities of daily living as needed to conserve energy.
Ineffective coping related to diagnosis of life-threatening illness, fatigue, and anxiety	Patient will marshal usual effective coping techniques to meet challenges of the illness	Establish rapport with the patient, the partner, and family. Assess past methods of effective coping. Assess patient's strengths. Schedule activities that may cause stress when the patient is most rested or has support person available. Review effective methods for problem solving.

CNS, central nervous system; *NSAIDs,* nonsteroidal anti-inflammatory drugs; *PRN,* as needed.

Continued

Table 11-5 Nursing Diagnoses and Interventions for the Patient with HIV/AIDS—cont'd

NURSING DIAGNOSIS	EXPECTED OUTCOMES	NURSING INTERVENTIONS
Disturbed sensory perception (visual) related to loss of visual fields and HIV damage to CNS	Patient will develop methods of dealing with visual changes within 1 mo	Assess amount of visual deficit. Orient patient to the environment. Speak to and touch patient frequently while in the room. Keep patient informed of what you are doing and what will be happening to decrease fear and anxiety. Instruct to report any further change in vision. Assist with methods to enhance remaining vision and to prevent injury.
Self-care deficit related to fatigue, deterioration of physical condition, mental changes, and neurologic impairment	Patient will accomplish as many activities of daily living as possible without undue fatigue. Patient will accept assistance with activities of daily living within 2 wk	Assess ability to perform own activities of daily living. Provide assistance for activities the patient is unable to perform. Refer to occupational and physical therapy for assistive devices and home equipment needed. Instruct significant other and family members how to assist with activities of daily living.

Box 11-5 Major Nursing Goals for Adults with HIV/AIDS

- Prevent secondary bacterial, viral, and fungal infections.
- Prevent wasting resulting from malnutrition.
- Maintain or improve the present level of immune function.
- Maintain adequate social functioning.
- Maintain or improve current mental status.

 Patient Teaching

The Patient with Compromised Immunity

- Perform hand hygiene frequently and particularly before eating, after toileting, after petting an animal, after touching or shaking hands, and when returning home from shopping or errands.
- Wash the armpits, groin, genitals, and anal area at least twice a day with an antimicrobial soap and dry areas thoroughly.
- Obtain adequate rest daily to allow the body to function as well as possible.
- Take the temperature at least once a day.
- Assess for signs of infection on a daily basis and report such signs immediately to the doctor.
- Take all prescribed medications per instructions.
- Refrain from mingling in crowds, especially during flu season.
- Avoid others who are displaying signs and symptoms of an infection.
- Avoid travel to areas with poor sanitation or inadequate health care facilities.
- Cook foods well and avoid eating raw, unwashed foods.
- Wash dishes in the dishwasher or with hot, soapy water.
- Cutting surfaces, knives, and food preparation areas where raw poultry, meat, and seafood were touching should be cleaned after use.
- Do not dig in the soil or work with houseplants.
- Use stress reduction techniques on a regular basis.

 Patient Teaching

Infection Control in the Home of the Person Who Is HIV Positive

GENERAL
- Consistent hand hygiene should be practiced by everyone in the home.
- Personal care items such as razors and toothbrushes should not be shared.

HOUSEKEEPING
- Clean up urine, blood, feces, vomitus, or other body fluids and the surrounding area with soap and warm water. Disinfect the area by wiping with a fresh 1:10 solution of household bleach (1 part bleach to 10 parts water). Dispose of solid wastes either by flushing down the toilet or placing in plastic trash bag and tying it closed.
- Soak rags, mops, and sponges used for cleaning in a fresh 1:10 bleach solution for at least 5 minutes to disinfect.
- Clean bathroom surfaces with regular household cleaners and then disinfect with a 1:10 bleach solution.

LAUNDRY
- Rinse clothes, towels, or linens of urine, blood, feces, vomitus, sputum, or other body secretions. Launder the items with hot water and detergent with 1 cup of bleach.
- Keep soiled clothes in a closed plastic bag before laundering.

BIOHAZARD DISPOSAL
- Dispose of "sharps" in a labeled puncture-proof container with a lid, using Standard Precautions. When the container is ¾ full, add a 1:10 bleach solution. Seal the container with tape and place it in a plastic biohazard bag. The home care nurse can dispose of it.
- Flush solid waste down the toilet. Place disposable diapers or contaminated paper towels and disposable gloves in tied plastic bags and dispose of them in the regular trash.

Adapted from Ignatavicius, D.D., & Workman, M.L. (2010). *Medical-Surgical Nursing: Critical Thinking for Collaborative Care* (6th ed.). Philadelphia: Elsevier Saunders, p. 384.

Wasting syndrome is defined as losing more than 10% of weight along with at least 30 days of either diarrhea or weakness accompanied by fever. There is loss of body fat and muscle mass. This syndrome has a strong correlation to progression of HIV disease, and leads to death. Contributing factors include decreased appetite; the inability to absorb enough nutrients through the small intestines because of the diarrhea; and an altered metabolism that may be associated with hormone levels. Referral to a nutritionist or dietitian and providing written materials, such as how to plan a nutritious balanced diet using the USDA MyPlate can be helpful.

 Nutrition Considerations

Improving Food Intake for the Patient with AIDS

Encourage the following measures:
- Eat small amounts frequently.
- Eat high-calorie snacks or commercially available liquid supplements or "power" bars.
- Eat foods at room temperature.
- Soften dry grain foods such as breads, crackers, and cookies in milk before eating them.
- Eat nonabrasive foods that are easy to swallow such as pasta, well-cooked eggs, baked fish, soft cheese, pudding, and ice cream.
- Suck on ice pops to numb or soothe mouth pain.

The patient should avoid:
- Raw fruits and vegetables unless they are thoroughly washed.
- Spicy, acidic, or salty foods.
- Alcohol and carbonated beverages.
- Excessively hot food.

Instruct the patient on how to take the medication and which medications should be taken with or without food. By consistently taking antimicrobials and antiretroviral medications as ordered, less resistance to the drugs occurs, and the effectiveness of the drugs is thus prolonged.

Encourage social interaction and independence in activities, as tolerated. Support groups can boost feelings of self-esteem and self-worth. Social interaction may reduce situational depression and can empower the patient. Promoting a positive attitude may reduce feelings of powerlessness. Referral to community-based AIDS organizations is appropriate, with the patient's consent.

■ Evaluation

A patient's expectations may not be the same as those of the health care team or the primary caregivers, so when outcomes are evaluated, variations in expectations should be addressed by all of those involved. Monitoring laboratory tests to determine immune status, viral load, blood cell status, and effects of medications is a large part of the evaluation process.

HIV Risk in the Over-50 Population

The life expectancy in the United States has increased to greater than 78 years (National Center for Health Statistics, 2009). A persistent myth is that older adults are no longer interested in sex. Many older adults are single as a result of divorce or death of a spouse or partner. Also, erectile dysfunction medications allow sexual activity for longer periods in some men. Because pregnancy is not a consideration, condoms are typically not used as they should be.

The media tend to report more on younger populations, including MSM, transgendered individuals, the homeless, and IV drug users. Many older adults are not aware of the risks, but old age is no barrier to becoming infected with HIV. The primary modes of transmission in the over-50 age-group are through heterosexual contact and sharing of contaminated needles in the IV drug population. The older adult may ignore symptoms, because of a belief that they are a normal part of aging. By the time an older at-risk adult is actually diagnosed, his survival rate is markedly less than that of a younger person (National Institute on Aging, 2009). This is probably because of comorbidities (simultaneous presence of two chronic diseases or conditions) common to the older population. Menopausal women are more vulnerable to HIV infection from sexual transmission, because decreased estrogen levels cause thinning of the tissue and decreased lubrication. Also a woman's male sex partner is statistically more likely to have had multiple other sexual contacts, increasing the likelihood of HIV infection. In the older population, the virus is spread easier because of the thinning and microscopic tearing of the anal mucosa.

Skin and mucous membranes are more fragile in the elderly person, possibly making transmission easier. To a small degree, the bone marrow is affected by the aging process; thus, after age 70, there is a definite decline in the functioning of the immune system. The nurse must educate and encourage this age group about the need for HIV testing in *both* partners before entering into a new sexual relationship, along with recommendations to use barrier techniques.

 Elder Care Points

New diagnoses of HIV infection are growing faster in the over-50 age group than in the under-50 age group. All sexually active adults should be assessed for at-risk behaviors, regardless of the age of the patient. Age-specific referrals to a geriatric nurse practitioner or counselor with experience working with older adults may also be appropriate.

Community Education and Care

All nurses should be alert to the possibility of transmission of HIV and the methods of prevention, and should share this information with at-risk populations.

Patients, their partners, families, and friends should all be included in the educational opportunities.

HIV Confidentiality and Disclosure Issues

With the implementation of the Health Insurance Portability and Accountability Act (HIPAA), if protected health information (PHI) is released inappropriately, there may be severe penalties such as legal or financial sanctions levied against the nurse or other health care providers. Therefore, when a patient signs a form to release medical information, the form must also state if the patient wants his HIV/AIDS diagnosis released. A lawsuit and the loss of the nursing license may be the penalty for the nurse who is indiscreet and discloses PHI without specific patient authorization. For the patient, the consequences may be the loss of a job, of housing or insurance benefits, and possible discrimination and rejection by families and friends.

 Legal and Ethical Considerations

Confidentiality and HIV

The diagnosis of AIDS is a medical diagnosis and can be discussed among health care personnel like any other medical diagnosis, for the purpose of rendering care to the patient, and does not require a patient's consent. The right to disclose HIV status is regulated by the state in which you are working. It is important for every licensed nurse to be aware of the state regulations and institutional policies. If the patient has given permission (preferably in writing) the family can be informed about the symptoms and what progress or lack of progress is occurring. (The nurse should reinforce the information provided by the physician.) It is always preferable for the patient to disclose diagnostic information and HIV status to the family.

Since 1983, all states have been required to report AIDS cases—including patient demographic information—to the local public health department. The information is ultimately sent to the federal government for tracking, as is the case with all infectious diseases. Most states have reported HIV status using a coded system allowing for anonymity of the patient. In July 2005 the CDC formally recommended that all states adopt a confidential name–based reporting system.

 Legal and Ethical Considerations

When a Nurse Is HIV Positive

If a health care worker is HIV positive, there is a risk of transmitting the virus to others. What are the ethical, moral, and legal responsibilities to patients in such a situation?

Blood-Borne Pathogen Exposure and Health Care Workers

Health care workers are at increased risk of exposure through needle sticks or contaminated blood and body fluids, especially if these fluids enter an open cut or the mucous membranes, such as the eyes or inside of the nose or mouth. The federal government has mandated guidelines that all health care workers are required to follow. Employers are also required, by law, to provide specially engineered devices and equipment at no charge to their employees. The proper use of personal protective equipment such as face masks, gloves, cover gowns, and safety engineered needles and syringes has greatly reduced the risk of exposure to blood-borne or other potentially infectious pathogens among health care personnel (see Figure 6-4).

 Safety Alert

Disposal of Sharps

- Place all disposable sharp instruments, or "sharps," directly into a special biohazard container immediately after use.
- Never place your fingers into a sharps container.
- Replace sharps containers when they are three-quarters full.
- Seal and send the full sharps container for disposal per facility protocol.
- If a needle stick occurs, wash the area of puncture thoroughly with soap and water, report to the charge nurse immediately afterward, complete an incident/occurrence report, and follow the agency-instituted protocol for treatment and follow-up.

The CDC and the Occupational Safety and Health Administration (OSHA), along with other health care agencies, have developed evidence-based guidelines to prevent exposure to blood, body fluids, and other potentially infectious microorganisms (OPIM). If the health care worker correctly implements these guidelines, the risk of being exposed is markedly reduced.

 Safety Alert

Possible Exposure to HIV

After an unintended exposure to blood or body fluids of a person who either is HIV positive or whose HIV status is unknown, the need for postexposure prophylaxis (PEP) must be assessed within 2 hours. Exposure can be from a large-bore needle stick, significant mucosal contact with body fluids, or contact with body fluids via a break in the skin. The facility's Infection Preventionist or infection control officer should be notified of the exposure. Two-drug or three-drug therapy, depending on the degree of determined risk, may be initiated as soon as possible after the exposure event. The medications may need to be taken until HIV status from the source patient has been determined; if known to be HIV positive, the drugs should be taken for 4 to 6 weeks. The drugs used are from a different class (NRTI, NNRTI, PI). If PEP is indicated, the nurse may be unable to work for the first few weeks while on the medications because of the significant side effects (i.e., headaches, nausea, vomiting, and diarrhea).

In many health care facilities across the United States, **disciplinary actions result from not following the CDC's Standard Precautions,** as well as the policies and procedures of the employer to prevent exposure to blood-borne pathogens. Consistent and correct use of personal protective equipment is required during every patient contact. Know what your rights and responsibilities are according to the state and institutional policy, should there be an accidental occupational exposure. Report any exposure to your manager or supervisor immediately and follow facility protocols that are in place. Infection prevention and control is the key to safety in any health care setting (see Chapter 6).

Get Ready for the NCLEX® Examination!

Key Points

- A barrier, such as a latex condom, should be used during insertive or receptive sexual intercourse to decrease the risk of acquiring HIV.
- HIV testing should be offered at the time of a complete physical examination for all sexually active patients.
- HIV disease in the United States is now usually a chronic controllable disease.
- Performing genotyping and phenotyping in the newly diagnosed HIV-positive person helps determine if the person has any drug-resistant strains of HIV.
- The diagnosis of AIDS is made by CD4 count less than 200 cells/μL or by the presence of specific OIs.
- Opportunistic infections secondary to AIDS cause increased morbidity and mortality.
- HIV medications can have severe side effects and can also have significant drug interactions. Long term effects are unknown.
- Wasting syndrome in an AIDS patient is defined as a weight loss of more than 10% of usual body weight.
- If a health care worker is exposed to blood or body fluids of an HIV-positive patient, the infection control officer should be notified to assist with treatment and follow up.

Additional Learning Resources

SG Go to your Study Guide for additional learning activities to help you master this chapter content.

evolve Go to your Evolve website (http://evolve.elsevier.com/deWit/medsurg) for the following FREE learning resources:
- Animations, audio, and video
- Answers and rationales for questions and activities
- Concept Map Creator
- Glossary with pronunciations in English and Spanish
- Interactive Review Questions and Exercises and more!

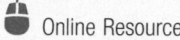
Online Resources
- Centers for Disease Control and Prevention, http://cdc.gov/hiv
- World Health Organization, www.who.int/hiv/en

Review Questions for the NCLEX® Examination

1. The nurse reinforces the physician's order to draw blood for HIV genotyping. The patient asks, "How does that help in my treatment?" What is the best explanation for the test?
   1. Confirms the presence of a viral autoimmune disease
   2. Informs how much of the virus has been replicated
   3. Determines the presence of any mutations in the virus
   4. Reveals the viral load or count of the virus

2. A patient known to be positive for human immunodeficiency virus is admitted with oral thrush, recurrent vaginal yeast infections, and skin infections. What do these signs indicate?
   1. Opportunistic infection
   2. Antimicrobial resistance
   3. Resistant strain of HIV
   4. Sentinel infection

3. Which laboratory test determines the stage of human immunodeficiency virus status, the timing of the initiation of therapy, and the prophylactic management of opportunistic infections?
   1. Blood culture and sensitivity
   2. Western blot test
   3. CD4 count
   4. Enzyme-linked immunospecific assay

4. The nurse explains the mechanism of action of a nucleoside reverse transcriptase inhibitor (NRTI) to a patient who is newly diagnosed with acquired immunodeficiency syndrome. What is the most accurate statement?
   1. "It prevents the virus from altering healthy CD4 cells."
   2. "It inhibits viral reproduction by disabling conversion of RNA to DNA."
   3. "It prevents the virus from maturing."
   4. "It prevents HIV genetic material from entering host cells."

5. A patient with AIDS and cytomegalovirus retinitis was prescribed foscarnet (Foscavir). Which finding requires immediate nursing attention before this medication is administered?

   1. Elevated serum creatinine
   2. Decreased CD4 lymphocytes
   3. Temperature 99.7° F
   4. Acyclovir viral infection

6. A patient has difficulty breathing associated with cough, fever, weight loss, and night sweats. What is an appropriate nursing action?

   1. Initiate airborne infection isolation precautions.
   2. Prohibit visitors.
   3. Administer antiparasitic medications.
   4. Monitor intake and output once a day.

7. A 59-year-old divorced woman comes to the clinic with complaints of weight loss, fatigue, and fever. Which question is irrelevant?

   1. Are you sexually active?
   2. How long have you had these symptoms?
   3. What have you changed in your diet?
   4. Have you been experiencing vaginal dryness?

8. A patient has just been newly diagnosed with HIV. What test will be performed that can indicate whether the patient will experience CNS difficulties if the CD4 count is $\leq 100 \, \mu L$?

   1. Toxoplasmosis
   2. Coccidioidomycosis
   3. Cryptococcus
   4. Histoplasmosis

9. Which statement(s) is/are true regarding human immunodeficiency virus transmission? *(Select all that apply.)*

   1. Breast milk can harbor the virus.
   2. Proper use of personal protective equipment reduces the risk of disease transmission.
   3. Needle exchange programs facilitate the spread of the virus.
   4. Being assessed 4 hours after a blood-borne pathogen (BBP) exposure decreases the risk of conversion.
   5. Monogamous relationships provide the best defense from the virus.

10. In determining the optimal therapy for a patient infected with the human immunodeficiency virus, what would the physician consider? *(Select all that apply.)*

    1. Clinical data
    2. Compliance with therapy
    3. Medication tolerance
    4. Insurance coverage
    5. Physician expectations

Critical Thinking Activities

Scenario A

Mark Johnson is an 80-year-old patient being admitted to the hospital for pneumonia. Five years ago he had a blood transfusion for treatment of injuries suffered in an automobile accident during a trip to Africa. He was recently found to be HIV positive. He has no other significant health problems. He is married and has three grown children and several grandchildren.

1. What symptoms are displayed by someone who is HIV positive?

2. What should be discussed with his family regarding his HIV status?

3. How should his HIV infection be treated?

Scenario B

A nursing assistant was instructed to clean up equipment that was used in a bedside procedure. She accidentally sustains a needle stick while putting a used syringe into an overly filled "sharps" container in the room of an HIV-positive patient. The nursing assistant is crying hysterically and unable to act in her own behalf.

1. What should you do first?

2. Outline the steps of treatment and reporting for this type of incident.

3. What factors may have contributed to the accident?

Care of Patients with Immune and Lymphatic Disorders

Objectives

Theory

1. Summarize the ideal actions of therapeutic immunosuppressive drugs.
2. Explain the importance of minimizing the administration of antimicrobial agents.
3. Describe effects of aging on the immune system.
4. Explain why an immune-suppressed patient, with infection, may not have an elevated body temperature.
5. Explain how an allergic reaction occurs during an excessive immune response.
6. Summarize the nurse's role in helping the patient to control allergies.
7. Discuss the three categories of autoimmune disorders and give examples of autoimmune disorders/diseases.
8. Evaluate and explain why the process of diagnosis and treatment for systemic lupus erythematosus would be difficult or frustrating for the patient.

9. Compare and contrast the two types of lymphoma and how they are diagnosed.

Clinical Practice

1. List nursing measures for the prevention of infection for an immunocompromised patient.
2. List key elements for data collection, if an immune-suppressant disorder is suspected.
3. Perform nursing assessment on a patient with a primary allergic condition.
4. List the usual measures for treating an anaphylactic reaction and locate the necessary emergency equipment on your clinical unit.
5. Perform nursing interventions for a patient with lymphedema.
6. Review a nursing care plan for a patient who has systemic lupus erythematosus.
7. List interventions that can be used for a patient with fibromyalgia.

Key Terms

allergy (p. 236)
allodynia (p. 254)
anaphylaxis (ă-nă-fă-LĂK-sĭs, p. 236)
angioedema (ăn-jē-ōh-ĕ-DĒ-mă, p. 241)
atopy (ĂT-ōh-pē, p. 237)
erythema (p. 245)
histamine (p. 236)
hyperalgesia (p. 254)
hypersensitivity reactions (p. 236)
iatrogenic (p. 234)

immunosuppression (p. 234)
lymphadenopathy (p. 250)
lymphedema (p. 253)
patch test (p. 237)
relapse (p. 250)
remissions (p. 254)
scratch test (p. 237)
syndrome (p. 243)
urticaria (ŭr-tĭ-KĀ-rē-ăh, p. 241)
wheals (wēlz, p. 241)

IMMUNE DISORDERS

Abnormal responses of the immune system are divided into two basic categories: immune deficiency disorders and autoimmune diseases. In immune deficiency disorders there is an insufficient production of antibodies, immune cells, or both and the disorders may be congenital or acquired. A deficiency in the immune system leaves the body unable to resist foreign microbes or toxins. Autoimmune disorders involve the overreaction or hypersensitivity to antigens from the external environment where the immune system is unable to tell the difference between "non-self" (foreign cells) and "self" (the body's own cells).

Common viral infections, such as influenza or infectious mononucleosis, can cause a short-term depression of an effective immune response. Other conditions that decrease the immune system include smoking, malnutrition, surgery, and stress. The immune system can also be therapeutically suppressed; for example, antirejection medications prevent a tissue transplant rejection.

THERAPEUTIC IMMUNOSUPPRESSION

A variety of disorders or conditions can be treated or controlled by medications or therapies such as corticosteroids, hemodialysis, organ transplantation, or

Box 12-1 **Ideal Actions of Immunosuppressive Drug Therapy**

- Wide margin of safety between therapeutic and toxic dosing.
- Selective effects on lymphoid cells while not harming the rest of the body.
- Suppress only the specific immune processes on the cells involved in causing the disease.
- Drug administration only needed for a limited amount of time so the body's immune response becomes familiar with the foreign antigen and sees it as a part of the "self."
- Once the new immune response has been developed, the drug should be effective against the immune processes of the body.

radiation. However, some of these treatments can lead to chronic medical conditions or iatrogenic complications such as diabetes mellitus, osteoporosis, chronic infections, and significant weight gain. Drug-induced **immunosuppression,** often referred to as therapeutically induced immunosuppression, requires a delicate balance between the control of the body's immune response and the side effects. The ideal balance of therapeutic immunosuppressive drugs would inhibit the normal immune system response; defend against invasion from assorted microbial agents; and control the occurrence of the usual side effects, such as stomach ulcers and tremors (Box 12-1).

An example of an **iatrogenic** (a side effect of medical treatment) immune suppression occurs with an organ transplant recipient. This type of patient is at increased risk of organ rejection if the patient's own immune system is activated to destroy this "foreign" organ. The patient must take multiple medications, as a lifetime therapy, such as azathioprine (Imuran) and cyclosporine (Sandimmune) (Table 12-1).

There is significant evidence that use of antirejection medications increases the survival rate of patients with certain organ transplants, but it does not completely eliminate the danger of organ rejection or other health complications. Immunosuppressant drugs may need to be adjusted according to the systemic and immune response of each patient and to prevent toxicity.

Immunosuppressive agents are used to manage autoimmune disorders such as multiple myeloma, non-Hodgkin's lymphoma, rheumatoid arthritis, and select neoplastic growths.

DIAGNOSTIC TESTS AND TREATMENT OF IMMUNE DEFICIENCIES

In the early stages of an autoimmune disorder, definitive diagnosis may be difficult. The health care provider must look at the complete health history, current complaints or symptoms, and physical examination findings so that the appropriate diagnostic studies can be performed (Box 12-2).

Some patients' immune systems have virtually no ability to respond to antigens (requires lymphocytes that are sensitized) or to synthesize antibodies, whereas

Table 12-1 **Types of Antirejection Medications**

NAME	ACTION
Antithymocyte globulin	Immunosuppressive agent that selectively destroys T lymphocytes.
Basiliximab	Binds and blocks T cells from replicating and from activating B cells, thereby decreasing the production of antibodies that can lead to rejection.
Daclizumab	Inhibits the function of interleukin-2 (IL-2) receptors on the T cells, which prevents the cells from activating and stimulating the formation of antibodies.
Lymphocyte immune globulin	Reduces the number of circulating thymus-dependent lymphocytes in the blood.
Methylprednisolone	A corticosteroid with anti-inflammatory properties.
Muromonab-CD3	Blocks the function of CD3 molecules in the membrane of human T cells.
Rapamycin	An antimicrobial that demonstrates antifungal, anti-inflammatory, antitumor, and immunosuppressive properties, which inhibits IL-2 so the T and B cells are not activated.

Box 12-2 **Examples of Diagnostic Tests to Determine Presence of Autoimmune Disorder**

- Complete blood count with differential
- Red blood cell count
- Creatinine level
- Antinuclear antibody (ANA)
- Bone marrow studies
- Serum protein
- Protein electrophoresis
- Immunoelectrophoresis
- T-cell and B-cell assays
- Enzyme-linked immunosorbent assays (ELISAs)

others have a temporary minor defect in the humoral or cell-mediated immune response. In some types of immune deficiency, passive immunity can be accomplished by transfusing specifically sensitized lymphocytes to help the patient resist infection. Injections of immune globulin may be given on a regular basis to provide passive immunity for those who are unable to produce their own antibodies. When impaired function of the bone marrow is involved, as in leukemia, the patient may receive a bone marrow transplant to provide the stem cells that will eventually become immune bodies. To help prevent or combat infection in immunosuppressed patients, granulocyte colony-stimulating factor—filgrastim (Neupogen)—can be used to promote the growth of neutrophils, especially in patients with AIDS or in certain types of cancer that produce significant immunodeficiency.

As soon as an infection is evident, antimicrobial agents are usually given. However, these drugs can also be immunosuppressive. One of the National Patient Safety Goals is to decrease the inappropriate use of antimicrobials, which can lead to the development of multidrug-resistant organisms (MDROs) leaving the patient more vulnerable to infection and other complications.

Ideally, treatment in an immunocompromised patient is aimed at controlling the disease or eliminating the condition that led to an inadequately functioning immune system. For example, with nephrosis, liver disease, drug toxicity, and viral infections, this may be possible. In other instances, treatment consists of minimizing the effects of the immune deficiency. Development of immune-specific drugs used in the treatment of HIV/AIDS has assisted in finding effective treatments in some other types of immunodeficiency disorders.

Elder Care Points

Aging does not affect the bone marrow to a significant degree. It does cause the thymus gland to become smaller, and T cells apparently diminish in the circulation; B-cell numbers usually remain the same. After age 70 there is a definite decline in the function of the immune system.

❖ NURSING MANAGEMENT
■ Assessment (Data Collection)

When an immune deficiency is suspected, information is gathered about the current physical status of the patient, such as her general state of health, infections she may have recently had, how the infections affected her, and how frequently they occur. It is also important to assess for risk behaviors such as intravenous drug use, multiple sexual partners, exposure to HIV, immunosuppressive drug therapy, alcohol consumption, and family history of genetic immune disorders. Assess for occupational or environmental exposure to assorted agents. Nutritional status should be assessed by measuring height and weight and inspecting the skin, hair, and overall appearance. If a significant decrease in weight is noted (usually greater than 10%), ask if it was intentional. If not, ask when the loss first started.

Physical assessment should include palpation of the superficial lymph nodes in the neck, axilla, and groin to detect any abnormalities, as well as assessing the body systems involved in the patient's chief complaints. For example, the patient tells the nurse that she feels a bulge around her stomach, so the nurse would palpate both upper quadrants of the abdomen.

Body temperature should be closely monitored for significant changes, **although immune-deficient patients may not have a temperature elevation even in the presence of infection.** The body may not be able to recognize that an infection is beginning until much later in the process because of the body's impaired immune response. Therefore the nurse must assess the whole patient and not just one or two areas, because important signs or symptoms of potential complications can be missed if not performed correctly.

■ Nursing Diagnosis and Planning

Nursing diagnoses for patients with immune deficiency should always include Risk for infection. The primary nursing goals when caring for a patient who has an immune deficiency are to (1) protect the patient from infection, (2) improve her health status, and (3) promote as high a degree of wellness as possible. Expected outcomes based on the nursing diagnoses might include:
- Patient will remain free from infection.
- White blood cell counts are within normal limits.

Planning care for the patient with an immune deficiency focuses on preventing exposure to pathogens. A patient whose immune deficiency is severe will likely need to be placed in transmission-based isolation precautions (formerly called reverse isolation or Neutropenic Precautions). (See Chapter 17 for additional information on neutropenia.) Working with patients in this type of isolation requires more time because of the need for donning and removing the personal protective equipment (PPE) before entering and on leaving the patient's room (see Chapter 6). Integrating care of this patient along with the rest of the patient assignments for the shift needs to be carefully planned.

■ Implementation

Proteins are needed to synthesize antibodies. If the patient has a condition or is on medications that suppress appetite or cause nausea, nutritional intake can be inadequate. Nutritional supplements may be added, and multiple small meals of high-protein foods chosen by the patient may need to be scheduled throughout the day. However, if the patient is on corticosteroid therapy, appetite control may be a challenge and the patient must be carefully monitored for weight gain. Providing low-calorie snacks such as vegetables and certain fruits to eat instead of high-calorie chips, cookies, and sodas would be helpful.

Think Critically

How would you explain to a patient why good-quality protein is important in the diet when an immunodeficiency is present?

Safety Alert
Preventing Infection Among Immune-Deficient Patients

Transmission-based isolation precautions may be indicated (see Chapter 6). In accordance with National Patient Safety Goals, scrupulous hand hygiene is the standard of care for all patients, but for the immunocompromised patient this basic measure could mean the difference between life and death. Disinfect any object, such as your stethoscope, that may serve as a source of infection. Observe strict surgical aseptic technique when performing invasive nursing care procedures such as catheterization, dressing changes, and intravenous infusions.

Excessive stress can further depress immune function. Many factors related to family, employment, finances, or transportation can significantly increase the stress level for the patient or loved ones. As illness progresses, many patients may have difficulties at school or work. Collaboration with a social worker is often indicated. Referrals to community resources can greatly assist the patient and family in dealing with the added stress. The nurse can also be instrumental in teaching the patient stress-reduction strategies, such as light exercise, meditation, relaxation techniques, and guided imagery (see Chapter 7).

Provide patient education regarding the immune disorder and any therapy that the patient is to receive. Teach the patient and family to assess for signs of infection and to report them immediately (see Chapter 11).

■ Evaluation

Ensure that strict hand hygiene is being performed and adhere to transmission-based isolation precautions. Check laboratory test results to assess whether immune function is improving. B-cell and T-cell assays are particularly important. Evaluate the patient for evidence of recovery from any infection that might have been present, as well as for general well-being, appetite, weight changes, and for side effects of medications or other therapies.

DISORDERS OF INAPPROPRIATE IMMUNE RESPONSE

ALLERGY AND HYPERSENSITIVITY

An **allergy** is an abnormal response to certain substances; it is considered to be a systemic immune disorder, rather than a localized one; and the reaction can be seen or expressed in multiple body systems. **Hypersensitivity reactions,** better known as allergic reactions, are the body's excessive response to a normally harmless substance. The severity of the condition can range from a mild rash to **anaphylaxis** (an extreme allergic reaction that is life threatening).

Etiology and Pathophysiology

As the environment has become cleaner over the past decades, there has been an increase in the development of allergies, especially among those in a higher socioeconomic status, living in an urban area versus rural, and being the first-born child (less exposure to other illnesses from siblings). There also appears to be a strong hereditary component to hypersensitive allergic reactions as well (Grammatikos, 2008).

Allergies are divided into two major categories: (1) immediate hypersensitivity reactions that are mast cell mediated (type I hypersensitivity) and (2) delayed-reaction allergies involving T cells (type II hypersensitivity). As with all types of normal and abnormal immune response, a reaction will not occur until an individual's body cells have been sensitized

to the specific substance that triggers the response. This means that on first contact with the allergen, the body's immune system is triggered to produce immunoglobulin E (IgE) antibodies to recognize the specific antigen. On the second and subsequent contacts with the allergen, the antibodies specific to the allergen are rapidly produced and released into the circulating blood or in the lymphoid tissues, in larger and larger quantities. Because of the increased amount of antibodies, they can be quickly transported to the location of the allergen, causing a more rapid, and sometimes virulent, allergic reaction. Type I or rapid inflammatory reactions result from the increased production of mast cells and basophils from IgE antibodies. During this reaction, **histamine** is released from a mast cell mediator. When histamine is released because of an immune response, it triggers increased mucus secretions, vasodilation, and increased vascular permeability, which leads to tissue edema. Dilated blood vessels transport the IgE antibodies, histamine, and other chemicals to the site of exposure to the allergen (Figure 12-1).

① Activation of B cells by the allergen (antigen)

② Production of clone with antibody-secreting plasma cell

③ Secretion of IgE antibodies

④ IgE antibodies bind to mast cells

⑤ Binding of allergen to the IgE antibodies on mast cells with the release of histamine

Bronchoconstriction

Vasodilation

FIGURE 12-1 Immediate-reaction allergy.

If the mast cells are IgE dependent, they typically produce only a localized allergic response. Examples of this are allergic conjunctivitis or allergy-induced asthma. A person who has atopy (a response that affects various parts of the body without being in direct contact with the allergen), such as seen in eczema, tends to be hypersensitive to a variety of allergens. Type II or delayed reactions result from increased production of IgG.

Signs and Symptoms

The body system most affected by the offending agent may present more specific symptomatology. For example, when the nose and eyes are exposed to a contact allergen, symptoms of itchy, red, watery eyes, soft palate pruritus, clear rhinorrhea, and sneezing are common. Should the allergen be inhaled, the release of histamine can cause the contraction of smooth-muscle tissues in the bronchioles of the lungs. These internal changes also produce an allergic response, notably erythema, edema, increased exudate, and breathing difficulties such as dyspnea and wheezing. Table 12-2 presents the four broad types of allergens.

Diagnosis

Identification of Allergens. Identification of allergens can be a tedious process. Many times more than one substance produces the symptoms of an allergy. Reactions to certain food products, animals, insect stings, drugs, and other substances that are out of the norm are noticeable because of the relationship between cause and effect. Therefore the patient must be asked about exposure to substances that appear to or are known to cause an adverse response. The nurse should help the patient to recognize that vague symptoms, such as consistently becoming "stuffed up" at night could be an allergic reaction to her pillow.

Diagnostic Tests. Two primary methods are used to test for allergy. One is performing a radioallergosorbent test, known as RAST. This test uses blood serum from the patient to see if the IgE to the suspected allergen is present. The major advantages to this type of allergy testing are that antihistamine medications can continue; it is safer for patients with serious heart and lung problems; there is no chance of an anaphylactic reaction; it is more useful to identify a true food allergy; and it can be used when severe skin conditions prevent skin testing. The disadvantages to the RAST are that it is more expensive than skin testing; it can take several days to weeks before results are known; and it is less specific, meaning this test tends to produce more false-positive and false-negative results to other allergens.

Skin testing is also used in the diagnosis of allergies. The scratch test has been considered to be the most reliable method of allergy testing for more than 100 years. The skin is pricked by a needle and then a drop of the suspected allergen is applied to the area. A needle is then used to slightly scratch the skin just below the epidermis. The patch test is similar to the scratch test except the allergen is simply placed on the surface of the skin and covered with an airtight dressing (patch). For both of these tests, a negative reaction occurs when there is no erythema, swelling, or complaints of itching by the patient. A positive reaction

Table 12-2 Four Broad Categories of Allergens*

CATEGORY	METHOD OF EXPOSURE	TRIGGERS	EFFECTS
Contactants	Direct contact with mucosa/skin/tissue	Dust, wool fabrics, detergents, soaps, lotions, cosmetics, plants such as poison ivy, dyes, metals in jewelry, latex	Irritation to the conjunctiva of the eyes, urticaria, rashes, hives, dermatitis, eczema
Ingestants	Swallowed	Food: citrus fruits, tomatoes, strawberries, cow's milk, wheat, eggs, dairy products, seafood, chocolate, nuts, monosodium glutamate (MSG), other preservatives, and artificial food coloring Drugs: aspirin, barbiturates, anticonvulsants, antimicrobials, but any drug may cause an allergic reaction	Abdominal pain, flatulence, nausea, vomiting, diarrhea Can also cause atopic dermatitis, rash, dyspnea
Inhalants	Entry through nose or mouth	Dust, molds, pollen, fragrances, animal dander, insect feces, and some chemicals	Edema of nasal mucosa, allergic rhinitis or sinusitis, rhinorrhea, sneezing, laryngeal edema, coughing, dyspnea, bronchoconstriction, wheezing
Injectables	Via needle (i.e., hypodermic, intramuscular, intravenous; animal or snake bites, insect stings)	Medications, vaccines, animal saliva, snake or insect venoms	Swelling and pain at injection site, bruising, discoloration, necrotic skin

*Any of the items mentioned can lead to severe allergic reactions including anaphylaxis and death if not recognized and treated immediately.

to either of these tests is indicated by the appearance of a small (usually dime-size) wheal at the site of contact with the allergen and possibly by complaints of itching by the patient.

Drug Allergy. A patient may have a confirmed medication allergy, yet the medication is required and there are no alternatives. Before administration, a test dose of the drug may be given. For IV medications, a very small dose can be given and then, at 10-minute increments, increasing amounts of the drug are infused until the full dose ordered by the health care provider is administered. The nurse must continuously stay with the patient and closely monitor for signs and symptoms of a reaction during this process. Resuscitation drugs and emergency equipment must be immediately available. This same process is repeated with each subsequent administration of the medication.

⚠ Safety Alert

Patients with Allergies

The medical record should be checked and the patient questioned about allergies before (1) giving medications or immunizations, (2) dispatching the patient for radiographic studies using contrast media, and (3) minor or major surgery.

Food Allergy. Even though other diagnostic methods are available to test for food allergies, a less expensive approach known as the elimination diet should be tried first. The patient should be taught to read product labels to identify offending substances used in the preparation or preserving of the food item. The patient is told to eliminate one food at a time and to keep a detailed diary, recording everything ingested each day, including the additives and preservatives in each food product. The patient should start with a food that is believed to be the cause of adverse reactions (e.g., itching, bloating). If symptoms persist for a week to 10 days after eliminating one food product (e.g., milk and dairy products), the patient would resume intake of that particular food, and choose another one for elimination. This process continues until the offending food source is identified.

Latex Allergy. Because many people have latex allergies, the nurse must be aware of whether the patient is allergic to latex. Most items routinely manufactured with latex are now being produced with non-latex alternatives, including gloves, Foley catheters, surgical drains, bandages, and condoms. The Occupational Safety and Health Administration (OSHA) requires that employers furnish personal protective equipment for their employees at no cost to the employee, and non-latex items should be made available for those with an allergy to latex. Severe latex allergies have caused some health care workers to change their work environment to one with little or no latex exposure.

Treatment

Drug Therapy. Drugs that help alleviate the systemic reactions to allergens include epinephrine, antihistamines, bronchodilators, corticotropin (adrenocorticotropic hormone), and cortisone (see Chapters 14 and 15 for specific drug information).

Antihistamines (histamine-blocking agents) help control the symptoms of hay fever and hives (Table 12-3) by preventing the release of histamine during an allergic reaction. The blocking action relieves itching, decreases swelling of mucous membranes and production of secretions, and reduces other symptoms of an allergic reaction. Diphenhydramine (Benadryl) is commonly used orally and topically to counteract many allergic symptoms.

Antihistamines can cause drowsiness and impaired coordination, so there are restrictions on driving an automobile and operating machinery at the beginning of therapy. Other common side effects include dry mouth, urinary retention, weakness, and blurred vision. Antihistamines and decongestants can aggravate hypertension and should be used with caution in patients who have high blood pressure. Elderly men taking antihistamines may experience hesitancy while voiding, urinary retention, and difficulty with ejaculation; the offending drug should be discontinued if the problem cannot be resolved.

Anti-inflammatory drugs such as corticotropin and cortisone are administered to reduce the inflammatory response that occurs in an allergic reaction. If the respiratory tract is involved, bronchodilators can be given to help relieve dyspnea and wheezing. Tranquilizers and sedatives may be ordered to promote the rest needed to successfully recover from a severe reaction and aid in relieving the stress that may have occurred. Local reactions involving widespread and deep skin lesions are treated with salves, wet compresses, and soothing baths. The patient must also be protected from a secondary bacterial infection.

Desensitization. When a patient cannot avoid exposure to allergens or if the symptoms cannot be managed successfully, the health care provider may suggest desensitization. The purpose is to decrease sensitivity to allergens. Regular injections of extremely small quantities of selected antigens are given daily, weekly, or monthly. The amount given is gradually increased until there is noticeable clinical improvement, and then a maintenance dosage is given. The program may last for years, but improvement should be noted in about 6 to 24 weeks after it is begun.

Table 12-3 Drugs Commonly Used in the Treatment of Allergy

CLASSIFICATION	ACTION	SIDE EFFECTS	NURSING IMPLICATIONS
Antihistamines			

First-Generation Agents
Ethanolamines
  Clemastine (Tavist Allergy)
  Diphenhydramine (Benadryl)
Ethylenediamine
  Tripelennamine (PBZ)
Alkylamines
  Brompheniramine maleate
    (Dimetane)
  Chlorpheniramine (Chlor-
    Trimeton)
  Dexchlorpheniramine
    (Polaramine)
  Triprolidine (Zymine)
Piperidine
  Azatadine (Optimine)
Phenothiazine
  Promethazine (Phenergan)
	Bind with H_1 receptors on target cells, blocking histamine binding
	Relieve acute symptoms of allergic response (itching, sneezing, excessive secretions, mild congestion)
		First-generation agents cross blood-brain barrier, bind to H_1 receptors in brain, cause *sedation* (diminished alertness, slow reaction time, somnolence) and *stimulation* (restless, nervous, insomnia).
		Some drugs (e.g., ethanolamines) are more likely to cause sedation.
		Patients vary in their sensitivity to these side effects.
		The next most common side effects involve the GI system and include loss of appetite, epigastric distress, constipation, and diarrhea.
		May cause palpitations, tachycardia, urinary retention or frequency.
			Warn patient that operating machinery and driving may be dangerous because of sedative effect; drowsiness usually passes after 2 wk of treatment
			Teach patient to report palpitations, change in heart rate, a change in bowel/bladder habits
			Instruct patient not to use alcohol with antihistamines because of additive depressant effect
			Rapid onset of action, no drug tolerance with prolonged use

Second-Generation Agents Loratadine (Claritin) Cetirizine (Zyrtec) Fexofenadine (Allegra) Desloratadine (Clarinex)	H_1-receptor agonist with minimal sedative side effects, blocks H_1 receptors and blocks effects of histamines (vasodilation, increased capillary permeability) Some also have anti-inflammatory properties Interfere with mediator released from mast cells	Second-generation agents have limited affinity for brain H_1 receptors. Cause minimal sedation, few effects on psychomotor activities or bladder function.	Teach patient to expect few, if any, side effects More expensive than classic antihistamines Rapid onset of action, no drug tolerance with prolonged use General interactions: Do not take with alcohol or any form of tranquilizer or sedative Do not take with any monoamine oxidase inhibitor
Decongestants			

Oral
  Pseudoephedrine (Sudafed)
  Phenylpropanolamine
	Stimulate adrenergic receptors on blood vessels, promote vasoconstriction, and reduce nasal edema and rhinorrhea	CNS stimulation, causing insomnia, excitation, headache, irritability, increased blood and ocular pressure, dysuria, palpitations, tachycardia.	Advise patient of adverse reactions
			Advise that some preparations are contraindicated for patients with cardiovascular disease, hypertension, diabetes, glaucoma, prostate hypertrophy, hepatic and renal disease

Topical (nasal spray)
  Oxymetazoline (Dristan)
  Phenylephrine
    (Neo-Synephrine)
  Azelastine (Astelin)
	Same as above
	Blocks action of histamine
		Same as above, plus rhinitis medicamentosa (rebound nasal congestion).
		Headache, bitter taste, somnolence, nasal irritation.
			Teach patient that these drugs should not be used for >3 days or >3-4 times/day; longer use increases risk of rhinitis medicamentosa

CNS, central nervous system; *GI,* gastrointestinal.

❖ NURSING MANAGEMENT

■ Assessment (Data Collection)

Identifying or isolating the allergens causing the patient's symptoms requires time and diligence.

 Focused Assessment

Indicators of Allergic Response

GENERAL
- History of food intolerances, colic, abdominal cramping, bloating, or pain, vomiting, and diarrhea in the absence of general illness
- History of unusual reaction to any drug, food, insect sting, odor, or fumes
- History of recurrent respiratory problems or seasonal flare-ups of any symptoms
- History of fatigue, wheezing, or shortness of breath on exertion
- Exposure to new personal hygiene products, or cleaning products

SKIN
- Itching, burning, dryness, scaling, irritations, inflammations, hives, rash (note symmetry and location), scratches, or urticaria

EYES
- Burning, itching, tearing, history of sties
- Redness, discoloration below eyes (allergic shiners), conjunctivitis, rubbing, or excessive blinking

NOSE
- History of nose twitching, stuffiness, recurring nosebleeds, sudden episodes of sneezing or snorting
- Allergic salute (pushing nose upward and backward with heel of hand), nasal polyps, nasal voice

MOUTH AND THROAT
- Open-mouth breathing, continual throat clearing, mouth wrinkling with facial grimaces, redness of throat, swollen lips or tongue

EARS
- History of hearing loss, drainage from ears

NECK
- Palpable, enlarged lymph nodes

Besides a food diary, the patient may need to keep track of any chemicals that are used (e.g., cosmetics, soaps, deodorants, household cleaners, garden products, etc.) for a few weeks. Recalling a family history of allergies and types of symptoms they displayed may also prove helpful. Repeated assessments may need to be planned over a period of weeks or months if the patient is reactive to a variety of allergens.

 Health Promotion

Nursing Goals for Patients with Hypersensitivity Reactions

- Assist in the diagnosis of hypersensitivity.
- Help the patient identify the particular substance or substances that trigger an allergic response.
- Assist the patient in devising ways to avoid or at least limit exposure to these allergens.
- Relieve the symptoms of an allergy.
- Decrease the exaggerated response to the allergen(s).
- Provide health teaching.

Households have common allergens, for example, pet dander, dust, dust mites, cosmetics, cleaning agents, and dyes in fabrics and materials used in home furnishings. Overstuffed furniture, heavy draperies, and thick carpets contribute by holding particulate matter. Removal of carpeting, routine cleaning as well as daily dusting and vacuuming, and elimination of dust-harboring furnishings can help remove some allergens. Compliance with daily dusting and vacuuming is more likely if the individual's allergy is severe, prompting every effort to control it. Electrostatic filters and top-quality vacuum cleaners with high-efficiency particulate air (HEPA) filters are essential for those with severe inhalant allergies. It may be necessary to part with a cherished family pet, or to overcome the habit of smoking and to ask others not to smoke. Purchase of an air-conditioning unit that effectively filters out airborne allergens may also be helpful. Wearing protective gloves or an apron when washing dishes, laundering clothes, or performing other chores that require contact with chemicals may help minimize the exposure and possible side effects. If there is an allergy to mold, houseplants should be removed. Molds grow in moist environments, so basements, building foundations, showers, and bathing areas are typically prone to mold growth. Routine cleaning and adequate ventilation can help reduce or eliminate mold growth in most homes. Good drainage and restricting moisture around foundations can help decrease structural mold. Dehumidifiers can reduce moisture in basements. Successful compliance with recommendations should reduce the frequency, severity, and symptoms of the allergic reaction.

Patients with allergy-induced skin conditions should be taught that a warm environment and sweating increase the sensation of itching. Advise the patient to keep cool without chilling and not to take excessively hot showers or baths. Over-the-counter topical lotions, as well as prescription medications and salves, can help relieve itching.

Avoiding exposure to allergens requires knowledge of the nature of the allergen, method of transmission, source or reservoir, and portal of entry. Alteration in habits and location may also help eliminate exposure. Successful management of hypersensitivity depends in large measure on the ability of the patient to understand the allergy and to follow the prescribed treatment regimen.

⬦ **Clinical Cues**

Nurses and others who handle certain drugs may develop allergies to these drugs. For example, penicillin and streptomycin can cause contact dermatitis in those who are regularly exposed to them. Hands should be washed thoroughly after handling antimicrobials.

? Think Critically

What actions would you suggest for removing allergens from the home environment for someone allergic to man-made fibers?

ANAPHYLACTIC REACTION AND ANAPHYLACTIC SHOCK

Etiology and Pathophysiology

Anaphylaxis is a serious, life-threatening, whole-body allergic reaction. The cardiovascular system, respiratory system, gastrointestinal system, and skin all contain copious amounts of mast cells. **Any agent that causes a severe hypersensitivity reaction can cause anaphylaxis.** Substances commonly known to cause hypersensitivity and possible anaphylaxis are listed in Box 12-3. For anaphylaxis to occur, the allergen usually needs to be delivered systemically before the sensitized mast cells are triggered to react. An example of this is the parenteral delivery of an antimicrobial agent such as penicillin. When the reaction occurs, the affected cells swell and rupture, with the subsequent release of histamine. Histamine causes dilation of small blood vessels, a pooling of blood, and release of fluid into tissues. This may lead to circulatory collapse and profound shock (Figure 12-2). A less severe reaction usually occurs if the allergen is delivered by direct contact, inhalation, or ingestion.

Non–IgE-Dependent Allergens. IgE-mediated immune responses typically require repeated exposures for a reaction to occur. In the non–IgE-allergen response, a single encounter can lead to anaphylaxis or even death if not recognized immediately. Examples include iodine-based dyes for select radiologic studies and certain narcotics such as morphine and vancomycin, especially if it is administered too rapidly.

Nurses must be alert for previous allergic reactions and identify patients who are likely to experience a serious reaction. Before administering any medication or drug, verify the patient's known allergies. Patients and families should be actively involved in knowing and reporting allergies. In accordance with National Patient Safety Goals, this active participation is viewed as a safety measure. Check all the areas in the medical record where allergies are usually documented. For example, the front of the chart may have an allergy alert label on it; the medical history obtained by the physician should contain information related to allergies; and the medication administration record (MAR), the multidisciplinary care plan, and the nurse's admission history may contain allergy information.

Box 12-3	Substances Known to Cause Hypersensitivity and Possible Anaphylaxis

DRUGS
- Aspirin
- Cephalosporins
- Chemotherapy agents
- Insulins
- Local anesthetics
- Nonsteroidal anti-inflammatory drugs (NSAIDs)
- Penicillins
- Sulfonamides
- Tetracyclines

DIAGNOSTIC AND TREATMENT AGENTS
- Allergenic extracts for desensitization
- Blood products
- Iodine-containing contrast media used for radiographs

ANTITOXIN SERA
- Diphtheria antitoxin
- Poisonous spider antitoxin
- Snake venom antitoxin
- Tetanus antitoxin

FOODS
- Chocolate
- Eggs
- Fish
- Milk
- Nuts (especially peanuts)
- Shellfish
- Strawberries
- Wheat

INSECT STINGS
- Ants (particularly fire ants)
- Bees, hornets, wasps, yellow jackets

Clinical Cues

Allergies to seafood indicate intolerance to iodine. This means there is potential for an allergic reaction to iodine-based contrast agents used in radiologic imaging studies. Be certain that the shellfish/iodine allergy is noted on the front of the chart, on the MAR, and in other locations where allergies are to be noted in the medical record.

Signs and Symptoms

An anaphylactic reaction requires immediate attention. The appearance of hives (urticaria) or swelling beneath the skin (angioedema) may signal the onset of an anaphylactic episode. Hives or sudden outbreaks of wheals (small areas of swelling) on the skin that itch and burn may appear without subsequent anaphylaxis.

Tachycardia, decreased pulses, and a rapid drop in blood pressure signal circulatory collapse, which can occur very rapidly. The patient will also exhibit increasing dyspnea because of the narrowing of the air passages (bronchoconstriction), accumulation of mucus, and wheezing. If an airway is not maintained, convulsions may occur. Treatment must be started immediately to avoid hypoxic brain injury or death within a matter of minutes.

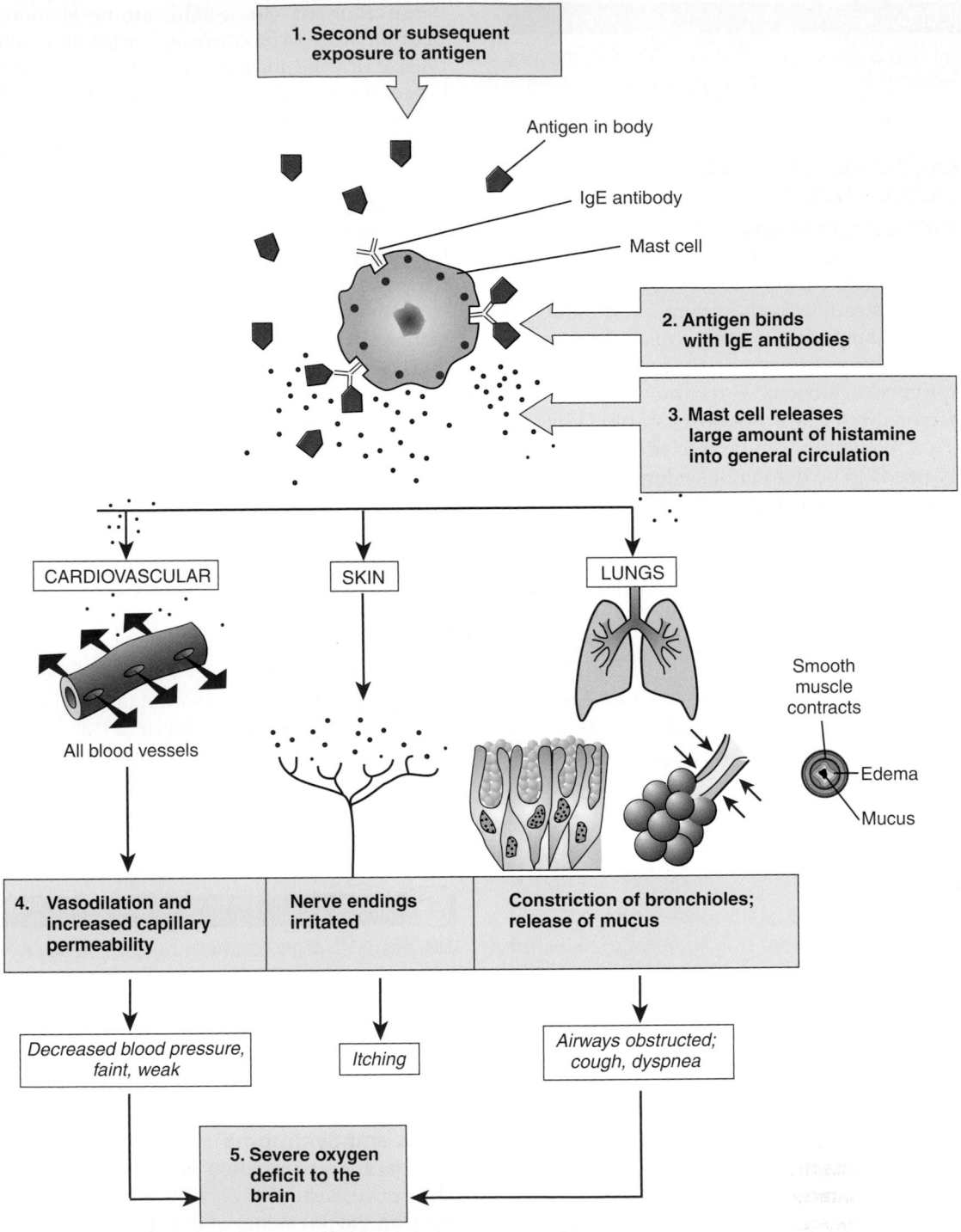

FIGURE 12-2 The effects of anaphylaxis.

Emergency supplies should be readily available whenever vaccines, serum for passive immunization, and highly allergenic drugs are administered. Symptoms from side effects can be treated and anaphylaxis may be avoided if complete information is obtained. Premedication with steroids and/or antihistamines can be administered if a substance needs to be given that the patient has shown sensitivity to in the past.

Clinical Cues

Many patients report allergies to medications that are actually manifestations of side effects, intolerance, or nonallergic adverse reactions. Nausea, constipation, diarrhea, coughing, or drowsiness may be side effects of medications, but reactions to drugs that do not involve the immune system are considered nonallergic adverse reactions. Careful questioning of the patient can help distinguish what kind of reaction the patient has experienced in the past.

Diagnosis

The clinical diagnosis of anaphylaxis is made from the presenting symptoms, including sudden onset involving one or more body systems, producing one or more symptoms such as itching, hives, stridor, wheezing, or shock. Once the patient's condition has been stabilized, laboratory and other diagnostic tests may be performed to rule out other possible causes for the symptoms, but there is no test to confirm the diagnosis of anaphylaxis.

Treatment and Nursing Management

Treatment of anaphylaxis includes the following:

- Establishing a patent airway and administering oxygen to relieve the symptoms of dyspnea and hypoxia.
- Administering intravenous epinephrine to counteract the effect of histamine: relax the bronchioles, increase the cardiac output, and elevate the blood pressure.
- Administering antihistamine (e.g., diphenhydramine hydrochloride [Benadryl]) to stop the effects of the histamine released by the body cells.
- Instituting measures to prevent or control shock.
- Providing psychological support during the course of the syndrome (a group of symptoms that characterize a disorder or condition) and its treatment.

When there is difficulty with breathing because of swelling in the airway, provide high-flow oxygen. Although the patient is still able to move air in and out, giving inhaled medications to relax the airways helps maintain breathing. If these measures are not effective, an emergency intubation, tracheotomy, or cricothyrotomy may need to be performed.

Epinephrine is given to counter the allergic reaction. It can be given intravenously, intramuscularly, subcutaneously, or through an established endotracheal tube. **If the patient is taking beta blockers, they will hinder the effectiveness of the epinephrine.** Diphenhydramine is also used to alleviate the symptoms of the allergic reaction. Corticosteroids may also be given to control the inflammatory response and reduce symptoms.

During the crisis, vital signs and respiratory effort must be monitored continuously. Adequate pharmacologic support and IV fluids are important to maintain perfusion and an adequate blood pressure. See Chapter 45 for additional information on treating shock.

? Think Critically

What is the first thing you would do if a patient starts complaining of shortness of breath and wheezing just after you have administered an antibiotic by injection?

People who have extreme sensitivities to certain allergens should carry a medical alert card or wear an identification bracelet or necklace that contains the information. Several companies offer "medical jewelry" that can relay pertinent information. It also is advisable for individuals who are highly allergic to stings from bees, wasps, or other insects, or severely allergic to nuts or some other food, to carry an EpiPen or a small kit containing epinephrine, syringe, needle, tourniquet, and diphenhydramine hydrochloride with them at all times. These pens and kits are available at pharmacies but require a prescription. They are strongly recommended by allergists because of how quickly an insect sting or inadvertent ingestion of a food can produce a fatal reaction in someone who is highly sensitive.

AUTOIMMUNE DISORDERS

Autoimmune disorders are thought to be caused by the immune system reacting against the body's own cells. The three categories of autoimmune disorders are classified according to how extensively the disorder affects body tissues: (1) *local*, in that this type affects only a single organ or tissue; (2) *systemic*, because these syndromes or diseases affect many organs or tissues; and (3) *mixed localized and systemic*, because these can cause problems in both a localized area and systemically.

Signs and Symptoms

Table 12-4 gives a partial list of diseases, with signs and symptoms, possibly caused by autoimmunity. Not all experts agree, but at this time more than 80 diseases are thought to be triggered by an alteration in immune function. Some of the diseases have other causes in addition to autoimmunity, and some may be primarily a disorder of the immune system.

Diagnosis

Diagnosing autoimmune disorders can be difficult. A detailed health history and complete physical examination must be conducted. Symptoms may be vague and intermittent and may occur over a period of years. Some health care providers may hesitate to initiate diagnostic studies on a patient's self-report because results are inconclusive in the earlier phase of the disease process. This can be frustrating for patients who "just have not felt well for some time" and are looking for an explanation or diagnosis. There are many tests that can be done to rule out conditions, but they can be costly and inappropriate.

Blood tests, such as a complete blood count with differential, will typically be performed (see Box 12-2). Some immune disorders are associated with a specific antibody that can be detected in the blood. Other laboratory tests evaluating inflammation, such as an erythrocyte sedimentation rate (ESR) and C-reactive

Table 12-4   Autoimmune Disorders and Body Systems Affected

DISORDER	AREA AFFECTED	SIGNS AND SYMPTOMS
Systemic Autoimmune Disease		
Autoimmune hemolytic anemia	Red blood cells	Anemia, splenomegaly, hyperbilirubinemia, fatigue
Bullous pemphigoid	Skin, more typically on arms, legs, and trunk	Large fluid-filled vesicles on a swollen erythematous base
Goodpasture's syndrome	Lungs and kidneys	Shortness of breath, hemoptysis, fatigue, edema, pruritus
Polymyalgia rheumatica	Large muscle groups, primarily neck, shoulders, upper arms, thighs, and hips	Moderate to severe aching and stiffness, fatigue, unintentional weight loss, anemia Can literally appear overnight; usually goes away on its own
Rheumatoid arthritis	Heart, lungs, joints, nerves, skin	Variety of symptoms depending on what is most affected: fever, fatigue, join pain and stiffness, deformity of the joints, shortness of breath, chest pain, edema, loss of sensation, rashes
Systemic lupus erythematosus (lupus)	Brain, heart, lungs, kidneys, joints, blood cells, and skin	Fatigue, weakness and light-headedness, shortness of breath, chest pain, pruritus, rash, butterfly rash on the face in some cases
Temporal arteritis/giant cell arteritis	Arteries of the head and neck	Can affect all vessels within the body Symptoms vary depending on location Can have headache, loss of vision, chest pain, dyspnea, kidney failure, abdominal pain, weight loss, skin rash
Wegener's granulomatosis (a form of vasculitis)	Nasal sinuses, lungs, and kidneys	Causes end-organ damage and can be life threatening if not treated Rhinitis is generally first sign in most patients
Localized Autoimmune Diseases		
Addison's disease	Adrenal glands	Slow progression Fatigue, dizziness, muscle weakness, diarrhea, diaphoresis, orthostatic hypotension, hyperpigmentation of the skin
Celiac disease Crohn's disease	Gastrointestinal tract	Intolerant of gluten products; nutrient absorption impaired, abdominal pain, chronic diarrhea, vomiting, weight loss *Celiac:* pale, foul-smelling or fatty stools *Crohn's:* bloody stools
Graves' disease (hyperthyroidism)	Thyroid gland	Tachycardia, tremors, nervousness, weight loss, intolerance to heat
Guillain-Barré syndrome	Peripheral nervous system	Ascending paralysis, starting in legs, then arms, and face Deep tendon reflexes disappear Some patients require mechanical ventilation until recovery occurs
Hashimoto's thyroiditis (hypothyroidism)	Thyroid gland	Weight gain, coarse skin, drowsiness, intolerance to cold
Multiple sclerosis	Brain and spinal cord	Abnormal sensations, weakness, vertigo, vision problems, muscle spasms
Myasthenia gravis	Connection between nerves and muscles (neuromuscular junction)	Muscles weaken and tire easily, especially the eyes
Pernicious anemia (vitamin B_{12} deficiency)	Select cells in stomach	Anemia results, inadequate production of mature blood cells and maintenance of nerve cells, leads to fatigue, weakness; nerves can be damaged with resulting loss of sensation

Data from Christensen, B. L. & Kockrow, E.O. (2011). *Adult health nursing* (6th ed.). St. Louis: Elsevier Mosby; Cohen, P. L. (2007). Autoimmune disorders. In *The Merck Manual of Medical Information*, Home Edition. Rahway, NJ: Merck. Retrieved from www.merck.com/mmhe/sec16/ch186/ch186a.html; Ignatavicius, D.D. & Workman, L.L. (2009). *Medical-surgical nursing; Critical thinking for collaborative care* (6th ed.). Philadelphia: Saunders.

Table 12-4 Autoimmune Disorders and Body Systems Affected—cont'd

DISORDER	AREA AFFECTED	SIGNS AND SYMPTOMS
Localized Autoimmune Diseases—cont'd		
Primary biliary sclerosis, primary sclerosing cholangitis, autoimmune hepatitis	Liver	Occurs more frequently in women Chronic cholestasis, which leads to destruction of the smaller bile ducts Fatigue, pruritus, hepatomegaly, jaundice, hyperpigmentation
Raynaud's disease (if occurs by itself) Raynaud's phenomenon (if accompanied by other autoimmune disorders [scleroderma, lupus])	Fingers, toes, nose, ears	Can be triggered by changes in temperature Numbness and tingling in digits, will then become pale, turn blue because of lack of oxygen, then as digits warm up, turn red because of influx of blood Restricts blood flow of the microvascular system, can cause pitting ulcerations In some cases, gangrene occurs and amputation is required
Type 1 diabetes mellitus	Islet (beta) cells of pancreas (insulin production)	Excessive thirst, appetite, and urination (initial symptoms) Can lead to significant multisystem disease (i.e., blindness, kidney failure, impaired circulation, amputations, especially of lower extremities)
Mixed Localized and Systemic Autoimmune Disorders		
Scleroderma	Localized: skin Systemic: heart, lungs, kidneys, and intestines	Skin and connective tissue tightens and hardens Skin will have patches of skin that are thick, white or pale in the center surrounded by a purple border Heart may develop dysrhythmias, congestive heart failure and pericarditis can also occur Lungs become scarred (pulmonary fibrosis) and pulmonary hypertension may also develop Kidneys will release more protein into the urine and can also trigger hypertension
Sjögren's syndrome	Salivary glands, lacrimal glands, joints	Dry eyes, mouth, gum disease, dental caries Can also affect lungs, lymphatic system, kidneys, and muscles

protein (CRP) levels, are not specific to immune disorders, but may help confirm the diagnosis when used with other information. For disorders that are organ specific, a biopsy of the affected tissue may be done to confirm or exclude the diagnosis.

Treatment and Nursing Management

Treatment falls into two categories: (1) replacement or support of lost or ineffective body function, and (2) therapies targeted to halt the destructive process. The goal of physical, occupational, speech, or even psychological therapeutic interventions is to help the patient learn how to effectively deal with the disorder and be able to function at the highest achievable level for as long as possible. In medication therapy for autoimmune disorders, the chemical treatment is aimed at altering cell function to prevent further harmful effects, not kill the cells. However, some medications are able to minimize side effects, whereas others can cause additional medical complications. Other autoimmune disorders are discussed in relevant chapters (multiple sclerosis, Chapter 25; rheumatoid arthritis, Chapter 33; and psoriasis, Chapter 43).

 Assignment Considerations

Protecting the Patient

Any health care team member that has a potentially infectious condition, such as a cold or the flu, should not be assigned to care for patients with alterations in immune function. If symptoms develop in the middle of the shift, the staff member should wear a mask and use gloves until the assignments are reorganized.

SYSTEMIC LUPUS ERYTHEMATOSUS

Systemic lupus erythematosus (SLE), also known as lupus, is an autoimmune disease. The term *erythematosus*, refers to the erythema (patchy congestion of capillaries of the skin with blood) that often accompanies the disease. As with most autoimmune disorders, the cause is unknown. Genetics, hormones, immunologic response, and environmental influences may play a role in the development of this disease; however, no specific link has been established. In SLE, the body begins to produce abnormal antibodies that attack the target tissues or cells instead of foreign agents such as bacteria, fungi, and viruses. Over time, the damage becomes more apparent.

There is a discoid form (skin is affected but internal organs are not), a systemic form (involves internal organs and is the most common type) and a drug-induced form (tends to be milder and less damaging to the body). Although SLE is incurable, symptoms can be treated.

Individuals of all ages have been diagnosed with SLE, but the typical age of onset appears to occur between 16 and 55 years, and it occurs more often in women than men (a ratio of 9:1). Most patients are diagnosed between ages 20 and 45. The overall rate is 40 to 50 new cases per 100,000 individuals in the United States. Of note, African Americans and Hispanic women of childbearing age in the United States are affected more often than other ethnicities. Before 1955, the 5-year survival rate was less than 50%. In 2006, the 5-year survival rate was around 97% and the 10-year survival rate was reported at 90% (Bernatsky et al., 2006).

Etiology and Pathophysiology

SLE occurs from an abnormal reaction of the body's immune system, especially against proteins found in the nucleus of body cells. Inflammation of the muscles, blood vessel abnormalities, and immune complex deposition in tissues occur throughout the body. SLE usually waxes and wanes throughout the course of the disease. Some individuals have a very mild form of the disorder and have infrequent flare-ups with minimal symptoms. Others have severe, debilitating symptoms that, if left untreated, can lead to death.

Prolonged exposure to sunlight can initiate a flare-up of SLE, therefore use of sunblock and covering of the skin are important. A variety of drugs exacerbate lupus, such as oral contraceptives (especially in women who test positive for the presence of antiphospholipid antibodies), sulfa-based antimicrobials, and penicillin. Additionally, hydralazine, procainamide, and minocycline are known to cause a lupus-like syndrome.

Signs and Symptoms

Signs and symptoms tend to come and go and include painful or swollen joints and muscle pain, unexplained fever, red rash usually on the face (Figure 12-3), unusual loss of hair, sensitivity to the sun, extreme fatigue, weakness, mouth ulcers, poor appetite, weight loss, abnormal menses, edema and swollen glands. All body systems can be affected (Figure 12-4). Weakness is a hallmark of the SLE disease process. It is not unusual to see skeletal abnormalities such as asymmetrical arthritis, especially in the fingers, hands, wrists, and knees. Azotemia, hematuria, proteinuria, and pyuria indicate renal involvement, such as nephrotic syndrome or acute or chronic renal failure (see Chapter 35). Neurologic symptoms may include headaches, seizures, psychosis, and other cognitive disorders. Pleurisy may develop in the lining of the lungs, which can lead to chest pain, shortness of breath, and pulmonary hypertension. Heart failure, pericarditis,

FIGURE 12-3 The characteristic "butterfly" rash of systemic lupus erythematosus.

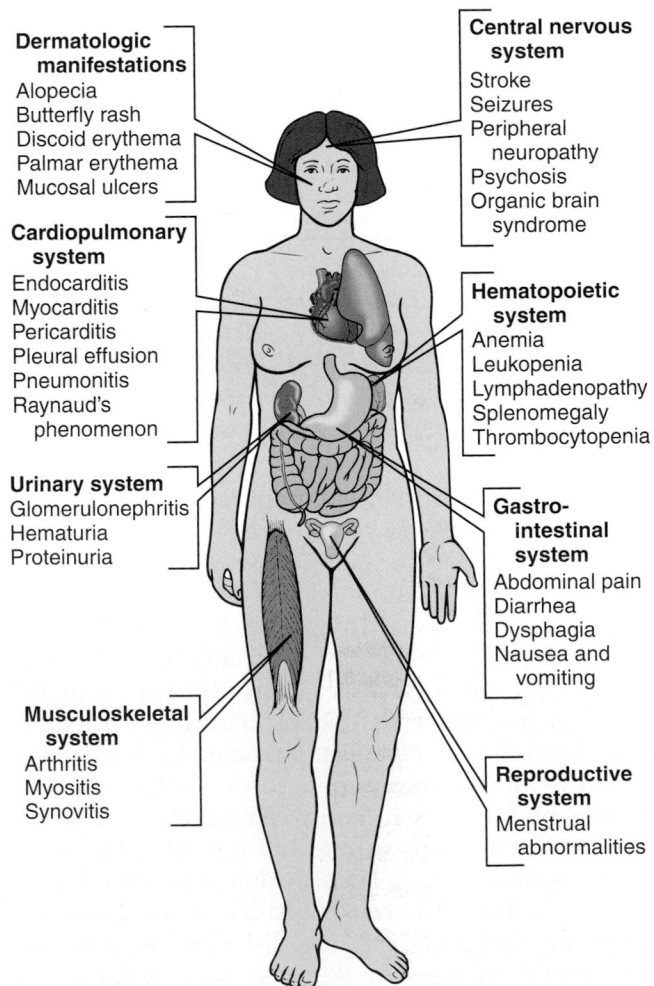

FIGURE 12-4 Multisystem involvement in systemic lupus erythematosus.

and coronary disease may also be symptomatic of SLE (see Chapters 20 and 21). Abnormal laboratory test results may also be seen, such as decreased C3, C4, CH50 (complement tests of proteins involved in inflammatory reactions) or elevated ESR.

Diagnosis

Currently, there is no single test that confirms a diagnosis of SLE. A complete medical history is necessary to guide the diagnostic studies. To confirm SLE, a patient must have at least 4 of the 11 clinical presentations or laboratory test results presented in Table 12-5. Typically the patient shows evidence of a multiorgan disorder. Initially, serum blood studies, along with a urinalysis and tests for renal and liver function, are performed. Levels are obtained for anticardiolipin antibody (ACA), antinuclear antibody (ANA), antiphospholipid antibody, autoantibodies (anti-DNA, anti-SM, anti-RNP, anti-Ro [SSA], and anti-LA [SSB]), and kidney and skin biopsies performed.

A syphilis test measures antiphospholipid antibodies in the blood, which are known to be present in lupus, so a false-positive syphilis test is another indicator of SLE. Tests for signs of inflammation include obtaining an ESR and CRP level. Current research is focusing on identifying biomarkers that would indicate if SLE is present.

Treatment

There is no cure. Current treatments are targeted toward symptom control to prevent exacerbations, treat flare-ups when they occur, and minimize organ damage and long-term complications. Hydroxychloroquine, an antimalarial drug, is currently approved by the Food and Drug Administration (FDA) for use in lupus. Glucocorticoids, such as prednisone are used for major flare-ups. Immunosuppressant may be given to decrease the need for steroids. Nonsteroidal anti-inflammatory drugs can be used to control pain. Rituximab, an anti–B-cell drug used to treat lymphoma, is showing promise in reducing the symptoms of lupus. Rest, balanced diet, and exercise are also primary treatments for patients with SLE.

Nursing Management

Assessment of the patient's ability to participate in activities of daily living (ADLs) is important. Joint pain is also common; therefore management of pain and assisting with mobility are priorities for the nurse. Ongoing assessment of body systems is important to determine if the disease process is affecting additional systems. Nursing Care Plan 12-1 presents interventions for the more common problems in most SLE patients.

The nurse must educate the patient about the disease and how to prevent possible complications. For example, any flulike illness lasting more than a few days should be reported to the health care provider. Review appropriate skin care, including the correct method of applying and reapplying sunblock with a sun protection factor (SPF) of 30 or higher. Infections can also exacerbate the symptoms, so the patient should avoid being around anyone who is showing signs or symptoms of a communicable disease.

Table 12-5	Diagnostic Criteria for Systemic Lupus Erythematosus
CRITERION	**DESCRIPTION**
Antinuclear antibody	Test is positive
Arthritis	Nonerosion of two or more peripheral joints, complains of swelling and tenderness, may also have evidence of effusions
Blood	Can have one or more: hemolytic anemia, leukopenia, lymphopenia, thrombocytopenia
Discoid rash	Patches on the skin that are red, scaly, and tend to scar
Immunologic	Anti-DNA (antibody to native DNA has abnormal titer); anti-Smith is positive if antibody to Sm nuclear antigen is present; positive antiphospholipid antibodies; false-positive serum test for syphilis
Malar rash	Erythematous rash that does not fade and covers both cheeks and the nose
Neurologic	Seizures or psychosis
Oral ulcers	In mouth and/or nasopharynx
Photosensitivity	Rash worsens when exposed to ultraviolet light
Renal	Proteinuria, casts in urine
Serositis	Pleuritis and/or pericarditis

Adapted from Edworthy, S.M., Zatarain, E., McShane, D.J., & Bloch, D.A. (1988). Analysis of the 1982 ARA lupus criteria data set by recursive partitioning methodology: New insights into the relative merit of individual criteria. *J Rheumatol, 15*(10), 1493–1498; and Schur, P. (2004). Approach to the patient with allergic or immunologic disease. In L. Goldman & D. Ausiello (Eds.), *Cecil Textbook of Medicine* (22nd ed., p. 1661). Philadelphia: Saunders.

Patient Teaching

Skin Protection for Patients with Systemic Lupus Erythematosus

- Avoid direct sunlight and any other type of ultraviolet lighting, including tanning beds.
- Use an SPF 30 or higher sunblock when outdoors.
- Wear long pants, a long-sleeved shirt, and a wide-brimmed hat when in the sun.
- Cleanse the skin only with a mild soap such as Ivory.
- Dry the skin thoroughly by patting rather than rubbing it.
- Apply lotion liberally to dry skin areas at least twice a day.
- Avoid using alcohol-based skin care products, face powder, or other astringent agents.
- Use cosmetics that contain moisturizers.
- Inspect the skin daily for rashes and open areas.

Adapted from Ignatavicius, D.D., & Workman, M.L. (2010). *Medical-Surgical Nursing: Critical Thinking for Collaborative Care* (6th ed.). Philadelphia: Elsevier Saunders, p. 350.

★ Nursing Care Plan 12-1   Care of the Patient with Systemic Lupus Erythematosus

Scenario
Julie Hansen, age 37, has just been diagnosed with systemic lupus erythematosus (SLE). She has flat erythema in a butterfly pattern over the face, is complaining of joint pain in her knees and elbows, and has experienced constant fatigue and weakness for the past 6 months. Her ESR is elevated and she has a positive ANA. Other tests helped confirm the physician's diagnosis. She lives with her husband and 12-year-old son and 14-year-old daughter.

Problem/Nursing Diagnosis
Weakness and fatigue/Activity intolerance related to inflammatory nature of the disease as evidenced by need for increased rest and sleep and inability to keep up with household chores along with work.

Supporting Assessment Data
Subjective: States she cannot keep the laundry done or the house clean as she is so tired when she comes home from work; has been using more and more "fast food" for family dinners.

Goals/Expected Outcomes	Nursing Interventions	Selected Rationale	Evaluation
Patient will manage household along with work with help within 6 wk.	Explore chores that other family members may be able to take over.	Husband and children could help with cleaning, laundry, errands, and meal preparation.	Daughter will wash the clothes and son will fold and put them away. Husband will do errands. All members will assist with meal preparation and cleanup.
	Assist to work out a schedule for rest periods at lunchtime, after work, and on the weekends.	Resting for 30 min at lunchtime eases fatigue.	Will try to find a place at or near her workplace where she can rest at lunchtime. Continue plan.
	Assist to plan meals for the week and to cook large quantities of items on the weekend that can be divided into individual meals and frozen for family dinners.	It is less fatiguing to cook large quantities of entrees once a week and to freeze portions than to prepare a dinner every day.	Will consider what meals might be cooked ahead on the weekends and frozen. Continue plan.

Problem/Nursing Diagnosis
Painful knees and elbows/Chronic pain related to inflammation from disease process.

Supporting Assessment Data
Subjective: "My knees and elbows ache whenever I have walked for more than a block or used my arms to lift things frequently during the day."
Objective: Tenderness around elbow and knee joints.

Goals/Expected Outcomes	Nursing Interventions	Selected Rationale	Evaluation
Patient will experience fewer days of pain with regular use of anti-inflammatory.	Instruct to take 400 mg of ibuprofen tid on a regular basis.	Keeping a steady blood level of the drug will help decrease and prevent inflammation.	States will begin taking the prescribed regimen of ibuprofen. Continue plan.
	Advise to let family lift heavy items and do chores requiring repetitive elbow motion or squatting.	Refraining from lifting, repetitive joint motion, and squatting helps prevent joint strain and added inflammation.	States will let family bring in groceries and put them away. Will remind family to pick up around the house every other day. Will refrain from gardening while bending down on her knees. Continue plan.

ANA, antinuclear antibody; *ESR,* erythrocyte sedimentation rate; *SPF,* sun protection factor.

Problem/Nursing Diagnosis
Reddened area over much of face/Risk for impaired skin integrity related to "butterfly" rash and sun sensitivity from disease process
Supporting Assessment Data
Subjective: States sunburns very easily.
Objective: Inflamed rash in butterfly pattern over large part of face.

Goals/Expected Outcomes	Nursing Interventions	Selected Rationale	Evaluation
Patient's skin will remain intact.	Instruct in proper skin care with mild soap and alcohol/astringent-free products.	Avoiding harsh skin care products will help prevent excoriation and breaks in the skin.	States will check her skin-care products for alcohol and astringents.
	Instruct to moisturize the skin twice daily.	Moisturizing products will help keep skin supple and prevent breaks.	Will begin moisturizing a second time a day before bedtime. Continue plan.
	Instruct to inspect the skin closely for any breaks or new lesions.	Finding breaks in the skin promptly and caring for them properly will help prevent infection.	Will begin to inspect skin after shower daily. Continue plan.
	Instruct to cover skin when out in the sun and to avoid ultraviolet rays as much as possible.	Protecting the skin from sunlight will help prevent flare-ups of the disease and will protect the skin from further damage.	Will wear suggested clothing of long sleeves, long pants, and a wide-brimmed hat when out in the sun.
	Instruct to use a sunblock product with an SPF of 30 or more when outdoors.	Sunblock helps prevent the damage that can occur from ultraviolet rays.	States will use sunblock on a daily basis on exposed parts of skin.
	Instruct to stop going to the tanning salon.	Ultraviolet light damages the skin and can cause a flare-up or progression of SLE symptoms.	States that she hates to give it up, but will refrain from going to tanning salon.

Critical Thinking Questions
1. What types of entrees could you suggest that could be fixed ahead in large quantities and then frozen in family-sized portions?
2. What might you suggest as ways to rest at lunchtime when the patient is at work on weekdays?

DISORDERS OF THE LYMPHATIC SYSTEM

LYMPHOMA

Lymphoma is a form of lymphatic cancer that primarily starts in the lymphocytes. These cells become malignant and multiply, crowding out the normal cells, which leads to the creation of solid tumors in the lymph nodes. The two main types of lymphoma are Hodgkin's lymphoma (HL) and non-Hodgkin's lymphoma (NHL). The primary differences between the two are the types of lymphocytes involved in the disease. If, under microscopic examination of tissue, Reed-Sternberg (R-S) cells are present, the patient has HL. If the R-S cells are not present, the patient is diagnosed as having NHL, which is further identified as B-cell and T-cell lymphoma. There are two main types of HL—classical Hodgkin's lymphoma with four subtypes and lymphocyte-predominant Hodgkin's lymphoma with two subtypes.

NHL has around 30 subtypes. Classification and staging of these two diseases is complicated. It relies heavily on microscopic examination of tissues and diagnostic studies, including serum blood testing and select types of scans in order to determine the type and true extent of the disease. Many of the NHL subtypes look similar, but they are quite different and respond to different therapies with varying degrees of success.

HODGKIN'S LYMPHOMA

Etiology
Hodgkin's lymphoma (HL), also known as Hodgkin's disease, is one of the more curable forms of cancer when diagnosed and treated early. It accounts for less than 1% of all cancers, including cancer-related deaths in the United States. HL primarily affects young adults, but it can occur in those over 55 years of age. The incidence rates are 25% higher in males and 21% higher in whites than African Americans (Dores et al., 2009). As of 2007, there were approximately 164,273 people in the United States with a history of HL (Altekruse et al., 2009). The National Cancer Institute reports that an estimated 8510 new cases were diagnosed in 2009 and 1290 deaths occurred in that same year and

were attributed to this disease. The overall survival rates are 85% at 5 years and 78% at 10 years (Jemal et al., 2005).

Pathophysiology

Initial presentation is enlarged, painless lymph nodes that can be felt just beneath the surface of the skin, in the neck, mediastinum, axilla, abdomen or groin. In addition to the lymphadenopathy (enlarged lymph nodes) the patient may also complain of abdominal fullness, fatigue, night sweats, unintentional weight loss, and pruritus. The cause of HL is not known, but there is a possible genetic as well as environmental component that, in combination, can initiate the onset of this disease. Other possible triggers are viral infections, such as Epstein-Barr and HIV. Previous exposure to various chemical agents has also been implicated.

The B cells in the immune system begin to develop atypical cells. The abnormal cells, called Reed-Sternberg (R-S), have two unique features: (1) they rapidly replicate more defective B cells, and (2) they do not die off as normal cells do. These R-S cells replace normal cells in the nodes and lymph tissue. The disease spreads from one area to another via the lymphatic system and can also invade various body systems. As it progresses, the ability of the body to fight off infection can become severely impaired.

Signs and Symptoms

The disorder often is discovered when swollen lymph nodes are found on a routine examination. High suspicion for HL exists when the patient has complaints of swollen lymph glands lasting for several weeks and no recent history of any type of infection. If these symptoms are also accompanied by conditions such as night sweats and weight loss, the patient will likely require a series of diagnostic studies. Some patients experience remittent fever, and severe pruritus is also an early sign. A small percentage of patients with HL will experience pain in the lymph nodes after consumption of alcoholic beverages. Although not a common finding, when present it is considered diagnostic for this disease. If there is a mediastinal mass of involved lymph tissue, the patient may have a nonproductive cough because of the narrowed airways from the swollen lymph glands. Many other organs can become affected, as displayed in Figure 12-5.

Diagnosis, Treatment, and Nursing Management

A definitive diagnosis for HL is confirmed by the presence of R-S cells in the tissues obtained by biopsy of the lymph nodes. Radiographs, computed tomography (CT) scans, and positron emission tomography (PET) scans can also be used to help determine the extent of the disease.

Treatment depends on the stage of the disease and whether involvement is above or below the diaphragm or both. Figure 12-6 presents the classification of four stages (I, II, III, and IV) for Hodgkin's lymphoma. Once the stage is known, the absence ("A") or the presence ("B") of one or more of the following symptoms is noted: unintentional weight loss of more than 10% of body weight over the previous 6 months; an unexplained fever greater than 100° F (38.5° C) for 3 days or longer; and profuse night sweats not related to weather conditions.

Chemotherapy can be given in all stages of the disease. Once it is completed, radiation therapy may be considered. Typically, radiation therapy is delivered only to the affected areas of the body. For stages I and II, administration of doxorubicin (Adriamycin), bleomycin, vinblastine, and dacarbazine (ABVD therapy); followed by radiation, has proven to be the most successful treatment. Stage III and IV disease shows better improvement with mechlorethamine, vincristine (Oncovin), procarbazine, and prednisone (MOPP therapy); in combination with ABVD therapy. The number of cycles of chemotherapy depends on the stage of the disease, the response of the patient to the therapies, and whether a relapse (reappearance of abnormal cells) occurs. Patients may experience many complications from HL and the treatments. Examples of some of the adverse effects include permanent sterility, temporary hair loss, and an increased risk of developing cancer in other organs years after completing radiation therapy.

Nursing care should focus on symptoms the patient is currently experiencing and the side effects of the therapies prescribed. Prevention of health care–associated infections is essential. The nursing diagnoses, expected outcomes, and interventions for the patient with Hodgkin's lymphoma are the same as those for the patient with leukemia (see Chapter 17).

NON-HODGKIN'S LYMPHOMA

Etiology and Pathophysiology

Non-Hodgkin's lymphoma (NHL) is the sixth most common cancer in males and the fifth most common cancer in females in the United States. The National Cancer Institute estimated that 66,360 new cases of NHL were diagnosed in 2011 and that at least 19,320 people with NHL died that same year (American Cancer Society, 2011). Part of the increase has been linked to the increased number of AIDS patients. But there is also an increase among those over age 65. This overall rise is thought to be related to the continued advances in the successful diagnosis and treatment of a variety of diseases.

NHL is similar to HL, but NHL is less predictable and tends to spread to other body sites much more rapidly. There is also an abnormal proliferation of defective B cells or T cells in NHL. The first form is a

Severe pruritus is an early sign
Cause: Unknown

Irregular fever usually present; temperature is elevated for a few days, then drops to normal or subnormal for several days; continuous high fever may indicate impending death
Cause: Apparently related to neoplastic involvement of internal nodes or viscera

Jaundice
Cause: Obstruction of the bile ducts as a result of liver damage causes bilirubin to accumulate in the blood and discolor the skin

Hepatosplenomegaly
Cause: Dissemination of the disorder from the lymph nodes to other organs

Renal failure
Cause: Ureteral obstruction by enlarged lymph nodes

Progressive anemia accompanied by fatigue, malaise, anorexia
Cause: Erythrocyte life span is shortened; erythropoiesis is unable to keep pace with erythrocyte destruction

Edema and cyanosis of the face and neck
Cause: Enlarged lymph nodes place pressure on veins, obstructing drainage of this area

Pulmonary symptoms, including nonproductive cough, stridor, dyspnea, chest pain, cyanosis, and pleural effusion
Cause: Mediastinal lymph node enlargement, involvement of the lung parenchyma, and invasion of the pleura

Alcohol-induced pain in the bones, in involved lymph nodes, or around the mediastinum occurs immediately after drinking alcohol and lasts for 30 to 60 minutes
Cause: Unknown

Bone pain, vertebral compression
Cause: Dissemination of disease from the lymph nodes to the bones

Paraplegia
Cause: Compression of the spinal cord resulting from extradural involvement

Nerve pain
Cause: Compression of the nerve roots of the brachial, lumbar, or sacral plexuses

FIGURE 12-5 Clinical manifestations and pathophysiologic basis of Hodgkin's lymphoma.

slow-growing indolent (follicular) lymphoma in which symptoms are usually not present until the advanced stages of the disease. This form has a better prognosis and at least a 10-year survival rate, if treatment is given in stage I or II of the disease. Usually radiation therapy is used, as most indolent forms of NHL are nodular in shape. The second form is aggressive; if treated with intensive chemotherapy, there is a survival/cure rate between 30% and 60% (National Cancer Institute, 2010). The symptoms manifest early in the aggressive form and with vigorous therapy, there is a potential for cure. The rate of cure is reduced if diagnosed in a late phase. Five risk factors are used to predict the outcome of patients with the more aggressive forms of B-cell lymphoma, which is the most common type. Having one or none of the risk factors suggests a good outcome, while having four or five indicates a poor prognosis: disseminated tumors, elevated levels of lactate dehydrogenase, poor functional ability of patient, older than 60 years, and spread beyond lymph nodes. If a relapse should occur, it usually appears within the

first 2 years after treatment. In some cases, patients may require a bone marrow or stem cell transplant.

Signs and Symptoms

NHL tends to have more widespread involvement of lymphoid tissue than found in HL. Unlike HL, NHL typically shows up in one node; then one or more nodes are skipped; and then another node is affected (referred to as *noncontiguous*). NHL usually manifests as a unilateral, painless enlargement of a lymph node that may progress to generalized, painless lymphadenopathy. NHL tumors can occur in the brain, respiratory system, spleen, GI tract, bone, or other parts of the body. As the disease progresses, the patient notices more symptoms, probably because of the increasing size of the affected lymph nodes. Symptoms related to other organs are site specific and can include complaints of high fevers, chills, night sweats, cough, dyspnea, chest pain, nausea, vomiting, a sense of fullness in the abdomen, and constipation. Hepatomegaly or splenomegaly occurs in about one third of patients.

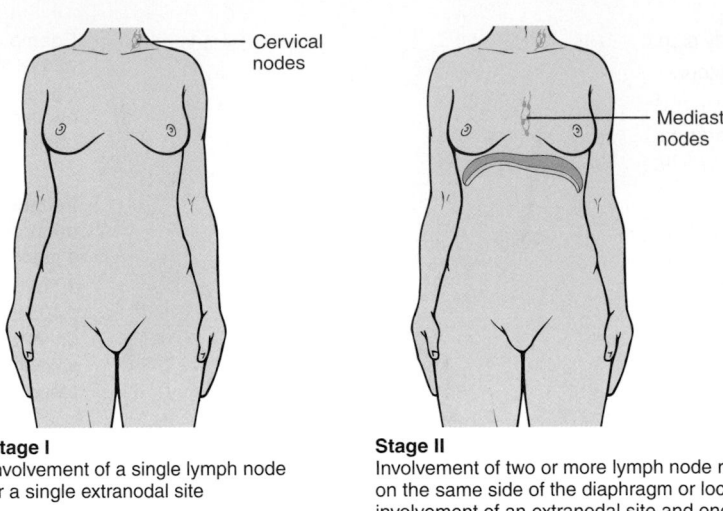

Stage I
Involvement of a single lymph node or a single extranodal site

Stage II
Involvement of two or more lymph node regions on the same side of the diaphragm or localized involvement of an extranodal site and one or more lymph node regions of the same side of diaphragm

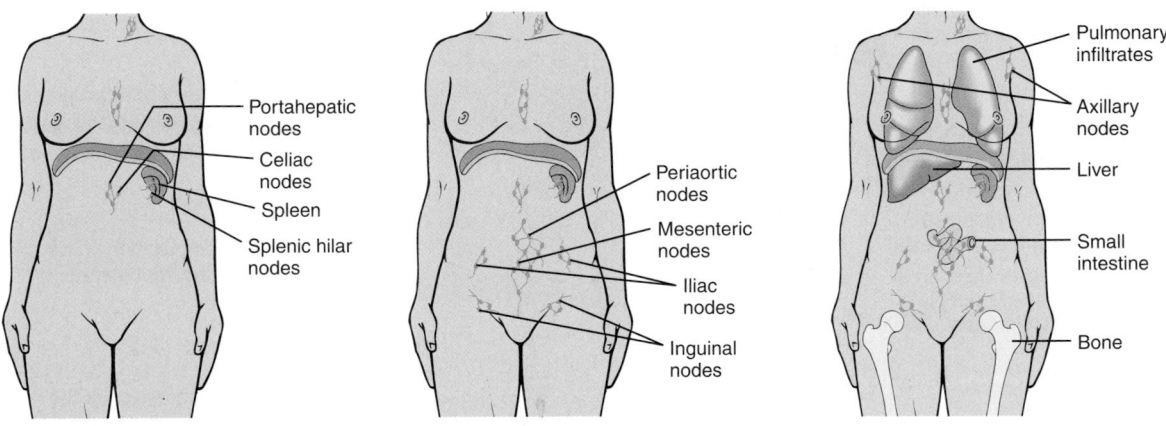

Stage III
Involvement of lymph node regions on both sides of the diaphragm. May include a single extranodal site, the spleen, or both; now subdivided into lymphatic involvement of the upper abdomen in the spleen (splenic, celiac, and portal nodes) (*Stage III$_1$*) and the lower abdominal nodes in the para-aortic, mesenteric, and iliac regions (*Stage III$_2$*)

Stage IV
Diffuse or disseminated disease of one or more extralymphatic organs or tissues with or without associated lymph node involvement; the extranodal site is identified as *H*, hepatic; *L*, lung; *P*, pleura; *M*, marrow; *D*, dermal; *O*, osseous

FIGURE 12-6 Staging of Hodgkin's lymphoma.

The nodes closer to the skin tend to be more easily palpated, very pruritic, and may be either red or purple in hue. Laboratory tests may show elevated liver enzymes. Physical examination may reveal a change in level of consciousness related to an elevation in intracranial pressure, especially in patients with aggressive NHL.

Diagnosis and Treatment

The effectiveness of treatment depends on the stage of the tumor at the time of diagnosis and the type of lymphoma (indolent or aggressive). Staging considers the number and location of affected lymph nodes, whether the nodes are on one or both sides of the diaphragm, and whether the disease has spread to other tissues. To aid in staging, CT, magnetic resonance imaging (MRI), PET, or ultrasound can be used to determine the extent of tissue involvement and to assess therapeutic response after therapy has been completed.

Biopsy of various body tissues may also be performed in one of three ways: (1) an excisional biopsy, in which an entire node is removed; (2) an incisional biopsy, in which only a piece of the node is removed; or (3) fine-needle aspiration (FNA), using a needle to aspirate tissue from the mass of cells. Bone marrow biopsy is usually performed after the diagnosis has been confirmed and it may also be done to determine if the disease has reached the bone marrow.

Treatment can be with chemotherapy or irradiation, depending on the stage of disease. Stage I or II or low-grade NHL may be cured with radiation therapy alone. Various combinations of drugs are used for other stages of the disease depending on the type and aggressiveness. Cyclophosphamide, hydroxy-daunomycin (doxorubicin), vincristine (Oncovin), and prednisone, (CHOP therapy) are commonly employed. Bone marrow transplantation, peripheral stem cell transplantation, and monoclonal antibodies are possible treatment options. Radiolabeled monoclonal antibody agents recognize and react to kill specific tumor cells. The drug used to "mark" the cells is called ibritumomab tiuxetan and is labeled with yttrium-90 (Zevalin). Other experimental therapies are under study.

Surgery may be employed if the tumor is localized. The use of highly active antiretroviral therapy (HAART) in conjunction with anticancer drugs seems to hold promise even for AIDS patients with advanced NHL. This therapy may be continued to prevent a recurrence of the disease after it has been treated with chemotherapy. Vaccines for this disease are currently in clinical trials. Overall, the 1-year relative survival rate for NHL is 70% and the 5-year survival rate is 51%.

Nursing Management

Nursing care is directed toward supporting the patient through the diagnostic process and observing for and treating the side effects of radiation and chemotherapy. If bone marrow or stem cell transplants are performed, nursing care and patient education must focus on prevention of infection and other complications. Chapter 8 provides information on specific nursing diagnoses and interventions for the patient with cancer. Common nursing diagnoses for the NHL patient include the following:

- Risk for infection related to neutropenia from chemotherapy or radiation
- Ineffective protection/risk for hemorrhage related to thrombocytopenia secondary to treatment
- Fatigue
- Imbalanced nutrition: less than body requirements

Expected outcomes might include the following:

- Patient will not experience infection.
- Patient will not experience hemorrhage.
- Fatigue will lessen after 6 weeks of treatment.
- Patient will gain 1 lb per week until desired weight is reached.

Nursing interventions are similar to those for the problems of leukemia (see Chapter 17).

LYMPHEDEMA

The lymphatic system drains water, proteins, lipids, and waste from the interstitial spaces throughout the entire body and returns it to the lymph nodes where waste materials and foreign cells, such as bacteria, are filtered out. Once "clean," the lymph fluid returns to the lymphatic vessels and the whole process is repeated. When the lymph system is unable to circulate normally, large amounts of fluid accumulate (lymphedema), causing swelling. If not controlled, this swelling can lead to further damage to surrounding nerves, blood vessels, and tissues.

There are two types of lymphedema: inherited and acquired. The inherited form (primary) is a congenital condition in which there is deficient growth of the lymphatic system, especially in a lower extremity. This condition chiefly affects females and most often becomes apparent during the middle teens to early twenties.

The acquired form (secondary) typically results from an obstruction caused by trauma to the lymph vessels and nodes, such as occurs during mastectomy when lymph nodes are removed, after radiation therapy, or after a liposuction procedure where some of the lymph nodes may have been damaged. Other causes of obstruction include extensive soft-tissue injury and scar formation and, in tropical countries, parasites that enter lymph channels and block them (i.e., elephantiasis). Patients may have a variety of symptoms, including restricted range of motion, heavy feeling, aching discomfort, recurrent infections, and thick, hard skin. Regardless of the cause, treatment goals are to minimize the impact of the disease process on the individual.

Lymphedema of an extremity can often be treated conservatively using simple nursing measures. For example, the patient can be taught to wrap the extremity with an elastic bandage, beginning at the most distal portion and working up the extremity. This compression bandage may help minimize the degree of lymphedema. Surgical intervention is palliative at best and is therefore controversial as a treatment option. There is no cure for the condition. Prevention and treatment of lymphedema of the arm and hand following mastectomy are covered in Chapter 39.

 Patient Teaching

Measures to Prevent or Decrease Lymphedema

Teach the patient to:

- Elevate the extremity to the level of the heart. This reduces hydrostatic pressure within the veins.
- Apply elasticized stockings or gloves when up and active. This increases pressure on vessels and encourages venous return. (Garments may be removed when the extremity can be elevated.)
- Avoid constrictive clothing.
- Do not cross your legs when sitting, or carry a heavy bag if an arm is affected.
- Perform active exercise of the skeletal muscles. This promotes massage of the lymph vessels and the movement of lymph.
- Cleanse and dry the skin thoroughly and regularly, applying mild skin moisturizers to prevent cracking.
- Try to avoid any minor trauma to the area (e.g., no blood pressure cuffs or blood draws on the affected extremity).

FIBROMYALGIA

In the 1970s, fibromyalgia was identified as a condition of chronic systemic pain and multiple symptoms that could not be explained as being caused by any other source or disease. This disorder affects women 10 times more than men and is seen in women ranging in age from 25 to 60 years. It is believed that stressors such as infection, trauma, drugs, hormonal influences, and psychological distress can trigger fibromyalgia and its related symptoms (Box 12-4). The most common feature of this disorder is musculoskeletal pain. It is typically described as diffuse or multifocal pain, with flare-ups and **remissions** (disease is under control), along with migration from one area of the body to another. Although not a true form of arthritis, fibromyalgia interferes with a person's ability to perform ADLs and can cause significant fatigue and pain.

Evidence-based research indicates that this disease is more likely the result of an inappropriate neural response to pain rather than inflammation. Patients typically have either **hyperalgesia** (heightened response to painful stimuli) or **allodynia** (pain response to nonpainful stimuli). This disorder may also be caused by a deficiency in the neurotransmitters dependent on serotonin and norepinephrine within the central nervous system. Research shows that patients with an autoimmune disorder such as SLE and rheumatoid arthritis also meet the American College of Rheumatology's criteria for fibromyalgia

(Wolfe et al., 1990). The criteria include assessing whether or not symptoms have been present for at least 3 months; whether they occur on both sides of the body; and determining if there are any tender points in at least 11 of 18 select tender points of the body (Figure 12-7).

Currently there is no specific diagnostic test that can confirm the diagnosis of fibromyalgia, so treatment is directed more toward symptom relief. A variety of antidepressants, such as amitriptyline (a tricyclic), fluoxetine or duloxetine (serotonin reuptake inhibitors), and milnacipran or pregabalin (reuptake inhibitors of serotonin and norepinephrine), can help in relieving some of the pain symptoms. Nonsteroidal anti-inflammatory drugs and long-term use of narcotic pain relievers are not as effective in treating the pain experienced in this disorder because of the abnormal reactions of pain receptors. Additional treatment is based on the symptomatology and could include exercise, massage therapy, guided imagery, dietary changes, and referral to a mental health provider. Nursing responsibilities include taking a detailed assessment of symptom history and measures that usually relieve symptoms. Family should be included in the education about disease process. Interventions are needed to help the patient to manage fatigue, pain, activity intolerance, sleep disruption, and stress.

Box 12-4 Fibromyalgia Symptoms

- Tension or migraine headaches
- Jaw and facial tenderness
- Insomnia or waking up feeling just as tired as when you went to sleep
- Vertigo
- Difficulty with concentration, memory recall, and performing simple mental tasks
- Anxiety, depression
- Stiffness on waking or after staying in one position for too long
- Chronic muscle pain, spasms or tightness, weakness in the limbs, and leg cramps
- Moderate to severe fatigue and decreased energy levels
- Reduced exercise tolerance and increased muscle pain after exercise
- Numbness or tingling in the face, arms, hands, legs, or feet
- A sensation of swelling (without actual swelling) in the hands and feet
- Abdominal pain, bloating, nausea, and constipation alternating with diarrhea (irritable bowel syndrome)
- Dysmenorrhea
- Increase in urinary urgency or frequency (irritable bladder)
- Sensitivity to one or more of the following: odors, noise, bright lights, medications, certain foods, and cold

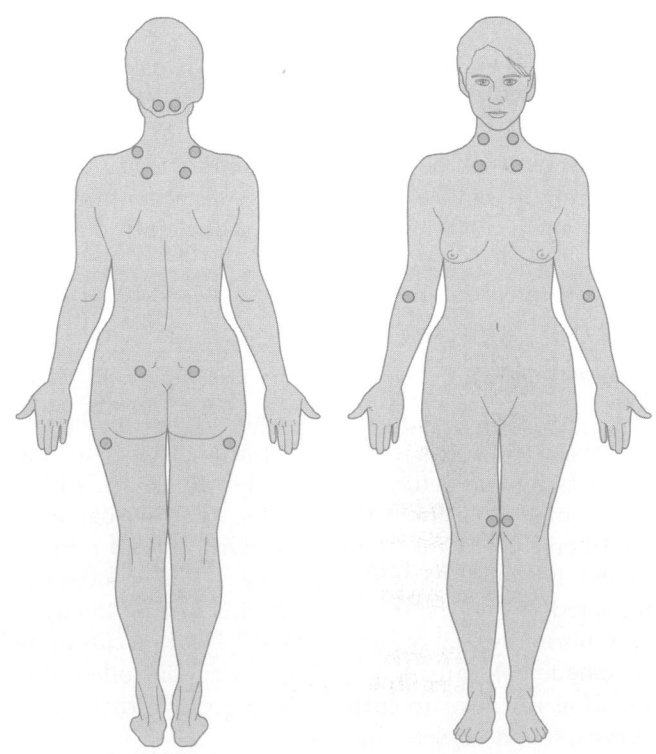

FIGURE 12-7 Tender points in fibromyalgia.

Get Ready for the NCLEX® Examination!

Key Points

- Immunosuppression may be used therapeutically for a variety of conditions, such as tissue transplants, rheumatoid arthritis, and non-Hodgkin's lymphoma.
- Nursing responsibilities in caring for patients with allergic conditions include: assisting in diagnosis of hypersensitivity, helping to identify substances that trigger an allergic response, assisting patient to avoid or limit exposure allergens, and relieving symptoms.
- Emergency equipment and medications must be available for an anaphylactic reaction which is a life-threatening condition.
- Autoimmune disorders are thought to be caused by the immune system reacting to the body's own cells and are typically treated by suppressing the immune system.
- In systemic lupus erythematosus, the body produces abnormal antibodies that attack the target tissues or cells. Inflammation of muscles, blood vessel abnormalities, and immune complex deposition in tissue occurs.
- Lymphoma starts in the lymph tissue when malignant lymphocytes multiply and crowd out normal cells; treatment depends on staging and the aggressiveness of the particular type of the disease.
- In Hodgkin's lymphoma, Reed-Sternberg (R-S) cells are seen on microscopic examination of tissue. In non-Hodgkin's lymphoma (NHL), the R-S cells are not present. NHL is further identified as B-cell or T-cell lymphoma.
- Nursing care for lymphomas focuses on preventing infection, managing the symptoms of the disease, and managing the side effects of the therapies.
- Patient education for lymphedema includes: elevating extremity, using elasticized stockings or gloves, avoiding constrictive clothing, not crossing legs when sitting, exercising, and avoiding minor trauma to the affected limb.
- In fibromyalgia, the most common feature is musculoskeletal pain that is diffuse, and multifocal with flare-ups and remissions.

Additional Learning Resources

SG Go to your Study Guide for additional learning activities to help you master this chapter content.

evolve Go to your Evolve website (http://evolve.elsevier.com/deWit/medsurg) for the following FREE learning resources:
- Animations, audio, and video
- Answers and rationales for questions and activities
- Concept Map Creator
- Glossary with pronunciations in English and Spanish
- Interactive Review Questions and Exercises and more!

 Online Resources
- SEER Stat Fact Sheets: Non-Hodgkin Lymphoma, http://seer.cancer.gov/statfacts/html/nhl.html
- National Fibromyalgia Association, www.fmaware.org/PageServer.html
- Systemic Lupus Erythematosus, www.ncbi.nlm.nih.gov/pubmedhealth/PMH0001471

Review Questions for the NCLEX® Examination

1. Which classes of drugs should be used with caution in patients with hypertension?
   1. Anti-inflammatory drugs and selective serotonin reuptake inhibitors (SSRIs)
   2. Prednisone and hydrocorticotropins
   3. Antihistamines and decongestants
   4. Bronchodilators and epinephrine

2. Which class of drugs hinders the effectiveness of epinephrine?
   1. Antihistamines
   2. SSRIs
   3. Beta blockers
   4. Tricyclics

3. The nurse is reviewing medication orders for a female patient with SLE, who is positive for the presence of antiphospholipid antibodies. The nurse would seek clarification from the physician about which medication?
   1. Oral contraceptives
   2. Hydroxychloroquine (antimalarial)
   3. Glucocorticoid medication
   4. Nonsteroidal anti-inflammatory medication

4. A patient has the medical diagnosis of fibromyalgia. Which nursing diagnosis is most likely to be used in this patient's care plan?
   1. Ineffective airway clearance
   2. Noncompliance
   3. Acute pain
   4. Risk for imbalanced fluid volume

5. The physician gives instructions to a patient with a transplant regarding the use of immunosuppressive drugs. Which patient statement indicates a need for further instructions?
   1. "These medications put me at risk for various types of infections."
   2. "Organ rejection is no longer my concern."
   3. "Some of my body's defenses would remain intact."
   4. "My physician would adjust the dosage of these medications, depending on my response."

6. The nurse admits an elderly man with Hodgkin's lymphoma. On initial assessment, the nurse notes that the patient is slightly confused, irritable, emaciated, has poor dentition, and is homeless. What is the priority nursing diagnosis?

   1. Risk for infection
   2. Ineffective coping
   3. Disturbed body image
   4. Deficient knowledge

7. A systemic autoimmune disease affects more than one type of body tissue or organ. Which would be considered systemic autoimmune disease(s)? *(Select all that apply.)*

   1. Non-Hodgkin's lymphoma
   2. Rheumatoid arthritis
   3. Systemic lupus erythematosus
   4. Goodpasture's syndrome
   5. Primary lymphedema

8. What are the advantages to performing a RAST? *(Select all that apply.)*

   1. The patient does not have to refrain from taking antihistamine medications.
   2. It is safer for patients with serious heart and lung problems.
   3. There is no chance of experiencing an anaphylactic reaction since it is performed on the blood.
   4. It can be used on patients whose skin condition is too severe to perform skin testing.
   5. The results can be obtained within several hours.
   6. It has greater specificity for allergens than other tests.

9. A patient with an immune disorder has a nursing diagnosis of Risk for infection. Which intervention(s) would be used in the care of this patient? *(Select all that apply.)*

   1. All health care workers should perform scrupulous hand hygiene.
   2. The patient should be instructed on how to wear personal protective equipment.
   3. The patient is placed in Contact Isolation as soon as possible.
   4. Caregivers with any type of infection should not be assigned to the patient.
   5. A high-protein diet with nutritional supplements is encouraged.

10. In which area(s) of the medical record would allergies usually be documented? *(Select all that apply.)*

    1. Allergy label on the front of the chart
    2. Medication administration record (MAR)
    3. Multidisciplinary care plan
    4. Nurse's admission history
    5. Nurses' notes
    6. Physicians' orders

Critical Thinking Activities

Scenario A

Mr. Watson is a 45-year-old patient admitted to the hospital for an abdominal hernia operation. You notice that he has cold symptoms and you ask him about them. Mr. Watson replies that he is allergic to something and often has these symptoms.

1. How might you help Mr. Watson determine the airborne substance(s) to which he is allergic?

2. What techniques are used to determine foods that may be allergens?

3. What role does histamine play in the symptoms of an allergic reaction?

4. Why are antihistamines helpful in managing allergy symptoms?

5. What measures should be taken to avoid a fatal allergic reaction to drugs that are administered in a hospital or clinic?

Scenario B

Marilyn Jost, age 15, is highly allergic to penicillin and bee stings. The last time she experienced a reaction to a bee sting on her leg, the entire limb became swollen. Marilyn is active in the teen church group and frequently goes on camping trips. Her physician has suggested that she wear an identification bracelet stating her allergies and that she carry an emergency kit when she is on a camping trip. Her mother sees no need for these precautions because Marilyn is a perfectly healthy girl. Marilyn says she would not know what to do with the kit if she did get stung by a bee or wasp.

1. How would you explain to Marilyn and her mother the need for the identification bracelet and the kit?

2. How would you go about teaching Marilyn to use the emergency kit?

Scenario C

Cindy Lee, a 45-year-old single mother of two, underwent left radical mastectomy 4 months ago. She works in an office full time and is having problems with lymphedema in her left arm.

1. What is the cause of lymphedema?

2. What will you recommend to Cindy to help reduce the problems she is having?

3. What resources are available for her?

The Respiratory System

Objectives

Theory

1. Recall the structure and function of the respiratory system.
2. Analyze three causative factors related to disorders of the respiratory system.
3. Provide instructions to patients on measures to prevent long-term problems of the respiratory system.
4. Summarize nursing responsibilities for patients undergoing diagnostic tests and procedures for disorders of the respiratory system.

Clinical Practice

1. Verify that nursing diagnoses chosen for patients with problems of the respiratory system are appropriate.
2. Propose interventions for a patient who has a problem with oxygenation.
3. Teach a patient about smoking cessation.
4. Employ proper techniques for assessing the respiratory system.

Key Terms

adventitious (ăd-věnt-TĬ-shŭs, p. 264)
antitussive (ăn-tĭ-TŬS-ĭv, p. 272)
aphonia (ă-FŌ-nē-ă, p. 262)
apnea (ĂP-nē-ă, p. 259)
bradypnea (brād-ĕp-NĒ-ă, p. 262)
compliance (kŏm-PLĬ-ăns, p. 259)
crackles (KRĂK-ŭlz, p. 263)
cyanosis (sī-ă-NŌ-sĭs, p. 262)
dyspnea (DĬSP-nē-ă, p. 259)
expectorate (ĕk-SPĔK-tō-rāt p. 257)

hypercapnia (hī-pĕr-KĂP-nē-ă, p. 273)
hypocapnia (hī-pō-KĂP-nē-ă, p. 273)
hypoxia (hī-PŎK-sē-ă, p. 274)
kyphosis (kĭ-FŌ-sĭs, p. 259)
orthopnea (ŏr-thŏp-NĒ-ă, pp. 263, 272)
perfusion (pĕr-FŪ-zhŭn, p. 260)
sputum (SPŪ-tŭm, p. 262)
stridor (STRĪ-dŏr, p. 264)
tachypnea (tăk-ĭp-NĒ-ă, p. 262)
wheezes (wēz-ĕz, p. 263)

OVERVIEW OF ANATOMY AND PHYSIOLOGY OF THE RESPIRATORY SYSTEM

WHAT ARE THE FUNCTIONS OF EACH OF THE STRUCTURES OF THE UPPER RESPIRATORY SYSTEM?

- Air passes through the nose, mouth, pharynx, larynx, and trachea and then into the lungs (Figure 13-1).
- The nasal cavity is lined with mucous membrane that warms and moistens the air as it passes through; moisture protects the cilia.
- The mucous membrane secretes mucus, which traps dust particles and bacteria.
- The *cilia* (small, hairlike projections) propel the mucus toward the larynx, so the person can swallow or expectorate it (cough up and spit out).
- The paranasal sinuses (maxillary, frontal, sphenoid, and ethmoid) are air-filled cavities lined with mucous membrane and situated among the facial bones around the nasal cavity (Figure 13-2).
- The sinuses reduce the weight of the skull, produce mucus, and influence voice quality.
- The pharynx is about 5 inches long and extends from the back of the mouth to the esophagus.
- The pharynx is a passageway for moving air to the lungs and food to the esophagus.
- The tonsils, which are part of the lymphatic system, are located in the pharynx; if they become inflamed and enlarged, they may interfere with breathing.
- The epiglottis forms a hinged "door" at the entrance to the larynx.
- The larynx sits between the pharynx and the trachea. The vocal cords are located in the larynx.
- The trachea is made up of cartilage, smooth muscle, and connective tissue and is lined with mucous membrane and extends from the larynx to the bronchi; it is the "windpipe" and carries air to the lungs.

FIGURE 13-1 Structures of the upper respiratory tract.

*Labels:* Nasopharynx, Sphenoid sinus, Auditory tube, Frontal sinus, Soft palate, Hard palate, External nares, Uvula, Palatine tonsil, Pharynx, Epiglottis, Glottis, Tongue, Vocal cord, Larynx, Esophagus, Trachea

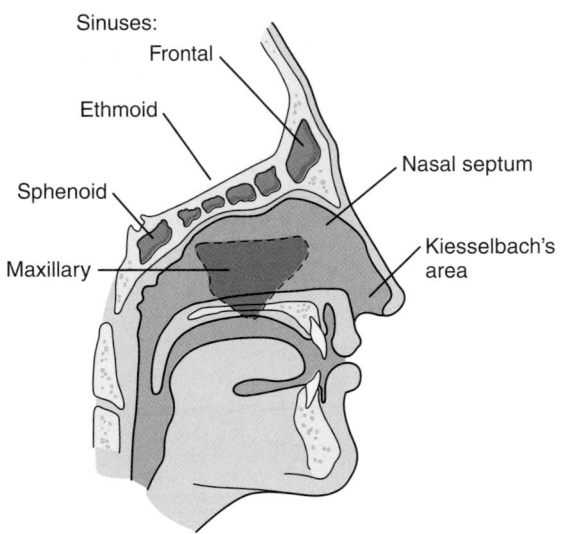

FIGURE 13-2 The paranasal sinuses.

*Labels:* Sinuses: Frontal, Ethmoid, Sphenoid, Maxillary, Nasal septum, Kiesselbach's area

HOW DOES THE EPIGLOTTIS PROTECT THE AIRWAY?

- When swallowing begins, the epiglottis closes over the larynx, preventing aspiration of food and secretions into the lungs. Food is then directed into the esophagus.
- When the swallowing reflex is weak or missing, aspiration is a risk.

HOW IS SPEECH PRODUCED IN THE LARYNX?

- The glottis is the space between the folds of the vocal cords, which are made up of mucous membrane attached to the front and back of the larynx.
- When air from the lungs exits through the larynx, it causes rapid opening and closing of the glottis. Movements of the mouth, lips, jaws, and tongue convert the sounds made by the rush of air through the glottis into speech sounds.

WHAT ARE THE FUNCTIONS OF THE STRUCTURES OF THE LOWER RESPIRATORY SYSTEM?

- On inhalation, after passing through the nose, pharynx, larynx, and trachea of the upper respiratory system, air enters the left and right bronchi, which branch off of the trachea.
- The bronchi carry air into the lungs; the right lung has three lobes, and the left lung has two lobes.

HOW IS OXYGEN DELIVERED TO THE ALVEOLAR MEMBRANE, WHERE IT CAN DIFFUSE INTO THE BLOOD?

- The main bronchi divide into smaller and smaller bronchi, and then divide into bronchioles that deliver the air to the alveoli (Figure 13-3). The right bronchus angles off to the right; inhaled foreign objects tend to lodge here.

HOW IS THE LUNG PROTECTED?

- The pleural sac, which encloses each lung and protects it, is an airtight compartment. **If the pleural sac is punctured, air will rush into the pleural cavity and collapse the lung.**
- The *pleura* is a serous membrane of two layers. One layer, the parietal pleura, covers each lung, and the visceral pleura lines the inner wall of the chest cavity.
- A small amount of fluid between the two layers of pleura lubricates the pleural cavity and prevents friction between the pleural layers when the lungs expand and deflate.

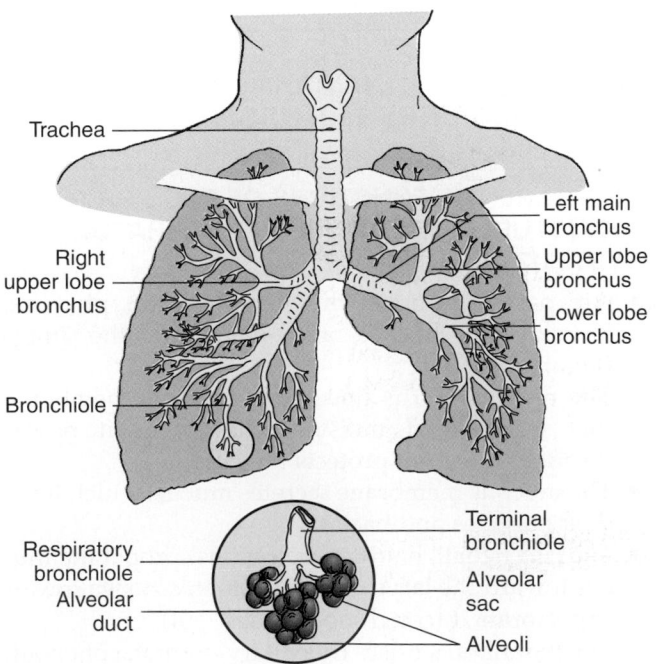

FIGURE 13-3 Structures of the lower respiratory tract and alveoli.

Labels: Trachea, Left main bronchus, Upper lobe bronchus, Lower lobe bronchus, Right upper lobe bronchus, Bronchiole, Respiratory bronchiole, Alveolar duct, Terminal bronchiole, Alveolar sac, Alveoli

- The pleural cavity is a potential space between the pleural layers where there is normally only a small amount of fluid.
- The mucous membrane lining the many small branches of the bronchial tree contains tiny hairlike projections (cilia) that trap and propel small foreign particles that are inhaled towards the entrance of the respiratory tract; the cough reflex works to expel the secretions.
- The alveoli contain macrophages that quickly destroy inhaled bacteria and other foreign particles.

HOW IS RESPIRATION CONTROLLED?

- The central nervous system controls both involuntary and voluntary respiration via the pons and the medulla. The vagus nerve supplies the pharynx, larynx, respiratory airways, and lungs.
- The brainstem chemoreceptors are sensitive to changes in carbon dioxide (CO_2) and hydrogen ions in the cerebrospinal fluid; the chemoreceptors in the aorta and the carotid arteries are sensitive to low oxygen (O_2) levels in the blood.
- The signals of changing levels of hydrogen ions (measured by pH), CO_2, and O_2 trigger the respiratory center to send signals through the spinal cord. The signals travel along the peripheral nervous system to the phrenic and intercostal nerves that control the diaphragm and respiratory muscle contractions.
- When CO_2 and hydrogen ion levels in the cerebrospinal fluid become higher than normal, the central receptors in the brainstem signal the nerves to initiate faster respiration to "blow off" the excess CO_2. Carbon dioxide levels give the primary signals for respiration.
- When arterial blood O_2 levels fall below normal, the respiratory centers in the aorta and carotid arteries signal the nerves to cause the lungs to inflate more fully, making the person breathe more deeply and at a faster rate.
- **When CO_2 levels are constantly high (as occurs with chronic lung disease such as emphysema) the respiratory drive comes from the receptors for low arterial O_2 instead of high levels of CO_2. If these patients are given too much oxygen, their respiratory drive is suppressed and they will stop breathing.** (Normal blood gas levels are listed in Table 13-3 on pp. 265-267.)

HOW DO THE BONES OF THE THORAX AND THE RESPIRATORY MUSCLES AFFECT THE RESPIRATORY PROCESS?

- Inspiration (inhalation) and expiration (exhalation) occur by movement of the diaphragm and the intercostal muscles in the chest wall. During normal breathing, about 500 mL of air moves in and out of the lungs with each breath.
- When the diaphragm contracts, it moves downward; the other chest muscles contract, pulling the rib cage up and out, expanding the lungs and creating a greater area of negative pressure. Air from the atmosphere, which has a positive higher pressure, flows into the lungs.
- When the muscles relax, the lungs are allowed to return to a resting position that has a smaller internal volume and air is pushed out in exhalation.
- **If damage to the spinal cord occurs above the level where the respiratory nerves are located (T1), voluntary respiration ceases.**
- If the muscles of the diaphragm and chest are paralyzed, apnea (absence of breathing) occurs.
- The thoracic cage—composed of the thoracic vertebrae, the sternum, and the ribs—forms a stable unit that allows the respiratory muscles to function correctly. If any bones of the thorax or chest wall are injured or fractured, breathing becomes harder and dyspnea (difficult breathing) occurs.
- Compliance describes the elasticity of the lungs or how easily the lungs inflate; when compliance is decreased, the lungs are more difficult to inflate. Chronic obstructive pulmonary disease (COPD) and aging alter compliance due to damage in the alveoli.
- **Weakness of the respiratory muscles, such as occurs with neuromuscular diseases, also causes decreased lung capacity.**
- Kyphosis (inward curvature and collapse) of the spine constricts the thoracic cavity and restricts the capacity of the lungs to expand fully.

WHAT FACTORS CAN AFFECT THE EXCHANGE OF OXYGEN AND CARBON DIOXIDE?

- Alveoli are tiny air sacs covered with a permeable membrane that come into contact with the pulmonary arterioles and venules; oxygen passes into the blood and carbon dioxide passes from the blood into the alveoli.
- Surfactant is secreted by cells in the alveoli; it decreases surface tension on the alveolar wall so that diffusion of O_2 and CO_2 can take place. Surfactant facilitates expansion with inspiration and prevents alveolar collapse on expiration. When surfactant levels are low, alveoli cannot properly expand and O_2 and CO_2 cannot cross the membrane adequately.
- When interstitial edema occurs in the lung tissue, the alveolar membrane is thickened and gases cannot diffuse across the membrane as easily. During inflammation if fluid fills the alveoli, gases cannot diffuse across the membrane. Tumors may create blockage.
- Edema in the lungs occurs with infectious processes such as pneumonia and in disorders such as congestive heart failure.

- The major portion of the O_2 (about 97%) attaches to the heme portion of the hemoglobin molecule carried by the *erythrocytes* (red blood cells) and forms *oxyhemoglobin*. The plasma also transports a portion of each gas; about 3% of O_2 is dissolved in the plasma.
- CO_2, a cellular waste product, combines with water in the red blood cell, forming carbonic acid; *dissociation* (uncombining) occurs, forming hydrogen ions and bicarbonate ions. About 77% of CO_2 is transported in the blood plasma in the form of bicarbonate ions. The remaining 23% of CO_2 combines with hemoglobin and is carried to the lungs. In the lung, the process reverses and the bicarbonate ions reenter the red blood cells and combine with hydrogen ions to form carbonic acid, which then dissociates into water and CO_2. The CO_2 diffuses across the alveolar membrane and is exhaled.

WHAT AGE-RELATED CHANGES AFFECT THE RESPIRATORY SYSTEM?

- The decrease in the immune system's efficiency makes the elderly more susceptible to upper respiratory infections.
- Aging results in a decreased cough reflex and an increased potential for aspiration.
- Osteoporosis may cause kyphosis, which impinges on lung expansion.
- Adults age 70 and older have some degree of change in connective tissue that causes decreased elasticity and affects lung function and ventilation.
- Total body water decreases to 50% after age 70, thus mucous and respiratory membranes are not as moist and mucous becomes much thicker.
- There is some impairment of the ciliary action, which makes it more difficult for the elderly to remove mucus, and retained mucus provides a breeding ground for bacterial infection.
- There is a loss of normal elastic recoil of the lung during expiration, and the patient must use muscle action to complete expiration. This increases the work of breathing.
- Muscle atrophy may affect the respiratory muscles, diminishing their strength.
- Connective tissue changes and loss of elastic tissue in the alveoli cause the alveolar membranes to become thickened. Oxygen saturation decreases for the elderly, with partial pressure of oxygen (P_{O_2}) dropping to 75 to 80 mm Hg from the usual 80 to 100 mm Hg.
- There is a decreased response to hypoxia (oxygen deficit in tissues) and hypercapnia (excessive amounts of carbon dioxide)

CAUSES OF RESPIRATORY DISORDERS

Trauma or disease can affect structures of the respiratory system, nerves controlling respiration, or diffusion of oxygen or carbon dioxide across the alveolar membranes into the capillaries. **Perfusion** (blood flow into cellular tissue) is essential because the bloodstream carries the oxygen to the cells of the body. Blood must be pumped past the alveolar membrane for oxygen and carbon dioxide *diffusion* to take place (Box 13-1). Cardiac disease, emboli, and other disorders of the heart and pulmonary blood vessels eventually cause problems in the respiratory system.

The respiratory system is particularly susceptible to harmful substances in the environment. Inhalation of bacteria and other organisms can quickly produce an infection in either the upper or lower respiratory tract. Tobacco smoke, allergens, poisonous gases, and other toxic substances cause irritation and inflammation of the air passages and can eventually lead to chronic inflammation, obstructive diseases, and tumors. There may be a familial tendency toward allergies, asthma, or other lung problems.

Box 13-1   Terms Commonly Used in Respiratory Care

- *Diffusion:* The movement of oxygen and carbon dioxide across the alveolar-capillary membrane. It takes place between the gas in the alveolar spaces and the blood in the pulmonary capillaries.
- *Elastance:* The extent to which the lungs are able to return to their original position after being stretched or distended.
- *Hypoxemia:* Deficient oxygenation of the blood.
- *Hypoxia:* A broad term meaning diminished availability of oxygen to the body tissues.
- *Lung compliance:* The ability of the lungs to distend in response to changes in volume and pressure of inhaled air. Lung compliance first increases and then decreases with age as the lungs become stiffer and the chest wall more rigid.
- *Perfusion:* The passage of a fluid through the vessels of a specific organ.
- *Pulmonary hygiene:* Methods used to clear secretions from the airways
- *Resistance:* The force working against the passage of air. The major determinant is the radius of the airway.
- *Respiratory failure:* An abnormality of gas exchange with either an excess of carbon dioxide or a deficit of oxygen, or both.
- *Shunting:* Intrapulmonary shunting is the diverting of blood so that it does not take part in the gas exchange at the alveolar sites. When intrapulmonary shunting occurs, blood enters the left side of the heart without being oxygenated. It is, therefore, a possible cause of hypoxemia.
- *Surfactant:* A complex lipoprotein produced by cells lining the alveoli, which lowers surface tension within the alveoli. It prevents collapse of the lung by stabilizing the alveoli and decreasing capillary pressures.
- *Ventilation:* The movement of air from the external environment to the gas exchange units of the lung. It can be spontaneous or done by a mechanical ventilator.

There are two major types of ventilatory diseases: *restrictive* and *obstructive*. *Restrictive diseases are characterized by decreased lung capacity.* They are not necessarily primarily lung disorders, but eventually the expansion of the lung and chest wall will be limited. Examples include scoliosis and kyphosis, both of which **decrease the size of the chest cavity.** Arthritis increases stiffness of the chest wall and results in a decreased ability of the chest cavity to expand and contract. *Pneumothorax* (collapsed lung) diminishes lung surface; neuromuscular disorders weaken the strength of the muscles of respiration (e.g., myasthenia gravis); and disorders of the lung (e.g., pneumonia, atelectasis, and fibrosis) increase stiffness and decrease lung volume.

Obstructive pulmonary diseases are characterized by problems moving air into and out of the lungs. Narrowing of the openings in the tracheobronchial tree increases resistance to the flow of air, making it difficult for oxygen to enter and contributing to air trapping; therefore exhalation is also difficult. Asthma, emphysema, and chronic bronchitis are examples of obstructive lung diseases. Tumor in the lung can also obstruct airflow to the alveoli.

RESPIRATORY DISORDERS

PREVENTION

The best ways to prevent infection and inflammation of the respiratory system are to practice hand hygiene frequently; stay out of crowds, especially during cold and flu season; refrain from smoking; avoid known allergens as much as possible; maintain adequate nutrition; and obtain sufficient rest to help keep the immune system healthy. Nurses should identify persons that have a high risk for infection (Box 13-2).

Allergy to airborne substances causes the mucous membranes of the nose and sinuses to become irritated and inflamed. When these membranes are inflamed, bacteria and viruses can more easily invade the cells and cause infection. By controlling inhaled allergens we can decrease the incidence of upper respiratory infection (URI).

Elder Care Points

The elderly should not be exposed to children with colds and coughs. If an elderly person is confined to the house or a long-term care facility, he or she will not have the immunity to common viruses and bacteria that younger, more socially active people do.

Elimination of such widespread respiratory diseases as the common cold and influenza is not possible; therefore nurses must practice good hand hygiene and use Standard Precautions and airborne or droplet precautions when working with patients with respiratory infections. For certain groups such as the elderly and the chronically ill, immunization against influenza is an effective means of reducing the incidence of respiratory

Box 13-2	Factors that Increase Risk for Respiratory Infection

- Older than 65 years of age
- Cigarette smoking
- Residing in extended-care facilities
- Chronic respiratory disorders (includes asthma)
- Congenital or chronic cardiovascular disorders
- Chronic renal disease
- Diabetes mellitus or a chronic metabolic disorder
- Compromised immune response

disease. Physicians, nurses, and others involved in providing health care should also be immunized. Among the more serious reactions to influenza vaccine are allergic reactions, fever, malaise, or muscle soreness. Guillain-Barré syndrome occurs in about 1 in 100,00 individuals. The vaccine is prepared from chicken embryos; therefore vaccination is contraindicated for anyone with an allergy to eggs, chicken, or feathers.

The U.S. Public Health Service Advisory Committee on Immunization also recommends immunization against pneumococcal infection for high-risk persons.

Perhaps one of the most important preventive measures is to avoid prolonged and repeated inhalation of irritating substances. Such substances include tobacco smoke, industrial gases, coal dust, soot and other carbons, and air polluted by automobile exhaust. Proposed *Healthy People 2020* objectives include reducing tobacco use by adults, adolescents, and pregnant women. Smoking cessation efforts are supported by increasing insurance coverage for evidenced-based interventions, increasing smoke-free environments, and strengthening tobacco laws. Beginning in early 2010, the Joint Commission began to develop and define Core Measures for the assessment and treatment of tobacco use. Nurses should participate by identifying patients at risk for tobacco-related disease and encourage cessation programs.

 Think Critically

Can you think of three changes in lifestyle that might prevent you or a family member from developing a chronic or serious respiratory disorder?

 Health Promotion

Smoking and Tobacco Cessation

There are "five As" for helping your patients to quit smoking: *Ask* about tobacco use. *Advise* about the health benefits of quitting. *Assess* readiness to quit. *Assist* in creating a cessation plan. *Arrange* follow-up. For those patients who are resistant to the five As model, an alternative model is the "Five Rights." Help the patient identify the personal *Relevance, Risks, Rewards,* and *Roadblocks,* and *Repeat* these at every visit (Agency for Healthcare Research and Quality, 2008).

❖ NURSING MANAGEMENT

■ Assessment (Data Collection)

History Taking

Observe respiratory function while you are talking with the patient and ask about frequency of URIs, known inhalant allergies, and sinus problems. Chest pain can occur with frequent coughing, pleurisy, or trauma to the lungs; however whenever there is a complaint of chest pain be vigilant for cardiac problems. Patients with sinus problems may complain of headache, malaise, a bad taste in the mouth, nasal congestion or obstruction, purulent drainage from the nose, and painful upper teeth. Those with pharyngitis often report a sore or "scratchy" throat, malaise, headache, and sometimes a cough. Dysphagia also might be a problem for patients with pharyngitis, because swallowing involves pushing the food back against the inflamed oropharynx. **Hoarseness and loss of the voice** (aphonia) **are common symptoms of laryngitis.** Hoarseness or a sore throat that lasts longer than 2 weeks, should be noted as this will assist in the early detection of throat malignancy. If the patient is in obvious respiratory distress, ask only a few

Focused Assessment

Data Collection for the Respiratory System

HISTORY TAKING
- Chief complaint and precipitating factors
- New onset of dyspnea or orthopnea
- Cough frequency with or without sputum production
- Measures used for symptom relief
- Medications, over-the-counter medicines, supplement use
- Smoking history
- History of respiratory disorders, such as asthma
- History of allergy or hay fever
- History of conditions such as sinusitis or bronchitis
- History of night sweats or tuberculosis
- History of other lung diseases
- History of alcohol consumption
- Occupational respiratory hazards
- Influenza and pneumonia immunization

PHYSICAL ASSESSMENT
- Nose: deviation, flaring of nostrils, discharge, patent nares
- Trachea position
- Sinus pain on palpation
- Skin color
- Posture: need to be upright or to lean forward
- Shape of chest and symmetry of chest expansion
- Use of accessory muscles for respirations: intercostal or supra-clavicular retractions
- Shape of fingers
- Rate of respiration, depth, rhythm, character
- Restlessness or agitation
- Cough: frequency, characteristics
- Sputum: amount, character, color, presence of blood
- Pulse oximetry readings
- Systematic pattern of auscultation
- Listen for abnormal breath sounds or absence of breath sounds
- Any wheezes, fine or coarse crackles, or "rubs"?
- Do abnormal sounds clear up when patient coughs?

questions about the present illness and chief complaint. Later, during a formal admission interview and informal discussions with the patient and family, obtain more information in order to plan individualized nursing care.

Elder Care Points

When assessing an elderly patient, it is important to obtain a thorough smoking history and a history of alcohol intake throughout adulthood. **Approximately 90% of throat cancer occurs in people who both smoke and immoderately drink alcohol** and is four times more common among men (American Cancer Society, 2010).

Physical Assessment

If the patient is not experiencing respiratory distress, start the assessment at the head and end with lung auscultation. There may be facial puffiness over the affected sinus. Palpation of the neck may reveal enlarged lymph nodes. Note skin color; cyanosis (bluish discoloration) of the skin is not a reliable indicator of hypoxemia. **Cyanosis occurs late in the process of oxygen depletion** and could indicate problems of circulation or hemoglobin deficiency.

Note the posture of the patient, the amount of effort exerted to breathe, the way abdominal muscles and other accessory muscles of respiration are used, the number of words that can be said between breaths, and the rate and character of respirations. Is respiration rapid (tachypnea) or slow (bradypnea)? Is chest expansion equal when a breath is taken? Are there retractions? Do you observe kyphosis or scoliosis, which may cause restriction of the thoracic cavity? Does the patient display or report coughing? A *productive* cough is moist and deep, often accompanied by bronchial crackles or wheezing, and ends in producing quantities of sputum. A *nonproductive* cough is dry and harsh and no sputum is produced. Sputum refers to material brought up from the bronchial tree. It is not mucus from the sinuses, nasal secretions, or saliva. Table 13-1 shows various characteristics and implications of sputum specimens.

A patient with chronic obstructive pulmonary disease (COPD) may lean forward in a sitting position and use the abdominal muscles to force air out of the lungs. Other movements during ventilation indicating difficulty are elevating the shoulders and ribs, tensing the neck and shoulder muscles, and flaring of the nostrils. Exhaling through pursed lips is another clue to obstructive disorders. A retraction of the spaces below and around the sternum also might be observed in a patient in respiratory distress. Obstructive disorders can cause enlargement of the front-to-back (anterior-posterior) measurement of the chest wall, giving a barrel-like appearance to the chest (Figure 13-4) because of the presence of trapped air

Table **13-1**	Characteristics of Sputum and Possible Causes*	

CHARACTERISTIC	POSSIBLE CAUSE
Thick, tenacious, and "ropey"; difficult to cough up	Chronic bronchitis, emphysema
Scant, sticky, rust colored	Pneumococcal pneumonia
Frothy, pinkish or blood tinged	Pulmonary edema
Yellow, yellow-green, or grayish yellow, with foul odor or taste	Pulmonary infection
Blood tinged, bloody, or blood streaked	Tuberculosis, or ulcerated pulmonary vessel, or bronchogenic carcinoma
Large amounts	Pneumonia or bronchitis
Scanty	Asthma
Very thick and viscous	Inadequate hydration

*Normal sputum is white and slightly viscous and has no odor or taste.

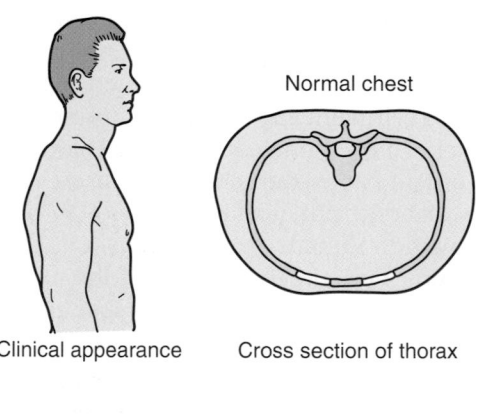

Normal chest

Clinical appearance   Cross section of thorax

Barrel chest

Clinical appearance   Cross section of thorax

FIGURE 13-4 Barrel chest typical of a patient with chronic obstructive pulmonary disease.

in the lungs and inadequate recoil. Over time there is a gradual elevation of the resting level of the diaphragm, which produces an increase in the size of the chest wall. Clubbing of the fingers (Figure 13-5) is frequently seen in patients with chronic respiratory or heart disease, because of inflammatory changes in the bones of the fingers from prolonged oxygen deficiency.

FIGURE 13-5 Clubbing of fingers.

Note the number of pillows the patient uses to prop up in bed or if the head of the bed needs to be raised to facilitate breathing. This position indicates **orthopnea.**

Clinical Cues

Restlessness, agitation, or mental confusion or an increase in pulse and heart rate are early indicators of inadequate oxygenation of the blood.

To auscultate the lungs, first turn off the radio or television and instruct the patient to sit up, if possible, so that the bed or back of the chair is not interfering with chest expansion. Ask the patient to remain quiet and to breathe slowly and deeply through the mouth. Listen to one full breath in each location (Figure 13-6). Place the stethoscope diaphragm against the skin with moderate pressure. Move from one side of the midline of the chest to the other side; compare the sounds. Begin above the clavicles and progress downward in the intercostal spaces to above the sixth rib. On the back, start above the scapula and progress downward along the sides of the spine, and then toward the lateral areas above the tenth thoracic vertebra. Laterally, listen in the midaxillary line in three descending locations to just above the diaphragm. If the patient is short of breath, begin posteriorly at the bases of the lungs and work upward as the patient may not be able to cooperate for the full sequence. Table 13-2 presents sounds normally heard in various locations.

Clinical Cues

Clean the diaphragm of your stethoscope with an alcohol swab between patients to decrease health care–associated infections.

Listen for abnormal sounds. **Wheezes** are a whistling, musical, high-pitched sound produced by air being forced through a narrowed airway. It is common in patients with asthma. Another type of coarse wheezing sound (formerly known as *rhonchi*) is coarse, low-pitched, sonorous, rattling sounds caused by secretions in the larger air passages. **Crackles** are produced

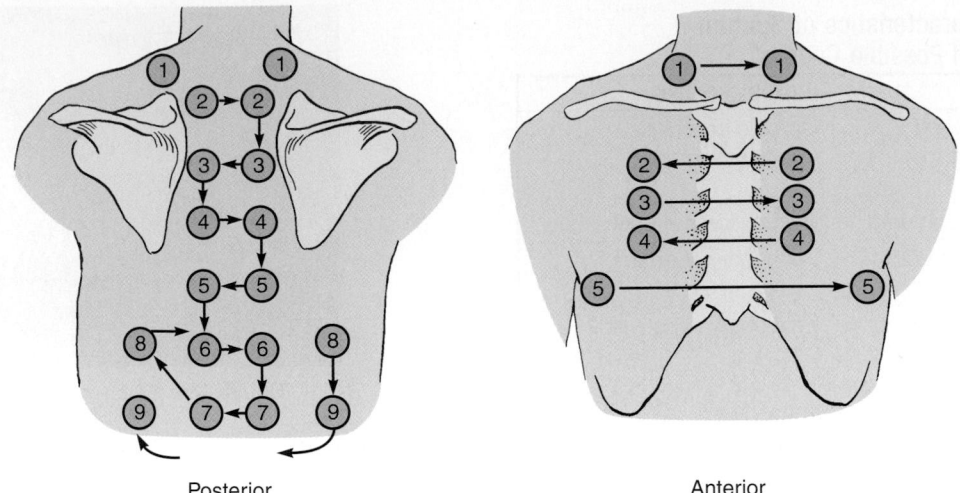

Posterior

Anterior

FIGURE 13-6 Sites for auscultation of the lungs.

by air passing through moisture in the smaller airways. **Fine crackles** are high in pitch and can be heard in patients who have atelectasis, fibrosis, pneumonia, or early congestive heart failure. **Coarse crackles** are louder and low in pitch and are heard in patients with bronchitis, pulmonary edema, and resolving pneumonia. **Crackles sound similar to the sound produced by rubbing hairs between the fingers close to the ear.**

Another abnormal, or adventitious, sound is that of a *pleural friction rub,* which is a grating or scratchy sound similar to creaking shoe leather or an opening, squeaky door that occurs when irritated visceral and parietal pleura rub against each other.

Stridor ("croaking" sounds) can be heard (without using a stethoscope) when there is partial obstruction of the upper air passages. These sounds are typically heard in children with croup, but can also occur in adults with some kind of obstruction. The inflammation that is producing the obstruction often also affects the larynx, producing hoarseness.

[?] Think Critically

How does shortness of breath affect a person's ability to speak?

Diagnostic Tests and Procedures

Table 13-3 presents the most common diagnostic tests performed for problems of the respiratory system. A complete blood cell count with hemoglobin and hematocrit determinations is done to detect any deficiency in oxygen-carrying capacity of the blood. An elevated white blood cell count may indicate the presence of infection. Anterior-posterior and lateral chest radiographs are usually ordered when the patient has a lower respiratory problem that does not quickly resolve.

Diagnostic Visual Examination of the Nose, Mouth, and Throat. The interior of the nose, mouth, and pharynx and the tonsils can be inspected by using a tongue blade and a good source of light. The nose is inspected for redness, swelling, discharge, and lumps. Using a nasal speculum, the head is tilted upward and the inside of the nares is inspected for pallor, redness, swelling, and polyps and for mucus color, consistency, odor, and amount. The hard and soft palates are inspected, and the mobility of the soft palate is evaluated by asking the patient to say "ah." The pharynx can be brought into view by asking the patient to say "ee." Presence of inflammation, lesions, plaques, or exudates is noted. The paranasal sinuses are assessed by observing

Text continued on p. 268

Table 13-2 Normal Lung Sounds		
TYPE OF SOUND	**LOCATION WHERE NORMALLY HEARD***	**DESCRIPTION OF SOUND**
Vesicular breath sounds	Over lung tissue to level of sixth intercostal space	Low to medium pitch with a soft whooshing quality; inspiration is two to three times the length of expiration
Bronchovesicular breath sounds	Over the mainstem bronchi, below the level of the clavicles, beside the sternum; posteriorly: between the scapulae	Moderate to high pitch with a hollow, muffled quality; equal time of inspiration and expiration
Bronchial breath sounds	Over the trachea above the sternal notch (these sounds are abnormal elsewhere and often indicate atelectasis)	High pitch with a loud, harsh, tubular quality; inspiration half as long as expiration

*See Figure 2-1.

Table 13-3 Diagnostic Tests for Respiratory Problems*

PURPOSE	DESCRIPTION	NURSING IMPLICATIONS
Oximetry (O₂ sat)		
To noninvasively monitor arterial oxygen saturation (SaO_2) To allow comparison of oxygenated hemoglobin to total hemoglobin	Device attaches to earlobe, pinna of ear, or fingertip Sensor warms skin, increasing capillary blood flow Light beam is used to obtain reading, which is displayed by number on oximeter monitor	Keep sensor intact on patient. Monitor and record SaO_2 readings. Report readings persistently below 95% to physician. Obstructions to blood flow, such as inflated BP cuff, peripheral artery disease, hypotension, or hypothermia, can cause false readings.
Arterial Blood Gas (ABG) Analysis		
To determine if there is adequate exchange of carbon dioxide and oxygen across alveolar membrane; to determine acid-base balance within the body; to determine hypoxemia	Useful for patients with respiratory disorders, problems of circulation and of blood distribution, body fluid imbalances, and acid-base imbalances Arterial blood sample is drawn and tested for pH, PaO_2, $PaCO_2$, and HCO_3^-	Explain procedure to patient; arterial puncture is briefly painful. Apply firm pressure for 5-10 min after specimen is drawn. Compare laboratory results to normal values: pH: 7.35-7.45 PaO_2: 80-100 mm Hg $PaCO_2$: 35-45 mm Hg HCO_3^-: 22-26 mm Hg
D-Dimer		
To assess thrombin and plasmin activity Useful for diagnosing pulmonary embolism and disseminated intravascular coagulation (DIC)	Blood test that provides assay of fibrin degradation	No fasting is required. Collect blood sample in a blue-top tube.
Sputum Analysis		
To examine sputum from lower respiratory tract for bacteria, bacilli, or malignant cells; to determine color, consistency, and sensitivity of bacteria to specific antibiotics	Sputum specimen is examined and cultured for bacteria; acid-fast stain and Gram stain are done for tuberculosis bacillus; cytologic studies may be done to search for malignant cells If bacteria are present, sensitivity studies to antibiotics are performed Nucleic acid amplification can detect *Mycobacterium tuberculosis* earlier than culture, and should be interpreted in correlation with acid-fast results	Explain that specimen is desired from lower areas of lungs; may require respiratory therapy to obtain proper specimen or coaching in proper coughing technique. Best specimen is obtained in A.M. before eating or mouth care. Provide mouth care after obtaining specimen. Specimen is expectorated into sterile container.
Sublingual CO₂ Level		
To detect early perfusion problems	Probe of handheld device is placed under the tongue	Reading takes 60-90 sec. Explain the procedure to the patient.
Capnography		
To detect hypoventilation	Monitors CO_2 in every breath by aspirating breaths from the airway using infrared technology Plots a waveform on the monitor	Uses a nasal cannula and a finger probe. Explain the procedure and purpose.
Pulmonary Function Tests (PFTs)		
To determine integrity of mechanical function and gas exchange function of the lungs: volume of air lung can hold, rate of flow of air in and out of the lung, and elasticity, or compliance, of lung	Patient breathes in as much air as possible and then breathes out as much air as possible into a spirometer, indicating the forced vital capacity (FVC); forced expiratory volume in 1 second (FEV_1) is measured Other measurements include total lung capacity (TLC), vital capacity (VC), tidal volume (TV), functional residual capacity (FRC), and residual volume (RV)	Should not be done within 1-2 hr of eating. No smoking for 4-6 hr before test. Patient is not to take any drugs causing sedation. Explain procedure to patient. *Post-test:* Monitor vital signs and allow patient to rest, as test can be fatiguing.

BP, blood pressure; HCO_3^-, bicarbonate ion; *IV*, intravenous(ly); *NPO*, nothing by mouth; $PaCO_2$, partial pressure of arterial carbon dioxide; PaO_2, partial pressure of arterial oxygen.
Note: For tuberculosis test, refer to Chapter 15.

Continued

| Table 13-3 | Diagnostic Tests for Respiratory Problems—cont'd | |

PURPOSE	DESCRIPTION	NURSING IMPLICATIONS
Chest Radiograph		
To determine pathologic conditions in the lungs, such as pneumonia, lung abscess, tuberculosis, atelectasis, pneumothorax, and tumor; also gives indication of heart size	Front, back, and lateral views are taken; fluoroscopy may be used to visualize lung and diaphragm movement	Tell patient to remove clothes down to the waist and put on an x-ray gown so that it ties in back. Will be asked to take a deep breath and hold it while the radiograph is taken.
Computed Tomography (CT)		
To visualize soft tissue densities, tumors, and blood clots	Chest CT with 5- to 10-mm cross-sectional views of the entire thorax with 1-mm scans of suspicious areas Contrast agent may be used	Check for sensitivity to iodine, shellfish, or the specific contrast medium. Provide information about the test.
Lung Ventilation and Perfusion Scan (V-Q scan)		
To assess lung ventilation and lung perfusion; to locate pulmonary embolism and diagnose tumor, emphysema, bronchiectasis, or fibrosis	*Perfusion scan:* An IV injection of radionuclide-tagged, macroaggregated albumin is given; decreased blood flow to any part of the lung is shown by decreased radioactivity in that area *Ventilation scan:* Radioactive gas is inhaled and, when scanned, presents a pattern of ventilation in the lungs	Assess for allergies. Ask patient to remove all metal jewelry from around the neck. Assure patient that amount of radioactivity used is very small and is not harmful. An IV access will be inserted. Patient will be asked to hold breath for a short period for the ventilation scan. Images are viewed by use of a scintillation scanner.
Pulmonary Angiography		
To visualize pulmonary vasculature; to locate pulmonary embolus or other abnormality	Radiopaque dye is injected via a catheter into the right side of the heart or the pulmonary artery Radiographs are taken; fluoroscopy is used	Check consent form. Assess for allergy to dye. Explain that patient may feel warm flush as dye is injected. *Post-test:* Monitor vital signs and check pressure dressing for signs of hemorrhage.
Bronchoscopy		
To inspect bronchi; to remove foreign objects or mucous plugs; to biopsy lesions	Preoperative sedation (benzodiazepine) is usually given Throat is sprayed with local anesthetic With neck hyperextended, a flexible fiberoptic bronchoscope is guided into bronchi; biopsies are taken if needed Oxygen is administered; a patent IV line is necessary in case emergency drugs are needed	Keep patient NPO for 6 hr before test. Check consent form; administer preoperative sedative. Give mouth care just before test. *Post-test:* For 24-48 hr, monitor vital signs, pulse oximetry readings and level of consciousness. Observe for bleeding, dyspnea, wheezing, discomfort, and swelling of face and neck; sputum will be slightly blood-tinged at first. Position patient on side until gag reflex has returned. Check for return of gag reflex by having patient take small sips of water. When gag reflex has returned, throat lozenges may be used for sore throat.
Laryngoscopy		
Direct: To detect or remove lesions, polyps, or foreign bodies in the larynx or to obtain biopsy specimens or tissue for culture	*Direct:* A fiberoptic laryngoscope is used; sedation and local or general anesthetic is administered	*Direct:* Patient should be NPO for several hours before procedure. Administer preprocedure medications; ensure that respiratory status will be monitored closely. Advise that the room will be darkened. An ice collar may be applied postprocedure. A mild sore throat and hoarseness may occur.

Table 13-3   Diagnostic Tests for Respiratory Problems—cont'd

PURPOSE	DESCRIPTION	NURSING IMPLICATIONS
Laryngoscopy—cont'd		
Indirect: To assess function of the vocal cords or obtain tissue by biopsy.	*Indirect:* A laryngeal mirror, head mirror, and light source are used Inspection is performed at rest and during phonation	*Indirect:* Patient will be upright for procedure. *Postprocedure:* Keep patient NPO until gag reflex has returned. Encourage fluid intake.
Mediastinoscopy		
To inspect the mediastinum and biopsy mediastinal lymph nodes Biopsies give information about lung metastasis, sarcoidosis, and granulomatous infections	Mediastinoscope is inserted via a small incision made at the suprasternal notch	Informed consent is required. Preoperative and postoperative care are the same as for other surgeries. Keep patient NPO after midnight the night before the procedure. Administer preoperative sedation 1 hr before the procedure. *Postprocedure:* Observe for crepitus around insertion site indicating air from pneumothorax. Observe for distended veins and pulsus paradoxus as a hematoma may be preventing cardiac filling.
Thoracentesis		
To remove pleural fluid, instill medication, or obtain fluid for diagnostic studies	With local anesthetic, a large-bore needle is inserted through the chest wall into the pleural space, and fluid is withdrawn with a large-bore syringe Aseptic technique must be used Specimens are obtained for culture, microscopic examination, and stains Medication may be instilled Usually done at the bedside	Requires signed consent. Explain procedure to patient. Take baseline vital signs. Position patient sitting, facing side of bed, and leaning over the overbed table with arms crossed on it; pillows or the back of a chair can also be used. Monitor respirations and skin color during procedure. Assist patient to remain still. Chest radiograph may be ordered after procedure. Monitor vital signs q 15 min for 1 hr or until stable, then routinely. Auscultate breath sounds frequently. Rapid breathing, cyanosis, hemoptysis, changes in breath sounds, and tachycardia should be reported immediately. Chart amount and appearance of fluid and condition of patient.

Ribs

Parietal pleura

Visceral pleura

Lung tissue
(parenchyma)

Pleural effusion

Diaphragm

Thoracentesis position.

for purulent discharge in the nares and by palpating over the sinus areas for tenderness. Sometimes sinus radiographs are ordered. Magnetic resonance imaging may be ordered to locate tumors and pathologic abnormalities of the esophagus and larynx.

Throat Culture. The most common reason for culturing pharyngeal secretions is to establish a definitive diagnosis of infection with *Streptococcus pyogenes* (strep throat). Rheumatic heart disease and glomerulonephritis can result if strep throat is not properly identified and treated. A "rapid strep test" is frequently done in the physician's office or ambulatory clinic. A throat culture also is sometimes done to establish a diagnosis of diphtheria, meningitis, or whooping cough. These diseases can be particularly harmful to elderly, debilitated, or very young patients.

Tuberculosis Tests. Sputum testing for acid-fast bacilli is ordered when tuberculosis is suspected. Sputum specimens should be collected just after the patient awakens in the morning. Suctioning may be required to obtain the specimen. A quicker, more accurate test for tuberculosis drug susceptibility is called microscopic-observation drug susceptibility (MODS). It is less expensive to perform than current culture-based tests (Moore, 2007). A new simple blood test may replace the tuberculin skin test used for tuberculosis screening. The QuantiFERON-TB Gold test is more reliable and has been indicated in the new guideline from the Centers for Disease Control and Prevention (CDC) on tuberculosis (TB) testing (CDC, 2009a). In recent updated guidelines from the CDC the recommendation is that nucleic acid amplification (NAA) testing should be performed when a patient is suspected of having TB and showing signs and symptoms (CDC, 2009b).

Lung Function Tests. Pulmonary function tests (PFTs) are useful in screening gross abnormalities in the respiratory system (Figure 13-7). The *forced vital capacity* (FVC) is affected by diseases that restrict lung motion. *Forced expiratory volume in 1 second* (FEV$_1$) gives some estimate of the amount of *obstruction* to the patient's airflow. The FEV$_1$ is lower in obstructive pulmonary diseases such as emphysema and chronic bronchitis.

The results of pulmonary function tests often are recorded in the following terms:

- *Total lung capacity (TLC):* The volume (amount) of gas the lung can hold at the end of a maximal inspiration
- *Vital capacity (VC):* The volume of gas that a person can exhale after inhaling as much air as possible (maximal inspiration)
- *Tidal volume (TV):* The volume of gas either inspired or exhaled during each breath
- *Functional residual capacity (FRC):* The volume of gas remaining in the lungs when the lungs and chest wall are at resting end-expiratory position (i.e., at rest at the end of a normal expiration)
- *Residual volume (RV):* The volume of gas remaining in the lungs after a person has exhaled as much air as possible (maximal expiration)

Figure 13-8 shows the various subdivisions of total lung capacity.

Peak Flowmeter. Asthma and COPD patients are often asked to check their peak expiratory flow with the use of a peak flowmeter (Figure 13-9). Normal peak flow values for adults are based on age, gender, height, and underlying lung disorder. Normal values range from 300 to 700 L/min but are assessed by comparison against a patient's baseline values. While standing or sitting upright, the patient exhales into the mouthpiece; a small arrow points to the maximum expiratory flow volume. The peak flowmeter is useful for knowing when additional medications are needed to prevent acute exacerbation of disease.

Lung Biopsy. When tumor is suspected, a lung biopsy may be obtained by bronchoscopy (Figure 13-10) or during open thoracotomy. Postprocedure care includes observing sputum for blood and monitoring vital signs closely. Nothing is given by mouth until the gag reflex returns. An open surgical biopsy will require usual postoperative care, including monitoring for bleeding, shortness of breath, and infection.

■ Nursing Diagnosis

Appropriate nursing diagnoses for patients with respiratory disorders, or respiratory surgery, depend on the type of problem and the stage of the disorder. The most commonly used nursing diagnoses include:

- Ineffective breathing pattern related to constricted airways
- Impaired gas exchange related to alveolar damage from chronic inflammation
- Ineffective airway clearance related to physical alteration in airway (presence of tenacious secretions or tracheostomy)

FIGURE 13-7 Patient undergoing pulmonary function testing administered by a respiratory therapist in the pulmonary laboratory.

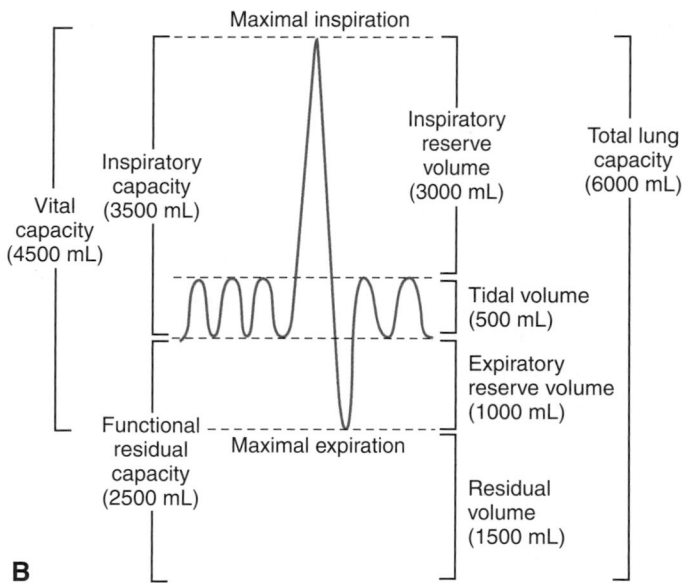

FIGURE 13-8 A, Comparison of respiratory volumes and capacities as measured by spirometry. **B,** Amounts of lung volumes and capacities. (Volumes can vary by age, sex, height, or weight.)

FIGURE 13-9 Use of a peak flowmeter to measure peak expiratory flow volume.

FIGURE 13-10 Fiberoptic bronchoscopy.

- Fatigue related to hypoxemia
- Activity intolerance related to hypoxemia
- Anxiety related to dyspnea
- Ineffective health maintenance related to inability to stop smoking
- Risk for infection related to chronic inflammation or surgical procedure
- Pain related to inflammation and constant cough
- Risk for imbalanced body temperature related to infection
- Impaired verbal communication related to surgical procedure (laryngectomy)
- Ineffective coping related to changes in body image and roles
- Disturbed body image related to loss of voice or disfiguring surgical procedure

Other diagnoses may be included in the care plan as they relate to secondary problems.

■ Planning

For the patient with a respiratory disorder, consider comfort measures, time needed for eating or feeding, use of strict asepsis for wound and tracheostomy care, provision of measures to provide a means of communication, time for patient education, and consideration of psychosocial needs. Working with patients who have dyspnea requires that the nurse plan extra time to accomplish treatments and care. A patient who is *hypoxic* (oxygen deficient) moves more slowly, takes more time to answer questions, and has less energy.

The nursing goals for the patient with a respiratory disorder are to:

- Promote oxygenation
- Prevent infection
- Prevent further lung damage
- Promote rehabilitation

Specific *expected outcomes* are individualized for each patient (see the nursing care plans in Chapters 14 and 15).

■ Implementation

Examples of interventions and teaching for the patient with respiratory disorders are presented in Table 13-4. Interventions are discussed later in this chapter and in Chapters 14 and 15.

■ Evaluation

Effectiveness of interventions for and treatment of the patient with a respiratory disorder is based on improved breathing pattern, pulse oximeter readings, arterial blood gas values, and lung sounds. Decreases in coughing, sputum production, wheezing, and signs of infection are other parameters that indicate improvements. Lessened dyspnea, as well as more energy and ability to perform more self-care and other activities, indicates that interventions are effective. Reassessment is an ongoing nursing activity for the patient with a respiratory problem.

Table 13-4	Common Nursing Diagnoses, Expected Outcomes, and Interventions for Patients with Respiratory Disorders	
NURSING DIAGNOSIS	**GOALS/EXPECTED OUTCOMES**	**NURSING INTERVENTIONS**
Impaired gas exchange related to decreased airflow and respiratory muscle fatigue	Patient will use modified breathing techniques to facilitate ventilation.	Instruct in techniques of pursed-lip breathing, diaphragmatic breathing, deep breathing, and effective coughing; teach relaxation techniques. Review medication dosages and schedule with patient and proper technique for use of measured-dose inhaler; assess effectiveness and compliance. Encourage use of incentive spirometer. Monitor pulse oximetry before, during, and after exertion. Begin stepped exercise program to improve plan for pacing activities of daily living.
Ineffective airway clearance related to viscous sputum	Thinner mucus that is easier to cough up. Fluid intake will increase to 3000 mL/day. Patient will demonstrate proper use of nebulizer.	Explain effect of inadequate fluid intake on liquidity of mucus; assess what fluids patient likes, advise to drink 8 oz of fluid every hour while awake, suggest use of room humidifier at home; review technique for using nebulizer and mucolytic agents. Obtain peak flow readings before and after nebulizer treatment.

Table 13-4	Common Nursing Diagnoses, Expected Outcomes, and Interventions for Patients with Respiratory Disorders—cont'd	
NURSING DIAGNOSIS	**GOALS/EXPECTED OUTCOMES**	**NURSING INTERVENTIONS**
Risk for respiratory infection related to compromised respiratory system and decreased resistance	Patient will have less than one respiratory infection per year.	Review ways to decrease contact with respiratory infectious organisms: avoiding people with colds, flu, and other infections; frequent hand hygiene. Teach to avoid respiratory irritants; stay in house when air pollution index is high; avoid smoke, dust, and cold air. Observe sputum for changes in color, consistency, odor, and amount; call clinic promptly if signs of infection occur and obtain culture for infective organism if indicated. Give influenza and Pneumovax vaccines. Encourage to maintain adequate nutrition.
Situational low self-esteem related to inability to do ordinary activities	Patient will express improvement in self-concept within 3 mo. Patient will be able to resume favorite hobby within 3 mo.	Allow to verbalize concerns; assist to focus on activities possible; explore ways of continuing favorite activities using modifications. Give encouragement and praise for efforts in stepped exercise program.
Activity intolerance related to dyspnea	Patient will be able to perform bathing and dressing without dyspnea within 3 mo. Patient will participate in and comply with stepped exercise program. Patient will display increased ability to tolerate activity by walking short distance without breathlessness.	Encourage use of pursed-lip and diaphragmatic breathing. Begin stepped exercise program as soon as acute respiratory infection has resolved. Alternate activity with rest periods, beginning with small increments of activity. Use oxygen as prescribed during acute episodes of dyspnea.
Anxiety related to hypoxia and dyspnea	Patient will verbalize that anxiety has lessened within 1 wk.	Allow to verbalize concerns within ability to speak without becoming dyspneic. Encourage use of pursed-lip and diaphragmatic breathing to decrease dyspnea. Teach best positions to decrease dyspnea. Teach relaxation techniques; encourage practice. Interact with calm, reassuring manner.
Ineffective health maintenance related to continued smoking	Within 1 wk patient will look at alternative ways to quit smoking. Patient will begin a smoking cessation program within 3 wk.	Explain the harmful effects of continued smoking. Motivate patient to quit smoking by emphasizing benefits of increased stamina and decreased dyspnea. Introduce to various methods and programs for quitting smoking. Introduce to people with equivalent lung disease who have quit smoking. Praise any effort at decreasing or quitting smoking.

COMMON RESPIRATORY PATIENT CARE PROBLEMS

INEFFECTIVE AIRWAY CLEARANCE

A cough is usually a reflex triggered by a foreign substance or some other irritant in the respiratory tract. Coughing can be beneficial and should be encouraged if it is effective in clearing the air passages and removing accumulations of stagnant mucus. The nurse should explain that deep-breathing and coughing maneuvers help to remove sputum and decrease likelihood of complications, such as pneumonia. (See Chapter 4 for deep-breathing and coughing maneuvers.)

If coughing is excessive, the patient will tire and the respiratory tissues and thoracic structures can be traumatized, so antitussive agents may be used to inhibit the cough reflex in the cough center in the brain. Many sedative cough mixtures contain codeine or other drugs that decrease the desire to cough. The liquefying agents and diluents thin secretions and help the patient to expectorate (cough up). Cough syrups are given to soothe the nerve endings in the upper respiratory mucosa. These medications are given in small doses to coat and protect the throat. **Water should not be taken immediately after a cough syrup.**

In bacterial infections and chronic respiratory diseases, the sputum often is foul smelling, leaving a bad taste in the mouth and offensive breath odor. Mouth care is especially needed before meals, when the taste or odor of the sputum may adversely affect appetite. **Frequent mouth care also helps remove pathogenic microorganisms from the oral cavity and thereby diminishes the possibility that they will be aspirated deep into the air passages.**

Mechanical suctioning is indicated when the patient cannot clear the airway of excessive amounts of secretions. Removing secretions from the nose, mouth, and throat (nasopharyngeal suctioning) is a relatively safe and simple procedure. However, deep tracheal suctioning—whether through the nose, mouth, or endotracheal tube—should only be performed using strict aseptic technique, and by someone experienced in the correct procedure.

The need for suctioning is based on patient assessment. Some patients may require suctioning only once or twice daily to remove deeply situated pools and plugs of mucus that cannot be coughed up. Others require suctioning every 10 to 15 minutes to clear their air passages. Remember: the purpose of suctioning is to facilitate breathing and to allow for an adequate exchange of carbon dioxide and oxygen in the lungs. Even though the procedure may be necessary, suctioning removes oxygen, and is uncomfortable for the patient.

Some basic guidelines should be helpful in avoiding the serious consequences of removing oxygen by suctioning:

- Select the proper size suction catheter; preoxygenate the patient before suctioning by (1) using a manual Ambu (resuscitator) bag attached to 100% oxygen for 2 minutes or (2) using the setting on the ventilator that will briefly hyperoxygenate the patient. Repeat this procedure after suctioning and between repeated sessions of suctioning.
- Suction no longer than 10 to 15 seconds; count silently while suction is applied to avoid suctioning too long. Apply suction only when withdrawing the catheter.
- The suction gauge pressure should be between 80 and 100 mm Hg when the tubing is unoccluded; no higher pressure should be used.
- If tachycardia or bradycardia develops during suctioning, stop and hyperoxygenate the patient unless the airway is badly occluded by secretions.

See Skill 14-1: Endotracheal and tracheostomy suctioning on Evolve.

INEFFECTIVE BREATHING PATTERNS

Dyspnea or Breathlessness

Administer oxygen as prescribed. Use a calm manner and assure the patient that everything possible is being done to bring relief of dyspnea. Coach the patient to perform pursed-lip and diaphragmatic breathing (see Chapter 15).

The high Fowler's position is best for patients with dyspnea. Proper positioning and support allow the respiratory muscles to function at maximum efficiency. For severe dyspnea, the orthopneic position is most effective. Orthopnea means that the patient has trouble breathing when supine. The patient should sit upright, lean over the overbed table, which is padded with pillows, and elevate and round the shoulders to allow maximum expansion of the lungs (Figure 13-11).

Another factor to consider is the pressure from organs below or near the lungs and diaphragm. A full stomach can contribute to dyspnea by limiting the amount of space available for expansion of the lungs. Abdominal distention due to edema or collection of flatus and fecal material can also make breathing more difficult.

Hypercapnia

Hyperventilation, hypoventilation, and the effect of these abnormal breathing patterns on the acid-base balance of body fluids are discussed in Chapter 3.

Pillows are used to support the back.

Other pillows are placed on an overbed table to support the weight of the arms, shoulders, and head.

FIGURE 13-11 Orthopneic position.

Hypercapnia (also called *hypercarbia*) is the retention of excessive amounts of carbon dioxide. It is the result of hypoventilation, during which the usual amount of carbon dioxide is not eliminated by exhalation.

Carbon dioxide is a respiratory stimulant; hence **the body responds to excessive levels of carbon dioxide by increasing the rate of respirations.** However, if the respiratory centers in the brain are exposed to higher than normal levels of carbon dioxide over a long time, they cease to react and a drop in the respiratory rate occurs. If the slow respiratory rate is not corrected, the accumulation of carbon dioxide continues, and coma can ensue.

Respiratory failure is defined by arterial blood gases: arterial oxygen (Pao$_2$) is below 50 mm Hg and the partial pressure of carbon dioxide (Pco$_2$) is equal to or greater than 50 mm Hg. The final outcome can be cardiac arrest from respiratory acidosis—a result of respiratory failure.

Hypocapnia

Hypocapnia, which is a deficit of carbon dioxide, occurs as a result of hyperventilation and eventually produces respiratory alkalosis. Conditions associated with hypocapnia include (1) those in which there is an increased metabolic rate, such as thyrotoxicosis, persistent fever, and acute anxiety; (2) salicylate overdosage; and (3) improper use of mechanical ventilation.

Clinical signs of respiratory alkalosis include hyperactive neuromuscular reflexes, tetany, carpopedal spasms, vertigo, blurred vision, and diaphoresis. Blood gas analysis will show a low partial pressure of arterial carbon dioxide (Paco$_2$) and a high pH (alkalinity).

Other Ineffective Breathing Patterns

Other abnormal respiratory patterns are as follows (Figure 13-12):

- *Kussmaul's respiration:* Respiration characterized by a distressing difficulty in breathing that occurs as increasing depth and rate of respiration with no expiratory pause; seen in patients with diabetic acidosis and coma.
- *Biot's respiration:* Respiration that is characterized by irregular periods of apnea alternating with periods in which four or five breaths of identical depth are taken; seen in patients with increased intracranial pressure.
- *Apneustic respiration (apnea):* Prolonged gasping inhalation, followed by short, ineffective exhalation. The pattern is indicative of damage to the respiratory centers in the brain.
- *Cheyne-Stokes respiration:* Breathing characterized by rhythmic waxing and waning of the depth of respiration, with regularly recurring periods of apnea; seen in patients in coma resulting from a disorder affecting the central nervous system.

? Think Critically

Can you name four nursing interventions that will help the patient suffering from dyspnea?

RISK OF INFECTION

Many acute URIs are transmitted by droplet infection; that is, the causative organisms are expelled along with the liquid secretions released during coughing and sneezing and cores of droplets continue to float in the air after the liquid evaporates. These *droplet nuclei* are teeming with bacteria or viruses when an infection is present.

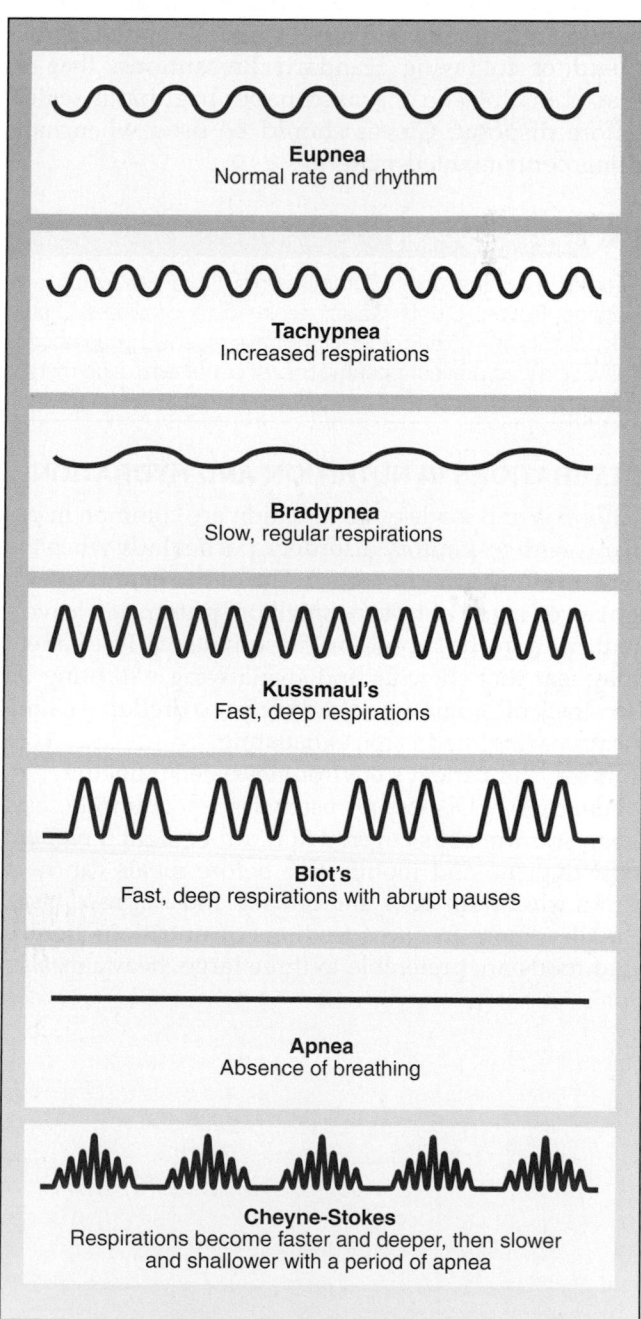

FIGURE 13-12 Respiratory patterns.

Patients with chronic respiratory disorders—and all health care personnel—should carefully avoid contamination. Avoiding crowded places, performing frequent hand hygiene, and, keeping the hands away from the face and mouth decreases the likelihood of infection. Standing to the side of a person who is coughing and sneezing reduces contamination. Hands should be washed after each contact with a person with a respiratory disorder that produces airborne or droplet secretions, or after contact with articles contaminated by secretions. Instruct patients to use a folded tissue over the nose and mouth while sneezing and to turn the head away when in close contact with others. An alternative is to sneeze or cough into the crook of the elbow so that the hands are not contaminated. Tissues should be disposed of following Standard Precautions, that is, placed in a plastic or waxed paper bag that is sealed before disposal. Gloves should be used when handling contaminated materials.

 Elder Care Points

According to the Joint Commission's Core Measures and National Patient Safety Goals, health care providers should ask patients age 65 and older if they have received pneumococcal vaccine, to prevent pneumococcal bacteremia and meningitis, and encourage vaccination if indicated.

ALTERATIONS IN NUTRITION AND HYDRATION

Anorexia and inadequate nutrition are common in patients with respiratory disorders, particularly when the disorder is chronic in nature. The patient may have an impaired sense of taste or smell or sputum can leave a bad taste in the mouth or cause nausea. The patient may fear that chewing and swallowing will bring on an attack of coughing, or he may be so tired that eating or preparing food is too exhausting.

Keep the patient's environment clean, uncluttered, and orderly. Dispose of used tissues promptly, and keep sputum cups covered and out of sight. Frequent oral hygiene and mouth care before meals can help diminish mouth odor and nausea and improve taste. Smaller, more frequent feedings of nutritious liquids and foods are preferable to three large, heavy meals.

Because there is increased energy expenditure when breathing is difficult, many patients have difficulty maintaining weight, even when they do take in normal amounts of calories. Supplements, such as Pulmocare, have an increased fat content and provide more calories in smaller quantities. **When a patient is receiving mechanical ventilation, caloric needs rise.** Sometimes total parenteral nutrition or lipid infusions are necessary to prevent malnutrition for patients with COPD.

A fluid deficit is likely in patients with respiratory disorders because there is an increased loss of fluid in respiratory secretions. The patient usually breathes through the mouth and exhales large amounts of moisture from the body. Unless contraindicated, an intake of at least 3000 mL of liquid should occur each day. This intake may include low-sodium bouillon, fruit juices, and other liquids in addition to water.

Humidifying the air breathed by the patient is an effective way to minimize dehydration and liquefy secretions in the air passages. Humidification is especially important to the patient whose secretions are thick and tenacious and difficult to cough up. Humidification of inhaled air is covered in Chapter 15.

FATIGUE

Hypoxia, which is an oxygen deficit in the tissues, produces a loss of energy because it causes a disturbance in cellular metabolism. Patients with respiratory disorders often have hypoxia and use their energy just to struggle for breath and cough up secretions.

Patients with respiratory disorders, whether acute or chronic, have some degree of intolerance to physical activity and therefore need periods of rest throughout the day. Treatments and medications should be scheduled so that the patient can rest without interruption. To rest the lungs, the patient should lie down for short naps. Deep-breathing exercises and coughing techniques should be planned whenever the patient is able to do them with or without some assistance. These activities should be followed by good mouth care and a short period of uninterrupted rest. The goal of nursing care should be to achieve a satisfactory balance of rest and activity because there are complications associated with excessive physical inactivity.

Get Ready for the NCLEX® Examination!

Key Points

- Inhalation of infectious organisms and chemical irritants causes respiratory problems.
- Cardiac disease can interfere with blood supply to the lungs and distribution of gases.
- There are two major types of ventilatory diseases: restrictive (decreased lung volume) and obstructive (narrowed air passages).
- Restrictive conditions, such as scoliosis and kyphosis, decrease lung capacity.
- Obstructive disorders cause problems moving air in and out of the lungs. Asthma, emphysema, and chronic bronchitis are obstructive disorders.
- Prevention of respiratory problems includes good health practices: rest, nutrition, and personal hygiene, and avoiding known allergens. At-risk persons should be immunized against influenza and pneumonia.
- The incidence of respiratory ailments decreases for people who stop smoking.
- Effectiveness of interventions and treatment is based on improvements in breathing pattern, pulse oximetry readings, arterial blood gas values, and lung sounds. Decreased cough, sputum production, wheezing, and dyspnea are other parameters.
- Positioning in high Fowler's position, or sitting with shoulders hunched and arms resting on knees with legs apart, eases breathing.
- Signs of respiratory acidosis are excessive P_{CO_2} and rapid respirations.
- Signs of respiratory alkalosis are tetany, carpopedal spasms, vertigo, blurred vision, diaphoresis, and low P_{CO_2} and high pH.
- Respiratory failure is defined as Pa_{O_2} below 50 mm Hg and P_{CO_2} equal to or greater than 50 mm Hg.
- Abnormal respiratory patterns include: Biot's respirations, Cheyne-Stokes respirations, Kussmaul's respirations, and apneustic respirations.
- Respiratory infections are transmitted by airborne or droplet secretions.
- Anorexia and inadequate nutrition are common with chronic respiratory disease.
- Patients should drink at least 3000 mL/day to help thin secretions. Humidification of air can help prevent fluid deficit.

Additional Learning Resources

SG Go to your Study Guide for additional learning activities to help you master this chapter content.

evolve Go to your Evolve website (http://evolve.elsevier.com/deWit/medsurg) for the following FREE learning resources:
- Animations, audio, and video
- Answers and rationales for questions and activities
- Concept Map Creator
- Glossary with pronunciations in English and Spanish
- Interactive Review Questions and Exercises and more!

 Online Resources
- Recommended Adult Immunization Schedule, www.cdc.gov/mmwr/PDF/wk/mm5753-Immunization.pdf for adult immunization schedule

- The Joint Commission, Tobacco and Alcohol Measures, www.jointcommission.org/tobacco_and_alcohol_measures

Review Questions for the NCLEX® Examination

1. Immediately after the physician intubates a patient who is in respiratory arrest, the nurse notes that there are no breath sounds in the left lung fields, but breath sounds are heard on the right side. The likely explanation is that the endotracheal tube:
   1. was placed in the esophagus.
   2. punctured the left lung.
   3. was inserted too far.
   4. is malfunctioning.

2. The nurse is caring for several patients who are scheduled for diagnostic testing for respiratory disorders. The patient who needs postprocedural care that includes frequent vital signs is the patient who had:
   1. capnography.
   2. a D-dimer test.
   3. a ventilation and perfusion scan.
   4. bronchoscopy.

3. The nurse is observing a nursing student who is suctioning a patient for excess secretions. The nurse would intervene immediately if the student:
   1. preoxygenated the patient with 100% oxygen for 2 minutes.
   2. applied suction while inserting the catheter.
   3. set the wall suction gauge at 80 mm Hg.
   4. monitored the patient frequently for tachycardia or bradycardia.

4. The nurse is caring for a patient who has asthma. Which lung sound would the nurse expect to hear when auscultating this patient's lung fields?
   1. Fine crackles
   2. Stridor
   3. Pleural friction rub
   4. Wheezes

5. The nurse knows to observe for and report which abnormal breathing pattern that is most likely to occur in patients with increased intracranial pressure?
   1. Cheyne-Stokes respirations
   2. Kussmaul's respirations
   3. Biot's respirations
   4. Apneustic respirations

6. The nurse attends to the nutritional needs of the patient with chronic respiratory disease by providing oral care. What is the best rationale for this nursing action?
   1. Low energy states diminish appetite.
   2. Respiratory secretions leave a bad taste.
   3. Chewing is believed to induce coughing spells.
   4. Nasal congestion reduces the flavor of food.

7. For a patient undergoing mechanical ventilation, which nursing intervention would reduce the insensible fluid loss?

   1. Suction frequently.
   2. Provide humidified air.
   3. Increase respiratory rate setting.
   4. Reposition every 2 hours.

8. The patient is instructed to take in a deep breath and slowly exhale while coughing three times in succession. What is the appropriate rationale for these instructions?

   1. Clears the nasal passages
   2. Mobilizes secretions and stimulates expectoration
   3. Increases the likelihood of atelectasis
   4. Decreases insensible fluid losses

9. While obtaining sputum for culture and sensitivity, the nurse notes that the specimen is thick, tenacious, and "ropey." This finding is most likely to be present in which disorder?

   1. Pneumococcal pneumonia
   2. Pulmonary edema
   3. Chronic bronchitis
   4. Tuberculosis

10. On initial assessment of a patient diagnosed with an acute exacerbation of chronic obstructive pulmonary disease (COPD), the nurse is likely to find which sign(s) and symptom(s)? *(Select all that apply.)*

    1. Tensing of the shoulder muscles
    2. Unable to tolerate sitting up
    3. Flaring of the nostrils
    4. Completes sentences with no effort
    5. Sternal retraction

Critical Thinking Activities

Scenario A

Mr. Keelog is an elderly man who may have cancer of the larynx. He will undergo diagnostic procedures to confirm this diagnosis. You observe that he is not currently having severe respiratory distress and can answer your questions. He appears willing and able to listen to information.

1. What questions should you ask to identify if Mr. Keelog has risk factors for cancer of the larynx?

2. Identify at least four questions that you would ask Mr. Keelog about his present status.

3. Describe the teaching plan that would be used for a patient undergoing a direct laryngoscopy.

4. What other diagnostic tests would have been done on this patient?

5. How can this type of cancer potentially be prevented?

Scenario B

Ms. Tiber has had frequent bouts of bronchitis. Her physician tells her that this disorder has caused some chronic obstructive pulmonary disease.

1. What measures would you teach her to make breathing easier?

2. Why is it important not to give a patient with COPD high-flow oxygen? What would happen?

Scenario C

Mrs. Clampett is an elderly woman who comes to the clinic for an annual flu vaccination. She would like a "good physical check of my lungs" and information about how to prevent respiratory disorders.

1. What questions should you ask in obtaining a history about potential respiratory problems?

2. Describe how you would auscultate her lungs.

3. If you heard an abnormal lung sound such as "fine crackles" what would you do?

Care of Patients with Disorders of the Upper Respiratory System

Objectives

Theory

1. Recognize symptoms of disorders of the sinuses, pharynx, and larynx.
2. Describe the postoperative care for the patient undergoing a rhinoplasty.
3. List emergency measures for the patient with an airway obstruction.
4. Review a nursing care plan for the patient who had a laryngectomy.

5. Analyze safety factors to be considered when caring for the patient with a tracheostomy.

Clinical Practice

1. Institute measures to stop epistaxis.
2. Provide tracheostomy care.
3. Devise interventions for the psychosocial care of the patient who has undergone a laryngectomy.
4. Visit a patient who has a permanent tracheostomy and ask her to share some of her successful coping strategies.

Key Terms

crepitation (KRĔP-ĭ-tā-shŭn, p. 283)
endotracheal intubation (ĔN-dō-TRĀ-kē-ăl ĭn-tyū-bā-shŭn, p. 284)
epistaxis (ĕp-ĭ-STĂK-sĭs, p. 280)
follicular pharyngitis (fōl-ĭk-yĕ-lĕr fĕr-ĭn-jī-tĭs, p. 280)
laryngectomy (lăr-ĭn-JĔK-tō-mē, p. 283)
laryngitis (lăr-ĭn-JĪ-tĭs, p. 280)
laryngoscope (lăr-ĭn-JĔ-skōp, p. 284)

lozenges (p. 280)
obturator (ŎB-tŭ-ră-tŏr, p. 285)
pharyngitis (fĕr-ĭn jī-tĭs, p. 280)
rhinitis (rī-NĪ-tĭs, p. 277)
rhinoplasty (RĪ-nō-plăs-tē, p. 283)
stoma (STŌ-mă, p. 283)
tracheostomy (trā-kē-ŎS-tō-mē, p. 284)

DISORDERS OF THE NOSE AND SINUSES

UPPER RESPIRATORY INFECTION (URI) (THE COMMON COLD) AND RHINITIS

The common cold—acute viral rhinitis—is an inflammation of the nose and upper respiratory tract. It is the most prevalent infectious disease among people of all ages. Many different strains of viruses can produce the symptoms of a common cold, thus total immunity is unlikely. Avoiding exposure to those who have a cold and maintaining a state of good health are the only ways one can avoid "catching" a cold.

Etiology and Pathophysiology

Viruses are spread by airborne droplet sprays from infected people during breathing, speaking, coughing, or sneezing, or by direct hand contact with a contaminated object. A chill, fatigue, physical or emotional stress, a compromised immune status or inflammation caused by allergic rhinitis makes one more susceptible to contracting an upper respiratory virus.

Signs, Symptoms, and Diagnosis

The common cold usually starts with a mild sore throat or a hot, dry, prickly sensation in the nose and back of the throat. Within hours after the onset of a cold, the nose becomes congested with increased secretions, the eyes begin to water, and sneezing, malaise, and an irritating, nonproductive cough appear. The invading organism causes inflammation and swelling of the mucosa. Muscle aches and headache may occur. There usually is no elevation of temperature; if a fever does develop, it is low grade (<101° F [38.3° C]). In most instances, a cold will last 10 to 14 days before all symptoms are gone.

Allergic rhinitis may have many of the symptoms of a cold, except there is no fever. It is caused by reaction of the nasal mucosa to an allergen, such as pollen or dust.

Treatment and Nursing Management

The treatment of allergic rhinitis is symptomatic. Antihistamines, steroids, and sprays that stabilize the mucous cell membranes are often prescribed (Table 14-1). The patient is taught to avoid the offending allergens

Table 14-1 Commonly Prescribed Drugs for Allergic Rhinitis and Sinusitis

CLASSIFICATION	ACTION	NURSING IMPLICATIONS	PATIENT TEACHING
Antihistamines			
First-Generation Agents Diphenhydramine (Benadryl) Clemastine (Tavist) Brompheniramine (Dimetane) Chlorpheniramine (Chlor-Trimeton)	Relieve sneezing, excessive secretions, itching, and nasal congestion. Block histamine binding by binding with H_1 receptor sites	Tend to cause sedation and slow reaction time May cause stimulation in some people May cause GI side effects: anorexia, constipation or diarrhea, or epigastric distress May cause urinary retention or frequency	Warn patient not to operate machinery and that driving may be dangerous due to sedation; this usually passes after the first 2 wk of treatment Ask patient to report changes in heart rate, palpitations, or urinary retention or frequency Warn that alcohol will have additive depressant effect
Second-Generation Agents Loratadine (Claritin) Fexofenadine (Allegra) Cetirizine (Zyrtec) Desloratadine (Clarinex) Azelastine (Astelin) nasal		Have limited attachment to H_1 receptors in the brain, do not cause sedation, and have less effect on reflexes; they do not affect bladder function	Do not take with alcohol or other CNS-active drugs Do not take with any monoamine oxidase inhibitor These drugs are more expensive than first-generation drugs
Corticosteroid Sprays			
Beclomethasone (Vancenase) Budesonide (Rhinocort) Flunisolide (Nasalide) Fluticasone (Flonase) Triamcinolone (Nasacort) Ciclesonide (Omnaris) Mometasone (Nasonex)	Inhibit inflammatory response Have low systemic absorption with normal doses	Encourage use as directed on a daily basis	Teach to use on a daily basis rather than PRN Discontinue if infection occurs May initially cause some burning in nostrils
Mast Cell Stabilizer			
Cromolyn sodium spray (Nasalcrom)	Stabilizes mast cells, preventing inflammatory reaction	Minimal side effects	Begin 2 wk before pollen season starts and use throughout pollen season to prevent allergy symptoms May be used prophylactically for isolated allergy (i.e., cat) Use 10-15 min before exposure
Decongestants			
Oral Pseudoephedrine (Sudafed) Oxymetazoline (Dristan) Phenylephrine (Neo-Synephrine) Saline nasal spray or rinse*	Promote vasoconstriction by stimulating adrenergic receptors on blood vessels; reduce nasal edema and rhinorrhea	May cause insomnia, headache, irritability, dysuria, palpitations, or tachycardia Can cause rebound nasal congestion	Some products are contraindicated for those with hypertension, cardiac disease, glaucoma, diabetes, prostatic hypertrophy, or liver or renal disease Use only three or four times a day for no more than 3 days

CNS, central nervous system; GI, gastrointestinal; H_1, histamine-1; PRN, as needed.
*Saline nasal sprays and rinses wash away pollen and dust, thin secretions, and soothe the nasal mucosa.

as much as possible. If the disorder is severe, an allergy evaluation is indicated so that a desensitization program can be started.

There is no cure for the common cold. However, zinc lozenges have proven effective in limiting a cold's duration and severity for many people, if started at the first signs of symptoms (Prasad et al., 2008).

 Complementary and Alternative Therapies

Alternative Treatment for a URI

Echinacea, goldenseal, or a combination of herbs, minerals, vitamins, and amino acids such as those contained in the product "Airborne" can be taken at the first sign of a cold, or before going into crowded areas during cold season. This product was developed by a schoolteacher and has been effective for many people.

A major goal in the care of a common cold is prevention of a secondary bacterial infection. Individuals with a cold should avoid contact with others so as to avoid picking up a bacterial infection or giving their viral infection to someone else. A person with a cold is contagious for about 3 days after symptoms first appear.

Colds are spread by droplet infection and most people realize that coughing and sneezing will spread viruses. Coughing and sneezing into tissues does limit the viruses' travel by air, but the viruses are also very likely to be on the person's hands, where they can be transferred to anything touched. Hand hygiene is important in the prevention of spreading infection to others and patients should also be taught not to share personal use items, such as drinking glasses.

The patient should stay indoors, preferably in bed or resting, during the first few days of the illness. Fluid intake should be increased. Fruit juices are recommended, especially citrus juices, because of their vitamin C content. Aspirin or another mild nonprescription analgesic can help relieve the muscle aches and headache of a cold.

 Elder Care Points

The elderly should be encouraged to stay away from people who have a cold or URI because of decreased immune function and if a cold develops a secondary infection is more likely. Older patients should continue the extra fluids and rest until symptoms are resolved.

Safety Alert

Caution with Aspirin

Aspirin should not be given to children. Aspirin has an association with Reye's syndrome, which occurs after a viral illness and may result in brain inflammation and possibly death. For children under 18, aspirin should only be given when prescribed by a physician (National Reye's Syndrome Foundation, 2009). Adults taking anticoagulants or nonsteroidal anti-inflammatory drugs should not take aspirin, because aspirin will further prolong the clotting time.

Decongestant nose drops or sprays such as oxymetazoline (for the relief of nasal congestion) can have a rebound effect, leaving the nose "stuffier" if used for more than 3 days. Frequent use of saline nasal spray decreases congestion without side effects. Antibiotics are not given because a cold is a viral infection.

A bacterial infection, which requires medical treatment, is present when a "cold" persists for more than a week to 10 days without improvement, or if the patient begins to feel worse, has a temperature of 101° F (38.3° C), and develops chest pains or coughs up purulent sputum.

 Think Critically

What are the various ways you can prevent contracting a cold?

SINUSITIS

Sinusitis is an inflammation of the mucosal lining of the sinuses. Pneumococci, streptococci, or *Haemophilus influenzae* are the usual pathogens and infection can spread from the nasal passages to the sinuses. The nasal passages can be blocked by a *deviated septum* which may occur congenitally, or from injury to the nose, or by nasal *polyps*. Polyps occur from repeated inflammation of the nasal mucosa and are tissue growths that obstruct airflow. Sinusitis often occurs after colds or other respiratory infections and during periods of uncontrolled allergic rhinitis. People with a deviated nasal septum or allergy problems tend to have recurrent sinusitis.

As exudate accumulates in the sinuses, pressure builds up causing pain. Symptoms include headache, fever, tenderness over the sinuses, malaise, purulent drainage from the nose, and sometimes a nonproductive cough. The upper teeth may become painful.

Treatment of sinusitis includes relieving pain, promoting sinus drainage, controlling infection, and preventing recurrence. Hot, moist packs over the sinus area can be helpful. Inhaling moist steam thins secretions and kits for sinus irrigation available at drugstores help to promote drainage. Medications are prescribed to promote decongestion or vasoconstriction and to reduce swelling, to promote drainage and to relieve pain. Infection may be treated with an antibiotic or anti-infective agent, often for at least 10 days. Rest, reduced stress, a balanced diet, and control of allergies can help prevent recurrence. Fluid intake should be increased. Dairy products increase the thickness of secretions, therefore are limited during the illness.

 Think Critically

How would you know if you or a patient has a sinus infection rather than just an ordinary cold?

Acute or chronic sinus infection can cause a variety of complications, including septicemia, meningitis, and brain abscess. When sinus infection is chronic, surgery to clean out the sinuses may be necessary. A deviated septum can be surgically repaired, and polyps can be removed by laser treatment.

EPISTAXIS

Epistaxis (nosebleed) is a common occurrence and usually results from crusting, cracking, or irritation of the mucous membrane covering the front of the nasal septum. Blood loss is usually minimal. Decreased humidity, excessive nose blowing, allergy with inflammation, and nose picking may cause nosebleeds. Overuse of nasal spray, street drug use (particularly "snorting"), and tumors are other causes. Any condition that prolongs bleeding time or lowers the platelet count may predispose to nosebleeds. Nosebleeds can also result from trauma, hypertension, and blood disorders such as leukemia. They are common in boys during pubescence.

Bleeding from the nose is the only sign of epistaxis. When epistaxis occurs, the patient should sit forward and apply direct pressure by pinching the soft portion of the nose for 10 to 15 minutes. This position prevents blood from running down the back of the throat. Cold compresses or ice may be applied to the nose to constrict the blood vessels. If there is still bleeding at the end of a 10- to 15-minute period, a small gauze pad may be inserted into the bleeding nostril and digital pressure applied (Figure 14-1). If bleeding continues, the patient should go to the emergency department, where a physician will cauterize the bleeding vessels or solidly pack the nose, or insert a small balloon device, to stop the bleeding (Figure 14-2). Once bleeding stops, the patient should rest quietly for a few hours and be warned not to blow the nose, pick at it, or rub it for 24 hours after the nosebleed has stopped.

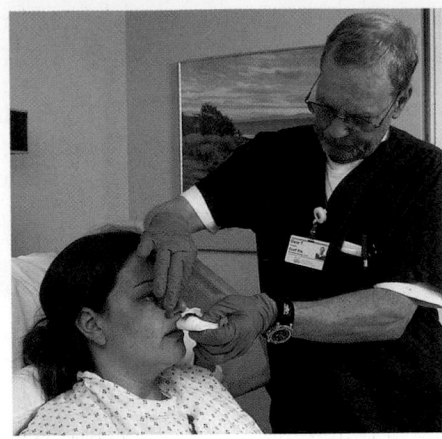

FIGURE 14-1 Stopping a nosebleed by applying pressure to the nose.

A   **B**

FIGURE 14-2 Placement of nasal packing to stop a nosebleed. **A,** Catheter is passed through the bleeding side of the nose and pulled out through the mouth with a hemostat. Strings are tied to the catheter and the pack is pulled up behind the soft palate and into the nasopharynx. **B,** Nasal pack in position in the posterior nasopharynx. A roll of dental packing placed at the nose helps maintain the packing in the correct position.

◉ Clinical Cues

If the patient is having an active nosebleed, instruct her to spit the blood into a basin or tissue rather than swallowing it. Accumulation of blood in the stomach will eventually cause nausea and vomiting and the patient's cooperation will help you to assess the amount of bleeding.

PHARYNGITIS

Etiology and Pathophysiology

Pharyngitis (inflammation of the pharynx), usually called a *sore throat*, may be caused by a virus, bacteria, or a fungus. The majority of cases are viral. Acute follicular pharyngitis ("strep throat") is caused by beta-hemolytic streptococcal infection. Fungal pharyngitis occurs with long-term use of antibiotics or inhaled corticosteroids, or in patients with immunosuppression, such as occurs with HIV or AIDS or during cancer treatment. Laryngitis (inflammation of the larynx with diminished voice or hoarseness) may occur if the infection progresses into the larynx. If the inflammation extends to the epiglottis, *epiglottitis* occurs; this is more common in children.

Signs, Symptoms, and Diagnosis

The symptoms include a dry, "scratchy" feeling in the back of the throat, mild fever, headache, and malaise. The throat, tonsils, palate, and uvula may be involved and will be reddened. Dysphagia causes discomfort when swallowing one's own saliva. With laryngitis, the voice may become hoarse or absent. The usual course for uncomplicated pharyngitis or laryngitis is 3 to 10 days. The diagnosis of pharyngitis is confirmed by clinical signs and symptoms. A throat culture is often done to confirm or rule out streptococcal infection.

Treatment and Nursing Management

Uncomplicated viral pharyngitis usually responds to conservative measures, such as rest, warm saline gargles (½ to 1 tsp of table salt to a glass of warm water), throat lozenges (small medicinal tablets that dissolve in the mouth), antiseptic sprays, plenty of fluids, and a mild analgesic for aches and pains.

Bacterial pharyngitis requires antibiotic therapy, particularly if the infecting organism is *Streptococcus*. Chronic pharyngitis may require diagnostic procedures to determine the underlying cause, and therapeutic measures such as humidification and filtering of environmental air. Fungal pharyngitis is treated with an antifungal agent, but may be difficult to control in immunocompromised individuals.

TONSILLITIS

Etiology and Pathophysiology

An infection with inflammation of the tonsils is usually caused by streptococci, staphylococci, or *H. influenzae* and is different from pharyngitis; however symptoms may be somewhat similar. Acute tonsillitis may occur repeatedly, especially in those who have a low resistance to infection.

Signs, Symptoms, and Diagnosis

Acute tonsillitis occurs more frequently in young children. There is high fever, sore throat, general malaise, pain referred to the ears, and chills. Inspection of the throat reveals redness and swelling of the tonsils and surrounding tissues with patches of yellow exudate. The white blood cell count becomes elevated.

Chronic tonsillitis usually produces an enlargement of tonsillar tissue and adenoidal tissue. Chronic infection produces less dramatic symptoms than acute tonsillitis but discomfort still occurs. A person with chronic tonsillitis and enlarged adenoids has frequent colds and appears to be in poor health.

Diagnosis is by physical examination and history. If a streptococcus infection is suspected, a throat culture may be performed, or a "rapid strep test" may be done.

Treatment

A throat culture is done before treatment to check for the presence of *Streptococcus*, which can cause rheumatic fever or glomerulonephritis if not treated promptly. Acute tonsillitis is treated with warm saline throat gargles and the administration of specific antibiotics (usually penicillin) to destroy the pathogen. Nursing measures include bed rest, fever management, and a liquid diet to minimize trauma to the tissues. After 24 hours on antibiotics, the patient is no longer considered contagious (Mayo Clinic, 2009).

Surgery is used to treat tonsillitis when it is recurrent or when enlargement of the tonsils and adenoids obstructs airways. Surgery is considered if the patient has more than seven episodes of tonsillitis per year, after acute infection has cleared.

 Think Critically

What would be appropriate foods to offer the patient with pharyngitis or tonsillitis?

Nursing Management

Preoperative Care. Tonsillectomy and adenoidectomy are generally done on an outpatient, same-day surgery basis. Preliminary laboratory testing and patient education begin before the patient is admitted. Physical preparation of the patient involves administration of preoperative medications as ordered and restriction of the patient's diet for 6 to 8 hours before surgery. An elevation of temperature or any signs of URI should be reported, because surgery is usually postponed if these signs are present. The patient also has an easier time swallowing postoperatively.

Postoperative Care. Although tonsillectomy and adenoidectomy patients usually recover rapidly and rarely suffer any complications, the nurse is vigilant for signs of hemorrhage. **Vital signs are checked frequently, and the patient is observed for frequent swallowing, which may indicate bleeding in the throat. Restlessness can be another clue to excessive bleeding.** Sneezing, coughing, and vomiting can cause bleeding. An ice collar may be placed around the neck to reduce swelling and prevent the oozing of blood from the operative site. The patient can be positioned on the side as long as there is drainage from the surgical wound. For comfort, the patient may sit up in a semi-Fowler's position after recovering from the anesthesia. The postoperative diet usually consists of ice-cold liquids, Popsicles, and gelatin (without red coloring), progressing to ice cream, custards, and other semisolid foods for the first 24 hours. Citrus fruits, hot fluids, and rough foods should be avoided until the throat has completely healed. Straws are not used because sucking may cause bleeding. Written instructions for routine care and emergency circumstances are reviewed with the caregiver and patient.

? **Think Critically**

What sign would alert you to the probability that the tonsillectomy patient was experiencing bleeding and that the blood was running down the throat where you cannot see it?

OBSTRUCTION AND TRAUMA

AIRWAY OBSTRUCTION AND RESPIRATORY ARREST

Laryngeal edema from inflammation of an infection or an allergic reaction may obstruct the airway. A crush injury of the larynx may cause airway obstruction. A foreign object or food that goes down the airway rather than the esophagus can cause obstruction. If the person seems to be choking, encourage forceful coughing if possible. If that person cannot breathe or speak, she may make the universal signal for choking, signaling for help by grasping at the throat with the hands (Figure 14-3). If breathing is obstructed,

FIGURE 14-3 The hands grasping the throat is the universal signal for choking.

abdominal thrusts (also known as the Heimlich maneuver) should be performed (American Heart Association, 2009). The arms are wrapped around the victim from behind. One hand makes a fist with the thumb inward, then position the fist just above the umbilicus. The other hand wraps around the fist. Upward thrusts are delivered into the abdomen to try to dislodge anything stuck in the airway (Figure 14-4) (see Chapter 45). **In the unconscious adult or child over 1 year of age, the most common cause of airway obstruction is the tongue.** An artificial airway may be orally or nasally inserted; it helps to keep the tongue in place (Figure 14-5).

FIGURE 14-4 Abdominal thrust.

FIGURE 14-5 Types of airways inserted during a respiratory emergency (endotracheal, nasal, oropharyngeal).

Clinical Cues

Nasal or oropharyngeal airways can be inserted by the nurse. In the event of respiratory arrest, an endotracheal tube would be inserted by a physician or a nurse anesthetist. The nurse's role in this emergency procedure would include obtaining the emergency airway equipment (e.g., laryngoscopy, 5- to 10-mL syringe, Ambu bag, endotracheal tube, and a securing device). The nurse may also be required to oxygenate the patient using the Ambu bag.

If the airway is obstructed for an extended period, the heart may stop due to hypoxia. If the obstruction is cleared, but the victim has no pulse, cardiopulmonary resuscitation must be started (see Chapter 45).

OBSTRUCTIVE SLEEP APNEA

Obstructive sleep apnea (OSA) is a condition in which the person stops breathing during sleep for 10 seconds or more, until there is a reflex gasp for air. Muscle relaxation at the back of the throat is the most common cause. Snoring is frequent with this condition and sleeping partners are usually the first to notice the problem. A sleep study should be performed to determine the specific type of disorder. Sleep apnea is treated with continuous positive airway pressure (CPAP) applied with a mask or nasal prongs. Untreated sleep apnea can contribute to myocardial infarction or stroke. It also causes constant fatigue. Research is being conducted on the use of capnography to monitor and identify patients with OSA. Capnography measures exhaled carbon dioxide, apneic events, and respiratory rates.

NASAL FRACTURE

Nasal fracture often results from sports injuries, motor vehicle accidents, or physical assault. If the cartilage or bone is not displaced, complications are unlikely and no treatment is needed. Displacement of the cartilage or bone can interfere with airflow, cause deformity of the nose, and become a potential spot for infection.

Diagnosis is by visual inspection for deformity, a change in nasal breathing, and presence of crepitation (grating sound or feeling of rough surfaces rubbing together) on palpation. If the patient is seen within the first 24 hours after injury, a closed reduction is most often performed using local or general anesthetic. Treatment includes pain relief and the use of ice or cold compresses to reduce swelling.

If the fracture is severe, rhinoplasty (surgical reconstruction of the nose) may be done to improve airflow and cosmetic appearance. After surgery, the patient will have packing in both nostrils and a small plaster splint or cast to provide support. A drip pad of folded gauze is secured as a "mustache" dressing beneath the nose.

The patient is observed for frequent swallowing postoperatively, which could indicate posterior nasal bleeding. Vital signs are monitored closely, and the amount of drainage on the dressing is observed. The patient should be encouraged to rest in a semi-Fowler's position. Cool compresses are used to decrease nose and facial swelling. Nonsteroidal anti-inflammatory drugs and aspirin are to be avoided as they may cause bleeding to occur in the early postoperative period. Forceful coughing and straining at stool (Valsalva maneuver) are to be avoided. A humidifier is used to decrease mucosal drying. After recovery from anesthesia, the patient is usually discharged to recuperate at home. It may take 6 to 12 months before the final result of the surgery is evident.

Cosmetic rhinoplasty is often performed on noses to improve physical appearance. Care is the same as for the procedure for a fractured nose.

CANCER OF THE LARYNX
Etiology and Pathophysiology
It was predicted that there would be 15,000 new cases of cancer of the larynx in 2011 (American Cancer Society [ACS], 2011). Approximately 90% of all patients who are diagnosed early and treated with radiation and/or surgery are cured. Although the cause of cancer of the larynx is unknown, there is some evidence that predisposing factors include cigarette smoking, alcohol abuse, diets rich in spicy foods, infection with human papillomavirus, chronic laryngitis, abuse of the vocal cords, exposure to radiation, and a familial tendency to cancer. Exposures over long periods to environmental pollutants, such as asbestos, paint fumes, or wood dust, are other risk factors (ACS, 2009c). The most common malignant tumor of the larynx is squamous cell carcinoma. It grows from the mucous membrane lining the respiratory tract. Metastasis may occur to the lung.

Signs, Symptoms, and Diagnosis
The larynx (sometimes called the voice box) is directly involved with the production of vocal sounds. A tumor of the larynx will quickly produce persistent hoarseness that does not respond to usual methods of treatment.

Health Promotion
Signs of Possible Throat Cancer
Tell patients to seek medical attention if the following signs of cancer of the larynx or throat occur:
- Hoarseness lasting more than 3 weeks.
- Sore throat that lasts more than 2 weeks.
- Consistent pain in or around the ear when swallowing.
- Difficulty swallowing.
- Dry, persistent cough for no known reason.
- Blood in phlegm or saliva lasting more than a few days.
- Lumps or knots on the neck indicating enlarged cervical lymph nodes.

After the cancer has spread beyond the vocal cords (and is much more difficult to treat), the symptoms may include difficulty in swallowing or breathing, halitosis, blood-tinged sputum, fatigue and weakness, a sensation of having a lump in the throat, cough, enlarged lymph nodes in the neck, pain in the region of the Adam's apple or an airway obstruction.

Diagnosis is established by visualizing the larynx via a laryngoscope, by a computed tomography scan of the larynx and throat, by magnetic resonance imaging, and by microscopic examination of a sample of tissues taken from the site.

Treatment
Once the type of cancer is determined, it is staged for appropriate treatment. Outpatient treatment is common. Radiation alone is 85% effective in treating early cancer of the larynx. Radiation may be combined with laser cordectomy for certain types of lesions. Brachytherapy along with external-beam irradiation is used for certain types of lesions. If the tumor is large or not restricted to the vocal cords, the surgeon may perform a partial laryngectomy in which the thyroid cartilage is split, and only the tumor and involved portion of the larynx and vocal cords are removed. A partial laryngectomy does not permanently eliminate voice sounds. A *tracheostomy* (surgical opening into the trachea) may be done to facilitate breathing temporarily, but the stoma (opening) is eventually closed, and the patient may resume talking after the affected area is completely healed.

Microlaryngoscopy combined with laser treatment is now the method of choice for removing vocal cord polyps and carcinoma that has not spread. Cure rates for malignancy of the true vocal cords treated by laser are about 90%. Other advantages include the absence of mechanical trauma and swelling when laser is used, which means that the patient returns to normal activities within about 3 days. There is no need for extended voice rest; 2 days is usually sufficient.

A total laryngectomy is performed if the tumor has progressed to the point of paralyzing the vocal cords. The surgeon excises the entire larynx, epiglottis,

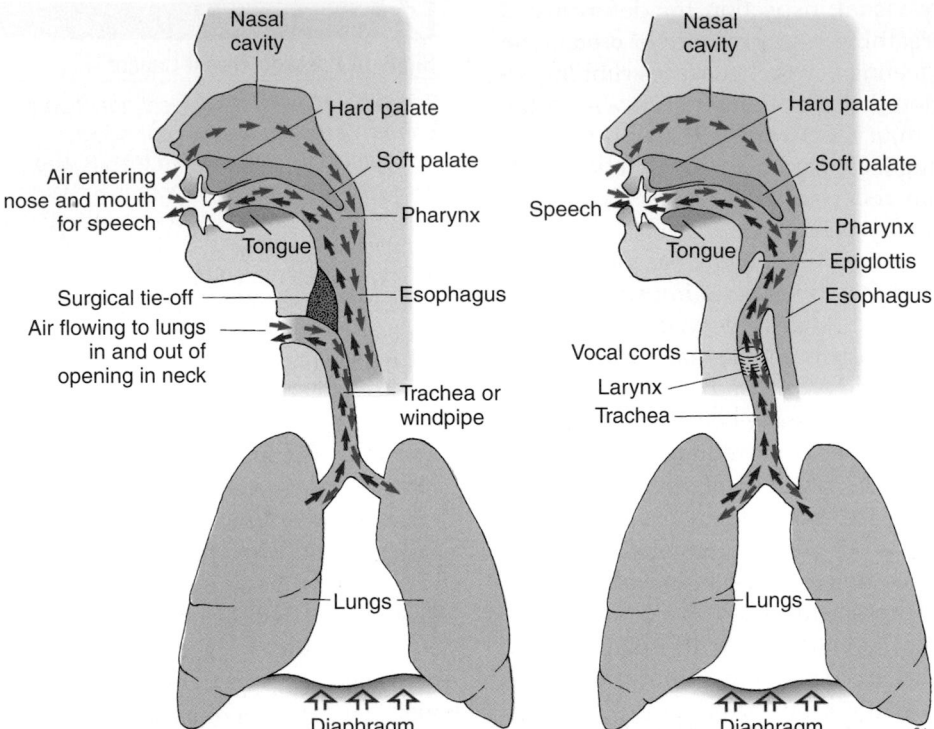

FIGURE 14-6 Airflow after laryngectomy *(left)* and in a normal respiratory tract *(right)*.

thyroid cartilage, hyoid bone, cricoid cartilage, and two or more rings of the trachea (Figure 14-6). A newer procedure, near-total laryngectomy, preserves voice production and swallowing in advanced disease.

If the tumor has extended to the lymph nodes, a radical neck dissection is performed on the side of the lesion. All the muscle, lymph nodes, and soft tissue from the lower edge of the mandible to the clavicle and from the top of the trapezius muscle to the midline are removed. Range-of-motion exercises are needed postoperatively to restore muscle movement. A permanent tracheostomy is performed at the same time. A laryngectomy tube, which is shorter and wider than a tracheostomy tube, is put into place before discharge. After the stoma is completely healed and matured, about 6 weeks after surgery, the tube can be taken out as long as there is no compromise of the airway.

A thin feeding tube is placed during surgery for postoperative use for about 10 to 14 days. The patient has only intravenous fluids initially but then progresses to regular tube feedings. With healing, the danger of contaminating the operative site is not a concern and training in eating and swallowing are initiated. With the appropriate encouragement and practice, most patients can master the techniques to avoid the sensations of choking and gagging.

When the patient is discharged from the hospital, a visiting nurse or clinic nurse will work with the patient on eating skills. Some patients have to rely on a feeding tube if they cannot master the swallowing procedure

without aspiration. The indwelling tube may then be replaced with a gastrostomy tube.

? Think Critically

How can nurses help decrease the incidence of cancer of the larynx?

Endotracheal Intubation and Tracheostomy. Endotracheal intubation means that an endotracheal tube is inserted into the trachea via the nose or the mouth with the use of a laryngoscope (Figure 14-7). An endotracheal tube is placed for airway protection against aspiration when there is upper airway obstruction and when mechanical ventilation is necessary. Endotracheal tubes are used for short-term respiratory support, such as for immediate relief of airway obstruction, during anesthesia, or for a few days postoperatively.

A tracheostomy is a surgical incision into the trachea for the purpose of inserting a tube for breathing. When the patient has a tracheostomy there is no connection between the nose and mouth and the lower respiratory system. Tracheostomy is done:

- To assist or control ventilation by mechanical means over a prolonged period of time.
- To facilitate suctioning of secretions in the air passages when the patient cannot cough.
- To prevent aspiration of oral and gastric secretions (as in unconscious or paralyzed patients).

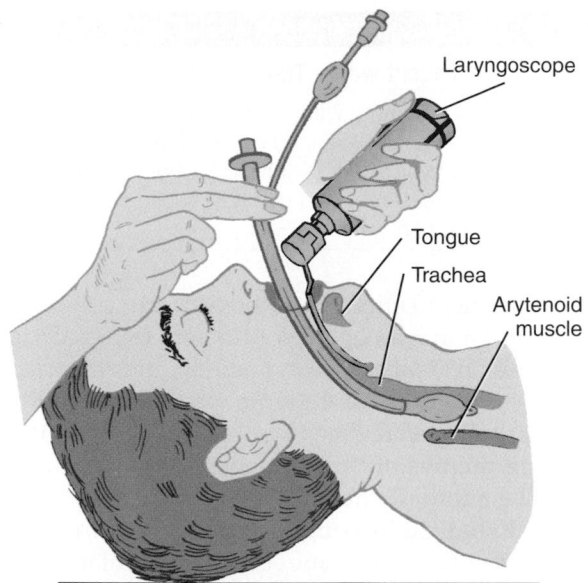

FIGURE 14-7 With the use of a laryngoscope, an endotracheal tube is inserted with the neck extended to align the airway.

- To bypass a constricted or obstructed airway (e.g., from edema of the larynx, presence of a foreign body or tumor, surgical procedures involving the neck, severe burns, facial trauma, or chest trauma).

Tracheostomy may be an emergency procedure or an elective operation. When passing an endotracheal tube through the nose or mouth is impossible or extremely difficult, a tracheostomy may be done to provide an airway. Some patients will need a tracheostomy tube for the rest of their lives because of anatomical changes in the throat. When a patient is expected to need an artificial airway for an extended period of time, tracheostomy may be preferred over prolonged endotracheal intubation (Charra et al., 2009) In the immediate postoperative period, the patient with a tracheostomy may need mechanical ventilation and/or oxygen therapy (see Chapter 15).

Types of Tracheostomy Tubes. Tracheostomy tubes are available in a variety of materials and styles. Most of the models are made of plastic (Figure 14-8). Tubes made of metal alloys are used chiefly for patients who need a permanent tracheostomy. The three styles of tracheostomy tubes are single-cannula, double-cannula, and fenestrated tubes. *Single-cannula tubes* are made of pliable materials that conform to the shape of the trachea more easily than do double-cannula tubes. In a *double-cannula tracheostomy tube,* the outer cannula acts as a sleeve for the inner cannula, which can be removed for cleaning. Newer tracheostomy tubes have no need for an inner cannula (the tube) or have a disposable inner cannula that can be replaced rather than cleaned. The **obturator** (insertion guide) is used during insertion as a guide (the tip, shaped like an olive, extends beyond the end of the tube) and to

FIGURE 14-8 Types of tracheostomy tubes. **A,** Tracheostomy tube in place with inflated cuff. **B,** Shiley and Portex fenestrated tracheostomy tubes with cuff, inner cannula, decannulation plug, and pilot balloon. **C,** Bivona Fome-Cuf tracheostomy tube with foam cuff and obturator (cuff is deflated on tracheostomy tube).

protect against scraping the sides of the trachea with the sharp edge of the tube.

Fenestrated tubes have a small opening in the outer cannula that allows some air to escape through the larynx. This helps prepare the patient for the time when the tracheostomy tube will be removed and breathing occurs normally again.

A one-way tracheostomy valve box can be fitted into the tube opening. It allows air to be inhaled through the tracheostomy opening, but the valve closes when the patient exhales. This diverts the exhaled air through the larynx and enables the patient to speak. Other types of speaking tracheostomy tubes are now available.

The *cuffed tracheostomy tube* has a small balloon encircling its tracheal end. It is sometimes called a *balloon tracheostomy tube.* When the balloon is inflated, it fills the space between the outside of the tracheostomy tube and the trachea, thereby providing a seal and preventing the escape of air around the tube. When positive-pressure artificial ventilation is administered, the air passes through the tracheostomy tube *only,* thus providing sufficient pressure to inflate the lungs. The cuffed tracheostomy tube may offer some protection against aspiration of mucus and fluids; however, the use of the cuffed tube does not replace careful nursing observation or interventions to prevent aspiration.

Foam-cuffed tracheostomy tubes have the cuff bonded to the tube and do not need to be inflated and deflated. They are disposable and cause minimal tissue necrosis.

Nursing Management

A patient with a new tracheostomy requires very specialized nursing care, especially if artificial ventilation through the tube is required. **Immediate postoperative care focuses on maintaining a patent airway** and observing for hemorrhage. During the first 24 hours, the patient is monitored continuously for signs of respiratory distress. If the patient is unable to cough to remove mucus and drainage, tracheal suctioning is necessary. If the lumen is not kept open, the patient will suffocate. Suctioning is done with strict sterile technique to prevent infection. Suctioning technique is presented in Skill 14-1 on Evolve and discussed in Chapter 13. See also Nursing Care Plan 14-1. Adequate humidification of the inhaled air helps to thin secretions.

 Clinical Cues

When you are performing suction on a tracheostomy or endotracheal tube and using a sterile suction kit, ask an assistant to accompany you to deliver oxygen before and during the procedure (as needed). Oxygenation of the patient will prevent desaturation, and the assistance of a helper allows you to maintain sterile technique.

The lungs should be auscultated (1) before suctioning to assess the need and (2) afterward to verify that the procedure successfully cleared the airways. Head-to-toe assessment is done as for any surgical patient (see Chapter 5).

When the patient has a tracheostomy tube with a cuff, the cuff must be inflated just enough to seal the trachea without causing extreme pressure against the tracheal wall, otherwise depression of the surface blood vessels in the tracheal wall will cause necrosis. Cuff pressure is checked each shift and each time the cuff is reinflated using a manometer.

 Assignment Considerations

Reporting on a Patient with a Tracheostomy

Instruct the UAP to immediately report coughing episodes or coarse gurgling sounds produced by a patient with a tracheostomy. Explain that you must be notified so that you can perform an immediate assessment and possible suctioning to alleviate an airway obstruction.

Preventing infection is another nursing responsibility. The incision is an open wound with minimal dressings and is an ideal entryway for infectious organisms. Tracheostomy care is a sterile procedure until the stoma is well healed. (See Skill 14-2 on Evolve.) **When changing the ties of the tracheostomy tube, the tube should be manually held in place, otherwise the tube may be dislodged by coughing.** (Coughing frequently occurs when the tube is moved or manipulated.)

If the patient is to go home with a tracheostomy, techniques for suctioning and providing the necessary tracheostomy care are taught to both the patient and a family member or caregiver.

 Patient Teaching

Home Care of a Tracheostomy

The patient and family should be taught the following points:
- Clean the stoma with normal saline, removing all secretions, on a daily basis.
- Replace the commercially slit gauze pad around the tube as frequently as needed when it becomes soiled. (Do not cut regular gauze pads, because the loose threads can be aspirated.)
- It is best to have two people help change the ties, because movement of the tube can easily cause the patient to cough and expel the tube from the stoma.
- Prepare the new ties before loosening the old ones.
- Hold the tube securely in place with thumb and forefinger while the ties are loose.
- Stand to the side of the stoma when providing care because if the patient coughs, mucus may be expelled.

Psychological support of the tracheostomy patient and family is essential. The patient has to learn to breathe in a totally different way and cannot speak or call out for help. Verbal reassurance will show awareness of apprehension and readiness to help. Explanations about what is being done and why it is being done are given each time tracheostomy care is provided. Teaching begins as soon as the patient is alert after the tracheostomy tube is placed. The patient may experience grief over losing her natural voice and the ability to eat normally if a total laryngectomy has been done. She will need help in facing a future in which she will not be able to speak normally. A radical neck dissection may create body image disturbance because the procedure is somewhat disfiguring. Initially, depression is common. Contact with others who have

★ Nursing Care Plan 14-1   Care of the Patient with a Laryngectomy

Scenario

Mr. Collins had a supraglottic laryngectomy 5 days ago. He is having difficulty adjusting to his tracheostomy and frequently chokes when trying to eat or swallow secretions. He indicates, with pencil and paper, that he does not feel he can learn to speak again and is very anxious about choking; he is withdrawn.

Problem/Nursing Diagnosis

Unable to cough up secretions/Ineffective airway clearance related to secretions resulting from surgery and tracheostomy.

Supporting Assessment Data

Objective: Unable to cough out secretions; becomes anoxic when secretions build up, decreasing airflow.

Goals/Expected Outcomes	Nursing Interventions	Selected Rationale	Evaluation
Tracheostomy will be cleared by suctioning as needed.	Assess respiratory effort and rate; auscultate upper airways to determine needs for suctioning. Observe ostomy site for secretions.	If rate or respiratory effort increases the airway may be obstructed. Coarse sounds heard in the upper airways or secretions at ostomy site indicate need for suctioning.	Respiratory rate varies; 18/min if patient is relaxed. Rate of 28–30/min when anxious or trying to cough out mucus. (Suctioning improves respiratory rate when mucus is cleared.)
	Suction as needed, at least q 4 hr.	Suctioning secretions clears airway.	Suctioning is effective.
Patient will learn to suction own tracheostomy effectively by discharge.	Encourage patient to assist with procedure (i.e., have patient hold water for moistening catheter).	Having patient assist with small steps helps him to develop confidence for home care.	Patient is making attempts to learn suctioning technique.
	Teach to attach catheter to suction tubing; teach to suction self using mirror.	Knowledge and practice are essential for self-care.	Beginning to attempt to cough out secretions and suction. Continue plan.
	Praise for all attempts.	Praise reinforces patient's efforts and learning.	Positive reinforcement given for any attempt.
	Point out advantages of not being dependent on others for care of airway.	Provides incentive to learn self-care.	States wants to be independent.
Patient will learn to clear tracheostomy by coughing effectively.	Medicate for discomfort and encourage patient to cough to remove secretions without suctioning.	Lessened discomfort makes it possible to cough effectively.	Analgesia provided q 4 hr.
	Assist to an upright position of at least 45 degrees.	Sitting upright allows for full expansion of chest cavity.	Is able to place self in an upright position and reposition self as needed.
	Remind to hold tissues in front of tube rather than the mouth.	Secretions will be coughed out of the tube.	Holding tissues in front of tube when coughing.
	Instruct to breathe deeply for several seconds and to forcefully cough 2 or 3 times using the abdominal muscles.	Use of abdominal muscles increases the force and depth of the cough.	Able to perform deep coughing with support and coaching.

Continued

Problem/Nursing Diagnosis

Surgical incision/Impaired skin integrity related to surgical incisions.

Supporting Assessment Data

Objective: Supraglottic laryngectomy and tracheostomy.

Goals/Expected Outcomes	Nursing Interventions	Selected Rationale	Evaluation
No infection at incision sites as evidenced by absence of redness, swelling, or purulent discharge.	Clean incision lines; apply antibiotic ointment as ordered q shift. Clean around tracheostomy stoma with normal saline; change gauze pad prn.	Cleans away bacteria and helps prevent infection.	No evidence of infection. Slight redness around tracheostomy stoma.
Skin integrity is intact within 6 wk.	Change tracheostomy ties at least q 24 hr. Observe for signs of infection.	Early recognition ensures prompt treatment.	Skin is intact; no redness or signs or irritation. No signs of infection. Continue plan.

Problem/Nursing Diagnosis

Unable to speak/Impaired verbal communication related to loss of larynx.

Supporting Assessment Data

Subjective: No verbal communication.
Objective: Laryngectomy and tracheostomy.

Goals/Expected Outcomes	Nursing Interventions	Selected Rationale	Evaluation
Patient will show interest in learning new style of speech within 6 wk.	Assist him to use Magic Slate or paper and pencil for communication; show patience.	Provides for some means of communication.	Using Magic Slate.
	Obtain order for visit from rehabilitated patient who has mastered some form of speech.	Seeing an example reinforces the possibility of regaining a form of speech.	Visit scheduled.
	Encourage affiliation with community support group	Support from people with a similar problem helps to decrease feelings of isolation and helplessness.	Advised about support group. Continue plan.

Problem/Nursing Diagnosis

Chokes when tries to swallow/Risk for aspiration related to choking when trying to swallow.

Supporting Assessment Data

Subjective: Writes that he does not feel he will be able to swallow or eat by mouth again.
Objective: Chokes when tries to swallow saliva; tends to aspirate.

Goals/Expected Outcomes	Nursing Interventions	Selected Rationale	Evaluation
Patient will not experience injury from aspiration of food or fluids.	Place in an upright position before eating or medication administration and maintain for at least 1 hour.	Gravity facilitates the downward movement of the food bolus.	Able to place self in an upright position; acknowledges need to remain upright for 1 hour after eating.
	Teach to hold his breath and perform the Valsalva maneuver while swallowing.	Valsalva maneuver closes the glottis over the tracheal opening in the throat, preventing food from entering the trachea.	Is practicing, but is having trouble coordinating the breathing and Valsalva maneuver and swallowing.
Patient will learn to swallow without aspirating within 6 wk.	Teach to keep neck relaxed forward, take small bite of food, keep chin towards chest, swallow, then forcibly exhale.	Exhaling forcibly after swallowing will expel particles that accidentally end up in the trachea.	Is still choking when he tries to swallow. Revise plan: Obtain consultation with speech therapist for swallowing exercises.

Critical Thinking Questions

1. What psychosocial problems might Mr. Collins experience?
2. How can you motivate Mr. Collins to participate in suctioning his tracheostomy?

🍎 Nutrition Considerations

Assisting the Partial Laryngectomy Patient with Swallowing

- Explain that swallowing food without choking is possible.
- Arrange a visit from a partial laryngectomy patient who has mastered the procedure.
- Begin practice with soft or semisolid foods.
- Supervise initial practice and explain that someone needs to be with the patient when she eats until swallowing without choking is mastered.
- Teach to swallow by asking the patient to:
  - Take a deep breath and bear down to close the vocal cords.
  - Place a small bite of food in the mouth.
  - Tip the chin toward the chest and swallow.
  - Emit a cough to rid the throat of any food particles.
  - Swallow again.
  - Cough again.
  - Begin breathing normally again.
- Offer encouragement for each effort.

---

had the surgery may help the patient focus on the benefits of lifesaving surgery.

The laryngectomy patient will need to be provided with a means of communication such as a pad and pencil, a Magic Slate, or a picture board device. She may be able to use a Passy-Muir speaking tracheostomy valve, or may learn to use esophageal speech (Figure 14-9).

FIGURE 14-9 Passy-Muir speaking tracheostomy valve.

Once the tracheal stoma is healed, protection of the tracheal opening from dust and lint can be accomplished through the use of a simple gauze covering or high-necked clothing. The patient also should be told to avoid swimming and to use care when taking a shower or tub bath so that water is not aspirated through the opening. To protect the patient from inhalation of extremely cold air (she no longer breathes through her nose and mouth, which normally warm the inspired air), the patient may wear a small scarf over the opening during the winter.

Rehabilitation. Proper rehabilitation is important in the acceptance of surgery and the consequences. The speech therapist helps the patient to master a new form of speech. Many people are able to learn esophageal speech; first they master the art of swallowing air and then moving it forcibly back up through the esophagus; then they learn to coordinate lip and tongue movements with the sound produced by the air passing over vibrating folds of the esophagus. The sounds may be somewhat hoarse, but are more natural than the sounds produced by an artificial larynx. For patients who cannot master esophageal speech, a tracheoesophageal prosthesis can be implanted. A fistula is made between the esophagus and trachea; a silicone prosthesis is inserted after the fistula heals. The patient covers the opening of the prosthesis with a finger or closes a special valve that diverts air from the lungs up through the trachea into the esophagus and out of the mouth. Lip and tongue movements form speech as the air is expelled.

An electronic artificial larynx is a battery-powered device that is externally applied to the skin of the esophagus to simulate speech. The sounds are not voicelike, but are understandable and make it possible for the patient to communicate (Figure 14-10).

Another option is an electronic speech aid that has a small tube device that can be inserted into the mouth. The patient can push a button device implanted in the throat that allows diaphragmatic speech.

In various parts of the United States, groups have been organized for laryngectomy patients who wish to get together for social and rehabilitation purposes. These clubs have names such as Lost Cord, New Speech, New Voice, and Esophageal Speech (see Online Resources).

❓ Think Critically

Can you identify all of the health care professionals who would be involved in the collaborative care of the patient undergoing a total laryngectomy and radical neck dissection?

COMMUNITY CARE

One of the primary aspects of community care for nurses is to promote immunization for influenza and pneumonia. Remind the public, that frequent hand hygiene and covering the mouth when coughing or sneezing are simple measures that prevent the spread of URIs.

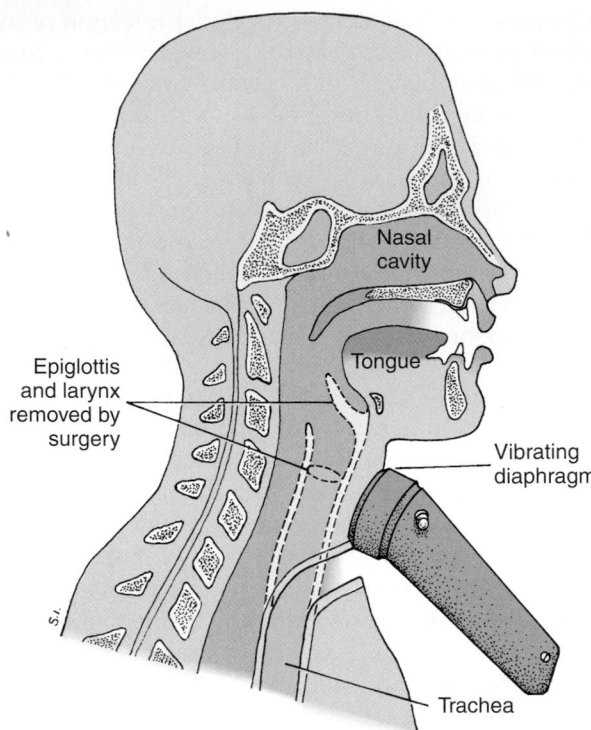

Epiglottis and larynx removed by surgery

Nasal cavity

Tongue

Vibrating diaphragm

Trachea

FIGURE 14-10 External electronic larynx. The vibrating cap of the electronic larynx is held against the throat with sufficient pressure to maintain firm contact. Sound vibrations are transmitted into the lower portion of the pharynx and transformed into speech by the normal movements of the tongue, lips, and teeth.

HOME CARE

Home care nurses can assist patients by reviewing the correct methods of deep breathing and coughing. **Reminding patients to take all prescribed antibiotics is very important in preventing the development of disease-resistant strains of bacteria** (Centers for Disease Control and Prevention, 2009). The home care nurse will also help patients with throat cancer; attention to nutritional concerns, wound care, supervision of self-care techniques for care of a tracheostomy, and psychosocial support are necessary.

Tracheostomy care in the home setting differs from hospital procedures. In the home, suction catheters may be used longer and can be disinfected for reuse. Once the stoma is healed, the patient learns to adapt supplies to her needs. The patient's economic status may dictate what type of supplies and which type of tracheostomy tube will be best.

EXTENDED CARE

Extended-care facility nurses must be vigilant for signs of URI among residents to prevent the spread of infection. If you have a contagious URI do not expose your elderly patients. Stay at home or diligently wear a mask and perform hand hygiene. Adequate protein stores and hydration will promote immunity for your patients. Timely immunization against influenza and pneumonia is a top priority. Assist residents with hand hygiene and remind everyone to cover sneezes and coughs to decrease the spread of URIs within the facility.

Get Ready for the NCLEX® Examination!

Key Points

- If a cold persists or high fever develops, the patient should obtain medical attention.
- Rhinitis may be allergic in origin. If it interferes with lifestyle or productivity, desensitization is an option.
- Sinusitis symptoms are headache pain, fever, tenderness over the sinuses, purulent drainage from the nose, painful upper teeth, and malaise. A nonproductive cough may be present.
- Epistaxis is caused by many factors such as irritation from nose blowing, hypertension, trauma, blood dyscrasias, decreased humidity, and nose picking. Apply direct pressure to the nose for 10 to 15 minutes to stop bleeding; cold compresses or ice are helpful.
- Pharyngitis is inflammation of the pharynx, or sore throat that is viral, bacterial, or fungal in origin. Treatment for viral pharyngitis is rest, warm saline gargles, throat lozenges, and a mild analgesic. A throat culture and antibiotics are usual for bacterial pharyngitis.
- Treatment and nursing interventions for tonsillitis consist of warm saline gargles, throat lozenges, rest, and antibiotics.
- When a tonsillectomy is performed, check vital signs frequently, keep the patient on her side or abdomen as long as there is drainage from the throat, and limit diet to soft, nonirritating foods until the throat is no longer sensitive. Observe for frequent swallowing, which may indicate blood running down the throat.
- Rhinoplasty is performed for severe nasal fracture; the postoperative priority is to monitor for and control bleeding.
- Cancer of the larynx risk factors include smoking, immoderate alcohol use, chronic laryngitis, and abuse of vocal cords. Persistent hoarseness is a first sign of cancer of the larynx; later signs are pain in the throat, coughing, dysphagia, a lump in the throat, or pain in the region of the Adam's apple. Surgical treatment for laryngeal tumor is laser treatment, partial or total laryngectomy, and possible radical neck dissection.
- Endotracheal intubation or tracheostomy provides an artificial airway. Major concerns of an artificial airway are maintaining an open airway and preventing infection.
- Promote immunization for influenza and pneumonia. Teach prevention of infection by hygiene measures—proper hand hygiene and covering the mouth when coughing or sneezing.

Additional Learning Resources

SG Go to your Study Guide for additional learning activities to help you master this chapter content.

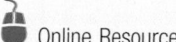 Go to your Evolve website (http://evolve.elsevier.com/deWit/medsurg) for the following FREE learning resources:
- Animations, audio, and video
- Answers and rationales for questions and activities
- Concept Map Creator
- Glossary with pronunciations in English and Spanish
- Interactive Review Questions and Exercises and more!

Online Resources
- American Speech-Language-Hearing Association www.asha.org/default.htm

Review Questions for the NCLEX® Examination

1. On initial assessment, the patient who just had tonsillectomy and adenoidectomy is restless and swallows frequently. What is the most likely explanation?
   1. Excessive thirst
   2. Swelling in the neck
   3. Bleeding
   4. Sore throat

2. A 45-year-old man who is eating steak suddenly rises from his seat. His hands are grasping his throat. What immediate action should be performed?
   1. Perform finger sweeps when food bolus is seen.
   2. Wrap the arms around the victim from behind.
   3. Position the open hand just above the nipple line.
   4. Deliver three downward squeeze thrusts.

3. When caring for the patient who had a rhinoplasty, the nurse should perform which intervention(s) in the immediate postoperative period? (*Select all that apply.*)
   1. Observe for frequent swallowing.
   2. Monitor amount of drainage on dressing.
   3. Position patient flat on the back.
   4. Apply warm compresses.
   5. Provide humidified oxygen.

4. The spouse of a patient with a tracheostomy asks, "Why did the physician order a fenestrated tracheostomy tube?" What is the best response?
   1. "It prepares the patient for long-term tracheostomy."
   2. "It allows gradual weaning before closure of the tracheostomy."
   3. "It prevents aspiration of mucus and fluids."
   4. "It reduces the risk for tracheal wall necrosis."

5. The patient has sinusitis. Which nonpharmacologic intervention(s) would be appropriate? (*Select all that apply.*)
   1. Apply ice packs over the sinus area.
   2. Suggest inhalation of moist steam.
   3. Increase fluid intake.
   4. Decrease dairy product intake.
   5. Rest, and reduce stress.
   6. Use a sinus irrigation kit.

6. While deciding whether to sign the surgical consent for tracheostomy, the patient's spouse asks, "What is the purpose of this procedure?" Which response(s) demonstrate(s) nursing knowledge regarding the procedure? (*Select all that apply.*)
   1. "The procedure facilitates suctioning of respiratory secretions."
   2. "The procedure prevents recurrence of respiratory arrest."
   3. "The procedure prevents hospital-acquired pneumonia."
   4. "The procedure bypasses an obstructed upper airway."
   5. "The procedure is a temporary airway for face and neck injuries."

7. A 55-year-old man with a new tracheostomy is unable to cough. Breath sounds are diminished. Pulse oximetry is 88% on 100% humidified air. What is the priority nursing action?
   1. Provide positive ventilation.
   2. Suction respiratory secretions.
   3. Administer pain medications.
   4. Humidify inhaled air.

8. A patient is newly diagnosed with a squamous cell carcinoma of the larynx. What is an early sign and symptom for this diagnosis?
   1. Crepitation
   2. Hoarseness
   3. Frothy sputum
   4. Drooling

9. The student nurse demonstrates endotracheal suctioning. Which action indicates a need for further instructions?
   1. Donning sterile gloves before suctioning
   2. Lubricating the suction catheter with lubricating jelly
   3. Assessing the need for suctioning
   4. Checking the suction hookup

10. The nurse is caring for a patient who is postoperative for tonsillectomy. Within the first 24 hours, which food item would be the most appropriate to offer the patient?
    1. Orange juice
    2. Warm tea
    3. Soda crackers
    4. Popsicles

Critical Thinking Activities

Scenario A

Mr. Kim has undergone diagnostic procedures to confirm suspected cancer of the larynx. He has been admitted to the hospital for a laryngectomy.

1. What is the primary issue related to Mr. Kim's nutritional status?

2. Identify interventions and teaching points that will allow Mr. Kim to eat and swallow safely.

3. Devise a postoperative nursing care plan for Mr. Kim, including interventions for psychosocial problems.

4. What resources in the community could be suggested to help Mr. Kim adjust to his laryngectomy?

Scenario B

Mr. George has undergone a total laryngectomy and radical neck dissection.

1. What structures would have been removed during this surgery and how would his life be affected?

2. When suctioning his tracheostomy, how long would you apply suction?

3. How might you facilitate communication with Mr. George during the postoperative period?

Scenario C

You are not scheduled to work today or tomorrow and you are glad, because you don't feel very well and suspect that you might have a cold.

1. What are the signs and symptoms of the common cold?

2. What measures will you take to prevent the spread of the virus to your family?

3. Describe the interventions that you will use to manage your own symptoms at home.

Care of Patients with Disorders of the Lower Respiratory System

Objectives

Theory

1. Compare and contrast commonalities and differences in nursing care for patients with bronchitis, influenza, pneumonia, empyema, and pleurisy.
2. List nursing interventions appropriate for care of patients with nursing diagnoses of: Ineffective airway clearance, Ineffective breathing pattern, Impaired gas exchange, and Fatigue related to hypoxia.
3. Analyze ways a nurse can contribute to prevention and prompt treatment of tuberculosis.
4. Summarize the pathophysiologic changes that occur during an asthma attack.
5. Evaluate problems that occur with aging that may cause a restrictive pulmonary disorder.

6. Describe the specifics of nursing care for the patient who has had thoracic surgery and has chest tubes in place.

Clinical Practice

1. Complete a nursing care plan, including home care, for the patient with chronic obstructive pulmonary disease.
2. Review nursing interventions for the tracheostomy patient on oxygen therapy.
3. Teach a patient how to use a peak flowmeter.
4. Observe a respiratory therapist (RT) who is responsible for a patient on a mechanical ventilator and identify how RTs and nurses work together to deliver safe care.

Key Terms

aerosols (ĂR-ō-sŏlz, p. 320)
asthma (ĂZ-mă, p. 305)
atelectasis (ă-tĕ-LĔK-tă-sĭs, p. 303)
bronchiectasis (brŏng-kē-ĔK-tă-sĭs, p. 301)
bronchodilators (brŏng-kō-DĪ-lā-tĕrz, p. 317)
cor pulmonale (kŏr pŭl-mō-NĂ-lē, p. 304)
emphysema (ĕm-fĭ-SĒ-mă, p. 303)
health care–associated pneumonia (HCAP) (p. 296)
hemoptysis (hē-MŎP-tĭ-sĭs, p. 299)
hemothorax (hē-mō-THŌ-răks, p. 313)
hospital-acquired pneumonia (HAP) (p. 297)
intrathoracic (ĭn-tră-thŏr-RĂ-sĭk, p. 315)
latent TB infection (LTBI) (p. 298)
leukotriene (lĕw-kō-trī-ēn, p. 320)

nebulizer (NĔ-bū-lī-zĕr, p. 320)
pleurisy (PLŪR-ă-sē, p. 302)
pneumonectomy (nū-mō-NĔK-tō-mē, p. 311)
pneumonia (nū-MŌ-nē-ă, p. 295)
pneumothorax (nū-mō-THŌ-răks, p. 313)
polycythemia (pŏl-ē-sī-THĒ-mē-ă, p. 303)
sarcoidosis (săr-koy-DŌ-sĭs, p. 302)
subcutaneous emphysema (sŭb-kū-TĀ-nē-ĕs ĕm-fĭ-SĒ-mă, p. 315)
thoracentesis (thŏ-ră-sĕn-TĒ-sĭs, p. 302)
thoracotomy (thō-ră-KŎT-ō-mē, p. 315)
thrombolytic (thrŏm-bō-LĬT-ĭk, p. 312)
tuberculosis (TB) (tū-BĔR-kū-LŌ-sĭs, p. 298)
ventilator-associated pneumonia (VAP) (p. 297)

RESPIRATORY INFECTIOUS DISEASES

ACUTE BRONCHITIS

Acute bronchitis frequently is an extension of an upper respiratory infection involving the trachea (*tracheobronchitis*) and is usually viral in origin. Other causes of acute bronchitis include inhalation of physical or chemical agents such as dust, automobile exhaust, industrial fumes, and tobacco smoke.

Early symptoms of acute bronchitis are similar to those of the common cold. In acute bronchitis, the symptoms progress to chest pain, fever, and a dry,

hacking, and irritating cough. Later the cough becomes more productive of mucopurulent sputum. The fever may be moderate (≤101° F [38° C]) and accompanied by chills, muscle soreness, and headache. The physician relies on history and signs and symptoms for diagnosis.

Symptomatic treatment includes humidification using either warm or cool moist air. Cough mixtures or bronchodilators are used to reduce coughing and soothe the irritated tracheal and bronchial mucosa. Nutrition and fluid balance should be maintained. Rest is recommended to avoid progression from an acute condition to a chronic one. Antibiotics are used if a sputum culture shows specific organisms.

INFLUENZA

Etiology

Influenza is an acute, highly infectious disease of the upper and lower respiratory tracts that occurs in isolated cases or in epidemics. Every year there are between 25 and 50 million cases resulting in more than 200,000 hospitalizations and between 30,000 and 40,000 deaths. Influenza is caused by three major types (A, B, and C) and numerous subtypes of influenza viruses. Type A is the most virulent and usually affects young adults first and then spreads to the very young and very old in the community. Influenza is spread by direct and indirect contact with infected people by coughing and sneezing and by virus transferred from contaminated hands to objects.

There are emerging infectious diseases that cause flu-like symptoms (Box 15-1). Severe acute respiratory syndrome (SARS) appears to be spread by person-to-person contact, whereas avian flu and West Nile virus are spread by vectors such as certain birds and mosquitoes (Centers for Disease Control and Prevention [CDC], 2010).

| Box 15-1 | Emerging Infectious Diseases that May Cause Influenza Symptoms |

AVIAN FLU

A pandemic of *avian influenza* that could kill millions of people is a worldwide fear. Vaccines are under development, but there is no effective vaccine yet. This type of bird flu had been restricted to poultry, but between 2003 and 2010 there were 495 confirmed cases and 292 deaths primarily in Southeast Asia and Africa (World Health Organization, 2010). All of these people had direct contact with infected poultry or secretions or excretions from poultry. Because there is no previous exposure to the virus, and consequently no built-up immunity, it can kill quickly. Symptoms are the same as for common influenza—fever, cough, sore throat, and muscle aches. Complications of pneumonia with acute respiratory distress syndrome have caused death. The drug oseltamivir (Tamiflu) is the only treatment available to decrease the severity of the disease. It is not known how effective this drug would be in a large outbreak.

To prevent the possibility of contracting avian flu, it is recommended to avoid areas where poultry are raised or kept; to not mingle with wild birds by feeding wild ducks, geese, or swans; and to be certain any poultry eaten is thoroughly cooked. Perform hand hygiene frequently and keep your hands away from your mouth, nose, and eyes.

H1N1

H1N1 (formerly known as swine flu) is a respiratory disease that occurs in pigs. The disease is usually passed from infected pigs to humans; however, human-to-human transmission has occurred when people are in close contact. The symptoms of swine flu are very similar to seasonal influenza. In spring 2009, there was public concern because Mexico reported deaths attributed to the H1N1 virus. At that time, travel to Mexico was not recommended. It was determined that the disease actually has a low mortality rate (1% to 4%); however, the possibility of a pandemic does exist if the virus were to become proficient at human-to-human transmission because most people do not have any natural immunity to H1N1.

The prevention measures are similar to avian flu. Avoid traveling to areas of known outbreaks. Avoid areas where swine are raised or kept. Cooking pork thoroughly will kill the virus. Perform hand hygiene and avoid touching the mouth, nose, or eyes. In September 2009, Novel H1N1 influenza A vaccine was approved by the Food and Drug Administration (FDA). Initial target groups for the vaccine included pregnant women, household contacts for children under 6 months of age, persons aged 6 months to 24 years, health care personnel, and adults 25 to 64 years old with underlying conditions that increase their risk for influenza.

WEST NILE VIRUS

West Nile virus (WNV) is transmitted by bites from infected mosquitoes. Most WNV infections are mild and inconsequential. The incubation period is 3 to 7 days. West Nile virus may cause flulike symptoms lasting up to 6 days. Symptoms include febrile illness with sudden onset malaise, anorexia, nausea, vomiting, headache, *myalgia* (muscle ache), eye pain, and lymphadenopathy. A rash may occur. The chances of becoming ill from one mosquito bite are very small. In about 1 in 150 instances of infection, the patient develops encephalitis, a severe neurologic disease. This occurs mostly in patients of advanced age. High fever and changing mental status are the initial signs. Treatment of severe disease is supportive, with hospitalization, intravenous fluids, respiratory support, and prevention of secondary infection.

Prevention of WNV is to avoid mosquito bites. Avoid being outdoors at dawn and dusk. When outside, wear a long-sleeved shirt, long pants, and socks with shoes and spray exposed skin and clothing with an insect repellent containing DEET. Keep containers around the yard empty of standing water. Use screens on open windows and doors.

SEVERE ACUTE RESPIRATORY SYNDROME

Severe acute respiratory syndrome (SARS) is caused by a previously unrecognized SARS-associated coronavirus (SARS-CoV). The disease first appeared as a global threat in 2003 and affected people ages 25 to 70 years. The illness begins with fever >100.4° F (>38° C) that may be accompanied by chills, headache, malaise, and body aches. For those infected, 10% to 20% develop diarrhea. Within 2 to 7 days, a dry cough or dyspnea occurs. Most patients develop pneumonia, and hypoxemia can progress to the need for mechanical ventilation.

SARS appears to be spread by close person-to-person contact, and is thought to be transmitted mostly by respiratory droplets via coughs and sneezes. It is possible that SARS is spread through the air, or by other ways not yet known. The severity of SARS ranges from mild illness to death. Supportive treatment and medications used for pneumonia are given. Antiviral agents may be added, but there is no known specific treatment for this disorder. Use of Standard Precautions and isolation precautions as specified by the facility would be initiated.

Pathophysiology

The influenza viruses affect the respiratory mucosa, causing inflammation and necrosis of tissue and shedding of the virus into the secretions. The inflammation may involve the lungs, pharynx, sinuses, and eustachian tubes. The necrotic tissue provides an environment for the growth of bacteria that cause secondary infection.

Signs and Symptoms

The first symptoms of influenza appear suddenly 2 to 3 days after exposure and include headache, fever (often 101° to 103° F [38° to 40° C]), chills, and muscle aches. Sore throat, hacking cough, runny nose, and nasal congestion and light sensitivity, nausea, vomiting, and diarrhea can also occur.

Diagnosis

Chest radiographs and auscultation usually show no abnormality. The white cell count is normal or slightly below normal. Diagnosis is usually based on clinical findings. To confirm the diagnosis, viral culture, serology, rapid antigen testing, or polymerase chain reaction and/or immunofluorescence assays must be performed.

Treatment and Nursing Management

Antibiotics are given only if there is evidence of bacterial infection secondary to the viral infection. If a person is known to be at high risk for influenza and has been exposed to type A influenza, the physician may choose to provide prophylaxis with an antiviral agent such as amantadine (Symmetrel), rimantadine (Flumadine), zanamivir (Relenza), or oseltamivir (Tamiflu). These drugs must be started within 48 hours of the start of symptoms.

Safety Alert

Warnings About Antiviral Medications

The U.S. Food and Drug Administration (FDA) has issued warnings that oseltamivir (Tamiflu) and zanamivir (Relenza) may cause neurologic and behavioral problems, such as hallucinations, delirium, abnormal behavior, and fatalities. Monitor for and report these changes to the primary care physician. Teach your patients to observe for and report problems. Be aware that additional research about these medications is planned.

Uncomplicated influenza usually is managed more effectively by nursing intervention than by drugs or other forms of medical treatment. Nursing interventions for patients with flu symptoms might include:

- Increase oral fluid intake to at least 3000 mL per 24 hours, unless contraindicated.
- Encourage patient to take analgesics when discomfort first appears.
- Saline gargles for a sore throat.
- Administer suppressant cough medicine at bedtime and during the night as prescribed.
- Perform mouth care at least every 4 hours, before each meal, and more frequently if patient reports bad taste in mouth or has halitosis from sputum.
- Cater to patient's food and drink preferences within limits of dietary restrictions.
- Give antipyretics and perform sponge bath and other measures to reduce high fever.
- Humidify inhaled air.
- Splint chest and abdomen with pillow during coughing attacks.
- Apply emollient to lips and nares as needed.
- Clear nostrils as much as possible to prevent mouth breathing.
- Provide for periods of uninterrupted rest.
- Protect from and monitor for secondary infections such as pneumonia, otitis media, and sinusitis, as the weakened immune system causes greater susceptibility.

Health Promotion

Protection from Influenza

The Advisory Committee on Immunization Practices (2009) recommends annual influenza vaccination for the following groups: (CDC, 2009).

- People at high risk for influenza-related complications and severe disease, including:
  - Children ages 6 to 59 months
  - Pregnant women
  - People age >50 years
  - People of any age with certain chronic medical conditions
- People who live with or care for persons at high risk, including:
  - Household contacts who have frequent contact with people at high risk and who can transmit influenza to those individuals
  - Health care workers

Complementary and Alternative Therapies

Alternative Therapy for the "Flu"

Elderberry extract has been used for centuries as a treatment to ease symptoms of the flu, colds, and sinus infections. It seems to prevent the influenza virus from latching onto cells. There are antioxidants found in the purple elderberry fruit that have an anti-inflammatory effect comparable to aspirin. This may explain why the juice produces symptom improvement (Long, 2011).

PNEUMONIA

Etiology and Pathophysiology

Pneumonia is an extensive inflammation of the lung with either consolidation of the lung tissue as it fills with exudate or interstitial inflammation and edema. It can affect one or both lungs or only one lobe of a lung (lobar pneumonia). In 2006, 55,477 people died of pneumonia; it is the eighth leading cause (combined with influenza) of death in the United States (American Lung Association, 2010a). Pneumonia is classified as community acquired or hospital acquired. Viral pneumonia does not produce exudate; it causes interstitial inflammation and it tends to be less severe than bacterial pneumonia. Bacterial pneumonia usually produces exudate leading to consolidation. It most commonly affects only one lung. *Streptococcus pneumoniae* (pneumococcus) is the most common cause of bacterial pneumonia. Pathogenic microorganisms are always present in the upper respiratory tract; pneumonia can occur when resistance is lowered by some other factor, such as chronic disease, alcoholism, debilitation, physical inactivity, or extremes in age (very young or very old). Pneumonia frequently occurs after an influenza infection. Concept Map 15-1 presents the pathophysiology of pneumonia.

Pneumonia also can result from inhalation of irritating gases (*chemical pneumonia*) or accidental aspiration of foods or liquids that cause a pneumonitis progressing to pneumonia (*aspiration pneumonia*). Hypostatic

pneumonia results from lying in bed for extended periods because of lack of physical exercise and inadequate aeration of the lungs. Fungi also may cause opportunistic pneumonia in immunocompromised patients. Cytomegalovirus has become a cause of pneumonia in immunocompromised patients, particularly those with AIDS or transplant patients on immunosuppressive drugs.

Prevention

People over age 65, and those with chronic respiratory disease, should receive Pneumovax, the pneumococcal pneumonia vaccine. A second dose may be needed 5 years after the first dose for immunocompromised patients or those over 65 years.

A variety of nursing interventions can help prevent pneumonia, including:

- Strengthening the patient's natural defenses and avoiding infection.
- Ensuring frequent turning, coughing, and deep breathing for postoperative patients or those who are otherwise unable to ventilate their lungs adequately.
- Watching for vomiting and initiating a side-lying position for patients with decreased consciousness, such as patients recovering from anesthesia.
- Elevating the head of the bed when assisting with meals or administering tube feedings and leaving the head elevated for 30 to 60 minutes afterward to prevent aspiration. Check residual before each feeding, or once every 4 hours (Eisenstadt, 2010).
- Avoiding thin liquids for patients who are at risk for aspiration.
- Faithfully following principles of cleanliness and asepsis when caring for debilitated patients and those most susceptible to infection.
- Encouraging pneumonia vaccine for those most at risk for developing the disease.
- Encouraging immunization against influenza.

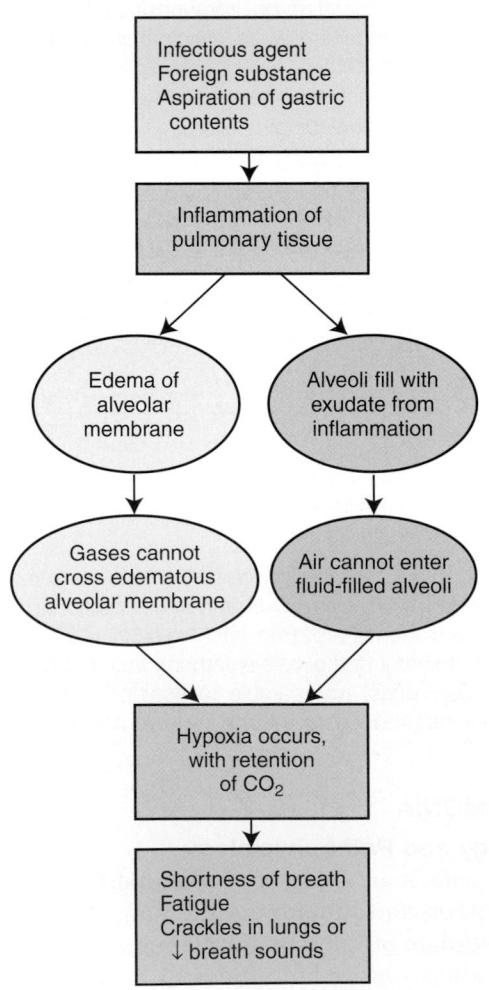

CONCEPT MAP 15-1 Pathophysiology of pneumonia.

Infectious agent / Foreign substance / Aspiration of gastric contents

↓

Inflammation of pulmonary tissue

↓ (branches to two ovals)

Edema of alveolar membrane

Alveoli fill with exudate from inflammation

↓

Gases cannot cross edematous alveolar membrane

Air cannot enter fluid-filled alveoli

↓

Hypoxia occurs, with retention of CO_2

↓

Shortness of breath / Fatigue / Crackles in lungs or ↓ breath sounds

⊕ Cultural Considerations

Ethnic Considerations for Pneumococcal Vaccine

The Advisory Committee on Immunization Practices (CDC, 2009) has recently clarified that routine use of pneumococcal polysaccharide vaccine is not recommended for persons of Alaskan Native or American Indian heritage unless they have underlying medical conditions such as chronic lung, liver, or renal disease. However, local public health authorities may consider recommending the vaccine for occurrences of increased risk.

Patients are at risk for health care–associated pneumonia (HCAP) (formerly known as *nosocomial pneumonia*). These at-risk circumstances include hospital-acquired pneumonia (HAP) where symptoms occur more than 48 hours after admission or ventilator-associated pneumonia (VAP) where pneumonia occurs 48 to 72 hours after endotracheal intubation. HCAP is also associated with nursing home or long-term care; intravenous therapy, chemotherapy, immunosuppressive treatment, or wound care; severe chronic obstructive pulmonary disease (COPD); or child care facilities, hospitals, or dialysis centers (Atkinson, 2010). HAP is a major problem that lengthens hospital stays and increases the cost of health care. VAP is the second most common hospital-acquired infection; however, vigilant and aggressive nursing and respiratory care can greatly decrease the incidence.

People who are on gastrointestinal acid–suppressive therapy should be educated that this may make them more susceptible to community-acquired pneumonia (Restrepo et al., 2010). Normal gastric acid helps prevent pathogens from colonizing the upper GI tract, where they can then be introduced into the respiratory tract.

Signs, Symptoms, and Diagnosis

In typical infectious pneumonia, there is usually a high fever accompanied by chills, a cough that produces rusty or blood-flecked sputum, sweating, chest pain that is made worse by respiratory movements, and a general feeling of malaise and aching muscles. Diagnosis is confirmed by chest radiograph, which reveals densities in the affected lung.

In atypical pneumonia, body temperature can be normal or subnormal, breath sounds can be normal with perhaps only occasional crackles and wheezes, and there may be no pleural involvement and therefore no pain, dry cough, or feeling of extreme fatigue. Chest radiography reveals diffuse, patchy areas of density.

Treatment

Typical pneumonia is treated with intravenous (IV) or oral antibiotic agents, such as erythromycin or the new macrolides (clarithromycin [Biaxin]), cephalosporins, aminoglycosides, or fluoroquinolones such as ciprofloxacin (Cipro).

Atypical pneumonia caused by *Mycoplasma* species usually is treated with either erythromycin, clarithromycin, or azithromycin. Viral, atypical pneumonia requires no anti-infective therapy, but antiviral medication may be administered. *Pneumocystis jiroveci* infection associated with AIDS is treated with aerosolized and intravenous pentamidine, trimethoprim-sulfamethoxazole (Bactrim), trimetrexate glucuronate (NeuTrexin), dapsone, clindamycin, or atovaquone.

According to the Joint Commission's Core Measures (2010), the first antibiotic dose should be administered within 6 to 8 hours of presentation whenever the admission diagnosis is community-acquired pneumonia. The timeliness of this therapy is related to decreased mortality rates. Supplemental oxygen is provided as needed. Some patients require mechanical ventilation.

 Complementary and Alternative Therapies

Treatment for Pneumonia

Barberry root bark is used against bacteria, fungi, and viruses as well as other organisms, (Clin-eguide, 2005) and is an alternative treatment for pneumonia. It has antimicrobial action against both gram-positive and gram-negative bacteria. It should not be used during pregnancy as it can cause spontaneous abortion.

 Think Critically

Can you identify five signs or symptoms found on assessment that might correlate with a diagnosis of pneumonia?

Nursing Management

The nursing care plan for a patient with pneumonia should include interventions to:
- Promote oxygenation
- Control elevated temperature
- Maintain nutritional and fluid intake
- Provide adequate rest
- Monitor vital signs and respiratory status
- Relieve pain and discomfort
- Provide good oral hygiene
- Prevent irritation of the lungs by smoke and other irritants
- Avoid secondary bacterial infections

 Clinical Cues

The first signs of decreasing oxygenation may be restlessness or confusion. The patient may want to sit upright to allow for better chest excursion. Respiratory rate will increase and later there will be flaring of the nares, then retraction of respiratory muscles if the condition worsens. Cyanosis is a very late sign.

The patient should deep breathe and cough 5 to 10 times each hour while awake. It is important that the nurse assess for signs of increasing impairment of gas exchange. Fluid intake, unless contraindicated, should be increased to 2500 to 3000 mL/day. Because abdominal distention, nausea, and vomiting also may accompany pneumonia, nursing interventions to deal with these problems may be indicated. Other problems include altered states of consciousness (delirium and confusion) or the development of such complications as empyema (see later) and congestive heart failure. For the young adult, convalescence with rest should extend for at least a week after acute symptoms subside. The older adult needs several weeks to do usual activities without undue fatigue.

Elder Care Points

The elderly are more at risk for influenza and pneumonia because of a less efficient immune system, decreased action of cilia, and decreased elasticity and muscle tone.

- Confusion often is the most obvious sign of atypical pneumonia in the elderly.
- It may take 6 to 12 weeks after a bout of pneumonia for an elderly patient to be able to resume normal activities without undue fatigue.
- The very elderly patient may never quite regain the former level of wellness after a serious episode of pneumonia.
- Teach the elderly to seek medical attention quickly if symptoms of pneumonia occur.

EMPYEMA

Empyema occurs when the fluid within the pleural cavity becomes infected and the exudate becomes thick and purulent. The organisms causing the infection may be staphylococci or streptococci. One or more chest tubes are inserted and a closed drainage system is established to remove excess fluid from the pleural cavity. A specimen of the fluid is sent for a culture and sensitivity, which determines the choice of antibiotic therapy.

FUNGAL INFECTIONS

The most common fungal lung infections are coccidioidomycosis and histoplasmosis. Coccidioidomycosis occurs primarily in the western United States and exposure occurs during desert recreational activities or when working in occupations that require digging in the earth. Typically, there are no symptoms or mild respiratory symptoms, but 40% will have cough, fever, pleuritic chest pain, myalgias, and arthralgias. Sometimes a flat red rash with dark red papules occurs. Histoplasmosis occurs in central and eastern portions of North America. The fungus lives in moist soil such as that in which mushrooms grow, on the floors of chicken houses and bat caves, and in bird droppings. Clinical signs are fever, fatigue, cough, dyspnea, and weight loss over 1 to 2 months.

The other fungal infections, such as blastomycosis, cryptococcosis, aspergillosis, and candidiasis, are seen mostly in immunocompromised people or those with cystic fibrosis. *Pneumocystis carinii* is now considered a fungus, renamed *Pneumocystis jiroveci*. It is found only in immunocompromised patients and is highly lethal (see Chapter 12). Fungal infections are diagnosed by history, signs and symptoms, and positive skin test reaction to the fungus. Treatment is IV amphotericin B for up to 12 weeks.

TUBERCULOSIS

Etiology

Pulmonary **tuberculosis (TB)** is an infectious disease, characterized by lesions within the lung tissue. The lesions may degenerate and become necrotic, or they may heal by fibrosis and calcification. The causative organism is the true tubercle bacillus *Mycobacterium tuberculosis*. **Latent TB infection (LTBI)** refers to an infection with *Mycobacterium tuberculosis* but no current active disease. LTBI may develop into active TB if the immune system is weakened by a serious illness such as HIV, or when the system is less efficient, as with advanced age.

Contrary to popular belief, TB is *not* highly contagious. Infection most often occurs after prolonged exposure, but not everyone contracts the disease, even after close and extensive contact with infected persons.

Cultural Considerations

Ethnic Occurrence of Tuberculosis

American Indians, Alaska Natives, Asian/Pacific Islanders, black non-Hispanics, and Hispanics have a high incidence of TB. The disease is most prevalent in people over 65 years of age in these groups. For the first few years of residence in the United States, new immigrants from areas where TB is prevalent have incidence rates similar to those of their former country.

Tuberculosis is a major health problem throughout the world. The increase in the number of immunodeficient people with AIDS, the influx of immigrants who are infected with TB, and an increase in the population of malnourished urban poor are major causes of the increase in the United States.

In countries where there are high rates of TB, the World Health Organization strongly recommends the widespread use of bacille Calmette-Guérin (BCG) vaccine, which seems to reduce the morbidity of TB. The vaccine's ability to increase resistance is in question, so it is not used in the United States.

Pathophysiology

Mycobacterium is an acid-fast, aerobic, slow-growing bacillus. When the organism enters the lungs, a local inflammatory reaction occurs, usually in the upper lobe. Bacilli migrate to the lymph nodes and activate a cell-mediated hypersensitivity response. This triggers granuloma formation with influx of macrophages and lymphocytes at the site of inflammation. The bacillus is walled off, forming a *tubercle*. Caseation necrosis (a core of cheeselike material) develops in the center of the tubercle. In a healthy person, the tubercles eventually calcify. In the unhealthy individual, the bacilli spread to other parts of the lung and to other organs. Bacilli may remain viable in a dormant state inside the tubercle for many years. The bacilli are difficult to eradicate when released into the environment because the bacillus is resistant to drying and to many disinfectants.

Signs and Symptoms

The onset of TB is gradual; a patient may have an active, progressive lesion before symptoms appear. Typical symptoms are cough, low-grade fever in the afternoon, anorexia, loss of weight, fatigue, night sweats, and sometimes hemoptysis (blood in sputum). Tight or dull chest pain and mucopurulent sputum may occur as the disease progresses. Persons with LTBI are asymptomatic and have a negative chest radiograph.

Diagnosis
Early detection of TB is of great importance because:
- The anti-TB drugs are more effective in the early stages of the disease.
- The period of disability is much shorter.
- The complications are fewer.

Tuberculin Skin Testing. Food handlers, those working with children, and health care workers must be periodically tested. Others who are symptomatic or have been exposed to someone with TB should be tested. Skin testing for TB is done by the Mantoux test. In this test, 0.1 mL of purified protein derivative (PPD) tuberculin is injected intradermally. The test is called the tuberculin skin test (TST) (formerly known as PPD test). The test is positive when the swelling at the site of injection is more than 5 mm in diameter 48 to 72 hours after injection in people who have a history of contact with infectious TB or in immunocompromised patients. Induration of more than 10 mm in diameter is positive in recent immigrants from countries where TB is prevalent, in medically underserved groups, and the homeless. For those persons at low risk, induration of more than 15 mm is considered positive. Skin testing is not used on people who have received BCG vaccine within the previous 10 years; this includes those in whom BCG has been used to treat bladder cancer.

A positive tuberculin test indicates that the person has been infected with the tubercle bacillus; however it does not indicate whether the disease is active or inactive, only that the body tissues are sensitive to tuberculin. A positive reaction indicates a need for further evaluation. Once positive, subsequent TSTs will always be positive.

A newer blood test, the QuantiFERON-TB Gold, is less likely to produce false-positive readings. It means one visit to the clinic or office for a blood draw, rather than the two required for the TST (the second visit is for reading the result). It is accurate even for people who have had BCG.

Radiographic Examinations and Sputum Cultures. A radiographic examination of the chest may or may not reveal tubercular lesions in the lung, but calcified and healed lesions can usually be seen on radiographs. **A diagnosis of active TB is established when the tubercle bacillus has been found in the sputum or gastric washings.** A sample of stomach contents may be examined if the patient cannot produce an adequate sputum specimen (*gastric analysis*). Sputum cultures are

slow growing, and culture results take 1 to 3 weeks to allow identification of the bacillus.

Treatment
Uncomplicated pulmonary TB is managed in the outpatient setting. Only those who are extremely debilitated or suffering from another chronic illness are hospitalized. Treatment consists of at least four drugs for an extended period of time (Table 15-1). The microscopic-observation drug susceptibility (MODS) test described in Chapter 13 is used to determine the best drugs. The drugs are given in varying combinations on varying numbers of days per week. Noncompliance is an issue because of side effects, the requirement to avoid alcohol, and the long duration of therapy. Two new drug combinations have made compliance easier for patients: Rifamate, containing rifampin and isoniazid, and Rifater, containing rifampin, isoniazid, and pyrazinamide. Rifapentine (Priftin) may make treatment easier as it is taken once a week during the last four months of therapy, in combination with other drugs. Effective cure can be obtained within 6 to 9 months for most patients with pulmonary TB.

Complementary and Alternative Therapies
Vitamin D to Prevent Tuberculosis
Vitamin D has been found to be successful in the prevention and treatment of TB (Talat et al., 2010). White blood cells convert vitamin D into an active form that helps make a protein that kills TB bacteria. This may be why moving to a sunny climate and a solarium environment helped people with TB in the past.

A new drug, PA-824, is in phase II clinical trials and holds promise for shortening the TB treatment regimen (National Institute of Allergy and Infectious Diseases, 2009), which could solve some problems related to compliance with TB therapy.

There is an increase in the incidence of multidrug-resistant TB, and patients with these infections do not fare well. For this reason, directly observed therapy (DOT) is recommended for patients who are known to be at risk of noncompliance with therapy (Mayo Clinic Staff, 2009). DOT involves the visual observation of the ingestion of each required dose of medication for the entire course of treatment. Often a public health nurse administers the medication at a clinic site. Follow-up visits are necessary for 12 months after completion of therapy to monitor for the presence of resistant strains.

Legal and Ethical Considerations
Noncompliance with Medication
When someone is found to have TB and the person is noncompliant with the treatment, is it legal or ethical to compel the person to come for treatment? What will happen if the person is allowed to remain in the community without treatment?

Table 15-1   **Drugs Commonly Used in the Treatment of Tuberculosis**

DAILY DOSAGE	TWICE-WEEKLY DOSAGE	MOST COMMON SIDE EFFECTS	TEST FOR SIDE EFFECTS	REMARKS
Primary Drugs				
Isoniazid (INH) 5-10 mg/kg up to 300 mg PO or IM	15 mg/kg PO or IM	Peripheral neuritis, hypersensitivity, jaundice	AST/ALT (not as a routine)	Bactericidal agent. Pyridoxine 10 mg as prophylaxis for neuritis; 50-100 mg as treatment.
Ethambutol (Myambutol) 15-25 mg/kg PO	50 mg/kg PO	Optic neuritis (reversible with discontinuation of drug; very rare at 15 mg/kg), skin rash	Red-green color discrimination and visual acuity	Use with caution with renal disease or when eye testing is not feasible.
Rifampin (RMP) (Rifadin) 10-20 mg/kg up to 600 mg PO	Not recommended	Hepatitis, febrile reaction, purpura (rare)	AST/ALT (not as a routine)	Bactericidal agent. Orange secretion color. Affects action of other drugs.
Streptomycin 15-20 mg/kg up to 1 g IM	25-30 mg/kg IM	VIIIth cranial nerve damage, nephrotoxicity, hypersensitivity	Vestibular function, audiograms; BUN and creatinine	Use with caution in older patients or those with renal disease.
Pyrazinamide 15-30 mg/kg up to 2 g PO	Not recommended for twice weekly dosage	Hyperuricemia, hepatotoxicity	Uric acid, AST/ALT	Under study as first-line drug in short-course regimens.
Secondary Drugs				
Kanamycin (Kantrex) 15-30 mg/kg up to 1 g IM	Secondary drugs are not recommended for twice-weekly dosage	Similar to streptomycin	BUN, creatinine	Increase hydration; evaluate hearing before therapy starts.
Capreomycin (Capastat) 15-30 mg/kg up to 1 g IM		Similar to streptomycin	BUN, creatinine	Periodic hearing evaluation needed.
Cycloserine (Seromycin) 10-20 mg/kg up to 1 g PO		Depression, psychosis, hypersensitivity	Neurologic examination	Warn to avoid alcohol; monitor serum blood levels of drug.
Ethionamide (Trecator) 15-30 mg/kg up to 1 g PO		Peripheral neuritis, GI distress, dermatitis	AST/ALT	Pyridoxine used for neuropathy. Give with meals; avoid alcohol.
Para-aminobenzoic acid (PABA) 150 mcg/kg up to 12 g PO		GI distress, hepatotoxicity, hypersensitivity	AST/ALT	Give with meals; monitor for hepatotoxicity.

Adapted from Lewis, S.L., Heitkemper, M.M., & Dirksen, S.R. (2011). *Medical-Surgical Nursing: Assessment and Management of Clinical Problems* (8th ed.). St. Louis: Mosby.

ALT, alanine aminotransferase; *AST,* aspartate aminotransferase; *BUN,* blood urea nitrogen; *GI,* gastrointestinal; *IM,* intramuscularly; *PO,* orally.

Nursing Management

A complete history and assessment of TB risk factors is needed. A focused assessment of the respiratory system is performed (see Focused Assessment on p. 263).

Nursing objectives are to control the spread of the infectious agent, promote immunity, and strengthen potential recovery in a patient with an infectious disease.

Nursing diagnoses for the patient with TB may include:

- Ineffective breathing pattern related to decreased lung capacity
- Noncompliance related to lack of knowledge of disease process and long-term requirements for treatment
- Activity intolerance related to fatigue, febrile status, and poor nutritional status
- Imbalanced nutrition: less than body requirements related to anorexia, fatigue, and productive cough

Control of Infection. Airborne Infection Isolation in addition to Standard Precautions (see Appendix B) is recommended for the hospitalized patient who has an active case of TB and is just beginning drug therapy. The patient is placed in a negative-pressure isolation room with an anteroom. A high-efficiency particulate air (HEPA) respirator mask that tightly fits the face is required for all personnel when caring for the patient. The home care patient does not need Airborne Infection Isolation because family members have already been exposed by the time of diagnosis. Patients and families should be educated about the importance of medication compliance and the basic principles of infection control: covering the mouth when coughing or sneezing, disposing of tissues in plastic bags, practicing good hand hygiene, and wearing a mask when in contact with crowds until medication effectively suppresses the infection. Sputum examinations are required every 2 to 4 weeks. When three consecutive sputum cultures are negative, the patient is considered no longer infectious and may resume work and other usual social activities.

Promotion of Immunity. Improving living conditions and carrying out sound health practices are essential to maintaining a natural resistance to TB. Close contacts are monitored with skin testing. Treatment of LTBI (previously called preventive therapy or chemoprophylaxis) is indicated for those at increased risk of progression to active TB. Isoniazid (INH) has a 90% effectiveness. The drug is taken once daily for 9 months; research suggests that a 4-month course of rifampin would improve compliance (Menzies et al., 2008). INH therapy is recommended for:

- Those living with—or closely associating with—a person who is newly diagnosed as having TB.
- People who have positive TST, but who have normal chest radiographs.
- People with positive TST who suffer from a chronic disease (e.g., diabetes mellitus), are taking steroids, or have had a gastrectomy.

- Those who have recently shown a positive TST, but no sign of active disease, and who have a history of previous negative TST.

A recombinant vaccine—rBCG30—has been developed at the University of California at Los Angeles, and the first clinical trials in humans began in 2004. It is hoped that this vaccine will provide a strong protective immune response against TB (Horowitz, 2010).

Support. When a person first learns that he has tuberculosis, he will need support in sorting out his feelings and overcoming any fears and misinformation he might have.

It is also important that the patient name all close contacts, so that they can be notified and appropriately tested and treated. Giving the names of contacts may be difficult for the patient because of the social stigma still attached to TB in certain cultural groups.

EXTRAPULMONARY TUBERCULOSIS

It is possible for the tubercle bacillus to attack and damage parts of the body other than the lungs. This is called *extrapulmonary* or *miliary tuberculosis.* The areas most frequently affected are the bones, meninges, urinary system, and reproductive system. Tuberculosis of the spine, called *Pott's disease,* can cause *kyphosis,* or "hunchback," but the condition is rare in the United States.

BRONCHIECTASIS

Bronchiectasis is a chronic respiratory disorder in which one or more bronchi are permanently dilated. It is thought to occur as a result of frequent respiratory infections in childhood.

Cystic Fibrosis

Cystic fibrosis (CF) is a major cause of bronchiectasis. It is a genetic disease (more frequent among whites) in which there is excessive mucus production because of exocrine gland dysfunction. The lungs, intestines, sinuses, reproductive tract, sweat glands, and pancreas are all affected. It is diagnosed by history, physical examination, and a positive sweat test.

Lung damage occurs in cystic fibrosis because of excessive secretion of abnormally thick mucus, impairment of ciliary action in the lungs, airway obstruction, and repeated infections, which cause scarring. It was once a pediatric disease, because children with cystic fibrosis died before reaching adulthood. Cystic fibrosis patients now live into their 40s and beyond with aggressive respiratory treatment and antibiotics. In 1989, the gene responsible for cystic fibrosis was identified (National Human Genome Research Institute, 2009). Work is continuing on ways to isolate and replace the missing gene to prevent or cure the disease.

Treatment includes bronchodilators, expectorants, oral pancreatic enzymes, double doses of fat-soluble vitamins, and mucolytics. A high-protein, high-calorie, moderate-fat diet is prescribed. Dornase alfa

(Pulmozyme) reduces the frequency of respiratory infections and improves pulmonary function for patients with CF. Breathing exercises and chest physiotherapy are used daily. A handheld device called the flutter valve; looks like a fat pipe. By exhaling actively into the pipe, the device causes vibrations of the airway walls, loosening secretions so that they can be coughed up. DNase, a recombinant deoxyribonucleic acid (DNA) medication is used to reduce the number of lung infections, to improve lung function, and to extend the average life span of the CF patient. Lung transplantation is a possible lifesaving measure.

OCCUPATIONAL LUNG DISORDERS

Coal dust, dust from hemp, flax, and cotton processing, and exposure to silica in the air all can cause work-related lung disorders. Asbestos exposure may cause mesothelioma, a rare cancer of the chest lining (Mesothelioma Research Foundation, 2010). Asbestos exposure also causes scarring of lung tissue. The other exposures cause obstruction of small airways or scarring and loss of elasticity and compliance. Occupational history is part of the respiratory assessment.

INTERSTITIAL PULMONARY DISEASE

Sarcoidosis

Sarcoidosis is a lung disease characterized by granulomas. This disease causes fibrotic changes in the lung tissue and other tissues over time. A cellular immune response seems to be responsible, but the exact cause is unknown. Sarcoidosis is 10 times more common in African Americans than in whites, and most cases occur between ages 20 and 40. The fibrotic changes cause a reduction in function in lung tissue. Although there is no specific treatment for sarcoidosis, occasionally patients recover without treatment.

Pulmonary Fibrosis

Pulmonary fibrosis occurs from severe infection, repeated infection, or inflammation that causes scarring of the lung tissue. The scarring decreases functional lung tissue. Occupational inhalation of lung irritants, smoking, and chronic aspiration are risk factors. Signs and symptoms are exertional dyspnea, nonproductive cough, and inspiratory crackles, and sometimes clubbed fingers. Diagnosis is by chest radiograph and pulmonary function testing. There is a 30% to 50% survival rate at 5 years after diagnosis. Treatment is with corticosteroids, immunosuppressants, and the antifibrotic agent colchicine. Lung transplantation is an option for some patients.

RESTRICTIVE PULMONARY DISORDERS

Restrictive pulmonary disorders are caused by decreased elasticity or compliance of the lungs, or decreased ability of the chest wall to expand. Disorders of the central nervous system or of the neuromuscular system can cause a restrictive lung disorder. Myasthenia gravis and arthritis are examples of extrapulmonary causes. *Kyphosis* of the spine or severe *scoliosis* may hamper lung expansion, but the lung tissue remains normal.

PLEURISY

Pleurisy—an inflammation of the pleura—could be caused by tuberculosis, pneumonia, neoplasm, or pulmonary infarction. Pleurisy pain is sharp and abrupt in onset and is most evident on inspiration. This causes shallow breathing. A pleural friction rub may be heard. Treatment is aimed at the underlying cause and providing pain relief. Lying on the affected side or splinting the affected side during coughing may provide some relief. An intercostal nerve block may be done for severe pleurisy pain.

PLEURAL EFFUSION

Pleural effusion is a collection of fluid in the pleural space. Transudate is a thin fluid containing no protein that passes from cells into interstitial spaces or through a membrane. A transudate occurs in noninflammatory conditions and is often a result of congestive heart failure, chronic liver failure, or renal disease. Exudate is thicker, contains cells, proteins, and other substances, and is slowly discharged from cells into a body space or to the outside of the body. Exudative pleural effusion is due to the increased capillary permeability characteristic of the inflammatory reaction. This type of effusion occurs with lung cancer, pulmonary embolism, pancreatic disease, and pulmonary infections.

When pleurisy is accompanied by effusion of serous fluid, the physician may perform a thoracentesis (removal of fluid from the pleural cavity) for diagnostic tests or symptom relief. It is not uncommon for as much as 500 mL to be removed during a thoracentesis (see Table 13-3).

OBSTRUCTIVE PULMONARY DISORDERS

Obstructive pulmonary disorders are characterized by problems with moving air in and out of the lungs. Narrowing of the openings in the tracheobronchial tree increases resistance to the flow of air, making it difficult for oxygen to enter; this contributes to air trapping, thus exhalation is also difficult. Asthma, emphysema, and chronic bronchitis are examples of diseases that cause chronic airflow limitation (CAL). The increase in the morbidity and mortality rates due to obstructive disorders is attributed to cigarette smoking and rising levels of air pollution. A third factor is genetic susceptibility to the destruction of lung tissue. *Alpha$_1$-antitrypsin* (AAT) is a serum protein which inhibits the activity of the enzyme *elastase*, which tends to break down lung tissue. In the absence of AAT, lung tissue is more easily destroyed by the enzyme. Patients with a deficiency of AAT may develop severe lung disease at an early age.

ATELECTASIS

Atelectasis is an incomplete expansion, or collapse, of alveoli. It may occur from compression of the lungs from outside, a decrease in surfactant, or bronchial obstruction that prevents air from reaching the alveoli. Postoperatively it occurs from retained secretions that accumulated during anesthesia, positioning on the operating room table for an extended period without movement, and hypoventilation related to surgical pain. It usually is a reversible condition. Breath sounds are diminished when the airways are collapsed, and oxygen saturation (SaO_2) will decrease. Treatment consists of expelling secretions by coughing. Deep breathing and use of the incentive spirometer helps to keep the alveoli open and functional.

CHRONIC OBSTRUCTIVE PULMONARY DISEASE

Chronic obstructive pulmonary disease (COPD) is the term used to describe a condition that includes two diseases, *emphysema* and *chronic bronchitis*. Approximately 12.7 million people in the United States have COPD and 24 million have impaired lung function with probable underlying COPD (American Lung Association, 2010b).

Etiology and Diagnosis of COPD

Smoking and AAT deficiency are the primary causes of emphysema and chronic bronchitis, with air pollution and occupational exposure being contributing factors. Diagnosis is by history, physical assessment, chest x-ray, pulmonary function testing, arterial blood gas analysis, and, if needed, lung biopsy.

Emphysema

Pathophysiology. In emphysema, there is destruction of alveolar and alveolar-capillary walls, as well as narrowed and tortuous small airways. This leads to large, permanently inflated alveolar air spaces. Air that is inhaled becomes trapped and it becomes harder to exhale air than to inhale it (Figure 15-1). As emphysema progresses, lung elasticity decreases.

FIGURE 15-1 Alveoli in emphysema.

Alveoli (air sacs)

Signs and Symptoms. Dyspnea is an early symptom of emphysema. There is minimal coughing with small amounts of mucoid sputum. As the disease progresses, dyspnea worsens and eventually interferes with activities of daily living. The diaphragm becomes permanently flattened by overdistention of the lungs, the muscles of the rib cage become rigid, and the ribs flare outward. The patient develops a "barrel chest" (see Figure 13-4).

To compensate for the loss of normal muscular action, the patient begins to use the neck and shoulder muscles. The shoulders are held high in an attempt to enlarge the space for lung expansion. The patient may look anxious or tense. The skin is a pink tone in whites even though hypoxia may be present. Carbon dioxide is usually not retained, and therefore an acid-base imbalance is unlikely.

Chronic Bronchitis

Pathophysiology. In chronic bronchitis there is excess secretion of thick, tenacious mucus that decreases ciliary function and interferes with airflow and causes inflammatory damage to the bronchial mucosa. Airways become edematous and narrowed, and air trapping occurs. Initially the larger airways are affected, and then the smaller airways also become obstructed. Inflammation of the bronchi is considered chronic when a recurrent cough is present for at least 3 months of each year for at least 2 years. Respiratory infections occur frequently because the thick mucus provides a growth medium for bacteria.

Signs and Symptoms. Symptoms can range from a mildly irritating "cigarette" cough in the morning with production of small amounts of sputum to a severe disabling condition. The latter extreme is characterized by increased resistance to airflow, hypoxia, and frequently hypercapnia (excess CO_2).

Pulmonary function testing reveals an increased residual volume due to the premature closure of the narrowed airways during exhalation. The patient has a marked increase in partial pressure of arterial carbon dioxide ($PaCO_2$) levels and a marked decrease in partial pressure of arterial oxygen (PaO_2) levels. **The retention of carbon dioxide and deficiency of oxygen give the skin and/or mucous membranes a reddish blue color.** The reddish color is also related to an increase in the red blood cell count (polycythemia) which is an attempt by the body to compensate for chronic hypoxia. Hemoglobin and hematocrit levels are elevated for patients with chronic bronchitis. Table 15-2 presents a comparison of emphysema and chronic bronchitis.

Treatment of COPD

COPD is treated with bronchodilators and anti-inflammatory agents. When bacterial infection is present, antibiotics, and sometimes steroid anti-inflammatory

Table 15-2 Comparison of Pulmonary Emphysema and Chronic Bronchitis

CLINICAL FEATURES/ CHARACTERISTICS	EMPHYSEMA	CHRONIC BRONCHITIS
Age of Onset (Years)	40-50	30-40
Pathophysiology	Destruction of alveolar walls Loss of elasticity, impaired expiration, hyperinflation	Increased mucous secretion, inflammation and infection, obstruction of airways
Health History	Generally healthy	Frequent URI, acute episodes
Smoking	Usually	Usually
Clinical Features		
Barrel chest	Yes	May be present
Weight loss	May be severe in late disease	Infrequent
Shortness of breath	Absent early; pronounced late in disease	Early symptom; especially with activity
Decreased breath sounds	Yes	Variable
Wheezing	Usually absent	Variable
Sputum	Absent or develops late in disease	Early sign; frequent infections with purulent sputum
Cyanosis	Usually absent; appears late in disease with low Pao_2	Yes; worsens as disease progresses
Cor pulmonale	Occasional	Common
Polycythemia	May appear in advanced disease	Frequently present
Blood gases	Normal until late in disease	May display hypercapnia Hypoxemia frequent

Pao_2, partial pressure of arterial oxygen; *URI*, upper respiratory infection.

agents, are used. In later stages of disease, when hypoxemia is present, oxygen therapy is initiated. **Oxygen is always used cautiously in patients with COPD, because they have adjusted to high levels of CO_2; they become dependent on low oxygen levels to stimulate breathing.** Smoking cessation is very important. Respiratory rehabilitation programs can help increase exercise tolerance and improve quality of life.

Nutrition is very important for the patient with COPD, because the extra work of breathing uses more calories and anorexia may be present. Extra protein is required to repair damaged tissues. It is beneficial to maintain as normal a weight as possible for height and age.

Nutrition Considerations

Nutritional Suggestions for the Patient with COPD

The following tips may prove helpful for the patient with COPD:
- Drink 6 to 8 glasses of noncaffeinated fluids per day to keep mucus thin and easier to cough up. Check with your physician if you are on fluid restrictions.
- Rest before eating.
- Avoid overeating, and avoid foods that cause gas or bloating as a distended stomach may make breathing more difficult.
- Eat four to six small meals a day rather than three regular meals, to decrease stomach fullness and reduce fatigue.
- Eat a well-balanced diet with adequate protein.

- Avoid lying down for an hour after eating.
- If you become short of breath while eating or right after meals:
  - Clear the airway 1 hour before eating.
  - Take small bites and chew food slowly.
  - Choose foods that are easy to chew.
  - Drink beverages at the end of the meal rather than during it.
  - Use your oxygen cannula while you eat.
- Take in sufficient calcium via dairy products, vegetables, and supplements—steroid medications put you at risk for osteoporosis.
- Cook when feeling most energetic; make extra portions and freeze them for easy, quick, frozen dinners.

Complementary and Alternative Therapies

Ginger, Cinnamon, Chili, and Garlic for Emphysema

Ginger and cinnamon are aromatic digestives that provide benefit for emphysema patients. Very small doses of *Capsicum annuum* (chili) or garlic can be useful as mucolytic agents (Glastonbury, 2009).

Complications of COPD

Cor Pulmonale. **Cor pulmonale** is enlargement of the right side of the heart as a result of pulmonary hypertension caused by constriction of the pulmonary vessels in response to hypoxia. Constant hypoxia stimulates erythropoiesis, with resulting polycythemia and increased viscosity of blood. Eventually right-sided heart failure causes systemic venous congestion which manifests as distended neck veins, right upper quadrant tenderness from an engorged liver, peripheral edema, weight gain, gastrointestinal distress, and ascites. Treatment is continuous low-flow oxygen and medications to treat both the heart failure and the fluid volume overload.

Pneumonia. Pneumonia is often a complication of COPD. Purulent sputum is the usual sign. Fever, chills, and elevated white blood cell count may or may not be present. Pneumonia is treated as previously discussed.

Peptic Ulcer and Gastroesophageal Reflux Disease. Peptic ulcer and gastroesophageal reflux disease (GERD) may occur due to long-term use of the bronchodilators and corticosteroid drugs used to treat COPD. GERD can worsen the symptoms of COPD; the reflux of acid in the esophagus stimulates a vagal reflex that causes bronchoconstriction (Rascon-Aguilar et al., 2006).

ASTHMA

Etiology

Factors implicated in the occurrence of asthma include allergens, viruses and other infectious agents, occupational and environmental toxins, exercise, perfumes, and emotional stress. Recent studies show a genetic correlation, along with environmental factors, predisposes to asthma. *Healthy People 2020* objectives include reducing deaths, hospitalizations, emergency department visits, and activity limitations related to asthma.

Pathophysiology

Asthma is a chronic lung disease characterized by reversible airway obstruction, airway inflammation from edema or swelling, and increased airway hypersensitivity to a variety of stimuli. With asthma, a precipitating factor creates inflammation of the airways, which causes bronchospasm. Cough usually indicates obstruction of the larger airways. Dyspnea, another common symptom, is indicative of inflammation of the airways, mucosal edema, and excessive secretion of mucus which cause a plugging of the small airways. With bronchoconstriction, there is further obstruction and narrowing of the airways, limiting airflow (Figure 15-2 and Concept Map 15-2).

Signs, Symptoms, and Diagnosis

Diagnosis is by history, physical examination, pulmonary function testing, arterial blood gas analysis, and chest radiograph. The symptoms may be continuous or episodic. Findings include wheezing, cough that is worse at night, difficulty breathing, and chest tightness.

FIGURE 15-2 Asthma.

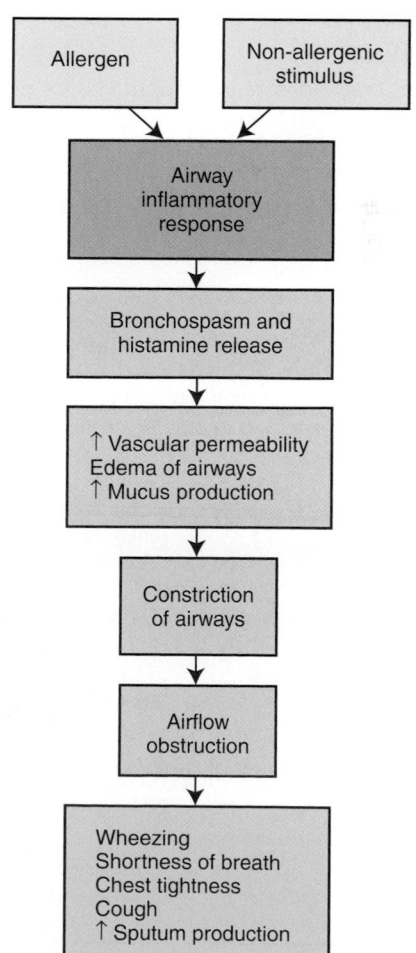

CONCEPT MAP 15-2 Pathophysiology of asthma.

Unrelieved asthma attacks become *status asthmaticus* and are very serious. **Respiratory distress without wheeze is an ominous sign for the asthma patient; this suggests further constriction with very little air movement.** Patients and nurses must know that a severe, acute asthma attack can cause death from hypoxia.

Clinical Cues

If your patient takes an angiotensin-converting enzyme (ACE) inhibitor, teach him to report a cough (which can be caused by this medication). Excessive coughing can trigger or worsen an asthma attack.

Treatment

Asthma is classified by a step system, based on the degree and frequency of symptoms (Table 15-3). The goals of medical treatment are to manage the underlying symptoms and include:

- Minimizing irritation of the air passages and relieving obstruction by secretions, edema, or bronchospasm
- Preventing or controlling infection and allergy
- Increasing the patient's tolerance for activity
- Determining the best drug combinations in the smallest dosages that will control symptoms

Table 15-3   The Step System of Asthma Treatment

CLINICAL MANIFESTATIONS	TREATMENT RECOMMENDATIONS
I. Mild Intermittent	
Symptoms or episodes occur less than once a week. Episodes/exacerbations are short, lasting only a few hours. Symptoms are present at night no more frequently than twice per month. PFTs are normal between episodes. During episodes/exacerbations, FEV_1 or PEF is at least 80% of normal. PEF variability is less than 20%.	No daily medication needed. Use of short-acting inhaled beta agonist during episodes (rescue inhaler). Increased use of rescue inhaler indicates the need to start long-term therapy.
II. Mild Persistent	
Symptoms or episodes occur more than once per week but not daily. Symptoms are present at night more than twice per month. During episodes/exacerbations, FEV_1 is at least 80% of normal. PEF variability is 20%-30%. Episodes affect sleep and activity	Use of a daily anti-inflammatory. Inhaled corticosteroid (ICS). Inhaled cromolyn. Leukotriene antagonist. Use of a rescue inhaler for relief during episodes.
III. Moderate Persistent	
Symptoms occur daily. Symptoms or episodes occur more than once per week. Symptoms are present at night at least once per week. During episodes/exacerbations, FEV_1 is only 60%-80% of normal. PEF variability is greater than 30%.	Daily use of ICS (low to moderate dose). Use of long-acting inhaled beta agonist (bronchodilator). Use of a rescue inhaler for relief during episodes (more than two days per week, the patient should be evaluated for progression to step IV).
IVa. Severe Persistent	
Episodes/exacerbations are frequent. During episodes/exacerbations, FEV_1 or PEF is less than 60% of normal. Physical activity is limited. Symptoms are frequently present at night. PEF variability is greater than 30%.	Daily use of ICS (medium dose) and long-acting inhaled bronchodilator or ICS (medium dose) and either a leukotriene receptor antagonist or theophylline.
IVb. Severe Persistent, Not Responsive to the Previous Step	
	High-dose ICS and long-acting beta agonist. Omalizumab for patients with exposure to nonseasonal allergens. High-dose ICS, and long-acting beta agonist lowest possible daily dose of oral corticosteroids. Omalizumab for patients with exposure to nonseasonal allergens.

Adapted from Ignatavicius, D.D., & Workman, L. (2010). *Medical-Surgical Nursing: Patient-Centered Collaborative Care* (6th ed.). Philadelphia: Elsevier Saunders. *FEV_1*, forced expiratory volume in 1 second; *ICS*, inhaled corticosteroid; *PEF*, peak expiratory flow; *PFTs*, pulmonary function tests.

Bronchodilators in the form of beta-adrenergic agonists, theophyllines, or anticholinergic agents such as ipratropium bromide (Atrovent) are mainstays of therapy. Corticosteroids, mucolytics, antibiotics, and oxygen may also be prescribed (Table 15-4). Ciclesonide is a new-generation, inhaled corticosteroid that improves lung function for patients with mild to moderate asthma (Manning et al., 2008).

 Clinical Cues

New inhalers use hydrofluoroalkane (HFA) rather than chlorofluorocarbons (CFCs). HFA is environmentally friendly and less damaging to the ozone layer; however, the price will increase. Teach your patient to expect a gentler puff and a different taste; also, HFA inhalers must be cleaned regularly or they will clog.

The asthma patient is taught to use a peak flowmeter to determine the drug dosage needed to control the asthma, to predict the effectiveness of therapy, and to detect airflow obstruction buildup before it becomes serious and requires hospitalization (see Figure 13-9). Peak flow monitoring is based on the greatest airflow velocity that can be produced during a forced expiration that starts from fully inflated lungs.

 Patient Teaching

Using a Peak Flowmeter

Peak flow should be monitored daily. Readings are recorded and compared to the baseline of the patient's personal best peak flow. If a reading is 60% below the patient's best, treatment should be adjusted. In the "green zone"—airflow is normal; in the "yellow zone"—usual airflow has decreased and routine medications should be increased; and in the "red zone"—rescue medications are needed and the health care provider should be notified. To properly use a peak flowmeter, instruct the patient to:

- Set the pointer to zero.
- While standing, take a deep breath.
- Put the mouthpiece in the mouth and clamp the lips firmly around it for a tight seal.
- Blow into the meter as hard and fast as possible.
- Record the value and reset the pointer.
- Rest for a couple of breaths.
- Repeat the procedure for a total of three readings.
- Record the highest reading on the peak flow sheet.

Oxygen is prescribed for moderate and severe hypoxemia. For acute episodes of hypoxemia, oxygen is given to raise the Sao_2 to 90 mm Hg or greater. Oxygen is used in patients with chronic obstructive disease who have consistent Pao_2 levels less than 55 to 59 mm Hg.

 Clinical Cues

When a patient has respiratory distress in an emergency situation, apply high-flow oxygen and monitor the saturation level with a pulse oximeter. **Observe and monitor continuously.** Immediately alert the RN and the physician. If there is a history of COPD, the oxygen rate should be changed, as ordered, to a lower flow of 1 to 3 liters per nasal cannula after the respiratory crisis has resolved.

Nursing Management and Rehabilitation

Rehabilitation and education of the patient and family are the chief long-term goals of nursing intervention. With proper home care, the patient with chronic lung disease can live longer and have a higher quality of life, reduce the number of hospitalizations and physician visits, and have fewer psychosocial problems related to inactivity and a feeling of hopelessness. This means working with the patient, identifying specific difficulties he is experiencing, assessing current ability to cope with them, and devising plans to accomplish specific goals for improvement. To prevent frequent hospitalizations for acute flare-ups of the disease, the patient should be taught how to avoid bronchial irritation and infection, and prevent such complications as right-sided heart failure (cor pulmonale).

It is very important for the family to be educated of the need for appropriate exercise and activity, and of the patient's natural desire for independence. Families may be overprotective because the episodes of dyspnea are very distressing.

Patient Teaching

Instructions for the Patient with Chronic Respiratory Disease

- To make mucus more liquid and easier to cough up, drink at least 2 and preferably 3 quarts of liquid every day.
- Normal sputum is white and slightly viscous and has no odor or taste. Changes in sputum should be reported to your health care provider.
- When you exert yourself, as in lifting something or getting up from your chair, exhale slowly through pursed lips. You should do the same thing when you are walking for exercise. It is natural to hold your breath during exertion, so you may need practice exhaling on exertion.
- Eat three or four small, balanced meals rather than one or two large ones each day.
- Practice your breathing exercises every day without fail.
- Try to avoid crowds during the flu and cold seasons.
- Do not take over-the-counter drugs. They can interact with your prescribed drugs. Antihistamines can dry out the mucus even more and make it more difficult for you to clear your air passages.
- Do not smoke or inhale the tobacco smoke of others.

Smoking Cessation. All patients should be encouraged to quit smoking; however, smoking cessation is critically important for those with asthma or COPD because quitting in the early stages of COPD can slow

Table 15-4 Commonly Prescribed Drugs for COPD and Asthma*

CLASSIFICATION	ACTION	NURSING IMPLICATIONS	PATIENT TEACHING
Bronchodilators			
Short-Acting Beta-Adrenergic Agonists			
Albuterol (Proventil, Ventolin) Pirbuterol (Maxair) Levalbuterol (Xopenex)	Stimulates beta-adrenergic receptors, producing bronchodilation. Increases ciliary action and mucus clearance. Selectively stimulates beta-adrenergic receptors, producing bronchodilation.	All may be administered by MDI. Some can be administered orally or by nebulizer. Monitor tachycardia, BP changes, nervousness, palpitations, muscle tremors, and dry mouth. May cause nausea, headache, insomnia, and hypokalemia. Acts in 5-10 min and lasts for 3-4 hr.	Should not be used in patients with cardiac disorders or angina. Increase fluid intake; watch for signs of potassium deficit. Wait 5 min before using a glucocorticoid inhaler (anti-inflammatory). Teach to use MDI correctly.
Long-Acting Beta-Adrenergic Agonists			
Salmeterol (Serevent) Formoterol (Foradil)	Relaxes bronchial smooth muscle, producing bronchodilation.	Monitor for tachycardia, muscle tremors, hypokalemia. Salmeterol should be combined with fluticasone (Advair). Formoterol should be combined with budesonide.	Not to be used for acute symptoms or exacerbations.
Methylxanthine Derivative			
Aminophylline (Theo-Dur, Slo-Bid, Uniphyl, Aerolate, Uni-Dur)	Relaxes bronchial smooth muscle, improves diaphragm contractility, increases ciliary action and mucus clearance, stimulates respiration and pulmonary vasodilation, improves exercise tolerance.	Administered orally or IV. CNS effects cause nervousness, irritability, headache, and insomnia. Causes tachycardia, BP changes, dysrhythmias, muscle twitching, flushing, anorexia, nausea and vomiting, epigastric pain, and diarrhea. Several drugs may increase theophylline levels. Monitor theophylline levels. (Therapeutic range is 10-20 mcg/mL.)	Length of drug action is decreased by smoking. Take with food to decrease GI effects. Lie down if dizziness occurs. Take medication regularly and only as prescribed. Teach to take pulse. Instruct not to use over-the-counter medications without checking with health care provider. Wear an ID bracelet stating asthmatic status. Check interactions with herbal products.
Anti-Inflammatory Agents†			
Beclomethasone (Vanceril, Beclovent) Triamcinolone (Azmacort) Flunisolide (AeroBid) Fluticasone (Flovent) Budesonide (Pulmicort) Ciclesonide (Alvesco) Mometasone (Asmanex)	Provides anti-inflammatory and immunosuppressive effect, decreasing edema in airways. Decreases mucus secretion.	All can be administered by MDI. Work synergistically with beta-adrenergic agonists. May affect potassium and glucose levels. Monitor weight. May mask infection. Monitor for edema. May have transient unpleasant taste.	Teach to carry ID indicating is a steroid user. Rinse mouth after each use of inhaler to prevent oral fungal infection. Do not discontinue use abruptly. Wash inhaler with warm water and dry after each use.
Cromolyn (Intal) Nedocromil (Tilade)	Stabilizes cell membranes possibly by inhibiting release of histamine and SRS-A by acting on mast cells.	Cromolyn nebulizer may be preferred for some patients if MDI is inadequate.	Therapeutic response may occur within 2 wk, but doctor may suggest a 4- to 6-wk trial. Some patients may experience a bad taste with nedocromil.

BP, blood pressure; *CNS,* central nervous system; *GI,* gastrointestinal; *IV,* intravenously; *MDI,* metered-dose inhaler; *OTC,* over the counter; *SRS-A,* slow-reacting substance of anaphylaxis.
*Many other drugs are also prescribed for asthma. †Systemic corticosteroids (hydrocortisone, methylprednisolone, or prednisone) may be administered orally or intravenously when severe or refractory asthma attacks occur.

Table 15-4 Commonly Prescribed Drugs for COPD and Asthma—cont'd

CLASSIFICATION	ACTION	NURSING IMPLICATIONS	PATIENT TEACHING
Anticholinergics			
Ipratropium (Atrovent)	Causes bronchodilation by blocking action of acetylcholine.	Do not mix with cromolyn sodium. Use cautiously in those with narrow-angle glaucoma, prostatic hypertrophy, or bladder neck obstruction.	Do not take more than two puffs at a time. Avoid excessive use of caffeine.
Ipratropium and albuterol (Combivent)	Causes bronchodilation by stimulating beta-adrenergic receptors, and blocking action of acetylcholine.		
Leukotriene Modifiers			
Zafirlukast (Accolate) Montelukast (Singulair)	Blocks action of leukotrienes in the lung once they are formed. Provides both bronchodilation and anti-inflammatory effects.	Administered orally. May cause headache, dizziness, nausea, vomiting, diarrhea, fatigue, or abdominal pain. Not to be used for acute asthma episodes.	Should take drug 1 hr before or 2 hr after meals daily. Increase fluid intake. Do not stop taking other asthma medications.
Leukotriene Inhibitor			
Zileuton (Zyflo)	Inhibits the synthesis of leukotrienes, providing bronchodilation and anti-inflammatory effect.	Administered orally. Monitor liver enzymes. May cause dizziness insomnia, dyspepsia, and abdominal pain. May interfere with warfarin (Coumadin) therapy and theophylline. Is not used to treat acute asthma attacks.	Check all medications and OTC drugs for ephedrine, which will increase stimulation. Teach to avoid alcohol. Notify health care provider of nausea, vomiting, anxiety, or insomnia. Continue to take even if symptom free.
Immunomodulators			
Omalizumab (Xolair) Subcutaneous injection	Decreases mast cell mediator release from allergen exposure.	Currently FDA is reviewing the possible association between omalizumab and an increased risk of heart attack, abnormal heart rhythm, heart failure, and stroke.	Subcutaneous dose is administered every 2-4 wk.
Mucolytic			
Acetylcysteine (Mucomyst)	Breaks down mucoproteins by enzyme action. Decreases viscosity and aids in mobilization of secretions.	Administered by nebulizer. Nausea and vomiting may occur. May cause bronchospasm or hemoptysis. Usually combined with bronchodilator. Monitor respirations.	Warn that secretions may become profuse. Teach that unpleasant odor will decrease with use. Discoloration of solution after bottle is opened does not impair its effectiveness.

the progression of the disease. After quitting smoking, pulmonary function gradually improves and after 10 to 20 years the chance of lung cancer is again equal to that of a nonsmoker. Explain the importance of smoking cessation to the patient and share

knowledge of community resources and the various programs designed to help people quit. There are nicotine patches, nicotine gum, nicotine nasal spray, and nicotine inhalers to help wean the patient off the addictive nicotine. Bupropion (Zyban) and varenicline tartrate (Chantix) are available by prescription and will help with smoking cessation. Chantix is taken for 12 weeks and has been shown to be effective; however, in 2008 the FDA issued a warning about Chantix: patients and family members should be alert for and report changes in mood or suicidal thoughts to their doctor.

Work with the patient to develop a plan that seems possible to achieve. Decreasing stress levels and improving coping techniques aid success for patients who are trying to quit smoking. Help patients to review what has helped or hindered past attempts to quit. Identify social settings that contribute to smoking, and explore substitute activities. Encourage patients to share their decision to quit with friends and family, and ask friends and family not to undermine the attempt to quit. Set a definite stop smoking date, and include specific ways to reach the goal. Exercise is a good distracter for the urge to use tobacco. A support group can be very helpful. Encouragement and praise for progress in quitting smoking are essential components of the treatment program. The American Lung Association has both literature and community programs directed to assist patients.

Psychosocial Care. The patient often needs help with adjustment to alterations in roles and lifestyle. He may have problems with self-esteem, body image, and sexuality that stem from his chronic disease. A trusting relationship between nurse and patient facilitates discussion of personal concerns and provides a means to explore possible solutions or adaptations for problems in these areas. Referral to community support groups also can be beneficial, as the patient then has an opportunity to see and hear how others in his situation have learned to cope and adapt.

Patient and Family Teaching. The teaching plan for the patient with an obstructive airway disease is extensive and includes:

- Management of medications and side effects
- Use of respiratory therapy measures and care of equipment
- Management of dyspnea
- Control of the immediate environment and avoidance of allergens
- Maintenance of nutrition
- Balancing exercise and adequate rest
- Awareness of signs of complications
- Need for close medical supervision

Education of the patient and family can be overwhelming; allow enough time for them to gain confidence in one aspect of care before introducing more information.

Most patients with chronic respiratory disease have difficulty getting sufficient rest and sleep because of dyspnea, anxiety, and decreased mobility. Sedatives and tranquilizers are contraindicated because they tend to depress respiration. Tension and anxiety often can be relieved if the patient is *taught* some relaxation techniques which can be learned, but it takes a bit of practice to use them whenever relaxation is needed (see Chapter 7). Simply telling him to relax or to stop worrying is not helpful; he is using almost every muscle in his body to struggle for breath or is extremely tense in anticipation of breathlessness. Some patients become very agitated and talkative. You should display a calm attitude, stay with the patient, hold his hand, and state, "Shh, we'll talk in a minute. Catch your breath first."

> **? Think Critically**
>
> Can you list five nursing interventions that might help your COPD patient avoid episodes of dyspnea?

LUNG CANCER

Etiology

Lung cancer is the leading cause of cancer deaths worldwide. In 2009 there were about 214,440 new cases of lung cancer and 159,390 deaths (American Cancer Society, 2010). Lung cancer is found most often in people 40 years of age or older. **Cigarette smoking is the primary cause (85%).** A person living with a smoker has twice the risk of lung cancer as someone not regularly exposed to smoke. Other risk factors are increasing air pollution, asbestos exposure, lung diseases such as TB and COPD, and radon exposure. About 15% of patients diagnosed with lung cancer survive more than 5 years (American Cancer Society, 2010).

Pathophysiology

Tumors arising from the bronchial epithelium are the most common lung malignancy. Squamous cell carcinoma and adenocarcinoma are both seen. Small cell or "oat" cell tumors grow rapidly and are often located near a major bronchus in the central part of the lung. Non–small cell tumors are usually found in the lung periphery and have undifferentiated cells that have slow growth and tend to metastasize.

Chronic irritation of the epithelial tissue in the lung causes changes in cell structure. This makes the tissue more vulnerable to the carcinogens and irritants inhaled when smoking. Dysplasia develops and the tumor grows. Common sites of metastases for cancer of the lung are the brain, bone, and liver.

Signs and Symptoms

At first there are few symptoms, usually only a cough and some wheezing. As the tumor grows larger, the patient may have some pain or discomfort in the chest, exertional dyspnea, and expectoration of blood-streaked sputum. More specific symptoms depend on the location and size of the malignant tumor and the areas to which it has metastasized. If, for example, the malignancy has involved the esophagus, there will be ulceration, bleeding, and dysphagia. Tumors pressing against the trachea can produce hoarseness and paralysis of the vocal cords. Fatigue, anorexia, and weight loss are common because lung cancer is usually advanced when discovered.

Diagnosis

Multiple tests are used to diagnose and stage lung cancer. These include chest x-ray; sputum cytology; low-dose computed tomography (CT); magnetic resonance imaging (MRI); cytology of specimens obtained by mediastinoscopy, bronchoscopy, or thoracentesis; fine-needle biopsy of the tumor; and video-assisted thoracoscopic surgery (VATS).

Treatment

Treatment is based on the type of cancer: small cell or non–small cell. It may be possible to remove the affected area of the lung by surgery if the malignancy is in its earliest stages and is localized. Surgical procedures include wedge resection, in which a small area of the lung is removed; segmental resection, which includes removal of lung tissue and surrounding blood vessels and bronchioles; lobectomy, with removal of an entire lobe of the lung; and **pneumonectomy**, in which an entire lung is removed. Lobectomy is the most common procedure used for small cell lung cancer. Radiation may be used before and after surgery; however, some types of lung cancers are radiation resistant. Small cell tumors respond dramatically to chemotherapy, but if the disease is extensive, the malignancy tends to recur because of metastasis that occurred before diagnosis. Four drugs are used in various combinations to treat small cell tumors: cyclophosphamide, doxorubicin, cisplatin, and etoposide. A drug once used to treat rheumatoid arthritis shows promise for some types of lung cancer. The drug aurothiomalate (ATM) is a targeted therapy that prevents normal cells from turning into cancerous tumor cells (American Lung Association, 2010c).

Non–small cell lung cancer is very aggressive and difficult to treat; unless caught in the very early stages, the prognosis for this cancer is not good. Combinations of one or two chemotherapy drugs, biotherapy agents, radiotherapy, and photodynamic therapy (PDT) are used, depending on the stage of the cancer and the symptoms of the patient. For PDT, the patient is given a drug that is taken up by the tumor cells, making them very sensitive to light and/or heat. The tumor is then exposed to a laser beam that destroys the malignant cells. The laser is introduced into the bronchi via a bronchoscope. Tumors in the main bronchi are particular targets for this type of therapy. In November 2004, the FDA approved the drug erlotinib (Tarceva) for types of non–small cell lung cancer that have not responded to other treatments. The drug seems to block tumor growth. In July 2009, the FDA approved pemetrexed (Alimta), the first drug available for maintenance therapy with advanced or metastatic lung cancer. The colon cancer drug bevacizumab (Avastin)—which acts to starve a tumor—was approved in 2006 for treating advanced lung cancer.

Nursing Management

Care of the patient undergoing thoracotomy for cancer of the lung follows later in the chapter. See Chapter 8 for nursing care of the patient with cancer. The nurse must educate the patient about tests and treatments; this may help to reduce the patient's and family's anxiety.

 Nutrition Considerations

Foods and Supplements that Offer Protection Against Lung Cancer

Research led by the National Cancer Institute (2010) indicates that leafy green vegetables, folate, and some multivitamins may offer some protective factors against lung cancer in current and former smokers.

PULMONARY VASCULAR DISORDERS

PULMONARY EMBOLISM

Etiology and Pathophysiology

Pulmonary embolism (PE) occurs when a pulmonary vessel is plugged with a mass or clot. Emboli can occur in solid, liquid, or gas forms and can occur from fracture of a long bone (fat embolus), from amniotic fluid during childbirth, from air introduced through a central line, and from clots formed elsewhere in the body (such as from a deep venous thrombosis or thrombi that form in the heart when the patient has dysrhythmias). Regardless of the origin of the embolus, there is interference with blood flow in the lung distal to the point where the embolus lodges. The obstruction causes shunting and blood flows past the alveoli without receiving oxygen or without giving up carbon dioxide. The consequences of pulmonary embolism can be minor or life threatening.

The elderly are especially prone to developing deep venous thrombosis (DVT) when they are immobilized from surgery or for a major illness. Many elderly patients can have atrial fibrillation, which when uncontrolled, is a direct cause of pulmonary emboli. The discovery of a new irregularity of heartbeat should be promptly reported to the physician. Long airplane flights, and sitting for long periods with the legs crossed, are other potential causes of DVT.

Signs and Symptoms

Symptoms depend on the size and location of the clot in the lung and whether it is one clot or multiple small clots. The general symptoms are respiratory distress with dyspnea, chest pain, cough, hemoptysis, and anxiety. Hypotension, tachycardia, or confusion may occur. A sudden onset of dyspnea in a patient at risk of thrombus formation is very suggestive of PE.

Diagnosis

Diagnosis is made by ruling out other problems, such as heart failure, and by tests to support a diagnosis of pulmonary embolus. The Institute for Clinical Symptoms Improvement (ICSI) (2010) offers guidelines. First, a clinical pretest probability score should be determined, based on presence of symptoms and risk factors. Plasma D-dimer testing is recommended when a PE is initially suspected (see Table 13-3). Computed tomographic pulmonary angiography is ordered (unless contraindicated—in which case a ventilation/perfusion scan is performed). Other tests include a chest radiograph, an echocardiogram, arterial blood gases (ABGs), and an electrocardiogram (ECG).

Treatment

Oxygen therapy is initiated to decrease hypoxia. Treatment depends on the size and location of the embolus. Intravenous heparin is usually begun and continued for 7 to 10 days. Warfarin (Coumadin) is initiated several days before discharge and is continued at home for up to 1 year. Some physicians are performing trials with thrombolytic (dissolves thrombi) therapy using streptokinase, urokinase, or tissue plasminogen activator. There is concern about whether the benefits of decomposing the clot outweigh the risk of bleeding complications. Pulmonary embolectomy is a last resort because the surgery carries a high mortality rate. An intracaval filter may be placed in the vena cava to prevent clots from traveling to the lungs in the future.

Nursing Management

Initial care for the patient who might be experiencing a PE is to remain calm, stay with the patient, raise the head of the bed to a high Fowler's position, begin low-flow oxygen therapy, assess vital signs, notify the physician of the patient's symptoms, start a peripheral IV and administer heparin when it is ordered. Prepare the patient for the diagnostic tests and for probable treatment. The patient is kept on bed rest in semi-Fowler's position initially, but turning, deep breathing, and coughing are important to prevent atelectasis.

PRIMARY PULMONARY HYPERTENSION

Pulmonary hypertension is elevated pressure in the pulmonary artery. It is rare as a primary disease, but has occurred after taking the appetite suppressant fenfluramine (Fen-Phen), which was removed from the market in 1996. The classic symptoms are dyspnea and fatigue. Other symptoms are chest pain with exertion, dizziness, and syncope. The disorder eventually causes right-sided heart enlargement (cor pulmonale), followed by heart failure.

There is no cure for primary pulmonary hypertension, but treatment can improve or relieve symptoms and increase the quality and length of life. Diuretics and anticoagulant therapy are used to reduce right ventricular overload and prevent thrombus formation and thrombosis. Calcium channel blockers may be used for their vasodilating effects. Epoprostenol (Flolan) promotes pulmonary vasodilation, but it must be continuously administered through a central IV line, and extensive education for the patient and family is necessary. Bosentan (Tracleer) and the new drug ambrisentan (Letairis) are oral forms of epoprostenol. An inhaled form is under investigation. A new drug, sildenafil citrate (Revatio), improves exercise tolerance, but must be used with caution as it can result in myocardial infarction or dysrhythmia. Research is also being conducted on the use of serotonin reuptake inhibitors to combat pulmonary hypertension. Lung transplantation is reserved for those pulmonary hypertension patients who do not respond to epoprostenol and who progress to severe right-sided heart failure.

LUNG TRANSPLANTATION

Lung transplantation is a viable option for a variety of end-stage lung diseases. Options include single lung, bilateral lung, and heart-lung transplantation. Patients must undergo extensive evaluation and psychological counseling, and meet stringent criteria. There must be no history of malignancy within 2 years, no presence of HIV, and no renal or liver impairment. The average wait for a suitable organ is 1 year. The most common cause of death after lung transplantation is infection, which often occurs within 4 to 6 weeks. Cytomegalovirus is the primary offender. Immunosuppressive therapy is lifelong to prevent organ rejection. After transplantation and stabilization, patients enter a rehabilitation program to improve physical endurance.

CHEST INJURIES

The major complications of chest trauma involve either the lungs and air passages or the heart and major blood vessels and the victim can rapidly deteriorate. Major concerns in the care of patients with chest injuries are:
- Maintenance of an airway
- Assurance of adequate ventilation
- Treatment of circulatory problems to ensure circulation of oxygenated blood

(See Chapter 45 for additional information about chest trauma.)

● PNEUMOTHORAX AND HEMOTHORAX

Pneumothorax and hemothorax frequently occur as a result of a blunt (nonpenetrating) or penetrating injury to the chest wall. These conditions can cause partial or total collapse of one or both lungs. The space within the pleural membranes is an airtight compartment with *negative pressure*. This negative pressure allows for the tidal movement of air in and out of the lungs. If, however, there is a break in the airtight compartment—either along the surface of the lung or from outside the pleural sac—air rushes in and collapses the lung. **Pneumothorax is a threat in chest injury, as well as in the period following chest surgery.** However, the

FIGURE 15-3 Insertion of a thoracostomy tube (chest tube).

condition also can occur spontaneously when there is a rupture of the alveoli. This is called spontaneous pneumothorax. Tall, thin people are more prone to spontaneous pneumothorax. Cases have occurred after scuba diving, flying, or mountain climbing.

A pneumothorax may require nothing more than rest and the administration of oxygen to relieve discomfort. If the amount of air in the pleural space is minimal, a large-bore needle may be used to aspirate it. For greater amounts of air or fluid, a thoracostomy tube (chest tube) may be inserted and connected to water-seal drainage to remove the air and allow reexpansion of the lung (Figure 15-3).

Hemothorax is the presence of blood within the pleural cavity due to laceration of the lung, heart, or blood vessels within the thorax. The accumulation of blood in the pleural cavity can cause partial or total collapse of the lung. There also is the possibility of mediastinal shift in hemothorax and the likelihood of impaired venous return in the pulmonary blood vessels. The blood is removed with a thoracostomy tube and chest drainage.

For a patient with pneumothorax, hemothorax, or a combination of the two—hemopneumothorax (Figure 15-4)—assess for a history of acute or chronic respiratory disease, accidental injury to the chest, or chest surgery. The patient may complain of sudden chest pain or a feeling of tightness in the chest. There is an increase in both pulse rate and rate of respirations, a drop in blood pressure, and the absence of normal chest movements and absent or diminished breath sounds on the affected side.

? Think Critically

You come upon an automobile accident and stop to assist. You have your stethoscope in your car. Name three assessment criteria that would lead you to believe that the driver of the vehicle has suffered a pneumothorax.

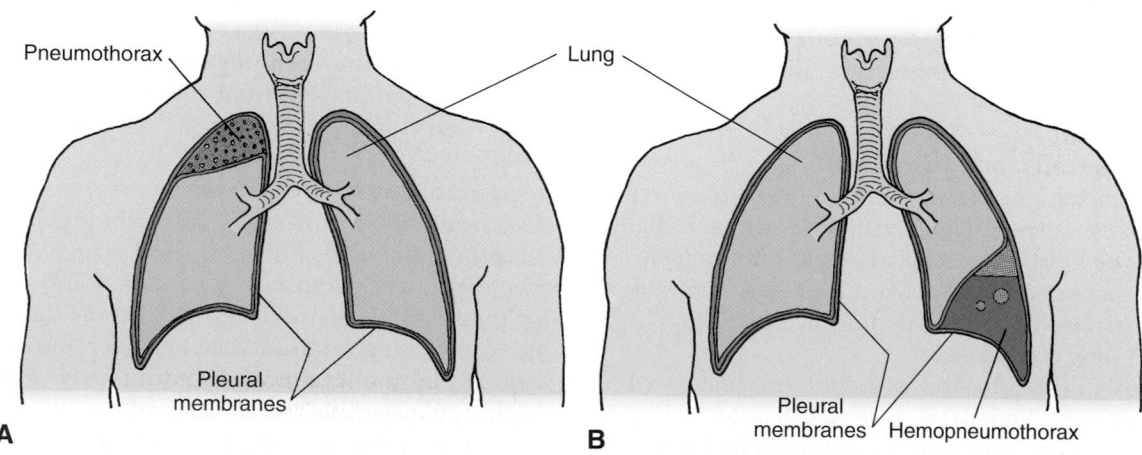

FIGURE 15-4 A, Pneumothorax. **B,** Hemothorax.

LUNG DISORDERS

PULMONARY EDEMA

Pulmonary edema is an abnormal collection of fluid in the interstitial spaces of the lung and inside the alveoli. Acute pulmonary edema is a medical emergency. Congestive heart failure is a major cause of pulmonary edema. Signs and symptoms include severe dyspnea, orthopnea, noisy respirations, pink frothy sputum, crackles heard on auscultation in the bases of the lungs extending upward, abnormal blood gases, restlessness, and possibly confusion. The patient will be very anxious and pale with cold, clammy skin. Diagnosis is based on ruling out other disorders, such as pneumonia, asthma, or pulmonary embolism, and on determining the cause. Treatment depends on whether the edema is a result of heart problems or from another cause. (See Adult [Acute] Respiratory Distress Syndrome below.)

Nursing care involves placing the patient in high Fowler's position. Oxygen is started immediately and continuous positive airway pressure (CPAP) may be necessary. Sodium and fluids are restricted. Furosemide is given for fluid diuresis and morphine reduces anxiety and the workload on the heart. Drugs for the underlying heart disorder also are administered. The nurse must closely monitor intake and output, and perform continuous respiratory and cardiac assessment to evaluate the effectiveness of treatment.

ADULT (ACUTE) RESPIRATORY DISTRESS SYNDROME

Etiology and Pathophysiology

Adult (acute) respiratory distress syndrome (ARDS) is a form of pulmonary edema that results from pulmonary changes that occur with sepsis, major trauma, major surgery, or any critical illness. When the alveolar capillary membrane is injured, it becomes more permeable to intravascular fluid. Alveoli fill with fluid, and oxygen and carbon dioxide cannot cross the membrane into and out of the capillaries. Pulmonary edema and lung stiffness occur, resulting in severe hypoxemia. ARDS is particularly dangerous when a patient has multisystem disorders; the mortality rate in these patients is 50% to 90%.

Signs, Symptoms, and Diagnosis

Dyspnea, tachypnea, cough, and restlessness occur. Auscultation may reveal fine, scattered crackles. Initially there may be mild hypoxemia and respiratory alkalosis from the tachypnea. As ARDS progresses, symptoms worsen, because of increased fluid accumulation and decreased lung compliance.

Diagnosis is by physical presentation, history of a disorder or event known to cause ARDS, arterial blood gas determination, and chest radiograph. **The hallmark for diagnosis is a Pao_2 below 70 mm Hg even with 100% oxygen delivery.** There is diffuse fluid and exudate infiltration that gives a "whiteout" appearance to lung radiographs.

Treatment and Nursing Management

Treatment for ARDS is ventilatory support with positive end-expiratory pressure (PEEP), treatment of the underlying disorder, careful fluid and electrolyte management, and total care for basic needs. Antibiotics, bronchodilators, and corticosteroids may also be necessary.

Complementary and Alternative Therapies

Adult (Acute) Respiratory Distress Syndrome (ARDS)

A nutritional supplement composed of borage seed oil, fish oil, protein, carbohydrates, and antioxidants was associated with a 35% reduction in mortality rate in patients with ARDS. The supplement is administered by enteral tube. Gamma-linolenic acid, a component of the borage seed oil, is thought to reduce inflammation and improve oxygen flow (Kaniecki, 2011).

Parenteral nutrition may be started to maintain nutritional status. The prone position may allow fluid to shift from the dorsal aspects, enabling undamaged alveoli to fill with oxygenated air, thereby decreasing hypoxemia. However, the efficacy of the prone position in lowering the risk of death has been challenged (Taccone et al., 2009). An intervention protocol for the prone position is currently under review (Bloomfield et al., 2009).

RESPIRATORY FAILURE

Respiratory failure is the result of insufficient oxygen or excessive carbon dioxide. **It has occurred when the Pao_2 is less than 60 mm Hg** (*despite supplemental oxygen*) **and the partial pressure of carbon dioxide (Pco_2) is more than 50 mm Hg.** There will be a high level of $Paco_2$, a high bicarbonate (HCO_3^-) level, and a low pH (acidosis) if the condition has been present for several days.

Hypoxemic respiratory failure can occur when insufficient oxygen passes from the alveoli to the capillaries. For example in pneumonia or with a massive pulmonary embolism, fluid fills the alveoli and interferes with gas exchange at the alveoli-capillary interface.

Hypercapnia (also called *hypercarbia*) is the result of hypoventilation, during which the usual amount of carbon dioxide is not eliminated by exhalation. Carbon dioxide is a respiratory stimulant and the normal response to excessive levels of carbon dioxide is an increase in respiratory rate. If, however, the respiratory centers in the brain are continuously exposed to higher-than-normal levels of carbon dioxide, as in COPD, they become less reactive, and a drop in the respiratory rate occurs. Indiscriminate use of sedatives and narcotics for COPD patients may also lead to respiratory depression.

Signs and symptoms of respiratory failure include restlessness, agitation or confusion. An increase in respiratory rate, pulse, and blood pressure signals a physiologic attempt to compensate for inadequate oxygenation. The patient may sit upright and bend forward and be unable to speak without pausing for breath. Diaphoresis and retraction of accessory respiratory muscles occurs as the work of breathing increases. Cyanosis is a late sign of hypoxemia that manifests at Pao_2 of ≥ 45 mm Hg. When patients retain excessive carbon dioxide, the respiratory rate may slow down. The final outcome can be cardiac arrest from respiratory acidosis.

Safety Alert

Recognition and Response to Changes in Patient Condition

An essential National Patient Safety Goal is to improve the recognition and response to changes in patient condition. Particularly for patients who are at risk for retaining carbon dioxide, do not assume that lethargy and drowsiness are secondary to the patient's having a "restless, sleepless night." Assess breathing patterns and respiratory rate and carefully compare the current mental status to baseline. Notify the physician if you suspect respiratory failure, and obtain an order for arterial blood gases.

Respiratory failure is treated with oxygen and respiratory therapy, including mechanical ventilation, measures to reduce and remove secretions, drugs to reduce bronchospasm and airway inflammation, and correction of acidosis. Treatment of the underlying cause is also necessary.

By vigilant observation and assessment of patients with respiratory problems and close attention to turning, deep breathing and coughing, the nurse can often prevent respiratory failure. Nursing measures are incorporated to relieve anxiety and agitation. Monitoring fluid balance is particularly important when there is concurrent heart or multiorgan failure.

COMMON THERAPEUTIC MEASURES

INTRATHORACIC SURGERY

Intrathoracic surgery requires opening the chest wall and entering the pleural cavity. For example, in addition to resection of lung tissue and other pulmonary structures, intrathoracic surgery also is necessary to repair the heart and great vessels or defects of the esophagus.

Today, video-assisted thoracoscopic surgery (VATS) is replacing the standard thoracotomy (incision with entry into the thorax) (Mayo Clinic, 2010). About 70% of thoracic procedures can be performed in this manner, including pulmonary resections, biopsy or

resection of mediastinal tumors or masses, and drainage of pleural effusions. An endoscope (equipped with a multichip mini-camera and intense lighting) magnifies the image of the cavity and its structures and transmits images to a video monitor. Instruments can be guided through the endoscope to biopsy or remove tissue and to place surgical staples. One to four 1-inch incisions are used to accommodate the endoscope, instruments, and suction.

Preoperative Care

Assessment of the patient's respiratory status before chest surgery depends on whether the surgery is elective or for accidental trauma. If there is time, a health history as well as subjective and objective assessment data should be obtained before the surgery (see Chapter 13).

Preoperatively, efforts are made to improve the respiratory status of the patient as much as possible. Special exercises may be prescribed to strengthen the chest, shoulder and accessory muscles of respiration and to remove accumulated secretions from the air passages.

When standard thoracotomy is to be performed, arm and leg exercises are taught preoperatively to avoid thrombophlebitis and problems with movement. Movement of the arm may be very painful, because of positioning during surgery, or the surgical involvement of muscles that control the arm. "Frozen" (immobile) shoulder can occur if the arm is not exercised. With VATS, this complication is less likely to occur.

Preoperative patient education focuses on teaching information to improve lung ventilation and to prepare for equipment such as chest tubes, suctioning, mechanical ventilation, and use of an incentive spirometer.

Postoperative Care

During the immediate postoperative period, nursing assessment and intervention focus on routine positioning, turning, coughing and deep breathing; procedure-specific observations; and attention to chest tubes and the closed drainage system. The patient with chest surgery usually must ambulate early. An advantage of VATS is that the patient is out of bed and into a chair within 4 to 6 hours of surgery; pain is less. The standard thoracotomy patient has a 4- to 6-week recovery, whereas the VATS patient resumes activities of daily living in 3 to 4 days and can even return to work within 1 week.

Special observations include watching for signs of pneumothorax, hemothorax, or both; observing for symptoms of respiratory distress; and auscultation and palpation of the upper chest and neck for swelling caused by subcutaneous emphysema (an accumulation of air or gas under the skin, which feels like bubble wrap on palpation). Subcutaneous emphysema can occur when air leaks into the tissues around chest tubes. It could be a sign of malfunctioning of the drainage system and should be reported. Inspecting the drainage system for air leakage is essential. Assessing for signs of infection, both respiratory and incisional, is also a nursing responsibility.

Gastric distention and paralytic ileus are possible complications of standard thoracic surgery. **Distention of the stomach and intestines is particularly hazardous for the post-thoracotomy patient, as distention can cause these organs to push up on the diaphragm and impair ventilation, which is already severely compromised by the surgery.**

Positioning for comfort, optimal ventilation, and adequate drainage of the operative site is important during post-thoracotomy care. In most cases the patient is allowed to lie on his back and operative side. Many surgeons do not permit lying on the unaffected side because this position diminishes the expansion of the good lung. When the patient has a tube inserted for drainage from the operative site, lying on the operative side facilitates the flow of drainage. Care must be taken when positioning the patient to prevent kinking the chest tubes.

A pneumonectomy patient is never turned onto his unoperated side, because tension pneumothorax and mediastinal shift could occur, or the bronchial stump where the lung was removed could leak and the patient could drown in accumulated fluid. For patients who have had chest surgery, it is always best to check the physician's orders before turning the patient or raising the head of the bed.

Care of Patients with Chest Tubes and Closed Drainage.

Monitor the patient who has a chest tube regularly and frequently. There are three major areas of assessment:

- The respiratory status of the patient
- The site at which the tube is inserted into the chest and the length of the tube (for kinks)
- The amount and character of the drainage in the collection chamber

The patient is assessed for ease of breathing, pain or discomfort, level of consciousness and orientation, and anxiety and restlessness. The rate and character of respirations are noted, as are breath sounds. The entry site is assessed for unusual drainage, infection, integrity of sutures, and the presence of subcutaneous emphysema.

The chest tube will be attached to a drainage system. Commercial disposable plastic water-seal drainage systems are the most common. The drainage system should (1) provide for drainage of air and blood from within the pleural cavity and (2) allow for gradual reexpansion of the lung (Figure 15-5). Figure 15-6 shows a disposable system. Note that the water in the left-hand chamber serves as a seal to prevent air from entering into the chest cavity. This chamber

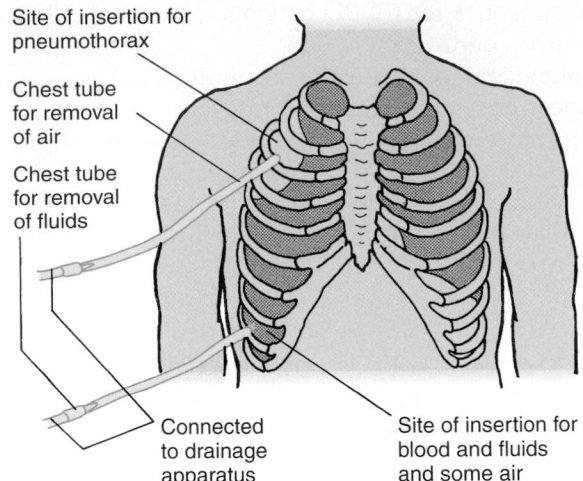

FIGURE 15-5 Location of sites for insertion of chest tubes for drainage of air and fluids.

FIGURE 15-6 Disposable water-seal drainage system; note the three chambers.

should not have bubbles, except when the suction is first turned on; the water level should fluctuate with breathing. The collection chamber—located on the far right of the device—is calibrated for more accurate measurement of drainage from the chest. It also contains float valves, which prevent the entry of air or fluid back up into the chest. Suction can be attached to the device to better facilitate removal of air and secretions from the lung. Gentle bubbling in this chamber will be continuous.

When caring for a patient with a three-chamber closed drainage system, the following precautions should be kept in mind:

- Remember that the pleural cavity is an airtight compartment. The apparatus and all connections must remain airtight at all times; all connections should be taped.
- Do not allow the tubing to become kinked or obstructed by the weight of the patient.
- Never pin the tubing to the bedclothes.
- Do not empty thoracotomy drainage containers. The system must remain closed. Replace the unit when the drainage chamber is full.
- The system operates by gravity and must remain below the patient's chest level at all times.
- Alert the surgeon if drainage exceeds 100 mL/hr (except for first 3 hours postoperatively).
- If the chest tube becomes unattached do not clamp the tube; place the end of the tubing in a cup of sterile water. This creates a "water seal" and can prevent tension pneumothorax. Temporary clamping may be performed by the surgeon to assess lung function or occasionally by the RN to check for the source of air leaks.
- Persistent bubbling in the water seal chamber indicates an air leak. Fluid in the chamber *should* fluctuate with inhalation and exhalation. Occasional bubbles may appear with breathing, sneezing, or coughing. If a pneumothorax is present, bubbling will occur with inspiration, as air is forced out of the area of the pneumothorax.
- A "puffed-up" appearance of the patient's chest or neck could be subcutaneous emphysema.
- Dressings may be reinforced but are not changed except by order of the surgeon.

There are other drainage systems that you might see such as bottle systems with one, two, or three bottles. In other systems, a flutter valve, or Heimlich valve, may be substituted in chest drainage systems. This valve permits the flow of air and fluid from the pleural space into a collection area, but prevents the return flow of air or fluid; the Heimlich valve is inserted between the chest tube and the drainage collection apparatus.

Ambulatory patients may be using a small portable chest drainage system that has only one chamber with a dry seal and does not contain water. The system is used for certain patients who have less than 500 mL of drainage daily. The collection chamber must be emptied when full. Two other devices, the Pneumostat and the Pleurx pleural catheter, are available for chest drainage for the home care patient. Each comes with specific care directions.

A dry-suction system is sometimes used in place of water-seal suction. It provides more consistent flow because the suction adjusts automatically to changes in the patient's pleural pressure or to fluctuations in wall suction pressure. The regulator within the unit is preset to -20 cm H_2O, but can be changed to range from -10 to -40 cm H_2O.

Specialized chest drainage systems are used to collect the patient's blood from the chest after surgery so that it can be reinfused in an autologous transfusion.

 Think Critically

Your patient is 1 day postoperative. What would you do if the fluid in the drainage chamber of the closed-chest drainage system had not increased over the past 4 hours?

The patient should be medicated 30 to 60 minutes before the removal of a chest tube. When the surgeon removes the chest tubes, the incision is covered with a dressing containing sterile petroleum jelly to close off the opening so that air does not enter the pleural space. This type of dressing is also applied if a chest tube is accidentally pulled out. Auscultate the lungs after chest tube removal to verify that a pneumothorax has not occurred. Eventually the incision will seal itself. A sample plan with interventions for a patient having thoracic surgery is shown in Nursing Care Plan 15-1.

 Think Critically

What would you do if you went to assess your first-day postoperative standard thoracotomy patient and the water in the closed drainage system was not fluctuating with the patient's breathing?

MEDICATION ADMINISTRATION

Bronchodilators are drugs that directly act on and relax the smooth muscle of the bronchi and thereby relieve bronchospasms. Box 15-2 lists general nursing implications for these drugs. Liquefying agents help to thin the bronchial secretions, making them less tenacious. Anti-infective agents include the tetracyclines, penicillin, cephalosporins, macrolides (clarithromycin [Biaxin]), fluoroquinolones (ciprofloxacin [Cipro]), and the sulfa drugs.

Corticosteroids are a major part of inhalation therapy for patients with chronic obstructive pulmonary disease. Acute respiratory problems are sometimes treated with oral corticosteroids. When corticosteroids are prescribed, the nurse and patient must be aware that steroids may mask infection. Steroids should not be abruptly discontinued; these drugs must be slowly tapered over several days. Potassium loss must be replaced and blood glucose is closely monitored for elevation.

⭐ Nursing Care Plan 15-1   Care of the Patient with Lung Cancer

Scenario
A 62-year-old female smoker with a diagnosis of early lung cancer is scheduled for a right thoracotomy and lobectomy. She has no other medical problems except mild arthritis, for which she occasionally takes aspirin.

Preoperative Problem/Nursing Diagnosis
Unfamiliar with surgery/Deficient knowledge related to postoperative care for thoracotomy.

Supporting Assessment Data
Subjective: "I've never had surgery before."

Goals/Expected Outcomes	Nursing Interventions	Selected Rationale	Evaluation
Patient will verbalize understanding of postoperative routine of frequent monitoring of vital signs, chest tube care, and respiratory treatments.	Explain purpose and show tubes, drainage apparatus, and oxygen equipment. Explain need for early ambulation. Describe methods of pain control.	Being familiar with equipment and what to expect after surgery decreases fear of the unknown.	Verbalizes understanding of what equipment is for. Says will try to ambulate this afternoon. States understanding of PCA pump for pain control. Outcomes met.
Patient will demonstrate use of spirometer and coughing and deep-breathing exercises.	Teach deep breathing, coughing, use of incentive spirometer, obtain return demonstration.	Learning the techniques before surgery facilitates postoperative performance.	Uses spirometer correctly and is able to demonstrate coughing and deep breathing.
Patient will be mobile and active after the surgery to prevent postoperative complications before discharge.	Teach leg exercises; flex and extend ankles and knees, circular rotation of ankles and gluteal tightening. Ambulate in the hall to determine preoperative abilities.	Teaching before surgery empowers patient and provides time to practice techniques and ask questions. Ambulating before surgery gives baseline information.	Is practicing leg exercises enthusiastically. "Hope I can keep this up after surgery." Ambulates independently in hall with steady gait. Easily walks full length of unit without distress.

Postoperative Problem/Nursing Diagnosis
Excision of lobe of lung/Risk of impaired gas exchange related to surgical removal of portion of lung and possible complications.

Supporting Assessment Data
Objective: Thoracotomy and lobectomy.

Goals/Expected Outcomes	Nursing Interventions	Selected Rationale	Evaluation
Patient will display normal respiratory rate and normal blood gas exchange before discharge.	Position on back or operative side; turn, cough, deep breathe and use incentive spirometer q 2 hr; splint incision with small pillow to minimize pain. Administer humidified oxygen as ordered. Monitor vital signs and respiratory effort, and auscultate lung fields q 4 hr; monitor blood gas levels. Pulse oximetry readings q 1 hr.	Position allows good lung to fully expand. Incentive spirometer use opens alveoli, promoting better gas exchange and prevents atelectasis. Oxygen saturation should be maintained. Respiratory rate, lung sounds, blood gas levels, and pulse oximetry readings provide data regarding respiratory status and can indicate decline or improvement.	Assisted to turn q 2 hr; using spirometer and coughing q 2 hr. Splints incision when coughing. Receiving humidified oxygen at 3L via nasal cannula. BP 134/82, P 85, RR 28/min. Left lung with normal breath sounds; right lung with diminished sounds in bases and absent over middle lobe area. Sao₂ 95% average.

BP, blood pressure; *CBC,* complete blood count; *IV,* intravenous; *P,* pulse; *PCA,* patient-controlled analgesia; *RR,* respirations; *Sao₂,* oxygen saturation; *SOB,* shortness of breath; *WBC,* white blood cell.

Goals/Expected Outcomes	Nursing Interventions	Selected Rationale	Evaluation
Patient will display normal respiratory rate and normal blood gas exchange before discharge.—cont'd	Encourage use of PCA to promote better cooperation with respiratory therapy, coughing, and deep breathing, but avoid oversedation and respiratory depression.	If pain is minimized, patient is able to more fully expand the lungs and to perform coughing and deep-breathing exercises.	Using PCA appropriately; pain at 4 on a scale of 1-10.
	Maintain intact, functioning closed-chest water-seal drainage system. Observe for signs of subcutaneous emphysema; assess for signs of pulmonary embolism.	Intact system prevents air from entering pleural space and collapsing lung.	Chest drainage system intact with 150 mL drainage. No subcutaneous emphysema; no signs of respiratory distress (i.e., labored, uneven respirations, no subjective SOB).
	Monitor abdomen for signs of distention or ileus.	Distention can cause pressure on diaphragm and, decrease lung expansion.	Abdomen soft and nondistended.

Postoperative Problem/Nursing Diagnosis

Surgical incision/Risk for infection related to surgical incision and chest tubes.

Supporting Assessment Data

Objective: Thoracotomy and lobectomy; chest tube in place.

Goals/Expected Outcomes	Nursing Interventions	Selected Rationale	Evaluation
No signs of infection as evidenced by clean incision, temperature in normal range, normal WBC count, and clear breath sounds during hospitalization.	Use aseptic technique for dressing changes and care of chest tube.	Prevents introduction of pathogenic organisms.	Very small amount of pink-tinged drainage on old dressing. Dressing changed, as ordered, with aseptic technique. Incision intact.
	Assess temperature trends q 24 hr; monitor WBC count. Observe wound for signs of infection.	Provides data that might indicate beginning infection.	Temp 99.4° F (37.4° C) CBC results pending. No redness, swelling, or pain to surrounding tissues. Dressing dry and intact.
	Protect from people with infections.	Helps prevent exposure to respiratory infection.	Note placed on door advising visitors, who may have infection, to check with nurses before entering.
	Maintain adequate nutrition and fluid intake.	Adequate fluid and nutrition are required for healing.	Taking clear liquids. IV line patent at 125 mL/hr.
	Auscultate lungs each shift and as needed for changes in respiratory status.	Auscultating at the beginning of the shift establishes baseline for comparison.	Breath sounds clear, but diminished in bases and absent over right middle lobe.
	Administer antibiotics as ordered.	Antibiotics may be ordered prophylactically because of weakened immune system.	Antibiotics are en route from the pharmacy, will be administered as soon as available. Continue plan.

Nursing Care Plan 15-1   Care of the Patient with Lung Cancer—cont'd

Problem/Nursing Diagnosis
Worry over diagnosis and treatment/Anxiety related to diagnosis of cancer of the lung, treatment, and prognosis.

Supporting Assessment Data
Subjective: "I'm scared. I don't want to die of cancer. Will I have to have chemotherapy? Will there be a lot of pain?"
Objective: Anxious look on face.

Goals/Expected Outcomes	Nursing Interventions	Selected Rationale	Evaluation
Patient will be less anxious about treatment and disease process by discharge.	Establish trusting relationship; use active listening. Encourage verbalization of fears and concerns, answer questions honestly. Engender hope; discuss what patient can do to optimize chances of survival: quit smoking, exercise program, diet, relaxation techniques, stress reduction. Advise that oncologist will discuss modes of treatment when pathology report is completed. Type of tumor, growth, and aggressiveness dictate treatment. Assure that pain control is possible.	A trusting relationship promotes sharing of feelings and fears. Hope allows patient to focus on the future. Active participation in her own survival is empowering and increases feelings of control over the disease. Giving correct information and explaining why more information is not immediately available helps to decrease anxiety. Fear of pain and uncertainty about ability to withstand pain is a major source of anxiety.	Using active listening, but patient is not verbalizing details. Reminded that many people have lived for many years after having lung cancer. Discussed aids for quitting smoking. Not willing to try relaxation exercise yet. Advised that oncologist would be in tomorrow morning to talk about options. States that she would like to have her family present for that discussion. Visibly relieved when reassured about pain management. Continue plan.

Critical Thinking Questions
1. Why should this patient not be positioned on the nonoperative side after surgery?
2. What would you do if you noticed that the amount of drainage in the disposable water-seal chest drainage system was not increasing?

Antihistamines are used to treat respiratory symptoms of an allergic disorder. They reduce the secretions of the nasal and bronchial mucosa. Decongestants are prescribed for symptoms of the common cold and sinusitis. Leukotriene inhibitors are the newest addition to the treatment for asthma. They help control symptoms by blocking the activity of those substances that mediate inflammation.

Metered-dose inhalers (MDIs) are used to deliver a variety of drugs to the respiratory patient. The patient should be taught to use an MDI properly. Bronchodilators, liquefying agents, and some anti-infective agents may be administered directly onto the mucous membranes of the respiratory tract by a nebulizer (device producing a fine spray) and mechanical ventilator.

HUMIDIFICATION

Aerosols are fine suspensions of very small particles of a liquid or solid that constitute a gas. Without adequate water and humidity, mucous secretions become extremely thick and tenacious, and the mucous membranes become dry, crusted, irritated and more susceptible to invasion by pathogenic microorganisms. Aerosols include a variety of bronchodilation or mucolytic drugs (see Table 15-4).

The four general purposes of aerosol and humidity therapy are:
1. Relief of edema and spasms of the bronchi
2. Liquefaction of bronchial secretions
3. Delivery of medication
4. Humidification of the respiratory mucosa

Aerosols are delivered by a nebulizer via face mask, face tent, or tracheostomy collar. Most aerosols are produced in a jet nebulizer in which a high-velocity gas shatters the liquid into small aerosol particles. Hand-held nebulizers are available for use at home. In the hospital, the nebulizer is attached to oxygen so that hypoxemia can be treated as medication is being administered. Nebulizer treatments are usually 20 to 30 minutes long and are given two, three, or four times a day.

The patient is taught to breathe through the mouth during the treatment. He should sit in a comfortable

Box 15-2   General Nursing Implications for the Administration of Bronchodilators

When giving a bronchodilator drug, you should:

- Follow the standard procedures for checking identification of patient, using the "five rights" verifying allergies, and monitoring for side effects and drug interactions.
- Auscultate the lungs to ascertain the types of lung sounds present.
- Take pulse and count respirations to establish ranges, before drug administration.
- Use these drugs cautiously in patients with cardiac disease, as they affect heart action.
- Consult the physician before administering a bronchodilator to a patient who has a current cardiac dysrhythmia.
- Give each dose of the drug as close to the ordered time as possible, in order to maintain a steady blood level of the drug.
- When the patient is taking theophylline, check drug serum levels; the therapeutic range is 10 to 20 mcg/mL. Withhold drug if the level is above 20 mcg/mL and notify the physician.
- Warn elderly patients that bronchodilators may cause dizziness and to take precautions when changing positions.

- Monitor the patient for effectiveness of the drug by performing a respiratory assessment.

Regarding possible side effects or adverse effects of the drug, you should:

- Warn the patient about the possibility of paradoxical bronchospasm and advise him to consult the physician if this happens before administering another dose.
- Tell the patient to chew sugarless gum or suck on hard candy to relieve dry mouth.
- Monitor the patient for specific side effects of each drug; general side effects of bronchodilators are dry mouth, insomnia, nervousness, dizziness, palpitations, gastrointestinal upset, and changes in blood pressure.

You should teach the patient taking a bronchodilator drug to:

- Take the drug with a full glass of water; if it causes gastrointestinal upset, take the drug with a meal.
- Take the drug 15 to 60 minutes before exercising (check specific time for individual drug as time depends on form of the drug [i.e., inhalant or oral tablet]).
- Follow correct procedure for inhaling the drug: shake the inhaler gently before using, clear the nose and throat, take a deep breath, relax, and completely exhale before inhaling drug.

Adapted from Lewis, S.L., Heitkemper, M.M., Dirksen, S.R., et al. (2011). *Medical-Surgical Nursing: Assessment and Management of Clinical Problems* (8th ed.). St. Louis: Mosby.

---

chair. Halfway through the treatment and after the treatment, deep breathing and coughing are performed to raise loose mucus. Equipment is cleaned and dried before storing.

PULMONARY HYGIENE

Patients with chronic pulmonary disease can benefit from a program of pulmonary hygiene that is designed to remove secretions, and to enable more efficient exchange of oxygen and carbon dioxide. Pulmonary hygiene programs include administering prescribed drugs, humidifying inhaled air, medication therapy via nebulizer or MDI, chest physiotherapy, and breathing exercises. A handheld flutter mucus clearance device may be used to provide positive expiratory pressure.

Chest physiotherapy includes postural drainage (when possible) and percussion and vibration. *Postural drainage* involves positioning the patient so that the forces of gravity can help remove secretions deep in the bronchi and lungs (Figure 15-7). Tapping, clapping, and vibrating techniques are used primarily for cystic fibrosis for the purpose of dislodging mucous plugs so that they can be coughed up more easily. The physician or physical therapist will give specific directions and therapy must be done by someone who has been instructed in the proper technique. Family members can be taught the procedures, if needed for home care.

Because there is likely to be some gagging during coughing episodes that take place during postural drainage, it is best to carry out the procedure before meals, when the stomach is relatively empty and vomiting is less likely. If the patient is to have postural

drainage only once a day, drainage should be done in the morning to remove secretions that have accumulated during the night. After postural drainage is completed, good mouth care—including brushing the teeth and using a refreshing mouthwash—will be appreciated.

 Elder Care Points

Elderly patients with osteoporosis are at risk for fractures of the vertebrae and ribs. Clapping should not be used on these patients; vibrating techniques are more appropriate.

 Patient Teaching

Pursed-Lip Breathing

- Sit up tall and move the back away from the chair; place the feet about shoulder-width apart. Lean forward slightly with hands or elbows on the knees.
- Close the mouth, and breath in through the nose.
- Purse the lips as though to gently whistle or blow out a candle; keep the lips and cheeks relaxed.
- Blow through relaxed pursed lips, exhale slowly, and do *not* force the air out of the lungs (this can bring about the collapse of the airway structures).
- Breathe out slowly without puffing out the cheeks; control the flow of exhaled air as if you wanted to cause a candle to flicker but not extinguish.
- Take twice as much time to let the breath out as it did to take it in.
- Tense the abdominal muscles to force as much air from the lungs as possible.
- Use pursed-lip breathing during any physical activity.
- Refrain from holding your breath when lifting objects or performing other physical activities.

Drains posterior basal segment of lower lobe

Drains lateral basal segment of lower lobe

Drains anterior basal segment of lower lobe

Drains superior segment of lower lobe

Drains lateral and medial segments of middle lobe

Drains superior and inferior lingular segment

Drains anterior segment of upper lobe

Drains posterior segment of upper lobe

Drains apical segment of upper lobe

FIGURE 15-7 Positions for postural drainage.

The purpose of performing breathing exercises is to strengthen the abdominal muscles so that they can push upward against the diaphragm and assist in the expiration of air from the lungs. These exercises also help overcome rigidity of the thorax so that the lungs can inflate and deflate more easily. Patients who follow the exercises prescribed for them often find that they can lead more active and useful lives than formerly possible because their exertional dyspnea is less severe (Troosters et al., 2010). The muscles of their body are stronger, thus there is less risk for complications that accompany immobility. The exercises also help patients to cough up secretions that would otherwise remain in the lower bronchi and serve as a growth medium for bacteria or a cause of atelectasis.

Patient Teaching

Abdominal (Belly) or Diaphragmatic Breathing

- Initially practice lying down.
- Lie on the back with the knees bent. Take a deep breath through the nose with the abdomen relaxed and, with the palm of one hand, feel the abdomen rise. Exhale slowly to a count of 4.
- Exhale slowly through pursed lips, tightening the abdominal muscles that push the diaphragm up, forcing more air out of the lungs.
- Once comfortable with the abdominal breathing technique, use it when standing or sitting. This type of controlled breathing will provide more endurance during physical activity.

Face mask   Tracheostomy collar   Face tent   Non-rebreathing mask   Venturi mask

FIGURE 15-8 *Various oxygen delivery devices.*

OXYGEN THERAPY

Oxygen is a drug and it must be prescribed and administered in specific doses to avoid oxygen toxicity. The dosage of oxygen is stated in terms of *concentration* and rate of *flow*. High concentrations (above 50%) may be prescribed to treat acute conditions in which the patient can benefit from prompt treatment of hypoxia, as in myocardial infarction and pulmonary edema. The rate of flow may be as high as 12 L/min. Methods of administration are divided into high-flow and low-flow systems (Figure 15-8 and Table 15-5).

Moderate concentrations of oxygen are prescribed when increased metabolic rate raises the consumption of oxygen, or when there is poor distribution of oxygen because of congestive heart failure. The concentrations of oxygen given in a moderate dosage are about 28% to 30% at a rate of flow of 4 to 7 L/min.

Low concentrations of oxygen of about 24% to 28% delivered at a rate of 1 to 3 L/min are indicated when the patient needs oxygen over an extended period. These percentages and rates of flow are approximate amounts. The exact dosage depends on the method of administration and the patient's individual need for additional oxygen supply. Even though oxygen is essential to life, excessive amounts are toxic. High concentrations of inhaled oxygen can bring about collapse of the

Table 15-5	Advantages and Disadvantages of Common Oxygen Delivery Devices

METHOD	O_2 DELIVERY	ADVANTAGES	DISADVANTAGES	NURSING IMPLICATIONS
Nasal cannula (nasal prongs)	Low concentrations; dependent on rate and depth of breathing *Flows:* 1 L = 24% O_2 2 L = 28% O_2 3 L = 32% O_2 4 L = 36% O_2 5 L = 40% O_2 6 L = 44% O_2	Patient can move about, eat, and talk while receiving oxygen. Most COPD patients can tolerate 2 L/min flow.	Restless patients can easily dislodge the prongs. Risk of skin irritation at nares, ears, and cheeks. Flow rate 3 L and above requires humidification as it will dry and irritate nasal mucosa.	Prongs should be facing down toward mouth when inserted in nose; check frequently as patients tend to replace the prongs incorrectly. Clean prongs every few hours.
Simple face mask	Low to medium concentrations; 35%-50% can be achieved with flow rate of 6-12 L/min.	Mask provides adequate humidification; delivers oxygen quickly for short-term therapy.	Discomfort and risk of pressure necrosis caused by tight seal between face and mask. Device must be removed for patient to eat, drink, or take medications. Muffles voice when talking. Requires at least 5-L flow to prevent accumulation of expired air in mask.	Wash and dry under mask and wipe out mask q 1-2 hr. Mask must fit snugly. May need to pad straps at ears to prevent necrosis.

COPD, chronic obstructive pulmonary disease; *Fio₂,* fraction of inspired oxygen.

Continued

Table **15-5** Advantages and Disadvantages of Common Oxygen Delivery Devices—cont'd

METHOD	O₂ DELIVERY	ADVANTAGES	DISADVANTAGES	NURSING IMPLICATIONS
Partial rebreathing mask	Higher concentrations; 40%-60% at flow rates of 6-10 L/min.	Mask is lightweight; reservoir bag traps portion of exhaled breath that is high in oxygen for rebreathing.	Risk of pressure necrosis with long-term use. Cannot be used with high humidity.	Bag should not be allowed to deflate during inspiration. Check skin under straps frequently.
Non-rebreather mask	Highest concentrations; 60%-90% can be achieved.	Delivers high concentration of oxygen accurately.	Cannot be used with high humidity. Flow rate must be sufficient to prevent bag from deflating during inspiration.	Mask should fit snugly; check skin contact areas for pressure necrosis.
Venturi mask	Delivers consistent Flo₂ regardless of breathing pattern. Concentration and liter flow marked on mask apparatus; available for 24%, 28%, 31%, 35%, 40%, and 50% O₂.	Mask can provide good humidification; good for delivering low, constant oxygen concentrations to patient with COPD.	Discomfort and risk of skin irritation. Must be removed for eating, drinking, and taking oral medications. Talking is muffled.	Air ports must not be occluded. Check skin contact areas frequently.
Transtracheal catheter	Delivers oxygen efficiently.	Flow requirement is reduced 60%-80%, increasing time oxygen is available from portable source. Catheter is less visible. Less nasal irritation occurs.	Catheter replacement is an invasive procedure. Not appropriate for someone with excessive mucus production.	Patient and family teaching about catheter replacement.
Tracheostomy collar	Delivers O₂ and humidification via tracheostomy; must be connected to a nebulizer with Flo₂ set at 24%-100%.	Adds humidity to help liquefy secretions. Lose some of O₂ flow since collar is not tight fitting.	Must drain condensation in tubing often. Risk of respiratory infection.	Drain condensation from tubing into receptacle, being careful not to allow fluid to go into tracheostomy. Remove and clean collar device and check skin under straps at least q 4 hr.
T-bar (Briggs adapter)	Delivers O₂ and humidification to tracheostomy; must be connected to a nebulizer with Flo₂ set at 24%-100%.	Fits more tightly than tracheostomy collar. Adds humidity to liquefy secretions.	Must drain condensation in tubing often. Risk of respiratory infection.	Drain condensation from tubing into receptacle; be careful not to get fluid into tracheostomy. Remove and clean T-bar device q 4 hr.

alveoli, because the oxygen displaces some of the nitrogen there. High oxygen concentration can also interrupt the production of *pulmonary surfactant,* a substance that stabilizes the alveoli and prevents atelectasis.

Short-term oxygen therapy, which is the administration of oxygen to treat hypoxemia, is indicated when:

- There is an inadequate intake of oxygen because of obstruction or restriction of airflow through the air passages.

- Oxygen is not distributed throughout the body because of circulatory failure.
- There is an inadequate supply of hemoglobin to transport the oxygen.
- Carbon dioxide or other gases displace the oxygen in the blood.

Objective criteria for oxygen needs include maintaining the Sao₂ greater than 90% and the Pao₂ greater than 60 mm Hg (for disorders such as COPD).

Outward signs of hypoxia vary in patients, but dyspnea and confusion are the most common signs. Blood gas analysis and determination of the blood pH are the most reliable indicators.

Long-term oxygen therapy for patients with asthma or COPD is used to:

- Relieve hypoxemia
- Reverse tissue hypoxia and its signs and symptoms
- Allow the patient to function better mentally and physically, thereby increasing self-reliance

Nursing Management

The nurse checks the oxygen delivery system at the beginning of the shift and then periodically to verify that the flow is set according to the physician's order. Tubing is checked to see that it is not kinked. Make sure that the patient is wearing the delivery device. Oxygen should be humidified, especially if the flow rate is more than 3 L/min. Oxygen is *not* explosive; however, oxygen does support combustion, which means that a spark or flame can cause a major fire. **Smoking is not allowed when oxygen is used. The tubing should be kept off the floor and the connections should be handled aseptically to prevent contamination of the system.**

When oxygen therapy is discontinued, it is usually done gradually. The patient is "weaned" from dependence on oxygen by first reducing the dosage, and then alternating periods of breathing room air with periods of breathing low concentrations of oxygen.

? Think Critically

Can you describe the assessment points you would cover at the beginning of the shift for a patient who is receiving oxygen therapy? Consider both the patient and the oxygen setup system.

MECHANICAL VENTILATION

Mechanical ventilation is needed when the patient cannot maintain adequate ventilation because of respiratory, neurologic, or neuromuscular problems or trauma. Two major types of ventilators are used to give support to patients with ventilatory problems: negative-pressure and positive-pressure ventilators. Negative-pressure ventilators are mainly used for patients with normal vital capacities who have neuromuscular disease, central nervous system disorders (e.g., spinal cord damage), and COPD. The iron lung is an example of a negative-pressure ventilator.

Positive-pressure ventilators are more commonly used. There are several types of positive-pressure ventilators and various modes of ventilation. The pressure delivered is greater than that within the airway and alveoli; therefore gas flows into the lungs, either assisting or controlling inhalation. When the pressure is released, exhalation is passive without effort by the machine or the patient. An endotracheal tube or tracheostomy tube is usually present (see Chapter 14).

Time-cycled ventilators deliver air into the lungs for a preset length of time. The Babybird and the Siemens Servo are examples of this type. These are mainly used for infants and children.

Volume-cycled ventilators deliver a preset volume of gas with preset pressure limits to the bronchi and lungs. This type of ventilator is most often used in critical care settings for severe chest disease or postsurgically for severely compromised respiratory function. Adequate tidal volumes will be delivered even when airway resistance is great (e.g., in patients suffering from severe obstructive lung disease). If the ventilator meets too much pressure, an alarm sounds to indicate that the correct tidal volume is not being delivered. This is commonly caused by excessive secretions in the lungs and suctioning is needed.

High-frequency jet ventilation provides good ventilation with the use of relatively small tidal volumes at very high respiratory rates. The oxygenation and ventilation are accomplished by gas diffusion and convection rather than a high flow of gas. Because the intrathoracic pressures needed for this type of ventilation are much lower, there are fewer complications (e.g., barotrauma, hypotension, and pneumothorax) than with other types of ventilation.

Modes of Ventilation

In *controlled-mode* ventilation, the machine is set to deliver a fixed number of breaths per minute, no matter how the patient is breathing. Controlled-mode ventilation is used during periods of central nervous system depression, such as during anesthesia and drug overdose.

The *assist-mode* ventilation decreases the work of breathing for the patient. When the patient takes a breath, the machine delivers a set tidal volume. Assist-mode ventilation is combined with the control function to provide an assist-control mode. If the patient's respiratory rate falls, the machine will deliver a set number of breaths per minute; if the patient is breathing within the set rate, the machine assists only by delivering the set tidal volume.

Intermittent mandatory ventilation (IMV) and *synchronized intermittent mandatory ventilation* (SIMV) are the most common modes of ventilation found in critical care settings. These allow the patient to breathe spontaneously and yet provide a preset number of ventilator breaths at a preset tidal volume, to ensure adequate ventilation without respiratory muscle fatigue. IMV can add more air at the end of a breath. SIMV is activated and therefore synchronized by the patient's breathing pattern. During mechanical ventilation, it is possible for a patient's lungs to weaken due to lack of use. One of the main advantages of assist ventilation modes is that the patient's respiratory muscles are partially at work during mechanical ventilation and this makes it easier to wean the patient from the ventilator.

In positive end-expiratory pressure (PEEP), the pressure in the airways never falls below a certain level (usually between 5 and 15 cm H_2O). This holds the smaller air passages open, thus limiting atelectasis. It also expands alveoli so that there is more time for gas to diffuse across the membrane and correct hypoxemia. PEEP is used for ARDS and respiratory failure when there is a Pa_{O_2} less than 50 and a P_{CO_2} greater than 50.

Pressure Support Ventilation. In pressure support ventilation (PSV), the patient controls both the duration and volume of inspiration, but PSV decreases the work of drawing airflow through the ventilator tubing; thus decreasing patient fatigue. PSV has proven very beneficial during weaning from IMV. PSV_{max} is also used during weaning and provides higher pressures to produce tidal breaths equivalent to conventional positive-pressure ventilation.

Continuous Positive Airway Pressure. Continuous positive airway pressure (CPAP) and bilevel positive airway pressure (BiPAP) can be used for patients who are breathing spontaneously but are showing signs of hypoxemia. It is used for infants with mild respiratory distress syndrome (RDS) and for adults in the early stages of respiratory failure. The patient does not have to be intubated for CPAP to be used. CPAP can be given with nasal prongs. These modes are also used for sleep apnea.

Noninvasive Positive Pressure Ventilation. Noninvasive positive pressure ventilation (NPPV) is safer, is more comfortable, and reduces the risk of ventilator-associated pneumonia. NPPV can be used successfully with carefully selected patients who have COPD or patients with cardiogenic pulmonary edema. With NPPV the patient is mechanically ventilated but receives oxygen via a nasal mask, facial mask, nasal prongs, or helmet. The nurse should carefully monitor for worsening of pH or carbon dioxide levels, hypoxemia, severe tachypnea, hemodynamic instability, decreasing level of consciousness, inability to clear secretions, or inability to tolerate the mask or helmet device. If these observations are noted, the physician must be alerted so that NPPV can be terminated and the therapy switched to invasive ventilation.

Nursing Management

Care for a patient who is receiving mechanical ventilation requires extensive training and supervised practice. The patient will require protection from infection, continuous monitoring of vital signs, observation for hypoventilation and hyperventilation, measurement of intake and output, and prevention of the disabilities of inactivity. When caring for a patient on mechanical ventilation, you should:

- Check the physician's order each shift and then check the ventilator for the proper settings: mode, FIO_2 (fraction of inspired oxygen, or the oxygen concentration that is delivered), respiratory rate, tidal volume, peak inspiratory pressure, and PEEP (Figure 15-9).
- Check alarms to see that they are turned on. Alarms should not be turned off when disconnecting the patient in order to suction, as the alarms may not be reactivated.
- Keep tubing clear of pooled water; empty the water into an appropriate receptacle as needed.
- Check for tension or stretching of the ventilator tubing every time a patient is repositioned.

The patient is observed for signs of complications, such as gastric distention, pneumothorax, and impaired cardiac output from decreased venous return, and the need for increasingly higher pressures to deliver the set tidal volume—which can indicate stiffening of the lungs (decreased compliance). Providing mouth care every 6 to 8 hours with chlorhexidine solution reduces the risk for ventilator-associated pneumonia (ICSI, 2009). Auscultate the lung fields to be certain

FIGURE 15-9 Check the ventilator settings against the orders each shift.

that both lungs are being ventilated. Monitor arterial blood gas levels to determine the effectiveness of ventilation treatment.

> **! Safety Alert**
>
> **Preventing Ventilator-Acquired Pneumonia**
>
> Use of a "ventilator bundle" helps prevent ventilator-acquired pneumonia. The Centers for Disease Control and Prevention recommends: (1) elevation of the head of the bed to 30 to 45 degrees; (2) continuous removal of subglottic secretions; (3) change of ventilator circuit no more often than every 48 hours; and (4) hand hygiene before and after contact with every patient. In addition, facility bundle policy may include checking the residual volume in the nasogastric tube, providing oral care with chlorhexidine, deep vein thrombosis prophylaxis, and peptic ulcer prophylaxis (Collins & Lipke, 2009; Tolentino-Delos Reyes et al., 2007).

For ventilation to be effective, the lungs must be kept clear of secretions. Many patients can cough up secretions and do not need to be suctioned; others may need suctioning as frequently as every 15 minutes. Endotracheal and tracheal suctioning must be done with strict aseptic technique because of the high risk of respiratory infection.

The intubated patient on the ventilator cannot talk, so alternative means of communication such as a Magic Slate, VitalVoice Communication device, or paper and pencil are offered.

Additional calorie intake is needed just to maintain weight when a ventilator is used. Continuous enteral feeding is the method most often used to prevent malnutrition in these patients. The nurse should monitor nutritional parameters.

If a ventilator alarm sounds and the problem cannot be located quickly, the patient should be disconnected from the machine and ventilated with a manual resuscitator bag and oxygen until the problem is solved.

Table 15-6 summarizes the dangers of mechanical ventilation.

> **[?] Think Critically**
>
> You have just assisted another nurse in turning a patient who is attached to a mechanical ventilator. The patient has been positioned on the left side and the ventilator is on the right side of the bed. What would you check before you leave the bedside?

COMMUNITY CARE

Home care nurses may be the first to notice that a patient needs home oxygen therapy; also chronic respiratory patients must be monitored for early signs of complications, such as pulmonary edema. Outpatient clinic nurses may be the first to notice that respiratory patients are having an increased number of sick days with an increased severity with each episode. Careful history and screening should be conducted to see if there is an occupational exposure to an irritant, or if the patient is developing hypersensitivity. The nurse can advocate for spirometry, because it is a good test for detecting nonmalignant occupational lung diseases. Community nurses participate in infection control by identifying and referring potential and active cases of tuberculosis within the community.

Working with patients to promote compliance with their exercise and medication regimen is a primary function of the nurse in the community. Teaching use of the peak airflow meter and the MDI can save health care dollars by decreasing serious episodes of acute respiratory dysfunction. *Rehabilitation* (see Chapter 9) of the chronic respiratory patient is directed at:
- Improving breathing
- Improving activity tolerance
- Decreasing infection
- Preventing acute episodes

Table 15-6	Dangers of Mechanical Ventilation
DANGER	**MANIFESTATIONS**
Barotrauma	Sudden increase in peak inspiratory pressure; absent breath sounds over one area of lung; pneumomediastinum; pneumothorax; subcutaneous emphysema; high-pressure alarm goes off frequently.
Oxygen toxicity	Parenchymal damage and absorption atelectasis; alveolar membrane damage; nonproductive cough; decreasing vital capacity; decreased compliance; increased peak inspiratory pressure.
Impaired cardiac output	Decreased blood pressure; poor peripheral perfusion; decreased level of consciousness.
Infection	Change in sputum color, quantity, and consistency; crackles and rhonchi; increased white blood cell count; fever; infiltrate on chest radiograph.
Fluid retention	Increasing body weight; fluid intake more than output; peripheral edema; crackles in lungs or diminished breath sounds.
Gastric distention	Increasing abdominal girth; complaint of distention; tender to palpation.
Gastrointestinal bleeding	Positive stool guaiac; "coffee-grounds" aspirate from gastric suction; dropping hemoglobin; black or bloody stool.

Get Ready for the NCLEX® Examination!

Key Points

- Symptoms of influenza are headache, fever, chills, and muscle aches, followed by hacking cough, runny nose and nasal congestion, and sensitivity to light.
- Hospital-acquired pneumonia can often be prevented by use of aseptic technique and good respiratory care. The elderly are at special risk for pneumonia.
- Symptoms of infectious pneumonia are high fever, chills, cough with rusty sputum, chest pain, diaphoresis, malaise, and aching muscles. There will be diminished or abnormal breath sounds.
- Fluids (unless contraindicated) should be increased for patients with respiratory infections.
- Treatment of tuberculosis requires multiple medications for a period of 6 to 9 months (see Table 15-1).
- Restrictive lung disorders include pleurisy, pleural effusion, kyphosis, severe scoliosis, and arthritis of the chest wall.
- Chronic obstructive lung disorders include emphysema and chronic bronchitis. Smoking cessation is one of the most important measures in the treatment of obstructive lung disease.
- Emphysema causes destruction of the terminal respiratory units and narrowed, stiff airways with loss of lung elasticity; it causes air trapping and CO_2 retention.
- Chronic bronchitis causes inflammation, excess secretion of mucus, chronic cough, increasing resistance to airflow, and hypoxia. Retention of carbon dioxide occurs, and polycythemia develops.
- In asthma, bronchospasm and excessive secretion of mucus with bronchoconstriction cause decreased airflow and hypoxia. A severe asthma attack can kill, if not relieved.
- COPD patients are taught diaphragmatic breathing and pursed-lip breathing techniques to assist aeration of the lungs.
- The primary cause of lung cancer is cigarette smoking. Symptoms of lung cancer include cough, wheezing, chest discomfort, exertional dyspnea, and expectoration of blood-streaked sputum. Treatment includes surgery, radiation, chemotherapy, and biotherapy agents.
- Signs and symptoms of pulmonary embolus are dyspnea, chest pain, cough, hemoptysis, and anxiety. Anticoagulant therapy is used for prevention or treatment of pulmonary embolus.
- Pneumothorax and hemothorax decrease lung capacity; treatment includes chest tubes and a closed drainage system.
- Pulmonary edema is a medical emergency. Symptoms include severe dyspnea, orthopnea, noisy respirations, pink frothy sputum, pale, cold, clammy skin, anxiety, restlessness, and possibly confusion.
- Adult respiratory distress syndrome is life threatening and is treated with ventilatory support with PEEP.
- Respiratory failure occurs when Pao_2 is below 50 mm Hg and Pco_2 is over 50 mm Hg.
- Frequent respiratory assessment is essential for the patient with chest tubes. Nursing care includes positioning on the back or on the operative side, or according to physician orders; checking tube for kinks; and reporting chest drainage of more than 100 mL/hr.
- Oxygen is a medication used to treat hypoxemia, and can be toxic. High concentrations of oxygen are not used for COPD patients as it can diminish their drive to breathe; use only low-flow oxygen of 1 to 3 L/min.
- Mechanical ventilation is necessary after chest surgery and for respiratory failure, ARDS, flail chest, and neuromuscular disorders that interfere with the respiratory muscles. Nursing care includes carefully checking ventilator settings each shift, ensuring that alarms are on, auscultating the lungs to be sure both lungs are being ventilated, suctioning as needed, administering nutritional therapy, and observing for complications.

Additional Learning Resources

SG Go to your Study Guide for additional learning activities to help you master this chapter content.

 evolve Go to your Evolve website (http://evolve.elsevier.com/deWit/medsurg) for the following FREE learning resources:
- Animations, audio, and video
- Answers and rationales for questions and activities
- Concept Map Creator
- Glossary with pronunciations in English and Spanish
- Interactive Review Questions and Exercises and more!

Online Resources
- American Lung Association, www.lungusa.org
- Centers for Disease Control and Prevention, www.cdc.gov
- Tuberculosis treatments and drugs, www.mayoclinic.com/health/tuberculosis/DS00372/DSECTION=treatments-and-drugs
- National Heart Lung and Blood Institute, www.nhlbi.nih.gov

Review Questions for the NCLEX® Examination

1. The nurse is caring for a patient with signs and symptoms of influenza. What home care for this respiratory condition would be appropriate?
   1. Schedule adequate periods of exercise and activity.
   2. Provide warming measures.
   3. Restrict fluid intake.
   4. Consider analgesics and antipyretics.

2. A 58-year-old man is admitted with bacterial pneumonia. He has high fever accompanied by chills, a cough productive of rust-colored sputum, and a general feeling of malaise. The medical diagnosis is confirmed by:
   1. blood cultures.
   2. chest radiographs.
   3. white blood cell count.
   4. bronchoscopy.

3. Which patient is at greatest risk for developing a pulmonary embolism?
   1. Peripheral IV that was started 2 days ago
   2. Three months pregnant with her first child
   3. Immobile for 1 week and is mildly dehydrated
   4. Ambulating 2 days after abdominal surgery

4. A frail 40-year-old woman is admitted with complaints of fever, fatigue, coughing, difficulty breathing, and weight loss. Which factor in the patient's history supports the probable medical diagnosis of histoplasmosis?

   1. Employment in a paint factory
   2. Exposure to bird droppings
   3. Recent desert expedition
   4. Exposure to asbestos

5. Which person should be advised not to have the tuberculosis (TB) skin test? The person who:

   1. is symptomatic after a short exposure to someone with TB.
   2. had a bacille Calmette-Guérin (BCG) vaccine 2 years ago.
   3. works with children at a large day care center.
   4. works as a waitress in a small local restaurant.

6. The nursing student is reviewing signs and symptoms with a group of persons who are at risk for lung cancer. The nurse would intervene if the student says:

   1. "Weight loss and fatigue are the first symptoms to manifest."
   2. "An occasional cough or wheezing would be the first signs."
   3. "Hoarseness could occur if a tumor presses against the vocal cords."
   4. "Deep bone pain could occur because the cancer may spread to the bones."

7. Which action is appropriate in the care of a patient who is on mechanical ventilation?

   1. Instruct the respiratory therapist to check the ventilator settings and alarms.
   2. Auscultate the lungs bilaterally to ensure that both lungs are being ventilated.
   3. Disconnect the alarms before suctioning or before turning the patient.
   4. Perform endotracheal suctioning every 15 minutes, using sterile technique.

8. A 55-year-old man was admitted for complaints of a recurring irritating "smoker's" cough with small amounts of sputum, and was diagnosed with chronic bronchitis. What is the most likely clinical finding?

   1. Blood-streaked sputum
   2. Decreased white blood cells
   3. Pale mucous membranes
   4. Elevated hemoglobin and hematocrit

9. The patient is immobilized and has been lying in bed for an extended period. What nursing intervention(s) should be done to prevent hypostatic pneumonia? (Select all that apply.)

   1. Avoid immunizations due to weakened state.
   2. Assist the patient to turn at least every 2 hours.
   3. Instruct the patient to cough and deep breathe.
   4. Maintain NPO to prevent aspiration.
   5. Practice scrupulous hand hygiene.

10. The nurse admits a patient who was diagnosed with active pulmonary tuberculosis. What nursing intervention(s) would help control the spread of the disease? (Select all that apply.)

    1. Implementing airborne isolation.
    2. Assigning the patient to a positive-pressure isolation room.
    3. Wearing an HEPA respirator mask when providing direct patient care.
    4. Explaining the importance of covering the mouth when smiling.
    5. Practicing good hand hygiene.

Critical Thinking Activities

Scenario A

You are assigned to take care of Janet Blair, a 26-year-old who has pneumococcal pneumonia. She is receiving humidified oxygen by nasal cannula at 3 L/min. She is on bed rest with bathroom privileges. She is receiving nebulization treatments from respiratory therapy and is receiving IV antibiotics. She is very weak and runs a temperature of 104.6° F (40.3° C) and sometimes experiences delirium.

1. What would be an appropriate plan of care for Janet?

2. How would you evaluate the effectiveness of the nursing interventions listed on the plan of care?

3. What psychosocial problems might Janet have? How would you help her with these?

Scenario B

Mrs. Wester is 62 years old. She has suffered from emphysema for several years but has not sought help in coping with the problems associated with the chronic lung disease. While in the hospital with an acute respiratory infection, she becomes very depressed and says she will never be able to take care of herself again because of her breathlessness. She has not been taught any techniques for pulmonary hygiene. She is not willing to give up smoking.

1. What do you think might be the attitude of some health care professionals in regard to Mrs. Wester's problems? What is your personal response to Mrs. Wester's situation?

2. Devise a teaching plan to help her with her problem of fatigue and breathlessness.

3. List interventions that would be appropriate in helping with her nutritional and hydration needs.

Scenario C

Mr. Cohen is admitted to the hospital for pneumonectomy. His diagnosis is early lung cancer. He is 56 years old and has worked in a cotton mill since he was 16. He is slightly underweight but is physically strong and has an optimistic outlook about his surgery and chances for recovery.

1. What special preoperative instruction would you expect Mr. Cohen to need?

2. What nursing interventions would you expect to be on his postoperative nursing care plan?

3. How would you help Mr. Cohen deal with the diagnosis of cancer, treatment, and prognosis?

Scenario D

Mr. Azale has recently been diagnosed with asthma. He is coming to the clinic for ongoing management of the condition. He wants to understand the disease and be an active participant in his own health care.

1. Prepare a teaching plan to help him understand his condition and self-care.

2. Describe what you would tell Mr. Azale about the possibility of having a severe, acute asthma attack.

chapter

16

The Hematologic System

evolve

http://evolve.elsevier.com/deWit/medsurg

Objectives

Theory

1. Describe the structures and functions of the hematologic system.
2. Differentiate between the various types of blood cells and their functions.
3. Discuss factors that may alter the function of the hematologic system.
4. Identify ways in which the nurse might help prevent blood disorders.
5. List at least five different kinds of information that can be obtained from a complete blood count (CBC).

6. Describe ways to accomplish hemostasis.
7. Apply the nursing process to patients with problems of the hematologic system.

Clinical Practice

1. Explain the procedure and care for a bone marrow aspiration to a patient about to undergo the procedure.
2. Perform a focused assessment on a patient with a problem of the hematologic system.
3. Choose nursing interventions for patients with problems of the hematologic system.

Key Terms

agranulocytosis (p. 335)
aplastic anemia (ā-plăs-tĭk ă-NĒ-mē-ă, p. 335)
dyscrasias (dĭs-KRĀ-zhē-ăz, p. 334)
erythropoiesis (ĕ-rĭth-rō-pō-Ē-sĭs, p. 332)
gingivitis (jĭn-jĭ-VĪ-tĭs, p. 339)
hemarthrosis (hē-măr-THRŌ-sĭs, p. 340)
hematocrit (hē-MĂT-ŏ-krĭt, p. 336)
hemolysis (hē-MŎL-ĭ-sĭs, p. 334)

iatrogenic (Ī-ă-trō-JĔN-ĭk, p. 334)
jaundice (JĂWN-dĭs, p. 339)
leukopenia (lū-kō-PĒ-nē-ă, p. 334)
melena (MĔL-ĕh-nă, p. 340)
petechiae (pĕ-TĒ-kē-ă, p. 339)
polycythemia (pŏl-ē-sī-THĒ-mē-ă, p. 339)
thrombocytopenia (thrŏm-bō-sīt-ō-PĒ-nē-ă, p. 335)

OVERVIEW OF ANATOMY AND PHYSIOLOGY OF THE HEMATOLOGIC SYSTEM

WHAT ARE THE FUNCTIONS OF BLOOD?

• Blood transports water, oxygen, nutrients, hormones, enzymes, and medications to the cells.
• Blood transports carbon dioxide and other waste products away from the cells.
• The 4 to 5 L of blood in the body help regulate fluid volume and electrolyte distribution.
• The blood regulates the pH and acid-base balance by its buffering ability.
• Blood assists in regulating body temperature.
• Blood provides clotting factors for hemostasis.

WHAT ARE THE COMPONENTS OF BLOOD?

• Blood is composed of formed elements and plasma (Figure 16-1).

• The formed elements are erythrocytes, neutrophils, lymphocytes, monocytes, eosinophils, basophils, and platelets.
• Plasma contains proteins, water, salts, dissolved gases (such as CO_2), bicarbonate (HCO_3^-), hormones, glucose, and wastes.
• The plasma proteins are albumin, globulins, and fibrinogen.

WHAT ARE THE FUNCTIONS OF THE PLASMA PROTEINS?

• Albumin raises osmotic pressure at the capillary membrane, preventing fluid from leaking out into the tissue spaces. (Osmotic pressure is covered in Chapter 3.)
• The alpha and beta globulins work as carriers for drugs and lipids by combining with them and transporting them throughout the body; gamma globulins act as antibodies.
• Fibrinogen is essential to the formation of blood clots.

FIGURE 16-1 Components of blood.

HOW DOES THE BODY PRODUCE BLOOD CELLS?

- Blood cells develop from stem cells located in the bone marrow through erythropoiesis (Figure 16-2).
- The kidney makes most of the body's erythropoietin-stimulating factor, which then prompts the liver to release erythropoietin for erythrocyte production.
- Erythropoiesis needs iron, vitamins B_{12}, C, and E, folic acid, and amino acids—all of which are obtained from proteins.

WHAT ARE THE FUNCTIONS OF THE RED BLOOD CELLS?

- Red blood cells (RBCs or erythrocytes, the most numerous of the blood cells), contain hemoglobin, which carries oxygen to the cells and a portion of carbon dioxide away from the cells.
- Each person has a hereditary blood type based on the antigens on the RBCs.
- The normal range for adults for RBCs is 4.2 to 6.2 million/mm^3.
- The normal range for hemoglobin in adults is 12 to 18 g/dL.
- Decreased numbers of RBCs or decreased hemoglobin results in a reduction in the amount of oxygen that can be carried to the cells of the body.

- RBCs live for approximately 120 days.
- Old, damaged red cells are removed by the spleen and the liver.

WHAT ARE THE FUNCTIONS OF WHITE BLOOD CELLS?

- White blood cells (WBCs or leukocytes) provide the first line of defense against microbial agents.
- The normal adult range for total leukocytes (WBCs) is 4500 to 11,000/mm^3.
- Leukocytes are divided into granulocytes (meaning *with granules*) and agranulocytes (meaning *without granules*) in the cell nucleus (see Figure 16-2).
- Leukocytes migrate from the bone marrow cells out into the tissues, and are carried by the bloodstream to locations where they are needed.
- Granulocytes are divided into neutrophils, eosinophils, and basophils and are produced in the red bone marrow.
- Neutrophils make up 54% to 62% of the WBC count and work by engulfing and destroying bacteria by the process of *phagocytosis.*
- An infection in the body stimulates increased production of neutrophils, resulting in a higher-than-normal WBC count, or leukocytosis.

FIGURE 16-2 Erythrocytes (RBCs), leukocytes (WBCs), and thrombocytes (platelets) are the end products of erythropoiesis.

- Eosinophils, which make up 1% to 3% of the total WBCs, help detoxify foreign proteins; eosinophils increase in number during allergic reactions and in response to parasitic infections.
- Basophils, which comprise up to 1% of the total WBC count, release histamine in response to allergens and help prevent clotting in the small blood vessels.
- Agranulocytes consist of lymphocytes and monocytes.
- Agranulocytes are produced in the red bone marrow and in lymphatic tissue.
- Lymphocytes, which comprise 25% to 33% of WBCs, are produced in the red bone marrow and the lymphatic tissue. Lymphocytes occur as B cells and T cells. B lymphocytes change into plasma cells that produce immunoglobulins responsible for the humoral immune response.
- Some T cells are killer cells that fight antigens and provide cell-mediated immune response (see Chapter 10).
- Monocytes comprise 3% to 7% of the WBCs and become macrophages (large mononuclear monocytes) migrating out into the tissues where they become phagocytes, fighting infection and ridding the body of foreign substances. They engulf bacteria and foreign substances and eliminate them from the body.
- A differential blood cell count gives information about the numbers of different types of leukocytes present in the blood and about the type of inflammatory process that is occurring.

WHAT ARE PLATELETS AND WHAT IS THEIR FUNCTION?

- Platelets, also called *thrombocytes*, are fragments of megakaryocytes that are produced by the bone marrow.
- Platelets provide the first line of protection, after vasospasm (contraction of a vessel), to prevent bleeding by promoting clotting when the wall of a blood vessel has been damaged.
- Platelets are involved in maintaining hemostasis by a complex process that balances the production of the clotting and dissolving factors.
- Fibrin strands derived from the plasma protein fibrinogen attach to aggregated platelets to help form a clot.

- Platelets are small formed elements of the blood active in the clotting process. Platelets tend to adhere to damaged or uneven surfaces and to clump together.
- The normal adult platelet count range is 150,000 to 400,000/mm^3; the life span of a platelet is about 10 days.
- Although the body can withstand a substantial drop in the number of platelets, when the platelet count is low, there is risk of spontaneous bleeding into the skin, kidney, brain, and other internal organs.

HOW DOES THE LYMPHATIC SYSTEM INTERACT WITH THE VASCULAR SYSTEM?

- The lymphatic system consists of lymph nodes, lymph channels, the spleen, and the thymus gland (see Chapter 10).
- The spleen, located in the upper left abdominal cavity below the diaphragm and behind the stomach, filters the blood, removing pathogens, old blood cells, and debris, and produces lymphocytes (see Figure 10-2).
- The spleen is a reservoir for extra blood; in response to hemorrhage, it contracts, and by contraction, the spleen releases some of its stored blood into the cardiovascular system.
- If the spleen is removed, its functions are taken over by other lymph tissue and by the liver.
- Lymph vessels collect excess fluid and protein from the interstitial spaces and return it to the bloodstream.
- Lymph nodes (bundles of lymphatic tissue) filter out leukocytes and cell debris from inflammations and infections before the lymph is returned to the bloodstream.

WHAT CHANGES OF THE HEMATOLOGIC SYSTEM OCCUR WITH AGING?

- Plasma volume decreases after age 60; the older person has less blood volume. This means less blood reserve in case of blood loss.
- Bone marrow activity decreases by about 50% as years advance; the marrow becomes infiltrated with fat and fibrotic tissue. Reduced bone marrow inhibits full production of blood cells, so the immune response is decreased, making the older person more susceptible to infection. There is less antibody response to foreign proteins.
- New cells are produced at a slower rate, and correction of anemia becomes a longer process.
- Antibody response to vaccines is decreased.
- When blood loss occurs, the elderly patient is at greater risk for hypovolemia and shock.
- Blood is more prone to coagulate, because platelets tend to aggregate more with advancing age, and there are alterations in clotting activity. The increased incidence of thrombosis in coronary and cerebral arteries may be related to changes in clotting activity. Daily low-dose aspirin sometimes is prescribed to counteract this phenomenon.
- There is progressive loss of body hair on extremities, which makes the use of this finding for a hematologic disorder unreliable in the elderly.
- Pigment loss and yellowish cast to the skin are common changes associated with aging; these routine skin changes make pallor and jaundice more difficult to discern in the elderly.

CAUSES OF HEMATOLOGIC DISORDERS

Hematology is the study of blood and blood-forming tissues. The lymphatic system, which drains the fluid from the spaces around each cell and channels it into the circulatory system, is discussed in Chapter 10. Several disorders that interfere with normal function of the blood are inherited. Hemophilia, sickle cell disease, and thalassemia types of anemias are examples. Accidental tearing or cutting of the vessels of the cardiovascular system and surgery cause bleeding and loss of blood. Blunt trauma to the spleen, such as might occur in an automobile accident, may cause tearing and massive internal hemorrhage. Chemicals and transfusions of the wrong blood type can cause **hemolysis** (destruction of red blood cells).

 Cultural Considerations

Genetic Hematologic Tendencies

- African Americans have the highest incidence of sickle cell disease.
- Pernicious anemia is more prevalent among those of Scandinavian descent and among African Americans.
- People of Middle-Eastern origin may have a genetic predisposition to thalassemia.

Some blood disorders are **iatrogenic;** that is, they are brought on by medical treatment. For example, blood **dyscrasias** (imbalance in numbers of types of cells) or other pathologic conditions of the blood can be induced through at least four kinds of actions:

- Bone marrow suppression, which interferes with the production of blood cells
- Interference with normal cell function
- Destruction of the blood cells by cytotoxic drugs
- Destruction of cells by a transfusion reaction of mismatched blood

Some antineoplastic drugs, for instance, act to depress the bone marrow, which inevitably causes a reduced supply of blood cells. Other drugs, such as phenytoin (Dilantin), primidone (Mysoline), and oral contraceptives, can produce anemia by interfering with the absorption and utilization of folic acid, a substance needed to produce RBCs. Diuretics such as furosemide (Lasix) and hydrochlorothiazide (Hydro-DIURIL) sometimes cause **leukopenia** (decreased numbers of white cells), aplastic anemia (deficient cell production due to a bone marrow disorder), and abnormally low counts of platelets and granulocytes. Procainamide hydrochloride (Pronestyl) and quinidine, which are used to correct dysrhythmias of the heart, also can cause thrombocytopenia (too few platelets), agranulocytosis (decrease in granulocyte production), and aplastic anemia. Most drugs are powerful chemicals that are capable of producing undesirable side effects, even though the drugs can be of great value.

Clinical Cues

If the patient is showing signs of a blood disorder, review the medications that are being taken, and note their side effects.

Nutritional deficiencies, such as low protein or lack of vitamin C, can interfere with erythropoiesis and normally functioning blood cells. Abnormal red cells are more prone to rapid destruction, which can result in anemia. Bone marrow damage from toxic substances may also interfere with the production of blood cells. Malignant conditions such as leukemia cause growth of abnormal blood cells and interfere with the production of normal cells. Box 16-1 presents factors that alter hematologic system function.

Nutrition Considerations

Nutrients Needed for Building Red Blood Cells (Erythropoiesis)

NUTRIENT	ROLE IN ERYTHROPOIESIS	FOOD SOURCES
Cobalamin (vitamin B_{12})	RBC maturation	Red meats, especially liver
Folic acid	RBC maturation	Green leafy vegetables, liver, meat, fish, legumes, whole grains
Iron	Hemoglobin synthesis	Liver and muscle meats, eggs, dried fruits, legumes, dark green leafy vegetables, whole-grain and enriched bread and cereals, potatoes
Vitamin B_6	Hemoglobin synthesis	Meats (especially pork and liver), wheat germ, legumes, potatoes, cornmeal, bananas
Amino acids	Synthesis of nucleoprotein	Eggs, meat, milk and milk products (cheese, ice cream), poultry, fish, legumes, nuts
Vitamin C	Conversion of folic acid to its active forms; aids in iron absorption	Citrus fruits, leafy green vegetables, strawberries, cantaloupe

RBC, red blood cell.

Box 16-1 Factors that May Alter Function of the Hematologic System

GENETIC DISORDERS
- Hemophilia
- Sickle cell disease
- Agranulocytosis
- Fanconi syndrome

HEMORRHAGE (ANEMIA)
- Surgical blood loss
- Blood loss from childbirth or spontaneous abortion
- Traumatic blood loss

ANEMIA
- Iron deficiency
- Folic acid deficiency
- Pernicious anemia
- Chronic slow blood loss
- Aplastic anemia

HEMOLYSIS
- Blood transfusion reaction
- Genetic types of anemia

BONE MARROW SUPPRESSION
- Antineoplastic agents used in treatment of cancer
- Radiation treatment used for cancer
- Excessive exposure to ionizing radiation
- Exposure to toxic chemicals that damage bone marrow
- Drugs that suppress the bone marrow

BONE MARROW PROLIFERATION OR ABNORMALITY
- Leukemia

PREVENTION OF HEMATOLOGIC DISORDERS

When considerable blood is lost through hemorrhage, the patient becomes anemic. Sometimes excessive blood loss can occur during menstruation. Prevent hemorrhage after surgery or childbirth by vigilantly assessing the amount of blood loss and by instituting measures to stop the loss if it is excessive.

Clinical Cues

The average amount of blood loss via menstruation is less than 80 mL. A better way to estimate that blood loss is to count the number of saturated pads or tampons. Each saturated pad is equal to about 50 mL of blood loss.

The nurse can help prevent anemia by promoting proper nutrition and by educating the public about the possibility of nutritional anemia. Nutritional anemia is a particular concern for individuals who subsist mostly on "fast food."

An elderly person, especially one who lives alone, is at high risk of poor nutrition. Problems with arthritis, vision, and chronic diseases make it more difficult for the elderly to shop for food and to prepare food. As a result, an elderly person may substitute cookies, toast, or cereal for a well-balanced meal. It is important to obtain a food intake history.

Secretion of intrinsic factor from the stomach and absorption of vitamin B_{12} is decreased in the elderly. The lack of these substances can lead to pernicious anemia from B_{12} deficiency (see Chapter 17).

Monitoring patients for drug side effects, and alerting the physician should blood-related side effects occur, can prevent a serious blood disorder from developing. Carefully monitoring blood transfusions and promptly reporting any untoward reaction may decrease the incidence of hemolysis from a reaction.

Health Promotion

Preventing Blood Disorders

- Caution the public about the dangers of exposure to ionizing radiation and harmful chemicals, in order to help decrease the incidence of blood disorders related to harmful substances.
- Suggest genetic counseling (for the possibility of transmitting a genetic blood disorder to offspring) to those adults who have such a genetic disorder.
- Inform patients about medications they are taking that can cause blood disorders; remind patients to be alert for signs of excessive bruising or easy bleeding. Suggest that CBCs be checked periodically, for monitoring purposes.

DIAGNOSTIC TESTS AND PROCEDURES

A surprising amount of information can be obtained from a stained blood film using only a 5-mL sample of uncoagulated blood. Each of the formed elements can be studied for shape, maturity, and number. Other kinds of studies include those done to measure the rate at which RBCs settle out from plasma (called the *sedimentation rate*) and to separate and classify various kinds of proteins, including antibodies, in the plasma. Explain the venipuncture procedure and the purpose of the test to the patient. Many patients have a great fear of needles. Others are concerned about having what seems like a lot of blood withdrawn. A few words of assurance and explanation can do much to relieve anxiety about a needle stick and to promote cooperation. Use Standard Precautions and aseptic technique for the venipuncture, and the correct tubes for each sample. Wear latex or impermeable gloves any time a venipuncture is performed, and dispose of phlebotomy equipment according to Standard Precautions (see Appendix B).

The CBC of your patient shows the following values:
- RBCs: 4.8 million/mm³
- WBCs: 6.7 million/mm³
- Hemoglobin: 10.2 g/dL
- Platelets: 250,000/mm³

What abnormalities, if any, do these results indicate?

Leukocyte counts provide information about infection and possible immune disorders (see Chapter 12). Data about the number of platelets are valuable in diagnosing a variety of diseases affecting—or affected by—the clotting of blood. There are at least 12 different types of hemoglobin in human blood. The types are designated by letters—for example, hemoglobin A is normal adult hemoglobin, hemoglobin F is normal fetal hemoglobin, and hemoglobin S is found in sickle cell disease. A **hematocrit** is a test that measures the volume of blood cells in relation to the volume of plasma. When there has been a loss of body fluids but no loss of cells (as in dehydration), the cell volume is high in proportion to the amount of liquid (plasma) in the bloodstream (i.e., the hematocrit rises). When either hemorrhage or anemia has depleted the supply of cells, the blood is "thinned" and the cell volume is low. Table 16-1 presents the most common diagnostic tests and related nursing care for the hematologic and lymphatic systems.

- Increased numbers of eosinophils often indicate allergy.
- A viral infection prompts the production of additional lymphocytes.
- Bacterial infection stimulates the production of neutrophils, and segmented neutrophils (segs) increase.
- Ongoing bacterial infections cause immature neutrophils to appear in the blood as *bands* (immature forms of segmented granulocytes). This is referred to as a "shift to the left."
- A "shift to the right" occurs when there are more mature neutrophils than usual; this occurs with anemia from vitamin B_{12} or folic acid deficiency.

❖ NURSING MANAGEMENT

■ Assessment (Data Collection)

History

The nurse assesses patients for signs and symptoms that indicate abnormalities in the blood. Abnormal symptoms result from too little circulating blood or too little hemoglobin, too few platelets, deficiency of normal neutrophils or lymphocytes, and too many abnormal blood cells. **When there is insufficient hemoglobin to carry oxygen to the cells, signs of oxygen deficit occur.** Perform a focused assessment to obtain an appropriate history. Inquire about renal disease as this may be a cause of anemia.

Table 16-1   Diagnostic Tests for Disorders of the Hematologic System

TEST AND NORMAL RANGE	PURPOSE	DESCRIPTION	NURSING IMPLICATIONS
Complete blood count (CBC)	Determine whether abnormalities are present in the numbers of blood cells or types of blood cells; assess the amount of hemoglobin present. Useful to diagnose anemia.	Fill a lavender-top tube containing EDTA with a venous sample of blood. Use a site where there is little chance of dilution from intravenous solution. Mix the blood and the EDTA by gently rotating the tube.	Warn the patient that a "stick" is about to occur, but that the pain will be short-lived. Apply pressure directly to the puncture site after withdrawing the needle; at the antecubital space, do *not* have the patient flex the arm as this tends to cause a hematoma.

Erythrocytes

Hemoglobin: females: 12.0-16.7 g/dL; males: 13.0-18.0 g/dL
Red blood cell (RBC) count: females: 4.2-5.4 million/mm^3; males: 4.6-6.2 million/mm^3
Hematocrit: females: 37%-47%; males: 40%-54%

Leukocytes

White blood cell (WBC) count: 4500-11,000/mm^3

Differential Count

Granulocytes
  Neutrophils: 54%-62% of WBCs
  Eosinophils: 1%-3% of WBCs
  Basophils: 0%-1% of WBCs
Agranulocytes
  Lymphocytes: 25%-33% of WBCs
  Monocytes: 3%-7% of WBCs
Thrombocytes (platelets): 150,000-400,000/mm^3 of blood
Mean corpuscular hemoglobin (Hb) (MCH): 26-34 pg/cell
Mean corpuscular Hb concentration (MCHC): 32-36 g/dL
Mean corpuscular volume (MCV): 80-96 μm^3

Erythrocyte Sedimentation Rate (ESR)

Wintrobe:
  Males: 0.5 mm/hr
  Females: 0-15 mm/hr
Westergren:
  Males: 0-15 mm/hr
  Females: 0-20 mm/hr
	To detect inflammation and infection.	Fill a blue-top tube with venous blood.
		The laboratory determines the rate at which the RBCs settle.
			Explain that this test helps diagnose an inflammatory process but is nonspecific.

Hemoglobin Electrophoresis

Hemoglobin A$_{1c}$:
  3%-5%
Hemoglobin A$_2$:
  1.5%-3%
Hemoglobin F: <1% of total
	Useful in diagnosing various types of anemia.
	Useful for diagnosis and monitoring of diabetes mellitus.
		Performed on venous sample using lavender-top tube with EDTA.	Same as for CBC.

Tests for Anemia

Ferritin, serum:
  20-200 ng/mL
Total iron-binding capacity:
  250-410 mcg/dL
Saturation 20%-55%
	Detect reason for anemia.	Obtain a venous blood sample of 5-7 mL in a red-top tube.	Same as for CBC.

Note: Normal values differ between laboratories.

Continued

Table 16-1 Diagnostic Tests for Disorders of the Hematologic System—cont'd

TEST AND NORMAL RANGE	PURPOSE	DESCRIPTION	NURSING IMPLICATIONS
Coagulation Tests			
Prothrombin time (PT): 12-14 sec Activated partial thromboplastin time (APTT): 20-25 sec Bleeding time, Ivy: 2.75-8.0 min	Determine abnormalities of clotting time.	Performed on a venous blood sample; use a blue-top tube.	Same as for a CBC; pressure may need to be applied longer than usual if the patient has an abnormal clotting time or is on heparin or warfarin therapy.
D-Dimer			
Negative: <0.5 mcg/mL	Blood test that provides assay of fibrin degradation to assess thrombin and plasmin activity. Useful for diagnosing pulmonary embolism and disseminated intravascular coagulation (DIC).	Collect blood sample in a blue-top tube.	No fasting is required.
Sickledex			
0	Tests for the presence of hemoglobin S.	Performed on a venous blood sample; use a lavender-top tube.	Client may be anxious about the result; be sensitive to patient emotions. Positive result indicates need for genetic counseling.
Bence-Jones Protein Test			
Presence of Bence-Jones proteins in the urine is abnormal	Assists in the diagnosis of multiple myeloma.	Obtain a 10-mL fresh morning specimen of urine in a clean container. Must be refrigerated or tested immediately.	Explain the procedure to the patient.
Schilling Test			
≥7% excreted within 24 hr	Determines ability to absorb vitamin B_{12}; used to diagnose pernicious anemia.	Radioactive B_{12} is given orally, followed in 2 hr by an intramuscular injection of B_{12}. A 24-hr urine specimen is collected.	Assess kidney function. Requires an 8- to 12-hr fast. No B vitamins for 3 days prior; no laxatives for 24 hr. Subnormal levels of B_{12} in the urine indicate the lack of intrinsic factor, which facilitates absorption of vitamin B_{12}.
Bone Marrow Aspiration and Biopsy			
Normal cell counts	Helps diagnose blood disorders.	Cells are withdrawn by needle from the sternum or iliac crest. Leukocytes, platelets, and erythrocytes are examined in the various stages of development to determine abnormalities. Assist in identifying certain anemias, leukemia, and thrombocytopenia.	Explain that the aspiration is done at the bedside. Seek an order for prebiopsy medication to decrease the discomfort. Explain that there is a feeling of pressure when the needle is inserted and sharp, brief pain when the marrow is aspirated. The area of aspiration is surgically prepped. The patient must hold perfectly still. Pressure is applied to the site afterward to prevent hematoma formation. Post-test, observe for swelling and tenderness, indicating continued bleeding or infection.

Focused Assessment

Data Collection for the Hematologic System

HISTORY TAKING

Ask the patient the following questions:

- Do you or anyone in your family have a genetic blood disorder (hemophilia, thalassemia, sickle cell trait or disease, aplastic anemia, agranulocytosis, or thrombocytopenic purpura)?
- What is your occupation?
- Have you ever been told you had anemia?
- Do you become easily fatigued?
- Do you have frequent sore throats or other infections?
- Do you frequently feel as though you have a fever?
- Do you ever have night sweats?
- Are your joints painful? Do they swell?
- Do you bruise easily or develop pinpoint blood spots?
- Do you suffer from itching?
- Do you have any swollen lymph nodes in the groin or armpits?
- Do you ever have tingling or numbness in the extremities?
- Do you have frequent headaches? Palpitations?
- Have you become more irritable than usual?
- Do you get dizzy frequently? Do you suffer fainting spells?
- Do you get short of breath when you walk a short distance or when you climb stairs?
- Do your gums bleed when you brush your teeth? Does your tongue get sore? Do you have frequent mouth sores?
- Do you have any difficulty eating?
- How much alcohol do you drink in a day?
- Do colds or infections seem to last a long time for you?
- Do you often feel fatigued even when not doing much?
- Have you been exposed to chemicals, such as pesticides, cleaning agents, or industrial chemicals of any kind?
- Have you ever noticed that you have black, tarry-looking stool? Smoky or brown urine?
- Do you have stomach pain or indigestion or ever had an ulcer?
- Are your menstrual periods unusually heavy?
- What do you usually eat for each meal?
- Are you often cold when others are not?
- Are there cultural factors you would like considered?
- What are your expectations of treatment?

PHYSICAL ASSESSMENT

Head and Neck

- Color of conjunctiva and sclera of eye
- Condition of gums, oral mucous membranes, and tongue
- Presence of enlarged cervical lymph nodes

Skin

- Color (pale) (check conjunctivae, palms of hands, and roof of the mouth in people with dark skin)
- Condition of fingernails (brittle, spoon-shaped)
- Presence of ecchymoses or petechiae
- Jaundice
- Nasal or gingival bleeding
- Hair (dry, brittle, thinning)

Chest and Abdomen

- Presence of swollen lymph nodes in armpits or groin
- Rapid respirations; shortness of breath on exertion
- Rapid pulse rate at rest
- Widened pulse pressure (greater distance between systolic and diastolic pressure)
- Epigastric tenderness
- Abdominal distention

Extremities

- Presence of swollen or painful joints
- Different lengths of fingers and toes

Urine and Stool

- Signs of blood

Physical Assessment

Skin. Although pallor may be a sign of anemia, it is not the most reliable sign. Many other factors can affect a person's complexion and skin color, including thickness of the skin, amount of skin pigment, and number and distribution of blood vessels near the surface of the skin. Pale mucous membranes or pale conjunctiva of the eye are better indicators of anemia. A very ruddy complexion with a red, florid appearance is typical of an excessive number of red blood cells (polycythemia).

Jaundice, or a yellowing discoloration of the skin and sclera of the eyes, can occur as a result of excessive destruction of red blood cells (hemolysis). When red blood cells are ruptured, bilirubin is released. The pigment eventually finds its way into the bloodstream, where it causes jaundice. If hemolysis is occurring, the urine will often contain bilirubin, giving urine a brown tea color.

Bruises and small, red, pinpoint lesions (petechiae) are typical of thrombocytopenic purpura, a hemorrhagic disease sometimes associated with a decrease in the number of circulating platelets. In dark-skinned people, check the palms of the hands and soles of the feet for petechiae. Bleeding under the skin and formation of bruises in response to the slightest trauma frequently occur in anemias, leukemias, and diseases affecting the bone marrow and spleen. These appear as darker areas on brown-skinned people.

Elder Care Points

- Elderly people bruise more easily because of thinner skin and greater fragility of blood vessel walls.
- Aspirin, omega-3 fatty acids, vitamin E, ginkgo biloba, and some prescription drugs also may make elderly people more prone to bruising.
- Bruising is not necessarily an unusual sign in this age group.

Cyanosis, or a bluish tint to the skin, can indicate hypoxia resulting from inadequate numbers of circulating erythrocytes. The gums or the roof of the mouth are the best places to check for a bluish color in dark-skinned people.

Mucous Membranes. Nutritional deficiencies contributing to anemia and resultant hypoxia may cause sore and painful gums and tongue. The patient may have difficulty chewing and eating. The tongue may be smooth and beefy red. Bleeding of the gums (gingivitis) may occur with toothbrushing when the platelet count is low.

Abdomen. Stomach pain or nausea can be caused by bleeding ulcers (a frequent cause of chronic blood loss). Black, tarry stools or coffee-ground emesis indicates gastrointestinal (GI) bleeding. Hiatal hernia also can cause a chronic blood loss.

Assignment Considerations

Observing for Blood

If a nursing assistant will be assisting the patient with toileting, remind that person to check stool for signs of **melena** (dark stool containing blood pigments) and the urine for a smoky color (indicating blood).

Clinical Cues

For the hospitalized patient with thrombocytopenia, abdominal girth should be measured daily to detect internal bleeding. Place marks on the lateral aspects of the abdomen where the measuring tape is placed and measure at the umbilicus. Put the measuring tape in the same place each day.

Swollen and Painful Joints. Bleeding into the joints (hemarthrosis) is not uncommon in certain kinds of anemia or in hemophilia. This might be evidenced by swelling and slight redness in the area of the joints, or the patient may move more slowly and with obvious discomfort.

Lymph Tissue Involvement. Enlarged lymph nodes occur in a number of different blood disorders, as well as in infections and immune disorders. The nodes most often inspected and palpated are those under the arm, in the neck, and in the inguinal (groin) region. Lymph node enlargement is often found while bathing a patient or helping her with activities of daily living (ADLs).

Assignment Considerations

Changes to Report

When assigning tasks to a certified nursing assistant (CNA) or unlicensed assistive personnel (UAP), ask the person to report any swellings he notices when assisting the patient with bathing. State that the patient may bruise easily and ask to report any new bruised areas or patient complaints of bleeding of gums or elsewhere.

Enlargement of the spleen, which also accompanies polycythemia and several other blood disorders, might be described by the patient as a feeling of fullness on the left side of the upper abdomen. Palpate the abdomen gently in a patient with a suspected blood disorder. Do not palpate deeply if there is tenderness in the area of the spleen, as this could cause rupture of the spleen.

Mental State. Irritability and mental depression are often found in patients with blood disorders. Irritability, dizziness, difficulty in concentrating, and headache may be caused by a decreased supply of oxygen to the brain. Depression often accompanies the chronic lack of energy, difficulty in eating and enjoying food,

and the many other problems from which patients with blood disorders often suffer.

Elder Care Points

An elderly person who has developed pernicious anemia may present with confusion and a loss of mental faculties. This state may be initially thought to be Alzheimer's disease. A blood count is important to establish the correct diagnosis.

Activity Intolerance. Physical activity increases the demand for oxygen, but if there are not enough circulating RBCs to carry the necessary oxygen, the patient becomes physically weak and unable to engage in physical activity without severe fatigue. Note whether the patient is able to do things for herself or needs help to complete specific ADLs.

Think Critically

- Can you name four signs or symptoms that you might encounter when taking a patient's history that could indicate your patient may be anemic?
- How can the conjunctiva and the sclera of the eye provide information about anemia or jaundice?
- What signs and symptoms might indicate that the patient is suffering a chronic blood loss?

■ Nursing Diagnosis

Nursing diagnoses for hematologic and lymphatic disorders are based on the problems the disorders cause for the patient. Nursing diagnoses commonly associated with hematologic disorders are listed in Table 16-2. They must be individualized for each patient.

Planning

Plan nursing care to provide rest periods for the patient. For patients with anemia, plan dietary teaching or consultation with the dietitian. **The patient with a blood abnormality is at higher risk for infection, so it is extremely important to use aseptic technique.** Patients with a blood abnormality should not be exposed to people who are ill with contagious diseases, such as colds or influenza. Nursing goals include:

- Prevent infection.
- Conserve patient's energy and prevent undue fatigue.
- Correct nutritional deficiencies.
- Provide treatment to halt or slow disease process.
- Control pain or discomfort.

Specific expected outcomes are written for individualized nursing diagnoses.

Table 16-2	Common Nursing Diagnoses, Expected Outcomes, and Interventions for Patients with Blood Disorders

NURSING DIAGNOSIS	GOALS/EXPECTED OUTCOMES	NURSING INTERVENTIONS
Imbalanced nutrition: less than body requirements, related to iron deficiency from inadequate intake, blood loss, vitamin B_{12} deficiency.	Protein levels will be within normal limits within 6 wk. Hemoglobin levels will be within normal range within 3 mo. CBC shows increasing RBCs and Hb within 3 wk. The patient will administer her own B_{12} injections on a regular schedule.	Teach the patient about foods that meet required needs. Obtain dietary consultation as needed. Administer iron preparation; if liquid, give through straw. Give iron with juice or food containing vitamin C. Warn that stool may be greenish black. Monitor CBC count for evidence of increase in RBCs and Hg. Administer vitamin B_{12} as ordered; advise that lifetime therapy is needed.
Impaired tissue integrity, related to inflammation of mucous membranes	The patient performs mouth care diligently on schedule. Patient displays normal-appearing mucous membranes.	Give gentle mouth care before meals and q 2 hr. Provide bland, easily chewed foods.
Activity intolerance, related to decreased RBCs or Hb	Patient uses oxygen as ordered. Patient alternates activities with rest. Patient seeks assistance with ambulation when dizzy.	Administer oxygen by nasal cannula at 3–6 L/min as ordered for patient with sickle cell crisis. Space activities, allowing rest periods for patient with fatigue. Assist with ADLs to prevent fatigue. If dizzy, caution to change position slowly; call for assistance with ambulation.
Pain, related to ischemia and swollen joints	Patient verbalizes that pain is controlled by analgesics. Patient verbalizes that pain has decreased within 48 hr.	Elevate swollen joints, and apply hot or cold packs. Teach to avoid strenuous exercise. Use bed cradle to support bed covers. Administer analgesics as ordered PRN.
Risk for injury, related to low platelet count	Platelet count will be within safe limits after platelet administration. Patient will have no new hematoma formation or other evidence of bleeding.	Assess for signs of internal bleeding (bruises, blood in urine or stool); measure abdominal girth q day. Minimize trauma; handle gently. Apply ice packs and gentle pressure if hematoma seems to be forming. Monitor administration of platelets PRN. Use small-gauge needle for injections; rotate sites. Apply pressure to puncture site for 10 min.
Risk for infection, related to decreased leukocytes	Patient will have no evidence of infection.	Observe for early signs of infection and report. Use strict aseptic technique for wound care and invasive procedures. Use protective isolation as needed. Teach patient good personal hygiene. Maintain integrity of skin and mucosa. Administer anti-infective drugs precisely as ordered.
Deficient knowledge, related to substances that damage bone marrow	Patient will verbalize knowledge of drugs and chemicals that are harmful to the bone marrow within 1 wk.	Assess for exposure to substances that could have damaged the bone marrow. Teach about drugs and chemicals that are harmful to bone marrow and how to prevent damage. Seek feedback to validate understanding of content taught.

ADLs, activities of daily living; *CBC,* complete blood count; *Hb,* hemoglobin; *PRN,* as needed; *RBCs,* red blood cells.

Continued

Table 16-2	Common Nursing Diagnoses, Expected Outcomes, and Interventions for Patients with Blood Disorders—cont'd	
NURSING DIAGNOSIS	**GOALS/EXPECTED OUTCOMES**	**NURSING INTERVENTIONS**
Anxiety, related to unknown outcome of diagnostic tests and knowledge of disease, treatment, and prognosis	Patient will verbalize purpose and expected experience for each diagnostic test ordered. Patient verbalizes fears regarding disease, treatment, and prognosis.	Provide teaching regarding each diagnostic test. Encourage verbalization of fears. Offer emotional support to patient and family.
Situational chronic low self-esteem, related to inability to perform usual activities	Patient will define ways to cope with physical limitations. Patient will verbalize strengths. Patient will discuss possibility of seeking counseling.	Assist to cope with limitations of the illness. Help plan ways to maintain appropriate activity. Help to focus on the things she can still do. Obtain counseling referral if psychological disturbance indicates need.
Risk of disabled family coping, related to expense of treatment and possible death of patient	Patient and family will seek assistance from community resources as needed. Patient and family will verbalize understanding of disease, treatment modalities, and their implications.	Refer leukemia patient and family to community resources, such as the American Cancer Society, for assistance. Assist family and patient to understand the disease, treatment modalities, and their implications. Encourage attendance for all family members in a support group. Obtain referral to social worker for further assistance. Encourage open communication within family.

■ Implementation

Handle patients with blood dyscrasias gently to prevent bruising and hematomas. Take care to apply pressure for 5 to 10 minutes after injections or venipuncture. Good skin care is essential, as the skin acts as a protective barrier against infection. Teach about nutrition and medication administration, prevention of infection, and measures to prevent bleeding. Pain control is important for the patient with sickle cell anemia in crisis, the hemophiliac with hemarthrosis, and for the advanced leukemia patient.

 Assignment Considerations

Report Oozing of Blood

Although the nurse is responsible for checking the patient for signs of bleeding, when a patient with a blood disorder has had blood drawn or an invasive procedure, ask the CNA or UAP to report any oozing noticed at the site or on bandages when he is providing basic care such as feeding or toileting.

 Think Critically

When caring for a patient who has been in an automobile accident and has sustained trauma to the trunk of the body, what laboratory values should the nurse check daily?

See Table 16-2 for specific interventions for patients experiencing blood disorders. Other interventions are included in the discussion of the various disorders in Chapter 17.

■ Evaluation

The evaluation process provides data to determine whether the specific outcome criteria are being met for each patient. Monitor laboratory values for blood counts and determine whether counts are improving to determine if treatment and nursing actions are meeting the patient's needs. Assess for side effects and evaluate how the patient is tolerating the medication or other treatment for the underlying disorder.

 Home Care Considerations

Evaluating Treatment

It is important that each home care nurse evaluate how closely the patient is following the prescribed treatment plan. Determine whether the treatment is effective, and if it is not effective, consult the physician about changing the plan.

 Clinical Cues

When a patient with leukemia is undergoing chemotherapy, evaluate the blood count results to determine that safe levels of leukocytes and platelets are present before administering another dose of a drug that inhibits their production.

COMMON PROBLEMS RELATED TO DISORDERS OF THE HEMATOLOGIC SYSTEM

EXCESSIVE BLEEDING

When injury has occurred, or spontaneous bleeding happens, you should immediately apply pressure to stop the bleeding (Figure 16-3). Severe bleeding can lead to irreversible hypovolemic shock and circulatory collapse from loss of intravascular fluid. Blood loss from an artery is bright red and will gush forth in spurts at regular intervals as the heart contracts. Blood from a severed or punctured vein leaks slowly and steadily and is dark red. Box 16-2 presents methods of controlling bleeding. If bleeding is due to absence of sufficient clotting factors, a transfusion of that factor or of platelets will be ordered. See Chapters 3 and 17 for information on transfusions.

Clinical Cues

Blood loss in the GI tract from an ulcer, tumor, or hiatal hernia can be in small amounts or in a large enough amount to make stool appear black (melena). Loss of 50 to 75 mL of blood from the upper GI tract is required before melena will appear.

FATIGUE

Help decrease fatigue by spacing activities throughout the day, with frequent rest periods. Assure the patient that her stamina will improve as her red cell count and hemoglobin rise. Work with the patient and family to decrease chores and expectations while fatigue is being experienced. Fatigue is common with anemia, and it affects all aspects of the patient's life (Agnihotri et al., 2007).

FIGURE 16-3 Locations of commonly used digital pressure points to stop hemorrhage. The screened areas are those within which hemorrhage may be controlled by pressure on a specific artery. **A,** Carotid artery. **B,** Temporal artery. **C,** External maxillary artery. **D,** Subclavian artery. **E,** Brachial artery. **F,** Femoral artery.

Box 16-2 Techniques to Control Bleeding*

- Position the body part that is bleeding over a firm surface and immobilize the part.
- Place a sterile dressing or clean cloth over the wound.
- With the flat palm of the hand or several fingers, apply direct pressure on the wound continuously for 5 minutes.
- Check whether bleeding has stopped after 5 minutes; if bleeding is occurring, apply pressure continuously for another 10 minutes.
- When bleeding has stopped, gently remove hand pressure and apply a pressure dressing over the cloth or dressing by folding another dressing or piece of cloth several times and tying it firmly over the wound.
- Check circulation distal to the wound to be certain that the pressure dressing is not so tight that circulation below the wound is cut off.
- Reinforce the dressing as needed by applying yet another layer of dressing as blood soaks through; do not remove previously applied dressings.
- If direct pressure will not stop the bleeding, and bleeding is considerable, apply pressure over the artery leading to the wound. **(Cut off arterial flow only as a last resort.)**
- Check for adequate pressure over the artery by determining a lack of pulse distal to the wound and patient report of a sensation of tingling and numbness in the wound area.

*Severe bleeding can lead to irreversible hypovolemic shock from loss of intravascular fluid and to circulatory collapse.

ANOREXIA

Serve small, frequent meals high in protein, vitamin C, and iron, unless contraindicated. Provide mouth care before each meal. Offer foods that are appealing to the patient. Keep the eating environment pleasant and free of odors. Ask family to sit with the patient, to offer socialization and encouragement during meals.

PAIN

If the patient is experiencing pain, all comfort measures should be employed. Assess pain level at least every 4 hours and medicate as ordered. Teach relaxation and imagery and assist the patient to perform these techniques (see Chapter 7). Pain may escalate quickly for the sickle cell anemia patient in crisis, so assess pain level at least every 2 hours.

INFECTION

When a patient is moderately to severely anemic, the oxygen-carrying capacity of the blood is considerably decreased. Less than optimal tissue perfusion and tissue hypoxia make it easier for pathogens to invade and cause infection. When WBCs are decreased or abnormal, there are fewer cells to fight infection. Patients with abnormalities of the blood need to be taught how to protect themselves from infection. Good hand hygiene is essential. Staying away from crowds and individuals with infections is necessary. Getting enough sleep and eating a well-balanced diet help keep the immune system as healthy as possible under the circumstances. Prophylactic antibiotics may be given in certain situations. Precautions for the patient who is prone to infection because of neutropenia are located in Chapters 8 and 17.

If the patient develops an infection, close monitoring of therapy and symptoms is needed. Rest, plenty of fluids, and sufficient protein and vitamin C are required to help the patient heal.

BONE MARROW FAILURE

Bone marrow failure occurs from abnormal cells overcrowding the normal cells or from inadequate production of normal cells. Leukemia causes overproliferation of abnormal cells in the bone marrow. Chemotherapy and radiation, thrombocytopenic purpura, and chemical toxicity can be factors in bone marrow failure. Predisposition to anemia, thrombocytopenia, and decreased WBCs occur. Sometimes bone marrow recovery occurs if the toxic agent is avoided, but usually a bone marrow transplant or stem cell transplant is necessary.

Get Ready for the NCLEX® Examination!

Key Points

- When there is a decreased number of RBCs or decreased hemoglobin, there is a reduction in the amount of oxygen that reaches the cells.
- Leukocytes are the first line of defense against microbial agents.
- Neutrophils perform phagocytosis.
- Lymphocytes such as B cells and T cells destroy foreign proteins.
- Platelets are the first line of cell protection to prevent bleeding when trauma has occurred.
- When the platelet count is low, spontaneous bleeding may occur.
- Bone marrow activity decreases by 50% in the elderly.
- Blood in the elderly coagulates more easily due to platelet *aggregation* (sticking together).
- Hemophilia, sickle cell disease, and certain types of anemias that cause blood disorders are inherited.
- Blood dyscrasias may be caused by drugs, radiation, or toxic substances (see Box 16-1).
- Nutritional deficiencies can cause anemia.
- The CBC with a differential count (count of the different types of white cells) can help diagnose many blood disorders (see Table 16-1).
- Bone marrow aspiration is used to diagnose a variety of blood disorders.
- A history is gathered and a focused physical assessment is performed for the patient with a suspected blood disorder.
- There are common nursing diagnoses appropriate for the patient with a blood disorder (see Table 16-2).
- Preventing infection, conserving energy, controlling pain, and correcting the underlying cause are the goals of care for the patient with a blood disorder.
- Patients with blood disorders must be handled gently.
- Checking serial CBCs is part of the evaluation process.
- Methods to stop bleeding should be taught to patients and families.
- Self-care measures are taught to each patient to prevent infection.

Additional Learning Resources

SG Go to your Study Guide for additional learning activities to help you master this chapter content.

evolve Go to your Evolve website (http://evolve.elsevier.com/deWit/medsurg) for the following FREE learning resources:
- Animations, audio, and video
- Answers and rationales for questions and activities
- Concept Map Creator
- Glossary with pronunciations in English and Spanish
- Interactive Review Questions and Exercises and more!

Review Questions for the NCLEX® Examination

1. For a patient with the clinical finding of leukocytosis, the nurse should:
   1. initiate transmission-based isolation precautions.
   2. inspect for signs of active bleeding.
   3. anticipate a possible physician order for antibiotic coverage.
   4. schedule periods of rest and activity.

2. For an elderly patient admitted for recent falls, which clinical finding(s) relative to the hematologic system would be associated with the aging process? *(Select all that apply.)*
   1. Decreased hematocrit and red blood cells
   2. Decreased antibody buildup from flu immunization
   3. Prolonged prothrombin time and sedimentation rate
   4. Increased neutrophils to fight infection
   5. Increased coagulability, which predisposes to clots

3. The physician informs the nurse that the patient has a "shift to the right." Which CBC laboratory result indicates a shift to the right?

1. 13.8, RBC 4.4 mm^3, WBC 12.4 mm^3, Neus 72%, Eos 1%, Lymphs 29%, Monos 1%, Platelets 268,000
2. 14.2, RBC 4.6 mm^3, WBC 4.4 mm^3, Neus 58%, Lymphs 36%, Platelets 285,000
3. 14.8, RBC 4.2 mm^3, WBC 10.8 mm^3, Neus 62%, Eos 2%, Lymphs 29%, Platelets 360,000
4. 10.8, RBC 3.2 mm^3, WBC 12.2 mm^3, Neus 56%, Lymphs 27%, Platelets 294,000

4. To confirm the diagnosis of pernicious anemia, the patient undergoes a Schilling test. This test involves a(n):

1. oral dose of vitamin B_{12} followed by collection of a 24-hour urine specimen.
2. oral dose of a multivitamin containing B_{12}, followed by an injection of B_{12}.
3. B_{12} injection followed by collection of a 24-hour urine specimen.
4. dose of radioactive vitamin B_{12} followed by an injection of B_{12} and collection of a 24-hour urine specimen.

5. The nurse describes the patient's skin as having a ruddy complexion with a red, florid appearance. The condition is most likely caused by:

1. increased red blood cells.
2. decreased platelets.
3. increased basophils.
4. decreased neutrophils.

6. The patient displays characteristic pinpoint red lesions. This assessment finding is called _____ and is often caused by _____.

1. ecchymosis; vitamin B_{12} deficiency
2. thrombocytopenic purpura; platelet deficiency
3. angioedema; iron deficiency anemia
4. petechiae; bruising of the skin

7. The nurse taking care of an elderly woman with pernicious anemia demonstrates understanding of the functional implications by:

1. promoting adequate rest.
2. actively listening to the patient's concerns.
3. monitoring for bleeding.
4. administering antibiotics.

8. The nurse initiates neutropenic precautions for a patient who has undergone chemotherapy. Which nursing action(s) would be considered appropriate? (Select all that apply.)

1. Use clean technique for wound care and invasive procedures.
2. Use transmission-based isolation precautions as needed.
3. Allow all visitors as desired.
4. Maintain integrity of skin and mucosa.
5. Provide analgesics, as needed.

9. The nurse formulates the following expected outcome for a patient admitted with hemarthrosis: "The patient will have no new hematomas or other evidence of bleeding." The most appropriate nursing intervention would be to:

1. suggest the patient use a soft toothbrush.
2. handle the patient very gently, protecting joints.
3. keep the skin well lubricated.
4. place the patient on a mechanical soft diet.

10. After removing a peripheral vascular access device, the nurse notes bleeding at the site. Put the following nursing actions in order of priority.

1. Tape a sterile dressing over the site.
2. Check for other areas of bleeding.
3. Apply direct pressure.
4. Elevate the extremity.

Critical Thinking Activities

Scenario A
You come upon an automobile accident and stop to help.

1. The first victim has a gash in his thigh and blood is spurting at regular intervals from the wound. What method would you use to stop the bleeding?

2. The second victim has a bleeding wound on the forehead. What method would you use to stop the bleeding?

Scenario B
Mr. Jones has a disorder that has caused leukopenia. He lives alone. To prepare him for discharge home, you would need to provide teaching for him.

1. What would you teach him about preventing infection?

2. What would you suggest regarding visitors who wish to see him?

3. What would you tell him about performing necessary errands?

Scenario C
Your 38-year-old male patient has a history of seizures and takes phenytoin. He has developed mild hypertension and takes hydrochlorothiazide to control the blood pressure.

1. What would you teach him about measures to prevent blood disorders?

2. What would you recommend to him for monitoring possible problems?

Objectives

Theory

1. Identify the causes of the various types of anemias.
2. Develop a plan of care for the patient with an anemia.
3. Explain the pathophysiology and care of sickle cell disease.
4. Compare cell abnormalities of polycythemia vera to those of leukemia.
5. Formulate a teaching plan for the patient with leukemia.
6. Comprehend why multiple myeloma is a disease affecting older people.
7. Discuss the problems and treatments the hemophilia patient faces.

Clinical Practice

1. Considering the goals of care, write expected outcomes for each of the appropriate nursing diagnoses for a patient with a blood disorder.
2. Prepare to provide preprocedure and postprocedure care for the patient undergoing a bone marrow aspiration.
3. Perform an assessment on a patient with a suspected hematologic disorder.
4. Assist with the development of a plan of care for an adult with leukemia.
5. Assess for signs and symptoms of disseminated intravascular coagulation.

Key Terms

allogeneic (ĂL-ō-JĔN-ĭk, p. 364)
anemia (ă-NĒ-mē-ă, p. 346)
autologous (ăw-TŎL-ŏ-gŭs, pp. 362, 364)
disseminated intravascular coagulation (DIC) (dĭ-SĔM-ĭ-nāt-ĕd ĭn-tră-VĂS-cū-lăr kō-ăg-ū-LĀ-shŭn, p. 362)
ecchymoses (ĕk-ĭ-MŌ-sēz, p. 359)
hemarthrosis (hē-măr-THRŌ-sĭs, p. 361)

hemolysis (hē-MŎL-ĭ-sĭs, p. 347)
hypovolemia (hī-pō-vō-LĒ-mē-ă, p. 346)
leukapheresis (lū-kă-fĕ-RĒ-sĭs, p. 356)
purpura (PŬR-pū-ră, p. 359)
splenomegaly (splē-nō-MĔG-ă-lē, p. 354)
stomatitis (stō-mă-TĪ-tĭs, p. 359)
thrombocytopenia (thrŏm-bō-sīt-ō-PĒ-nē-ă, p. 359)

DISORDERS OF THE HEMATOLOGIC SYSTEM

ANEMIA

In the human body, healthy red blood cells (RBCs) carry oxygen to tissues. A balance is maintained between the production of new RBCs and the disposal of old "worn-out" RBCs. Anemia occurs when something interferes with this balance or interferes with the maturation of cells. Anemia is a state in which there are insufficient numbers of functioning RBCs, or a lack of hemoglobin, to meet the demands of the tissues for oxygen.

Etiology

There are three major classifications of anemia, according to cause:
- Anemia resulting from blood loss
- Anemia resulting from a failure in blood cell production

- Anemia associated with an excessive destruction of red cells

Rapid, severe bleeding leads to anemia from blood loss, hypovolemia (decreased volume of circulating blood), and, potentially, shock. A blood loss that leads to anemia may result from severe trauma to the blood vessels and massive hemorrhage or the blood loss may be more gradual, as from a small, bleeding peptic ulcer that causes a chronic blood loss.

The amount of blood loss that leads to hypovolemic shock varies, depending on the ability of the patient's body to compensate for the lost fluid volume. A blood loss of even 500 mL in an adult who had normal circulating volume may cause hypovolemic shock. See Chapter 45 for the treatment of shock. Table 17-1 shows the amount of blood loss and consequent clinical manifestations.

Anemia caused by a failure in cell production is the result of either a deficiency of certain substances

Table 17-1	Clinical Manifestations of Acute Blood Loss
VOLUME LOST	**CLINICAL MANIFESTATIONS**
10%	None
20%	At rest, no signs or symptoms; slight postural hypotension when standing; tachycardia with exercise
30%	Blood pressure and pulse normal when supine; postural hypotension and tachycardia with exercise
40%	Below-normal blood pressure, central venous pressure, and cardiac output at rest; rapid, thready pulse and cold, clammy skin
50%	Shock and potential death

Adapted from Lewis, S.L., Heitkemper, M.M., Dirksen, S.R., et al. (2007). *Medical-Surgical Nursing: Assessment and Management of Clinical Problems* (7th ed.). St. Louis: Mosby, p. 695.

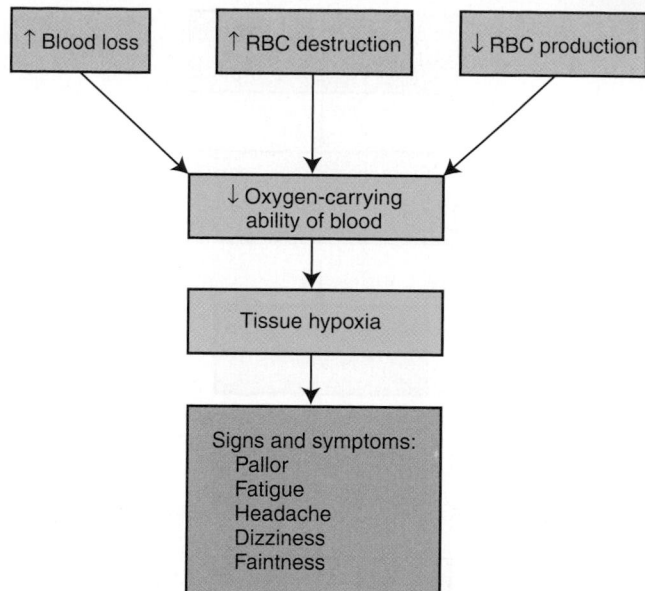

CONCEPT MAP 17-1 Pathophysiology of anemia.

necessary for the formation of RBCs, or results from the abnormal function of bone marrow. Examples of this type of anemia are:

- Nutritional anemia, in which there is an inadequate intake of foods containing proteins, folic acid, and iron
- Anemia resulting from bone marrow suppression caused by toxic substances
- Pernicious anemia, in which there is faulty absorption of specific nutrients, such as vitamin B_{12}

Iron or folic acid may not be well absorbed in people who have an intestinal malabsorption syndrome.

Hemolytic anemias, in which red cells are destroyed prematurely in the body, have many causes. Hemolytic anemia can be a result of genetic defects that affect cell structure, causing the cells to disintegrate quickly. Some of the hemolytic anemias, such as *thalassemia*, are inherited, whereas others are acquired when erythrocytes are exposed to poisonous agents, such as chemicals or certain bacterial toxins.

Immune reactions can cause blood cell **hemolysis** (destruction of red cells). The presence of toxins in the blood, infections such as malaria, transfusion reactions, and changes in blood chemistry may cause red cell hemolysis. Blood incompatibility in the newborn (*erythroblastosis fetalis*) is another cause.

Elder Care Points

There is about a 20% incidence of anemia among the elderly, most often because of poor nutrition. Shock may develop with smaller blood loss in this group because of decreased vascular tone and impaired cardiac function.

Pathophysiology

Iron deficiency anemia occurs when total body iron is insufficient and erythropoiesis is diminished. The lack of iron impedes the formation of hemoglobin (Hb) (Concept Map 17-1). In *pernicious anemia*, an autoimmune disease, the intrinsic factor is missing from the gastric juices, and vitamin B_{12} is not absorbed without it. Vitamin B_{12} acts as a coenzyme in conjunction with folate metabolism and is important in the utilization of iron and protein for the manufacture of RBCs. The result of the missing intrinsic factor is that the red cell production is decreased, and those red cells that are produced are abnormal in their structure and function (Concept Map 17-2). To correct this condition, the physician will order the administration of vitamin B_{12}. A folic acid deficiency also contributes to anemia (Gentili et al., 2009).

Hemolytic anemias associated with excessive destruction of RBCs are quite rare. When red cells are not normal, they break up easily or are destroyed by the body more quickly than are normal red cells. This RBC destruction causes the anemia.

Anemia occurs in end-stage renal disease patients when there is a deficiency of production of *erythropoietin*, a substance necessary to stimulate the production of RBCs in the bone marrow. This problem is usually corrected by the administration of epoetin alfa (Epogen), which stimulates red cell production (Singh, 2006). **Oxygen transport depends on the number and condition of the red cells and the amount of hemoglobin they contain.**

Clinical Cues

If your patient has had gastric bypass surgery or a gastrectomy, there is a risk of pernicious anemia as there will be a decrease of available intrinsic factor. Observe for signs of pernicious anemia in this patient.

Patients who take medications over a long period of time that suppress gastric acid secretion (histamine-2 inhibitors, proton pump inhibitors) must be watched for signs of pernicious anemia. Supplementation with vitamin B_{12} injections or sublingual vitamin B_{12} may help avoid this problem.

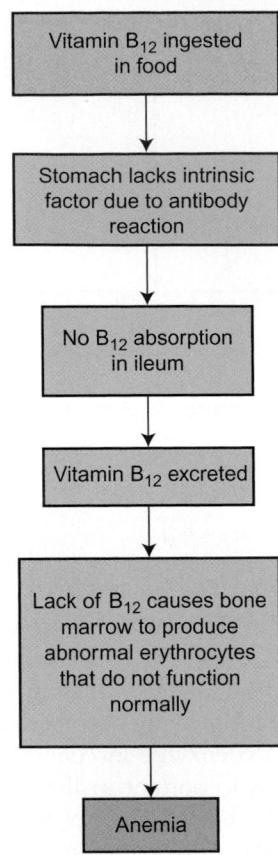

Vitamin B$_{12}$ ingested in food

↓

Stomach lacks intrinsic factor due to antibody reaction

↓

No B$_{12}$ absorption in ileum

↓

Vitamin B$_{12}$ excreted

↓

Lack of B$_{12}$ causes bone marrow to produce abnormal erythrocytes that do not function normally

↓

Anemia

CONCEPT MAP 17-2 Pathophysiology of pernicious anemia.

Signs and Symptoms

Signs and symptoms of anemias from causes other than rapid bleeding depend on whether the anemia is mild, moderate, or severe. Signs and symptoms of mild anemia (Hb 9.5 to 13 g/dL) are mild headache, palpitations, and dyspnea on exertion. Moderate anemia (Hb 6 to 10 g/dL) may include brittle nails, sore tongue, pallor, chronic fatigue, headache, and dizziness or faintness. Table 17-2 presents the many signs and symptoms of severe anemia. Tachypnea and tachycardia may develop with severe anemia due to the decreased ability of the blood to transport sufficient oxygen to the tissues.

Diagnosis

The microscopic appearance of the red cells in a film of blood that has been spread over a slide (a peripheral smear) gives information about abnormalities in size, shape, and color of erythrocytes circulating in the patient's bloodstream. The complete blood count (CBC) and differential cell count results are used to diagnose the presence of anemia. Measuring the quantity of hemoglobin tells whether the cells have sufficient amounts of hemoglobin to carry adequate oxygen to the body.

The prefix *normo-* refers to normal; the suffix *-cyte* refers to cells; the suffix *-chrom* refers to color; and the suffix *-ic* means "having the quality of" or "characterized by." Thus a normocytic, normochromic anemia is

Table **17-2**	Signs and Symptoms of Severe Anemia
BODY SYSTEM	**SIGNS AND SYMPTOMS**
General	Sensitivity to cold, lethargy, weight loss
Eyes	Blurred vision, blue colored sclera, yellowing of conjunctiva or pale conjunctiva, retinal hemorrhage
Skin	Pallor of face and palms, pruritus, jaundice, pale nail beds, pale mucous membranes, stomatitis, brittle nails, cheilitis
Cardiovascular	Palpitations, tachycardia, angina, systolic murmur, widened pulse pressure, intermittent claudication, CHF, possible MI
Respiratory	Tachypnea, orthopnea, dyspnea at rest
Gastrointestinal	Anorexia, difficulty swallowing, glossitis, enlarged liver, enlarged spleen, smooth tongue
Musculoskeletal	Bone pain
Neurologic	Headache, dizziness, impaired thinking, irritability, depression, fatigue

CHF, congestive heart failure; *MI,* myocardial infarction.

characterized by cells that are normal in size and color, but that have a deficiency in the number of RBCs and a low hematocrit. **This type of anemia usually occurs as a result of sudden blood loss.**

A hypochromic, microcytic anemia is characterized by decreased levels of hemoglobin (not enough color) and small (micro) cells. **This type of anemia is typical of an iron deficiency anemia.**

Nutrition Considerations

Common Foods High in Iron and Folic Acid

FOODS HIGH IN IRON

- Beef liver
- Blackstrap molasses
- Chicken liver
- Cooked oatmeal
- Cooked prunes
- Cooked shrimp
- Dried apricots
- Egg yolks
- Kidney beans
- Lean beef
- Lima beans
- Whole grains
- Prune juice
- Raisins
- Spinach and green leafy vegetables
- Turkey

Adding raw spinach to dinner salads and snacking on raisins or dried apricots can quickly improve iron intake. Iron-enriched cereals and breads also can be added to the diet.

FOODS HIGH IN FOLIC ACID

- Asparagus
- Beef
- Fish
- Cabbage
- Brussels sprouts
- Broccoli
- Legumes (kidney beans, etc.)
- Liver
- Eggs
- Whole grains

Note: Many of the foods high in iron also are high in folic acid.

Treatment

Anemia from chronic, slow blood loss is treated by correcting the underlying problem and then building replacement blood cells. Anemia caused by inadequate iron, folic acid, or protein intake is managed with oral iron supplements, vitamins, and diet adjustment. If the anemia is serious, blood transfusions may be given, or iron supplementation may be administered intravenously (IV) with iron dextran (Imferon), sodium ferrous gluconate, or iron sucrose.

Pernicious anemia is treated by regular injections of vitamin B$_{12}$, or by weekly use of an intranasal form of cyanocobalamin (Nascobal), as the deficiency of intrinsic factor prevents adequate absorption of this vitamin from food. There should be sufficient folic acid in the diet or by supplement. Table 17-3 presents the medications most commonly prescribed for hematologic disorders.

For *hemolytic* anemia, the underlying cause is found and corrected (if possible) and then the blood volume is rebuilt with added iron and appropriate diet. If the anemia is severe, blood transfusion may be indicated.

 Think Critically

Your patient who has suffered a blood loss and is now anemic complains that he is short of breath. Can you explain how blood loss might affect respiration?

❖ NURSING MANAGEMENT

■ Assessment (Data Collection)

Whenever a patient complains of fatigue, headaches, or shortness of breath, anemia should always be considered. Besides the CBC results, data regarding physical signs and symptoms are collected.

Table 17-3 Medications Commonly Prescribed for Disorders of the Hematologic System*

CLASSIFICATION	ACTION	NURSING IMPLICATIONS	PATIENT TEACHING
Mineral			
Ferrous sulfate (Feosol, Fer-In-Sol) Ferrous gluconate (Fergon) Ferrous fumarate (Feostat, Ircon) Iron dextran (Imferon) IM or IV Iron sucrose IV (Venofer) Sodium ferric gluconate IV	Increases elemental iron as a component in the formation of hemoglobin. Used to treat iron deficiency anemia.	May cause GI upset: nausea, diarrhea, or constipation; monitor for constipation. Tell patient that oral form will turn stool black. Do not give with milk as it reduces absorption. Dilute elixir in juice and give through a straw to prevent staining of the teeth. Do not crush enteric-coated or sustained-release tablets or capsules. For IM form, give with at least a 3-inch, 19- to 20-gauge needle and use Z-track technique to prevent staining of the skin. Change needles after drawing up the solution. When given IV, monitor closely for anaphylactic reaction. Give with epinephrine; have Solu-Medrol on hand. Flush line with 10 mL saline postinfusion.	Take oral form with orange juice or other vitamin C–rich food. Avoid taking iron with milk products. Keep out of reach of children as it is toxic. Have Hb checked according to physician's schedule to check response to medication. Eat foods high in iron. Increase fluids and roughage if constipation occurs.
Vitamins			
Folic acid (Folvite)	Promotes normal erythropoiesis; used in certain types of anemia.	May interfere with anticonvulsant blood levels. Chloramphenicol interferes with absorption. Increase foods high in folic acid.	Have blood count monitored according to physician's schedule to determine effectiveness of therapy.

BP, blood pressure; *CBC*, complete blood count; *GI*, gastrointestinal; *Hb*, hemoglobin; *HIV*, human immunodeficiency virus; *IM*, intramuscularly; *IV*, intravenously; *RBCs*, red blood cells; *Subcut*, subcutaneously; *WBC*, white blood cell.
*Chemotherapy drugs are presented in Chapter 8.

Continued

Table 17-3   Medications Commonly Prescribed for Disorders of the Hematologic System—cont'd

CLASSIFICATION	ACTION	NURSING IMPLICATIONS	PATIENT TEACHING
Vitamins—cont'd			
Vitamin B$_{12}$ Cyanocobalamin (Rubramin, Anacobin); methylcobalamin	Acts as coenzyme for cell replication and hematopoiesis. Used in pernicious anemia, other GI disorders that decrease vitamin B$_{12}$ absorption, and cases of dietary deficiency.	Give Subcut or IM daily for 5-10 days and then once monthly for maintenance. Can cause anaphylactic reaction when given IV. Deficiency more common in strict vegetarians.	Teach importance of maintaining monthly injections for life, in order to prevent further episodes of pernicious anemia. Encourage increased intake of vitamin B$_{12}$ in diet if deficiency is diet related.
Antimetabolite			
Hydroxyurea (Hydrea)	Inhibits DNA synthesis. Used to reduce episodes of sickling in sickle cell anemia. Used to eradicate abnormal cells in leukemia, myeloma, and some solid tumors.	Discontinue if WBC count is <2500/mm^3 or platelet count is >100,000/mm^3. Capsule granules may be mixed with water if taken immediately. May cause GI problems: stomach upset, stomatitis, vomiting, diarrhea.	Use cautiously in presence of renal dysfunction. Radiation therapy increases toxicity. Monitor intake and output. Monitor for infection. Monitor blood counts for neutropenia and thrombocytopenia; bone marrow suppression. Caution to avoid exposure to infection and to report signs or symptoms of infection promptly. Increase fluid intake to maintain adequate hydration. Give mouth care q 4 hr to prevent stomatitis. Report bleeding to the physician.
Biologic Response Modifiers			
Epoetin alfa; erythropoietin (Epogen, Procrit)	Controls rate of red cell production; a natural hormone produced by recombinant DNA techniques. Stimulates the bone marrow, functioning as a growth factor. Used to combat reduced production of erythropoietin in end-stage renal disease. Used as adjunct therapy in HIV-infected patients with anemia secondary to drug therapy.	Also used for patients with anemia secondary to chemotherapy and in rheumatoid arthritis patients who experience anemia from therapy. May be used to increase RBCs in anticipation of autologous blood transfusion before surgery.	May cause seizures. Monitor blood count closely; dosage may need to be reduced if hematocrit rises too rapidly. Monitor blood pressure closely; may cause rise. May cause pain in limbs and pelvis. Explain the purpose of the injections. Remind that the drug must be refrigerated; discard after 6 hr at room temperature.
Filgrastim (Neupogen)	Stimulates production, maturation, and activation of neutrophils.	CBC with differential before beginning therapy and twice weekly thereafter. Monitor BP as may cause transient increase.	Teach to inform physician if fever, chills, severe bone pain, chest pain, or palpitations occur.
Pegfilgrastim (Neulasta)	Regulates production of neutrophils within bone marrow. Increases phagocytic activity.	CBC and differential before therapy and routinely thereafter. Monitor for allergic reaction (i.e., peripheral edema). Assess muscle strength. Observe mouth for stomatitis, mucositis.	Inform of possible side effects and how to watch for allergic reaction. Remind that regular blood counts are important.

Focused Assessment

Data Collection When Anemia Is Suspected

HEALTH HISTORY

Ask the patient the following questions:

- Have you had any recent blood loss or trauma?
- Do you have chronic liver, endocrine, gastrointestinal, or renal disease?
- What medications, vitamins, supplements, or herbal products do you take?
- What surgeries have you had and when?
- Have you ever had radiation treatments or chemotherapy?
- Is there a history of genetic blood disorders in your family?
- Has your appetite or weight changed?
- Have you noticed any changes in your urine or stool?
- Are you experiencing shortness of breath, weakness, or fatigue?
- Have you noticed any heart palpitations?
- Do you get frequent headaches?
- Have you noticed any changes in vision or dizziness?
- Do you have pain or itching anywhere?
- Do you become cold when others are not?

PHYSICAL ASSESSMENT

Check for the following:

- *Skin:* Pale skin and mucous membranes; pale conjunctiva, yellowing of sclera; cracks in lips; brittle, spoon-shaped fingernails (Figure 17-1); jaundice; petechiae; ecchymoses; dry, brittle, thinning hair
- *Respiratory:* Tachypnea, orthopnea, dyspnea on exertion or at rest
- *Cardiac:* Tachycardia, systolic murmur, angina, ankle edema
- *Gastrointestinal:* Sore mouth, stomatitis, beefy red tongue, abdominal distention, enlarged liver or spleen
- *Neurologic:* Headache, dizziness, confusion, irritability, ataxia (unsteady gait), paresthesia

PERTINENT LABORATORY VALUES

- CBC, serum iron, ferritin, folate, cobalamin (vitamin B_{12}), stool for guaiac, urinalysis, serum erythropoietin

■ Nursing Diagnosis

Nursing diagnoses are chosen based on the clinical findings and problems identified. Common nursing diagnoses include:

- *Activity intolerance,* related to weakness and fatigue
- *Impaired gas exchange,* related to decreased hemoglobin

FIGURE 17-1 Thin, concave (spoon-shaped) nails with raised edges may be seen on people with iron deficiency anemia.

- *Nutrition: less than body requirements,* related to poor nutritional intake and anorexia
- *Ineffective therapeutic regimen management,* related to lack of knowledge about appropriate nutrition and medication regimen

■ Planning

Expected outcomes are written for the specific individual nursing diagnoses chosen to resolve the patient's problems. For the nursing diagnoses listed above, outcomes might include:

- Within 1 month patient will be able to perform hygiene, dressing, and grooming activities without needing to rest between activities.
- Within 2 months patient will be able to carry out usual daily activities without shortness of breath or fatigue.
- Patient will eat three nutritious meals, containing sufficient iron, folic acid, vitamin C, and protein daily.
- Patient will verbalize understanding of dietary and medication regimen within 1 week.

■ Implementation

Intervention is based on an understanding of the particular kind of anemia affecting the patient. Anemia from blood loss presents problems quite different from those related to chronic—and possibly incurable—aplastic or hemolytic anemia. For patients with anemias that interfere with clotting and that tend to cause bleeding episodes, nursing actions are directed toward preventing the episodes. For any patient with anemia severe enough to cause fatigue, assist with daily living activities, and provide planned rest periods.

Nursing functions include administering blood, iron, vitamin B_{12}, and folic acid and monitoring for desired effects. Patients are educated about needed dietary adjustments. Patients should be taught that iron is absorbed more readily if vitamin C is simultaneously present in the gastrointestinal (GI) system. Taking iron medication with orange juice provides the necessary vitamin C.

Analgesia for headache or joint pain is given as ordered, and the patient is monitored for adverse side effects. More nursing diagnoses commonly associated with hematologic problems, including anemia, and lists of appropriate interventions are included in Table 16-2.

Elder Care Points

- Iron supplements should be taken 1 hour before or 2 hours after a meal, as long as they do not cause GI distress.
- Many elderly people have chronic conditions that require daily medication. Antacids and many other drugs interfere with iron absorption.
- Check all drugs a patient is receiving, in order to determine whether drug interactions might interfere with iron absorption.

■ Evaluation

Evaluation data are gathered to determine whether expected outcomes are being met. Laboratory values are particularly important when evaluating the care of the patient with anemia. However, equally important are data showing that the problems caused by the anemia are resolving.

APLASTIC ANEMIA

Aplastic anemia (a rare disorder) may develop after a viral infection, as a reaction to a drug, or because of an inherited tendency. The disease is characterized by bone marrow depression and is thought to probably be an immune-mediated disease. Red cells, white cells, and platelet levels are decreased. The toxic effects of certain substances can be responsible for aplastic anemia. Some of these agents include benzene; insecticides; drugs, such as chloramphenicol (Chloromycetin), phenylbutazone (Butazolidin), and sulfonamides; some anticonvulsants; gold compounds used to treat rheumatoid arthritis; and alkylating agents or antimetabolites used in chemotherapy. Many other drugs can cause aplastic anemia, but this adverse effect is rare. Radiation exposure is another factor in the development of the disorder.

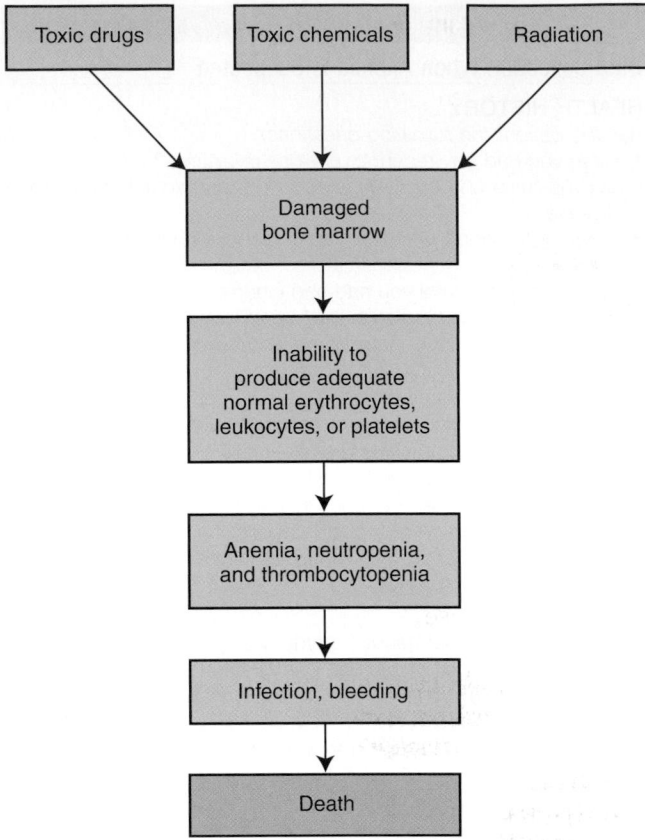

CONCEPT MAP 17-3 Pathophysiology of aplastic anemia.

! Safety Alert

Monitor Drug Side Effects

It is your responsibility to monitor blood studies carefully for all patients who are receiving any drug that is potentially damaging to the bone marrow.

? Think Critically

What chemical products in your home or garage are capable of causing bone marrow depression?

Impairment or failure of bone marrow function leading to the loss of stem cells is the cause of aplastic anemia (Concept Map 17-3). With aplastic anemia, the bone marrow has decreased cells and increased fatty tissue. In addition to the signs and symptoms of iron deficiency anemia, ecchymosis, petechiae, and hemorrhage related to low platelet count also occur. Infection is frequent and may not cause an inflammatory response because of the very low leukocyte count. There is often frequent bleeding in the mouth.

Diagnosis is by blood count with differential, bone marrow biopsy, and ruling out other disorders. **Aplastic anemia causes an emergency situation.** Treatment must eliminate any identifiable underlying cause. Packed red cells and platelets are administered. Antibiotics are given for identified infection; oxygen is sometimes administered to patients with low

erythrocyte counts. Bone marrow transplantation (BMT) is the treatment of choice for those under 45 years of age with severe bone marrow depression, but there must be an identical human leukocyte antigen (HLA) match. Immunosuppressive therapy with antithymocyte globulin (ATG) and cyclosporine is showing promise at improving outcomes. ATG contains polyclonal antibodies against human T cells.

Prevention of hemorrhage and infection is a top priority. Psychological support of the patient and family is important when they are faced with this life-threatening condition. Safety measures are priorities. Actions for problems of weakness and fatigue are the same as those presented for anemia earlier in the chapter. Other common nursing interventions are included in Table 16-2. See Chapter 8 and the Evolve website for precautions and actions for the patient with leukopenia and neutropenia and for safety measures when thrombocytopenia is present.

🏃 Health Promotion

Dangers of Toxic Agents

All nurses should promote public education about the dangers of toxic agents. It is vitally important that people read and follow the label instructions on all cleaning agents, insecticides, and chemical compounds.

Table 17-4	Comparison of Four Types of Anemia		
ANEMIA	**CHARACTERISTIC RBC**	**ETIOLOGY**	**ADDITIONAL EFFECTS**
Iron deficiency anemia	Microcytic, hypochromic Decreased hemoglobin production	Decreased dietary intake, malabsorption, blood loss	Only effects of anemia
Pernicious anemia	Megaloblasts, immature nucleated cells	Deficit of intrinsic factor due to immune reaction	Neurologic damage Achlorhydria
Aplastic anemia	Often normal cells Pancytopenia	Bone marrow damage or failure	Excessive bleeding and multiple infections
Sickle cell anemia	RBC elongates and hardens in "sickle" shape when O_2 levels are low—short life span	Recessive inheritance	Painful crises with multiple infarctions Hyperbilirubinemia

From Gould, B.E. & Dyer, R. M. (2011). *Pathophysiology for the Health Professions* (4th ed., p. 259). Philadelphia: Saunders.
RBC, red blood cell.

SICKLE CELL DISEASE

Etiology

Sickle cell disease is a genetic disorder in which the gene is inherited from both parents (homozygous gene) (Table 17-4). Sickle cell disease is characterized by erythrocytes that contain more hemoglobin S than hemoglobin A. Sickle cell disease is found in less than 1% of African American newborns, but also affects some people whose ancestors are from the Mediterranean region, the Middle East, and India. Approximately 8% of African Americans carry the gene.

Sickle cell trait, in which only about 50% of an individual's total hemoglobin is affected, is present in about 10% of the African American population of the United States. The trait is heterozygous, meaning that the person has an inherited gene for the trait from one parent only. People with the heterozygous trait for sickle cell are carriers; they can transmit the gene to their children even when they themselves do not show signs of the disease. Therefore, genetic counseling and adequate screening for early detection of the disease are considered extremely important to control sickle cell anemia. In the United States, many patients with sickle cell anemia live into their mid-40s. The most common cause of death is acute chest syndrome, where damage occurs to the lungs.

Pathophysiology

When the patient with sickle cell disease experiences lower oxygenation than normal, the defective S hemoglobin forms clumps in the red cells, causing them to assume a sickle shape, blocking blood vessels, breaking apart, and forming thrombi that cause organ damage. Sickle cells are destroyed by the body very quickly, causing anemia.

Sickle cell trait occurs in people who have only one gene, rather than a pair of genes, for sickle cell anemia. They usually do not have problems with cells assuming a sickle shape unless they experience severe oxygen deficiency.

Signs and Symptoms

The signs and symptoms of sickle cell disease are those that indicate lack of oxygen and blood flow, such as pallor, lethargy, and pain. The problems from interrupted normal blood flow affect many organs (Figure 17-2). Painful swelling of the hands and feet related to bone infarction from the sickled cells (hand-foot syndrome) may occur. After sickle cell crisis, signs typical of anemia occur because the abnormally shaped cells are very fragile, break easily, and are destroyed. The RBC and hemoglobin counts can drop very quickly during a crisis.

Diagnosis

A peripheral blood smear can show sickled cells. The sickling test, which exposes RBCs to a deoxygenating agent, is diagnostic. Hemoglobin electrophoresis identifies the presence of abnormal hemoglobin. During crisis, there will be elevations of serum bilirubin because of the hemolysis of the abnormal red cells. Bone and joint abnormalities are revealed by skeletal x-rays.

Treatment

There is no cure or specific treatment for sickle cell anemia; treatment is primarily symptomatic and preventive. Patients should be taking folic acid regularly and

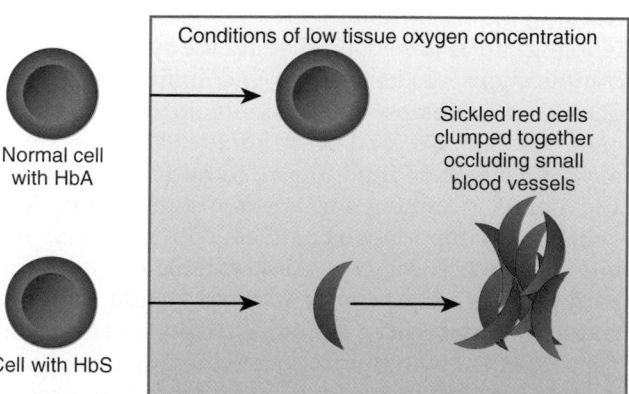

FIGURE 17-2 Sickling of red cells occurs when tissue oxygen is low.

eating a diet with sufficient protein to help build red cells. Infection is to be avoided, and the patient should receive all recommended immunizations against influenza, hepatitis A and B, pneumonia, tetanus, and the like. **Adequate intake of fluid on a daily basis is important to keep the blood as fluid as possible.** Alcohol and recreational drugs are to be avoided as they can cause complications. Quick attention for illness should be sought.

The drug hydroxyurea (Hydrea) has been found to reduce the frequency of sickling episodes. Patients on this drug have shown a 50% decrease in the number of hospitalizations for crisis (Platt, 2008). Sodium cromoglycate given by inhalation or via nasal route has been shown to significantly reduce the percentage of cells that sickle in venous blood (Bizumukama et al., 2009). If a crisis occurs, the patient may be treated at home with bed rest, adequate fluid intake, and analgesics. Pain control is important during a crisis. Narcotic analgesia with morphine is administered on a continuous basis, usually by patient-controlled analgesia pump. If the patient's hemoglobin drops considerably or his condition suddenly deteriorates, he is hospitalized, given oxygen, and transfused with packed red cells; in addition, IV fluids are given. An attempt is made to mobilize the sickled cells and to prevent damage to major organs. Infection is treated with appropriate antibiotics.

There are many complications of sickle cell disease, including cholecystitis, stroke, congestive heart failure, and damage to all major organs (Figure 17-3). One of the most common problems is leg ulcers, from impaired circulation to the legs and feet. Protecting the feet and lower legs from injury is important, since small wounds tend to develop into difficult-to-heal ulcers.

BMT is the only available treatment that can cure some patients. The scarcity of donors, the cost, and the risks involved greatly limit the use of this option. Gene therapy is offering hope for future treatment of sickle cell disease.

Nursing Management

Nursing care is aimed at relieving the symptoms from complications of the disease and minimizing organ damage. Patients are taught to avoid high altitudes, vigorous exercise, and iced liquids. Patients are to maintain adequate fluid intake, refrain from smoking, and obtain treatment for infections promptly. Adequate rest is important as patients with sickle cell anemia experience fatigue. **Assessment for adequate pain relief is a top priority** (Arnold & Besa, 2010). Intake and output will be monitored to prevent overloading the patient with fluid. Oxygen therapy is instituted if the patient is hypoxic (oxygen therapy helps prevent further cellular damage).

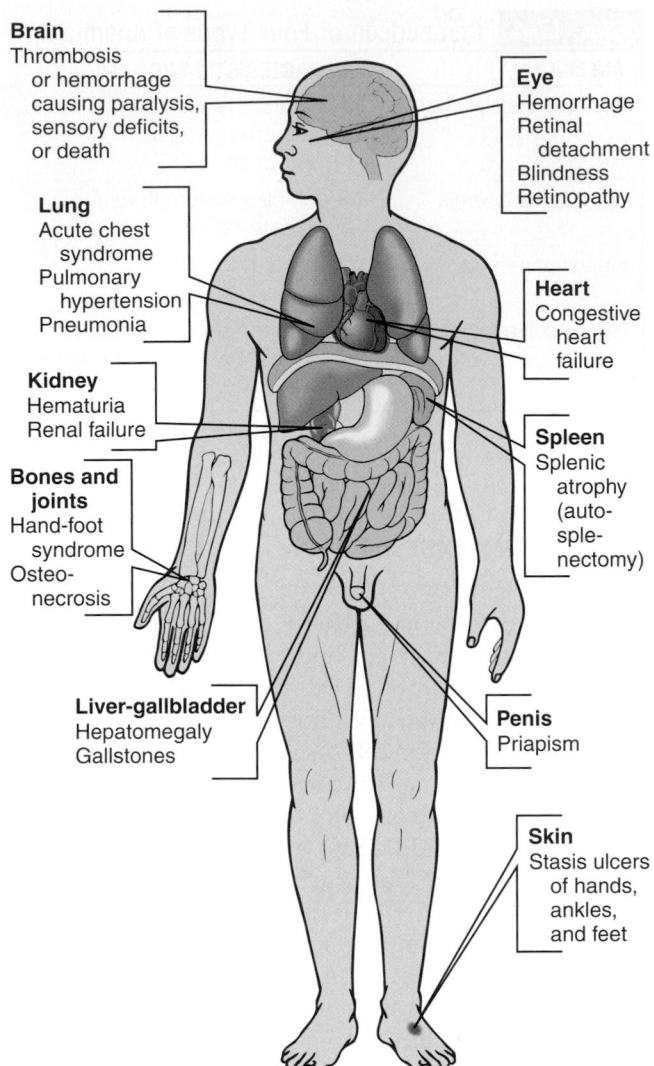

FIGURE 17-3 Clinical manifestations and complications of sickle cell disease.

POLYCYTHEMIA VERA

Excessive production of RBCs results in polycythemia vera. White cell numbers also increase, but not to the degree that they do in leukemia. The cause of polycythemia vera is unknown, but the disease is considered a neoplastic disorder. The blood becomes thick from the increased numbers of cells, blood vessels become distended, and blood flow is sluggish. Because of the sluggish flow, there is a tendency to develop blood clots. Blood pressure is elevated and the heart hypertrophies. Hemorrhage is frequent in areas of distended blood vessels. Signs and symptoms of polycythemia vera include a reddish face with deep-red purplish lips, fatigue, weakness, dizziness, headache, enlarged spleen (splenomegaly), and congested liver. Minor injury may result in excessive bleeding.

Treatment is aimed at reducing the number of blood cells. Phlebotomy, antineoplastic agents, and radiation therapy are all used. In phlebotomy, a blood vessel is pierced, and blood is drawn off. As much as 500 mL of blood at a time may be withdrawn every 2 to 3 months. **Increased fluid intake is essential to decrease blood viscosity, and aspirin is used to decrease platelet clumping and clot formation.**

A secondary polycythemia may develop in response to prolonged hypoxia and increased erythropoietin secretion. Secondary polycythemia does not have the same effects as primary polycythemia.

LEUKEMIA

The word *leukemia,* translated literally, means "white blood." Actually, the white blood cells (WBCs) would have to number $1,000,000/mm^3$ before the blood would have a milky white appearance, and, although leukemia is characterized by an increase in the number of leukocytes, their number rarely rises above $500,000/mm^3$. In addition to the increase in number, however, the leukocytes of the patient with leukemia are abnormal cells that do not function as normal white cells do.

Etiology

Leukemia is a cancer, and as with other types of cancers, the exact cause of leukemia is not known. There are factors considered to be closely linked with the development of leukemia. **Exposure to ionizing radiation in relatively large doses is one such factor. Another is exposure to certain chemicals, such as benzene, that are toxic to bone marrow.** Benzene is an ingredient in lead-free gasoline, and the incidence of leukemia has risen since lead-free gasoline has been in use. The amount of exposure to benzene and other chemicals that causes bone marrow suppression is unknown, and this amount possibly varies among individuals. **The point is to be careful about breathing gasoline fumes and using household chemicals and pesticides.** The third factor is the retrovirus known as human T-lymphotropic virus 1 (HTLV-1), which causes human T-cell leukemia. People with an abnormal number of chromosomes and chromosomal translocations are at a greater risk for developing acute lymphocytic leukemia. About 90% of patients with chronic myelogenous leukemia have the Philadelphia chromosome.

Malignant production of WBCs is the actual cause of the disease. DNA become damaged. Table 17-5 shows the clinical manifestations of leukemia and the factors linked to their development.

Pathophysiology

An acute leukemia is one in which there are a large number of primitive cells, called blasts. In chronic leukemia, the predominant cells are more developed than blasts. Leukemias are also classified by the origin of the abnormal cells. Myeloid leukemia arises from the bone marrow, whereas lymphoid leukemia has its origin in the lymphatic system. There are four main types of leukemia: acute myelogenous leukemia (AML), chronic

Table 17-5	Causes of Clinical Signs of Leukemia
MANIFESTATIONS	**CAUSES**
Severe infections	Immature and abnormally functioning leukocytes, even though there is an increased number of them.
Symptoms of anemia	Rapidly proliferating white cells apparently "crowd out" developing red cells and platelets.
Enlarged spleen, liver, and lymph nodes	Excess white cells accumulate within organs, causing distention of tissues.
Weakness, pallor, and weight loss due to elevated metabolic rate	Increased production of white cells requires large amounts of amino acids and vitamins. Increased destruction of cells leads to more metabolic wastes that must be disposed of by the body.
Renal pain, urinary stones and obstruction to flow of urine, and urinary tract infection	Large amounts of uric acid are released when white cells are destroyed by antileukemic drugs.
Headache, disorientation, and other central nervous system symptoms	Abnormal white cells infiltrate the central nervous system.

myelogenous leukemia (CML), acute lymphocytic leukemia (ALL), and chronic lymphocytic leukemia (CLL).

About 43,050 people developed leukemia in 2010 and 21,840 people in the United States will have died from it (National Cancer Institute, 2010). In acute leukemia there is a sudden, rapid growth of immature blast or stem cells, rapid progression of the disease, and a short survival if the disease is not treated.

Chronic forms of leukemia have a more gradual onset, slower disease progression, and a relatively longer survival time. CLL is common in men over age 50 and accounts for one third of the new cases of leukemia annually. CML is most common in young and middle-aged adults. Over time CML progresses to the acute form, and eventual death is common.

Leukemia has three major effects:
1. Increased numbers of abnormal, immature leukocytes
2. Accumulations of these cells within the lymph nodes, spleen, and other organs
3. Eventual infiltration of the malignant cells throughout the organs of the body

Signs, Symptoms, and Diagnosis

Patients with chronic leukemias are often asymptomatic, and the disease is detected during a regular physical examination and routine CBC. Other signs and symptoms of leukemias include fever, malaise, frequent or persistent infections (sore throat, flu, etc.), swollen lymph nodes, enlarged spleen, bone pain, weight loss, and easy bleeding or thrombosis. Diagnosis is made by using the history, physical examination, CBC with differential, and bone marrow studies to rule out other disorders.

Treatment

Treatment is aimed at:

- Slowing down the growth of the malignant blood cells
- Maintaining a normal level of red cells, hemoglobin, and platelets
- Managing the symptoms and meeting the special needs of each patient

Acute leukemia treatment consists primarily of chemotherapy with a combination of antineoplastic agents targeted at different phases of the cell cycle. The drug therapy is divided into three phases: induction, consolidation, and maintenance. *Remission induction* therapy is initiated at the time of diagnosis and consists of an intensive combination chemotherapy aimed at achieving a complete remission of symptoms. *Consolidation* therapy is another course of the same agents, or others, at a different dosage level, and the goal is to achieve cure. *Maintenance therapy* is usually oral chemotherapy at lesser doses taken for 2 to 5 years to maintain remission.

Elder Care Points

Patients over age 65 require reduced dosages of chemotherapeutic drugs (to prevent toxicity) because they have decreased kidney and liver function and the drugs are not metabolized as quickly as they are metabolized in a younger person.

Before chemotherapy is started, the patient should be well hydrated and given a drug orally to prevent hyperuricemia and kidney stones. Radiation therapy is used supplementally to increase the success of treatment and to decrease discomfort from enlarged organs (spleen, liver). Cure is sometimes possible, as has been evidenced in children with ALL. Results in adults have not been as good. BMT is a possibility for patients who have had an initial remission with chemotherapy. Eventually it is hoped that stem cell treatment, or monoclonal antibody treatment combined with BMT, will provide lasting remission. If an enlarged spleen does not respond to radiation, splenectomy may be performed. *Chronic lymphocytic leukemia (CLL)*—the most common leukemia seen in the elderly—is not treated until the patient experiences symptoms. At that time a combination of chemotherapy agents is used.

Chronic myelogenous leukemia (CML) is currently treated with imatinib (Gleevec) or a combination of imatinib with other agents. Recombinant human alpha interferon has been shown to reduce the growth and division of leukemic cells in 55% to 60% of patients (Besa & Woermann, 2009). Hydroxyurea (Hydrea) may be used as a single chemotherapeutic agent. Leukapheresis (separation of white cells) may be done to reduce the massive number of circulating leukocytes that clog organs and cause damage. Blood is drawn and the unwanted white cells are separated out, and the remainder is returned to the patient. A small percentage of CML patients are likely candidates for BMT.

Transfusions of blood components are prescribed for leukemia patients to maintain a near-normal blood

---

Box 17-1   Chemotherapeutic Agents Used to Specifically Treat Leukemia

CHRONIC LYMPHOCYTIC LEUKEMIA
- Chlorambucil
- Fludarabine
- Cyclophosphamide
- Vincristine
- Prednisone
- Rituximab
- Alemtuzumab
- Pentostatin
- Cladribine

CHRONIC MYELOGENOUS LEUKEMIA
- Imatinib
- Dasatinib
- Bisulfan
- Hydroxyurea
- Interferon alfa

ACUTE MYELOGENOUS LEUKEMIA
- Cytosine arabinoside
- Anthracycline
- Daunorubicin
- Doxorubicin
- Anthrocenedione
- Arabinosyl cytosine

ACUTE LYMPHOCYTIC LEUKEMIA/ACUTE LYMPHOBLASTIC LEUKEMIA
- Daunorubicin
- Vincristine
- Prednisone
- L-Asparaginase
- Cyclophosphamide
- Cytarabine
- 6-Mercaptopurine
- Methotrexate
- Cytosine arabinoside
- Clofarabine
- Doxorubicin
- Fludarabine
- Pentostatin
- Rituximab

picture. Platelet transfusion during or after chemotherapy often is necessary. Antibiotics may be given prophylactically during chemotherapy and are started immediately on signs of infection because the body's defense mechanisms are seriously compromised. Box 17-1 lists the chemotherapy agents used to treat the various types of leukemia.

Nursing Management

A thorough health assessment is performed and specific problems are identified. Nursing diagnoses for the patient with leukemia include those appropriate for anemia, leukopenia, and thrombocytopenia. Patient problems to be addressed are:

- Potential for infection
- Abnormal bleeding
- Anemia
- Nutritional alteration with severe anorexia and weight loss
- Increased levels of uric acid in the urine and blood (resulting from chemotherapy)
- Psychosocial problems related to the effects of the disease, as well as the prescribed treatment

Collaboration with the dietitian and the pharmacist is a key point in nursing care of the leukemic patient. Nursing Care Plan 17-1 presents care for common problems of the patient with leukemia.

Infections from bacteria, viruses, and fungi are the most common cause of death in people with leukemia. Infection is a threat either because of abnormal function of bone marrow that is characteristic of the disease or because of suppression of bone marrow function as a result of therapy. Nursing measures to prevent infection are essential, as is vigilant assessment for early signs (see Chapter 8 for the patient at risk for infection due to the effects of chemotherapy or radiation).

Abnormal bleeding as a result of a very low platelet count is the second most common and dangerous complication of leukemia. Observation of the patient, awareness of the patient's current platelet count, and prevention of trauma to body tissues and blood vessels as a result of low platelets are primary concerns in nursing management. See the Patient Teaching box on p. 169 for guidelines for the patient prone to bleeding.

✳ Nursing Care Plan 17-1   Care of the Patient with Leukemia

Scenario

James Cathcart, a 42-year-old man, has acute myelogenous leukemia (AML). He is undergoing outpatient chemotherapy and is being followed at home by a home care agency nurse.

Problem/Nursing Diagnosis

Very low white blood cell count/Risk for infection related to low WBCs.

Supporting Assessment Data

Objective: WBCs 2000/mm^3

Goals/Expected Outcomes	Nursing Interventions	Selected Rationale	Evaluation
Patient will remain free of infection.	Monitor temperature daily. Report elevation >100.4° F (>38° C) that lasts for more than 4 hr.	Temperature elevation may indicate beginning infection.	Temp remains at 99.2° F (37.3° C).
	Teach patient and family to perform hand hygiene frequently.	Hand hygiene helps prevent infection.	Hand hygiene used consistently.
	Use meticulous hand hygiene when caring for patient.	Helps prevent transmission of microorganisms.	
	Have patient deep breathe q 2 hr while awake.	Respiratory exercises help prevent respiratory infection from pooled secretions.	Using incentive spirometer regularly.
	Administer transfusion of granulocytes as needed.	Granulocyte transfusion provides WBCs to help fight infection.	Transfusion not ordered yet. Continue plan.
	Caution to eat only cooked fruits and vegetables.	Raw foods often carry bacteria that could cause infection.	States understands need to only eat cooked foods.

ADLs, activities of daily living; *CBC,* complete blood count; *RBCs,* red blood cells; *WBCs,* white blood cells.

Continued

Problem/Nursing Diagnosis
Has no energy/Fatigue related to chemotherapy side effects.

Supporting Assessment Data
Subjective: States has no energy; frequently falls asleep.
Objective: RBCs 3.2 million/mm³, Hct 33 mL/dL.

Goals/Expected Outcomes	Nursing Interventions	Selected Rationale	Evaluation
Patient will be able to bathe and dress self without assistance.	Provide bathing assistance daily.	Conserves patient's energy.	Bathing assistance given daily.
	Encourage resting between care activities.	Prevents undue fatigue.	Is resting between activities.
	Encourage to perform ADLs in small segments.	Preserves energy.	Is combing hair and brushing teeth.

Problem/Nursing Diagnosis
Patient cannot work/Disabled family coping related to loss of patient's income.

Supporting Assessment Data
Subjective: Patient too weak to work; wife seeking full-time employment.

Goals/Expected Outcomes	Nursing Interventions	Selected Rationale	Evaluation
Patient's wife will cope effectively as primary wage earner.	Assist wife with defining alternatives for employment.	Helps focus direction for employment.	Wife is considering possible alternatives.
	Arrange consultation with social worker to coordinate patient's care when wife returns to work.	Social worker can arrange in-home assistance.	Social Services appointment made.
	Suggest community resources that might help wife find employment.		Wife given list of community resources for employment. Continue plan.

Problem/Nursing Diagnosis
Low platelet count/Risk for injury related to decreased platelets.

Supporting Assessment Data
Objective: Platelets 106,000/mm³.

Goals/Expected Outcomes	Nursing Interventions	Selected Rationale	Evaluation
Patient will not experience episodes of bleeding.	Monitor CBC and platelet counts.	Will detect further decrease in platelets.	CBC remaining stable, but platelets down to 104,000/mm³.
	Instruct to report oozing of blood from the gums.	Alerts to potential for impending bleeding episode.	No oozing of blood.
	Instruct to observe stool and urine for signs of bleeding.		
	Administer stool softener to prevent constipation.	Soft stool will not injure rectal mucosa, causing bleeding.	Stool soft without signs of blood.
	Instruct to use soft toothbrush or toothettes to clean teeth.	Helps prevent small breaks in mucosa or skin that might cause bleeding.	Using soft toothbrush and electric razor. Continue plan.
	Instruct to use an electric razor to shave.		

Critical Thinking Questions
1. What measures are necessary for a patient who is immunosuppressed from chemotherapy and is susceptible to infection?
2. How could you help boost Mr. Cathcart's self-esteem now that he has to give up his role as the family wage earner?

Clinical Cues

The classic signs and symptoms of hypovolemic shock are falling blood pressure; rapid, weak pulse; cool, damp skin; thirst; decreased urine output; and restlessness progressing to decreased consciousness.

? Think Critically

Why is it common for the leukemia patient to have frequent infections? What causes this problem? When caring for a leukemia patient, what parameters would you need to assess to detect early signs of infection?

Elder Care Points

- The elderly patient already has decreased immune system function. When leukemia develops, or is treated, this patient is at very high risk for infection.
- The elderly patient cannot tolerate hemorrhage, and so hemorrhage must be carefully guarded against.
- Other conditions may affect appetite. Emphasis on an appropriate diet, supplements, good nutritional status, and excellent mouth care can make a marked difference in the quality of life of the elderly leukemia patient.

Anemia and its associated problems of fatigue, hypoxia, GI upsets, and cardiovascular complications affect the patient with leukemia. The anemia can result from the disease itself, from excessive bleeding, or from the therapy administered. Nursing measures previously described for the patient with anemia are appropriate to the care of the patient with leukemia. Colony-stimulating factor drugs sometimes are used to counteract the anemia and neutropenia caused by treatment for leukemia. However, these drugs may stimulate the growth of abnormal cells, making the patient's condition worse, and so are used with caution.

Nutritional problems arise from any of a number of conditions. **Extreme weight loss and cachexia are nearly always seen in patients with advanced cancer.** Failure to eat sufficient amounts of nutritious foods is not the only reason this is so. As explained in Chapter 8, metabolic changes that occur with the proliferation of malignant cells in the body also are responsible for weight loss and emaciation. If nursing measures to alleviate or minimize stomatitis (inflammation of the mouth), nausea, and vomiting are not effective, parenteral nutrition may be necessary (DeRanieri, 2008).

The increased level of uric acid that results from rapid cell destruction during chemotherapy often causes the uric acid crystals to settle out in the kidney structures, causing impaired renal function. Maintaining adequate hydration and administering drugs to decrease the production of uric acid are important nursing measures, as is close observation of fluid intake and urinary output. The emotional impact of a diagnosis of cancer and the psychosocial needs of the cancer patient and his family are discussed in Chapter 8.

THROMBOCYTOPENIA

Thrombocytopenia occurs when the platelet count drops to less than 150,000/mm^3 and can be a life-threatening condition. Causes include bone marrow depression from chemotherapy or radiation, autoimmune diseases, bacterial and viral infections, disseminated intravascular coagulation (DIC), and overfunction of the spleen. Certain drugs, such as nonsteroidal anti-inflammatory drugs (NSAIDs) and thiazides, also can result in platelet deficiency.

Immune thrombocytopenic purpura (ITP) is the most common acquired thrombocytopenia. It is an autoimmune disease in which there is abnormal destruction of circulating platelets. In ITP the platelets are covered with antibodies. In the spleen, these platelets are recognized as foreign, and are destroyed by macrophages. This disorder commonly occurs in women between 20 and 40 years of age. The chronic form of ITP has a gradual onset, with transient remissions. Heparin therapy sometimes causes a type of thrombocytopenia that can be life threatening. Porcine-prepared heparin seems to cause less of this problem than other types of heparin.

Many patients with thrombocytopenia are asymptomatic. Signs and symptoms of thrombocytopenia include purpura (small areas of multiple petechiae in the skin and mucous membranes) or large bruised areas caused by hemorrhage that are called ecchymoses (Figure 17-4). Bleeding can occur in any part of the body. Hemorrhage is the major danger.

Some patients recover spontaneously. Otherwise, transfusion of platelets is used to control hemorrhage.

FIGURE 17-4 Ecchymoses of the hand from thrombocytopenia.

Splenectomy is done when the cause of the thrombocytopenia is unknown and the patient does not respond to other therapy, with the hope that this will remove the cause of platelet destruction. A new drug, eltrombopag (Promacta), has been approved by the Food and Drug Administration (FDA) to treat the disease.

Nursing care is focused on prevention of bleeding by careful handling of the patient, close observation for signs of spontaneous bleeding, and quick intervention. Invasive procedures are used only when essential. Patients are taught to avoid activities that might induce bleeding (see Chapter 8).

 Safety Alert

Prevent Bleeding

For a patient with a low platelet count, whenever venipuncture is performed, an injection is administered, or an intravenous catheter or needle is discontinued, pressure over the site must be maintained for 10 minutes to prevent continuous oozing.

MULTIPLE MYELOMA

Multiple myeloma is a disease in which neoplastic plasma cells infiltrate the bone marrow and destroy bone. It occurs in about 4 in 100,000 people. Men are affected twice as often as women, and the disease occurs in African Americans twice as often as whites. The disease usually occurs after age 40, with the average age at diagnosis being 65 years.

Etiology and Pathophysiology

The cause of multiple myeloma is unknown. Risk factors include a family tendency toward the disease, ionizing radiation, and exposure to herbicides, insecticides, and chemicals (particularly benzene). Genetic factors and viral infections may play a role.

In multiple myeloma, abnormal plasma cells multiply out of control in the bone marrow. These abnormal cells produce excessive amounts of abnormal immunoglobulin and cytokines. The accumulation of the abnormal cells (tumors) in the bone marrow disrupts normal RBC, leukocyte, and platelet production. The disruption of normal cell production leads to anemia, impaired immune response with susceptibility to infection, and bleeding tendencies. The tumors disrupt normal bone marrow function and weaken the bone, predisposing the patient to frequent fractures.

Signs, Symptoms, and Diagnosis

The onset of multiple myeloma is gradual, and symptoms appear when the skeletal system is heavily involved. The patient may experience backache, bone pain that is worse with movement, or pathologic fractures and severe pain. Multiple myeloma is diagnosed by x-ray studies, bone marrow biopsy, and blood and urine tests. The appearance of light chains from the abnormal immunoglobulins in the urine, or Bence-Jones

proteins, is a diagnostic sign. Because the bone destruction during multiple myeloma releases calcium, a hypercalcemia occurs that may lead to kidney stone formation and renal impairment. The CBC will show anemia, leukopenia, and thrombocytopenia. For the patient with multiple myeloma, bone marrow studies show large numbers of immature plasma cells.

Treatment

Chemotherapy or palliative radiation is used to combat the disease. Pain control is a primary concern. Hypercalcemia and osteoporosis often develop, and patients must be monitored and treated for these complications. Measures must be taken to prevent pathologic fractures.

The most common chemotherapy regimen is melphalan and prednisone. It is given orally for 4 to 7 days and repeated at 4- to 6-week intervals. Bortezomib (Velcade) is another successful, targeted therapy for multiple myeloma. Thalidomide (Thalomid), an immune-modulating drug, has proven very successful alone or in combined treatment. Interferon alfa may be used to prolong a remission. Other chemotherapy agents may be used as needed. Bisphosphonates such as etidronate (Didronel), pamidronate (Aredia), or zoledronic acid (Zometa) inhibit bone breakdown and thereby decrease skeletal pain and hypercalcemia. The drug is given IV once a month. Measures are instituted to reduce blood calcium levels. There is no cure for multiple myeloma, but stem cell transplantation can prolong life for some patients.

Nursing Management

Supportive care for the many complications of the disease and treatment is provided. Encouraging adequate hydration with an intake of 3 to 5 L of fluid a day to minimize problems from hypercalcemia is a priority. Pain assessment and management are crucial to the quality of life for the patient. Acetaminophen and NSAIDs are used along with narcotic analgesics. Care is taken in moving the patient due to the potential for fractures.

 Assignment Considerations

Assisting Patients with Blood Disorders

When enlisting the aid of a nursing assistant to help with positioning, moving, or toileting the patient, remind the person that the patient is very prone to bruising, bleeding, or fractures (as the case may be). Do not assign ambulation of a patient with multiple myeloma to assistive personnel, because any slight bump or twist of the body may cause a fracture.

Psychosocial care is essential as the disease has remissions and exacerbations, and is eventually fatal. The nursing care for the patient with a neoplastic disorder is covered in Chapter 8. The patient and family must be taught about the signs and symptoms of hypercalcemia and instructed to report these signs and symptoms immediately to the physician. Measures to prevent falls must be instituted, both in the hospital and in the home. Mental status is monitored closely, and measures to protect the patient are instituted if confusion arises.

● HEMOPHILIA

Etiology

Hemophilia is an inherited X-linked disorder in which there is a deficiency of specific clotting factors. Classic hemophilia, or hemophilia A with a factor VIII deficiency, affects 1 in 5000 male births in the United States. Hemophilia B, or Christmas disease, causes a deficiency of factor IX. Christmas disease affects 1 in 30,000 male births. Both types of hemophilia are characterized by a delayed blood coagulation time that produces a prolonged period of bleeding after injury or surgery. These types of hemophilia almost always occur in males, and are genetically transmitted through the female. Although the female does not have the disease herself, she and all her female descendants can transmit classic hemophilia to their offspring. Acquired hemophilia can affect both men and women, but the disease is rare. Hemophilia can develop as a result of formation of antibody to the clotting factors in blood transfusions, in patients with collagen vascular disease, or after a drug reaction. Idiopathic occurrence may be seen in people older than 50 years of age.

Pathophysiology

The hallmark of hemophilia is bleeding into joints, causing loss of mobility and unequal extremity lengths. In all types of hemophilia, there is a decrease in the amount of activity of one of the 11 different clotting factors normally present in blood and essential to the formation of clots. The blood of a hemophiliac patient forms a clot immediately after injury, but the clot breaks down and does not effectively stop bleeding. In von Willebrand's disease, there is a decrease in the activity of factor VIII, even though the factor is present in normal amounts in the plasma.

There are varying degrees of severity in the types of hemophilia, depending on the amount of the factor present and the role of the factor in clot formation. For patients with mild cases (those who have 25% to 50% of the deficient factor present in the serum), symptoms may not appear at all until a severe injury or surgery is followed by prolonged bleeding, and the hemophilia is thus discovered. In very severe cases (those in which less than 1% of the factor is present) the affected individuals may bleed spontaneously without injury, and severe hemorrhage can develop very quickly whenever an injury does occur.

Signs and Symptoms

The most obvious symptom of hemophilia is bleeding. Bleeding most often occurs internally, with leakage of blood into the joints, into the intestinal wall or peritoneal cavity, and into the deeper tissues of the body. Hemarthrosis—bleeding into the joints—produces swelling, pain, warmth, and limitation of movement similar to that suffered by the patient with rheumatoid arthritis (Figure 17-5). Hemarthrosis is the primary problem for most hemophiliac patients. If the bleeding occurs in the intracranial spaces and thereby increases intracranial pressure, the patient may experience convulsions and brain damage that can be fatal. Other serious complications from internal bleeding in the person with hemophilia include obstruction of the airway as a result of hemorrhage into the neck or pharynx, and intestinal obstruction resulting from bleeding into the intestinal wall or peritoneum.

Diagnosis and Treatment

Diagnosis is by history, physical examination, CBC, and tests for the various clotting factors in the blood. In the more common types of hemophilia, transfusion of the blood factors replaces the missing factors and prevents bleeding. Recombinant forms of factor VIII and factor IX are now available; both decrease the risk of transmitting undetected viruses and prions as can occur with donor blood.

For mild hemophilia A and for some subtypes of von Willebrand's disease, desmopressin acetate (DDAVP), which is a synthetic form of vasopressin, may be given to stimulate an increase in factor VIII and von Willebrand factor. Tranexamic acid (Cyklokapron) and aminocaproic acid (Amicar) are administered to inhibit fibrinolysis by increasing clot stability.

Analgesic drugs and corticosteroids may be used to treat the joint inflammation and pain caused by hemarthrosis and by the frequent resultant arthritis. Safe analgesics include acetaminophen, oxycodone, propoxyphene, and pentazocine. Prophylactic factor

FIGURE 17-5 Aspiration of the knee to relieve the hemarthrosis common in hemophilia.

treatment may be administered before dental procedures or in advance of other invasive diagnostic tests and unavoidable surgery.

 Safety Alert

Avoid Taking Aspirin

Aspirin must never be taken by hemophiliac patients, as aspirin increases the bleeding problems. Patients must read the labels on every over-the-counter preparation to be certain that drug products do not contain aspirin or acetylsalicylic acid.

Many patients with hemophilia have been receiving blood products for a number of years. Unfortunately, many older patients have been infected with the human immunodeficiency virus (HIV) and/or hepatitis C virus from contaminated plasma concentrates. The problem of contamination has created additional psychological stress for the patient with hemophilia. About 90% of older people with severe hemophilia are HIV positive. Death from AIDS has been common. Fortunately, adequate screening is in place now and the problem is resolving.

Nursing Management

In addition to administering the necessary clotting factors, interventions include elevating the injured body part, applying cold packs, controlling pain, observing for further bleeding, and providing psychological support for the patient and family. The nurse should also encourage genetic counseling for family members, if this counseling has not occurred previously.

DISSEMINATED INTRAVASCULAR COAGULATION

Disseminated intravascular coagulation (DIC) is a complicated disorder that usually occurs in conjunction with tissue destruction. It accompanies serious problems, such as severe trauma, gram-negative sepsis, shock, respiratory distress syndrome, malignancy, transfusion reaction, amniotic embolus, and abruptio placentae (separation of the placenta from the uterine wall).

Damaged tissue liberates tissue thromboplastin, creating a state of excessive clotting in the microcirculation throughout the body. When excessive clotting depletes the body's clotting factors, hemorrhage follows, leading to hypotension or shock. DIC is always life threatening.

The first signs of DIC are usually continued bleeding from an injection or IV site, extensive bruising in areas of injury, ecchymoses where there has been no trauma, and petechiae. There may be oral, vaginal, or rectal bleeding. Laboratory studies will reveal a decreased hemoglobin and low platelet count. The prothrombin and activated partial thromboplastin times will be increased. The fibrinogen level is reduced, and the fibrin degradation products level is increased. The D-dimer result is elevated.

Treatment consists of correcting the underlying problem (e.g., trauma, infection). Vascular volume is maintained with fluid replacement; vasopressor medications are given to decrease bleeding, and mechanical ventilation is needed for ventilatory support and tissue perfusion. Fresh frozen plasma—packed RBCs—and other blood coagulation factors are administered, in order to restore blood volume and control clotting (Becker & Wira, 2009).

As a nursing priority, be alert to the possibility of the development of DIC whenever a patient has a condition that predisposes to it. Early detection of external bleeding and monitoring sensorium and vital signs for indications of internal bleeding are both extremely important.

THERAPIES FREQUENTLY USED IN THE MANAGEMENT OF HEMATOLOGIC DISORDERS

TRANSFUSIONS

A blood transfusion involves the administration of a blood component. To minimize the risks of circulatory overload, HIV, hepatitis, transfusion reaction, and other problems related to the administration, blood usually is transfused only when there has been a large blood loss, when the patient has a deficiency of a blood component, or when there must be a total blood exchange in a newborn. Table 17-6 shows some commonly used blood products, the usual amount given per transfusion, and reasons why each is used.

Autologous (originating in one's self) blood transfusion is commonly used when the patient's own blood can be collected and reinfused. Blood is collected either during or after surgery (such as from chest drainage) or blood is donated by the patient during the weeks before surgery, for later use. Laboratory procedures that separate the various components by centrifuge or other means allow for the administration of only the particular element of blood needed by a particular patient.

Dextran—a plasma expander similar to human albumin—is often used to replenish volume quickly, until needed blood products are obtained from the blood bank. Several artificial substitutes for human blood that eliminate the need for cross-matching are being tested. So far, no artificial substitutes for human blood have been released for use by the FDA. Special precautions are always taken when any blood component is given. Blood banks have written procedures and policies for withdrawing and dispensing blood for transfusion.

 Legal and Ethical Considerations

Consent for Blood Administration

The patient must have signed a consent form to receive a blood transfusion. If the patient is unable to sign, and the condition is life threatening and no family member is reachable, the physician may make the decision to transfuse the patient.

Table 17-6 Blood Products and Their Use

COMPONENT	VOLUME	INFUSION TIME	INDICATIONS
Packed red blood cells (PRBCs)	200-250 mL	2-4 hr	Anemia; hemoglobin <6 g/dL, depending on symptoms
Washed red blood cells (WBC-poor PRBCs)	200 mL	2-4 hr	History of allergic transfusion reactions Bone marrow transplantation patients
Platelets Pooled	About 300 mL	15-30 min	Thrombocytopenia, platelet count <20,000/mm^3 Patients who are actively bleeding with a platelet count <80,000/mm^3
Single donor	200 mL	30 min	History of febrile or allergic reactions
Fresh frozen plasma	200 mL	15-30 min	Deficiency in plasma coagulation factors Prothrombin or partial thromboplastin time 1.5 times normal
Cryoprecipitate	10-20 mL/unit	15-30 min	Hemophilia A or von Willebrand's disease Fibrinogen levels <100 mg/dL
White blood cells (WBCs)	400 mL	1 hr	Sepsis, neutropenic infection not responding to antibiotic therapy

Adapted from Ignatavicius, D.D., & Workman, M.L. (2010). *Medical-Surgical Nursing: Critical Thinking for Collaborative Care* (6th ed.). Philadelphia: Elsevier Saunders, p. 917.

Blood products are always checked by two nurses before administration (Figure 17-6). An LPN who is not qualified to transfuse blood may be asked to assist in checking the blood with the RN and to help *monitor* the patient during the infusion.

Legal and Ethical Considerations

Check the LPN/LVN Role

Some states have expanded their LPN practice act to include the administration of blood products. Check your nurse practice act to see if that procedure is within legal practice in your state.

All blood bank and agency policies must be strictly followed to decrease the possibility of an adverse reaction or the administration of wrong blood to the wrong patient.

FIGURE 17-6 Two nurses must check the label on the blood product bag, the blood administration form of the blood bank, and the patient's armband and blood bracelet.

Nursing Management

Determine whether the patient has an IV site already established, and note what size catheter is in place. It is best to give blood through an 18-gauge or larger catheter. Best practices and safety require blood to be administered through a Y-type infusion set, with 250 mL of 0.9% saline on the other side of the Y. If a reaction to the blood occurs, the blood can be quickly shut off and the normal saline opened to maintain patency of the IV site. A special blood filter is included in the Y-type infusion set, and the drop factor is different from that of a regular IV tubing set. This infusion system is usually set up before the blood is obtained from the blood bank.

Elder Care Points

- Vessels in elderly people are fragile. A 22-gauge cannula may be used for transfusion to the elderly, rather than an 18-gauge cannula.
- Blood products should be transfused more slowly, to allow an elderly person's body time to adjust to the added fluid.
- Careful assessment for fluid overload during and after the transfusion is essential. Signs of fluid overload are rapid bounding pulse, hypertension, and visibly swollen veins.

A lag period of 2 hours can be observed between each unit transfused, in order to prevent fluid overload. The blood bag should be handled very gently to prevent damage to the cells. After obtaining the blood from the blood bank, immediately inform the nurse in charge of the patient that the blood is ready to be infused. The blood must be started within 30 minutes of arrival on the scene and should never be left at room temperature for more than 4 hours because blood is an excellent medium for bacterial growth; it takes from 1.5 to 4 hours for a unit of packed cells to infuse.

⚠ Safety Alert
Blood Product Safety

Blood bags should never be heated in a microwave oven or placed in hot water. No other solution or drug is ever administered through the same line or to the same site through which blood is infusing because destruction of the cells might occur or a precipitate might be formed that could cause emboli.

❓ Think Critically

If there has been carelessness in the proper identification method used to ensure that the right blood is given to the right patient, and the patient has a reaction, could the nurse be sued for negligence?

Transfusion Reaction

The word *reaction* means sensitivity to the blood itself, or sensitivity to the preservatives or other substances that have been added to a solution. Reactions to RBCs are the result of incompatibility between blood types. There are antigens on the surfaces of RBCs that can bring about a reaction when exposed to blood that is not the same type and is incompatible. The antigen-antibody reaction causes the cells to clump together and obstruct the flow of blood through the capillaries.

⚠ Safety Alert
Signs and Symptoms of a Transfusion Reaction

The symptoms of a transfusion reaction may be so mild that they go unnoticed, or so severe that death is the outcome (Table 17-7). In milder cases, the patient may develop a rash, hives, itching, or facial flushing. In more severe reactions, the patient may experience a variety of problems, including shock. A delayed reaction such as hepatitis, syphilis, malaria, or other infectious agents might not be evident until 4 to 6 weeks or longer after the blood has been given.

👁 Clinical Cues

If there is *any* sign of reaction, the blood transfusion is stopped immediately, saline is started, vital signs are taken, and the physician and charge nurse are notified.

Diphenhydramine hydrochloride (Benadryl) may be ordered by injection, if an allergic reaction is suspected. In severe anaphylactic reactions the treatment is the same as for anaphylaxis due to any extreme hypersensitivity. Should the patient's temperature rise above 100.4° F (38.0° C), the infusion is stopped, the saline started, and the physician notified. Follow the policies of the facility if a reaction occurs. As long as there are no signs of adverse reaction, the patient is assessed and vital signs are taken every 30 to 60 minutes until the transfusion is completed, depending on agency policy.

❓ Think Critically

Your patient is receiving a unit of packed RBCs. When you assess him after the first hour of the transfusion, his pulse rate has increased from 78 to 84, he is slightly restless, and he is complaining of discomfort in his back. His temperature has risen from 98.4° F to 99° F. He has no skin rash and denies nausea. What would you do?

LEUKAPHERESIS

Leukapheresis is a procedure performed to clear excessive WBCs from the blood. Leukapheresis may be performed directly on the patient, or the procedure may be performed on separated blood products. When performed directly, the patient is connected to a blood separator machine. Blood is drained a bit at a time from the patient, the WBCs are washed out of the blood, and the red cells and plasma are returned to the patient. This treatment is used to lower the WBC count in CML patients and is sometimes used to treat certain immune disorders, such as myasthenia gravis.

BIOLOGIC RESPONSE MODIFIERS: COLONY-STIMULATING FACTOR THERAPY

Research with DNA-recombinant techniques has developed drugs that stimulate the bone marrow to produce erythrocytes or neutrophils. Erythropoietin (Epogen) is given parenterally to patients who have decreased erythropoietin resulting from end-stage renal disease, or who have suppressed bone marrow from the toxicity of chemotherapy given for malignancy, rheumatoid arthritis, or HIV.

Granulocyte colony-stimulating factor (G-CSF; Neupogen, Neulasta) is given parenterally to combat neutropenia. It is used for patients with bone marrow suppression from chemotherapy, particularly for those with non–blood-related malignancies. Granulocyte-macrophage colony-stimulating factor (GM-CSF; Leukine), accelerates the recovery of bone marrow after autologous BMT in ALL, Hodgkin's disease, or non-Hodgkin's lymphoma patients who have undergone total destruction of the bone marrow during therapy.

BONE MARROW AND STEM CELL TRANSPLANTATION

Bone marrow transplantation (BMT) is aimed at providing healthy bone marrow when the patient's own bone marrow is faulty or has been destroyed by chemotherapy and/or irradiation during attempts to rid the body of leukemic or other cancer cells. The bone marrow used for transplantation can be allogeneic (from another person) or autologous (from the patient).

Table 17-7 Acute Transfusion Reactions

CAUSE	CLINICAL MANIFESTATIONS	MANAGEMENT	PREVENTION
Acute Hemolytic Reaction			
Infusion of ABO-incompatible whole blood, RBCs, or components containing 10 mL or more of RBCs Antibodies in the recipient's plasma attach to antigens on transfused RBCs, causing RBC destruction	Chills, fever, low back pain, flushing, tachycardia, tachypnea, hypotension, vascular collapse, hemoglobinuria, acute jaundice, dark urine, bleeding, acute renal failure, shock, cardiac arrest, death	Treat shock if present. Draw blood samples for serologic testing slowly to avoid hemolysis from the procedure. Send urine specimen to the laboratory. Maintain BP with IV colloid solutions. Give diuretics as prescribed to maintain urine flow. Insert indwelling urinary catheter or measure voided amounts to monitor hourly urine output. Dialysis may be required if renal failure occurs. Do not transfuse additional RBC-containing components until blood bank has provided newly cross-matched units.	Meticulously verify and document patient identification from sample collection to component infusion.
Febrile, Nonhemolytic Reaction (most common)			
Sensitization to donor WBCs, platelets, or plasma proteins	Sudden chills and fever (rise in temperature of >1° C [>1° F]), headache, flushing, anxiety, muscle pain	Give antipyretics as prescribed—avoid aspirin in thrombocytopenic patients. *Do not restart transfusion* unless physician orders.	Consider leukocyte-poor blood products (filtered, washed, or frozen) for patients with a history of two or more such reactions.
Mild Allergic Reaction			
Sensitivity to foreign plasma proteins	Flushing, itching, *urticaria* (hives)	Give antihistamine as directed. If symptoms are mild and transient, transfusion may be restarted slowly. *Do not restart transfusion* if fever or pulmonary symptoms develop.	Treat prophylactically with antihistamines. Consider washed RBCs and platelets.
Anaphylactic and Severe Allergic Reaction			
Sensitivity to donor plasma proteins Infusion of IgA proteins to IgA-deficient recipient who has developed IgA antibody	Anxiety, urticaria, wheezing, progressing to cyanosis, shock, and possible cardiac arrest	Initiate CPR, if indicated. Have epinephrine ready for injection (0.4 mL of a 1:1000 solution Subcut or 0.1 mL of 1:1000 solution diluted to 10 mL with saline for IV use). *Do not restart transfusion.*	Transfuse extensively washed RBC products, from which all plasma has been removed. Use blood from IgA-deficient donor. Use autologous components.
Circulatory Overload			
Fluid administered faster than the circulation can accommodate	Cough, dyspnea, pulmonary congestion, headache, hypertension, tachycardia, distended neck veins	Place patient upright with feet in dependent position. Administer prescribed diuretics, oxygen, and morphine. Phlebotomy may be indicated.	Adjust transfusion volume and flow rate based on patient size and clinical status. Have blood bank divide unit into smaller aliquots for better spacing of fluid input.
Sepsis			
Transfusion of bacterially infected blood components	Rapid onset of chills, high fever, vomiting, diarrhea, marked hypotension, or shock	Obtain culture of patient's blood and send bag with remaining blood and tubing to blood bank for further study. Treat septicemia as directed—antibiotics, IV fluids, vasopressors.	Collect, process, store, and transfuse blood products according to blood banking standards and infuse within 4 hr of starting time.

From Lewis, S.L., Heitkemper, M.M., Dirksen, S.R., et al. (2007). *Medical-Surgical Nursing: Assessment and Management of Clinical Problems* (7th ed.). St. Louis: Mosby, p. 733.
BP, blood pressure; *CPR,* cardiopulmonary resuscitation; *IgA,* immunoglobulin A; *IV,* intravenous; *RBC,* red blood cell; *Subcut,* subcutaneously; *WBCs,* white blood cell.

Peripheral stem cells or stem cells from umbilical cord blood can also be used for transplant, if there is a good match with the patient. If the transplant is to be autologous, cells are taken from the patient during a period of remission of disease—either by bone marrow aspiration, or by pheresis (for peripheral stem cells). Allogeneic bone marrow is harvested from an HLA-matched person. The HLA match is determined by tissue typing. Finding a good HLA match is difficult, and there is only a 25% chance of matching with the patient's own sibling.

🌐 Cultural Considerations

Bone Marrow Donations

Most people willing to donate bone marrow are white. There is a 30% to 40% chance of a human leukocyte antigen (HLA) match for a white patient and donor marrow. Far fewer African Americans have signed up at the bone marrow registry, and the chance for an HLA match for an African American patient is less than 20%. Efforts are being made to encourage African Americans to become bone marrow donors.

Bone marrow harvest is done in the operating room, where multiple aspirations from the iliac crests are performed. About 500 to 1000 mL of marrow is harvested. The marrow is filtered and may be purged to rid autologous marrow of cancer cells or to rid the allogeneic marrow of T cells. Autologous marrow is then frozen (National Cancer Institute, 2010). Nursing care after harvest consists of monitoring the dressings for bleeding and medicating the donor for pain in the hip area. Nonaspirin analgesics often are sufficient to control pain.

The patient undergoes a conditioning regimen to rid the body of malignancy or to obliterate the diseased bone marrow. This usually takes 5 to 10 days. The process involves intensive high-dose chemotherapy, and often includes total body irradiation. The patient experiences all the side effects of these treatments: bone marrow suppression, diarrhea, stomatitis, severe nausea, and vomiting. The patient is at extreme risk for infection. Meticulous supportive and preventive nursing care is essential during and after this phase.

At least 2 days after the end of chemotherapy, the BMT infusion takes place, through a central line, over approximately 30 minutes. If the bone marrow or stem cells are from an allogeneic donor, the infusion takes place right after harvest. The process of engraftment begins as the cells find their way to the marrow-forming locations in the patient's bones and establish themselves there. Engraftment takes 2 to 5 weeks and is considered successful when the patient's erythrocyte, leukocyte, and platelet counts begin to rise. Until engraftment is complete, the patient is at dire risk of infection and hemorrhage. Other complications include failure of engraftment and graft-versus-host disease, wherein the cells see the patient's tissues as foreign and mount an immune attack. Thrombosis and phlebitis in the liver also can occur; either will cause liver damage if not resolved.

OXYGEN THERAPY

The administration of low concentrations of oxygen may be employed to relieve severe dyspnea and hypoxia during the acute phase of a blood disorder. The treatment is mostly symptomatic, but it does offer some relief if there is sufficient hemoglobin to carry the oxygen to the tissues. With sufficient hemoglobin transportation, oxygen administration may prevent a myocardial infarction. The care of a patient receiving oxygen therapy and the need for careful monitoring of blood gases are discussed in Chapter 15.

IRON THERAPY

Iron is one of the principal elements in the production and maturation of RBCs. When the body lacks iron, the amount of hemoglobin is decreased in the red cells, making them very small and pale in color. In simple iron deficiency anemia, the condition is relieved by administering iron salts. The iron preparations most often used are ferrous sulfate and ferrous gluconate. Ferrous sulfate is thought to be absorbed the best.

Although iron salts are absorbed better from an empty stomach, they are irritating to the GI tract. There will be fewer gastric upsets if this medication is given in divided doses and immediately after meals. The patient should be warned that taking iron salts by mouth produces greenish black stools and that there is no cause for alarm if this change in the color of stools occurs. Because iron salts may form deposits on the teeth and gums, causing a discoloration, the liquid forms of this medication should be given through a straw. Following administration of each liquid dose, the teeth should be thoroughly cleansed and the mouth well rinsed.

Some patients suffer such severe gastric disturbances from the oral intake of iron salts that the medication must be given by another route. Patients who are anemic because of gastric or intestinal bleeding cannot take iron by mouth because the irritation aggravates their condition. The drug of choice in these cases is iron dextran (Imferon), an iron preparation that is given IV or is injected deep into the muscle. Such intramuscular (IM) injections must not exceed 2 mL at each site, and the sites of injection should be rotated to allow for proper absorption and to minimize the hazards of local inflammation. The Z-track technique for IM injection is recommended. Patients receiving an IV infusion of iron dextran must be watched closely for anaphylactic and other adverse reactions.

Vitamin C usually is given with iron because it enhances iron's absorption. If a pharmaceutical preparation of vitamin C is not prescribed, the patient can take the iron salts with orange juice or another juice that is a good source of vitamin C.

 Think Critically

What would you teach a home care patient who is complaining that the iron medication is causing a mild nausea, stomach discomfort, and constipation?

VITAMIN B₁₂ THERAPY

Vitamin B_{12} has two main functions in the body. First, vitamin B_{12} is needed for RBCs to develop into mature, normally functioning cells; second, vitamin B_{12} is necessary for nerve cells to function normally. Another B-group vitamin, folic acid, also is needed for RBC maturation, but it has no effect on the nervous system. Vitamin B_{12} is used to treat pernicious anemia.

Injections of vitamin B_{12} are given daily for the first few weeks and later may be spaced a week apart. As the patient improves, vitamin B_{12} injections may be necessary only once a month, but injections must continue for the duration of life for patients with pernicious anemia.

In addition to administration of supplemental iron and vitamins, the patient with nutritional anemia should eat nutritionally balanced, high-protein meals.

 Nutrition Considerations

Hints for Adding Protein to the Diet

- Mix dry skim milk into the milk called for in recipes.
- Provide between-meal shakes made with commercial protein powder available at the grocery or health food store.
- Add dry skim milk to hot or cold cereal, scrambled eggs, soups, gravies, meal loaf or meatballs, casseroles, and desserts.
- Add diced or ground meat to soups and casseroles.
- Drink commercial canned high-protein drinks (available from pharmacies) between meals, or use instant breakfast drink mix.
- Add cream cheese or peanut butter to breakfast breads.
- Eat peanut butter on crackers, apple, celery, or toast for snacks.
- Mix cooked diced shrimp, tuna, crab, or ham with sliced boiled eggs in cream sauce and serve over cooked rice, pasta, biscuits, or toast.
- Eat desserts made with eggs.
- Eat commercial high-protein bars for snacks, available at the grocery, health food store, or sporting goods store.

SPLENECTOMY

Indications for surgical removal of the spleen include:
- Severe trauma to and rupture of the spleen
- Splenomegaly due to rapid destruction of blood cells

- Splenomegaly from blood disorders, such as leukemia

If the spleen is removed, the other organs of the monocyte-macrophage system take over many of its chores. Individuals who no longer have a functioning spleen are at a very high risk to develop life-threatening infections, especially those caused by pneumococci. It is recommended that these persons receive vaccination with the Pneumovax vaccine. They are advised to consult a physician and take preventive antibiotics as prescribed when they experience even a seemingly trivial respiratory infection.

The patient with a ruptured or torn spleen is in immediate danger of hemorrhage and shock. Whenever an accidental blow, stab wound, or gunshot wound occurs in the vicinity of the spleen, the patient must be watched closely for signs of internal bleeding, such as an expanding abdomen and increased pain. After surgery, the patient is observed for early signs of infection, abdominal distention, and other more general complications of abdominal surgery.

COMMUNITY CARE

Patients with blood disorders are treated in many different places in the community. Patients undergoing chemotherapy may attend an outpatient clinic to receive the doses of the drugs they need. Support groups for patients with the various disorders may meet in hospitals, clinics, churches, or schools, or at other community locations. Patients with sickle cell disease or hemophilia may attend ambulatory clinics.

Patients with blood disorders are frequently treated as home care patients. The elderly patient with pernicious anemia who is home-bound may need a nurse, who gives vitamin B_{12} injections and draws laboratory specimens for periodic blood counts. The leukemia patient frequently is followed at home during chemotherapy and recovery periods. The patient with sickle cell problems is more likely to be treated in the home setting, after the initial crisis period is over. In some instances blood products are administered at home. Some types of chemotherapy agents are given in the home setting, and the nurse must monitor the patient for all of the adverse effects that such therapy can cause.

The home care nurse must do considerable patient and family teaching about prevention of infection, prevention of and treatment for bleeding episodes, appropriate nutrition, and regulation of medication. The home care nurse manager will coordinate care for the patient with the physician, pharmacist, home infusion company, home health aide, and family.

Get Ready for the NCLEX® Examination!

Key Points

- Anemia results in insufficient oxygen carried to cells for the body's needs.
- Anemias result from blood loss, failure in blood cell production, or excessive destruction of red cells.
- Hypovolemia from blood loss may result in shock.
- Blood cell production requires protein, folic acid, and iron.
- Pernicious anemia results from lack of intrinsic factor and faulty absorption of vitamin B_{12}.
- There are a variety of causes of hemolytic anemia, some of which are genetic.
- A CBC and differential (peripheral smear) are used for diagnosis of blood disorders.
- Sickle cell disease is a genetic inherited disorder wherein the affected gene is transmitted from both the father and the mother.
- Abnormal hemoglobin causes red cells to sickle when oxygen tension in the blood is lowered.
- There are many signs and symptoms and problems for those with sickle cell disease (see Figure 17-3).
- Nursing care for sickle cell disease and crisis is aimed at relieving the symptoms of complications and minimizing organ damage.
- Treatment of anemia is aimed at curing the underlying disorder and providing nutrients or supplements needed for building red blood cells.
- Aplastic anemia can be life threatening and may require a bone marrow or stem cell transplant.
- Polycythemia vera causes blood to become too thick and predisposes to blood clots.
- Thrombocytopenia affects the platelets and causes bleeding that can be life threatening.
- Nursing care for thrombocytopenia focuses on preventing bleeding.
- There are four major types of leukemia.
- Agents that are toxic to the bone marrow are a key factor in the development of leukemia.
- Leukemia is acute or chronic, according to the phase of cell development present and the symptoms.
- The leukemia patient may be asymptomatic or may have fever, malaise, and frequent infections.
- Treatment is aimed at slowing the growth of malignant blood cells and maintaining normal levels of red cells, hemoglobin, and platelets.
- Bone marrow or stem cell transplantation is an option for certain types of leukemia.
- Infection and hemorrhage are two major complications of leukemia.
- Hemophilia is mostly an inherited disorder affecting the blood's ability to clot.
- Bleeding into the joints is the major problem of hemophilia.
- Blood factor replacement is the treatment for hemophilia.
- Disseminated intravascular coagulation occurs in conjunction with many disorders.
- There is clotting in the microcirculation and bleeding in DIC.
- Blood transfusions must be administered very carefully as reactions can be serious or fatal.
- Patient consent is needed before blood component transfusion.
- There are many signs and symptoms of a blood transfusion reaction (see Table 17-7).
- If there is any sign of a transfusion reaction, the transfusion is stopped immediately.
- Bone marrow transplantation requires an HLA match and is a dangerous procedure.
- Iron, vitamin C, folic acid, and vitamin B_{12} supplementation are used to treat anemias.

Additional Learning Resources

SG Go to your Study Guide for additional learning activities to help you master this chapter content.

evolve Go to your Evolve website (http://evolve.elsevier.com/deWit/medsurg) for the following FREE learning resources:
- Animations, audio, and video
- Answers and rationales for questions and activities
- Concept Map Creator
- Glossary with pronunciations in English and Spanish
- Interactive Review Questions and Exercises and more!

 Online Resources
- Acute lymphoblastic leukemia, http://emedicine.medscape.com/article/207631-overview
- Acute myelogenous leukemia, http://emedicine.medscape.com/article/197802-overview
- Aplastic anemia, http://emedicine.medscape.com/article/198759-overview
- Chronic myelogenous leukemia, http://emedicine.medscape.com/article/197802-overview
- Disseminated intravascular coagulation in emergency medicine, http://emedicine.medscape.com/article/779097-overview
- Hemophilia, www.ncbi.nlm.nih.gov/pubmedhealth/PMH0001564
- Leukemia & Lymphoma Society, www.leukemia-lymphoma.org
- Multiple myeloma, http://emedicine.medscape.com/article/204369-overview
- National Cancer Institute, www.cancer.gov
- National Hemophilia Foundation, www.hemophilia.org
- Sickle Cell Disease Association of America, www.sicklecelldisease.org
- Sickle cell anemia, http://emedicine.medscape.com/article/205926-overview; www.scinfo.org; www.nhlbi.nih\gov/new/sicklecell.htm
- Stem cell transplant, www.mayoclinic.com/health/stem-cell-transplant/MY00089/METHOD=print

Review Questions for the NCLEX® Examination

1. While reviewing the laboratory results for a patient who had gastric bypass surgery last year, the nurse notes that the amount of red blood cells has remarkably decreased. The nurse suspects that the anemia is related to:
   1. vitamin B_{12} deficiency.
   2. chronic renal failure.
   3. iron deficiency.
   4. bone marrow suppression.

2. An emergency department patient has a suspected gunshot wound to the abdomen. The nurse who finds a profusely bleeding abdominal wound should anticipate which signs(s) and symptom(s) of profuse blood loss? (*Select all that apply.*)
   1. Increased blood pressure
   2. Rapid, weak pulse
   3. Cold, clammy skin
   4. Urine output >50 mL/hr
   5. Decreased blood pressure

3. The patient is prescribed Feosol oral medication for a mild anemia. Which patient statement indicates a need for further teaching about this medication?
   1. "The medication is absorbed best on an empty stomach."
   2. "The medication is more effective if I drink orange juice as well."
   3. "I should take the medication with milk."
   4. "I should increase fluids and fiber to prevent constipation."

4. _____ refers to the painful swelling of the hands and feet related to bone infarction from sickled red blood cells.
   1. Hemarthrosis
   2. Hand-foot syndrome
   3. Ecchymosis
   4. Thrombocytopenia

5. The patient with multiple myeloma may display which signs and symptoms on assessment?
   1. Ruddy complexion and elevated RBCs
   2. Joint pain and low platelet count
   3. Leukocytosis and frequent sore throat
   4. Bone pain and a positive Bence-Jones protein test

6. Which measure(s) should the patient with leukopenia institute to prevent infection? (*Select all that apply.*)
   1. Avoid eating salads, raw fruits, and raw vegetables.
   2. Stay within the home.
   3. Wash hands after handling the mail.
   4. Do not get close to pets.
   5. Stay away from crowds and crowded places.
   6. Do not reuse dishes or eating utensils without washing them first.

7. The nurse starts a peripheral venous access site on a patient who had multiple traumatic injuries. The nurse notes blood in the urine and the feces. Suspecting disseminated intravascular coagulopathy, the nurse expects which laboratory result?
   1. Increased hematocrit
   2. Elevated platelet count
   3. Increased activated partial thromboplastin time
   4. Decreased D-dimer

8. After the first few minutes of transfusing packed red blood cells, the patient has a temperature of 101.5° F (38.6° C), heart rate 120 beats/min, and blood pressure 90/50 mm Hg with complaints of back pain. The priority nursing action would be:
   1. flush the line with normal saline.
   2. stop the transfusion.
   3. notify the physician.
   4. administer diphenhydramine (Benadryl).

9. A patient with cancer who has undergone bone marrow transplant, chemotherapy, and total body irradiation continues under close observation. The nurse would continue with transmission-based precautions isolation for _____ until the patient begins to show signs of improvement when engraftment takes place. (*Fill in the blank.*)

10. An elderly woman was admitted with complaints of fever, malaise, frequent sore throat, swollen lymph nodes, enlarged spleen, bone pain, weight loss, and easy bleeding. The nurse understands that which intervention(s) would be *best* to plan for this patient? (*Select all that apply.*)
    1. Institute aseptic measures for all procedures and care.
    2. Encourage mobility activities.
    3. Apply pressure to any puncture site for 5 to 10 minutes.
    4. Encourage oral care at least four times a day.
    5. Place the patient in protective isolation.
    6. Medicate as ordered for bone pain.

Critical Thinking Activities

Scenario A

Mrs. Hutton is a young mother who has three small children. She is admitted to the hospital with a severe anemia. Her hemoglobin is 7.5 g/dL, and her red cell count also is very low. Mrs. Hutton confides in you that she has never eaten as she should, especially when she was a teenager. With the added strain of having the children to care for at home, she doesn't take the time to cook the meals she knows they should have, because she is so tired all the time. Her husband makes a fairly good salary, but Mrs. Hutton is under the impression that an adequate diet would cost more than they can afford at present.

1. How can you teach the patient the value of nutritious food and help her with shopping practices that would provide her family with food items that are not expensive?

2. Which foods that are high in iron would you suggest she include in her diet?

3. What practical suggestions could you make to help Mrs. Hutton cope with fatigue?

Scenario B

Mr. Tate is a 24-year-old who has acute lymphocytic leukemia. He is receiving chemotherapy with cyclophosphamide, vincristine, prednisone, and daunorubicin. He is experiencing many of the problems associated with a blood disorder, as well as the problems caused by the side effects of the potent drugs he is receiving.

1. Describe the physiologic problems Mr. Tate is likely to experience as a result of the disease and the therapy.

2. Identify psychosocial concerns that Mr. Tate might have.

Scenario C

Mr. Harris, a 72-year-old white man, has just been diagnosed with chronic myeloid leukemia (CML). He has started chemotherapy with hydroxyurea and imatinib. If this is unsuccessful, he will begin treatment with interferon alfa.

1. What do you need to teach Mr. Harris about the drugs he is taking? Will he be on other drugs to control the side effects of this chemotherapy?

2. His wife asks whether he would be eligible for bone marrow transplantation. What should you answer?

Scenario D

Mrs. Solter, age 82, is to receive a transfusion of packed red cells as she is very anemic and not responding to oral medication. You are assigned to assist with the transfusion and to monitor the patient.

1. What are the priorities of care for this patient at this time?

2. Mrs. Solter asks what this transfusion will do for her. How would you respond?

3. What is the proper sequence of actions you would take if Mrs. Solter experiences a transfusion reaction while the blood product is infusing?

The Cardiovascular System

Objectives

Theory

1. Describe the normal anatomy and physiology of the cardiovascular system.
2. Discuss the risk factors and incidence of cardiovascular disease.
3. Explain ways to modify risk factors for the development of cardiovascular disease.
4. State ways in which nurses can contribute to the prevention of cardiovascular disease.
5. Describe the diagnostic tests, specific techniques, and procedures for assessing the cardiovascular system.

6. Identify three likely nursing diagnoses for patients who have common problems of cardiovascular disease and list the expected outcomes and appropriate nursing interventions for each.

Clinical Practice

1. Teach patients about the more common diagnostic tests and procedures to diagnose and evaluate cardiovascular diseases.
2. Assist patients to form plans to modify cardiovascular disease risk factors.

Key Terms

arteriosclerosis (ăr-tē-rē-ō-sklĕ-RŌ-sĭs, p. 375)
atherosclerosis (ăth-ĕr-ō-sklĕ-RŌ-sĭs, p. 374)
cardiac output (p. 373)
cardiomyopathy (kăr-dē-ō-mī-ŎP-ăth-ē, p. 385)
cellulitis (sĕl-ū-LĪ-tĭs, p. 388)
coarctation (kō-ărk-TĀ-shŭn, p. 375)
dysrhythmia (dĭs-RĬTH-mē-ă, p. 375)
ejection fraction (p. 373)
endocarditis (ĔN-dō-kăhr-DĪ-tĭs, p. 376)
hypertension (hī-pĕr-TĔN-shŭn, p. 375)

infarct (p. 375)
intermittent claudication (ĭn-tĕr-MĬT-ĕnt klăw-dĭ-KĀ-shŭn, p. 385)
ischemia (ĭs-KĒ-mē-ă, p. 375)
palpitations (păl-pĭ-TĀ-shŭnz, p. 394)
pericarditis (pĕr-ē-kăhr-DĪ-tĭs, p. 376)
rubor (rū-bŏr, p. 388)
stroke volume (p. 373)
syncope (SĬN-kō-pē, p. 387)

OVERVIEW OF ANATOMY AND PHYSIOLOGY OF THE CARDIOVASCULAR SYSTEM

WHAT ARE THE STRUCTURES OF THE HEART AND THEIR FUNCTIONS?

- The heart wall consists of three layers. The epicardium is the outer layer of tissue; the myocardium is the middle layer of muscle fibers that contract to pump blood; and the endocardium is the lining of the inner surface of the heart chambers.
- A membranous sac, the pericardium, surrounds the heart.
- The pericardium is a double-layered sac. The double layer helps provide a barrier to infection, prevents displacement of the heart, and contains pain and other receptors that elicit reflex changes in heart rate and blood pressure.

- The pericardial space contains a thin layer of fluid (5 to 20 mL).
- The four chambers of the heart make up two coordinated pumps: the right-side pump is a low-pressure system; the left-side pump is a high-pressure system.
- The right atrium and right ventricle receive deoxygenated blood from the vascular system and pump it through the lungs.
- The left atrium and left ventricle receive oxygenated blood from the lungs and pump it through the systemic circulation (Figure 18-1).
- A septum separates the right and left sides of the heart.
- The cardiac valves direct the flow of blood through the heart chambers.
- Blood enters the right atrium via the superior and inferior vena cava and goes to the right ventricle through the tricuspid valve.

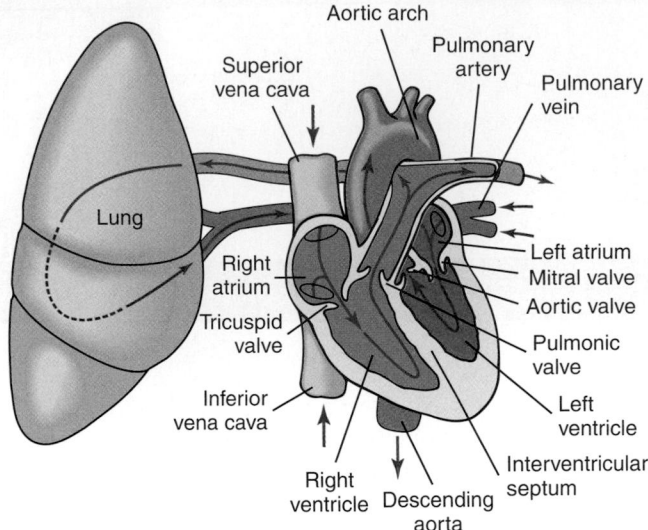

FIGURE 18-1 Heart structures and path of oxygenated blood flow out of the left ventricle and into the aorta.

- Blood leaves the right ventricle through the pulmonic valve and goes into the pulmonary artery to circulate in the lungs, exchanging carbon dioxide for oxygen. Other arteries in the body carry oxygenated blood.
- The left atrium receives oxygenated blood from the pulmonary veins, and the mitral valve controls the flow from the atrium into the left ventricle. Other veins in the body carry blood containing carbon dioxide.
- The left ventricle ejects the blood through the aortic valve into the aorta and the systemic circulation.
- The coronary arteries branch from the aorta and supply the cardiac muscle with blood (Figure 18-2).
- The left coronary artery divides into the anterior descending and the circumflex arteries providing blood for the left atrium and the left ventricle.
- The right coronary artery supplies the right atrium, right ventricle, and part of the posterior wall of the left ventricle, as well as the atrioventricular node of the cardiac conduction system (see Figure 18-2).
- The heart is located within the mediastinum and is tilted forward and to the left side of the chest.
- The point of maximal impulse (PMI) can normally be felt between the fifth and sixth ribs on a line dividing the left clavicle in half. Listen to the apical heart rate at this location.

WHAT CAUSES THE HEART TO CONTRACT AND PUMP BLOOD?

- The heart's pumping action is sparked by specialized pacemaker cells and conduction fibers that initiate spontaneous electrical activity, causing muscle contractions that result in a heartbeat.
- The conduction pathways are located in the myocardium and transmit the electrical impulse throughout the heart.

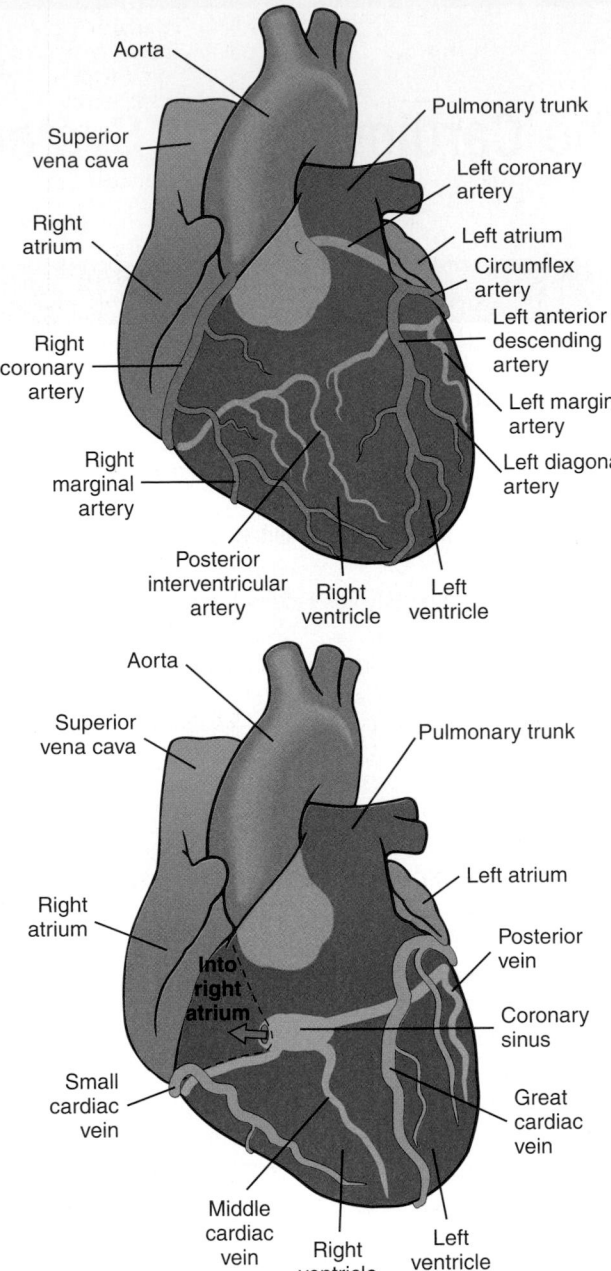

FIGURE 18-2 A view of the coronary arterial system. *Top,* Arteries. *Bottom,* Veins.

- The sinoatrial (SA) node is located in the right atrium and is called the "pacemaker" of the heart because it normally initiates the electrical impulses.
- The atrioventricular (AV) node is located in the lower part of the right atrium. It relays the impulse from the SA node to the bundle of His and throughout the ventricles via the Purkinje fibers (Figure 18-3).
- The heart rate and rhythm also are influenced by the autonomic nervous system; factors affecting the autonomic nervous system can speed up or slow down the heart rate.

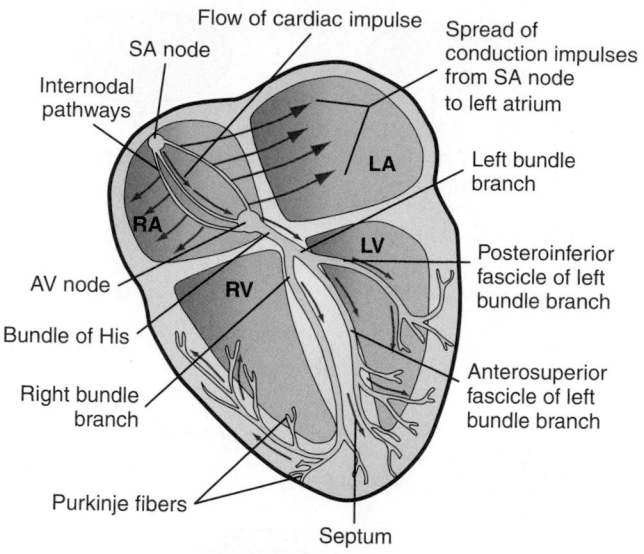

FIGURE 18-3 The cardiac conduction system.

WHAT IS THE CARDIAC CYCLE?

- The cardiac cycle consists of contraction of the muscle (systole) and relaxation of the muscle (diastole).
- The heart pumps out about 5 L of blood every minute.
- The amount of cardiac output depends on the heart rate, the amount of blood returning to the heart (venous return), the strength of contraction, and the resistance to the ejection of the blood (pressure in the arterial system)

WHAT IS THE EJECTION FRACTION?

- The ejection fraction is the percentage of blood that is ejected from the heart during systole.
- A normal ejection fraction is 50% to 70%.
- As ejection fraction decreases with heart failure, tissue perfusion diminishes.
- A decreased ejection fraction causes backup of blood into the pulmonary vessels.
- Too much blood and the increased pressure in the pulmonary vessels can cause pulmonary edema.
- Stroke volume equals the amount of blood ejected by a ventricle during contraction.
- Cardiac output equals stroke volume multiplied by the heart rate.

HOW DOES THE VASCULAR SYSTEM FUNCTION TO CARRY BLOOD THROUGHOUT THE BODY?

- Three types of blood vessels make up the vascular system: arteries, veins, and capillaries; these vessels conduct the blood from the body tissues to the heart and from the heart back to the tissues.
- Arteries carry oxygenated blood away from the heart (Figure 18-4). Veins carry oxygen-depleted blood back to the heart for reoxygenation by the lungs (Figure 18-5).
- Small veins, *venules,* and small arteries, *arterioles,* are connected by the capillaries.

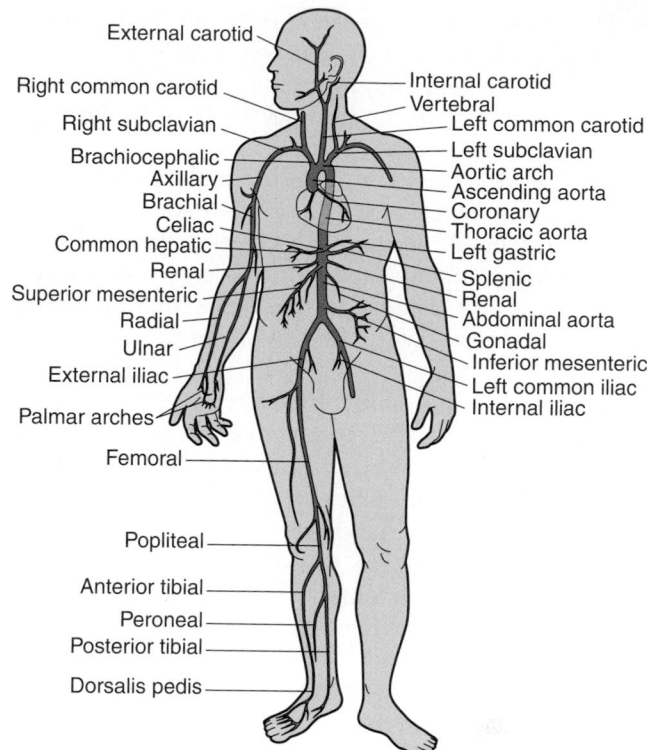

FIGURE 18-4 Major arteries in the body.

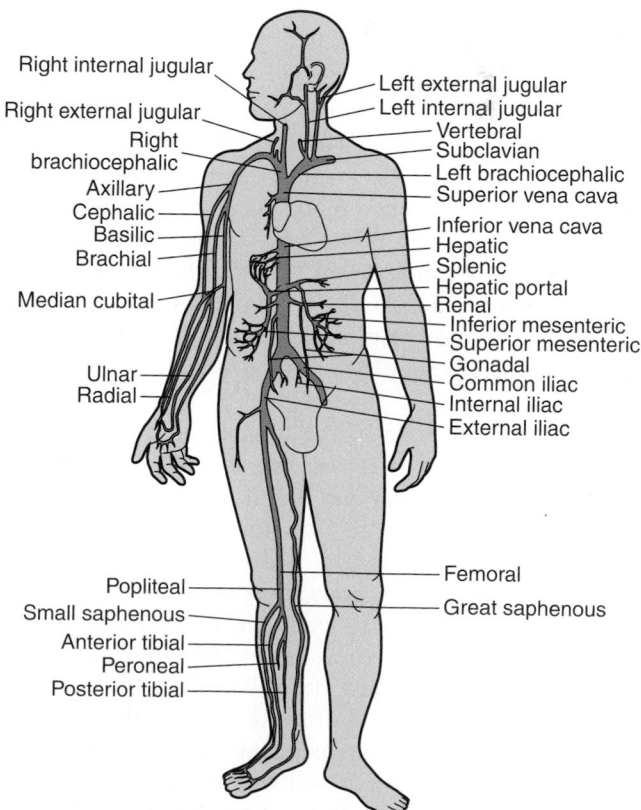

FIGURE 18-5 Major veins in the body.

- The aorta is the largest artery in the body, and it receives blood from the left ventricle.
- The inferior and superior vena cava are the largest veins in the body and empty blood into the right atrium of the heart.
- Arteries are elastic and accommodate changes in blood flow by constricting or dilating.
- Three layers of tissue make up the artery wall: The outer layer (the *tunica adventitia*) is connective tissue; the middle layer (the *tunica media*) is smooth muscle; and the inner layer (the *tunica intima*) consists of endothelial cells.
- Veins have the same three layers but with less smooth muscle and connective tissue. The veins are thinner and less rigid, and for that reason the veins can hold more blood.
- The heart pumps blood through the arterial system with each contraction. Skeletal muscle contraction, respiratory movements that change pressures in the chest, and constriction of the veins propel blood back to the heart.
- Sets of valves in the medium and large veins open and close, keeping blood flowing toward the heart.
- For blood to circulate the arteries must be unobstructed, and they must be able to dilate and constrict as necessary to regulate the blood flow. Veins also must be patent, their valves must function normally, and surrounding muscles must contract so that venous blood is continually being moved in the direction of the heart.

WHAT IS THE BLOOD PRESSURE AND WHAT AFFECTS IT?

- Arterial blood pressure is the force that the blood exerts against the walls of the aorta and its branches.
- The blood pressure is greatest during ventricular contraction, *systole*, when blood is ejected into the aorta.
- Diastolic pressure is the pressure when the ventricles are in the relaxation phase, *diastole*, just before the next contraction of the ventricles.
- The difference between the systolic blood pressure and the diastolic blood pressure is called the *pulse pressure.*
- If the diameter of blood vessels becomes smaller because of atherosclerosis, blood pressure increases in an effort to force the blood through the smaller opening. Atherosclerosis is the condition in which fibrous plaque with fatty deposits forms in the interior layers of the arteries, causing narrowing.
- If there is an increase in the volume of fluid in the blood vessels, the pressure within the vessels increases, and the heart must work harder to pump the increased volume of fluid through the vessels.
- If blood volume decreases, the kidneys secrete the enzyme renin in the blood (Figure 18-6).
- Renin acts on certain blood proteins to produce angiotensin I.

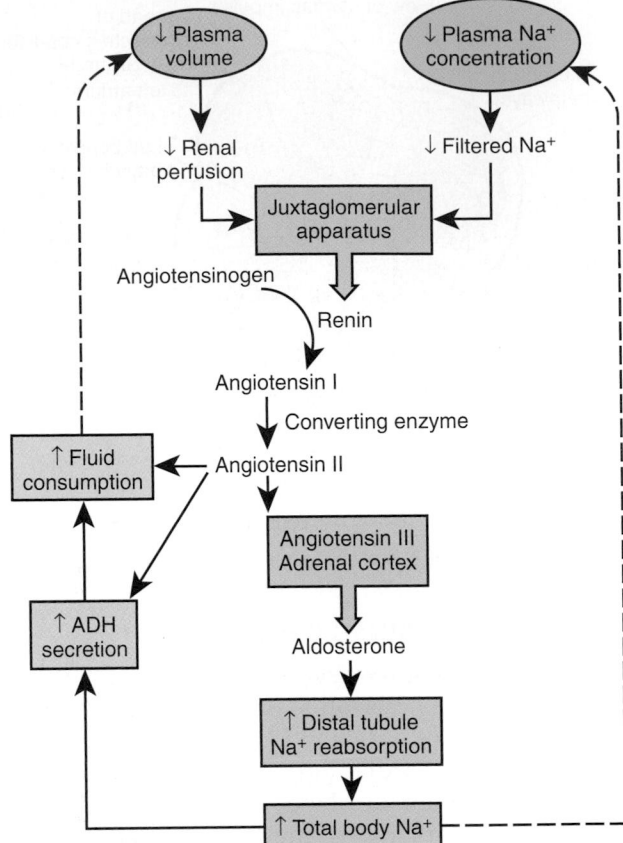

FIGURE 18-6 The renin-angiotensin-aldosterone system.

- Angiotensin I is converted to angiotensin II by the angiotensin-converting enzyme from the lungs.
- Angiotensin II acts directly on the blood vessels, causing them to constrict, and stimulates the adrenal gland to release aldosterone. Angiotensin increases resistance to blood flow in the peripheral vessels and causes sodium and water retention by the renal tubules through its influence on secretion of aldosterone.
- The retained sodium and water increase the blood volume, causing increased cardiac output and blood pressure elevation.
- Blood flow is affected by the amount of resistance in the vessels and by the viscosity of the blood.
- Vascular resistance is controlled by the nervous system, hormones, blood pH, and some ions that regulate the diameter of the vessels.
- **When the vessel diameter increases, resistance falls and blood flow increases. When vessel diameter decreases, resistance rises and blood flow decreases.**
- The sympathetic nervous system plays a major role in regulating vessel diameter because it prompts the release of the hormones norepinephrine and epinephrine that cause vasoconstriction.
- Blood viscosity is affected by the hydration status of the body. When dehydration occurs, blood viscosity increases; thicker blood causes an increase in blood pressure.

WHAT CHANGES OCCUR IN THE CARDIOVASCULAR SYSTEM WITH AGING?

- The aging heart becomes stiffer and contractile ability decreases, resulting in decreased stroke volume in the elderly.
- The coronary arteries become tortuous and dilated and have areas of calcification.
- The cardiac valves become thickened, particularly the mitral and aortic valves, which are subject to higher pressures. A systolic murmur is common in those older than age 80.
- The SA node loses about 40% of the pacemaker cells over time predisposing to cardiac **dysrhythmia** (abnormal rhythm) or SA node failure.
- The aorta becomes stiffer, contributing to an increase in systolic blood pressure because the left ventricle must pump against greater resistance.
- Atherosclerosis is a natural part of the aging process, and atherotic plaque begins to occur after age 20.
- The arterial walls thicken and lose elasticity, making them less able to adjust to changes in volume and to comply with sympathetic stimulation.
- Varicose veins develop in the elderly as veins lose their elasticity, valve function lessens, and the leg muscles weaken and atrophy from decreased exercise.
- Platelet aggregation and increased coagulation potential lead to a greater incidence of thrombus formation, deep vein thrombosis, and thrombophlebitis in those of advanced age.
- Chronic health problems and failing eyesight often lead to less activity in the elderly, predisposing to vascular problems.

CARDIOVASCULAR DISEASE

Cardiovascular disease (CVD) affects one in three people in the United States, and more than 800,000 people die in the United States as a result of cardiovascular problems each year. Cardiovascular disease is responsible for the largest portion of Medicare funds spent each year. Together with the heart, the vascular system provides the body with nutrients and oxygen needed for life. The vascular system also transports metabolic wastes that are excreted by the lungs and the kidneys. When a disorder of the cardiovascular system occurs, homeostasis is upset. Many of the disorders that afflict the cardiovascular system can be prevented or controlled.

WOMEN AND HEART DISEASE

Heart disease in women has been increasing. Nearly 42 million women live with heart disease. It is the number one killer of women. Low blood levels of "good" cholesterol (high-density lipoprotein [HDL]) appear to be a stronger predictor of heart disease in women than in men, particularly in the over-65 age group. High blood levels of triglycerides are another particular risk factor in women. Although it was once thought that postmenopausal hormone replacement therapy (HRT) was heart protective, it was discovered that there were more cardiovascular events in women who were on HRT (Hlatky et al., 2002). Women with CVD may experience subtle symptoms such as shortness of breath, fatigue, or changes in sleep patterns.

 Health Promotion

Preventing Cardiovascular Disease in Women

- *Public awareness should be increased:* Obtain regular physical activity—at least 30 minutes four or five times a week.*
- Maintain HDL >50 mg/dL, low-density lipoprotein (LDL) <129, and triglyceride levels <150 mg/dL.
- Refrain from smoking.
- Do not consume more than 1 alcoholic drink per day.
- Obtain and maintain a healthy weight as it reduces the chance of type 2 diabetes.* Type 2 diabetes increases the risk of cardiovascular disease.
- Maintain a body mass index (BMI) of <25.
- Discontinue use of estrogen contraception/supplementation as soon as possible.
- Reduce the amount of *trans* fat in the diet.
- If diabetes is present, keep blood sugar <100 mg/dL.
- If hypertension is present, take medication regularly to keep pressure within 130/80 mm Hg (<115/75 mm Hg is optimal).
- Incorporate stress reduction techniques into the daily lifestyle, as increased stress is a risk factor for cardiovascular disease.

*These factors play an even larger role in prevention of heart disease in women than in men.

 Think Critically

Can you think of two physiologic reasons why the elderly are more at risk for hypertension?

CAUSES OF CARDIOVASCULAR DISORDERS

Causes of cardiovascular disorders can be congenital or acquired. Narrowing of the aorta **(coarctation)**, holes in the septum, or abnormal formation of a cardiac valve can occur congenitally. Acquired defects include narrowing or hardening of the blood vessels from **arteriosclerosis** (thickening and loss of elasticity) or atherosclerosis and aneurysms of the large vessels. Inflammation of the valve structure may cause narrowing (stenosis) or incomplete closure (insufficiency) of the valve. Alteration of the myocardial muscle tissue by extra growth with thickening (hypertrophy) or fibrosis may occur as a result of systemic **hypertension** (persistently elevated blood pressure), pulmonary hypertension, or valve problems. Lack of adequate blood supply **(ischemia)** or **infarct** (area of tissue that has died from lack of blood supply) may occur from coronary artery stenosis. Deterioration of the pacemaker cells and conduction fibers related to hypertrophy or inflammation of tissues may cause conduction disorders.

Several disorders involving either the heart or the vessels through which it pumps blood can eventually weaken and damage the heart muscle and lead to pump failure. This condition, called *heart failure,* is a complication of many cardiovascular diseases, as discussed in the following chapters.

Disturbances in any part of the heart's conduction system can result in an increase in heart rate (tachycardia), a slowing down of the heart rate (bradycardia), and disturbances in the rhythm of the heartbeat (dysrhythmias).

Infection and inflammation also can take their toll on the structure and function of the heart. Endocarditis, inflammation within the lining and valves of the heart, and pericarditis, an inflammation of the sac surrounding the heart, can occur as primary diseases, but they are more often secondary to infection and inflammation elsewhere in the body. An example is rheumatic heart disease, which occurs after a streptococcal infection.

Substances in the blood, such as excess carbon dioxide and certain drugs, can affect the rate and rhythm of the heart through their effect on the autonomic nervous system. The heart also responds to physiologic changes that indicate a need for more or less oxygen.

The arterial walls can be injured by several factors. Hypertension causes a mechanical injury by applying increased pressure continuously on the arterial walls. For each increment of 20/10 mm Hg above a pressure of 115/75, the risk of CVD doubles (National Heart, Lung, and Blood Institute, 2003). Elevated levels of LDLs and decreased levels of HDLs predispose to the deposition of fatty deposits in the arterial walls, causing a narrowing of the vessels. Chemical toxins such as carbon monoxide (present in the blood) when a person smokes, and the toxins caused by renal failure, cause injury to the arterial walls. Substance abuse with alcohol, stimulants, and nicotine are damaging to the cardiovascular system (see Chapter 47).

Physiologic disorders such as diabetes mellitus and metabolic syndrome directly cause physical changes in the vessel walls, leading to more rapid arteriosclerosis, possibly from elevated blood glucose levels, an increased rate of atherosclerosis, and an earlier onset of hypertension. Some inherited disorders, such as hyperlipidemia, contribute to atherosclerosis.

Obesity, a sedentary lifestyle, and stress are all directly related to the increased incidence of atherosclerosis and hypertension. Smoking, and the changes it causes in the vessel walls, is directly related to arteriosclerosis of the peripheral vessels and decreased circulation in the lower extremities. Long-term hypertension causes arteriosclerosis and is a direct factor in the development of aortic aneurysm in many patients. Hypertension cannot be prevented, but it can be managed with diligent therapy and cooperation of the patient.

PREVENTION OF CARDIOVASCULAR DISEASE

Cardiovascular diseases claimed 864,480 lives in 2005 in the United States (American Heart Association, 2009). Heart disease remains the major cause of death in the United States. Cardiovascular diseases also account for a large percentage of the chronic illnesses that disable, to some degree, a large portion of the U.S. population.

There are many kinds and degrees of heart disease. Advances in medical science have made it possible either to cure or successfully manage a large number of cardiovascular problems. Reasons for the decline in deaths from heart disease since the mid-1980s include improved emergency treatment of persons experiencing a coronary occlusion or "heart attack," improved education of the public regarding ways to prevent heart disease, and teaching about the warning signs of a heart attack. Every nurse has a responsibility to assist with public education about heart disease.

Health Promotion
Know the Warning Signs of a Heart Attack

- **Chest discomfort:** A feeling of tightness, pressure, or a crushing or squeezing pain lasting more than a few minutes, or it comes back. In women, discomfort in the middle of the chest.
- **Pain or discomfort in other areas of the upper body:** Arms, shoulder, back, neck, jaw, or the top of the stomach. Women often have jaw or back pain.
- **Shortness of breath:** May occur with or without chest discomfort.
- **Breaking out in a cold sweat,** nausea, or light-headedness with or without chest discomfort.
- **Feeling of impending doom** that does not go away.
- **Chest pain** unrelieved by prescribed doses of nitroglycerin. ***Call 911 or emergency number immediately—get help!***

Nonmodifiable risk factors are those that cannot be prevented by an individual. However, control of diseases such as hypertension and diabetes mellitus and the reduction of high cholesterol are possible. Since hypertension and diabetes are factors in the development of atherosclerosis, controlling them can help prevent the early onset of heart disease. If a person with diabetes can keep the hemoglobin A_{1c} below 6% the risk of atherosclerosis is lessened (Matsushita, et al., 2010). Management of hypertension is one of the major tools for heart disease prevention.

Table 18-1 presents the risk factors for cardiovascular disease. Metabolic syndrome is particularly an indicator of cardiovascular risk and is diagnosed when three or more of the components in Box 18-1 are present (Gami et al., 2007). More than 50 million Americans have it. Modifiable risk factors are the major focus for education to prevent heart disease.

The use of cocaine and methamphetamine has added to the problem of heart disease (American Heart Association, 2011). Cocaine causes vasoconstriction and is thought to speed up the atherosclerosis process. Also, cocaine has been known to cause sudden cardiac death, or stroke, in susceptible individuals. Research is

Table 18-1 Risk Factors for Cardiovascular Disease

UNMODIFIABLE RISK FACTORS	SIGNIFICANCE
Heredity	Children of parents with cardiovascular disease are more likely to develop the same problem.
Race	African Americans experience high blood pressure two to three times more frequently than whites. Consequently the risk of heart disease in this group is higher.
Sex	Males experience more heart attacks than females earlier in life. After age 65, the death rate from heart disease increases in women.
Age	Four out of five people who die of a heart attack are age 65 or older. Increasing age increases risk.

MODIFIABLE RISK FACTORS	MEANS OF MODIFICATION
Obesity	Keep weight within normal limits by diet and exercise.
High cholesterol >200 mg/dL	Low-fat diet and exercise; medication.
Hypertension	Encourage blood pressure <120/80 mm Hg.
Diabetes	Good control by keeping blood sugar within normal limits (<110 mg/dL).
Cigarette smoking	Quit smoking.
Sedentary lifestyle	Exercise program of 30-min sessions three to five times a week.
Excessive stress	Use stress-reduction techniques regularly, such as exercise, relaxation techniques; reduce hostility; maintain a positive support system.
Excessive alcohol intake	Limit alcohol consumption to no more than recommended levels: men, 2 drinks/day; women, 1 drink/day.
Cocaine use	Do not use cocaine.

Box 18-1 Metabolic Syndrome Components

- Elevated waist circumference indicating abdominal obesity; men >40 inches (102 cm), women >35 inches (88 cm)
- Elevated triglycerides >150 mg/dL
- Reduced HDL cholesterol; men <40 mg/dL and women <50 mg/dL
- Elevated blood pressure at or above 130/85 mm Hg
- Elevated fasting glucose indicating insulin resistance; glucose ≥100 mg/dL

finding that the ingestion of both alcohol and cocaine greatly increases the chance of cardiac death. Methamphetamine increases heart rate, causes vasoconstriction that can lead to hypertension, and speeds up electrical conduction, potentially causing dysrhythmias and myocardial infarction (MI). Cigarette smoking–related health problems are heavy contributors to heart disease, and smoking is a key factor in sudden cardiac death.

? Think Critically

Can you identify two risk factors you can modify to decrease your risk of heart disease?

Nurses can play an important role in teaching others about hypertension and can support patient efforts to avoid the disease and its long-term consequences.

Although systolic blood pressure rises as a natural process of aging because arteries become less elastic, systolic hypertension should be treated in the elderly patient. Hypertension in the elderly is associated with an even higher risk of heart disease, stroke, and death from coronary thrombosis (Aronow et al., 2011). Hypertension has been associated with more rapid memory loss and loss of cognitive function in some research studies.

Contribute to reducing the incidence of the harmful effects of hypertension by participating in community screening programs and education. Nurses and other health care professionals have an obligation to serve as models for a healthy lifestyle.

DIAGNOSTIC TESTS AND PROCEDURES

In addition to a routine physical examination and medical history, the physician has access to a number of procedures and tests to help diagnose cardiovascular disease (Figure 18-7). Noninvasive procedures usually are performed first

Specific cardiovascular diagnostic tests and their nursing implications are listed in Table 18-2. In women,

Text continued on p. 384

FIGURE 18-7 Cardiac treadmill stress test.

Table 18-2 **Common Diagnostic Tests for the Cardiovascular System**

TEST	PURPOSE	PROCEDURE	NURSING IMPLICATIONS
Chest radiograph	Shows size and shape of heart and mediastinal structures	Performed standing in a gown or in high Fowler's position in bed.	No special requirements.
Electrocardiography (12-lead electrocardiogram [ECG])	Records electrical impulses of the heart to determine rate, rhythm of heart, site of pacemaker, and presence of injury at rest	Small electrodes are placed on the chest and extremities, to show conduction patterns in different directions of electrical flow. *Signal-averaged ECG* can be used for patients at high risk for serious ventricular arrhythmias.	Inform patient that there is no discomfort with this test. Maintain electrical safety. Normal finding: normal ECG.
Holter monitor (ambulatory ECG)	Correlates normal daily activity with electrical function of the heart to determine whether activity causes abnormalities	Patient wears a small ECG recorder for 6, 12, or 24 hr while going about usual tasks. A diary is kept to show at what time the various activities were performed and any symptoms experienced. The tape is analyzed to correlate any dysrhythmia with the activity at that time.	Remind patient that all activities must be recorded in the diary: brushing teeth, climbing stairs, sexual intercourse, bowel movements, sleeping, etc. Caution patient not to remove the electrodes and not to get the recorder or wires wet. Have patient wear a loose shirt during test.
Exercise ECG stress test (treadmill)	Records electrical activity of the heart during exercise Insufficient blood flow and oxygen show up in abnormal waveforms	Small electrodes are placed on the chest, and a tracing is made while the patient exercises on a treadmill, bicycle, or stairs. The degree of difficulty of the exercise is increased as the test continues to see how the heart reacts to increasing work demands. Vital signs are continuously recorded. May be combined with radionuclide imaging or echocardiograph. Physician is present.	Requires a signed consent form. Have patient wear comfortable clothes and walking shoes. Light meal 2-3 hr prior, then NPO. Regular medications are given. Chest is shaved as needed for electrode placement. Inform patient that the test will be stopped if chest pain, severe fatigue, or dyspnea develops.
Chemical stress test with dipyridamole, adenosine, or dobutamine	Used for those who cannot exercise for an ECG stress test	An ECG is done and the drug is injected. Blood pressure and pulse are taken and recorded q 15 min while the drug takes effect by diverting blood flow from the coronary arteries, causing cardiac ischemia. Thallium or technetium-99m (^{99m}Tc) may be injected during exercise at maximum heart rate. Scanning images are taken with a gamma camera over a period of 40 min. A repeat scan may be done in 3-4 hr. The patient is NPO during the test.	Mild nausea or headache may occur. Explain that patient will lie on back for the imaging. If BP drops too low, phenylephrine is given.
Nuclear imaging (thallium perfusion imaging)	Evaluates blood flow in various parts of the heart; determines areas of infarction	Thallium-201 is injected IV, radioactive uptake is counted over the heart by a gamma scintillation camera.	Explain that the radioactivity used is a very small amount and lasts only a few hours. Explain that a camera will be positioned over the heart.

BP, blood pressure; *NPO*, nothing by mouth.

Table 18-2   **Common Diagnostic Tests for the Cardiovascular System—cont'd**

TEST	PURPOSE	PROCEDURE	NURSING IMPLICATIONS
Nuclear imaging (thallium perfusion imaging)–cont'd		May be done in conjunction with an exercise ECG stress test.	ECG electrodes are placed on the chest; scanning is done 10-15 min after injection; can be done as an outpatient procedure. May be done in two parts a few hours apart.
Technetium pyrophosphate scan and multiple-gated acquisition (MUGA) scan	Determines area and extent of myocardial infarction Assesses left ventricular function	^{99m}Tc is injected IV and is taken up by areas of infarction, producing hot spots when scanned. Multiple serial images are obtained. Best results occur when done 1-6 days after a suspected MI.	Inform patient that radioisotopes will be given IV and that it will be necessary to lie still while the machine scans the heart. The patient's glucose must be between 60-140 mg/dL. If scan is combined with exercise, patient will need to be NPO and must refrain from tobacco and caffeine for 24 hr before the test.
Ventilation-perfusion scan (V-Q scan)	Detects blood clots, particularly pulmonary emboli	A radioisotope is injected, and after a waiting period for uptake, a scintillation scanning camera is used to measure the amount of radioactivity present in the area in question.	Determine whether patient has an allergy to the dye. After the test encourage large fluid intake to flush the dye through the kidneys.
Positron emission tomography	Evaluates myocardial perfusion	IV nitrogen-13-ammonia is injected and a scan performed to show myocardial metabolic function. Then fluoro-18-deoxyglucose is injected and a scan performed. In a normal heart, the scans will match; in an ischemic heart, the scans will differ.	Inform patient that radioisotopes will be given IV and that it will be necessary to lie still while the machine scans the heart. The patient's glucose must be between 60-140 mg/dL. If scan is combined with exercise, patient will need to be NPO and must refrain from tobacco and caffeine for 24 hr before the test.
Echocardiography	Useful in evaluating size, shape, and position of structures and movement within the heart Test of choice for valve problems	A metal wand that emits sonar waves is guided over the chest wall while the patient is supine or turned on the left side. Takes 30-60 min. May be done in combination with the exercise (stress) test.	Inform patient that there is no discomfort, although conduction jelly may feel cool. Normal finding: no abnormalities of size or location of heart structures; normal wall movement.
Stress echocardiogram	Detects differences in left ventricular wall motion before and after exercise	Resting echocardiogram images are obtained. The patient exercises, and then within 1 min, postexercise images are obtained.	Explain the procedure and the importance of returning to the examining table immediately after exercising. No heavy meal beforehand, no smoking or caffeine for 6-8 hr before test. Tell patient to wear walking shoes.
Dobutamine echocardiogram	A substitute for an exercise stress test when individual cannot exercise Detects abnormal heart wall motion	IV dobutamine, a positive inotropic agent, is infused. The dosage is increased at 5-min intervals during the echocardiogram.	Administer IV dobutamine as ordered. Monitor vital signs; watch for symptoms of distress.

Continued

Table 18-2 Common Diagnostic Tests for the Cardiovascular System—cont'd

TEST	PURPOSE	PROCEDURE	NURSING IMPLICATIONS
Transesophageal echocardiogram (TEE)	Provides images of the heart, mitral valve, atrial septum, and thoracic aorta	Pharynx is anesthetized with topical agent. With patient in left side-lying position, an endoscope and a transducer are placed in the esophagus behind the heart. Recordings of the images are made. Test takes about 20 min.	NPO for 4-6 hr before test. Initiate IV access before test for sedation. Apply ECG leads for monitoring during test. Monitor pulse oximetry and BP. Observe after test until sedation has worn off.
Angiogram (venogram)	Identifies thrombi within the venous system	A tourniquet may be placed on the extremity and dye is injected into the affected extremity. Radiographs are taken at timed intervals. Also used to identify venous stenosis.	Requires a signed consent form. Assess for allergies to radiopaque dye. Hydrate the patient prior to the procedure. Tell patient it takes 30-90 min and that a warm flush may be felt when the dye is injected.
Arteriogram	Visualizes arterial anatomy and vascular disease in carotid, vertebral, aorta, renal, coronary, and peripheral arteries	A catheter is placed via the femoral artery into the desired artery. Radiopaque contrast is injected while x-ray images are obtained. Digital subtraction techniques obliterate bony structures from the views. CO_2 gas may be used in place of dye if the patient is allergic to the dye. A balloon may be used during the procedure to open constricted areas. A stent may be placed in the vessel to keep it open. *Magnetic resonance angiography* may also be used to visualize vessels.	Requires a signed consent form. NPO for 2-8 hr before test. Mark peripheral pulses before procedure. Check renal function studies before test and alert physician of abnormal values. Mucomyst may be administered a day before and after the test to prevent dye induced nephropathy. Warn that dye may cause some bladder distention during the test.
Cardiac catheterization with coronary angiography	Assesses pumping action of both sides of the heart Measures pressure within the heart chambers Measures cardiac output Calculates differences in oxygen content of arterial and venous blood Assesses size and patency of coronary arteries and presence of collateral circulation	Catheter is inserted into vein or artery, depending on which side of the heart is to be tested. Femoral artery or brachial vein is often used. With local anesthetic and sedation, the catheter is threaded up into the heart, and pressure readings and oxygen saturation determinations are taken. Contrast media may be injected to visualize the size and shape of the chambers and structures. Takes 1½-3 hr. Fluoroscopy is used during the procedure. Angiography performed by dye injection during cardiac catheterizations. Computed tomographic angiography used to enhance images.	Requires a signed consent form. Patient is NPO for 6-8 hr before test. Assess for allergy to iodine, shellfish, or contrast dye. Have patient void before giving preoperative medication. Record baseline vital signs and mark location of pedal pulses. Inform patient that procedure involves being strapped to a table that tilts, will have an IV, and patient must lie still during test. ECG leads will be in place during the test. If dye is used, patient will feel a hot flush for a minute after the dye is injected. Patient may be asked to cough during the procedure. Patient will be constantly monitored and emergency equipment is at hand.

BP, blood pressure; *NPO,* nothing by mouth.

Table 18-2   Common Diagnostic Tests for the Cardiovascular System—cont'd

TEST	PURPOSE	PROCEDURE	NURSING IMPLICATIONS
Cardiac catheterization with coronary angiography–cont'd		Video recording made during procedure for later review.	Post-test: vital signs q 15 min × 4, q 30 min × 4, then q 1 hr × 4, or until stable. Assess peripheral pulses with vital signs and question patient about numbness or tingling. Inspect insertion site for bleeding or sign of hematoma. Pressure dressing or clamp, or sandbag weight are left in place for 1-3 hr. If femoral insertion site was used, keep patient flat and leg extended for 6 hr. If brachial site was used, immobilize arm for 3 hr. If dye was used, encourage fluids unless contraindicated. Mark location of distal pulses before the procedure. Postprocedure, prevent hip flexion on affected side.
Ultrasound			
Coronary	Determines patency of coronary arteries and presence of collateral circulation	Performed during cardiac catheterization. A flexible catheter with a miniature transducer at the tip is introduced into a peripheral vessel and advanced into a coronary artery. The transducer emits high-frequency sound waves, which create a two- or three-dimensional image of the vessel lumen.	Consent form required. See cardiac catheterization for post-test care.
Lower extremity	Assesses occlusion or thrombosis in an artery or vein	Skin is bared and a water-soluble gel is applied to the area to be assessed. A Doppler transducer is passed over the area of the vessel. A gray-scale image of the vessel is obtained. A computer provides a two-dimensional image of the vessel along with an image of blood flow.	Instruct to abstain from smoking for 30 min before the test.
Carotid duplex examination	Studies blood flow in external carotid arteries	Patient is positioned supine with neck extended. The probe is moved up and down each side of the neck over the external carotid arteries.	Explain that plaque in the arteries can be visualized in this manner. This test assists in determining need for endarterectomy surgery.
Computed tomography (CT) scan	Determines size and condition of aortic aneurysm	Noninvasive, unless dye contrast used. Patient is positioned on scanning table and moved under the scanner.	Instruct patient in necessity of holding still during scan.

Continued

Table 18-2	Common Diagnostic Tests for the Cardiovascular System—cont'd		
TEST	**PURPOSE**	**PROCEDURE**	**NURSING IMPLICATIONS**
Magnetic resonance imaging (MRI) Magnetic resonance angiography (MRA)	Evaluates cardiac tissue integrity, detects aneurysms, determines ejection fraction and cardiac output, and determines patency of proximal coronary arteries	Noninvasive magnetic resonance is used to depict tissue images. IV gadolinium is injected as a contrast medium for the MRA.	Explain about the cylinder within which the patient will be positioned. Warn that there will be loud noises from the machine. Administer antianxiety medication if needed and ordered; provide music if patient desires it.
Electrophysiology studies	Measures and records electrical activity from within the heart to determine the area of origin of the dysrhythmia and the effectiveness of the antidysrhythmic drug for the particular dysrhythmia	Three to six electrodes are placed in the heart through the venous system. They are attached to an oscilloscope that records the intracardiac and ECG waveforms simultaneously. After baseline tracings are taken, the cardiologist tries to trigger the dysrhythmia that is to be studied by programmed electrical stimulation through the electrodes. Once the dysrhythmia is triggered, an antidysrhythmic drug is administered to determine its effectiveness in stopping the abnormal rhythm. Studies may take from 1½-4 hr; serial studies may be done on different days.	Provide psychological support for the patient, who is often scared of having dysrhythmias induced. Antidysrhythmic drugs may be stopped 24 hr or more before the test to eliminate them from the patient's system. Assure the patient of constant monitoring and that emergency equipment and staff will be on hand. Keep patient NPO after midnight. Patent IV line is maintained. Electrodes are placed using fluoroscopy. Patient will be supine on an x-ray table. Chest surface electrodes will be placed before the electrodes are threaded into the heart. The femoral vein is most commonly used; the groin is shaved, and local anesthesia is used. Post-test care: much the same as for cardiac catheterization.
Impedance plethysmography	Estimates blood flow in a limb based on electrical resistance present before and after inflating a pneumatic cuff placed around the limb Detects deep vein thrombosis	Measurements of electrical resistance are taken before and after a pneumatic cuff placed around the limb is inflated. Electrodes are placed on opposite sides of the limb.	Instruct to wear loose clothing. Explain that some discomfort may occur during inflation of the cuff. The patient is placed on an examination table and positioned supine in a relaxed, comfortable position. The limb is properly positioned, and electrodes and the pneumatic cuff are applied.
Hemodynamic monitoring via Swan-Ganz catheter	Determines pressure, flow, and oxygenation within the cardiovascular system *Normal values:* *Preload:* RAP 2-8 mm Hg PAWP 6-12 mm Hg PADP 4-12 mm Hg *Afterload:* MAP 70-105 mm Hg *Oxygenation:* Arterial Hgb Sao$_2$ 95%-99%	A special catheter, infusion system, transducer, and a monitor are prepared and the catheter is placed in the heart or great vessels by the physician.	The system must be calibrated to perform properly. Readings are taken for right atrial, pulmonary artery, and pulmonary wedge pressures. Other data can then be calculated regarding stroke volume, cardiac output, and oxygenation. Triglycerides contribute to arterial disease. As triglycerides rise, so do low-density lipoproteins, which are a factor in atherosclerosis. The lipoproteins (LDL, VLDL, and HDL) are increased in hyperlipidemia.

BP, blood pressure; *CO$_2$,* carbon dioxide; *EDTA,* ethylenediaminetetraacetic acid; *HDL,* high-density lipoprotein; *HF,* heart failure; *LDL,* low-density lipoprotein; *MAP,* mean arterial pressure; *NPO,* nothing by mouth; *PAWP,* pulmonary artery wedge pressure; *PADP,* pulmonary artery diastolic pressure; *RAP,* right atrial pressure; *VLDL,* very-low-density lipoprotein.

Table 18-2   Common Diagnostic Tests for the Cardiovascular System—cont'd

TEST	PURPOSE	PROCEDURE	NURSING IMPLICATIONS
Hemodynamic monitoring via Swan-Ganz catheter–cont'd	Mixed venous Hgb Sao₂ 69%-80%		Lipoprotein fractions are determined by electrophoresis and are used to assign a "risk" factor in cardiovascular disease. High levels for HDL appear to protect against coronary artery disease and MI, whereas increased levels of LDL are associated with increased atherosclerosis and MI.
Laboratory Tests*			
B-type natriuretic peptide (BNP)	Determines degree of HF.	Obtain 5-7 mL of venous blood in an EDTA lavender-top tube.	No fasting is required.
C-reactive protein (CRP)	Assesses cardiac risk; increased with inflammation Low risk <1 mg/dL High >3 mg/dL	Obtain one red-top tube of venous blood.	Some laboratories require fasting; water is permitted.
Serum lipids	Determines level: *Normal values:* Cholesterol: 150-200 mg/dL HDL: 32-75 mg/dL LDL: 73-200 mg/dL (with two or more risk factors, <73 mg/dL) Triglycerides: 50-250 mg/dL	Elevation of cholesterol is a risk factor for atherosclerotic heart disease.	Patient is NPO except for noncaloric liquids for 12 hr.
Vertical auto profile (cholesterol)	Provides more comprehensive cardiac risk assessment	Requires a blood draw and can be done along with total lipid profile.	Should fast for 12 hr
Myoglobin	Detects damage to the myocardium from a myocardial infarction. *Normal range:* <90 mcg/L	Requires a blood draw of 5 mL in a red-top tube. Apply pressure to venipuncture site.	Explain procedure. No fasting is required.
Troponin I (Tn I) Troponin T (Tn T)	<0.3 mcg/L <0.1 mcg/L	Specific to heart muscle damage. Levels may elevate within 4-6 hr after MI, peak within 10-24 hr, and return to normal within 10 days.	
Creatine phosphokinase (CPK)	Men: 55-170 IU/L Women: 30-135 IU/L	Elevated within 4-8 hr following heart attack (may also rise with injury to other muscles). Peaks within 12-24 hr, returns to normal levels within 3-4 days.	
Homocysteine	Men: 5.2-12.9 µmol/L Women: 3.7-10.4 µmol/L	Elevation is considered an independent risk factor for ischemic heart disease.	Blood sample in blue- or purple-top tube; 10- to 12-hr fast required.
CK-MB (creatine kinase)	<3 ng/mL	Elevates within 2-6 hr after an MI, peaks within 12-24 hr, and returns to normal within 3 days. CK-MB is specific to myocardial injury.	
Myeloperoxidase antigen (MPO)	<6 U/mL	Detects or assists in ruling out microangitis of the arteries.	Requires 0.5 mL blood in a yellow-top tube. No fasting required.

*Electrolyte values are listed in Table 3-3, p. 41.

an electron-beam computed tomography for coronary artery calcium scoring may be better than the standard treadmill test for detecting heart disease. A stress echocardiogram also is helpful.

Cardiac Monitoring

Continuous monitoring of cardiac rate and rhythm often is done by *telemetry*. Disposable electrodes and wire leads from a bedside monitor or battery-operated transmitter unit are applied to the patient. The wave pattern signals are sent to a monitor in a central station, where they are continually observed. This allows patients to walk around the nursing unit while being monitored. The wave pattern signals may also be displayed on a bedside monitor.

Cardiac monitors can detect specific *dysrhythmias* (abnormal variations of heart rhythm), automatically store the wave pattern, and alert the nurse to the abnormality with an alarm. Cardiac monitoring is used for patients experiencing an acute cardiac disorder, after cardiac surgery, and after pacemaker insertion. Figure 18-8 shows proper placement for telemetry leads.

Specific Tests for Vascular Disorders

Diagnosing a vascular problem begins with a history and physical examination that includes a variety of tests for risk factors for vascular disorders. A complete blood count (CBC), urinalysis, blood lipid and cholesterol assessment (including HDL and LDL), or sequential multiple analyzer (SMA) panel that screens liver and kidney function, electrolytes, and blood glucose are ordered. If blood pressure is elevated, tests of thyroid, adrenal glands, kidneys, and renal arteries are done to rule out the possibility of another disease that might cause secondary hypertension. Hyperthyroidism, Cushing's syndrome, pheochromocytoma, nephrosclerosis, and renal arterial stenosis all elevate blood pressure.

Doppler flow studies are performed to detect a thrombus when one is suspected and to assess the patency of the carotid arteries. Angiography may be performed to determine areas of narrowing in arteries or to detect a lodged embolus. Nuclear medicine scans are performed to detect emboli in the lungs.

The ankle-brachial index (ABI) is an inexpensive, noninvasive screening test to evaluate arterial status in the lower extremities. A regular blood pressure cuff is placed above the malleolus. Another blood pressure cuff is positioned over the brachial artery. A Doppler probe is used to check the systolic end point at the dorsalis pedis and the posterior tibial sites. The brachial blood pressure is measured. The ABI is calculated by dividing the ankle pressure by the brachial pressure. An ABI of 1 or more is considered normal. An abnormal ABI indicates arterial

A Three-electrode placement

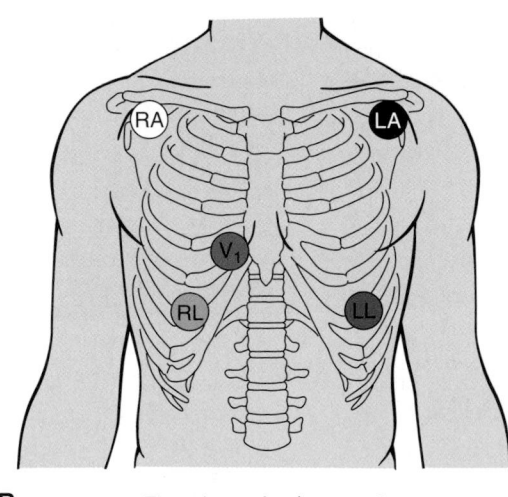

B Five-electrode placement

FIGURE 18-8 Placement of the most commonly used telemetry leads. **A,** Two leads (three-electrode system); **B,** Five leads (five-electrode system).

disease and can confirm a vascular cause for ischemic pain in the legs at rest and *claudication* (cramping pain in the calves) when walking. See Table 18-2 for diagnostic tests used to detect other problems in the vascular system. Serum cholesterol and lipids are discussed more fully in Chapter 19.

 Think Critically

Can you identify four teaching points to be covered for the patient who is to undergo an arteriogram?

❖ NURSING MANAGEMENT
■ Assessment (Data Collection)
History Taking

It is important to determine whether the patient has risk factors for cardiovascular disease.

Much of this information is obtained by the physician or nurse practitioner during history-taking and

Focused Assessment

Data Collection for the Cardiovascular System

HISTORY TAKING

Ask the following questions:

- Do you ever have any chest discomfort or pain? What does it feel like? What, if anything, seems to bring it on? What makes it worse? How long does it last? Is it worse when you breathe in deeply? What gives relief? Does the pain radiate (spread) to other parts of the body, for example, down the arm or up into the neck or jaw, or to the upper abdomen? Is it localized, or does it cover a large area? On a scale of 1 to 10, with 10 being the worst and 1 being the least, how do you rate your pain? Do you have numbness, tingling, nausea, sweating, shortness of breath, anxiety, or dizziness when you have chest pain?
- Have you or any member of your family ever been told that you have diabetes mellitus; cardiovascular, thyroid, or renal disease; arteriosclerosis; hyperlipidemia; atherosclerosis; peripheral vascular disease; a blood disorder; gout; kidney disease; or an immune disorder such as lupus erythematosus?
- Do you become easily fatigued? Dizzy or light-headed?
- Do you become short of breath? When? Do you sleep on more than one pillow? Is your shortness of breath worse after physical activity? What kind of activity? Walking up steps? Does it occur when you are at rest? Does resting relieve it? Do you wake up at night short of breath or feeling like you are suffocating? Does sitting up on the side of the bed or getting up give you relief?
- Do you have a cough? What kind? Dry and hacking, or wet and productive? What does the sputum look like? Is there ever any blood in your sputum?
- Do you notice your heart beating very fast or pounding in your chest (palpitations)? Does it skip a beat?
- Have you ever fainted or felt like you were going to faint?
- Do you get up in the night to urinate? How many times do you get up each night?
- Have you noticed any sudden weight gain or swelling in the feet and legs?
- Do you experience pain in your legs when walking?
- Are your feet always cold?
- Have you ever had a bad injury to either leg?
- Have you ever had a deep vein thrombosis (DVT) or thrombophlebitis?
- What medications do you take that are prescribed by your physician? What over-the-counter medications do you take? Do you take herbals? Do you use recreational drugs?
- Do you smoke? Have you ever smoked? How much and for how long?
- Do you drink alcohol? What do you usually drink? How many drinks do you have? About how many times a week do you drink something alcoholic?
- What do you usually eat? Can you tell me what you generally eat for breakfast, lunch, and dinner? Do you have a midmorning, midafternoon, or evening snack? What do you eat for a snack? Do you eat fast food often? What type of fast food? What do you usually drink at meals? Do you drink liquids between meals?
- Do you regularly add salt to your food?
- Do you have leg pain at night?
- Have you ever had a sore on your foot or lower leg that was slow to heal?
- How would you rate your stress levels? What do you do to cope with or reduce stress?

by the admitting nurse during a complete nursing assessment. Some additional information, however, will be gathered in less formal interactions when the patient becomes more relaxed and comfortable with the nurses who care for her.

Information concerning the patient's actual eating habits, such as snacking on "junk" food or daily consumption of several drinks containing caffeine, is more likely to be obtained during nursing care activities than during the initial assessment. Data concerning stressors in the patient's life and her response to them are more easily assessed while interacting over time.

An understanding of the patient's perception of her disorder and overall health are necessary to plan appropriate teaching. The effectiveness of your communication with the patient will determine the quality of subjective data obtained. Many drugs can cause vasoconstriction and elevate blood pressure. Cold remedies, decongestants, and diet pills are particularly noted for having this effect. Other prescription medications that may affect the heart are bronchodilators, anticoagulants, contraceptives, psychotropic medications, and street drugs. A careful, specific diet history should be gathered. Fast-food intake is significant because it is often high in fat and sodium. **Excessive alcohol intake is a factor in the development of hypertension and cardiomyopathy.** Questions are asked that relate to changes from damage to the cardiovascular system, such as congestive heart failure (CHF), angina, or kidney failure. Intermittent claudication (cramping pain in the muscles brought on by exercise and relieved by rest) is a common symptom of arterial insufficiency to the lower extremities. This pain most frequently occurs in the calves of the legs, but it also can affect the muscles of the thighs and buttocks. Often chronic occlusive arterial disease will cause pain described as burning and tingling, with numbness of the toes. It is most noticeable at night when the patient is in bed.

 Think Critically

How would you phrase questions about alcohol intake or drug use so that the patient would answer the questions honestly?

Physical Assessment

Significant findings include abnormal or extra heart sounds, crackles in the lungs, or pink frothy sputum indicating pulmonary edema.

 Cultural Considerations

Dyspnea as the Major Symptom

African Americans often experience dyspnea as the most acute symptom during an MI. Dyspnea is more common than the more classic chest discomfort in this group. For this reason, they may delay seeking assistance.

Chest pain, if present, should be further assessed using the "PQRST" memory device (Table 18-3). Other

Table 18-3 PQRST for Pain Assessment*

FACTOR	QUESTIONS TO ASK
Precipitating events	What events or factors precipitated or caused the pain or discomfort?
Quality of pain or discomfort	What does the pain or discomfort feel like? Is it aching, dull, sharp, tight, heavy pressure, etc.?
Radiation of pain	Where is the pain located? Does it radiate to the back, arms, jaw, teeth, shoulder, or elbow?
Severity of pain	On a scale of 1 to 10, with 10 being the most severe, how do you rate the pain?
Timing	When did the pain or discomfort begin? Has it changed since it started? Has this type of pain occurred before?

*This memory device is used to assist in obtaining information from any patient experiencing chest pain or discomfort.

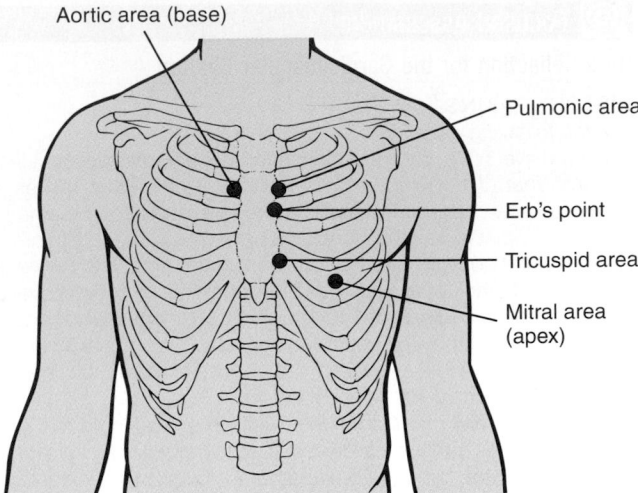

FIGURE 18-9 Sites for auscultation of heart sounds. S_1 is loudest at mitral and tricuspid areas. S_2 is loudest at aortic and pulmonic areas. Listen in the mitral area for S_3 and S_4 sounds.

significant findings might be a bluish cast to skin; pallor or diaphoresis (sweating); clubbing of the fingers; or pitting edema of the feet, ankles, or sacral area (see Figure 3-4). There may be distended jugular veins, an abnormal rate or volume of pulses, or a pulse deficit. A pulse deficit is the difference between the apical and radial pulse rate when they are counted at the same time.

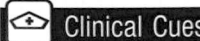

Focused Assessment

Physical Examination of the Cardiovascular System

When assessing the cardiovascular system, check for:
- Skin color, temperature, and texture
- Facial expression; signs of pain or anxiety
- Vital signs
- Heart sounds; S_1, S_2, abnormal sounds, murmurs
- Apical pulse rate and rhythm; presence of pulse deficit
- Quality of peripheral pulses; compare them bilaterally
- Breath sounds, presence of crackles in lung bases
- Shape of fingers; presence of clubbing
- Appearance of neck veins; presence of venous jugular distention
- Abdomen; presence of distention; abdominal pulsation
- Degree of body tension
- Ankles and feet; presence of edema and degree
- General body appearance; presence of edema
- Weight; gain of 2 lb or more over a few days
- Varicosities in lower extremities

Clinical Cues

Chest pain should be considered cardiac in origin until such a cause can be ruled out. Many things can cause chest pain, but it is important to always think "cardiac first."

An apical pulse rate should be taken for all patients on admission. Privacy should be provided before baring the chest and the room should be warm. Heart sounds are auscultated at least every 8 hours on all patients who have a known dysrhythmia or a potential for dysrhythmia, a valve problem, or heart failure (Figure 18-9). The diaphragm of the stethoscope is placed over the bare skin at the mitral area to listen to the apical pulse. S_1 (lub) and S_2 (dub) should be distinguished. S_1 occurs with the closing of the AV valves during systole. S_2 is the closure of the pulmonic and semilunar valves during diastole. Extra sounds or gallops may occur as S_3 sounds. Splitting of the S_2 sound may be normal in children and young adults, but may be abnormal in adults. S_4 is usually heard just before S_1 and can indicate various heart diseases.

The bell of the stethoscope is used to listen for heart murmurs. **It must be placed lightly on the skin for the sounds to be heard.** Murmurs usually have a "swooshing" sound from turbulent blood flow. Murmurs are commonly from damaged valves, causing abnormal blood flow in the heart. As heart sounds often are very soft, ask the patient to refrain from talking, and turn off the television or radio while listening. (Just remember to turn it back on.) Having the patient roll to the left side or lean forward may make the sounds louder and clearer.

Elder Care Points

The thickening of valve leaflets with age may cause a systolic murmur common in persons older than age 80.

Pulses. Check the arterial pulses and determine the pulse rate, rhythm, and character (force) of the pulse (Box 18-2). When performing a cardiovascular assessment, the radial pulse should be assessed and compared with the apical pulse. **The apical pulse should be counted for a full minute.** The carotid, femoral,

Box 18-2   Scale for Grading Pulse Quality

0—Absent
1—Weak, thready
2—Light volume
3—Normal volume
4—Full, bounding

popliteal, and pedal pulses should also be palpated and compared bilaterally, noting quality and character (Figure 18-10). The pulse may be described as *normal* or *absent, regular* or *irregular, strong, weak,* or *thready.*

If pulsations are weak or undetectable, use a Doppler stethoscope to check them. A Doppler stethoscope measures the velocity of blood flow through a vessel with ultrasound waves. It can sense weak pulsations even in severely narrowed arteries (Figure 18-11).

? Think Critically

Can you recall the correct way to locate a dorsalis pedis and a posterior tibial pulse? Could you demonstrate the technique to a classmate?

Examine the abdomen with the patient lying supine for a visual abdominal pulsation from the aorta. This sometimes indicates the presence of an aneurysm.

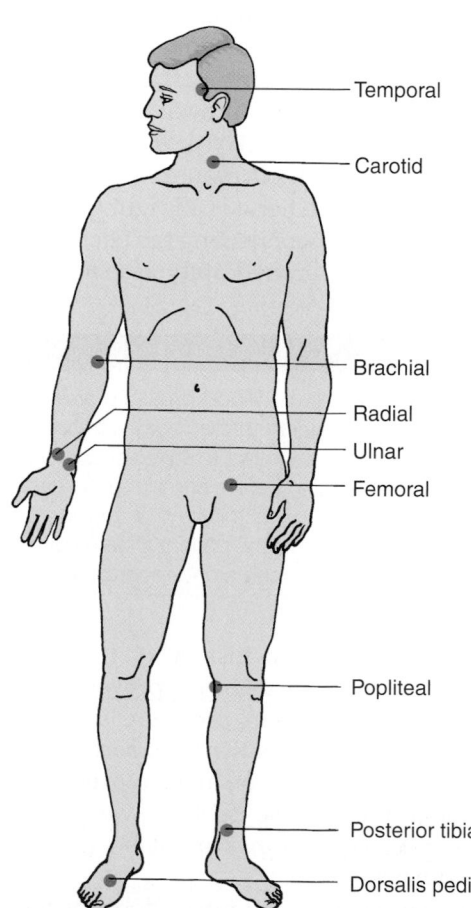

FIGURE 18-10 Palpation sites for arterial pulse.

- Temporal
- Carotid
- Brachial
- Radial
- Ulnar
- Femoral
- Popliteal
- Posterior tibial
- Dorsalis pedis

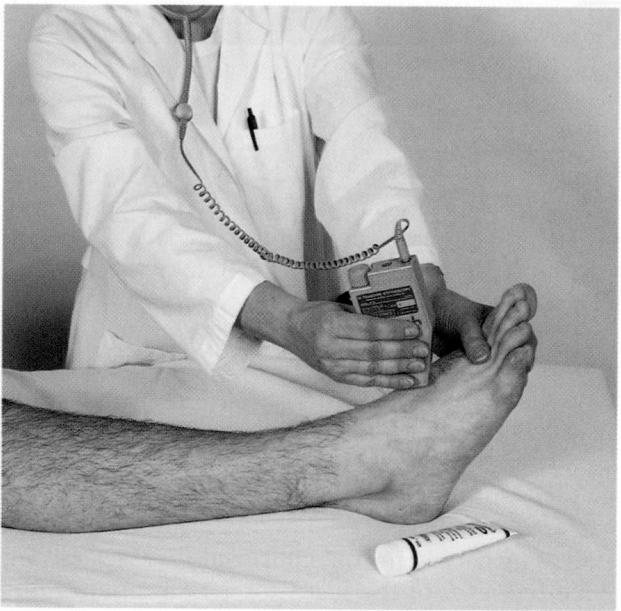

FIGURE 18-11 The Doppler stethoscope is used to detect a faint pulse.

Bruits. A whooshing or purring sound (a bruit) is made when blood passes through a partially obstructed artery. To detect bruits, listen with the bell of the stethoscope applied lightly over the skin of the carotid arteries, abdominal aorta, and femoral arteries.

Blood Pressure. For more accurate readings, be certain the patient has not had a cigarette or any caffeine for the past 30 minutes. Blood pressure should be carefully measured with the correct size cuff. The cuff should fit the upper arm with the lower edge 2.5 cm (1 inch) above the antecubital space. If the cuff is too narrow, the pressure will be falsely elevated. Cuffs are available in child, normal adult, and large adult sizes. The bladder must be centered over the brachial artery, and its length should cover at least 80% of the extremity's circumference when positioned correctly. The pressure should be taken sitting, lying supine, and standing for a thorough assessment. Standing blood pressure measurements also are important when a patient is started on a new medication, particularly an angiotensin-converting enzyme (ACE) inhibitor. Blood pressure should be measured on both arms. The patient's arm on which the cuff is placed should be supported at heart level and the feet should be supported or be on the floor. The patient should be resting quietly for 5 minutes before the measurement is taken. The equipment used should be calibrated, and the valve should open and close smoothly. The cuff should be deflated slowly and smoothly to obtain a correct diastolic reading. Automatic blood pressure machines must be properly calibrated and checked for accuracy regularly.

Orthostatic or postural hypotension occurs when the blood pressure drops when a person stands. Orthostatic or postural hypotension is a common cause of **syncope** (fainting) in older patients.

The blood pressure of the elderly patient will be lower right after a meal. For accurate readings, assess blood pressure between meals.

Skin. Tissues in light-skinned people that are receiving an adequate supply of oxygenated blood appear pink and rosy, whereas tissues deprived of normal amounts of arterial blood appear pale and mottled. In dark-skinned people, the mucous membranes will be rosy and pink if oxygenation is adequate. However, the environment must be taken into account. Pale and mottled skin also can indicate that the patient is just cold. Reddish blue color can indicate venous insufficiency.

One way to assess arterial blood flow more accurately is by having the patient elevate her feet and legs above the level of the heart for 1 to 3 minutes until pallor occurs. Have the patient lower the legs to a dangling position while sitting. Compare both feet, noting the time necessary for pinkness to return (usually about 10 seconds). Note the time it takes for the veins of the feet and ankles to fill (usually about 15 seconds). For those with dark skin, inspect the soles of the feet for color change and use a light shining at an angle to visualize vein filling.

Return of color to the lowered feet is delayed in arterial insufficiency. If there is severe peripheral arterial disease the dangling feet soon take on a dusky red color (rubor). The skin may be shiny and taut.

A cold environment and immobility will cause the extremities to feel cold to the touch. However, when a patient experiences persistent coldness of an extremity in a warm environment, peripheral arterial disease should be suspected. When observing a patient for signs of arterial disease, the nurse should note differences in skin temperature in various areas of the same limb, as well as differences between limbs.

Skin that is chronically malnourished because of decreased blood supply has a characteristic appearance: the skin appears smooth, shiny, and thin, and there is little or no hair on its surface. The nails are thick with deposits of cornlike material under them.

If there is severe malnutrition of the tissues for several days, the tissues become necrotic. This causes the skin to assume a purple-black color. This is a deep cyanotic condition indicative of gangrene. Gangrene of the toes is not an uncommon complication in the diabetic patient who has poor circulation in the feet.

Chronic venous insufficiency is accompanied by chronic edema. This in turn leads to inflammation of the tissues (cellulitis) and eventually to the formation of ulcers. Edema is either present, absent, pitting, or nonpitting. Pitting means that a fingertip pressed into the area for 5 seconds leaves an indentation. Increased pigmentation of the skin, dryness and scaling, and excoriations are objective signs of venous insufficiency.

The capillary refill test has traditionally been used to check peripheral circulation. A fingernail or a toenail is squeezed over the bed of the nail sufficiently to cause blanching; the pressure is removed and an observation is made of how quickly the color returns. Normally the color returns immediately. Although it is a good gross assessment of circulation to the extremity, this test is unreliable as many factors can cause a decrease in time for color to return. This test is most useful for determining whether circulation is occluded by constriction or thrombosis above the area. Review Chapter 3 for assessment and staging of edema.

■ Nursing Diagnosis, Planning, Implementation

Table 18-4 presents general nursing diagnoses, expected outcomes, and nursing interventions for patients experiencing cardiovascular problems. Nursing diagnoses may be added to the care plan for problems secondary to treatments, such as drug side effects or complications from surgery.

A goal of community nursing is the promotion of healthful living to prevent cardiovascular disease. A concerted effort is being made to decrease childhood obesity as a method of decreasing later possibilities for cardiovascular disease in adulthood.

When planning care for cardiovascular patients, it is important to schedule nursing activities to conserve the strength of the patient and prevent excessive fatigue. Patients undergoing telemetry monitoring should not be disconnected from their monitor for any extended time. Check to see whether it is all right to have the patient shower before disconnecting the telemetry device. **Reconnect the leads immediately afterward.**

Know what the patient's last blood pressure and pulse measurements were before going to the room with cardiovascular medications. Often you will need to take an apical pulse rate and blood pressure reading before administering certain medications. You need to know what those measurements had been previously in order to evaluate the patient's status properly. Plan time to take these measurements and record them.

When a patient has a history of thrombosis, the nurse must plan measures to prevent recurrence regardless of what patient problem is currently the focus of treatment. If the patient has peripheral arterial disease, the nurse should be alert to prescribed medications that may cause further vasoconstriction. Specific expected outcomes must be written on an individual basis.

A large part of what the nurse does for the patient with a cardiovascular disorder is to monitor the
Text continued on p. 392

Table 18-4   Common Nursing Diagnoses and Interventions for Patients with Heart Disorders

NURSING DIAGNOSIS	GOALS/EXPECTED OUTCOMES	NURSING INTERVENTIONS
Cardiac Disorders		
Activity intolerance related to decreased perfusion	Patient will not experience undue fatigue performing activities with changes in vital signs.	Space activities of daily living and nursing procedures to prevent undue fatigue. Encourage use of oxygen as ordered. Implement actions to promote rest.
Risk for injury related to dysrhythmia or complications of myocardial infarction (MI) or heart failure (HF)	Patient will not experience serious dysrhythmia and will have a stable ECG. Patient will not experience complications from MI or HF.	Monitor ECG or telemetry tracings, observing for changes and life-threatening dysrhythmias. Assess for complications: • Monitor lungs for crackles. • Check for jugular venous distention. • Auscultate for changes in heart sounds, extra sounds, changes in rhythm. • Assess respirations for increasing dyspnea. • Assess for signs of inflammation or infection; check temperature trend, white blood cell (WBC) level. • Assess for chest pain on exertion or at rest. • Monitor for central and peripheral edema. • Assess trends in daily weight. • Assess trends in 24-hr intake and output. • Monitor vital signs.
Decreased cardiac output related to dysrhythmia or ineffective cardiac muscle action	Patient will demonstrate adequate cardiac output with normal pulses, vital signs, skin color, and urine output.	Assess apical pulse q shift. Administer antidysrhythmic and cardiotonic medications, as ordered. Observe for side effects of medications. Assess for adequate perfusion: • Check peripheral pulses. • Assess color of extremities and around mouth. • Assess mentation. • Monitor urine output (related to perfusion of kidneys). • Auscultate lungs for crackles q shift. • Assess level of fatigue. • Treat impaired oxygenation and fluid imbalance. • Give stool softeners or laxatives, as ordered, to prevent straining at stool (Valsalva maneuver) and slowing of pulse or stopping of heart.
Impaired gas exchange related to cardiac failure	Patient will not experience impaired oxygenation; Spo_2 within normal limits and Po_2 between 80 and 100.	Place in high Fowler's position. Administer oxygen, as ordered. Feed frequent small meals to decrease oxygen demand. Administer diuretics as ordered. Monitor intake and output. Enforce fluid restrictions. Assist with activities of daily living (ADLs). Promote relief of anxiety. Give morphine, as ordered, to ease breathing and decrease anxiety. Monitor lung sounds, pulse oximetry, and blood gases. Assist to use incentive spirometer q 2 hr, as ordered. Provide measures to drain pulmonary fluid, as ordered (i.e., postural drainage, suction, nebulizer treatments).
Self-care deficit, bathing/hygiene, toileting, dressing/grooming, related to fatigue, weakness, or dyspnea	Patient will increase performance of own ADLs of 1-3 metabolic equivalents (METs) within 1 wk.	Assist with all ADLs as needed. Plan nursing treatments to provide rest periods. Encourage to do small tasks of ADLs as condition improves. Assist to turn in bed q 2 hr. Assess skin q shift and when turning. Provide mouth care before meals to stimulate appetite.

Continued

Table 18-4   Common Nursing Diagnoses and Interventions for Patients with Heart Disorders—cont'd

NURSING DIAGNOSIS	GOALS/EXPECTED OUTCOMES	NURSING INTERVENTIONS
Cardiac Disorders—cont'd		
Fear related to life-threatening illness	Patient will verbalize feelings and fears regarding life-threatening condition. Patient will identify own best coping mechanisms.	Perform a spiritual assessment. Determine usual coping style. Support in coping mechanisms. Obtain clergyman if patient desires contact. Provide privacy for prayer and devotions. Assist to ventilate fears to reduce anxiety. Keep informed of what is being done for treatment and what to expect. Inform of positive gains toward wellness. Allow state of denial in acute stage as denial may be protective. Provide time with loved ones. Provide therapeutic touch if patient is accepting. Assess cultural meanings of events to patient. Actively listen to the patient's fears and concerns. Offer realistic reassurance as appropriate.
Impaired home maintenance related to fatigue, dyspnea, and activity intolerance	Appropriate home services will be in place before discharge.	Refer for social services consultation. Consider home health care services. Offer information on homemaker aide services. Consult with family regarding ongoing care of patient at home. Collaborate with patient regarding plans for home care.
Vascular Disorders		
Ineffective tissue perfusion related to: Vascular damage from elevated blood pressure	Patient's blood pressure will be within normal range within 3 mo.	Assess blood pressure; determine effectiveness of therapy. Administer medications to lower blood pressure. Discourage intake of caffeine and excess sodium. Discourage smoking. Teach to arise slowly and stabilize before walking to counteract postural hypotension effect from medication. Teach anxiety- and tension-reduction techniques to decrease blood pressure. Encourage regular rest, relaxation, and exercise program.
Obstructed blood flow	Patient will not develop emboli. Thrombosis will resolve within 10-14 days.	Assess for signs and symptoms of deep vein thrombosis and impaired blood flow. Maintain activity restrictions as ordered. Elevate affected extremity as ordered. Increase fluid intake to 3000 mL/day unless contraindicated. Administer anticoagulants as ordered; monitor for side effects. Teach to prevent future episodes by encouraging not to sit with legs crossed, not to sit for long periods, and not to put pressure on the back of the knees. Apply elastic stockings or sequential pneumatic devices to promote venous return.
Surgical revascularization	Patient will not develop thrombosis.	Check incisions for bleeding q 1-2 hr × 24 hr then q 4 hr × 6, then q shift. Assess for internal hematoma by checking sensation below surgical area. Assess for adequate blood flow by checking pulses distal to incision on same schedule. Assess skin color and temperature above and below incision when checking for bleeding. Reinforce dressing as needed; change dressing per orders, using strict aseptic technique.

Table 18-4	Common Nursing Diagnoses and Interventions for Patients with Heart Disorders—cont'd	
NURSING DIAGNOSIS	**GOALS/EXPECTED OUTCOMES**	**NURSING INTERVENTIONS**
Vascular Disorders—cont'd		
Pain related to decreased blood flow and edema	Patient will verbalize adequate pain control attained from analgesics and comfort measures provided.	Assess type and location of pain experienced. Handle gently and avoid jarring the bed. Use a bed cradle or footboard to prevent pressure from bed linens. Administer analgesics and anti-inflammatory agents as ordered. Apply heat as ordered; monitor closely to prevent burns. Teach relaxation techniques, imagery, or distraction to decrease pain. Elevate edematous extremity. Apply elastic stockings or sequential pneumatic devices to encourage venous return and decrease edema. Medicate for sleep as ordered if discomfort is interfering with rest.
Activity intolerance related to pain in legs when walking	Patient will develop own activity program within 3 wk. Patient will exercise regularly according to devised program.	Collaborate with physical therapist to encourage prescribed exercises. Assist to plan walking, swimming, or cycling program.
Disturbed body image related to: Diagnosis of chronic illness Edema and dilated veins in the legs Loss of limb by amputation Inability to maintain former lifestyle	Patient will verbalize feelings regarding diagnosis, body changes, and needed lifestyle changes. Patient will identify personal strengths and coping mechanisms within 3 wk. Patient will become as independent as possible in tasks of daily living within 2 mo.	Allow to ventilate feelings about illness and disease process. Assist through the grief process. Assist to identify personal strengths. Reinforce coping mechanisms that have been helpful before. Be with patient for first dressing change. Clarify misconceptions about physical limitations after amputation. Involve patient in care of the wound after initial period of adjustment. Foster independence in tasks of daily living. Assist to explore lifestyle changes. Encourage significant others in their support of the patient. Teach ways to decrease risk of further amputation.
Impaired tissue integrity related to: Ulcer from decreased circulation Surgical wound (Risk for infection may be used here also)	Patient will not develop a wound infection.	Use strict aseptic technique for wound care. Treat and dress wound per physician's orders. Promote adequate nutrition to promote healing. Administer medication, as ordered, to prevent infection. Position affected limb, as ordered. Maintain correct body alignment.
Risk for impaired tissue integrity related to bed rest and impaired circulation	Patient will not develop impaired tissue integrity.	Inspect pressure points q 2 hr. Turn at least q 2 hr. Maintain smooth linens on bed, provide appropriate padding to prevent pressure areas. Keep skin clean and dry. Refrain from raising the knee section of the bed. Encourage foot and ankle exercises q hr while patient is awake. Prevent shearing when patient is moving in bed by using a lift sheet and two people to turn the patient. If skin breakdown occurs, notify physician immediately and provide appropriate wound care.

Continued

Table 18-4	Common Nursing Diagnoses and Interventions for Patients with Heart Disorders—cont'd	
NURSING DIAGNOSIS	**GOALS/EXPECTED OUTCOMES**	**NURSING INTERVENTIONS**
Vascular Disorders—cont'd		
Deficient knowledge related to inadequate information about disease process, medications, and self-care	Patient will verbalize knowledge of disease process and ways to prevent further damage. Patient will verbalize how to take medications and side effects to report. Patient will demonstrate self-care techniques.	Explain what is happening in the body to cause the decreased blood flow. Allow time for questions. Instruct in ways to decrease risk factors. Teach self-care methods, including exercises, skin care, foot care, dietary changes, and lifestyle changes. Teach about medications, including schedule of administration, action, side effects, what to report to the physician. Encourage regular visits to the physician.
Noncompliance related to refusal to follow treatment regimen	Patient will verbalize frustrations and problems in complying with treatment regimen and lifestyle changes. Patient will demonstrate compliance with treatment regimen.	Reinstruct about disease process. Explore problems with treatment regimen. Allow patient to express feelings about lifestyle changes. Explore ability to obtain and afford medications. Explore any difficulty in swallowing medications. Explain progression of disease and consequences of poor control; discuss complications and impact on lifestyle. Seek support system for compliance with treatment program. Give praise for each attempt at compliance. Respect the patient's right to make decisions about compliance.
Risk for injury related to: Embolus or bleeding from anticoagulant medication	Coagulation times will remain within safe therapeutic range. Patient will have no signs of bleeding. Patient will have no signs of embolus.	Do not massage affected extremity. Encourage activity restrictions as ordered. Monitor laboratory values: international normalized ratio (INR) or activated partial thromboplastin time (APTT) and notify physician when values are outside of accepted therapeutic limits. Assess urine and stool for signs of blood. Assess patient for excessive bruising; bleeding gums, nosebleeds, bleeding at puncture sites. Check injectable anticoagulant dosages and IV admixtures with another nurse before administration to verify correct ordered dosage and rate of infusion.
Circulatory occlusion from embolus		Assess for signs of embolus: chest pain, shortness of breath, change in level of consciousness, sudden headache, or other neurologic signs.

ADLs, activities of daily living; *METs,* metabolic equivalent.

condition and determine whether treatment is effective. Considerable time is spent on teaching patients about the disease, self-care, and medications. It is very important to monitor side effects or adverse effects of medication.

Remember that any patient experiencing fatigue or weakness takes longer to accomplish the tasks of daily living. Space nursing actions appropriately. Watch the patient receiving cardiac drugs for postural hypotension; have her hold on to the bed rail and steady herself for a couple of minutes after arising, before beginning to walk. This will help prevent falls. Specific nursing interventions are discussed with the various disorders in the following chapters.

Collaboration

Cardiovascular patients often are being treated by the physical therapist, dietitian, and respiratory therapist, as well as by the physician and nurse. It is important that the nurse consult with the other health professionals involved in the patient's care. Early collaboration with the discharge planner is important to provide continuity of care after discharge. The nurse's work will go more smoothly if it is possible to plan when other health professionals will see the patient. Providing others on the health care team with information useful to them promotes a good working relationship.

■ Evaluation

Evaluation involves both subjective and objective data. Use good communication skills to ask the right questions in order to gather the required information from the patient. Ask the patient to describe any "different" feelings she has experienced. Inquire about changes in appetite and bowel movements that could indicate possible medication toxicity. Check laboratory values for therapeutic drug levels before giving doses of medication, and note the latest blood levels of electrolytes. Assess for signs and symptoms of drug toxicity, and for fluid or electrolyte imbalance. Ask yourself whether the patient is showing signs indicating that the medication you are giving is effective. The nursing care plan should be checked daily to evaluate whether each nursing action is effective. If an action is ineffective over time, it should be deleted and a new action should be devised to resolve the problem.

It is important to look at serial blood pressure readings to evaluate the effectiveness of treatment and of nursing interventions. Pressures that are consistently higher than normal in between medication doses indicate a need to change either the dosage schedule or the medication.

Carefully evaluating pulses and comparing them bilaterally is an important part of nursing care for patients with problems of the cardiovascular system. Writing a good description of the quality and character of the pulses monitored in the nurse's notes will give coworkers an accurate assessment baseline on which to evaluate changes in the pulse.

It is important to determine if skin color and temperature have changed since the last assessment. Accurately measure and document areas of discoloration in the nurse's notes. Monitor ulcerated areas closely and measure and photograph the areas to determine whether healing is occurring. Evaluate the color of the healing tissue and presence of exudate. If the wound is growing or not improving, the nursing actions or treatment must be changed.

Often the nurse must rely on subjective data from the patient to evaluate whether treatment and nursing actions are effective. Increases in peripheral circulation may be evident only by a decrease in pain or an ability to walk farther without pain.

COMMON PROBLEMS OF PATIENTS WITH CARDIOVASCULAR DISORDERS

FATIGUE AND DYSPNEA

When the coronary arteries fail to supply adequate oxygen to the cells of the heart muscle, the heart is unable to perform as it should, especially when extra demands are placed on it. The result is a general hypoxia of the tissues throughout the body, which causes fatigue and dyspnea on exertion. In the early stages of heart disease, the patient may be only slightly aware of the inability to do as much physical work as she formerly could.

Bed rest with bedside commode privileges is ordered for the first 24 to 72 hours for MI and severe CHF. The patient may feed herself and assist with her sponge bath. She should be cautioned against any isometric activity, such as pushing up in bed. Stool softeners are given to prevent straining at stool (Valsalva maneuver), which causes a sudden increase in cardiac workload (Felker et al., 2006). Straining while coughing or repositioning in bed can cause the Valsalva as well, and such straining is to be avoided. Progress patient activity to chair sitting, ambulating to the bathroom, and then ambulating down the hall. Monitor patients via telemetry units to watch for dysrhythmias or excessive heart rate changes during ambulation. The amount of energy used in activity is expressed in *metabolic equivalents* (METs). The patient is guided from 1 to 3 METs before discharge. Sitting, eating, washing hands and face, and conversing are 1 to 3 MET activities. Table 21-4 on p. 464 shows the metabolic equivalents for various activities.

Criteria used to determine whether the cardiac patient is tolerating the activity include the following:
- The heart rate does not rise more than 20 beats per minute over baseline rate.
- Systolic blood pressure does not drop.
- There is no complaint of chest pain, dyspnea, or severe fatigue.
- There is no abnormal heart rate or rhythm.

The progress of activity often is jointly supervised by a physical therapist and a nurse. More information on cardiac rehabilitation is presented in Chapter 9.

FLUID OVERLOAD (EDEMA)

Edema is an accumulation of fluid in the interstitial fluid compartment. It becomes a problem in heart disease when blood flow into or out of the heart is inhibited, causing a slowing down of the normal movement of body fluids and their eventual excretion.

Continually assess the fluid balance of a patient with cardiac disease by looking for signs of abnormal collections of fluid in the body tissues. Daily weight change is considered the best indicator of fluid buildup. Check the feet and ankles of ambulatory patients for signs of dependent edema, and watch bed rest patients for signs of swelling in the area of the sacrum, buttocks, and thighs. Observe for progressive signs of shortness of breath, and auscultate lung fields each shift to detect crackles—a sign of beginning pulmonary congestion. Observe the jugular veins for prominence when the patient is in an upright position; prominent veins may indicate fluid overload and CHF.

Clinical Cues

A weight gain of 3 lb or more in a 24-hour period indicates fluid retention.

Nursing responsibilities include recording the patient's weight daily before breakfast, supervising fluid restriction, accurately measuring intake and output, and assessing for signs of both fluid deficit and fluid overload. Elderly patients on fluid restriction and diuretics can easily become dehydrated.

Therapeutic measures to control edema include the administration of diuretics and restriction of sodium and, possibly, the restriction of fluid. You must observe for adverse effects of medication, such as electrolyte imbalance and postural hypotension. Potassium supplementation may be ordered for the patient who is experiencing hypokalemia.

 Safety Alert

Signs of Hypokalemia

Be alert for the following signs of hypokalemia: fatigue, muscle weakness, muscle cramps, drowsiness, confusion, new onset of bradycardia, or postural hypotension. Hypokalemia may cause life-threatening dysrhythmias.

PAIN

Pain can be a symptom of a life-threatening heart event. Each episode of pain is carefully assessed by noting when it started, the location and radiation pattern, degree of pain on a scale, activity before onset, associated symptoms such as nausea, diaphoresis, or palpitations, and vital signs.

Severe pain is most often associated with heart disease of an acute nature (e.g., MI). Anginal pain caused by narrowed coronary arteries can interfere with the patient's lifestyle, as well as cause discomfort. Acute anginal pain is treated with nitroglycerin, oral nitrates, oxygen, reassurance, and careful monitoring for relief. Nitrates and other medications that dilate coronary arteries to promote better blood flow and decrease ischemia are used to control or prevent anginal pain.

 Clinical Cues

If chest pain is not relieved after administering three nitroglycerin sublingual tablets 5 minutes apart, notify the physician. Institute oxygen therapy according to agency protocol, monitor vital signs, and stay with the patient. The patient may be experiencing an MI. (Do check to make certain that the nitroglycerin causes tingling under the tongue. If not, the tablets are too old and will not work.)

If pain is not relieved, the analgesic drug used most often in an emergency situation is morphine sulfate, as it decreases both anxiety and cardiac workload, as well as alleviates pain (Fenton, 2010). The drug is given IV initially for quick pain relief. As the acute phase and severe pain subside, these drugs may be replaced with oral dosages or milder sedatives that promote relaxation and freedom from anxiety.

The patient's pain may be increased because of nervousness and anxiety, and you can do much to help relieve pain by providing a restful environment, interacting therapeutically with "active listening," and balancing rest with prescribed physical activity.

Sleep deprivation and fatigue can increase the pain. Turning, administration of medications, visiting, exercise, and other procedures should be coordinated so that the patient is not disturbed more than necessary.

Determining those factors that seem to trigger an attack can identify stressors that the patient may be able to avoid. Relaxation and other noninvasive techniques to manage pain are discussed in Chapter 7.

ALTERED TISSUE PERFUSION

In peripheral vascular disease, blood flow may be sluggish or altered by constriction of the vessels. The smooth muscles of the arterial walls respond to temperature by constricting in the presence of cold and extreme heat and relaxing in the presence of warmth. Therefore the nurse's care plan should include (1) providing a warm environment for the patient; (2) covering the hospitalized patient with warm blankets or dressing her in warm clothing; and (3) instructing the patient to avoid extremes of cold and heat.

The constricting effect of extreme heat rules out the use of local applications in the form of hot water bottles. In addition to the danger of burning the patient because of decreased sensitivity to extremes of temperature, local heat increases metabolic activity in the tissues to which it is applied and therefore upsets even more the balance of supply and demand for blood flow to all the tissues.

The goal in application of additional warmth is even distribution throughout the body.

 Think Critically

What would you recommend to the elderly home care patient to keep her lower extremities warm during the winter? The patient does not have the funds to keep the house heated above 68° F (20° C).

A second consideration is that of *pressure* against the walls of the blood vessels. Constricting clothing is avoided, particularly circular garters and elastic materials in underclothing. Frequent position changes are essential; position must be changed at least every 2 hours.

The patient with poor venous circulation can benefit from periodic elevation of the lower extremities to facilitate venous return of blood to the heart. Elevation above the level of the heart is preferred.

Even, well-distributed support of the vessels near the surface of the body will help improve venous return. To provide this kind of support, the physician may prescribe an elastic bandage or fitted elastic stockings. The stockings or elastic bandage should be applied early in the morning, before the legs are placed in a dependent position, because the blood vessels are less congested after a prolonged rest. Bandages and hose should be applied by beginning at the feet and working upward to avoid trapping blood in the lower leg. The patient should have two pairs of elastic hose and should wash the hose after each day's wearing. Elastic hose should be replaced every 6 months as they lose their elasticity. When stockings are removed, the heels should be checked for pressure areas. **Elastic stockings are not used for patients with arterial disorders.**

Exercise is especially beneficial to patients with decreased blood flow. Walking is ideal exercise for the ambulatory patient. Bedridden patients will need range-of-motion (ROM) exercises and the other kinds of muscular movements described in Chapter 9. Use of a treadmill for patients who cannot exercise by walking outside is very beneficial. An Exercycle is another alternative.

In addition to mechanical factors, certain chemical factors affect the constriction of blood vessels. *Nicotine*, which is inhaled with tobacco smoke, has the effect of producing spasmodic narrowing of the peripheral arteries. Patients with arterial insufficiency are encouraged to stop smoking. Used in conjunction with a community stop smoking support program, the booklet *You Can Quit Smoking*, available from the Agency for Health Care Research and Quality Publications Clearinghouse (540 Gaither Rd., Rockville, MD 20850), can be very helpful.

Alcohol is a mild vasodilator when taken in moderate amounts. Unless the patient has moral or religious convictions against its use, the physician may approve a daily intake of a specific, small amount of wine or liquor. It is important to find out whether alcohol will interfere with the action of medications being taken.

Health Promotion

Drink in Moderation

Promote proper use of alcohol for those who consume alcoholic beverages. Moderate alcohol intake for a man is two drinks in any one day. For a woman, the appropriate amount is one drink per day. One drink is 1½ ounces of alcohol, 4 ounces of wine, or 12 ounces of beer.

Drugs that are helpful to relieve vasoconstriction and improve blood flow are prescribed. These drugs are of value only when the arteries are still capable of dilating. Severely sclerosed vessels respond very poorly to therapy of this kind. Some think that vasodilators may actually be harmful because they shunt blood away from the zone of ischemia to well-perfused tissues.

IMPAIRED TISSUE INTEGRITY

Tissues that have a diminished blood supply are subject to severe and permanent damage from the slightest injury, because the normal processes of healing and repair are impaired. Arterial and venous stasis often lead to chronic leg ulcers.

These ulcers are particularly distressing to the patient because they heal very slowly and many never completely heal. Patients must be taught to avoid conditions that contribute to injury of the extremities and to report any injury, no matter how minor.

Prevention of leg ulcers includes (1) wearing elastic bandages or support hose; (2) proper positioning and exercise; (3) avoiding injury to the feet and legs; and (4) avoiding extremes of heat and cold and other mechanical and chemical factors that contribute to obstruction of blood flow. Information on care of the patient with a venous stasis ulcer is provided in Chapter 19.

Get Ready for the NCLEX® Examination!

Key Points

- Cardiovascular disease is the leading cause of death in the United States.
- The heart and vessels become stiffer with age and there is less cardiac reserve.
- Atherosclerosis and arteriosclerosis are major contributors to cardiovascular disease.
- Close to one third of the population in the United States has elevated blood pressure.
- Control of hypertension and obesity could lower the incidence of cardiovascular disease.
- Peripheral pulses should be compared bilaterally.

- Blood pressure should be taken—using correct technique—lying, sitting, and standing.
- Comprehensive nursing care plans should be holistic and may need to include problems secondary to the cardiovascular disease.
- Planning should include time management, as many heart medications need to be given as close to the prescribed time as possible to maintain a steady blood level of the drug.
- Collaboration with other health care team members assists in providing consistent, thorough care for the patient with a cardiovascular disorder.

- Evaluation involves checking blood levels of electrolytes, obtaining laboratory values for cardiac drugs to determine adequate dosing or toxicity, and monitoring blood counts for adequate red cells and hemoglobin to carry sufficient oxygen to the tissues of the body.
- Fatigue and dyspnea occur when the heart cannot pump sufficiently to carry adequate oxygen and nutrients to the tissues.
- Activity during cardiac rehabilitation is measured in metabolic equivalents; activity is started slowly and may progress according to the body's response.
- Heat therapy is applied cautiously to extremities of patients with peripheral vascular disease.
- When blood flow out of the heart is inhibited, there is a slowing of normal movement of body fluids and their excretion, causing edema.
- Daily weight change is the best indicator of fluid buildup.
- Watch patients who have fluid imbalances for accompanying electrolyte imbalances.
- Measures to reduce or prevent edema are often needed for the patient with peripheral vascular disease.
- Pain from an MI may be acute or described as discomfort.
- Nitroglycerin, morphine, aspirin, and oxygen are the drugs of choice for myocardial pain.
- Anginal pain is treated with nitroglycerin and other drugs to promote arterial vasodilation.
- Decreasing anxiety and promoting rest may decrease anginal pain.
- It is very important to encourage the patient with cardiovascular disease to quit smoking, as nicotine is a vasoconstrictor.
- Patients with peripheral vascular disease have difficulty healing lower leg and foot wounds.

Additional Learning Resources

SG   Go to your Study Guide for additional learning activities to help you master this chapter content.

evolve   Go to your Evolve website (http://evolve.elsevier.com/deWit/ medsurg) for the following FREE learning resources:
- Animations, audio, and video
- Answers and rationales for questions and activities
- Concept Map Creator
- Glossary with pronunciations in English and Spanish
- Interactive Review Questions and Exercises and more!

 Online Resources
- Cardiovascular assessment, www2.kumc.edu/instruction/ cardiologyphysical2.htm

Review Questions for the NCLEX® Examination

1. Which statement(s) regarding drug use and the risk of cardiac disease is/are true? *(Select all that apply.)*
   1. The vasodilation effects of cocaine hasten atherosclerosis.
   2. Sudden cardiac death is associated with cocaine use.
   3. Methamphetamine dilates blood vessels.
   4. Cigarette smoking contributes heavily to heart disease.
   5. Methamphetamine can cause myocardial infarction.

2. The ankle-brachial index test is ordered for a patient experiencing signs of peripheral vascular disease. Which patient statement indicates that further teaching about the test needs to occur?
   1. "I'll be lying down for this exam."
   2. "The test is noninvasive."
   3. "My brachial and pedal pulses will be checked and compared."
   4. "My brachial and ankle blood pressure will be taken."

3. Morphine 6 mg is ordered for a man admitted with chest pain and a probable myocardial infarction. On hand is morphine 10 mg/mL. The nurse should give _____ mL to the patient. *(Fill in the blank.)*

4. During initial assessment of an older adult, the nurse finds that the skin appears smooth, shiny, and thinned with little or no hair on the surface. Which nursing diagnosis should be on the care plan?
   1. Ineffective tissue perfusion
   2. Risk for infection
   3. Pain, related to decreased perfusion
   4. Deficient fluid volume

5. When taking care of a patient with cardiac disease, the nurse teaches the importance of preventing dysrhythmia. Which nursing intervention should be included in patient instructions?
   1. Use the feet and arms to push against the mattress when moving up in bed without assistance.
   2. Take stool softener to prevent straining at stool.
   3. Encourage coughing regularly to clear secretions.
   4. Lightly exercise and slowly increase activity.

6. The nurse weighs a patient with congestive heart failure and determines that there is a net weight gain of 3 pounds within the last 24 hours. Which nursing intervention should be carried out?
   1. Administer ordered diuretics.
   2. Restrict potassium intake.
   3. Monitor pulse oximetry.
   4. Administer potassium supplement.

7. The nurse administered two consecutive sublingual nitroglycerin tablets to a patient complaining of moderate chest pain. If the patient's blood pressure is 148/88 mm Hg with continued chest pain, the next nursing action would be to:
   1. administer morphine sulfate.
   2. get an IV cannula inserted.
   3. give another sublingual nitroglycerin.
   4. provide emotional support.

8. When interviewing a patient complaining of moderate chest pain, what question(s) should be asked? *(Select all that apply.)*

   1. Who witnessed the pain?
   2. What does the pain or discomfort feel like?
   3. What relaxation strategies were implemented?
   4. Where is the pain located?
   5. Where does the pain radiate?

9. The nurse assesses an 83-year-old and finds a diastolic murmur on auscultation of the heart. The priority action for the nurse should be to:

   1. stop the examination and call the physician.
   2. document the finding in the chart.
   3. inquire if other members of the family have a murmur.
   4. realize that such a murmur is normal in this age group.

10. The patient is receiving a drug that may cause postural hypotension. For safety, the nurse should instruct the patient to do what? *(Select all that apply.)*

    1. Increase fluid intake to prevent dehydration.
    2. Arise slowly from a lying to a sitting position.
    3. Sit on the side of the bed until not light-headed before standing.
    4. Stand holding onto the bed rail to stabilize before walking.
    5. Always ask for assistance when up and about.

Critical Thinking Activities

Scenario A

Debra Johnson, a 20-year-old African American college student on your campus, comes to the health center complaining of frequent headaches. The assessment data show that she is 5' 4" tall, weighs 149 lb, temp 98.8° F (37° C), P 82, RR 14, and BP 138/84 mm Hg. She smokes about half a pack of cigarettes a day. She has a heavy academic schedule and rarely exercises. She eats a lot of "food on the run" at the local fast-food places. Her mother and uncle both have hypertension.

1. Which of her data is abnormal for her age?

2. What risk factors does she have for cardiovascular disease?

3. Which risk factors are modifiable?

Scenario B

Akio Sukura, a 64-year-old man, comes into the emergency department after experiencing chest pain and diaphoresis. His ECG is abnormal. He is scheduled for a cardiac catheterization.

1. Is a permit required for this procedure? If so, would he be able to sign it?

2. What questions would you need to ask him when preparing him for this diagnostic test?

3. What would be the priorities of care related to this diagnostic test after the procedure is finished?

Scenario C

Jackson Smith, a construction worker, comes into the clinic. The physician suspects that he has chronic venous insufficiency.

1. What are the risk factors for this type of cardiovascular disease?

2. What diagnostic tests might be ordered for him?

3. Why would it be important to assess for signs of diabetes mellitus as well?

Care of Patients with Hypertension and Peripheral Vascular Disease

Objectives

Theory

1. Diagram the pathophysiology of hypertension.
2. Predict the complications that can occur as a consequence of hypertension.
3. Briefly describe the treatment program for mild, moderate, and severe hypertension.
4. Contrast the pathophysiology of arteriosclerosis with that of atherosclerosis.
5. Review four factors that contribute to peripheral vascular disease.
6. Recognize the signs, symptoms, and treatment of aneurysm.
7. Prepare a teaching plan for a patient with Raynaud's syndrome.
8. Compare the etiology and care for thrombophlebitis and deep vein thrombosis.
9. Summarize how venous insufficiency may lead to a venous stasis ulcer.

10. Compare venous stasis ulcer with arterial leg ulcer.
11. List types of surgery performed for problems of the peripheral vascular system.

Clinical Practice

1. Develop and implement a teaching plan for a patient who has hypertension.
2. Choose the points to be included in the teaching plan for the patient who has experienced thrombophlebitis.
3. Institute a teaching plan for the patient undergoing anticoagulant therapy.
4. Differentiate between venous and arterial insufficiency during a physical assessment.
5. Prepare a nursing care plan for the patient with arterial insufficiency.
6. Identify three likely nursing diagnoses for patients who have common problems of vascular disease and list the expected outcomes and appropriate nursing interventions for each.

Key Terms

bruit (BRŬ-ē, p. 413)
embolus (ĔM-bō-lŭs, p. 406)
gangrene (găng-GRĒN, p. 413)
hypertension (p. 398)
intermittent claudication (ĭn-tĕr-MĬT-ĕnt klăw-dĭ-KĂ-shŭn, p. 407)

rubor (RŪ-bŏr, p. 407)
scleropathy (sklĕr-ŎP-ă-thē, p. 420)
stent (p. 409)
thrombophlebitis (thrŏm-bō-flĕ-BĪ-tĭs, p. 406)
thrombus (THRŎM-bŭs, p. 409)
varicose veins (VĂR-ĭ-kōs vānz, p. 416)

HYPERTENSION

Hypertension is defined as persistently high blood pressure. This means a systolic pressure that is equal to or greater than 140 mm Hg and a diastolic pressure that is equal to or greater than 90 mm Hg when taken at least twice and averaged on two different occasions 2 weeks apart. The diastolic pressure is the main focus of treatment. It reflects the amount of pressure being exerted against the vessel walls while the heart is in its phase of relaxation and there is no added pressure from blood being forced out of the left ventricle and into the arteries. Table 19-1 presents ranges for the classification of hypertension.

Hypertensive individuals usually die of long-term damage to the end organs or target organs, that is, from damage to the brain, heart, and kidney. More than half

the deaths associated with persistent and unrelieved hypertension are caused by myocardial infarction. Immediate causes of death related to high blood pressure include cerebral hemorrhage and heart failure.

 Elder Care Points

Can you think of two physiologic reasons why the elderly are at greater risk for hypertension?

Etiology

The etiology of hypertension is unknown, but there are several contributing factors. Secretion of excess sodium-retaining hormones and vasoconstriction substances, high sodium intake, obesity, diabetes mellitus, excessive alcohol intake, and sympathetic nervous system activity all contribute to elevated blood pressure.

Table 19-1	Blood Pressure Classification			
CLASSIFICATION	**SYSTOLIC**	**DIASTOLIC**	**PATIENT ACTION**	
Normal	Less than 120	Less than 80	Monitor if risk factors are present.	
Prehypertension	120-139	or 80-89	Modify diet, increase exercise, lose weight, stop smoking.	
High Stage 1 Stage 2	 140-159 160 or higher	 or 90-99 or 100 or higher	 Antihypertensives and diuretics may be prescribed. Additional antihypertensive drug(s) may be prescribed. Continue lifestyle modifications.	

There are two major types of hypertension: primary (idiopathic or essential) and secondary hypertension. Persons with a family history of hypertension are at risk for developing primary hypertension. Approximately 90% to 95% of all cases of hypertension are primary.

In 5% to 8% the hypertension is secondary to another disorder. Acute stress, excessive alcohol intake, sickle cell disease, arteriosclerosis, coarctation of the aorta, eclampsia of pregnancy, renal disorders, endocrine disorders, and neurologic disorders are examples of secondary causes. Amphetamine use, chronic nonsteroidal anti-inflammatory drug (NSAID) use, and tyramine-containing foods such as beer and wine taken with monoamine oxidase (MAO) inhibitors contribute to secondary hypertension. Female hormone therapy and nicotine use appear to be contributing factors in some people. If the underlying disorder can be detected and treated successfully, the problem of secondary hypertension is eliminated or more easily controlled. If no underlying disease can be identified as elevating the patient's blood pressure, the patient is said to have primary hypertension.

Table 19-2 presents the nonmodifiable and modifiable risk factors for hypertension. Many times a loss of excess weight alone can return a slightly elevated blood pressure to normal. A moderate reduction of salt intake has been effective in lowering the blood pressure of some persons with mild or moderate hypertension. There is continuing research on the relationship of race, gender, and ethnicity on the incidence and effects of hypertension.

Table 19-2	Nonmodifiable and Modifiable Risk Factors for Primary Hypertension
Nonmodifiable Risk Factors	
Age	Systolic blood pressure (SBP) rises with age. After age 50 SBP >140 mm Hg is a cardiovascular risk factor.
Gender	Until age 55, hypertension is more prevalent in men; after age 55, it is more prevalent in women.
Ethnicity/race	Incidence is much higher in African Americans.
Family history	A close relative with hypertension increases a person's risk for developing it.
Modifiable Risk Factors	
Alcohol	Excessive alcohol intake is strongly associated with hypertension. Daily intake should be limited to 1 oz for those with hypertension.
Cigarette smoking	Nicotine contributes to arteriosclerosis and thereby to hypertension. People with hypertension who smoke are at greater risk of cardiovascular disease.
Diabetes	Diabetes accelerates atherosclerosis and leads to damage to the large vessels. Hypertension is twice as prevalent in diabetics as nondiabetics.
Obesity	Central body obesity in particular is associated with the development of hypertension. When combined with other factors in metabolic syndrome, the risk of hypertension is increased even more.
Stress	Stress increases peripheral vascular resistance and stimulates sympathetic nervous system activity. If stress responses become excessive, they can contribute to the development of hypertension.
Elevated serum lipids	Elevated cholesterol and triglycerides are risk factors for atherosclerosis. Atherosclerosis contributes to hypertension in many individuals.
Excess dietary sodium	High sodium intake contributes to hypertension in some patients.
Lower socioeconomic status	Hypertension is more prevalent among lower socioeconomic groups and among the less educated.

Hypertension and African Americans

African Americans tend to have a higher incidence of hypertension than do other minority groups and whites; African Americans also have higher noncompliance, complication, and mortality rates. Economic issues, access to health care, dietary practices, weight, and diabetes have been identified as possible reasons for the disparities (American Heart Association, 2011).

The rising incidence of childhood obesity has resulted in an increase in the incidence of hypertension. Health promotion activities targeting nutrition and exercise habits of children are increasing.

Pathophysiology

Blood pressure equals the amount of blood pumped out of the heart multiplied by the systemic vascular resistance. If the diameter of blood vessels becomes smaller because of atherosclerosis or vasoconstriction, blood pressure increases in an effort to force the blood through the smaller opening. If there is an increase in the volume (amount) or viscosity (thickness or consistency) of fluid in the blood vessels, the pressure within the vessels increases and the heart must work harder to pump the fluid through the vessels. A pathologic response to stress can result in an elevation in blood pressure by stimulating the sympathetic nervous system and causing peripheral vasoconstriction and increased heart rate.

Insulin, glucose, and lipoprotein abnormalities are common in primary hypertension. High blood insulin concentration stimulates sympathetic nervous system activity contributing to vasoconstriction.

In some instances of hypertension, an excess of renin is secreted by the kidneys. Renin acts on a substance called *angiotensinogen,* converting it to angiotensin I. Angiotensin I is converted to angiotensin II by angiotensin-converting enzyme (ACE). Angiotensin II acts directly on the blood vessels, causing them to constrict, and stimulates the adrenal gland to release aldosterone. Angiotensin thereby increases resistance to blood flow in the peripheral vessels and causes retention of sodium and water by the renal tubules through the influence of aldosterone (see Figure 18-6). The retained sodium and water increase the blood volume, causing increased cardiac output and elevation of blood pressure. Concept Map 19-1 shows the pathophysiology of hypertension.

Elder Care Points

The stiffening of arteries occurring with arteriosclerosis is a natural part of aging. The baroreceptors that normally help adjust blood pressure become less sensitive with age. The lack of elasticity of the vessels and the decreased sensitivity of the baroreceptors cause the elderly to be at risk for orthostatic (postural) hypotension when changing position. An elevation of systolic pressure above normal should be treated in this age group.

Signs, Symptoms, and Diagnosis

Hypertension has been called the "silent killer" because in early stages it does not usually cause discomfort or any other subjective signs and symptoms to indicate its presence. About one third of those who have hypertension are not aware of it. Signs may appear only in the later stages when damage has been done to the target

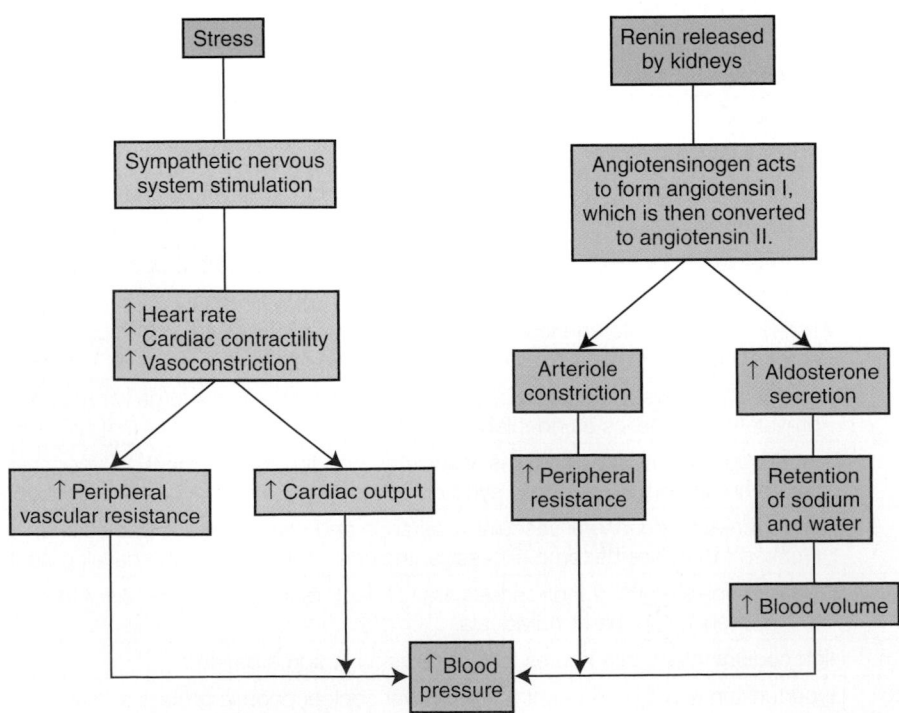

CONCEPT MAP 19-1 Pathophysiology of hypertension.

organs—that is, the kidney (renal ischemia and nephrosclerosis), brain (arteriosclerosis and microaneurysms), aorta (aortic aneurysm), eyes (retinal damage), and heart (left ventricular hypertrophy and reduced cardiac output). **Patients with symptoms may complain of headache, dizziness, blurred vision, blackouts, irritability, angina, dyspnea, or fatigue.**

Hypertensive patients develop coronary heart disease at a rate two to three times greater than that of persons with normal blood pressure. Examination of the blood vessels of the retina will reveal any damage to the retinal vessels. This retinal assessment gives an indication about how much damage the high blood pressure has done to vessels throughout the body. If retinal damage has occurred, it is an indication that the person's hypertension is moderate to severe.

Diagnosis is by blood pressure readings on at least two occasions 2 weeks apart. An electrocardiogram (ECG) and cardiac stress test may be ordered to determine whether any damage has been done to the coronary arteries or to the heart muscle.

Treatment

The goals of treatment are (1) reduction of high blood pressure and (2) long-term control to decrease the risk of stroke, heart attack, loss of vision, and kidney disease. The target is to control blood pressure at or below 120/80 mm Hg. Treatment is individualized, using a stepped-care approach. For mild hypertension, smoking cessation, weight reduction, sodium restriction, alcohol restriction, exercise, a low-fat diet, and stress control are instituted. Sodium should be kept to less than 2400 mg/day with the DASH (Dietary Approaches to Stop Hypertension) eating plan. Alcohol intake should not exceed one serving of liquor, wine, or beer for women per day or two servings for men per day. Aerobic exercise of 30 to 45 minutes most days of the week is recommended. If blood pressure is still high, a diuretic is added. If the blood pressure does not fall within normal limits, the second step is initiated, and an antihypertensive drug is prescribed.

Other drugs are added, if needed, to keep the blood pressure consistently within normal limits. Patients with more severe hypertension often require more than two drugs to attain control. The third step is to add additional drugs. The dose of each drug is increased as needed to achieve the desired blood pressure level unless side effects occur. In the event of side effects, another drug is substituted. Newer blood pressure medications are very expensive, and cost is a concern for many patients. Some drug companies have programs to help patients who cannot afford their medications. If a potassium-wasting diuretic is prescribed, the patient is taught to increase the potassium intake. A potassium supplement is added to treatment, and electrolyte levels are monitored regularly.

Patients should monitor their blood pressure at home and keep records of the readings. Periodic visits to the physician's office for regular examinations are necessary. The better the blood pressure is controlled and kept within normal limits, the less damage there will be to the target organs.

Antihypertensive Therapy. The drugs prescribed to reduce blood pressure work by decreasing blood volume, cardiac output, or peripheral resistance. Table 19-3 and Box 19-1 list examples of the drugs most commonly prescribed for hypertension and relevant nursing interventions.

The blood pressure of the elderly patient who is taking antihypertensive medication should be measured when the patient is sitting and when standing. Many of these medications can cause orthostatic hypotension; measuring blood pressure with the patient standing will reveal whether the medication is reducing the blood pressure too much. Assess patients receiving antihypertensives for dizziness, confusion, syncope, restlessness, and drowsiness, which may indicate hypotension.

 Patient Teaching

Safety Measures to Prevent Falls for Patients with Orthostatic Hypotension

Teach the patient who experiences the side effect of orthostatic hypotension from medication to:

- Rise slowly from a lying to a sitting position; do not hold your breath as you arise. Sit for 1 minute before standing; stand slowly holding on to a stable object. Stand for 1 minute before walking.
- While seated, flex and rotate the feet several times before attempting to stand; have feet firmly planted on the floor before standing.
- When walking, do not turn your head or body abruptly.
- When feeling unsteady while standing, call for assistance before walking.
- Report light-headedness or sudden dizziness.
- Use the bathroom before meals and try to avoid getting up for 30 to 60 minutes after meals.

Complications

Malignant hypertension is a term describing rapidly progressive moderate to severe hypertension that is difficult to control. Diastolic pressure ranges from 140 to 170 mm Hg, and unless effective intervention is found, the patient may suffer eye, heart, kidney, and brain damage.

Hypertensive Crisis

Hypertensive emergency is a life-threatening situation in which the blood pressure rises higher than 180/120 mm Hg and there is indication of target organ damage. Symptoms may include severe headache, blurred vision, seizures, nausea, and change in level of

💊 **Table 19-3** **Drug Classifications Used for Patients with Vascular Disorders**

TYPE OF DRUG	ACTION
Diuretics	
Thiazides and Related Drugs Hydrochlorothiazide (Esidrix, HydroDIURIL, Dyazide) Metolazone (Zaroxolyn) Indapamide (Lozol)	These drugs increase the excretion of water, sodium, potassium, and chloride by blocking the reabsorption of sodium and chloride.
Loop Diuretics Bumetanide (Bumex) Furosemide (Lasix) Torsemide (Demadex)	These drugs work in the loop of Henle to block reabsorption of sodium and chloride. This prevents passive reabsorption of water and promotes its excretion. These drugs produce the greatest amount of diuresis.
Potassium-Sparing Diuretics Spironolactone (Aldactone) Triamterene (Dyrenium)	These drugs block the action of aldosterone in the distal nephron. This prevents the promotion of sodium uptake in exchange for potassium secretion usually caused by aldosterone, and potassium is "spared" (not secreted) and sodium is excreted. These drugs cause very little diuresis.
Antihypertensives	
Adrenergic Inhibitors *Beta Blockers* Atenolol (Tenormin) Propranolol (Inderal) Metoprolol (Lopressor, Toprol XL) Timolol (Apo-Timol) Bisoprolol (Zebeta) Carvedilol (Coreg)	It is not certain how these drugs work to reduce blood pressure. Blockade of the beta$_1$ receptors lowers cardiac output by decreasing heart rate and contractility. Action on the beta$_1$ receptors in the kidney decreases the release of renin, which is a factor in rising blood pressure.
Alpha Blockers Doxazosin (Cardura) Prazosin (Minipress) Terazosin (Hytrin)	These drugs block alpha$_1$ stimulation on arterioles and veins, preventing sympathetic vasoconstriction. This action results in vasodilation, reducing peripheral vascular resistance and venous return to the heart.
Alpha-Beta Blocker Labetalol (Normodyne, Trandate)	This drug blocks both alpha$_1$ and beta$_1$ receptors, producing decreased heart rate, contractility, peripheral vascular resistance, and venous return.
Angiotensin-Converting Enzyme (ACE) Inhibitors Benazepril (Lotensin) Captopril (Capoten) Enalapril (Vasotec) Fosinopril (Monopril) Lisinopril (Prinivil) Quinapril (Accupril)	These agents lower blood pressure by inhibiting the conversion of angiotensin I into angiotensin II, thereby preventing vasoconstriction. They also restrict volume expansion mediated by aldosterone.
Calcium Channel Blockers Diltiazem (Cardizem) Nicardipine (Cardene) Nifedipine (Procardia) Verapamil (Calan, Isoptin)	These drugs reduce blood pressure by causing dilation of arterioles. Calcium channels are blocked, preventing the influx of calcium that promotes contraction.
Central-Acting Agents Clonidine (Catapres) Guanabenz (Wytensin) Methyldopa (Aldomet)	These agents act within the brainstem to suppress sympathetic impulses to the heart and blood vessels. This action decreases the release of norepinephrine by sympathetic nerves, reducing activation of peripheral adrenergic receptors, and promotes vasodilation. The agents also decrease heart rate and cardiac output.
Peripherally Acting Adrenergic Blockers Guanethidine (Ismelin) Reserpine (Serpaline)	These agents reduce blood pressure by blocking adrenergic receptors in the postganglionic sympathetic neurons and causing decreased sympathetic stimulation of the heart and blood vessels.
Direct-Acting Vasodilators Hydralazine (Apresoline) Minoxidil (Loniten)	These agents reduce blood pressure by promoting arteriole vasodilation.
Direct Renin Inhibitors Aliskiren (Tekturna)	This new class of drugs inhibits renin secretion from the kidney, reducing angiotensin I and angiotensin II, inhibiting vasoconstriction.

Box 19-1   General Nursing Interventions for the Administration of Diuretics and Antihypertensive Drugs

DIURETICS

- Follow the "Five Rights" and "five rules" of medication administration to prevent errors and injury to the patient: *right* patient, *right* drug, *right* dose, *right* route, *right* time; instruct the patient, take a drug history, assess for drug allergies, check for possible interactions, and document after administration.
- Check for sulfa allergy. Thiazide and thiazide-like diuretics are related to sulfonamides. Patients allergic to sulfas may have adverse reactions.
- Monitor intake and output to determine amount of diuresis and the drug's effectiveness.
- Track the patient's weight daily to determine the drug's effectiveness; evaluate for decreased edema.
- Check all drugs the patient is receiving for drug interactions with the diuretic drug to prevent toxicity or lack of absorption. Several diuretics are ototoxic, and this adverse effect may be potentiated by other ototoxic drugs.
- If possible, administer diuretic dose in the morning, and if a second dose is required, give it mid-afternoon to avoid sleep interference by need to urinate.
- Provide assistance with urination in a timely manner (answer call bell quickly).
- Assess for signs of dehydration and hypotension; take blood pressure on a set schedule. The elderly are prone to excessive diuresis and can quickly become dehydrated.
- Monitor diabetic patients for increased blood glucose levels when taking loop or thiazide diuretics, as these drugs may cause hyperglycemia.

Regarding possible side effects or adverse effects of the drug, the nurse should:

- Monitor potassium levels frequently if the patient is taking a potassium-wasting diuretic; assess for signs of hypokalemia: weakness, tremor, muscle cramps, change in mental status, cardiac dysrhythmia.
- If the patient also is taking digoxin, consult the physician before administering the dose if the potassium level is below 3.5 mEq/L or if the patient exhibits signs of hypokalemia, as hypokalemia increases risk of fatal cardiac dysrhythmia in patients taking digoxin.
- If a patient is taking a potassium-sparing diuretic and potassium level is above 5 mEq/L, or if signs of hyperkalemia develop (abnormal cardiac rhythm), consult the physician before administering the dose.
- Monitor blood pressure. If blood pressure drops considerably, speak with physician before giving another dose of the drug.
- Monitor the patient for signs of constipation, as diuresis may cause this problem.
- Monitor patients with a history of deep venous thrombosis (DVT) for recurrence, as diuretics reduce circulating fluid volume.
- Monitor the patient for side effects or adverse effects of the particular drug taken. The most common general side effects are constipation, electrolyte disturbance, gastric upset, and hypotension. Adverse effects are dehydration, ototoxicity, hyperglycemia, and hyperuricemia.
- Monitor the patient for signs of allergic reaction, such as rash or itching.

Teach the patient taking a diuretic to:

- Expect frequent need to urinate, and an increased volume of urine.
- Report any new heartbeat irregularity.
- Report any signs of ringing of the ears, roaring sounds, a feeling of fullness in the ears, or decreased hearing.
- Eat foods high in potassium, such as bananas, orange juice, cereals, meats, tomatoes, potatoes, and raisins, daily, unless taking a potassium-sparing diuretic.
- If taking a potassium-sparing diuretic, restrict foods high in potassium.
- Take potassium supplement regularly if one is prescribed.
- Increase fiber in the diet if prone to constipation; consult physician if constipation occurs. The elderly patient who is inactive is more prone to constipation.
- Watch for signs of postural hypotension, such as dizziness or light-headedness, when changing position. Encourage patient to arise slowly from a supine position and to sit a minute before standing. (The elderly are particularly prone to this side effect.)
- Avoid the sun or take precautions; do not use a sunlamp when taking a loop or thiazide diuretic, as the medication may cause photosensitivity.
- Watch for signs of gout (tenderness or swelling of joints) when taking a loop or thiazide diuretic and notify the physician if these occur. Loop diuretics may cause an increase in uric acid levels.
- When taking spironolactone, menstrual irregularities or impotence may occur; report these occurrences to the physician.

ANTIHYPERTENSIVE DRUGS

- Establish that the patient is not hypotensive before giving a dose of an antihypertensive drug. If the patient's blood pressure is below normal levels, consult the physician before giving the dose.
- Monitor the heart rate for bradycardia or tachycardia. Follow specific parameters for administration of the specific drug; some drugs may cause bradycardia, others may cause tachycardia.
- Follow the "Five Rights" and "five rules" of medication administration, and check the patient's ID by two methods before *each* dose.
- Inquire about any dizziness. If dizziness has been occurring, measure blood pressure standing and sitting to determine whether the patient is experiencing orthostatic hypotension; several antihypertensives may cause orthostatic hypotension.
- Note contraindications and precautions for each specific drug the patient is taking. Angiotensin-converting enzyme (ACE) inhibitors are contraindicated during pregnancy.
- Check all drugs the patient is receiving for drug interactions to prevent toxicity or increased severity of side effects. Many of the antihypertensive drugs have a depressant effect on the heart.
- Monitor blood pressure readings to evaluate effectiveness of the drug.

Continued

Box 19-1 | General Nursing Interventions for the Administration of Diuretics and Antihypertensive Drugs—cont'd

ANTIHYPERTENSIVE DRUGS—cont'd

Regarding possible side effects or adverse effects of the drug, the nurse should:

- Monitor the patient for the side effects of each drug administered.
- Monitor serum glucose levels in patients with diabetes who are taking a beta-blocker drug, as the drug may mask hypoglycemia.
- Monitor lipid levels for changes in patients taking beta-blockers, as these drugs interfere with lipid metabolism.
- Observe for hypersensitivity reactions such as rash; ACE inhibitors may cause hypersensitivity.
- Monitor patients for signs of congestive heart failure, such as edema; beta blockers, calcium channel blockers, and other drugs that decrease cardiac output may precipitate heart failure in patients with borderline cardiac function.
- Check the skin of the patient using a clonidine patch for signs of irritation, a potential side effect of the patch. Be certain the old patch is removed when applying a new one.
- Give the first dose of an ACE inhibitor at bedtime, as it often causes hypotension.
- Monitor the potassium level of the patient taking an ACE inhibitor. Because it suppresses the release of aldosterone, it increases potassium retention.
- Monitor liver function tests for patients taking centrally acting drugs, such as clonidine, as these drugs may cause liver damage in some patients.
- Monitor renal function tests in patients taking hydralazine, as this drug may cause renal impairment.

Teach the patient taking an antihypertensive to:
- Monitor blood pressure regularly and record the readings.
- Alter lifestyle factors that contribute to hypertension, such as smoking, excess weight, excessive stress, excessive alcohol ingestion, high-salt diet, and lack of exercise.
- Rise slowly from a lying position and stabilize before standing for a couple of minutes.
- Report alteration in sexual response, as some of the antihypertensive drugs may cause impotence.
- Report persistent side effects and any adverse effects of the drug.
- Monitor for weight gain from retention of sodium and water by weighing at least twice a week; report weight gain of more than 2 lb to the physician.
- Report signs of ankle edema, as several of the antihypertensive drugs can precipitate congestive heart failure.
- Be aware that methyldopa may cause dark urine for the first few weeks of therapy.
- Avoid abruptly discontinuing centrally acting antihypertensives, such as clonidine, as rebound hypertension may occur.
- Check with the physician before taking over-the-counter drugs, as many are contraindicated in hypertension.
- Comply with medication therapy even when blood pressure is normal, as long-term compliance is the key to preventing the organ damage that hypertension can cause.
- Set own goals for lifestyle changes and medication therapy; a patient-directed program has a better chance of success.

consciousness. It may occur if a patient has stopped taking antihypertensive medication, or it may be secondary to another disease process such as renal stenosis. The patient is placed in the intensive care unit and treated with intravenous (IV) emergency drugs, such as IV sodium nitroprusside (Nipride), nicardipine (Cardene IV), fenoldopam (Corlopam), or labetalol (Normodyne), to lower the blood pressure. A reduction in blood pressure to 160/100 mm Hg is desired over the first 2 hours. Blood pressure is monitored every 5 to 15 minutes. Medication is adjusted to reduce the pressure slowly to prevent renal, cerebral, or coronary ischemia. *Hypertensive urgency* occurs when the blood pressure rises to 180/120 mm Hg but there are no signs or symptoms of target organ damage. This is the more common occurrence. The patient is observed in the emergency department and treated with oral medication. The patient is directed to follow up with the primary care physician.

❖ NURSING MANAGEMENT

■ Assessment (Data Collection)

The patient should be assessed for indications of modifiable and nonmodifiable risk factors for cardiovascular disease. Physical assessment of the cardiac system should be performed. Assessment of blood pressure and documentation of levels and potential influences on values is an important aspect of nursing care. The patient's blood pressure should be taken sitting, lying supine, and standing for a thorough assessment. Standing blood pressure measurements also are important when a patient is started on a new medication, particularly an ACE inhibitor, because orthostatic hypotension may occur.

 Elder Care Points

The blood pressure of the elderly patient will be lower immediately after a meal. For accurate readings, assess blood pressure between meals.

■ Nursing Diagnosis and Planning

Common nursing diagnoses for a patient with hypertension include:
- Risk for injury related to complications of hypertension
- Deficient knowledge (disease process, medications) related to new diagnosis of hypertension
- Imbalanced nutrition: more than body requirements, related to obesity, high-fat diet, or high sodium intake
- Anxiety related to potential complications of disease process

Expected outcomes for a patient with hypertension may include:

- The patient will not experience retinopathy.
- The patient's blood pressure will return to normal limits.
- The patient will verbalize an understanding of teaching related to medications and disease process.
- The patient will lose 10% of body weight in a designated period.
- The patient will be able to choose low-fat and low-sodium items from a variety of menus.

■ Implementation

Nursing interventions consist of assisting the patient to make necessary lifestyle changes that will help control the blood pressure and slow further atherosclerosis. Diet changes are often the most difficult for the patient. It is best to work with the patient's current dietary likes and dislikes, modifying methods of food preparation to decrease sodium and fat content.

Sources of hidden sodium should be learned, and the patient should be taught how to read food labels.

 Nutrition Considerations

Decreasing Sodium in the Diet

For the patient who must reduce sodium in the diet, instruct to:

- Avoid "convenience" foods: ready-mixed sauces, frozen dinners, cured or smoked meats (including lunch meats), canned soups, and prepared salad dressings, unless the label truly indicates low sodium content.
- Be aware that regular canned vegetables often contain a large amount of sodium; in some instances rinsing will greatly decrease the sodium content. Use fresh or frozen vegetables or those canned without sodium when possible.
- Check soft drink labels for sodium content; avoid those that contain more than 140 mg of sodium.
- Check cereal box labels for sodium content; switch to a lower sodium cereal, such as shredded wheat.
- Use one fourth to one half the amount of salt that a recipe calls for.
- Avoid adding salt to food after cooking.
- Make a salt substitute seasoning of ½ tsp garlic powder, mixed with 1 tsp each of basil, black pepper, marjoram, onion powder, parsley, sage, savory, and thyme; or use a product such as Mrs. Dash or lemon pepper instead of salt.
- When ordering at restaurants, ask which dishes are low in sodium; or ask that the cook refrain from adding salt to your meal.
- Ask fast food restaurants to supply you with a list of their available foods showing sodium content of each item.
- Do not eat preserved or commercially prepared smoked meats, such as bacon, hot dogs, salami, pastrami, ham, smoked turkey, or sausage.
- Read all labels on food containers looking for the words *salt* and *sodium,* and the letters *NaCl.*
- Check condiments for amount of sodium. Catsup, soy sauce, steak sauce, and others are high in sodium.

⊕ **Cultural Considerations**

Cultural Diet Variations

Working with patients from diverse cultures who have very different diets is a challenge. Encouraging fat and sodium restriction in the cultural diet requires working with the patient to discover food preferences and food preparation patterns inherent in the family.

Patients who need to increase potassium intake are taught to include citrus fruits and juices, beef and turkey, tomatoes, and potatoes in the diet. The person who does the shopping and food preparation must be included in the diet instruction process. **Weight loss is the most important lifestyle change in obese clients.** The goal is a weight that is within 15% of ideal body weight.

If caffeine restriction is recommended, teach the patient to gradually decrease his caffeine consumption so that he will not experience withdrawal symptoms, such as headache and nervousness. Remind the patient that many types of soft drinks, as well as coffee, tea, and chocolate, contain caffeine. Some of these beverages are available in decaffeinated formulas. Because it produces vasoconstriction, nicotine has a major impact on blood vessels and blood pressure. Stopping smoking can be a difficult task for many patients. Core Measures call for counseling and an information packet on smoking cessation to be given to the patient. An exercise program that fits the patient's personality, ability, and preference should be designed. Walking to work from a parking lot a few blocks away, climbing stairs instead of using elevators, and a daily walk in the neighborhood often are sufficient. Other patients might prefer to use a stationary bicycle or treadmill. The object is to work on something that the patient will continue to do for the rest of his life.

Weight loss will begin to occur if the patient is faithful to the prescribed diet and exercise program. As his weight decreases, remind the patient of the direct effect these efforts have had on the blood pressure. Even a moderate weight loss of 7 to 12 lb (3 to 5 kg) can reduce blood pressure. Positive reinforcement should be given for even small amounts of weight loss.

Stress reduction requires an evaluation of lifestyle. Meditation, yoga, leisure activities, or just saying no to extra obligations can all decrease stress. Help the patient determine where his stressors are and what can practically be done to manage them. Lifetime compliance with diet, exercise, stress reduction, and medication plans is difficult for most patients. Alternative therapy may help.

 Complementary and Alternative Therapies

Grapeseed Extract for Hypertension

Grapeseed extract is an alternative medicine treatment for hypertension that also helps decrease cholesterol.

Many do not understand or accept that it is up to them to control their disease. They do well for several months or a few years, but then, because they feel well (while their blood pressure has been controlled), they stop taking their medication and gradually return to previous lifestyle patterns. By teaching them what high blood pressure does to the blood vessels and the heart, brain, eyes, and kidneys, you can do much to encourage patients to follow the treatment plan for life. Each patient needs continuing praise for maintaining blood pressure control.

Patient Teaching

Complications of Uncontrolled Hypertension

The following information should be included in the teaching plan of the patient at risk for noncompliance with treatment of hypertension:

- Hypertension can cause damage to arteries, making them less elastic. This places an increased workload on the heart. This may cause myocardial infarction, left ventricular hypertrophy, and congestive heart failure.
- Small vessel damage to the brain disrupts circulation and may lead to transient ischemic attacks (TIAs) and stroke.
- Hypertension may cause damage to the small vessels of the kidney and may lead to kidney failure.
- Hypertension damages the arteries of the eye, causing the formation of clots or occurrence of hemorrhage that may lead to blurred vision or blindness.

There are many resources to help hypertensive patients manage their illness more effectively. The American Heart Association, Heart Center Online, the National Institutes of Health, and many others offer educational materials for patients with hypertension. *Healthy People 2020* goals and objectives have been written for hypertension.

Health Promotion

Assessment for and Management of Hypertension

Blood pressure should be assessed every time there is contact with a health care provider. All adults should have their blood pressure assessed at least once a year, even if it has always been within normal limits. The patient with hypertension requires intense teaching to assist in achieving health management goals. Blood pressure should be monitored regularly at home with an arm-type monitor. Ensure that the patient understands the needed lifestyle changes and how to accomplish behavior modification. The patient may be referred to a local support group as a resource in the management of his health.

▪ Evaluation

Consistent maintenance of blood pressure within prescribed limits is a primary indicator of effectiveness of disease management. Evaluate the patient's knowledge of prescribed medications, including use, side effects, and administration. Knowledge of dietary management, exercise activities, stress management, and smoking cessation should be discussed at follow-up sessions. The patient's compliance with the management of hypertension is critical to preventing or minimizing complications of the disease process.

ARTERIOSCLEROSIS AND ATHEROSCLEROSIS

Arteriosclerosis (hardening of the arteries) is a general term for a variety of arterial changes. Arteriosclerosis occurs with aging as degenerative changes occur in the small arteries and arterioles. The disorder is characterized by thickening of the artery walls that progresses to hardening as calcium deposits form. Vessel elasticity is lost. The thickening and calcification reduce the diameter of the vessels and cause slowing of blood flow. This may lead to ischemia and necrosis in various tissues. *Atherosclerosis* is another form of artery narrowing. Lipids are deposited along the vessel walls and combine with cells, fibrin, and cell debris to form plaques. The plaque grows and extends into the lumen of the artery where inflammation or erosion causes the plaque to be exposed to the blood. This triggers clotting and subsequent blocking of the vessel by a clot. Atheromatous plaque with thrombi form primarily in the larger arteries and the carotid arteries. Diabetes mellitus, particularly when uncontrolled, speeds the development of arteriosclerosis and atherosclerosis. Hypertension is a major factor in arteriosclerosis.

PERIPHERAL VASCULAR DISEASE

Peripheral vascular disease involves narrowing or obstruction of peripheral blood vessels, and loss of function. These vessels may be in the arms, neck, abdomen, or lower extremities (Figure 19-1). Diabetes, particularly when uncontrolled, contributes to vascular disease.

Other causes of problems include spasm of the smooth muscles in the arterial walls (e.g., Raynaud's disease), structural defects in the arteries (aneurysms), trauma, or embolus (blood clot or debris that travels and lodges in a blood vessel) that causes occlusion. Peripheral venous problems are caused by defective valvular function and formation of *venous thrombosis* (blood clots), which may be accompanied by thrombophlebitis (inflammation of a vein).

Prevention of peripheral vascular disease is focused on decreasing atherosclerosis and arteriosclerosis, controlling diabetes mellitus, controlling hypertension, and preventing smoking. Smoking cessation is important because nicotine causes vasoconstriction resulting in elevation of blood pressure and decreased blood flow through the vessels.

FIGURE 19-1 Diagram of the peripheral vascular system. Veins and arteries of the lower extremities.

PERIPHERAL ARTERIAL DISEASE (ARTERIAL INSUFFICIENCY)

Etiology and Pathophysiology

The most common etiology of peripheral arterial disease (PAD) is atherosclerosis. The vessel walls become narrowed or the lumen obstructed, leading to loss of blood flow to the extremity. Restriction or cessation of blood flow in the arteries leads to ischemia and tissue death (necrosis). Arterial ulcers may result. PAD may be acute or chronic. Embolism is the most common etiology of acute interruption of arterial blood flow. PAD may occur in any peripheral artery, and often occurs in the carotid arteries.

Signs, Symptoms, and Diagnosis

Obtain a complete history and physical examination of the patient. Table 19-4 summarizes the signs and symptoms of arterial disorders. Signs and symptoms of PAD of the lower extremities include intermittent claudication (pain when walking that diminishes at rest), pain at rest, tightening pressure in calves or buttocks, and ischemic changes. Blood pressure in the extremity affected by PAD is lower.

Patients with PAD have pallor in the affected extremity when the leg is elevated and rubor (dark redness) when the leg is dependent. The skin may appear tight and shiny. Hair is usually absent on the affected extremity and the toenails are thickened. Pulses are diminished or absent. There also is a temperature change distal to the occlusion. Wounds on the lower leg are difficult to heal. The severity of these symptoms depends on the extent of the lesion, degree of occlusion, and amount of collateral circulation that has been established.

If severe ischemia occurs from occlusion of arterial blood flow, tissue distal to the occlusion blanches, becomes cold, hurts, and eventually becomes numb as necrosis occurs. Ischemic areas of the lower leg and foot may develop skin breakdown without injury. *Arterial ulcers* with a sharp edge and a pale base may form that are quite painful. These ulcers are very slow

Table 19-4 Differences in Signs and Symptoms of Arterial and Venous Disease

CHARACTERISTIC	ARTERIAL DISEASE	VENOUS DISEASE
Pulses	Diminished, weak, or absent	Strong and symmetrical; may be difficult to palpate if edema is present
Skin	Pallor, dependent rubor; thin, dry, shiny, cool	Mottling with brown pigmentation at ankles, veins may be visible; legs or feet bluish when dependent; dermatitis; warm at ankle
Edema	Absent or mild	Present, particularly around ankle and in foot
Ulceration	On toes or at pressure points on feet	At bones of ankle
Necrosis and gangrene	Likely	Unlikely
Pain	Intermittent claudication when walking; sharp, stabbing, gnawing; lessens when at rest	Aching, cramping, particularly when dependent; may have nocturnal cramps
Nails	Thick, brittle (normal in elderly)	Normal
Hair	Hair loss distal to area of occlusion (hair loss normal in elderly)	Normal

FIGURE 19-2 Patient with PAD. Arterial ulcers of the lateral malleolus and distal and lateral portion of the leg. Note round, smooth shape.

FIGURE 19-4 Patient with gangrene of toes.

FIGURE 19-3 Patient with cellulitis of the legs.

and difficult to heal (Figure 19-2). This is particularly true for diabetic patients. The affected part may develop cellulitis, edema, and become gangrenous, necessitating amputation (Figures 19-3 and 19-4). The toes and foot are most often affected.

An arterial thrombosis can occur as a vessel is narrowed by atherosclerosis. Atherosclerotic plaque ruptures, platelets aggregate at the roughened area, and a clot forms. If the clot breaks loose and travels it becomes an arterial embolus and may cause acute occlusion of an artery. An embolus more commonly is caused by a thrombus formed in the heart by atrial fibrillation. **Signs and symptoms of embolus occlusion of an extremity artery are the six *P*s: pain, pulselessness, poikilothermia (coldness), pallor, paresthesias, and paralysis.**

 Elder Care Points

Hair loss is a natural occurrence with aging, as is thickening of fingernails and toenails. These signs alone are not reliable indicators of vascular problems on the extremities in the elderly.

Diagnosis of PAD is made using the ankle-brachial index (ABI). The normal value is 1 (i.e., the systolic pressure is the same at the ankle and brachial artery sites). Radiographic and ultrasound procedures also may be performed.

Treatment

The best treatment for arterial occlusive disease is regular exercise. Walking vigorously for 20 minutes twice a day will encourage growth of collateral circulation and reduce the severity of claudication in the majority of patients. The exercise program is started slowly, working up to a faster pace and the full 20 minutes (Karthikeyan & Eikelboom, 2009). Some dietary supplements have proven helpful in increasing circulation.

 Complementary and Alternative Therapies

L-Carnitine

Several research studies have shown that L-carnitine, a natural substance found in muscle, heart, brain, and nerve cells, may be beneficial in improving the exercise capacity of individuals with peripheral artery disease. L-Carnitine, especially in the form of proprinylcarnitine, improves muscle recovery following exercise. L-Carnitine can be found in many foods, with higher concentrations in red meat and dairy products. It is supplied as a dietary supplement in 50- to 500-mg tablets. Recommended dosage for individuals with PAD is 600 to 1200 mg three times per day or 750 mg twice daily. Side effects are few; however, these dosages in the upper range may cause diarrhea, hyperactivity, and insomnia.

Areas of ulceration are kept clean and free from pressure. Bed rest may be prescribed. Dry eschar is left in place. Debridement is performed only by a qualified health professional. Moist dressings are used on the clean and granulating ulcer to promote healing. The goal of treatment of PAD is directed toward increasing blood flow through the peripheral arteries and decreasing the risk of clot formation in the vessels. Antiplatelet agents and platelet inhibitors may be used alone or in combination with other drugs. Aspirin is the most commonly used antiplatelet agent. It prevents the aggregation of platelets in the arteries. Platelet inhibitors, such as clopidogrel (Plavix), may be prescribed. Patients experiencing intermittent claudication may achieve relief of symptoms when prescribed pentoxifylline (Trental) or cilostazol (Pletal). These drugs increase blood flow by inhibiting clot formation in the vessel. Patients experiencing acute ischemia may receive thrombolytic therapy. Urokinase, alteplase (t-PA, Activase), and tenecteplase (TNKase) are the drugs of choice for thrombolysis. Cholesterol-lowering drugs (e.g., atorvastatin [Lipitor], simvastatin [Zocor], ezetimibe [Zetia]) have been shown to be effective by decreasing low-density lipoprotein (LDL) and increasing high-density lipoprotein (HDL) levels, thus reducing plaque deposits in the arteries.

 Clinical Cues

Medications to treat PAD or thrombosis may cause serious adverse reactions. The major adverse reaction is bleeding. Observe the patient for and report immediately evidence of excessive bruising or bleeding, prolonged clotting after a needle stick, hematuria, changes in vital signs, or changes in neurologic signs.

Percutaneous transluminal angioplasty (PTA) may be done to open an occluded artery. A catheter is introduced into the artery, and when the proper spot is reached, a balloon is inflated multiple times to dilate the vessel, promoting better blood flow. A metal or mesh **stent** (tubular device to give support to a vessel interior) may be placed to prevent narrowing or closure of the artery (see Chapter 21 for a similar stent illustration).

Laser angioplasty is now used more commonly to open clogged arteries. This procedure is done in a fashion similar to percutaneous balloon angioplasty. The surgeon enters the artery with a catheter and uses the laser to destroy the plaque buildup that is occluding the artery.

Surgical treatment of PAD is a palliative measure only. It does not cure the disease or halt the atherosclerotic process. It can, however, relieve ischemic pain, help avoid amputation, and add years to a patient's life. The purpose of vascular surgery is to revascularize and nourish cells in the affected area. Atherectomy with the Rotablator may be used to improve blood flow to a limb. It can scrape hardened plaque from the arterial wall without damaging the wall itself.

An aortoiliac bypass or a femoropopliteal bypass is performed to correct arterial occlusion of the leg to prevent the need for amputation. A synthetic graft is placed to divert blood around the obstructed area, or the occluded portion is dissected and replaced by a graft from the patient's saphenous or other vein. Figure 19-5 shows a schematic of a femoropopliteal bypass graft surgery. Postoperative care is the same as for other operative procedures but includes careful assessment of pulses distal to the graft to detect **thrombus** (clot) formation. As with any vascular surgery, extra attention is paid to assessment for signs of bleeding. An aortoiliac bypass requires both an abdominal and a groin incision. A hyperbaric oxygen chamber is sometimes used for patients with severely compromised circulation to a lower extremity to increase tissue oxygen and avoid amputation.

❖ NURSING MANAGEMENT

■ Assessment (Data Collection)

Perform a physical assessment of the patient's affected extremity at least every 4 hours or per facility protocol. Feet should be assessed for warmth, paresthesia, pain,

Superficial femoral artery

Popliteal artery

Superficial femoral artery

Popliteal artery

Anterior tibial artery

Peroneal artery

Posterior tibial artery

Anterior tibial artery

Peroneal artery

Posterior tibial artery

A **B**

FIGURE 19-5 Femoropopliteal bypass graft. **A,** Femoropopliteal bypass graft around an occluded superficial femoral artery. **B,** Femoropopliteal bypass graft around occluded superficial femoropopliteal and proximal tibial arteries.

and pulses. All findings must be documented, including any changes. If ulcers are present, assessment and documentation of skin integrity should be included. A major role of the nurse is early detection and prevention of complications. Acute changes in assessment of patients with arterial insufficiency are unlikely; however, maintain a record of the patient's condition in the event of complications.

■ Nursing Diagnosis and Planning

The major nursing care goals for patients with PAD are (1) maintaining arterial blood flow to the lower extremities; (2) protecting tissues from further injury from pressure and constriction of blood flow; and (3) preventing wound infection.

Nursing diagnoses may include:
- Ineffective tissue perfusion related to narrowed vessels
- Impaired skin integrity related to ulcers on lower extremities
- Injury related to loss of peripheral circulation
- Acute pain related to ischemia to lower extremities

Expected outcomes may include:
- The patient will not experience loss of skin integrity.
- Peripheral pulses will remain palpable.
- The patient will report reduction in pain level in the lower extremities.

Rehabilitation of the patient requires instruction and guidance in special exercises to increase collateral circulation to the legs. See Table 18-4 for other common nursing diagnoses and interventions appropriate for patients with peripheral arterial occlusive disease.

■ Implementation

The nurse can encourage blood flow by keeping the patient and the environment warm. Constricting clothing is to be avoided, and the legs should not be raised in the bed as this puts added pressure on the back of the knees and further occludes blood flow. The nurse should encourage the patient to change position frequently while awake. The lower extremities should be positioned below heart level to facilitate arterial blood flow. The legs are elevated only if edema is impeding circulation. See Evolve for a nursing care plan for the patient with PAD.

Clinical Cues

Assess the affected extremity; document and report significant changes in pain level, pulses, sensation, and skin temperature. Additional medical intervention may be needed to prevent complications that could result in amputation of all or part of an extremity.

Encouraging exercise is especially beneficial to patients with decreased blood flow. Walking regularly every day is best for the ambulatory patient. Swimming also is good because it applies light pressure to the surface of the legs and requires muscle action that encourages venous return. Bed rest patients should be encouraged to do foot and leg exercises at least once each hour.

Think Critically

Rhonda, a 63-year-old executive, is experiencing worsening intermittent claudication. Describe how you would interact with her to develop an exercise program that could lessen her symptoms.

Patients should be dressed in warm, nonrestrictive clothing and should avoid becoming cold. Blankets or throws may be added for additional warmth. The room temperature should be maintained at the patient's comfort level.

Elder Care Points

Elderly adults are less tolerant of cold temperatures because of decreased subcutaneous fat tissue as a result of the aging process. Room temperatures must be maintained at the patient's comfort level. Chilling can result in vasoconstriction and contribute to discomfort of patients with vascular disorders.

Tobacco use, especially smoking, contributes to peripheral vascular disease because of the vasoconstrictive effect of nicotine. If appropriate, patients should be referred to a smoking cessation program. Information concerning the effects of alcohol on vascular disorders, surgical interventions, patient teaching, and interventions to prevent leg ulcers can be reviewed in Chapter 18.

 Think Critically

Can you describe the specific actions you would take to help a patient recognize the need to establish a smoking cessation program?

▪ Evaluation

Evaluation of the effectiveness of the plan of care involves assessing changes in peripheral pulses and skin integrity. Improvement or extension of vascular ulcers should be documented in writing and photographed periodically (e.g., weekly). Note changes in color, sensation, and temperature of the lower extremities. The patient's perception of pain level should be documented using a scale of 0 to 10. Evaluate the patient's level of compliance with establishing an exercise routine. Include type, frequency, and tolerance of exercise activities. Evaluate the patient's ability to meet established goals and revise the plan as needed.

ANEURYSM

Etiology

Aneurysms—outpouching of the wall of the artery resulting from a structural defect in the layers of the arterial wall—occur in a weakened area of a blood vessel. Aneurysms usually are the result of plaque formation, genetic predisposition, or hypertension. Aneurysms may also occur in areas weakened by trauma or surgical procedures. Aortic aneurysms can occur in the area below the stomach (abdominal aneurysm) or on the ascending aorta in the chest (thoracic aneurysm). An abdominal aortic aneurysm is usually located below the kidneys. Long-term hypertension and smoking are risk factors, particularly in men.

Congenital malformations, diabetes mellitus, and hyperlipidemia predispose to various types of aneurysm. However, atherosclerosis and hypertension are thought to be the major factors in their development. Atherosclerotic plaque weakens the vessel wall, and hypertension puts extra pressure on the weakened walls. Cerebral aneurysm is covered in Chapter 24.

Pathophysiology

An aneurysm can occur along any artery. Blood flow may become stagnant along the wall of the aneurysm, and clots can form. The clots can cause occlusion by thrombosis; alternatively, a clot may break away from the thrombosis to become an embolus that travels and lodges elsewhere. Once an aneurysm develops, it continues to grow larger. Aneurysms may eventually rupture if not repaired. *Aortic dissection* of the medial layer of the arterial wall can occur causing bleeding between layers of the wall with increasing pressure on surrounding structures. As the dissection extends, blood flow through the arterial branches of the aorta become blocked. Blood flow slows to the organs those branches feed. This occurs more frequently than aneurysm, particularly in men who are hypertensive.

Signs, Symptoms, and Diagnosis

Aneurysm rupture is common in the cerebral vessels, causing intracerebral bleeding and stroke (see Chapter 24). A ruptured aneurysm often leads to sudden death. Aneurysms often display no obvious symptoms. Patients with an abdominal aortic aneurysm (AAA) may report back pain or a feeling of pressure and may have a visible pulsation of the abdomen. An aortic aneurysm in the thoracic area may cause substernal or tracheal pressure and difficulty with breathing. Diagnosis of aneurysms is difficult because of lack of symptoms. Physical examination and screening of patients with a family history may be the best means of early detection. The presence of an aneurysm can be verified by chest or abdominal radiograph, ultrasound, magnetic resonance imaging (MRI), or computed tomography (CT) scans. Men who have hypertension and a smoking history should undergo ultrasound screening for abdominal aortic aneurysm.

Aortic dissection or rupture causes abrupt, excruciating pain. The pain radiates to the back, chest, abdomen, or extremities. Peripheral pulses are diminished. Chest radiographs and transesophageal echocardiogram are used for diagnosis.

Treatment

If an aortic aneurysm is detected early, it often can be surgically repaired before it dissects or ruptures. The size and location of the aneurysm guides the need for surgical intervention. Aneurysms in the ascending aorta are life threatening; therefore, emergency surgery is performed. Those located in the descending thoracic and abdominal aorta may not warrant immediate action. The patient is evaluated every few months with ultrasound tracking of the size of the aneurysm. Surgery may be performed when the aneurysm is greater than 3 cm in diameter. Patients may be prescribed antihypertensive drugs, such as beta blockers, to reduce the pressure on the arterial walls. If symptoms occur, surgical intervention may be necessary to prevent rupture of the aneurysm.

Surgery for aortic aneurysm involves replacing the area of the vessel wall that is weakened with a graft or inserting a stent graft into the vessel. The use of a stent graft is a minimally invasive procedure and is used for patients who are not good candidates for open surgical repair of the aneurysm. A mesh stent is placed in the area of the aneurysm percutaneously. Small incisions in the groin are used to access the femoral artery. The graft provides support to the vessel wall and allows blood to flow through the stent, thus reducing pressure on the vessel wall. The aneurysm is then monitored frequently. Treatment for aortic dissection focuses on lowering blood pressure and treating the pain.

❖ NURSING MANAGEMENT

■ Assessment (Data Collection)

Careful physical assessment is needed to detect the presence of an aneurysm. Immediately report findings of pulsations in the abdomen or other structures in which this is abnormal. Information concerning family history of aneurysm should be gathered during the patient history interview. Assessment of pain patterns—especially changes in intensity and location—is needed to identify progression of the patient's condition, one that may be life threatening.

■ Nursing Diagnosis and Planning

The main goal for a patient with an aneurysm is the prevention of rupture. Rupture of an aneurysm is a medical emergency and causes rapid hypovolemic shock, which can lead to death. Advise the patient to report any change in symptoms, such as pain intensity, apprehension, light-headedness, or any unusual sensation. Nursing diagnoses may include:

- Risk for injury from potential rupture or dissection of aneurysm
- Acute pain related to pressure of aneurysm on body structures and nerves
- Deficient knowledge related to management of medical condition

Other nursing diagnoses will depend on the location of the aneurysm and whether there is leaking. Expected outcomes might be:

- The patient will not experience rupture or dissection of the aneurysm
- The patient will report absence of pain
- The patient will verbalize understanding of management of medical condition

■ Implementation

Presurgical patient education is important. The patient must be taught signs and symptoms that should be reported to the health care provider immediately. Teaching concerning the medical and surgical treatment regimen should be included along with what to expect postoperatively.

> **? Think Critically**
>
> You detect a pulsation in the patient's abdomen during physical examination. He states that it has been present for several years and the physician is "watching it." List indications that could indicate a need for surgical intervention.

The surgical procedure and nursing care depend on the location of the aneurysm and the procedure performed. If aortic aneurysm is treated by thoracotomy or abdominal surgery, the care is similar to that of other types of thoracic and abdominal surgery. The main difference is that you must also carefully assess pulses and function distal to the repair site. Renal function must be watched closely as blood flow to the kidneys is briefly cut off when the aorta is clamped for surgical repair.

> **⌂ Clinical Cues**
>
> Attentive postsurgical care is very important. Monitor urinary output at least every 30 minutes in the immediate postoperative period, then every 2 hours. The urinary output should be at least 30 mL/hr. Report falling urinary output immediately.

The patient spends 24 to 48 hours in an intensive care unit postoperatively. Assist the patient to deep-breathe and use an incentive spirometer every 1 to 2 hours. Coughing is not encouraged, but should it occur the incision should be splinted with a pillow or folded bath blanket. Paralytic ileus occurs for a few days after abdominal surgery and a nasogastric tube will be in place. Auscultate the abdomen every shift for the return of bowel sounds. Adequate pain medication is needed.

The patient undergoing thoracic aortic aneurysm repair will undergo chest surgery with use of the cardiopulmonary bypass machine. The care is the same as for other chest surgery patients. Chest tubes will be in place. This patient is especially at risk for atelectasis and pneumonia. Pain management is necessary to promote adequate respiratory effort. Cardiac dysrhythmias may be a problem depending on the location of the repair.

■ Evaluation

Objective data—including vital signs, neurologic status, distal pulses, and respiratory status—should be assessed. Subjective data—including pain level and loss of sensation—should also be determined. Evaluation of the patient's understanding of teaching related to the disease process, potential complications, follow-up appointments, medications, and recommended lifestyle changes should be assessed and appropriate revisions made to the nursing care plan.

CAROTID OCCLUSION

When atherosclerosis has narrowed the carotid arteries leading to the brain, the signs and symptoms include carotid bruit (a purring sound heard with a stethoscope), confusion, visual abnormality in one eye, fainting, extremity weakness or paralysis, or other signs of decreased blood flow to the brain. The condition is treated by carotid endarterectomy or carotid artery angioplasty with stenting. Surgery is performed when the artery is 70% occluded (Singh et al., 2009). Both procedures are done to prevent the occurrence of stroke (see Chapter 24).

Specific postoperative care for endarterectomy includes assessing for signs of bleeding, for pressure from hematoma on the trachea (evidenced by increasing hoarseness), and for neurologic problems caused by thrombosis or embolus. Neurologic signs are monitored every 2 to 4 hours.

 Clinical Cues

There is risk for cerebrovascular accident (stroke) following carotid endarterectomy. Assess the patient for signs of disorientation, hoarseness, impaired speech, impaired swallowing, hemiparesis, facial asymmetry, aphasia, and hypertension. These findings should be reported immediately to the surgeon. Because there may be swelling in the neck that may occlude the airway, observe for difficulty breathing.

If surgery is not indicated, the patient is taught to maintain adequate hydration and to comply with drug therapy for hypertension and diabetes, if applicable. Teaching is provided regarding prescribed antiplatelet aggregation or anticoagulant drugs. Signs and symptoms of further problems are reviewed and the patient is advised to call 911 for emergency assistance if sensory or motor deficits appear.

BUERGER'S DISEASE (THROMBOANGIITIS OBLITERANS)

Etiology and Pathophysiology

Thromboangiitis obliterans, or Buerger's disease, involves the small and medium-size arteries. Inflammation, thickening of the arterial walls, and occlusion of the vessels in the hands and feet occur. The disease occurs more often in men than women and is commonly found in people from the Middle East, the Far East, India, and Southeast Asia. There is increasing incidence of the disease in women older than age 50. Moderate to heavy cigarette smoking is directly linked to the progression of the disease. It may be classified as an allergic response in some people in which the body reacts to properties in nicotine.

Signs, Symptoms, Diagnosis, and Treatment

The signs and symptoms include numbness and tingling of the toes or fingers in cold weather, pain in the feet, and intermittent claudication that progressively becomes more severe. The pain is intense. Ulcerations and gangrene (death of tissue) may occur. Diagnosis is made through patient history and symptoms. **Cessation of smoking is the single most important treatment factor.** Cigarette smoking must be stopped immediately. Those who do not stop smoking are at great risk for gangrene and amputation of fingers or toes. Exercise may be used to increase circulation in the legs and feet.

❖ NURSING MANAGEMENT

■ Assessment (Data Collection), Nursing Diagnosis, Planning, and Evaluation

The most important role of the nurse is patient teaching and reinforcement of the need for smoking cessation. Assessment of the extremities for skin impairment is essential. Nursing care and teaching is the same as for PAD.

RAYNAUD'S DISEASE AND RAYNAUD'S PHENOMENON

Etiology and Pathophysiology

The etiology of Raynaud's disease is unknown. Raynaud's disease is characterized by spasm of the arteries of the upper and lower extremities. The body has an exaggerated response to cold and stress, resulting in bilateral vasospasm. The disease is seen more often in young women. It mostly affects the fingers and toes. Raynaud's disease can be a primary disorder or may occur secondary to another disease such as lupus erythematosus, rheumatoid arthritis, or scleroderma. In the latter instance it is known as Raynaud's phenomenon and often occurs on only one side of the body.

Blood vessels normally constrict in cold environments; however, with Raynaud's disease, this process is excessive. The affected body part changes color. When the spasm stops, there often is burning pain and throbbing. In about 10% of those affected, the disease progresses to the point at which ischemia from arterial spasm is so severe that gangrene occurs and amputation is necessary.

Signs and Symptoms

Signs and symptoms of Raynaud's disease include:
- Fingers and toes may display a series of color changes from white to blue to red; these changes are evident on the dorsal surface of the hands and feet (Figure 19-6).
- The patient may experience numbness or a prickly sensation on warming and relief of stress.
- There may be decreased sensory perception.
- Edema may be present.
- Discomfort may occur in the extremity.

FIGURE 19-6 Raynaud's disease.

Diagnosis and Treatment

Diagnosis of Raynaud's disease is usually made by evaluation of patient symptoms. The physician may order laboratory studies such as erythrocyte sedimentation rate (ESR) to determine the presence of autoimmune disorders, or antinuclear antibody (ANA) test to determine the presence of immune responses. Medical therapy consists of stress control, avoidance of exposure to cold, and smoking cessation. Calcium channel blockers may be used to dilate capillaries in the hands and feet. Other drugs such as alpha blockers and vasodilators may be used to achieve vasodilation in the small blood vessels in the hands.

Nursing Management

The major nursing intervention for Raynaud's disease is teaching the patient to protect extremities and prevent injury. The patient should be taught to dress warmly when in cold environments. Clothing should be layered and hat and gloves should be worn. Warm socks should be worn to protect feet. The patient should be taught to wear protective gloves when reaching into ovens and when handling extremely cold items. Teach the patient to avoid cold temperatures when possible, to manage stress, and to stop tobacco use. Caffeine intake should be limited. If appropriate, the patient should be referred to a smoking cessation program.

Health Promotion

Smoking Cessation

Encourage smokers with vascular disorders to seek smoking cessation programs in their communities. The American Lung Association program "Freedom from Smoking" is offered free of charge online at the American Lung Association website, http://ffsonline.pub30.convio.net/. Discuss other programs such as nicotine replacement therapy. Group programs are offered in many communities, hospitals, American Lung Association affiliates, and community-based health programs. A variety of products are available to decrease and prevent nicotine cravings during the cessation process. Assessment of progress with smoking cessation should occur at each visit with a health care provider.

Evaluate the progression of symptoms, including changes in skin color and sensation. Any changes in skin integrity should be noted. The patient's compliance with recommended lifestyle changes should be evaluated and the plan revised as needed to assist the patient to meet established goals.

VENOUS DISORDERS

VENOUS THROMBOSIS

Venous thrombosis occurs in association with inflammation of the vein. Either a superficial or a deep vein is affected. Superficial thrombophlebitis occurs in approximately 65% of all patients receiving IV therapy. It is usually easily treated and resolved. Deep vein thrombosis (DVT) occurs most frequently in the iliac and femoral veins. DVT occurs in about 5% of all surgical patients. It is more serious because DVT can lead to embolization from the thrombus to the lungs.

Etiology and Pathophysiology

Three factors (Virchow's triad) for venous thrombosis are (1) venous stasis, (2) damage of the inner lining of the vein (endothelium), and (3) hypercoagulability of the blood. Venous stasis occurs when the vein valves are damaged or when muscles of the extremities are inactive. People who are immobile for a long time are very susceptible to DVT. Prolonged surgeries, spinal cord damage and paralysis, and chronic heart failure all contribute to venous stasis. Trauma or external pressure may damage the endothelium. Inflammation of the vessel leads to aggregation of blood components at the site of the inflammation. A clot forms at the inflammation site, leading to obstruction of blood flow. If not treated, the clot may become an embolus that may travel to the lungs resulting in pulmonary embolus.

Infusion of caustic IV substances is a high-risk factor for DVT. An IV catheter in place for more than 72 to 96 hours at the same site causes vein irritation and damage. Smoking, female hormone replacement, estrogen-based contraceptives, corticosteroids, and various blood disorders are contributing factors to blood hypercoagulability. Obesity and dehydration contribute to coagulability also.

Elder Care Points

Elderly patients who have problems with mobility or stress incontinence tend to drink less fluid so that they do not have to visit the bathroom so often. This can lead to dehydration and more viscous blood, which in turn can predispose to thrombus formation in those susceptible to this disorder. Encourage adequate fluid intake to promote circulation, and provide a means for convenient toileting for these patients. The occurrence of DVT or thrombophlebitis increases with advanced age.

Patients particularly at risk for DVT are those having orthopedic surgery, those who smoke, or those who have diabetes, lung disease, blood disorders, peripheral vascular disease, sepsis, and cancer. If a DVT is not resolved, increased pressure in the vein could result in destruction of venous valves and development of venous insufficiency. *Embolism* may be caused when a portion of a DVT in a leg breaks loose and travels to the lungs. The embolus lodges in small vessels, especially those in the pulmonary system. Blood flow is interrupted and loss of oxygenation and interruption of blood flow to the lung may occur. The condition can be life threatening (see Chapter 15). When a pulmonary embolus is suspected, place the patient in a high Fowler's position, provide oxygen and reassurance, notify the physician, and stay with the patient. Medication for pain and anxiety may be ordered; tests to determine if a pulmonary embolus has occurred will be ordered.

SUPERFICIAL THROMBOPHLEBITIS

Continuous IV therapy and contaminated IV drug needles are frequent causes of superficial thrombophlebitis.

Signs, Symptoms, and Diagnosis

Signs and symptoms of thrombophlebitis include swelling, redness, warmth, and considerable tenderness and pain on touching. Diagnosis is by ultrasound studies or venography. Physical examination, patient history, and evaluation of signs and symptoms are important in diagnosing thrombophlebitis.

Treatment and Nursing Management

Treatment for thrombophlebitis includes discontinuing the source of irritation and modifying risk factors; applying warm, moist heat; elevating the extremity; and administering NSAIDs and antibiotics if infection is present. If the IV is implicated as a cause, the IV catheter site will be changed to a new location. Patients are encouraged to stay off their feet and to elevate their legs. Support stockings are to be worn after the acute phase.

Nursing management of the patient with thrombophlebitis includes assessment and documentation of the color, warmth, circumference, and pulses of the affected extremity. Explain the importance of adhering to the prescribed level of physical activity, and explain the potential complications if noncompliant. Make certain that the patient receives medications as prescribed. Warm, moist compresses to the affected extremity may be ordered. Emphasize the importance of this treatment. Develop a discharge teaching plan related to the disease process, medications, activity level, home care, and follow-up. Components of teaching may include:

- Avoidance of sitting for long periods with the legs down
- Avoidance of standing in one place for long periods

- Management with NSAIDs
- Application of compression stockings
- Activity limits
- Preventive measures

? Think Critically

What teaching points would you cover for a 52-year-old female hairdresser who is being discharged after hospitalization for thrombophlebitis of the right leg?

Decreased redness, swelling, and pain indicate resolution of the thrombophlebitis. Evaluation of patient success in meeting goals would include compliance with medications and demonstrated evidence of understanding of discharge teaching. Often, subjective data from the patient must be relied on to evaluate whether treatment and nursing actions are effective.

DEEP VEIN THROMBOSIS

Signs, Symptoms, and Diagnosis

The main sign of a DVT is edema in one extremity (Figure 19-7). The area over the thrombosis may feel warm. Never rub or vigorously palpate the area, as this can dislodge the clot and send it into the circulation, which can cause severe damage or death.

The most common method of diagnosing DVT is duplex sonography. Sound waves detect blood flow through the veins and identify areas of abnormality. If sonography is not clear, an MRI may be done. Activated clotting time (ACT), activated partial thromboplastin time (aPTT), international normalized ratio (INR), hemoglobin (Hb), hematocrit (Hct), and D-dimer laboratory tests are done to detect blood dyscrasias or abnormal clotting times. A venogram sometimes is performed, but it requires injection of a dye to identify areas of obstruction which may further irritate the vessel. Obtain the patient's allergy history before this procedure.

FIGURE 19-7 Patient with DVT.

Treatment

Medical treatment for DVT usually consists of intravenous infusion of heparin or administration of a fibrinolytic agent to dissolve the clot followed by subcutaneous injections of low-molecular weight heparin (LMWH) such as enoxaparin (Lovenox) injection and then by oral anticoagulation with warfarin sodium (Coumadin), plus compression stockings. When pain and swelling are controlled ambulation is encouraged. Warfarin is continued for 3 to 6 months (Torpy et al., 2008). Anticoagulants will not dissolve the clot but may prevent new ones. The body dissolves the clot on its own over time.

Thrombolytic therapy may be used to dissolve the thrombus if vessel obstruction is severe; urokinase, reteplase (Retavase), and alteplase (t-PA) are some of the agents used. There is a high risk of bleeding with these drugs. If the patient does not respond to treatment, a thrombectomy may be performed to prevent necrosis.

A thrombolytic agent is followed by a few additional days of heparin while the patient is started on warfarin. Warfarin takes at least 3 days to build to an effective blood level. Other drugs used for DVT include direct thrombin inhibitors (lepirudin [Refludan] and bivalirudin [Angiomax]). Factor Xa inhibitors (fondaparinux [Arixtra]) do not require coagulation monitoring. These drugs are administered subcutaneously and are used when the patient is unable to use heparin.

Sequential compression devices (SCDs) may be prescribed or compression stockings are fitted for daily use. Stockings must be proper fitting and kept smooth. The compression forces blood from the superficial veins into the deep veins, decreasing venous stasis. Compression stockings are only removed for bathing, and are changed and laundered daily. They must be replaced after 6 months as the elastic quality decreases. Special Jobst compression stockings individually fit to the patient are prescribed for long-term therapy to prevent further DVT (Anderson & Audet, 2010)

If a patient is considered at risk for further embolus formation from DVT and is not a candidate for anticoagulation, a *vena caval filter* will be inserted. The umbrella-shaped strainer device is placed in the inferior vena cava below the kidneys to prevent pulmonary emboli. The umbrella is collapsed, and with the use of a special catheter, is threaded into the vena cava. The umbrella catches the emboli and the body slowly dissolves and disposes of them.

Postthrombotic syndrome is a potential complication. Some blockage remains in the vessel and there is increased swelling, pain, hyperpigmentation, and possibly skin ulcers. It is treated with anticoagulation therapy, compression stockings, and extremity elevation. For patients undergoing surgery or on bed rest, research shows that a combination of anticoagulation and the use of graduated elastic compression stockings reduces the incidence of postthrombotic syndrome the best (Vazquez & Kahn, 2010).

Heparin-induced thrombocytopenia (HIT) may occur when unfractionated heparin is used for several days to weeks. It is heralded by a sudden decrease in platelet count. If HIT occurs, heparin administration must be stopped.

❖ NURSING MANAGEMENT

■ Assessment (Data Collection)

Assess patients at risk for DVT each shift for signs and symptoms. Assessment should include:
- Observation of the extremity for asymmetrical size
- Areas of warmth and redness over a vein
- Calf pain and/or tenderness
- Pitting edema of the affected extremity
- Measurement of calf circumference
- Body temperature greater than 100.4° F (38° C)

■ Nursing Diagnosis, Planning, and Implementation

Early ambulation postoperatively helps promote circulation and reduces the risk of clot formation. Encouraging patients on bed rest to change position and perform leg and ankle exercises each hour while awake can do much to decrease the incidence of DVT. Venous thrombosis occurs fairly often during long plane flights or car trips. Staying well hydrated, exercising the leg and calf muscles frequently during the trip, and walking every 1 to 2 hours helps to prevent clots from occurring. Wearing support hose at work aids venous return and helps prevent thrombosis in those who have varicose veins (Lew, Weaver, & Feied, 2010).

Nursing diagnoses and expected outcomes are presented with interventions in Nursing Care Plan 19-1. Information and nursing care for the administration of anticoagulants is presented in Chapter 20.

■ Evaluation

Decrease in leg circumference and adequate blood flow to the extremity as evidenced by color, warmth, and lack of edema indicate that interventions for DVT are working. Evaluation of interventions for thrombophlebitis include checking for increases in peripheral circulation and a decrease in pain or an ability to walk further without pain.

VARICOSE VEINS

Varicose veins are enlarged and tortuous veins that are distorted in shape by accumulations of pooled blood. Veins that develop varicosities have incompetent valves that allow reflux of blood from the deep to

Nursing Care Plan 19-1   Care of the Patient with a Deep Vein Thrombosis

Scenario

Mrs. Hanson, age 72, sustained multiple bruises and a concussion in an automobile accident. She has cardiac dysrhythmia and was admitted 2 days ago for observation and recuperation. She has now developed pain in her right calf, and her lower leg is swollen, with a hot, tender area in the midcalf region. She has been placed on a continuous heparin drip.

Problem/Nursing Diagnosis

Circulatory compromise/Ineffective tissue perfusion related to presence of clot in vein and inflammation.

Supporting Assessment Data

Subjective: "My leg really hurts." Complains of pain in right calf.
Objective: Reddened, warm, tender area on midcalf. Temperature, 101.2° F (38.4° C). Leg circumference increased compared to left leg.

Goals/Expected Outcomes	Nursing Interventions	Selected Rationale	Evaluation
Thrombus will resolve within 2 weeks as evidenced by Doppler flow studies.	Maintain on bed rest with bathroom privileges; keep right lower leg elevated.	To avoid potential embolus from clot.	Maintaining bed rest with right leg elevated.
Thrombosis will begin to resolve by discharge as evidenced by normal temperature and no calf tenderness, redness, or swelling.	Active range of motion (ROM) of left ankle, knee, and hip.	Maintain venous circulation.	Exercising foot and leg q 2 hr.
	Administer analgesia for aching and tenderness.	Promotes comfort.	Analgesic administered × 2. States is more comfortable.
	Warm packs to right leg; handle right leg gently.	Provide comfort, decrease edema.	Warm packs applied × 3. Edema slightly decreased.
	Auscultate lung sounds every shift; be alert for signs of pulmonary emboli.	Early detection of pulmonary emboli for immediate intervention.	Lung sounds clear to auscultation.
	Monitor level of consciousness (LOC) and neurologic status every shift.	Change in central nervous system status could indicate cerebral embolism.	Alert and oriented × 3.

Problem/Nursing Diagnosis

Risk for thrombus formation or bleeding/Risk for injury related to heparin drip, thrombus formation, or embolus.

Supporting Assessment Data

Objective: Heparin drip 50,000 U in 500 mL at 50 mL/hr. Deep venous thrombosis (DVT) in right leg.

Goals/Expected Outcomes	Nursing Interventions	Selected Rationale	Evaluation
Patient will not experience embolus or other DVT during hospitalization.	Maintain heparin drip on IV pump at ordered rate; assess IV site q hr for infiltration.	Prevent formation of additional thrombi.	Heparin drip continuous; IV site without redness or swelling.
	Caution not to rub leg.	Rubbing may dislodge a clot and cause an embolus.	States understands not to rub the leg.
	Monitor level of consciousness and neurologic status every shift.	Change in neurologic status could indicate cerebral embolism.	Alert and oriented × 3. Pupils equal, round, and reactive to light and accommodation (PERRLA) without headache, alert and oriented.
	Encourage increase in fluid intake.	Assists in reducing blood viscosity.	Intake 2000 mL this shift.
	Apply compression stockings smoothly, removing only for bathing.	Assist with venous return and prevent blood pooling.	Compression stockings in place; smoothed q 2 hr.

Continued

Goals/Expected Outcomes	Nursing Interventions	Selected Rationale	Evaluation
No hemorrhage from heparin as evidenced by no sign of bleeding internally or externally.	Observe for bleeding of gums, excessive bruising, blood in urine or stool, nosebleeds, and abdominal pain with rigidity.	Heparin can cause bleeding.	Slight bleeding of gums. Bruising from previous needle sticks; buttocks bruised from bed rest. No evidence of blood in urine or stool; bowel sounds present all four quadrants, abdomen soft.
	Monitor Hb and hematocrit to detect blood loss.	May indicate need to change infusion rate or administer protamine sulfate if excessive blood loss occurs.	No change in Hb and hematocrit.
	Monitor ACT or aPTT and advise physician immediately if values rise above 2½ times the control value or above therapeutic range.	Allows for adjustment of heparin dosage to keep it within therapeutic range.	aPTT 2 × control value.
	Hold pressure over any needle stick for 5 minutes.	Heparin can extend bleeding time.	No excessive bleeding with lab draws.
	Begin warfarin (Coumadin) therapy as ordered 3 days before heparin is stopped.	Anticoagulant therapy will continue when discharged home.	Coumadin administered today.
	Handle patient very gently.	Prevents bruising.	Handling gently; no new bruising.

Problem/Nursing Diagnosis

Lack of knowledge about medication and disorder/Deficient knowledge related to precautions necessary when taking warfarin and about treatment regimen.

Supporting Assessment Data

Will go home on warfarin for at least 6 to 12 months. Has never taken this medication.

Goals/Expected Outcomes	Nursing Interventions	Selected Rationale	Evaluation
Patient will verbalize danger signs to report to physician and proper dosage of medications before discharge.	Teach the following: Avoid foods high in vitamin K (give list).	Vitamin K interferes with the action of warfarin.	Began teaching regarding dangers of warfarin; needs time to absorb information; will continue teaching tomorrow; gave written instruction sheet.
	Avoid over-the-counter medications and drugs that might extend clotting time or interfere with action of warfarin (e.g., aspirin, etc.).	Some over-the-counter drugs have anticoagulant actions that may increase risk of complications of drug therapy.	States understands to check with physician before using over-the-counter medications.
	Move around carefully, trying not to hit head on anything or bump into things.	Injury could cause bruising and hematoma formation.	Slight bruising noted on buttocks. Continue to monitor.
	Observe urine and stool for signs of bleeding.	May indicate elevated international normalized ratio (INR).	No signs of bleeding in urine or stool.
	Maintain good hydration by drinking at least 10 glasses of fluid a day.	Hydration supports blood flow and reduces risk of additional clot formation.	Oral intake 2000 mL/day.
Patient will verbalize understanding of need for regular medical follow-up and periodic lab clotting times before discharge.	Instruct her to maintain close contact with physician to monitor clotting times.	Monitoring of INR important to evaluate effectiveness of warfarin therapy.	Verbalizes need to keep appointments for follow-up laboratory studies.
	Explain dosage schedule. Give written instruction sheet.	Provides reference for safe administration of drug.	Given written instructions to be followed when taking warfarin.

ACT, anticoagulant therapy ; *aPTT,* activated partial thromboplastin time.

Goals/Expected Outcomes	Nursing Interventions	Selected Rationale	Evaluation
Patient will completely stop smoking within 1 mo.	Stop use of cigarettes.	Cigarette smoking constricts vessels and contributes to blood coagulability.	Has been trying to stop smoking. Gave smoking cessation packet of information and encouraged smoking counseling.
Patient will establish a walking program when acute stage has resolved.	Assist to establish walking schedule.	Walking promotes venous return by calf muscles compressing the veins.	Is thinking about a walking schedule.
	Caution not to sit with legs crossed or to sit for long periods without elevating legs.	Crossing the legs decreases venous return and promotes blood pooling in the extremity. Sitting causes dependent pooling in legs.	States understands not to sit with legs crossed or for long periods with legs dependent.
	Caution not to wear constricting clothing.	Tight clothing can decrease venous return and cause pooling in extremities.	States she understands not to wear tight clothing items.

Critical Thinking Questions
1. List the signs and symptoms of pulmonary embolism.
2. What additional assessment data would you expect to find during the physical examination of a patient with deep vein thrombosis?

the superficial veins. The increased blood flow and resultant pressure on the vein walls cause the vessels to dilate and become tortuous.

Varicosities usually occur in the saphenous veins and perforator veins in the ankle. Congenital or family disposition that leads to loss of vessel wall elasticity is a primary cause. Standing for long periods, obesity, and pregnancy are possible contributing factors. Trauma, DVT, and inflammation that results in vein valve damage are secondary causes. Individuals who must be on their feet a great deal are encouraged to wear support stockings to encourage venous return.

 Think Critically

Can you identify two lifestyle changes you could personally make that would decrease your risk of a vascular disorder later in life?

Elder Care Points

Varicose veins develop in the elderly as the veins lose their elasticity and the leg muscles weaken and atrophy from decreased exercise.

Signs and symptoms of varicose veins include dilated, twisted-appearing, superficial vessels on the legs. Swelling of the foot and ankle on the affected leg may occur by the end of the day, and swelling is often accompanied by aching. The patient may complain of pain, itching, or both along varicose veins

(Figure 19-8). The legs may feel full and heavy during walking or exercise. Diagnosis is made by thorough physical assessment and patient history.

Treatment

Treatment of varicose veins includes using elastic support hose, exercising the legs and feet periodically throughout the day, and elevating the legs whenever possible. Prolonged standing, sitting, or crossing the legs is to be avoided. Weight reduction is recommended for obese patients. Exercises such as walking or swimming are beneficial because the muscle contraction encourages venous return to the heart. Some herbs are helpful for varicose veins.

 Complementary and Alternative Therapies

Herbs for Varicose Veins

Several herbs have been found to be helpful for patients with varicose veins (but should not be used during pregnancy and lactation):

Bilberry: may cause constipation; affects blood glucose levels, may increase the action of anticoagulants; check drug and herbal interactions

Butcher's broom: not to be used for patients with hypertension or prostatic hypertrophy

Gotu kola: also helpful for hypertension

Horse chestnut: check for interactions with other drugs the patient is taking; do not use with hypoglycemics, salicylates, or anticoagulants

Patients need to be aware of potential side effects of herbs, as well as prescribed medications.

FIGURE 19-8 Varicose veins.

Knee-length elastic stockings or elastic wraps should be applied early in the morning, before the legs are placed in a dependent position, because the blood vessels are less congested after a prolonged rest. If wraps are used, the legs should be wrapped twice daily to maintain appropriate pressure. Bandages should be applied by beginning at the feet and working upward to avoid trapping blood in the lower leg. The patient should have two pairs of elastic hose and should wash them after each day's wearing. Elastic hose should be replaced every 6 months as they lose their elasticity. When stockings are removed, the heels should be checked for pressure areas.

Clinical Cues

Follow directions carefully and measure the patient's calves and legs before choosing a pair of elastic stockings. Accurate fit is crucial to effective treatment. If standard sizes do not coincide with the measurements, custom stockings may need to be purchased.

Exercise is especially beneficial to patients with decreased blood flow. Walking is the ideal exercise for the ambulatory patient. If a patient is unable to ambulate, promote venous return through range-of-motion (ROM) exercises and other kinds of muscular movements. Use of a treadmill for patients who cannot exercise by walking outside is very beneficial. A stationary exercise bicycle is another alternative.

Medications such as NSAIDs (e.g., aspirin) may be used for aching. Surgical procedures may be used when medical treatment is ineffective. Small varicosities can be treated by **scleropathy**, which involves injecting an agent that will sclerose the vessel, causing it to dry up and wither. Veins with multiple, severe varicosities (more than 4 mm in diameter) are treated by vein stripping, done as an outpatient procedure. Generally there will be multiple incisions along the leg to ligate and strip out the vein. Bed rest and leg elevation the night after surgery are recommended. Newer, less invasive procedures include endovenous occlusion using laser, radiofrequency closure, or transilluminated powered phlebectomy (Lew, Weaver, & Feied, 2010). The legs are wrapped with elastic bandages postoperatively to decrease bleeding and hematoma formation. ROM exercise of the legs is done every hour to help prevent thrombosis and the patient is ambulatory. Prevention of infection after surgery is essential. Instruct to limit sitting and avoid standing in one place and to elevate the legs when sitting.

CHRONIC VENOUS INSUFFICIENCY

Etiology and Pathophysiology

This condition is common among the elderly. It occurs when the venous valves are damaged such as occurs with severe cases of DVT. When valves are damaged, there is retrograde venous blood flow and blood pools in the legs. Swelling results with increasing venous pressure and stasis of blood flow. The condition may lead to venous stasis ulcers.

Venous return occurs by the pumping action of the calf muscles against the venous walls. When valves are incompetent, venous return is compromised and flow goes both ways in the vessel. The increased pressure leads to leakage of red blood cells into the tissues. The breakdown of the red cells releases hemosiderin, which causes a brownish skin color (Weiss, & Feied, 2009). Fibrous tissue replaces subcutaneous tissue around the ankle. The skin becomes thick and hardened.

Signs, Symptoms, and Diagnosis

Signs and symptoms of chronic venous insufficiency include chronically swollen legs; thick, brownish skin around the ankles; and itchy, scaly skin (Figure 19-9). Stasis dermatitis is common. Venous stasis ulcers often occur (Figure 19-10). Infection and cellulitis occur if an ulcer is untreated. Diagnosis is made through physical assessment and patient history.

FIGURE 19-9 Characteristic skin changes in the patient with venous insufficiency.

FIGURE 19-10 Venous stasis ulcer.

Treatment and Nursing Management

Treatment is the use of knee-length elastic support stockings and elevation of the legs for 8 out of 24 hours each day. Teach the patient to avoid prolonged standing or sitting and to sleep with the foot of the bed elevated 6 inches. Legs should not be crossed when sitting and tight clothing, garters, and girdles are to be avoided. Legs should be elevated above heart level whenever possible.

VENOUS STASIS ULCERS

The diabetic patient with venous insufficiency is at high risk for this disorder because of compromised circulation in the extremities and a slow rate of healing. The ulcers may extend deeply into the tissue and are very slow and difficult to heal because of tissue congestion and edema that prevent nutrients from reaching the cells. The ulcer may begin as a small, tender, inflamed area and becomes very painful. With the slightest trauma, the skin breaks and the ulcer enlarges. It is imperative that the patient with venous insufficiency be taught the extreme importance of good foot and leg care. An inflamed skin area can be preventively treated with a clear occlusive dressing, such as Tegaderm or OpSite, to help prevent ulcer formation. These transparent dressings allow monitoring of the site for signs of infection or complications of healing. Teach the patient about proper self-care and signs of beginning skin breakdown. The slightest injury to an ischemic area can take a very long time to heal and can easily become infected, as the blood supply is inadequate to provide the usual leukocyte defenses. Any injury to an affected extremity, no matter how minor, should be reported to the physician immediately.

Treatment for an ulcer consists of leg elevation, a moist dressing, and compression. A culture is done to determine if infection is present. Saline or mild soap is used to clean around the ulcer. A lanolin-type lotion is used to keep skin moist and supple. The dressing to be used depends on the condition of the ulcer and the amount of exudate produced. A vacuum-assisted drainage device may be needed for excessive drainage. The wound may need a graft to heal completely. Venous stasis ulcers can take weeks to months to heal. Compression dressings are not used if arterial insufficiency is also present. Compression therapy options include compression stockings, elastic tubular support bandages, intermittent compression devices, a paste bandage such as Unna boot, or placement of two to four layers of compression dressings to the affected area. Venous return is accomplished as the patient moves his leg and achieves pressure on the calf muscles. Compression dressings can be placed over wound dressings. The dressings help to reduce ulcer pain, keep the wound moist, and assist debridement. The dressing is changed from every 2 to 3 days to every few weeks depending on the type of dressing applied.

For success, the underlying venous problem must be treated. If a graft is necessary to heal the ulcer, it is debrided and varicosities in the area are removed. A split-thickness graft or bioengineered skin may be used. Advise the patient to avoid injury to the graft site. Patients are placed on bed rest for several days after grafting to protect the site. Give the patient considerable support, as treatment is long, recurrent, and tedious. Patients with stasis ulcers frequently become depressed. Praise for compliance with instructions and for any small gains made toward healing can do much for a patient's morale.

❖ NURSING MANAGEMENT

▪ Assessment (Data Collection)

Subjective information is gathered during history taking. A nutritional assessment is essential. Objective assessment data should include status of the skin, noting color, warmth, and moisture. Stasis dermatitis may be present, and pruritus and edema are common. Document the location, size, and presence of exudate, its color and odor, and include a photograph. Obtain a patient statement of pain at the site on a scale of 0 to 10. Assess the patient's experience with pain, including intensity, when pain occurs, and how it is relieved. Assess arterial pulses and determine the pulse rate, rhythm, and character (force) of the pulse. For diagnostic tests refer to Table 18-2.

◎ Focused Assessment

Data Collection for Vascular Disorders

Gather data on the following while interviewing the patient.

HEALTH HISTORY
- Family history of hypertension, cardiovascular disease, stroke, hyperlipidemia, aortic aneurysm, diabetes mellitus, or peripheral vascular disease
- History of trauma to the lower extremities
- Personal history of any peripheral vascular disease
- All medications taken on a regular basis (prescribed and over-the-counter medications)
- History of tobacco use, especially smoking
- History of alcohol use
- Dietary practices, especially sodium and fat intake
- Current or history of central nervous system occurrences, such as dizziness, headaches, or loss of consciousness
- Occurrence of edema in the legs, feet, or ankles
- Occurrence of leg pain during walking (When? How is it relieved?)

PHYSICAL ASSESSMENT
- Color of skin of the neck
- Observe for jugular vein distention
- Auscultate carotid arteries for presence of bruit
- Auscultate heart sounds and note any abnormalities
- Any visible abdominal pulsation over aorta?
- Auscultate over aorta in abdomen for presence of bruit
- Assess peripheral pulses and compare bilaterally
- Assess blood pressure on both arms, sitting and standing
- Assess skin for temperature, color, appearance, lesions, dryness, presence or absence of hair on legs
- Note presence of varicosities
- Assess capillary refill

▪ Nursing Diagnosis and Planning

Nursing diagnoses are chosen based on those assessment data that indicate problems for the patient. Common nursing diagnoses associated with vascular disorders are listed in Table 18-4. Nursing diagnoses may be added to the care plan for problems secondary to treatments, such as drug therapy or surgery. Other nursing diagnoses sometimes used include:

- Insomnia related to pain in the legs while at rest
- Situational low self-esteem related to inability to perform usual roles because of chronic leg ulcers

Appropriate exercise is important to treat vascular disease. Collaborate with the physician and physical therapist about activity, exercises, and the reinforcement of teaching (WOCN, 2010). Collaborate with the dietitian to promote the patient's adequate nutrient intake for healing. Specific expected outcomes must be written on an individual basis (see Table 18-4).

▪ Implementation

A major role of the nurse caring for a patient with venous insufficiency is to monitor the condition and determine whether treatment is effective. Table 18-4 lists helpful interventions for the most common nursing diagnoses associated with problems of the vascular system. Nursing interventions for selected problems in a patient with a venous stasis ulcer are summarized in Table 18-4.

▪ Evaluation

Evaluate the patient's response to treatment to determine effectiveness and potential development of complications. Carefully evaluating pulses and comparing them bilaterally is an important part of nursing care for patients with problems of the vascular system. Documenting a good description of the quality and character of the pulses monitored in the nurse's notes will give coworkers an accurate assessment baseline on which to evaluate changes in the pulse.

It is important to determine if skin color and temperature have changed since the last assessment. Ulcerated areas are monitored closely, measured, documented in writing, and photographed to determine whether healing is occurring. The color of the healing tissue and presence of exudate also are evaluated. Documentation of the characteristics of any exudate should be included. If the wound is enlarging or not improving, the nursing actions or treatment must be changed.

Subjective data from the patient helps evaluate whether treatment and nursing actions are effective. Increases in peripheral circulation may be evident only by a decrease in pain or an ability to walk farther without pain. The patient should be able to demonstrate understanding of the disease process, preventive measures, medications, signs and symptoms to report to the health care provider, and follow-up care.

COMMUNITY CARE

Many patients with vascular disease are treated in outpatient clinics and their homes. Patients who have venous stasis ulcers are often treated by the home health nurse. With early discharge after surgery, many patients receive postoperative care in the home. Patients with arterial bypass may be referred for rehabilitation exercise programs at a rehabilitation center. Your role in these settings is focused on ongoing assessment, coordination of care with other members of the health care team, monitoring progress and compliance with treatment, and patient education.

Include careful monitoring of the blood pressure for the presence of hypertension. Patients should be aware of expected blood pressure levels and critical levels to report to the health care provider. Evaluate the home care patient's understanding of medication, diet, and exercise to accomplish optimal management of hypertension.

Some patients may have the capability of monitoring their coagulation status through home monitoring devices. This is especially important for patients who are taking drugs such as warfarin. The international normalized ratio (INR) can be monitored by use of the AccuCoag device. The patient then has more information to manage his coagulation status and avoids missed lab appointments. Be aware of patient use of these devices and ensure that the patient is using them correctly.

Get Ready for the NCLEX® Examination!

Key Points

- Hypertension is more prevalent and more severe in African Americans than in other minority groups and whites.
- Treatment of hypertension involves measures to assist the patient to maintain blood pressure at or below 120/80 mm Hg.
- Antihypertensive drugs work by decreasing blood volume, cardiac output, or peripheral resistance.
- Nursing care of patients with hypertension includes counseling and education about lifestyle changes, diet, weight control, stress relief, and exercise.
- Noncompliance with medical regimen for hypertension can result in heart problems, blindness, stroke, and kidney failure.
- Obesity, stress, and sedentary lifestyle contribute to the incidence of atherosclerosis and hypertension.
- Atherosclerosis is the most common etiology of peripheral vascular disease.
- Arterial wall injury may be caused by hypertension, deposit of fatty plaque, chemical toxins, or diabetes mellitus.
- Disorders of peripheral arteries invariably lead to ischemia.
- Quitting smoking, following a low-fat diet, controlling diabetes mellitus, and following an exercise program decrease the incidence of PAD.
- Signs and symptoms of PAD include intermittent claudication, pain at rest, and ischemic changes. The six P's are pain, pulselessness, poikilothermia (coldness), pallor, paresthesias, and paralysis.
- The best treatment for arterial insufficiency is exercise—specifically, walking.
- Long-standing hypertension and atherosclerosis are factors in the development of aneurysms.
- Aneurysms may be repaired by surgical resection and graft or stent insertion.
- An aneurysm rupture frequently causes death.

- The etiology of Raynaud's disease is an exaggerated response to cold environment and stress.
- Carotid occlusion is signified by a carotid bruit, confusion, blackouts, extremity weakness or paralysis, visual abnormality in one eye, or other neurologic symptoms.
- Treatment includes carotid endarterectomy or stenting.
- Thrombophlebitis is the development of a clot and inflammation of a vessel.
- DVT is a clot in a deep vein occluding blood flow.
- The effects of a thrombus depend on the location and size of the clot and the degree of obstruction to blood flow.
- The etiology of DVT includes immobility, trauma, surgery, cancer, dehydration, and abnormal clotting.
- Treatment of DVT may include IV heparin, subcutaneous enoxaparin, oral warfarin, and hydration.
- Medical management: elevation of extremity when seated, compression stockings ambulation, warm moist packs, NSAIDs, and sometimes antibiotics.
- Varicose veins are enlarged, tortuous veins engorged with pooled blood.
- The symptoms of varicose veins include fatigue, a feeling of heaviness in the legs after prolonged standing or sitting, pain, and itching along the course of the blood vessel.
- Medical management involves compression stockings treatment of obesity, and exercise.
- Surgical treatment may include scleropathy, vein stripping, ligation, or endovenous laser treatment.
- Venous insufficiency occurs from damaged valves in veins and pooling of blood.
- Venous stasis ulcers are skin lesions, usually on the lower leg, from venous insufficiency.
- Treatment includes acute debridement, dressings, compression, and prevention of infection.

Additional Learning Resources

SG Go to your Study Guide for additional learning activities to help you master this chapter content.

 Go to your Evolve website (http://evolve.elsevier.com/deWit/medsurg) for the following FREE learning resources:

- Animations, audio, and video
- Answers and rationales for questions and activities
- Concept Map Creator
- Glossary with pronunciations in English and Spanish
- Interactive Review Questions and Exercises and more!

Online Resources

- Blood thinners, www.ahrq.gov/consumer/btpills.htm
- American Heart Association, www.heart.org
- Peripheral Arterial Disease Coalition, www.padcoalition.org
- Peripheral arterial disease, www.nhlbi.nih.gov/health/public/heart/pad/index.html
- National Heart, Lung, and Blood Institute, "Lowering Your Cholesterol with TLC," www.nhlbi.nih.gov/health/public/heart/chol/chol_tlc.pdf
- Society for Vascular Surgery, www.vascularweb.org
- Vascular Disease Foundation, www.vdf.org/diseaseinfo/pad

Review Questions for the NCLEX® Examination

1. A 40-year-old woman complains of leg pains that are associated with fullness during walking. She describes itching on the lower leg and on inspection has a twisted-appearing swelling in her legs. The patient most likely will be treated for:
   1. venous stasis ulcers.
   2. deep vein thrombosis.
   3. arterial insufficiency.
   4. varicose veins.

2. The nurse reinforces discharge instructions to a patient who is diagnosed with chronic venous insufficiency. Which instruction(s) should be included? *(Select all that apply.)*
   1. "Take a low-dose aspirin every day."
   2. "Consider swimming for exercise."
   3. "Avoid wearing tight clothing."
   4. "Reapply elastic wraps in the afternoon."
   5. "Decrease fluid intake to help prevent edema."
   6. "Elevate the legs above the level of the heart as much as possible."

3. If a patient complains of intermittent claudication, the nurse would expect which clinical finding?
   1. Strong, symmetrical peripheral pulses
   2. Skin mottling
   3. Rubor when legs are dependent
   4. Continual pain

4. A patient diagnosed with a venous disorder asks, "What is sclerotherapy?" An accurate explanation would be:
   1. "An instrument is inserted into the blood vessel to remove tissues."
   2. "An injection of a medication that shrinks the vein."
   3. "A surgical procedure that cuts through the vein to remove clots."
   4. "An insertion of a filter to prevent the spread of blood clots."

5. A patient is started on antihypertensive medications. Which patient statement indicates effectiveness of teaching?
   1. "I will be able to perform sit-ups in the morning."
   2. "I need to take the medication when I feel dizzy."
   3. "It helps reduce the incidence of a blood clot."
   4. "Sudden changes in position may cause dizziness."

6. The nurse is receiving a patient who had femoropopliteal bypass surgery. Which nursing intervention would take priority in the immediate postoperative period?
   1. Assessing the pulses proximal to the graft
   2. Monitoring for signs of bleeding
   3. Determining range of motion
   4. Checking bowel sounds

7. The nurse is reinforcing the physician's instructions to an elderly woman who is newly diagnosed with hypertension. The patient does not speak the nurse's language and is legally blind. What is the best nursing action?
   1. Recruit a translator to provide instructions.
   2. Speak slowly.
   3. Use a loud voice.
   4. Provide written instructions for the family.

8. A 54-year-old man complains of pain when walking and numbness of his lower extremities. On examination, the nurse notes that both extremities are pale and cool to touch. The highest priority nursing diagnosis would be:
   1. Ineffective peripheral tissue perfusion.
   2. Activity intolerance.
   3. Deficient fluid volume.
   4. Risk for injury.

9. A patient with peripheral arterial disease is prescribed a daily dose of aspirin. The nurse accurately explains the prescription by stating:
   1. "Aspirin controls the body temperature to reduce vasoconstriction."
   2. "Aspirin helps prevent formation of clots."
   3. "Aspirin reduces local inflammation."
   4. "Aspirin reduces pain associated with inadequate tissue perfusion."

10. The nurse promotes lifestyle modifications to a 39-year-old man who is diagnosed with prehypertension. Which lifestyle modification(s) should be recommended? *(Select all that apply.)*
    1. Smoking cessation
    2. Restrict sodium intake to 4000 mg/day
    3. Exercise 30 minutes per day most days of the week
    4. Limit alcohol intake to two drinks per day
    5. Low-fat diet
    6. Stress reduction measures

Critical Thinking Activities

Scenario A
Mrs. Dunn is being discharged from the hospital after being treated for arterial insufficiency in both lower extremities. Her physician requests that Mrs. Dunn receive instruction in the care of her feet and legs before discharge.

1. What findings do you expect on physical examination of Mrs. Dunn's legs?
2. What medication and treatment do you expect the physician to prescribe? Why are these prescribed?
3. List five priority teaching points for Mrs. Dunn.

Scenario B
Ms. Yao, age 27, developed a DVT in her left thigh after surgery to repair a fractured right femur. She is receiving heparin IV and will begin enoxaparin subcutaneously the following morning.

1. Describe the pathophysiology of DVT. How does Ms. Yao's diagnosis relate to development of DVT?
2. Identify essential information you need to safely administer the medications prescribed.
3. Develop a teaching plan for Ms. Yao.

Scenario C
Mr. Tompkins, age 66, who is hypertensive and only recently quit smoking, has been diagnosed with a 3-cm abdominal aortic aneurysm.

1. What treatment would you expect for him?
2. What signs and symptoms of complications would you teach him?
3. What measures could he take to help prevent the aneurysm from growing and rupturing?

Care of Patients with Cardiac Disorders

Objectives

Theory

1. Compare left-sided and right-sided heart failure.
2. Describe the nursing assessment specific to the patient who is admitted with heart failure.
3. Identify life-threatening heart rhythms from a selection of cardiac rhythm strips.
4. Describe usual treatment for atrial fibrillation, third-degree heart block, and ventricular tachycardia.
5. Discuss how nursing interventions for patients with a valvular disorder differ from those for a patient with a cardiac dysrhythmia.
6. State nursing responsibilities in the administration of cardiac drugs.
7. Describe under what circumstances cardiac surgery is appropriate treatment.

8. Discuss the nurse's role in caring for patients with heart disorders in the long-term care facility or the home.
9. Develop a teaching plan with dietary recommendations for heart disease.

Clinical Practice

1. Develop a plan of care for a patient who has heart failure.
2. Perform a basic physical assessment on a patient who has a mitral valve stenosis and dysrhythmia.
3. Use the nursing process to care for assigned patients who have cardiovascular disorders.
4. Safely administer medications for patients with cardiac disorders.
5. Provide support to patients undergoing diagnostic testing and treatment for cardiac disorders.
6. Develop a teaching plan for patients with cardiac disorders.

Key Terms

ablation (ăb-LĀ-shŭn, p. 442)
arrhythmia (ă-RĬTH-mē-ă, p. 435)
atrial fibrillation (p. 437)
cardiac tamponade (KĂR-dē-ăk tăm-pŏn-ĀD, p. 443)
cardiomyopathy (kăr-dē-ō-mī-ŏp-ă-thē, p. 444)
cardioversion (kăr-dē-ō-VĔR-zhŭn, p. 440)
dysrhythmia (dĭs-RĬTH-mē-ă, p. 435)
effusion (ĕ-FŪ-zhŭn, p. 443)

ejection fraction (p. 428)
endocarditis (ĔN-dō-kăhr-DĪ-tĭs, p. 442)
friction rub (FRĬK-shŭn, p. 443)
infarct (ĭn-făhrkt, p. 435)
palpitations (păl-pĭ-TĀ-shŭnz, p. 435)
pericardiocentesis (pĕr-ĭ-KĂR-dē-ō-sĕn-TĒ-sĭs, p. 444)
pericardiotomy (pĕr-ĭ-KĂR-dē-ŏt-ō-mē, p. 444)
pulsus paradoxus (p. 444)

DISORDERS OF THE HEART

HEART FAILURE

There are about 5 million Americans with heart failure (HF), and approximately 670,000 are newly diagnosed each year. Approximately 1 in 100 people will develop HF. The prevalence of HF is increasing and it is a major chronic condition. Half of patients diagnosed with HF will die within 5 years. African Americans have a higher incidence of HF and have higher mortality rates than other populations. Heart failure can occur at any time the heart muscle is prevented from fulfilling its function as a pump and circulator of blood. Heart failure may be acute or chronic, mild or severe. There are four stages of HF classed according to exercise tolerance (Table 20-1).

Etiology

The most common causes of HF are coronary artery disease and uncontrolled hypertension. Other factors that contribute to weakness of the heart muscle are toxins, infection, anemia, myocarditis, dilation from blood backup behind diseased valves, and damage from myocardial infarction (MI) (Concept Map 20-1). Toxins include cocaine, excessive alcohol, certain chemotherapy

 Elder Care Points

Heart failure is the most common reason for hospitalization among adults age 65 or older. As life spans continue to extend, more and more elderly adults will develop HF related to hypertension and CAD.

Table 20-1 Classification of Heart Failure

CLASS	ACTIVITY TOLERANCE
I	Ordinary physical activity with no symptoms
II	Dyspnea with long-distance walking, climbing 2 flights of stairs or strenuous activity
III	Dyspnea and fatigue with short-distance walking or climbing 1 flight of stairs
IV	Dyspnea at rest or with very little activity

Adapted from the New York Heart Association Heart Failure Symptom Classification System. Retrieved from www.clevelandclinicmeded.com/medicalpubs/diseasemanagement/cardiology/heart-failure.

Box 20-1 Factors that Can Precipitate Heart Failure

- Anemia
- Systemic infection (sepsis)
- Fluid overload
- Pulmonary embolism
- Thyroid disorders
- Dysrhythmias
- Pericarditis, myocarditis, or endocarditis
- Thiamine deficiency
- Chronic pulmonary disease
- Physical, emotional, or environmental stress

CONCEPT MAP 20-1 Pathophysiology of HF after an MI.

drugs, nonsteroidal anti-inflammatory drugs (NSAIDs), thiazolidinediones used for diabetes, and doxazosin (Cardura) (Coviello, 2009). Cardiac dysrhythmias also can contribute to HF. (Coronary artery disease [CAD] and MI are covered in Chapter 21, along with cardiac surgery.)

Pathophysiology

The key words to understanding HF are *congestion* and *increased pressure.* Congestion develops because the heart is unable to move blood as quickly as it should.

This may occur because the heart muscle is too weak or because the blood vessels throughout the body are narrowed and constricted (due to atherosclerosis or arteriosclerosis). Therefore the vessels cannot accommodate a normal supply of blood, causing the heart muscle to become exhausted trying to overcome the resistance (pressure) in the vessels. Poorly functioning valves may cause the chambers to dilate from blood backup, causing thinning of the myocardium and decreased pumping ability. Box 20-1 lists factors that precipitate HF.

Elder Care Points

Aging processes also contribute to arteriosclerosis and stiffening of the heart muscle. The combination of high blood pressure, diabetes, and age greatly contributes to the number of older patients who develop HF.

Heart failure may be classified as right-sided HF or left-sided HF. The heart has two pumps: a right-sided and a left-sided pump. The right-sided pump receives blood from the body and pumps it to the lungs for oxygenation. The left-sided pump receives blood from the lungs and pumps it out to the body. Left-sided failure typically occurs first. Normally, the ventricles of the heart contract, while the atria relax, allowing for the filling and emptying of each chamber. If the muscle wall of the left ventricle cannot contract effectively, some of the blood is left in the ventricle—this residual blood prevents part of the blood in the left atrium from progressing into the ventricle. The blood that cannot leave the left atrium prevents the entrance of some blood from vessels, and, in turn, blood backs up into the pulmonary vessels. The pressure within those vessels increases, and fluid leaks into the lung tissue—producing congestion and, eventually, pulmonary edema. If not corrected, left-sided failure, because of the backup of blood and increased pulmonary artery pressure, will soon lead to failure of the right side of the heart. Table 20-2 compares the signs and symptoms of left-sided and right-sided HF.

Primary right-sided heart failure is often caused by chronic pulmonary disease. If the right ventricle does

Table 20-2   Comparison of Left-Sided and Right-Sided Heart Failure

	RIGHT-SIDED HEART FAILURE	LEFT-SIDED HEART FAILURE
Selected etiology	Pulmonary stenosis, pulmonary hypertension Severe emphysema, right ventricular MI	Hypertension, coronary artery disease, MI, mitral or aortic valvular disease
Pathophysiology	Increased pump pressure needed to eject blood into pulmonary arteries. The myocardium of the right atrium and ventricle becomes thickened, and contraction strength weakens	Weakness of the left ventricle resulting in reduced cardiac output and backup of blood into the atrium and the pulmonary system
Signs and symptoms	Fatigue; edema in sacrum, legs, feet, ankles; hepatomegaly; abdominal distention as a result of ascites; weight gain; dyspnea	Fatigue; dyspnea; wheezing; orthopnea; sleep apnea; pulmonary edema (pink, frothy sputum); pallor; clammy skin

MI, myocardial infarction.

not contract as strongly as it should, the ventricle cannot completely empty and becomes engorged with blood. More blood flow into the engorged ventricle causes overfilling and dilation of the chamber, slowing movement of blood out of the atrium. As blood in the atrium backs up, it prevents normal movement of blood flow from the vena cava, thus increasing the pressure in the vena cava, the neck veins, and all other veins of the body.

As the rate of blood flow slows down and pressure in the vessels increases, the fluid from the intravascular fluid compartment begins to leak into the interstitial compartment. This produces retention of fluid and edema. When the right side of the heart fails, the edema is first evident in the lower extremities (*dependent* or *pitting* edema; Figure 20-1). There also is an accumulation of fluid in the liver and abdominal organs, as the portal circulation becomes involved. Congestion of blood flow to and from the kidneys may lead to impaired renal function, preventing normal excretion of urine and causing more accumulation of body fluids. Inadequate circulation to and from the brain may cause mental confusion and irritability, which sometimes progresses to delirium and coma.

The systemic backup of blood that occurs in right-sided HF may eventually lead to left-sided heart failure, as the heart will have to pump against increasing

FIGURE 20-1 Dependent/pitting edema.

pressure in the aorta and systemic circulation. The circulatory system is exactly that: a system. Failure of one component affects the entire system.

 Think Critically

Can you describe the changes that occur with chronic hypertension that may cause heart failure?

Left-sided heart failure is subdivided into systolic and diastolic heart failure. In the cardiac cycle, atria fill and allow blood flow to the ventricles; the ventricles fill and then eject blood into the circulatory system. Different problems cause failure of this process. Here the problems occur in the upper or the lower chambers of the heart.

Systolic Failure. Systolic failure is caused by anything that interferes with ejection of blood from the ventricles. Muscle loss problems from MI, dilated cardiomyopathy, and aortic or pulmonic stenosis may lead to systolic failure.

Diastolic Failure. Diastolic failure occurs when conditions prevent the filling of the heart with blood. Tricuspid and mitral stenosis, cardiac tamponade, or constrictive cardiomyopathy can cause diastolic failure. Decreased filling results in decreased stroke volume and cardiac output. Ejection fraction is normal in primary diastolic failure. Ejection fraction is the percentage of the filling volume pumped out with ventricular contraction. A hallmark of diastolic failure is neck vein (jugular) distention.

Think Critically

Can you explain to a patient in simple terms what happens in the body when systolic HF occurs?

Signs, Symptoms, and Diagnosis

Initially, compensatory mechanisms prevent symptoms of HF. Heart rate rises to increase output and the ventricles hypertrophy in order to pump out more blood with each contraction. In left-sided failure compensatory mechanisms eventually weaken the heart and the blood backs up into the pulmonary vessels, pressure within those vessels increases, and fluid leaks into the lung tissue, producing congestion. Fatigue and shortness of breath (SOB) are first noticed with activity and when lying down. If failure progresses, pulmonary edema occurs. Diagnosis is made on the basis of history, examination, signs and symptoms, chest x-ray, echocardiogram, electrocardiogram (ECG), magnetic resonance imaging (MRI), electrolytes, complete blood count (CBC), and brain natriuretic peptide (BNP). BNP measures the level of a protein released when myocardial cells are stretched. A level greater than 500 pg/mL is consistent with HF when other symptoms are present (see Table 20-2).

Advanced systolic HF signs are S_3 and S_4 heart sounds. Weight gain of 2 lb in 24 hours or 5 lb in 1 week occurs as fluid is retained. Dyspnea and crackles or wheezes are heard in the lungs.

> **[?] Think Critically**
>
> You auscultate the lung sounds of a patient with HF. You hear crackles. Which side of the heart is failing?

Treatment

Treatment of the underlying cause of HF should be initiated. Dysrhythmias are controlled. Surgical correction of valve or septal abnormalities may reverse HF.

Medical treatment is largely symptomatic and depends on the type and degree of HF present. Drugs and other therapies are used to reduce or eliminate the symptoms and complications of HF, but they only control the condition; they do not cure it. Efforts are made to (1) reduce the demand for oxygen and the workload of the heart; (2) strengthen the heart's pumping action; (3) relieve venous congestion in the lungs; and (4) minimize sodium and water retention in the tissues (Jessup et al., 2009).

To accomplish the goals of medical intervention, the following may be prescribed:

- Angiotensin-converting enzyme (ACE) inhibitors and angiotensin-receptor blockers (ARBs) decrease the workload of the heart by causing vasodilation; as a result, blood pressure is reduced (Table 20-3). ACE inhibitors and ARBs also play a role in reducing fluid retention.
- Beta-adrenergic blockers (e.g., metoprolol [Toprol XL]) are used to slow the heart rate if tachycardia is causing the HF, thereby decreasing oxygen demand. Beta blockers are used cautiously as they can also cause HF.
- Diuretics, especially loop diuretics, are prescribed to reduce fluid retention in the lungs and lower extremities. Watch for ototoxicity with these drugs. Thiazide diuretics such as hydrochlorothiazide (Diuril) may also be prescribed.

Table 20-3   Drugs Used to Treat Heart Failure*

CLASSIFICATION	EXAMPLES	USE

Diuretics
  Loop
  Potassium sparing
  Thiazide
	
	Furosemide (Lasix), bumetanide (Bumex)
	Triamterene (Dyrenium), amiloride (Midamor)
	Hydrochlorothiazide
		Remove excess fluid
		
		Remove fluid but not potassium
		Removes fluid but wastes potassium

Angiotensin-converting enzyme inhibitors	Enalapril (Vasotec), captopril (Capoten), lisinopril (Zestril)	Prevent vasoconstriction
Angiotensin-receptor blockers	Losartan (Cozaar), valsartan (Diovan), irbesartan (Avapro)	Produce vasodilation and salt and water excretion
Beta-adrenergic blockers	Atenolol (Tenormin), metoprolol (Lopressor), nadolol (Corgard)	Reduce blood pressure
Calcium channel blockers	Amlodipine (Norvasc), diltiazem (Cardizem), nifedipine (Procardia), verapamil (Calan)	Vasodilation and reduced heart rate
Vasodilators (nitrates)	Nitroglycerine (Nitrostat, Nitro-Bid), isosorbide (Isordil), nitroprusside (Nipride)	Dilate blood vessels; decrease preload and relieve shortness of breath; relieve myocardial ischemia
BNP analog	Nesiritide (Natrecor)	Alleviate dyspnea
Inotropics Beta-adrenergic agonists	 Dobutamine (Dobutrex), dopamine (Intropin)	 Increase cardiac contractility and cardiac output
Phosphodiesterase inhibitors Digitalis	Milrinone (Primacor) Digoxin	Reduce preload and afterload; vasodilation; increase cardiac contractility

BNP, brain natriuretic peptide.
*The choice of drugs depends on the type of heart failure and whether the left ventricle function is normal.
See Table 19-3, Box 19-1, and Table 20-4 for further information and nursing implications for these drugs.

Measures are taken to prevent electrolyte imbalances from the use of these drugs.

- Digitalis is occasionally used to increase the force of heart contraction (i.e., an inotropic agent) and slow the rate, thereby increasing cardiac output. The most commonly used drug in this category is digoxin (Lanoxin). Several large doses of the drug are given initially, followed by a lower, regular-maintenance dosage. This drug is not recommended for elderly white women because it increases mortality rates in this group.
- Venous vasodilators such as isosorbide dinitrate (Isordil) and nitroglycerin (NTG), which relax and dilate blood vessels, allow the vessels to accommodate larger percentages of the total blood volume.
- Morphine is prescribed if pulmonary edema is present to relieve anxiety and make breathing easier.
- Benzodiazepines may be used for anxiety and reduction of emotional stress.
- Limited physical activity or bed rest in semi-Fowler's or high Fowler's position.
- Oxygen therapy.
- Lifestyle modifications, including regular exercise as tolerated, and possible limitation of sodium intake to 2 to 3 g/day; in severe cases, restriction of fluid intake (Heart Failure Society of America, 2009).
- Dobutamine (Dobutrex) or milrinone (Primacor) may be used intravenously (IV) for acute HF to improve cardiac contractility.

⬤ Nutrition Considerations

Guidelines for a Heart-Healthy Diet

- Limit foods high in saturated fat, *trans* fat, and cholesterol. Limit meat intake to no more than 6 oz of cooked *lean* meat, and skinless poultry (singly or in combination) per day. Fix main dishes with pasta, rice, beans, or vegetables mixed with small amounts of lean meat, poultry, or fish to create "low-meat" dishes. Restrict intake of organ meats, such as liver, brains, chitterlings, kidney, gizzards, and sweetbreads, as they are very high in cholesterol.
- Avoid as much *trans* fat as possible. Read product labels. Limit food high in saturated fat, including tropical oils and partially hydrogenated vegetable oils.
- Cook using little or no fat; broil, bake, roast, poach, stir fry, microwave, or steam foods rather than frying them.
- Eliminate as much fat as possible by trimming meat and skinning poultry before cooking. After browning meats, drain off all fat. Chill soups, stews, and so on, and then skim off fat before reheating to serve.
- Use fats with no more than 2 g of saturated fat per tablespoon. Olive, canola, corn, or safflower oil and liquid and tub margarines are good choices.
- Eat fish at least twice a week. Fatty fish such as salmon, mackerel, and tuna are best.

- Eat five to seven servings of fruit and vegetables per day. Use fresh or frozen vegetables and fresh fruit or fruit canned in juice rather than high-fructose corn syrup.
- Increase intake of fiber and carbohydrate by eating six or more servings of whole-grain products, such as cereals and breads, per day. Check labels to see that the product really contains *whole* grains.
- Use skim or 1% fat milk and nonfat or low-fat yogurt, cheeses, and ice creams.
- Limit consumption of egg yolks to three or four per week, including those in baked or cooked items. Check store packages for listing of eggs or egg yolk as an ingredient.
- Eat less than 1500 mg of salt (sodium chloride) per day.
- Have no more than one alcoholic drink per day if you are a woman and no more than two per day if you are a man. Examples of one drink are 12 oz of beer, 4 oz of wine, or 1½ oz of 80-proof spirits.

Note: The heart-healthy diet is promoted by the American Heart Association.

Other treatments may include:

- The pumping action of the atria and ventricles may be synchronized for more efficient pumping by use of the *biventricular pacemaker.* This procedure is cardiac resynchronization therapy (CRT), in which wires attached to an impulse generator are placed in the heart to send electrical impulses to the right and left ventricles. It is the treatment of choice when drug therapy does not control HF.
- A left ventricular assist device (LVAD) may be used to help with the heart's pumping action. This device is implanted in the patient's abdomen and attached to the heart. These devices have proven to be beneficial to adults diagnosed with severe HF. The device may be used while the patient is awaiting transplant and, with continued research, may possibly eliminate the need for transplant in some patients (Figure 20-2).

FIGURE 20-2 Heartmate left ventricular assist device.

- Surgery to reduce the size of an enlarged heart (ventricular restoration surgery) may be effective for some patients. The less effective portions of the left ventricle are removed and the remaining muscle is reattached and shaped to form a more efficient pump. Sometimes the heart enlarges again.
- Heart transplant may be the only alternative for patients with advanced HF who do not respond to other medical or drug treatment. Heart transplant is discussed in Chapter 21.
- At least one herb is thought to be helpful for heart failure.

▨ Complementary and Alternative Therapies

Hawthorn Use in Heart Failure and Coronary Artery Disease

The herb hawthorn is thought to improve performance of damaged myocardial tissue and to improve myocardial perfusion. Hawthorn is said to reduce the symptoms of mild to moderate HF. Hawthorn should be used cautiously in the elderly. Hawthorn may increase hypotension when used in combination with antihypertensive drugs. This herb may increase the effects of cardiac glycosides. Cardiovascular status should be monitored closely (Heart Center Online, 2007).

Short-term treatment for HF after an MI or open heart surgery is accomplished with the intraaortic balloon pump (IABP). The IABP is positioned in the descending aorta. The IABP is designed to increase blood supply to the myocardium and allow it to rest. The balloon will inflate during diastole, thus increasing perfusion to the coronary arteries. The balloon deflates during systole, making it easier for the left ventricle to eject blood (Figure 20-3).

FIGURE 20-3 Intraaortic balloon pump. Balloon is inflated during diastole. Balloon is deflated at beginning of systole to decrease afterload.

Acute Pulmonary Edema. Acute pulmonary edema is a medical emergency that must be treated promptly. The patient with this condition has severe dyspnea; a cough productive of frothy, pink-tinged sputum; tachycardia; and moist, bubbling respirations with cyanosis. Nursing interventions for acute pulmonary edema include placing the patient in high Fowler's position to relieve the dyspnea; administering oxygen, diuretics, morphine, and other prescribed drugs; limiting and monitoring activity; and assessing cardiopulmonary status.

❖ NURSING MANAGEMENT

▪ Assessment (Data Collection)

The effects of HF can range from very mild to extremely serious. A thorough nursing assessment can help identify specific patient care problems. Data guide the physician in the evaluation of the patient's response to medical treatment and the decision to continue or change prescribed drugs and other therapies. It is important to ask the patient if her clothes, rings, or shoes fit tighter than previously, indicating edema. Is pedal edema worsening or improving? Obtain an accurate weight. What has the trend of weight been? Feelings of breathlessness or having to catch the breath in midsentence may indicate fluid in the lungs and left-sided HF. Are crackles present in the lungs? Inquire how much activity causes SOB. Does the patient have paroxysmal nocturnal dyspnea (wakes up at night with SOB)? Ask about medication compliance and any problems or side effects noted. Assess the diet to determine usual sodium, fat, and calorie intake and obtain a smoking history.

▨ Clinical Cues

For the patient who has been diagnosed with HF, but is well controlled *(compensated)*, it is very important to weigh daily at home and to write down the weight. If the patient can see that fluid weight gain is occurring, she may be able to avert a trend back into *decompensated* HF by adjusting diuretic medication, lowering sodium intake, treating infection, and decreasing activity and resting.

Significant Findings Indicating Heart Failure Is Occurring

Left-Sided Failure
- Increasing fatigue
- Dyspnea and a dry, hacking cough.
- Crackles heard on auscultation of the lungs.
- Pale, cool, and clammy skin, which are signs of poor peripheral circulation.
- Diminished peripheral pulses.
- Dizziness, confusion, restlessness, and difficulty concentrating and remembering due to diminished blood flow to the brain.
- Gradually increasing heart rate, even when the patient is at rest; increased heart rate occurs when

the heart attempts to remove blood from a distended ventricle.
- Extra heart sound (S_3, S_4).
- Decreased blood pressure as ventricle fails.

Right-Sided Failure
- Weight gain without a change in caloric intake.
- Dependent, pitting edema (assess feet and ankles in ambulatory patient or one sitting up most of the time). Assess thighs and sacral region in patient confined to bed. Patient may feel "bloated" and experience a loss of appetite and nausea due to diminished venous return from abdominal organs, liver enlargement resulting from increased pressure in the portal veins, edema in the intestine, and accumulations of fluid in the abdominal cavity.
- Jugular venous distention; visible jugular vein pulsation more than 4.5 cm above the clavicle when patient is in semi-Fowler's position. Complaint of feeling "warm" when others are comfortably cool because of vasoconstriction and poor circulation, which prevents removal of body heat.
- Reduced urinary output, which reflects the kidney's response to poor perfusion by retaining sodium and water.
- Blood pressure increased from fluid overload.

 Elder Care Points

Elderly patients who have little cardiac reserve can be at risk for HF from any condition that increases the body's demand for blood or oxygen. Pneumonia, generalized infection, severe trauma, or other conditions that increase the metabolic rate and demand for oxygen can be the precipitating factor, because the heart that is already having difficulty meeting normal body oxygen demands cannot respond. When the elderly patient has an infection, carefully assess the lungs for signs of crackles that might indicate beginning HF. Your quick action can save the patient from considerable problems. Assess urinary output of elderly patients. Renal function is decreased due to the aging process. Loss of perfusion related to HF will place the patient at greater risk of renal insufficiency or failure.

■ Nursing Diagnosis and Planning

The main nursing diagnoses for the patient with HF are listed in Nursing Care Plan 20-1 (see also Table 18-4). Plan extra time when caring for the patient with HF because fatigue, possible lack of mobility, and oxygen deficit cause the patient to move slowly and need more time to accomplish the activities of daily living. Specific outcome criteria are written for each individual's nursing diagnoses.

 Nursing Care Plan 20-1   Care of the Patient with Heart Failure

Scenario
Miguel Garcia, age 60, is admitted to the nursing unit with exacerbation of left- and right-sided heart failure. Physical examination reveals 3+ pitting edema of the right lower extremity and 4+ pitting edema of the left lower extremity. He is in acute respiratory distress and is positioned in high Fowler's to facilitate breathing. He has oxygen per simple mask at 8 L/min. T 98° F (36.6° C), P 96, R 28, BP 160/90, Po$_2$ 90%, Wt. 255 (20-lb increase).

Problem/Nursing Diagnosis
Dyspnea/Impaired gas exchange related to fluid in lung tissue, Po$_2$ 90% on 8 L oxygen.

Supporting Assessment Data
Subjective: States has difficulty breathing while lying down.
Objective: Po$_2$ 90%, elevated respiratory rate, sitting up to facilitate breathing.

Goals/Expected Outcomes	Nursing Interventions	Selected Rationale	Evaluation
Po$_2$ 95% on room air.	Assess vital signs and Spo$_2$ q 2 hr. Report increase in respiratory rate or decrease in oxygen saturation.	Change in vital signs and oxygen saturation may indicate improvement or deterioration of condition.	Spo$_2$ remains within 93%-95%. The respiratory rate is 12-22/min. The heart rate remains between 60 and 100.
	Increase oxygen to maintain Spo$_2$ at level specified by physician.	Maintain oxygen saturation at levels that indicate effective gas exchange.	Spo$_2$ 94%. O$_2$ at 5 L/min.
	Assess lung sounds at least q 4 hr.	Changes in lung sounds indicate positive response to therapy or need to modify treatment plan.	Lung sounds clear on right, fine crackles on left.
	Maintain high Fowler's position as needed for comfort.	Promotes optimum expansion of thoracic cavity to facilitate breathing and improve gas exchange.	Head of bed at 45 degrees. Continue plan.
	Teach patient pursed-lip breathing.		

Problem/Nursing Diagnosis
Fatigue: unable to complete activities of daily living without assistance/Activity intolerance related to fluid in lungs, fluid retention in lower extremities.

Supporting Assessment Data
Subjective: States feet have become more swollen over the past 3 days.
Objective: Pitting edema both lower extremities, dyspnea on exertion, crackles in bases bilaterally.

Goals/Expected Outcomes	Nursing Interventions	Selected Rationale	Evaluation
Patient will be able to complete activities of daily living and personal hygiene without fatigue.	Assess activity tolerance. Assist with personal hygiene initially. Monitor oxygen saturation. Provide frequent rest periods. Coordinate care with other health care providers to conserve energy.	Provide guideline for planning care activities. Conserve patient energy. Avoid overtiring by scheduling activities to maximize energy use. Prevents fatigue.	Able to complete partial bath. Becomes fatigued, requires assistance. Patient remains fatigued. Continue plan; reassess readiness to meet goals.

Problem/Nursing Diagnosis
Fluid retention lower extremities, crackles in lung fields/Fluid volume excess related to pulmonary and venous congestion.

Supporting Assessment Data
Subjective: Patient reports nonproductive cough.
Objective: 3–4+ edema both lower extremities; crackles in lung bases on auscultation.

Goals/Expected Outcomes	Nursing Interventions	Selected Rationale	Evaluation
Lung fields will be clear, pitting edema in lower extremities 0–1+.	Assess lung sounds q 4 hr. Assess lower extremities each shift. Administer diuretics as prescribed by the physician. Maintain accurate intake and output. Daily weights.	Identifies changes in condition. Identifies effectiveness of drug therapy. To reduce fluid retention through diuresis. Identify positive or negative response to treatment.	Fine crackles on auscultation. Less distress. 2+ pitting edema bilaterally. Urinary output 2500 mL q 8 hr. Continue plan. Weight 245 lb.

Critical Thinking Questions
1. List three additional nursing diagnoses that are appropriate for this patient.
2. List five items to be included in the discharge teaching plan for this patient.
3. What assessment data might indicate a worsening of this patient's condition?
4. What assessment data might indicate improvement of this patient's condition?

■ Implementation

Heart failure is a chronic disease. Patients with mild HF may not be hospitalized, but they do require instruction in self-care. Instruction includes balancing rest with physical activity, limiting sodium intake, and following other dietary restrictions. The entire family should be included in dietary teaching. Teach self-administration of medications and awareness of adverse side effects that must be reported. Review the dangers of drug-drug interaction when taking nonprescription drugs, particularly NSAIDs. Reconcile medications. Immunize the patient against seasonal flu and pneumonia. Modify lifestyle, as needs indicate (diet, smoking, physical activity). Teach symptoms that should be reported to the physician if they become worse or appear for the first time. An objective of *Healthy People 2020* is to reduce hospitalizations of elderly adults with HF as the principal diagnosis. Thorough patient teaching and nursing follow-up helps achieve this objective.

Patient Teaching

Instructions for the Patient Taking Warfarin (Coumadin)

Teach the patient who has been prescribed warfarin to:

- Take Coumadin at the same time every day.
- Keep appointments for international normalized ratio (INR) blood test or perform the test at home.
- Take a missed dose as soon as it is remembered on the day it is due. Do not double up on the dose the next day if the previous dose was totally forgotten.
- Check all medications, all over-the-counter preparations, and all herbs for interactions with Coumadin.
- Wear a Medic-Alert bracelet stating you take Coumadin. Carry a wallet ID card indicating Coumadin use.
- Tell all medical personnel that Coumadin is being taken.
- Foods containing vitamin K should be eaten consistently in the diet week to week; asparagus, beans, broccoli, cabbage, spinach, cauliflower, Brussels sprouts, kale, and mustard greens are high in vitamin K and should not be eaten in large quantities. Fish, rice, and yogurt also contain vitamin K.
- Avoid consuming more than one or two drinks of alcohol per day.
- Use an electric razor if prone to nicking the skin when shaving.
- Use a soft toothbrush.
- Blow the nose gently.
- Report unusual bleeding or bruising to the physician.
- Report signs of intestinal bleeding and blood in the urine.

Elder Care Points

The elderly patient who is experiencing HF often is taking many medications. With decreased kidney function, it is especially important to look for drug interactions and to monitor for signs and symptoms of toxicity. Loop diuretics continue to work even after excess fluid is eliminated. Monitor the elderly patient for signs of dehydration such as decreased urine output and confusion.

It is of vital importance to monitor patients with HF for electrolyte imbalances, especially imbalance of sodium or potassium. **Electrolyte imbalances may cause serious cardiac dysrhythmias** (MayoClinic.com, 2011).

Patients with chronic HF will need encouragement to follow the prescribed regimen. A chronic disease management program is advised (Willacy, 2011). If treatment does not stop the progress of the disease, the patient may be admitted to the hospital for reevaluation and a change in therapies. Sometimes the patient's heart continues to fail in spite of aggressive therapy, and pulmonary edema, liver, and renal failure occur.

Think Critically

Why does weighing the patient daily help you evaluate the treatment for HF? How would you know that the treatment is not effective?

Assisting the hospitalized patient with activities of daily living will decrease oxygen demand. Scheduling all activities to promote as much rest as possible is a high priority. Activity is alternated with rest throughout the day. Several pillows may be required to achieve a comfortable bed position. Accurate recording of intake and output is very important. Daily weight is recorded at the same time each day, preferably before breakfast. Careful attention to turning and skin care is essential, as edematous tissue breaks down easily. Particular attention should be given to the sacral area due to pressure points of the patient on bed rest. Bed rest causes venous pooling, and active or passive leg exercises should be performed every 1 to 2 hours to help prevent thrombosis. Elastic stockings or sequential compression devices to prevent venous pooling may be prescribed. Careful ongoing physical assessment is essential. Nursing interventions for selected problems in a patient with HF are summarized in Nursing Care Plan 20-1. Box 20-2 presents the Joint Commission's Core Measures for HF. Instructional materials regarding smoking cessation are sent home with all smokers and they are counseled about the importance of quitting smoking (Joint Commission, 2009). Discharge instructions include (1) activity level, (2) diet, (3) discharge medication, (4) follow-up appointment, (5) weight monitoring, and (6) what to do if symptoms worsen.

HF patients with left ventricular dysfunction (ejection fraction <40%) should receive a prescription for an ACE inhibitor or an ARB medication. Providing education about warning signs of worsening condition (decompensation), exercise needs, diet compliance, and lifestyle changes greatly helps symptom control (Willacy, 2011).

■ Evaluation

The patient with HF requires extensive treatment with medication and lifestyle changes. Evaluate objective and subjective data to determine if expected outcomes are being met. Note subjective data related to activity tolerance, respiratory status, comfort, and understanding of teaching related to the disease process and self-management. Understanding of the medication regimen is key to the patient's progress. The cardiovascular system should be monitored for improvement

---

Box 20-2 | **The Joint Commission Core Measures for Heart Failure**

These topics are to be addressed before discharge:
- Discharge instructions
- Evaluation of left ventricular function
- ACE inhibitor or ARB for left ventricular systolic dysfunction
- Smoking cessation advice/counseling

Retrieved from www.jointcommission.org/assets/1/6/Heart%20Failure.pdf. *ACE,* angiotensin-converting enzyme; *ARB,* angiotensin receptor blocker.

of status. Observe the patient for the improvement of symptoms including edema, respiratory quality, and activity tolerance. Improvement is an indication of patient progress.

CARDIAC CONDUCTION DISORDERS (DYSRHYTHMIAS)

A normal heart generates electrical impulses that are essential to contraction of the heart's ventricles and atria. If impulses are not generated normally, an abnormal heart rhythm occurs. The goal for the beginning nurse is to be able to determine when the tracing is not a normal sinus rhythm.

Etiology

Alterations in the conduction of cardiac electrical impulses that create heart rate and rhythm may occur due to congenital abnormalities, electrolyte disturbances, too much caffeine, illegal drug use, stress, and medication side effects. Valvular disorders, damage to the heart from **infarct** (area of necrosis caused by ischemia), thyroid problems, infective endocarditis, and problems in the autonomic nervous system also cause conduction disorders.

Pathophysiology

The sinoatrial (SA) node generates impulses 60 to 100 times per minute. Each impulse travels through the atria to the atrioventricular (AV) node, which relays the impulse via the bundle of His and the Purkinje fibers to the ventricles, causing them to contract (Figure 20-4). Box 20-3 provides the procedure for evaluating an ECG strip. If the SA node fails to produce an electrical impulse, the AV node will initiate an impulse at 40 to 60 beats per minute. If neither the SA nor the AV node is functioning, the Purkinje fibers in the ventricles will initiate an impulse at a slower rate. When

| Box 20-3 | Evaluating an ECG Rhythm Strip |

- Obtain a strip with at least 10 large graph squares.
- Calculate the rate. Count the number of 0.2-sec divisions between two consecutive QRS complexes and divide this into 300 to determine the rate. For irregular rhythms, count the number of cycles or complexes in 6 sec and multiply by 10.
- Measure the distance between the P waves. Is the distance the same? If so, the rate is regular. Calculate the atrial rate by counting the number of small boxes between the P waves and dividing that number into 1500. If the atrial rate is irregular, are there premature atrial beats?
- Measure the P-R interval. Is it normal (0.12–0.20 sec)? Does it vary?
- Measure the QRS duration. Is it normal (0.04–0.12 sec)? Measure with calipers from R wave to R wave throughout the tracing to determine whether the rate is regular. Are there premature QRS complexes? Do all the QRS complexes look the same? Calculate the ventricular rate by counting the number of small squares between R waves and dividing that number into 1500. Are the atrial and ventricular rates the same? A rough calculation can be made by counting the number of complexes in a 6-sec tracing and multiplying by 10.

there is disruption of the normal electrical conduction in the heart, abnormal heart rhythm occurs. This is called an **arrhythmia** or **dysrhythmia.**

Signs and Symptoms

Normal pulse rate is 60 to 100 beats per minute (bpm). Figure 20-5 shows the ECG pattern of normal sinus rhythm. A pulse below 60 indicates *bradycardia*, one type of dysrhythmia. Bradycardia may drop cardiac output enough to cause the patient to have symptoms of decreased blood flow. Athletes often have a bradycardia without a pathologic condition. Symptomatic bradycardia is treated with atropine or a pacemaker.

If the heart rate rises above 100, the patient has a dysrhythmia known as *tachycardia*. When the heart beats this fast, the ventricles do not have adequate time to fill with blood and therefore cannot pump effectively. As a result, cardiac output falls. Sinus tachycardia with a rate of 100 to 150 bpm can be caused by pain, fever, stress, hypovolemia, or hypoxia. It is usually managed by treating the underlying condition. If removing the underlying cause does not correct the problem, a beta blocker may be prescribed.

When the heart's electrical conduction system fails, adequate blood is not pumped out to the body. Symptoms the patient may experience include dizziness, **palpitations** (abnormally rapid throbbing or fluttering of the heart), fatigue, chest pain, and loss of consciousness; death may occur. The severity of the symptoms depends on whether the abnormal rhythm is atrial or ventricular in origin, the amount of cardiac output, and whether the dysrhythmia is persistent.

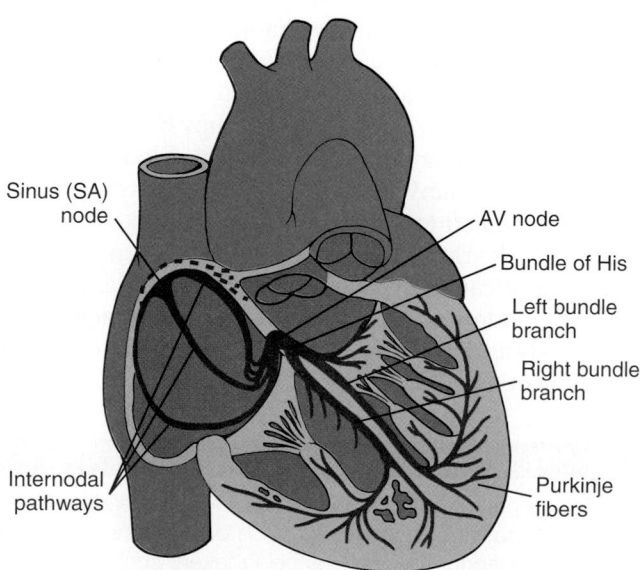

Sinus (SA) node
AV node
Bundle of His
Left bundle branch
Right bundle branch
Internodal pathways
Purkinje fibers

FIGURE 20-4 Cardiac conduction system.

FIGURE 20-5 ECG tracing of normal sinus rhythm.

Premature atrial contraction (PAC) happens when an ectopic electrical focus fires before the next SA node impulse is due, thereby depolarizing the atria. An abnormally shaped P wave appears on the ECG before the QRS wave. The impulse is routed to the AV node and then to the ventricles causing ventricular contraction. The PAC is followed by a compensatory pause. The heart rhythm will be slightly irregular. PACs are common and do not often produce symptoms. PACs result from sympathetic nervous system stimulation as occurs with anxiety, hypoxia, or ischemia.

Supraventricular tachycardia (SVT) is a rhythm that originates in or above the bundle of His. SVTs include sinus tachycardia, atrial flutter, and atrial fibrillation. The rate will be greater than 100 bpm.

In *first-degree heart block* impulse conduction between the atrium and the ventricle is lengthened beyond 0.2 seconds. The P-R interval is consistently greater than 0.2 seconds. First-degree block can be temporary or permanent. It often occurs after open heart surgery or an MI. Digoxin, calcium channel blockers, and beta blockers may cause this arrhythmia.

Second-degree heart block (Mobitz I or Wenckebach) displays on the ECG with normal P-R interval followed by increasingly lengthened P-R intervals until a P wave appears without a QRS complex because the impulse was not conducted to the ventricles. The cycle then begins again after the AV node has rested for that one beat. Parasympathetic tone or drug effect from digoxin, calcium channel blockers, or beta blockers is the culprit. The arrhythmia is most often transient and rarely progresses to third-degree heart block; it is considered benign.

Type II second-degree block (Mobitz II) is a more severe heart block. The AV node blocks certain beats through to the ventricles in a fixed ratio. Every second or third impulse is blocked. The P-R interval is constant throughout. The atrial rate may be two, three, or possibly four times the ventricular rate. The rhythm can be regular or irregular. This rhythm is dangerous as it may progress to third-degree heart block and is most often due to ischemia. This arrhythmia often occurs after open heart surgery. Bradycardia may be the result and the patient may or may not be symptomatic depending on the ventricular rate. If the patient is symptomatic, a temporary transvenous pacemaker may be inserted followed by a permanent pacemaker if needed.

There are many types of cardiac dysrhythmias. Nurses assigned to a coronary care unit take a special course in dysrhythmia recognition to learn the patterns, significance, and treatment of each type. Cardiac arrest is evidenced by a straight-line ECG tracing. All nurses should be able to recognize life-threatening dysrhythmias.

Clinical Cues

Any time a person notices an irregular or rapid heartbeat, ask how much caffeine is consumed each day. If consumption is minimal, ask about medications being taken, such as decongestants. Ask about the person's stress levels. The problem may disappear when the precipitating factor is removed.

Life-Threatening Cardiac Dysrhythmias

Atrial Flutter/Fibrillation. The atrial depolarization occurs at 250 to 350 times a minute causing ineffective atrial contraction. Only some impulses are conducted to the ventricles with a ventricular response of 60 to 150 bpm; this causes a drop in cardiac output because not as much blood goes to the ventricles to be pumped out to the body (Figure 20-6, *A*). Atrial flutter may occur with high blood pressure, HF, coronary artery disease, hyperthyroidism, or chronic obstructive pulmonary disease (COPD). Impulses in **atrial fibrillation** are from multiple reentry circuits in the atria and occur at rates of 400 or more per minute. The atria do not fully depolarize and instead of atrial contraction there

is quivering. P waves are not visible on the ECG tracing. There are only a lot of tiny, erratic spikes visible. Since the AV node cannot respond to the huge number of impulses, it conducts impulses to the ventricle in an erratic manner resulting in irregular ventricular contractions. The rhythm is *irregularly irregular*. The patient becomes dizzy and short of breath. Treatment is with loading doses of diltiazem (generic) or digoxin, amiodarone, a beta blocker, and calcium channel blockers such as diltiazem. An antidysrhythmic such as quinidine may be added. If drug treatment is unsuccessful, cardioversion is performed to convert to a normal sinus rhythm. A new drug, dronedarone (Multaq), is useful but has serious side effects

FIGURE 20-6 ECG patterns of abnormal and life-threatening dysrhythmias. **A,** Atrial fibrillation. **B,** Premature ventricular contractions. **C,** Complete (third-degree) heart block. **D,** Ventricular tachycardia. **E,** Ventricular fibrillation.

Atrial fibrillation predisposes the patient to clot formation in the atria. Ineffective pumping of the atria allows blood to pool leading to formation of small clots. Patients with chronic atrial fibrillation are usually placed on oral anticoagulant therapy. This medication is taken by the patient at home. Teach the patient the importance of taking the medication as directed by the physician. Dislodged clots can cause an embolus to the lungs, heart, or brain and possibly result in stroke, MI, or death.

Premature Ventricular Contractions.

The premature ventricular impulse originating in the right or left ventricle causes ventricular contractions before the contraction of the atria are complete (Figure 20-6, *B*). Blood is not received from the atria, and so is not added to the ventricular blood that is to be pumped out to the body. The premature ventricular contraction (PVC) appears on the ECG as an early beat without a P wave and with a wide QRS complex. A long pause occurs after the premature beat. The ventricle does not have a chance to fill completely and less blood is pumped out with that beat. The patient perceives a PVC as a skipped beat. An apical and radial pulse deficit may be detected. The ventricular irritability causing PVCs may be from caffeine, drugs, or increased emotional stress. Hypoxia, hypokalemia, and myocardial ischemia may trigger PVCs too. A few PVCs are not abnormal, but when there are more than six or seven in a minute, cardiac output may fall. Dysrhythmia also makes the heart more likely to develop ventricular tachycardia or ventricular fibrillation, if the myocardium is ischemic; this can be life threatening. If PVCs are persistent and symptomatic, antidysrhythmic drugs are used to control them (Table 20-4).

Complete Heart Block.

In complete heart block (third-degree heart block) (Figure 20-6, *C*), separate impulses cause uncoordinated contraction in the atria and in the ventricles. The AV node does not conduct atrial impulses to the ventricles. An "escape" stimulus from the ventricle provides a slow ventricular rhythm. There is noncoordination between the atria and ventricles and blood is not received normally from the atria, which decreases the amount of blood available for pumping out to the body. Cardiac output falls drastically. This dysrhythmia can be life threatening, but it depends on the rate and how the patient is tolerating it. Atropine may be given until a pacemaker can be implanted.

Ventricular Tachycardia.

Ventricular tachycardia (VT) consists of three or more PVCs in a row with a ventricular rate greater than 100 bpm. It is usually caused by cardiac ischemia and the same causes as for PVCs. Cocaine use is another cause. This life-threatening dysrhythmia is generated from one or more focal points in the bundle of His in the ventricle at a very fast rate

Table 20-4 Antidysrhythmic Drug Therapy

CLASSIFICATION AND ACTION	EXAMPLES*	NURSING IMPLICATIONS	PATIENT TEACHING
Class I Antidysrhythmics (Antidysrhythmics)			
Uses: Atrial and ventricular dysrhythmias *Actions:* Slows the sodium channel, prolongs time of depolarization, and increases refractory period	**1A** Quinidine sulfate Procainamide (Pronestyl, Procan) Disopyramide (Norpace) **1B** Lidocaine (Xylocaine) Phenytoin (Dilantin) Tocainamide (Tonocard) Mexiletine (Mexitil) Moricizine (Ethmozine) **1C** Flecainide (Tambocor) Propafenone (Rythmol)	*Quinidine:* monitor for cinchonism: tinnitus, headache, nausea, vertigo, and disturbed vision. Observe for changes in ECG pattern. If patient is taking *digitalis,* monitor for digitalis toxicity as quinidine can double digoxin levels. *Cimetidine* increases effects of *quinidine. Quinidine* may enhance action of anticoagulants. Monitor for diarrhea. Monitor drug level. *Procainamide:* monitor for systemic lupus erythematosus–like syndrome: joint pain; hepatomegaly; unexplained fever; soreness of the mouth, throat, or gums. Discontinue medication if this occurs. Observe for side effects or adverse effects of particular drug administered. Monitor electrolyte levels; watch for postural hypotension, especially if patient is taking antihypertensives.	Instruct to report signs of adverse effects of the drug. Report noticeable changes in cardiac rhythm to the physician. Advise to take quinidine with meals to prevent gastrointestinal (GI) upset. Advise to minimize citrus fruit intake as it changes the urine pH and decreases excretion of quinidine. Procainamide is absorbed best on an empty stomach; if GI upset occurs, take immediately after a meal.

Table 20-4 Antidysrhythmic Drug Therapy—cont'd

CLASSIFICATION AND ACTION	EXAMPLES	NURSING IMPLICATIONS	PATIENT TEACHING
Class II Antidysrhythmics (Beta Blockers)			
Uses: Atrial and ventricular dysrhythmias *Action:* Slows sinoatrial nodal impulses	Propranolol (Inderal) Acebutolol (Sectral) Atenolol (Tenormin) Carvedilol (Coreg) Esmolol (Brevibloc) Nadolol (Corgard) Sotalol (Betapace) Metoprolol (Lopressor, Toprol XL) Esmolol (Brevibloc)	Monitor for signs of congestive heart failure (CHF); monitor pulse and blood pressure, watching for bradycardia and hypotension. Monitor electrolytes. Carefully monitor blood sugar in diabetic patients.	Instruct not to discontinue the drug abruptly. Notify physician if skin rash, confusion, fever, sore throat, or unusual bleeding or bruising occurs. Monitor weight and report gain of >2 lb/wk. Report edema or shortness of breath.
Class III Antidysrhythmics			
Uses: Control supraventricular and ventricular dysrhythmias *Actions:* Increases the refractory period and action potential duration	Amiodarone (Cordarone) Bretylium (Bretylol) Dofetilide (Tikosyn) Ibutilide (Corvert)	Check for drug interactions and for side or adverse effects of specific drug administered. Monitor heart rhythm, blood pressure, and pulse. Monitor renal function.	Instruct to report adverse reactions to specific drug being taken. Advise of need for physician supervision. Report any new heart rhythm irregularities.
Class IV Antidysrhythmics (Calcium Channel Blockers)			
Use: Paroxysmal supraventricular tachycardia (PSVT) *Action:* Converts PSVT to normal sinus rhythm by slowing conduction time through the nodes	Verapamil (Calan, Isoptin, Verelan) Diltiazem (Cardizem)	Monitor heart rate and rhythm; watch for signs of CHF. Observe for hypotension and edema. Use very cautiously with beta blockers.	Instruct to report signs of edema, shortness of breath, or weight gain of >2 lb in 1 wk. Notify physician of new changes in heart rhythm. Explain the rationale for the administration of heparin. For patients receiving oral anticoagulants, instruct about the drug being given; the hazards of hemorrhage; the reason for frequent blood tests, safety precautions, foods that affect clotting, and not to take over-the-counter medications without consulting the physician as they may alter the drug's effect. Warn specifically not to take aspirin or other salicylates.
Other Agents			
	Atropine	Used to raise the heart rate, monitor rate and rhythm.	Explain goal of use.
	Digoxin (Lanoxin)	Monitor heart rate for expected decrease.	Teach signs and symptoms of toxicity: visual changes, anorexia, nausea, vomiting, diarrhea, headache, confusion, new dysrhythmia.
	Adenosine (Adenocard)	Monitor for expected decreased heart rate.	Monitor for dizziness, blurred vision, facial flushing, nausea, dyspnea, bronchospasm, new dysrhythmia, and chest pressure.
	Magnesium	Used to correct digitalis toxicity, to aid in correction of ventricular dysrhythmias, and in cardiac arrest.	Monitor for muscle weakness, flushing, confusion, nausea, cramps, diarrhea, and circulatory collapse.

*Generic drugs are listed first, followed by brand name(s) in parentheses.

(150 to 200 bpm) (Figure 20-6, *D*). VT occurs in bursts, short runs, or as a sustained rhythm. The length of time this rhythm continues and the underlying condition of the heart determine how well the body can tolerate it. The atria do not have a chance to contract and push blood into the ventricles. The ventricles contract too fast to allow time for adequate filling with blood. Cardiac output falls drastically, and death may occur. **The ECG tracing will not tell if the patient has a pulse; feel for the pulse.** VT can quickly deteriorate into ventricular fibrillation or cardiac standstill. Treatment depends on whether the dysrhythmia is sustained and how well the patient is tolerating the rhythm. Intervention with drugs such as amiodarone (Cordarone) is used to stabilize VT. If the patient is symptomatic with changes in BP, pulse, and level of consciousness, the VT is unstable; synchronized cardioversion starting at 100 joules is the treatment. Cardioversion attempts continue at 200 joules and then at 360 joules. If the patient is pulseless, defibrillation is performed. If the patient is not symptomatic, treatment is with oxygen and lidocaine or amiodarone. Procainamide may be started if the dysrhythmia is not resolved.

Ventricular Fibrillation (VF). Ventricular fibrillation (VF) frequently occurs before cardiac arrest. Multiple areas in the ventricles initiate impulses at random, producing a chaotic uncoordinated rhythm. The ventricles quiver rather than contract; there is no cardiac output, and without cardiopulmonary resuscitation (CPR) and defibrillation, death will occur (Figure 20-6, *E*). There is no pulse and no blood pressure. The ECG shows coarse electrical waveforms varying in size and shape. There are no measurable waveforms from which intervals can be determined. Patients who are successfully converted to a rhythm providing adequate cardiac output often will have an automatic implantable cardioverter-defibrillator (AICD) surgically inserted.

Elder Care Points

With age the left ventricle and cardiac valves thicken and the amount of fibrous tissue and fat in the SA node increases, which decreases the number of pacemaker cells the SA node contains. These changes make those older than age 75 more prone to cardiac dysrhythmias as changes occur in the conduction system. Failure of the SA node and the need for a pacemaker occur fairly frequently. Thyroid studies should be performed for patients over age 65 who have atrial fibrillation as thyroid problems can be a cause. Hypothyroidism or hyperthyroidism may also aggravate heart failure.

Diagnosis and Treatment

Disorders of the cardiac conduction system are diagnosed by a 12-lead ECG, by continuous ECG monitoring (Holter monitoring), and by patient history (see Table 18-2). Drug therapy is effective in correcting or controlling dysrhythmias in many cases. A variety of antiarrhythmic agents may be used alone or in combination to regulate the heartbeat (see Table 20-4). Oxygenation, acid-base status, and electrolyte balance are watched carefully and corrected as needed. Deviations from normal limits in any of these areas can precipitate a dysrhythmia. Early recognition and correction of abnormalities decreases life-threatening dysrhythmia (Zipes et. al., 2006).

Cardioversion. Patients who experience supraventricular tachycardia or atrial fibrillation that does not respond to drug therapy may be treated with **cardioversion**. A mild electrical shock is delivered to the heart at a specific time in the cardiac cycle to interrupt the abnormal rhythm and begin a new, normal rhythm of electrical impulse and contraction. The patient is given a sedative before the procedure. Signed consent is required. The procedure may be performed in the cardiac catheterization laboratory, or in the emergency department by the physician. Resuscitation equipment must be at hand. The patient must be monitored for response to treatment, including heart rate, rhythm, and blood pressure.

Cardiac Pacemakers. Cardiac pacemakers may be used to manage chronic and life-threatening dysrhythmias and are used to support heart rate when bradycardia occurs. Advances in pacemaker technology have made available units that are programmable for single- and dual-chambered control. A pacemaker can be used to pace the atria and one or both ventricles. Some units can override a dysrhythmia and keep the heart at a more steady rhythm. There are rate-responsive pacemakers, in which the pacemaker automatically adjusts to the patient's level of activity. When the patient exercises, the heart rate increases (similar to the normal SA node response).

Pacing can be a temporary measure if the problem is an emergent, transient condition, such as drug toxicity. An external pacemaker often is used in the emergency department. A temporary transvenous pacemaker is placed if transient complete heart block (i.e., no impulse travels from the atria to the ventricles) develops after an MI. Transvenous pacemakers are inserted by fluoroscopy with local anesthesia. The leads are attached to an external power source. Patient consent is required, and a sedative is given to the patient before the procedure. Epicardial pacemaker wires are often placed during cardiac surgery for quick use should the patient need to be "paced" in the postoperative period. The wires are brought through the chest wall and are attached to an external power source. When the need for the wires is past, the surgeon will pull them out. A transcutaneous pacemaker is used in an emergency situation and is noninvasive. A transcutaneous pacemaker utilizes two electrode pads and a power source.

One pad is placed on the front of the chest and the other pad is positioned on the back between the spine and the left scapula. It causes uncomfortable muscle contractions as current passes through the chest.

Clinical Cues

The patient is at risk for cardiac tamponade when the pacer wires are pulled. Monitor the patient for signs and symptoms of bleeding into the pericardial sac, including sharp chest pain, dyspnea, hypotension, cyanosis, tachycardia, paradoxical pulse and distended neck veins.

A permanent pacemaker is implanted for SA node dysfunction or heart block. All pacemakers have the same function: to produce effective heartbeats. A permanent pacemaker is inserted in the operating room or cardiac catheterization laboratory to ensure an aseptic environment, even though the procedure is relatively minor (Figure 20-7). The pulse generator is placed in a pocket below the right or left clavicle. Set-rate pacemakers are still used in patients with atrial fibrillation, as sensors have a problem interpreting the chaotic electrical activity of the atrium.

Nursing Management

If inserting a pacemaker is not an emergency procedure, there will be opportunities to assess the patient's knowledge of and feelings about having her heart rate regulated. Assess the patient's learning needs, seek to identify the source of any fear, and gauge the level of anxiety.

? Think Critically

How would you approach discussion with an elderly patient who is fearful of getting a permanent pacemaker?

Both the American Heart Association and the manufacturers of pacemakers provide illustrated booklets to help patients learn more about their cardiac pacers. You can go over these booklets with the patient and perhaps show her a demonstration model and explain how it works to her advantage.

Elder Care Points

Older patients who have SA node disease and resulting cardiac dysrhythmias can achieve a far better quality of life with an implanted pacemaker. Many patients are fearful of the surgery required and can benefit from talking to another patient who has had a successful pacemaker implantation.

Postoperative nursing care for the permanent pacemaker patient includes continuous monitoring of heart rate, rhythm, blood pressure, and temperature. Patients are also monitored for hematoma formation at the site of insertion. Prophylactic antibiotic therapy may be prescribed for a short time. The battery in a pacemaker should last 6 to 9 years, depending on the type, but it can weaken prematurely.

Patient Teaching

Instructions for the Patient with a Permanent Pacemaker

The patient who has a permanent pacemaker implanted should receive these instructions before discharge:
- Avoid lifting the arm and shoulder on the pacemaker side until your physician says you may progress to normal activity. Lifting may dislodge the leads from their positions.
- Keep the incision dry for at least 4 days after the surgery.
- Check for redness, swelling, drainage or fever and report such findings to your physician immediately.
- Refrain from activities that might cause a direct blow to the pacemaker.
- Use a cell or cordless phone on the ear opposite the pacemaker.
- Stay away from high-output electrical generators or large magnets such as a magnetic resonance imager. Such devices can interfere with pacemaker function.
- Monitor your pulse daily and report to the physician if it drops below the set rate.
- Carry a pacemaker information card with you at all times.
- Wear a Medic-Alert bracelet or necklace at all times.
- Keep follow-up appointments with your physician to check the insertion site and to check pacemaker function.
- *Microwave ovens are safe to use, and airport security screening should not cause a problem with the function of the pacemaker. Travel is not restricted.*

FIGURE 20-7 Thoracic placement of permanent pacemaker and transvenous catheter. **A,** Pacemaker. **B,** Placement of pacemaker and wires.

The patient must understand the importance of periodic evaluations of her condition for the rest of her life. Some pacemakers have a telephone monitoring device that allows calling a monitoring station to have the pacemaker checked. Instructions for the use of the pacemaker and monitoring device are included in the owner's manual.

Because of the sensors implanted in the chambers of the heart, the patient is at risk for infection of the lining of the heart (endocarditis). She should be given prophylactic antibiotics before many invasive dental or other procedures.

Radiofrequency Catheter Ablation. When drugs will not control supraventricular or ventricular tachydysrhythmia, the irritable focus can sometimes be destroyed with radiofrequency catheter ablation. Electrophysiologic studies are done in a specially equipped cardiac catheterization laboratory to pinpoint the irritable focus. A specially trained physician then uses radiofrequency waves to destroy the irritable focus via heat and subsequent scarring. The procedure may affect the normal conduction system, requiring the implantation of a permanent pacemaker.

Automatic Implantable Cardioverter-Defibrillators. Automatic implantable cardioverter-defibrillators (AICDs) are used for patients who have repeated episodes of life-threatening ventricular fibrillation or cardiac asystole (arrest). The defibrillator is implanted in the operating room. The pulse generator is larger than for a regular pacemaker. This device monitors the heartbeat and provides an electrical shock similar to that delivered in cardiac defibrillation when a life-threatening rhythm is detected. Most AICDs have the ability to pace as well as defibrillate. The patient is warned to avoid exposure to microwave towers, transformers and electrical transmitters, electrical generators, handheld security devices at airports, and arc welding equipment. The patient should not lean over the alternator of a running car or boat motor.

INFLAMMATORY AND INFECTIOUS DISEASES OF THE HEART

The tissues of the heart are subject to the same inflammatory conditions that affect other parts of the body. The inflammation may be present in the inner lining (endocarditis), the heart muscle (myocarditis), or the sac surrounding the heart (pericarditis). Inflammation may be from an infectious source or from a noninfectious cause.

INFECTIVE ENDOCARDITIS
Etiology
Infective endocarditis (IE) is an infection of the endocardial surface of the heart. It may affect the heart valves, the walls, or a septal defect in the heart. IE

was formerly called bacterial endocarditis (BE), or subacute bacterial endocarditis (SBE), depending on the cause. When the wall of the heart is affected, *myocarditis* is present. Myocarditis is most often caused by the Coxsackie virus, but can be caused by a toxin or inflammation from an autoimmune disorder.

Infective endocarditis may be caused by bacteria, viruses, or fungi. Ports of entry are the oral cavity, particularly with dental procedures, the skin, from surgery or invasive procedures, and from infections in the body. Intravenous drug use with unclean needles is a major cause of endocarditis.

Elder Care Points

In the elderly, systemic infections of the respiratory tract, urinary tract, gastrointestinal tract, or skin often are the causes of endocarditis. The immune system function decreases with age, making the elderly more susceptible to IE. Diagnosis is difficult because symptoms are frequently vague. The aortic valve is most often affected.

Although antibiotics—particularly penicillin—have decreased the incidence of rheumatic fever, the danger is still present. Throat culture should be performed any time there is a question that beta *Streptococcus* A is the organism responsible for a sore throat. If the streptococcal infection is treated early with antibiotics, inflammation in the heart is usually avoided. In susceptible adults circulating microorganisms in the bloodstream may attack the endocardium.

Pathophysiology
The inflamed tissues of the heart become rough and swollen. The inflamed tissue traps organisms. The small deposits that develop on the valves are called *vegetations.* Vegetations decrease the effectiveness of the valve and are frequently the reason for valve replacement. The mitral valve is the most frequent location of infection (Figure 20-8). Vegetations can grow and arterial emboli may occur as pieces of the vegetation break off and travel. Where an embolus lodges depends on the side of the heart from which it emerges. Emboli from the right side of the heart become pulmonary emboli. From the left side of the heart, emboli can lodge in the brain or coronary vessels, or can affect other organs of the body.

Signs, Symptoms, Diagnosis, and Treatment
The signs and symptoms of IE vary considerably. The sedimentation rate and leukocyte count are elevated, and signs of low-grade intermittent fever are evident. A blood culture will be positive. The spleen becomes enlarged. Splinter hemorrhages (thin black lines) can occur under the nails, and there may be petechiae (pinpoint red spots) inside the mouth, in the conjunctivae, and above the clavicles. Echocardiography

FIGURE 20-8 A, Thickening and valve leaflet distortion from infection and inflammation of the endocardium. **B,** Mitral stenosis.

confirms the diagnosis. Fatigue, chills and sweats, malaise, anorexia, muscle aches, and headache may occur.

An existing cardiac murmur may worsen, or a new murmur may appear as a valve is damaged. Cardiac dysrhythmia may appear. There may be complaints of sharp, stabbing chest pain. Cardiac inflammation (endocarditis) may be recurring. Each instance of endocarditis further damages the heart valves. The scar tissue that occurs as the inflammation subsides may cause the valve to leak, resulting in regurgitation (lack of closure), or the valve leaflets may become thickened and calcified, causing narrowing or stenosis. The mitral and aortic valves are most often affected. When mitral or aortic stenosis or regurgitation causes symptoms sufficient to interfere with the patient's usual lifestyle, surgery becomes necessary. Stenosis and regurgitation of cardiac valves may eventually cause heart failure.

Elder Care Points

The valve leaflets thicken with age; this gives rise to the common systolic murmur heard in persons over age 80. This murmur does not indicate cardiac inflammation.

Treatment for IE is with antibiotics for underlying infection. NSAIDs are used to decrease inflammation. Pain medication is provided. Medications for dysrhythmia and heart failure are administered for those complications. Repair of congenital cardiac problems, such as atrial or ventricular septal defect, may be performed.

Safety Alert

Infective Endocarditis

Streptococcus viridans, bacteria found in the mouth, is responsible for about 50% of cases of infective endocarditis. Regular dental care is very important. The health care provider should be advised of all cardiac history before any invasive procedure so that appropriate prophylactic treatment can be provided.

PERICARDITIS

Pericarditis is inflammation of the pericardium (the sac that encloses the heart). Pericarditis may be caused by cancer and its treatment, systemic connective tissue disease, infectious organisms, renal failure, trauma, or tissue damage from an MI. The serous fluids that typically are produced by inflammation may cause an **effusion** (accumulated fluid) in the pericardium. If the effusion becomes large, it can affect the filling of the heart and the cardiac output. Should the fluid become excessive, **cardiac tamponade** may occur as the fluid restricts the filling and pumping of the heart (Figure 20-9). If unresolved, the heart cannot supply the body with needed oxygen and nutrients and death occurs.

Symptoms of pericarditis include fever, tachycardia, chest pain eased by sitting up and leaning forward, dyspnea, and a pericardial **friction rub**. The rub is a high-pitched scratchy sound heard with the diaphragm of the stethoscope placed at the left sternal border at the third intercostal space. The ECG will show changes.

Dressler's syndrome is pericarditis with effusion occurring from inflammation after an MI. It appears 1 to 12 weeks after infarct. When effusion is present, there may be malaise and fatigue related to decreased

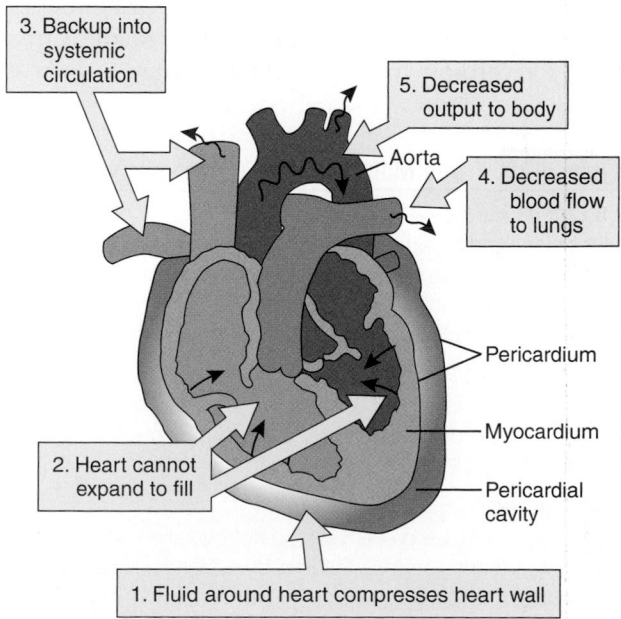

FIGURE 20-9 Effects of pericardial effusion.

cardiac output and decreased perfusion of the tissues with oxygen. Assess for fever, muffled heart sounds, tachycardia, restlessness, anxiety and confusion, distended neck veins, and **pulsus paradoxus**—a drop in systolic blood pressure greater than 10 mm Hg on inspiration. This can be noted when measuring the blood pressure.

Diagnosis of pericarditis is made by history and physical examination and confirmed by ECG, echocardiogram, computed tomography (CT) scan or MRI, and laboratory studies of C-reactive protein (CRP), CBC, and erythrocyte sedimentation rate (ESR). **Pericardiocentesis** will be performed at the bedside if effusion is interfering with cardiac output. The fluid extracted is analyzed to determine a cause of the inflammation. Restrictive pericarditis may be treated by **pericardiotomy** and creation of a window in the pericardium. Pain is controlled with medication.

 Think Critically

Which patients should you watch for signs of pericarditis?

CARDIOMYOPATHY

Cardiomyopathy is a group of diseases that affect the structure or function of the heart. The risk of cardiomyopathy is increased in systemic hypertension, with chronic excessive alcohol intake, during pregnancy, and in those who have had a systemic infection. The heart enlarges and becomes an inefficient pump. There are three main types of cardiomyopathy (Box 20-4).

The major problems exhibited by patients with cardiomyopathy are heart failure and dysrhythmias. Signs and symptoms of cardiomyopathy include dyspnea, activity intolerance, angina, dizziness, hypertension, and palpitations. Diagnosis is made through history plus chest x-ray, cardiac catheterization, echocardiography, ECG, or MRI/CT scans. Medical treatment for cardiomyopathy includes drugs to increase

Box 20-4	Three Main Types of Cardiomyopathy

DILATED
Characterized by extensive enlargement of the ventricles with impairment of contraction. Causes include chemotherapy, alcohol abuse, infection, inflammation and poor nutrition, and connective tissue disorders. Advances to heart failure.

HYPERTROPHIC
Increased growth of left ventricle muscle. May be hereditary as autosomal dominant gene, caused by hypertension, or hypoparathyroidism. Sudden death may occur.

RESTRICTIVE
Stiffened ventricles prevent adequate relaxation after systole, affecting ventricular filling. Caused by systemic diseases such as amyloidosis or sarcoidosis. Progresses to right-sided heart failure.

contractility (such as digoxin), antihypertensive drugs, diuretics, antiarrhythmic drugs, and anticoagulants. Severe cardiomyopathy can be rapidly fatal. These patients are possible candidates for a heart transplant. Because of the possibility of cardiac arrest, families are taught CPR. In later stages, a left ventricular assist device (LVAD) may be used to rest the heart or as a bridge to heart transplant. An LVAD can be external or it can be implanted. When implanted, the pump is placed in the upper abdomen. A tube from the left ventricle pulls blood into the pump and the pump sends the blood into the aorta. The patient may have an AICD implanted.

Nursing Management for Infectious and Inflammatory Heart Disease

Complete a thorough history and physical examination and document all data as a baseline assessment. Any abnormalities should be noted and included in the nursing care plan. Assess heart sounds carefully. Assess vital signs on a regular basis and note abnormalities. The patient may experience an elevation in temperature in addition to changes in heart rate and rhythm. Attention to prescribed medications is essential to care. Ordered medications must be given on schedule. The teaching plan should include information about the drugs, as well as detailed information about the specific disease process. Some patients may require complete bed rest. Make the patient as comfortable as possible and reinforce the rationale for the prescribed activity level. Oxygen administration may be required; discuss the importance of this treatment with the patient. Include evaluation of the patient's physical status, assessment of the patient's understanding of the home care requirements, and teaching related to medications and treatment in discharge planning. Advise that prophylactic antibiotic therapy is necessary before dental procedures that involve gingival manipulation or bleeding. If the patient is at high risk for IE, prophylaxis may be needed before other invasive procedures.

 Think Critically

Can you describe why it is important to assess the patient with infective endocarditis for lung, brain, and abdominal organ abnormalities?

CARDIAC VALVE DISORDERS

Mitral and aortic valve disorders are the most common cardiac valve disorders. Tricuspid and pulmonic valve problems are rare. Tricuspid problems are usually from IV drug abuse. Pulmonic stenosis is congenital. Besides congenital abnormalities, rheumatic fever, and IE, rheumatoid arthritis and the Parkinson's drug pergolide (Permax) can cause cardiac valve disorders. More cardiac valve problems are being seen in AIDS patients.

Mitral valve prolapse (MVP) occurs when the valve leaflets are enlarged and prolapse into the left atrium during systole. This is most often a benign condition. MVP is most often asymptomatic, but can cause chest pain, palpitations, exercise intolerance, or fainting. A midsystolic click heard at the apex is characteristic of MVP.

MITRAL STENOSIS

Mitral stenosis is most commonly caused by rheumatic fever. This disorder is occurring less frequently since the incidence of rheumatic fever from *Streptococcus A* has declined. Other causes are systemic lupus erythematosus, rheumatoid arthritis, and related conditions. Valve leaflet thickening and calcification cause stiffening. Left atrial pressure rises and the left atrium dilates. The left atrium must work harder to pump blood through the narrowed valve into the left ventricle. Pulmonary pressure increases and consequently the right ventricle hypertrophies.

The first symptom may be dyspnea on exertion. Paroxysmal dyspnea (sudden dyspnea at night), palpitations of atrial fibrillation, and a dry cough may occur. If untreated, right-sided heart failure may eventually occur. Atrial fibrillation may be present. A diastolic murmur that is rumbling is heard on auscultation.

MITRAL REGURGITATION (INSUFFICIENCY)

Rheumatic heart disease is the main cause of mitral regurgitation. Papillary muscle rupture from ischemic heart disease, a congenital anomaly, and infective endocarditis are other causes. Fibrosis and calcification prevent the valve from closing completely during systole. Backflow of blood into the left atrium occurs as the ventricle contracts. In diastole, the blood flows back into the left ventricle along with the normal blood flow from the atrium. This increased volume must be ejected with the next contraction. The left ventricle and left atrium dilate and hypertrophy to accomplish the ejection. More women than men develop mitral regurgitation.

Symptoms take decades to emerge. Fatigue and weakness from reduced cardiac output begin. Dyspnea on exertion and orthopnea are later developments. There may be complaints of palpitations, anxiety, and atypical chest pain. Peripheral pulses are thready and the extremities may be cool and clammy. Atrial fibrillation may occur. Right-sided heart failure causes jugular venous distention, hepatomegaly, and pitting edema. Auscultation at the apex reveals a high-pitched systolic murmur. A third heart sound occurs when regurgitation is severe.

AORTIC STENOSIS

Aortic stenosis is the most common valve disorder in the United States. Atherosclerosis with degenerative calcification of the valve is a common factor in older adults. Congenital valve malformations and rheumatic

fever are causes in younger patients. The aortic valve opening narrows and obstructs left ventricular outflow during systole. The increased pressure required to eject the blood causes left ventricular hypertrophy. Eventually cardiac output is decreased to the point that the body's demands cannot be met during exertion. Systolic heart failure begins and pulmonary congestion produces symptoms. **When the valve opening becomes less than 1 cm, surgery is urgent.**

Dyspnea, angina, and syncope on exertion are classic symptoms of aortic stenosis. Later, extreme fatigue, weakness, and peripheral cyanosis become apparent. A narrowed pulse pressure is found when blood pressure is measured. Auscultation reveals a systolic crescendo-decrescendo murmur.

 Elder Care Points

Elderly people with long-term hypertension are at risk for aortic stenosis because of increased atherosclerosis and stiffening of the aorta. Carefully assess aortic valve sounds of the elderly patient, especially if hypertension is not well controlled.

AORTIC REGURGITATION (INSUFFICIENCY)

Infective endocarditis, congenital abnormalities, long-term hypertension, and Marfan syndrome (a rare genetic connective tissue disease) are factors in aortic regurgitation. The valve leaflets do not close properly during diastole allowing backflow of blood from the aorta into the left ventricle. The left ventricle dilates and hypertrophies from the greater blood volume.

Symptoms do not appear until left ventricular failure happens. Dyspnea on exertion, orthopnea, and paroxysmal nocturnal dyspnea begin. Nocturnal angina with diaphoresis and palpitations particularly when lying on the left side occur late in the disease. The pulse is bounding and pulse pressure is widened with increased systolic pressure and decreased diastolic pressure. On auscultation there is a high-pitched, blowing diastolic decrescendo murmur.

TREATMENT OF VALVE DISORDERS

Treatment depends on the valve affected and the degree of impairment. Yearly monitoring and drug therapy for symptoms is standard when disease is not severe. Later, heart surgery may be needed. Rest is an important part of therapy.

Medical Treatment

Diuretics, beta blockers, digoxin, and oxygen along with rest are used to improve symptoms of heart failure and dysrhythmias. Nitrates may be used cautiously for aortic stenosis. Vasodilators such as calcium channel blockers may be employed for aortic or mitral stenosis. Before many invasive procedures, prophylactic antibiotics are necessary for all patients with valve disease. Atrial fibrillation is corrected with drug therapy and/or cardioversion. If atrial fibrillation cannot be converted to a normal sinus rhythm, drugs such as amiodarone (Cordarone), procainamide (Pronestyl), or a beta-blocking agent may be prescribed to slow ventricular response rate. The patient with chronic atrial fibrillation is placed on regular anticoagulant therapy.

Surgical Treatment

When valvular disease becomes severe, surgery is required to correct the problem. Reparative procedures are becoming more common. Balloon valvuloplasty is sometimes used to open stenosed valves. It is performed with a balloon-tipped catheter. The catheter is threaded via the femoral artery into the heart and to the diseased valve. The balloon is inflated to enlarge the opening, then is deflated and removed. However, it is questionable as to how long the valve will stay open. Often the stenosis recurs before 6 months.

Direct commissurotomy occurs during cardiopulmonary bypass with open heart surgery. Thrombi are removed from the atria and the leaflets are incised, along with calcification debridement. This opens the valve orifice.

Mitral valve annuloplasty (reconstruction) is performed for acquired mitral regurgitation. The valve ring (annulus) that attaches to the leaflets and supports them is made smaller with sutures or tucks. Leaflets are repaired as well to provide good closure of the valve at systole.

Valve Replacement

Replacement may be done as an open heart procedure with cardiopulmonary bypass, or as minimally invasive surgery. Many mechanical (prosthetic) and biologic (tissue) valves are available (Figure 20-10). Some tissue valves are used from human cadavers. Mechanical valves require lifetime anticoagulation postoperatively, due to the possibility of clot formation. Biologic valves may be from a pig (porcine) or from a cow (bovine). Biologic valves do not require postoperative anticoagulation therapy. Biologic valves tend to wear out in about 15 years, requiring replacement. Mechanical valves are more durable. The aortic valve is always replaced with a mechanical valve because of the high pressure in the aorta.

Nursing Management for Cardiac Valve Disorders

The primary nursing goals for patients with cardiac valve disease are to maintain adequate cardiac output, to control dysrhythmias, and to prevent or control HF. Assessing the patient for signs of developing heart failure, teaching the patient about prescribed medications, and preparing the patient for surgical procedures should all be included in the nursing plan of care. See Chapter 18 for common nursing diagnoses

FIGURE 20-10 Examples of mechanical and biologic tissue valves for valve replacement. **A,** Bileaflet mechanical valve. **B,** Porcine heterograft. **C,** Carpentier-Edwards aortic pericardial valve.

and interventions for complications related to valve problems.

Valve surgery is most often an elective procedure. Preoperative and postoperative care are very similar to that of coronary artery bypass graft surgery (see Chapter 21). Patients on anticoagulation drugs preoperatively must stop taking them about 72 hours before the procedure. Any needed dental work is obtained before the valve replacement to decrease the chance of infective endocarditis.

Patients with mitral stenosis may have pulmonary hypertension and stiff lungs. Postoperatively, respiratory status must be monitored very closely during weaning from the ventilator. Patients undergoing aortic valve replacement are at higher risk of postoperative hemorrhage. Be particularly alert for bleeding. Monitor cardiac output closely and watch for signs of heart failure. Fatigue is a common problem during convalescence. Rest and activity must be balanced carefully. For those with a mechanical valve, teach about care needed when taking an anticoagulant.

CARDIAC TRAUMA

Blunt chest trauma often causes myocardial contusion, but it also can cause tears in the great vessels and massive bleeding. Contusion may result in cardiac dysrhythmia. Symptoms may mimic those of an MI since cardiac tissue has been damaged. Treatment is much the same as for an MI. Monitor the patient's cardiac rhythm closely when such trauma has occurred.

Penetrating trauma usually causes a hemothorax. Cardiac tamponade can occur from either type of wound if bleeding into the pericardial sac occurs. Blood collects in the pericardial sac, which will not stretch, compressing the myocardium; the heart cannot fill or pump effectively. Heart sounds become muffled and distant, and hypotension occurs along with increased central venous pressure evidenced by neck vein distention. Shock and death will result if the bleeding is not stopped and the fluid removed. Surgical repair may be necessary.

COMMON THERAPIES AND THEIR NURSING IMPLICATIONS

The medical treatments most commonly used to manage heart disease include (1) oxygen therapy, (2) pharmacologic agents, and (3) dietary controls. Education and rehabilitation of the cardiac patient also must be included in the plan of care. Surgical treatment of cardiac conditions most often is used to correct structural defects of the heart and great vessels.

OXYGEN THERAPY

Administering supplemental oxygen to relieve the dyspnea and hypoxemia of a cardiac patient is a routine therapeutic measure. Any patient experiencing chest pain is started on low-dose oxygen. Responsibilities regarding oxygen therapy for a cardiac patient are primarily concerned with observation to determine a patient's need for supplemental oxygen, maintenance of the ordered flow rate, and the response to therapy once oxygen has been initiated. It is important to be alert for signs of changing oxygen needs, such as increased pulse rate and symptoms of cerebral anoxia, including irritability, confusion, and disorientation. The patient's oxygen saturation can be monitored by pulse oximetry or by blood gas analysis.

Clinical Cues

The patient's P_{O_2} should be maintained between 95% and 100%. If P_{O_2} falls lower than 93% consistently, notify the physician. Oxygen saturation by blood gas determination should be 80 to 100 mm Hg. Patients with history of pulmonary disease such as emphysema may normally exhibit an oxygen saturation between 85% and 90%.

PHARMACOLOGIC AGENTS

Many types of drugs are used to treat heart disorders (see Tables 20-3 and 20-4). Digitalis in its various forms is a widely prescribed drug. However, it is a potent drug that can produce serious toxicity. **Classic symptoms of digitalis toxicity are yellow-green halos around lights, nausea, diarrhea, and confusion.**

Digitalis can be very effective in treating certain kinds of cardiac disorders, but its therapeutic range is quite narrow. A therapeutic dose is only about one third less than the dose that will induce toxicity. Moreover, physiologic changes resulting from age, electrolyte imbalances (particularly hypokalemia or hypercalcemia), renal impairment, metabolic disturbances, and certain heart conditions can predispose a patient to digitalis toxicity. Other drugs given simultaneously, including erythromycin, also can alter the effects of digitalis and make it more toxic. Learn each physician's guidelines regarding a pulse rate lower than 60 bpm and check the nursing unit protocols. Both beta blockers and calcium channel blockers will lower the heart rate, and beta blockers may cause pedal edema.

Clinical Cues

Remember that digitoxin has a slower and more prolonged action and is 10 times more potent than digoxin. **For this reason, digitoxin and digoxin are not interchangeable.**

Some physicians may not want a dose of digitalis held if the patient's pulse rate is below 60 bpm, as long as there are no signs of digitalis toxicity. If the pulse rate is less than 60, check the physician's order sheet before administering the medication.

When life-threatening complications arise from digitalis toxicity, digoxin immune Fab is given to counteract the excess digitalis. This drug is used cautiously, as side effects include hypotension, hypokalemia, worsening of HF, and rapid ventricular rates if the patient is experiencing atrial fibrillation.

? Think Critically

Can you list four signs and symptoms that might indicate your patient is experiencing digitalis toxicity?

Anticoagulants are prescribed to inhibit the formation of clots within blood vessels and the heart. Anticoagulants do not dissolve clots that have already formed, but they can prevent existing ones from growing larger and can interfere with the development of new clots. Long-term anticoagulant therapy is necessary for patients with chronic atrial fibrillation or mechanical valve replacement.

DIETARY CONTROL

The National Heart, Lung, and Blood Institute cites obesity as a risk factor for cardiac disorders. When obesity is present in conjunction with other factors, such as metabolic syndrome, hypertension, high cholesterol levels, diabetes mellitus, smoking, or family history of heart disease, the likelihood of cardiovascular problems is increased.

Many health professionals consider the self-help groups to be most successful in assisting people to lose pounds and then to keep their weight within normal range once the excess is lost. These groups include Weight Watchers, TOPS (Take Off Pounds Sensibly), and Overeaters Anonymous. Results of studies have shown that the behavior-modification techniques these groups use are very successful. To prevent heart disease and decrease the factors that predispose one to cardiovascular disease, the American Heart Association recommends the following measures.

Health Promotion

Heart-Healthy Lifestyle Recommendations

- With daily activities plus exercise, use up as many calories as you consume. To calculate, multiply current weight by 15 if moderately active; if sedentary, multiply weight by 13.
- Follow a heart-healthy diet:
  - Eat less nutrient-poor foods such as soft drinks and candy.
  - Keep saturated fat at 8% to 10% of each day's total calories with 30% or less calories from all fats.
  - Keep cholesterol at or below 200 mg per day.
  - Limit sodium intake to 1500 mg per day. Read labels for sodium content of foods.
  - Avoid intake of monosodium glutamate (MSG), excessive caffeine, and other food additives.
- Exercise with physical activity at least 30 minutes a day.
- Avoid smoking tobacco and avoid tobacco smoke.

Increased fiber will lower cholesterol even without cutting down on dietary fat. Adults should consume about 35 g of fiber per day; the national average consumption is about 12 g. Increasing fiber in the diet also lowers the risk of cancer.

Foods containing *trans* fats increase the cholesterol level, especially low-density lipoprotein. A tub, soft-style margarine that lists water or liquid vegetable oil as its first ingredient contains less *trans*-fatty acids than other types (American Dietetic Association, 2006). Patients should be taught to read food labels for the presence of *trans* fat. There are excellent resources for information and support for patients who have a cardiovascular disease and are attempting to follow a dietary regimen as part of their overall treatment plan. Many community hospitals sponsor weight management programs. Local chapters of the American Heart Association provide pamphlets and other sources of information about diet.

A high intake of sodium is thought to contribute to the development of high blood pressure. Limiting sodium intake is an important part of preventing and treating hypertension. Several cookbooks that make low-sodium, low-cholesterol meals easier to plan and prepare are sponsored by the American Heart Association and others. The fact that the tendency to develop cardiovascular disease is familial gives the patient and the family good reason to develop good eating habits

and to change to more heart-healthy foods. Restriction of sodium, prescribed because of sodium's association with retention of water in the tissues, is discussed in Chapter 3.

Dietary programs to reverse coronary heart disease have been introduced by many proponents of severe restriction of saturated fat in the diet. These programs (e.g., the Pritikin Diet, Dr. Dean Ornish Diet) claim that arteriosclerosis and other factors that lead to heart disease can be reversed if a diet high in complex carbohydrates, fiber, and limited fat is followed. In addition, exercising consistently, managing weight, managing emotional stress, and maintaining positive relationships are emphasized to reduce modifiable risk factors. These programs take considerable personal motivation. The entire family and support system must be involved to achieve optimum success.

Think Critically

How could you specifically change your eating habits in a way that would help you follow a more heart-healthy diet?

COMMUNITY CARE

Patients with infectious and inflammatory disease of the heart are sent home after a few days in the hospital. A home care nurse is usually assigned to supervise any ordered IV antibiotic infusion and to carefully assess the patient on a regular basis. The importance of taking prescribed NSAIDs for inflammation is discussed. A thorough heart and lung assessment is performed at every visit. The nurse teaches the patient or family how to infuse the antibiotics and how to care for the IV or peripherally inserted central catheter (PICC) line. The importance of tracking temperature daily is stressed. Signs and symptoms to report to the physician are reviewed, including new or increased chest pain, dysrhythmia, fatigue, shortness of breath, change in level of consciousness, sharp abdominal pain, or dependent edema. Assessment for signs and symptoms of adverse reactions is performed. Repeat blood cultures and CBCs are drawn at intervals to determine effectiveness of treatment.

The nurse in long-term care must be vigilant for beginning signs of heart failure as many elderly residents have had chronic hypertension, previous MIs, or previous episodes of heart failure. Whenever a resident has an infection, an increased demand is placed on the heart and heart failure can develop quickly if the heart is already compromised. Episodes of vomiting or diarrhea, or of dehydration, cause electrolyte imbalances that can lead to dysrhythmias. Heart rates and rhythms should be monitored closely and fluid and electrolyte replacement should begin early in the course of the illness.

Get Ready for the NCLEX® Examination!

Key Points

- HF is the inability of the heart to pump as it should, and pressure changes cause blood to back up into lungs and systemic circulation.
- Common systolic HF symptoms are fatigue, dependent edema, dyspnea, cough, and crackles in lungs.
- Common symptoms of diastolic HF are pitting peripheral edema, abdominal distention, weight gain, and fatigue.
- Medical treatment of HF includes limited activity initially; oxygen therapy; medications such as ACE inhibitors or ARBs, digoxin, loop diuretics, and antihypertensive drugs; restricted sodium intake; and smoking cessation.
- Recording daily weight and keeping accurate intake and output records are essential.
- Assist the patient to maintain fluid restrictions as required.
- Disruption of normal SA node conduction leads to dysrhythmias; lack of normal regular myocardial contraction decreases cardiac output.
- Life-threatening dysrhythmias include ventricular tachycardia, ventricular fibrillation, and asystole.
- Dysrhythmias causing decreased cardiac output include severe bradycardia, atrial fibrillation, complete heart block, and frequent PVCs.
- Dysrhythmias are diagnosed using 12-lead ECG, continuous ECG monitoring, patient history, and electrophysiologic testing.
- Failure of the heart's natural pacemaker may require an artificial pacemaker.
- Artificial pacing can be temporary or permanent, external, transvenous, or internal.
- AICDs may be used in patients with repeated episodes of ventricular tachycardia, ventricular fibrillation, or asystole.
- Inflammation of the heart may occur as endocarditis, myocarditis, or pericarditis.
- Medical treatment includes rest to reduce workload of the heart, anti-infective drugs to control infection, and surgery to replace or repair valves damaged by the inflammatory process.
- Severe cardiomyopathy is treated by heart transplant.
- Cardiac valve disorders are caused by congenital defect, rheumatic fever, endocarditis, or long-term hypertension.
- Valve disorders include stenosis and regurgitation (insufficiency).
- Valve disease, if left untreated, often progresses to heart failure.

Additional Learning Resources

SG Go to your Study Guide for additional learning activities to help you master this chapter content.

evolve Go to your Evolve website (http://evolve.elsevier.com/deWit/medsurg) for the following FREE learning resources:
- Animations, audio, and video
- Answers and rationales for questions and activities
- Concept Map Creator

- Glossary with pronunciations in English and Spanish
- Interactive Review Questions and Exercises and more!

 Online Resources
- American Association of Heart Failure Nurses, www.aahfn.org
- American Heart Association, www.americanheart.org
- Heart Failure Society of America, www.hfsa.org
- Hypertrophic Cardiomyopathy Association, www.4hcm.org
- Mended Hearts, www.mendedhearts.org

Review Questions for the NCLEX® Examination

1. The nurse is about to administer the first dose of torsemide (Demadex) to a patient diagnosed with heart disease. Which assessment finding(s) indicate(s) a possible side effect of this drug? *(Select all that apply.)*
   1. Facial tic
   2. Difficulty hearing
   3. Muscle weakness
   4. Light-headedness
   5. Increased blood pressure

2. The patient is admitted with a cardiac dysrhythmia. The morning lab values show potassium as 5.8 mg/dL. What action is most important to take?
   1. Encourage intake of extra fluid.
   2. Notify the physician immediately.
   3. Check the breakfast tray for sodium-containing foods before serving.
   4. Check the patient's vital signs.

3. _____ is the delivery of a mild electrical shock at a specific time of the cardiac cycle to interrupt an abnormal rhythm and to possibly initiate a normal rhythm.
   1. Cardioversion
   2. Defibrillation
   3. Pacemaker initiation
   4. Electrophysiology study

4. After pacemaker implantation, it is important to teach the patient to:
   1. stay away from microwave ovens.
   2. count her pulse regularly.
   3. refrain from swimming.
   4. use a safety razor to shave her legs.

5. A 48-year-old patient is admitted for tachycardia, shortness of breath, and chest pain eased by sitting up and leaning forward. The nurse auscultates a high-pitched scratchy sound at the left sternal border of the chest. The patient most likely has:
   1. heart failure.
   2. pericarditis.
   3. pneumonia.
   4. aortic stenosis.

6. Which assigned patient would take priority for immediate attention?

    1. The patient with infective endocarditis who has an antibiotic dose due
    2. The patient awaiting aortic stenosis surgery who is complaining of pain
    3. The patient with systolic heart failure whose weight is up 1.5 lb today
    4. The patient with dysrhythmia whose heart rate has dropped to 42 bpm and is dizzy

7. The patient has heart failure and atherosclerosis. Which patient statement regarding healthy food choices demonstrates a need for further teaching?

    1. "I can have an egg two to three times per week."
    2. "I need to watch red meat intake, but can have all the cheese I want."
    3. "I should read labels to see how much sodium a serving contains."
    4. "Canned goods are often high in sodium."

8. The nurse explains the importance of reducing salt in the diet to a Hispanic man who was recently diagnosed with heart failure. The nurse realizes that the relatives are at the bedside with the patient. An appropriate nursing action would be to:

    1. involve the youngest male in the family to translate.
    2. ensure patient privacy by directing the relatives out of the patient room.
    3. determine who does the cooking in the family.
    4. include all the relatives in the diet teaching.

9. In discussing heart failure with a patient, the physician explains that the underlying weakness of the left ventricle results in reduced cardiac output and backup of fluid in the pulmonary system. The nurse anticipates which sign/symptom?

    1. Edema in sacrum, legs, feet, ankles
    2. Hepatomegaly
    3. Crackles in the lungs
    4. Ascites

10. The patient asks, "Why am I taking lisinopril (Zestril)?" An accurate statement by the nurse would be:

    1. "The medication increases the force of contraction of the heart."
    2. "The medication increases the heart rate."
    3. "The medication helps prevent vasoconstriction."
    4. "The medication causes excretion of extra fluid."

Critical Thinking Activities

Scenario A

Mr. Jenkins, age 56, is admitted to the telemetry unit with a diagnosis of atrial fibrillation. Physical assessment reveals a restless, apprehensive man with an irregular heart rate of 145 and dyspnea.

1. Describe the rhythm you expect to note on the telemetry monitor.

2. What treatment do you expect the physician to prescribe for Mr. Jenkins?

3. List five priority teaching points you should establish for Mr. Jenkins.

Scenario B

Mr. Zulic, age 76, received a permanent pacemaker to correct complete heart block. He is 1 day postoperative and preparing for discharge home.

1. What are indications for a pacemaker?

2. Describe the types of pacemakers and indications for their use.

3. Describe preoperative and postoperative nursing interventions when caring for a patient receiving a pacemaker.

Scenario C

Mr. Postma, age 72, is diagnosed with systolic heart failure. He has been experiencing fatigue and shortness of breath when walking the dog for a mile, and has gained 5 lb over the past 2 weeks.

1. What stage of heart disease is Mr. Postma in?

2. What would you expect to be prescribed for him?

3. What topics should your teaching plan cover?

Care of Patients with Coronary Artery Disease and Cardiac Surgery

Objectives

Theory

1. Discuss the causes of coronary artery disease.
2. Describe the pathophysiology of coronary artery disease.
3. Outline nursing interventions to care for a patient experiencing angina, including medication administration and patient teaching.
4. Discuss the pathophysiology of myocardial infarction.
5. Compare and contrast the symptoms of and care for unstable angina with those of myocardial infarction.
6. Develop a nursing care plan for a patient experiencing a myocardial infarction.
7. Describe the nursing care of a patient undergoing cardiac surgery.
8. List five complications of cardiac surgery.

Clinical Practice

1. Develop a teaching plan for a patient with coronary artery disease.
2. Identify signs and symptoms that indicate a patient may be experiencing a myocardial infarct.
3. Administer medications to patients experiencing cardiac disorders.
4. Collaborate with other health care providers to care for patients after cardiac surgery.
5. Contribute to discharge planning for a patient after cardiac surgery.

Key Terms

angina pectoris (ăn-JĪ-nă-PĔK-tŏr-ĭs, p. 453)
atherosclerosis (ăth-ĕr-ō-sklĕ-RŌ-sĭs, p. 451)
coronary artery bypass graft (CABG) (p. 464)
coronary insufficiency (KŎR-ō-nĕr-ē
  ĭn-să-FĬSH-ăn-sē, p. 452)
drug-eluting stent (stĕnt, p. 464)

infarction (ĭn-FĂRK-shŭn, p. 458)
metabolic equivalent (MET) units (p. 463)
myocardial infarction (MI) (mī-ō-KĂR-dē-ăl
  ĭn-FĂRK-shŭn, p. 451)
necrosis (nē-KRŌ-sĭs, p. 452)

CORONARY ARTERY DISEASE

Coronary artery disease (CAD) is a progressive disease leading to narrowing or occlusion (blockage) of the coronary arteries. The coronary arteries are responsible for supplying oxygen and nutrition to the myocardium (see Figure 18-2). As the coronary vessel narrows, the patient may experience symptoms of ischemia, such as chest tightness and angina. When a sudden obstruction to blood flow through one or more major coronary arteries occurs and cuts off oxygen and nutrients to the cardiac cells, a **myocardial infarction (MI)** occurs.

Etiology

A major factor in the development of CAD is atherosclerosis, in which plaque containing cholesterol and lipids is laid down inside the arteries as fatty streaks. Plaque can occur in the cerebral vessels, the aorta, and arteries other than the coronaries. **Atherosclerosis** is one form of arteriosclerosis. *Arteriosclerosis* is a general term for disorders that cause thickening and loss of elasticity of the arteries.

Factors such as age (over 40), gender, and race contribute to the disease; however, these susceptibilities cannot be modified. Those who have had one or more immediate family members die of coronary artery disease during middle age are considered to be at high risk for the disorder. Postmenopausal women and women who use oral contraceptives or hormone replacement therapy are at greater risk of coronary artery disease than are women outside these categories.

 Cultural Considerations

Ethnicity and Coronary Artery Disease

The incidence of coronary artery disease is disproportionately higher in African Americans, especially African American males. Research continues to determine the etiology of this finding and the approaches to decrease the incidence. Ethnicity-based treatment of heart disease is also explored, as research has demonstrated that some classifications of medications are more effective for persons of diverse ethnicity.

Pathophysiology

The process of atherosclerosis begins during late childhood, when streaks or islands of fatty material are laid down on the inner walls of the arteries. Low-density lipoprotein (LDL) is the major contributing factor to the formation of this fatty material. Plaques accumulate, particularly where there has been irritation or inflammation of the blood vessel from smoking, hypertension, diabetes, or infection. Later, the plaques become fibrous as a result of inflammation and healing. The plaque area protrudes into the artery, decreasing the vessel's size (Figure 21-1). When plaque areas rupture, the rough edges cause platelet clumping and clotting (thrombosis). Over time, the plaque begins to calcify, causing rigidity of the vessel wall. The further narrowing of the coronary arteries causes **coronary insufficiency** (decreased or insufficient blood flow). Obstruction occurs from this process and from thrombosis. Arterial spasm may contribute to deficient blood flow and consequent heart muscle damage.

Elder Care Points

When compared to the coronary blood flow in a 25-year-old, coronary blood flow in a 60-year-old is decreased. Elderly people have less cardiac reserve, meaning that any added oxygen demands may compromise the coronary circulation and the heart's ability to pump properly.

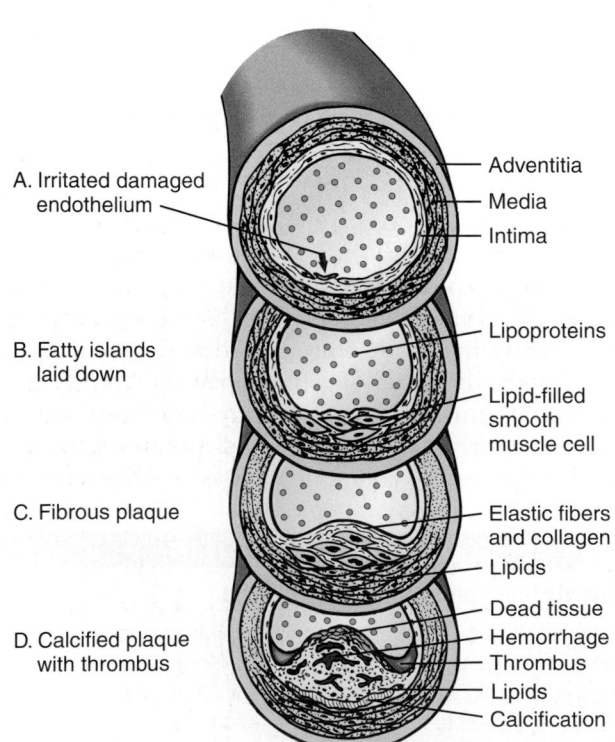

A. Irritated damaged endothelium

B. Fatty islands laid down

C. Fibrous plaque

D. Calcified plaque with thrombus

Adventitia
Media
Intima

Lipoproteins

Lipid-filled smooth muscle cell

Elastic fibers and collagen
Lipids

Dead tissue
Hemorrhage
Thrombus
Lipids
Calcification

FIGURE 21-1 Progression of atherosclerosis.

There is a proven link between hyperlipidemia or high levels of LDL and triglycerides and atherosclerosis. High levels of homocysteine and episodes of inflammation causing an elevated level of C-reactive protein (CRP) are also factors in the development of atherosclerosis.

As coronary artery disease progresses, the coronary vessels become narrower, decreasing blood supply to the myocardium. This lack of blood supply leads to ischemia and eventually **necrosis** (cell death) of the myocardium. If loss of muscle tissue occurs (MI), the heart muscle is unable to pump effectively and cardiac output is reduced. Cardiac dysrhythmias and death may occur if medical intervention is not obtained.

Signs and Symptoms

Signs and symptoms of coronary artery disease are related to the lack of oxygen supply to the myocardium and inability of the heart to pump blood effectively to oxygenate tissues and cells (Box 21-1). Angina pectoris, acute coronary syndrome (ACS), or sudden cardiac death may occur.

The condition is called *stable angina* when symptoms only appear with activity. *Unstable angina* occurs when symptoms occur even at rest. *Acute coronary syndrome* occurs when ischemic symptoms are prolonged and are not quickly relieved. It is an umbrella term for unstable angina and acute ischemic MI with or without ST-segment elevation on the electrocardiogram (ECG).

Diagnosis

Diagnosis of coronary artery disease is accomplished through tests, such as ECG, echocardiogram, cardiac stress test, cardiac angiography (cardiac catheterization), cardiac computed tomography (CT) for calcium index, or magnetic resonance angiogram.

Treatment

A low-fat diet, weight control, and exercise are prescribed to lower cholesterol and total lipids (American Heart Association, 2009a). If elevated cholesterol and

Box 21-1	Signs and Symptoms of Coronary Artery Disease

- Chest discomfort, including feeling of tightness, aching, burning
- Chest pain (angina pectoris) radiating to the arm, jaw, or back
- Dyspnea (shortness of breath)
- Palpitations or tachycardia
- Nausea and vomiting
- Cold, clammy skin
- Undue fatigue (particularly in women)
- Weakness and inability to complete usual activities without chest pain or dyspnea.

triglyceride levels cannot be lowered by a low-fat diet and exercise, lipid-lowering drugs are prescribed (Table 21-1). These medications are not effective alone and may not reduce cholesterol levels to a point of eliminating the risk for coronary artery disease. Several herbs and supplements have shown the ability to lower cholesterol. Advise patients to consult with their physician before taking over-the-counter medications or herbs.

 Complementary and Alternative Therapies

Herbs and Supplements that Naturally Lower Cholesterol

The following have been found to lower cholesterol in patients with hyperlipidemia.
- Garlic
- Omega-3 fatty acids
- Red rice yeast
- Milk thistle
- Fiber
- Phytosterols
- Soy
- Coenzyme Q_{10}

Patients who choose to use these substances should check for interactions with other medications they are taking. Some of the substances only lower cholesterol and LDL; others raise high-density lipoprotein (HDL).

Nursing Management

Patients should be encouraged to adopt a healthy lifestyle, including exercise and a diet low in saturated fat. Obtain a referral to a dietitian and assist the patient by reinforcing the need for changes in dietary habits. A cardiac rehabilitation program referral is very helpful. The program will help the patient choose an exercise regimen that he can manage on a long-term basis. Emphasize the importance of maintaining a normal body weight.

 Health Promotion

Aspirin to Prevent Myocardial Infarction

New guidelines from the U.S. Preventive Services Task Force recommend daily aspirin therapy for men ages 45 to 79 to prevent a heart attack; 75 mg has proven as effective as higher doses. Patients must be screened for risk of gastrointestinal bleeding before starting aspirin therapy. Patients taking an anticoagulant must not take aspirin.

If the patient is on a statin drug to lower cholesterol, remind him that he needs to have blood drawn periodically to determine if the drug is effective and to monitor for serious side effects.

 Nutrition Considerations

Ways to Lower Fat and Cholesterol in the Diet

Teach the patient to:
- Avoid all fried foods; trim fat from meat and stick to 3-oz portions of meat per meal (a piece the size of a deck of cards). Remove skin from poultry.
- Eat fish with omega-3 fatty acids at least twice a week (salmon, mackerel, tuna).
- Use egg whites or Egg Beaters as cholesterol-free egg substitutes, both for breakfast cooking and in recipes.
- Decrease or eliminate all commercial baked goods containing *trans* fat, saturated fat, or high levels of fat. Check the labels. Pies, doughnuts, croissants, and pastries are very high in fat.
- Use unsaturated fats for home baking and cooking. Avoid palm oil, coconut oil, lard, bacon fat, and hydrogenated vegetable shortening. Use olive oil whenever possible in salad dressings and for cooking. Do not use cube margarine that contains *trans* fats.
- Microwave bacon on paper towels to decrease the amount of fat; use turkey bacon rather than regular bacon.
- Check the amount of fat in cheeses and choose the lower-fat varieties. Eat only small amounts of cheese.
- Drink nonfat milk and use a nondairy, no-cholesterol creamer if you must have creamer in your coffee.
- Decrease the use of all dairy products and use only the low-fat or nonfat varieties.
- Eat more high-fiber whole grains, fruits, and vegetables.

Clinical Cues

- Because statins can injure muscle tissue and are toxic to the liver in some patients, blood should be drawn for levels of CK (an enzyme released from damaged muscle) and for liver enzymes. Elevated liver enzymes may indicate toxic damage to the liver.
- Patients should be told to report any unexplained muscle tenderness or pain persisting for more than a few days. When a statin drug is begun, baseline blood values should be obtained before therapy. Repeat laboratory tests for liver enzymes every 1 to 3 months for the first 18 months of therapy.
- Grapefruit juice should not be consumed when taking a statin drug. Grapefruit juice interferes with the metabolism of the drug, which can lead to increased serum levels and risk of toxicity (Skidmore, 2011).

ANGINA PECTORIS

Angina pectoris (chest pain) occurs when blood supply to the heart is decreased or totally obstructed. The ischemia (inadequate blood and oxygen supply) of the heart tissue causes pain. Angina may be caused by atherosclerosis or arterial spasm. The decreased blood flow is caused by atherosclerotic plaque narrowing the artery or by arterial spasm (sudden constriction). Any activity that increases the heart's workload increases its need for oxygen. When the occluded coronary arteries cannot deliver adequate

Table 21-1   Drugs Commonly Used to Treat Hypercholesterolemia

DRUG	ACTION	COMMON SIDE EFFECTS	USUAL ADULT DOSAGE	NURSING INTERVENTIONS
Bile Acid Sequestrants				
Cholestyramine (Questran) Colestipol (Colestid) Colesevelam (Welchol)	Bind bile acid in the GI tract, resulting in decreased absorption of cholesterol	Abdominal pain, constipation, nausea	4 g PO once or twice per day	Instruct patient to take before meals. Instruct to mix with 4-6 oz liquid. Advise drug may cause constipation and to increase fluid intake if not contraindicated. Counsel patient to continue low-fat diet and exercise.
Fibric Acid Derivatives				
Gemfibrozil (Lopid) Clofibrate (Atromid) Fenofibrate (Tricor) Lovaza	Reduce triglyceride production by the liver	Abdominal pain, diarrhea, epigastric pain	600 mg PO bid	Encourage to keep appointments for follow-up lab studies. Encourage to notify physician if symptoms of side effects occur.
HMG-CoA Reductase Inhibitors (Statins)				
Atorvastatin (Lipitor) Lovastatin (Mevacor) Fluvastatin (Lescol) Simvastatin (Zocor) Rosuvastatin (Crestor) Pitavastatin (Livaio)	Inhibit the enzyme HMG-CoA reductase, which is responsible for synthesis of cholesterol	Abdominal pain, constipation, diarrhea, flatus, heartburn, rash	Individual drug dependent	Teach to notify physician if severe muscle pain and weakness occur. Encourage to keep follow-up appointments and have periodic lab work performed. Pregnancy category X. Advise female patients to notify physician immediately if pregnancy is suspected. Notify physician of alcohol intake. May be at risk for liver disease.
Cholesterol Absorption Inhibitor				
Ezetimibe (Zetia)	Inhibit intestinal absorption of cholesterol	Possible headache and mild GI distress; infrequent	10 mg daily	Can be used along with other antilipemics. Do not use for those with active liver disease. Take bile acid sequestrant 2 hr before or 4 hr after this drug. Obtain periodic lipid levels and liver function enzymes.
Niacin				
Niacin (Nicobid, Nicotinex) Nicotinic acid (Slo-Niacin, Novo-Niacin)	Inhibit formation and secretion of VLDL and LDL	Flushing and itching of face and upper body, nausea and vomiting, indigestion, orthostatic hypotension	500-1500 mg/day in divided doses Start with 50-100 mg bid for 7 days and then gradually increase	Monitor liver function when patient is taking high doses. Instruct to take aspirin or NSAID 30-60 min before dose to decrease flushing. Take niacin with food. Increase folic acid intake if homocysteine levels rise.

bid, twice a day; *GI*, gastrointestinal; *LDL, HMG-CoA*, 3-hydroxy-3-methylglutaryl coenzyme A; low-density lipoprotein; *NSAID*, nonsteroidal anti-inflammatory drug; *VLDL*, very low-density lipoprotein.

amounts of blood to meet normal needs, the patient experiences an angina attack. Attacks can be precipitated by physical exertion, emotional excitement, eating a heavy meal, exposure to cold, infection, or any disorder or activity that increases the oxygen demand and consumption or decreases the availability of oxygen to the myocardial tissue. When the patient's angina is no longer adequately controlled by medication and the attacks become more frequent or severe, surgery may be indicated to prevent a life-threatening MI.

Signs, Symptoms, and Diagnosis

Anginal pain or discomfort may vary in individuals, but in most cases it is described as a dull pressure or ache under the sternum or pain that radiates to the neck or jaw. The pain may also radiate down one or both arms. Angina sensation is seldom sharp or stabbing. The feeling may be described as suffocating. The pain can occur between the shoulder blades. In women, there may be no chest pain, but just a tenderness to touch or a burning or tingling sensation. Patients may think they are experiencing indigestion or esophageal reflux.

There are three types of angina:

1. *Stable or exertional angina:* Triggered by physical activity or stress, and is related to atherosclerosis. Goal of therapy is to reduce intensity and frequency of attacks.
2. *Variant or vasospastic angina:* Caused by coronary artery spasms which restrict the blood flow to the myocardium. The goal of treatment is to reduce the number and severity of attacks.
3. *Unstable angina:* Usually caused by occlusion of coronary arteries. Angina pain occurs even at rest. May not respond well to drug therapy. May require immediate surgery.

Medical diagnosis is established on the basis of history, clinical signs and symptoms, and whether rest and nitroglycerin provide relief during an acute attack. Response of the heart muscle to increased oxygen demands can be determined by exercise stress testing. Cardiac catheterization with coronary angiography may be performed (Figure 21-2). Echocardiography may be ordered to rule out a valve disorder or to evaluate left ventricular function. Laboratory levels of blood lipids will be ordered, and cardiac enzymes may be ordered to rule out an MI. An electrocardiogram is a standard diagnostic procedure.

FIGURE 21-2 Stenosis *(arrow)* of the left anterior descending coronary artery.

Treatment

The treatment of angina pectoris is mostly symptomatic, with emphasis on eliminating those factors that are known to precipitate an attack in the individual patient. With guidance and teaching, the patient may soon be able to correlate certain activities with an attack and thereby learn to avoid one whenever possible. Nitroglycerin, nitrates, calcium antagonists, and beta blockers are used in combination with drugs to lower cholesterol and prevent platelet aggregation. A low daily dose of aspirin (81 mg or 325 mg) may be prescribed for the treatment of CAD. Aspirin helps prevent clotting and may prevent a thrombus that could cause an MI. If the patient is allergic to aspirin, clopidogrel (Plavix) is prescribed. Nitroglycerin administered sublingually is the most common drug for treatment of angina. An aerosol spray and a buccal form of the drug are also available.

Nursing Management

Collect data that assist in determining the type of angina the patient is experiencing. Patients with a history of angina may experience increased episodes when exposed to very cold environments. Externally cold temperatures result in vasoconstriction. The patient should be instructed to wear warm clothing when exposed to cold and may consider remaining indoors when the weather is extremely chilly. Nursing interventions for selected problems related to angina pectoris are summarized in Nursing Care Plan 21-1.

🔼 Clinical Cues

Sublingual nitroglycerin tablets should be kept in a cool, dark place and should be carried by the patient at all times. If the mouth is dry, a sip of water should be taken before placing the tablet under the tongue. If possible, the patient should lie down when using nitroglycerin. In the hospital, a baseline blood pressure should be measured, a tablet given, and then the pressure should be checked again in 5 minutes. If the pain has not eased or the pressure has risen, another tablet is placed under the tongue. Check the blood pressure again in 5 minutes. The blood pressure should decrease. If it has not or if the pain is still present, administer a third sublingual tablet at the end of 15 minutes since the first tablet. Notify the physician immediately if the pain worsens or does not resolve after the three tablets. If oxygen is available, administer it according to hospital policy while waiting for communication from the physician. Patients should frequently check the expiration date on the bottle and replace the nitroglycerin tablets accordingly. See the Evolve website for *Healthy People 2020* objectives to lower heart disease.

ACUTE CORONARY SYNDROME AND MYOCARDIAL INFARCTION

If ischemia is prolonged and not quickly reversed, acute coronary syndrome (ACS) occurs. ACS includes unstable angina, non–ST segment elevation myocardial infarction (NSTEMI) and ST segment elevation myocardial infarction (STEMI). All patients with heart disease should be taught the signs of MI and be advised that the best survival rate is directly related to obtaining medical attention as quickly as possible. About 1,200,000 Americans experience an MI annually. Although males outnumber females, females die more frequently after an MI. According to the American Heart Association, heart disease is the leading cause of death among American women, claiming about 500,000 lives each year. The incidence of heart disease, including MI, continues to rise among women. Women are more likely to experience heart attacks after reaching menopause; however, poor dietary habits, sedentary lifestyle, and increased levels of stress contribute to the development of cardiovascular disease earlier in life for an increasing number of women.

★ Nursing Care Plan 21-1   Care of the Patient with Angina

Scenario

Mrs. Ralston, age 63, is admitted to the telemetry unit. She has a history of chest pain and dyspnea precipitated by physical or emotional exertion. Her BMI is 30, and she has a history of smoking two packs of cigarettes per day for 40 years. She is admitted for control of chest pain and evaluation of cardiac status. Cardiac enzymes are negative for MI.

Problem/Nursing Diagnosis

Chest pain unrelieved by sublingual nitroglycerin/Acute pain related to cardiac ischemia.

Supporting Assessment Data

Subjective: States she took five nitroglycerin tablets before admission with no relief of chest pain.
Objective: BP 100/70, HR 90, R 26. O_2 sat 92% on 5 L oxygen via nasal cannula.

Goals/Expected Outcomes	Nursing Interventions	Selected Rationale	Evaluation
Pain will be relieved within 15 min by sublingual nitroglycerin.	Assess level and duration of angina.	Determines severity of pain and need for additional intervention.	Pain relieved after two nitroglycerin tablets 5 min apart.
	Teach to notify nurse and lie down and rest when pain occurs.	Early intervention for pain relief and assessment of change in condition.	Blood pressure maintained within 4 mm Hg of beginning of episode.
	Assess vital signs during episodes of angina and medication administration.	Recognize side effects, such as hypotension and patient's response to treatment.	Continue plan.

Problem/Nursing Diagnosis

Apprehensive concerning upcoming tests and possible change in condition/Anxiety related to diagnostic tests and recurrent chest pain.

Supporting Assessment Data

Subjective: Asks, "Are you sure I didn't have a heart attack this time?"
Objective: Scheduled for cardiac catheterization in the A.M.

Goals/Expected Outcomes	Nursing Interventions	Selected Rationale	Evaluation
Patient will verbalize that anxiety has decreased within 12 hr.	Assess level of anxiety. Administer medication if appropriate.	Increased anxiety can precipitate episodes of angina.	Required diazepam (Valium) 5 mg PO for anxiety.
	Allow patient opportunity to express concerns.	Active listening will help to reduce patient's anxiety.	Patient verbalized fear of dying from heart attack or complications of procedures.
Patient will verbalize understanding of cardiac catheterization.	Provide information related to cardiac catheterization.	Adults desire straightforward information concerning their medical status.	Verbalized understanding of procedure. Some anxiety.
	Answer questions or refer to appropriate health care provider as needed.	Provides level of control for decision making.	Reevaluate and continue plan.

BMI, body mass index; *MI*, myocardial infarction; *PO*, orally.

Problem/Nursing Diagnosis

BMI 30, cholesterol level 235/Deficient knowledge related to lack of understanding impact of diet on medical condition or methods to improve cardiac health.

Supporting Assessment Data

Subjective: "I just can't exercise, and I don't understand how to choose and cook foods without salt or frying."
Objective: Wt. 195 lb, elevated cholesterol, resting HR 98.

Goals/Expected Outcomes	Nursing Interventions	Selected Rationale	Evaluation
Within 2 weeks after discharge, patient will be able to verbalize how to choose and prepare foods that are low in fat and sodium.	Assess current knowledge of food content and reading food levels. Refer for outpatient dietitian consult.	Provides starting point for teaching. Expert knowledge of dietitian needed to determine caloric needs and develop nutrition plan.	Patient able to choose low-fat and low-sodium foods from a menu list. States has dietitian consultation appointment.
Patient will establish regular exercise program. Patient will learn a new method of stress reduction.	Determine if patient is candidate for cardiac rehabilitation program. Make referral after collaboration with physician.	Provide structured, monitored exercise program that also includes dietary and emotional counseling. Reevaluate plan, refer to social services for assistance with financial concerns. Collaborate with patient and physician about evaluation of emotional status that may interfere with ability to remain compliant.	States she will consider participation in a cardiac rehabilitation program if funds are available. Contacted social services for consultation.

Problem/Nursing Diagnosis

Has not quit smoking and has recurrent episodes of angina/Risk for injury related to continued cigarette smoking.

Supporting Assessment Data

Subjective: "I have tried to quit smoking but it just doesn't work."

Goals/Expected Outcomes	Nursing Interventions	Selected Rationale	Evaluation
Patient will agree to enter a community smoking cessation program.	Assess willingness to reduce amount of or stop smoking. Teach complications related to heart disease and smoking. Refer to social services for community programs available; give a smoking cessation packet of information.	Patient must be internally motivated for optimal success. Provide understanding of role of smoking and vasoconstriction that lead to episodes of angina. Social services personnel are aware of community resources that can benefit patient care.	Patient states she had tried many times to stop smoking with limited success. States she understands need to quit smoking and the impact smoking has on her health. Identified smoking cessation program within patient's neighborhood in nearby church. Patient states she will contact program before discharge. Gave smoking cessation packet.

Critical Thinking Questions

1. What are five risk factors for coronary artery disease? What are complications?
2. List the three types of angina. In which category would you place Mrs. Ralston? Why?
3. Provide a teaching plan for a patient with angina. Include commonly used medication administration and side effects.
4. What is the most commonly used medication for angina/chest pain? How should it be administered?

Patient Teaching

Guidelines for the Patient with Angina

Patients who experience anginal attacks are taught to:
- Avoid eating heavy meals.
- Avoid physical activity for an hour after meals to prevent excessive oxygen demands.
- Take nitroglycerin before heavy physical activity that is known to cause an attack, such as intercourse or sports activities.
- Avoid exposure to cold; do not walk into a cold wind.
- Decrease controllable risk factors, such as lifestyle stress, obesity, hypertension, and improper diet.
- Adopt a graduated exercise program.
- Stop smoking.
- Learn meditation or other deep relaxation techniques.
- Take a sublingual nitroglycerin tablet and lie down at the beginning of an anginal attack. Make certain that the tablet produces a tingling sensation where it contacts mucous membrane. Nitroglycerin may be repeated twice more at 5-minute intervals for a total of three tablets if the pain persists. If the pain has not eased within 15 minutes, call 911, and notify the physician.
- Check pulse rate once daily if taking a calcium channel blocker or a beta-adrenergic blocker. These drugs should never be stopped abruptly; call physician if heart rate drops below 60 beats per minute.
- Rise slowly from a supine or sitting position because of potential postural hypotension.
- Cleanse area of previous application of nitroglycerin paste when applying a new dose.
- Keep appointments for regular checkups.
- Obtain sufficient rest daily.
- Avoid high environmental temperatures and high humidity; stay in air-conditioned areas when such conditions occur as they increase cardiac workload.
- Nitrates may initially cause a headache and hypotension.

Etiology and Pathophysiology

An MI may be caused by thrombosis resulting from atherosclerosis, an embolus from the heart that blocks a coronary artery, or sustained arterial spasm and prolonged ischemia in a coronary artery. An embolus may result from atrial fibrillation or valvular disease. Whatever the cause, blood flow is stopped to a portion of the myocardium. MI occurs most often in those older than age 45.

An infarction is an area of necrosis in tissue caused by an obstruction to the flow of blood to that area for a prolonged period (Figure 21-3). In an MI, there is an area of necrosis (cell death) in the heart muscle. That portion of the heart muscle cannot contract normally to help pump blood out of the heart. Dead tissue does not return to normal and scar tissue forms and interferes with the normal functions of pumping and electrical conduction. Most MI cases are related to obstruction from atherosclerosis.

The prognosis of the patient who suffers an acute MI depends on the size of the artery obstructed, the location, and the amount of heart tissue that is damaged. If a large area of the heart is affected, instant death may

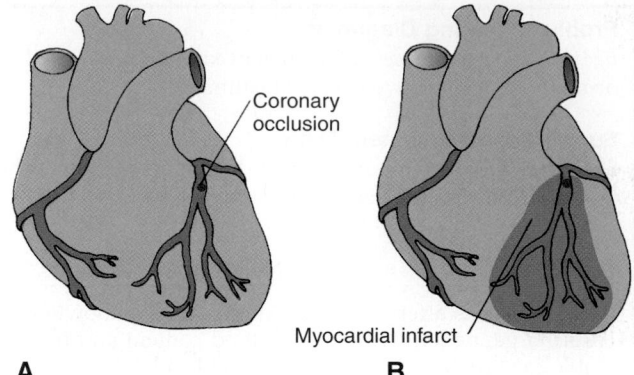

FIGURE 21-3 Occlusion of a major coronary artery **(A)** leads to area of infarct **(B)** resulting from ischemia.

occur. Smaller ischemic areas may heal if treated promptly and effectively. As the coronary vessels narrow, small blood vessels are formed that supply oxygen to the myocardium. A patient with a well-established collateral circulation may experience a milder heart attack with fewer complications. Most MIs occur in the left ventricle, the main "pump."

Signs and Symptoms

Classically, during an MI there is a sudden, severe pain in the chest, usually described as tightness, pressure, squeezing, or crushing, that is not relieved by nitrates or rest. Sometimes the pain is mistaken for anginal pain the patient has experienced before. The patient also shows symptoms of dyspnea, nausea with or without vomiting, wheezing, and ashen, clammy, cool skin. Signs of shock with pallor, profuse sweating, clammy skin, and anxiety, may occur. The heart rate may be very fast (tachycardia) or very slow (bradycardia), or the pulse may be irregular. In older adults, the attack may manifest as fatigue, syncope (temporary loss of consciousness), or weakness. Women often complain of recent episodes of extreme fatigue, with inability to complete daily activities without prolonged rest periods. These episodes may be accompanied by chest pressure, followed by eventual return to a full energy state. Feelings of "indigestion" are common. **A woman may never experience typical chest pain during an MI.** Denial is a real factor in not seeking quick treatment (Bird, 2009).

Although these symptoms are usually present in an acute MI, they are not always severe, and in some cases patients have described their pain as mild. Sometimes the patient only experiences pain in the left arm, jaw, or back. Some people experience a "silent" MI where no symptoms are perceived. **It is paramount for the patient to seek quick medical attention when experiencing any new onset of chest pain.** The window of time to prevent significant myocardial damage is narrow (about 6 hours) and the quicker medical treatment is started for an MI, the greater the chance of saving myocardium and preserving life.

Elder Care Points

Elderly patients may never complain of chest pain when having an MI. Associated symptoms such as indigestion, nausea, dyspnea, and confusion are more common complaints.

Diagnosis

The ECG may or may not show evidence of an MI initially. For this reason ECGs are repeated serially every 8 to 12 hours for three times or on a daily basis for 3 days. Changes slowly evolve and will occur in the QRS complex, ST segment, and T wave when ischemia or damaged tissue occurs. The severity of the symptoms will depend on the size of the area of ischemia or infarction. When there is necrotic tissue anywhere in the body, the white cell count increases and the sedimentation rate rises. Within 24 hours of an acute attack, the temperature of the patient with MI rises slightly, and mild leukocytosis appears.

In addition to the clinical manifestations, ECG changes, and other diagnostic tests, laboratory determinations of specific enzymes are used to establish a diagnosis of MI and evaluate the extent of damage done to the heart muscle (Table 21-2). Troponin levels are the preferred biomarker for diagnosis. Serum troponin T and troponin I are accurate within a few hours. Troponin is found only in cardiac tissue. CK isoenzymes, lactic dehydrogenase (LDH), and LDH isoenzyme levels are observed over a 72-hour period. The CK is fractionalized into CK-MB, an enzyme that is only found in heart muscle. The level of CK-MB rises in 4 to 8 hours and begins to decline in 12 to 24 hours; LDH level increases 24 to 48 hours after an MI and stays high for up to 2 weeks. The most significant laboratory finding for diagnosis of MI is an elevated troponin level, especially if accompanied by an elevated CK-MB. Myoglobin levels rise with cardiac damage.

Cardiac catheterization and angiography may be done soon after the patient is admitted to the emergency department if MI is the probable diagnosis.

This provides immediate, definitive diagnosis and treatment for occluded vessels. The nurse must thoroughly assess the status of the patient after cardiac catheterization. The patient may be up and about within about 2 hours when an arterial closure device is used for the procedure. Distal pulses on the affected leg must be assessed frequently and the groin area must be assessed for presence of hemorrhage or a hematoma. Renal function should be monitored because of potential adverse effects of contrast dyes used during the procedure.

Safety Alert

Contrast Dye

If the patient is diabetic and takes metformin, hold the drug before the contrast-dye procedure. If the procedure is done as an emergency, metformin should be held for 3 days afterward. Metformin and contrast dye have an adverse effect on kidney function. When any patient has received a contrast dye for a diagnostic test, promote good hydration either by oral or IV fluids. Keeping the patient hydrated will increase the rate of urine flow, dilute the urine, and help prevent kidney damage as the dye is excreted.

After the patient is stabilized, further testing will be done. Chest radiography, magnetic resonance imaging (MRI), echocardiography, and a technetium-99m sestamibi scan may be performed to determine the full extent of the infarction.

Think Critically

How would you prepare the patient who has experienced a probable MI for the diagnostic tests he will most likely undergo? What teaching is required?

Treatment

In many areas of the United States, there are specially designed and equipped mobile units staffed with trained personnel to give immediate care to the patient who has had a heart attack. Chewing and swallowing an aspirin when signs of an MI occur has been adopted

Table 21-2	Tests Performed to Determine Myocardial Infarction	
	NORMAL VALUE	**SIGNIFICANCE OF ABNORMAL VALUE**
Troponin I (TnI) Troponin T (TnT)	<0.3 mcg/L <0.1 mcg/L	Specific to heart muscle damage. Levels may elevate within 4-6 hr after MI, peak within 10-24 hr, and return to normal levels within 10 days.
CPK (creatine phosphokinase)	Men: 55–170 IU/L Women: 30–135 IU/L	Elevated within 4-8 hr following heart attack (may also rise with injury to other muscles). Peaks within 12-24 hr, returns to normal levels within 3-4 days.
CK-MB	<3 ng/mL	Elevates within 2-6 hr after an MI, peaks within 12-24 hr, and returns to normal within 3 days. CK-MB is specific to myocardial injury.
Myoglobin	0-85 ng/mL	Detects muscle damage to myocardium.

Other laboratory tests are listed in Table 18-2.

as part of the emergency treatment protocol to decrease or prevent heart damage by decreasing platelet aggregation (American Heart Association, 2010).

Outside the hospital, a trained emergency medical team should be called immediately. If the patient shows signs of cardiac or respiratory arrest, help should be called and cardiopulmonary resuscitation (CPR) with defibrillation, if indicated, should be started immediately. Many public areas, such as airports and shopping malls, have automated external defibrillators (AEDs) available. These AEDs can be used by individuals trained in CPR to detect and treat possible convertible rhythms until emergency personnel are on the scene.

As soon as a patient with an acute MI is brought to the emergency department, measures are taken to relieve pain, decrease ischemia, and prevent further circulatory collapse and shock. The MONA (morphine, oxygen, nitrates, aspirin) regimen is initiated (The Cochrane Library, 2010). Oxygen via nasal cannula or mask is started, intravenous (IV) access is obtained for administration of fluids and emergency drugs, and the patient is placed on a cardiac monitor. A thorough cardiac history is obtained. The Joint Commission has Core Measures in place for patients admitted with an MI (Box 21-2).

? Think Critically

A patient has chest pain. The physician orders lab studies. Which results may indicate MI versus an episode of angina?

Sublingual nitroglycerin is given unless contraindicated. Drugs administered to control pain in a patient with acute MI are morphine sulfate or hydromorphone hydrochloride (Dilaudid). One of these is given IV to provide immediate relief; morphine is the drug of choice because of its vasodilation property. **Pain medication given IV has a shorter duration, and doses must be repeated more frequently to keep the patient comfortable.** A nitrate infusion also may be started.

Box 21-2 | The Joint Commission Core Measures for Myocardial Infarction

- Aspirin administered within 24 hours of arrival at the hospital or within 24 hours before arrival.
- Beta blocker started within 24 hours of arrival.
- Thrombolytic agent administered within 30 minutes of hospital arrival.
- Aspirin therapy at discharge.
- Beta-blocker therapy continued at discharge.
- Angiotensin-converting enzyme (ACE) inhibitor therapy at discharge for left ventricular ejection fraction <40%.
- Patients with a history of cigarette use within past year given smoking cessation advice or counseling during hospitalization.

Antidysrhythmia drugs are given as indicated by abnormal ECG rhythms. Antianxiety agents, such as lorazepam (Ativan), are administered to relieve anxiety. Oxygen is administered. Close assessment of respiration is essential, as the drugs for pain can depress respiration at a time when the heart's oxygen demand is increased. Pulse oximetry is instituted quickly to measure oxygen saturation.

If the patient sought immediate medical attention on experiencing the symptoms of MI, he may be given thrombolytic agents in an attempt to dissolve a clot obstructing the coronary artery. Thrombolytic therapy must be started preferably within 6 hours but up to 12 hours of onset of symptoms to prevent necrosis of the myocardium and is indicated when the ECG shows ST segment elevation (Rivera-Bou, 2010). Agents used IV to dissolve the clot include alteplase (t-PA, Activase), tenecteplase (TNKase), reteplase (Retavase), and anistreplase (Eminase). These drugs are contraindicated in patients who have severe, uncontrolled hypertension or a history of a hemorrhagic stroke, gastrointestinal (GI) bleed, intracranial or intraspinal surgery within the past 2 months, a brain tumor, arteriovenous malformation, or aneurysm. After one of these agents is infused, a heparin drip may be started to prevent reocclusion. When a patient is not a candidate for thrombolytic therapy, heparin and low-dose aspirin may be administered to prevent further thrombosis.

If there is ST segment elevation and the clinical picture indicates that there is complete occlusion of a coronary artery, the patient may immediately undergo cardiac catheterization and balloon angioplasty with placement of stents to restore blood flow.

? Think Critically

How would you explain the thrombolytic therapy used when a patient has acute coronary occlusion?

Nursing Management
Nursing care is directed toward:
- Relieving pain.
- Promoting rest.
- Administering ordered medical therapy and observing for side effects.
- Assisting with activities of daily living (ADLs) and ambulation.
- Monitoring physical status by performing a thorough cardiovascular assessment every 4 to 8 hours, and monitoring vital signs every 2 to 4 hours.
- Recording daily weight and comparing with previous weight. Intake and output are accurately recorded and compared with previous amounts and urine output is closely monitored.
- Maintaining a patent IV access at all times.

- Limiting visitors and monitoring the heart rate closely during visits.
- Monitoring for signs of complications of MI, such as dysrhythmia, heart failure (HF), pulmonary edema, pericarditis, cardiogenic shock, or cardiac arrest (Table 21-3). Quick identification and treatment of complications is lifesaving and greatly reduces the cost of treatment during recovery.
- Decreasing anxiety and stress for the patient. Explain the function of all equipment and tests in simple terms. Explain the routine of frequent assessment and tests so the patient will know what to expect. Decreasing the family's anxiety by reinforcing what the physician has told them about the patient's condition and treatment.
- Assisting with rehabilitation activities.

The patient with damage to the myocardium is admitted to the intensive care unit (ICU) or coronary care unit (CCU). The patient is placed in bed and kept on bed rest with assistance for toileting for 24 to 48 hours.

Table 21-3	Signs and Symptoms of Complications After Myocardial Infarction
COMPLICATION	**SIGNS AND SYMPTOMS**
Dysrhythmia	Irregular pulse; abnormal ECG pattern. Ventricular fibrillation is the most common complication after MI. Report more than three PVCs per minute, heart rate of >120 or <40 bpm.
Heart failure	Dyspnea; pedal edema; sacral edema; crackles in lung bases; distended neck veins; enlarged, tender liver; weight gain of more than 2 lb in 24 hr; pulmonary edema.
Cardiogenic shock	Significant drop in systolic blood pressure (>20 points); diaphoresis; rapid pulse; cold, clammy skin; gray skin; restlessness.
Papillary muscle dysfunction	Mitral valve regurgitation with systolic murmur; dyspnea, pulmonary edema and decreased cardiac output.
Ventricular aneurysm	Outpouching of ventricular wall may cause HF, dysrhythmias, and angina. May cause formation of thrombi that lead to a stroke.
Pericarditis	Pericardial friction rub on auscultation; chest pain aggravated by movement and lessened by sitting up and leaning forward.
Dressler syndrome	Occurs 4-6 weeks after MI. Chest pain, fever, friction rub, pleural effusion, and arthralgia.

bpm, beats per minute; *ECG*, electrocardiographic; *HF*, heart failure; *MI*, myocardial infarction; *PVCs*, premature ventricular fibrillations.

Physical activity is gradually increased according to the patient's individual condition and response to activity. An IV line or a saline lock is inserted to provide a route for administration of emergency drugs to control blood pressure and dysrhythmias.

Vital signs and Po_2 are continuously monitored by electronic means and are assessed every 15 minutes to 2 hours. The temperature may be slightly elevated. Continuous ECG (cardiac telemetry monitoring) is essential to provide an accurate evaluation of the status of the heart. Death occurs most frequently within the first 24 hours of an MI and is caused by ventricular fibrillation.

While in the ICU or CCU, a pulmonary artery flow-directed catheter (Swan-Ganz type) may be inserted to read central venous pressure (CVP), pulmonary artery pressure (PAP), and pulmonary capillary wedge pressure (PCWP), which give a better picture of the injured heart's ability to pump. The patient may be placed on nothing-by-mouth (NPO) status or on a liquid diet for the first 24 hours. Then a low-sodium, low-fat diet is ordered when the patient's vital signs have stabilized. A stool softener is given to decrease the risk of bradycardia, which can be caused by straining to have a bowel movement. Potassium and magnesium are monitored closely as imbalances can cause dysrhythmias. Medication to correct dysrhythmia is ordered as needed (see Table 20-4). Measures to correct acid-base imbalance are begun. A beta-adrenergic blocker, such as metoprolol (Toprol XL, Lopressor), may be ordered to decrease the heart's workload. An angiotensin-converting enzyme (ACE) inhibitor such as captopril (Capoten) may also be prescribed. Continuous oxygen via mask or nasal cannula is administered at a rate of 2 to 5 L/min. Various IV drugs may be used to regulate blood pressure or to control dysrhythmias; these include sodium nitroprusside (Nitropress) to lower blood pressure or dobutamine (Dobutrex) to raise blood pressure. Cardiac catheterization to determine degree of occlusion is scheduled.

A temporary pacemaker may be inserted if the patient's heart rate drops below 40 beats per minute and remains there, or if he experiences complete heart block (whereby the electrical impulse does not go through the atrioventricular [AV] node to the ventricles and the ventricles are not signaled to contract) (see Chapter 20). If the MI has caused a ventral septal defect, a ventricular aneurysm, or papillary muscle rupture, open heart surgery is necessary.

CARDIOGENIC SHOCK

If the left ventricle is badly damaged, cardiogenic shock may occur. Signs and symptoms are those that accompany decreased cardiac output, such as confusion, restlessness, diaphoresis, rapid and thready pulse, increased respiratory rate, cold and clammy skin, and diminishing urinary output to less than 20 mL/hr. The best position for the patient is with the head of the bed elevated to 45 degrees to help breathing and oxygenation. The patient is cared for in the ICU, where a variety of drugs aimed at improving cardiac output may be administered.

The intraaortic balloon pump (IABP) may be used to ease the heart's workload while it begins to heal. This device uses a balloon catheter positioned in the aorta that inflates during diastole and deflates during systole, effectively decreasing the workload of the heart and increasing blood flow through the coronary arteries. This procedure is done while the patient is in the ICU or CCU. Only registered nurses who are certified in the care of the patient on an IABP are assigned to care for these patients. See Chapter 45 for further information on shock.

Intermediate Care

When very frequent assessment and monitoring are no longer essential and the patient is able to participate in his personal hygiene activities without detrimental effects on the healing heart tissues, he is transferred out of the ICU or CCU into a telemetry, or "step-down," medical unit. For some patients, this move is frightening because they know they will no longer have a nurse giving constant attention. Every effort is made to assure the patient that he is making progress toward recovery and no longer needs intensive care. While the patient is on the telemetry unit, physical activities are gradually increased according to ability to tolerate exercise, as evidenced by stable heart rate, blood pressure, and respiratory rate. There is close monitoring for symptoms of excessive strain on the heart, such as dysrhythmia or dyspnea, or for the development of complications. These measures may minimize damage from an MI, but the patient still has CAD, requires treatment, and must attend to lowering his risk factors.

Rehabilitation

A variety of emotional and behavioral responses may occur after an MI (Box 21-3). The patient and his family will need much help and support as they work to make the necessary adjustments. Many hospitals offer an outpatient cardiac rehabilitation program to help the patient make lifestyle changes to reduce future risk of cardiac problems. The program provides counseling on dietary changes for a heart-healthy diet; stress-reduction techniques; reduction of risk factors, such as avoiding tobacco use; controlling hypertension and diabetes; and a supervised exercise program with continuous ECG monitoring for 4 to 6 weeks. Such programs have been found to be effective in decreasing cardiac death and heart failure (Patient.co.uk, 2011). Progressive, supervised exercise is continued for an additional 6 to 8 weeks, and then a maintenance program is devised that the patient can do independently. A support group consisting of other individuals who have the same condition or have had similar surgery often is available. Most insurance coverage will pay for the program, as it has been highly successful in helping people to develop and maintain a healthier lifestyle and to reduce risk factors.

One area of major concern is sexuality. The patient may be fearful of resuming intercourse, thinking that it may cause a heart attack. The partner often has these fears also. Both partners need reassurance that resumption of normal sexual activities will be possible. The patient may need to take a more passive role during intercourse, at least for a while, using alternate positions that cause less strain and less oxygen demand. The patient should be told that the workload of

---

Box 21-3 Emotional and Behavioral Responses to Acute Myocardial Infarction

DENIAL
- May have history of ignoring symptoms related to heart disease
- Minimizes severity of medical condition
- Ignores activity restrictions
- Avoids discussing MI or its significance

ANGER
- Is commonly expressed as, "Why did this happen to me?"
- May be directed at family, staff, or medical regimen

ANXIETY AND FEAR
- Fears death and long-term disability
- Overtly manifests apprehension, restlessness, insomnia, tachycardia
- Less overtly manifests increased verbalization, projection of feelings to others, hypochondriasis
- Fears activity, recurrent heart attacks, and sudden death

DEPENDENCY
- Is totally reliant on staff
- Is unwilling to perform tasks or activities unless approved by heath care provider
- Wants to be monitored by ECG at all times
- Is hesitant to leave ICU or hospital

DEPRESSION
- Experiences mourning period concerning loss of health, altered body function, and changes in lifestyle
- Realizes seriousness of situation
- Begins to worry about future implications of health problem
- Shows manifestations of withdrawal, crying, anorexia, apathy
- Depression may be more evident after discharge

REALISTIC ACCEPTANCE
- Focuses on optimum rehabilitation
- Plans changes compatible with altered cardiac function

From Lewis SL, Heitkemper MM, Dirksen SR, et al. (2011). *Medical-Surgical Nursing: Assessment and Management of Clinical Problems* (8th ed.). St Louis: Mosby.
ECG, electrocardiogram; *ICU*, intensive care unit; *MI*, myocardial infarction.

intercourse with a known partner is equal to climbing a flight of stairs. If a flight of stairs can be climbed without much change in heart rate, respirations, or blood pressure, intercourse should not cause harm. The physician should discuss this area with the patient and his partner, but if the physician does not, see that the proper information is given. Sexual dysfunction may occur at first, but with patience on the part of both partners, it usually passes.

Patients should be taught to plan sexual activity for times when they are well rested and to avoid an environment that is too hot or too cold. It is best to space such activity at least 2 hours after eating a meal or drinking any alcohol. Nitroglycerin should be used prophylactically if intercourse causes angina symptoms. If angina does occur, the patient should cease activity, place a nitroglycerin tablet under his tongue, lie down, and rest.

Levels of physical activity are designated through metabolic equivalent (MET) units. One MET is the amount of oxygen needed by the body at rest. The patient's rehabilitation program slowly progresses stepwise to higher energy expenditures over a period of months (Table 21-4).

Rehabilitation involves three major aspects: (1) a program of increasing activity based on the patient's individual progress and needs; (2) instruction of the patient and family about the nature of the illness and the rationale for every aspect of its management; and (3) assistance to the patient and family as they work toward the goal of accepting the limitations imposed and the changes in lifestyle that may be required.

The main purpose of instruction is to provide the patient with the information needed to avoid the problems and complications that can occur once the structured program is finished. The rationale for the therapy and necessary lifestyle changes must be understood.

Patient Teaching

Guidelines for Recovery from an MI

Teach the patient to:
- Recognize the signs of recurrent MI and to seek immediate medical attention should they occur. These are chest pain, diaphoresis, nausea, and anxiety.
- Adopt a lifetime regular, graduated exercise program.
- Alter controllable risk factors: reach and maintain a normal weight; cease smoking; keep alcohol consumption at a moderate level (no more than 1.5 oz per day); keep cholesterol within normal limits; control hypertension.
- Reduce stress and learn relaxation techniques.
- Observe for complications, such as irregular pulse rate, dyspnea and fatigue, chest pain, and fever.
- Continue on a low-fat, low-sodium diet individualized to taste.
- Take medications as ordered and monitor for side effects.

It is important to stress to the patient that he has control over his rehabilitation and prognosis. He alone has

Table 21-4	Energy Expenditure in Metabolic Equivalents
	CALORIES BURNED
Low-Energy Activities (Fewer than 3 METs or 3 cal/min)	
Activities in Hospital	
Resting supine	1.0
Sitting	1.2
Eating	1.4
Conversing	1.4
Washing hands, face	2.5
Activities Outside Hospital	
Sewing by hand	1.4
Sweeping floor	1.7
Painting, sitting	2.5
Driving car	2.8
Assembling a radio	2.7
Sewing by machine	2.9
Moderate-Energy Activities (3-6 METs or 3-6 cal/min)	
Activities in Hospital	
Sitting on bedside commode	3.6
Walking at 2.5 mph	3.6
Showering	4.2
Using bedpan	4.7
Walking at 3.75 mph	5.6
Activities Outside Hospital	
Bricklaying	4.0
Tractor plowing	4.2
Ironing, standing	4.2
Mopping floor	4.2
Bowling	4.4
Cycling at 5.5 mph on level ground	4.5
Golfing	5.0
Dancing	5.5
High-Energy Activities (6-8 METs or 6-8 cal/min)	
Ambulating with braces and crutches	8.0
Performing carpentry	6.8
Mowing lawn by hand	7.7
Playing singles tennis	7.1
Riding on trotting horse	8.0
Walking at 5 mph	6.5
Ascending stairs	7.0

Adapted from Lewis SL, Heitkemper MM, Dirksen SR, et al. 2011. *Medical-Surgical Nursing* (8th ed.). St Louis: Mosby.

full control over his lifestyle changes and the treatment program. When the patient feels that he, rather than the physician, is in control, he is much more likely to remain on the treatment program.

Through its local chapters, the American Heart Association provides an abundance of written material designed for the person recovering from an MI (see Online Resources on p. 470). Patients and their families should know about this valuable source of information and support as they work toward the goal of rehabilitation.

SURGICAL AND NONSURGICAL TREATMENT OPTIONS

PERCUTANEOUS TRANSLUMINAL CORONARY ANGIOPLASTY

If only a few areas of stenosis are identified, a percutaneous cardiac intervention may be performed. The patient may have a percutaneous transluminal coronary angioplasty (PTCA) rather than coronary artery bypass graft (CABG) to improve blood flow. Although not an open heart procedure, PCTA is invasive and similar to the procedure used for cardiac catheterization. It is performed on patients with only one or two occlusions. PTCA is a nonsurgical interventional technique to open blocked coronary arteries. It is performed in the cardiac catheterization laboratory using fluoroscopy. A catheter with a balloon attachment is threaded into the blocked artery, and when the narrowed area is reached, the balloon is inflated, flattening the plaque and widening the interior of the artery. A percentage of patients experience reocclusion about 6 months after PTCA and will eventually require a CABG. If no myocardial damage has occurred from ischemia, the patient is discharged in about 24 hours.

A metal or drug-eluting stent (continually releases an anticoagulant/antiplatelet drug) usually is placed in the artery to help maintain the opening (Figure 21-4). A stent is made of stainless steel and acts as a brace for the artery wall. Research has shown that the drug-eluting stents may reduce the need to restent the vessels over time because of cellular hyperplasia as the body adjusts to the foreign body. When a clot has been

FIGURE 21-4 Placement of coronary artery stent. **A,** The stent is positioned at the site of stenotic lesion. **B,** The balloon is inflated, expanding the stent. The balloon is then deflated and removed. **C,** The implanted stent is left in place.

present, a glycoprotein (GP) IIb/IIIa inhibitor such as abciximab (ReoPro), tirofiban (Aggrastat), or eptifibatide (Integrilin) is given to reduce platelet aggregation for up to 48 hours to prevent cardiac ischemia. When a stent is placed, the patient must take antiplatelet agents, such as aspirin, and/or clopidogrel (Plavix) for up to 1 year following placement. Injecting vascular endothelial growth factor (VEGF) during angioplasty helps initiate new blood vessel growth, which results in increased blood supply to the myocardium. The patient must be prepared to undergo CABG if angioplasty is unsuccessful.

 Safety Alert

Proton Pump Inhibitors

Proton pump inhibitors may interfere with the action of clopidogrel (Plavix); proton pump inhibitors should not be taken when clopidogrel is prescribed (Juurlink, 2009).

Other procedures to remedy clots are laser angioplasty, thrombectomy, and atherectomy. Laser angioplasty breaks up the clot. Rheolytic thrombectomy uses low-pressure, high-speed saline jets to break up the clot. Atherectomy devices either excise and retrieve plaque or destroy it. These procedures are sometimes used when a patient has reocclusion after CABG and PTCA. CABG surgery is covered in the section on cardiac surgery.

Studies are ongoing to determine whether a regimen consisting of a very-low-fat diet, regular exercise, reduction of stress, and practice of relaxation techniques can reverse CAD without surgery. These methods have been effective in people who can maintain the discipline to stick to the program.

TRANSMYOCARDIAL LASER REVASCULARIZATION

For patients who are critically ill and are not candidates for PTCA or CABG, transmyocardial laser revascularization (TMR) is an option. This procedure may be available to patients with severe chest pain that limits their ability to perform ADLs, who have a history of CABG, and who have no other treatment options. A carbon dioxide laser is used to drill tiny holes in the heart's left ventricle. These channels heal on the outside of the heart, but remain open on the inside, allowing blood to flow into the myocardium, where it was previously diminished because of blocked coronary arteries.

CARDIAC SURGERY

Open heart surgery is made possible by the heart-lung machine. The machine functions as an artificial heart (pump) and lung (oxygenator). Because all this is done outside the patient's body, the procedure is called *extracorporeal circulation*. The surgeon inserts large tubes in the vena cava and reroutes the unoxygenated venous blood through the heart-lung machine. There, the blood is exposed to an atmosphere of oxygen in which an exchange of gases takes place (carbon dioxide is released and oxygen is taken up), and the oxygenated blood is returned to the patient via the femoral artery. The blood may be cooled so that the patient's body temperature is lowered (hypothermia), thereby reducing the body's metabolic needs during surgery.

Open heart surgery is performed by extracorporeal circulation or off pump using hypothermia. Congenital heart defects, valve replacements, bypass of clogged coronary arteries, and heart transplant are accomplished by open heart techniques.

Coronary Artery Bypass Graft Surgery

CABG is performed (1) when angina cannot be controlled medically or (2) to prevent greater occlusion and consequent MI. The CABG surgery bypasses the artery that is blocked, replacing it with sections of a vein or artery taken from another part of the patient's body. Usually the mammary artery or sections of saphenous vein or radial artery are grafted. The mammary artery is left attached to the subclavian artery and the other end is sewn distal to the blockage in a coronary artery. Saphenous vein grafts are sewn to the aorta and then distal to the blockage in a coronary artery. These new vessels supply blood to the myocardium. Although the heart is not "opened," its activity often is stopped for the procedure. The patient will have a midsternal incision and, if saphenous veins were used for the grafts, will have leg incisions as well (Figure 21-5). Figure 21-6 shows CABG procedures using vein grafts or the internal mammary artery.

Elder Care Points

Elderly patients tolerate CABG surgery well, but the recovery period is longer because of the slower healing rate and lessened ability of the body to handle this degree of physical stress.

FIGURE 21-5 **A,** Sternal incision for CABG. **B,** Leg incision for removal of saphenous vein for grafting to coronary arteries.

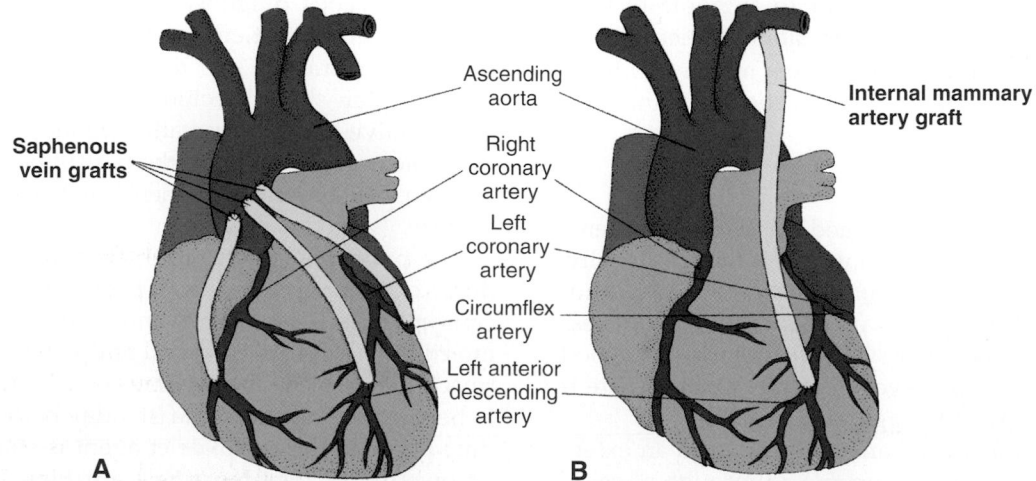

FIGURE 21-6 Two methods of coronary artery bypass grafting. **A,** Saphenous vein grafts. **B,** Internal mammary artery graft.

An off-pump coronary artery bypass technique for CABG procedures—minimally invasive direct coronary artery bypass (MIDCAB)—does not require stopping the heart's activity and therefore does not require using the heart-lung machine. MIDCB procedures are done on about 25% of patients who undergo coronary artery bypass. The MIDCAB procedure requires only a 3-inch incision, is performed with the use of drugs to slow or stop the heart briefly, uses special instruments, and takes approximately one third the time to complete as traditional CABG. Patients may be discharged home in less than 36 hours. However, only patients with one or two lesions in an easily accessible area of a major coronary artery are candidates for this simplified procedure. The main advantage of the MIDCAB procedure is to the patient in the areas of cost, time spent in the hospital, recovery time, and avoidance of large surgical incisions. Studies have not shown that there is significant difference in outcome or prognosis between the various procedures (Brown, 2011).

Coronary bypass surgery is expensive, averaging $25,000 to $35,000 for surgery, anesthesia, and in-hospital care. Less invasive approaches average $3000 to $5000 less. CABG does not cure the disease, it only relieves the symptoms and may prevent myocardial damage from total occlusion of a coronary artery. After the surgery, anginal chest pain disappears in about 65% of patients, and another 25% show improvement. Many of those patients who had a coronary artery bypass in the past 10 years are returning for a second operation because the new arteries have become occluded. A greater emphasis is being placed on the need for adherence to lifestyle changes to prevent a second operation. Nursing Care Plan 21-2 summarizes care of the patient following cardiac surgery.

The grafts have an average life of 10 years before occlusion begins, unless the patient truly makes the commitment to a heart-healthy diet, lowers stress, and exercises regularly. Recent research suggests that patients in stable condition with minimal cardiac disease demonstrate results similar to angioplasty with conservative medical treatment alone. Patients managed medically did not experience a higher incidence of MI, stroke, or other complications (Skinner & Cooper, 2009).

Heart Transplant

Heart transplants are performed for selected patients who have end-stage left ventricular failure. Ideally, candidates must be younger than age 65, have end-stage cardiac disease with predicted survival of less than 1 year, have no other systemic disease, have good renal function, and be psychologically stable. There is some flexibility with the age requirements.

Candidates for heart transplant undergo an extensive psychological evaluation and a thorough physical assessment. Patients must also be evaluated for the ability to remain in compliance with health care instructions and for the ability to obtain and administer antirejection medications. Transplant patients must take immunosuppressants and other medications for the remainder of their lives. Very few donor hearts are available, and the waiting lists are long. A heart transplant operation takes 5 to 8 hours.

Patients who receive a heart transplant face considerable financial cost, a life of taking immunosuppressive drugs that have many serious side effects (including risk for infection), and the constant threat of organ rejection. However, the benefits are considerable, with an average 1-year survival rate of about 82%, a 3-year survival rate of about 78%, and a 5-year survival rate of 70% (American Heart Association, 2009b). A significant number of heart transplant patients survive beyond 10 years.

Transplant patients must adhere to strict dietary and exercise regimens to prevent the new heart from becoming affected with problems that led to the original heart failure. Heart transplants are performed in highly specialized medical centers. Patients who are too unstable for care in the home may remain in the hospital for an extended period until a heart is available. Other patients may be given a special pager for notification of an available heart. These patients must be available for immediate admission to the hospital. Patients awaiting a heart transplant are placed on a national waiting list. A heart may be available within 24 hours, or one may be months away. Unfortunately, some patients die before a suitable heart is available. There has been limited success with use of xenograft and mechanical artificial hearts, but research continues. The left ventricular assist device has been of benefit in providing needed perfusion for patients awaiting transplant surgery.

Nursing Care of the Patient Having Cardiac Surgery

Preoperative Care. Before cardiac surgery, the patient undergoes diagnostic tests and examinations, mostly on an outpatient basis. Teaching and psychological preparation are done before surgery. The teaching plan should include expectations during the preoperative and postoperative periods. There is considerable apprehension on the part of both the patient and the patient's family when faced with open heart surgery.

The patient is given information about the procedure, explaining what to expect and what kind of equipment will be used. Admission occurs early the morning of surgery. If an oral antiplatelet agent (aspirin, clopidogrel) has been being taken, a switch is made to heparin by injection at least 1 day before surgery. If time permits, the antiplatelet agent is stopped 7 days preoperatively. See Nursing Care Plan 21-2 for care of the patient following cardiac surgery.

★ Nursing Care Plan 21-2 | Care of the Patient Following Cardiac Surgery

Scenario
Mr. Jacobi, age 57, was admitted to the telemetry unit following a coronary artery bypass graft (CABG) and is 2 days postoperative. Mr. Jacobi is married and has three teenage children. He plans to return to his job as a truck driver after surgical recovery.

Problem/Nursing Diagnosis
Unable to ambulate 50 feet in the hallway without complaints of dizziness and dyspnea/Activity intolerance related to postsurgical hemodynamic changes.

Supporting Assessment Data
Subjective: States, "I'm feeling faint and short of breath" after ambulating 30 feet.
Objective: RR 32, Po_2 90% after ambulating short distance, Po_2 increases to 95% to 100% when returned to chair, RR decreased to 24.

Goals/Expected Outcomes	Nursing Intervention	Selected Rationale	Evaluation
Patient will be able to ambulate 50 feet in hallway without complaints of dizziness and dyspnea.	Assess Po_2 and vital signs before and after ambulation.	Provides baseline values for evaluation.	Po_2 96%, no complaints of dizziness by third postoperative day.
	Provide safety during ambulation (e.g., follow with wheelchair, use gait belt, instruct to use handrails).	Prevent falls if hemodynamic changes occur.	Patient did not sustain fall.
	Provide rest periods every 15 feet.	Improve success of ambulation.	Patient able to ambulate 100 feet without rest period by third postoperative day.
	Gradually increase distance of ambulation as condition stabilizes.	Decrease workload on heart and facilitate patient recovery.	Patient ambulated 100 feet tid without complaints of dizziness and dyspnea by third postoperative day. Continue plan.

Problem/Nursing Diagnosis
Midsternal and left lower leg surgical incision/Impaired skin integrity related to thoracotomy and saphenous vein graft.

Supporting Assessment Data
Subjective: Patient asks about care of wounds to chest and left lower leg.
Objective: Incisions to midsternum and left lower leg. Both incisions intact, no areas of redness noted.

Goals/Expected Outcomes	Nursing Intervention	Selected Rationale	Evaluation
Surgical incisions will remain intact and free of signs of infection.	Assess and document status of incision at the beginning of each shift.	Determine changes in status of wound, such as development of redness, edema, opening of suture lines.	Midsternal incision intact, no signs of infection. Incision to left lower leg slightly edematous, ½-inch opening of wound on fourth postoperative day. Documented and reported. Continue to monitor.
	Assess vital signs.	Elevated temperature and heart rate may indicate beginning of wound infection.	HR 72, T 100° F (37.8° C). Continue to monitor.
	Include wound management in discharge teaching plan.	Provides knowledge to prevent and recognize complications associated with wound healing.	Demonstrated appropriate wound care. Verbalized signs and symptoms of infection.

ADLs, activities of daily living; *tid,* three times a day.

Continued

Nursing Care Plan 21-2   Care of the Patient Following Cardiac Surgery—cont'd

Problem/Nursing Diagnosis

Complains of incisional pain during deep-breathing exercises and use of incentive spirometer/Acute pain related to midsternal surgical incision.

Supporting Assessment Data

Subjective: States, "It hurts too much to do these breathing exercises."
Objective: Unable to reach incentive spirometer goals; Po_2 94%.

Goals/Expected Outcomes	Nursing Intervention	Selected Rationale	Evaluation
Patient will verbalize decreased pain during deep-breathing exercises.	Assess pain level before deep-breathing exercises and use of incentive spirometer. Provide pain medication as needed. Teach to splint incision during respiratory exercises.	Patient will be more likely to complete exercises if he is pain free.	Completes breathing exercises without pain medication by third postoperative day.
Patient will reach incentive spirometer goals within 24 hr.	Encourage patient to use incentive spirometer at least q 2 hr. Gradually increase goal.	Prevent postoperative respiratory complications.	Reaches 90% of incentive spirometry goal by third postoperative day.
Po_2 will remain at or above 98%.	Monitor O_2 Sat before and after use of incentive spirometer.	Baseline values to determine effectiveness of treatment.	Po_2 98% before and after use of incentive spirometer. Continue plan.

Problem/Nursing Diagnosis

Patient expresses concern about home care management/Deficient knowledge related to postoperative care after discharge from hospital.

Supporting Assessment Data

Subjective: States, "I don't know how I can manage all this at home. When can I return to work?"
Objective: Patient anxious, irritable during discussion of discharge planning.

Goals/Expected Outcomes	Nursing Intervention	Selected Rationale	Evaluation
Patient will demonstrate knowledge of home care instructions including: wound management, medications, exercise, diet, ADLs, and when to return to work.	Assess level of understanding of discharge instructions.	Baseline for developing discharge plan.	Verbalized understanding of discharge instructions.
	Provide opportunity to verbalize concerns.	Reduces patient anxiety.	Verbalized concerns openly, stated some anxiety relieved.
	Provide instructions concerning medications, wound care, ADLs.		Demonstrated understanding of instructions.
	Refer to dietitian/nutritionist for dietary requirements.	Knowledge of expectations increases confidence and reduces anxiety.	States understands diet instructions and will attempt to follow them.
	Collaborate with physician concerning additional instructions, such as return to work and cardiac rehabilitation recommendations.	Expert knowledge may be needed to provide appropriate information. Reinforce information as provided by physician.	Verbalized disappointment that he will be unable to return to work for at least 8 wk. May require part-time basis for longer period. Continue plan.

Critical Thinking Questions

1. List five additional nursing diagnoses that are appropriate for a patient after cardiac surgery.
2. List five additional priority assessments you should complete for this patient.

Postoperative Care. During the early postoperative period, the patient remains in an ICU, where specialized cardiac monitoring equipment is used and highly skilled personnel are in constant attendance. Cardiac rate and rhythm are monitored closely. For the patient who had an open heart procedure, chest tubes for drainage and proper reexpansion of the lungs need special attention. The patient often continues to receive mechanical ventilation for a few hours after surgery. Once consciousness has fully returned, weaning from the ventilator is begun if oxygenation is adequate. Autologous blood transfusion is performed with blood drained from the chest cavity. Chest tubes are usually removed before the patient is moved out of the ICU. Temporary epicardial pacemaker leads will be in place and may or may not be connected to a pacemaker. Usually, at least two IV lines are in place for medication delivery and fluid maintenance, as well as an arterial line for hemodynamic monitoring. If saphenous vein grafts were used rather than the mammary artery, there will be leg incisions to care for along with the chest incision. Urine output is initially monitored hourly and thereafter every 2 hours to detect signs of decreased perfusion to the kidneys and cardiogenic shock.

After the first 24 to 48 hours, the surgeon will assess the patient's condition and decide whether transfer to a step-down unit is possible. The patient will continue to need very special nursing care with continuous ECG monitoring. Vital signs must be taken and recorded at frequent intervals; urinary output is monitored closely. Fluid intake may be restricted for a brief period. Daily weight is monitored to assess fluid balance.

Clinical Cues

Priorities for care of the postsurgical patient must be established. Plan on frequent assessment of respiratory and cardiac status, care of invasive lines and chest tubes, wound assessment and care, fluid and electrolyte balance, pain management, and assessment of emotional status.

Coronary artery bypass surgery can produce many special problems related to rehabilitation of the patient. Among the physiologic symptoms that can persist into the home recovery period are fatigue and weakness, incisional discomfort, edema in the donor leg, dysrhythmias, loss of appetite, and unusual physical sensations. There also is the possibility of closure of the graft and the reappearance of original symptoms. Sometimes the patient develops Dressler syndrome, a type of pericarditis causing chest pain, which is treated with nonsteroidal anti-inflammatory drugs (NSAIDs).

Depression for weeks to months is not uncommon after heart surgery. Patients should be alerted to this possibility and referred for assistance if this occurs. Women are more likely than men to experience depression following heart surgery, and their cases are more severe.

Most patients do not experience all these problems during the home recovery period after coronary artery bypass surgery, and some have relatively trouble-free recovery periods. It is important that bypass surgery patients and their families realize that bypass surgery is not a cure for CAD. Bypass surgery is simply one form of therapy for a chronic condition that will require continued management in order to slow the disease process and reduce the incidence of life-threatening events in the person's life. Other specific postoperative care is directed at preventing infection to the surgical sites, managing wounds, monitoring for complications, and promoting rehabilitation.

Usually after the first 48 hours, minimal medication is needed for pain. The patient often is very fatigued and tends to have mood swings. With an uncomplicated recovery, the patient is usually discharged home within 3 to 7 days and referred to a cardiac rehabilitation outpatient program.

Cardiac transplant patients are threatened by organ rejection, infection, development of CAD in the new heart, and development of a malignant tumor as a result of immunosuppressive therapy to prevent transplant rejection. Antiviral therapy is administered to decrease the incidence of post-transplant malignancy. Many viruses are linked to neoplastic growth. Heart biopsies are performed regularly.

COMMUNITY CARE

With early discharge from the hospital after surgery, many patients have continuing care from home health nurses. Patients recovering from cardiac surgery, MI, atherosclerotic heart disease, angina, or valvular heart disease all may be referred to a cardiac rehabilitation program. The goal of such programs is to reduce risk of further heart problems or death. The program is directed toward restoring and maintaining optimal physiologic function. Improving psychological outlook, maintaining ability to work, and social well-being are other components of the program.

Home care nurses have many patients diagnosed with heart disease. The goal of home care is to monitor the patient's condition and to prevent complications, such as life-threatening dysrhythmias, MI, and CHF. Nurses supervise the medication regimen, monitor weight gain, draw blood for laboratory tests to determine drug levels and electrolyte status, and assess for beginning signs of complications. By detecting complications early, patients can be treated at home rather than at the hospital, thereby decreasing costs of care.

Many residents in long-term care facilities have cardiac disorders. Assessing changes in condition is a high priority. If changes can be found quickly, the severity of a complication can be reduced in this population. It is important to know each resident's history.

Get Ready for the NCLEX® Examination!

Key Points

- High levels of cholesterol (LDL) contribute to development of atherosclerosis, a major factor in occlusion of coronary vessels.
- Ischemia occurs as blood supply is lost to the myocardium.
- A cardinal sign of myocardial ischemia is angina pectoris (chest pain).
- Angina may be classified as stable, variant, or unstable.
- *Acute coronary syndrome* is an umbrella term for a group of symptoms indicating severe myocardial ischemia.
- Nitrates (nitroglycerin) are the most commonly used drugs to treat angina.
- Patients should be monitored for hypotension and development of a throbbing headache while taking nitroglycerin.
- When a coronary artery becomes completely obstructed, necrosis of myocardial tissue occurs (MI).
- Necrotic myocardial tissue cannot perform its function of pumping.
- Diagnosis of MI is made by patient history, ECG, and serum cardiac enzyme levels.
- A patient may be given an aspirin tablet if an MI is suspected. Aspirin helps prevent further clot formation.
- Emergency care for a patient suspected of experiencing an MI includes oxygen; IV access; cardiac monitoring; pain management, usually morphine sulfate IV; ECG; and management of dysrhythmias.
- Medications following MI may include nitrates, antihypertensive drugs, anticoagulants, beta blockers, ACE inhibitors, and antidysrhythmic drugs.
- Cardiac catheterization is likely to be performed on a patient experiencing an MI.
- Nursing care after cardiac catheterization includes cardiac monitoring, maintaining the patient in a supine position with the legs straight for at least 2 hours, monitoring the femoral area for hematoma formation, assessing peripheral pulses frequently, and monitoring urinary output.
- Stents may be placed to maintain patency of coronary vessels in an attempt to avoid CABG. Stents may be placed during PTCA.
- CABG may be needed when a patient's angina cannot be controlled by medical means or when there is myocardial damage due to occlusion of one or more coronary vessels.
- An alternative to CABG is MIDCAB performed off pump.
- A heart transplant may be needed for a patient with end-stage left ventricular heart failure.
- Patients must receive extensive physical and psychological assessment before acceptance into a cardiac transplant program. Family counseling is also advisable.
- Donor hearts are not readily available; therefore patients must be carefully screened to determine the most appropriate recipient.
- Patients must be advised of potential complications, the need to follow through on dietary and exercise recommendations, and the need to continue medications, such as immunosuppressants, for the remainder of their lives.

- Nursing care of patients after heart transplant includes intense monitoring in the CCU or ICU; assessing for signs of complications; wound management; administration of emergency, antirejection, and appropriate cardiac drugs; pain management; assessment of respiratory function; and initial return to physical activity such as out of bed to chair.
- Discharge planning should prepare the patient for return home and the beginning of care in the community.
- Monitoring the patient's understanding of and compliance with prescribed medications is an important responsibility of the home health nurse.

Additional Learning Resources

SG Go to your Study Guide for additional learning activities to help you master this chapter content.

 Go to your Evolve website (http://evolve.elsevier.com/deWit/medsurg) for the following FREE learning resources:
- Animations, audio, and video
- Answers and rationales for questions and activities
- Concept Map Creator
- Glossary with pronunciations in English and Spanish
- Interactive Review Questions and Exercises and more!

 Online Resources
- American Heart Association, www.heart.org
- Mended Hearts, www.mendedhearts.org
- National Cholesterol Education Program, www.nhibi.nih.gov/aabouat/ncep/ncep_pd.htm

Review Questions for the NCLEX® Examination

1. After reviewing risk factors for cardiac disease, the patient is prescribed atorvastatin (Lipitor) to reduce cholesterol levels. The nurse must include which instruction(s)? *(Select all that apply.)*
   1. Report any muscle weakness.
   2. Avoid exposure to sunlight.
   3. Keep appointments for lab work.
   4. Drink grapefruit juice.
   5. Maintain a low-protein diet.

2. The patient asks, "What causes angina pectoris?" An accurate response by a nurse would be:
   1. "It is caused by the decreased blood flow to the coronary arteries due to shunting of the blood."
   2. "It is caused by a decreased blood flow to the myocardium due to partial obstruction of the coronary arteries."
   3. "It is caused by poor oxygenation of the coronary arteries due to poor gas exchange across the alveolar basement membrane."
   4. "It is caused by the inflammation of the sternal cartilage."

3. A patient is diagnosed as having attacks of angina pectoris. As part of the discharge instructions, the patient is instructed on the appropriate storage and use of sublingual nitroglycerin. Which of the following patient statements indicates a need for further instructions?

   1. "The tablets should be kept in a cool, dark place."
   2. "I need to lie down after I take the medication."
   3. "I can take the tablet every 15 minutes for angina pains."
   4. "The expiration date on the bottle is important."

4. A 44-year-old patient is admitted with a sudden, severe chest tightness unrelieved by rest or nitroglycerin, and profuse sweating. Which test would exhibit an elevated level only if the patient has had an MI?

   1. Serum troponin
   2. Blood urea nitrogen
   3. Myoglobin level
   4. Prothrombin time

5. Immediate therapeutic measures provided for a patient entering the hospital with an acute myocardial infarction include which measure(s)? *(Select all that apply.)*

   1. Morphine sulfate
   2. Oxygen therapy
   3. Furosemide
   4. Nitroglycerin
   5. Aspirin

6. Which food has been found to reduce cholesterol levels?

   1. Garlic
   2. Onion
   3. Ginger
   4. Nutmeg

7. The physician explains the treatment options to a Hispanic woman diagnosed with occlusion of multiple coronary vessels. Before signing an informed consent, the patient is most likely to defer her health care decisions to her:

   1. oldest adult son.
   2. oldest adult daughter.
   3. brother-in-law.
   4. husband.

8. The patient has experienced an MI and has ST-segment elevation on the ECG. The priority nursing diagnosis would be:

   1. Impaired oxygenation.
   2. Ineffective coping.
   3. Ineffective tissue perfusion.
   4. Activity intolerance.

9. Immediate postoperative nursing care of a patient who has undergone coronary artery bypass grafts includes which intervention(s)? *(Select all that apply.)*

   1. Assessing cardiac rate and rhythm
   2. Checking chest tubes for drainage
   3. Monitoring liver enzymes
   4. Assessing bowel sounds
   5. Managing pain

10. After change-of-shift report, which of the following assigned patients should the nurse attend to first? The patient with:

    1. stable vital signs who returned 40 minutes ago after a PCTA.
    2. an MI complaining of a headache who was transferred from the coronary care unit earlier.
    3. stable angina whose chest pain was relieved by 2 nitroglycerin tablets 2 hours ago.
    4. unstable angina who is having chest pain, shortness of breath, nausea, and anxiety.

Critical Thinking Activities

Scenario A
Ms. Trotter, a 62-year-old woman, comes to the clinic for her annual examination results. Her cholesterol level is 260 mg/dL, with HDL 30 mg/dL and LDL 220. She has a family history of atherosclerosis and heart disease. She asks about the danger of her high cholesterol level.

1. Describe to her how atherosclerosis can lead to heart problems.
2. Help her identify ways to decrease her cholesterol level and raise her HDL level.
3. Describe to her the symptoms of heart problems she should report to her doctor.
4. Have her identify the symptoms that might indicate a heart attack and what she should do if they occur.

Scenario B
Mrs. Yee, a 50-year-old woman, comes to the emergency department complaining of a burning, squeezing sensation in her chest, and a feeling of nausea. She is diaphoretic and apprehensive.

1. Compare and contrast the symptoms of heart attack between men and women.
2. Describe the probable emergency treatment of Mrs. Yee in the emergency department.
3. What lab tests may be ordered to evaluate for possible MI? What is a significant ECG finding indicating MI?

Scenario C
Ms. O'Hare, a 45-year-old, is on the list for a heart transplant. She has a left ventricular assist device and is waiting at home.

1. What are the criteria for heart transplant? List contraindications.
2. Describe the purpose of the left ventricular assist device.
3. Develop a discharge teaching plan for Ms. O'Hare after transplant.

The Neurologic System*

Objectives

Theory

1. Define the vocabulary particular to problems of the nervous system.
2. Discuss the differences in the action of sympathetic and parasympathetic nervous systems.
3. Identify four specific ways in which a nurse can contribute to preventing neurologic disorders.
4. State the appropriate preparation and postprocedure care for patients undergoing lumbar puncture (spinal tap), electroencephalogram (EEG), and radiologic studies of the brain and cerebral vessels.

5. Become familiar with the techniques used for assessment of the nervous system.
6. Compare and contrast the various signs and symptoms of the common problems experienced by patients with nervous system disorders.

Clinical Practice

1. Gather a pertinent history for a patient with a nervous system problem.
2. Demonstrate a "neuro" check.
3. Score the neurologic status of a patient with a nervous system disorder according to the Glasgow Coma Scale.

Key Terms

accommodation (p. 488)
aphasia (ă-FĀ-zhă, p. 495)
Babinski's reflex (p. 480)
calculi (KĂL-kū-lī, p. 494)
caloric testing (kăl-Ō-rĭk, p. 480)
clonus (KLŌ-nŭs, p. 480)
decerebrate posturing (dē-SĔR-ē-brāt, p. 487)
decorticate posturing (dē-KŎR-tĭ-kāt, p. 487)

delirium (dĕ-LĬR-ē-ŭm, p. 495)
dysphagia (dĭs-FĀ-jē-ă, p. 493)
hemiparesis (hĕm-ē-pă-RĒ-sĭs, p. 492)
hemiplegia (hĕm-ĭ-PLĒ-jă, p. 492)
nystagmus (nĭs-TĂG-mŭs, p. 487)
quadriplegic (kwŏd-rĭ-PLĒ-jĭk, p. 492)
tetraplegia (TĔT-ră-PLĒ-jă, p. 492)

OVERVIEW OF ANATOMY AND PHYSIOLOGY OF THE NEUROLOGIC SYSTEM

HOW IS THE NERVOUS SYSTEM ORGANIZED?

- The functional unit of the nervous system is the neuron, which consists of a cell body, dendrites, and an axon (Figure 22-1). Neurons react to stimuli, conduct impulses, and influence other neurons. There are afferent and efferent neurons.
- The nervous system consists of the central nervous system (CNS) and the peripheral nervous system (PNS).
- The CNS is made up of the brain and spinal cord (Figure 22-2).
- The brain is divided into the cerebrum, diencephalon, cerebellum, and brainstem, which each perform

various functions. Table 22-1 lists the functions of the various divisions of the brain.
- The brainstem consists of the midbrain, pons, and medulla.
- The different parts of the brain control various functions (Figure 22-3).
- The PNS is composed of the sensory organs—eyes, ears, taste buds, olfactory receptors, and touch receptors—12 pairs of cranial nerves, and 31 pairs of spinal nerves and ganglia that link the sensory organs, muscles, and other parts of the body to the brain and spinal cord. The distribution pathways of the spinal nerves are called *dermatomes* (Figure 22-4).
- There are 12 pairs of cranial nerves, some of which are sensory nerves and others of which are motor nerves (Table 22-2).
- The spinal cord extends from the medulla to the level of the first lumbar vertebra.
- The spinal cord is a conduction pathway for impulses going to and from the brain and also serves

*Refer to an anatomy and physiology text for a thorough review of the complex nervous system.

FIGURE 22-1 Structure of a neuron.

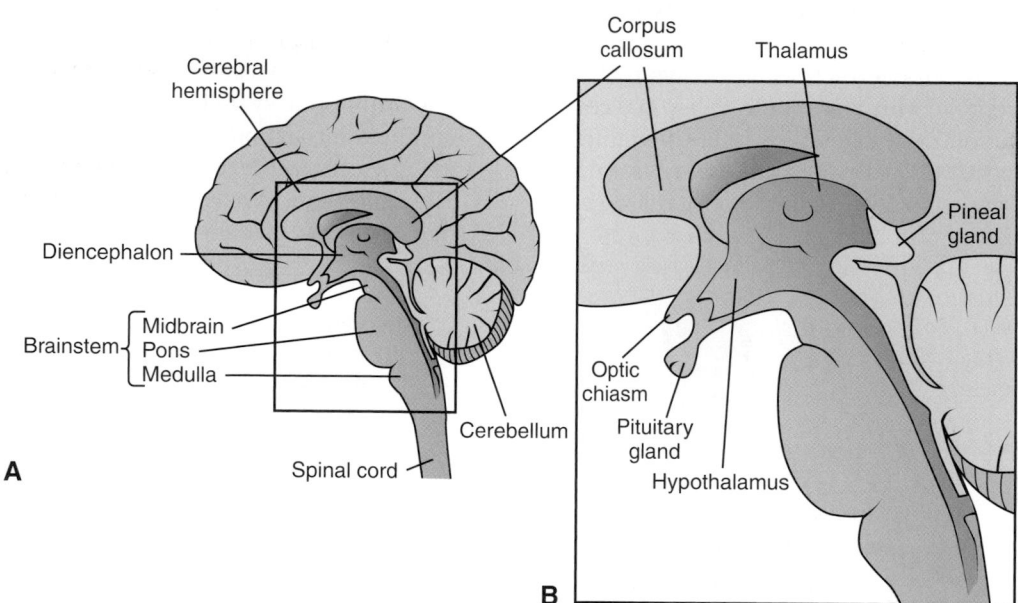

FIGURE 22-2 A, Main divisions of the central nervous system. **B,** Diencephalon (thalamus and hypothalamus).

Table 22-1 | Functions of the Divisions of the Brain

DIVISION	FUNCTION
Cerebrum	Center of intellect and consciousness. Receives and interprets sensory information; controls voluntary movements and certain types of involuntary movements; responsible for thinking, learning, language capability, judgment, and personality; stores memories.
Cerebellum	Responsible for coordination of movement, posture, and muscle tone that are the mechanisms of balance.
Diencephalon	Consists of two parts.
Thalamus	Relay center between spinal cord and cerebrum.
Hypothalamus	Controls body temperature, appetite, and water balance; links nervous and endocrine systems.
Brainstem	Consists of three parts.
Midbrain	Mediates visual and auditory reflexes; controls cranial nerves III and IV and certain eye movements.
Pons	Links connecting various parts of the brain; helps regulate respiration.
Medulla oblongata	Contains reticular formation that regulates heartbeat, respiration, and blood pressure; controls center for swallowing, coughing, sneezing, and vomiting; relays messages to other parts of the brain.

FIGURE 22-3 Specialized functions of the lobes of the cerebrum.

as a reflex center for nerve impulse transmission. Sensory impulses travel to the brain on ascending conduction pathway tracts; motor impulses travel on descending tracts.

- Pyramidal tracts are conduction pathways that begin in the cerebral cortex and end in the spinal cord. These tracts control skeletal muscle movement. All other conduction pathways are extrapyramidal tracts, and they control muscle movements associated with posture and balance.

HOW DOES THE PERIPHERAL NERVOUS SYSTEM INTERACT WITH THE CENTRAL NERVOUS SYSTEM?

- The PNS is subdivided into an afferent division and an efferent division. The afferent division carries impulses to the CNS; the efferent division carries impulses away from the CNS.
- The reflex arc is a simple conduction pathway that utilizes a receptor (a sensory neuron centered in the spinal cord) and a motor neuron located in an effector (skeletal muscle). A stimulus travels from the sensory receptor through the spinal cord and back to the effector, causing action (Figure 22-5).
- Reflex arcs are important to most functions of the body, including maintaining an upright position.
- The cranial and spinal nerves are part of the somatic subsystem and respond to changes in the outside world. Because these nerves initiate voluntary action, the somatic system often is called the *voluntary system.*
- The autonomic system of the PNS is active in maintaining internal body balance *(homeostasis)* and is automatic (involuntary) in its actions.
- The autonomic system is divided into the sympathetic nerves, which mobilize energy to initiate

FIGURE 22-4 Dermatomes (cutaneous innervation of spinal nerves). Stimulation of the skin in the depicted area for each nerve causes reflex activity. *C,* cervical spinal nerves; *T,* thoracic spinal nerves; *L,* lumbar spinal nerves; *S,* sacral spinal nerves.

Table 22-2   The Cranial Nerves and Their Functions

	CRANIAL NERVE (CN)	TYPE AND FUNCTION
O	Olfactory (CN I)	*Sensory:* smell
O	Optic (CN II)	*Sensory:* visual acuity, field of vision, pupillary response (afferent impulse)
O	Oculomotor (CN III)	*Motor:* eyelid elevation, extraocular eye movement, pupil size, convergence, pupillary constriction (efferent impulse)
T	Trochlear (CN IV)	*Motor:* extraocular eye movement (inferior and lateral)
T	Trigeminal (CN V)	*Sensory:* corneal reflex *Motor:* facial sensation; chewing, biting, lateral jaw movement
A	Abducens (CN VI)	*Motor:* extraocular eye movement (lateral)
F	Facial (CN VII)	*Sensory:* taste *Motor:* facial muscle movement, including muscles of expression; lacrimal gland and salivary gland control
A	Acoustic (CN VIII)	*Sensory:* hearing, sense of balance
G	Glossopharyngeal (CN IX)	*Sensory:* sensations of the throat, taste (posterior tongue) *Motor:* gagging and swallowing movements
V	Vagus (CN X)	*Sensory:* sensations of posterior tongue, throat, larynx; impulses from heart, lungs, bronchi, and gastrointestinal tract
S	Spinal accessory (CN XI)	*Motor:* shoulder movement and head rotation
H	Hypoglossal (CN XII)	*Motor:* tongue movement, articulation of speech

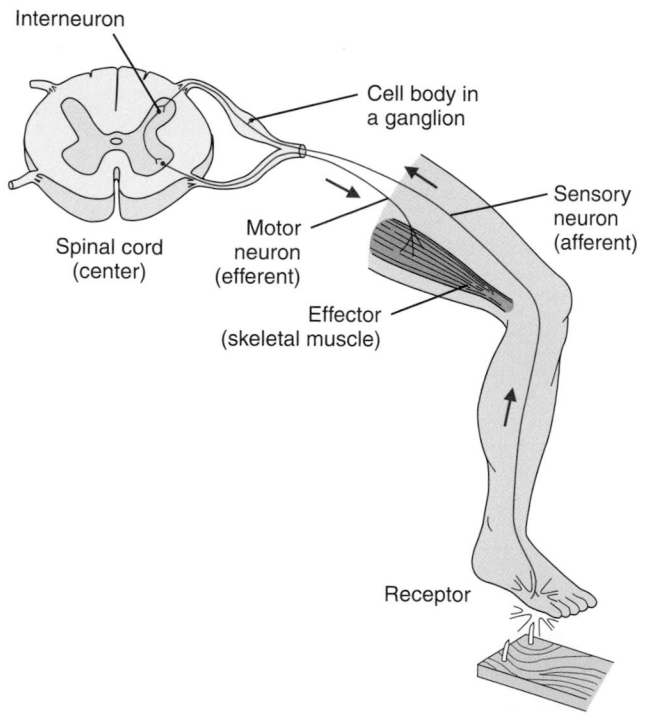

FIGURE 22-5 Components of a generalized reflex arc.

changes aimed at maintaining or restoring homeostasis, and the parasympathetic nerves, which conserve and restore energy that has been used to maintain homeostasis.

- **Sympathetic and parasympathetic nerves have opposite effects on many organs** (Table 22-3).

HOW IS THE CENTRAL NERVOUS SYSTEM PROTECTED?

- The bones of the skull and the vertebral column form the outer layer of protection for the brain and the spinal cord.
- The meninges are protective membranes that cover the brain and are continuous with the membranes covering the spinal cord. The meninges consist of the pia mater, which covers the brain; the arachnoid, which encases the entire CNS; and the dura mater, which is a tough membrane protecting the brain and spinal cord.
- The subarachnoid space is located between the pia mater and the arachnoid membrane and is where the cerebrospinal fluid (CSF) circulates (Figure 22-6).
- CSF serves to cushion and protect the brain and spinal cord. It is formed continuously as a filtrate from the blood in specialized capillary networks in the choroid plexus, located in the ventricles of the brain. It is reabsorbed by the arachnoid villi of the arachnoid membrane at the same rate at which it is formed. The volume of CSF normally stays constant (see Figure 22-6).
- **Normal CSF pressure is 70 to 125 cm water pressure (cm H_2O).** When there is an excess of fluid in the subarachnoid space, the CSF pressure rises above normal.

HOW DO NERVES CONDUCT IMPULSES?

- The axons of many neurons, bundled together and wrapped in connective tissue, make up a nerve. Ganglia are collections of nerve cell bodies outside the CNS.

Table 22-3   **Autonomic Effects on Various Organs of the Body**

ORGAN	EFFECT OF SYMPATHETIC STIMULATION	EFFECT OF PARASYMPATHETIC STIMULATION
Eye		
Pupil	Dilated	Constricted
Ciliary muscle	Slight relaxation (far vision)	Constricted (near vision)
Glands: nasal, lacrimal, parotid, submandibular, gastric, pancreatic	Vasoconstriction and slight secretion	Stimulation of copious secretion (containing many enzymes for enzyme-secreting glands)
Sweat glands	Copious sweating (cholinergic)	Sweating on palms of hands
Apocrine glands	Thick, odoriferous secretion	None
Blood vessels	Most often constricted	Most often little or no effect
Heart		
Muscle	Increased rate Increased force of contraction	Slowed rate Decreased force of contraction (especially of atria)
Coronaries	Dilated (β_2); constricted (α)	Dilated
Lungs		
Bronchi	Dilated	Constricted
Blood vessels	Mildly constricted	Dilated
Gut		
Lumen	Decreased peristalsis and tone	Increased peristalsis and tone
Sphincter	Increased tone (most times)	Relaxed (most times)
Liver	Glucose released	Slight glucose synthesis
Gallbladder and bile ducts	Relaxed	Contracted
Kidney	Decreased output and renin secretion	None
Bladder		
Detrusor	Relaxed (slight)	Contracted
Trigone	Contracted	Relaxed
Penis	Ejaculation	Erection
Systemic arterioles		
Abdominal viscera	Constricted	None
Muscle	Constricted (α-adrenergic) Dilated (β-adrenergic) Dilated (cholinergic)	None
Skin	Constricted	None
Blood		None
Coagulation	Increased	None
Glucose	Increased	None
Lipids	Increased	None
Basal metabolism	Increased up to 100%	None
Adrenal medullary secretion	Increased	None
Mental activity	Increased	None
Piloerector muscles	Contracted	None
Skeletal muscle	Increased glycogenolysis Increased strength	None
Fat cells	Lipolysis	None

From Guyton, A.C., & Hall, J.E. (2006). *Textbook of Medical Physiology with Student Consult Access* (11th ed.). Philadelphia: Elsevier Saunders, p. 754.

- When in a state of polarization, neurons have the capacity to become excited (stimulated). They also have the ability to conduct that stimulus along the nerve pathways.
- A stimulus is a physical, chemical, or electrical event that changes the cell membrane and initiates

- conduction of the stimulus as an electrical impulse along the nerve pathway.
- The stimulus travels from one neuron to another across a *synapse* (the space between two neurons).
- A neurotransmitter secreted by the neuron is necessary for transmission of an impulse across the

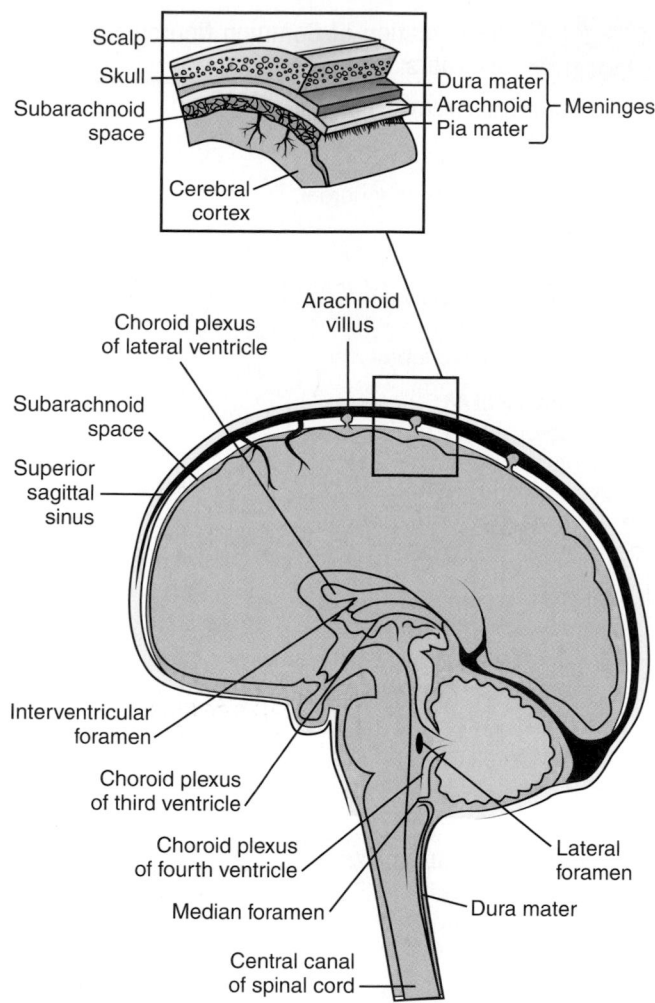

FIGURE 22-6 Flow of the cerebrospinal fluid. *Inset*, Meninges covering the brain.

synapse (Table 22-4). Acetylcholine, dopamine, and norepinephrine are the major neurotransmitters.

- Neurotransmitter substances are secreted at the synapse, and these diffuse across the synapse to stimulate the postsynaptic membrane on the next neuron. **When the neurotransmitter is absent or decreased at the synaptic junction, the stimulus cannot travel along the nerve pathways normally.**
- Impulses either travel in a reflex arc, going to the spinal cord and traveling back to an effector site, or they travel along nerve pathways to the brain to be interpreted.
- After impulse interpretation, a message may be sent out from the brain via the spinal cord or cranial nerves (PNS) for appropriate action to be taken. In other words, a stimulus produces a response.
- Many axons are surrounded by a myelin sheath that is a white, fatty covering. The myelin sheath is an excellent electrical insulator and it speeds the conduction of nerve impulses. **When myelin is destroyed, as in multiple sclerosis, impulse transmission is slowed or stopped.**

WHAT ARE THE SPECIAL CHARACTERISTICS OF THE NERVOUS SYSTEM?

- Although some cells in the PNS have an outer membrane called the *neurolemma* that may regenerate after damage, cells of the CNS do not have this capability. **Once destroyed, cells in the brain cannot be replaced** but other brain cells may pick up their function.
- In the PNS, the Schwann cells can regenerate. The Schwann cells form myelin sheaths that wrap around the axons in the PNS.

Table 22-4	Neurotransmitters that Affect Transmission of Nerve Impulses		
NEUROTRANSMITTER	**LOCATION**	**FUNCTION**	**COMMENTS**
Acetylcholine	CNS and PNS	Generally excitatory but is inhibitory to some visceral effectors	Found in skeletal neuromuscular junctions and in many ANS synapses
Norepinephrine	CNS and PNS	May be excitatory or inhibitory depending on the receptors	Found in visceral and cardiac muscle neuromuscular junctions; cocaine and amphetamines exaggerate the effects
Epinephrine	CNS and PNS	May be excitatory or inhibitory depending on the receptors	Found in pathways concerned with behavior and mood
Dopamine	CNS and PNS	Generally excitatory	Found in pathways that regulate emotional responses; decreased levels in Parkinson's disease
Serotonin	CNS	Generally inhibitory	Found in pathways that regulate temperature, sensory perception, mood, onset of sleep
Gamma-aminobutyric acid (GABA)	CNS	Generally inhibitory	Inhibits excessive discharge of neurons
Endorphins and enkephalins	CNS	Generally inhibitory	Inhibit release of sensory pain neurotransmitters; opiates mimic the effects of these peptides

ANS, autonomic nervous system; *CNS*, central nervous system; *PNS*, peripheral nervous system.
From Applegate, E. (2010). *The Anatomy and Physiology Learning System* (4th ed.). Philadelphia: Elsevier Saunders, p. 177.

- Neurons are very sensitive to oxygen and die quickly when deprived of oxygen. **The brain's neurons cannot survive anoxia for more than 4 to 6 minutes.**

WHAT CHANGES OCCUR IN THE NERVOUS SYSTEM WITH AGING?

- There is a loss of neurons with aging, and brain weight may drop considerably after age 70; there is no loss of intellectual function attributable to this loss of neurons.
- The number of functioning dendrites decreases with aging. This decrease causes slower impulse transmission and resultant slower reaction time in the older person.
- Blood flow to the brain is decreased with advanced age; this makes the elderly more susceptible to permanent damage if blood flow to the brain is further compromised.
- Loss of neurons and slower nerve conduction cause a decrease in efficiency of the autonomic nervous system in advanced age.
- In late adulthood, changes can cause slower movement, slower response time, and decreased sensation. Tremors may occur without rigidity and tendon reflexes may be hypoactive.
- Body homeostasis is more difficult to maintain or regain in the elderly. Exposure to prolonged cold or to excessive heat may cause death. Adaptation to physiologic stress takes much longer, and recovery often is incomplete.
- Recent, short-term memory is affected by the aging process, but long-term, distant memory is often not affected. The ability to learn is not affected by aging, but the learning process is slower. It takes longer to process new information. Abstract reasoning ability slowly diminishes with advancing age, and perception may become impaired.
- Decreases in secretion of the neurotransmitters norepinephrine and dopamine occur with advanced age, and there is an increase in monoamine oxidase, which can affect cognitive function, gait, and balance.
- The number of posterior root nerve fibers and sympathetic nerve fibers of the autonomic nervous system declines with aging of the spinal cord. In the PNS, the motor nerve fibers and the myelin sheath degenerate with advancing age; reflexes may become diminished or absent with advanced age.
- Pupils decrease in size with advanced age, and more light is needed for reading.
- The elderly person may need more time to process questions, solve problems, or learn new information.
- Using the brain and keeping it active promotes continued intellectual function in the healthy elderly individual.

Box 22-1   Classification of Common Neurologic Disorders

GENETIC/DEVELOPMENTAL DISORDERS
- Cerebral palsy
- Muscular dystrophy
- Huntington's disease (chorea)

TRAUMA
- Head injury
- Penetrating brain injury
- Spinal cord injury
- Ruptured intervertebral disk

CEREBROVASCULAR
- Cerebrovascular accident
- Ruptured aneurysm
- Arteriovenous malformation
- Migraine, cluster headache

TUMOR
- Brain tumor
- Spinal cord tumor

INFECTION
- Meningitis
- Encephalitis
- Brain abscess
- Poliomyelitis
- Guillain-Barré syndrome

NEUROMUSCULAR DISORDERS
- Multiple sclerosis
- Myasthenia gravis
- Amyotrophic lateral sclerosis

DEGENERATIVE DISORDERS
- Parkinson's disease
- Alzheimer's disease

CRANIAL NERVE DISORDERS
- Bell's palsy
- Trigeminal neuralgia

CAUSATIVE FACTORS INVOLVED IN NEUROLOGIC DISORDERS

Many factors can affect neurologic function, including genetic and acquired developmental disorders. Infections and inflammation, benign and malignant tumors, vascular or neuromuscular degeneration, and metabolic and endocrine disorders all can cause damage to or interfere with normal function of the nervous system. Chemical or physical trauma often causes permanent damage to the brain or spinal cord. Box 22-1 lists by category the most common neurologic disorders in the adult.

PREVENTION OF NEUROLOGIC DISORDERS

The nervous system coordinates all sensory and motor activities by receiving, interpreting, and relaying messages that are vital to the proper performance of all the body's activities. Respiratory, circulatory, digestive, and endocrine functions all depend on an intact and normally functioning autonomic nervous system.

Nurses can help prevent neurologic problems in many ways. The goals for *Healthy People 2020* encourage health protection through education about safety and responsible self-care.

Health Promotion

Protecting the Nervous System

- Encourage people to wear helmets when biking, in-line skating, skateboarding, or riding motorcycles, and when involved in other sports activities that may lead to head injury.
- Remind people that wearing safety hats or helmets when in a workplace where head injury is a danger does reduce the number of injuries.
- Review safety precautions when diving and swimming. To help prevent spinal cord injury, never dive into water of unknown depth.
- Encourage people to fasten their seat belts before putting the car into gear.
- Be certain that children are fastened into appropriate restraints.
- Wear mask, gloves, long pants, and long-sleeved shirt when spraying with insecticide; wash up immediately afterward and change clothes.
- Refrain from using recreational drugs, because they can affect the cardiovascular system and can cause a stroke.

Teaching the dangers of recreational drug use, such as the possibility of stroke from the use of "crack" cocaine and the potential for accidents while under the influence of some drugs, are other areas for public education. Informing the public about the damaging effect of too much alcohol on brain cells, as well as the increased incidence of alcohol-induced accidents, is another area for education.

Promoting immunizations to protect from tetanus, measles, poliomyelitis, and infectious diseases that may cause high fever and resultant brain damage is an area in which nurses can be effective. **Control of hypertension and cholesterol can reduce the number of strokes and the damage they cause.** Teaching people to recognize the symptoms of stroke and to seek early treatment may prevent permanent disability.

Pesticides and various chemicals in household and work environments can cause neurologic toxicity and damage. Parkinson's disease has been particularly more prevalent in farm workers and others who handle pesticides or work where pesticides are frequently used (*Science Daily Ed.*, 2009). Read information on containers of pesticides carefully. Wear long-sleeved clothing and gloves when spraying pesticides in the garden. Spray in quiet, nonwindy conditions. Wash hands and exposed skin with soap and water afterward. Change clothes and launder the clothing worn after pesticide spraying.

EVALUATION OF NEUROLOGIC STATUS

The complete neurologic examination performed by the health care provider systematically measures the ability of the body to perform its myriad motor and sensory functions. Mental acuity, memory, and emotional stability also are assessed. A complete neurologic examination is a very long procedure and may be performed in stages over several days. However, gross assessment of the cranial nerves, coordination and balance, muscle strength, and reflexes is standard for every patient with a neurologic complaint. Nurses sometimes do all or part of the examination.

CRANIAL NERVES

The 12 cranial nerves (CNs; designated as CN I through CN XII) control both sensory and motor activities within various parts of the body (see Table 22-2). Table 22-5 tells how to perform a basic assessment of cranial nerve function.

Clinical Cues

A mnemonic for remembering the cranial nerve names is as follows:

"On Old Olympus's Towering Top A Finn And German Viewed Some Hops" (**O**lfactory, **O**ptic, **O**culomotor, **T**rochlear, **T**rigeminal, **A**bducens, **F**acial, **A**coustic, **G**lossopharyngeal, **V**agus, **S**pinal accessory, **H**ypoglossal).

COORDINATION AND BALANCE

This portion of the neurologic examination evaluates functions controlled by the higher centers of the brain, the cerebrum and cerebellum. The patient is asked to stand with her feet together and to close her eyes (Romberg's test). If the sense of balance is normal, a steady posture will be maintained and there will not be swaying from side to side. Next ask the patient to walk across the room, and assess the gait. Next stand in front of the patient, hold up a finger, and ask the patient to touch your finger and then her own nose; move your finger to different locations in front of the patient. This tests both the ability to follow directions and coordination.

NEUROMUSCULAR FUNCTION TESTING

Groups of large muscles are tested for strength and coordination. Evaluate the patient's gait while walking, hand grip strength, and arm and leg strength as the patient pushes against resistance. More sophisticated tests include electromyography (Table 22-6 on pp. 481 to 484).

REFLEXES

A *reflex* is an action or movement that is built into the nervous system and does not need the intervention of conscious thought to take place. In other words, it is an

Table 22-5 | **Quick Gross Assessment of Major Cranial Nerves**

CRANIAL NERVE TESTED	QUICK METHOD OF TESTING*
Olfactory	Have patient smell a sample of ground coffee, perfume, and pickle juice.
Optic	Test visual acuity with a Snellen eye chart. Test visual fields by asking patient to hold the head still and identify items on various areas of a chart.
Oculomotor, trochlear, and abducens	Assess pupil size, direct and consensual constriction, and accommodation. Assess the cardinal fields/directions of gaze.
Trigeminal	Ask patient to clamp jaw shut, open the mouth against resistance, open the mouth widely, move the jaw from side to side, and make chewing motions. Test sensation by placing a hot and then a cold item on various portions of the face. Ask whether item is warm or cold.
Facial	Observe the face for symmetry; ask patient to smile, frown, raise the eyebrows, tightly close the eyes, whistle, show the teeth, and puff out the cheeks.
Vestibulocochlear (or acoustic)	Whisper from varying distances and locations behind the patient and ask what was said. Test equilibrium with Romberg's test: ask patient to stand with feet only slightly apart and eyes closed. See if there is swaying of the body.
Glossopharyngeal and vagus	Ask patient to open mouth wide and say "Ah." Place tongue depressor on first third of tongue to flatten it and observe movement of the uvula and palate. They should rise symmetrically with the uvula at midline. Assess gag reflex by touching each side of the pharynx; there should be a brisk response. Have patient swallow a bit of water.
Spinal accessory	Ask patient to elevate the shoulders with and without resistance, turn the head to each side, resist attempts to pull the chin back toward the midline, and push the head forward against resistance.
Hypoglossal	Ask patient to open mouth wide, stick out tongue, and rapidly move it from side to side and in and out. Watch for deviation from midline. Apply pressure to cheek and ask patient to push tongue against hand to check for strength.

*These maneuvers do not check for every function of these cranial nerves, but will provide data indicating whether a more thorough assessment is needed.

automatic response. The knee jerk is an example of the simplest type of reflex. When the knee is tapped, the nerve that receives this stimulus sends an impulse to the spinal cord, where it is relayed to a motor nerve. This causes the quadriceps muscle at the front of the thigh to contract and to move the leg upward. This reflex, or simple reflex arc, involves only two nerves and one synapse. The leg begins to jerk up while the brain is just becoming aware of the tap on the knee (see Figure 22-5).

The knee jerk, or patellar reflex, tests nerve pathways to and from the spinal cord at the level of the second through fourth lumbar nerves. In addition to testing the patellar reflex, a neurologic examination might include testing the biceps reflex (pathways for the fifth and sixth cervical nerves), triceps reflex (seventh and eighth cervical nerves), brachioradialis reflex (fifth and sixth cervical nerves), and Achilles tendon reflex (first and second sacral nerves). Reflexes are graded as follows: $0/5$ = absent; $1/5$ = weak response; $2/5$ = normal; $3/5$ = exaggerated response; and $4/5$ = hyperreflexia with clonus. **Clonus** is a continued rhythmic contraction of the muscle while there is continuous application of the stimulus.

Another reflex action widely used as a diagnostic aid in CNS disorders is **Babinski's reflex,** which is elicited by scraping an object such as a key along the sole of the foot. In a normal response to this stimulus, the toes will bend downward. In a *positive* Babinski's reflex, the great toe bends backward (upward) and the smaller toes fan outward. A positive Babinski's reflex in the adult not under the influence of chemical substances indicates an abnormality in the motor control pathways leading from the cerebral cortex (Figure 22-7 on page 485).

In the unconscious person, tests are performed to determine brainstem function. After ruling out spinal cord injury, the oculocephalic ("doll's eye") and oculovestibular reflexes are assessed. For the doll's eye reflex, the examiner places a hand on each side of the patient's head, using the thumbs to gently hold open the eyelids. While watching the patient's eyes, the head is rotated briskly to one side and eye movement is observed in relation to head movement. If the brainstem pathways are intact, the eyes appear to move in a direction opposite to that of the head movement; that is, if the head is rotated to the right, the eyes appear to move to the left. After ensuring that the tympanic membrane is intact, the oculovestibular reflex is assessed by **caloric testing.** With the patient's head elevated at least 30 degrees, 20 to 200 mL of cold or ice water is instilled into the ear with a

Text continued on p. 485

Table 22-6   Diagnostic Tests for Neurologic Disorders

TEST	PURPOSE	DESCRIPTION	NURSING IMPLICATIONS
Skull and spine radiographs	To detect fractures, bone loss, and other bony abnormalities	Radiographs are taken of the desired area from various angles.	Explain that the test is noninvasive. Advise that various positions will need to be assumed.
Lumbar puncture (spinal tap) (see Figure 22-11)	To determine if CSF pressure is elevated; to determine if there is a blockage to the flow of CSF; to inject medications; to obtain fluid for chemical analysis and culture	Physician performs a sterile puncture into the arachnoid space, using local anesthetic, between L3 and L4 or L4 and L5; opening pressure is obtained; fluid is aspirated and placed in sterile test tubes labeled 1, 2, and 3. Fluid is analyzed for color, pH, cell count, protein, chloride, and glucose; a culture is usually done. Local anesthetic is used.	Procedure requires a signed consent form. Obtain sterile lumbar puncture tray, local anesthetic, sterile gloves, and tape. Assist patient into position with back bowed, head flexed on chest, and knees drawn up to the abdomen. Patient may be lying or sitting. Assist patient to maintain position and to hold still during procedure. Reassure patient and provide emotional support. Personnel must wear a mask during procedure. *Postprocedure:* Appropriately label tubes with patient data afterward and transport them to the laboratory immediately. Keep patient flat in bed to reduce headache for 1 hr or longer after procedure and encourage fluid intake unless contraindicated. Observe the site for signs of drainage and inflammation.
Electroencephalography (EEG)	To detect abnormal brain wave patterns that are indicative of specific diseases, such as seizure disorder, brain tumor, CVA, head trauma, and infection; to determine cerebral death	May be performed while patient is asleep, drowsy, or undergoing stimulation such as hyperventilation or rhythmic bright light. Test may be done at the bedside or in the EEG lab. Tracing is taken with patient in reclining chair or lying down. Electrodes are applied to the scalp with an electrode paste. Test takes 45 min–2 hr.	Explain purpose of test to the patient; assure her she will not receive an electrical shock, the test is not painful, and that the machine does not determine intelligence or read her mind. Hair should be clean and dry. No sleeping pills or sedatives the night before test; check with physician regarding other drugs to be held; restrict coffee, tea, caffeine, and alcohol for 24-48 hr. If a sleep EEG is ordered, patient may need to be kept up most or all of the night before the test; do not keep NPO, as hypoglycemia can affect the test. *Postprocedure:* Wash hair to remove the electrode paste. *Nothing touches the patient during the procedure.*
Magnetoencephalography (MEG)	To pinpoint the area of the brain damaged by a stroke, where seizure activity is originating, or location of other injury or disorder	A biomagnetometer machine detects the small magnetic fields generated by neurons.	*Postprocedure:* Care is the same as for Electroencephalography (see above).
Electromyography (EMG)	To measure electrical activity of skeletal muscle at rest and during voluntary activity to determine abnormalities in muscular contraction; helpful in diagnosing neuromuscular, peripheral nerve, and muscular disorders	With the patient sitting in a chair or lying on a table, needle electrodes are inserted in selected muscles. Tracings of electrical activity are taken with the muscles at rest, then with various voluntary activities that produce muscle contraction. The test takes 1–2 hr depending on how many muscles are tested.	Procedure requires a signed consent form. Explain the procedure to the patient; tell her that there is discomfort when the electrodes are placed. Check with physician regarding medications to be withheld; muscle relaxants, cholinergics, and anticholinergics can influence test result. There is no food or fluid restriction. If serum enzymes are ordered, they should be drawn before the EMG.

Continued

CN, cranial nerve; *CNS,* central nervous system; *CSF,* cerebrospinal fluid; *CVA,* cerebrovascular accident; *ICP,* intracranial pressure; *IV,* intravenous; *NPO,* nothing by mouth; *VS,* vital signs; *WBCs,* white blood cells.

Table 22-6   Diagnostic Tests for Neurologic Disorders—cont'd

TEST	PURPOSE	DESCRIPTION	NURSING IMPLICATIONS
Myelography	To detect spinal lesions, intervertebral disk problems, tumors, or cysts	Contrast medium is injected into the spinal canal, and fluoroscopic examination and radiographs are made. The study is contraindicated if the patient has increased ICP. The patient is placed prone and strapped to the x-ray table for the spinal puncture; as the contrast medium is injected, the table is tilted. After the test, if oil-based medium was used, it is withdrawn. The patient is kept in bed with head of bed elevated 60 degrees or flat depending on the contrast medium used. Procedure takes 1 hr. Rarely performed.	Procedure requires a signed consent form. Explain what to expect. Patient may feel a warm flush when contrast medium is injected. Bowel evacuation regimen may be ordered the night before. Keep NPO for 4-8 hr before procedure. Check for medications to be withheld before and for 48 hr after test. Assess for allergy to iodine or shellfish. Dress in myelogram pajamas; administer preoperative sedative or analgesic if ordered. *Postprocedure:* Monitor VS q 30 min × 2 hr, then q 1 hr × 4 hr. Assess pulses and sensation in extremities; monitor urinary output; catheterize as ordered if patient cannot void in 8 hr; encourage increased fluid intake. Observe for signs of meningitis.
Computed axial tomography (CAT or CT scan) Xenon CT Intrathecal contrast-enhanced CT	To examine the brain from many different angles, obtaining a series of cross-sectional images that provide views from three dimensions To identify hematomas, tumors, cysts, hydrocephalus, cerebral atrophy, obstruction to CSF flow, and cerebral edema	May be done with or without contrast dye enhancement. Patient lies on a narrow table with her head cradled and is moved so that her head is inside the circular opening of the machine. A security strap is wrapped snugly around her. CT scanner produces a narrow x-ray beam. Various clicking and whirring noises are heard as the machine rotates the scanner for different views. The test takes 45 min-1½ hr. A lumbar puncture is needed for an intrathecal contrast-enhanced CT.	Procedure requires a signed consent form. Explain the procedure and what patient will see, hear, and feel. If contrast dye is used, the patient will feel a warm flush and have a metallic taste in her mouth as it is injected. If contrast dye is used, patient should be NPO for 3-4 hr before test to prevent vomiting. Assess for allergy to iodine or shellfish. Remove all hairpins, jewelry, and metal from the head and neck. Patient may need to be sedated if she is prone to claustrophobia; the table can be uncomfortable for those with arthritis or back problems. She will be able to communicate with the machine's operator. *Postprocedure:* Care is the same as for lumbar puncture (see above).
Cerebral angiography	To visualize the structure of the cerebral arteries to determine the presence of stricture, tumor, aneurysm, thrombus, or hematoma	Radiopaque liquid is injected through a catheter inserted into the common carotid artery, and a series of radiographs is taken. Fluoroscopy is used during the procedure. Digital subtraction angiography (DSA) is done by using a computer along with the angiography procedure. Test takes 1-2 hr.	Procedure requires a signed consent form. Assess for allergy to iodine and shellfish. Explain procedure; patient will be supine on x-ray table; local anesthetic will be used to introduce the catheter; an IV line will be started in case of need for emergency drugs; patient will feel a flush as the dye is injected. Patient should be NPO 8-12 hr before test; anticoagulants are discontinued beforehand. May be given preprocedure sedative, antihistamine, or steroid to decrease possibility of allergic reaction to dye. *Postprocedure:* Assess for bleeding at catheter site; assess distal pulses; perform neurologic checks; monitor VS q 15 min × 2 hr, then q 1 hr × 4 hr or until stable. Assess for dysphagia and respiratory distress that could indicate internal bleeding in the neck. Activities are restricted for 24 hr.

Test	Purpose	Description	Nursing Care
Radionuclide imaging (brain scan)	To detect an intracranial mass: tumor, abscess, hematoma, or aneurysm	A radioisotope is administered IV. Abnormal tissue usually absorbs more of the isotope than normal tissue. After a 1- to 3-hr waiting period for absorption, a scintillation scanner is used to image the brain. The test takes 30 min–1 hr.	Explain the procedure; patient will sit or lie on a table; the scanner makes clicking noises; the amount of radioactivity is very low and is not dangerous to the patient or others. Patient will need to lie or sit still during the scanning. A drug may be given the night before to block uptake of the radioactive element by the thyroid and salivary glands. There is no food or fluid restriction; no special aftercare.
Magnetic resonance imaging (MRI)	To visualize soft tissue without the use of contrast media or ionizing radiation; provides excellent images of soft tissue, eliminating bone; can visualize lesions undetected by CT scan To detect white matter areas in nervous system that represent demyelination, as in multiple sclerosis	An electromagnet is used to detect radiofrequency pulses produced by alignment of hydrogen protons in the magnetic field. Computer produces tomographic images with high contrast of area studied. Cannot be used in the presence of metal. Is quite expensive. A contrast agent often is used for better visualization and definition of specific structures.	Inform patient that the test is painless; no dietary restrictions. Remove all metal objects before test. Screen the patient for hidden sources of metal, such as bullet fragments, iron filings, aneurysm clips. MRI is contraindicated for patients with pacemakers. Patient must be still during test. Explain that body part to be imaged is moved inside large machine; some patients become claustrophobic. Patient will be able to communicate with the machine operator. Requires a signed consent for use of contrast media.
Magnetic resonance angiography (MRA)	To evaluate intracranial and extracranial blood vessels and for diagnosing cerebrovascular disease; is rapidly replacing cerebral angiography	Similar to MRI. Uses differing signals of flowing blood to collect data. May be enhanced with use of contrast media.	Explain the need for lying completely still for 1 hr. May require sedation. Screen patient for any metal on body before test. Requires a signed consent for use of contrast media.
Magnetic resonance spectroscopy (MRS)	To determine loss of neurons with markers of neuronal integrity (e.g., N-acetyl aspartate) and to study brain diseases	Uses MRI to gather information about chemical composition of brain tissue.	Same as for MRI (see above).
Positron emission tomography (PET)	To assess for cell death, damage in brain tissue	Radioactive material is given and provides differing color in areas of cellular activity.	Procedure requires a signed consent form. Explain that two IV lines will be inserted. Patient is to avoid sedatives or tranquilizers before test. Ask to empty bladder before test. Patient may be asked to perform various activities during the test.
Single-photon emission computed tomography (SPECT)	To visualize glucose or oxygen metabolism in the brain and to visualize blood flow	Radiolabeled compounds are injected and their single-photon emissions are scanned. Images are made of the accumulated radiolabeled compounds.	Same as for PET (see above).
Ultrasound arteriography (Doppler flow studies)	To study flow and determine areas of constriction or obstruction in cerebral arteries. To detect arterial spasm	Noninvasive test. Doppler image scanning device is used with computer to visualize anatomy of major cerebral arteries.	Tell patient that the test is noninvasive and painless. A small Doppler wand is positioned over particular "window" areas on the skull (temples), and with the computer, sound waves are directed so as to produce an image of the interior arteries and their blood flow. No special preparation or aftercare.

Continued

Table 22-6 Diagnostic Tests for Neurologic Disorders—cont'd

TEST	PURPOSE	DESCRIPTION	NURSING IMPLICATIONS
Carotid duplex Doppler studies	To determine if blood flow in carotid arteries is decreased or blocked	Sound waves graph a picture of blood flow in the carotid arteries.	Explain that the test is noninvasive and painless. Patient will lie flat with head turned to one side and then the other as metal wand passes along the artery.
Evoked potential studies	To measure response of the CNS to visual, auditory, or sensory stimulus and helpful in detecting tumor of CN VIII, blindness in infants, or brainstem lesions. Also useful in diagnosing multiple sclerosis	May be done in conjunction with EEG. Electrodes are used to pick up and transmit impulses to a computer while a stimulus is delivered to the patient. Signals are displayed on an oscilloscope, and data are stored for later interpretation.	Explain the procedure to the patient. Visual-evoked potentials: stimulus may be a bright flashing light or checkerboard patterns. Somatosensory-evoked potentials require stimulation of a peripheral sensory nerve with a mild electric shock. Auditory brainstem-evoked potentials use various noises or tone bursts through earphones. Discomfort is minimal. Test takes 30-60 min.
Cerebrospinal fluid analysis and culture	To detect abnormalities that are indicative of specific neurologic problems and determine which organism is responsible for infection	CSF is obtained by lumbar puncture. It is analyzed for color, cell count, protein, chloride, and glucose. The fluid is cultured to detect the presence of organisms; if present, an antibiotic sensitivity test is done to determine which drug will best kill the organism. CSF pressure also is measured. Normal CSF values for the adult are: Color: clear Cell count (WBCs): 0-8 mm^3 Protein: 14-45 mg/dL Chloride: 118-132 mEq/L Glucose: 40-80 mg/dL Pressure: 70-150 cm H_2O or < 20 mm Hg	Follow lumbar puncture procedure. Label the test tubes as 1, 2, and 3 and be certain they are filled with at least 3 mL of CSF in this order. Do not refrigerate the tubes; transport to the laboratory immediately. Maintain Standard Precautions (see Appendix B).
PLAC (lipoprotein-associated phospholipase A$_2$; Lp-PLA$_2$)	To detect enzyme marker for increased ischemic stroke risk	This substance is thought to be partly responsible for atherosclerosis formation.	Explain that this is a simple blood test. Results take 7-10 days.

Line of
stimulation:
outer sole,
heel to
little toe

Plantar (normal) reflex
Toes curl inward

Positive Babinski's
reflex (always
abnormal)
Great toe bends
upward; smaller
toes fan outward

FIGURE 22-7 Normal and Babinski's reflexes.

catheter-tipped syringe. While the external ear canal is irrigated, the patient's eye movements are observed. Normally the eyes will show nystagmus, darting away from the irrigated ear. Absence of eye movement may indicate a brainstem lesion.

❖ NURSING MANAGEMENT

 ### ■ Assessment (Data Collection)

Neurologic nursing requires special training and experience in observation, critical judgment, and specific skills to help patients cope with a myriad of problems. The nurse not only must be aware of subtle changes in the patient's condition but also must recognize the significance of these changes and act promptly when medical attention is needed. The LPN/LVN assists the RN with the gathering of data for the neurologic assessment.

Assignment Considerations

Reporting Observations

If a patient with a neurologic problem that may affect level of consciousness is assigned to a certified nursing assistant (CNA) for bathing and morning care, remember to remind the assistant to report to you any change in wakefulness, irritability, speech, eye appearance, gait, or balance. It is best not to assign a patient who has already shown some signs of deteriorating level of consciousness to a CNA.

Patient History

Because neurologic disorders can be present in conjunction with or in addition to disorders of other body systems, include questions about neurologic status in the initial and ongoing assessments of all patients. For example, a surgical patient could have had a previous stroke, or could have a history of seizures or an existing neuromuscular disease such as multiple sclerosis. Although these may not be the primary reason for admission to a hospital, they will certainly influence the course of the illness or injury for which admission occurred.

 ### Focused Assessment

Data Collection for the Neurologic System

When gathering a history for a patient who may have a neurologic problem, ask the following questions.
- Do you or does any member of your family have any genetic disorder of the nervous system?
- Have you ever had a seizure or been told you have epilepsy?
- Have you ever had difficulty in speaking, concentrating, remembering, or expressing thoughts? Have you noticed any changes in these functions?
- Have you had any changes in muscle strength or coordination?
- Have you ever injured your head?
- Have you ever had a really high fever?
- Have you had any severe sinus, ear, tooth, or facial skin infection?
- Do you recall any episodes of tremors, muscle spasms, fainting, dizziness, ringing in the ears, or blurred vision?
- Have you had any "blackout" spells?
- Have you noticed any changes in taste or smell?
- Do you have any numbness or tingling in the extremities?

Physical Assessment

A basic nursing assessment of neurologic function is performed on any patient who is suspected of experiencing a neurologic problem. Nurses often need to assess for the occurrence of cerebrovascular accident (CVA, or stroke) or of a neurologic deficit after a surgical procedure. Basic neurologic assessment includes assessment of the following areas.

Vital Signs. Assessing and recording temperature, pulse, respirations, and blood pressure are essential. The patient's temperature is important and may be elevated for a number of reasons. Infection or damage to the temperature control mechanisms within the brain from increasing intracranial pressure (ICP) may be present.

Changes in blood pressure, particularly a rise in systolic pressure and a widening pulse pressure, may indicate an ICP increase. The pulse may become slow and bounding, and breathing may become irregular and labored as ICP rises. Changes in breathing pattern often indicate a problem with neurologic control of respiration. Any identified change must be reported to the physician promptly.

Clinical Cues

When the systolic and diastolic pressure readings are farther apart, a widening pulse pressure has occurred. For example, if the blood pressure was 128/78 mm Hg earlier and is now 136/64 mm Hg, there is a widened pulse pressure. Notify the physician when the pulse pressure widens.

Current vital signs should be compared to those from the previous several days to determine any changes or trends. Look for changes in blood pressure, pulse rate and quality, and respiratory pattern, and for rising temperature.

Mental Function and Level of Consciousness. Patients experience varying levels of consciousness and ability to respond. It is necessary to determine where the patient is in relation to level of consciousness (LOC), the extremes being alert wakefulness and deep coma (no responsiveness at all).

When observing a patient to determine LOC, the best assessment is based on established criteria or standards that are understood by the observer as well as by others who will be reading the results of the observations. The Glasgow Coma Scale (GCS) is a tool that is universally used in one form or another for this purpose (Table 22-7). The patient's LOC is scored in three different categories. The first category is eye opening, the second is best motor response, and the third is best verbal response. A number is assigned for each category depending on what the assessment reveals. Assessment in the first and last category determines whether the patient can respond to voice commands or to pain or does not respond at all. Verbal responses are evaluated according to whether the patient is oriented and "making sense," confused, making inappropriate remarks, incomprehensible, or silent. **The score in each area is added together, with the optimal score being 15, which indicates a fully alert patient. A score of 3 indicates a totally comatose patient.** Coma level is indicated by a score of 8 or less. Some of the criteria for assessing LOC include: Does the patient awaken easily? Is she oriented to person (herself as well as others), place, and time? Is she able to

follow commands? Does she fail to respond to any stimulus, even physically painful ones? Is she restless? Combative? Does she respond to pain with abnormal posturing?

The FOUR (Full Outline of UnResponsiveness) score developed by Dr. Eelco Wijdicks, a neurologist at the Mayo Clinic, is becoming preferred for comatose or intubated patients who cannot speak. A score of 0 to 4 is assigned in each of four categories: eye, motor, brainstem, and respiratory function. A score of 0 indicates no function and a score of 4 indicates normal function (Murthy, 2009).

? Think Critically

If your patient's blood pressure was 138/84 mm Hg and is now 146/76, what is happening? Is the ICP probably increasing or decreasing?

In the alert patient, note changes in mental function by asking questions to determine orientation to person, place, and time: "What day is today? What month is it? Where are you now?" Assessing memory lapses may be done by asking when the patient was born, what state she resides in, what the last major holiday was, and so on. Thinking can be evaluated by asking the patient to add three numbers together; to count by 6s; or to solve a simple puzzle, such as "If a man goes to the store and purchases four oranges at 40¢ each, two apples at 60¢ each, and two bananas for 46¢, how much did he spend?" (Allow pencil and paper to be used.) If the patient can read English, hand her a card with a command written on it, such as "walk to the sink" or "turn on your right side" (assuming she is physically capable of performing such a task).

Judgment can be grossly tested by assessing whether the patient has been making rational choices in her day-to-day life and by asking her what she would do in a particular situation. Asking specifically what she would do should there be a fire in the trash can will provide information about her judgment.

Neurologic and Neuromuscular Status. Basic assessment of cranial nerves and motor function can be performed by watching the patient perform morning activities of daily living (ADLs). Assess the following: Does the face move symmetrically when she smiles? Is speech clear when she answers questions? Does she move left and right extremities without noticeable problems? Is there anything abnormal about her gait as she moves across the room or down the hall? Does she have difficulty eating or swallowing? Observe the pupils of the eye for size and equality. Pupils should be equal size and should constrict and dilate readily when the environmental light changes (Figure 22-8). Can the patient hear you if you speak to her when her back is turned? Does she seem as alert as usual? Is she having any trouble with balance?

Table 22-7 Glasgow Coma Scale

	SCORE*
Eye Opening	
Spontaneous	4
To sound	3
To pain	2
Never	1
Motor Response	
Obeys commands	6
Localizes pain	5
Normal flexion (withdrawal)	4
Abnormal flexion posturing	3
Extension posturing	2
None	1
Verbal Response	
Oriented	5
Confused conversation	4
Inappropriate words	3
Incomprehensible sounds	2
None	1

*A score of 8 or less indicates coma. The highest possible score is 15.

FIGURE 22-8 Pupil gauge (mm).

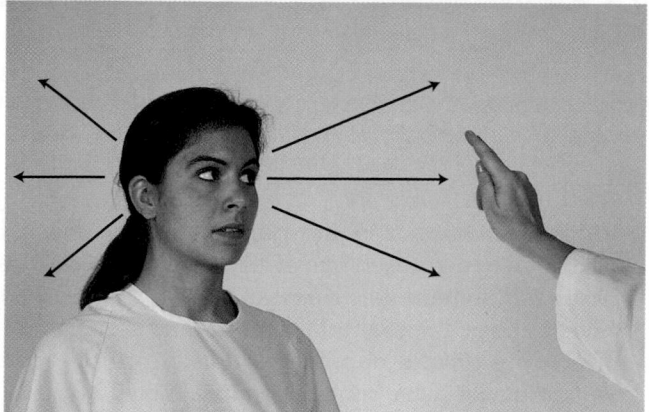

FIGURE 22-9 Checking the cardinal positions of eye movement.

Evaluate the extraocular muscle movements. Ask the patient to follow your finger while you move it through the cardinal positions of gaze (Figure 22-9). Note whether both eyes move together (conjugate) or one deviates. If there is deviation, it is important to note the direction of the deviation. Note any quick back-and-forth oscillation (nystagmus) of the eye at the end points of each direction. Nystagmus can indicate abnormality, such as multiple sclerosis, or can be a side effect of medication, such as phenytoin (Dilantin).

Neuromuscular assessment is concerned with the function of the motor pathways. Test each of the upper and lower extremities. Ask the patient to follow verbal commands such as "raise your left leg," "bend your right knee," "touch your left elbow with your right hand," and "touch your face with your left hand." Have her push against the palms of your hands first with one foot and then the other to test the strength of the leg muscles. To test muscle strength, have the patient extend her arms in front of her, and press down on each arm one at a time, while asking her to try to raise her arm. If the patient has an extremity that is not responding, another stimulus may be necessary to test it. If the patient does not respond to voice commands at all, and deafness is not an issue, test the degree of unconsciousness. First use a louder voice to try to arouse the patient; then, if she does not respond, gently shake her as you would to awaken a child. If that is not successful, painful stimuli are applied for 20 to 30 seconds. First try applying pressure above the eye by placing a thumb under the orbital rim beneath the middle of the eyebrow and pushing upward. If there is no response, pinch the trapezius muscle at

the angle of the shoulder and neck; twist the fingers slightly. If there is no response, apply pressure to the angle of the mandible with the index and middle fingers. If there is still no response, the sternum is rubbed with the knuckles in the form of a fist; a twisting motion is used. **The sternal rub is performed on subsequent assessments only if there is good reason to believe that the patient's comatose status is changing, as it causes bruising.**

The levels of response are:
- Purposefully withdrawing from the stimulus or an attempt to push it away
- Nonpurposeful response, in which the patient may frown or move her arm or leg in a random fashion
- Failure to respond at all

Nonpurposeful responses to pain occur in two ways. Decorticate (flexor) posturing, which is the extension of the legs and internal rotation and adduction of the arms with the elbows bent upward, occurs with damage to the cortex. In decerebrate (extensor) posturing, the arms are stiffly extended and held close to the body, and the wrists are flexed outward. This response means there is damage to the midbrain or brainstem, which indicates a very serious injury (Figure 22-10). The response may be "lateralization," wherein one side of the body shows typical decorticate or decerebrate posturing. An important aspect of neurologic assessment is to look for changes in the patient from each day to the next. Bilateral flaccidity is usually present when there is no response at all.

Pupillary Reactions. Changes in pupil size in response to a bright light are frequently used to determine whether the areas of the brainstem that help control consciousness are functioning normally.

DECORTICATE POSTURING

Flexed
Plantar flexed
Adducted
Flexed
Internally rotated

DECEREBRATE POSTURING

Plantar flexed
Adducted
Extended
Flexed Pronated

FIGURE 22-10 Decorticate and decerebrate posturing indicating brainstem injury.

Cranial nerves II and III control pupil movement. When ICP rises beyond a certain point, pressure on these nerves causes changes in the pupils. If at all possible, find out the normal pupil size for the patient. Although pupils of equal size are considered normal, some people have pupils that are unequal in size. The size of the pupils also may vary from person to person (see Figure 22-8). It is best to measure pupil size rather than estimate it.

Examine the pupils in a room with low light, when the pupils would usually be dilated. Direct a bright light into each eye from the side while the other eye is covered. Observe whether the pupil into which the light shines constricts and whether it does so briskly or sluggishly (direct reflex). Finally, shine the light into each eye while watching to see if the pupil constricts in the other eye (consensual reflex) (Table 22-8). **When pupils have been previously reactive, changes in pupil size or reactivity may signal an emergency, and the physician must be notified immediately.** To test for accommodation (eyes able to focus on both near and far objects) ask the patient to look at an object across the room away from the light source, and then to look at your fingers held about 6 inches from the eyes. The lenses should change shape and the pupils constrict. If a flow sheet is not being used for charting, normal pupil responses often are charted as "PERRLA," meaning "pupils equal, round, and reactive to light with accommodation."

Pupils that remain dilated and fixed in the presence of a bright light indicate brain damage as long as there are no drugs in the system that affect the pupils. One pupil that remains fixed and dilated indicates increased ICP. If both pupils remain constricted, there probably is damage to the pons.

! Safety Alert
Report Changes Immediately
If changes in data indicate a rise in ICP or a decrease in LOC, it is important to alert the charge nurse and physician. This is even more important when possible intracranial bleeding is suspected as it may indicate an emergency situation.

Although changes in the pupils, such as unequal constriction or decreased rate of constriction, indicate increased ICP, sometimes changes in pupils can be caused by medications. For example, atropine and scopolamine can produce dilated pupils, and opiates, miotics, and street drugs can cause constriction (see Table 22-8).

The "Neuro" Check. Monitoring the neurologic status of a patient with a known neurologic disorder includes a "neuro" check on a set schedule. It is performed to determine whether increased ICP is present or ICP is rising. For example, monitoring is necessary after a traumatic head injury, after ingestion of an overdose of a drug or other chemical, when a stroke has occurred or is suspected, or for any other condition in

Table 22-8 Pupillary Abnormalities and Possible Causes

ASSESSMENT DATA	APPEARANCE	POSSIBLE CAUSES
Unilateral, fixed, dilated pupil. Unreactive to light. May be accompanied by ptosis and deviation to side and downward.		Damage to oculomotor nerve related to increased intraocular pressure, compression of oculomotor nerve, head trauma with epidural or subdural hematoma
Bilateral dilated and fixed pupils that do not react to light.		Hypoxia associated with cardiopulmonary arrest. Pressure on midbrain. Severe CNS disorder. Anticholinergic drug overdose
Bilateral small, fixed pupils that do not react to light. Accompanied by motor deficits, drowsiness, confusion, headache, vomiting, incontinence when due to damage to diencephalon.		Side effect of opiates such as morphine. Miotic eyedrops. Hemorrhage into the pons. Damage to the diencephalon
Unequal pupil size; both pupils react to light unless there is underlying pathology.		Ocular inflammation. Congenital aberration. Adhesion, as of iris to cornea or lens. Disturbance of neural pathways

CNS, central nervous system.

which the patient has lost or may lose consciousness. A neurologic assessment flow sheet is used to chart assessment data so that the trend in function of each area can be quickly identified. Four areas are monitored: vital signs, LOC, pupil reaction, and motor function. Neuro checks may be ordered as frequently as every 15 minutes or at intervals from 2 to 8 hours.

Assignment Considerations
The "Neuro" Check

Although the measuring of vital signs can be assigned to assistive personnel, the gathering of data for the "neuro" check should not be delegated. It is important to compare current data with previous data and to carefully assess neuromuscular and pupillary response.

Think Critically

You arrive at the home of an elderly woman who has severe heart disease and atherosclerosis and is very weak. Her spouse says she is confused and lethargic and that she would not eat breakfast. He is worried. As her nurse, what specific assessments would you perform in an attempt to determine whether she has suffered a CVA?

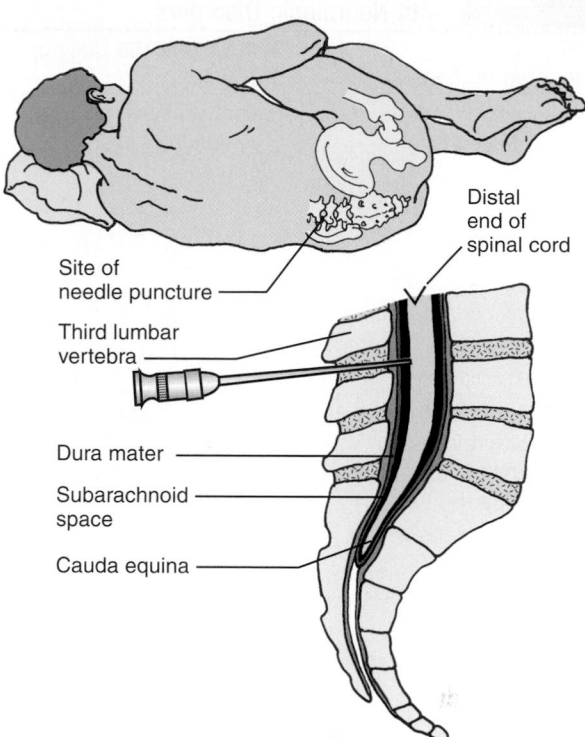
FIGURE 22-11 Lumbar puncture technique.

Diagnostic Tests. The major diagnostic tests most commonly used to evaluate the neurologic system are presented in Table 22-6. Basic physiologic testing is also done to rule out disease in some other system that might be affecting the nervous system. A nerve or muscle biopsy may be done to determine pathologic changes in these tissues. Figure 22-11 shows the technique used for lumbar puncture.

■ Nursing Diagnosis

The most common nursing diagnoses for patients with neurologic disorders are listed in Table 22-9. Each nursing diagnosis chosen for the patient should be individualized to fit the situation. Nursing diagnoses in a care plan vary according to whether the patient is in the acute stage, recovery stage, or rehabilitative stage of the disorder. General expected outcomes for each nursing diagnosis are presented in Table 22-9 along with appropriate interventions.

■ Planning

Overall goals for patients with neurologic disorders depend on whether there is a physiologic possibility that full function may be regained or not. When permanent neurologic deficit occurs, as may occur with some spinal cord injuries, the ultimate goal is for the patient to function at the highest physiologic level. This requires adjusting to limitations imposed by the neurologic deficit so that the patient may live life in a meaningful way. A goal for all patients with neurologic disorders is to

prevent injury, whether from complications of immobility, accidents related to lack of sensation, aspiration from difficulty in swallowing, or any of the other problems that the neurologic deficit may cause.

Caring for patients with neurologic deficits can be very time consuming and requires considerable patience and understanding. If the patient has any weakness, paralysis, or decreased sensation in the extremities, or is confused, disoriented, aphasic, or otherwise incapacitated, providing care will take more time than usual. Extended time must be included in the daily work plan. When a patient is comatose or paralyzed, it is best to team up with another helper to provide care and to turn or reposition the patient. By working together, care is smoother and less taxing.

■ Implementation

Interventions for each nursing diagnosis concerning common problems of neurologic disorders are listed in Table 22-9. Patients should be given information about the disorder and taught about diagnostic tests and self-care. Positive coping skills should be reinforced and ongoing support offered. Interventions are discussed in the following sections on common care problems and with the specific neurologic disorders in Chapters 23, 24, and 25.

■ Evaluation

Evaluation of interventions is performed to determine whether goals are being met. Are the interventions chosen helping to meet the specific expected outcomes

Table 22-9 Common Nursing Diagnoses, Expected Outcomes, and Nursing Interventions for Patients with Neurologic Disorders

NURSING DIAGNOSIS	GOALS/EXPECTED OUTCOMES	NURSING INTERVENTIONS
Risk for injury related to decreased level of consciousness, paralysis, or decreased sensation	Patient will have no evidence of injury or trauma.	Side rails up at all times patient is unattended. Bed in low position when patient is unattended. Pad side rails if seizure activity or restlessness indicates need. Provide eye care for unconscious patient and if corneal (blink) reflex is absent; lubrication and eye patch or shield as needed. Position carefully, protecting extremities from contact with side rails. Maintain correct body alignment. Administer anticonvulsants as ordered to prevent seizure activity. Protect from thermal injury. Use hand mitts to prevent injury from dislodging tubes.
Ineffective breathing pattern related to neurologic disruption of respiration	Maintain a patent airway. Maintain a Po_2 of 80-100 mm Hg. Patient will have no evidence of pulmonary infection.	Assess respiratory status q 2-8 hr depending on patient condition. Position to maximize open airway and to promote chest expansion. Insert oropharyngeal airway as ordered. Suction secretions PRN as ordered. For controlled ventilatory support: auscultate to verify that both lungs are inflating. Check ventilator settings with those ordered. Keep alarm set to "on" at all times. Remove excess water gathering in ventilator tubing as needed. Suction patient using sterile technique as ordered PRN. Monitor blood gas values for changes. Provide frequent mouth care (i.e., q 2-4 hr). Monitor hydration status.
Impaired physical mobility related to CNS deficit, weakness, paralysis, or fatigue	Patient will maintain mobility of all joints. Patient will have no evidence of contractures. Patient will regain optimal physical mobility neurologically possible.	Perform passive ROM or supervise active ROM qid. Teach ROM exercises to patient and family. Teach transfer techniques to hemiplegic patient and family. Collaborate with physical therapist to maximize activity.
Risk for impaired skin integrity related to impaired mobility, decreased sensory awareness, or decreased sensation	Patient's skin will remain intact.	Inspect pressure points for redness, warmth, tenderness, or edema each time patient is turned. Thoroughly inspect skin every shift. Position and pad joints to prevent pressure ulcers. Formulate regular turning/repositioning schedule and stick to it. Use special mattress or special bed to enhance skin protection. Teach patients in wheelchairs to shift weight q 15 min. Teach patient and family to inspect pressure areas and skin for beginning signs of breakdown.
Self-care deficit related to neurologic impairment: paresis, paralysis, decreased LOC, or confusion	Patient will meet self-care needs of hygiene, toileting, feeding, and grooming. Patient will resume self-care at level physiologically and neurologically possible.	Assist with hygiene, toileting, feeding, and grooming as needed. Assist patient to set small, attainable goals for self-care. Explain and demonstrate specific ADL in small, one-task segments. Obtain and demonstrate adaptive devices to assist with ADLs. Offer patience, support, and encouragement for each attempt at self-care. Maintain chart of self-care improvement to track achievement so that patient can see progress.
Imbalanced nutrition: less than body requirements related to inability to swallow or danger of aspiration	Patient's nutritional status will remain adequate as evidenced by normal weight and adequate levels of serum protein.	Institute tube feeding as needed. Check tube placement before initiating each feeding; aspirate stomach contents; test acidity if there is doubt about origins of aspirated fluid. Check residual before each intermittent feeding or q 4 hr for continuous feedings; if greater than 150 mL or more than half of previous feeding, replace and delay next feeding for 1-2 hr. Position patient with head of bed up at least 30 degrees when feeding and for 30-60 min after feeding. Monitor for adverse side effects such as diarrhea. Flush tube with 30-60 mL water after each feeding.

ADLs, activities of daily living; *CNS*, central nervous system; *LOC*, level of consciousness; *Po_2*, partial pressure of oxygen; *PRN*, as needed; *qid*, four times a day; *ROM*, range of motion.

NURSING DIAGNOSIS	GOALS/EXPECTED OUTCOMES	NURSING INTERVENTIONS
Imbalanced nutrition: less than body requirements related to inability to swallow or danger of aspiration– cont'd		Instill water between feedings to maintain hydration. Monitor glucose levels after initiation of feedings until blood glucose is stable. Check weight at least twice a week. Monitor intake and output. *For patient with dysphagia who can take oral feedings:* Serve semisoft foods. Provide six small meals per day; provide nonstressful atmosphere with few distractions for mealtime. Teach to sit upright with head slightly forward and neck flexed; encourage to place food on strongest side of mouth and tongue; encourage to take small bites at a time. Remain with patient to decrease fear of choking; keep suction at hand and turned on during meal. Ensure privacy for meal to decrease embarrassment about drooling, dropping food, or choking. Provide appropriate tube care (see Chapter 29).
Constipation/diarrhea/ bowel incontinence related to decreased level of consciousness, neurogenic impairment, or side effects of medications	Patient will have normal bowel movements as evidenced by soft, formed stool. Patient will attain bowel continence.	Monitor bowel movements and evaluate regularity based on nutritional intake. Administer stool softeners, rectal suppository, or enemas as ordered for constipation. Check for and remove fecal impaction if it occurs, guarding against spinal dysreflexia in the paralyzed patient. Institute bowel training program if needed (see p. 494). If diarrhea occurs, determine cause and alleviate if possible. Administer antidiarrheal if ordered. Keep rectal area clean and dry; protect rectal mucosa. Monitor hydration status; evaluate intake and output.
Disturbed sensory perception related to decreased level of consciousness	Patient will respond to family interaction as evidenced by movement, hand squeezing, eye opening, or speech. Patient will return to alert state as evidenced by proper orientation to person, time, and place.	Speak of current events or daily happenings while providing care. Encourage family members and friends to speak to patient of day's occurrences or fun times in past. Play music on the radio that is to the patient's taste. Play videotapes on topics of interest to the patient. Turn on the patient's favorite television shows. Ask questions and patiently listen for a response. With a tape recorder, introduce sounds from the patient's home and work environment.
Social isolation related to immobility and intellectual limits imposed by neurologic impairment	Patient will have social interaction with visiting friends. Patient will maintain relationships with family members and loved ones. Patient will make new friends among support group members.	Encourage friends and family to visit. Instruct friends and family on how to interact with the patient. Encourage patient to discuss her feelings regarding social contact. Encourage participation in an appropriate support group. Encourage development of a social network. Encourage participation in church, civic, volunteer, and social groups in community. Provide referrals to community job retraining resources if patient is unable to resume former employment or lifestyle.
Interrupted family processes related to role changes, uncertainty of the future, and financial constraints	Each family member will demonstrate appropriate coping methods. Each family member will regain an optimistic outlook. Each family member will accept the patient in her changed state. Each family member will use referrals to support groups and community resources.	Assess strengths of each family member; look for signs of stress. Provide opportunity for verbalization of fears and concerns and feelings about patient's changed condition. Refer to social worker and community resources for support services. Arrange for psychological counseling or family therapy as needed. Encourage contact with appropriate support group. Initiate interaction and honest communication between patient and family members when patient and each member is ready. Teach problem-solving methods if coping skills are weak.

written? If not, the plan needs to be changed. Progress in the patient experiencing a neurologic deficit is often slow. It may take a considerable time for improvement to be noted. Long-term goals of a realistic nature are appropriate. Keep in mind that certain types of neurologic deficits, such as those caused by spinal cord severance, may not improve.

COMMON NEUROLOGIC PATIENT CARE PROBLEMS

Neurologic disorders and illnesses cause many of the same problems. Whether the patient has encephalitis, has a head injury, is recovering from cranial surgery, has suffered a stroke, or has multiple sclerosis or Parkinson's disease, she may need nursing intervention in one or more of the following areas.

INEFFECTIVE BREATHING PATTERN

Weakness of the diaphragm or respiratory muscles or interruption of normal brain function may occur with a variety of neurologic disorders. Monitor the adequacy of respiratory effort and promote a patent airway and chest expansion. Elevating the head of the bed 30 degrees allows the diaphragm to drop more easily and promotes chest expansion. This is only done when there is no spinal injury or severe head injury. When consciousness is depressed, the tongue may be flaccid and fall back, blocking the airway. Positioning the patient on the side allows the tongue to fall to the side and opens the airway. Insertion of an oropharyngeal tube or oral airway is helpful.

Assisting the patient with deep breathing and the use of an incentive spirometer can help prevent atelectasis and improve ventilation. Respiratory assessment is performed every shift and includes auscultating the lungs for signs of atelectasis or retained secretions and judging the quality of respiratory effort. If respiratory efforts are considerably impaired, the patient may need intubation and mechanical ventilation. Interventions for the patient undergoing mechanical ventilation are presented in Chapter 15.

IMPAIRED MOBILITY

The nurse, the physical therapist, and the patient work together to help the patient cope with muscle weakness or paralysis. Activities such as proper positioning and range-of-motion (ROM) exercises are started immediately to preserve proper alignment of joints and limbs and prevent contractures and muscle atrophy. Assistive devices, such as splints and slings, may be used. The patient who suffers hemiplegia (paralysis and loss of sensation in an extremity) is taught to become aware of arm or leg placement when she turns or transfers to a chair to avoid injury to the affected extremity.

For example, the patient with left hemiplegia from a CVA may neglect her paralyzed side. She must therefore be taught to attend to the affected side of her body by scanning it frequently. To prevent discomfort in the shoulder and arm on the affected side and to prevent dislocation of the shoulder, take care not to pull on the affected arm or shoulder during transfers or ambulation. Support the affected arm with pillows or an armrest to keep it from dangling when the patient is seated. Use a sling for comfort and to promote better balance when ambulating and transferring the patient.

The patient with hemiplegia is taught, step by step, the safest way to transfer from the bed to a wheelchair and back, and how to use assistance from others. She is also taught how to care for and protect her skin in areas of decreased sensation.

The patient who has hemiparesis (one-sided weakness) is taught how to strengthen her muscles and use assistive devices, such as walkers, crutches, or canes, to walk. She is taught the best ways to get out of bed and into and out of a chair. The quadriplegic patient (four limbs paralyzed) is helped in learning to cope with this drastic alteration in her life and how she might direct her energies toward different, but attainable, goals. (A newer term for quadriplegia is tetraplegia.)

All patients who have suffered an impairment of mobility need assistance with the grieving process, help in establishing healthy and effective coping patterns, and assistance with depression.

Attention to pain relief and muscle spasm is necessary for the patient to achieve the highest level of rehabilitation possible. Paralyzed extremities are susceptible to edema and to decrease this problem extremities should be elevated when the patient is at rest. The patient needs to be turned frequently to prevent complications from pressure and sluggish circulation.

Elderly patients may suffer joint stiffness from arthritis. Assess joints for tenderness and pain before performing ROM, and be gentle and considerate when turning and repositioning.

Take measures to promote skin integrity. Place the patient on a special bed or protective mattress cover or pad, inspect pressure points frequently, and keep the skin clean and dry. Chapter 9 discusses the effects of immobility on each body system, along with the nursing activities necessary to avoid disabilities resulting from inactivity. The principles and practices presented in that chapter are relevant to the nursing care of a patient with a neurologic disorder that produces some type of paresis or paralysis, and for the patient who is unconscious.

SELF-CARE DEFICIT

Neuromuscular impairment may interfere with the patient's ability to perform hygiene activities or other ADLs. She may need assistance with bathing, grooming, oral hygiene, dressing, eating, and toileting. Work with the patient as her condition dictates, assisting with techniques to perform self-care in spite of disability when possible, offering encouragement, and praising any effort at accomplishing a self-care task.

Inability to carry out the most basic of self-care activities can erode a person's sense of independence and self-esteem. The ability to feed, clothe, and take care of toileting is an important part of independence. Regaining some level of self-care in these areas is of particular concern to the adult who, because of neurologic dysfunction, may have to relearn ways to perform the simplest of daily activities.

If the patient is unconscious, the mouth must be kept clean to avoid infection of the parotid gland. The lips, tongue, and gums are cleansed and lubricated at frequent intervals as mouth breathing makes them excessively dry. This cleansing may be done by turning the patient to the side, turning on the oral suction device, and—with a toothbrush or a tongue depressor with gauze taped to it—wiping the oral surfaces. A solution of 50% water/50% mouthwash, or water with a small amount of hydrogen peroxide and sodium bicarbonate, may be used to moisten the gauze. Too much hydrogen peroxide will cause excessive foaming. Using an irrigation syringe filled with water in one hand and the oral suction device in the other allows rinsing of the mouth while preventing aspiration of the liquid. It is easiest for two caregivers to work together to rinse and suction the mouth. Each time the mouth is cleansed, the patient should be positioned on the opposite side to ensure thorough cleansing of each side of the mouth. Oral suction should be available and turned on any time mouth care is given to a patient who has a weakened gag reflex, cannot swallow normally, or has weakness of the facial muscles. Studies show that tooth and tongue brushing decreases iatrogenic infection significantly.

When the patient cannot shut her eyes, the nurse or caregiver must provide care to prevent keratitis or corneal ulceration. The eyelids are cleansed with warm sterile water or normal saline every few hours to remove discharge and debris. Artificial tears or a lubricant is instilled as prescribed to prevent dryness. If the corneal reflex is absent, an eye shield or patch is placed over the eye. The eyelid is closed before a patch is applied. The eyes are examined each day for signs of inflammation.

The ability of relatives to learn how to care for the patient, and their willingness to do so, are important parts of assessing and planning for rehabilitation. Goals for rehabilitation must be realistic and mutually agreed on by the patient, her family, and the nurse.

Assistive devices help patients with neurologic deficits to feed and dress themselves. Occupational therapists can help the patient relearn how to perform elementary tasks necessary for daily living. Patients are retaught how to feed themselves, how to get in and out of a bed or a chair, how to select and put on clothes and fasten them, and how to bathe, brush teeth, and comb hair.

Provide assistance when the patient cannot do a task completely, and—most of all—provide encouragement and praise for efforts made. **When pursuing self-help rehabilitation, the nurse needs to remember that the patient tires easily; tasks must be spaced apart so that energy is available to achieve them.** Pushing the patient to try another task when she is too tired only sets her up for failure and frustration.

DYSPHAGIA

Every patient who has suffered a neurologic insult (damage) from head injury, stroke, or intracranial surgery should have the swallowing reflex assessed: have the patient try to sip plain water before attempting to eat food. Check periodically that the patient automatically swallows saliva, before offering water. Patients who have paresis from a stroke or who suffer from myasthenia gravis or other neurologic disorders often have difficulty swallowing (dysphagia). Those patients who have difficulty eating are at risk for nutritional disorders and aspiration pneumonia. Patients with dysphagia should be sitting upright or in a high Fowler's position to eat. The position should be maintained for at least 30 minutes after a meal (Paik, 2008). A nonstressful meal environment without distractions is best, as stress makes dysphagia worse.

When the patient cannot swallow without choking or aspirating, tube feeding is necessary. When the patient is receiving nutrients by tube, the caloric intake should be assessed frequently. Tube-fed patients are weighed twice a week and intake and output are recorded and evaluated. Interventions for the patient receiving tube feedings are outlined in Chapter 29.

INCONTINENCE

Many patients with CNS disorders experience temporary or permanent urinary or fecal incontinence. Some patients experience constipation. The patient must be kept clean and dry. A condom catheter for the male patient or incontinence briefs or pads are used for urinary incontinence.

Perhaps the first step in planning and implementing either a bladder or a bowel training program is to convince the nursing staff and the patient and her family that something can be done to improve, if not completely relieve, the situation. A negative attitude and lack of persistence can doom a program to failure before it is started. Be content with small successes at first, setting short-term goals that will eventually lead to a satisfactory resolution of the problem.

Bladder Training Program

Bladder training is a program designed to help a patient with some degree of loss of normal bladder function and a resulting disturbance of voiding and bladder control. Loss of control can occur in a variety of neurologic disorders, including stroke, spinal cord injury, and tumors and lesions of the spinal cord.

The purposes of a bladder reconditioning program are to prevent urinary complications such as infection and calculi (stones) and to allow the patient freedom from fear of embarrassment and loss of self-esteem. Calculi are less likely to develop when there is a high fluid intake and frequent, complete emptying of the bladder.

Bladder function is assessed to determine the optimal neural and muscular control that can be realistically expected in view of the physiologic cause of loss of control. In developing a bladder reconditioning program, the patient's mental and emotional ability to cooperate and take an active part in carrying out the program is evaluated.

The cause of urinary incontinence must be known, and the specific symptoms manifested by the patient must be clearly defined. Significant data include information about:

- Difficulty in starting to void
- Any methods the patient uses to initiate voiding (e.g., pressure on the bladder)
- Degree of awareness of the need to void
- Ability to empty the bladder completely, and amount of residual urine
- Signs of bladder distention and dribbling or overflow
- Nighttime incontinence
- Stress incontinence
- Usual times for voiding

Spinal cord injuries and lesions produce what is known as a cord bladder or neurogenic bladder. Patients with disorders of this type are not aware of the need to void and must be trained in techniques to initiate voiding and emptying the bladder.

The second step in a bladder training program is to keep an accurate record of actual voiding times for a 2- to 3-day period. Some problems of incontinence can be corrected by a simple scheduling of voiding times. Offering a bedpan or getting the patient up to the bathroom one-half hour before times she is usually incontinent may remedy the problem.

A bladder training program usually begins with a 2-hour schedule for toileting. The patient should attempt to drink 2000 to 3000 mL of fluid between waking up and 6 P.M. Coffee, tea, alcoholic beverages, and soda with caffeine should be avoided after dinner, because they have a diuretic effect. The patient is toileted before retiring for the night. The maintenance of an accurate training record is essential. A trial of 6 weeks is necessary before determining whether the training is successful. Various drugs that affect the voiding process, such as oxybutynin chloride (Ditropan), flavoxate hydrochloride (Urispas), or solifenacin (VESIcare), may be helpful for certain types of patients. The nurse assesses whether the medication is beneficial.

Patients who have nerve damage and paralysis are trained in specific techniques to empty the bladder. Credé's maneuver, in which the open hand is pressed over the bladder area and directed toward the suprapubic area, can facilitate emptying a flaccid bladder. Self-catheterization is taught to paraplegic patients so that they are not dependent on an indwelling catheter or on other people for their urinary elimination (Rackley, 2009) (see also Chapter 35).

Some patients are candidates for the implantation of an artificial sphincter to control bladder release of urine. More and more types of successful devices are developed each year, but these are primarily for the patient who has no neurologic control over the bladder.

Every patient undertaking a bladder retraining program needs a great deal of understanding and encouragement and a positive attitude to be successful. Praise for each small achievement should be given. Accidents should be expected and not looked on as "failures." Achieving total continence takes considerable time and effort, but is possible for many patients.

Bowel Training Program

Bowel training for the neurologic patient is done to correct incontinence or prevent constipation and impaction. The bowel training program begins with an assessment of the specific patterns of elimination. It also helps to know the patient's former bowel pattern before illness or injury. Did she regularly rely on the use of enemas or laxatives? Has she been prone to constipation? Next, the nurse needs to establish whether the patient is aware of the urge to defecate or has any warning of evacuation.

Bowel training for either constipation or incontinence should incorporate an exercise program that is within the patient's ability, a high-fiber diet, and adequate liquid intake during the day. An accurate recording of bowel movements correlated with times of oral intake over a 2- to 3-day period will help establish the most opportune times to try to stimulate evacuation and thus establish a habit. If incontinence occurs at specific times after eating, toileting 30 minutes sooner and using a rectal suppository or a gloved finger to stimulate the urge to defecate may alter the pattern. Gradually the use of the suppository is discontinued.

For the patient who is prone to constipation and incontinence, increasing liquid intake and administering a stool softener can be effective. If this does not work, a planned regimen of suppository or enema use may be necessary to assist with evacuation at a desired time, thus preventing incontinence.

All patients need to be comfortable when attempting to evacuate the bowel. A raised, padded toilet seat, handrails, and perhaps a footstool can provide enough comfort to allow the patient to relax so that evacuation can occur naturally. Privacy is essential. Remember to provide privacy for the bedridden patient. Most of all, a positive attitude is needed by staff members. Many times, if the nurse and the patient are optimistic and patient, success can be achieved.

PAIN

Many patients with neurologic disorders experience pain. The pain often is chronic in nature. The nurse must work with the patient to identify the characteristics of the pain, its location and spread, its intensity, and how it is affecting the patient's life. When the patient has suffered a head injury or is experiencing increasing ICP, narcotic analgesics may not be given, as they mask the signs of rising ICP. Other methods of analgesia must be employed.

A trusting relationship between the patient and the nurse is necessary for teaching to be assimilated. Teaching the patient about pain and its relief, the adverse effect of stress, anxiety, and unpleasant stimuli, and the benefits of distraction from the pain become part of the plan. Pain may cause difficulty in sleeping. Pharmacologic agents and alternative methods for pain control are used (see Chapter 7).

 Think Critically

How would you determine if a patient who has a decreased level of consciousness is experiencing pain?

Depression often occurs with chronic pain and lack of sleep. The combination of an antidepressant and pain medication often is more effective for chronic pain control than either type of drug used alone.

CONFUSION

Patients with brain tumors, head injuries, and strokes, as well as degenerative diseases, may experience confusion and deficits in memory, intellectual ability, or judgment. Confusion may be acute and short term, or it may be a permanent state. Confusion also may be mild or severe and may be accompanied by anxiety, agitation, and refusal to cooperate. The person is in a state of disorientation, and until the symptoms subside, she cannot behave rationally. She must be supported and protected, or she may injure herself. In states of severe (acute) confusion (delirium) the patient may experience hallucinations, delusions, and severe agitation. This is usually an acute, short-term state caused by fever or metabolic imbalance. Patients who experience confusion after a head injury often become combative as their ICP rises. It is not advisable to restrain these patients; be very careful to stay out of range of flailing arms.

The nurse should be alert to signs of confusion in any patient with a CNS problem. Subjective and objective assessment data include the following:

- Loss of orientation to person, place, or time
- Inability to cooperate fully with simple tasks and requests, such as eating and bathing
- Inappropriate statements or inappropriate answers to questions
- Restlessness and agitation
- Hostility and anxiety
- Hallucinations or delusions
- Other signs of inability to maintain control over thought processes and behavior

The patient who is confused needs above all else a stable and calm environment. Her thought processes are, in a sense, "fractured" and somewhat beyond her control. Stimuli entering her brain are frightening and threatening to her, and she simply cannot make sense out of most of what is going on around her. A calm, consistent, and orderly approach combined with a set daily routine is most helpful.

Attention to safety of the patient is a priority. Family members must be taught measures to protect the patient who wanders, is disoriented, or lacks judgment (see Chapter 48).

Confused patients need a dependable, consistent schedule. If agitation or confusion causes undesirable behavior, the use of distraction can be beneficial. Handing the patient an item, leading her from the area, or decreasing environmental stimuli (turning off the television or radio) can calm the patient.

The patient with memory loss who can still read benefits from written instructions and from a posting of the day's schedule of activities. Measures to protect the patient and deal with confusion are presented in Chapter 48.

APHASIA

Aphasia is a defect in the ability to express oneself in speech or writing, or an inability to comprehend spoken or written language. Aphasia is caused by disease or injury of the brain centers controlling language comprehension and expression, located in Wernicke's area of the left cerebral hemisphere.

Aphasia may be *receptive, expressive,* or *global.* The person with receptive aphasia has difficulty interpreting communications to her in either spoken or written form. In expressive aphasia, the person has difficulty expressing herself in speech or writing. Global aphasia is when the person has a combination of receptive and expressive aphasia. Aphasias vary in degree and in type of deficit. For example, a person may be able to write a message but cannot form the words to say it.

A comprehensive assessment of the patient who has some type of aphasia usually is a team effort carried out under the leadership of a specially trained speech therapist. Nurses and others responsible for the care of the aphasic patient can assist by noting specific abilities or inabilities of the patient to communicate with them.

Focused Assessment

Determining Type of Aphasia Problem

Questions to ask when evaluating the type and degree of aphasia a patient is experiencing include:

- Can the patient understand yes/no questions? Are her responses of "yes" and "no" reliable (does that seem to be what she means)?
- Can she point to or look toward objects you have named that are in her line of vision?
- Can she name the objects?
- Is she able to follow simple directions (e.g., "Turn your head.")?
- Can she repeat simple words? Complex words?
- Can she repeat sentences?
- Can she follow simple written requests?
- Can she write answers to questions?
- Can she write requests?
- Can she read questions or directions?

The patient who suddenly has a problem speaking or understanding words or signs is likely to feel isolated and extremely frustrated unless an effort is made to establish some means of communicating with her as quickly as possible. Once the patient's specific problem is identified, which could be relatively simple or extremely complex, measures are taken to help the patient communicate as fully as her condition will allow.

Goals for the care of the aphasic patient are focused on stimulating communication without undue frustration and gradually guiding her to appropriate responses and requests. Reaching these goals may take weeks or months, but there are helpful principles and techniques that can be used by all members of the health team and by family members and friends.

Perhaps the most important rule of all is to avoid talking to the aphasic person as if she were mentally incompetent. Her inability to communicate does not mean a lack of intelligence. She should be spoken *to,* not spoken *about* as if she cannot hear and understand what others are saying in her presence.

Speak slowly and distinctly in a normal voice as you are facing her. Use body language and sign language to communicate if it seems to help the patient. Your facial expressions, posture, and gestures can often say more than the words you are saying.

Give the aphasic patient time to respond to questions. Do not ask more than one question at a time. It takes longer for an aphasic person to process what is being said. If you need to repeat a statement or question, use *exactly* the same words. She may have comprehended only half of the sentence the first time. Only one person should speak at a time. Be certain to establish eye contact with the patient before speaking. Keep the environment orderly, relaxed, and relatively free from distractions that make it difficult to concentrate on communicating.

The speech therapist will plan the patient's speech therapy program and will share with the nurse the details of how best to work with each individual patient. Some general guidelines include:

- Give praise for attempts at communication and for each correctly expressed word or sentence.
- Do not correct the patient's pronunciation, as she is liable to become too frustrated and give up speaking.
- Be very patient.

Problems with aphasia sometimes resolve spontaneously in 3 or 4 months after a CVA. Total speech rehabilitation can take many months and may never reach the pre-aphasia level.

Think Critically

Can you identify three specific techniques you might use to assist a patient with aphasia to communicate her needs?

Among the techniques used to stimulate communication and help the patient deal with her problem of aphasia are self-talk, parallel talk, expansion, and modeling. *Self-talk* helps the aphasic person associate activities with specific words and phrases. The caregiver talks about what he is doing while performing a task (e.g., making the bed). Self-talk is done in the presence of the patient so she can make the connection between what is being said and what she sees being done (Royal-Evans & Marcus, 2004).

Parallel talk describes for the patient what she is doing while she is performing some activity. In *expansion,* the person communicating with the patient completes the patient's sentences when she is able to verbalize but cannot yet speak in complete sentences. No new information is added during expansion. In *modeling,* the patient's sentences are completed, and new information is added.

All of these techniques are helpful in improving communication. They are forms of therapy, however, and are used only in a planned program that has been designed to meet a patient's individual needs. Whatever techniques are chosen, they should not be used in a condescending manner; the adult patient should always be treated respectfully.

The plan of care for the aphasic patient should not neglect the physical condition of her mouth and tongue. Good oral hygiene is needed to keep the oral mucosa clean and moist and in optimal condition so that it is easier for the patient to form words.

SEXUAL DYSFUNCTION

Sexual dysfunction from a lesion in neural pathways should be dealt with by allowing expression of the patient's concerns, beliefs, and feelings. Sexual counseling by someone skilled in working with patients with neurologic deficits should be initiated. Alternative techniques for meeting sexual needs must be explored. Many patients can, with teaching, lead a sexually satisfying life.

PSYCHOSOCIAL CONCERNS

The multiple stresses, alteration in roles, and changes in body image and self-esteem that result from a chronic neurologic disorder can be overwhelming. The patient will need time and assistance in adapting to an altered body image. The nurse must be accepting of the patient's expression of anxiety, anger, denial, regression, and depression. Work to support the patient emotionally, attempting to establish realistic hope for quality of life. Exploring the patient's previous methods of coping with adversity, as well as her support systems, talents, and desires, helps to provide clues for how best to help her. Jointly establishing small, accomplishable goals can do much to rebuild self-esteem.

Collaboration with the social worker concerning referral to support groups and interaction with others with similar disabilities who are coping well can prove most beneficial. Contact with community agencies that offer support services and job retraining, if pertinent, is essential. The patient needs a way to be a productive member of society and to contribute to the welfare of her family. The county or state office of vocational rehabilitation may help with funding.

Reentry into the community and a normal social life are other areas for intervention. Often the patient has been out of touch with her normal social circles for many months during the illness and recovery process. Plans should be made before discharge for social contact to be reinstated.

INEFFECTIVE FAMILY COPING

A chronic neurologic disorder that disrupts normal function for the patient also disrupts normal roles within the family. Family lifestyle is altered, and changes in roles may lead to family conflict. Family members often feel powerless, ambivalent toward the patient, angry, and guilty for having angry feelings. Family members need to be included when educating the patient about her disorder, the possibility of remissions and exacerbations, and the self-care measures necessary. Everyone needs time to adjust to the situation. Referrals to counseling and support groups can be very helpful.

Get Ready for the NCLEX® Examination!

Key Points

- When deprived of oxygen, neurons die quickly.
- Many changes occur with aging, and after age 70 the brain atrophies somewhat.
- Reflexes diminish or are lost as age advances.
- Preventing accidents and head injuries by teaching safety practices reduces the number of neurologic injuries.
- Discouraging recreational drug use helps prevent neurologic damage.
- Teaching patients how to reduce risk factors for stroke can prevent the devastation that a stroke can inflict.
- Nurses routinely perform gross assessment of the cranial nerves, coordination and balance, muscle strength, and reflexes.
- Vital signs, mental function, neuromuscular status, papillary reactions, and level of consciousness are parts of the physical assessment and are always performed as part of the "neuro" check.
- A thorough history is gathered focusing on areas of neurologic function (see Focused Assessment).
- Nursing care is individualized, with nursing diagnoses, outcome objectives, and interventions chosen to alleviate the various problems (see Table 22-9).
- Every effort is made to maintain effective breathing for the neurologic patient.

- Many neurologic patients experience impaired mobility, and nurses attempt to prevent the associated potential problems.
- Assisting with ADLs when patients have self-care deficits is a major part of nursing care for patients with neurologic disorders.
- Specific techniques are needed for the patient who experiences dysphagia to prevent aspiration.
- Many patients with bowel or bladder incontinence can regain continence through bowel and bladder retraining programs.
- Pain control can be a difficult issue because most pain medications dull the sensorium and will interfere with accurate neurologic assessment and signs of decreasing level of consciousness.
- Many patients with neurologic disorders become confused, and there are special techniques nurses use to assist these patients.
- Learning to work with an aphasic patient is essential to providing care for her.
- When appropriate, neurologic patients should be referred for sexual counseling.
- When a family member has a neurologic deficit, it affects the whole family and can disrupt normal family functioning; families need help to learn to cope.

Additional Learning Resources

SG Go to your Study Guide for additional learning activities to help you master this chapter content.

evolve Go to your Evolve website (http://evolve.elsevier.com/deWit/medsurg) for the following FREE learning resources:
- Animations, audio, and video
- Answers and rationales for questions and activities
- Concept Map Creator
- Glossary with pronunciations in English and Spanish
- Interactive Review Questions and Exercises and more!

 Online Resources
- Aphasia Help, www.aphasiahelp.org
- The National Aphasia Association, www.aphasia.org

Review Questions for the NCLEX® Examination

1. While performing an initial assessment, the nurse notes that the patient provides inappropriate responses to verbal communication. When showing the patient a key and asking "What is this?" The response was, "Argh ooh." This clinical finding is referred to as:
   1. dysphagia.
   2. expressive aphasia.
   3. dysarthria.
   4. receptive aphasia.

2. When giving instructions to a patient with some dysphagia, further teaching is needed if the patient states:
   1. "I must sit upright when I eat."
   2. "I can watch my crime show on TV while I eat."
   3. "I should stay upright after eating for at least 30 minutes."
   4. "I should be calm and unhurried when eating."

3. While assisting the patient with feeding, the nurse describes every step in meal preparation in simple language. This is referred to as:
   1. parallel talk.
   2. self-talk.
   3. expansion.
   4. modeling.

4. The nurse is providing discharge instructions to an elderly Iranian man who experienced a stroke. The nurse notices that the patient seems indifferent to teaching. The nurse must consider:
   1. talking to the wife or daughter.
   2. involving the entire family in the care of the patient.
   3. sending the patient to a long-term care facility.
   4. stopping and trying again later.

5. With an open hand, the nurse presses over the flaccid bladder of a patient. When questioned regarding the nursing action, an appropriate response would be:
   1. "The technique increases the muscle tone of the bladder."
   2. "The maneuver facilitates removal of urinary sediments."
   3. "The technique assists with complete bladder emptying."
   4. "The technique reduces the incidence of bladder irritation."

6. To assess _____ the nurse shines a light on the right eye and watches the left pupil.
   1. accommodation
   2. consensual reflex
   3. direct reflex
   4. blink reflex

7. The nurse uses the Glasgow Coma Scale to evaluate the neurologic responses of a patient. The patient opens eyes to pain, makes incomprehensible verbal sounds, and extends extremities with pain. The score would suggest:
   1. locked-in syndrome.
   2. brain death.
   3. coma.
   4. lethargy.

8. The nurse demonstrates understanding of the physiologic changes in the nervous system associated with aging by:
   1. providing extra time for the patient to process and answer questions.
   2. reminding the patient how to perform activities of daily living.
   3. finishing the patient's sentences when responding to questions.
   4. communicating slowly and loudly with low-pitched tones.

9. The nurse scrapes an object along the sole of the patient's foot and notes that the great toe bends upward and the smaller toes fan outward. The clinical finding is suggestive of:
   1. sensory abnormality of the cortex.
   2. motor abnormality of the cortex.
   3. cerebellar tissue destruction.
   4. a normal finding.

10. Which nursing intervention(s) would be appropriate when providing care for a patient with right hemiplegia from a stroke? *(Select all that apply.)*
    1. Reminding the patient to pay attention to the left side
    2. Protecting the right extremities during transfers
    3. Supporting unaffected arm with pillows
    4. Using a sling on the affected arm to promote better balance
    5. Initiating range-of-motion exercises

Critical Thinking Activities

Scenario A

Mr. Lawson is to have several diagnostic tests done to determine the cause of his neurologic symptoms, which include headache, visual disturbance, muscular weakness, and personality change.

1. How would you explain an electroencephalogram to Mr. Lawson? A computed tomography scan? Magnetic resonance imaging?

2. If you are to assess Mr. Lawson's "neuro signs" and he is using eyedrops for glaucoma that constrict the pupils, how would you evaluate his pupillary responses?

Scenario B

Mr. Horton has experienced a CVA and has incontinence of urine.

1. How would you institute a bladder training program for him?

2. What would you do to protect his skin, and his dignity, during the bladder training?

3. If bladder training cannot be accomplished, what is the best way to handle his urinary elimination?

Care of Patients with Head and Spinal Cord Injuries

Objectives

Theory

1. Describe the types of injuries that result from head trauma.
2. Compare and contrast the signs and symptoms of subdural hematoma and epidural hematoma.
3. Explain why an epidural hematoma causes an emergency situation.
4. Discuss the type of procedure performed to relieve a subdural hematoma.
5. Illustrate the pathophysiology of increasing intracranial pressure in a patient who has experienced a severe head injury.
6. Identify the reasons why an elderly person is more at risk for an intracranial bleed from a head injury.
7. Explain the possible ramifications of spinal cord injury.

8. List appropriate nursing interventions necessary to provide comprehensive care for a patient who has suffered a C5 spinal cord injury.
9. Analyze the symptoms of low back pain and correlate them with their causes.

Clinical Practice

1. Teach a family member how to properly assess and care for a patient who has suffered a concussion.
2. Perform a neurologic check on a patient who has suffered head trauma.
3. Participate in a collaborative care planning conference for a patient who has sustained a spinal cord injury.
4. Prepare a plan for teaching self-care measures to a patient who suffers from low back pain.

Key Terms

concussion (kŏn-KŬ-shŭn, p. 500)
contralateral (kŏn-tră-LĂT-ĕr- ăl, p. 502)
contusion (kŏn-TŪ-zhŭn, p. 501)
coup-contrecoup injury (koo kŏ-trĕ-koo, p. 501)
epidural hematoma (Ĕ-pĭ-DŪ-rŭl hē-mă -TŌ-mă, p. 501)
hydrocephalus (hī-drō-SĔF-ă-lăs, p. 508)
intracerebral hematoma (ĭn-trăh-sĕ-RĒ-brăl, p. 501)

ipsilateral (ĭp-sĭ-LĂT-ĕr-ăl, p. 502)
nuchal rigidity (p. 502)
papilledema (p. 506)
quadriplegia (kwŏd-rĭ-PLĒ-jă, p. 509)
subdural hematoma (sŭb-DŪ-rŭl, p. 501)
subluxation (sŭb-lŭk-SĀ-shŭn, p. 509)

HEAD INJURIES

Head injuries are a frequent cause of death. About 1.5 million people sustain head and brain injury in the United States each year. Approximately 52,000 die, and 1.2 million are treated for traumatic brain injury and released. Those who survive initial head injury require meticulous observation and care so that damage to the brain cells can be kept at a minimum and death averted. There are about 5.6 million people in the United States who have need of lifelong help with activities of daily living because of residual disabilities from brain injury (Dawodu, 2009).

Etiology

A blow to the head may cause a laceration of the skin or scalp and fracture of the skull, or may only cause a minor contusion. The injury may cause movement of the brain within the skull, tearing blood vessels. Accidents are the most common cause of head injury, with motor vehicle accidents being the leading cause of head injury.

Pathophysiology

When a depressed skull fracture occurs, there is bruising, contusion, or laceration of the underlying brain tissue, with the inflammatory changes that occur with any wound. A minor head injury may cause concussion. Concussion is the term used to describe a closed head injury in which there is a brief disruption in level of consciousness (LOC), amnesia regarding the occurrence, and headache. A concussion's seriousness is based on the length of time there was loss of consciousness. There can be long-term neurologic deficits from concussion, particularly if an individual suffers repeated concussions from accidents or sports.

Skull fractures are described as:
- Linear or depressed
- Simple, comminuted, or compound
- Closed or open

A *closed* injury is one in which the scalp and skull remain intact, but the underlying brain tissue is damaged. There may be contused areas or hematoma. In an *open* injury there is laceration of the scalp and fracture of the skull with damage to brain tissue.

Elder Care Points

The brain atrophies with age and does not take up as much space in the cranial vault. This allows for more movement and more potential for torn vessels and contusions on the brain when an accident occurs that involves a head injury.

In a **contusion**, the brain tissue is bruised, blood from broken vessels accumulates, and edema develops, causing increased intracranial pressure (ICP).

A **coup-contrecoup injury**, or an *acceleration-deceleration injury,* occurs when the head is moving rapidly and hits a stationary object, such as a windshield. The contents within the cranium hit the inside of the skull (coup) and then bounce back and hit the bony area opposite the site of impact, causing a second injury (contrecoup) (Figure 23-1).

Subdural hematoma is a common result of head injury. It often happens in the elderly as a result of a fall. Anticoagulant therapy puts a patient at greater risk for a subdural hematoma (blood-filled swelling) after even a minor blow to the head. When a blow is delivered to the head, it may rupture the blood vessels

FIGURE 23-1 Coup-contrecoup (acceleration-deceleration) injury.

that lie between the delicate arachnoid membrane covering the brain and the tough, fibrous dura mater. As the blood leaks under the dura mater (subdural), the hematoma grows in size, pressing against the softer arachnoid and the brain tissue it is covering (Figure 23-2, *A*).

Diffuse axonal injury occurs from a rapid acceleration-deceleration injury in which there is lateral movement. There is diffuse injury to the white matter of the brain.

Elder Care Points

Because the brain of the older person tends to move more in the cranial vault when head trauma occurs, small vessels may be torn and the patient is more at risk for a slow-developing subdural hematoma. When such injury occurs, the person should be watched for several months for signs of personality change, decreasing LOC, increased irritability, and other signs of increased ICP.

An **epidural hematoma** occurs more rarely, but when it does, there is rapid leakage of blood from the middle meningeal artery, which quickly elevates ICP (see Figure 23-2, *B*). This constitutes a medical emergency. A craniotomy is needed to repair the damaged vessel and relieve the rapidly rising pressure, before death occurs from the increased ICP. An **intracerebral hematoma** may occur within the brain from a blow to the head (see Figure 23-2, *C*).

Signs and Symptoms
The severity of brain damage from a head injury is best judged by the symptoms presented by the patient, a neurologic assessment, the history of the type of blow received, and whether and for how long the victim lost consciousness. The outward symptoms of head injury are fairly obvious: these include bruising, swelling, lacerations, and bleeding. There may be a skull fracture with ecchymoses (raccoon eyes), or ecchymoses behind the ear (Battle's sign) (Figure 23-3). There may be otorrhea (fluid from the ear), rhinorrhea (fluid from

A Subdural hematoma   **B** Epidural hematoma   **C** Intracerebral hematoma

FIGURE 23-2 A, Subdural hematoma. As a result of trauma to the head, small ruptured blood vessels leak blood into the space under the dura mater (slower than an epidural bleed). **B,** Epidural hematoma, the result of a head injury that tears a large meningeal artery, has caused a rapid bleed with a large amount of blood above the dura mater. If not relieved, subdural and epidural hematomas can be fatal. **C,** Intracerebral hematoma. Small vessels within the brain have torn and bled.

FIGURE 23-3 Battle's sign.

the nose), tinnitus (ringing in the ear) or hearing difficulty, facial paralysis, and conjugate deviation of gaze wherein both eyes deviate to one side. Otorrhea and rhinorrhea should be tested to determine if there is a cerebrospinal fluid (CSF) leak. Testing with a Dextrostix will determine whether glucose is present; the presence of glucose indicates cerebrospinal fluid. A bleeding into the subarachnoid space may be evidenced by **nuchal rigidity** (neck pain with flexion).

Whenever a moderate or severe head injury has occurred, cervical spine injury is assumed, until proven otherwise.

Clinical Cues

If the fluid from the ear or nose is tinged with blood, a Dextrostix will not give accurate results. Collect about a teaspoon of the fluid on a white gauze pad. Within a few minutes blood will move to the center and a yellow ring (halo) will form around it if the fluid is CSF (Figure 23-4).

A concussion can cause a brief disruption of the normal LOC, amnesia regarding the event, and headache. A contusion can cause an alteration in LOC and may cause seizures. Box 23-1 shows the downward progression of decreased LOC.

A subdural hematoma may be acute, subacute, or chronic, building up over time. An acute intracerebral bleed causing hematoma formation is accompanied by unconsciousness, hemiplegia on the **contralateral** (opposite) side, and a dilated pupil on the **ipsilateral**

(same) side. However, the symptoms indicating a slow buildup of pressure within the skull are more subtle and less easily detected.

Signs of epidural hematoma may include unconsciousness at the time of the injury, a brief lucid interval followed by decreasing LOC, headache, nausea and vomiting, and dilation of the ipsilateral pupil. The patient is observed for signs of increased ICP, as well as other focal changes (see Increased Intracranial Pressure later in this chapter).

Diagnosis

The diagnostic tests and examinations commonly used to determine the extent of head injury include a radiograph of the skull, a computed tomography (CT) scan, magnetic resonance imaging (MRI) with contrast, positron emission tomography, evoked potentials, and electroencephalography (Figures 23-5 and 23-6) (see Table 22-6).

? Think Critically

Why should every patient who has sustained a head injury be monitored closely for 24 to 48 hours?

Treatment

The patient with a head injury usually is treated conservatively, at first. If the injury causes an increase in ICP or is a compound fracture of the skull, surgical debridement of the wound and removal of splintered bone from the brain tissues or elevation of the skull fragment is performed. All measures to keep ICP from rising are instituted for serious head injuries.

A patent airway must be secured, and the head raised 20 to 30 degrees with the body in correct alignment. Elevation helps reduce ICP. Neurologic signs are monitored closely. An intravenous (IV) line is inserted for access for diuretic drugs, if needed, and for administration of fluid. Intravenous fluids are infused very slowly to prevent fluid overload that would increase the ICP. Diuretics are used to decrease vascular volume and keep ICP as low as possible.

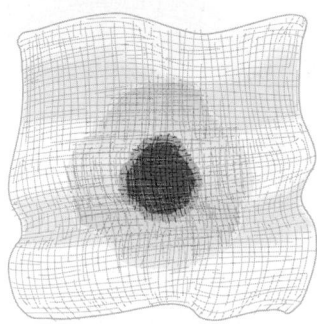

FIGURE 23-4 Assessing for the halo sign on fluid from the nose or ear after a head injury. The blood will draw together in the middle of the gauze pad, leaving a yellow ring (halo) around the blood, indicating the presence of cerebrospinal fluid.

FIGURE 23-5 MRI midline sagittal view of the brain.

FIGURE 23-6 Electroencephalogram (EEG).

? Think Critically

Why would a nurse check for a patent airway before performing a neurologic assessment on a patient with a head injury?

Surgical Intervention. Subdural hematoma is removed surgically either via burr holes or by craniotomy incision. The hematoma is evacuated by suction or surgical instruments. Epidural hematoma necessitates immediate, emergency craniotomy to prevent death from increased ICP. The craniotomy procedure is described in Chapter 24 along with surgeries of the brain.

Preoperative Period. The patient with a hematoma is quickly prepared for surgery. The operative site is shaved after the patient is under anesthesia. For planned surgery, a shampoo may be ordered the evening before surgery. Preoperative preparation is the same as for other surgeries. Any scalp lesions or other unusual conditions that are noted at this time should be reported. Usually the entire head is not shaved, only the operative area, and—if the patient has long hair—any hair that is cut off may be saved to be used as a hairpiece until the patient's hair grows back.

Postoperative Period. During the immediate postoperative period, the patient who underwent a craniotomy is in the intensive care unit for continuous monitoring. Essentially, care will be the same as that for any patient in danger of increasing ICP. Additional postoperative care of the patient who has undergone intracranial surgery includes:

- Positioning the patient according to written orders from the attending surgeon. **Make no exceptions.** Positioning is important to prevent added increases in ICP.
- Keeping the neck in midline and preventing excessive hip flexion to promote venous drainage from the head and keep ICP from rising (American Association of Neuroscience Nurses, 2007).
- Using nasal suctioning *only* if there is a written order allowing this as there may be a fracture that allows a pathway to the brain tissue.
- Watching carefully for signs of leakage of CSF from the nose, ear, and operative site, and report evidence of leakage immediately. Use aseptic technique in applying dressings to catch the drainage and prevent microorganisms from entering.
- Providing a quiet, nonstimulating environment.
- Administering only those treatments, comfort measures, and medications for which there are specific written orders.
- Reporting promptly any changes in the neurologic status of the patient.

Nursing Management

If it has been determined that there is indeed leakage of spinal fluid through the nose, ear, or an open head wound, special precautions must be taken to prevent infection and the physician must be notified. These precautions include the following:

- Keep the patient on absolute bed rest with the head of the bed elevated 20 to 30 degrees to promote venous drainage from the head.
- Cover a draining ear with a sterile gauze pad, changing the pad periodically to look for drainage.
- Instruct the patient *not* to blow his nose or pick at it; blowing may increase ICP, and picking may allow entry of microorganisms.
- Do not plug the nose or ear if there is drainage of CSF, as blockage may increase ICP.
- Remind the patient that he is not to change his position *in any way* unless he has been told it is all right to do so, in order to prevent ICP from rising.

Continued neurologic assessments are an integral part of care. Specific nursing diagnoses are listed in Nursing Care Plan 23-1. Specific instruction is required for the observation of a patient treated in an emergency department for head injury and released to go home. The long-term outcome for patients who have suffered a severe head injury is unpredictable. Recovery is a long process, and improvement may occur over many months for some patients. Disabilities may be lifelong.

Nursing Care Plan 23-1   Care of the Patient with a Head Injury and Increased Intracranial Pressure

Scenario
An 18-year-old boy who suffered a head injury in an automobile accident is groggy, but arousable.

Problem/Nursing Diagnosis
Blow to skull/Ineffective cerebral tissue perfusion related to increased intracranial pressure from head injury.

Supporting Assessment Data
Subjective: Hit right side of head on dashboard.
Objective: Nondepressed skull fracture, alteration in LOC, confused as to where he is, what day it is; somewhat combative.

Goals/Expected Outcomes	Nursing Interventions	Selected Rationale	Evaluation
Patient will not display further increase in ICP.	Monitor neurologic status q 1 hr using Glasgow Coma Scale (GCS); notify physician of any pupil changes or signs of increasing ICP, such as widening pulse pressure, change in respiratory pattern, slowing of pulse, increase in temperature, or decrease in LOC.	GCS provides good estimate of neurologic status.	GCS maintaining at 12.
	Monitor for seizure activity; institute seizure precautions. Administer ordered anticonvulsant.	Increased pressure on brain tissue may cause cellular irritability and seizure activity.	No sign of seizure activity. Precautions in place; padded tongue blade at bedside.
	Keep head of bed (HOB) at 30 degrees and body in correct alignment; turn side to side q 2 hr if condition warrants.	Keeping head slightly elevated and in proper alignment helps promote venous drainage from the head.	HOB at 30 degrees; positioned in correct alignment with neck midline. Turned q 2 hr.
	Maintain IV infusion at 50 mL/hr.	Decreasing IV rate helps prevent increased ICP and maintains IV access.	IV infusion at 50 mL/hr; patent without redness or swelling at site.
	Administer diuretic as ordered.	Diuretic decreases vascular volume and intracranial volume, lowering ICP.	Mannitol administered.
	Keep room calm and softly lit; do not disturb more than necessary; talk to patient while giving care; allow rest periods between any invasive procedures; monitor intake and output; reorient patient frequently.	Invasive procedures raise ICP.	Room is tidy and softly lit; care procedures grouped at intervals allowing rest; I > 400 mL, O > 375 mL.

Problem/Nursing Diagnosis
Unable to bathe and dress self/Self-care deficit related to confusion, grogginess, and increased ICP.

Supporting Assessment Data
Objective: Falls asleep during attempts at bath, etc.; confused about how to use ordinary objects such as toothbrush.

Goals/Expected Outcomes	Nursing Interventions	Selected Rationale	Evaluation
Patient will have adequate assistance with hygiene and dressing.	Provide assistance with all ADLs.		Assisted with morning care.
	Inspect skin when turning; place foam pad on bed.	Pressure-relieving device helps prevent pressure ulcer formation.	No signs of reddened areas on skin. Foam pad on bed.
Patient will resume self-care by discharge.	Encourage self-care as LOC improves.		Continue plan. Not ready for self-care yet.

ADLs, activities of daily living; *I,* input; *ICP,* intracranial pressure; *IV,* intravenous; *LOC,* level of consciousness; *O,* output.

Problem/Nursing Diagnosis
*Mother is very anxious/*Disabled family coping related to patient's decreased LOC and hospitalization.

Supporting Assessment Data
Subjective: Mother states she is afraid son is going to die.
Objective: Mother keeps trying to rouse the patient when she is in the room.

Goals/Expected Outcomes	Nursing Interventions	Selected Rationale	Evaluation
Mother's anxiety will decrease as she gains information about her son's condition and prognosis.	Explain to family that confusion and grogginess are usual after head injury.	Knowledge decreases fear of the unknown.	Explained patient's condition to family and measures to keep ICP down. Mother seems less anxious. Discussed need for calm and positive talk in room. Continue plan.
	Explain that the danger is if the ICP keeps increasing; tell what measures are being done to minimize increasing ICP; explain all procedures; explain that calm, rest, and positive talk in the room will help.	Knowing the treatment plan decreases anxiety.	
	Call hospital chaplain or own minister if family desires.	Presence of spiritual advisor can decrease anxiety.	
	Keep family informed of changes in patient's condition.		

Critical Thinking Questions
1. Why would it be contraindicated for this patient to strain to have a bowel movement?
2. Why is it important to decrease stimuli and provide a calm, soothing environment for this patient? (Be specific.)

Patient Teaching

Instructions for Care of a Patient with a Head Injury

Teach the family or significant other to do the following:
- For the first 24 hours, awaken the person every 2 to 3 hours to be certain he can be easily aroused.
- Question the person about where he is, who you are, what happened, and so on, to check orientation.
- Check the pupils to see that they are equal in size and that they will constrict; use a flashlight.
- Patient should avoid strenuous activity for 48 hours.
- Apply an ice bag to areas of swelling for 20 minutes out of an hour while awake—continue for 24 hours.
- For 48 hours, watch for and report the following signs:
  - Change in level of consciousness (e.g., becoming more groggy, difficult to awaken, confused)
  - Projectile vomiting (vomit travels a distance) without nausea
  - Unusual dizziness, sleepiness, loss of balance, or fall
  - Change in vision (i.e., seeing double, blurred vision)
  - Jerking movements of the eyes
  - Increasing headache that is worse when moving
  - Any twitching that cannot be controlled (seizures)
  - A change in speech or ability to find words or converse
  - Behavior that is odd for the individual

Legal and Ethical Considerations

Documenting Patient Teaching

Because there are legal ramifications of inadequate patient/family teaching, document all teaching in the medical record and send home clearly written instructions. It is best to have the patient or family sign a form for the record that indicates that teaching and written instructions have been received.

Think Critically

Why is the patient with a head injury positioned with the head of the bed elevated 20 to 30 degrees with the head and neck in proper alignment?

INCREASED INTRACRANIAL PRESSURE

Etiology and Pathophysiology

Because the skull is a closed bony structure in the adult, it is unable to expand. **Any lesion or fluid accumulation that begins to take up space within the cranial cavity causes an increase in the pressure within the cavity.** Therefore any swelling of the brain tissue from injury or surgery, leakage of blood from ruptured cerebral vessels, excessive production of CSF, or tumors, abscesses, or any other space-occupying lesion within the skull presents an increased ICP risk. Pressure against cerebral veins and arteries interferes with the flow of blood, producing a local ischemia and hypoxia. Pressure against the cells themselves can interfere with their vital functions. If the ICP rises very high and remains high for very long, death can result from inadequate cerebral perfusion or cerebral herniation. Brainstem injuries or pressure on the brainstem from increased ICP cause respiratory depression from pressure on the medulla oblongata—carbon dioxide accumulates, causing vasodilation and further increases in ICP. *Normal ICP is 0 to 15 mm Hg.* Concept Map 23-1 shows the relationship between the causes and the pathologic occurrences of increased ICP.

Signs, Symptoms, and Diagnosis

When the body can no longer compensate for the increase in volume in the cranial vault, decompensation begins and clinical signs of increasing ICP become apparent. **The earliest sign of increasing ICP is lethargy and decreasing consciousness, accompanied by a slowing of speech and delay in response to verbal cues.** Papilledema (swelling of the optic disc) viewed with an ophthalmoscope is a classic sign of increased ICP.

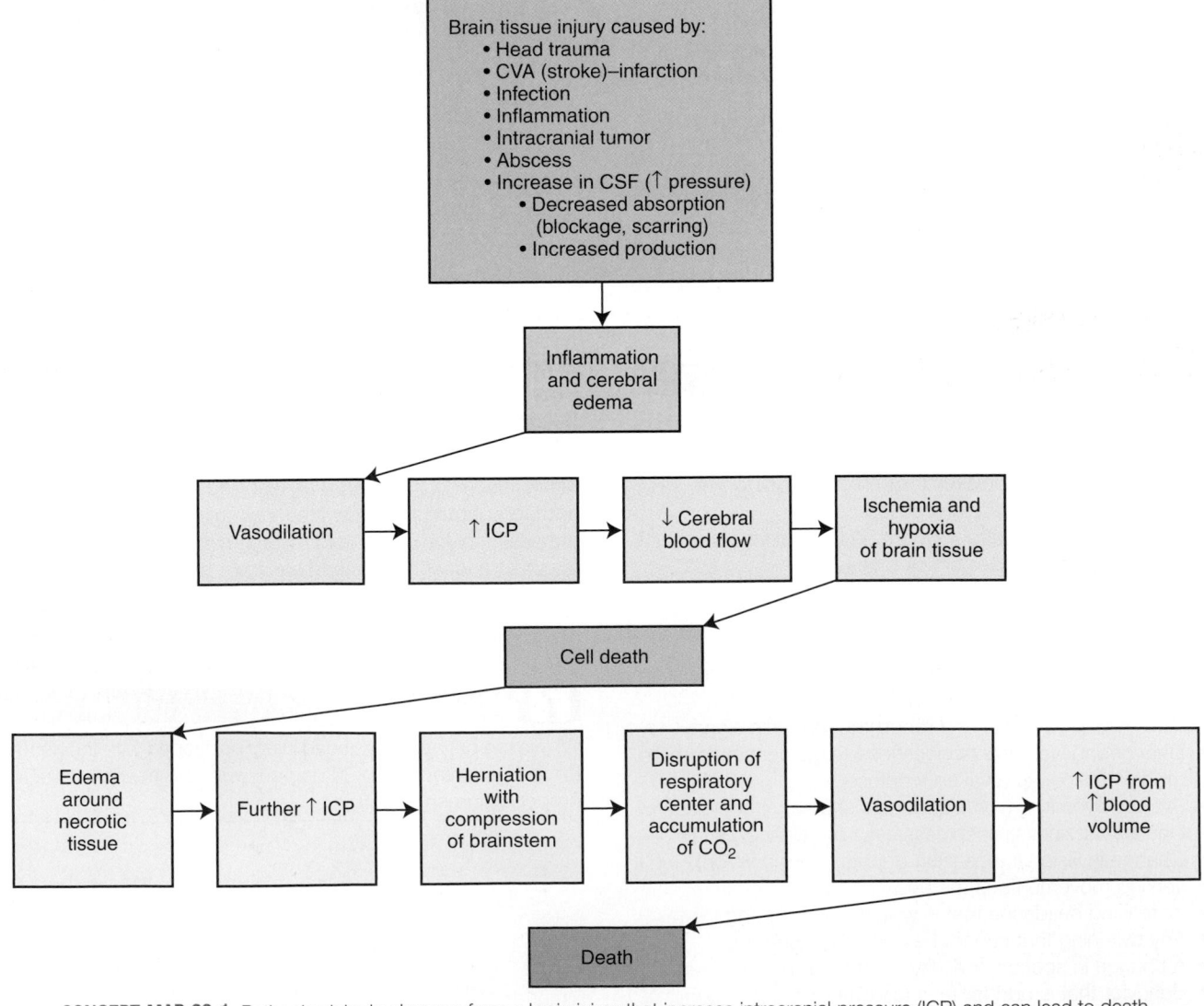

CONCEPT MAP 23-1 Pathophysiologic changes from a brain injury that increase intracranial pressure (ICP) and can lead to death.

When ICP rises, it affects the oxygenated blood perfusion of the brain and tissue hypoxia occurs. Nerve cells are particularly sensitive to hypoxia and cannot be replaced once they have been destroyed. Extended periods of hypoxia cause brain cell death. The body tries to compensate for hypoxia by raising blood pressure, to force more oxygenated blood through the brain tissue. If ICP continues to rise, the brain tissue will herniate through the tentorial notch at the midline of the foramen magnum. This herniation results in pressure on the vital structures of the midbrain, pons, and medulla, and causes changes in the vital signs and pupil reactions characteristic of increased ICP.

As brain tissue swells or fluid volume increases in the cranium, pressure is placed on the optic nerve. Pupils begin to react slowly; pupil size becomes unequal, progressing to dilation, and then the pupil size becomes fixed as reflexes disappear.

Clinical Cues

Abnormal pupillary responses can reverse to normal if the cause of increased ICP can be resolved in time.

The classic signs of increased ICP, with the first three called *Cushing's triad*, are:
- Rising systolic blood pressure
- Widening pulse pressure
- Bradycardia with a full, bounding pulse
- Rapid or irregular respirations (Figure 23-7)

These signs tend to be late, as are pupil changes, and signal a severe emergency and the need for immediate action to try to prevent the patient's death.

Think Critically

Why does increasing intracranial edema cause a double threat to the brain?

Treatment

The patient with greatly increased ICP is usually placed in an intensive care unit. Increased ICP is treated with supportive care to keep the pressure from rising further and with interventions to decrease the cranial blood or CSF volume. Osmotic diuretics (mannitol, glycerol, urea) are administered to remove fluid from the body, thereby reducing fluid in the brain. Dosage is determined by body weight, and electrolytes are monitored every 6 hours, as mannitol and diuretic action can cause electrolyte imbalances. Furosemide (Lasix) is sometimes also given. An indwelling urinary catheter is inserted to monitor output. Electrolytes and fluid balance are watched closely.

Dexamethasone (Decadron) may be given to decrease the inflammation and cerebral edema if the ICP is caused by a brain tumor or abscess (Garde, 2009). Histamine (H_2)-receptor blockers or proton pump

Pattern	Location of Lesion	Description
1. Cheyne-Stokes	Bilateral hemispheric disease or metabolic brain dysfunction	Cycles of hyperventilation and apnea
2. Central neurogenic hyperventilation	Brainstem between lower midbrain and upper pons	Sustained, regular rapid and deep breathing
3. Apneustic breathing	Mid or lower pons	Prolonged inspiratory phase or pauses alternating with expiratory pauses
4. Cluster breathing	Medulla or lower pons	Clusters of breaths follow each other with irregular pauses between
5. Ataxic breathing	Reticular formation of the medulla	Completely irregular with some breaths deep and some shallow. Random, irregular pauses, slow rate

FIGURE 23-7 Common abnormal respiratory patterns associated with coma.

inhibitors are given to protect the gastric mucosa. With the head of the bed at 20 to 30 degrees, the head and neck must be kept positioned midline so that venous drainage into the body is not restricted. Hip flexion should be less than 90 degrees. Rolled washcloths, towels, or trochanter rolls can be used for positioning.

If ICP is dangerously high as indicated by a Glasgow Coma Scale score of 9 or less and an abnormal CT scan, the surgeon may insert an intraventricular catheter into the lateral ventricle, through which CSF can be drained in small amounts to relieve the pressure. A probe can also be positioned in the epidural area, to monitor the pressure. Cerebral perfusion pressure (CPP) must be maintained at 50 to 70 mm Hg to ensure oxygenation of the brain tissue (CPP = mean arterial pressure − intracranial pressure) (National Guideline Clearing House, 2009). Normal CPP is 70 to 100 mm Hg. A monitoring device connected to the inserted probe may be used to measure cerebral blood flow. There are some new devices used to monitor cerebral oxygenation and blood flow.

If the patient is on a ventilator and is extremely agitated, pancuronium bromide (Pavulon) to paralyze skeletal muscles, in combination with sedation, may be used to prevent further increases in ICP. Because carbon dioxide is a vasodilator and can increase blood volume within the cranial cavity, hyperventilation is sometimes used short term to combat the increased ICP. This is accomplished by increasing the rate of controlled respiration. A CO_2 level between 25 and 30 mm Hg will improve oxygenation to the brain by causing vasoconstriction. Box 23-2 provides general guidelines for the care of patients with increased ICP.

Barbiturates are sometimes used along with continuous brain wave monitoring when patients do not respond to the more common therapies for reduction of ICP. Their purpose is to induce heavy sedation and slow metabolism, thereby decreasing ICP. In general, the short-acting barbiturates are used (e.g., pentobarbital [Nembutal] and thiopental [Pentothal]). Phenytoin (Dilantin) may be used to prevent seizures for the first 7 days after injury.

Temperature control is achieved by placing the patient on a hypothermia blanket for cooling if increased ICP has affected temperature regulation by pressure on the hypothalamus and the patient is feverish. Fever increases cerebral metabolism and cerebral edema.

Warmed blankets and tepid baths can be used to raise the temperature of the hypothermic patient and prevent shivering. Deep vein thrombosis prophylaxis is started early. Intravenous insulin may be titrated if the blood glucose rises above 110 mg/dL.

Complications

Damage to brain cells from injury and during periods of increased ICP may cause residual scarring and seizures. Hydrocephalus (excessive accumulation of CSF) may occur (see Chapter 24), causing motor deficits, cranial nerve deficits, or decreased cognitive ability. Rehabilitation efforts are focused on eliminating or decreasing deficits and promoting as much cognitive and physical function as possible (see Chapter 9).

Diabetes Insipidus. Diabetes insipidus may occur from injury or edema of the pituitary gland. Antidiuretic hormone is released in inadequate amounts, resulting in polyuria, and the awake patient may complain of *polydipsia* (excessive thirst). Intravenous vasopressin and fluid replacement are the preferred treatments. Carefully monitor intake and output and electrolyte balance.

❖ NURSING MANAGEMENT

▪ Assessment (Data Collection)

Early recognition of increasing pressure is extremely important. Careful neurologic assessment with monitoring of the patient's LOC, pupillary reactions, level of neuromuscular activity, and vital signs is essential to accurately evaluate the patient's progress. "Neuro checks" are performed every 15 minutes to every 2 hours for the acute patient (see Chapter 22). The following indications that ICP may be rising should be reported immediately:

- Extreme restlessness or excitability following a period of apparent calm
- Deepening stupor and decreasing LOC
- Headache that is unrelenting and increasing in intensity
- Vomiting, especially persistent, projectile vomiting
- Unequal size of pupils and other abnormal pupillary reactions
- Leakage of CSF from the nose or ear
- Changes in the patient's blood pressure, pulse, or respiration; widening pulse pressure; a slow, bounding pulse

---

Box 23-2 Guidelines for Patients with Increased Intracranial Pressure (ICP)

DO
- Conduct neurologic checks at least once every hour unless more frequent monitoring is indicated.
- Report changes immediately.
- Maintain a patent airway and adequate ventilation to ensure proper oxygen and carbon dioxide exchange.
- Elevate the head of the bed 20 to 30 degrees to facilitate return of blood from the cerebral veins.
- Use measures to maintain normal body temperature. Elevations of temperature raise blood pressure and cerebral blood flow. Shivering also can increase ICP.
- Monitor intake and output. Restrict or encourage fluids according to physician's order.
- Give passive range-of-motion exercises.
- Space activities apart.

DO NOT
- Allow patient to become constipated or perform Valsalva maneuver.
- Hyperextend, flex, or rotate the patient's head.
- Flex the patient's hips (as in female catheterization).
- Place patient in Trendelenburg's position for any reason.
- Allow patient to perform isometric exercises.

❓ Think Critically

Why do you think an elderly person is at greater risk when a head injury or other cause of increased ICP occurs?

▪ Nursing Diagnosis, Planning, and Implementation

The appropriate nursing diagnosis is Ineffective cerebral tissue perfusion related to effects of increasing intracranial pressure. Goals of nursing care are to:

- Maintain cerebral perfusion
- Reduce ICP
- Maintain adequate respiration
- Protect from injury
- Maintain normal body functions
- Prevent complications

The expected outcome would be Patient will not experience brain damage from increased intracranial pressure.

Maintaining an open airway and adequate respiration may require suctioning and possibly intubation with mechanical ventilation. (If the patient has sustained a head injury, x-rays to rule out a basilar fracture are necessary before suctioning the nonintubated patient to prevent the possibility of the suction catheter entering the cranial vault.) The patient whose consciousness level is decreased and whose gag and swallowing reflexes are impaired is in danger of aspirating blood, vomitus, mucus, and other material into the air passages.

Position the patient on his side and ask him to exhale as you turn him to prevent a Valsalva maneuver, which could raise ICP. Instruct the patient not to grip the side rails or push with his feet or elbows against the mattress during repositioning for the same reason. Plan uninterrupted rest periods between activities that cause an increase in ICP; preferably, plan rest for 1 hour at a time. Provide a soothing environment free of noxious odors and noise. Keep the room temperature adjusted to normalize the patient's temperature and to prevent shivering (American Association of Neuroscience Nurses, 2007).

Nutrition supplied early improves outcomes after brain injury and increased ICP, as nutrition promotes healing (Hartl et al., 2008). If the patient is unable to take food orally, supplementation is begun within 3 days after injury. Full nutritional supplementation should be in place by day 7. Nutrition is planned according to determined metabolic needs and the fluid and electrolyte status. Metabolic needs are calculated based on age, weight, and height.

Unless the patient has a tracheostomy or an oral airway in place, he should be positioned on his side—not on his back—as the tongue may occlude the airway, and mucus cannot drain naturally. **The unconscious patient requires care for all basic needs.** See Table 22-9 and pp. 490 to 491.

▪ Evaluation

Data are gathered regarding the success of the nursing interventions. If the interventions are not helping the patient meet the expected outcomes, the interventions should be changed.

⦿ INJURIES OF THE SPINE AND SPINAL CORD

Etiology

A person may suffer from injury to the spinal cord in a number of ways. Injury in the cervical and lumbar areas is more frequent because these segments are more mobile. Automobile accidents, gunshot wounds, diving accidents, and other forms of trauma often inflict severe damage to the spinal cord, but tumors, degenerative disease, and infections also can impair the functions of the spinal cord and its branches. Generally speaking, spinal cord injuries are classified according to their anatomic location—that is, cervical, thoracic, lumbar, or sacral (Figure 23-8). There are 12,000 spinal cord injuries per year in the United States (National Spinal Cord Injury Statistical Center, 2011). Whatever the cause of spinal cord injury, motor and sensory losses may occur. The amount of loss of function and sensation depends on the level and extent of injury to the spinal cord.

Pathophysiology

Fracture, dislocation, or subluxation (partial dislocation) of the vertebral column often results in spinal cord damage. Cord injury is caused by compression, pulling and twisting, or tearing of the cord, with four types of injuries occurring. Penetrating trauma from gunshot or knife wounds or other types of accidents may cause severance, compression, or contusion of the spinal cord. Extreme flexion or hyperextension of the neck, or falling on the buttocks (which causes flexion of the lower thoracic and lumbar spine), all may cause spinal cord damage (Figure 23-9). Tumor growth may compress or destroy spinal cord tissue. Whatever the cause of injury to the spinal cord, nerve transmission to the brain or from the brain may no longer occur below the level of the damage, resulting in paralysis.

Microscopic bleeding occurs in the gray matter immediately after spinal cord injury. Irritation of the cells causes edema to develop and spread along the next one or two cord segments. The edema peaks in 2 to 3 days and subsides in about 7 days after injury. The edema causes temporary loss of function and sensation. Hemodynamic instability with drops in blood pressure may cause decreased blood flow, and hypoxia in the cord increases the initial damage. The inflammatory process may injure the myelin covering the axons, and the chemical and electrolyte changes interrupt nerve impulse transmission.

Signs, Symptoms, and Diagnosis

A complete severance of the spinal cord, or damage to the cord's entire thickness, results in a total loss of sensation and control in the parts of the body below the point of injury. If the cord is damaged in the cervical region, the paralysis and loss of sensory perception may include both arms and both legs (*tetraplegia*), also called quadriplegia. Severe injury to the cord above the level of the fifth cervical vertebra often is fatal if emergency care is not immediate, because the phrenic nerves that innervate the diaphragm originate in the third, fourth, and fifth cervical segments. Branches of these nerves play a major role in the control of respiration, and when they are severed, respiration must be maintained by artificial means. If the damage is only partial (incomplete) there will be some losses, but not all motor and sensory innervation is lost.

FIGURE 23-8 Divisions of the spinal column and designations of spinal nerves.

Interruption of the thoracic spinal cord through L1 and L2 causes *paraplegia* (paralysis of both legs). Table 23-1 presents activities possible at varying levels of cord injury.

Injury to the spinal cord that does not involve complete severance of the cord may result in a temporary paralysis, which may subside as the spinal cord recovers from the swelling and initial shock of the injury.

Diagnosis is by made by physical examination and testing of reflexes. CT scan or MRI may be performed to determine the extent of the damage and to see whether the cord is completely *transected* (severed). This helps determine if neurologic deficits are likely to be permanent. A myelogram may be performed when other tests do not reveal sufficient information.

Treatment

There are four main objectives in the treatment and nursing care of the patient with an injury of the spinal cord:

1. To save the victim's life
2. To prevent further injury to the cord by careful handling of the patient
3. To repair as much of the damage to the cord as possible
4. To establish a routine of care that will improve and maintain the patient's state of health and prevent complications, so that eventual physical, mental, and social rehabilitation is possible

As soon as an injury to the spinal cord occurs, the patient must be handled with extreme care.

COMPRESSION

Compression
fracture

Force

FIGURE 23-9 Accidents can cause vertical compression on the cervical or lumbar spine.

Safety Alert

Prevent Further Spinal Injury

Anyone with a head injury is treated as if he has also suffered a spine injury until proven otherwise. The neck must be stabilized to prevent any movement. When no cervical collar is available, use a shirt, towel, coat, or other material rolled and placed around the neck as a collar to keep the neck as straight as possible, preventing it from flexing or hyperextending. If the victim must be moved to safety, he should be rolled like a log, as one straight piece, onto a flat surface, such as a board of plywood or a door removed from its hinges. Roll the patient as one piece onto his side, the flat surface placed beside him, and then carefully roll him back onto the board. This is done slowly and carefully to avoid twisting or bending the spinal column. The victim is kept still.

Because a nurse or physician may not be at the scene of the accident to supervise the moving of the victim, laypersons should learn the proper emergency care of such injuries. When an accident victim complains of neck or back pain, or cannot move the legs or has no feeling in them, treat the victim as if he has a spinal cord injury. **To avoid flexion of the neck,** *no pillow or other kind of support is placed under the head. Do not move the victim unless life-threatening conditions require it.*

Table 23-1	Level of Spinal Cord Damage, Function Present, and Activities Possible	
LEVEL OF INJURY	**FUNCTION PRESENT/NEUROLOGIC DEFICIT**	**ACTIVITY POSSIBLE**
C1-C3	No respiratory function; usually fatal unless immediate emergency help is available to establish respiration Quadriplegia	Respirations stimulated with phrenic pacemaker. Can manipulate electric wheelchair with breath, chin, or voice control.
C4	Loss of diaphragm movement; breathe with assistance Quadriplegia	May live if assisted respiration is begun immediately. Can use a mouthstick to turn pages, type, or write.
C5	Partial shoulder movement; partial elbow movement	Can turn head. Able to feed self with special adaptive devices. Able to move wheelchair for short distances, moves well with electric wheelchair. Can assist a bit with self-care.
C6	Retains gross motor function of arms; partial shoulder, elbow, and wrist movement possible Paraplegia	Needs adaptive devices; may be able to propel wheelchair. Independent in feeding and with some grooming with adaptive devices. Can roll over in bed. Can drive a car with hand controls. Can assist in transfer. Can self-catheterize the bladder.
C7	Shoulder, elbow, wrist, hand partial movements possible Paraplegia	Manipulates wheelchair with arms; transfers to and from chair; may drive specially fitted car. Excellent bed mobility. Independent in most ADLs.
C8	Normal arm movement; hand weakness Paraplegia	Bed and wheelchair independent. Can perform most ADLs and may achieve vocational and recreational goals. Performs self-catheterization.
T1-T10	Normal arm movement and strength; loss of bowel, bladder, and sexual function	May achieve walking with braces. Able to perform ADLs and achieve vocational and recreational goals.
T11 and below	Loss of bowel, bladder, and sexual function	Wheelchair not essential. Able to perform ADLs, work, and recreational activities.

ADLs, activities of daily living.

Transfer of the patient to the hospital should be done only by trained emergency medical technicians. In the emergency department of the hospital, the patient's condition is stabilized and a thorough examination is conducted to establish the extent of his injuries. Methylprednisolone, a corticosteroid, may be given as soon as the examination and diagnosis of cord injury are made. If given within 8 hours of injury, it is thought to minimize further damage and improve the return of both motor function and sensation (Schreiber, 2009). Use of a corticosteroid is controversial due to recent research about the lack of evidence of benefit versus the many side effects of the drug.

FIGURE 23-10 Crutchfield tongs for cervical traction.

Clinical Cues

Drug metabolism is altered in spinal cord injury. Drug interactions are more frequent. Be vigilant in checking for signs and symptoms of drug interactions.

Normal saline is used for fluid replacement, and drugs such as dopamine (Intropin) may be given to sustain a sufficient blood pressure to prevent cord hypoxia. Pulmonary edema and increased ICP if a head injury is present are potential problems, and fluid balance is watched carefully.

Respiratory Management. Intubation and mechanical ventilation are often required to sustain life in patients with an injury at C5 or above. Patients with intact phrenic nerve innervation may receive a phrenic nerve stimulator that assists them to breathe by stimulating action of the diaphragm. Patients who can breathe when they first arrive at the hospital may be intubated because as cord edema progresses, respiration may become impaired. Mechanical ventilation relieves the muscle work of breathing and conserves the patient's energy during the emergent phase of the injury. An oral airway may be placed if a tracheostomy is unnecessary.

Immobilization and Surgery. Surgery on the spine with removal of bone fragments is performed to relieve pressure, provide stabilization, and prevent further injury. **Cervical spinal cord injury is usually treated with traction to immobilize the affected vertebrae and maintain alignment.** Traction can be accomplished by skeletal traction using Crutchfield or Gardner-Wells tongs with ropes, pulleys, and weights (Figure 23-10); or a halo ring and fixation pins (Figure 23-11). The halo is often used for cord injury not requiring surgery and allows for early ambulation.

Selecting the type of bed to be used for a patient with spinal cord injury depends on many factors. Some physicians and nurses prefer placing the patient in a special lateral rotation bed that is designed to prevent the problems of immobility while maintaining traction

FIGURE 23-11 Halo traction vest for cervical stabilization. Note the rigid shoulder straps and encompassing vest. Various vest sizes are available prefabricated. The halo ring superstructure and the vest are magnetic resonance imaging (MRI) compatible.

(Figure 23-12). If halo traction is used and the patient has an incomplete spinal cord injury, a standard orthopedic bed may be used. All measures to prevent the problems of immobility are instituted (see Chapter 9).

Urinary Management. An indwelling urinary catheter is inserted to prevent bladder distention and protect the skin from reflex bladder emptying. After the first week, a bladder management program will be initiated (see Chapter 22).

Psychological Care. The short-term and long-term psychological changes brought about by spinal cord injury and paralysis are difficult, if not impossible, to measure. Adjustment to such a drastic change in one's lifestyle is a continuous process that may well last a lifetime (see Chapter 9).

FIGURE 23-12 RotoRest Delta Advanced Kinetic Therapy system.

Grief and mourning response. Sustaining a spinal cord injury that causes permanent neurologic deficit brings with it many losses. Most patients experience grief and mourning of the losses experienced and the changes that such losses bring to their roles and lifestyle. Table 23-2 presents a review of the stages of grief

Table 23-2	Stages of Grief and Associated Behaviors
STAGE OF GRIEF OR MOURNING	**FREQUENT BEHAVIORS SEEN**
Shock and denial	Complete dependence, withdrawal, excessive sleep, struggle for survival, unrealistic expectations.
Anger	Hostility toward caregivers and family, manipulative behavior, abusive language, refusal to discuss paralysis and losses, decreased self-esteem.
Bargaining	Bargaining with a higher power or fate: "If you'll let me walk again, I'll pray every day."
Depression	Sadness, "blue" mood, withdrawal, insomnia, agitation, refusal to participate in education for self-care, suicidal thoughts and comments.
Adjustment	Begins active participation in therapy and education for self-care, planning for future, expresses hope for future functioning, finds meaning in whole experience of injury and therapy, return of usual personality.

and the behaviors that might be seen. In caring for these patients, use active listening, be supportive, and help the patient to focus on positive strengths and the possibilities for the future.

Sexual Concerns. One area of concern to the patient and his family members that sometimes receives inadequate attention is that of sexual function and sexuality following spinal cord injury. Many individuals have difficulty discussing sexual matters. The nurse who wishes to help a patient deal with problems of sexuality must first come to terms with her own feelings and attitudes and clarify her own values. She should not be critical or judgmental in her discussions about the patient's sexuality. The patient and his partner must be encouraged to verbalize concerns and questions and should be given guidance about alternative ways to express sexuality and meet sexual needs.

Complications

Spinal Shock and Neurogenic Shock. The disruption in the nerve communication pathways between upper motor neurons and lower motor neurons may cause spinal shock. Spinal shock is characterized by flaccid paralysis and loss of reflex activity and of sensation below the level of the injury. Spinal shock occurs immediately after injury and lasts 48 hours to several weeks.

Neurogenic shock may occur within 24 hours and is caused by loss of vasomotor tone caused by the injury; neurogenic shock is characterized by bradycardia, hypotension, venous pooling with decreased cardiac output, and occasionally paralytic ileus. Vital signs become labile. Treatment is aimed at maintaining adequate blood pressure and heart rate. Neurogenic shock may occur with a cervical or high thoracic injury.

Muscle Spasms. Immediately after a spinal cord injury, the patient will usually have a flaccid type of paralysis. Later, as the cord adjusts to the injury, the paralysis will become spastic, and there will be strong, involuntary contractions of the skeletal muscles. These muscle spasms, which may be violent enough to throw the patient from the bed or wheelchair, must be anticipated, and the patient must be secured so that accidents can be avoided. If the upper extremities are involved, he is likely to tip over glasses, water pitchers, or anything within reach of his arms when seized with uncontrollable muscle spasms.

The patient and family may interpret these spasms as a return of voluntary function of the limbs and will have false hopes of complete recovery. The nurse or the physician must explain to them that these spasms are frequently seen in patients with spinal cord injuries. To avoid stimulating the muscles when moving the patient and thereby precipitating a spasm of the muscles, avoid grasping the muscle itself. The palms of the hands are used to support the joints above and below the affected muscles. The administration of antispasmodic medications such as baclofen (Lioresal) orally or intrathecally may decrease the severity of the spasms (Table 23-3).

Autonomic Dysreflexia (Hyperreflexia). Autonomic dysreflexia (AD) is an uninhibited and exaggerated reflex response of the autonomic nervous system to some form of stimulation and it occurs in 85% of all patients who have spinal cord injury at or above the level of the

Table 23-3 Medications Commonly Used for Patients with Head and Spinal Cord Injury

CLASSIFICATION	ACTION	NURSING IMPLICATIONS	PATIENT TEACHING
Corticosteroid			
Methylprednisolone (Solu-Medrol)	Decreases inflammation by suppression of leukocyte migration to injury site; decreases capillary permeability	Give as IV bolus. May cause insomnia, increased susceptibility to infection, and GI distress. May delay wound healing. Monitor electrolyte levels. H_2-receptor blocker or proton pump inhibitor often given concurrently to prevent stress ulcer.	Advise to report heartburn or stomach pain.
Skeletal Muscle Relaxant			
Baclofen (Lioresal)	Inhibits synaptic responses in CNS by decreasing GABA, thereby decreasing frequency and severity of muscle spasms	Monitor for seizure activity. Observe for muscle weakness and fatigue. Assess for allergic symptoms: rash, fever, respiratory distress.	Advise not to drink alcohol as it increases CNS depression. Do not discontinue medication quickly or abruptly.
Adrenergic Action Vasoconstrictor			
Dopamine (Intropin)	Acts on alpha receptors causing vasoconstriction in blood vessels, thereby raising blood pressure	Monitor vital signs closely; assess for chest pain. Monitor I&O. Place patient on a cardiac monitor during therapy. May cause nausea, vomiting, or diarrhea. Be certain that IV access is patent as drug will cause necrosis if extravasation into the tissue occurs.	Explain purpose of drug is to raise blood pressure so that brain has adequate perfusion and oxygen. May cause headache.
Osmotic Diuretic			
Mannitol	Increases osmotic pressure of glomerular filtrate; promotes diuresis	Monitor vital signs closely. Track I&O, assess skin turgor and mucous membranes for signs of dehydration. Monitor electrolytes. Observe for nausea, backache, hives, and chest pain.	Explain that the drug will cause increased urine output and that this is its intended action.
Neuromuscular Blocking (Paralyzing) Agent			
Pancuronium (Pavulon)	Inhibits transmission of nerve impulses, producing skeletal muscle relaxation for surgery, endotracheal intubation, and mechanical ventilation when patient is fighting the ventilator	Be certain that alarms are properly set on the ventilator. Observe patient frequently. Keep Ambu bag at bedside. Monitor electrolytes and I&O. Observe for urinary retention. Observe for allergic reaction: rash, fever, pruritus. Protect the eyes with artificial tears and keep lids closed.	Explain that patient will be paralyzed and unable to move. Assure patient that he will be monitored at all times and that there are backup measures in place in case of power outage when ventilator would not work.

CNS, central nervous system; *GABA,* gamma-aminobutyric acid; *GI,* gastrointestinal; *H_2,* histamine-2; *I&O,* intake and output; *IV,* intravenous.

sixth thoracic vertebra (T6). The AD response is potentially dangerous to the patient, because it can produce vasoconstriction of the arterioles with an immediate elevation of blood pressure. The sudden hypertension can, in turn, cause a seizure, retinal hemorrhage, or stroke. Less serious effects include severe headache, changes in pulse rate, sweating and flushing above the level of the spinal cord lesion, and pallor and "goose bumps" below the level of injury.

AD occurs most often with spinal cord disorders at or above the T6 level. The problem can occur any time after a spinal cord injury; in some cases it has first appeared as late as 6 years after the injury.

Many kinds of stimulation can precipitate AD. Most are related to the bladder, bowel, and skin of the patient. For example, catheter changes, a distended bladder, the insertion of rectal suppositories, enemas, and sudden changing of position can provide the stimulation which results in AD (National Spinal Cord Injury Association, 2009).

🔱 Clinical Cues

Careful attention must be paid to keeping the bladder from becoming overdistended. If the patient is on bed rest, check the catheter and drainage tubing for the indwelling catheter every couple of hours. When voiding has not occurred, monitor output and time of voiding for the patient who does not have an indwelling catheter, and palpate the bladder for distention every few hours.

Once the patient exhibits symptoms of AD, an emergency exists. Efforts should be made to lower blood pressure by placing the patient in a sitting position or elevating his head to a 45-degree angle. If the cause of the stimulation is known—for example, an impacted bowel, overdistended bladder, or pressure against the skin—the stimulus should be removed as gently and quickly as possible. The physician should be notified immediately so that the appropriate medications can be prescribed and administered. Patients who experience repeated attacks of AD may require surgery to sever the nerves responsible for the exaggerated response to stimulation (Agency for Healthcare Research and Quality, 2007).

Orthostatic Hypotension. Vasoconstriction is impaired after spinal cord injury, and the lack of muscle function in the legs causes pooling of blood in the lower extremities. Sudden change in position from supine to sitting or sitting to standing may cause dizziness and fainting. Compression stockings, moving slowly, and use of a reclining wheelchair may help prevent this problem.

Deep Venous Thrombosis. Decreased blood pressure combined with lack of muscle movement slows venous return to the heart. Thrombosis may occur.

Compression stockings, sequential compression devices, and/or heparin injections may be needed to prevent deep venous thrombosis.

Infection. Impaired respiratory muscles with decreased cough and shallow respirations predisposes the patient with a high spinal cord injury to respiratory infection. Mechanical ventilation with intubation provides an avenue for microorganisms to enter the lungs, and so mechanical ventilation is a risk factor for infection. Urinary catheterization for loss of bladder control is a risk factor for infection as well.

Skin Breakdown. Lack of sensation and inability to move for repositioning places the patient at great risk for skin breakdown and pressure ulcers. Pressure-relieving devices, meticulous skin care with regular inspection, and manual repositioning are essential to prevent this problem.

Renal Complications. Urinary reflux from the bladder to the kidney often occurs due to impaired bladder function. Catheterization and immobility predispose to bladder infection; the infection may travel up the ureters to the kidneys. Permanent kidney damage may eventually occur from such infections.

❓ Think Critically

Can you name three care interventions that might trigger an episode of AD? How could you possibly avoid causing this reaction?

Heterotopic Ossification. Heterotopic ossification may occur with long-term immobility. *Heterotopic ossification* is bony overgrowth that may invade muscle. Assess for swelling, warmth, redness, and decreased range of motion of the extremities to detect ossification.

❖ NURSING MANAGEMENT

There often is a tendency to treat a physically disabled patient as if he were less than a "whole" person with the same desires, hopes, and anxieties that all humans share. The nurse can serve patients by reacting to and interacting with physically disabled patients in an open and honest manner. If unprepared to handle a certain problem, readily admit embarrassment, confusion, or lack of information, and seek assistance from other members of the health care team. Rehabilitation of patients with spinal cord injuries is discussed in detail in Chapter 9.

■ Assessment (Data Collection)

Continued assessment for signs of decreased oxygenation, blood pressure instability, infection, skin breakdown, gastrointestinal or nutrition problems, and urinary problems is essential. Perform a daily review of systems and collection of data regarding physical status. Assess the tracheostomy tube, traction devices and pins, correct placement and use of sequential compression devices or compression stockings, indwelling catheter, IV cannula, feeding tube, and the like each shift.

■ Nursing Diagnosis

Nursing diagnoses appropriate for the patient with a spinal cord injury may include:

- Impaired gas exchange related to diaphragm paralysis, diaphragm fatigue, or retained secretions
- Impaired physical mobility related to vertebral column instability, disruption of the spinal cord, and traction
- Decreased cardiac output related to hypotension and decreased muscle action causing venous pooling
- Imbalanced nutrition: less than body requirements related to increased metabolic demand from healing injuries, slowed gastrointestinal motility, and inability to feed self
- Constipation related to lack of bowel enervation, decreased fluid intake, and immobility
- Impaired urinary elimination related to decreased innervation of the bladder
- Constipation related to loss of nerve stimulation to the bowel and due to immobility
- Pain related to muscle spasms
- Risk for autonomic dysreflexia related to reflex stimulation of sympathetic nervous system
- Risk for impaired skin integrity related to immobility and loss of sensation
- Risk for ineffective coping related to loss of control over bodily functions and altered lifestyle secondary to paralysis
- Disturbed body image related to paralysis and loss of control over bodily functions
- Interrupted family processes related to change in role within the family because of neurologic deficits
- Grieving related to neurologic deficits and to changes in roles and lifestyle

■ Planning, Implementation, and Evaluation

Specific, individual expected outcomes are written for each nursing diagnosis supported by data gathered. Long-term goals are considered, and planning for rehabilitation begins with hospitalization. The patient will often be transferred to a rehabilitation facility for intensive rehabilitation and retraining for activities of daily living.

Care for the patient with a spinal cord injury can be very complex, depending on the level of the injury. Often a head injury accompanies the trauma to the spinal cord. When a stabilization device is in place on the head, assessment and care of the pin sites are

performed every shift initially and then twice a day. Sterile technique is used and is performed according to agency policy. Solutions such as sterile normal saline are used for cleansing and an antibiotic ointment is applied. Weights used for cervical traction must be kept hanging freely to be effective. Traction pull should never be interrupted. Tongs may stay in place for 4 weeks. If the patient is wearing a halo fixation device, skin care must be given frequently and the skin checked to see that the jacket or cast is not causing pressure ulcers. One finger should be able to slip easily beneath the cast or jacket to be sure it is not too tight. The patient is never moved or turned by holding or pulling on the halo device. **The halo jacket is never unfastened unless the patient is supine because head movement will immediately occur.** "Log rolling" must be done with extreme care to avoid twisting the vertebral column and further damaging the spinal cord (Figure 23-13).

Assignment Considerations

Inappropriate Delegation

Although many tasks may be delegated to the certified nursing assistant (CNA) or unlicensed assistive personnel (UAP), moving or positioning the patient with neurologic injury or surgery should *not* be delegated. If given proper, complete instructions, the CNA or UAP may help log roll the patient with the nurse's help and supervision.

All the nursing measures designed to prevent the disabilities that may result from immobility, to promote healing, and to avoid complications are used to help the patient achieve the goals of rehabilitation. Bladder and bowel training programs, as well as instruction in moving from bed to chair—and other aspects of self-care—may be necessary. Realistic goals should be set for the patient, and every effort made to achieve them.

FIGURE 23-13 Log-rolling procedure using a lift sheet and three people.

Encourage the patient to do whatever he can for himself as soon as is feasible. The overall goal is to promote as much independence as possible. A great deal of encouragement and praise are required. Evaluation is ongoing to see if the interventions have been successful in achieving the expected outcomes. If they have not been successful, the plan is rewritten.

Rehabilitation

A full team of professionals will be involved in the care and rehabilitation of the patient with a spinal cord injury. The physical therapist, occupational therapist, psychologist, physician, respiratory therapist, pharmacist, and ancillary personnel will collaboratively plan the patient's care. The patient and family are often invited to participate in the planning process.

The use of robotics and computers is providing hope for some patients to walk again (Rehabilitation Institute of Chicago, 2009). A system called functional electrical stimulation (FES) is used to generate neural activity and overcome lost function. The system stimulates muscles to make walking motions. The patient is suspended in a harness to support body weight and is retrained to walk using a treadmill. The antidepressant escitalopram, a selective serotonin reuptake inhibitor (SSRI), has improved results of the therapy for some patients. Research is underway on a neuroprosthetic microchip implant that would help certain patients to walk again. The ReWalk brace support suit that is combined with computerized technology is in clinical trials in Israel (Neiman, 2008). It allows an otherwise healthy paraplegic to walk using Canadian crutches. It runs on a power pack carried on the back. A pacemaker for the bladder is under study for the treatment of urinary incontinence.

Communication between team members is crucial to the success of the individual plan. When the patient is discharged, all plans and specifics required for the patient's care must be shared with home caregivers and home care nurses who will be involved in his care. His primary physician must be fully briefed.

BACK PAIN AND RUPTURED INTERVERTEBRAL DISK ("SLIPPED DISK")

Etiology

Back pain occurrence is surpassed only by headaches. Emergency physicians treat more than 6 million cases of back pain annually. In people under age 45, back pain is the most common cause of work absence and is the most costly health condition for employers. Carelessness and incorrect methods of lifting contribute to a large percentage of back problems. On-the-job accidents and resultant trauma to the spine are another cause. Obesity and lack of exercise, and poor lifting and moving techniques, contribute to the stress placed on the back muscles and to the occurrence of injury or the severity and duration of pain. Exercise promotes

good muscle tone. Other risk factors leading to back pain include lack of exercise (causing poor muscle tone), poor posture, cigarette smoking (which decreases oxygenation to the disks and predisposes to degenerative disease), and stress. Repetitive heavy lifting also may cause back pain. This is often a factor for health care workers. Causes of musculoskeletal back pain include:

- Acute lumbosacral strain
- Instability of lumbosacral spine
- Osteoarthritis of the spine
- Intervertebral disk degeneration and spinal stenosis
- Herniation of the intervertebral disk

Preventing back pain and disorders begins with proper posture and the use of correct lifting techniques. Maintaining one's weight within normal limits also helps decrease back strain. Sufficient physical exercise that maintains the condition of the back muscles and specific exercises to strengthen the abdominal and back muscles can greatly decrease the repeated incidence of injuries that lead to back pain.

Pathophysiology

The bodies of the spinal vertebrae lie flat on one another like a stack of coins. Between the vertebral bodies there is a disk of fibrous cartilage filled with gelatinous substance (in the nucleus) that acts as a cushion to absorb shocks to the spinal column. This gelatinous disk may be ruptured by an injury, such as by the strain caused when lifting a heavy object or by wrenching the spinal column or by falling on the back. When the disk ruptures, part of the contents squeeze out from between the vertebrae and disk fragments may lodge in the spinal canal. The disk compression on the adjacent nerve root causes the pain (Figure 23-14). When protein from the disk content leaks out into the canal, the body perceives it as a foreign substance, causing an

Herniated nucleus pulposus

FIGURE 23-14 Herniated disk (nucleus pulposus) with compression of spinal cord.

inflammatory response, with pain. Thus the person suffers from what is sometimes called a "slipped disk." Another name for this condition is *herniated nucleus pulposus.*

 Elder Care Points

The older person has decreased flexibility of the spine and, as age increases, degeneration of the spine. Many elderly individuals suffer from osteoporosis and osteoarthritis. These factors make the elderly person more prone to back pain, especially if regular exercise is not performed to maintain flexibility and bone density.

Acute back pain usually occurs from activity that puts stress (hyperflexion) on the tissues of the lower back. Back pain that is a result of muscle spasm is usually self-limiting and often resolves within 4 weeks. Chronic back pain is pain that lasts for more than 3 months or is a repeat episode. Chronic back pain may be due to degenerative disk disease or osteoarthritis, but lack of exercise, prior injury, and obesity are frequent factors. The most common sites of disk rupture are L4-L5 and L5-S1. Herniation may also occur at C5-C6 or C6-C7.

Signs, Symptoms, and Diagnosis

Sometimes a lumbar herniated disk causes pain radiating down the sciatic nerve into the buttock and below the knee. Muscle weakness and paresthesias may occur. Cervical herniated disk causes pain in the neck and shoulder, radiating down the arm with numbness and tingling in the hand. Muscle tightening and spasm in the area of injury are common.

Diagnosis requires a history and physical examination. The straight-leg-raising test is often used for low back pain. While supine, the leg is raised off the bed or examination table with the whole leg straight. If back pain occurs, the test confirms a disk problem (presence of pain in the low back). Reflexes may be decreased or absent. The patient may experience muscle weakness or paresthesias in the legs or feet.

If conservative therapy does not relieve the pain, diagnostic radiographs, MRI, or CT scanning is performed. An electromyogram may be ordered to determine the degree of nerve irritation and to rule out other pathologic conditions.

Treatment

The physician will treat back pain initially with conservative measures in the hope that surgical correction will not be necessary. If there is no sciatic pain, bed rest is not recommended as research has shown that walking provides a quicker recovery. When sciatic pain is present, bed rest for 2 to 3 days is helpful (Miller, 2010). Ice packs are applied for 5 to 10 minutes at a time each hour for the first 48 hours to reduce muscle spasm in the back. After 48 hours, heat may

be more helpful, as heat relaxes strained muscles. Ultrasound treatments are often helpful. Heating pads, hot packs, and hot showers work well to relax the muscles.

 Complementary and Alternative Therapies

Help for Pain

Acupuncture, acupressure, and massage therapy have all proven beneficial for back pain. Research from the National Institutes of Health has proven that acupuncture is effective for back pain. For those with chronic back pain, acupuncture is worth trying. Massage and acupressure help relieve muscle spasm, especially when heat is applied to the affected muscles first.

A study done at Johns Hopkins showed that wearing a portable heat wrap for 8 hours on 3 consecutive days decreased pain by 60% in a group of patients with back pain (American Pain Society, 2010). Transcutaneous electrical nerve stimulation may help relieve the patient's pain. Acupuncture has proven useful to help relieve back pain. Back strengthening exercises are prescribed as soon as acute symptoms subside; these exercises are initially supervised by a physical therapist. The exercises are encouraged for a lifetime, as muscles need to be toned to prevent back strain. Specially designed corsets or back braces are sometimes used to maintain proper alignment of the spine when the patient is allowed out of bed. The patient is cautioned not to lift anything heavier than 2 to 5 lb and not to twist when reaching for things. The patient should be up and moving about frequently rather than sitting for long periods. High heels should be avoided.

Swimming or walking for short distances frequently is very beneficial for patients suffering back pain. Standing for long periods is to be avoided, and when standing, the patient should shift weight from one foot to the other frequently. Adjustments and treatments by a chiropractor may also help relieve pain, although chiropractic treatment is not appropriate for all types of back injuries. Chiropractic help seems most effective if the pain has been present for less than 16 days. If pain continues beyond 3 to 4 weeks, or if pain is worsening, there is evidence of neurologic deficit, and surgery may be indicated.

For many patients, gentle yoga movements have been more successful than prescribed back exercises for relieving pain. For others, core body stretching and muscle strengthening work well.

Surgical Procedures. For those patients who cannot find relief through conservative measures, surgical removal of the damaged disk may be the only alternative. A diskectomy is performed to decompress the nerve root. This is a microsurgical technique that uses a very small incision through which the herniated intervertebral disk material is dissected and extracted. A minimally invasive electrothermoplasty or radiofrequency diskal nucleoplasty may be performed. If the area cannot be handled with microsurgery, an open incision diskectomy or laminectomy, which involves removal of the posterior arch of the vertebra along with the disk, is done. A laminectomy may be done in conjunction with spinal fusion.

A percutaneous laser diskectomy is an outpatient procedure. A tube is passed through the retroperitoneal soft tissues to the disk's lateral border. Local anesthesia and fluoroscopy are used during the procedure. A laser is used to cut away and destroy the herniated portion of the disk. Small stab wounds are used, there is minimal blood loss, and rehabilitation time is shorter. An artificial Charité disk may be inserted after diskectomy when there is degenerative disk disease.

A spinal fusion is necessary in some patients to stabilize the spine. In a spinal fusion, a piece or pieces of bone from the iliac crest or cadaver bone are grafted onto the vertebrae to strengthen them. Fixation with metal rods and screws may be employed to decrease spinal motion and irritability. A device, the InFuse Bone Graft/LT-CAGE, is an option to avoid the need to use bone from the patient for grafting (Patel & Slipman, 2009). Genetically engineered protein contained in the device stimulates new bone growth at the site.

A laminectomy may be done for conditions other than a ruptured disk—for example, for such degenerative diseases of the spine as Pott's disease (tuberculosis of the spine), for fractures of the spine, and for spinal dislocation. Once a laminectomy with a fusion has healed, the fused vertebrae are immobile.

Nursing Management

Preoperatively, a baseline neurologic assessment is performed and documented. Other preoperative care is the same as for other types of general surgery. Postoperatively, the major concern after spinal fusion, laminectomy, or diskectomy is to keep the spinal column in alignment so that healing can take place and no further injury occurs to the spinal cord. Pillows are placed under the thighs when the patient is on his back and between the legs when on the side, to maintain correct spinal alignment and decrease the pressure to the back. If the surgeon allows the patient to be turned to the side, log rolling is used to avoid twisting the spine (see Figure 23-13). Sometimes the surgeon will allow the patient to be positioned only on the back or sometimes the abdomen. Whenever the patient's position is changed, an ample number of people should be available to help move him. The patient who has had cervical spine surgery is placed in a cervical collar and continues to wear a collar for several weeks.

 Focused Assessment

Data Collection Following Spinal Surgery

Immediately postoperatively, assess every 15 to 30 minutes; after first 4 hours, assess every 2 to 4 hours postoperatively. Assess the following areas and compare findings with preoperative data:

SENSATION
- Check extremities for numbness and tingling.
- Check all anatomical surfaces of forearms and hands, upper and lower legs, and feet.

MOVEMENT
- Check for ability to move shoulders, arms, hands, legs, and feet.

MUSCLE STRENGTH
- Check each extremity for weakness by having the patient push against your hands while you apply downward pressure to the extremity.

WOUND
- Assess surgical (and donor) site for drainage, noting amount, color, and characteristics.
- Check carefully for signs of CSF leak at surgical site.
- Determine adequacy of analgesia.

PAIN
- Assess for site of pain, characteristics of the pain, and degree of pain on a scale of 1 to 10, with 10 being the worst pain.
- Reevaluate pain after administering analgesia for effectiveness.
- Monitor respirations and vital signs.

SKIN PRESSURE POINTS
- Check for reddened areas on bony prominences when turning patient.

CSF, cerebrospinal fluid.

When the laminectomy or spinal fusion patient is allowed out of bed, a back brace or corset may be ordered to support the spinal column until complete healing has occurred. For several weeks the patient is not allowed to sit for any length of time. He must walk or lie down. Standing for long periods is discouraged. The microdiskectomy patient is usually up and about the day after surgery. However, weeks to many months of exercises and physical therapy are necessary before recovery is complete.

 Clinical Cues

At the time of discharge, the instructions about not sitting or standing for any length of time should be reinforced. Patients tend to overdo sitting or standing when they get home and become very fatigued, have more pain, and become discouraged.

An IV opioid via patient-controlled analgesia pump may be ordered for pain control the first 24 to 48 hours after surgery. Additional boluses for adequate pain control may be needed. Assess frequently for effectiveness of the pain medication. Once fluids are being taken, oral analgesia is started with acetaminophen with codeine, hydrocodone (Vicodin), or oxycodone (Percocet). Muscle relaxants may be given as well.

After spinal surgery a small fracture bedpan is used for toileting if the patient is not to be allowed up. The patient's back must be firmly supported while he is resting on the pan. When the patient is steady enough to be allowed out of bed, a bedside commode (or for the male patient, standing at the bedside) is encouraged to promote complete bladder emptying. Provide privacy for toileting activity. If difficulty with voiding occurs, intermittent catheterization or an indwelling catheter will be required.

Interference with bowel function and paralytic ileus may occur after laminectomy or spinal fusion. Observe for constipation, nausea, abdominal distention, and return of bowel sounds. Stool softeners are used to help prevent constipation. Incontinence or difficulty with bowel evacuation may indicate nerve damage, and should be reported to the surgeon.

Activity allowed varies according to the underlying pathology and the patient's progress. Be clear about activity orders, whether a brace or corset is to be worn, and whether such is to be put on while lying down, sitting, or standing.

If a bone graft has been performed, the donor site must be assessed regularly and care provided. Pain is usually greater at the donor site than at the spinal fusion site. If the fibula is the donor site, neurovascular assessments of the limb must be performed on a regular schedule, as edema can occur.

Depending on the type of spinal surgery performed, many weeks to months are needed for complete recovery. The patient must learn to perform activities without twisting the spine.

Patient Teaching

Guidelines for the Patient with Low Back Pain or Spinal Surgery

DO
- Bend knees, with back straight, and crouch to lift an item off the floor.
- Carry items close to the center of your body.
- Perform your back exercises twice a day; periodically review the correct way to do them.
- Maintain appropriate body weight; lose weight if overweight.
- Use a lumbar pillow or roll when sitting and particularly when driving for long distances.
- Stop and walk around at least every 2 hours when on long trips.
- Consider how to safely perform a task before starting to do it.

DO NOT
- Lean over without bending the knees.
- Reach to lift items or lift heavy items higher than the elbows.
- Stand or sit for long periods.
- Sleep with legs out straight without pillow cushioning under the thighs or between the legs when on the side.
- Bend from the waist to pick up an item.
- Twist to the side to lift things (e.g., groceries or things in the car or trunk).

Get Ready for the NCLEX® Examination!

Key Points

- Head injuries are open or closed and result in concussion, contusion, acceleration-deceleration injury, skull fracture, or tearing of cranial vessels.
- Subdural or epidural hematoma may result from a head injury; epidural hemorrhage is a life-threatening event.
- A significant head injury causes disruption in normal LOC.
- Drainage from the ear or nose should be evaluated to determine the presence of CSF.
- Any lesion or extra fluid that begins to take up space in the cranial vault causes an increase in ICP.
- The earliest sign of increased ICP is decreasing LOC.
- Treatment of increased ICP includes maintaining a patent airway, administering diuretic agents to decrease edema, monitoring neurologic signs for increased ICP, regulating temperature, maintaining adequate blood pressure, and instituting nursing measures to prevent further increases in ICP (see Table 22-9 and Nursing Care Plan 23-1).
- Neurologic assessment is performed every 15 minutes to 2 hours for the acute patient with injury to or surgery on the brain.
- For maintenance of a patent airway, intubation or a tracheostomy and mechanical ventilation may be necessary.
- Early nutritional support is very important for both head injury and spinal cord injury patients.
- The unconscious patient requires care for all basic needs; the eyes must be protected from injury since the blink reflex may be absent.
- Complications of head injury and increased ICP include hydrocephalus and diabetes insipidus.
- The extent of permanent cord damage often cannot be assessed until many days after injury because of edema and resulting pressure that edema causes on the spinal cord.
- The degree of neurologic impairment and activities that the patient will still be able to perform depend on the level and extent of the injury (see Table 23-1).
- Autonomic dysreflexia is potentially very dangerous to the patient as it can severely elevate blood pressure.
- Traction provided by Crutchfield or Gardner-Wells tongs, or a halo ring and fixation pins, immobilizes the spine while healing takes place.
- Back pain can be caused by muscle strain or herniated or ruptured intervertebral disk.
- Back pain should be treated conservatively before surgery is considered.
- Treatment depends on whether or not a disk rupture is present and on the severity of the pain and disability.
- Conservative treatment includes rest, gentle exercise, ice or heat, analgesics, and muscle relaxants.

- Surgical procedures include minimally invasive procedures, microdiskectomy or laminectomy (with or without fusion), percutaneous laser diskectomy, and spinal fusion.
- Postoperative care depends on the type of procedure performed.

Additional Learning Resources

SG Go to your Study Guide for additional learning activities to help you master this chapter content.

 evolve Go to your Evolve website (http://evolve.elsevier.com/deWit/medsurg) for the following FREE learning resources:
- Animations, audio, and video
- Answers and rationales for questions and activities
- Concept Map Creator
- Glossary with pronunciations in English and Spanish
- Interactive Review Questions and Exercises and more!

Online Resources
- American Association of Neuroscience Nurses, www.aann.org
- American Pain Society, www.ampainsoc.org
- Brain Injury Association of America, www.biausa.org
- Brain Trauma Foundation, www.braintrauma.org

Review Questions for the NCLEX® Examination

1. A 75-year-old patient who fell and hit his head a week ago is admitted for apparent personality changes, decreased level of consciousness, and irritability. The physician suspects a possible subdural hematoma. A family member asks about the condition. An accurate explanation would be:
   1. "It is the presence of bleeding in the brain parenchyma."
   2. "Bleeding occurs between the skull and the dura mater."
   3. "It is the collection of blood between the brain and the inner surface of the dura mater."
   4. "It is the intermittent blockage of circulation in various areas of the brain."

2. The nurse is admitting a patient with a possible skull fracture. Which clinical finding(s) would likely confirm the diagnosis? *(Select all that apply.)*
   1. Battle's sign
   2. Partial blindness
   3. Ecchymosis around eyes
   4. Rhinorrhea
   5. Swallowing difficulty

3. Which statement by a patient being discharged after experiencing a concussion indicates a need for more teaching?
   1. "I can resume most activities after 12 hours."
   2. "I need to report a worsening headache to the physician."
   3. "I'll have to be awakened every few hours when asleep."
   4. "I can expect to be more fatigued for a while."

4. The nurse keeps the postcraniotomy patient's neck in midline position and ensures that there is no excessive hip flexion. The rationale for the nurse's action would be that this position:
   1. restores neutral position of the joints.
   2. prevents a further increase in intracranial pressure.
   3. promotes comfort and rest.
   4. prevents the formation of blood clots.

5. The nursing assistant is attending to the needs of a patient with head injury who is lethargic and has increased intracranial pressure. Which action by the nursing assistant indicates a need for further instruction?
   1. Stopping the patient from coughing up secretions
   2. Monitoring blood pressure every 2 hours
   3. Dangling the patient on the side of the bed
   4. Reporting blood on the dressing

6. The classic signs of increased intracranial pressure include rising systolic blood pressure, widening pulse pressure, and _____.

7. The surgeon inserts an intraventricular catheter into the lateral ventricle of a patient with increased intracranial pressure. When asked by a relative about the procedure, an accurate response by the nurse would be:
   1. "The catheter allows direct visualization of the brain tissue."
   2. "The catheter is used to monitor brain waves."
   3. "The catheter is used to remove excess fluid inside the brain."
   4. "The catheter is used to infuse fluids and medications into the brain."

8. A 40-year-old man with a T4 spinal cord injury suddenly complains of severe headache, increased pulse rate, sweating, and flushing above the level of the spinal cord lesion, and "goose bumps" below the level of injury. Which immediate nursing action(s) should be included? *(Select all that apply.)*
   1. Place flat in bed.
   2. Identify the cause of stimulation.
   3. Decrease blood pressure.
   4. Provide measures to facilitate bowel movement.
   5. Clamp indwelling catheter.

9. A 30-year-old man is admitted to the emergency department after a motor vehicle accident. On examination, the patient is diagnosed with a T6 spinal cord injury. He has flaccid paralysis, slowed heart rate, low blood pressure, and no bowel sounds. The patient must be developing:
   1. autonomic dysreflexia.
   2. muscle spasms.
   3. spinal shock.
   4. diabetes insipidus.

10. Instructions for the patient with a "slipped disk" with acute pain and sciatica should include:

   1. using ice packs on the area of back pain for 5 to 10 minutes each hour while awake for the first 48 hours.
   2. resting in bed for 2 to 3 days and walking every hour even if walking causes more pain.
   3. obtaining a massage each day to loosen the muscle spasms in the back.
   4. not lifting anything heavier than 10 lb for several weeks.

Critical Thinking Activities

Scenario A

Mary is a 22-year-old college student who has suffered a head injury in an automobile accident. She was healthy before her accident. The emergency medical services team brought her to the emergency department (ED). She is stabilized in the ED, cervical spine injury is ruled out, and she is admitted to the neurologic intensive care unit. She is confused and groggy and has leakage of cerebrospinal fluid (CSF) from one ear and irregular respirations.

1. What assessments would you perform?

2. What specific nursing measures would you include in your care plan concerning the leaking CSF?

3. What measures would you take to provide appropriate respiratory care?

Scenario B

Gus Berrini is a 40-year-old truck driver who received a severe spinal injury when he was shot in the back by a hitchhiker. The bullet severed the spinal cord at the sixth thoracic vertebra.

1. What kinds of activities should Mr. Berrini eventually be able to perform?

2. How would you plan his care during the acute stage of his illness so that efforts at rehabilitation might be successful?

3. What other members of the health care team might participate in his care and rehabilitation?

Scenario C

Henry Jones, a 35-year-old construction worker, comes to the clinic with low back pain. He states that this is not the first time he has had a problem with the back pain. He says that this time it is worse and that he can hardly move. He is unable to work.

1. What tests will the health care provider probably perform or order?

2. What is likely to be recommended in the way of treatment?

3. What should Mr. Jones be taught before he leaves the clinic?

Objectives

Theory

1. Describe the appropriate nursing actions and observations to be carried out for a patient experiencing a seizure.
2. Explain why seizure may be a consequence of a stroke, tumor, or infection in the brain.
3. Compare the subjective and objective findings of thrombotic stroke and intracerebral bleed.
4. Devise a nursing care plan for the patient who has suffered a cerebrovascular accident (CVA, stroke).
5. Discuss nursing actions to assist the patient who has developed a complication after a cerebrovascular accident.
6. Describe subjective and objective findings indicative of a brain tumor.
7. Explain the pathophysiology behind the symptoms of a brain tumor.
8. Diagram the mechanism by which infection in the brain may cause increased intracranial pressure.

9. Recall the signs of increasing intracranial pressure from early to late signs.
10. Compare and contrast symptoms of meningitis and encephalitis.
11. Explain the assessment data that differentiate migraine headaches from cluster headaches.
12. Compare the signs, symptoms, and treatment of trigeminal neuralgia and Bell's palsy.

Clinical Practice

1. Teach a teenage patient recently diagnosed with epilepsy what she needs to know about her disorder and care.
2. Perform neurologic checks on a patient who is admitted with a suspected CVA.
3. Assist with the care of a patient who has had intracranial surgery.
4. Devise a teaching plan for the patient who has suffered a CVA and has right-sided hemiplegia.

Key Terms

agnosia (ăg-NŌ-zhă, p. 532)
aneurysm (ĂN-ūr-ĭ-zĭm, p. 528)
aphasia (ă-FĀ-zhă, p. 532)
apraxia (ă-PRĂK-sē-ă, p. 532)
ataxia (ă-TĂK-sē-ă, p. 532)
aura (ĂW-ră, p. 524)
automatisms (ăw-TŌM-ă-tĭsmz, p. 524)
dysarthria (dĭs-ĂHR-thrē-ă, p. 532)
dysphasia (dĭs-FĀ-zhă, p. 532)
embolus (ĔM-bō-lŭs, p. 528)

epilepsy (Ĕ-pĭ-lĕp-sē, p. 524)
homonymous hemianopsia (hō-MŎN-ĭ-mŭs hĕ-mē-ă-NŎP-sē-ă, p. 532)
hydrocephalus (hī-drō-SĔF-ă-lăs, p. 542)
infarct (ĭn-făhrkt, p. 528)
nuchal rigidity (NŪ-kăl, p. 542)
postictal (PŌST-ĭk-tĕl, p. 524)
ptosis (TŌ-sĭs, p. 546)
scotoma (skō-TŌ-mă, p. 545)
status epilepticus (STĂ-tŭs ĕp-ĭ-LĔP-tĭ-kŭs, p. 524)

SEIZURE DISORDERS AND EPILEPSY

Etiology

Seizures can be symptomatic of a large number of disorders. Brain injury from a stroke, pressure from a brain tumor, infectious diseases with high fever, end-stage renal disease with uremia, toxicity (such as that occurring in eclampsia during pregnancy or in drug poisoning), epilepsy, and tetanus are but a few examples of seizure-producing disorders. **Seizures also can occur any time the brain is deprived of oxygen.**

Seizures may be symptoms of an underlying illness. Metabolic disturbances such as acidosis, electrolyte imbalances, hypoglycemia, hypoxia, and water intoxication may cause seizures. Alcohol or barbiturate withdrawal can cause seizures. In children, a high temperature is a frequent cause of seizures. There are at least 40 types of seizure disorders linked to genetic defects. Epilepsy is present when correcting the metabolic problem does not stop the seizures. Epilepsy affects 4 to 8 in 1000 people in the United States (Ko & Sahai-Srivastava, 2009). Incidence increases in those 60 to 80 years of age.

Pathophysiology

Epilepsy is a chronic disturbance of the nervous system characterized by various types of recurrent seizures that are the result of abnormal electrical activity of the brain. Epilepsy is characterized by spontaneous recurring seizures. It is thought that in epilepsy a group of abnormal neurons fire spontaneously. Some unknown stimulus causes the cell membranes to depolarize. The depolarization of the neurons causes abnormal sensory or motor activity and may cause unconsciousness. The neurons involved have a low threshold for excitation. The excitation spreads to surrounding cells, spreading the activity to a small area or throughout the brain. Seizures are classified as *partial* or *generalized*. Each seizure lasts a few seconds or a few minutes. The abnormal electrical activity generated can be captured by an electroencephalogram (EEG).

Signs and Symptoms

Partial Seizures. Partial seizures are further divided into three subgroups: simple partial seizures, in which consciousness is not impaired but there are other motor, sensory, autonomic, or psychological symptoms; complex partial seizures, in which there is some impairment of consciousness with or without automatisms (repetitive, automatic actions such as lip smacking); and partial seizures that become generalized as the seizure continues.

Partial seizures also are called simple or focal seizures and result from an abnormal localized cortical discharge. Partial seizures with complex symptomatology may also be called temporal lobe seizures because they usually originate in the temporal lobe of the brain. Partial seizures can be unilateral, with involvement on only one side of the brain and activity only on one side of the body.

Generalized Seizures. Generalized seizures are bilaterally symmetrical (affecting both sides of the body equally) and do not have a local onset; that is, they do not typically begin in one part of the body. Generalized seizures have symptoms or activity that is bilaterally symmetrical and include absence, myoclonic, clonic, tonic, tonic-clonic, and atonic seizures and infantile spasms (usually caused by increased temperature).

Generalized seizures are characterized by bilateral synchronous electrical discharges in the brain. The whole brain is affected and there is no warning or aura (preceding sensation). The patient usually quickly loses consciousness lasting for a few seconds up to several minutes.

The manifestations of epilepsy depend on the area of the brain where the abnormal firing occurs. **Absence or petit mal seizures last only a few seconds. The onset is sudden, with no aura or warning and no postictal symptoms.** Seizures of this type tend to affect children between 5 and 12 years of age and disappear during puberty. There usually is a twitching about the eyes and mouth. The person remains standing or sitting and appears to have had no more than a lapse of attention or a moment of absentmindedness.

With tonic convulsions, there is continued contraction of all muscles and the body becomes rigid. Grand mal or tonic-clonic seizures usually begin with bilateral jerks of the extremities or focal seizure activity. There is loss of consciousness with both tonic and clonic convulsions. The patient may be incontinent during the attack, and there is danger of biting the tongue. In the postictal (after a seizure) phase, the person is confused and drowsy.

Atonic or akinetic seizures are characterized by loss of body muscle tone that results in nodding of the head, weakness of the knees, or total collapse and falling ("drop attacks"). The person usually remains conscious during the attack.

The third major group, unclassified seizures, simply means that not enough data have been obtained to determine which type of seizure the patient is experiencing.

The fourth designation, status epilepticus, indicates prolonged partial or generalized seizure without recovery between attacks. Status epilepticus is a grave condition in which there is a rapid, unrelenting series of convulsive seizures without intervening periods of consciousness, and an absence of respiration. **Irreversible brain damage can occur if the seizures are not controlled.**

In classifying epileptic seizures on the basis of origin, seizures are grouped as either idiopathic or symptomatic. Idiopathic epilepsy has no known cause. Symptomatic epilepsy has a known physical cause (e.g., brain tumor, injury to the head at birth, a wound or blow to the head, toxicity, or an endocrine disorder).

Diagnosis

Diagnosis of epilepsy is based on the history and the actual signs and symptoms observed during a seizure. A thorough physical examination and tests for underlying disease are ordered based on the history and physical findings. Confirmation of the diagnosis is by EEG and magnetic resonance imaging (MRI). These tests help locate the site, or *locus,* and possibly the cause of the seizures. Electrolyte levels are determined as imbalances may predispose to a seizure.

Treatment

When the cause of seizures is known, as in cases of high fever or drug toxicity, medical treatment is aimed at controlling or eliminating whatever is responsible for the seizures. For recurrent seizures, as in epilepsy, the condition usually is managed with anticonvulsant drug therapy. An implanted vagus nerve stimulator is proving helpful for generalized epilepsy for many patients with uncontrolled seizures.

The major antiepileptic drugs are presented in Box 24-1. Patient education is extremely important,

Box 24-1 **Medications Commonly Used for Seizure Control**

DRUGS FOR GENERALIZED TONIC-CLONIC AND PARTIAL SEIZURES
- Phenytoin (Dilantin)
- Fosphenytoin (Cerebyx)
- Carbamazepine (Tegretol)
- Primidone (Mysoline)
- Lacosamide (Vimpat)
- Lamotrigine (Lamictal)
- Phenobarbital (Luminal)
- Felbamate (Felbatol)
- Gabapentin (Neurontin)
- Levetiracetam (Keppra)
- Oxcarbazepine (Trileptal)
- Pregabalin (Lyrica)
- Rufinamide (Banzel)
- Tiagabine (Gabitril)
- Topiramate (Topamax)
- Valproic acid (Depakene)
- Zonisamide (Zonegran)
- Vigabatrin (Sabril)

DRUGS FOR ABSENCE, AKINETIC, AND MYOCLONIC SEIZURES
- Valproic acid (Depakene)
- Ethosuximide (Zarontin)
- Clonazepam (Klonopin)
- Divalproex (Depakote)
- Phenobarbital

GENERAL NURSING IMPLICATIONS
- Educate patient about the importance of taking the drug exactly as it is prescribed.
- All these drugs cause some degree of sedation, drowsiness, and lethargy. Warn about driving or operating machinery when these effects are significant. Advise not to drink alcohol or use other central nervous system depressants.
- The patient should not stop taking an anticonvulsant abruptly without consulting the physician.
- Check interactions with other drugs before administering any of these drugs. Interaction with anticoagulants, oral contraceptives, digoxin, aspirin, certain antibiotics, antacids, folic acid, and other drugs are significant. Some anticonvulsant drugs interact with each other (e.g., phenobarbital).
- Periodic blood work, every 1 to 3 months, should be done when taking an anticonvulsant.
- Dosages of each drug are based on therapeutic blood level of the drug.
- Anticonvulsants have a narrow therapeutic range; toxicity occurs if too much of the drug is taken.
- Patient should be under the close supervision of the health care provider.
- All of the anticonvulsant drugs can produce some unpleasant side effects, such as fever and leukopenia and, in the case of phenytoin, gingival hyperplasia and rash.
- Physical dependence can become a problem for patients taking either phenobarbital or primidone, which is largely converted to phenobarbital in the bloodstream.
- Toxic side effects such as ataxia, drowsiness, nausea, sedation, and dizziness are not uncommon.

because the patient will need to report any untoward effects to the physician or nurse clinician so the dosage can be adjusted or the drug changed. All anticonvulsant drugs cause some central nervous system (CNS) depression with grogginess, dizziness, fatigue, and cognitive changes.

A ketogenic diet is beneficial in younger patients with refractory (difficult to control) generalized seizures. A ketogenic diet provides sufficient calories from fats and proteins, but produces a ketotic (acidotic) state that seems to prevent seizure activity.

Biofeedback techniques are geared toward teaching the patient to maintain a certain brainwave frequency that is not susceptible to seizure activity.

Treatment of status epilepticus depends on its cause. Many times patients who are known to have epilepsy arrive in the emergency department with status epilepticus because, for one reason or another, they stopped taking the medication that controls their seizures. Treatment in this instance would involve administering lorazepam, phenytoin, and/or phenobarbital in a dose sufficiently high to stop the seizures (Cavazos, 2009). Care is focused on supporting vital signs and preventing injury. Intubation may be required for respiratory support. If seizures will not stop, an anesthetic agent may be required. Rectal diazepam has been approved by the U.S. Food and Drug Administration (FDA) in a system called Diastat AcuDial. It can be used at home by nonprofessional caregivers, and clinical studies have shown that the system resolved seizures in 85% of patients (Epilepsy Action, 2010).

Surgical Treatment. Surgical procedures involve removing the epileptic focus or preventing the spread of epileptic activity by sectioning the corpus callosum. A temporal lobe resection may eliminate seizures in more than 70% of patients with temporal lobe seizures. For patients with extensive damage in one side of the brain that causes intractable seizures, a hemispherectomy may be performed. Surgeries are not without danger and are reserved for those patients whose seizures cannot be managed by medical treatment and in whom the focus of the seizures is accessible.

For intractable partial seizures, a NeuroCybernetic Prosthesis (vagal nerve stimulator) can be implanted in the chest cavity with a wire tunneled to stimulate the vagus nerve. The device acts like a pacemaker and provides a tiny electric jolt every 5 minutes that stimulates the brain to interrupt seizures (Carroll & Berbadis, 2009).

Uncontrolled seizures secondary to hypoglycemia (as in improperly controlled diabetes mellitus) can be relieved by IV administration of 50% dextrose. If the unrelenting seizures are caused by chronic alcoholism or withdrawal, treatment consists of IV administration of thiamine.

When phenytoin is ordered to be administered intravenously (IV), mix it in 0.9% saline solution and flush the line before and after administration if a glucose IV solution is running. Glucose is incompatible with phenytoin. **Never administer IV phenytoin faster than 50 mg/min because of the risk of cardiac dysrhythmia.** For patients with a history of heart problems, administer the solution no faster than 25 mg/min.

❖ NURSING MANAGEMENT

■ Assessment (Data Collection)

Patients with a known seizure problem usually are treated on an outpatient basis, but may be encountered in the hospital or long-term care facility. Assess the patient carefully to provide optimal safety and care. Significant history information includes the kind of seizures they experience, whether they have any sensation just before the appearance of clinically observable signs, what medications they are taking, and what measures are known to be helpful either to prevent a seizure or to assist while they are having a seizure and afterward. Assessment should include any factors that could have triggered the seizure (e.g., hyperventilation, bright lights [photosensitivity], alcohol and other drugs, fluid and electrolyte imbalances, lack of sleep, and emotional stress).

 Focused Assessment

Observations to Make During a Seizure

Observe as much of the following as possible and document your findings.
- Time the seizure began and the time it ended
- What the patient was doing just before the seizure (was the patient picking at clothing?)
- Where in the body the seizure began, what parts of the body are involved
- Which way eyes are moving, whether they constrict or dilate, deviate to the right or the left, or roll upward
- Which side the head turns toward
- Whether the patient cries out or screams as the seizure begins
- Whether there is evidence of repetitive movements: lip smacking, chewing, grimacing, tapping, or "pill rolling"
- Whether movements are bilateral and symmetrical
- Incontinence of urine or stool, vomiting, frothing at the mouth, or bleeding
- Whether the patient becomes apneic or cyanotic
- Changes in skin color or profuse perspiration

Postictal assessment, after a patent airway is ensured, includes determining:
- Length of time before regaining awareness
- Presence of lethargy or confusion
- Presence of headache
- Presence of speech impairment
- Presence of muscle soreness
- Whether there was an aura before the seizure began
- Effects of the seizure on the patient's vital signs

When caring for a patient who is likely to experience a seizure during an acute illness, periodically observe the patient for tremors, unexplained sensory or motor changes, mental changes that indicate confusion or disorientation, and restless or agitated behavior. In many cases, a change in the neurologic status of a patient can signal the possibility that a seizure might occur.

■ Nursing Diagnosis, Planning, and Implementation

The main nursing diagnosis for the patient who experiences seizures is *Risk for injury related to seizure activity.* Expected outcomes are written for the individual patient and the type of seizure disorder, possible triggers, and manifestations.

Nursing care of patients with epileptic seizures is concerned with immediate care during and after a seizure and long-term management and control of seizures and their psychosocial implications. Witnessing a seizure for the first time can be a frightening experience. The nurse's first responsibility is to stay calm, remain with the patient, and call for assistance.

The environment of a patient at risk for seizure should be made as safe as possible. If the patient is very likely to have seizures, the side rails and headboard of the bed are padded. **Never try to pry open the patient's mouth or insert something into it once the jaw is clamping down, as teeth may be broken and the airway may become obstructed.**

If a seizure comes on without warning and the patient drops to the ground, leave her wherever she is lying. If she is on a hard surface, her head should be protected from injury by placing a rolled blanket or coat under it. The head should be turned to the side, if possible, to prevent aspiration of secretions. Do not attempt to restrain the patient's movements or to move her to a bed or chair during the seizure. If supplemental oxygen is near, it should be administered, if possible. Call for help and provide privacy, if possible. When the seizure is over, turn the patient to the side, and suction the airway if needed. Check oxygen saturation with a pulse oximeter. Check the glucose level, if possible, and assess for injuries. Stay with the patient until she is completely conscious. When consciousness is regained, reorient and reassure her. The patient should be allowed to rest or sleep after the seizure. Thoroughly document the event in the medical record with time, duration of the seizure, and observations of the seizure activity and any aura that occurred before its start.

 Clinical Cue

If a patient who is receiving phenytoin is receiving tube feedings, stop the tube feeding for 2 hours before and 2 hours after administering phenytoin to ensure proper drug concentration and absorption.

The long-term management of epileptic seizures is primarily focused on providing the patient with the information and support she needs to care for herself and to avoid recurring and debilitating seizures. Psychosocial support is necessary to encourage the patient to talk about her fears and concerns. Lifestyle changes will have to be made if she is not permitted to drive. Most states allow resumption of driving when a patient has been seizure free for 1 year. A referral to the local epilepsy society for connection with a support group can be very helpful for both the patient and her family.

Most individuals who suffer from epileptic seizures are perfectly normal between seizures; they are not mentally retarded and are quite capable of becoming contributing members of society if only they are given the chance to prove their worth.

 Patient Teaching

The Patient with Epilepsy

Cover these points in the teaching plan:
- Treatment and side effects of anticonvulsant therapy.
- Triggers for seizures and how to avoid them (lack of sleep, alcohol and recreational drugs, stress, photosensitivity).
- Necessity of taking medication daily and as close to the same time each day as possible.
- Greatest trigger for a seizure is not taking the medication.
- Handling a missed dose or inability to retain medication.
- Not using over-the-counter or prescription medication without consulting the physician who prescribed the anticonvulsants.
- Schedule for laboratory work to determine drug therapeutic levels.
- Need for medical alert bracelet, necklace, and wallet card listing physician's phone number and drugs being taken.
- Resources for assistance available in the community.
- Need for proper nutrition; dangers of erratic meals.
- Avoiding alcohol and excessive fatigue.
- Relaxation therapy for stress reduction.
- Danger of swimming alone.
- Refraining from driving or operating dangerous machinery until seizures are well controlled.
- Keeping follow-up appointments with the physician.

FOR WOMEN
- Risk of seizure during menstruation.
- Should consult physician before becoming pregnant; some anticonvulsant drugs may cause congenital abnormalities.

FOR THE FAMILY
- What to do in the event of a seizure.
- How to protect the patient during a seizure:
  - For tonic-clonic generalized seizure: assisting to the floor, protecting the head, loosening clothing, turning to the side.
- When medical assistance is necessary.

Patient Education

Self-care for the epileptic patient requires that she understand the nature of her disorder, the purpose of her prescribed medications, their side effects, and the signs of toxicity that should be reported to the physician. The patient must understand the necessity for compliance with the prescribed regimen to avoid recurrent seizures. She will need assistance in developing coping mechanisms to deal with the psychosocial impact of having epilepsy.

■ Evaluation

Evaluation is based on whether the expected outcomes are being achieved. This will include whether the patient is seizure free, or whether the number of seizures has decreased. Patient compliance with the medication regimen and avoidance of triggers for seizure activity is evaluated as well. Patient teaching may need to be reinforced. If progress toward the achievement of outcomes is not occurring, the plan must be revised.

 Think Critically

What safety measures would you teach a 22-year-old man who has just been diagnosed with grand mal seizures?

TRANSIENT ISCHEMIC ATTACK

Between 200,000 and 500,000 Americans experience what are called *transient ischemic attacks* (TIAs) each year. TIAs are caused by a brief interruption in blood flow. Narrowed arteries and vascular occlusion, perhaps by small emboli or vasospasm, cause the interruption. Recreational drugs that constrict vessels are another cause of TIAs. TIAs are warnings that a more serious neurologic event may occur; 11% of patients who experience a TIA have a stroke within 90 days. During the TIA, the person may feel a sudden weakness or numbness on one side of the body, slurring of speech or inability to talk, visual disturbances such as blindness or double vision, confusion, diminished coordination or ability to balance, and a headache. Symptoms are similar to those of a stroke. These symptoms generally last no more than an hour and completely resolve without residual deficits (Goldstein, 2011). It is very important that the person be evaluated by medical personnel, as the same symptoms may indicate a stroke that will not resolve without treatment.

A thorough history of the event is essential: how it began, the symptoms experienced, and how long it lasted. If carotid obstruction is suspected, carotid duplex ultrasound studies are done to determine if obstruction in the carotid arteries is preventing normal blood flow from reaching the brain. Multiple tests may be performed if carotid occlusion is ruled out, including blood tests, MRI, and EEG. If there is near-total occlusion of the carotid artery, either an angioplasty procedure with stent implantation or a carotid endarterectomy is considered. If occlusion from plaque obstruction is less than 60%, medical treatment with diet and lifestyle modification and medication to prevent platelet aggregation (i.e., aspirin, clopidogrel [Plavix], dipyridamole [Persantine]) is prescribed.

CEREBROVASCULAR ACCIDENT (STROKE, BRAIN ATTACK)

Etiology

More than 795,000 first and repeat strokes occur in the United States each year. Stroke is the leading cause of disability and the third leading cause of death (Stroke Center, 2010). The incidence is about 19% higher in males than in females. About 25% of cases occur in people younger than age 65 (American Heart Association, 2009). An increase in public education about the risk factors for and signs of stroke could result in lessened disability and death from stroke.

Health Promotion

Risk Factors for Stroke

Educate all patients about the risk factors for stroke and encourage measures to alter those factors that can be changed.

MODIFIABLE RISK FACTORS
- Cigarette smoking
- Using cocaine or other recreational drugs
- Drinking more than two drinks per day
- Heart disease (especially atrial fibrillation)
- Diabetes
- High blood pressure
- High cholesterol
- Sedentary lifestyle
- High red blood cell count (polycythemia)
- Transient ischemic attacks (TIAs)
- Use of oral contraceptives or hormone replacement therapy

NONMODIFIABLE RISK FACTORS
- Age over 65
- Asymptomatic carotid bruit (indicates atherosclerosis, which increases stroke risk; a bruit is a swishing sound in an artery)
- Heredity (family history of stroke increases individual risk)
- Prior stroke
- Race (African Americans have a 60% higher risk rate)
- Sex (incidence is 30% higher in men)

Cultural Considerations

Greater Incidence of Stroke in African Americans and Hispanic Americans

It is known that African Americans have about a 60% greater incidence of stroke than whites. A study at the University of Michigan found that Hispanic Americans have a far greater chance of suffering a stroke than non-Hispanic whites. It is thought that untreated hypertension may be the risk factor involved (American Heart Association, 2009).

Control of high blood pressure, quitting cigarette smoking, decreasing intake of cholesterol and

controlling blood lipids, maintaining a normal blood sugar level, avoiding excessive alcohol intake, getting sufficient exercise, avoiding obesity, and living a lifestyle that helps prevent heart disease can help reduce the risk of stroke. Atherosclerosis is a major cause of stroke, as it can predispose to thrombus formation in the brain vessels or plaque in other arteries that can break off and become emboli.

Pathophysiology

A cerebrovascular accident (CVA) is the result of an interruption of blood flow to a specific area of the brain (i.e., *cerebral ischemia*). Ischemia of cells directly causes cellular *necrosis* (death) and infarct (area of tissue that has become necrotic from lack of blood supply) (Figure 24-1). Ischemia can be caused by:
- Cerebral thrombosis (formation of a blood clot in a cerebral artery)
- An embolus (a traveling clot, fat, bacteria, or tissue debris that lodges in a vessel, occluding it)
- Intracerebral hemorrhage (the blood vessel ruptures and leaks blood into brain tissue, or an aneurysm or arteriovenous malformation in the brain leaks or ruptures)
- Pressure on a blood vessel (tumor)

Health Promotion

Dangers of Cocaine or Methamphetamine Use

Caution people about the dangers of using cocaine or methamphetamine. Both of these drugs can cause vasoconstriction and brain ischemia. Cocaine may also cause hemorrhage. Using these drugs causes a fivefold increase in the incidence of stroke. The incidence of this type of stroke has greatly increased in young adults (Agarwal, 2011).

The carotid arteries supply a major portion of the blood that goes to the brain (Figure 24-2). **If plaque forms in these arteries as a result of atherosclerosis, the person is at risk for a stroke as blood supply to the brain is diminished or stopped.** Less common causes of stroke are arterial spasms, compression of cerebral vessels by a tumor, local edema, rupture of a cerebral aneurysm, or another disorder.

Think Critically

How many risk factors for stroke are present for each member of your family?

Cerebral Aneurysm and Arteriovenous Malformation.

Structures that can cause an intracerebral hemorrhage are an aneurysm and an arteriovenous malformation. An aneurysm is an abnormal ballooning of an artery wall (Figure 24-3). It may be congenital or caused by a weakening of the artery wall from chronic hypertension. Rupture of a brain aneurysm causes bleeding

FIGURE 24-1 A, Events causing stroke. **B,** Magnetic resonance imaging showing hemorrhagic stroke in the left cerebrum.

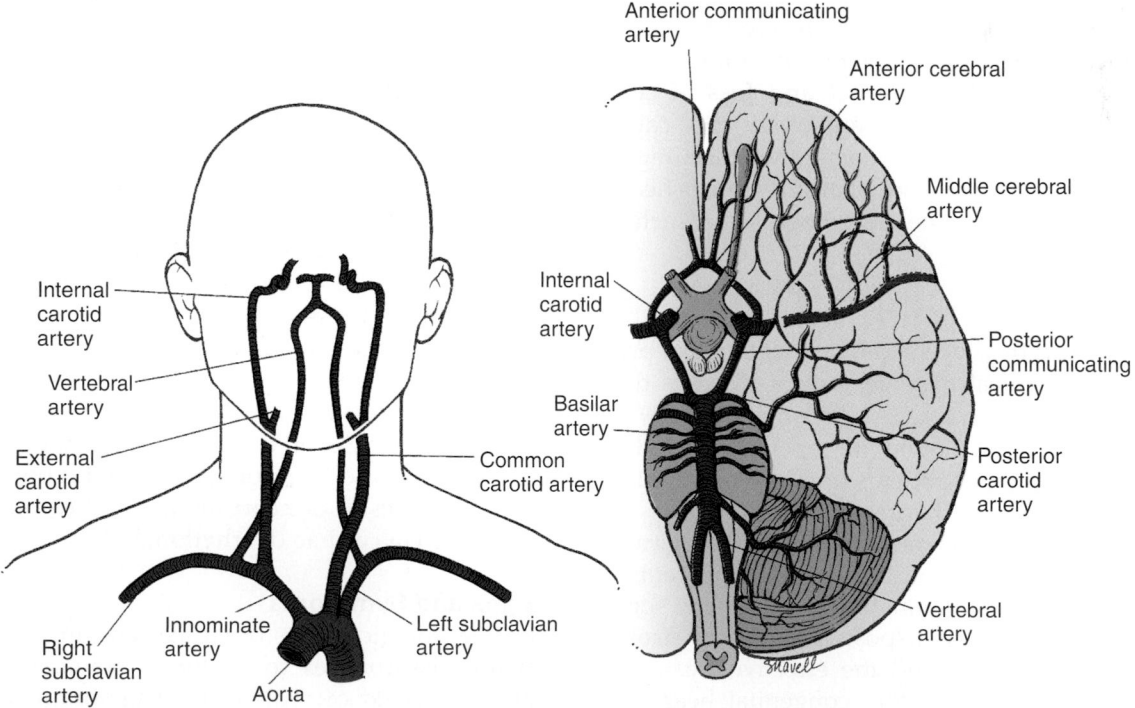

FIGURE 24-2 Major arteries supplying blood to the brain. Blockage of any major artery precipitates a cerebrovascular accident (CVA).

FIGURE 24-3 Dissected circle of Willis showing a large cerebral aneurysm.

Patient Teaching

Warning Signs of Stroke

Teach people to seek immediate medical attention in an emergency department if any of the following warning signs of stroke appears:

- Sudden weakness, numbness, tingling, or loss of feeling in the face, arm, or leg
- Sudden trouble seeing in one or both eyes; double vision
- Sudden confusion, slurred speech, trouble talking, or difficulty understanding what others are saying
- A sudden, severe headache for no known reason
- Sudden trouble walking, dizziness, or a feeling of spinning around
- Loss of balance or coordination
- Blackouts

Should any of the above signs occur, ask the person to:

- Smile
- Shrug the shoulders
- Repeat a sentence or saying what you say first
- Tell you who she is and where she is

Clinical Cues

Valve disorders and arrhythmias such as atrial fibrillation predispose to stroke from emboli. Emboli form in the chambers of the heart when blood flow is abnormal and these emboli can be ejected into the cerebral circulation.

into the subarachnoid space or into the ventricles. An *arteriovenous malformation* (AVM) is a congenital abnormality and is a tangled mass of malformed, thin-walled, dilated vessels that form an abnormal communication between the arterial and venous systems. An AVM can leak, causing an intracerebral hemorrhage. Vasospasm often occurs after intracerebral bleeding, leading to further ischemia of the brain tissue and more neurologic impairment. Resultant deficits are the same as for other kinds of strokes.

Subarachnoid hemorrhage, which refers to bleeding in the brain below the arachnoid, often causes rapid onset of neurologic deficit and loss of consciousness. A leaking cerebral aneurysm may cause a severe headache. However, sometimes bleeding is slower, producing a more gradual progression of headache, neck stiffness, and other neurologic signs, such as blurred vision.

Stroke Prevention

Many strokes can be prevented by either surgical procedures or by medical management of diseases that predispose a person to a CVA. An angioplasty with stent placement is an option for opening occluded carotid arteries. Care for patients undergoing vascular surgery is presented in Chapter 21.

Aneurysms and AVMs can sometimes be surgically corrected, if found before rupture. Medical preventive measures are aimed at eliminating or managing some of the conditions that predispose a person to stroke. Control of hypertension and the effective treatment of inflammatory heart disease, congenital heart defects, cardiac dysrhythmias, and atherosclerosis have significantly reduced the incidence of stroke. Teaching people to seek assistance immediately when signs of stroke occur may allow medical intervention that will decrease permanent neurologic deficit.

Aspirin or another drug to reduce platelet aggregation and decrease the chance of thrombosis often is prescribed to prevent the recurrence of stroke from thrombosis (Table 24-1). A combination of two inflammatory marker blood tests is showing promise in predicting which middle-aged people are at risk of a stroke. Researchers reported that C-reactive protein and lipoprotein-associated phospholipase A_2 (LP PLA$_2$) were higher in those who later had an ischemic stroke than in those who did not have a stroke (Wright et al., 2009).

Cerebral ischemia caused by thrombosis causes signs that progress slowly. Thrombosis develops in an area of the vessel where there is atherosclerotic plaque. Lodging of an embolus in a major cerebral vessel causes sudden neurologic deficit. Emboli most often are the result of heart disease and resultant atrial fibrillation, a cardiac dysrhythmia.

Signs and Symptoms

The neurologic effects of stroke can range from mild motor disturbances to profound coma. Figure 24-4 shows selected control zones of the brain and motor and sensory functions likely to be affected by a stroke. Signs and symptoms will depend on the type of event that has caused the stroke and the location of the clot or bleed. There may be weakness (*hemiparesis*) or paralysis (*hemiplegia*), difficulty or inability to speak or

Table 24-1 | **Medications Commonly Used for Patients after a CVA**

DRUG	ACTION	NURSING IMPLICATIONS	PATIENT TEACHING
t-PA (alteplase; tissue plasminogen activator)	Converts fibrin to plasminogen, causing lysis of thrombus or embolus of CVA	Frequent VS; monitor for dysrhythmias; frequent neurologic checks; assess for bleeding until 24 hr after infusion. Monitor for hypersensitivity; monitor clotting/bleeding studies. Do not give concurrently with anticoagulants, antiplatelet aggregation drugs, or NSAIDs.	Explain that the intermittent IV infusion is for the purpose of breaking up the clot stopping blood flow to part of the brain.
Aspirin (Ecotrin)	Decreases platelet aggregation	Administer with food; observe for signs of intestinal bleeding, tinnitus. Monitor blood count and liver enzymes.	Instruct to take with a full glass of water and when in an upright position. Ask to report any blood in stool, bleeding gums, nose bleeds, or excessive bruising. Report ringing in the ears or skin rash. Caution not to crush the pill. Do not take OTC products containing aspirin or salicylic acid.
Phenytoin (Dilantin)	Alters ion transport, inhibiting spread of seizure activity to motor cortex	Assess for skin rash; monitor drug levels, CBC; observe for respiratory depression. Shake suspension well; dilute before giving via feeding tube. Flush IV line with NS before and after administering slowly by IV piggyback. May cause Stevens-Johnson syndrome.	Teach that PO doses should be taken with meals; urine may turn pink; not to stop taking drug abruptly; take as directed; brush teeth and floss thoroughly and regularly, and visit dentist every 3-6 mo; do not use alcohol. Do not use antacids within 2 hr of the drug. Adjust to drug before operating machinery or performing hazardous activities.
Nimodipine (Nimotop)	Inhibits calcium ion flux across cellular membrane; decreases or prevents cerebral vasospasm	Frequent neurologic assessment and VS; monitor liver enzymes; assess BP and apical pulse immediately before administration. Hold if systolic BP is <90 mm Hg. Monitor for hypotension.	Advise that the drug may cause hypotension and dizziness with movement.

BP, blood pressure; *CBC,* complete blood count; *CVA,* cerebrovascular accident; *IV,* intravenous; *NS,* normal saline; *NSAIDs,* nonsteroidal anti-inflammatory drugs; *OTC,* over the counter; *PO,* oral; *t-PA,* tissue plasminogen activator; *VS,* vital signs.
See Chapter 21 for information on warfarin (Coumadin).

FIGURE 24-4 Each area of the brain controls a particular activity.

understand (*dysarthria* or *aphasia*), difficulty with vision, loss of balance or poor coordination (ataxia), decreased level of consciousness, and confusion. Incontinence may occur. Bleeding into the brain or edema around necrotic tissue causes intracranial pressure (ICP) to increase (see Chapter 23 regarding increasing ICP).

Motor function deficits affect mobility, respiratory function, swallowing, speech, gag reflex, and self-care abilities. Because the pyramidal pathways cross at the level of the medulla, injury to brain cells in the right hemisphere affects the left side of the body and damage to cells in the left hemisphere affects the right side of the body. There may be hemiplegia or hemiparesis. Muscle tone is usually flaccid at first, and then there may be spasticity and hyperreflexia. Keeping the body in good alignment to prevent contractures is very important.

Language disorders involve expression and comprehension of both written and spoken words. Aphasia or **dysphasia** (minimal speech activity) or a mixed type of aphasia may occur (see Chapter 22). Many stroke patients experience *dysarthria* (difficulty in speaking) due to lack of muscular control of the tongue. A speech therapist works with the patient to improve speech capability. There are computer software programs for rehabilitation of the aphasic patient that have been beneficial to many.

The frustration of trying to perform a function that has always been easy before the stroke may cause the patient to cry. Alternatively, the patient may display an angry emotional outburst, and sometimes foul language.

Clinical Cues

Because of the damage to the nervous tissue, fatigue is another problem for the stroke patient. When working with the patient to relearn walking, dressing, or other activities, keep the session short and allow for adequate rest periods between activities.

Memory and judgment may be affected by the stroke. The ability to learn may be affected, which makes relearning activities to promote independence a slow process. A great deal of patience and encouragement is needed from the staff working with the patient.

Spatial-perceptual deficits may cause the patient to totally neglect input from the affected side of the body (*unilateral neglect*). She must be taught to attend to the body parts on that side of the body in order to protect them from injury. **Homonymous hemianopsia** (blindness in part of the visual field of both eyes) adds to the spatial-perceptual problems by making it difficult to judge distances (Figure 24-5). The patient is taught ways to deal with the problems of the particular type of visual defect developed. **Agnosia** (inability to recognize an object by sight, touch, or hearing) makes it difficult to do ordinary tasks. **Apraxia** (the inability to

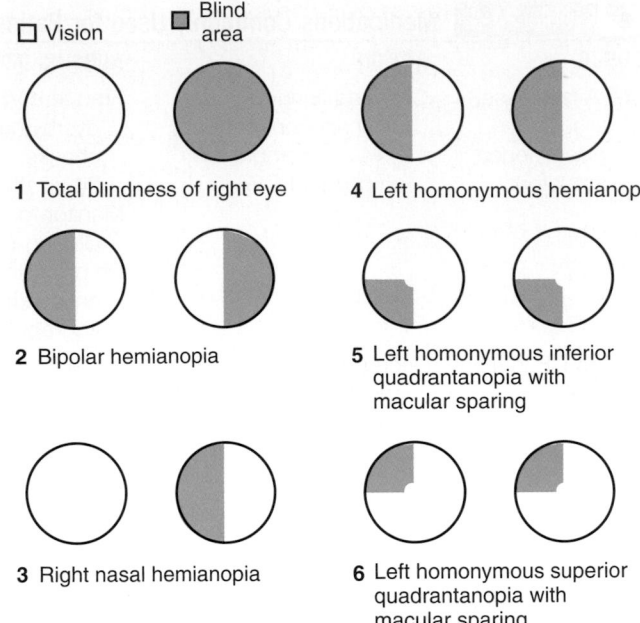

FIGURE 24-5 Homonymous hemianopsia: visual field defects that can occur after a stroke.

carry out learned sequential movements on command) adds to the difficulty in regaining independence.

Bladder and bowel incontinence are often temporary after a stroke. Constipation does occur because of immobility, weakened abdominal muscles, dehydration, and diminished response to the defecation reflex. The patient's inability to express needs and her difficulty in managing clothing contribute to bladder and bowel incontinence and constipation. With time, these problems can be overcome.

Diagnosis

In addition to a complete physical and neurologic examination, the physician may order an MRI or cerebral angiogram to determine the specific cause of the stroke. An EEG is performed; brain scans or transcranial Doppler flow studies and carotid artery Doppler studies may also be ordered. Testing for blood levels of glutamate, which will increase and damage brain tissue during a progressive ischemic stroke, may alert physicians to patients whose condition is likely to rapidly deteriorate. If a hemorrhagic stroke is suspected, a lumbar puncture will be performed to see if there is blood in the cerebrospinal fluid.

Treatment

When a stroke is suspected, the first priority is to maintain an open airway. All constricting clothing around the patient's neck should be removed, and the patient should be turned to one side to prevent aspiration of saliva and obstruction of the air passages. When outside of the hospital, no attempt should be made to move the person until an ambulance has arrived. Reassure the patient, regardless of whether or not she is able to respond. Elevate the head slightly to reduce ICP.

Once under medical care, supplemental oxygen is started. If breathing is impaired or the patient is comatose, an artificial airway is inserted to maintain a patent airway, and the patient may be mechanically ventilated. Hypovolemia is treated with fluids, and hypertension of greater than 220/130 mm Hg is treated. Vital signs may be unstable. Two IV lines for drug and fluid access are inserted, and normal saline is administered. Electrolytes are assessed frequently to prevent imbalances. If the temperature is elevated and rising, a hypothermia blanket may be used to keep the temperature down (Jauch, 2011). Measures to prevent deep vein thrombosis are instituted.

 Clinical Cues

There is a fine line between keeping blood pressure high enough to perfuse the brain when an obstruction is present, and keeping blood pressure low enough to prevent vessel rupture or increased bleeding from a rupture that has occurred.

Once the specific cause of the stroke has been determined, the physician is able to plan a more effective regimen of care. Alteplase or systemic tissue plasminogen activator (t-PA) is used to dissolve clots and emboli in ischemic stroke. It must be administered within 3 to 6 hours of the onset of symptoms and clot location (Jauch, 2011). The drugs are effective in about one of eight patients treated. Sometimes the fibrinolytic drug is directed to the clot via a catheter positioned during angiography. A new drug, caffeinol, improves the outcome in ischemic stroke, when administered IV. It is a combination of caffeine and ethanol. Platelet inhibitors and anticoagulants may be given to prevent further clot formation. If t-PA has been given, no anticoagulants or antiplatelet aggregation drugs are given for 24 hours. **The drug is *not* administered to anyone with a known risk of bleeding or who has had an intracerebral bleed.** Antihypertensive drugs are ordered as appropriate. Oral warfarin may be started after the acute stage of a thrombotic stroke.

! Safety Alert

Cranberry Juice Interaction

The consumption of cranberry juice while taking warfarin (Coumadin) can produce an interaction that increases the serum level of the drug, extending clotting time. Patients who drink cranberry juice should consult their physicians. Off-and-on intake of cranberry juice will affect the prothrombin time and international normalized ratio (INR).

A recombinant human interleukin-1 receptor antagonist has been shown to be effective in patients with acute stroke symptoms in reducing the amount of injury and residual deficits; research is continuing. Use of a natural growth factor, neuregulin-1, which protects brain cells from the damage caused by stroke, is also under study. The biggest benefit of neuregulin-1 is that its therapeutic window is much longer than t-PA and it can be administered up to 13 hours after the onset of the stroke. This drug has shown no adverse side effects to date. Desmoteplase is a genetically engineered version of a protein in a vampire bat's saliva that prevents clotting. The drug can break down a clot without affecting the coagulation system, thereby decreasing the risk of intracerebral bleeding. It works when given within 9 hours of a stroke and is in Phase III clinical trials.

Nimodipine or nifedipine may be given to decrease arterial spasm if the stroke is from subarachnoid hemorrhage. Testing of new drugs continues in an effort to find a way to decrease the resultant damage from a stroke. Another neuroprotective drug being tested, citicoline, is thought to speed recovery and improve the patient's mental functioning (Dugdale & Hoch, 2009). Hypertonic saline infusion is being studied as a treatment for hemorrhagic stroke to improve oxygenation of the brain and to decrease ICP. The patient is given sedation and analgesia for the headache and neck pain. Blood glucose levels are monitored and controlled.

Surgical Procedures. About one third of all strokes can be traced to obstruction of any one of the four arteries in the neck that supply blood to the brain. These arteries are generally accessible, so the surgeon can open the artery and remove the obstruction, which is usually from plaque buildup. The vessel wall is then sutured or a Dacron patch is sewn at the incision, leaving the vessel larger than before.

The Mechanical Embolus Removal in Cerebral Ischemia (MERCI) Retriever can be used up to 8 hours after the onset of an ischemic stroke to remove a thrombus. A catheter is threaded up through the femoral artery to the brain and a wire device is guided through the catheter to the brain. The end of the wire resembles a corkscrew and ensnares the clot, which is pulled out through the catheter (Lutsep, 2009). The interventional radiologist performs this procedure during angiography. If successful, blood flow can be restored to the brain within 20 minutes. Several mechanical methods for clot dissolution or retrieval are undergoing trials. Clot aspiration is another retrieval method. Several methods of mechanical removal of a clot are undergoing trials. There are risks of bleeding with these procedures that must be considered.

A cerebral aneurysm may be repaired during a craniotomy by placing a clip around the stalk of the aneurysm. The aneurysm may be wrapped with a material that prevents the wall from rupturing if it cannot be clipped or resected. A radiologic procedure wherein

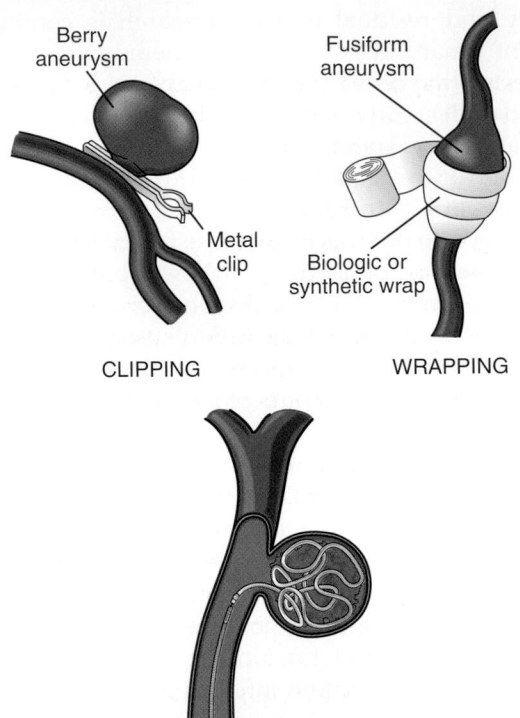

CLIPPING   WRAPPING

COILS CAUSE THROMBOSIS

FIGURE 24-6 Techniques used for aneurysm repair.

a small platinum wire is guided carefully into the aneurysm is another option. Coils of wire are curled into the aneurysm sac, filling it (Figure 24-6). Electricity is sent down the wire to break the wire off and leave the coils in the aneurysm. Thrombosis completes the solidification of the aneurysm, effectively eliminating it. AVMs are treated in much the same way, but may be eliminated using radiosurgery. More than one type of intervention may be used.

Neurologic assessments are performed often to monitor closely for signs of increasing ICP (see Chapter 23). Measures are instituted to prevent or alleviate a rise in ICP. Increased ICP occurs most frequently with a subarachnoid hemorrhage.

Complications

Extension of Hemorrhage or Rebleed. If initial symptoms were caused by a leaking cerebral aneurysm, rupture is a danger until the aneurysm is repaired. Neurologic signs and level of consciousness are watched closely to detect deterioration of the patient's condition due to further bleeding and a rise in ICP. The patient is kept as quiet as possible, with outside stimuli kept to a minimum. An aneurysm that is repaired by wrapping or embolization has a greater chance of bleeding again than one that is repaired with a clip.

Seizures. Seizures are a common complication of a stroke because neural pathways are interrupted when blood flow is blocked or there is irritation of the cerebral cortex from an intracerebral bleed. The type of seizure depends on the area of the brain involved and the extent of the intracerebral bleed or blockage of blood flow. Generalized seizures may occur. The patient may be started on an anticonvulsant to prevent seizure occurrence. The tensing of muscles during a generalized seizure increases ICP. Anticonvulsant therapy may be continued for many months to 2 years after the last seizure occurs.

Hydrocephalus. If blood has leaked into the ventricular system, it interferes with the resorption of cerebrospinal fluid (CSF), causing hydrocephalus. This is more common when a subarachnoid hemorrhage has occurred. It may be necessary to prevent increased ICP by shunting the fluid out of the brain; a catheter is placed into the lateral ventricle and then tunneled down to the right atrium or the peritoneal cavity to drain the excess fluid.

❖ NURSING MANAGEMENT

When the stroke patient is first admitted to the hospital, the general state of health is assessed as well as effects of the stroke. The Agency for Healthcare Research and Quality (2009) has issued clinical practice guidelines for post-stroke rehabilitation. Standardized, validated assessment tools are used to determine deficits and to measure progress toward recovery.

Care of the stroke patient can be divided into three phases: *phase 1,* or initial care; *phase 2,* which is concerned with rehabilitation efforts; and *phase 3,* during which plans are made for continuity of care once the patient returns home. These are not phases in the sense that one begins only after another is finished. There is overlapping of activities in each phase. Because about 80% of all stroke victims survive the first or initial phase of their illness, rehabilitation and plans for self-care are of the utmost importance. The Joint Commission's Core Measures require that the patient receive venous thromboembolism prophylaxis, be discharged on antithrombotic therapy and statin medication, receive thrombolytic therapy if appropriate that is discontinued by day 2, receive stroke education, and be assessed for rehabilitation. Chapter 9 discusses concepts of rehabilitation.

Assess stroke patients for risk of falls and institute appropriate interventions to prevent falls. Assess pain regularly using an appropriate validated pain scale. A nutritional and dysphagia screening should be done within 24 hours of being awake and alert (Registered Nurses Association of Ontario, 2010).

Phase 1

■ Assessment (Data Collection)

Immediate assessment of breathing and respiratory rate is essential. Level of consciousness (LOC) is assessed next. Initial care of the stroke patient includes careful assessment to determine the extent to which neurologic functions have been affected. Complete hemiplegia is a common effect of stroke. Aphasia often indicates ischemia of the brain cells on the left side of the brain and is usually accompanied by right-sided hemiplegia. Figure 24-7 illustrates deficits often experienced by damage to the left or right side of the brain.

🔳 Clinical Cues

If any change in the patient's thought processes or LOC appear, or the patient becomes more restless, notify the physician immediately as these may be early signs of increasing ICP. Treatment to decrease ICP may prevent disability and may prevent death from herniation of the brain.

After the acute stage of the stroke has passed and there is physiologic stability, an assessment of functional abilities is performed so that rehabilitation goals and plans can be devised. Assessment of and nursing intervention for the patient with problems of immobility, incontinence of urine and feces, aphasia, delirium or confusion, and altered LOC are discussed in Chapter 22. Because the patient who has suffered a stroke is at risk for a second occurrence, assessment for new signs of neurologic impairment is ongoing.

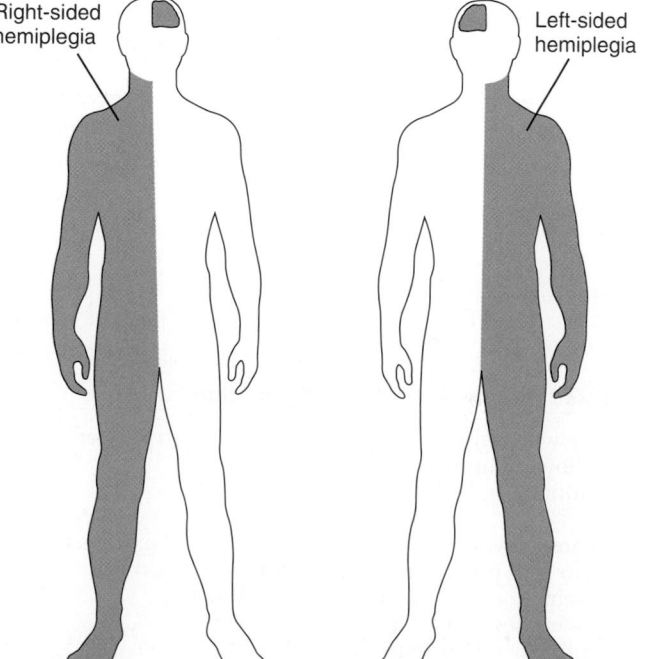

LEFT-SIDED BRAIN DAMAGE
• Slow and cautious in behavior
• Speech problems, aphasia
• Difficulty in following verbal commands
• Apraxia
• Difficulty in performing simple tasks

Right-sided hemiplegia

RIGHT-SIDED BRAIN DAMAGE
• Quick and impulsive in behavior
• Short attention span
• Neglects left side
• Easily distracted

Left-sided hemiplegia

FIGURE 24-7 Comparison of deficits and behavior related to damage to the left and right sides of the brain.

■ Nursing Diagnosis and Planning

Nursing diagnoses for the patient who has experienced a CVA commonly include:
• Risk for injury related to weakness, paralysis, confusion, decreased consciousness, or unilateral neglect
• Impaired physical mobility related to weakness or paralysis
• Imbalanced nutrition: less than body requirements related to impaired swallowing and hemiparesis or hemiplegia
• Self-care deficit related to inability to perform activities of daily living (ADLs—feeding, bathing, grooming) without assistance
• Functional urinary incontinence related to neurologic deficits
• Bowel incontinence related to impaired mobility and neurologic impairment
• Risk for impaired skin integrity related to decreased mobility, paresis, or paralysis
• Impaired verbal communication related to inability to clearly verbalize or inability to comprehend communication
• Disturbed body image related to neurologic damage and hemiplegia
• Disturbed sensory perception: visual—related to loss of vision in parts of visual field; *kinesthetic*—related to decreased sense of touch on one side of the body
• Situational low self-esteem related to alteration in body image and to dependence on others
• Ineffective coping related to loss of usual lifestyle, neurologic deficits, and dependence on others
• Unilateral neglect related to lack of sensation in extremity

Planning for specific goals must take into account the individual patient's previous lifestyle, age, general health or illness status, and specific problems of care. The 80-year-old retired person will not have the same goals for rehabilitation and recovery as the 47-year-old mother of three who had been working full time as a schoolteacher before her attack.

Major nursing goals during the first phase are to:
• Maintain an adequate airway
• Establish baseline data regarding vital signs, LOC, neuromuscular function, and neurologic status
• Preserve joint and muscle function
• Prevent complications that may interfere with rehabilitation

Specific individual expected outcomes are written for each identified problem or nursing diagnosis (see Nursing Care Plan 24-1).

■ Implementation

The amount of activity permitted a stroke patient during the initial acute stage of her illness depends on the cause of the stroke. If there is danger of continued hemorrhage from a ruptured artery and resultant increase in ICP, physical activity will necessarily be limited. When there is no danger of further damage to the brain, the patient usually is encouraged to become active as soon as her condition has stabilized.

Think Critically

What interventions would you employ to help the patient with unilateral neglect?

Many patients have *dysphagia* (difficulty swallowing) as a result of the stroke. The speech therapist should be called to do a swallowing study and to devise a plan to improve swallowing. Be certain the patient has a gag reflex by having her sip a small amount of water before feeding orally. When the patient has dysphagia, aspiration when eating is a real danger.

Measures to prevent complications, such as subcutaneous low-molecular-weight heparin injections and elastic stockings to prevent deep venous thrombosis,

---

Nursing Care Plan 24-1 | Care of the Patient Who Has Experienced a Stroke

Scenario
Mr. Lewis, age 68, suffered an ischemic stroke (CVA) 4 days ago. He is experiencing left-sided paresis, decreased alertness, and difficulty swallowing.

Problem/Nursing Diagnosis
Groggy, but arousable/Ineffective cerebral tissue perfusion related to obstruction from a thrombus.

Supporting Assessment Data
Subjective: "What day did you say it was?"
Objective: Requires shaking his shoulder and calling his name to arouse him. Thrombotic ischemic CVA.

Goals/Expected Outcomes	Nursing Interventions	Selected Rationale	Evaluation
Patient will show no further decrease in LOC.	Monitor neurologic status q 2 hr. Notify physician of decreasing LOC, pupil changes, change in respiratory pattern, widening pulse pressure, slowing of pulse, or increase in temperature.	Changes in neurologic signs may indicate rising intracranial pressure.	No changes in neurologic signs. Difficult to arouse, but orients quickly.
	Monitor for seizure activity.	Seizure activity is common after a brain injury or CVA.	No signs of seizure activity.
	Administer medications to prevent clot formation as ordered.	Aspirin is effective to help prevent clot formation.	Managed to swallow the enteric-coated aspirin tablet.
	Monitor for bleeding gums, blood in urine or stool.	Anticoagulants may cause bleeding.	No signs of blood in urine or stool; gums not bleeding.

Problem/Nursing Diagnosis
Trouble swallowing food and large pill/Impaired swallowing related to weakness of swallowing muscles.

Supporting Assessment Data
Subjective: "I almost choked on that capsule."
Objective: Coughing when trying to swallow capsule.

Goals/Expected Outcomes	Nursing Interventions	Selected Rationale	Evaluation
Patient will not aspirate food or pills.	Place in high Fowler's position for meals, snacks, and oral medication administration.	Gravity will assist swallowing in this position.	Raised to high Fowler's for oral intake.
	Instruct to tilt head and neck forward when attempting to swallow.	Facilitates elevation of the larynx and posterior movement of the tongue allowing food to go into esophagus rather than trachea.	Is tilting head and neck forward when swallowing.

CVA, cerebrovascular accident; *LOC*, level of consciousness; *ROM*, range of motion.

Goals/Expected Outcomes	Nursing Interventions	Selected Rationale	Evaluation
Patient will not aspirate food or pills—cont'd	Have swallow a sip of water before eating or taking an oral medication.		Swallows sip of water without much difficulty now.
	Assist to choose foods for meals that are easily swallowed.	Custard, eggs, canned fruit, mashed potatoes, and other soft foods are more easily swallowed.	Choosing soft foods for tomorrow's meals.
	Encourage to take small bites of food.	Small amounts are more easily swallowed than large amounts.	Is taking small bites of food.
	Use a thickening agent in liquids if they are particularly hard to swallow.	Thickening makes liquids easier to swallow without aspirating.	Thickening agent not needed.
	Avoid putting foods of different texture in the mouth at the same time.		Is eating one type of food at a time.
	Reinforce swallowing techniques/exercises recommended by speech therapist.	Muscle strengthening exercises may improve swallowing if done regularly.	Is practicing techniques suggested by speech therapist to improve swallowing.

Problem/Nursing Diagnosis
Left arm and leg weakness/Risk for injury related to muscle weakness in left extremities.

Supporting Assessment Data
Subjective: "I can't put full weight on my left leg."
Objective: Left leg unable to push much against resistance; when trying to stand, left leg will not support full weight.

Goals/Expected Outcomes	Nursing Interventions	Selected Rationale	Evaluation
Patient will not fall or sustain injury before or after discharge.	Assist to stand and walk to the bathroom.	Assistance prevents falling.	Using gait belt and cane to walk to bathroom.
	Instructed not to get up without assistance.		Asking for assistance to go to the bathroom.
	Place call bell within reach each time he is repositioned.	Allows patient to call for help when wishing to arise.	
	Encourage ROM exercises and strengthening exercises taught by physical therapist.	Working the muscles may improve muscle tone.	Performing ROM and strengthening exercises 3 times/day.

Problem/Nursing Diagnosis
Is left-handed and cannot shave himself or comb his hair well/Self-care deficit related to weakness and fatigue.

Supporting Assessment Data
Subjective: "I'm too weak to hold the razor properly to shave."
Objective: Hand shakes when trying to grip razor and shave.

Goals/Expected Outcomes	Nursing Interventions	Selected Rationale	Evaluation
Patient will resume some self-grooming by discharge.	Assist with bathing, dressing, and grooming.	Assistance prevents undue fatigue. Assistance helps accomplish daily hygiene activities.	Assistance with bathing, dressing, and grooming provided.
	Encourage patient to attempt to comb hair and brush teeth.	Small accomplishments provide hope of independence.	Attempted to comb hair with right hand; praise given.
	Praise for every successful attempt at self-care.	Praise reinforces desired behavior.	
	Help to practice shaving with electric razor using right hand.	New skills improve with practice.	Wife will bring in an electric razor for him tomorrow. Continue plan.

Continued

★ Nursing Care Plan 24-1	Care of the Patient Who Has Experienced a Stroke—cont'd

Problem/Nursing Diagnosis
Left extremity weakness, difficulty in remembering things/Ineffective coping related to memory impairment, difficulty swallowing, and paresis of left extremities.

Supporting Assessment Data
Subjective: "I don't want to be a burden to my wife."
Objective: Tends to forget what wife or nurses have told him; eyes fill with tears at times.

Goals/Expected Outcomes	Nursing Interventions	Selected Rationale	Evaluation
Patient will express hope of full recovery before discharge.	Assure that it is too early to tell if there will be any permanent disability from the stroke.	Validates that the future is not known at this time.	Assurance given during bathing discussion.
	Help patient explore his fears and anxieties about his condition and his future.	Expressing fears decreases anxiety.	Spoke about fear of being dependent on wife for daily care.
	Actively listen with patience when patient shares his thoughts.	Actively listening establishes trust and provides emotional support.	Sat with patient, established eye contact, and listened to his concerns.
	Do not express negative thoughts or opinions about his condition or progress in his or his wife's presence.	Negative thoughts can destroy hope.	No negative comments made.
	Point out each small bit of progress in self-care, eating, and mobility.	Acknowledging progress toward recovery helps dispel fear of permanent dependence.	Acknowledged improvement in swallowing at noon meal. Continue plan.

Critical Thinking Questions
1. How would you incorporate Mrs. Lewis into the care of her husband?
2. What might be accomplished with a social services consultation for this patient?
3. How could a social services consult be helpful for this patient and his wife?

skin care to minimize the risk of skin breakdown, physical therapy and splinting to prevent contractures and spasticity, and measures to prevent falls, are included in the complete plan of care. To reduce the possibility of recurrence of a stroke, risk factors are identified and teaching is begun to modify them.

Listening to music after a stroke seems to improve recovery, according to studies done in Finland (Gutierrez, 2008).

■ **Evaluation**

Evaluation is based on whether the interventions are effective in achieving the expected outcomes. Assess whether the overall goals have been met. If the outcomes are not being met, the care plan must be revised.

Phase 2

■ **Rehabilitation**

Plans for rehabilitation should begin the moment the patient is admitted. This means maintenance of an adequate airway and aeration of the lungs, proper positioning, range-of-motion exercises for affected limbs,

adequate nutrition and fluid intake and output, prevention of pressure ulcers, use of devices to keep extremities in anatomical position, and all other nursing measures directed toward maintaining normal body functions until the patient is able to maintain them on her own.

If the patient suffers from homonymous hemianopsia, she has a visual defect affecting the same half of the visual field in each eye. She will not be able to see past the midline toward the side opposite the lesion and must turn her head to scan that side (see Figure 24-5). The problem may cause accidents when ambulating. The patient must be taught ways to deal with this visual problem. Teach the patient with unilateral neglect to bathe both sides of the body. Demonstrate how to dress the affected side first. The weakened arm and/or leg must be positioned in correct alignment when the patient moves. A sling may be used to prevent shoulder subluxation of the affected upper extremity.

If disabilities from inactivity are avoided, rehabilitation has a much better chance of success. During phase 2, various members of the health care team collaborate

Nutrition Considerations

The Patient Who Has Dysphagia

To help prevent aspiration, tell the patient to:

- Sit up straight to eat, and tilt your head slightly forward.
- Place only one teaspoon of food in your mouth at a time.
- If you have paresis from a stroke, the food should be placed on the unaffected side of your mouth.
- Place your chin on your chest and swallow; wait a few seconds and swallow again.
- Refrain from taking liquids and solids at the same time.
- Sip from the cup or glass rather than use a straw.
- Remain in an upright position for 45 to 60 minutes after a meal.

Interventions to assist the patient to eat without aspirating include:

- Plan a 30-minute rest and relaxation period before each meal.
- Allow plenty of time for a relaxed meal.
- Serve food cold or well warmed; lukewarm foods are more difficult to swallow.
- Serve foods in the consistency ordered; some patients find semisolid food easier to swallow.
- Avoid serving peanut butter, syrup, and bananas because they are sticky and difficult to swallow.
- Avoid serving dry foods such as rice, popcorn, toast, or crackers as they tend to be more difficult to swallow and can stick in the throat.
- Keep the container for liquids less than two-thirds full so that the patient does not have to tilt the head back too far to drink. Tilting the head back tends to cause fluid to go into the trachea.

with the patient and her family to help resolve both psychosocial and physical problems. Among the team members helping the stroke victim may be the physical therapist, speech pathologist, social worker, psychologist, and occupational therapist. The patient usually is transferred from the hospital to a rehabilitation facility. The patient is encouraged with physical therapy to strengthen her muscles as well as her resolve to help herself. She will need to exercise her muscles actively and retrain them.

There are many ways to encourage the patient. Instead of feeding her every item on her tray, let her hold bread and other "finger foods," suggesting that she feed herself these things. Chewing may be slow at first; the patient should not be hurried, nor should she be allowed to chew to the point of exhaustion. Eating often is difficult and messy, and privacy must be provided. If hemiplegia is causing the patient to "pocket" food in the folds of the mouth, the mouth should be checked after meals.

Combing and brushing the hair is good exercise for the arm and shoulder, as are brushing the teeth and washing the face and hands. The patient may not be able to carry all these procedures through to completion at first, but with occupational therapy and encouragement she can gradually improve until she is able to

perform much of her own personal care. **The patient who has suffered brain injury becomes fatigued very quickly, and this must be kept in mind when performing self-care activities.** Encouragement and praise for the smallest accomplishment can help the patient's tattered self-esteem.

The stroke patient can be prone to rapid mood swings and spontaneous weeping. All health care workers must be patient and accepting, and an explanation to the patient and family that this is common after a stroke can ease the patient's embarrassment.

Various rehabilitation techniques are undergoing trials to see if more function can be regained in the extremities. Further information on rehabilitation programs is located in Chapter 9.

Phase 3

■ Continuum of Care

In phase 3, plans are made for discharge and referral to individuals and agencies outside the hospital that will help the patient and her family adjust to her new way of life. A visiting nurse often is assigned for a period of time to coordinate rehabilitation efforts, assist with teaching, and assess the patient's status. The patient continues rehabilitation as an outpatient under the physician's supervision. In some rural areas, Tele-Health services using the Internet and telephone are available to provide continued speech therapy.

BRAIN TUMOR

Etiology and Pathophysiology

About 200,000 new brain tumors are discovered each year in the United States. About 40,000 of those are primary tumors and the rest are metastatic tumors from a different site of origin (Table 24-2). It is not known how brain tumors begin, and there are over 120 different types. Low-grade astrocytomas are more common in young people than in older adults (Kennedy, 2009). High-grade gliomas are more prevalent in the elderly. Cerebellar tumors are more common in children.

Neoplasms within the confines of the skull are space-occupying lesions, and thus create problems of increasing ICP by compressing adjacent tissues. If the tumor arises from brain cells, the cranial nerves, or the pituitary gland, the neoplastic cells can infiltrate and destroy these structures; other types of tumor can destroy tissue through pressure. Many brain tumors are benign, such as a meningioma or acoustic neuroma. However, because of increased ICP that tumors cause and the way they can invade brain tissue, a benign tumor also presents a serious condition.

Intracranial tumors may begin in the brain itself, or they may begin in the meninges, cranial nerves, or pituitary gland. Primary malignant brain tumors

Table 24-2 Different Types of Brain Tumors*

TUMOR	TYPE OF TISSUE
Gliomas (malignant)	
Glioblastoma multiforme	Primitive stem cells (glioblasts)
Astrocytoma	Astrocytes and glial cells
Medulloblastoma	Primitive neuroectodermal cells
Oligodendroglioma	Oligodendrocytes
Ependymoma	Ependymal epithelium
Pituitary adenoma (usually benign)	Pituitary gland cells
Acoustic neuroma (usually benign)	Myelin sheath cells of cranial nerve VIII
Meningioma (most often benign)	Cells of the meninges
Hemangioblastoma (benign)	Cells from blood vessels in the brain
Metastatic tumors (malignant)	Mostly from lung, breast, kidney, thyroid, and prostate carcinomas

*Primary brain tumors are classified by the type of tissue from which they derive.

rarely metastasize outside the brain. Tumors in the cerebral hemispheres are termed *supratentorial* and those located beneath the tentorium (fold of dura mater) are termed *infratentorial*. This area of the cerebral hemisphere contains the structures of the brainstem and the cerebellum.

Signs, Symptoms, and Diagnosis

There can be as many symptoms of intracranial tumors as there are functions of the structures within the skull. The symptoms depend on location and may appear gradually, or—if the tumor is a highly malignant, fast-growing type—they may appear suddenly. In a slow-growing type of tumor, the patient may first show personality changes, disturbances in judgment and memory, loss of muscular strength and coordination, or difficulty in speaking clearly. Headache awakening the patient is a key sign. Vomiting, visual problems, and other signs of increased ICP also may occur. Approximately 20% to 50% of adults with brain tumors develop seizure activity. Diagnostic procedures to identify the site and extent of intracranial tumors include skull x-rays, MRI, computed tomography (CT) scan, and arteriography.

Treatment

The three modes of therapy for intracranial tumors are the same as those for neoplastic diseases elsewhere in the body: surgery, radiation therapy, and chemotherapy. Radiation is usually given 5 days a week for 6 weeks. With brachytherapy, tiny radioactive particles are inserted into the tumor tissue via an implanted catheter. This treatment extends over about 5 days. Radiation precautions are needed during this period. If the tumor is found while it is still very small, a

stereotactic Cyberknife or gamma knife procedure may destroy it. Gamma knife procedures use a steel frame attached to the head with ports through which radiation is directed from several angles. Cyberknife procedures use a molded head mask or body mask to keep the patient from moving during treatment. Measurements are calculated by a computer to precisely locate the tumor, and the radiation is delivered only to the tumor, which spares surrounding tissue. These procedures also can be used for small recurrent tumor growth (see Figure 8-4).

Most chemotherapy drugs cannot cross the blood-brain barrier. To get the drugs into the brain circulation, an Ommaya reservoir may be implanted between the scalp and the skull. An Ommaya reservoir consists of a port attached to a catheter that is placed in the lateral ventricle of the brain (Figure 24-8). Chemotherapy drugs can be injected into the port and instilled into the CSF in the ventricle. In this way the chemotherapy drug is carried to the tumor cells in greater quantity than can be achieved by infusion of the drugs into the bloodstream. The FDA has approved a wearable device that blasts glioblastoma brain tumors via an electrical field (Walker, 2011).

In patients for whom chemotherapy and radiation have previously failed, implantation of carmustine (BiCNU; Gliadel) wafers into a glial cell tumor slows growth. The drug is inserted into brain tissue after removal of the glioma, to fight the malignancy and slow or prevent regrowth. Temozolomide (Temodar) is an oral chemotherapeutic drug that does cross the blood-brain barrier. Trials with local hyperthermia, biologic therapy, electrochemotherapy, and immunotherapy are underway. Molecularly targeted drugs include erlotinib (Tarceva), gefitinib (Iressa), and

FIGURE 24-8 Implantation of an Ommaya reservoir for chemotherapy of a brain tumor.

bevacizumab (Avastin). Treatments are discussed more thoroughly in Chapter 8. If there are signs of increased ICP, measures are instituted to try to lower the ICP and to provide supportive care (see Chapter 23).

Surgery. Surgery is used to remove intracranial tumors and then other modes of treatment are used to destroy remaining cells. Sometimes, however, the tumor has infiltrated vital parts of the brain that must not be traumatized by surgical procedures. If the tumor is located in the cerebrum, a *craniotomy* is done. A "window flap" of scalp and bone is cut and pulled down, the dura is opened, and the tumor is removed. Tumors in or near the *cerebellum* are removed through an incision under the occipital bone. If all of the tumor cannot be removed, a portion of the tumor may be removed to relieve compression of the brain against the skull. This procedure is only a temporary measure to relieve the patient's symptoms. Care of the patient after brain surgery is presented in Chapter 23.

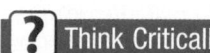 **Think Critically**

How should the patient who has had a craniotomy for a supratentorial tumor be positioned?

Nursing Management
Routine neurologic assessments are performed, as well as assessment of ability to perform ADLs. Pain assessment and control are important. Helping the patient and family to communicate fears and cope with the situation should be part of the care plan. Nursing diagnoses commonly used for the patient with a brain tumor are:

- Ineffective tissue perfusion related to tumor pressure and cerebral edema
- Pain related to cerebral edema and increased ICP
- Self-care deficit related to altered neuromuscular function, sensory deficits, or decreased LOC
- Anxiety or fear related to diagnosis and prognosis
- Risk for injury related to seizure activity caused by the tumor
- Risk for injury related to increasing ICP from tumor growth
- Impaired memory related to damaged cells from pressure
- Impaired home maintenance related to physical impairments
- Disturbed personal identity related to inability to work

Specific outcomes appropriate for the individual are written and interventions are planned to help the patient meet the outcomes. Evaluation is based on data that indicate the outcomes are being met. (See Chapter 22 for care for common problems and interventions for various nursing diagnoses related to neurologic problems; see Nursing Care Plan 23-1 and pp. 504 to 505 for further interventions.)

FIGURE 24-9 Ventriculoperitoneal shunt to drain excess cerebrospinal fluid into the peritoneal cavity, where it is absorbed through the mucosa.

Complications
Hydrocephalus. Obstruction of CSF flow may require placing a shunt to reduce CSF pressure and prevent increased ICP. A shunt is a tube placed in a ventricle and attached to a small manual pump that moves excess CSF fluid from the ventricles to the peritoneal cavity or into the atrium of the heart, from where it is absorbed (Figure 24-9).

Intracerebral Hemorrhage. Bleeding in the brain may occur as the tumor erodes blood vessels. Depending on the condition of the patient, the size of the tumor, and prognosis, various measures to stop the bleeding and reduce ICP will be employed.

INFECTIOUS AND INFLAMMATORY DISORDERS OF THE NERVOUS SYSTEM

BACTERIAL MENINGITIS
Etiology and Pathophysiology
Meningitis is an inflammation of the membranes covering the brain and spinal cord and is caused by an infectious agent. Viruses, bacteria, and fungi can cause meningitis. Fungal meningitis occurs mostly in patients with AIDS. The membranes can become infected in a number of ways, because infectious agents can be carried through the bloodstream to the membranes, or brain tissue can become affected as an infection in a particular area of the brain spreads. Infection can spread from the spinal cord or sinuses to the brain. Two examples of how infectious organisms may enter the cranial vault other than via the bloodstream are (1) through an opening in the skull in a head injury or from surgery or (2) by accidental introduction of infectious agents into the spinal canal during spinal puncture.

Many different strains of bacteria can cause meningitis, but the causative organisms are usually the bacteria *Streptococcus pneumoniae* and *Neisseria meningitidis.* In children the causative organism may be *Haemophilus influenzae* type B. Bacterial meningitis frequently follows an upper respiratory infection. Immunization of all young adults against bacterial meningitis is recommended.

 Health Promotion

Meningitis Immunization

Meningitis vaccine is available and is required for all students entering college. It should be encouraged for adults living in a communal situation. Meningitis can spread quickly when people are in proximity, such as in classrooms or dormitory rooms.

A consequence of bacterial meningitis can be an increase in circulating CSF due to obstruction of normal mechanisms of CSF absorption. Bacteria, white blood cells, and debris block the arachnoid villi, resulting in an obstructive **hydrocephalus** (increased CSF in the ventricles of the brain) that increases ICP. Meningitis can cause permanent neurologic damage and may cause severe vasoconstriction that requires amputation of part of a limb.

Signs and Symptoms

The most outstanding symptom of meningitis is the **sudden onset of fever and a severe and persistent headache that is greatly aggravated by moving the head.** Other signs of meningeal irritation include pain and stiffness of the neck when flexing the neck (**nuchal rigidity),** as well as exaggerated deep tendon reflexes, irritability, photophobia, and hypersensitivity of the skin. A positive Brudzinski's sign can be elicited by placing a hand behind the patient's head and, with the other hand on the chest, gently flexing the patient's neck forward by moving her chin toward her chest. If there is flexion of the knees and hips when you try to flex the neck, Brudzinski's sign is positive and indicates meningeal irritation. For Kernig's sign, have the patient supine and, with the hip and knee flexed at 90-degree angles, slowly extend the knee (Figure 24-10). If there is pain, not just discomfort, behind the knee, Kernig's sign is positive, indicating meningeal irritation. Meningococcal meningitis often is accompanied by a petechial rash covering the chest and extremities. Seizures frequently occur, as well as nausea and vomiting, in the patient with meningitis. Quick medical attention is needed to prevent death.

Diagnosis

When meningitis is suspected, a spinal tap is performed, and the CSF is examined for the number and type of organisms present. The CSF pressure is elevated (see Chapter 22). A Gram stain identifies

FIGURE 24-10 A, Positive Brudzinski's sign: Passive flexion of the head and neck causes flexion of the thighs and legs. **B,** Positive Kernig's sign: Inability to extend the leg from a position of 90-degree flexion at the hip due to pain and spasms in the hamstring muscle.

the causative organism. Blood tests may be performed to rule out other disorders that can mimic meningitis.

 Clinical Cues

When meningitis is present, the spinal fluid may appear milky as a result of the increased number of white cells suspended in the fluid. Other abnormal findings in the CSF include the presence of protein and decreased amounts of glucose.

Treatment

Successful treatment of meningitis and prevention of permanent disability depend on early recognition and prompt treatment. Antibiotics are started immediately for bacterial meningitis, and when the causative organism has been identified, specific antibiotics to which the organism is sensitive are administered. A combination of two antibiotics is common. The disease usually responds well to IV antibiotic therapy followed by oral doses given for a total of 10 days. Dexamethasone along with the antibiotics has proven beneficial to decrease inflammation for many patients (Razonabie & Keating, 2009). Anticonvulsive drugs are administered to control seizures, and ibuprofen, aspirin, or acetaminophen is given for headache.

 Clinical Cues

Narcotics are rarely used for pain control in patients with increased ICP, as they cause sedation and prevent accurate neurologic assessment.

Prophylactic antibiotics are usually given to those in close contact with the patient to prevent the spread of the disease. Death occurs in about 25% of cases.

VIRAL MENINGITIS

Several viruses can cause meningitis, and the most common ones are enteroviruses, arboviruses, HIV, and herpes simplex virus. Viral meningitis tends to be milder than bacterial meningitis. The initial signs and symptoms include a headache, fever, photophobia, and stiff neck. Brain involvement symptoms are not usually present.

Examination of the CSF is performed to confirm the diagnosis. A complete blood count will show increased lymphocytes *(lymphocytosis)*. A polymerase chain reaction (PCR) test to detect virus-specific DNA or RNA can diagnose CNS viral infection.

The disease is self-limiting and is managed symptomatically. Full recovery of the patient is usual within 7 to 10 days. Sometimes residual effects such as persistent headaches, mild mental impairment, and lack of coordination occur.

❖ NURSING MANAGEMENT

■ Assessment (Data Collection) and Nursing Diagnosis

In addition to noting the specific signs and symptoms of meningitis, assess the patient for subjective and objective data relevant to each of the patient care problems that might accompany the disease. Examples include convulsive seizures, elevated body temperature, nausea and vomiting, delirium, pain, increased ICP, and fluid and electrolyte imbalances. Ongoing, vigilant neurologic assessment is a high priority in monitoring for signs of increasing ICP, changes in condition, and response to treatment. An ongoing assessment should be done each shift.

 Focused Assessment

Assessment of the Patient with Brain Infection

An assessment (data collection) should be performed each shift for the following areas:
- Neurologic check for increasing intracranial pressure
- Stiff neck or paralysis
- Temperature and monitoring of temperature trend
- Assessment for electrolyte and fluid imbalance; skin turgor, mucous membranes, condition of lips; intake and output
- Gastrointestinal assessment: bowel sounds, distention, constipation, diarrhea, nausea, vomiting
- Intravenous access site
- Skin condition
- Psychosocial concerns

Nursing diagnoses are written for the specific problems identified via data collection (see Table 22-9, Nursing Care Plan 23-1, and Nursing Care Plan 24-1).

■ Planning, Implementation, and Evaluation

Expected outcomes are written for the nursing diagnoses chosen. Specific nursing interventions in the care of the patient with meningitis are primarily concerned with measures to:
- Conserve the patient's strength
- Prevent seizures
- Promote healing

Preventing the spread of infection includes use of Standard Precautions and droplet precautions.

The patient's room should be quiet and dimly lit. Sudden noises or bright flashes of light can cause a seizure because the sensory input activates nerve impulses. Care and treatments are coordinated to allow as much rest as possible. Meningitis often produces mental confusion and delirium, as well as the possibility of seizures. *Herpes simplex* (fever blister) frequently accompanies meningitis.

 Clinical Cues

The presence of herpes lesions, plus drying of the lips and mouth from fever and dehydration, requires special mouth care. Using Standard Precautions (see Appendix B), the lips and mouth should be cleansed and lubricated at least every 2 hours during the acute stage of the disease.

Fluid volume deficit is often a problem. Monitor the patient's intake and output and prevent dehydration. Report excessive vomiting or outward signs of early dehydration promptly so that IV fluids may be given to correct fluid volume deficits. Administration of corticosteroids, mineralocorticoids, estrogens, and progesterones can increase ICP because they cause fluid retention.

Irritation of the neural centers in the brain may cause a decrease in the peristaltic action of the intestines in the patient with meningitis and can lead to an accumulation of flatus and fecal material with severe abdominal distention. Check the patient's abdomen for distention, and note bowel sounds and record them in the medical record. Rectal suppositories, simethicone, or small-volume enemas (less than 150 mL) may be ordered for relief.

The patient will need support and reassurance from the nurse, because the severity of this illness is frightening. If confusion occurs, frequent orientation is necessary. The family needs information and reassurance as well.

Once the acute stage of the disease is over, the patient is allowed to gradually resume her former activities. Side effects of the disease, such as paralysis, deafness, and visual defects, sometimes occur, but these *sequelae* (results) of meningitis do not usually occur if the disease is diagnosed and treated in the early stages. Gather evaluation data regarding the effect of the interventions performed. Determine if the expected outcomes are being met. If outcomes are not being met, the plan must be revised.

ENCEPHALITIS

Etiology and Pathophysiology

Encephalitis is less common than meningitis. It is an acute inflammation of the brain that is serious and sometimes fatal. Some of the viruses responsible for encephalitis are associated with particular seasons of the year or with geographic locations. Ticks and mosquitoes are the vectors that transmit the disease. Examples of viruses in the United States that cause encephalitis are eastern equine encephalomyelitis, western equine encephalomyelitis, La Crosse encephalitis, St. Louis encephalitis, and West Nile viruses. Encephalitis may occur as a complication of the viral diseases chickenpox, measles, and mumps. Postviral encephalitis is an immune-mediated disorder and follows the end of the viral infection by 2 to 12 days. Herpes simplex virus 1 (human herpesvirus 1) is frequently the cause of non–vector-transmitted encephalitis. Cytomegalovirus encephalitis is a complication in patients with AIDS.

 Health Promotion

Protect Against Mosquitoes and Ticks

During mosquito season, wear insect repellent and protective clothing. Prevent water from standing in containers around the home and property to discourage the breeding of mosquitoes. Avoid being out of doors for recreational purposes at dusk and at night, when mosquitoes are more likely to be about. Use insect repellent and protective clothing when out in wooded areas. Skin should be inspected for ticks after the outing.

 Clinical Cues

Whenever a patient is admitted with symptoms of a brain infection, check the skin thoroughly and question the patient about a recent history of herpes lesions. If you find any herpes lesions, or are told that they were present within the past several days, notify the physician immediately. Herpes encephalitis can be fatal if not treated early.

Once the virus crosses the blood-brain barrier and enters neural cells, disrupting normal neural function, hemorrhage and an inflammatory response occur in the gray matter.

The severity of the illness may be mild or fatal. The most common type of viral encephalitis in the United States is that caused by herpes simplex virus 1. West Nile virus has emerged as a cause of encephalitis since 1999.

Neurologic impairment is caused by direct infection of neural cells. Western equine encephalitis is usually seen in June and July. Herpes simplex encephalitis spreads from neural tissue to the CNS. It can be a primary or secondary infection and can occur from reactivation of latent virus. **If treatment for the herpes simplex is not started before coma occurs, death is almost certain.**

Signs, Symptoms, and Diagnosis

The onset of encephalitis may be either sudden or insidious. There may be behavioral and personality changes and a decreased LOC. **Stiff neck, photophobia, and lethargy are classic symptoms of encephalitis. Seizures, acute confusion, and flaccid paralysis may occur.** CNS signs usually appear 1 to 4 hours after the onset of other symptoms. Lethargy may progress to coma. The patient with herpes simplex encephalitis may exhibit flulike symptoms that rapidly progress.

Encephalitis symptoms differ from those of meningitis in that with encephalitis there is altered mental status, motor or sensory deficits, and speech or movement disorders.

Diagnosis is confirmed by the presence of the virus in the CSF or bloodstream. The CSF in herpes simplex encephalitis will show a slightly elevated white blood cell count, a small increase in protein, and normal glucose levels. PCR tests for herpes simplex virus DNA and RNA levels in CSF allow for early diagnosis. MRI, positron emission tomography scanning, and an EEG may be performed to demonstrate inflammation and the disruption of normal neural impulses. A brain biopsy may be required to verify the responsible organism so proper treatment can begin.

Treatment and Nursing Management

The treatment of encephalitis is primarily symptomatic, with general supportive measures to maintain cardiac and respiratory function, maintain the patient's strength, promote healing, and prevent complications. Herpes simplex type 1 encephalitis is treated with antiviral IV acyclovir. There is no specific drug treatment for other types of encephalitis.

Specific nursing measures are essentially the same as for any patient who is subject to seizures, high fever, delirium, or altered LOC (see Table 22-9). The nursing care plan must be individualized to the patient's needs.

Complications

Permanent neurologic disabilities may occur, such as problems with walking, paralysis, cognition, memory, and self-care. About 65% of survivors of encephalitis have long-term problems.

BRAIN ABSCESS

A brain abscess is a collection of purulent material in a cavity within the brain. A bacterial infection that has traveled from the gums or teeth, sinus, ear, or mastoid region to the brain usually is the cause. An abscess can form from bacteria introduced at the time of any type of head injury or cranial surgery. **Signs and symptoms are headache, fever, and progression to lethargy and confusion.** If the abscess is not treated, ICP will rise as the size of the abscess increases. Teach patients who experience sinus infections with purulent drainage to seek treatment if symptoms last for more than a few days. A combination of antibiotics is used to eradicate the abscess. Surgery may be required to drain the abscess or relieve ICP.

HEADACHES

Headaches are the most common cause of complaints of pain. Headaches are commonly caused by allergy and related sinus problems or by tension, or are vascular in origin. Arthritis, cervical spondylitis, and temporomandibular joint syndrome may also cause headaches. The pain of a headache may be minor or severe. Persistent headache requires testing to rule out organic problems such as anemia, brain tumor, or cerebral aneurysm.

Treatment for severe, recurrent headaches begins with determining the cause, if possible, and identifying factors that seem to precipitate the headache. Mild headaches usually are relieved by rest and a mild analgesic.

MIGRAINE HEADACHES

Approximately 23 million Americans have at least one migraine headache a year. Women experience them more than men. It is thought that constriction and subsequent dilation of cerebral arteries cause migraine headaches. Attacks usually occur irregularly and may begin with an aura such as visual disturbances or "spots before the eyes" (scotoma). Many patients with migraine do not have an aura preceding the attack. Pain usually begins on one side of the head and is described as throbbing in character. A migraine headache is often accompanied by nausea and vomiting. Symptoms may last for 4 to 72 hours. Light or sound cause irritation and sensitivity, and for some sufferers, certain types of light set off the headache. Frequent migraine headaches are very debilitating.

⚠ Safety Alert

Triptans and Antidepressant Use

Patients who are taking triptans as migraine medication should not also take antidepressant/mood disorder medications that are selective serotonin reuptake inhibitors (SSRIs) or selective serotonin/norepinephrine reuptake inhibitors (SNRIs). There is a greater risk of increased serotonin levels occurring if triptans are combined with SSRIs or SNRIs, and the resulting serotonin syndrome can be life threatening. Signs and symptoms of serotonin syndrome include restlessness, hallucinations, loss of coordination, tachycardia, rapid changes in blood pressure, hyperthermia, overactive reflexes, nausea, vomiting, and diarrhea. Consult with the physician rather than abruptly stopping the SSRI or SNRI medication.

Lying in a darkened, quiet, odor-free room with eyes closed decreases the symptoms. Sometimes doing this at the very beginning of symptoms can prevent a full-blown migraine headache. Metoclopramide (Reglan), droperidol (Inapsine), or chlorpromazine (Thorazine) is often prescribed for the nausea that accompanies a migraine. Various behavioral treatments such as biofeedback, acupuncture, and relaxation therapy, combined with lifestyle adjustments and medication, seem to offer the best result (Emedicinehealth, 2010).

Clinical Cue

Patients should be told that long-term use of metoclopramide may cause tardive dyskinesia (a neurologic disorder) (FDA, 2009).

Treatment consists of using one or more of the agents listed in Box 24-2 (Chawla, 2009). A cold compress to the temple, eye, and occiput areas is helpful. Identifying food or other substances that seem to trigger an attack is very important.

If migraine headache tends to occur around the time of menses, taking a prescribed diuretic for 3 to 5 days before onset of menstruation may be effective in preventing the headache.

Nutrition Considerations

Finding Foods that Trigger a Migraine Headache

Ask patients who suffer from migraine headaches to keep a food diary and see if any of the following foods or additives are triggering the attacks:
Alcohol
Caffeine
Chocolate
Artificial sweeteners (aspartame, sucralose, saccharin)
Monosodium glutamate (MSG)
Citrus fruits
Meats with nitrites (bacon, salami, etc.)
Salt
Foods containing tyramines: peanuts, raisins, vinegars, soy sauce, aged cheese, yogurt, sour cream, chicken livers, sausages, bananas, avocados, pickled herring, freshly baked breads, pork, beans

Occipital nerve stimulation is under study to control migraine and other headache pain. An electrode is placed close to the occipital nerve at the base of the skull. The neurostimulator control is implanted in the abdomen. The stimulator impulse can be adjusted depending on the level of stimulation that blocks pain. It is hoped that the device will diminish pain perception and the person will be able to function normally again (Gever, 2009). The FDA has approved Botox for the prevention of migraines (Frieden, 2010).

Box 24-2 Medications Used for Migraine Headache Treatment

DRUGS THAT ABORT MIGRAINE SYMPTOMS
- Sumatriptan (Imitrex, Imigran)
- Zolmitriptan (Zomig, Zomig ZMT)
- Naratriptan (Amerge, Naramig)
- Rizatriptan (Maxalt, Maxalt MLT)
- Almotriptan (Axert)
- Frovatriptan (Frova)
- Eletriptan (Relpax)
- Ergotamine tartrate (Cafergot)
- Methysergide (Sansert)
- Acetaminophen-isometheptene-dichloralphenazone (Midrin)
- Dihydroergotamine (D.H.E. 45 injections, Migranal Nasal Spray)

PREVENTIVE DRUGS (TAKEN DAILY)
- Valproic acid (Depakote)
- Topiramate (Topamax)
- Amitriptyline (Elavil)
- Nortriptyline (Pamelor)
- Propranolol (Inderal) and other beta blockers
- Timolol (Blocadren)
- Verapamil (Covera) and other calcium channel blockers
- Cyproheptadine (Periactin)

Complementary and Alternative Therapies

Vitamin B$_6$, Herbs, and Vitamin B$_2$

If taking a diuretic drug is contraindicated for some reason, taking time-release vitamin B$_6$ tablets for 3 to 5 days before the start of menses will often cause enough diuresis of fluid buildup to be helpful. Vitamin B$_6$ should not be taken continuously as toxic levels can occur that cause neuropathy. All herbs should be approved by the health care provider, as they may interfere with other medications the patient is taking. Herbs that have been found to help prevent or alleviate migraine headache are:
- Feverfew
- Willow
- Bay
- Ginger
- Lemon balm
- Purslane
- Red pepper

A supplement that is beneficial for some patients in preventing migraine headaches is vitamin B$_2$ 400 mg/day.

CLUSTER HEADACHES

Cluster headaches occur more frequently in men, and are not as common as migraine headaches. A cluster headache causes the most severe headache pain. The pain is abrupt in onset and usually lasts 30 to 90 minutes. It may start during sleep. The headache may recur several times a day, and the clusters usually last 2 to 3 months. The cause and pathophysiology are not clearly known, but the trigeminal nerve is implicated. Vasodilation occurs, causing the headache. It is thought that

the disorder may be caused by dysfunction of the biologic clock mechanisms of the hypothalamus. Alcohol can trigger this type of headache.

Signs and symptoms include severe unilateral orbital, supraorbital, or temporal pain along with one of the following: redness of the conjunctiva of the eye, tearing, nasal congestion, dripping nose, facial swelling, pupil constriction, or **ptosis** (drooping) of the eyelid. The person becomes restless and often paces the floor, and is sensitive to touch.

History usually is sufficient to diagnose a cluster headache, but CT scan, MRI, or magnetic resonance angiography may be performed to rule out tumor, aneurysm, or infection. Treatment for cluster headache includes a combination of analgesic and 100% oxygen by face mask, sumatriptan succinate (Imitrex) and other triptans, internasal lidocaine 4% aqueous solution, or intranasal capsaicin. Opiates are to be avoided as they can cause rebound headache.

 Safety Alert

Caution When Taking Analgesics

Fiorinal should be avoided for long-term use as it contains a barbiturate and is habit forming. Drugs containing acetaminophen should be used within the dosage guidelines and not used daily as this drug can cause liver failure and impaired renal function. The guidelines are to refrain from taking more than 4 g of acetaminophen per 24 hours. Remind patients who take acetaminophen not to combine it with alcohol as doing so can cause liver damage in some people. Those taking aspirin, ibuprofen, or a drug containing either should monitor themselves for peptic ulcer and gastric bleeding. Signs and symptoms to report are epigastric pain, dyspepsia, black stool, or vomiting of blood. Fatigue, headache, and dizziness may indicate anemia from a slow gastric bleed.

TENSION HEADACHES

Tension headaches are quite common, but are not as severe as migraine or cluster headaches. This type of headache usually involves the head along with neck stiffness and limitation of range of motion of the neck. Analgesic medication, muscle relaxants, tension-reducing medication or relaxation techniques, massage, yoga, and biofeedback are often helpful. Biofeedback can be very effective in preventing or averting headaches for many people.

CRANIAL NERVE DISORDERS

TRIGEMINAL NEURALGIA (TIC DOULOUREUX)
Etiology and Pathophysiology
Trigeminal neuralgia is a relatively rare facial pain syndrome. The cause of trigeminal neuralgia is not known, although it can be related to pressure on the nerve root by a tumor, or to a lesion of the blood vessels. Multiple sclerosis can be a factor. Often, no cause can be found and the disorder is considered

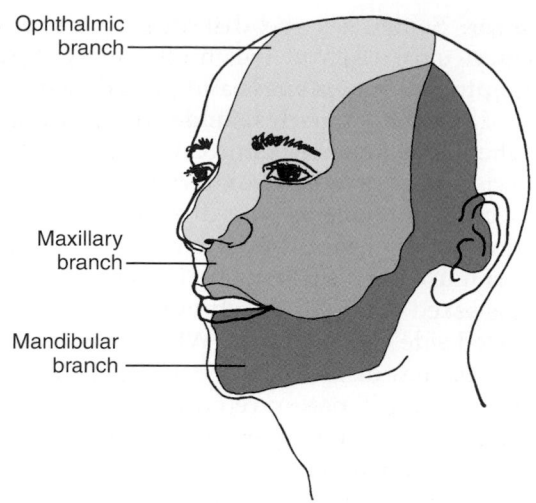

Ophthalmic
branch

Maxillary
branch

Mandibular
branch

FIGURE 24-11 Areas of innervation by each of the three branches of the trigeminal nerve.

idiopathic. This disorder most commonly affects people over age 60.

This disorder involves one or more branches of the fifth cranial (trigeminal) nerve. The three branches of this nerve are the ophthalmic, the mandibular, and the maxillary (Figure 24-11). In most cases of trigeminal neuralgia, the ophthalmic nerve is not involved. The mechanism of pain production is controversial. It may be due to increased afferent firing in the nerve or failure of inhibitory mechanisms.

Signs, Symptoms, and Diagnosis

The most notable symptom of trigeminal neuralgia is severe facial pain, which is described as sharp and intense, lasting for 1 to 2 minutes, and located along the pathway of one of the branches of the trigeminal nerve. The pain is localized on one side of the face, rarely affecting both sides. It can extend from the midline of the face across the cheek and jaw to the ear.

Attacks are usually triggered by exposure to drafts, light touch or vibration, drinking cold or very hot liquids, chewing, brushing the hair, shaving, or washing the face. The pain causes a brief muscle spasm of the facial muscles—the tic. Between acute flare-ups the patient may experience no pain, or may report a dull ache. The pain during the acute phase is so severe that many patients live in constant fear they will do something to provoke an attack.

Diagnosis is based on the patient's history and chief complaint and tests to rule out a cerebellopontine angle tumor that is affecting the nerve. There is no test to confirm the diagnosis, and there are no observable pathologic changes.

Treatment

Medical management usually is preferred to surgical intervention, because the latter involves dissection of nerve rootlets with resultant loss of motor and sensory function. The drugs most frequently prescribed to prevent or relieve spasmodic pain are the anticonvulsants carbamazepine (Tegretol) and phenytoin (Dilantin) and the muscle relaxant baclofen (Lioresal). Other anticonvulsants are effective in some patients. Intranasal spray of lidocaine or calcitonin may be effective for temporary relief. Relief of severe pain usually can be obtained by injecting glycerol into the terminal branch of the trigeminal nerve (glycerol rhizotomy). Percutaneous stereotactic rhizotomy or microvascular decompression are neurosurgical choices.

❖ NURSING MANAGEMENT

■ Assessment (Data Collection) and Nursing Diagnosis

Observing the patient between acute attacks can help identify clues to affirm the presence of trigeminal neuralgia. The patient may not want to wash her face (male patients may not want to shave), and the patient will guard her face or hold it immobile to avoid an attack. The patient is very sensitive to any contact with her face and will indicate the area of pain by pointing to but never touching it.

The nursing diagnosis for patients with trigeminal neuralgia is, of course, pain. Because chewing can provoke an attack of pain, the patient may be susceptible to nutritional deficit. Small, frequent feedings consisting of food that is moderately warm can help provide adequate nutrition and at the same time avoid precipitating an acute attack.

■ Planning, Implementation, and Evaluation

Specific expected outcomes are written for the patient regarding the control of pain and its triggers. Nursing intervention for the patient who is being treated medically includes instruction about the expected actions and adverse side effects of the drug she is taking. Phenytoin can produce *ataxia*, skin eruptions, overgrowth of the gums, nystagmus, and Stevens-Johnson syndrome (a serious immune reaction). Carbamazepine can damage the bone marrow and produce such hematologic reactions as leukopenia, aplastic anemia, and decreased platelet count. Skin eruptions also can occur as a reaction to carbamazepine or baclofen. The patient's blood count and liver function must be closely monitored to detect early signs of drug toxicity. Baclofen may cause transient drowsiness, nausea, weakness, or fatigue.

Surgical treatment of trigeminal neuralgia brings about problems related to potential for damage to the cornea when the ophthalmic branch is dissected. The patient must be taught to avoid rubbing her eyes or exposing them to foreign objects because the normal protective corneal reflex is no longer functional. She should get into the habit of wearing protective goggles when there is the possibility of getting dust and debris in her eyes, and should try to blink her eyes often to cleanse their surfaces.

Dissection of the second or third branches of the trigeminal nerve produces problems of potential damage to the oral mucosa and teeth. The patient cannot feel hot liquids and foods and could be burned, could bite the inside of the mouth without realizing it, or may have dental caries that will not cause pain. Good oral hygiene and periodic dental examinations are particularly important when the body's natural warning system is not operative. Immediately postoperatively, an ice pack is applied to the cheek for 3 to 4 hours to prevent swelling.

Evaluation data are gathered to see if the specific expected outcomes are being met.

BELL'S PALSY

Bell's palsy is weakness or paralysis of the muscles supplied by the facial nerve. It usually affects only one side of the face, and usually occurs in people over age 30. The disorder affects about 23 per 100,000 people and affects the right side of the face most often. The etiology of Bell's palsy is controversial. It is thought to be caused by edema and ischemia that compresses the facial nerve. The herpes simplex virus is thought to be a cause. Stress can be a factor also. Exposure to cold is a risk factor. Sometimes the disorder occurs during pregnancy, most often in the third trimester. **Signs and symptoms are numbness and partial or total paralysis of the facial muscles suddenly or over a few days.** There may be taste disturbances. The eyelid on the affected side loses its blink reflex and the mouth droops, causing problems with drooling.

Diagnosis is by history and exclusion of other neurologic or muscular disorders, and Lyme disease. If the patient is asked to raise the eyebrows, the eyebrow on the affected side will not move. When asked to smile, the face becomes distorted as the affected side of the mouth and face will not move normally.

Treatment consists of closing and patching the eye if it loses the blink reflex. Artificial tear eyedrops also are used to prevent dryness of the cornea. Corticosteroids are given if they can be started right after the beginning of symptoms. They are ineffective if delayed more than 7 days. Acyclovir may be prescribed as well, since herpesvirus may be a causative organism (Monell, 2009). Recovery is individual; some patients with total paralysis may not achieve full recovery but will improve as inflammation declines. Eighty percent to 90% of patients recover completely within 6 weeks to 3 months. Bell's palsy recurs in 10% to 15% of patients.

Get Ready for the NCLEX® Examination!

Key Points

- Many conditions can cause a seizure. Epilepsy is a chronic condition in which abnormal electrical activity is triggered in the brain without an underlying metabolic cause.
- Seizures are classified as generalized or partial.
- Irreversible brain damage can occur if seizures are unrelenting and uncontrolled.
- Treatment of epilepsy is by drugs and/or surgery (see Box 24-1).
- Close observation of a seizure with documentation by the nurse is very helpful (see Focused Assessment box on p. 526).
- Patient education is extremely important for safety and for the prevention of recurrent seizures.
- A cerebrovascular accident is caused by a thrombus, embolus, or an intracranial hemorrhage that interrupts circulation to an area of the brain.
- Risk factors for stroke are high blood pressure, atherosclerosis, cigarette smoking, excessive alcohol intake, insufficient exercise, high cholesterol, obesity, and diabetes.
- t-PA is best given within 3 to 6 hours of the onset of symptoms to be effective for thrombotic stroke.
- Cerebral aneurysms and arteriovenous malformations may leak or burst and cause a stroke.
- Subarachnoid hemorrhage is a medical emergency.
- A thrombosis causes cerebral ischemia that progresses slowly; an embolus causes sudden neurologic deficits.
- Homonymous hemianopsia, hemiplegia or hemiparesis, agnosia, apraxia, aphasia, and dysphagia are some of the problems caused by a CVA.
- Fatigue and emotional lability with crying or outburst may be common after a stroke or other injury to the brain, depending on the area of the brain involved.
- Hydrocephalus may be a complication of several disorders of the brain; a shunt can be placed to divert the excess CSF to the peritoneal cavity (see Figure 24-9).
- Rehabilitation for the stroke patient is extremely important and takes extensive work.
- Brain tumors may be benign or malignant; many are metastatic from a different malignant site (see Table 24-2).
- Brain tumors compress adjacent tissue, causing problems and increased ICP.
- Some common signs of brain tumors are personality change, disturbance in judgment and memory, loss of muscular strength and coordination, and difficulty speaking clearly. Headache, projectile vomiting, visual problems, and signs of increased ICP may be present.
- Depending on the site and type of brain tumor, treatment is by surgery, radiation, and/or chemotherapy.

- Viral and bacterial infections cause the inflammation of the membranes covering the brain and spinal cord in meningitis.
- Severe and persistent headache with nuchal rigidity are classic signs of meningitis, but a spinal tap is needed for diagnosis.
- Meningitis causes an increase in ICP.
- West Nile virus is a cause of encephalitis and is spread by mosquitoes.
- Encephalitis is most often the result of a viral infection or the toxins produced by viral organisms such as measles, chickenpox, and mumps.
- Stiff neck, photophobia, and lethargy are classic symptoms of encephalitis.
- Nursing care is geared toward the problems of seizures, high fever, and delirium of altered LOC (see Table 22-9).
- A brain abscess can develop from a severe sinus, ear, tooth, or gum infection.
- Headaches are common, and approximately 23 million Americans suffer from migraine headaches.
- Tracking triggers for migraine, avoiding them, and taking medication helps prevent migraine attacks (see Nutrition Considerations box on p. 545).
- Migraine may be preceded by an aura and most often causes pain on one side of the head.
- Cluster headaches cause severe pain and tend to be periodic in nature.
- Trigeminal neuralgia is a painful disorder affecting the fifth cranial nerve and the muscles of the face. Only one side of the face is usually affected.
- Bell's palsy is thought to be caused by edema and ischemia that compress the facial nerve. It causes weakness or paralysis of the muscles supplied by the nerve.
- Numbness and partial or total paralysis of the facial muscles, usually on one side, occur with Bell's palsy.
- Corticosteroids and acyclovir are the drugs used to treat Bell's palsy.

Additional Learning Resources

SG Go to your Study Guide for additional learning activities to help you master this chapter content.

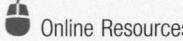volve Go to your Evolve website (http://evolve.elsevier.com/deWit/medsurg) for the following FREE learning resources:
- Animations, audio, and video
- Answers and rationales for questions and activities
- Concept Map Creator
- Glossary with pronunciations in English and Spanish
- Interactive Review Questions and Exercises and more!

Online Resources
- American Speech-Language-Hearing Association (ASHA), www.asha.org
- American Stroke Association, www.strokeassociation.org
- Brain Tumor Center, http://btc.mgh.harvard.edu
- Meningitis Foundation of America, www.meningitisfoundationofamerica.org
- National Aphasia Association, www.aphasia.org
- National Brain Tumor Foundation, www.braintumor.org

- National Rehabilitation Information Center (NARIC), naricinfo@heitechservices.com, www.naric.com
- National Stroke Association, www.stroke.org
- Stroke Patient Education pamphlets, www.strokefoundation.com.au/component/option,com_docman/Itemid,132/task,cat_view/gid,64

Review Questions for the NCLEX® Examination

1. The nurse determines that the appropriate nursing diagnosis for a patient with status epilepticus would be *Risk for injury related to seizure activity.* An appropriate expected outcome would be:
   1. everyone will stay calm during the episodes.
   2. the caregiver will stay with the patient during the episodes.
   3. the patient will be free from any injuries associated with the seizures.
   4. standing orders will be obtained to medicate acute seizure episodes.

2. Nursing care of a patient who *just* had a seizure includes which nursing intervention(s)? *(Select all that apply.)*
   1. Assess for injuries.
   2. Check the glucose level.
   3. Reassure and reorient patient.
   4. Provide uninterrupted periods of sleep and rest.
   5. Provide a 24-hour sitter.

3. Which patient statement indicates a need for further teaching regarding the prevention of seizures?
   1. "I need to avoid situations that could potentially trigger a seizure."
   2. "Alcohol can lower the seizure threshold."
   3. "I must avoid becoming overly fatigued and should pace activities."
   4. "I am less likely to have seizures during menstruation."

4. An _____ is a tangled mass of malformed, thin-walled, dilated blood vessels that form a connection between arterial and venous systems.

5. Which are *true* regarding an ischemic stroke? *(Select all that apply.)*
   1. The onset may evolve over a period of hours.
   2. A fibrinolytic drug may be given.
   3. Aspirin therapy may be started within 48 hours.
   4. Increased intracranial pressure occurs immediately.
   5. May occur as a complication of atrial fibrillation.

6. A patient has had a cerebrovascular accident. The nurse assesses the patient's readiness for transfer to another level of care. The patient continues to have agnosia and apraxia. These clinical findings indicate that the patient would:
   1. require assistance with undertaking activities of daily living.
   2. demonstrate independence in performing ordinary tasks.
   3. prompt self to complete sequential tasks.
   4. not understand verbal communication.

7. An appropriate nursing intervention for a patient with homonymous hemianopsia is:
   1. considering bold print editions.
   2. turning the head to scan both sides.
   3. avoiding bright lights.
   4. wearing prescription glasses.

8. A 21-year-old man complains of a sudden onset of fever, severe headache, and stiffness of the neck. The nurse notes a petechial rash over the chest and extremities. Which nursing action(s) would be appropriate? *(Select all that apply.)*
   1. Institute Standard Precautions and droplet precautions.
   2. Administer antibiotics as ordered.
   3. Maintain a quiet and dimly lit patient room.
   4. Encourage active range-of-motion exercises.
   5. Administer narcotic analgesics for headache and neck pain.

9. A patient is admitted to the urgent care center for complaints of an abrupt onset of severe headache. Clinical history indicates that symptoms started during sleep and recurred several times during the day. These symptoms suggest:
   1. brain tumor.
   2. migraine.
   3. cluster headaches.
   4. tension headaches.

10. The nurse providing care to a 60-year-old Chinese patient with trigeminal neuralgia identifies that pain is the priority nursing diagnosis. The nurse anticipates:
    1. assessing the level of pain based on facial expressions.
    2. administering an anticonvulsant class of medication.
    3. placing warm cloths on the face.
    4. preparing the patient for surgery.

Critical Thinking Activities

Scenario A
Jack Thompson, age 36, suffered a seizure while walking down the hall at work. He fell to the ground and demonstrated jerking motions of his body.

1. What type of seizure is this most likely to be?

2. What observations should be made if he has another seizure?

3. How would you care for Mr. Thompson after the seizure is over?

4. If Mr. Thompson is diagnosed with epilepsy, what patient teaching will he need?

Scenario B
Part I
Mr. Foster is a 77-year-old retired teacher who complained of a severe headache during dinner and then slumped over the table, unconscious. He was rushed to the hospital, and a tentative diagnosis of cerebrovascular accident (CVA) was made.

1. What diagnostic tests might be appropriate for Mr. Foster?

2. What emergency care could you have given Mr. Foster if you had been present at dinner?

Part II
Mr. Foster's diagnostic tests indicate a subarachnoid hemorrhage from a ruptured aneurysm. He is comatose; his pupils are equal and reactive to light; and he responds to pain with decorticate posturing, opens his eyes at random, and seems to be paralyzed on the right side.

3. What are the priorities of care for Mr. Foster?

4. If Mr. Foster survives, what potential complications might he experience if he has had an intracerebral hemorrhage?

Scenario C
Janice Pringle, age 19, has been experiencing headaches more frequently over the past 6 months. She comes to the student health center on her college campus to seek help. This headache is really bad and she is nauseated.

1. What subjective and objective assessment data would you gather regarding this young lady and her headaches?

2. What are your priorities of care for Janice?

3. What interventions would you suggest at this time?

Care of Patients with Peripheral Nerve and Degenerative Neurologic Disorders

Objectives

Theory

1. Compare and contrast the pathophysiology of Parkinson's disease and myasthenia gravis.
2. Discuss treatments for Parkinson's disease.
3. Describe the nursing care needed for the patient with Parkinson's disease.
4. Explain why multiple sclerosis might be difficult to diagnose.
5. Devise a home care plan for the patient with multiple sclerosis.
6. Compile a nursing care plan for the patient with Guillain-Barré syndrome.

7. Identify the differences between Huntington's disease and amyotrophic lateral sclerosis.
8. Illustrate the signs and symptoms of myasthenia gravis.
9. Compare and contrast the complications of Parkinson's disease with those of myasthenia gravis.

Clinical Practice

1. Teach a newly diagnosed patient about the medications for Parkinson's disease.
2. Teach a patient about the diagnostic tests that might be ordered if multiple sclerosis is suspected.
3. Write a nursing care plan for the myasthenia gravis patient who is hospitalized with a respiratory infection.

Key Terms

bradykinesia (brā-dē-kǐ-NĒ-zē-ă, p. 552)
chorea (kǎ-RĒ-ă, p. 562)
demyelination (dě-MĪ-ě-lǐ-nā-shǔn, p. 557)

diplopia (dǐ-PLŌ-pē-ă, p. 562)
hyperesthesia (hī-pěr-ěs-THĒ-zē-ă, p. 560)

PARKINSON'S DISEASE

Parkinson's disease (PD) is named after James Parkinson, who first described the syndrome in 1871. PD is considered a major health problem because of its crippling effects. It is a progressive disorder, beginning rapidly at first and then advancing more slowly. It affects more men than women and occurs most frequently after age 60. Approximately 1 million people in the United States are affected with PD, and about 50,000 people in the United States are diagnosed with PD each year.

Etiology

The specific cause of PD is unknown, but it involves degeneration of the dopamine-producing neurons in the substantia nigra of the midbrain, and the presence of Lewy bodies (cytoplasmic inclusions). Genetic susceptibility and environmental toxins appear to play a role. The most common type of PD is *idiopathic,* that is, the primary or specific cause is not known. Secondary PD can be drug induced, especially by reserpine-type antihypertensives such as methyldopa, phenothiazines, some tranquilizers such as the butyrophenones (e.g., haloperidol [Haldol]), some antiemetics, methamphetamine, and a few other drugs. These drugs block the uptake of dopamine at the receptors in the brain cells, and

so may induce PD symptoms. Pesticide and herbicide exposure is largely implicated as a cause of PD.

Pathophysiology

PD affects the extrapyramidal system, in particular the motor structures in the basal ganglia. This is the part of the brain that controls balance and coordination. The basal ganglia are gray matter that is scattered throughout the white matter of the cerebrum beneath the cerebral cortex. Stimulation of the basal ganglia causes muscle tone in the body to be inhibited and allows refined voluntary movements. Two neurotransmitters accomplish this action: dopamine and acetylcholine (ACh) (see Table 22-4 for the action of the common neurotransmitters). ACh-producing neurons transmit excitatory messages throughout the basal ganglia. Dopamine inhibits the function of these neurons so that there can be control of voluntary movement (Figure 25-1). There is usually a balance between these neurotransmitters. The degenerative changes in the basal ganglia lead to a decrease in dopamine. The ACh-secreting neurons remain active, creating an imbalance between excitatory and inhibitory neuronal activity. The excessive excitation of neurons prevents a person from controlling or initiating voluntary movements.

FIGURE 25-1 Dopaminergic synaptic activity is mediated by dopamine. Cholinergic synaptic activity is mediated by acetylcholine. A balance between the two kinds of synaptic activity produces normal motor function. A relative excess of cholinergic activity produces akinesia and rigidity. A relative excess of dopaminergic activity produces involuntary movements.

FIGURE 25-2 Parkinson's disease causes abnormalities of movement. Movements are jerky in nature.

Signs and Symptoms

The onset of PD is gradual and may involve only one side of the body initially. A triad of symptoms is characteristic of PD: tremor, bradykinesia, and rigidity. The first, *tremor*, occurs when the body is at rest, decreases when there is voluntary movement, and is absent when the patient is asleep. The tremor is most often a "pill-rolling" motion of the thumb against the fingers. This is when there is a circular rubbing of a finger or two as if rolling a piece of string or fuzz into a "pill." If the patient suffers stress and emotional tension, the tremor becomes more pronounced.

Bradykinesia (condition exhibiting slow movement and speech) produces poor body balance, a characteristic gait, and difficulty initiating movement. The gait is shuffling, with short steps that become quicker (Figure 25-2). There is decreased swinging of the arms when walking. A foot may drag or may be stiff, producing a limp. Earlier in the disease process, the patient may lean slightly to one side, propel forward uncontrollably, or fall backward. In advanced stages there is a stiff, bent-forward posture when walking.

The third symptom is *rigidity* affecting the skeletal muscles and contributing to postural changes and difficulty in movement. Postural changes affect coordination and balance. The face becomes blank or masklike in appearance with little or no expression. Speech becomes low in tone, monotonous sounding, and slow; enunciation becomes difficult due to the decreased dopamine and the excitatory response from the increased acetylcholine. Drooling may occur. The patient may experience decreased tearing, constipation, incontinence, excessive perspiration, heat intolerance, and decreased sexual ability. PD does not usually affect intellect; however, a percentage of patients do develop a dementia similar to that of Alzheimer's disease. Mood disturbance does occur, and depression is a problem. Stress tends to make symptoms worse.

? Think Critically

A patient comes into the clinic complaining about hand tremors and "stiffness" of the joints that started recently, excessive sweating, and some urinary incontinence. You notice that his gait is abnormal. What would be a priority question you would ask him as you start history taking?

Diagnosis

The characteristic symptoms of the disease are used to diagnose the disorder. Laboratory tests usually reveal findings within normal ranges. However, magnetic resonance imaging (MRI) scans of the brain may be performed to rule out other neurologic disorders. Single-photon emission computed tomography (SPECT) can display the reduced uptake of dopamine (Figure 25-3).

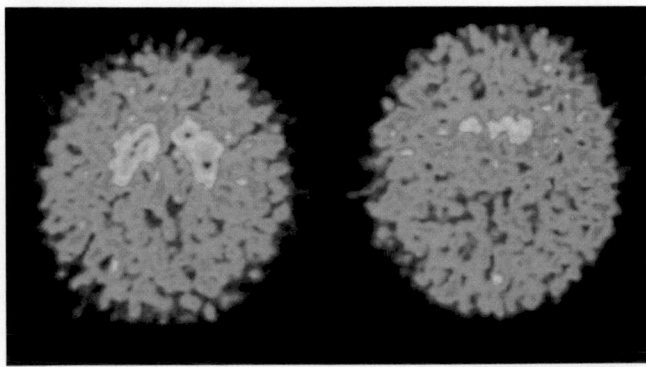

FIGURE 25-3 Positron emission tomography scan showing reduced uptake of dopamine in a patient with Parkinson's disease.

Treatment

Treatment of PD usually includes drug therapy, physical therapy, and considerable emotional support. Drug therapy aims to provide dopamine to the basal ganglia and thus reduce symptoms. Anticholinergics, dopamine agonists, and monoamine oxidase inhibitor (MAOI) drugs are used to control symptoms. MAOIs block the metabolism of dopamine, leaving more dopamine in circulation.

In the early stages of the disease when disability is not evident, selegiline (Eldepryl), a drug that increases dopamine's action, may be given. When disability is present, L-dioxyphenylalanine (L-dopa, or levodopa) or a combination of levodopa and carbidopa (Sinemet) is given. Sinemet is given in increasing doses until control of the symptoms is achieved; however, side effects can be troublesome (Box 25-1) Various drugs are used either alone or in combination with L-dopa (Table 25-1).

 Safety Alert

Caution When Administering MAOIs

When a patient with Parkinson's disease has been prescribed selegiline (an MAOI), caution him against eating foods containing tyramine such as aged cheeses, anything fermented, smoked fish or meat, yeast extract, some imported beers, Chianti wine, dietary protein supplements, and soy sauce. Giving meperidine to someone taking an MAOI can cause *hyperpyrexia* (excessive elevation of temperature) and possible death. Many drugs interact adversely with MAOIs, and the health care provider or pharmacist should be consulted before taking any other drug with an MAOI.

 Complementary and Alternative Therapies

Supplements Helpful for Parkinson's Disease

Nutritional supplements that are helpful for slowing the progression of Parkinson's disease include the enzyme NADH (nicotinamide adenine dinucleotide; 10 mg), coenzyme Q-10 (100 to 200 mg), phosphatidylserine (200 to 300 mg), and the antioxidants ester-C (1000 mg twice a day), vitamin E as mixed tocopherols (800 to 1200 mg), and alpha-lipoic acid (100 mg twice a day). Physicians sometimes prescribe these supplements in addition to the treatment medications.

Box 25-1   Nursing Implications for Drugs Commonly Used for Parkinson's Disease

WHEN GIVING A DRUG FOR PARKINSON'S DISEASE

- Pay close attention to dosage amount as therapy is individualized to each patient.
- Check other medications patient is receiving to see if there may be interactions with the antiparkinsonian drug, contraindicating administration of the drug.
- Administer the drugs as close to the time ordered as possible to maintain a consistent blood level of each drug.
- Carbidopa-levodopa may cause many neurologic disturbances, including psychiatric problems; discuss any onset of new symptoms that occur with the physician.
- Administer anticholinergic medications with meals to decrease gastrointestinal irritation.
- Selegiline may increase the side effects of carbidopa-levodopa. If this occurs, seek an order to decrease the dosage.
- Monitor for effectiveness of each drug by observing for a decrease in Parkinson's symptoms, such as tremor, rigidity, or drooling; assess for decrease in side effects of carbidopa-levodopa when anticholinergic drugs are given for that purpose.
- Continually assess the patient for worsening of symptoms that may be due to disease progression, side effects of medication, or failure of medication.

REGARDING POSSIBLE SIDE/ADVERSE EFFECTS OF THE DRUG

- Monitor patients taking carbidopa-levodopa, amantadine, bromocriptine, or pergolide for orthostatic hypotension and urinary retention.
- Assess patients who are taking carbidopa-levodopa for excessive or inappropriate sexual behavior.
- Bromocriptine may cause changes in mental status; report observed changes.
- Amantadine and pergolide may cause insomnia and should not be administered at bedtime.

- Many of these drugs can cause nausea, dyspepsia, and abdominal pain.
- Anticholinergics are contraindicated in patients with acute narrow-angle glaucoma.
- Anticholinergics cause dry mouth and constipation; increase fluids to 3000 mL/day; treat constipation as needed per orders; add fiber to diet.
- Monitor blood pressure and pulse during initiation and adjustment of anticholinergic medication; report tachycardia.
- Consult pharmacology book or drug insert for specific side effects of each particular drug.

TEACH THE PATIENT TAKING ANTIPARKINSONIAN DRUGS

- Selegiline may cause dizziness; warn patient to move cautiously during initiation of therapy.
- Orthostatic hypotension causes dizziness and can precipitate falls; it is important to allow the blood pressure to stabilize with the patient in a sitting position before standing, to rise slowly and to have the patient stabilize while holding on to something when standing before walking.
- Carbidopa-levodopa will turn the urine dark.
- Ropinirole (Requip) may cause drowsiness; advise patient not to operate machinery or drive until adjusted to the drug.
- When taking a catechol-O-methyltransferase (COMT) inhibitor, it is important to have liver function checked regularly.
- Constipation is a problem with the anticholinergic drugs; increases in dietary fiber, plenty of fluid, and exercise can help control constipation; bowel movement frequency should be monitored to prevent impaction.
- Adjustment of dosages and combination of medications that will control symptoms with the fewest of side effects may take weeks or months to accomplish.

Table 25-1 **Drugs Commonly Used for Patients with Parkinson's Disease**

DRUG CLASSIFICATION	USE
Antiparkinsonian/Adrenergic	
Levodopa (L-dopa) Levodopa-carbidopa (Sinemet) Bromocriptine mesylate (Parlodel) Pergolide (Permax) Pramipexole (Mirapex) Ropinirole (Requip) Apomorphine (Apokyn)	Decrease presence of tremor, rigidity, and bradykinesia and improve motor function
Antiviral	
Amantadine (Symmetrel)	Decreases presence of rigidity, bradykinesia
Anticholinergic	
Trihexyphenidyl (Artane) Biperiden (Akineton) Benztropine (Cogentin)	Decrease tremor
Monoamine Oxidase Inhibitor (MAOI)	
Selegiline (Eldepryl, Carbex) Rasagiline (Azilect)	Decrease presence of tremor, rigidity, and bradykinesia, and improve motor function
Monoamine Oxidase Inhibitor B (MAOI-B)	
Rasagiline (Azilect)	Blocks breakdown of dopamine; initial monotherapy or as adjunctive therapy to levodopa.
Catechol-_O_-Methyltransferase (COMT) Inhibitor	
Tolcapone (Tasmar) Entacapone (Comtan)	Slow the breakdown of dopamine, thereby prolonging the action of levodopa

 Think Critically

What would be appropriate nursing interventions for the patient who is beginning to experience dysphagia?

Surgical Treatment. Stereotactic neurosurgery may be done if the drug therapy fails to assist the patient with PD symptoms. In one such procedure the area in the thalamus that is causing the involuntary movements is destroyed. Microsurgical procedures such as pallidotomy improve rigidity and bradykinesia (Clarke, 2007; WebMD, 2010b).

Other procedures with some success in relieving symptoms include transplanting tissue from the adrenal medulla into the brain, or implanting fetal tissue or stem cells. Stem cells are transplanted into the caudate nucleus of the brain. This is still experimental, but the procedure has shown substantial clinical improvements in motor function (Susman, 2010).

Deep brain stimulation (DBS) uses electrode implants to provide electrical shocks that control tremors by blocking them. The device that delivers the shocks

can be adjusted as the patient's symptoms change or worsen (National Institute of Neurological Diseases and Stroke, 2007). There has been considerable success with DBS, but it is expensive at $10,000 for the implant unit and another $8000 every few years for battery replacement.

Depression is frequent in Parkinson's patients, but most respond well to a selective serotonin reuptake inhibitor (SSRI) antidepressant.

Complications

Dysphagia may develop and mobility becomes severely limited as the disease progresses. Problems of immobility occur (see Chapter 9). Constipation, urinary incontinence, and insomnia are also common.

❖ NURSING MANAGEMENT

■ Assessment (Data Collection) and Nursing Diagnosis

A thorough history is gathered and a physical examination is performed for the patient who has or is thought to have PD. Nursing Care Plan 25-1 contains the common nursing diagnoses, expected outcomes, and specific interventions for the patient with PD.

 Focused Assessment

Data Collection for the Patient with Parkinson's Symptoms

Gather data regarding history by asking the following questions:
- Have you ever had a head injury, meningitis, encephalitis, or cerebrovascular disorder?
- Have you ever been exposed to metals, pesticides, or carbon monoxide for extended periods?
- What medications do you take? (Particularly important are major tranquilizers such as haloperidol [Haldol], phenothiazines, reserpine, methyldopa, and amphetamines.)
- Do you have a problem with fatigue?
- Have you noticed excessive salivation and problems handling secretions?
- Do you have any trouble swallowing?
- Have you been steadily losing weight?
- Do you suffer with constipation or urinary incontinence?
- Do you sweat excessively?
- Do you have difficulty initiating walking or other movements? Do you fall frequently?
- Has your dexterity decreased? Has your handwriting deteriorated?
- Do you have insomnia?
- Do you experience pain or cramping?
- Do you have mood swings? Are you depressed? Do you have hallucinations?

Points to cover in physical examination:
- Presence of drooling
- Ability to swallow
- Facial expression or lack thereof
- Presence of ankle edema
- Evidence of postural hypotension
- Presence of tremor at rest; pill-rolling movements
- Rigidity of body and jerky movements of extremities
- Slow start, then quick short steps when ambulating; shuffling gait with bent-forward posture
- Difficulty stopping once ambulating

Assignment Considerations

Feeding the Dysphagic Patient

Unlicensed assistive personnel (UAP) should not be assigned to feed the dysphagic patient if at all possible. If an aide must be used to help feed a patient with dysphagia, be certain that suction is turned on and at hand and that the aide has been trained in helping a dysphagic patient to eat. Remind the UAP that the patient should be positioned as upright as possible, to give small bites, to wait for that bite to be swallowed before offering another one, and not to rush the patient. Coaching the patient to drop the chin when swallowing helps prevent choking.

▪ Planning, Implementation, and Evaluation

Nursing care focuses on preventing complications of PD, drug therapy, enhancing voluntary movement, and safety. Constipation is a problem and requires the addition of fiber to the diet and an increase in fluids to at least 3000 mL per 24 hours. Grasping coins or other objects may help decrease tremors because it is an intentional action. Walking may be improved by having the patient think about imaginary lines across the pathway on which to walk. Imagining stepping over something helps prevent "freezing" when walking. Teach the patient to consciously assume correct posture. Not using a pillow when resting helps prevent flexion of the spine. Learning to sleep prone also is beneficial for posture correction. The physical therapist will institute an exercise program to help the patient maintain muscle function and promote joint mobility.

Remember that the PD patient needs extra time to finish tasks. A warming tray can be used to keep food hot during meals so that the patient can take rest periods while eating. Considerable patience and understanding are necessary to help the patient deal with the frustration of deteriorating body control and inability to do things that he formerly could easily do. Degeneration of cognitive skills occurs in the late stages of PD.

Falls are common, and safety is a major factor. Using a cane or walker will increase stability and decrease the incidence of falls. Leg braces or foot braces may help to maintain balance. Loose carpets should be removed from the home. Grab bars should be installed in the shower and tub; a raised toilet seat should also be installed. Patients with tremor must be cautioned against carrying hot liquids, as spills may cause burns. Chapter 22 discusses measures to help with the problems typical of many neurologic disorders. Patient and family teaching is an important part of nursing care for patients with PD.

⭐ Nursing Care Plan 25-1 | Care of the Patient with Parkinson's Disease

Scenario
A 63-year-old man is admitted to your unit because of increasing incidence of falling. He is diagnosed with Parkinson's disease. He is beginning to have trouble swallowing and his speech has slowed. He has a tremor in his left hand and upper extremity.

Problem/Nursing Diagnosis
Has trouble swallowing/Imbalanced nutrition: less than body requirements related to dysphagia.

Supporting Assessment Data
Subjective: "I can't chew and swallow very well."
Objective: Difficulty chewing; difficulty getting food to go down.

Goals/Expected Outcomes	Nursing Interventions	Selected Rationale	Evaluation
Patient will not aspirate food.	Monitor swallowing during drug administration and meals to assess degree of swallowing difficulty.	Allows assessment of swallowing ability.	Swallowing pills one by one without problem. No choking or difficulty during meal as long as eats slowly.
	Keep suction equipment at hand to remove pooled secretions and prevent aspiration; turn on before meal.	Readies suction and allows removal of secretions.	Suction on and at hand during meals.
	Maintain upright position for drug administration and meals.	Gravity helps food go down to the stomach, and helps prevent aspiration.	Sitting fully upright for medications and meals.
	Provide semisoft foods and thickened liquids for diet.	Semisoft foods and thickened liquids are easier to swallow.	Has a semisoft diet. Thickener used for liquids.

Continued

Problem/Nursing Diagnosis

Repeated falls/Impaired physical mobility related to abnormal posture, rigidity, bradykinesia, and difficulty in initiating movements.

Supporting Assessment Data

Subjective: "I seem to have trouble with balance. I've fallen four times this month."
Objective: Rigidity of joints, jerky movements, shuffling gait, stooped posture.

Goals/Expected Outcomes	Nursing Interventions	Selected Rationale	Evaluation
Patient will ambulate safely. Patient will maintain joint mobility and muscle strength.	Physical therapist to work with patient on joint mobility, muscle strengthening, and ambulation.	Physical therapy helps to decrease rigidity and muscle weakness.	Physical therapist is working with the patient. Patient is performing prescribed exercises with spouse's help.
	Administer antiparkinsonian medication as ordered. Monitor for side effects and effectiveness of medication.	Decreases tremor, rigidity, and bradykinesia.	Receiving ordered medications with no signs of side effects as yet. Rigidity slightly improved.
	Cane or walker provided if necessary.	Assistive device promotes safety.	Using walker when ambulating.
	Teach to perform active ROM exercises bid.	Techniques improve gait and movement.	Performing ROM exercises bid.
	Teach to walk as if over an imaginary line and to rock back and forth to initiate movement.		Physical therapist is coaching the patient in how to walk.

Problem/Nursing Diagnosis

Having difficulty with swallowing; decreased appetite/Risk for imbalanced nutrition related to eating difficulties.

Supporting Assessment Data

Subjective: "I haven't had much appetite lately and I've choked on food a few times."
Objective: Slight drooling, weight down 4 lb this month.

Goals/Expected Outcomes	Nursing Interventions	Selected Rationale	Evaluation
Patient will not aspirate food.	Obtain consultation with speech therapist for swallowing studies.	Detects dysphagia.	Consultation with the speech therapist is ordered.
	Reinforce teaching regarding methods to be used for swallowing.	Various maneuvers can assist with correct swallowing and prevent choking.	Teaching plan is in place and teaching is ongoing.
	Obtain consultation with dietitian.	Assists with nutritional problems.	Dietitian will come tomorrow.
	Offer six small meals per day.		Offering between-meal small snacks.
	Serve hot meals on warming tray and do not rush patient with eating.	Keeps food warm while patient rests during meal.	Reheating food as needed during meal.
	Offer nutritional supplements between meals if needed.	Increases caloric intake.	Taking a protein shake in the afternoon.
	Administer anticholinergic medication as ordered.	Decreases drooling.	Medication is showing effect in decreased drooling.
	Monitor for side effects and effectiveness of medication; observe for urinary retention.	Identifies side effects patient experiences.	No urinary retention or other side effect as yet.
	Increase fiber intake and increase fluids to 3000 mL/day to prevent constipation.		Drank 2800 mL today. Fiber in diet increased.

Critical Thinking Questions
1. What are the side effects of Sinemet?
2. What would you suggest be done around the house to help prevent falls?

bid, twice daily; *ROM,* range-of-motion.

Patient Teaching

Parkinson's Disease

The following points should be covered in teaching the patient with Parkinson's disease how to cope with the illness. Keep teaching lessons short to prevent excessive fatigue.

MEDICATIONS
- How to take them per a written schedule.
- Purpose of each medication.
- What side effects to expect and what reactions to report.

DIET AND EATING
- Eat smaller, frequent meals.
- How to keep food warm while eating.
- Add more fiber to the diet to prevent constipation.
- Increase fluids to help prevent constipation.
- When attempting to swallow, keep lips closed and teeth together; put food on the tongue, lift the tongue up and back, and then swallow.
- Eat slowly and take small bites.

MOVEMENT AND EXERCISE
- Exercise and stretch regularly to prevent rigidity and contractures.
- Exercise in the morning when energy levels are higher.
- Wear good, sturdy shoes.
- Avoid soft, deep chairs; to get up from a chair, bend over slowly so that your head is over your toes.
- If bradykinesia is present, rock back and forth to begin walking.
- Use a cane or walker if balance is unsteady.
- Concentrate on standing upright.
- Imagine that you are stepping over a series of imaginary lines when walking.
- Count to yourself while walking.
- Visualize your intended movement.
- To calm tremor of the hands, hold change in your pocket or squeeze a small rubber ball.

FOR EXCESSIVE SALIVATION
- Make a conscious effort to swallow saliva frequently.
- Keep the head in an upright position so saliva will collect in the back of the throat and stimulate the swallowing reflex.
- Swallow excess saliva before speaking.

Adapted from Black, J.M., & Hawks, J.H. (2009). *Medical-Surgical Nursing: Clinical Management for Positive Outcomes* (8th ed.). Philadelphia: Elsevier Saunders, p. 1906.

Evaluation includes gathering data about the results of the interventions implemented. Next, determine if the expected outcomes are being met. If progress toward the outcomes is not occurring, revise the care plan.

MULTIPLE SCLEROSIS

Etiology

Multiple sclerosis (MS) is a chronic inflammatory disease causing demyelination in the central nervous system. The most common type of MS is characterized by periods of remission and exacerbation. Another type is progressive without remission periods. The cause of MS is not known, but it is thought that an environmental factor (bacteria, virus, or chemical) combined with a genetic predisposition for the disease is responsible.

Table 25-2	The Four Clinical Progressions of Multiple Sclerosis
TYPE OF PROGRESSION	**CHARACTERISTICS AND CLINICAL COURSE**
Relapsing-remitting (most common type)	Clearly defined relapses of acute worsening neurologic function. Partial or complete recovery occurs in remission period.
Primary progressive	Slow but almost continuous worsening with occasional plateaus and temporary minor improvements.
Secondary progressive	Initial period of relapsing-remitting disease followed by a steadily worsening course. May or may not have occasional relapses, minor remissions, or plateaus.
Relapsing-progressive	Disease steadily worsens from onset, but there are clear acute relapses with or without recovery. Disease progresses between relapses.

There are four clinical progressions of MS (Table 25-2). There is no cure. The disease appears mostly in people of northern European ancestry. It affects females more frequently than males. Symptoms most often appear between 15 and 50 years of age, but can occur at any age. A genetic factor can be involved as the disease is sometimes seen in more than one family member. There are about 350,000 people in the United States with MS.

Pathophysiology

Lymphocytes and macrophages infiltrate the central nervous system; immunoglobulin G (IgG) levels increase in the cerebrospinal fluid (CSF), indicating a humoral response with B-cell activation. T cells become reactive to a single myelin protein. Myelin is a protective sheath that insulates axons and assists impulse transmission. Axons transmit electrical impulses from one neuron to the next. In patients with MS, plaques form along the myelin sheath, causing inflammation. When myelin is eroded by inflammation and replaced by scar tissue (demyelination), nerve impulses cannot travel along the damaged neurons (Figure 25-4). Thus the muscles served by the affected nerves do not receive the impulses they need to perform in a well-coordinated and useful manner. When inflammation subsides, some remyelination occurs, but it is often incomplete and nerve transmission is not normal.

Signs and Symptoms

Clinical signs and symptoms reflect the pathologic changes that occur as a result of inflammation and subsequent scarring of myelin covering the nerves. MS typically follows a course of unpredictable flare-ups that are followed by periods of partial or complete remission. The very nature of the disease affects a

FIGURE 25-4 Effects of multiple sclerosis. **A,** Normal nerve cell with myelin sheath. **B,** Normal axon. **C,** Myelin breakdown. **D,** Myelin totally disrupted; axon not functioning.

patient's life in terms of ability to make a living, maintain satisfying interpersonal relationships with family and friends, and maintain a positive self-image.

The more common manifestations of MS are as follows:

- *Motor dysfunction* can include weakness or paralysis of limbs, trunk, and neck; diplopia caused by oculomotor weakness; and spasticity of the muscles.
- *Sensory dysfunction* may include numbness, tingling, burning, and painful sensations; patchy or total blindness or blurring of vision in one or both eyes; dizziness; ringing in the ears and hearing loss.
- *Problems of coordination* include ataxia (unsteady gait), intention tremor of limbs and eyes, slurring of speech, and dysphagia (difficulty swallowing).
- *Mental changes* usually are limited to depression and cognitive problems such as impaired judgment, decreased ability to solve problems, and memory loss, which occur late in the disease.
- *Fatigue* is a characteristic of MS and is worsened by heat (e.g., a hot shower, hot weather, or high humidity may induce or worsen symptoms).
- Other problems that occur late in the disease are related to urinary and bowel incontinence and altered sexual function: loss of male and female self-esteem, physical impotence in the male, and diminished sensation in the female.

The neuromuscular dysfunctions characteristic of MS are unique to each person and can vary greatly from time to time in the same person. Symptoms may disappear for a while.

Diagnosis

No laboratory test will definitively establish a diagnosis of MS, although most patients have elevated IgG levels in their CSF, with the presence of oligoclonal bands (bands of IgG produced by electrophoresis of the CSF). An MRI study usually shows characteristic white matter lesions scattered through the spinal cord and/or brain, which confirms the diagnosis of MS. However, the clinical signs and symptoms presented by a patient usually are sufficiently characteristic of the disorder to allow the neurologist to make a diagnosis that the patient possibly or probably has MS. The clinical manifestations of the disease reflect the extent to which inflammation and scarring of the myelin have occurred (Figure 25-5). Diagnosis may take several years, occurring only after a second attack.

Treatment

One of the biologic response modifier drugs, such as interferon beta-1b (Betaseron), is effective for many ambulatory patients with relapsing-remitting MS. It is given by injection. It reduces MS attacks by one third and decreases the number of severe attacks. It is not a cure, and not all patients respond to it. Interferon beta-1a (Avonex) causes fewer injection site reactions than interferon beta-1b. These drugs are very expensive and are used to prevent relapses. Acute attacks are treated with intravenous (IV) methylprednisolone for 5 days followed by oral prednisone in tapering doses. Adrenocorticotropic hormone (ACTH) may be given for its ability to suppress immune system activity. Most therapeutic efforts are centered on supportive measures to maintain resistance to infection, reduce muscle spasticity, and manage specific symptoms, such as diplopia, speech disorders, muscle weakness, fatigue, and depression. The drug regimen is geared to each patient's symptoms. Central nervous system stimulants may be prescribed to combat fatigue. Sometimes the antiparkinsonian drug amantadine (Symmetrel) is used for fatigue.

FIGURE 25-5 Chronic multiple sclerosis. Demyelination plaque *(P)* at gray matter–white matter junction and adjacent partially remyelinated shadow plaque *(V).*

An exercise program is very beneficial for the MS patient to relieve spasticity and improve coordination (WebMD, 2010a). Swimming provides considerable benefits as exercising in water is less fatiguing than exercising out of water. Because of fatigue, it is often difficult to convince MS patients to exercise.

In addition, the patient should be provided the support and physical and psychological means necessary to develop a positive and hopeful outlook. There is an understandable tendency to become depressed and pessimistic about the future when confronted with the realities of muscle weakness, incontinence, sexual impotence, and any combination of disabilities likely to be experienced during the course of MS. Antidepressants may be helpful.

❖ NURSING MANAGEMENT

■ Assessment (Data Collection), Nursing Diagnosis, and Planning

A careful history can provide many clues to the possibility that the patient has MS. Testing extremity strength, looking for visual problems, and checking reflexes are part of the physical examination.

Nursing diagnoses are based on the assessment findings and may include:

- Fatigue related to improper transmission of neural impulses
- Impaired physical mobility related to muscle weakness, spasticity, or *paresthesias* (tingling or numbness)
- Self-care deficit related to muscle spasticity and neuromuscular deficits
- Reflex urinary incontinence related to sensory motor deficits
- Sexual dysfunction related to neuromuscular deficits
- Risk for impaired skin integrity related to immobility
- Interrupted family processes related to potential financial problems, changing roles, and fluctuating physical abilities
- Ineffective coping related to loss of usual abilities and roles

Expected outcomes are written for each nursing diagnosis specific to the individual's problems.

■ Implementation and Evaluation

Appropriate care for the patient with MS depends on the severity of the disease and the symptoms. Care is individualized for each patient. During the diagnostic phase, the patient and family need a great deal of emotional support as they realize there is no cure.

Ongoing care by an interdisciplinary team focuses on safety, prevention of complications, assistance with physical therapy, and emotional support. The patient should not be exposed to excessive heat or hot baths, as this causes weakness to become much worse

(Roberts & Harper-Bennie, 2010). Care of the common problems of the neurologic patient is covered in Chapter 22. The importance of proper nutrition with adequate fluids and fiber in the diet should be stressed to maintain proper bowel function and decrease the likelihood of urinary tract infections. Calcium and vitamin D should be included in the diet to help prevent osteoporosis that may result from the IV steroid treatments. Medications to decrease stomach acid and prevent ulceration from the steroids may be administered (histamine [H_2]-receptor blockers or proton pump inhibitors).

Help the patient and family establish a consistent daily routine that will promote optimum levels of functioning for the patient. The routine should include daily physical exercise balanced by rest periods to prevent fatigue. Patient teaching involves:

- Education about the unpredictability of the disease and the need to avoid stress, infections, and fatigue to maintain independence as long as possible.
- Referral to the National Multiple Sclerosis Society and local support groups. (Additional information and local sources of help for the patient with MS and the family can be obtained from the Internet at www.nationalmssociety.org or by writing to the National Multiple Sclerosis Society, 733 Third Avenue, 3rd Floor, New York, NY 10017.)

Evaluation of care is based on whether the expected outcomes are being achieved. If they are not, the plan is revised.

ALZHEIMER'S DISEASE

Alzheimer's disease, a form of dementia caused by pathologic changes in the brain tissue of the patient, is covered in Chapter 48. Diagnosis is by history and examination as the specific diagnostic changes can be detected only at autopsy. The cause of Alzheimer's disease is unknown, and considerable research is in progress to better define this disease. It can occur during middle age or during the later decades of life and causes devastation to the patient and family. The disease has a slow onset, progresses at varying rates of speed through several stages, and is eventually fatal.

AMYOTROPHIC LATERAL SCLEROSIS

Etiology and Pathophysiology

Amyotrophic lateral sclerosis (ALS), also called *Lou Gehrig's disease,* is a progressive neuromuscular disease characterized by degeneration of the gray matter in the anterior horns of the spinal cord and the lower cranial nerves. After degeneration, electrical and chemical messages generated in the brain cannot reach the muscles to activate them. Incidence of ALS is 1 per 100,000 people. It most often occurs in people between the ages of 40 and 70 years and affects men more than women. Although some people with ALS can survive for many years, the disease usually progresses rapidly, producing a prognosis of death within about 3 years of the onset of symptoms.

Signs and Symptoms

One of the first clinical manifestations of ALS is weakness of the voluntary muscles, especially of the distal muscles of the extremities. Some patients may notice difficulty swallowing and speaking clearly because of oropharyngeal weakness. As the disease progresses, there is atrophy of the muscles. Until atrophy is complete, however, there may be spontaneous contractions or spasticity of the muscles and abnormal sensations *(paresthesias),* such as tingling or prickling. The patient also may report pain, which is probably caused by undue strain on weakened muscles.

Only the motor neurons are affected in ALS; therefore the patient remains mentally alert and does not have sensory impairment. Mental depression is relatively common as a result of the unrelenting progression of muscle weakness and atrophy. Death is usually due to respiratory infection and dysfunction as weakness and atrophy of the respiratory muscles impede normal respiration and mechanisms to clear bacteria and secretions from the lungs.

Diagnosis and Treatment

There is no laboratory test to confirm a diagnosis of ALS; electromyelography in combination with muscle biopsy and a creatine kinase level provide data for positive diagnosis. Other neuromuscular disorders such as MS, myasthenia gravis, and progressive muscular dystrophy must be ruled out.

There is no cure for ALS. Eventually the muscle paralysis renders the patient totally dependent because of inability to move, swallow, speak, and, ultimately, breathe. The drug riluzole (Rilutek), a glutamate antagonist, has been shown to slow the progression in certain patients (Armon, 2010). Eventually impaired breathing requires a tracheostomy and mechanical ventilation.

Nursing Management

During the first contact with the ALS patient, conduct a thorough neurologic assessment. As the disease progresses, periodic assessments can identify specific needs. Nursing diagnoses likely to be associated with ALS are those related to difficulty with respiration, all problems of immobility, dysphagia, impaired ability to communicate, pain, ineffective coping, and depression.

In the latter stages of ALS, the patient and family will need more assistance and guidance to maintain some level of independence and comfort for the patient. Rehabilitation includes obtaining equipment and devices such as a walker, wheelchair, hospital bed, suction machine, and nasogastric or gastrostomy tube feeding supplies.

Because of the nature of the disease, issues related to terminal illness, death, and the grieving process are likely to be present (see Chapter 8). Toward the end of life, the services of a visiting nurse or a hospice program can provide appropriate instruction and physical and emotional support.

GUILLAIN-BARRÉ SYNDROME

Etiology and Pathophysiology

Guillain-Barré syndrome (GBS) is a relatively rare disease that affects the peripheral nervous system, especially the spinal nerves outside the spinal cord. It also can affect the cranial nerves. The cause of GBS is not known, but it usually follows a viral respiratory infection or gastroenteritis in adults within 10 to 21 days. There have been a few cases of Guillain-Barré syndrome in recipients of meningococcal conjugate vaccine (Centers for Disease Control and Prevention, 2008). Authorities believe that the disease is a cell-mediated immunologic response preceded by stimulation from a viral infection, trauma, surgery, viral immunizations, HIV, or neoplasm of the lymphatic system. Cytomegalovirus and Epstein-Barr virus are two viruses that have been linked to GBS.

Pathologic changes include demyelination, inflammation, edema, and nerve root compression. These changes bring about the paresthesia, pain, and progressive, ascending paralysis typical of the syndrome. Autonomic nervous system dysfunction with alterations in both sympathetic and parasympathetic systems may occur, causing orthostatic hypotension, hypertension, abnormal vagal responses, bowel and bladder dysfunctions, facial flushing, and diaphoresis. When the lower brainstem becomes involved, the cranial nerves are affected.

Signs and Symptoms

Objective and subjective symptoms of GBS include mild sensations of numbness and tingling in the feet and hands, followed by muscle pain, tenderness, and aching, especially in the shoulder, pelvis, and thighs. There is progressive muscle weakness, usually starting in the lower extremities and moving upward over 24 to 72 hours. However, it also can affect the cranial nerves and facial muscles first and move downward. Symptoms peak in about 14 days. Sensory loss can also occur, but is not as common as motor loss. If respiratory function is affected, ventilatory support may be needed.

Pain is common and may be evidenced as paresthesias, muscular aches and cramps, and hyperesthesia (abnormal sensitivity to stimuli). Pain often is worse at night when there is less distraction in the environment.

Diagnosis

Diagnosing GBS is difficult because its characteristic signs and symptoms are similar to those of several other diseases. Analysis of the CSF is helpful. Typically there is an elevated CSF protein content that tends to rise as the disease progresses, peaking in 4 to 6 weeks. The number of leukocytes remains within normal limits, as does CSF pressure. Electromyelography and nerve conduction studies show reduced conduction velocity. For the most part, the physician must depend on the clinical picture presented by the patient to diagnose GBS.

Treatment

Medical treatment is mainly supportive. Within the first 2 weeks, plasmapheresis, in which the patient's plasma is removed and "washed" to remove antibodies, hastens recovery in some patients and decreases the time ventilatory support is needed. The use of IV immune globulin (IVIG) to hasten recovery is also effective (Davids et al., 2009).

Nutritional support via tube feedings may be required due to dysphagia. If paralytic ileus (halt to bowel peristalsis) occurs, parenteral nutrition will be necessary.

 Clinical Cues

Signs and symptoms of paralytic ileus are absence of bowel sounds, abdominal pain, and considerable abdominal bloating with lack of passage of stool.

❖ NURSING MANAGEMENT

■ Assessment (Data Collection), Nursing Diagnosis, and Planning

Assessment is the most important aspect of care during the acute stage. Monitor progression of ascending paralysis, assess respiratory function carefully, and assess gag, corneal, and swallowing reflexes closely. Monitor arterial blood gases and oxygen saturation. Observe vital sign trends and watch for orthostatic hypotension and cardiac dysrhythmia, which can indicate the degree of autonomic nervous system dysfunction.

Nursing diagnoses depend on the degree of nervous system involvement, but may include:

- Impaired spontaneous ventilation related to disease progression affecting respiratory nerves
- Impaired physical mobility related to paralysis of muscles by disease progression
- Risk for aspiration related to dysphagia
- Imbalanced nutrition: less than body requirements related to dysphagia and inability to feed self
- Acute pain related to paresthesias, muscle aches and cramps, and hyperesthesias
- Self-care deficit related to inability to use muscles to accomplish activities of daily living

- Fear related to seriousness of disease and unknown outcome
- Impaired verbal communication related to paralysis of speech muscles or intubation

Expected outcomes must be written for each nursing diagnosis. Overall goals of care are:

- Maintain adequate ventilation.
- Control pain adequately.
- Prevent damage from aspiration.
- Maintain communication.
- Maintain adequate nutritional status.
- Return patient to normal function.

■ Implementation and Evaluation

There are three phases of GBS: the acute phase, the static phase, and the rehabilitation phase. Each demands different kinds of monitoring and intervention. During the *acute* phase, the goals are to sustain life, prevent complications related to immobility, and promote rest and comfort. Respiratory problems are particularly troublesome and may require suctioning, tracheostomy care, artificial ventilation, and other life-support measures.

Vital signs must be checked frequently. Alterations in the autonomic nervous system can cause drastic changes in blood pressure, particularly hypotension. Cardiac arrhythmias also frequently occur, and the patient is continuously monitored.

The paralysis and loss of control that take place with GBS come on so suddenly and are so overwhelming that the patient becomes very frightened. Because the course of the disease usually extends for months with a very slow recovery, the patient begins to have feelings of hopelessness, despair, and isolation.

The *static* phase is a kind of plateau the patient reaches 1 to 3 weeks after the onset of the illness. During this time the motor loss and paresthesias no longer progress, and the patient's condition becomes somewhat stabilized; he gets no better or no worse. This phase can last from a few days to months.

? **Think Critically**

What problems requiring specific nursing interventions would you expect to encounter for the patient with Guillain-Barré syndrome who is now stable but has paralysis of the lower extremities and paresis of the upper extremities?

During the static phase, nursing care is concentrated on preventing complications of immobility and helping the patient deal with his feelings of anger, depression, and anxiety. Exercises are usually begun, but are limited to passive and gentle range-of-motion and stretching exercises. There must be a balance of rest and exercise and no sudden changes in posture or position, in case blood pressure suddenly drops.

Meticulous skin care is essential because of immobility. Monitoring for thrombophlebitis is important, as this is a frequent complication. Elastic stockings or sequential compression devices are applied to the legs, along with anticoagulant therapy, to try to prevent thrombophlebitis.

 Clinical Cues

Signs of thrombophlebitis are warmth, swelling, and pain in the extremity. Temperature may be elevated.

The final phase, *rehabilitation,* is one of gradual recovery. The patient may become elated over the change in his condition and must be prevented from overexertion, which can lead to a relapse. As muscle function returns, the level of exercise and activity is slowly increased (Davids et al., 2009). It may take up to 2 years for maximal improvement with return to normal functioning. Approximately 80% to 90% of patients have little residual deficit.

POLIOMYELITIS AND POSTPOLIO SYNDROME

Poliomyelitis destroys the motor cells of the anterior horn of the spinal cord, the brainstem, and the motor strip located in the frontal lobe. It is caused by a virus and can be prevented by immunization with the Salk (killed-virus) or Sabin (attenuated live-virus) polio vaccine. It is rare in the United States as immunization is given in childhood, but outbreaks still occur in other parts of the world. It is mentioned here because some people who had poliomyelitis have developed postpolio sequelae or postpolio syndrome. A new onset of weakness, pain, and fatigue occurs in people who had the disease over 30 years ago. Disability may be temporary or permanent. Treatment is geared toward making lifestyle modifications to preserve energy and physiologic function. Swimming in warm water has been found to promote comfort and help maintain flexibility.

HUNTINGTON'S DISEASE

Huntington's disease or Huntington's chorea is a rare, genetically transmitted degenerative neurologic disorder characterized by abnormal movements (chorea). It is accompanied by a decline in intellectual capacity and emotional disturbances. Signs of Huntington's disease usually become evident during the fourth or fifth decade of life, but may occur earlier. Women and men are equally affected. The disorder is progressive and causes disability and then death within 15 to 20 years after signs appear. Death is from neurologic degeneration affecting all body systems. Genetic transmission is by an abnormal gene on the short arm of chromosome 4. It is an autosomal dominant disorder,

meaning that 50% of the children of a person who has the disease will inherit it. If a child does not inherit the disease, the gene is not passed on to the next generation.

The person with Huntington's progresses from being fidgety and restless to a state of constant movement. Voluntary movement deteriorates until the patient is totally helpless. Intellectual decline causes depression, suspiciousness, and eventual dementia. There is no specific test for the disease, but genetic testing can determine the possibility of it developing; there is no known treatment to alter its course.

MYASTHENIA GRAVIS

Etiology and Pathophysiology

The words *myasthenia gravis* (MG) literally mean "grave muscle weakness." The disease is a chronic disorder. Skeletal muscles, respiratory muscles, and muscles enervated by cranial nerves are affected. The muscular weakness can be so mild that it causes a minor inconvenience or so severe that it is life threatening because of its effect on the muscles used for breathing and swallowing.

In 80% to 90% of MG patients there is an autoimmune disease in which circulating autoantibody is directed against the postsynaptic acetylcholine (ACh) receptors at the neuromuscular junction (the point at which nerve impulses are transmitted to muscle tissue) (Shah, 2009). The antibody reduces the number of functional receptor sites, and restricts the neuron uptake of ACh. As a result, nerve impulses are not transmitted and the muscle cannot contract properly. Other types of antibodies are present in the remaining percentage of MG patients.

There is a suggested connection between overgrowth of the thymus gland tissue and MG. An association between MG and hyperthyroidism, treatment with D-penicillamine, interferon alfa and bone marrow transplantation also exists.

Signs and Symptoms

Symptoms of myasthenia gravis include diplopia (double vision), difficulty chewing and swallowing, and ptosis (Figure 25-6). The patient's voice tends to be hoarse or nasal in quality, and voice volume decreases toward the end of a sentence. Severe muscle weakness that improves with rest is the outstanding symptom of the disorder. Any of the skeletal muscles might be involved; intestine, bladder, and heart muscles are not affected.

Ocular myasthenia may occur first and be demonstrated by diplopia and ptosis. In a small percentage of patients the disease progresses no further. If cranial nerves become more involved, bulbar myasthenia occurs with facial and oropharyngeal muscle weakness causing a blank facial expression and a smile resembling a snarl. Swallowing and speaking become

FIGURE 25-6 Ptosis (drooping upper lid) characteristic of the muscle weakness of myasthenia gravis.

difficult. Further progression to generalized myasthenia involves the muscles of the neck, shoulders, limbs, hands, diaphragm, and abdomen. The disease does not affect the level of consciousness. Muscles are strongest in the morning and become weaker with activity. Respiratory muscle weakness may require mechanical ventilation.

Diagnosis

Diagnosis is established by history and physical examination. A Tensilon test may be ordered to confirm the diagnosis. Two divided injections of edrophonium (Tensilon) are administered; a marked increase in muscular strength is noted within 1 minute of the second injection if the patient has myasthenia gravis. The first injection is a test dose to see if the patient will have an adverse reaction to the medication. Atropine is kept on hand to reverse the effects of the Tensilon if necessary. A blood test for antibodies to ACh receptors is ordered. Electrodiagnostic testing is performed to check muscle function. A chest radiograph and chest computed tomography (CT) scan will be ordered to check the thymus gland.

Treatment

There are two main modes of therapy, the choice depending on the severity of the symptoms. In milder cases the physician may manage the disease by dealing with the specific symptoms, rather than trying to induce a remission of the disease. In more severe cases, efforts are made to manage the underlying cause of the symptoms by inducing remission.

Because 80% to 90% of myasthenia gravis patients have autoantibodies against ACh receptors, plasmapheresis (plasma exchange) can be an effective treatment for the patient in crisis. It is particularly helpful in restoring muscle function when the patient is dependent on a ventilator. The purpose of the plasma exchange is to remove the circulating autoantibodies from the patient's blood. This mode of therapy may bring clinical improvement in some patients, but it is not a cure for myasthenia gravis.

Anticholinesterase therapy is the primary treatment for myasthenia gravis. Acetylcholine must be present at the point where nerve impulses are transmitted to muscle for sustained repetitive muscle contraction to occur. Anticholinesterase agents inactivate acetylcholinesterase, a substance that prevents accumulations of ACh at the neuromuscular junction. Anticholinesterase agents temporarily increase muscle strength by allowing ACh to work, but they do not cure the problem. Two drugs commonly used as anticholinesterase agents are neostigmine (Prostigmin) and pyridostigmine (Mestinon). Pyridostigmine is more commonly used because it can be taken orally. Corticosteroids and immunosuppressant drugs such as azathioprine (Imuran), rituximab (Rituxan), or cyclophosphamide (Cytoxan) may be used to suppress the immune response. Intravenous immune globulin (IVIG) infusion is sometimes prescribed.

The dosage of anticholinesterase drugs is precisely calculated for each patient. The aim is to achieve a delicate balance between too much and too little ACh at the neuromuscular junction. Stress can quickly alter a patient's need for ACh; hence overmedication or undermedication can occur rather suddenly. Unfortunately, the symptoms of too much medication are quite similar to those of too little medication, so it is often difficult to adjust the dosage correctly.

Another method of treatment is to remove the thymus gland, which decreases the antibody production (Shah, 2009). Treatment with IVIG for 5 days may produce a favorable response for 30 to 60 days.

❖ NURSING MANAGEMENT

▪ Assessment (Data Collection), Nursing Diagnosis, and Planning

The severity of myasthenia gravis is assessed by asking about the degree of fatigue, what body parts are affected, and how severe the problem is. Observe for ptosis of the eyelid and inquire about diplopia. Knowledge of the disorder should be determined, and the patient's coping abilities assessed. Assessment of respiratory function is a top priority. Assess muscle strength of the face, swallowing, speech volume and clarity, and cough and gag reflexes. Check the strength of the shoulder muscles and of the limbs.

Clinical Cues

When assessing status of a myasthenia gravis patient, have the patient look up at the ceiling. Watch to see if the eyelids start to move downward. This is often an early sign of the disease or that the medication is insufficient.

Nursing diagnoses will depend on the severity of the disease and may include:

- Ineffective breathing pattern related to diaphragm and intercostal muscle weakness
- Ineffective airway clearance related to weakness of intercostal muscles, and impaired cough and gag reflexes
- Disturbed visual sensory perception related to ptosis and diplopia
- Imbalanced nutrition: less than body requirements related to impaired swallowing ability
- Activity intolerance related to fatigue and muscle weakness
- Impaired verbal communication related to intubation or weakness of larynx, mouth, and pharynx muscles
- Ineffective coping related to inability to maintain usual roles and lifestyle

Expected outcomes are written for each nursing diagnosis based on the specific problem the patient is experiencing.

Patient Teaching

Teaching for the Patient with Myasthenia Gravis

Use your anticholinesterase medication correctly:
- Take the drug with food or fluid.
- Take the drug 45 minutes before meals to permit maximum effect for chewing and swallowing.
- Adjust drug dosage and times of administration as instructed according to your individual pattern of weakness and daily activities.
- Do not take over-the-counter or other prescribed medications without the approval of your health care provider or pharmacist.
- Report signs of cholinergic crisis to the health care provider quickly.
- Modify the diet for ease of chewing and swallowing; soft foods are easier to consume.
- Eat slowly in a calm environment and take small bites.
- Balance rest and activity throughout the day.
- Figure out ways of conserving energy while doing usual activities.
- Compensate with extra rest during periods of extra stress, illness, hormone swings during menstruation, and environmental temperature extremes.
- Wear a medical alert bracelet or necklace at all times; carry a card in your wallet stating that you have myasthenia gravis and list contact numbers for next of kin or significant other.
- Be aware of the signs and symptoms of myasthenic crisis and report them immediately.

■ Implementation and Evaluation

Infection, surgery, and other physical and emotional stresses can precipitate a myasthenic crisis and cause hospitalization. During the crisis, frequent monitoring is essential. The patient's ability to swallow and breathe on his own can be seriously compromised. Suctioning, tracheostomy, and artificial ventilation may be necessary to maintain life until the crisis is over.

Education of the patient and his family must include instruction about the nature of the illness and the adverse effects of emotional upsets, respiratory infections, and similar stresses. Care focuses on the neurologic deficits and their effect on daily activities. Rehabilitation goals include education and support for the patient and family so that the patient remains as independent as possible.

Because he can become critically ill and need immediate medical attention at any time, the patient with myasthenia gravis should at all times wear a medical alert emblem that identifies him as having the disease. The patient, as well as members of the family and the nurses who care for him in the hospital or at home, should know the symptoms of overdosage of anticholinesterase medication. The symptoms of myasthenic crisis caused by underdosage of anticholinesterase agents, a precipitating illness, or stress factors are equally important to know (Box 25-2). If any of these symptoms occurs, the physician should be notified immediately.

? Think Critically

What immediate action would you take if you found your patient in cholinergic crisis?

In addition to being affected by problems arising from the anticholinesterase drugs, the myasthenic patient also can suffer from exaggerated and bizarre

Box 25-2	**Signs and Symptoms of Cholinergic Crisis and Myasthenic Crisis**

CHOLINERGIC CRISIS
- Generalized weakness within 1 hour of the dose
- Dyspnea and increased bronchial secretions
- Poor tongue control producing difficulty in chewing
- Difficulty swallowing and excessive salivation
- Restlessness, anxiety, and irritability
- Diaphoresis
- Abdominal cramps, nausea or vomiting, diarrhea

MYASTHENIC CRISIS
- Increase in myasthenia gravis symptoms after failure to take drug as prescribed or following a precipitating illness or increased stress:
  - More difficulty swallowing
  - Diplopia
  - Ptosis
  - Dyspnea

Notify the physician immediately if these signs and symptoms appear.

effects from a variety of drugs. These include the steroids and thyroid compounds; sedatives and respiratory depressants, such as morphine; tranquilizers, such as the phenothiazines; many antibiotics; beta blockers; and some cardiac drugs, such as verapamil, procainamide, chloroquine, and quinidine. Because so many drugs are potentially dangerous to a patient with myasthenia gravis, it is imperative that the nurse check with the physician ordering a medication to be sure there is awareness that the patient has myasthenia gravis. **Always check each drug the patient is to receive for interactions and contraindications.**

COMMUNITY CARE

After leaving the hospital, patients with neurologic problems often are cared for in long-term care facilities, rehabilitation programs, outpatient clinics, and the home. Nurses who work in long-term care facilities must be confident in caring for patients with Parkinson's disease, as a large percentage of residents in these facilities have this disorder. Because elderly patients often have more than one chronic illness, it is essential that nurses be knowledgeable about medication interactions and side effects. Each patient's

medications must be continually assessed for possible adverse effects and side effects, as well as for data indicating that each medication is producing a sufficient therapeutic effect to warrant continued administration. A close working relationship with the pharmacist can assist the nurse in judging these matters. Collaborative care between the pharmacist, nurse, nurse aides, physical therapist, social worker, and others who interact with the patient is needed to provide the best plan of care for these patients who require complex care.

The nurse who works with patients who have neurologic deficits that cause some degree of immobility must constantly try to prevent the complications of immobility and to achieve as high a level of function for the patient as possible.

The home care nurse interacts with the entire family and needs to continually offer support as the difficulties of learning to live with someone who has a neurologic deficit are met. Family roles often are altered and strained, and the period of adjustment for the patient and family is lengthy. It often is difficult for the family to cope with the personality changes that occur in the patient who has a degenerative neurologic disorder. Referral to community support groups is often helpful for both the patient and the family members.

Get Ready for the NCLEX® Examination!

Key Points

- The characteristic triad of symptoms of Parkinson's disease (PD) is tremor, bradykinesia, and rigidity.
- Treatment of PD is with drug therapy, physical therapy, and emotional support (see Table 25-1).
- When drug therapy for PD fails, surgical treatment may be warranted.
- Multiple sclerosis (MS) is a chronic inflammatory disease causing demyelination of the myelin sheath in the central nervous system (see Table 25-2).
- Common manifestations of MS are motor dysfunction, sensory dysfunction, problems of coordination, mental changes, fatigue, bowel and bladder problems, and altered sexual function.
- MS is treated with biologic response modifier drugs and drugs to treat the problems caused by the disease.
- Alzheimer's disease is a form of dementia and is covered in Chapter 48.
- Amyotrophic lateral sclerosis (ALS) is a rare but devastating disease that usually results in death within 3 years after diagnosis.
- ALS affects the motor neurons and causes weakness of the voluntary muscles.
- Nursing care for the ALS patient focuses on preventing complications and dealing with the problems the disease has caused, particularly immobility, dysphagia, inability to communicate, pain, and depression.
- Guillain-Barré syndrome (GBS) affects the peripheral nervous system and the cranial nerves.

- GBS is a cell-mediated immunologic response to a stimulus from a viral infection, trauma, surgery, viral immunization, HIV, or neoplasm of the lymphatic system.
- GBS usually causes an ascending paralysis and considerable pain.
- Nursing care for GBS is directed at maintaining adequate ventilation, nutrition, and supportive care for immobility and activities of daily living.
- Postpolio syndrome is the reappearance of polio symptoms many years after the initial polio illness.
- Huntington's disease (HD) is a genetic disease characterized by chorea.
- HD causes a decline in intellectual capacity, emotional disturbances, and total dependence, with death occurring in 15 to 20 years.
- Myasthenia gravis (MG) is an autoimmune disease affecting the neuromuscular junction.
- MG is chronic and is manifested by fatigue and muscular weakness (both symptoms improve with rest).
- Ptosis, diplopia, a weak nasal-quality voice, a blank expression, and a smile resembling a snarl are signs and symptoms of MG.
- MG may affect the intercostal muscles and the diaphragm, causing inadequate respiration.
- Anticholinesterase therapy is the common treatment for MG.
- Nurses must know the signs of overdosage of anticholinesterase drugs.

Review Questions for the NCLEX® Examination

1. During a neurologic examination, the patient demonstrates difficulty initiating movement. The steps are short with quick cadence. Arm swings are decreased with subsequent steps. The clinical findings are referred to as:
   1. muscle atrophy.
   2. akinesia.
   3. rigidity.
   4. tremors.

2. A patient is admitted due to progressive muscle weakness in the lower extremities. The patient complains of tingling and numbness in the hands. The patient recovered from the flu a week ago. Which intervention(s) should be anticipated in the care of this patient? (*Select all that apply.*)
   1. Medication for pain and discomfort
   2. Immediate need for physical therapy exercise
   3. Possible need for ventilatory assistance
   4. Need for airway suctioning
   5. Administration of muscle relaxants

3. The physician discusses the treatment options with a patient newly diagnosed with Parkinson's disease. The patient asks, "What will happen to me?" An appropriate response would be:
   1. "You seem worried. Let's talk about your concerns."
   2. "Your physician can fully explain your condition."
   3. "You will be all right."
   4. "We all eventually get there."

4. A 45-year-old patient newly diagnosed with multiple sclerosis asks about the nature of the illness. Teaching about the condition would include stating:
   1. "The condition is a progressive degeneration of the gray matter in the anterior horns of the spinal cord and the lower cranial nerves."
   2. "The condition can only be diagnosed during an autopsy."
   3. "The condition affects the spinal nerves outside the spinal cord and usually follows a viral infection."
   4. "The condition is a chronic demyelinization of the central nervous system with possible periods of remissions and exacerbations."

5. A female patient with myasthenia gravis is admitted with dyspnea and increased bronchial secretions, difficulty swallowing, abdominal cramps, and diaphoresis. The probable cause of these symptoms is

   _____.

6. The nurse observes a nursing assistant feed a dysphagic patient. Which action by the nursing assistant indicates a need for further instruction and guidance?
   1. The wall suction is turned on and readily available.
   2. The patient is propped up with one pillow.
   3. The food is cut into small, bite-size pieces.
   4. The nursing assistant coaches the patient to drop the chin.

7. The nurse reinforces pharmacy instructions regarding safe use of pyridostigmine (Mestinon), an anticholinesterase, by a patient newly diagnosed with myasthenia gravis. Which statement indicates a need for further teaching?
   1. "I need to take the medication after meals on a full stomach."
   2. "I can adjust the drug dosage and times depending on daily activities."
   3. "I shouldn't take over-the-counter medications without physician approval."
   4. "I should balance rest and activity throughout the day."

8. Thirty seconds after the administration of edrophonium (Tensilon), the patient is observed to have slowed heart rate, sweating, and cramping. An appropriate nursing action would be to:
   1. start chest compressions.
   2. notify the physician.
   3. administer atropine.
   4. give pyridostigmine (Mestinon).

9. The priority nursing assessment of a patient with myasthenia gravis would be to:
   1. determine the degree of fatigue.
   2. assess the level of knowledge regarding the disease.
   3. monitor the adequacy of respiratory function.
   4. check the patient's swallowing, speech, and protective reflexes.

10. The nurse determines that risk for injury is the priority nursing diagnosis for a patient diagnosed with Parkinson's disease. Which nursing intervention(s) would help prevent occurrence of falls? *(Select all that apply.)*
    1. Encourage use of wheelchair.
    2. Apply leg braces.
    3. Remove loose carpets or throw rugs.
    4. Install grab bars in the shower and tub.
    5. Install low toilet seats.

Critical Thinking Activities

Scenario A
Your patient had a bout of the "flu" about a week ago. Today he noticed he was having trouble walking. When he got home from an errand, he had trouble pulling his sweater over his head. His wife brought him to the emergency department.

1. Which neurologic problem within this chapter do you think he might have?

2. What might be done to establish a diagnosis?

3. What would be a top priority in his care at this time?

4. What further problems do you think could occur?

Scenario B
Mrs. Jones seems less animated than she has been over the past several months. Her husband tells you she has fallen three times since her last office visit. You notice that she seems more stooped over and her movements are "jerky." The physician examines her and after a thorough history and physical tells the couple that he thinks Mrs. Jones has Parkinson's disease. He prescribes Sinemet for her.

1. What can you anticipate that Mr. and Mrs. Jones will need to be taught?

2. What are the potential complications of Parkinson's disease?

Scenario C
A fellow student in your clinical group confides that she has myasthenia gravis. She takes Mestinon for control of the disease.

1. What factors could cause her symptoms to worsen?

2. What might happen if she forgets to take her medication before reporting for her clinical rotation?

Scenario D
A man comes to the clinic complaining of difficulty enunciating, of having tingling and prickling in the extremities, and of having more difficulty walking. After diagnostic testing it is determined that he has amyotrophic lateral sclerosis.

1. What is the focus of interdisciplinary care?

2. What is the prognosis for the patient?

The Sensory System: Eye and Ear

evolve

Objectives

Theory

1. Identify ways in which nurses can help patients preserve their sight and hearing.
2. Identify signs and symptoms of eye and ear problems.
3. Discuss tests and examinations used to diagnose eye and ear disorders.
4. Perform nursing activities associated with assessing the eye and ear.
5. Use the nursing process for patients with disorders of the eye or ear.

Clinical Practice

1. Provide teaching for a patient who is to undergo tests for a vision problem.
2. Perform focused assessments for disorders of the eyes and ears.
3. Assist visually impaired patients to find resources to maximize their vision.
4. Instruct a spouse in ways to effectively communicate with a hearing-impaired partner.

Key Terms

cerumen (sĕ-RŪ-mĕn, p. 579)
ectropion (ĕk-TRŌ-pē-ŏn, p. 571)
entropion (ĕn-TRŌ-pē-ŏn, p. 576)
exophthalmos (ĕk-sŏf-THĂL-mŏs, p. 576)
keratitis (kĕr-ă-TĬ-tĭs, p. 571)
nystagmus (nĭs-TĂG-mŭs, p. 583)
otorrhea (ō-tō-RĒ-ă, p. 585)

photophobia (fō-tō-FŌ-bē-ă, p. 576)
presbycusis (prĕz-bē-KŪ-sĭs, p. 589)
presbyopia (prĕz-bē-Ō-pē-ă, p. 570)
ptosis (TŌ-sĭs, p. 571)
refraction (rē-FRĂK-shŭn, p. 569)
sensorineural loss (sĕn-sō-rē-NŪ-răl, p. 581)
xanthelasma (zăn-thĕ-LĂZ-mă, p. 576)

OVERVIEW OF ANATOMY AND PHYSIOLOGY OF THE EYE

WHAT ARE THE STRUCTURES OF THE EYE?

- The eyeball is spherical in shape and 2 to 3 cm in diameter (Figure 26-1).
- The sclera, which is part of the wall of the eyeball, is opaque white and covers the posterior five sixths of the eyeball.
- The transparent cornea is part of the wall of the eyeball and covers the anterior one sixth of the eyeball.
- The choroid is part of the middle layer of the eyeball. It is a highly vascular layer containing brown pigment located between the sclera and the retina.
- The ciliary body is part of the middle layer of the eyeball and contains finger-like ciliary processes that produce aqueous humor. The ciliary body helps change eye shape for near and far vision.
- The iris is the third part of the middle layer of the eyeball; it is the colored portion of the eye and is a doughnut-shaped diaphragm with the pupil as the central opening. The iris contains two groups of smooth muscles that constrict and dilate the pupil to regulate the entrance of light.
- The biconvex, transparent lens, together with the suspensory ligaments and the ciliary body, forms a partition that divides the interior of the eyeball into two chambers. The anterior chamber between the lens and the cornea is filled with aqueous humor. The posterior chamber, between the lens and the retina, contains vitreous humor.
- The suspensory ligaments connect the ciliary body to the lens.
- The retina is the inner coat of the eyeball and is found in the posterior portion of it. The retina contains several layers. The layer with rods and cones acts as the receptor for light images.
- The optic nerve carries messages from the nerve cells in the retina to the brain.
- The optic disc is formed by the axons of the ganglion cells of the retina.

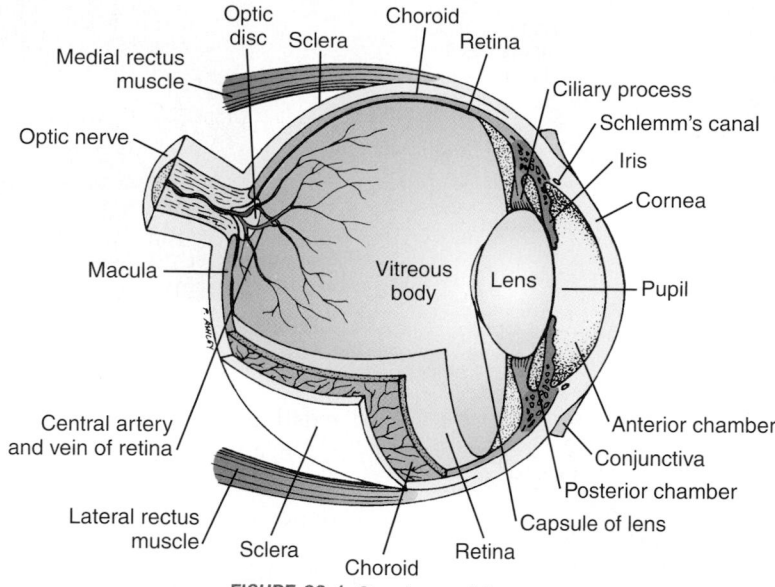

FIGURE 26-1 Structures of the eye.

- The macula lutea is a yellow spot just lateral to the optic disc that allows for visual detail.
- The fovea centralis is the area of the retina that produces the sharpest image.
- The eyelids are composed of skin, connective tissue, and conjunctiva. The conjunctiva is a thin mucous membrane that lines the eyelid and covers the anterior portion of the eyeball, except for the cornea.
- Eyelashes line the edge of the eyelid.
- Sebaceous glands are situated with the eyelashes.
- The lacrimal glands are located in the upper outer area above the eyes. The lacrimal ducts and canals carry tears from the eye to the nose.
- Six muscles attach to the eyeball and allow for movement. The muscles come from the bones of the orbit and insert on the outer layer of the eyeball.

WHAT ARE THE FUNCTIONS OF THE EYE STRUCTURES?

- The bony orbit protects the eyeball.
- The eyelashes help trap foreign particles, keeping them from landing on the eyeball.
- The eyelids protect the eyes from foreign matter and help distribute moisture on the eye surface.
- The sebaceous glands secrete an oily fluid that lubricates the lids.
- Blinking of the eyelid 6 to 30 times a minute stimulates the lacrimal glands to produce tears.
- The lacrimal gland secretes tears that moisten, lubricate, and cleanse the surface of the eye. Tears contain an enzyme that helps destroy bacteria and prevent infections.
- The transparent cornea allows light to hit the lens. It assists with the bending of light rays **(refraction),** so that the rays will hit the retina in the right location for images to be transmitted to the brain.

- The choroid's brown pigment absorbs excess light rays that could interfere with vision.
- The ciliary processes secrete aqueous humor that helps maintain the shape of the anterior chamber; it also nourishes the structures in this part of the eye. The aqueous humor assists with refraction of light onto the retina. **The amount of aqueous humor present determines the internal pressure of the eye.** The aqueous humor is reabsorbed by the blood vessels located at the junction of the sclera and the cornea.
- Muscles in the iris control dilation and constriction of the pupil.
- The suspensory ligaments connected to the ciliary body and lens allow light to focus on the lens and retina, which is necessary for close vision.
- The retina's rods and cones are photoreceptors for light and color. The nerves of the retina transmit the images perceived to the brain.
- The optic nerve conducts nerve impulses from the retina to the brain.
- Visualization of the optic disc provides information about the pressure within the eye and within the skull. When intracranial pressure gets higher, the optic disc appears "swollen" or "choked."
- Visual impulses travel along the optic nerve to the optic chiasma just anterior to the pituitary gland; at this point some of the axons cross over to the other side. Images from the medial portion of the left eye and from the lateral portion of the right eye are carried by the right optic tract. Images from the medial portion of the right eye and from the lateral portion of the left eye are carried by the left optic tract (Figure 26-2). Images are conducted to the visual cortex in the occipital lobe of the brain.
- Six muscles control movement of the eyeball. Table 26-1 lists these muscles and the nerves that control them.

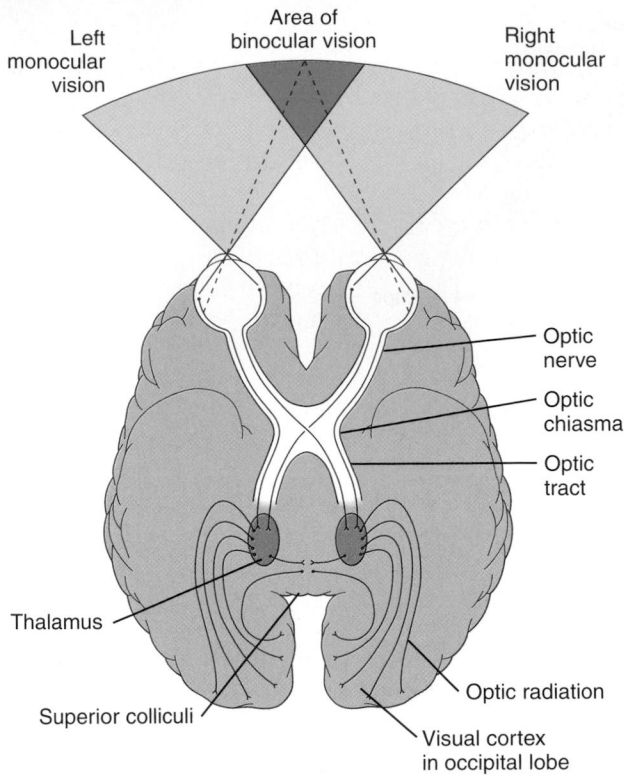

FIGURE 26-2 Visual pathway.

Left monocular vision

Area of binocular vision

Right monocular vision

Optic nerve

Optic chiasma

Optic tract

Thalamus

Superior colliculi

Optic radiation

Visual cortex in occipital lobe

FIGURE 26-3 Arcus senilis, a white ring around the cornea.

WHAT CHANGES OCCUR IN THE EYE WITH AGING?

- Subcutaneous fat and tissue elasticity decrease, and the eyes appear to be sunken.
- *Arcus senilis*, an opaque ring outlining the cornea, sometimes results from the deposition of fatty globules (Figure 26-3).
- The cornea flattens and develops an irregular curvature after age 65, causing astigmatism or making an existing astigmatism worse; vision becomes blurred. Cornea transparency also decreases.
- The sclera develops a yellowish tinge due to fatty deposits; thinning of the sclera may cause a bluish tinge.
- The ability of the iris to dilate decreases, causing difficulty for the older person in going from a bright area into a darkened area.
- The lens of the eye changes after age 40, gradually losing water and becoming harder. Cataracts may form.
- The ciliary muscle has less ability to allow the eye to accommodate, a process responsible for the gradual extension of distance from the eyes at which an item to be read is held (presbyopia). This change begins around age 40.
- The farthest point at which an object can be identified decreases, and the older person has a narrower visual field.
- Pupil size becomes smaller, reducing the ability to see in dim light.
- Color discrimination decreases with advancing age and may cause problems.

Table 26-1 Muscles of the Eye

MUSCLE	CONTROLLING NERVE	FUNCTION
Extrinsic (Skeletal) Muscles		
Superior rectus	Oculomotor (CN III)	Elevates eye or rolls it superiorly and toward the midline.
Inferior rectus	Oculomotor (CN III)	Depresses eye or rolls it inferiorly and toward the midline.
Medial rectus	Oculomotor (CN III)	Moves eye medially, toward the midline.
Lateral rectus	Abducens (CN VI)	Moves eye laterally, away from the midline.
Superior oblique	Trochlear (CN IV)	Depresses eye and turns it laterally, away from the midline.
Inferior oblique	Oculomotor (CN III)	Elevates eye and turns it laterally, away from the midline.
Intrinsic (Smooth) Muscles		
Ciliary	Oculomotor (CN III): parasympathetic fibers	Causes suspensory ligament to relax, so lens becomes more convex for close vision.
Iris, circular muscles	Oculomotor (CN III): parasympathetic fibers	Decreases the size of the pupil to allow less light to enter the eye.
Iris, radial muscles	Sympathetic fibers from spinal nerves	Increases the size of the pupil to allow more light to enter the eye.

Adapted from Applegate, E.J. (2011). *The Anatomy and Physiology Learning System* (4th ed.). Philadelphia: Saunders, p. 205.
CN, cranial nerve.

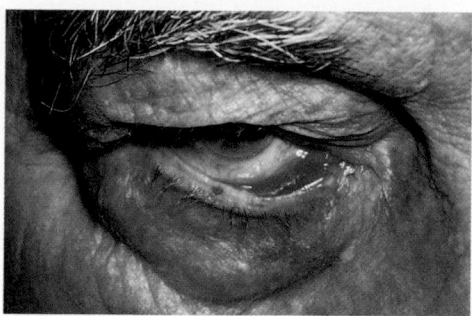

FIGURE 26-4 Ectropion.

- Moisture secretion decreases during the senior years, placing the eyes at greater risk for irritation and infection. This is especially common after age 70. Repeated episodes of keratitis (inflammation of the cornea) may seriously compromise vision and can lead to loss of independence for an elderly person.
- Eversion of the lower lid (ectropion) occurs because of loss of muscle tone and elasticity (Figure 26-4).
- Decreased muscle tone and decreased elasticity may cause drooping of the upper lid to a point where it interferes with vision (ptosis).

THE EYE

EYE DISORDERS

There are two general kinds of patients with impaired vision: those who were born blind, and those who develop some degree of visual impairment later in life. This chapter focuses on the latter type of visually handicapped patient.

Eye disorders are caused by injury or disease, or are disorders for which there is a genetic predisposition. Diabetes mellitus and hypertension contribute greatly to visual loss in the United States. Untreated glaucoma causes blindness. Macular degeneration is another major cause of impaired vision. It is now known that smoking has a direct link to the incidence of macular degeneration. Cataracts eventually cause blindness, if they are not removed.

There are approximately 15 million visually impaired or blind people in the United States. Of those, 7.3 million are over 65 years of age (Braille Institute of America, 2010). There are many new surgical techniques and medical treatments that offer hope for eyesight preservation to increasing numbers of people. Efforts also have been made to educate the public about eye care, prevention of eye disease, and periodic examinations to detect eye disorders in their earliest and treatable stages.

Acquired immunodeficiency syndrome (AIDS) can cause blindness as a result of opportunistic infections that the AIDS patient contracts. Ocular problems of the AIDS patient are discussed in Chapter 11.

Prevention

As health care providers, nurses share responsibility for preserving vision throughout the patient's life span. Three major nursing goals to promote good vision are:
- Health education to inform the general public about basic eye care
- Prevention of accidental injury to the eye
- Prevention of visual loss

Healthy People 2020 goals contain 10 objectives related to preventing vision loss and improving vision.

BASIC EYE CARE

To prevent eye strain, rest the eye muscles periodically when working at the computer, watching television, doing needlework, or performing any activity that demands intensive visual effort. If the eyes tire easily or if there is headache or burning, itching, or redness of the eyes, the eyes should be examined. Good nutrition is important to eye health, and certain nutrients such as lutein and zeaxanthin are especially beneficial to vision.

 Nutrition Considerations

Vitamins and Antioxidants Beneficial to Vision

Vitamin A protects against night blindness, slow adaptation to darkness, and glare blindness. The carotenoids are the precursors for vitamin A and are found in green leafy and yellow vegetables. Carrots, greens, spinach, orange juice, sweet potatoes, and cantaloupe are rich sources of the carotenoids (Linus Pauling Institute, 2010). Lutein and zeaxanthin, both antioxidants, may help prevent macular degeneration and cataracts. They are found in yellow fruits and vegetables, red and purple fruits, and greens. Lutein is particularly high in tomatoes, carrots, broccoli, kale, spinach, and romaine lettuce. Corn, cornmeal, kale, Japanese persimmons, and turnip greens have large quantities of zeaxanthin, with corn containing the highest amount. Many vitamin supplements have added lutein to their formulation (National Eye Institute, 2010).

Normal secretions of the conjunctiva and tear glands should be sufficient to lubricate the eye and wash away small particles of dust. **Accumulations of purulent material or excessive tearing usually indicate the need for an eye examination.** Dry eye syndrome in people younger than 60 years could be symptomatic of underlying disease.

 Elder Care Points

Older persons sometimes suffer from "dry eyes." This is due to decreased production of tears and is treated by instilling "replacement tears," which are commercial preparations or prescriptions of solutions similar in composition to real tears.

Adults should have an eye examination once between ages 20 and 29, twice between ages 30 and 39, and a baseline screening at age 40. After age 65, eyes should be examined by an eye specialist every 2 years (Eyecareamerica, 2010). It is particularly important to test for glaucoma because this disease usually is asymptomatic until damage to vision has occurred. People with a family history of glaucoma should be especially careful to have their eyes tested frequently for increased pressure within the eyeball, as this is the basic pathology of glaucoma, and the disorder tends to be hereditary.

PREVENTION OF EYE INJURY

Accidental injury to the eye is a major cause of diminished or total loss of vision. Adults should be cautioned to wear protective eyewear when engaging in sports such as racquetball and squash, in which small balls travel at high speeds. Protective eyewear should be worn when using machinery that might cause debris to fly into the eye, such as lawn mowers, weed trimmers, sanders, or power saws.

The rate of occupational accidents has gone down since the establishment and enforcement of rules for wearing goggles and other protective devices by people working in a hazardous environment. The National Institute of Occupational Safety and Health (NIOSH) in Rockville, Maryland, provides information about eye safety and hazards in the workplace.

Cosmetics for the eyelids, eyelashes, and eyebrows can be a source of infection and allergy. Eye makeup should be discarded every 6 months to help prevent infection. Most dyes used for hair on the scalp are not intended for use on the eyelashes and eyebrows.

Saliva should not be used to moisten eye pencils, eye shadow, or mascara, as it may contain organisms that can cause eye infection. Apply eye cosmetics with

Health Promotion

Danger Signals of Eye Disease

- Persistent redness of the eye. Infections and inflammations of the structures of the eye that are not treated may leave scars that can produce loss of vision.
- Continuing pain or discomfort especially following injury.
- Disturbance of vision. Although these symptoms may simply indicate a need for eyeglasses, blurred vision, loss of side vision, double vision, and sudden development of many floating spots in the field of vision may be symptomatic of more serious systemic diseases.
- Colored light flashes, or a feeling that a curtain has been pulled across the line of vision or a shade has been pulled down. This can indicate a retinal detachment and requires prompt attention.
- Crossing of the eyes, especially in children.
- Growths on the eye or eyelids or opacities visible in the normally transparent portion of the eye.
- Continuing discharge, crusting, or tearing of the eyes.
- Unequal size of the two pupils or distorted shape.

a steady hand to avoid accidentally scratching the cornea and eyelids. Cosmetics should never be shared, as this can transmit organisms.

PREVENTION OF VISUAL LOSS

Diabetes mellitus and hypertension are chronic diseases that—when uncontrolled—may cause visual loss. Patients with these disorders are more susceptible to retinopathy. Nurses should encourage good control over these diseases.

Cultural Considerations

Latinos and Eye Disease

The Los Angeles Latino Eye Study found that Latinos had high rates of diabetic retinopathy and of open-angle glaucoma. The study interviewed and examined 6300 Latinos age 40 and older from the Los Angeles area. Many of those Latinos involved in the study were found to have previously undiagnosed diabetes. Almost half of the individuals in the study who had diabetes had diabetic retinopathy. Seventy-five percent of Latinos with glaucoma were undiagnosed before participating in the study (National Eye Institute, 2010).

To help prevent infections that might cause corneal scarring and loss of vision, encourage people who experience an accident causing a corneal abrasion to seek medical attention quickly. Promptly seeking medical attention when the eye is inflamed, is secreting purulent discharge, or is sore assists in treatment of infection that may cause a residual visual loss.

Think Critically

Can you identify four specific ways in which you might prevent eye disorders among your relatives and patients?

Assessing patients for the presence of cataracts and recommending regular periodic eye examinations should be a part of every nurse's practice. Cataract removal can greatly improve vision. Screening for glaucoma reduces the incidence of blindness from that condition. Free screening clinics often are available in communities. Nurses can inform patients of when and where such screenings are available. The Tono-Pen is often used for such screenings. It is also used in the emergency department when a patient complains of symptoms that might be from increased intraocular pressure (Figure 26-5).

Nurses must be aware that there are many types of visual loss. Some may affect only one area of the field of vision in one eye, whereas others affect parts of the field of vision in both eyes. The degree of visual impairment varies greatly.

FIGURE 26-5 The Tono-Pen is used to check intraocular pressure.

DIAGNOSTIC TESTS AND EXAMINATIONS

Diagnostic tests are performed to test visual acuity, prescribe prescription lenses, inspect the interior of the eye, check intraocular pressure, and assess the health of the retinal blood vessels (Figure 26-6). Computed tomography, optical coherence tomography, and magnetic resonance imaging may also be used to diagnose eye disorders. Table 26-2 provides further information about diagnostic tests.

❖ NURSING MANAGEMENT

The nursing care of patients with severe visual handicaps demands a special awareness of the unique problems encountered by someone who has either a partial or a total loss of vision. You must be sensitive to these patients' special needs. Patient education is especially important to these patients' acceptance of their visual disorder, their participation in diagnostic and therapeutic measures, and their adjustment to their new

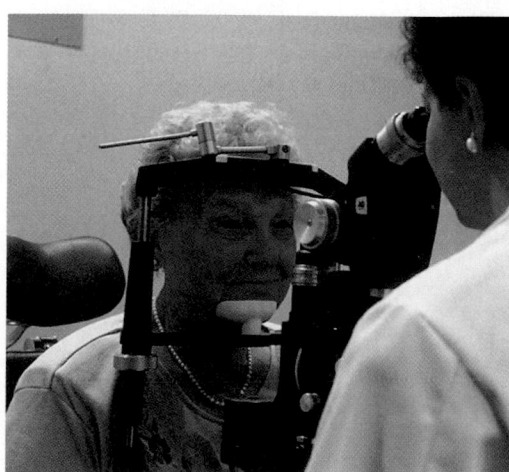

FIGURE 26-6 Slit-lamp ocular examination.

surroundings when they are hospitalized or admitted to a long-term care facility.

■ Assessment (Data Collection)

All nurses should be able to perform a basic eye examination, inspecting the eye for signs of redness or discharge, and checking visual acuity with a Snellen eye chart. Only nurses who have had special training are qualified to conduct a complete eye assessment (Figure 26-7). Significant data can be obtained by nurses who lack specialized education, by taking an adequate history.

History Taking

Many systemic diseases, including AIDS, hypertension, and diabetes mellitus, secondarily affect the eye and its functions. In the general assessment of any patient, you should be aware of the more obvious indications of an ophthalmic pathology, whether it be primary or secondary.

A history of neurologic disorders should be noted. Neuromuscular diseases are especially likely to cause diplopia, blurred vision, or inability to move the eyes. Endocrine disorders that secondarily affect the eyes include thyroid disease and diabetes mellitus. Acute hyperglycemia can alter the shape of the lens and temporarily cause blurred vision. **Prolonged hyperglycemia can adversely affect the blood vessels of the retina, causing bleeding, and leading to loss of vision.** Liver and kidney failure can produce pathologic changes in both neural and vascular structures within the eye. Retinal changes also can be caused by hypertension and atherosclerosis.

Some drugs are capable of producing either transient or permanent ocular changes that lead to disturbances in color vision and visual acuity, and to the formation of cataracts, retinopathy, and glaucoma. Among common drugs that have possible ocular side effects are digitalis leaf, corticosteroids, indomethacin (Indocin), and sulfisoxazole (Gantrisin).

A family history of eye disorders can be significant because disorders such as strabismus, retinitis pigmentosa, glaucoma, and cataracts tend to run in families, or follow a pattern of inheritance.

FIGURE 26-7 Examination of the eye with an ophthalmoscope.

Table 26-2 Diagnostic Tests for Eye Problems

TEST	PURPOSE	DESCRIPTION	NURSING IMPLICATIONS
Ophthalmoscopy (retinoscopy)	To inspect the fundus (back portion) of the eyeball to detect abnormalities of the retina, macula, optic disc, and retinal vessels	The examiner uses an ophthalmoscope (see Figure 26-7) to focus light through the pupil onto the fundus.	The room is darkened before the examiner approaches the patient with the ophthalmoscope. Drops may be placed in the eye before this examination to dilate the eye and offer a wider area through which to view the fundus.
Visual acuity	To determine status of vision	The Snellen eye chart is used. It is placed 20 feet from the patient, and first one eye is occluded and then the other eye is occluded. The person begins reading lines of letters that decrease in size. Visual acuity is expressed as a fraction for each eye. The numerator (first) figure indicates the distance between the patient and the chart. The denominator (second) figure expresses the distance at which the person with 20/20 vision could read the letters in the line correctly. Visual acuity of 20/20 in each eye is normal; vision of 20/200 (with correction) is legally defined as blindness.	Explain the procedure to the patient. Have the patient hold the occluding card close to the nose so that the entire eye is covered. Start with the third line. If the patient cannot read that, progress upward; if the line is correctly read, go to the next line down; etc. Test the other eye. Record the findings.
Near vision test	To determine status of near vision	The patient is given a Jaeger's Test Type card with different sizes of type on it. One eye is occluded while the patient reads the lines of type. Determination of vision status is made on the basis of what a person with normal vision can read.	Explain that this is a simple test of vision to determine whether there are any problems that might require further testing.
Visual fields test (confrontation test)	To examine the patient's visual fields, detecting problems with peripheral vision	The examiner faces the patient and asks her to look directly into his eyes. The examiner covers his right eye, and the patient covers her left eye. Then the examiner's finger is moved from an area outside of the peripheral vision into the line of vision. The patient should detect the finger about the same time as the examiner. The test is repeated with the other eye covered.	Explain the test to the patient and remind her to keep looking directly into your eyes.
Extraocular muscle function test	To test the function of the extraocular muscles	Ask the patient to hold her head still and to move the eyes to follow a small object such as a pen to each of the six cardinal points: right; upward and right; down and right; left; upward and left; down and left.	Observe for parallel eye movements and any deviation of movement. Nystagmus is a normal finding for the far lateral gaze. Record your findings.
Color vision test	To determine if the patient has any color blindness	Use the Ishihara chart book, which shows numbers composed of dots of one color within an area of dots of a different color. Ask the patient what she sees on the page for each chart. Test each eye separately. Reading the numbers correctly indicates normal color vision.	Explain the purpose of the test. Tell the patient to tell you what number appears on the chart. Record your findings.

Test	Purpose	Description	Patient Teaching
Refraction	To determine amount of lens correction necessary to restore person's vision to as near normal as possible with glasses	A series of glass lenses are placed in front of the patient's eyes to determine which lens provides the best vision correction. Each eye is tested separately.	A prescription for glasses will be written depending on the findings of the refraction test. The test may be performed for both near and far vision.
Intraocular pressure test	To determine the amount of pressure within the eye; aid in diagnosis of glaucoma	A tonometer is used to measure the pressure. This may be a handheld instrument, but it usually is a device that measures pressure by taking a reading while air is directed at the eye by a pneumotonometer. Another type of tonometer is the applanation tonometer. Normal intraocular pressure is 10-21 mm Hg.	Explain that this is a test to determine whether a patient might have glaucoma. More than one reading on different days is necessary to confirm a diagnosis of glaucoma. If a diagnosis of glaucoma is made, medication can be prescribed to help control the intraocular pressure and preserve vision.
Slit-lamp biomicroscopic examination	To examine the surface of the eye	A beam of light is reduced to a narrow slit that illuminates only a small section of the eye, allowing examination of a thin section of the eye structures at a time.	Explain that this device helps detect "floaters" in the vitreous humor, and abnormalities of the cornea and other structures of the eye. The eyes may be dilated with mydriatic drops for this test.
Topical dye (corneal staining)	To detect abrasions of the cornea or the presence of a foreign body on the cornea	Fluorescein dye drops are administered to the affected eye. The dye remains on the injured tissue or surrounds a foreign body. Such areas usually appear as green spots.	Explain the procedure and the rationale for the test. Warn that the drops may sting slightly for a few minutes. Give the patient a tissue to absorb the excess drops as they may stain clothing.
Fluorescein angiography (retinal angiography)	To detect tumors of the interior of the eye and to help diagnose and measure the extent of retinopathy	An IV injection of sodium fluorescein is given. A short time later, photographs of the fundus are taken with a special camera.	An IV injection is necessary. A signed consent form is required to perform the procedure.
Electroretinography	To test the functional integrity of the retina; evaluates degeneration of the photoreceptor cells	Electrodes embedded into a contact lens are placed directly on the anesthetized eye. A light stimulus is introduced. The change in electrical potential of the eye caused by the flash of light is measured.	Instruct the patient that she must fixate on the target and not move her eyes during the test.
Optical coherence tomography (OCT)	To record images of retinal structures; To differentiate the anatomical layers within the retina and allow measurement of retinal thickness; To detect macular holes, epiretinal membranes, cystoid macular edema, and other pathologies	Focused beams of light are directed into the eye that scan the structural features of the retina. A cross-sectional image similar to a topographic map is produced.	The patient's eyes must be dilated. Tell the patient that she will be looking into a machine. The test takes from 10-20 min.
Amsler grid test	To detect macular degeneration	Using a handheld card printed with a grid of black lines similar to graph paper, the patient fixates on a center dot and records abnormalities of the grid lines.	Test should be performed every week or two. Instruct the patient to record seeing wavy or missing lines, or distorted areas.
Ultrasonography	To evaluate the characteristics of a lesion, and its size and growth over time, or to determine the presence of a foreign body	A probe is placed directly on the eyeball. Sound waves are transmitted into the eye, bounce back off the various tissues, and are collected by a receiver and amplified on an oscilloscope screen.	Explain the procedure to the patient.

IV, intravenous.

Data Collection for Eye Disorders

The following questions should be asked when gathering history regarding an eye disorder:

- Have you noticed a change in your vision?
- Do you have any pain or discomfort in the eyes? Itching? Burning? Stinging? Excessive tearing or watering?
- Have you had any episodes of blurred vision? Double vision? A loss in the field of vision? Blind spots? Floating spots?
- Do you have difficulty with vision at night?
- Is there any pain in the eyes when you are in bright light?
- Do you have headaches in the brow area?
- Do you see halos around lights?
- Have you ever injured an eye in any way?
- Do you experience frequent reddening of the eye (conjunctivitis)?
- Do you ever experience discharge or sticky matter in the eye?
- Do you find that your lids are crusty when you awaken?
- Do your eyes feel dry? Do you frequently use eyedrops?
- Do you wear contact lenses? Use glasses?
- What medications do you take regularly?
- Is there any history of glaucoma in your family?
- Have you ever been told you have diabetes? Hypertension?
- When did you have your last eye examination?
- *For those patients who have a previous visual loss:* How do you cope with your loss of vision?

Sometimes patients are not aware of gradual changes in vision, but have noticed that they have had more minor accidents lately, seem to be more easily fatigued, or are less interested in doing things that once gave them pleasure, such as sewing or some other hobby.

Physical Examination

Observe the patient's eyes and eye area for redness of the conjunctiva, swelling of the eyelids or in the periorbital space, excessive tearing, change in visual acuity, secretions and encrustations on the eyelids, abnormal position of the eyelid, and exophthalmos (protrusion of the eyeball). Abnormalities of lid position are described in Table 26-3. Xanthelasma, or soft, raised, yellow areas, sometimes appear on the eyelid after age 50 (Figure 26-8). Signs and symptoms of selected eye diseases are listed in Table 26-4. In addition to the more obvious signs of eye disease, visual impairment also can be assessed by noting the patient's head, hand, and eye movements. Tilting the head to one side to improve vision could mean that the patient has double vision or that one eye is much stronger than the other. Squinting could mean poor vision. Shading the eyes with the hands may indicate an increased sensitivity to light (photophobia).

Observation of the patient's ability to move the eyebrows and eyes can be helpful in diagnosing nerve damage. Inability to raise the eyebrows indicates damage to the facial nerve. Movement of the eyeball to direct the gaze is controlled by no less than six muscles, which are themselves under the control of three cranial nerves: the oculomotor nerve (third cranial), the trochlear nerve (fourth cranial), and the abducens nerve (sixth cranial) (see Table 26-1).

Table 26-3 Abnormalities of Lid Position

ABNORMALITY	CAUSES	SYMPTOMS	TREATMENT
Entropion: Inversion of lid margin; eyelids are turned inward toward eyeball so that lashes rub against eyeball	Scarring and contraction of skin near eyelid (cicatricial entropion); or aging of skin with laxness of tissues supporting the lid and contraction of orbicularis muscle (spastic entropion)	Pain, tearing, redness, and corneal ulceration due to lid margin and eyelashes rubbing against cornea	Splinting the lid, using a pressure patch, or taping lid into everted (turned outward) position Surgical correction by tightening musculature and everting lid margin
Ectropion: Eversion or outward turning of the lower lid	Aging and laxness of skin and muscle tissues, facial paralysis, edema of conjunctiva lining the lid, or contraction of scar tissue	Irritation of palpebral conjunctiva, spilling of tears down the cheeks due to blocked outlet, irritation of skin of cheeks, symptoms of conjunctivitis	Usually responds to patching of the eye Surgical correction necessary if paralysis of orbicularis muscle is permanent or if there is severe scarring and contraction of skin near the lid
Ptosis: Drooping of the eyelid so that it partially or completely covers the cornea	Congenital weakness of the levator superioris muscle or long-term presence of foreign body; one of first signs of myasthenia gravis	Obvious drooping of eyelid If not corrected in infants, can lead to blindness because light rays cannot enter and stimulate development of the eye Patient may be observed tilting head back or raising eyebrows in an effort to see from under eyelids	Surgical correction Removal of foreign body, if that is the cause

FIGURE 26-8 Xanthelasma.

▪ Nursing Diagnosis

Nursing diagnoses are based on the data obtained from assessment. The LPN/LVN collaborates with the RN in formulating the nursing care plan and selecting the nursing diagnoses. Some of the nursing diagnoses most frequently encountered in the care of patients with eye disease are:

- Disturbed sensory perception related to decreased visual acuity
- Risk for injury related to decreased visual field
- Fear of blindness related to consequences of diabetic retinopathy

Table 26-4 Clinical Signs and Symptoms of Selected Eye Diseases, Medical Treatment, and Nursing Interventions

DISEASE	SIGNS AND SYMPTOMS	MEDICAL TREATMENT AND NURSING INTERVENTIONS
Blepharitis: Infection of glands and lash follicles along lid margin	Itching, burning, sensitivity to light Mucus discharge and scaling; eyelids crusted, glued shut, especially on awakening Loss of eyelashes	Warm compresses to soften secretions; scrub eyelids with baby shampoo; stroke sideways to remove exudate and scales Antibiotic eyedrops; systemic and topical antibiotics if skin is infected
Chalazion: Internal stye; infection of meibomian gland	Astigmatism or distorted vision, depending on size and location of chalazion Small, hard tumor on eyelid	Chalazion may require surgical excision and antibiotics to avoid chronic state and cyst formation
Hordeolum: External stye; infected swelling near the lid margin on inside	Sharp pain that becomes dull and throbbing Rupture and drainage of pus bring relief Localized redness and swelling of lid	Hordeolum usually resolves spontaneously Warm compresses qid for 10-15 min to bring stye to a head and hasten rupture Caution patient never to squeeze swelling, as this could spread infection; poor health status can predispose a person to recurrence of styes
Conjunctivitis: Inflammation of the conjunctiva; "pink eye" is a specific type caused by chemical irritants, bacteria, or virus	Varying degrees of pain and discomfort Increased tearing and mucus production Itching; sensation of a foreign body in the eye	Depends on type of infecting organism; antibiotic eyedrops and ointments Special care when handling infective material
Keratitis: Inflammation of the cornea	Varying degrees of pain and discomfort Photophobia; blurred vision if center of cornea is affected	Depends on specific causes; could be allergy, microbes, ischemia, or decreased lacrimation. Most superficial lesions are self-healing. Antibiotic eyedrops or ointment used for bacterial infections. Steroids can reduce inflammation and discomfort; however, herpes infection can rapidly worsen keratitis unless an antiviral agent is given simultaneously Patient is encouraged to use good personal hygiene, frequent hand hygiene
Corneal abrasion or ulceration	Moderate to severe pain and discomfort aggravated by blinking History of trauma, contact lens wear	Change or discontinue use of contact lens Teach patient proper way to insert, remove, and care for contact lens Caution patient not to moisten lens with saliva

- Impaired home maintenance management related to impaired or lost vision
- Deficient diversional activity related to visual limitation
- Deficient knowledge related to proper method and schedule for instilling eyedrops

■ **Planning**

Expected outcomes for the above nursing diagnoses might be:

- Patient will compensate for decreased visual acuity and not suffer sensory deprivation.
- Patient will not experience injury.
- Patient will verbalize decreased fear as treatment begins to help condition.
- Patient will seek assistance with home maintenance within 7 days.
- Patient will explore other means of diversion than reading and watching television.
- Patient will demonstrate proper installation of eyedrops and will verbalize the schedule for the eyedrops.

When a patient is visually impaired, the nurse must plan extra time to assist with personal care, to allow the patient to perform as much self-care as possible. The instillation of preoperative eyedrops is a very time-consuming nursing task (Box 26-1). The nurse must plan for this when creating the work plan for the shift. Hands must be washed before and after instilling eyedrops. Often an eye patch must be removed, and then a new one placed, after instilling eye medication. Planning also must be done to incorporate patient teaching on the administration of medication, self-care instructions for the patient with glaucoma, and postoperative instructions.

■ **Implementation**

Many problems with the eye require eyedrops or ophthalmic ointment applied to the eye, several times a day. A new contact lens delivery system is being tested to dispense an antibiotic directly to the surface of eye in a time-release manner. The lens stays in the eye for 1 month. A prototype is in trials (Bankhead, 2009).

Nursing Interventions for the Visually Impaired Patient

Those who are deprived of optimum sight must make considerable adjustments. People who have lost their eyesight may experience hopelessness and despair. The visually impaired patient goes through stages of grief in much the same way the dying person does. A different lifestyle must be learned, but it is not necessarily less meaningful.

When communicating with these patients, remember that the person has a vision impairment; she is not deaf. Speak normally. Speak to the person and identify yourself as you enter the room, and do not touch her until after you have spoken to her—this

| Box 26-1 | Instillation of Eyedrops and Eye Ointment | |

Check the medication label and be certain which eye is to receive the medication. Follow the "Five Rights" of medication administration. Perform hand hygiene and apply gloves.

EYEDROPS
- Remove the cap and place it on the table on its side or upside down.
- With the patient sitting or reclining, ask the patient to look up at the ceiling and tilt the head slightly toward the eye receiving the drop.
- With a tissue beneath the fingers, retract the lower lid downward, exposing the conjunctival sac.
- Stabilize the eyedrop container above the eye and drop the designated number of drops directly into the conjunctival sac. Do not place drops on the cornea. Block the entrance to the lacrimal gland by placing a finger over it.
- Carefully replace the cap on the container without contaminating the dropper tip.
- Ask the patient to close the eyelids gently and move the eyes from side to side under the lids to distribute the medication.

EYE OINTMENT
- Remove the cap from the tube and set it down on the table upside down.
- Expose the conjunctival sac.
- Apply a thin ribbon of ointment along the entire length of the conjunctival sac.
- To end the ribbon, twist the tube with a lateral movement of the wrist without touching the eye.
- Recap the tube.
- Ask the patient to gently close the eyelids and roll the eyes around under the lids to distribute the medication.

prevents startling or frightening the patient when she may not have heard you enter the room. Be certain that she is oriented to the room and can easily locate the call bell.

Prevention of accidents is an important part of the care of a blind person. Aside from the physical effects of bumping into objects or falling over them, the visually impaired person also suffers from a loss of self-confidence and security if movement is not safe and independent. Doors should be kept closed or left completely open. They must never be left ajar. Always return things to their places when working in the room. If it is necessary to move any object in the room, ask for the patient's consent, and state the object's new location. When you leave the room, tell the visually impaired person that you are going. This will prevent her from becoming frustrated by resuming a conversation, only to find that no one is there. When ambulating with the visually impaired patient, lead with the patient holding your arm, as she follows.

Pity is neither expected nor appreciated by the visually impaired. They only want to be treated as normal people and would prefer to ask for your help when they need it rather than have you do everything for them. If you are assigned to the care of a visually impaired person, determine the amount of assistance the patient needs and wants, by asking. Do not assume that the person is helpless, but avoid neglect when help is needed.

When a visually impaired patient is admitted, she will require special orientation to the room and surroundings. If there is total blindness, describe the size of the room and the placement of furniture, using the bed as the focal point. An ambulatory patient can be walked around the room and to the bathroom to develop familiarity with the location of the commode, bath, and sink. As with any patient, explain how to locate and use the call system, the radio, and the telephone (if there is one at the bedside).

Most patients prefer to feed themselves, if at all possible. However, it usually is necessary to set up the meal tray of the visually impaired patient, using the "clock" method for placement of food on the plate. The patient is told what food is in which area (i.e., "The potatoes are at 2 o'clock"). Setting up the meal tray includes opening containers of milk and juice, pouring coffee or tea, and cutting meat into bite-sized pieces, unless the patient is accustomed to doing these things.

👥 Assignment Considerations

Assisting the Visually Impaired Patient

If a certified nursing assistant (CNA) or unlicensed assistive personnel (UAP) is assigned to help feed, ambulate, or care for a visually impaired patient, be certain that the person understands what the visual impairment is and whether one or both eyes are affected. Ask that the aide announce his presence with a knock on the door and to speak before touching the patient. Review how to feed the blind patient and how to assist with ambulation. Gently remind the CNA or UAP that the patient is blind and not deaf, unless deafness is also a patient problem.

Do not give a visually impaired person a straw or drinking tube unless you are asked to, because it may be awkward to use. If you must feed the patient all of a meal, work slowly and calmly. Indicate about hot and cold foods on the tray, and alternate dishes rather than feeding all of one thing before offering another. Avoid talking too much, thus forcing the patient to either stop eating or answer you with a mouth full of food. Whenever possible, help the patient select finger foods such as sandwiches and raw fruit or vegetables from the menu. The goal is to help the patient maintain dignity and self-respect while meeting her personal needs.

If a guide dog is present, do not interfere with it or pet it as it is working. Do not feed the dog; let the patient feed at the appropriate time. Be sure the dog is near the bed on its own mat. Ask if the mat may be on the side of the bed that the staff are less likely to use.

❓ Think Critically

Can you think of three specific ways in which you can assist a blind patient who is admitted to the hospital to maintain as much independence in this setting as possible?

▪ Evaluation

Evaluation is based on reassessing data and determining whether expected outcomes have been met. This is an ongoing process. Some questions to be asked when gathering data for evaluation include: Is the patient compliant with the use of eye medications? Is an infection resolving? Is vision improving? If interventions have not been effective in helping the patient achieve expected outcomes, the plan of care should be altered.

COMMUNITY CARE

Nurses in all settings should be conscious of eye safety for themselves and those around them. Public education about using sunhats, visors, and dark glasses when out of doors to protect the eyes from ultraviolet A and B (UVA and UVB) rays is another function of all nurses.

Nurses working in home care often find that patients have not had eye care in many years; prescriptions have not been changed, and their quality of vision has decreased. Arrange for referral to an appropriate agency to set up an eye examination when the patient cannot afford an eye exam. Glaucoma testing should be encouraged every 2 to 3 years for all adults over age 40.

OVERVIEW OF ANATOMY AND PHYSIOLOGY OF THE EAR

WHAT ARE THE STRUCTURES OF THE EAR?

- The external ear consists of the pinna (auricle) and the canal (auditory meatus). The pinna is the fleshy part of the ear situated on the side of the head (Figure 26-9).
- The auditory meatus is a tube about 2.5 cm long extending from the pinna to the tympanic membrane.
- The meatus is lined with numerous hairs and glands that secrete a waxy substance called cerumen (earwax).
- The middle ear contains the auditory bones (ossicles), and opens into the eustachian tube.
- The auditory ossicles are three small bones: the malleus (hammer), the incus (anvil), and the stapes (stirrup).
- The malleus attaches to the tympanic membrane.
- The stapes attaches to the oval window.
- The incus links the malleus and the stapes.
- The tympanic membrane (eardrum) separates the middle ear from the external ear.
- The eustachian tube connects the middle ear with the throat.

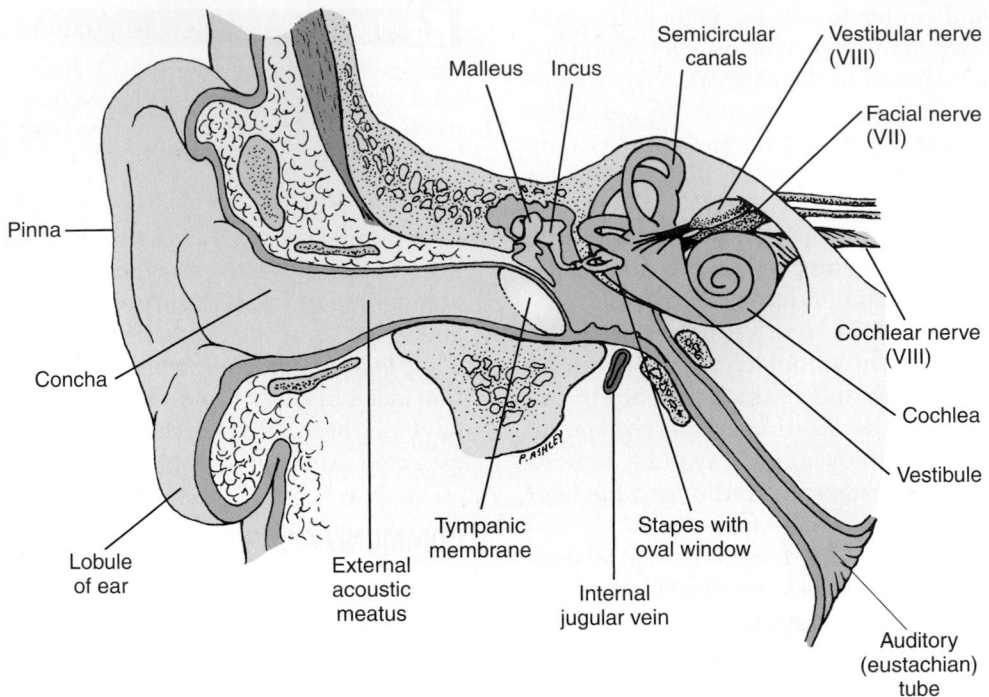

FIGURE 26-9 Structures of the ear.

- The oval window and the round window connect the middle ear to the inner ear.
- The inner ear is divided into the vestibule, the semicircular canals, and the cochlea.
- The inner ear contains a bony labyrinth with a membranous labyrinth lining; the inner ear is located in the temporal bone of the skull.
- A clear fluid, endolymph, fills the membranous labyrinth.
- The cochlea contains the organ of Corti, which is composed of sound receptors.

WHAT ARE THE FUNCTIONS OF THE EAR STRUCTURES?

- The pinna collects sound waves and channels them into the auditory meatus.
- The hairs and cerumen in the canal help prevent foreign objects from reaching the tympanic membrane.
- The tympanic membrane vibrates when sound waves hit it; the sound vibrations are conducted to the malleus.
- The bones of the middle ear transmit the sound vibrations to the inner ear. The malleus transmits them to the incus, and the incus transmits sound vibrations to the stapes. The stapes transmits the sound vibrations to the oval window, which transfers the motion to the fluid in the inner ear.
- Fluid motion in the inner ear stimulates the sound receptors in the cochlea and the organ of Corti.
- The organ of Corti transmits impulses to the cochlear branch of the vestibulocochlear nerve

(cranial nerve VIII). This nerve carries the impulses to the medulla oblongata, the thalamus, and then to the temporal lobe of the brain, which contains the auditory cortex.
- The eustachian tube helps equalize pressure in the middle ear.
- Receptors responsible for equilibrium (balance) are located in the inner ear, within the bony vestibule and at the base of the semicircular canals.
- Impulses from the equilibrium receptors are transmitted to the brain via the vestibular branch of the vestibulocochlear nerve (cranial nerve VIII). The cerebellum is important in mediating the sense of equilibrium and balance.

WHAT CHANGES OCCUR IN THE EAR WITH AGING?

- Cerumen becomes harder, containing less moisture, and its buildup within the ear may contribute to a hearing loss in the low-frequency range.
- The tympanic membrane loses elasticity.
- The joints between the auditory bones become stiffer; the stiffness interferes with the transmission of sound waves, but is not clinically significant by itself.
- There is a gradual loss of the receptor cells in the organ of Corti after age 40.
- With increasing age, the number of nerve fibers in the vestibulocochlear nerve decreases, contributing to hearing loss and sometimes affecting balance and equilibrium.

THE EAR

Approximately 26 million adults in the United States have some degree of hearing loss (National Institute on Deafness and Other Communication Disorders, 2010a). The number has risen dramatically in the last three decades. About 26 million Americans between the ages of 45 and 69 have high-frequency hearing loss due to exposure to loud sounds. Social withdrawal is not unusual when hearing becomes severely impaired. The inability to hear causes difficulty with communication. Approximately 2 in 1000 babies born in the United States have some form of congenital hearing problem. After age 75, about 47% of the population has some degree of hearing loss. It is thought that the trend of playing very loud music—causing damage to the acoustic nerve—will result in considerably more hearing loss in the coming decades.

⚡ Health Promotion

Coping with Hearing Loss

The sooner the person with a hearing loss obtains and learns to use a hearing aid, the greater the hearing improvement. The brain does better at integrating the hearing aid transmissions when hearing has not been gone for a very long time. Encourage those individuals with any hearing loss to be tested and to try a hearing aid if one is recommended. The person should be told that there is an adjustment curve with new hearing aid use, and it often takes several trips back to the hearing aid center for minor adjustments to the instrument to be made. It also takes practice in using the aid to achieve better hearing.

There are two types of hearing loss related to problems in the ear: *sensorineural* and *conductive.* About 80% of hearing loss is due to a disorder of the hearing nerve **(sensorineural loss).** Conductive hearing loss is caused by a problem transmitting sound impulse through the auditory canal, the tympanic membrane, or the bones of the middle ear. Causes of sensorineural and conductive hearing impairment are listed in Box 26-2.

Arteriosclerosis can cause decreased blood flow to the otic nerve (eighth cranial nerve), resulting in sensorineural hearing loss. This often contributes to hearing loss in the elderly.

A loss of hearing—like a loss of sight—burdens its victims with physical, emotional, psychosocial, and financial problems. Hearing allows for communication with others in everyday conversations, in the classroom, and in business transactions. Without the ability to hear, one can be deprived of many of the joys and pleasures of life: music, drama, exchange of ideas, and the thousands of sounds in one's environment. Because hearing warns one of danger, an inability to hear can cause anxiety and fear. Adults who have a hearing deficiency might lose jobs and alienate friends because of their communication handicap. Nurses must learn

---

| Box 26-2 | Common Causes of Sensorineural and Conductive Hearing Loss |

CONDUCTIVE LOSS
- Obstruction by impacted cerumen
- Infection with labyrinthitis
- Otosclerosis
- Trauma and scarring of the tympanic membrane
- Congenital malformation of the outer or middle ear

SENSORINEURAL LOSS
- Presbycusis
- Heredity with congenital loss
- Ototoxic drugs
- Loud noise exposure
- Tumor (acoustic neuroma)
- Ménière's disease
- Severe infection such as measles, mumps, meningitis
- Rubella in utero

---

ways to help prevent hearing loss, and to assist patients who already have such a loss.

Inner ear disorders can cause problems with balance. Dizziness, vertigo, and ataxia can greatly interfere with an individual's ability to work or to perform usual activities of daily living. Accidental injury and fractures from falls may occur. To understand the problems affecting the ear, it is necessary to recall the ear's normal structure and functions.

HEARING LOSS

Causes and Prevention

A glance at the causes of hearing loss listed in Box 26-2 will help identify some of the ways the nurse can help prevent hearing loss. Not all cases of hearing disability can be prevented, but education of the general public about causes of hearing loss can reduce its incidence. *Healthy People 2020* includes many objectives to prevent hearing loss and improve hearing among the American public. Adequate treatment of severe ear infections helps preserve hearing. Loud noise is a major cause of sensorineural hearing loss, and the use of headphones or earbuds contributes considerably to hearing damage (Table 26-5) (National Institute on Deafness and Other Communication Disorders, 2010b).

Hairpins, the ends of pencils, and other assorted objects should never be used to relieve tickling or itching in the ear, or to remove cerumen. Earwax normally moves on its own out of the ear canal to the outer ear, where it can be removed without danger of damaging the delicate lining of the ear canal or the tympanic membrane (eardrum). Obstructing cerumen should be removed by using drops that dissolve it or by a physician or nurse skilled in removing impacted cerumen. Foreign objects, such as beans, peas, and other organic substances, also should be removed by

Table 26-5	Range of Sounds Audible and Hazardous to the Ear
LEVEL IN DECIBELS (dB)	**EXAMPLE**
0	Lowest sound audible to the human ear
30	Quiet library, soft whisper
40	Living room, quiet office, bedroom away from traffic
50	Light traffic at a distance, refrigerator, gentle breeze
60	Air conditioner at 20 feet conversation, sewing machine
70	Busy traffic, noisy restaurant; at this decibel level, noise may begin to affect hearing if exposure is constant
Hazardous Zone for Hearing Loss	
80	Subway, heavy city traffic, alarm clock at 2 feet factory noise; these noises are dangerous if exposure to them lasts for more than 8 hr
90	Truck traffic, noisy home appliances, shop tools, lawn mower; as loudness increases, the "safe" time exposure decreases; damage can occur in 8 hr
100	Chain saw, stereo headphones, pneumatic drill; even 2 hr of exposure can be dangerous at this decibel level; with each 5-dB increase, the safe time is cut in half
120	Rock band concert in front of speakers, sandblasting, thunderclap; the danger is immediate; exposure of 120 dB can injure ears
140	Gunshot blast, jet plane; any length of exposure time is dangerous; noise at this level may cause actual pain in the ear
160	Rocket launching pad; without ear protection, noise at this level causes irreversible damage; hearing loss is inevitable

Adapted from Lewis, S.L., Heitkemper, M.M., Dirksen, S.R., et al. (2011). *Medical-Surgical Nursing: Assessment and Management of Clinical Problems* (8th ed.). St. Louis: Mosby.

someone who is experienced and aware of the potential for ear damage.

Conductive hearing loss most often occurs from stiffening of the bones of the middle ear or from scarring of the tympanic membrane. Continued exposure to excessively high levels of sound can produce sensorineural loss called *noise-induced hearing impairment*. This condition is particularly likely to occur in industrial settings where machinery operation creates loud noise. The standards of the Occupational Safety and Health Administration (OSHA) require the wearing of ear protectors in such settings.

A more recent phenomenon is the potential damage to the inner ear caused by amplified music. **Sustained exposure to noise levels of 90 to 95 dB may result in hearing loss.**

Many drugs can be toxic to the inner ear. This is especially true if a very high dose of the drug is given or if it is given incorrectly. Commonly administered drugs that can be ototoxic are many of the antibiotics, nonsteroidal anti-inflammatory drugs, chemotherapy agents, and potent diuretics, such as furosemide (Lasix) (Box 26-3). Aspirin and other salicylates can produce loss of hearing of high frequencies and ringing in the ears *(tinnitus)*.

Nurses should be aware of the potential for damage to the ear by potent drugs. Nonsteroidal anti-inflammatory drugs are more toxic in the elderly, and when used at maximum dosages over an extended period of time.

 Elder Care Points

The older the patient, the greater the chance of ototoxicity occurring from analgesic medications because many older patients have chronic conditions that cause chronic pain. The liver and kidneys in the elderly generally have decreased function because of aging, and so they cannot degrade and eliminate drugs as easily as they can for the younger person. For that reason drugs and drug metabolites can build up to toxic levels when medication is taken on a continuing basis.

 Safety Alert

Dangers of Ototoxic Drugs

Know the toxic effects of the drugs you administer. Patients should be assessed frequently while receiving a potentially ototoxic drug. Any signs of ototoxicity, such as ringing in the ears, subtle changes in hearing ability, and difficulty in hearing, should be reported immediately. Many times ototoxicity occurs because patients are taking more than one drug that can be toxic to the ear. Teach patients who are taking daily doses of aspirin or nonsteroidal anti-inflammatory drugs for arthritis or other chronic pain conditions to immediately report the signs of ototoxicity.

Diagnostic Tests and Examinations

Visual Examination of the Ear. The two instruments most commonly used to examine the ear canal and tympanic membrane are the otoscope and the aural speculum. The otoscope is fitted with a light and a

Box 26-3   Ototoxic Drugs and Environmental Chemicals

Ototoxicity (ear poisoning) is caused by drugs or chemicals that damage the inner ear or the vestibulocochlear nerve. The vestibulocochlear nerve sends balance and hearing information from the inner ear to the brain. Ototoxicity may result in temporary or permanent disturbances of hearing, balance, or both. Environmental chemicals can be toxic from inhalation of fumes or powder residue or from skin contamination.

DRUGS THAT MAY CAUSE OTOTOXICITY
Antibiotics
- Tobramycin
- Gentamicin
- Streptomycin
- Kanamycin
- Amikacin
- Neomycin
- Netilmicin
- Dihydrostreptomycin
- Erythromycin (IV)
- Vancomycin
- Chloramphenicol
- Minocycline
- Capreomycin
- Dibekacin
- Etiomycin

Antineoplastic Drugs
- Cisplatin
- Carboplatin
- Bleomycin
- Nitrogen mustard

Loop Diuretics (IV)
- Furosemide
- Torsemide
- Bumetanide
- Ethacrynic acid

Salicylates
- Aspirin

Nonsteroidal Anti-inflammatory Drugs
- Ibuprofen
- Naproxen sodium

Quinidine Derivatives
- Quinidex
- Atabrine
- Plaquenil
- Quinine sulfate
- Mefloquine
- Chloroquine

ENVIRONMENTAL CHEMICALS
- Metals (lead, mercury, gold, arsenic)
- Aniline dyes
- Toluene
- Carbon monoxide
- Trichloroethylene
- Xylene
- Povidone-iodine
- Nicotine
- Potassium bromate

IV, intravenous.

FIGURE 26-10 Examination of the ear with an otoscope.

magnifying lens to facilitate inspection (Figure 26-10). The aural speculum is used with a special circular, slightly concave head mirror that has a hole in its middle. The head mirror is positioned so that the central hole lies in front of one eye of the examiner. A source of light, such as a lamp, is placed behind the examiner so that it shines on the head mirror and is reflected into the ear.

The simple speculum can be modified by attaching a special tube and inflatable bag (pneumatic otoscope), thereby creating an airtight system. This allows the examiner to determine whether the tympanic membrane responds to positive and negative pressure. The normal eardrum moves in response to pressure. Healed perforations and scars on the eardrum can be seen when the tympanic membrane is moved.

A simple hearing test is the *whisper test.* The examiner stands behind the patient and whispers a question to the patient. If the patient hears the question, an answer is forthcoming. The examiner backs up a step and whispers another question, and so on.

Tuning Fork Tests. Tuning forks measure hearing by air conduction or by bone conduction (Weber's test and Rinne test). A tuning fork is activated by holding it by the stem and striking the tines softly on the back of your hand (Table 26-6).

Test for Nystagmus. To test for nystagmus (involuntary rhythmic jerking of the eyes), the nurse holds a finger directly in front of the patient at eye level. The patient is asked to follow the finger without moving the head. The nurse moves the finger slowly from the midline toward the right ear about 30 degrees. Then the finger is moved back to the midline and then slowly toward the left ear about 30 degrees.

Table 26-6	Diagnostic Tests for Ear Problems		
TEST	**PURPOSE**	**DESCRIPTION**	**NURSING IMPLICATIONS**
Weber's test	To determine loss of hearing in one ear or both	Tuning fork is struck, and then the handle is placed on the patient's forehead. Normal hearing or equal loss in both ears is demonstrated by hearing the sound in the middle of the head.	Explain purpose and procedure to patient.
Rinne test	To determine whether hearing loss is sensorineural or conductive	Tuning fork is struck, and then the handle is placed on the mastoid bone; the fork is removed and struck again and held beside the ear. The patient is asked in which position she heard the sound better or longer.	Explain procedure to patient.
Audiometry	To determine degree of hearing loss in each ear	Earphones are placed on the patient's ears and, with the use of an audiometry machine, the audiologist channels sounds of different decibels and pitch into one ear and then the other of the patient. The patient signals when she hears the tone.	Explain procedure to patient.
Caloric test	To check for alteration in vestibular function in each ear	With patient in a seated or supine position, each ear is separately irrigated with a cold and then a warm solution to determine vestibular response. Normal response is nystagmus, vertigo, nausea, vomiting, falling; decreased response indicates abnormality.	Explain procedure to patient; tell patient she may experience nystagmus, vertigo, nausea, and vomiting, but these will indicate a normal response.
Electronystagmography (ENG)	To assess for disease of vestibular system	Electrodes are placed near the patient's eyes. Caloric test is performed; movement of the eyes is recorded on a graph. Decreased response is abnormal.	Explain procedure and equipment to patient. Tell her that nausea, vertigo, etc. indicate a normal response.
Evoked-response audiometry (ERA); auditory brainstem response (ABR)	To determine abnormality of nerve pathways between eighth cranial nerve and brainstem	Electrodes are attached to the client's head in a darkened room; similar to EEG. Auditory stimuli are directed to the patient, and a computer is used to track and separate the auditory electrical activity of the brain from other brain waves.	Explain procedure and equipment to patient. Tell her the room will be darkened.
Magnetic resonance imaging (MRI)	To detect tumor of the eighth cranial nerve, acoustic neuroma	Huge electromagnet is used to detect radiofrequency pulses from the alignment of hydrogen protons in the magnetic field. A computer translates the pulses into cross-sectional images. Provides high-contrast views of soft tissue.	Explain to patient that her head will be placed in a machine that looks like a large tube. She will need to lie very still during the test; all metal must be removed before the test.
FTA-ABS blood test	To test for syphilis	Blood is drawn and sent to the lab for determination of presence of syphilis. Syphilis can cause problems with nerve transmission from the ear.	Explain that a blood sample is needed.

EEG, electroencephalography; *FTA-ABS,* fluorescent treponemal antibody absorption.

The patient's eyes are watched for any jerking movements. Nystagmus other than at the extremes of lateral gaze is abnormal and may indicate an inner ear problem, intracranial tumor, or paralysis of an eye muscle.

Romberg Test. This is a test of equilibrium. The patient stands with the feet together, the arms out to the sides, and the eyes open. The nurse notes ability to maintain an upright posture without swaying. The patient is then asked to close the eyes and posture is observed again. If the patient loses balance, it may indicate a problem with the inner ear or the cerebellum.

❖ NURSING MANAGEMENT

■ Assessment (Data Collection)

Patients over age 60 should always be assessed for hearing loss. If a patient has a known hearing impairment, the nurse should assess how the patient is coping with it. Hearing and balance are subjective problems and require a good history from the patient.

Focused Assessment

Data Collection for Ear Disorders

Ask the following questions:
- Have you had any pain in the ear?
- Have you had a recent temperature elevation?
- Do you suffer from allergies?
- Do you have frequent upper respiratory infections?
- Have you ever been exposed to very loud noise? Do you work in an area that is noisy? Do you listen to loud music?
- Have you ever had a head injury?
- Do you scuba dive, hunt or shoot skeet, or fly in small airplanes?
- Do you ever have ringing, buzzing, or odd sounds in the ears?
- Do you feel your hearing ability has decreased? Do people you live with think that you do not hear as well as you used to hear? Do you frequently have to ask people to repeat things that have been said to you?
- Is there a history of hearing loss in your family?
- Have you ever had a really high fever?
- What medications are you taking regularly? Are there other medications that you have taken for an extended period in the past? Do you take aspirin?
- How do you clean your ears?
- Do you ever suffer with dizziness, vertigo, or loss of balance?

Diagnosis of infection requires an otoscopic examination. It should be noted that the color, texture, and amount of cerumen varies among individuals. In whites and African Americans cerumen tends to be moist and rust-brown colored. Native Americans and Asians have cerumen that is lighter in color and drier. Normally, the top of each pinna is aligned with the corner of the eye on each side of the head. Lesions on the pinna may indicate skin cancer, particularly in the elderly patient. There should be no secretions other than cerumen from the ear. Ear pain may be referred from other parts of

the head and neck and may occur from sinusitis, dental problems, or temporomandibular joint syndrome.

Focused Assessment

Physical Assessment of the Ear

- Compare the pinna from one side to the other for symmetry and placement.
- Palpate the pinna for the presence of nodules.
- Observe for the presence of lesions on the pinna.
- Check for drainage (**otorrhea**) from the ear; note color and odor.
- Observe the gait to detect any problem with balance.
- Observe for wavering when arising from a supine or seated position that might indicate dizziness or equilibrium problems.
- Observe for signs of bruising on the body from falls that may indicate problems with balance.
- Observe to see whether the person speaks in a voice louder than necessary.
- Observe to see whether facial expression indicates difficulty in understanding what is being said.
- Determine whether responses to statements are inappropriate.
  Note: Someone qualified and experienced in using an otoscope should inspect the auditory meatus and the tympanic membrane.

The ears of elderly in long-term care facilities should be checked with an otoscope at regular intervals for cerumen. Many long-term care residents have a correctable hearing loss related to impacted cerumen. Cerumen can be removed by using cerumen softener drops, and then irrigating the external ear canal (Figure 26-11).

■ Nursing Diagnosis and Planning

Nursing diagnoses are chosen based on the data provided during the assessment (Table 26-7). General goals for the patient with problems of the ear or hearing are:
- Promote knowledge to protect hearing
- Prevent infection and injury
- Promote effective communication
- Promote coping with hearing loss

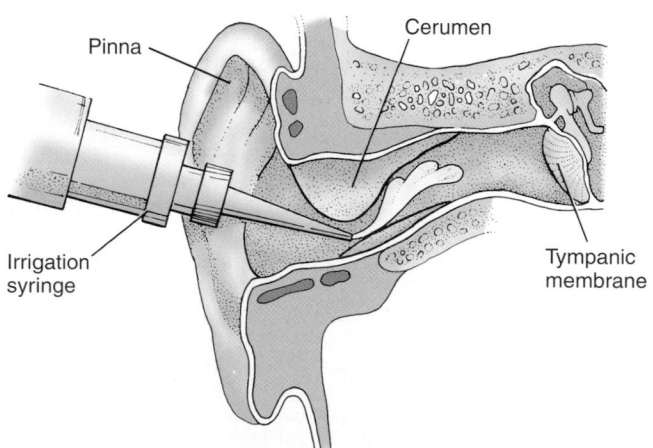

FIGURE 26-11 Irrigating the external ear canal. Warm water is used to remove cerumen and debris from the canal. Aim the stream of water above or below the impaction to allow back pressure to push it out rather than farther down the canal.

Table 26-7   Nursing Diagnoses, Expected Outcomes, and Nursing Interventions for Patients with Ear Disorders

NURSING DIAGNOSIS	GOALS/EXPECTED OUTCOMES	NURSING INTERVENTIONS
Disturbed sensory perception related to damage from infection or obstruction	Patient will verbalize ways to prevent further hearing loss. Patient will be free of ear infection within 10 days.	If cerumen is obstructing the auditory canal, irrigate as ordered; warm the irrigation solution to body temperature. If infection is present, instruct regarding antibiotic medication and encourage to take entire prescription. Instruct in use of hearing aid if one is prescribed. Advise of ways to prevent further hearing loss: avoid loud noise or wear ear protectors; seek treatment immediately for signs of ear infection.
Pain related to inflammation in the ear	Pain will be controlled with analgesia within 8 hr. Pain will be resolved within 7 days.	Administer analgesics as ordered as needed. Warm analgesic eardrops to room temperature before administration. Have patient rest head on heating pad turned on "low" setting if this seems to decrease pain.
Impaired verbal communication related to inability to receive messages or to decode and interpret them	Patient will assist in choice of methods to improve ability to communicate. Patient will try hearing aid for 2 wk if there is an indication that this device would help hearing.	Plan with patient the best way to communicate so that instructions and information are comprehended; explore tone of voice, level of volume, distance from patient when speaking, writing out communication, etc. Establish a routine procedure to confirm patient's understanding. Refer for evaluation by audiologist. Encourage daily use of hearing aid if one is prescribed. Explain that time and adjustments are necessary to obtain the optimum result. Give praise for efforts to use hearing aid.
Anxiety related to inability to hear warnings, perform at work, or communicate in social settings	Patient will explore methods of maintaining safety within 2 wk. Patient will verbalize ways in which assisted hearing devices might assist in performance in the work environment.	Encourage verbalization of fears. Utilize means to enhance communication. Advise of assisted-hearing devices, hearing aids, and availability of "hearing ear" dogs. Introduce means of learning alternative communication methods, such as sign language and speech reading. Explore methods of enhancing attention to visual cues of dangers in the environment (i.e., close attention to signal lights, or observing others at street crossings). Discuss problems of communication in social settings and explore possible solutions (i.e., masking devices for use in crowds, having interaction with only one or two people at a time, avoiding noisy restaurants, or using hearing aid).
Risk of injury related to impaired equilibrium	Patient will verbalize methods to ensure safety within 3 days. Patient will not experience a fall or injury.	Administer medication for vertigo as ordered. Encourage a low-sodium diet. Instruct to change positions very slowly. Encourage to hold on to something solid or to someone when rising from a sitting to a standing position. If vertigo is present, do not ambulate without assistance. Teach or reinforce vestibular/balance exercises as prescribed. Assist to identify any aura (presence of symptoms that precede an attack). Instruct to lie down and keep the eyes open and focused straight ahead when experiencing vertigo.
Deficient knowledge related to the nature of disability, self-care, and availability of community resources for the hearing impaired	Patient will verbalize ways to enhance safe self-care within 2 wk.	Explain nature of hearing loss or vertigo and possible causes. Describe measures to assist the hard-of-hearing person to adapt; refer to support groups and sources for information. Refer to community agencies and resources for the hearing impaired.
Social isolation related to difficulty in communicating	Patient will establish an adequate social network within 2 mo.	Assist patient to consider possibilities for social contact despite hearing problems. Help patient obtain a telephone for the hearing-impaired person. Encourage the use of computer e-mail for contact with friends and family and social interaction with others.

Expected outcomes are written for each nursing diagnosis chosen for the patient's care plan. Writing the outcomes should be done in collaboration with the patient and other health team members. In addition to the nurse and physician, an audiologist, hearing aid specialist, and speech therapist may be involved in the patient's care. Both long- and short-term goals for the patient should be considered.

When a patient is severely hearing impaired, communication with the patient for treatments and activities of daily living may take longer than with patients who hear normally. The nurse should take this into consideration when creating the daily work plan. If the patient does not have adequate aids for hearing, the nurse must devise an acceptable method of two-way communication with the patient.

■ **Implementation**

Interventions for the patient with a hearing or balance problem are geared toward patient education, treatment of infection, preoperative and postoperative care and instructions, measures for communication (Box 26-4), and referral to resources. The hearing aid must be cared for properly (Box 26-5).

Instillation of Ear Medication

Eardrops may be ordered to dissolve cerumen, relieve pain, or combat infection in the auditory meatus. The patient should be positioned in a supine lateral position so that the affected ear is uppermost. The

---

Box 26-4   Communicating with the Hearing-Impaired Person

- If the person uses a hearing aid, encourage its use and see that it is situated, turned on, and adjusted before beginning speaking.
- Be certain you have the person's attention before beginning speaking.
- Sit facing the person with the light on your face rather than from behind you.
- Ask permission to turn down the volume or turn off the television or radio.
- The best distance for speaking to a hearing-impaired person is 2½ to 4 feet. Place yourself on eye level with the person. Do not speak directly into the person's ear as this prevents the person from obtaining visual cues while you are speaking.
- Do not smile, chew gum, or cover the mouth while speaking.
- Use short, simple sentences. If the patient does not appear to understand or responds inappropriately, state the message again using different words. Try to limit each sentence to one subject and one verb.
- Give the person time to respond to questions.
- Ask for oral or written feedback to make certain your message is understood.
- Avoid using the intercom system as it may distort sound.

Box 26-5   Caring for a Hearing Aid

When a hearing aid does not work:
- Check that the switch is "on."
- Examine the ear mold for attached wax or dirt; clean the sound hole.
- Check the battery to see that it is inserted correctly.
- Check the connection between the ear mold and the receiver.
- Replace the battery. Batteries last an average of 12 to 14 days depending on type of aid.
- Check placement of the ear mold in the ear; it should fit snugly.
- Adjust the volume.
- If all else fails, take the hearing aid to an authorized service center for repair.

To clean the hearing aid:
- Turn the hearing aid off.
- Wash the ear mold with mild soap and warm water; do not submerge in water.
- Use a pipe cleaner or toothpick to gently cleanse the opening or short tube that fits into the ear.
- Dry the mold completely before turning on the aid or before reattaching it to the hearing aid (if it is separate).

---

medication should be at room temperature. Cold eardrops may cause discomfort or dizziness. For the adult, the ear canal is straightened by drawing the pinna upward and toward the back of the head (Figure 26-12). For a child under age 3, the pinna is pulled down and back. Following the "Five Rights" of medication administration, draw up the correct amount of medication. Insert the tip of the dropper into the external ear canal and instill the medication (Box 26-6). Place cotton in the external meatus to prevent the medication from escaping. Have the patient remain in the lateral position for 5 to 10 minutes.

Communicating with the Hearing-Impaired Patient

The patient who is hearing impaired has unique problems of communication when in the hospital or long-term care facility. If she cannot hear well and misunderstands or misinterprets the voices and sounds in the unfamiliar surroundings, she is likely to be

FIGURE 26-12 Straightening the ear canal to instill eardrops.

Box 26-6 | Instilling Otic Medication

- Follow the "Five Rights" of medication administration.
- Read the order carefully to determine which ear is to receive the medication.
- Position the patient supine and in the lateral position so that the affected ear is uppermost.
- Draw medication into the medicine dropper by depressing the bulb and letting it go.
- Straighten the ear canal by drawing the pinna upward and toward the back of the head. For children younger than 3 years, draw the earlobe slightly down and back.
- Insert the tip of the medicine dropper into the external ear canal and depress the bulb to dispense the medication. Withdraw the dropper.
- Place cotton in the external meatus to prevent the medication from escaping.
- Have the patient remain in the lateral position for 5 to 10 minutes.

---

frustrated, fearful, and anxious. Unless a special effort is made to have frequent contact with the patient, social isolation may occur.

When speaking to a hearing-impaired patient, sit at eye level facing the patient. Gain eye contact and speak slowly and enunciate clearly. When trying to communicate with a person who is hearing impaired, bear in mind that attempts to answer questions without fully understanding what is asked may occur. Past experience has taught many hearing-impaired persons that to ask for repetition of questions irritates people and causes them to think the person is stupid. **For this reason, many people who cannot hear well frequently smile and say "Yes," when such an answer is either incorrect or inappropriate.** Another problem is that the individual may fill in parts of sentences with similar-sounding words. For example, the words "Knott's Berry Farm" may be interpreted as "not very far." Some guidelines to help the hearing-impaired patient and improve the nurse's ability to communicate are given in Box 26-4.

? Think Critically

What three techniques of communication with a hearing-impaired patient do you think would be the most helpful?

A piece of tape or sign of some kind should be placed over the terminal on the intercom system that designates the room of a hearing-impaired patient. This serves to remind the person answering the light to go to the patient's room rather than try to talk over the intercom system.

■ **Evaluation**

Evaluation involves reassessment to determine whether the expected outcomes are being met. Determining whether hearing has improved is the criterion by which

effectiveness of treatment is evaluated. Improvement is verified by audiometry. Fading or resolution of dizziness and vertigo indicate that actions and treatments for these problems have been effective. Resolution of infection is determined by the appearance of the eardrum, absence of pain, and normal temperature.

COMMON PROBLEMS OF PATIENTS WITH EAR DISORDERS

Hearing Impairment

Hearing impairment ranges from difficulty in hearing certain ranges of tones or in understanding certain words to total deafness. Persons with sensorineural hearing loss typically have more difficulty hearing high-pitched tones than low-pitched ones; thus they frequently can understand the speech of men better than that of women. Another characteristic of sensorineural hearing loss is difficulty hearing softly spoken and poorly enunciated words. Speaking slightly louder to the person with sensorineural hearing loss may help, but it is especially important to speak slowly and clearly and to face the person when communicating with her. Because people with sensorineural hearing loss do not hear their own voices as well as a person with normal hearing, they tend to speak louder than necessary.

Assignment Considerations

Caring for the Hearing Impaired

When assigning tasks for a hearing-impaired patient to UAP and CNAs, remind the person how to effectively communicate with the patient: face the patient and obtain the patient's attention before speaking; speak slowly and enunciate clearly in a normal voice. If the patient wears a hearing aid, it should be in the ear and the patient should be reminded to turn it on before communication begins.

Hearing aids help some people with sensorineural hearing loss. Aids designed to amplify some pitches and block out others that do not need amplification are most helpful. Hearing aids are not always the answer to a problem of hearing loss, and for some people the most effective therapy is focused on rehabilitation to facilitate acceptance of the loss and learning of new ways to communicate in spite of some degree of deafness. Most hearing aid professionals and companies will offer a 30-day money-back guarantee on any hearing aid so that the patient can try it.

 Clinical Cues

The earlier a hearing-impaired person who can benefit from a hearing aid obtains and uses one, the better her brain will adjust and the better the quality of hearing that can be achieved (Healthy Hearing, 2010).

Central hearing loss occurs in the brain as a result of some pathologic condition above the junction of the eighth cranial nerve and the brainstem. Central hearing loss can be due to a problem of transmission of stimuli in the brain, an inability to decode and sort signals received from one or both ears, or a failure in the transmission of sounds from one hemisphere of the brain to the other. Causes include brain tumors, vascular changes that suddenly deprive the middle ear of its blood supply, and cerebrovascular accidents.

Many people have a combination of two or more types of hearing impairment. Often there is a combination of sensorineural and conductive loss.

It should be noted that when a person is fitted with a hearing aid, it takes considerable time of working with the audiologist on adjustments to the device to obtain the best result. Too many people give up on a hearing aid because they have not taken the time to work through the adjustment process.

 Think Critically

How would you go about working with a hearing-impaired patient who is a candidate for a hearing aid, but adamantly refuses to consider trying out one?

Dizziness and Vertigo

The sense of balance and equilibrium is governed by the vestibular system in the inner ear. Increases in fluid pressure in the inner ear, inflammations, and vascular disorders that interrupt blood supply to the cochlea can produce dizziness, loss of balance, and nausea and vomiting. These symptoms can range from mildly annoying to completely incapacitating and should always be assessed whenever a person has an ear disorder and loss of hearing. Ménière's disease and labyrinthitis cause vertigo.

The patient who experiences dizziness and positional vertigo should be cautioned to avoid suddenly turning her head or making other movements that aggravate the vertigo. She should be told to call for assistance whenever she needs to move from her bed or chair. When helping the patient to her feet, move slowly and give her time to stand for a moment before beginning to walk. **Typically, patients with this kind of vertigo feel that the room is spinning around during an attack, and any motion makes the sensation even worse.** While the patient is having an attack of vertigo, she should lie in bed and remain as motionless as possible. Stabilizing her head with a pillow on either side may encourage immobility. Attacks can last from a few minutes to hours.

Medications to reduce motion sickness and nausea should be given precisely as ordered. These are usually given every 3 to 4 hours or on a preventive basis *before* the patient's symptoms become severe. A series of head movements called Epley maneuvers or Brandt-Daroff exercises can be helpful.

When increased fluid pressure in the inner ear is suspected as the cause of dizziness, the physician may order a low-sodium diet and limit fluid intake. Patients with recurrent attacks of vertigo are encouraged to stop smoking if they are habitual tobacco smokers. Tobacco is vasoconstrictive and can affect the blood supply to the inner ear and nerves. **Stress may affect the frequency of attacks of vertigo in patients with inner ear disorders.** Teaching the patient effective coping mechanisms to handle stress or adding rest periods into the work schedule may be helpful.

Tinnitus

Ringing, buzzing, or other continuous noise in the ear (*tinnitus*) can be mildly annoying or so severe that it interferes with activities of daily living and prevents the patient from getting sufficient sleep and rest. Common causes of tinnitus include presbycusis (hearing loss associated with aging), constant exposure to loud environmental noise, inflammation and infection in the ear, otosclerosis, Ménière's disease, and labyrinthitis. Systemic disorders such as hypertension and other cardiovascular disorders, neurologic disease (including head injury), and hyperthyroidism and hypothyroidism also can cause ringing in the ears. **Tinnitus may be one of the first symptoms produced by an ototoxic drug.** Symptoms of tinnitus are subjective, and diagnosis is by patient history.

 Clinical Cues

Because of the overload of sensory input to the brain, the patient with tinnitus will become more fatigued than others when in a noisy location such as a social gathering, a restaurant, or the like. Family and friends should be informed of this situation.

Medical treatment begins with efforts to determine the underlying cause and treat it. When the cause cannot be found, symptomatic relief is tried. However, some cases of intractable tinnitus resist all modes of conventional therapy. Less traditional measures that have varying degrees of success include biofeedback training and "masking." Sometimes substances that increase circulation are helpful (Niacin). The benzodiazepines, such as diazepam (Valium) or chlordiazepoxide (Librium), seem to help some people. Oral Lipoflavinoid has provided relief for many patients with tinnitus.

Biofeedback training is especially helpful in those cases in which emotional stress and anxiety are thought to be the underlying causes of tinnitus. Through visual or auditory signals, the person learns to relax and exert some degree of control over her autonomic nervous system. This can lower blood pressure and pulse rate and relax muscles that are very tense.

Masking simply provides a low-level noise to block out, or "mask," the head noise heard by the person complaining of tinnitus. Some examples include playing soft music or a tape of sounds of nature, such as a waterfall, while the person is resting or sleeping; providing "white noise" in the working environment, using a hearing aid to amplify sound from the outside and overcome head noise; and wearing a special tinnitus instrument, which is a combination hearing aid and tinnitus masker for people who have both hearing loss and tinnitus. The therapeutic effect of masking is highly individualized. Some people find instant relief, some have partial abatement of the head noise, and some do not benefit from attempts to mask the sounds of tinnitus. Earplugs or ear protection should be worn when noise exposure cannot be avoided.

REHABILITATION FOR HEARING LOSS

Specific measures to rehabilitate a patient with hearing loss depend on the age and aptitude of the patient. Adults who have acquired the skills of speech and language before their loss of hearing occurred are better able to pick up language cues and understand what is being said to them, and therefore should have fewer problems with communication by language.

Lip-Reading (Speech Reading)

Instruction in reading lips is one mode of therapy for the hearing impaired, but it is not a remedy for all difficulties. Only about 60% of the sounds in the English language can be identified by watching the lips. Most experienced lip-readers do not catch more than half of the words spoken to them. Communication by lip-reading is enhanced by other nonverbal clues, such as facial expressions and hand gestures. Learning to lip-read is difficult. It requires at least average intelligence, exceptional language skills, excellent eyesight, and much persistence and patience.

Sign Language

Many deaf people learn to communicate with sign language. American Sign Language (ASL) is the third most commonly used language in the United States. There are online dictionaries for ASL and several websites that provide tutorials (see Online Resources). Most major hospitals have someone on staff who can act as an interpreter for ASL.

Hearing Aids

An evaluation by a reputable audiologist provides a prescription for a hearing aid designed to provide the best possible improvement of hearing. Hearing aids can improve hearing for a variety of types of hearing loss. For the person who does not have a defect in the middle ear, a hearing aid can transmit amplified sound from the receiver through the eardrum to the inner ear. This is accomplished by amplifying sound waves transmitted by air conduction and bone conduction. There are many types of hearing aids on the market. Newer digital types can amplify the tones needed while masking other levels of noise. It takes time to adapt to the use of a hearing aid, and the audiologist must make repeated adjustments to the device to achieve optimum function.

The design of a hearing aid varies. Some are worn in the ear, others behind the ear, and still others are built into the frame of eyeglasses. Persons with binaural hearing loss (both ears are affected) must wear a hearing aid in each ear. Regardless of the type of hearing aid, it will have a microphone, an amplifier, a receiver, and a battery (Figure 26-13).

The hearing aid should not be handled roughly or dropped. The ear mold can be cleaned with soap and water, but the other parts of the aid should not get wet (see Box 26-5). Hair spray can damage the microphone of a hearing aid. Regular servicing by a dealer can keep the aid in good working order. When an incapacitated patient has a hearing aid, the nurse is responsible for the security of the hearing aid.

Cochlear Implant

Cochlear implants are now available for some patients who have no hearing at all. The device is a small computer that changes spoken words into electrical impulses that are transmitted via an implanted coil to the nerve endings in the cochlea. Success with the

FIGURE 26-13 Parts of a typical in-the-ear hearing aid.

FIGURE 26-14 Cochlear implant.

Microphone

Implant

Headpiece

Electrode system

Auditory nerve

Cochlea

Sound processor

surgical implant varies considerably from one person to the next (Figure 26-14). Bone hearing devices and semi-implanted devices are under development. A speech therapist works with the patient once the cochlear implant is in place.

Hearing-Assistive Devices

Many devices on the market use hearing aid technology. These devices assist people to hear telephone conversations, television, and sound systems, such as those in church or the theater. A telecommunication device for the deaf (TDD) is available. It is a combination typewriter and telephone and can be used to communicate with someone else who has a TDD, or can be used to call a relay center that then communicates the message to the intended person. There are alarm clocks that activate a flashing light, smoke detectors that flash light, and doorbells and telephones that flash a light when a sound is produced. "Hearing ear" dogs are trained to alert their owners to particular sounds and to keep their owners safe when around traffic.

COMMUNITY CARE

Public education about the dangers of loud noise and music could do much to prevent thousands of people from becoming hearing impaired. Teaching people to seek medical attention for symptoms of otitis media quickly prevents damage to the tympanic membrane and preserves hearing ability.

Encouraging those with hearing impairment to have a thorough evaluation and to try a hearing aid could do much to improve the quality of their lives. There is little economic reason for refusing to *try* a hearing aid. Veterans should be told that the Veteran's Administration Health Clinics will perform hearing tests and supply a hearing aid. The Office of Vocational Rehabilitation may provide this service as well. Nurses in home care and in long-term care settings should frequently assess the function of the patient's hearing aid.

The elderly person with arthritis or poor vision may have difficulty properly inserting the battery into a hearing aid. If the aid is not working, it may be that the battery simply is not inserted correctly.

Get Ready for the NCLEX® Examination!

Key Points

- Eye disorders are caused by injury, disease, or genetic predisposition.
- Everyone older than age 40 should have a complete eye examination.
- After age 65, an eye examination is recommended every 2 years.
- Control of diabetes mellitus and hypertension can help preserve vision.
- Obtaining a good history is important to data collection regarding vision.
- The tympanic membrane must be able to vibrate when sound is received in order for the sound waves to be transmitted to the middle ear.
- The bones of the middle ear transmit the sound waves to the inner ear.

- Sound is transmitted from the inner ear to cranial nerve VIII.
- Changes in the ear structures with aging may cause hearing impairment.
- Exposure to loud noise causes sensorineural hearing loss.
- A variety of drugs are ototoxic (see Box 26-3).
- There are several diagnostic tests and examinations for problems of the ear (see Table 26-6).
- Learning to communicate with the hearing-impaired person is important for nurses (see Box 26-4).
- Labyrinthitis and Ménière's disease cause dizziness and vertigo.
- Decreasing stress often decreases dizziness and vertigo.
- Tinnitus is common with a variety of ear disorders.
- A variety of treatments are available to help the patient with tinnitus; biofeedback and masking help many people.

- Lip-reading or speech reading is helpful to the hearing-impaired person but is difficult to learn.
- Various types of hearing aids are available, but using one takes practice.
- Cochlear implants are available for the patient who is totally deaf.
- Nurses should actively educate in the community about ways to prevent hearing loss.

Additional Learning Resources

SG Go to your Study Guide for additional learning activities to help you master this chapter content.

Evolve Go to your Evolve website (http://evolve.elsevier.com/deWit/medsurg) for the following FREE learning resources:
- Animations, audio, and video
- Answers and rationales for questions and activities
- Concept Map Creator
- Glossary with pronunciations in English and Spanish
- Interactive Review Questions and Exercises and more!

 Online Resources
- American Foundation for the Blind, www.afb.org
- American Sign Language, www.lifeprint.com/asl101/.com; www.ddeafworld.com
- American Speech-Language-Hearing Association, www.asha.org
- Association for Education and Rehabilitation of the Blind and Visually Impaired, www.aerbvi.org
- Bookshare, www.bookshare.org
- Exercises for vertigo, http://ivertigo.net/vertigo/vertherapy2.html
- Guide Dogs for the Blind, Inc., www.guidedogs.com
- Hearing Loss Association of America, www.shhh.org
- International Hearing Dog, Inc., www.ihdi.org
- National Association of the Deaf, www.nad.org
- National Braille Association, www.nationalbraille.org
- National Institute on Deafness and Other Communication Disorders, www.nidcd.nih.gov

Review Questions for the NCLEX® Examination

1. When a patient is receiving Lasix for a problem with edema, which assessment relative to this drug is important to the patient's health?
   1. Measuring the blood pressure
   2. Determining if the patient is nauseated
   3. Inquiring about constipation
   4. Checking for hearing loss

2. When administering eardrops to an adult, the nurse would:
   1. draw the pinna upward and toward the front of the head.
   2. draw the pinna upward and toward the back of the head.
   3. pull the pinna downward and toward the front of the head.
   4. pull the pinna downward and toward the back of the head.

3. When communicating with a hearing-impaired patient, the nurse should: (Select all that apply.)
   1. Sit at eye level facing the patient.
   2. Use a slightly higher tone than usual.
   3. Enunciate clearly.
   4. Speak directly into the patient's ear.
   5. Use simple, short sentences.

4. The nurse evaluates the visual acuity of the patient using the Snellen chart. Which statement is true regarding the use of the Snellen chart?
   1. The chart is placed 40 feet away from the patient.
   2. The patient reads the letters using one eye at a time.
   3. The numerator (top number) indicates the smallest line that the patient could read.
   4. The denominator (bottom number) refers to the patient's distance from the chart.

5. While looking at a card with a geometric grid of identical squares, the patient is asked to focus on a central dot and to describe any distortions of the surrounding boxes. Which patient statement indicates a need for further diagnostic testing?
   1. "I get dizzy staring at these boxes for so long."
   2. "I am beginning to see color differences in the squares."
   3. "I can see all the boxes surrounding the dot."
   4. "There are wavy lines around the central dot."

6. During a physician visit, a 65-year-old man complains of pain in his right eye associated with excessive tearing. The nurse notes that the eye is red with lashes rubbing against the cornea. A likely condition would be:
   1. ptosis.
   2. ectropion.
   3. hordeolum.
   4. entropion.

7. The nurse applies a vibrating tuning fork to the middle of the patient's forehead. The patient reports hearing the sound in the middle of the head. The patient's response indicates:
   1. sensorineural hearing loss.
   2. conduction hearing loss.
   3. normal hearing.
   4. inconclusive findings.

8. The nurse observes another nurse administering eye ointment. Which action indicates a need for further instructions about technique? The nurse administering the ointment:
   1. places the cap from the tube upside down on the table after removal.
   2. applies the ointment to the lower part of the eyeball.
   3. twists the tube slightly to end the ribbon of ointment.
   4. closes the eye and has the patient move the eyes side to side to distribute the medication.

9. While ambulating, the patient with Ménière's disease complains of dizziness and vertigo. An immediate nursing action would be to:

   1. provide oxygen.
   2. assist patient to supine position.
   3. administer nausea medication.
   4. notify the physician.

10. Which nursing action(s) demonstrate(s) appropriate care of a visually impaired patient? *(Select all that apply.)*

   1. Introduce self before touching.
   2. Speak slowly with a loud voice.
   3. Keep the door ajar.
   4. Ensure ready access to the call button for assistance.
   5. Assist with feeding using the clock method.

Critical Thinking Activities

Scenario A

Mr. Hartman comes to the ambulatory clinic because he "got something in my eye" while using the weed trimmer.

1. What type of examinations would you expect the health care provider to perform?

2. What would you teach Mr. Hartman about eye safety before he leaves?

3. What questions would you ask him about basic eye care while you are interviewing him before the physician sees him?

Scenario B

Mrs. Como is admitted to the hospital for management of her hypertension. She has had sensorineural deafness for several years, and it is much worse in her left ear than in her right. Her inability to hear well causes additional stress for Mrs. Como, and she is especially anxious about being in the hospital among strangers. Mrs. Como also suffers from tinnitus, which adds to her stress and inability to relax and rest. Tinnitus and the stress of not being able to hear adversely affect Mrs. Como's hypertension.

1. What evidence would you expect to find that would indicate that Mrs. Como has a hearing impairment?

2. What can the nurses do to improve communication with Mrs. Como and help allay her anxiety about being in the hospital?

3. Why could her hearing problem make her blood pressure rise?

Scenario C

Mrs. Martinez is scheduled for a cochlear implant and states that she "really doesn't understand" how the device works.

1. What should she be told?

2. What should she expect she will need to do after the cochlear implant surgery?

Care of Patients with Disorders of the Eyes and Ears

Objectives

Theory

1. Discuss errors of refraction and their treatment.
2. Devise nursing care for the patient who is undergoing a corneal transplant.
3. Compare measures used to provide assistance after a chemical eye burn with measures for an eye injury with a foreign object.
4. Describe the signs and symptoms of selected disorders of the eye and appropriate medical treatment and nursing interventions for each.
5. Choose nursing interventions for the patient having a scleral buckle or a cataract extraction.
6. Identify aids and resources for people with vision loss.
7. Explore the impact of hearing or vision loss on an individual and his family.

8. List the signs and symptoms of selected disorders of the ear, appropriate medical or surgical treatment, and nursing interventions for each.
9. Teach the patient with tinnitus or vertigo measures that may decrease the symptoms.
10. Research aids and resources for people with impaired hearing or tinnitus.

Clinical Practice

1. Provide appropriate care for a patient who is preoperative for eye surgery.
2. Properly administer eye medications.
3. Teach a patient to properly administer ear medication.
4. Provide appropriate care for a postoperative ear surgery patient.
5. Assist a patient to find resources for low-vision assistance.

Key Terms

accommodation (ă-kŏm-ō-DĀ-shŭn, p. 594)
astigmatism (ă-STĬG-mă-tĭsm, p. 594)
drusen (drū-zĕn, p. 609)
enucleation (ē-nū-klē-Ā-shŭn, p. 597)
exophthalmos (ĕk-sŏf-THĂL-mŏs, p. 595)
hyperopia (hī-pĕr-Ō-pē-ă, p. 594)

myopia (mī-Ō-pē-ă, p. 594)
nystagmus (nĭs-TĂG-mŭs, p. 613)
photodynamic therapy (fō-tō-dī-NĂM-ĭk, p. 609)
photophobia (fō-tō-FŌ-bē-ă, p. 598)
presbyopia (prĕz-bē-Ō-pē-ă, p. 594)
tympanoplasty (tĭm-pă-nō-PLĂS-tē, p. 613)

COMMON DISORDERS OF THE EYE

ERRORS OF REFRACTION

The most common visual defects are those of refraction. This means that light rays entering the eye are not "refracted," or bent, at the correct angle (Figure 27-1, *A*) and therefore do not focus on the retina. Errors of refraction may be caused by a number of structural defects within the eyeball itself. For example, if the distance between the lens and retina is too short, the light rays focus behind the retina. This causes difficulty in seeing objects close at hand and is called *farsightedness* (hyperopia) (Figure 27-1, *B*).

If the opposite is true, and the eyeball is too elongated, the light rays will converge and focus in front of the retina. The individual then has difficulty seeing objects at a distance and is referred to as being nearsighted. *Nearsightedness* is called myopia (Figure 27-1, *C*).

Light rays from distant objects do not enter the eye at the same angle as light rays from near objects. When

looking off into the distance and then quickly looking down at a book, the eyes must make an adjustment to the difference in the light rays entering the eye. This adjustment, which is called accommodation, is accomplished by ciliary muscles and ligaments that change the shape of the lens, making it more rounded or flatter, thereby allowing light rays to fall on the retina (Figure 27-2).

With age, the ciliary muscles become less elastic and cannot readily accommodate the needs of distant and near vision. Hardening of the ciliary muscles occurs in many people over 40 years of age and is known as presbyopia. Bifocal glasses are usually prescribed for this condition because they allow for two sets of lenses in one pair of glasses, one for viewing distant objects and one for seeing close objects.

Astigmatism is a visual defect resulting from a warped lens or an irregular curvature of the cornea; either condition will prevent the horizontal and vertical rays from focusing at the same point on the retina. Actually, very

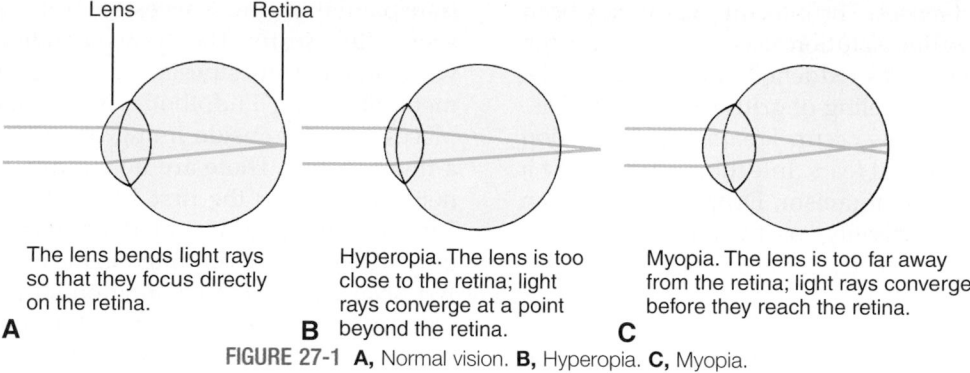

FIGURE 27-1 **A,** Normal vision. **B,** Hyperopia. **C,** Myopia.

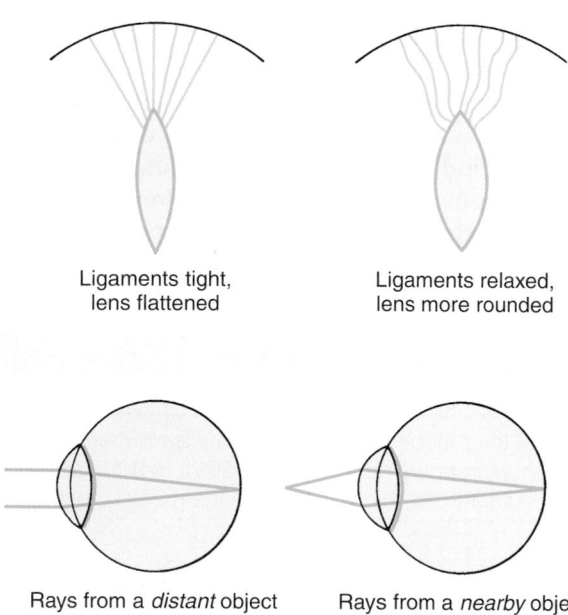

FIGURE 27-2 Flattening and rounding of the lens during accommodation.

few people have perfectly shaped eyeballs, and thus there are very few who do not have some degree of astigmatism. If the astigmatism is very slight, the eye can accommodate for its imperfection by changing the shape of the lens. If there is a serious error of refraction, the eyes will tire very easily or the person will have defective vision because the eyes cannot change the shape of the lens enough to compensate for the abnormality.

Serious errors of refraction are treated with prescription eyeglasses or contact lenses that are fitted so that the light rays are brought into proper focus on the retina. In recent years, advances have been made in refractive surgery that permit correction of refraction problems for some people. Those who are nearsighted (myopic) can undergo one of three procedures. In photorefractive keratectomy (PRK), an excimer laser is used to remove a thin layer of tissue from the cornea. This corrects the excessive curvature of the cornea that is interfering with the proper focus of

light rays through the lens. The preparation takes 30 minutes and the actual procedure takes less than a minute to perform; visual improvement is apparent within 3 to 5 days. LASIK (laser in situ keratomileusis) is the most common procedure for nearsightedness in the United States. The middle layer of the cornea is reshaped with a laser after a very thin outer layer of the cornea is peeled back. The outer layer is replaced. Postoperative recovery is very rapid with little discomfort. The procedure takes about 10 to 15 minutes per eye and is done as an outpatient procedure.

Radial keratotomy is used to correct both nearsightedness and astigmatism. Tiny cuts are made in the cornea that flatten it. It is another outpatient procedure. LASIK and PRK have mostly replaced this procedure.

UVEITIS

The uveal tract consists of the iris, the ciliary body, and the choroid. Uveitis is inflammation of the uveal tract. The cause is unknown; uveitis may be due to allergens, trauma, infectious agents, or systemic disease (rheumatoid arthritis, herpes simplex, herpes zoster, or bacterial infection). Signs and symptoms are tearing, blurred vision, photophobia, aching around the eye, a bloodshot sclera, or a small, nonreactive, irregular pupil. Treatment involves resting the ciliary body with a cycloplegic drug. The pupil is dilated to prevent adhesions of the involved structures. Analgesics, antibiotics, and ocular steroid injections may be employed. Cool or warm compresses are used for discomfort. Sunglasses should be worn to reduce photophobia. Low light indoors is advisable.

CORNEAL DISORDERS

Keratitis

Keratitis is an inflammation of the cornea caused by irritation or infection. Patients who have had a stroke may develop irritation of the cornea because the eyelid does not close normally. Keratitis may occur in a comatose patient who is not receiving proper eye care. Some people with **exophthalmos** (protruding eyeballs) develop this disorder. Infection is not uncommon in those who wear contact lenses. The infecting agent may be in home-prepared saline solution used for cleaning the lenses. The eye becomes reddened, and there may be tearing, along with a feeling of grittiness or pain. Discharge from the eye may occur. Treatment of irritation is instillation of artificial tears. Infection is treated by a medication to kill the organism. Drugs may be given topically, subconjunctivally, or by intravenous (IV) infusion.

Corneal Ulcer

A corneal ulcer may occur from irritation, infection, or injury. The ulcer is cultured to determine whether there is a causative organism when there is no history of injury. Antibiotic medication is usually supplied. Scarring from corneal ulcers or severe infection is treated by keratoplasty.

Corneal Transplantation (Keratoplasty)

Corneal transplants replace corneas that have been damaged by genetic disorders, trauma, ulcers, or disease such as *keratitis* (inflammation of the cornea); transplants help restore corneal clarity. Two types of procedures are done: a full-thickness keratoplasty (corneal transplant), or a lamellar keratoplasty, which replaces only a superficial layer of corneal tissue. The full-thickness keratoplasty restores vision in about 95% of patients (Figure 27-3, *A*). Corneas for

transplantation are harvested from donor cadavers soon after death. The transplantation is performed with regional anesthesia. A new procedure, Descemet's Stripping Endothelial Keratoplasty (DSEK) replaces only the inside lining of corneal cells through a tiny incision. There are no sutures and the cells are held in place for the first 24 hours by an air bubble. Vision is improved in a matter of weeks. DSEK is used only when disease is limited to the endothelial surface. Artificial cornea transplantation studies are showing success in both adults and children and reduces the chance of rejection of human tissue.

The patient must be "on call" to come for the transplantation, as it is unpredictable when a matching donor cornea will become available. The surgery is an outpatient procedure. The patient must realize beforehand that it takes 1 to 2 weeks before any improvement in vision is noticeable and that improvement will continue for several months. Because the cornea does not have an abundant blood supply, healing is very slow and is not complete for about 1 year. **Prevention of infection is extremely important.** Preoperative care is much the same as for other eye surgeries.

> ### ⚠ Safety Alert
> #### Correctly Mark the Surgical Site
> As part of the preoperative preparation, clearly mark the operative site, verifying verbally with the patient that the site is correct. Document that this was done in the medical record.

After surgery, the keratoplasty patient remains in recovery for 1 to 2 hours and then is discharged home. A pressure dressing and eye shield are applied in the surgical suite after the procedure and should be removed only by the physician the next day. The shield is then worn at night for at least a month, and when around small children or pets. The pressure dressing helps keep the donor tissue in contact with the eyeball. Nursing actions focus on caring for a patient with disturbed sensory perception (visual). Instructions regarding safety are provided before discharge. The patient may lie only on his back and nonoperative side postoperatively. Graft rejection is a possibility and is heralded by inflammation beginning near the graft edges (see Figure 27-3, *B*). This finding must be reported promptly. Should the first transplant fail, the procedure can be redone.

Sometimes an eye excimer laser is used to polish the cornea, restoring vision. A scleral lens has been developed. It is like an oversized contact lens that arches over the cornea. The space between the lens and the cornea is filled with artificial tears, providing lubrication, and thus the scleral lens fulfills the optical functions of the damaged cornea. These innovations may eventually make corneal transplants unnecessary for many people.

A

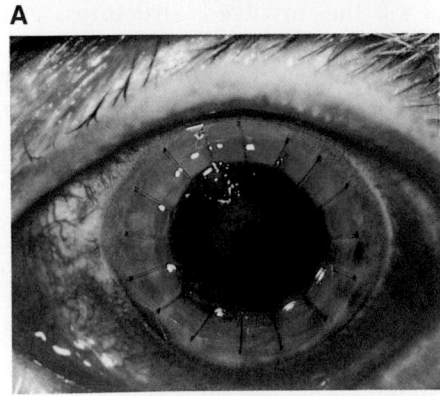

B

FIGURE 27-3 A, Keratoplasty (corneal transplant). **B,** Acute transplant rejection.

The elderly patient who is visually impaired temporarily or permanently may experience a loss of independence and a change in self-perception. This patient will need specific suggestions on ways to maintain independence. After an eye surgery which is often done on an outpatient basis, the person will need someone to help at home for a few days, at least.

EYE TRAUMA

Eye trauma occurs from accidents and from debris in the air. Not using safety goggles or glasses when sanding or operating weed trimmers and various types of power equipment accounts for most incidents of foreign bodies landing in the eyes.

Removal of Foreign Bodies from the Eye

If the foreign body is not deeply embedded in the tissues of the eye, it can easily be removed by irrigation. Irrigation with clear, lukewarm water or sterile water or saline is used to remove a foreign body sticking to the cornea. Continuous irrigation can be done with small tubing, and a bottle of solution or an irrigating syringe or bottle can be used. The nurse must be very careful not to touch the eye with the tip of the irrigating device. Sometimes a speck of foreign matter on the cornea can be removed with a moistened, sterile cotton swab. Have the patient tilt the head back. Hold the eyelids open to prevent blinking.

If a foreign body is sticking out of the eye, no attempt to remove it should be made. Both eyes should be patched to prevent further eye movement, and the patient should be transported to the emergency department or to an ophthalmologist. If the patient continues to complain of a sensation that a foreign body is still in the eye after it appears to have been removed by irrigation, or complains of continuing pain, refer to a physician immediately, as there may be a corneal abrasion.

The physician will apply a stain to the eye to assess whether the cornea is abraded. If there is an abrasion, medicated ointment will be prescribed, and the eye will be patched. The patient must be given instructions on how to instill the ointment (see Box 26-1). A thin line of eye ointment is applied from the inner canthus to the outer canthus along the lower eyelid inside the conjunctival sac (Figure 27-4). The patient closes the eyelid and moves the eyeball around in the socket to distribute the ointment. Excess medication is gently wiped away with a tissue, moving from the inner to the outer canthus. If an eye patch is not applied, the patient is warned that the ointment may blur vision for a while. A corneal abrasion is painful; a nonsteroidal anti-inflammatory drug may be used for discomfort.

Chemical Burns

Chemical burns should be treated by lengthy, continuous irrigation. An IV bag of normal saline is the preferred solution; otherwise, tap water will do. Place

FIGURE 27-4 Applying eye ointment.

Twist tube to release ointment

the patient supine with his head turned to the affected side. With gloves on, direct the stream of fluid to the inner canthus so that the stream flows across the cornea to the outer canthus, holding the lids apart with your thumb and index finger. At intervals, stop and have the patient close his eyes to move secretions and particles from the upper eye to the lower conjunctival sac; then begin again. The patient should be seen by a physician as soon as possible. All commercial businesses where exposure to chemicals is a possibility must comply with Occupational Safety and Health Administration (OSHA) standards and have an eyewash station within the facility as close as possible to the area where chemicals are likely to be used.

Enucleation

If the eye is too damaged by trauma to be salvaged, or is irreparably damaged by disease or tumor, enucleation (removal of the eye) is performed. An implant is created to maintain the orbital anatomy while a matching artificial eye is created. The implant is sutured to the muscle structures. When the artificial eye is placed, the muscle attachments allow for coordinated eye movement.

Postoperatively, observe for signs of complications such as excessive bleeding, swelling, increased pain, elevated temperature, or displacement of the implant. Losing an eye is a devastating experience even when there has been a long period of painful blindness preoperatively. Understanding of the emotional impact and support of the patient are prime nursing responsibilities. The permanent prosthesis is placed about 6 weeks after the surgery.

Care of an Artificial Eye. The procedure for cleansing and caring for an artificial eye is similar in many ways to the care of dentures. Both require basic principles of cleanliness, careful handling, and proper storage. An artificial eye is very expensive and must be handled very carefully.

The artificial eye is cleansed with gentle soap and water, unless the patient, his family, or the physician directs otherwise. Keep it in a safe place to avoid damage. When the eye is to be reinserted, it should be cleansed again with soap and water. When inserting or removing the prosthesis, have the head over a padded surface. The patient's upper lid is lifted, and the eye is inserted with the notched end toward the nose. After the prosthesis is placed as far as possible under the upper lid, the lower lid is depressed, allowing the eye to slip into place.

CATARACT

A *cataract* is opacity of the lens that produces an effect similar to one a person would get when looking through a sheet of falling water (Figure 27-5). A cataract causes a blurring of vision because the lens, which is normally transparent, becomes cloudy and opaque.

Etiology and Pathophysiology

Congenital cataracts are most often due to maternal infection with rubella or *Toxoplasma gondii.* Most often cataracts occur as a result of aging and are found in people over age 50 (adult-onset [senile] cataracts).

Traumatic cataracts may occur from a physical blow, extreme heat, or chemical toxins. Cigarette smoking increases the risk of developing cataracts. Heavy drinking also is implicated. Chronic use of corticosteroids predisposes to the development of cataracts.

🏃 Health Promotion

Cataract Prevention

Encouraging the habit of wearing sunglasses that protect from ultraviolet light and a hat when outdoors can help prevent the development of cataracts. Cumulative exposure to ultraviolet light is the greatest risk factor for cataracts.

❓ Think Critically

What would you teach the person with rheumatoid arthritis about eye care, if that person is on corticosteroids most of the time?

FIGURE 27-5 Cloudy appearance of eye with cataract.

Signs, Symptoms, and Diagnosis

In addition to the blurred vision typical of opacity of the lens, with cataracts there may be decreased color perception. Uncomplicated cataracts are usually painless, but the patient may have **photophobia** (intolerance of light). Assessment may reveal the following symptoms:

- Hazy, blurred, or double vision *(diplopia)*
- Increasing complaints about glare
- Increasing nearsightedness
- Complaints that colors are faded or appear yellowish or brownish
- Desire for increased light by which to read
- Difficulty with night vision
- Frequent need for eyeglass prescription change

The loss of vision associated with cataracts is progressive and sometimes is partially due to secondary glaucoma. As an untreated cataract progresses, the lens of the eye becomes cloudy or milky white, then may turn yellow, and eventually may become brown or black (see Figure 27-5).

Diagnosis of a cataract is confirmed by examining the dilated pupil with a slit lamp, which enables the examiner to see opacities more clearly. Glaucoma should first be ruled out as a possible cause of the symptoms. Tonometry is used to determine intraocular pressure (IOP). For screening purposes, the Tono-Pen may be used.

Treatment

Cataract surgery is performed when the loss of vision greatly affects the quality of the person's life. The only effective method of treating cataracts is surgical removal of the affected lens with clear lens implantation; cataract surgery is the most commonly performed surgical procedure in the United States. Surgical techniques are (1) *extracapsular extraction,* in which the lens is removed along with the anterior portion of the lens capsule; and (2) *intracapsular extraction,* in which both the capsule and the lens are removed. Extracapsular extraction is most frequently performed because it allows an intraocular lens to be inserted inside the remaining capsule. Lenses are now available that allow for multifocal vision rather than monovision where vision is good at only one distance without glasses. One type of lens is hinged to the ciliary muscle, allowing for accommodation of vision for various distances (Harvard Eye Associates, 2010). If a monovision lens is chosen, vision is corrected for nearsightedness or farsightedness by the lens implant and further correction of vision is achieved with regular eyeglasses or contact lenses. Vision is improved within 2 weeks and is usually fully recovered within 3 months of surgery (Nursing Care Plan 27-1).

One technique for intracapsular cataract extraction (ICCE) utilizes *cryosurgery,* in which the lens is frozen by a super-cooled probe and then removed. *Phacoemulsification,* in which the tissue is pulverized

Nursing Care Plan 27-1 | **Care of the Patient Undergoing a Cataract Extraction**

Scenario

Mrs. Fort, age 79, is admitted to the outpatient surgery unit for extraction of a cataract of the left eye with lens implant. The vision in her right eye also is affected by a cataract, but the visual loss is not as severe in that eye. Mrs. Fort suffers from a crippling osteoarthritis of the hands, but her general health is good. She is well oriented, outgoing, and physically active. She lives alone in an apartment building for retired senior citizens. Her daughter and son-in-law live nearby and are in daily contact with her. Mrs. Fort has only been in the hospital once in her life for pneumonia and is concerned about what to expect preoperatively and postoperatively.

Problem/Nursing Diagnosis

Lack of knowledge/Knowledge deficient related to preoperative and postoperative procedures and care.

Supporting Assessment Data

Subjective: "I have never had surgery before."

Goals/Expected Outcomes	Nursing Interventions	Selected Rationale	Evaluation
Patient will verbalize preoperative routine activities and postoperative procedures and expectations.	Teach patient and daughter about eye medications to be used at home and how to instill them; how to dress and shield eye properly, how to remove bandage without contaminating eye.	To comply with instructions, teaching must occur on how to instill drops and how to dress and shield the eye and perform care needed.	Provided teaching for patient and daughter. Will ask for return demonstration before discharge. Left printed instructions.

Problem/Nursing Diagnosis

Potential postoperative complications/Risk for injury related to postoperative complications such as hemorrhage and increased intraocular pressure.

Supporting Assessment Data

Objective: Undergoing cataract extraction; hemorrhage and increased intraocular pressure are potential complications.

Goals/Expected Outcomes	Nursing Interventions	Selected Rationale	Evaluation
Intraocular hemorrhage will not occur, and there will not be an increase in intraocular pressure.	Teach signs and symptoms of complications that are to be reported to physician immediately: increasing eye pain, purulent discharge, decreasing vision, fever or chills, increasing brow headache.	Patient must know what to look for in order to report complications.	Gave instructions and left printed list. Will ask for feedback before discharge.
	Instruct to refrain from straining at stool; encourage to use milk of magnesia or stool softener to prevent straining as needed.	Preventing the Valsalva maneuver will help prevent an increase in intraocular pressure.	Verbalizes the ways to prevent raising intraocular pressure.
	Perform hand hygiene thoroughly before instilling eye medications or changing dressing; teach patient and daughter to wash hands before approaching eye area. Demonstrate how to put on eye shield for sleep.	Aseptic techniques help prevent infection. Maintaining asepsis aids in protecting the surgical site from infection and prevents complications.	Patient and daughter state that they understand hand hygiene and aseptic techniques for postoperative eye care.
	Instruct patient to avoid rapid or sudden movements and bending from the waist.	Bending from the waist increases intraocular pressure.	Instructed to crouch rather than bend at the waist and to avoid sudden movements.

Continued

⭐ Nursing Care Plan 27-1   Care of the Patient Undergoing a Cataract Extraction—cont'd

Goals/Expected Outcomes	Nursing Interventions	Selected Rationale	Evaluation
Intraocular hemorrhage will not occur, and there will not be an increase in intraocular pressure—cont'd	Instruct patient to take medication immediately for nausea and vomiting. Remind patient not to lie on affected side. Encourage patient to seek assistance with ambulation while vision is blurred.	Quickly medicating for nausea may avert vomiting.	Instructions given and a written instruction sheet at bedside.

Problem/Nursing Diagnosis
Limited use of hands/Self-care deficit related to disabilities imposed by osteoarthritis.

Supporting Assessment Data
Objective: Severe osteoarthritis of the hands with limited dexterity.

Goals/Expected Outcomes	Nursing Interventions	Selected Rationale	Evaluation
Assistance with administration of postoperative eye medications and eye care will be given by daughter.	Teach daughter techniques needed for postoperative eye care and give her a written schedule for that care.	Written instructions and a schedule reinforce the teaching and help care to occur on time.	Daughter observed care and administration of eye medications today; will demonstrate postoperative eye care when meds are next due.

Critical Thinking Questions
1. Why should one wait 5 minutes between instilling one type of eyedrop and the next type of eyedrop?
2. What is one of the most important things to teach someone who is to instill eyedrops or ointment postoperatively?

and the debris is removed by suction, is often used for extracapsular cataract extraction (ECCE). These outpatient surgical procedures are performed under procedural sedation and local anesthesia. An intraocularlens implant is placed after cataract extraction. Postoperative care is covered later in this chapter.

👥 Patient Teaching

General Care After Eye Surgery

Instructions for the patient and/or family caregiver:

- Always wash the hands before instilling medication. Check the label of the container to be certain it is the right medication.
  Do not contaminate the applicator tip of the medication.
- Instill only the number of drops ordered; apply pressure at the inner canthus to prevent systemic absorption; close the eye gently (do not squeeze the eye shut).
- Change the eye patch dressing at least once a day; change as needed to keep the area clean.
- Follow the medication schedule prescribed by the physician exactly. (Send home a written schedule.)
- Maintain designated head position and activity restrictions.
- Report signs of complications: sudden, increasing pain in the eye, which can indicate hemorrhage; purulent drainage; decreasing vision; signs of increased intraocular pressure, such as brow headache.
- Keep the follow-up appointment with the surgeon.
- Use caution to prevent getting water in the eye.
- Protect the eye during the day with glasses; use sunglasses for outside wear; wear a protective eye shield at night.

Nursing Management
The patient must be told that there is a period of visual adjustment after cataract surgery. The surgeon may prescribe miotic eyedrops after surgery to constrict the pupil and lessen the danger of lens dislocation. **Patient adherence to the schedule for postoperative medications is critical to preventing complications and promoting healing.**

❓ Think Critically

Can you identify patients who should be carefully assessed for signs and symptoms of cataract?

GLAUCOMA

Etiology
The term *glaucoma* comprises a complex group of disorders that involve many different pathologic changes and symptoms, but have in common an optic neuropathy that damages the optic disc, causing atrophy and loss of peripheral vision. The neuropathy often is caused by increased IOP (National Eye Institute, 2011). Glaucoma may come on slowly and cause irreversible visual loss without presenting any other noticeable symptoms, or it may appear abruptly and produce blindness in a matter of hours. Glaucoma can be present at birth, or can develop at any age. It can result from genetic predisposition, trauma, or

another disorder of the eye. Glaucoma frequently is a manifestation of diseases and pathologies in other body systems. The amount of increased IOP that causes damage differs from one person's eye to another. **Blindness is preventable if the disorder is treated early.**

[?] Think Critically

How can you include inquiries about family history or predisposing risk factors for glaucoma into your patient care?

Pathophysiology

The IOP is determined by the rate of *aqueous humor* production and the outflow of the aqueous humor from the eye. Aqueous humor is produced in the ciliary body and flows out of the eye through the canal of Schlemm into the venous system (Concept Map 27-1). An imbalance may occur from overproduction by the ciliary body or by obstruction of outflow. Increased IOP greater than 22 mm Hg requires thorough evaluation. Increased IOP restricts the blood flow to the optic nerve and the retina. Ischemia causes these structures to lose their function gradually. **The vision impairment from damage to the optic nerve or retina is permanent.** Glaucoma may be secondary to eye infection, trauma, eye surgery, or ocular tumor.

There are three types of glaucoma: narrow-angle or angle-closure (acute) glaucoma, open-angle (chronic) glaucoma (Figure 27-6), and associated or secondary glaucoma. The terms *narrow angle* (angle closure) and *open angle* refer to the angle width between the cornea and the iris. *Acute* and *chronic* refer to either the onset

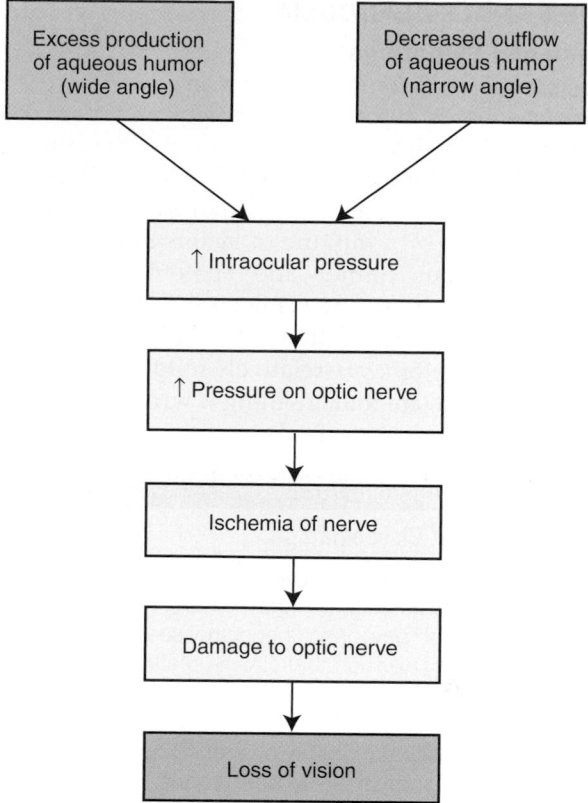

CONCEPT MAP 27-1 Pathophysiology of glaucoma.

or duration of the problem. These two major types differ in their clinical signs and symptoms, treatment, and effects on vision. *Associated glaucoma* may occur with diabetes mellitus, hypertension, or extreme myopia, or after retinal detachment.

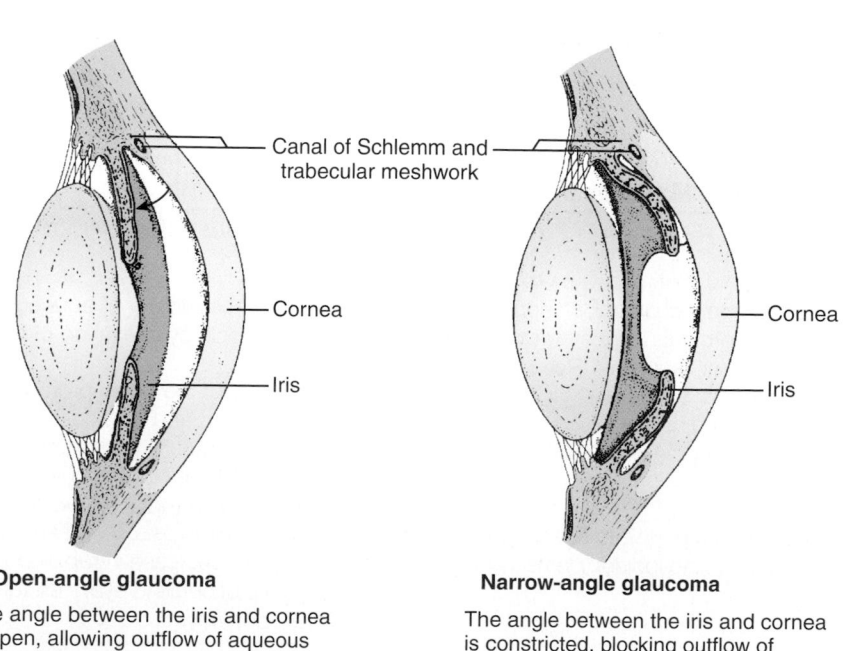

Open-angle glaucoma

The angle between the iris and cornea is open, allowing outflow of aqueous humor through the canal of Schlemm and the trabecular meshwork

Narrow-angle glaucoma

The angle between the iris and cornea is constricted, blocking outflow of aqueous humor

FIGURE 27-6 Comparison of open-angle (wide, chronic) and narrow-angle (closed, acute) glaucoma.

OPEN-ANGLE GLAUCOMA

Signs and Symptoms

Open-angle, or chronic, glaucoma, in which there is no angle closure, is much more insidious and more common, occurring in about 90% of people with glaucoma. It often is an inherited disorder that causes degenerative changes in the aqueous humor outflow tracts. It may be caused by a mixture of factors of overproduction of aqueous humor and anatomical problems within the eye. It usually is bilateral and can progress to complete blindness without ever producing an acute attack. Its symptoms are relatively mild, and many patients are not aware that anything is wrong until vision has been seriously impaired.

 Health Promotion

Danger Signals of Glaucoma

The National Society for the Prevention of Blindness lists the following symptoms as danger signals of open-angle glaucoma:
- Glasses, even new ones, that do not seem to clarify vision
- Blurred or hazy vision that clears up after a while
- Trouble in getting used to darkened rooms, such as in movie theaters
- Seeing rainbow-colored rings around lights
- Narrowing of vision at the sides of one or both eyes

Encourage a complete eye examination if any of these signs is present.

Diagnosis

People at high risk for glaucoma are:
- Diabetics
- African Americans (at least four times as many African Americans as non–African Americans have glaucoma-related blindness)
- Individuals with a family history of glaucoma

A commonly used screening technique for early detection of glaucoma is to measure IOP with an air tonometer. A puff of air is directed at the cornea, which

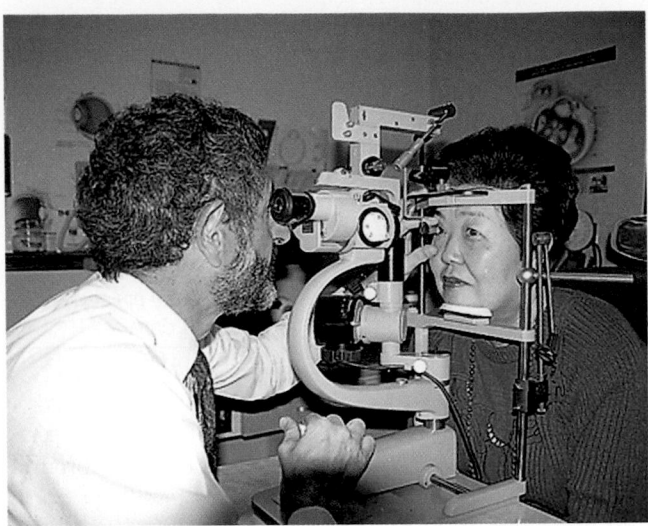

FIGURE 27-7 Applanation tonometer.

causes a momentary indentation while a pressure reading is taken (WebMD, 2010). The test is painless, and nothing but the air touches the eye. Verification of the diagnosis of glaucoma may require the use of a more complex instrument called an *applanation tonometer* (Figure 27-7). The cornea is flattened and pressure is measured with a slit-lamp biomicroscope.

Treatment

The initial treatment of choice for chronic (open-angle) glaucoma is medication rather than surgery. If drugs are not effective, or if they produce worrisome side effects, surgery is performed.

Drugs prescribed are intended to enhance aqueous humor outflow, decrease its production, or both (Table 27-1). They do this by constricting the pupil (miotics) or by inhibiting the formation of aqueous humor. Miotics cause blurred vision for 1 to 2 hours after use. Adjustment to dark rooms is difficult because of

Table 27-1	Pharmacologic Management of Eye Disorders	
CLASSIFICATION	**EXAMPLES**	**ACTION/NURSING IMPLICATIONS**
Drugs Used for Glaucoma		
Miotics	*Prostaglandin analogs:* latanoprost (Xalatan), bimatoprost (Lumigan), travoprost (Travatan) Unoprostone isopropyl (Rescula)	Increase outflow of aqueous fluid through the ciliary muscle by relaxation of the muscle.
	Cholinergics: pilocarpine HCl (Isopto Carpine), pilocarpine nitrate (Ocusert Pilo-20, Ocusert Pilo-40), carbachol (Miostat)	Constrict the pupil, promote outflow of aqueous humor, and reduce intraocular pressure. Reduce visual acuity in dim light; advise patient to avoid driving at night. Ocusert is placed in conjunctival sac and replaced weekly.
	Cholinesterase inhibitors: echothiophate iodide (Phospholine iodide), demecarium bromide (Humorsol)	Produce miosis, increase aqueous humor outflow, and decrease intraocular pressure. Avoid touching tip of bottle to eye; moisture may interfere with drug potency.

💊 Table 27-1   **Pharmacologic Management of Eye Disorders—cont'd**

CLASSIFICATION	EXAMPLES	ACTION/NURSING IMPLICATIONS
Miotics—cont'd	*Beta-adrenergic blockers:* timolol maleate (Timoptic), betaxolol (Betoptic), levobunolol (Betagan), metipranolol (OptiPranolol), carteolol (Ocupress)	Reduce production of aqueous humor, thereby reducing intraocular pressure. Betoptic reduces intraocular hypertension. Monitor pulse and blood pressure during initiation of therapy. Blurred vision decreases with continued use. Use beta blockers cautiously in patients with a history of asthma.
Carbonic anhydrase inhibitors	Acetazolamide (Diamox), dorzolamide (Trusopt), brinzolamide (Azopt)	Interfere with carbonic acid production, thereby decreasing aqueous humor formation and decreasing intraocular pressure. Taken orally or as eyedrops (TruSopt). When taken orally, these drugs have a diuretic action; observe for dehydration and postural hypotension. Monitor electrolytes. Confusion may occur in the elderly. Check interaction with other drugs patient is receiving.
Sympathomimetics	Epinephrine (Epifrin), dipivefrin (Propine), apraclonidine (Iopidine)	Reduce intraocular pressure by increasing aqueous outflow. May cause brow headache, headache, eye irritation, and blurred vision. Used for open-angle glaucoma only. May cause tachycardia and rise in blood pressure.
Alpha-2 adrenergic agonist	Brimonidine tartrate (Alphagan) L	Acts on alpha receptors in the blood vessels, decreasing the production of aqueous humor. Do not use with soft contact lenses. Contraindicated in heart disease.
Anti-inflammatories	*Corticosteroids:* Pred Forte, Ocu-Pred, Ophtho-Tate *NSAIDs:* ketorolac (Acular), flurbiprofen (Ocufen) *Prostaglandin analog:* latanoprost (Xalatan)	Decrease inflammation and swelling; reduce miosis. Interact with contact lens materials.
Drugs Used to Facilitate Diagnosis and Surgery of the Eye		
Cycloplegics and mydriatics anticholinergic agents	Atropine (Atropisol), cyclopentolate (Cyclogyl), homatropine (Isopto Homatropine), scopolamine (Isopto Hyoscine), tropicamide (Mydriacyl)	Dilate the pupils and paralyze the muscles of accommodation, causing mydriasis and cycloplegia. Mydriasis facilitates observation of the eye's interior during an examination. Cycloplegia prevents movement of the lens during assessment of the eye.
Adrenergic agonist	Phenylephrine (Ocu-Phrin)	Induces mydriasis by action on the muscle of the iris. Causes blurred vision. Photophobia may be eased by using dark glasses.
Staining solution	Fluorescein	Turns corneal scratches bright green; a green ring surrounds foreign bodies. Dye will filter through the lacrimal duct into the nasal secretions.
Topical anesthetics	Proparacaine (Alcaine, AK-Taine), tetracaine (Pontocaine)	Anesthetize the eye. Caution patient not to rub the eye while it is anesthetized. Patch eye when patient leaves the office if medication is still in effect.
Anti-infective Optic Medications		
Antibiotics	Gentamicin sulfate (Garamycin ophthalmic), erythromycin (Ilotycin), polymyxin B sulfate, neomycin sulfate, bacitracin, sulfonamides (Sodium Sulamyd, Gantrisin), ciprofloxacin (Ciloxan), chlortetracycline (Aureomycin), ofloxacin (Ocuflox),	Used to treat infection or for prophylaxis. Caution patient to use a clean washcloth and towel on the face each time to prevent reinfection.
Antifungal	Natamycin (Natacyn ophthalmic)	To treat *Fusarium*. Caution as above.
Antivirals	Idoxuridine (IDV, Stoxil, Herplex), trifluridine (Viroptic) Vidarabine (Vira-A ophthalmic)	Store in refrigerator. Do not use with boric acid. If no improvement, discontinue after 1 wk. Effective against DNA viruses; used for keratoconjunctivitis.

pupil constriction. Pilocarpine is available in an eye medication disk that resembles a contact lens. The disk is inserted into the conjunctival sac in a patient's lower eyelid, where it can remain for up to 7 days. The medication is slowly released. Use of the disk does not prevent the wearing of contact lenses. Diuretics may be prescribed to reduce the production of aqueous humor fluid. Not all diuretics reduce IOP, and a substitute should not be used for the specific drug prescribed.

Whenever glaucoma is being managed by medication, the patient must continue the eyedrops and oral medications on an uninterrupted basis. Patients admitted to the hospital for disorders other than glaucoma often are allowed to keep their glaucoma medication at the bedside if they are able to administer it themselves.

🔲 Clinical Cues

When admitting a patient with a history of glaucoma, check to see that he has his eye medication with him and that there is an order on the chart for leaving it at the bedside. Otherwise, verify that there is an order on the chart for his usual glaucoma medications. If there is no order, call the physician for one.

When drugs do not control glaucoma and increased IOP persists, surgery is an alternative. The goal is to create openings so that excess fluid can escape. A laser is used to create evenly spaced openings in the collecting meshwork (*trabeculoplasty*) to facilitate aqueous humor drainage in open-angle or chronic glaucoma. Microsurgery filtering procedures create a drainage hole in the iris between the anterior and posterior chambers. A tiny shunt may be placed to drain excess aqueous humor if other surgeries do not produce the desired result. When surgical procedures fail, the ciliary body may be treated by applying a freezing probe tip (*cyclocryotherapy*). This permanently damages cells in the ciliary body and decreases the production of aqueous humor.

Laser surgery is performed with procedural sedation. The patient may experience a mild headache and blurring of vision during the first 24 hours. There is a possibility that IOP may increase because of an inflammatory response. **Increasing pain in the eye should be reported to the ophthalmologist immediately.** The patient should be instructed to prevent increasing the venous pressure in the head, neck, and eyes by avoiding the Valsalva maneuver (straining with a closed glottis), not bending over, keeping the head up, and not making any sudden movements. A stool softener is given to prevent constipation. Strenuous exercise is to be avoided for 3 weeks. The head of the bed should be elevated 15 to 20 degrees to decrease pressure within the eyes during sleep. Elevated IOP will persist for a week or so in some patients. Glaucoma medications are continued to meet the patient's individual needs. The patient must understand the importance of frequent checkups and the necessity of consistently following instructions; the

surgical procedure does not always eliminate the need for medication.

Nursing Management

Education of the patient and his family is a major aspect of care. Failure to follow the prescribed treatment regimen to control glaucoma and neglecting to maintain regular contact with the physician can result in progressive loss of vision and eventual blindness (Figure 27-8).

FIGURE 27-8 Glaucoma causes a progressive loss of peripheral vision.

The patient who has glaucoma needs to be fully informed about the nature of this disorder, how it can affect vision, the treatments available, and the expected result of those treatments. An analogy that can be used to explain the nature of the disorder is to compare the eye to a sink with an open faucet (the ciliary processes), a drain (angle), and pipes (trabecular structures). As long as water flows into and out of the sink at the same rate, there is no problem. If something blocks the drain or the pipes, the water will fill the sink beyond its holding capacity. Treatment with miotics helps keep the pipes open so that drainage is possible; beta blockers and diuretics can slow down the rate at which water flows from the tap. If the medications do not work, or if the sink suddenly is blocked by a clogged pipe, it may be necessary for the surgeon to clear the drainage system so that the water can drain from the sink.

In addition to learning about the nature of glaucoma and the expected results of prescribed treatments, the patient also must be made aware of the possibility of vision loss if the condition is not managed. **Teaching should emphasize that glaucoma medications prevent further vision loss, but medications cannot restore vision.** Teaching must be done with tact and sensitivity for the patient's feelings. The information should never be presented in such a way that the patient feels threatened or becomes so fearful that he is unable to participate in the management of his disorder.

Patient Teaching

Points to Cover in the Glaucoma Teaching Plan

- Signs of IOP include pain in the eye, redness, tearing, blurred vision, halos around lights, and frequent need for change in eyeglasses.
- Measures to prevent increase in IOP include low-sodium diet, little caffeine, preventing constipation and Valsalva maneuver, and decreasing stress.
- Need to take prescribed medications and refrain from taking over-the-counter or other medications without physician's knowledge. Glaucoma medication must be taken regularly for life.
- Use good aseptic technique when instilling eye medication.
- Wear ID tag or bracelet stating "Glaucoma" and carry card in wallet that states what medications are being taken.
- Keep extra bottle of eye medication on hand. Carry eyedrops.
- Maintain close medical follow-up with physician.
- Practice safety habits; avoid night driving if possible.

ID, identification; *IOP*, intraocular pressure.

NARROW-ANGLE (ANGLE-CLOSURE) GLAUCOMA

Signs, Symptoms, and Diagnosis

Narrow-angle, or acute, glaucoma is a medical emergency in which there is severe pain in the eye accompanied by the appearance of colored halos around lights, blurred vision, and pain in and around the eye. Nausea and vomiting may occur. The cause of narrow-angle glaucoma is the position of the iris, which lies too close to the drainage canal and bulges forward against the cornea, blocking the drainage of aqueous humor (see Figure 27-6). The IOP rises suddenly, sometimes reaching a pressure of 50 to 70 mm Hg. Relief of the situation must be prompt, or damage to the optic nerve will cause blindness in the affected eye. Diagnosis is by history, testing of IOP, and dilated eye examination.

Treatment and Nursing Management

Emergency treatment in narrow-angle glaucoma consists of measures to reduce IOP as quickly as possible. During the attack, drugs such as pilocarpine, topical epinephrine, and IV acetazolamide are used. Surgery is performed as soon as inflammation subsides to relieve pressure against the optic nerve endings. *Laser iridotomy, trabeculectomy, laser trabeculoplasty,* or other procedures that allow filtering of the aqueous humor from the anterior chamber into the subconjunctival space are performed. If these procedures fail, sometimes *cyclocryotherapy* (the application of a freezing tip) may be used on the ciliary body to decrease the aqueous production.

Nursing management is the same as for other eye surgeries: teaching about activity precautions during healing, schedule for eyedrops, symptoms to report to the surgeon, and aseptic handling of the eyedrops and eye shield.

RETINAL DETACHMENT

Etiology

Retinal detachments often are classified as either primary or secondary. Primary retinal detachment is the result of spontaneous or degenerative changes in the retina or the vitreous humor. Secondary retinal detachment is associated with mechanical trauma, inflammation within the eye, or some other ophthalmic disorder, such as diabetic or hypertensive retinopathy. Retinal detachments frequently occur in people with a high degree of myopia. The incidence of retinal detachment increases dramatically after 40 years of age and is most common between ages 40 and 70. Fifteen percent of people with retinal detachment in one eye develop detachment in the other eye.

Cultural Considerations

Incidence of Retinal Detachment in People of Jewish Descent

Retinal detachment is seen more frequently in people of Jewish ethnicity. The condition is relatively infrequent in African Americans. The reason may be that the Jewish population has more incidence of myopia, and that condition tends to be inherited. Severe myopia is a risk factor for retinal detachment.

Detached retina

FIGURE 27-9 Retinal detachment.

Pathophysiology

Retinal detachment is actually not a detachment of the whole retina, but a separation of the sensory layers of the retina from the pigmented epithelial layer, the choroid. Retinal detachment can cause vitreous fluid to leak under the retina, separating a portion of it from the vascular wall and thereby depriving the retina of its blood supply (Figure 27-9).

Signs, Symptoms, and Diagnosis

Onset can be either gradual or sudden, depending on the cause and extent of the detachment and the location of the area involved. The patient may see flashes of colored light accompanied by showers of floaters (black spots), or may feel as if a curtain has been drawn over a portion of the visual field. Later, cloudy vision or loss of central vision is noticed. In severe cases, there may be complete loss of vision.

 Think Critically

What would you say to your friend if you are having a meal together in a restaurant and he comments that he is seeing flashes of colored light in his left eye? What would you tell him to do?

Diagnosis of detached retina can be made with a direct ophthalmoscope, but diagnosis is greatly simplified by a stereoscopic indirect ophthalmoscope. This instrument permits visualization of the entire retina, and produces an image of the retina with less magnification and distortion than the direct ophthalmoscope. Ultrasound can be used to detect retinal detachment when the eye is clouded by opacity from cataract or hemorrhage.

Treatment

Retinal holes and tears sometimes can be repaired on an outpatient basis with laser therapy that creates an inflammatory reaction, causing the layers to adhere during healing. Tears located in the posterior fundus can be coagulated and sealed with a laser beam or photocoagulator. Peripheral retinal holes through which no fluid has leaked can be closed by applying a freezing probe tip (cryotherapy). The frozen area scars over in a few days, and the hole is thus sealed. A third procedure, called *scleral buckling*, requires more extensive surgery. In effect, scleral buckling places the retinal breaks in contact with the pigmented epithelial layer. Adhesions are formed that bind the sensory and epithelial layers and the choroid together. Before the procedure, gas may be injected into the eye to apply pressure on the retina from the interior of the eye. This application of pressure helps hold the layers together during healing.

In instances when hemorrhage into the vitreous obstructs vision, the surgeon may perform a closed vitrectomy during retinal repair. The purpose of the vitrectomy is to remove the cloudy vitreous humor and stabilize the retina against the choroid. Inert gas or oil is used to fill the space, until aqueous humor eventually refills the area.

Nursing Management

Positioning of the patient and the level of activity allowed after surgery are prescribed by the surgeon. The head is positioned so that the area repaired is dependent, preventing the pull of gravity from disrupting the surgical site. The designated position for the head also is calculated to position the oil or gas bubble—if one was used—in the best place to apply pressure to the retina. Position the patient according to the physician's orders. IOP is monitored closely for at least 24 hours. Vision does not return immediately because of postoperative swelling and the effects of the dilating drops. Vision improves on a gradual basis over several weeks to months. The eyes may both be patched, or just the operative one may be patched. Eye patches are changed at least once a day (Box 27-1). A shield is worn when napping and at night. Several types of eyedrops may be ordered for postoperative use, as well as an antibiotic ointment. Strict asepsis is observed when instilling eyedrops and ointment.

There usually is some degree of pain after all types of retinal surgery. Acetaminophen with oxycodone or codeine often is prescribed for pain. If the patient is allergic to these medications, extra-strength Tylenol may be sufficient to control the pain.

Flashing lights are common for the first few weeks after retinal surgery. These decrease over 2 to 6 months; if they worsen within several weeks of surgery, the physician should be notified. Light sensitivity is common in both eyes after surgery, and may cause tearing. This gradually lessens over a period of 4 to 6 weeks. Wearing dark sunglasses when outdoors helps eliminate this problem. A moderate amount of discharge from the eye is not unusual; it should be yellowish or pink-tinged. If the amount of discharge increases

Box 27-1 Applying an Eye Patch

- Perform hand hygiene, and cleanse the skin of the patient's forehead and cheek with a skin prep solution or pad.
- Prepare strips of nonallergenic paper or other tape to secure the patch.
- Ask the patient to close both eyes and position the pad over the lid of the eye to be patched.
- Secure the patch by placing strips of tape diagonally over the patch from the cheek to the forehead. Use several strips of tape to ensure adhesiveness.
- After surgery, the shield is used for 2 to 6 weeks, depending on the surgeon's instructions.

FOR A PRESSURE PATCH
- Use two eye patches. Fold the first one in half; place it over the closed lid and then place the other patch on top of the folded one. Apply tape as above.

FOR SLEEPING
- A plastic or metal eye shield may be placed over the eye and secured to further protect the eye. Often, the patch can be left off when the shield is placed for sleeping.

markedly or is accompanied by severe pain, or if discharge has a foul smell or a greenish tinge, infection may be present; notify the surgeon. Cleanse the eyelid with a gauze pad or cotton ball moistened with irrigating solution or tap water. Wipe from the inner to the outer area of the eye. A separate clean pad or cotton ball should be used for each eye.

The patient is allowed to sponge-bathe, brush the teeth, shave, and comb the hair as long as care is taken not to get water in the affected eye (see discussion later in this chapter).

At discharge, the patient is cautioned to avoid heavy lifting, straining at stool, and vigorous activity for several weeks. Eyeglasses are worn during the day for protection, and the eye shield is worn at night after an eye patch is no longer necessary.

Home Care Considerations

Home Care Instructions for Retinal Surgery or Vitrectomy

Instructions will vary if the patient has a gas bubble that was injected intraocularly. Positioning and activity are more restricted in this instance.

ACTIVITY
- Restrict activity according to physician's instructions. Bed rest with bathroom privileges for the first few days is usual. The head may need to be positioned to the left or right most of the time. A head-down or semiprone position to the right or left will be required for the majority of the time if a gas bubble was injected into the eye.
- The following activities are allowed immediately after discharge unless a gas bubble has been injected into the eye as part of the procedure:
  - Watching television from a distance of at least 10 feet.
  - Tub bath or shower, using extreme care not to get soap or water into the eyes. Take care not to fall.
  - Walking outdoors with the guidance of a companion.
  - Reading for brief periods.
  - Gentle shampooing of hair with head tilted backward and care not to get soap or water into the eyes.
  - Riding in a car as a passenger.

EYE CARE
- The operated eye is to be patched at all times and protected by an eye shield or glasses until you are told you may leave the eye uncovered. A patch or shield may still be recommended for use while sleeping. The eye patch is removed only to administer eyedrops or ointment. The eyelid may be cleansed with cotton or gauze moistened with irrigating solution. Each time the patch is changed, check the movement of the eyeballs under the lids. Gently retract the upper lid, and look down as far as possible. Next, look up while retracting the lower lid. This helps break adhesions of the eyeball to the lids.
- The following are expected and should not cause alarm: tearing, a small amount of blood on the eye patch, a scratchy sensation, blurred vision, unusual visual images, a few light flashes, and floaters. Do call the physician if these symptoms *significantly* increase after discharge.
- Have someone else administer the eye medications. Assume a reclining position for eyedrop or eye ointment placement. Pull down the lower lid and, with the patient looking up, place the correct number of drops into the center of the conjunctival sac. Let the lid gently close. The patient should try not to squeeze the eye shut or blink excessively. Wait 3 to 5 minutes between types of eyedrops so that they do not wash each other out and dilute the intended effect. Patch the eye after each set of drops or ointment is administered. If a shield is to be used, it is placed on top of the taped-down eye pad.

COMFORT
- Take a prescribed analgesic or extra-strength acetaminophen to relieve pain. A cool washcloth or ice pack to the forehead may provide comfort. Report pain that grows markedly worse or is accompanied by nausea and vomiting.

PRECAUTIONS
- In case of cough, take cough syrup. Do not try to hold back sneezes. Do not strain at stool; take a stool softener or milk of magnesia if needed to prevent this.

RESTRICTIONS
- Avoid driving a car until visual acuity is 20/40 or better; your physician will tell you when you may resume driving.
- Avoid lifting heavy objects (those over 20 lb) for at least 4 months.
- Refrain from work for 2 to 6 weeks (depending on type of work); your physician will tell you when you may return to work. Light housework that does not require bending over or vigorous scrubbing may be resumed within 1 to 2 weeks depending on the type of surgery performed.
- Avoid vigorous or strenuous activity for 4 months.
- Do not bend with your head down; keep the head upright, and bend at the knees.
- Avoid sports for 3 to 4 months.

Think Critically

How do the signs and symptoms of glaucoma and cataract differ?

RETINOPATHY

Etiology

The two major causes of retinopathy are diabetes mellitus and hypertension. Years of elevated blood pressure cause retinal vasospasm, which damages and narrows the retinal arterioles, thereby decreasing the blood supply to the retina. Contributing factors are excessive use of nicotine and caffeine, and high stress levels.

Pathophysiology

Diabetic patients experience two different forms of retinopathy: proliferative and nonproliferative retinopathy. In the nonproliferative type of retinopathy, microaneurysms develop on the retinal blood vessels. These eventually swell and rupture, causing hemorrhage into the vitreous humor, which interferes with vision. The proliferative form of retinopathy occurs later in the course of diabetes. New blood vessels grow from the existing retinal vessels in a process called *neovascularization.* The new vessels are thinner and rupture more easily, causing hemorrhage. The blood from the hemorrhage causes scarring, which also interferes with vision. High blood pressure creates blockages in retinal blood vessels. Retinal hemorrhages and macular swelling may cause vision impairment.

Signs, Symptoms, and Diagnosis

It is important that diabetic patients have regular, frequent eye examinations, since the early stages of retinopathy present no symptoms. As the retinopathy progresses, there are alterations in vision such as blurring, missing areas in the field of vision, and seeing red or black lines or spots. These signs can be observed on ophthalmologic examination of the retina and by fluorescein angiography. When the macula is involved, there is a loss of vision that may progress to blindness. Retinal detachment may occur as a result of proliferative retinopathy.

Treatment

Tight control of blood glucose levels (100 to 115 mg/dL) is very important to prevent excessive diabetic retinopathy. There is no other known way to halt the process. The microaneurysms and the neovascularized vessels are treated with laser photocoagulation therapy to prevent hemorrhage and the consequent scarring and loss of vision. Vitrectomy also can be done if hemorrhage has caused serious impairment of vision. Hypertension must be kept under good control.

Research is underway to determine whether a deficiency of insulin-like growth factor (IGF)—a hormone that helps maintain nerve function—rather than uncontrolled glucose levels is the cause of diabetic retinopathy. If so, IGF injections may prevent the problem.

Nursing Management

Within 15 years of becoming diabetic, nearly all patients with type 1 diabetes and 80% of patients with type 2 diabetes develop some retinopathy; therefore the nurse can be instrumental in promoting glucose control and regular eye examinations. Nurses must encourage glucose testing in patients who have a family history of diabetes, or who are in a high-risk category, so that the disease may be discovered early before vascular effects have occurred.

 Think Critically

What would you teach your diabetic patient about the prevention of retinopathy? What factors enter into the development of retinopathy?

MACULAR DEGENERATION

Etiology

The macular region of the retina gives us color vision, acute vision, and central vision. Macular degeneration (also called age-related macular degeneration [AMD]) occurs with aging and is the most common cause of visual loss in the elderly. Inflammation may be a factor as the presence of *Chlamydia pneumoniae* has been found in the eye tissue of some people with the wet form of AMD. Although it has been proposed that both statin drug users and aspirin users may have less incidence of macular degeneration, a study has shown that statins have no effect on wet AMD (Maguire et al., 2009). There is a genetic tendency for the disease, and diabetes and hypertension are associated risk factors. Wearing sunglasses regularly when outdoors may help protect against AMD. Certain vitamins, minerals, and antioxidants seem to help prevent or slow AMD.

 Health Promotion

Tobacco and Alcohol and AMD

Teaching people to quit smoking and to abstain from immoderate drinking (four or more alcoholic drinks a day) can decrease the incidence of AMD. Smoking is thought to double the risk of AMD (National Guideline Clearinghouse, 2008). In Britain there is a movement to add the warning about the risk of vision loss to the other warnings on cigarette packages.

 Complementary and Alternative Therapies

Preventing or Slowing Progression of AMD

The antioxidants acetyl-L-carnitine, concentrated omega-3, and coenzyme Q-10 have been shown to improve vision in AMD patients in a recent Italian study (Mayer, 2010). The combination is available in Europe in a supplement called Phototrop. Fish oil, which acts as an anti-inflammatory, may protect the retina from AMD. It contains docosahexaenoic acid that protects photoreceptors (*Science News*, 2010).

A new genetic test performed on saliva, Macula Risk, is available for patients at increased risk of macular degeneration.

Pathophysiology

There are two types of atrophic macular degeneration: dry and wet. Exudative macular degeneration may occur at any age. In the dry form, gradual blockage in the retinal capillaries leads to death of rod and cone photoreceptors in the macula of the retina. This form accounts for 85% to 90% of cases. Dry AMD may progress to wet AMD. In the wet form, abnormal vessels develop in or near the macula. Central vision is affected. The fragile vessel network grows into the subretinal space and may bleed into the macular region, causing central visual impairment. Exudative macular degeneration is caused by a serous detachment of pigment epithelium in the macula. Sudden central vision loss occurs.

Signs and Symptoms

AMD is bilateral and progressive. Early symptoms may be an inability to see the vividness of colors or to see details. Blurred vision, presence of scotomas, or distortion of vision gradually occurs. Objects may appear to be the wrong size or shape, or straight lines may appear crooked or wavy. As central vision deteriorates, there may be a large dark spot or empty place over the center of what is viewed. The patient retains peripheral vision and can walk, dress, cook, and sometimes drive if impairment is minimal, but cannot read when the disorder becomes severe. Exudative MD may occur in only one eye.

Diagnosis

Ophthalmologic examination of the retina and macula is the first step in diagnosis. In dry AMD yellow exudates called drusen are found beneath the retinal pigment epithelium. Drusen represent extracellular debris. In wet AMD fluid and blood are detected by the examination. Patients at risk for macular degeneration, or extension of the problem, are taught to use an Amsler grid (a small card with lines in a grid formation) at home to assess for progression of the disorder (Figure 27-10). If macular degeneration is occurring, the lines appear wavy. Fluorescein angiography or optical coherence tomography shows the specific areas of the retina involved.

Treatment

There is no specific treatment for dry AMD that restores vision, but a novel inhibitor of a protein involved in inflammation that contributes to vision loss is being developed and is in Phase 1 trials. A Phase 3 clinical trial with oral fenretinide to slow or halt the progression of the disease is underway (AMD.org, 2011). For wet AMD, prompt laser treatment to destroy the fragile blood vessels can sometimes be done to prevent further bleeding and visual deterioration. Photodynamic therapy using verteporfin (Visudyne) intravenously, followed by a low-light-level laser that destroys only the cells that absorbed the dye, is another therapy. This therapy destroys abnormal blood vessels, without permanent damage to the photoreceptor cells and the retinal pigment epithelium. Because direct exposure to sunlight or other intense forms of light can activate the dye in

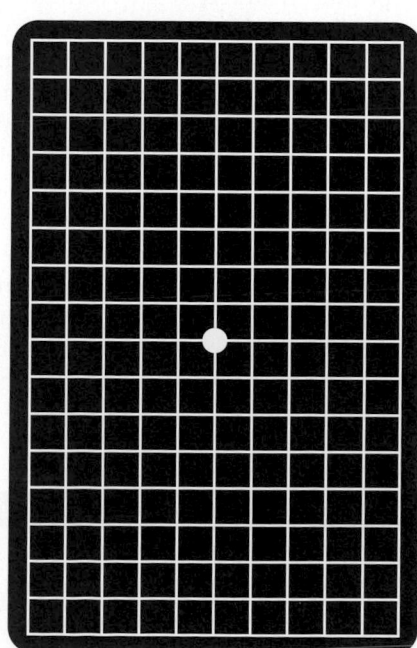

USE ONLY AS INSTRUCTED BY YOUR OPHTHALMOLOGIST

REMINDERS:

• Cover one eye—Hold card directly in front of the uncovered eye

• Look at center spot

• Note any irregularities (e.g., wavy, gray, fuzzy)

• Rotate 90 degrees and repeat

• Test other eye

Contact your ophthalmologist as instructed, if necessary

Name _____

Address _____

_____

Phone _____

The Yannuzzi Card (Modified Amsler Grid)
Copyright © 1981 BMI, A service from The Macula Foundation, Inc.

FIGURE 27-10 Amsler grid used to check for macular degeneration.

the cells, the patient must avoid those forms of light for 5 days, after which the remaining dye will have been fully excreted.

Pegaptanib sodium injection (Macugen) has received Food and Drug Administration (FDA) approval for the treatment of wet AMD. It is injected into the eye, under local anesthesia, once every 6 weeks. During clinical studies, this drug has limited the progression to legal blindness by 50% compared to the controls.

Ranibizumab (Lucentis) has been approved by the FDA for wet AMD, but it is very expensive at $1950 per treatment. Intravitreal injections are necessary monthly with Lucentis. A derivative of bevacizumab (Avastin) has been used "off label" and has shown promise in improving wet macular degeneration. Avastin costs $50 to $75 per dose. Clinical trials are underway. The drug is injected intravenously and is effective within 1 week. Long-term studies are needed to determine if the benefits outweigh the risks. Some patients have experienced a stroke after the treatment. Anecortave acetate (Retaane) is another drug undergoing review by the FDA for the treatment of AMD. It inhibits the abnormal growth of blood vessels in the back of the eye. It is administered onto the outer surface of the back of the eye at 6-month intervals.

A technique under investigation is transplantation of healthy cells of retinal pigment epithelium to replace or enhance degenerating epithelium. It is hoped that transplantation of such cells before vision has greatly deteriorated will slow or eliminate the progression of AMD.

A device called ForeseeHome Monitor is available to monitor vision changes at home for those with dry macular degeneration. Treatment is most effective when changes in vision are detected early.

Nursing Management

Help patients with permanent vision loss learn to use low-vision aids. A referral to a low-vision device specialist and low-vision support group often is needed. Devices are available to illuminate and magnify reading material. Books with large print are easier to read. Learning to turn the head and move the eyeballs to work around the central scotoma may help. A closed-circuit television system that magnifies a printed page on screen can be used for reading or doing crossword puzzles. Telescopic lenses can help for watching movies, attending the theater, reading street signs, and seeing traffic lights. A head-mounted low-vision enhancement system provides both distance and close-up enhancement. Easy-to-read watches with large numerals, television screen magnifiers, and guides that fit over checkbooks to assist with writing on them are some of the less expensive low-vision aids that are available.

NURSING CARE OF THE PATIENT HAVING EYE SURGERY

PREOPERATIVE CARE

Most eye surgery procedures are done on an outpatient basis, unless the patient has other serious disorders such as cardiac dysrhythmias, severe diabetes, or a chronic disability. Therefore a large part of nursing care is directed at discharge teaching for home care. One surgery that is performed as an inpatient procedure is a scleral buckle for retinal detachment (see Retinal Detachment on pp. 605 to 607).

Stool softeners may be started a day or two before surgery to prevent constipation and the Valsalva maneuver postoperatively. The Valsalva maneuver can increase IOP. Some physicians direct the patient to wash the face with surgical soap several times the evening and morning before surgery. The patient may be given instructions on the administration of eyedrops the night before and the morning of surgery.

After admission, the patient is fully oriented to the outpatient surgery unit and given instructions about the layout of the room and area and the ways in which the nurse can be summoned. Side rails are usually necessary to prevent falls, and the patient should be cautioned against getting up without assistance. Preoperative eyedrops and medications are instilled by the nurses in the outpatient surgery center the morning of surgery. Drugs must be given with extreme care and accuracy, especially if only one eye is affected. **Be sure that the medication is applied to the correct eye.**

Preoperative dilating (*mydriatic*) eyedrops often are administered every 5 minutes for six doses. Other eyedrops may be administered in between these doses. An IV infusion is started shortly before surgery.

Because the great majority of patients undergoing eye operations are elderly and therefore are most likely to be suffering from some additional chronic disease, the nurse must remember to apply the principles of geriatric nursing in administering care. Fear, anxiety over surgery, and confusion about the expected results of the surgery are all factors to be considered when preparing the patient for the operation. Instructions and information should be given both verbally and in writing. Measures to ensure patient safety are very important both preoperatively and postoperatively since vision is impaired.

 Safety Alert

Prevent Falls from Impaired Vision

The elderly person who has an eye patched, has low vision, and is in a strange environment is subject to falls. The patient may need to be reoriented to place, time, and surroundings frequently to decrease confusion and agitation.

POSTOPERATIVE CARE

In caring for a patient undergoing any type of eye surgery, the key word is *gentleness*. The patient's head should not be jarred when transferring from the operating table or stretcher to the bed. Remember to speak before touching a patient who is blind or who is wearing bandages over the eyes.

Patients are usually kept in the recovery area of the outpatient surgery department for 2 to 3 hours postoperatively. Nausea and subsequent vomiting can wreak havoc with delicate suture lines in the eye. **If the patient becomes nauseated, antiemetic medication should be administered immediately and all food and liquids withheld.**

An eye patch is often placed over the eye that was operated on (Figure 27-11). If it is necessary to restrict movement of the eyes, both eyes are patched.

Instructions regarding postoperative medications and how they are to be instilled are given before discharge (Figure 27-12). Different types of eyedrop medications come with color-coded tops for easy identification. Eyedrop bottles also can be "labeled" by wrapping one, two, or three rubber bands around them so that the vision-impaired patient can differentiate one type of drop from another.

FIGURE 27-11 Patient with eye patch to protect surgical site and prevent eye movement. The head is kept elevated in the immediate postoperative period.

FIGURE 27-12 Instilling eyedrops.

Should the patient need to stay in the hospital because of other problems, the nurse must be thoroughly familiar with his individual care needs. It should be known whether the patient can be turned on one or both sides or must remain flat on the back, whether pillows are allowed under the head, and how high the head of the bed may be raised. For certain types of retinal surgery, the head may need to be raised and positioned toward a particular side. If a gas bubble has been injected intraocularly, the patient is positioned prone or supine with the head toward one side or the other, according to orders. If the patient is allowed out of bed, care must be taken not to jar the head or move too suddenly.

Sexual activity can usually be resumed in 1 to 8 weeks postoperatively, depending on the procedure performed. The surgeon will explain this to the patient. Make certain that the patient understands the time of the next appointment with the ophthalmologist. The patient and family should be encouraged to follow the physician's directions faithfully during the healing period at home so that nothing will jeopardize the success of the surgery.

Discharge planning for the patient having surgery from the outpatient department or the hospital is of utmost importance. Refer to Home Care Considerations on p. 607 for home care of the patient following retinal surgery or vitrectomy.

COMMUNITY CARE

RESOURCES FOR THE VISION IMPAIRED

Loss of vision need not be devastating for a person if support and encouragement are given for coping with the impairment. There are resources to help the visually impaired person learn to care for himself, find employment, and enjoy educational and recreational activities. Many colleges provide special funds to enable blind students to hire readers and tape recorders to help them with their studies.

Both home care nurses and those working in long-term care should be alert to signs of progressing macular degeneration. The Amsler grid can assist in identifying this problem. Patients with known eye disorders should be periodically assessed to see how much vision has deteriorated and how much the patient's ability to perform activities of daily living and partake in usual hobbies is affected. Nurses should be instrumental in helping patients obtain low-vision aids.

All nurses should encourage the donation of corneas at death. Signing a donor card for organ harvest should be a consideration for all, as well as indicating "tissue donor" on the driver's license. The nurse may be the person to approach the terminal patient or the family about the possibility of donating corneas after death and giving the gift of sight to another. The

Library of Congress in Washington, D.C., lends records and recording machines without charge to the blind and maintains a wide selection of recordings. Recordings of required textbooks may be obtained free of charge from Recording for the Blind and Dyslexic (see Online Resources on p. 618).

COMMON DISORDERS OF THE EAR

EXTERNAL OTITIS

Etiology and Pathophysiology

Infection of the external ear is common and often occurs in the ears of swimmers. It is caused by either bacterial or fungal pathogens, with staphylococci being the most frequent cause. Other infections of the skin may affect the external ear (see Chapter 43). A moist environment, or disruption of the skin from trauma, provides a place for pathogens to grow.

Signs and Symptoms

Pain occurs with the infection. An early sign may be pulling at the pinna or itching in the canal. If swelling occurs in the ear canal, hearing may be impaired as sound waves cannot reach the tympanic membrane.

Diagnosis, Treatment, and Nursing Management

Redness is evident on otoscopic examination, and there may be drainage. A culture of the drainage may be performed. Antibiotic or fungal eardrops and ointments are the usual treatment. A severe infection may require oral antibiotics as well. Teaching patients to use drops of an alcohol solution in the ears after drying them helps to prevent external otitis. A mild analgesic may help decrease the discomfort during healing.

IMPACTED CERUMEN AND FOREIGN BODIES

Normally the ear canal is self-cleaning, but in certain individuals cerumen may become impacted. Foreign objects such as insects or organic matter may obstruct the canal. A feeling of fullness in the ear combined with a hearing loss can indicate that obstruction has blocked the canal, preventing sound waves from reaching the tympanic membrane. If otoscopic examination reveals hardened cerumen blocking the canal, irrigation of the canal is performed to remove it.

> **Elder Care Points**
>
> With age, the auditory canal narrows and the hairs become coarser and stiffer. The cerumen glands atrophy, causing cerumen to be drier. This combination may result in impaction of cerumen that causes a conductive hearing loss and tinnitus. Elders with this problem should be taught to use cerumen softening drops and an ear syringe to wash out the cerumen periodically. Those who are unable to cleanse the ears themselves should have regular ear checks by their health care provider.

> **Clinical Cues**
>
> When irrigating an ear canal, the water should be tepid. Cold water and too much irrigation pressure can cause dizziness and nausea as well as pain. Check the temperature of the water each time the syringe or irrigation container is refilled. Drape the patient so that the clothing does not become wet.

OTITIS MEDIA

Etiology

This condition is an inflammation of the middle ear caused by various types of bacteria or viruses. Although it is mostly seen in infants and young children, it does occur in adults. It results in the accumulation of fluid behind the eardrum and some temporary impairment of hearing.

Pathophysiology

The inflammation of otitis media usually follows an upper respiratory tract infection or trauma to the ear. It is usually viral in origin, but may be complicated by bacteria. Obstruction of the eustachian tube usually precedes the disorder and is caused by an upper respiratory infection or allergy. Middle ear inflammation occurs when the eustachian tube that usually drains that area becomes blocked. The obstruction changes the pressure within the middle ear. The inflammation may provide an environment for *Streptococcus pneumoniae, Haemophilus influenzae, Moraxella catarrhalis, Streptococcus pyogenes,* or other pathogens to invade the tissue.

When the infection is sudden in onset and of short duration, it is termed *acute otitis media.* The eardrum is retracted inward because of negative pressure due to a closed eustachian tube. The pain can be severe. When the infection is repeated, often causing perforation of the eardrum and drainage, it is called *chronic otitis media.*

Otitis media sometimes is accompanied by an allergy and may be aggravated by enlarged adenoids. Fluid may build up in the middle ear. This disorder is called *serous otitis media.*

Signs, Symptoms, and Diagnosis

Symptoms may be mild and may consist only of a feeling of fullness in the ear and evidence of impaired hearing and tinnitus. There may be pain in the infected ear, headache, fever, and pulling on the ear. If the fluid remains over an extended time, it causes tympanic membrane contraction and can permanently impair its movement.

Depending on the stage of infection, otoscopic examination may show retraction of the eardrum, redness and bulging, or pus behind the eardrum. Perforation may occur with drainage of the pus. This type is termed *suppurative otitis media.*

Treatment

There is great controversy about using antimicrobials for otitis media because so many strains of pathogens are becoming antimicrobial resistant. If there is otitis media with fluid behind the eardrum, and no acute systemic or local evidence of severe infection, antimicrobials are withheld. The condition is treated conservatively with antihistamines and decongestants.

For repeated episodes of otitis with fluid, or when the fluid will not resorb, a *myringotomy* (incision into the eardrum) is done, and a ventilating tube is inserted to drain the excess fluid in the middle ear and to equalize pressure while the eustachian tube is blocked. The tympanic membrane is anesthetized locally. The procedure is painless and takes about 15 minutes. The incision heals within 24 to 72 hours unless a tube is placed in the opening. Tubes remain in place for 6 to 18 months before they are naturally expelled. The hole then heals. If allergy is thought to be responsible for the fluid buildup, antihistamines are prescribed.

Acute otitis media occurs when pus-producing bacteria infect the middle ear. Treatment consists of systemic therapy with antibiotics for at least 5 to 7 days, topical therapy with eardrops, and oral analgesics to reduce pain and fever. With repeated episodes, tympanoplasty to repair a ruptured eardrum and damaged ossicles, and, sometimes, mastoidectomy may be needed to eliminate all sources of infection and prevent further degeneration of bone.

Nursing Management

Keeping the patient comfortable at home, encouraging compliance with the medication regimen, and requesting return for an examination when medication is finished are usual nursing actions. Show a family member how to instill eardrops properly (see Box 26-6). Temperature should be taken each day during the course of acute otitis media to track improvement.

Infections in the middle ear always have the potential for spreading to the meninges and causing meningitis, or to the mastoid bone, causing mastoiditis. With the advent of antibiotics, surgery to scrape and clean infected mastoid bone is performed far less frequently than it was previously. Although otitis media is a fairly common occurrence, it should always be treated immediately.

LABYRINTHITIS

Etiology and Pathophysiology

Labyrinthitis is an inflammation involving the vestibular portion of the labyrinth in the inner ear. It most commonly occurs from a viral respiratory infection, but can be a complication of bacterial meningitis or chronic otitis media.

Signs, Symptoms, and Diagnosis

The symptoms include sensorineural hearing loss in the affected ear, tinnitus, severe dizziness with nausea and vomiting, and nystagmus (abnormal jerking movements of the eyes). If the disorder is viral, there usually is no tinnitus and resolution occurs within 7 to 10 days. Diagnosis is made from the symptoms and by ruling out tumor or other disease.

Treatment and Nursing Management

Treatment is aimed at removing the source of infection and controlling symptoms. Meclizine (Antivert, Bonine) or another antihistamine that assists in decreasing vertigo and its associated nausea and vomiting is used. Scopolamine patches behind the ear can be used after the acute phase to control vertigo. Antibiotics may be given in massive doses to control a bacterial infection.

 Clinical Cues

Remind the patient to wash his hands again after applying the scopolamine patch. If the eye is touched after touching the patch, severe eye irritation may occur.

Initially the patient is kept on bed rest to prevent falls and injury. The family is cautioned not to let the patient get out of bed without assistance. Nursing management consists of safety measures to prevent falling and instructions about the medications. Attention to hydration is important if the patient is nauseated to the point of repeated vomiting.

MÉNIÈRE'S DISEASE (MÉNIÈRE'S SYNDROME)

Etiology and Pathophysiology

The exact cause is unknown, but Ménière's disease occurs most often in people who have had chronic ear disorders and allergic symptoms involving the upper respiratory tract. There is a genetic link, and about 50% of those with the disorder have family members who are also afflicted.

An increase of endolymph within the spaces of the labyrinth, with swelling and congestion of the mucous membranes of the cochlea, occurs. Resultant pressure in the labyrinth of the inner ear results in permanent damage to both the cochlear and vestibular structures. The disorder is usually unilateral. Long-term stress may be a factor.

Signs, Symptoms, and Diagnosis

The symptoms include attacks of dizziness, ringing in the ear (tinnitus), and unilateral sensorineural hearing loss. Poor balance makes walking difficult or impossible. **Any sudden movement of the head or eyes during an attack usually produces severe nausea and vomiting.** Diagnosing Ménière's disease usually is not difficult, but because these symptoms could indicate a tumor of the auditory mechanism, a *caloric test* (electro-nystagmogram [ENG]) may be performed, which involves instilling very warm or cold fluid into the auditory canal. A patient with Ménière's disease will experience a severe attack; a normal person will complain of only slight dizziness. A person with a tumor of the auditory mechanism will have no reaction at all. Tympanometry and audiometry are ordered, and a brainstem-evoked response (BSER) test is performed to rule out an acoustic neuroma or problem in the brain.

 Think Critically

How would you check for nystagmus when assessing a patient who has vertigo?

Treatment

Treatment of Ménière's disease focuses on relieving symptoms; there is no cure for this condition, although the disorder does disappear spontaneously in some cases. For an acute attack with disabling vertigo, atropine may be given subcutaneously, followed by diazepam (Valium), dimenhydrinate (Dramamine), meclizine (Antivert), or other drugs for motion sickness. To control edema and reduce pressure in the inner ear, the patient may be placed on a low-sodium diet, his fluid intake may be restricted, and diuretics may be ordered. Anticholinergic drugs, such as propantheline (Pro-Banthine) or glycopyrrolate (Robinul), may be given to help control the vertigo and nausea. To improve circulation in the ear, papaverine (Vasospan) or niacin may be prescribed. Some patients find that *Ginkgo biloba,* which acts as a vasodilator, helps. The patient is kept quiet and in bed to avoid aggravating his symptoms. He may be very irritable and withdrawn and may refuse to eat or drink because of fear of vomiting. Care should be taken to avoid increasing his irritation by jarring the bed, turning on bright overhead lights, or making loud noises.

If attacks continue and are very severe despite medical treatment, the endolymph sac from the inner ear can be removed with microsurgical techniques. When hearing loss is total on the affected side, surgical destruction of the eighth cranial nerve may be done to resolve the symptoms. Although this produces permanent deafness in the affected ear, the severe attacks are eliminated. In most persistent cases of Ménière's disease, the patient will eventually suffer a serious or even total loss of hearing regardless of the treatment used.

For those with dizziness and unsteadiness who do not wish to undergo surgery, vestibular rehabilitation therapy may decrease the dizziness and balance problems resulting from inner ear damage (Hain et al., 2011). The Meniett low-intensity alternating-pressure generator that is self-administered at home displaces fluid from the inner ear and relieves or prevents symptoms (Benson, 2009).

 Think Critically

What would you teach the patient with Ménière's disease about a low-sodium diet?

Nursing Management

If the patient uses nicotine products, encourage him to quit, as nicotine constricts blood vessels and will decrease inner ear circulation as well. If allergy seems to be a factor in the onset of attacks, encourage consultation with an allergist to obtain control of allergens. Decreasing stress is a helpful intervention when there has been a pattern of attacks after particularly stressful times in the patient's life.

ACOUSTIC NEUROMA

An acoustic neuroma is a rare benign tumor on the eighth cranial nerve and is usually unilateral. It occurs in 0.7 to 1.0 per 100,000 people. Symptoms are gradual hearing loss and tinnitus. This tumor is usually curable with surgery or stereotactic (Gamma Knife, CyberKnife) radiotherapy. If untreated it causes deafness. Treatment is surgical and nursing care is the much the same as for other intracranial surgeries, using measures to decrease intracranial pressure.

OTOSCLEROSIS AND HEARING LOSS

Etiology and Pathophysiology

Otosclerosis is a hereditary degeneration of bone in the inner ear. It occurs twice as often in females and begins in the late teens or early 20s. It may become worse during pregnancy. Hearing is decreased if there has been damage to the tympanic membrane (eardrum) from trauma or infection.

The sense of hearing depends in part on the vibration of very small bones of the inner ear. The *stapes,* or stirrup, is particularly important, because it conducts sound waves to the fluid in the semicircular canals in the inner ear. Otosclerosis is a disease process that causes the formation of excess bone. This causes the footplate of the stapes to be fixed so that it no longer vibrates to transmit sound waves received via the tympanic membrane.

Signs, Symptoms, and Diagnosis

The patient often complains of difficulty hearing the voices of others, yet his own voice sounds unusually loud. In response to this, he may lower his voice to the point that he can scarcely be heard by others. Diagnosis is by otoscopic examination, Rinne and Weber's tests, and audiogram.

Treatment

The hearing loss of otosclerosis can sometimes be corrected by using a hearing aid. Care for a hearing aid is presented in Box 26-5. Microsurgical intervention can restore air-conductive hearing by providing a new movable pathway for the sound waves. During the operation, called a *stapedectomy*, the stapes is removed and is replaced with a prosthetic device. This device may be a steel wire and fat implant, a wire and a segment of vein, or a vein graft with polyethylene tubing. In any case, the prosthesis is attached to one end of the *incus* (anvil of the middle ear) so that sound can be transmitted to the inner ear. The surgical procedure is extremely delicate and would not be possible without the dissecting binocular microscope and other modern surgical instruments that allow visualization and manipulation of the very small structures of the middle ear. Outpatient surgery with local anesthesia is usual. Hearing improvement may not occur for about 6 weeks.

Tympanoplasty reconstructs the middle ear and improves conductive hearing loss. Tympanoplasty involves the surgical reconstruction of the tympanic membrane and ossicles to restore middle-ear function. There are several types of procedures ranging from simple closing of a tympanic membrane perforation to extensive repair of the middle-ear structures. The procedure is performed with an operating microscope via the external auditory canal or through a postauricular incision. Although performed as an outpatient procedure, tympanoplasty requires general anesthesia.

Nursing Management

Postoperative care involves keeping the patient quiet and flat in bed for at least 12 hours. The head is turned so that the affected ear is uppermost. When the patient is allowed to move about, he must be warned that dizziness is likely to occur, especially if he turns his head suddenly. Position changes should be accomplished slowly. Coughing and sneezing should be avoided, or if unavoidable, should be accomplished with the mouth open to decrease pressure in the ear (Nursing Care Plan 27-2).

NURSING CARE OF THE PATIENT HAVING EAR SURGERY

Most ear surgeries are performed as outpatient procedures. Nursing care is focused on the immediate preoperative and recovery periods and on instructions for home care.

PREOPERATIVE CARE

Nursing care of the patient during the preoperative period is rather routine, except for the administration of eardrops or other special medications. Physical preparation for ear surgery may or may not involve removing some of the hair from the scalp. Male patients

---

⭐ Nursing Care Plan 27-2 | Care of the Patient Having a Tympanoplasty

Scenario

Miss Cook, age 38, is a high school teacher who has had progressive hearing impairment as a result of recurrent otitis media of the right ear. She is admitted to outpatient surgery for tympanoplasty. During her initial assessment, the nurse found Miss Cook to be well informed about the nature of her disorder but somewhat anxious about the outcome of surgery. Her physical health status is good; her only previous hospitalization was for an appendectomy when she was 19 years old. Care is for the postoperative period.

Problem/Nursing Diagnosis
*Possible disruption of graft/*Risk for injury related to graft displacement.

Supporting Assessment Data
Objective: Tympanoplasty.

Goals/Expected Outcomes	Nursing Interventions	Selected Rationale	Evaluation
Graft will be successful as evidenced by restored hearing in affected ear.	Position patient side-lying on nonoperative side.	Prevents collection of fluid behind graft and reduces pressure.	Positioned on nonoperative side or back with HOB raised 30 degrees.
	Reinforce preoperative instructions to remain in bed for 4 hr, avoid sudden movements, blowing nose, or sneezing.	These measures help prevent graft disruption.	Compliant with instructions. Continue plan.
	Check vital signs, for evidence of infection, bid.	Elevation in temperature may indicate beginning infection.	Temperature within normal range. No sign of infection.
	Give analgesic/sedative as ordered.	Analgesic/sedative will promote rest.	Patient resting comfortably; pain at 2/10.
	Provide quiet environment.		

bid, twice daily; *HOB*, head of bed.

Continued

★ Nursing Care Plan 27-2   **Care of the Patient Having a Tympanoplasty—cont'd**

Problem/Nursing Diagnosis
May experience vertigo and dizziness/Risk for activity intolerance related to vertigo and instability.

Supporting Assessment Data
Subjective: After tympanoplasty, states she is very dizzy and nauseated.

Goals/Expected Outcomes	Nursing Interventions	Selected Rationale	Evaluation
Falls and head trauma will be avoided.	Up with assistance only. Repeat explanation for safety precautions.	Helps to prevent falls.	Asking for assistance when needs to get up.
	Caution patient to change positions and turn her head very slowly.	Abrupt changes in position are likely to cause vertigo and nausea.	Compliant with instructions.
	Provide well-lighted room when ambulating.	Good lighting prevents tripping over obstacles when ambulating.	Room lighting is adequate.
	Administer medication prescribed for vertigo.	Medication can help control vertigo.	Medication for vertigo is effective.

Problem/Nursing Diagnosis
Lack of knowledge about postoperative care/Deficient knowledge regarding postoperative care.

Supporting Assessment Data
Subjective: Asks about restrictions and self-care.
Objective: Cannot verbalize knowledge of medications.

Goals/Expected Outcomes	Nursing Interventions	Selected Rationale	Evaluation
Patient will verbalize knowledge of home self-care before discharge.	Instruct to avoid loud noises and pressure changes for 6 mo, especially avoiding flying and diving.	Loud noise and pressure changes can disrupt the graft.	Instructions gone over verbally and printed instructions left with patient.
	Stress importance of not blowing her nose for at least 1 wk, to avoid an upper respiratory infection; if at all possible, protect her ear against cold; and refrain from any activity that might provoke dizziness or disturb the graft (e.g., straining at stool, bending, and heavy lifting).	Preventing pressure changes helps protect the integrity of the graft.	Provided correct feedback on postoperative precautions.
Patient will demonstrate dressing change correctly before discharge.	Teach patient how to change dressing on the external ear.	Will prepare patient for self-care.	Patient has not changed bandage as yet. Continue plan.
	Reiterate importance of taking full course of prescribed antibiotic and reporting to surgeon at scheduled times.	Taking the full course of antibiotics correctly will help prevent infection.	Acknowledges importance of taking antibiotics as directed. Reassurance given.
	Reassure patient that because of swelling of tissues and presence of surgical pack, it may be several weeks before she can fully evaluate effectiveness of the surgery.	Inflammation at the surgical site will cause swelling that interferes with hearing initially.	States she understands that it may be a while before hearing is as good as it will get.

Critical Thinking Questions
1. Why can dizziness and vertigo occur after a tympanoplasty?
2. What level of noise would be considered "too loud"?

FIGURE 27-13 An ear surgery dressing. The patient is positioned with the head elevated or side-lying on the unaffected side.

should be clean shaven the morning of surgery. The external ear and surrounding skin should be thoroughly cleansed, preferably with a surgical soap. Female patients with long hair should have it braided or pinned back securely so that it will not become soiled by drainage from the ear or serve as a source of infection at the operative site.

POSTOPERATIVE CARE

The patient will often return from major ear surgery with an ear dressing (Figure 27-13). Positioning of the patient after ear surgery depends on specific instructions from the physician. Often the patient is placed flat in bed, and his head is supported so that he does not turn it from side to side. In addition to noting the vital signs, the nurse should watch for signs of injury to the facial nerve, including inability of the patient to close his eyes, wrinkle his forehead, or pucker his lips. The patient and family are advised to report such symptoms to the surgeon. If they appear later than 12 hours after surgery, they may be due to edema, and the physician may order a loosening of the dressings.

Safety precautions, such as raising side rails, should be taken to avoid injury due to dizziness and loss of balance during the recovery period. Balance is temporarily affected as a result of disturbance to the mechanism that maintains equilibrium. When the patient is allowed to get up and move about, assistance should be provided to prevent falls. The patient should arise slowly to a sitting position and sit for a few minutes. Then the patient stands while holding on to something or being supported by another. Dizziness must pass before the patient attempts walking.

Because the ear is so near the brain, a special effort must be made to avoid contamination of the surgical site. Dressings may be reinforced to keep them dry, but excessive drainage must be reported to the surgeon.

The patient should be instructed beforehand about what is to be expected from the surgery. Hearing is usually slightly impaired immediately after surgery because of edema or bandages, but is expected to improve in time.

🏠 Home Care Considerations

Instructions After Ear Surgery

The following instructions are given to the patient after ear surgery at the time of discharge:

- Sneezing, coughing, and nose blowing are all ways in which the operative site may be disturbed. If necessary, blow the nose gently one side at a time. Cough or sneeze with the mouth open. Continue this for 1 week after surgery.
- Do not drink through a straw for 2 to 3 weeks. Avoid drinking directly from the mouth of a plastic bottle as negative pressure occurs if the bottle opening is sealed.
- Limit physical activity for 1 week after surgery. Refrain from exercising and sports for 3 weeks or until the surgeon discharges you.
- Avoid heavy lifting for 3 weeks. Avoid bending over from the waist or moving the head rapidly for 3 weeks.
- Keep the ear dry for 4 to 6 weeks after surgery by placing a cotton ball covered with petroleum jelly (such as Vaseline) in the ear canal; refrain from shampooing hair with water for 1 week after surgery.
- After the initial dressing is removed, keep a cotton ball in the ear to protect it; change the cotton ball daily.
- Avoid people with colds.
- Do not fly until the surgeon allows it.
- Wear ear protectors when exposed to a loud environment.
- A return to work is usual after 3 to 7 days; strenuous work may not be resumed for 3 weeks.

Note: The surgeon will explain the specific time limitations for each activity based on the type of surgery.

Myringotomy (incision of the eardrum) with placement of tubes is a lesser outpatient procedure and the only dressing may be a cotton ball in the ear. There is less occurrence of dizziness or nausea with this surgery.

COMMUNITY CARE

Cautioning people about the dangers of listening to loud music through earpieces can help curb hearing loss. Teaching adults to seek medical attention for symptoms of otitis media quickly prevents damage to the tympanic membrane and preserves hearing ability.

A hearing assessment should be part of any thorough health assessment. Encouraging those who have any difficulty with hearing to have a thorough evaluation and to try a hearing aid, if the need is indicated, could help improve the quality of their lives. Nurses in home and long-term care settings should frequently assess the function of the patient's hearing aid.

Various accommodations can be found to help the hearing impaired. There are even assistance dogs to help keep the hearing-impaired person safe both in the home and on the streets.

Get Ready for the NCLEX® Examination!

Key Points

- A problem with refraction is the most common eye disorder.
- Cataracts cause a blurring or loss of vision and usually occur slowly.
- Cataract surgery with lens implant usually restores vision.
- The increase in intraocular pressure, unless treated, will eventually cause blindness.
- Glaucoma medication most often must be used for the rest of the patient's life.
- Acute narrow-angle glaucoma is a medical emergency.
- Retinal detachment symptoms are flashing colored lights followed by the appearance of "floaters."
- Unless treated quickly and successfully, retinal detachment causes vision loss.
- Positioning and restriction of amount of movement are crucial after eye surgery.
- Retinopathy is a disorder that occurs most frequently with diabetes or hypertension.
- Tight glucose control helps prevent diabetic retinopathy.
- Retinopathy is frequently treated by laser.
- Keratoplasty may be performed for damaged corneas.
- Macular degeneration is a frequent problem in the elderly, but can occur at an earlier age.
- There is presently no cure for macular degeneration, but new drugs and treatments may be able to slow it or reverse some of the vision loss.
- Eye trauma should be treated by a health care provider promptly.
- Keep the eye surgery patient quiet and treat nausea immediately.
- Otitis media is a common malady and may be induced by allergy or upper respiratory infection.
- Impacted cerumen or foreign bodies in the ear interfere with hearing.
- Otosclerosis is generally hereditary.
- Tympanoplasty may be performed for otosclerosis or for tympanic membrane dysfunction.
- Labyrinthitis and Ménière's disease cause vertigo and tinnitus.

Additional Learning Resources

SG Go to your Study Guide for additional learning activities to help you master this chapter content.

evolve Go to your Evolve website (http://evolve.elsevier.com/deWit/medsurg) for the following FREE learning resources:
- Animations, audio, and video
- Answers and rationales for questions and activities
- Concept Map Creator
- Glossary with pronunciations in English and Spanish
- Interactive Review Questions and Exercises and more!

 Online Resources
- American Foundation for the Blind, www.afb.org
- American Printing House for the Blind, www.aph.org
- American Tinnitus Association, www.ata.org
- Better Hearing Institute, www.betterhearing.org
- The Center for the Partially Sighted, http://low-vision.org
- Helen Keller International, www.hki.org
- Hearing Loss Association of America, www.hearingloss.org
- Lighthouse International, http://lighthouse.org
- Macular Degeneration Foundation, www.eyesight.org
- National Eye Institute, www.nei.nih.gov
- National Library Service for the Blind and Physically Handicapped (NLS), www.loc.gov/nts
- Recording for the Blind & Dyslexic, www.rfbd.org

Review Questions for the NCLEX® Examination

1. A male patient was informed that he would need to wear a pair of corrective lenses for astigmatism. When asked about the condition, the patient demonstrates understanding when he states that:
   1. "Astigmatism is hardening of the ciliary muscles."
   2. "Astigmatism is an irregular curvature of the cornea."
   3. "Astigmatism enables focusing of light in front of the retina."
   4. "Astigmatism is an increased opacity of the lens."

2. Which instruction must be included in the discharge teaching of a patient who has undergone corneal transplant?
   1. Increase physical activity.
   2. Wear an eye shield when in close contact with children or pets.
   3. Remove pressure dressing as needed.
   4. Lie only on the operative side.

3. A woman complains of eye itching, tearing, halos around lights, and decreased central vision. Which symptom most clearly relates to macular degeneration?
   1. Eye itching
   2. Tearing
   3. Halos around lights
   4. Decreased central vision

4. An elderly patient is admitted for cataract extraction. Which sign or symptom is associated with this condition?
   1. Increased tearing
   2. Increasing farsightedness
   3. Increasing complaints about glare
   4. Bluish discolorations

5. _____ is a condition common in diabetic patients that causes impairment of vision and if not controlled leads to blindness.

6. Following eye surgery, the patient is instructed to avoid movements that increase the venous pressure in the head, neck, and eyes. Which movement(s) increase(s) venous pressure? *(Select all that apply.)*

   1. Straining
   2. Bending over
   3. Keeping the head up
   4. Sudden head movements
   5. Strenuous exercises

7. Before eye surgery, the patient is instructed to take stool softeners. When asked about the rationale for taking the stool softener, the nurse appropriately responds:

   1. "The medication reduces the possibility of straining at stool postoperatively."
   2. "The medication prevents constipation caused by anesthetic agents."
   3. "The medication cleanses the gastrointestinal tract."
   4. "The medication enhances surgical recovery."

8. Older adults are more prone to conductive hearing loss and tinnitus because of:

   1. hypertrophy of the cerumen glands.
   2. hardened cerumen.
   3. widening of the auditory canal.
   4. hair loss in the auditory canal.

9. The nurse emphasizes safety precautions to a 60-year-old Hispanic female patient with Ménière's disease. An appropriate nursing approach would be to:

   1. use first name when addressing the patient.
   2. include family members in instructions.
   3. address decision making to the patient.
   4. set specific schedule for providing instructions.

10. Which instruction(s) would be appropriate postoperative teaching for a patient who has had ear surgery? *(Select all that apply.)*

    1. Cough or sneeze with the mouth open.
    2. Resume routine exercises.
    3. Avoid bending or heavy lifting.
    4. Keep ear dry by plugging with cotton covered with petroleum jelly.
    5. Drink with a straw.

Critical Thinking Activities

Scenario A

Mr. Lavant, age 52, and his wife, who has diabetes, have heard about a glaucoma screening clinic being held in their community. They are interested in attending the clinic but are very apprehensive about the kind of tests that will be done. They ask you about the tests and whether you think they should go to the screening clinic when they have no symptoms of glaucoma or any other eye disease.

1. How would you explain a test with a tonometer?

2. How would you explain glaucoma in terms Mr. and Mrs. Lavant could understand?

3. Who are among the people at high risk for glaucoma?

4. What is the usual treatment for chronic, open-angle glaucoma?

Scenario B

Mr. Wilson, age 78, is scheduled for a right cataract extraction and intraocular lens implant. He has bilateral cataracts that have made him legally blind for years. He did not consult a physician until recently, because he had always heard that cataracts had to be "ripe" before they could be treated, and he felt he could not afford frequent trips to a physician when nothing could be done for his condition. Mr. Wilson enters the outpatient surgery area, and you are assigned as his nurse.

1. How would you approach and orient Mr. Wilson to his surroundings?

2. What would you tell Mr. Wilson about the preoperative routine and medications at this time?

3. What nursing diagnoses would be appropriate for Mr. Wilson at this time?

4. What are the advantages of intraocular lens implants over cataract glasses and/or contact lenses?

Scenario C

Mr. Thompson is suffering from a severe attack of Ménière's disease and vertigo. He is severely nauseated, and his vertigo prevents him from getting out of bed. The physician wants to rule out the possibility of tumor as a cause of Mr. Thompson's vertigo, so he is scheduled for an electronystagmogram (ENG) with a caloric test and a magnetic resonance imaging (MRI) scan.

1. What nursing actions would be appropriate for him?

2. How would you explain this disorder to Mr. Thompson?

3. How would you explain these tests to Mr. Thompson?

chapter

28

The Gastrointestinal System

℮volve

http://evolve.elsevier.com/deWit/medsurg

Objectives

Theory

1. Analyze major causative factors in the development of disorders of the gastrointestinal system.
2. Summarize measures to prevent development of disorders of the gastrointestinal system.
3. List nursing responsibilities in the pretest and post-test care of patients undergoing diagnostic tests for disorders of the gastrointestinal system.
4. Describe the assessment of a patient with a possible gastrointestinal disorder.
5. Evaluate the care of the patient who is having a liver biopsy.

Clinical Practice

1. Perform an assessment of gastrointestinal status.
2. Provide pretest and post-test care of patients undergoing tests of the liver, gallbladder, and pancreas.
3. Evaluate the outcomes of care for a patient who is experiencing diarrhea.
4. Teach a patient strategies to alleviate constipation.

Key Terms

absorption (ăb-sŏrp-shŭn, p. 623)
adhesions (ăd-HĒ-shŭnz, p. 623)
anabolism (ă-NĂB-ŏ-lĭzm, p. 623)
anorexia (ăn-ŏ-RĔK-sē-ă, p. 633)
ascites (ă-SĪ-tēz, p. 631)
catabolism (kă-TĂB-ō-lĭzm, p. 623)

chyme (KĪM, p. 621)
flatus (FLĀ-tŭs, p. 635)
mastication (măs-tĭ-KĀ-shŭn, p. 620)
metabolism (mĕ-TĂ-bō-lĭzm, p. 623)
pancreatitis (păn-krē-Ă-TĪ-tĭs, p. 624)
peristalsis (pĕr-ēs-TĂL-sĭs, p. 623)

OVERVIEW OF ANATOMY AND PHYSIOLOGY OF THE GASTROINTESTINAL SYSTEM

WHAT ARE THE ORGANS AND STRUCTURES OF THE GASTROINTESTINAL SYSTEM?

- Organs of the gastrointestinal (GI) system are the mouth, pharynx, esophagus, stomach, small intestine, large intestine, rectum, and anus (Figure 28-1).
- The accessory organs are the liver, gallbladder, and pancreas (Figure 28-2).
- The gastroesophageal sphincter (cardiac sphincter) controls the opening from the esophagus into the stomach; it prevents reflux from the stomach into the esophagus.
- The stomach lies in the upper left portion of the abdominal cavity (see Figure 28-1).
- The pyloric sphincter controls release of food substances into the small intestine (Figure 28-3).
- The small intestine is divided into the duodenum, jejunum, and ileum and is about 6 m long.
- The ileocecal valve controls the progress of substances into the large intestine.

- The large intestine is divided into the cecum, colon, rectum, and anal canal; the colon is about 1.5 m long.
- The colon has four portions: the ascending, transverse, descending, and sigmoid colon.
- The appendix is attached to the cecum and has no known function in the digestive process.
- The walls of the digestive tract have four layers: mucosa, submucosa, muscular layer, and a serous layer called serosa.
- The peritoneum is a serous sac that lines the abdominal cavity and encloses the intestines, stomach, liver, and spleen and partially encloses the uterus and uterine tubes.

WHAT ARE THE FUNCTIONS OF THE GASTROINTESTINAL SYSTEM?

- The teeth and tongue are instrumental in the chewing (mastication) process, and they help break down food into smaller pieces that can be acted on by various enzymes.
- Food moves from the mouth through the pharynx down the esophagus to the stomach, where mixing movements occur.

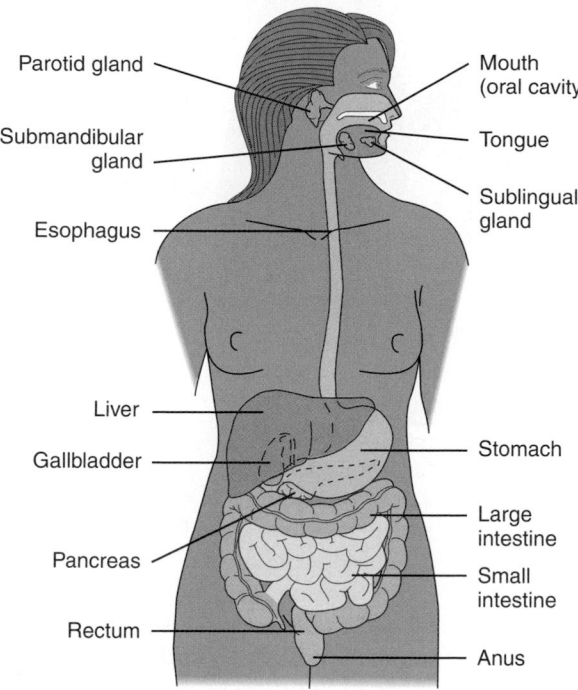

FIGURE 28-1 Organs of the digestive system.

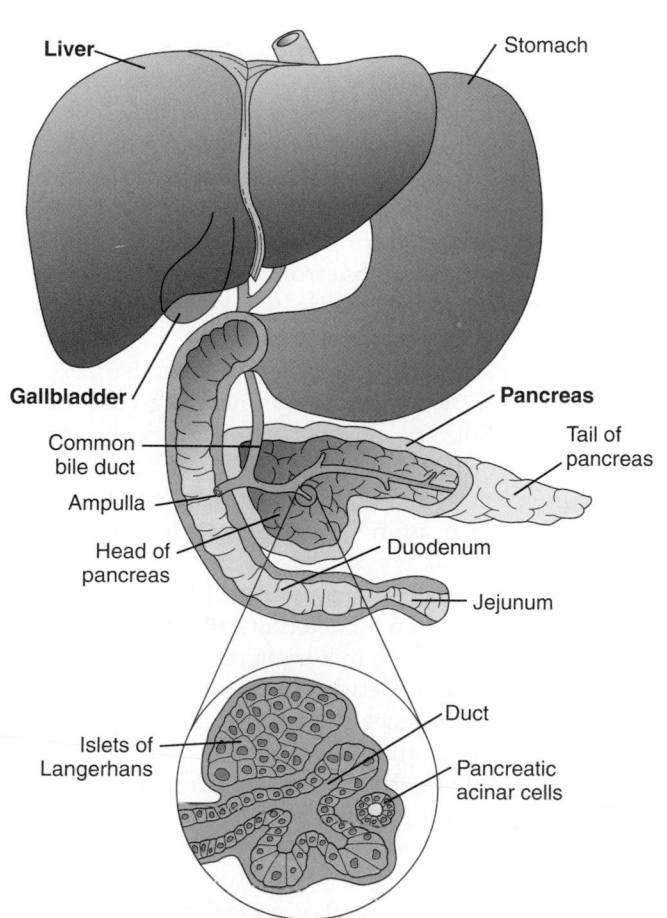

FIGURE 28-2 Accessory organs of the digestive system.

- Mucus, hydrochloric acid (HCl), intrinsic factor, pepsinogen, and gastrin are secreted into the stomach from cells within its walls and are mixed into the food to break down further the particles for absorption. The mixture produced is called **chyme.**
- The small intestine receives the chyme from the stomach, adds more digestive enzymes and fluids, receives bile and pancreatic enzymes from the common duct, and further digests the chyme into a more liquid state.
- Substances are moved along the intestinal tract by the peristaltic action of the intestinal smooth muscle.
- Digested food particles are absorbed into the bloodstream from the villi on the walls of the small intestine.
- The large intestine reabsorbs water and electrolytes, formulates some vitamin K, and eliminates waste products (Figure 28-4).
- The large intestine is populated with bacteria that aid in the breakdown of waste products.
- The rectum stores fecal material until it is eliminated through the anus.
- The internal anal sphincter at the top of the anal canal is under involuntary control; the external anal sphincter at the end of the anal canal is under voluntary control.
- The gastrocolic reflex initiates elimination; it is stimulated by the ingestion of food. By tightening the voluntary anal sphincter, the reflex emptying of the rectum can be stopped.

WHAT EFFECTS DOES AGING HAVE ON THE GASTROINTESTINAL SYSTEM?

- Dentures or partial plates and bridges are common in those over 65. Ill-fitting dentures cause eating problems and can lead to nutritional deficits.
- With advanced age, muscles used for swallowing may become weaker and less coordinated and food particles are retained in the cheek pouches or pharynx.
- The esophageal sphincter becomes less efficient at opening and closing and risk for aspiration increases.
- Taste buds atrophy, causing inability to distinguish between flavors, particularly between salty and sweet.
- After age 70, the parietal cells in the stomach decrease their secretion of hydrochloric acid; enzyme and intrinsic factor secretion also decrease. The lack of intrinsic factor may cause pernicious anemia.
- The mucosa of the small intestine becomes less absorptive, and the large intestine may develop diminished motility.

WHAT ARE THE STRUCTURES AND LOCATIONS OF THE ACCESSORY ORGANS?

- The *gallbladder* is a small sac attached to the lower portion of the liver.
- The *liver* is a large reddish brown organ located in the upper right quadrant of the abdominal cavity under the diaphragm; it is protected by the rib cage.

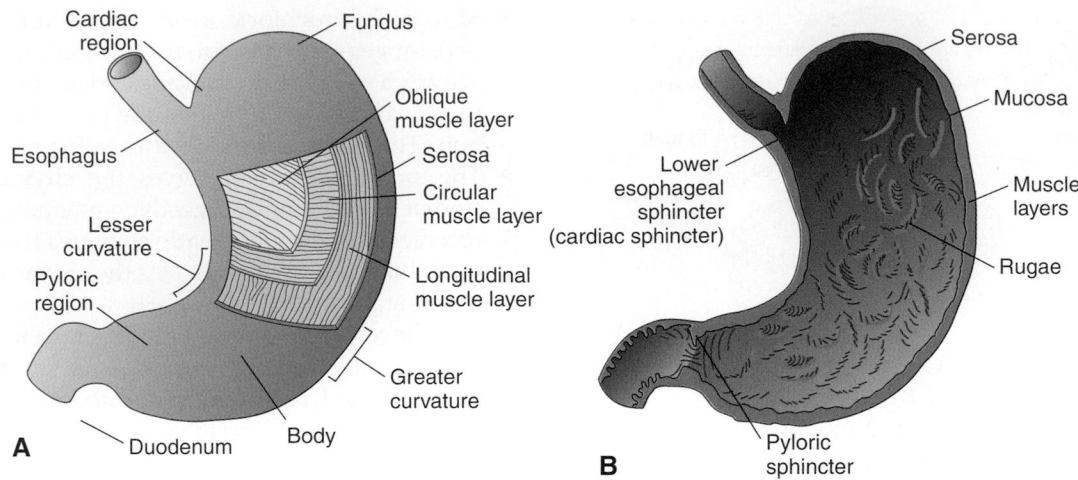

FIGURE 28-3 The stomach. **A,** External view. **B,** Internal view.

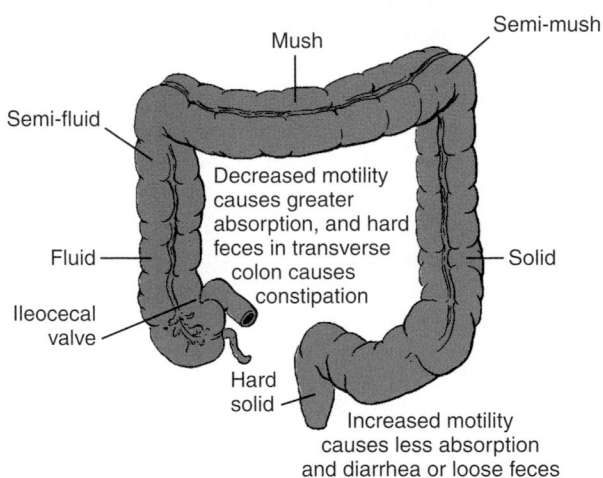

FIGURE 28-4 Absorptive and storage functions of the large intestine.

- The portal vein transports venous blood and nutrients absorbed from the small intestine to the liver.
- The *pancreas* is an elongated, flat organ that sits behind the stomach and consists of a "head" and a "tail" (see Figure 28-2).
- The gallbladder connects to the common bile duct that leads from the liver to the duodenum.
- The pancreatic duct extends the length of the pancreas and connects with the common bile duct, conducting its secretions into the duodenum.

WHAT ARE THE FUNCTIONS OF THE GALLBLADDER, LIVER, AND PANCREAS?

- The gallbladder stores bile produced in the liver and delivers it as needed to the small intestine; the gallbladder can store up to 50 mL of bile.
- The liver manufactures and secretes bile and bile salts necessary to digest fat.
- The liver synthesizes albumin, fibrinogen, globulins, and clotting factors.

- The liver is a storage area for glucose (in the form of glycogen); vitamins A, D, E, K, and B_{12}; and iron.
- The liver receives blood directly from the digestive tract via the hepatic portal vein. All nutrients and oral medications pass through the liver before being distributed to other parts of the body.
- The liver is responsible for how drugs are metabolized.
- The liver detoxifies and breaks down many compounds and drugs, preparing them for excretion; it alters ammonia, a by-product of protein metabolism, so that it does not harm the body.
- The liver helps break down and excrete hormones, drugs, cholesterol, and hemoglobin from worn-out red blood cells.
- The liver plays a major role in glucose metabolism, removing excess glucose from the blood, converting it to glycogen, and then, as glucose is needed, converting glycogen back to glucose.
- The liver plays key roles in lipid metabolism, breaking down fatty acids and synthesizing cholesterol and phospholipids, and in converting excess carbohydrates and proteins into fats.
- The liver is instrumental in protein metabolism, converting certain amino acids into different ones as needed for protein synthesis.
- The liver is a large filter containing phagocytic Kupffer cells that remove bacteria, damaged red blood cells, and other toxic materials from the blood.
- The liver may store between 200 and 400 mL of blood.
- The liver synthesizes the prothrombin needed for normal blood clotting.
- The islets of Langerhans, which are regions of endocrine tissue in the pancreas, secrete the hormones insulin and glucagon into the blood; insulin is essential to the metabolism of carbohydrates.
- The pancreatic acinar cells secrete digestive enzymes into ducts that connect with the pancreatic duct.

- The major pancreatic enzymes are amylase, protease, trypsin, and lipase; these enzymes are essential to the digestion and absorption of nutrients from the small intestine.
- Secretion of pancreatic enzymes is controlled by secretin and cholecystokinin, two substances secreted by the intestinal mucosa.

HOW DOES AGING AFFECT THE ACCESSORY ORGANS OF DIGESTION?

- Gallstone incidence is higher in the older person, possibly due to an increase in biliary cholesterol related to diet and to a tendency toward dehydration.
- Secretion of lipase from the pancreas decreases, altering fat digestion, and may contribute to a depressed nutritional state in the elderly.

THE GASTROINTESTINAL SYSTEM

The intestinal tract and accessory organs of digestion perform the intake, absorption, and assimilation of food to provide nourishment for the body. The transfer of nutrients from the intestine into the blood is referred to as absorption. Food substances are moved along the intestinal tract by peristalsis (wavelike motions of involuntary muscles within the walls of the organs). Metabolism is the sum of many physical and chemical processes of the absorbed nutrients. Metabolic activities involve the synthesis of substances needed to build, maintain, and repair body tissues (anabolism). Metabolism is also responsible for the breakdown of larger molecules into smaller molecules so that energy is available (catabolism).

GASTROINTESTINAL SYSTEM DISORDERS

Causes

The gastrointestinal tract is subject to infection, inflammation, physical and chemical trauma, and structural defects. An intestinal tract problem may occur due to blockage of movement of food through the intestine (intestinal obstruction). Postoperative adhesions sometimes cause intestinal obstruction. Adhesions are bands of scar tissue that bind two anatomical surfaces together that are normally separate. Tumor may also cause intestinal obstruction. Obstruction of the bile or pancreatic ducts can cause interference with the flow of digestive juices and of the enzymes needed for digestion. Continued irritation and inflammation of the GI mucosa can lead to intestinal bleeding and to increased peristalsis, causing inadequate absorption of nutrients.

Psychological and emotional stresses greatly influence appetite and motility of the stomach and intestines. The secretion of digestive juices in amounts sufficient for the breakdown of food is regulated in part by the emotions. Excessive stimulation of digestive acid and enzymes can cause a breakdown

in the integrity of the mucous membrane lining the digestive tract. The damage to the mucous membrane can result in gastric or duodenal ulcers and chronic colitis.

Some disorders, such as Crohn's disease and ulcerative colitis, are correlated with a genetic predisposition. Both disorders are more common among the Jewish population. Certain forms of colon cancer have been identified as having a genetic link and there is a familial tendency for the occurrence of colon cancer. Esophageal and stomach cancer are linked to consumption of charred foods and those containing nitrites. Cigarette smoking is linked to stomach cancer.

Patient Teaching

Foods that May Contribute to Colon Cancer

The patient should be taught that the following foods may contribute to the development of colon cancer.

NITRATES AND NITRITES
- Hot dogs
- Bologna and other luncheon meats
- Bacon
- Ham
- Smoked fish
- Some imported cheeses (check labels)

Nitrates and nitrites are used extensively as food preservatives. Check labels on "deli" products. Charred grilled foods or meat cooked at high temperatures also contain substances that are potentially cancer-causing.

Autoimmune diseases often affect the GI system, causing inflammation or fibrosis of organs. Treatments such as drug and radiation therapy may cause GI problems as a side effect. Some people who have undergone chemotherapy for cancer develop a mechanical form of sprue, a malabsorption problem that remains even after chemotherapy is complete. Lactose intolerance, which is not uncommon in the older adult, may cause continuous diarrhea and malabsorption.

Think Critically

Can you identify any GI problems that seem to run in your family? What measures can family members take to prevent such problems?

Causes of Gallbladder Disorders. The formation of stones within the gallbladder can cause irritation and create areas susceptible to inflammation and infection. Stones can lodge in the common duct, causing obstruction to the flow of bile. Liquid weight loss diets or very rapid weight loss appears to be associated with developing gallstones. Women develop gallstones more frequently than men. The incidence increases with age;

obesity and having several children. People who have diabetes mellitus or Crohn's disease are at higher risk for the disorder.

 ## Cultural Considerations

Genetic Gallstone Risk

Native Americans secrete high levels of cholesterol in bile. A majority of Native American men have gallstones by age 60, and 70% of the women of the Pima Indians in Arizona have gallstones by age 30. Mexican Americans of both sexes and all ages also have high rates of gallstones (National Digestive Diseases Information Clearinghouse, 2007).

Causes of Liver Disorders. The liver filters out many toxic substances and is constantly exposed to any infectious organisms circulating in the bloodstream. The hepatitis virus in particular attacks the liver, causing inflammation and damage to the tissue. Hepatitis B and C are implicated in liver cancer (Clin-eguide Guideline, 2010). *Healthy People 2020* objectives include not only reducing the number of hepatitis infections, but also increasing the percentage of people who are actually aware that they have a hepatitis infection.

Many drugs and chemicals are toxic to the liver, and the nurse should always be aware of the drugs a patient is taking that may cause liver damage. Alcohol and other toxic substances are major factors in the development of cirrhosis of the liver (Box 28-1) (Mehta & Rothstein, 2009).

Liver trauma or laceration may cause massive internal hemorrhage. However, the liver is resilient and will regenerate, if part of the liver remains functional and repair is performed quickly.

Parasites may cause cirrhosis, cysts or abscesses. Most parasites that damage the liver enter the body when people wade or swim in contaminated water in tropical countries, or eat contaminated food.

Cancer in the liver may be primary, or may be secondary to metastasis from a site elsewhere in the intestinal tract.

Causes of Pancreatic Disorders. Pancreatitis (inflammation of the pancreas) is associated with alcoholism, obstructive cholelithiasis, peptic ulcer, hyperlipidemia, and trauma. Pancreatic cancer incidence rises steadily with age. Although the cause of pancreatic cancer is not known, the incidence is higher in cigarette smokers. Obesity, chronic pancreatitis, and diabetes mellitus are also risk factors for this cancer. (See Chapter 38 for information on diabetes mellitus.)

Prevention of Gastrointestinal System Disorders

Eating a normal, well-balanced diet aids digestion. Maintaining good oral health is important to the health of the rest of the body (Kullberg et al., 2009). Consuming sufficient bulk in the diet helps maintain a healthy colon by enhancing passage of waste. A diet lacking in fiber is one factor in the development of diverticulosis, in which pockets form along the colon where waste material can lodge. Drinking at least eight glasses of fluid a day prevents constipation by helping to keep the stool moist.

Heeding the need to defecate promptly aids in keeping the gastrocolic reflex functioning well and prevents constipation and hemorrhoids. Straining at stool increases intra-abdominal pressure which causes the hemorrhoidal vessels to engorge and contributes to

---

Box 28-1 Drugs and Substances Toxic or Harmful to the Liver

TOXIC DRUGS AND SUBSTANCES
- Acetaminophen (Tylenol)
- Carbon tetrachloride
- Ethyl alcohol
- Mushroom: *Amanita phalloides*
- Polychlorinated biphenyls (PCBs)
- Toluene
- Trichloroethylene
- Yellow phosphorus
- Many pesticides

DRUGS AND SUBSTANCES THAT MAY BE DAMAGING TO THE LIVER
Drugs
- Acetylsalicylic acid (aspirin)
- Amiodarone
- Amitriptyline
- Amoxicillin-clavulanic acid
- Chloroform
- Chlorpromazine (Thorazine)

- Diazepam (Valium)
- Erythromycin
- Ethambutol
- Fluconazole
- Gold compounds
- Halothane (Fluothane) anesthetic agent
- Ibuprofen
- Imipramine
- Indomethacin
- Isoniazid (INH)
- Ketoconazole
- 6-Mercaptopurine
- Methotrexate
- Methyldopa (Aldomet)
- Nifedipine (Verapamil)
- Nitrofurantoin
- Oral contraceptives
- Phenobarbital

- Phenytoin (Dilantin)
- Propylthiouracil
- Rezulin
- Rifampin
- Serzone
- Statin drugs
- Thiazide diuretics
- Tricyclic antidepressants

Chemical Substances
- Acetaldehyde
- Aerosolized paint
- Cadmium
- Ethylene oxide
- Mercury
- Nitrosamines
- Paint thinner
- Many cleaning solvents

hemorrhoid formation. Decreased mobility in the elderly patient often leads to digestive problems; therefore ambulation is encouraged

🏃 Health Promotion

Maintaining Abdominal Tone

Obtaining sufficient daily exercise maintains abdominal muscle tone and contributes to peristalsis and the ability to defecate normally. Defecating at more or less the same time each day aids the defecation process and helps promote continued ability to control defecation.

Maintaining body weight within normal limits helps prevent hiatal hernia and esophageal reflux. Developing healthy coping mechanisms and keeping stress within acceptable limits may prevent ulcers and chronic irritability of the bowel.

Mechanical and chemical irritants that produce inflammation often can be identified by elimination diets to determine the foods that cause GI upsets. Once the offending foods are identified, the patient can learn to avoid those foods and to maintain adequate nutrition.

Following general rules of good hygiene and sanitation can prevent many infectious GI upsets: wash the hands before eating and clean cooking and eating utensils properly. Food poisoning can be prevented by adequate refrigeration and by proper canning, freezing, and food-handling methods. Meats, and foods containing mayonnaise or dairy products, should be kept chilled. When not in the refrigerator, food should be kept covered.

❓ Think Critically

Can you teach your family and friends about ways to decrease the risk of colon cancer? What would you recommend to your parents regarding screening for colorectal cancer?

Prevention of Gallbladder Disorders. Maintaining a normal body weight, eating a low-fat, low-cholesterol, high fiber and high calcium diet, avoiding rapid weight loss diets, consuming alcohol moderately, and maintaining an active lifestyle all help prevent gallstones (Clin-eguide, 2009). If gallstones are irritating the gallbladder, prompt surgery might help to prevent cancer.

Prevention of Liver Disorders. Obtaining immunization against hepatitis A and hepatitis B helps to prevent these viral diseases. A vaccine against hepatitis C is under study at present. Using Standard Precautions (see Appendix B) when handling any body fluids, particularly blood, greatly reduces the risk of infection with hepatitis B and C, which may decrease the chance of developing liver cancer. Refraining from consuming excessive amounts of alcohol decreases the risk of

developing cirrhosis of the liver. Avoiding exposure to known toxic or carcinogenic chemicals helps prevent liver damage and liver cancer.

🏃 Health Promotion

Avoiding Contraction of Hepatitis

Practicing good hygiene and avoiding contact with substances that harbor the hepatitis virus, such as raw oysters and shellfish from contaminated waters may prevent infection with hepatitis A. Avoiding unprotected sex with people who are drug users, or those known to be carriers of hepatitis B or C, helps prevent the contraction of both types of hepatitis.

Prevention of Pancreatic Disorders. Avoiding consumption of large quantities of alcohol may prevent pancreatitis. Removing a gallbladder that has gallstones can help prevent obstruction of the pancreatic duct with stones. Removal prevents backup of pancreatic enzymes that are thought to be a cause of pancreatitis. Compliance with therapy for a peptic ulcer helps prevent irritation of the pancreas and resultant pancreatitis. Smoking cessation decreases the risk of pancreatic cancer.

Diagnostic Tests, Procedures, and Nursing Implications

Diagnostic tests for disorders of the intestinal tract and accessory organs consist of x-rays, computed tomography (CT) scans, nuclear medicine scans, magnetic resonance imaging, ultrasound studies, endoscopy, biopsy, laboratory tests, tests of gastric secretions, and stool and urine studies (Table 28-1).

The patient often is scheduled for a series of tests, some of which use a contrast medium. Check the patient's allergies to make certain that a particular contrast medium or injectable marker is not contraindicated. For women of childbearing age, a pregnancy test might be ordered. It is important that GI tests be done in the correct order, so that the contrast media do not interfere with other tests. For example, if the patient is scheduled for an upper GI series, a gallbladder sonogram, and a barium enema, she should have them done in this order: sonogram, barium enema, and then the upper GI series.

A relatively new test, virtual colonoscopy, is available for colon cancer screening. The procedure combines images from a high-tech spiral CT scan to create a computer-generated three-dimensional picture of the colon. The procedure is less costly than standard colonoscopy and requires no sedation. However, if a polyp or suspicious area is seen, the patient must undergo a regular colonoscopy for tissue specimens to be obtained. For screening, a yearly fecal occult blood test, or fecal immunochemical test (FIT), is recommended. Stool DNA is a new primary screening test for colorectal cancer. Multiple stool take-home

Text continued on p. 631

Table 28-1   Diagnostic Tests for Gastrointestinal (GI) Disorders

TEST	PURPOSE	DESCRIPTION	NURSING IMPLICATIONS
Radiologic Examinations			
Upper GI series (UGI)	Radiographic examination with fluoroscopy to locate obstruction, ulceration, or growths in the esophagus, stomach, and duodenum	Patient drinks a contrast medium and is placed in various positions on the x-ray table.	Keep patient NPO for 8-12 hr before the test. Explain what happens during test. After radiographs, increase fluids and give ordered laxatives to clear GI tract of contrast medium and prevent impaction. Stool may be white up to 3 days after test.
Barium enema (BE)	Radiographic examination of the colon using fluoroscopy to locate tumors, obstruction, and ulceration	A radiopaque substance is instilled into the colon by enema. After evacuation of this substance, air may be instilled for contrast studies.	Keep patient NPO for 8 hr before test. Give ordered laxatives and enemas. Bowel must be clear of stool. Explain what will happen during the test. Post-test care is same as for upper GI series.
Computed tomography (CT)	To visualize soft tissue and density changes when sonography is inconclusive To detect tumors, abscesses, trauma, cysts, inflammation, and bleeding	Radiography is combined with computer techniques to provide a series of sectional pictures of the gallbladder.	Patient is kept NPO for 4 hr when oral contrast is to be used. Verify presence of signed informed consent form for this procedure. Assess for allergy to iodine or shellfish. Explain to patient that she will be positioned supine on a special, narrow table and her body will be in the circular opening of the scanner. She will have a strap over her waist to secure her to the table. Clicking noises will be heard from the machine. The test takes about 30 min. An IV contrast agent that causes a transitory warm feeling may be given to enhance images. Patient will be asked to hold her breath at certain points in the test. The machine uses narrow x-ray beams.
Virtual colonoscopy	Noninvasive method of determining if there are polyps or abnormalities in the colon Does not allow for biopsy of suspicious areas	Helical CT scan of the colon is performed. An oral contrast agent may be given 1 day before the scan.	Patient must lie still during the procedure. Remove all metal from the body surface. Usually takes about 30 min. Encourage large quantities of fluid postprocedure if barium contrast material was swallowed.
Ultrasonography	To obtain images of soft tissue that indicate density changes To diagnose gallstones, tumor, cysts, abscess, etc.	Sonograms are produced with high-frequency sound waves that pass through the body. Echoes vary with tissue density.	Patient is kept NPO after midnight. Explain procedure: will be supine on table, lubricant will be applied to the skin surface, and a handheld metal probe is passed back and forth with light pressure. Test takes about 30 min. Patient needs to remain still.

Test	Purpose	Description	Nursing Implications
Magnetic resonance imaging (MRI)	To evaluate abnormalities in the liver	Places the patient in a magnetic field. Uses radiofrequency signals to determine how hydrogen atoms behave in the magnetic field. Provides better contrast than CT between normal tissue and pathologic tissue.	Explain that there is no exposure to radiation. Antianxiety medication may be administered to those patients who are claustrophobic. There are no food or fluid restrictions before the test. The test takes 30-90 min. Remove all metal objects from the body, including dental bridges. Inform patient that she will be required to remain motionless during this study. A thumping sound will be heard during the test. There may be a tingling sensation in metal fillings. A contrast medium may be injected into a vein.
Hepatobiliary scintigraphy (hepatoiminodiacetic acid [HIDA] scan)	To determine blood flow distribution in the liver, biliary tree, gallbladder, and proximal small bowel. To confirm cirrhosis, neoplasm, and acute cholecystitis	^{99m}Tc is injected. Patient is positioned under imaging camera and images are taken as radioactive material is distributed.	Only traces of radioactivity are administered and there is little radioactivity danger. Patient will lie flat during scanning.
GI scintigraphy	To determine site of active GI bleeding	Radioactive tracer is administered IV and attaches to red blood cells. Images of the abdomen are obtained at intermittent intervals.	Same as for hepatobiliary scan.

Endoscopic Studies

Test	Purpose	Description	Nursing Implications
Esophagogastroduodenoscopy	To visualize the esophagus, stomach, and duodenum with a lighted tube (endoscope) to detect tumor, ulceration, or obstruction. Separate study of esophagus, stomach, or stomach and duodenum may be done	Patient is given preoperative sedation. IV sedation may be given for the test. A local spray or gargle may be used to anesthetize the throat. The patient lies on a table with head extended, and the endoscope is introduced through the mouth.	Keep patient NPO for 8 hr. Verify presence of signed informed consent form for procedure. Explain what she will experience during the test. Give preoperative medication. After procedure, keep patient NPO until gag reflex has returned. Take vital signs q 15-30 min as ordered. Watch for signs of perforation: rising temperature, pain, changes in vital signs.
Endoscopic retrograde cholangiopancreatography (ERCP)	Performed when common radiologic studies do not reveal the cause of the problem. To identify obstruction and other pathologic conditions in the biliary and common ducts	An endoscope is passed through the mouth into the duodenum with the use of fluoroscopy. A cannula is positioned in the common bile duct, and a contrast medium is injected. Radiographs are then taken.	Verify presence of signed informed consent form for procedure. Patient is kept NPO after midnight. Explain the procedure to the patient (same as for esophagogastroduodenoscopy). A pretest sedative may be ordered. Postprocedure care is same as for esophagogastroduodenoscopy.

Continued

Table 28-1 Diagnostic Tests for Gastrointestinal (GI) Disorders—cont'd

TEST	PURPOSE	DESCRIPTION	NURSING IMPLICATIONS
Endoscopic Studies—cont'd			
Flexible sigmoidoscopy	To examine the lining of the rectum and sigmoid colon to detect polyps, tumor, obstruction, or ulceration	The patient is placed in the knee-chest position, often on a special table. A sigmoidoscope is introduced through the anus. Biopsies can be taken from areas of suspect tissue; polyps can be removed. The patient will experience some cramping during the procedure.	Give laxatives and enemas the evening before as ordered. Give clear liquids for dinner the night before, then keep patient NPO until after examination. Explain what she will experience. Encourage use of deep breathing and relaxation techniques to decrease cramping. Observe for rectal bleeding after biopsy or polyp removal.
Colonoscopy	To directly view the lining of the colon with a flexible endoscope	Patient is moderately sedated for this procedure, which takes about 1½-2 hr. Polyps can be removed or biopsies taken.	Give clear liquid diet 1-3 days before test. Patient is kept NPO for 8 hr before test. Give laxatives for 1-3 days before test and enemas the night before. Explain procedure and what she will experience. Verify presence of signed informed consent form for procedure. Give preoperative sedation. After procedure, observe for rectal bleeding and signs of perforation: abdominal distention, pain, elevated temperature.
Gastric analysis	To determine the rate of secretion of gastric juices and degree of acidity	A nasogastric tube is inserted, and the stomach contents are aspirated. A substance may be given to stimulate the flow of gastric secretions, and another sample is aspirated in 30 min. Increased secretion can indicate peptic ulcer or pancreatic tumor. A low degree of acidity may indicate gastric ulcer. An absence of acid can accompany cancer of the stomach or pernicious anemia.	Withhold drugs affecting gastric secretion for 24-48 hr before test. No smoking the morning of test (nicotine stimulates secretions). Keep patient NPO for 8 hr before test. Explain use of NG tube and procedure.
Liver biopsy	To remove a tissue sample for microscopic examination and diagnosis of various liver disorders	Under local or general anesthesia, a special biopsy needle is inserted through the abdominal wall into the desired area of the liver, and a tissue sample is aspirated.	Verify presence of signed informed consent form for procedure. Patient must be kept NPO 4-8 hr before procedure. Place patient in supine or left lateral position. Patient will need to hold very still if performed under local anesthesia. The needle is introduced during sustained exhalation. She will feel pain similar to a punch in the shoulder lasting only a minute or so. Procedure takes about 15 min. Take baseline vital signs. Assess for allergy to local anesthetic. Have patient empty the bladder before the procedure.

Continued

Test	Purpose	Description	Nursing actions
			Check coagulation studies for abnormalities. After biopsy, place a small dressing over puncture site; position patient on right side with support to provide pressure over biopsy site for 1-2 hr. Observe for bleeding. Monitor vital signs q 15 min for 1 hr; then q 30 min for 4 hr; then q 4 hr for 24 hr. Assess for tenderness at biopsy site. Observe for respiratory problems, such as dyspnea, cyanosis, or restlessness, which might indicate pneumothorax. Instruct patient to avoid coughing or straining that might increase intra-abdominal pressure. She should refrain from heavy lifting or strenuous activities for 1-2 wk.
Tubeless gastric analysis	To determine of presence or absence of hydrochloric acid in the stomach secretions	The patient is given special granules in 240 mL of water. Urine specimens are collected at specific intervals. If HCl is present in the stomach, the urine will be blue; if none is present, the urine will be normal color.	Explain test and procedure to patient.

Laboratory Tests

Test	Purpose	Description	Nursing actions
Fecal analysis (stool examination)	To analyze for presence of mucus, elevated fat content, blood (guaiac), bacteria, or parasites	Stool specimen is obtained in bedpan or container in commode. Small smear is made on special paper and tested with special solution for guaiac or with Hemoccult test. Specimen is placed in container and sent to laboratory for testing.	Explain test to patient. Provide means for collection of stool. Promptly retrieve stool, obtain sample for guaiac test, place specimen in laboratory container, and dispatch to laboratory immediately (bacteria will multiply if specimen is left at room temperature for extended period; parasites may disintegrate). Patient must have red meat-free diet for at least 3 days before a stool guaiac test can be considered accurate.
Serum bilirubin *Normal values:* Total: 0.1-1.2 mg/dL Indirect: 0.2-0.8 mg/dL Direct: 0.1-0.3 mg/dL	To detect abnormal bilirubin metabolism Jaundice is present when bilirubin is >2.5 mg/dL	Collect 5-7 mL venous blood in red-top tube. Protect sample from bright light.	Explain that a blood sample will be taken. Some laboratories require an 8-hr fast.
Alanine aminotransferase (ALT) *Normal value:* 1-45 IU/L	An enzyme used to detect liver disease With viral hepatitis, ALT/AST ratio is >1.0 With other liver disease, ALT/AST ratio is <1.0.	Collect 7-10 mL venous blood in a red-top tube. Injury of liver cells causes release of this enzyme.	Explain that a blood sample will be collected. No fasting is required.
Aspartate aminotransferase (AST) *Normal range:* 1-36 units/L	An enzyme found in heart, liver, and muscle tissue To detect acute hepatitis or biliary obstruction	Collect 7-10 mL venous blood in a red-top tube. Diseases affecting hepatocytes cause this enzyme to rise in the blood.	Explain that a blood sample will be drawn. Avoid hemolysis of sample. IM injection will affect level.

Table 28-1 Diagnostic Tests for Gastrointestinal (GI) Disorders—cont'd

TEST	PURPOSE	DESCRIPTION	NURSING IMPLICATIONS
Laboratory Tests—cont'd			
Alkaline phosphatase (ALP) *Normal range:* 35-150 units/L	Enzyme found in bone, liver, and placenta To detect liver tumor in conjunction with other clinical findings Rises when there is obstruction of biliary tree	Collect 5-7 mL venous blood in a red-top tube.	No fasting is required.
Ammonia *Normal range:* 10-80 mcg/dL	Is a product of protein metabolism To support diagnosis of severe liver disease with encephalopathy	Collect 4-7 mL venous blood in a green-top tube. May need to ice the specimen.	No fasting is required.
Gamma-glutamyl transpeptidase (GGT) *Normal range:* 510 g/dL	To detect liver cell dysfunction, biliary obstruction, cholangitis, or cholecystitis	Collect 7-10 mL venous blood in a red-top tube.	Explain that a blood sample will be taken. Drugs that affect this test are alcohol, phenytoin, phenobarbital, clofibrate, and oral contraceptives.
Protein *Normal range:* 6.0-8.0 g/dL	To detect altered protein metabolism Decreased in liver failure	Collect 5-7 mL venous blood in a red-top tube.	Explain that a blood sample will be drawn. No fasting is required.
Albumin *Normal range:* 3.5-5.5 g/dL	To detect deficiencies in clotting mechanisms (activators have been added to PTT tests reagents: APTT)	Collect 5-7 mL venous blood in a red-top tube.	No fasting is required.
Prothrombin time (PT) *Normal range:* 12.0-14.0 sec	Protein produced by the liver and used in blood clotting Depends on adequate intake and absorption of vitamin K Reduced in patients with liver disease, causing a prolonged clotting time	Collect 5-7 mL venous blood in a blue-top tube.	No fasting is required. Apply pressure to venipuncture site. INR used to determine therapeutic level of anticoagulant medication.
Partial thromboplastin time (PTT) *Normal PTT:* 60-70 sec	To detect deficiencies of stage II clotting mechanisms Prolonged in liver disease	Collect 5-14 mL venous blood in one or two blue-top tubes.	No fasting is required. Apply pressure to venipuncture site.
Activated PTT (APTT) *Normal APTT:* 20-35 sec	Decreased in liver failure	Collect 5-14 mL of venous blood in a blue-top tube.	If patient is receiving heparin injections, draw specimen 30-60 min before next dose.
Helicobacter pylori antibody test *Normal:* none present	To detect antibodies to *H. pylori* bacterium in the stomach *H. pylori* is a risk factor for gastric and duodenal ulcers, chronic gastritis, or ulcerative esophagitis	Collect a sample of venous blood according to the laboratory's instructions.	Explain to patient that a blood sample will be drawn. No fasting is required.

IM, intramuscular; *INR*, international normalized ratio; *IU*, international units; *IV*, intravenous; *NG*, nasogastric; *NPO*, nothing by mouth; ^{99m}Tc, technetium-99m.

tests should be done; positive results indicate the need for colonoscopy (American Cancer Society, 2010).

The patient needs specific instructions about preparing for a diagnostic test. Many of the studies require cleansing of the GI tract and inadequate bowel prep may cause a delay or necessitate a repeat of the test. When laxatives are administered in liquid form, the patient can drink them more easily if they are chilled or poured over ice.

 Assignment Considerations

Assisting with a Bowel Prep

When an unlicensed assistive personnel (UAP) is assigned to care for a patient who is undergoing a bowel prep for a diagnostic test, ask the assistant to be prompt in answering a call bell for assistance to the bathroom. The need to defecate may be urgent. When a patient is consuming large quantities of fluid, such as with GoLYTELY, ask the UAP to promptly report any degree of confusion, shortness of breath, extra weakness, or muscle cramping. Remember that delegation is never a substitute for good nursing assessment.

 Elder Care Points

The older patient is especially at risk for problems of electrolyte imbalance, fluid overload, or dehydration when undergoing preparation for diagnostic tests that require a fasting state and/or bowel cleansing.

 Clinical Cues

If a patient has trouble with nausea, sucking on an ice cube first and then using a straw to drink the solution for colon "prep" helps to decrease the taste sensation.

For many GI tests, the patient is kept on nothing-by-mouth (NPO) status the night before. In the hospital, mouth care should be offered in the morning, and the door of the room should be kept closed so that food odors do not enter and increase hunger. A food tray should be obtained immediately on return to the floor, as long as NPO status is no longer in effect. You can provide juices and coffee or tea while waiting for the meal tray to be delivered. Frequent assessment for signs of dehydration is necessary. Cleansing enemas and lack of oral intake can quickly dehydrate a patient who has already been ill with nausea, vomiting, or diarrhea.

❖ NURSING MANAGEMENT

 ■ **Assessment (Data Collection)**

Assessment for problems of the accessory organs of the digestive system begins during history taking. Ask questions regarding family history, diet, dietary intolerances, pain, exposure to toxins or chemicals and problems with blood clotting. Verify immunization status. Because of the many functions of the liver, assessment of the patient with liver disease must include all systems of the body.

 Focused Assessment

Data Collection for the Gastrointestinal System and Accessory Organs

When obtaining a GI history, ask the following questions:
- Have you gained or lost weight recently?
- Do you have any difficulty chewing or swallowing?
- When did you have your last dental examination?
- Do you ever experience indigestion? Do certain foods disagree with you? Do you have known food intolerances?
- Do you drink alcohol? About how often do you drink? How many drinks do you average?
- Has your appetite changed in any way?
- Have you been experiencing any abdominal pain or nausea and vomiting? Do you experience any regurgitation or reflux? Is pain related to your eating patterns?
- Can you describe your usual diet? How much of each item do you eat? (Ask about what is eaten at each meal typically, and then ask about between-meal snacks and drinks.)
- What drugs do you take on a regular basis? (aspirin, nonsteroidal anti-inflammatory drugs [NSAIDs], and corticosteroids are particularly important.)
- Are you able to shop and prepare meals? Is there any problem with obtaining sufficient food (if patient is known to have economic constraints)?
- Do you have any cultural preferences for food?
- What is the typical frequency of your bowel movements? Have you noticed any changes in color, frequency, or form of stools?
- How do you handle stress? How do you relax?

Additional questions pertinent to the accessory organs:
- Does eating fatty or fried food give you pain or diarrhea?
- Does your blood take a long time to clot when you cut yourself?
- Have you had any rapid weight loss from dieting?
- Have you been immobile for a long period of time?
- Have you been exposed to chemical toxins such as cleaning agents, pesticides, or industrial chemicals?
- Have you had hepatitis B and/or hepatitis A immunizations?
- Have you ever had a blood transfusion?
- Have you had any surgeries? If so, what year were they?
- Do you use recreational drugs?
- Do you have any tattoos or body piercings?
- Do you smoke? If so, how much do you smoke? How many years have you smoked?
- Have you experienced any abdominal trauma?
- Do you have a sexual partner? Are you monogamous? Has any sexual partner been a carrier of hepatitis B or hepatitis C?

Physical Assessment

Inspect the patient's teeth, gums, and oral mucosa for obvious problems. Examine the skin for color and lesions, and note any discolorations on the abdomen. Assess for the presence of edema and ascites (fluid in the abdominal cavity) by observing for marked abdominal distention and by taut, glistening skin. Check the contour of the abdomen, and note any outpouchings indicating a hernia.

Auscultate bowel sounds for each quadrant of the abdomen using the diaphragm of the stethoscope

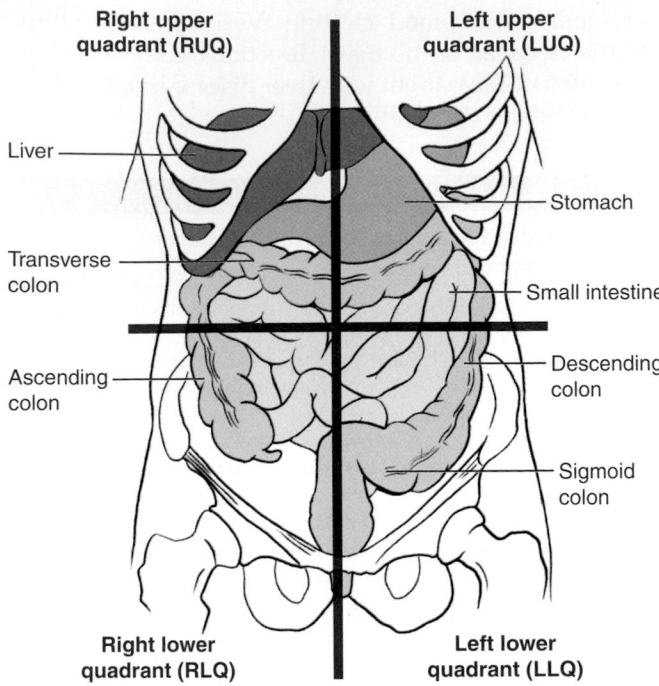

Right upper quadrant (RUQ) — Liver, Transverse colon, Ascending colon

Left upper quadrant (LUQ) — Stomach, Small intestine, Descending colon, Sigmoid colon

Right lower quadrant (RLQ)

Left lower quadrant (LLQ)

FIGURE 28-5 Auscultate bowel sounds in all four quadrants.

(Figure 28-5). **Perform auscultation before palpation or percussion because palpation may cause peristaltic movement that otherwise would not have occurred. Bowel sounds are caused by air and fluid moving through the intestinal tract, and are heard as soft gurgles and clicks every 5 to 15 seconds.** The normal frequency for these sounds is about 5 to 30 in 1 minute. Note both the character and frequency of sounds. Loud, frequent sounds occur when there is excessive motility in the bowel.

Clinical Cues

For bowel sounds to be considered absent, it is necessary to verify that no sounds are heard after listening in each of the four quadrants for 5 minutes. Hypoactive bowel sounds can be noted in the medical record when no sounds are heard after listening in each of the four quadrants for 30 seconds.

If hyperactive, high-pitched sounds are heard in one quadrant, and decreased sounds are heard in another quadrant, assess for nausea and vomiting, as the patient may have an intestinal obstruction.

Lightly palpate over each quadrant of the abdomen to detect areas of tenderness and any masses that might be present. Watch the patient's face during palpation to detect signs of discomfort. If a pulsating abdominal mass is present, do not perform palpation; this pulsation could signal an abdominal aneurysm with a potential danger of sudden rupture.

Percussion is performed by placing the middle finger of one hand on the abdomen and striking the finger

lightly below the knuckle and listening for the pitch of sound produced. A resonant sound is heard over areas filled with air and a dull, thudding sound is heard over solid organs. **Percussion detects excessive air in the intestinal tract, which occurs with irritation and inflammation.**

Assess ascites by placing the patient supine and exposing the abdomen. With the patient's arms at the sides and knees flexed, observe for *bulging flanks,* indicating fluid accumulation. If ascites is present; measure abdominal girth. Place a tape measure around the fullest part of the abdomen, usually at the umbilicus. Place small ink marks at the sides of the tape on the axillary lines, so that future measurements may be taken at the same place for comparison. If ascites is continuous, the abdominal girth will increase with subsequent measurements. Percuss from the umbilicus to the flanks to detect shifting dullness caused by air rising and fluid shifting to the dependent areas.

Check the laboratory values and diagnostic test results (see Table 28-1). Evaluate the urine for presence of bilirubin, which makes the urine dark or the brown color of tea. Inspect stool for the presence of fat and urobilinogen. If undigested fat is present, the stool will float in the toilet bowl. If bile is not reaching the intestine, the stool appears clay-colored or whitish.

Focused Assessment

Physical Assessment of the Gastrointestinal System and Accessory Organs

- Inspect the mouth for condition of teeth, gums, and mucous membranes.
- Inspect swallowing ability.
- Inspect the skin for color, areas of discoloration, and presence of surface vessels and easy bruising.
- Inspect the sclera and mucous membranes for signs of icterus.
- Inspect the contour of the abdomen.
- Auscultate for bowel sounds in all four quadrants.
- Lightly palpate each quadrant of the abdomen
- Percuss each quadrant of the abdomen if there seems to be a problem with intestinal irritation or inflammation.
- If there is evidence of ascites, measure abdominal girth.
- Inspect stool, if available, for characteristics; test for occult blood if indicated.
- Inspect color of urine.
- Inspect anus for presence of external hemorrhoids.
- If vomiting has occurred, inspect vomitus for characteristics; test vomitus for blood if indicated.

Elder Care Points

Recording all the medications the elderly patient is taking, both prescription and over-the-counter drugs, is very important when assessing the digestive system. Many drugs affect digestion, bowel motility, and appetite in these patients, and can cause constipation or diarrhea.

■ Nursing Diagnosis and Planning

Common nursing diagnoses and examples of expected outcomes for problems of the GI tract are located in Table 28-2. More time is often needed to care for a patient who has diarrhea or is incontinent of feces. It is important to consider the time it takes for toileting and cleaning up after loose bowel movements. A bowel retraining program takes patience and time. These time-consuming tasks are also assignment considerations for UAPs. Diapered or incontinent patients may need to be treated using isolation precautions. Administering enemas can be quite time consuming as well.

■ Implementation

Institute nursing interventions to control and eliminate pain, maintain fluid and electrolyte balance, promote adequate nutrition, rest, and healing, and prevent complications (see Table 28-2). All nurses must ask each patient each day about bowel movements to prevent constipation and possible impaction in hospitalized patients.

■ Evaluation

Analyze laboratory values to see whether problems are resolving with treatment. Ideally, the patient should demonstrate normalization of eating habits and bowel patterns; however **you should continually evaluate whether the patient is experiencing adverse side effects of therapy or complications of the disease process.** For legal reasons and for continuity of care, your evaluation findings and your follow-up actions must always be documented.

COMMON PROBLEMS RELATED TO THE GASTROINTESTINAL SYSTEM

Anorexia

Anorexia is the absence of appetite. Physical causes for a diminished interest in eating include poorly fitting dentures, stomatitis, decaying teeth, halitosis, and a bad taste in the mouth. Pain or nausea related to surgical procedures or the presence of a mouth or GI infection or irritation decreases appetite.

Appetite depends on complex mental processes having to do with memory and mental associations that can be pleasant or extremely unpleasant. Appetite is stimulated by the sight, smell, and thought of food. The physical and social environment in which a person is eating stimulates appetite. The enjoyment of eating can be inhibited by unattractive or unfamiliar food, by surroundings or company, and by emotional states such as anxiety, anger, and fear. Mental depression also may cause anorexia.

Nursing Management. Loss of appetite is to be expected when a person becomes ill. However, persistent anorexia must be dealt with to avoid the consequences of inadequate nutrition. Because of the complex nature of anorexia, it may be necessary for the nurse to talk with the patient, family, and significant others and to consult the medical record to learn why appetite has diminished.

Elder Care Points

Both taste and smell sensation diminish with age. Sometimes this is due to a zinc deficiency. Elderly persons may lose teeth because of gingival or dental disease, making eating more difficult. Dental plates may not fit correctly, making eating painful. Many elderly patients take a variety of medications for various conditions. The combination of these medications may greatly affect appetite and digestion. *Polypharmacy* (taking many medications) is a frequent cause of anorexia in the elderly patient.

Nursing interventions include mouth care before each meal to eliminate or minimize oral causes of poor appetite. Laboratory results regarding albumin and electrolyte levels should be monitored. The percentage of each meal eaten should be noted and documented.

If psychosocial or cultural factors are involved, the nurse might try offering preferred foods if possible and not detrimental to health. Meals that are planned to include a variety of colors, textures, and tastes are more appealing and enjoyable than those that are monotonous and bland.

Assignment Considerations
Assisting with Meals

Be sure and instruct the UAP who is assisting with meals to encourage patients to eat slowly and enjoy the meal. If it is necessary to feed the patient, this should be done cheerfully and in a manner that encourages the social aspect of eating.

Elder Care Points

If weight loss and loss of appetite occur in an elderly patient without evidence of any specific cause, the possibility of depression should be investigated. The depressed elderly patient may give up hope and just stop eating much.

The nurse, a family member, or a friend can provide companionship while the patient eats. If there is a patient cafeteria or gathering place for patients to eat together, and the patient is able to go there for meals, this can sometimes alleviate or minimize anorexia.

Any time a patient has continual problems with eating, a dental care history and an oral cavity examination should be performed. Some people may be embarrassed by physical limitations that cause them to be awkward with eating, and so will eat very little in the company of others. Others who have difficulty

Table 28-2 Common Nursing Diagnoses, Expected Outcomes, and Interventions for Patients with Gastrointestinal Disorders

NURSING DIAGNOSIS	GOALS/EXPECTED OUTCOMES	NURSING INTERVENTIONS
Deficient fluid volume related to nausea and vomiting or diarrhea	Vomiting will be controlled within 24 hr; diarrhea will be controlled within 24 hr. Fluid volume will be within normal limits within 48 hr as evidenced by adequate skin turgor and urine output >50 mL/hr.	Assess urine output for signs of fluid deficit. Provide mouth care after vomiting to decrease nausea. Medicate for nausea and vomiting as ordered. Provide quiet environment and rest. Medicate for diarrhea as ordered; keep patient clean and dry. Give only small sips of clear liquids by mouth until vomiting subsides. Continue clear-liquid diet until diarrhea is controlled.
Imbalanced nutrition: less than body requirements related to anorexia, nausea, and vomiting	Patient will ingest at least 1200 calories per day after vomiting subsides.	Offer mouth care before meals. Provide six small meals a day plus small, high-calorie snacks between meals. Weigh q 3 days and record. Keep room odor free. Provide company and quiet atmosphere for mealtime.
Diarrhea related to intestinal infection or inflammation	Infection or inflammation episode will resolve within 72 hr. Diarrhea will be controlled to prevent fluid imbalance within 24 hr.	Medicate with antibiotics, anti-inflammatories, and antidiarrheals as ordered. Rest bowel with clear-liquid diet or bland diet as ordered. Protect anal mucosa with barrier ointment. Keep anal area clean and dry. Provide warm sitz bath to soothe anal tissues as needed. Medicate for discomfort from abdominal cramping as ordered. Provide restful environment.
Constipation related to side effects of medication, loss of ability to initiate defecation, or improper diet	Patient will have normal bowel movements regularly within 2 wk.	Increase fluid intake to 2500 mL/day unless contraindicated. Add fruit juices to diet. Increase fiber in diet; add slowly to prevent excessive gas formation. Increase exercise on a daily basis. Encourage patient to heed gastrocolic reflex and not delay defecation. Administer stool softener or bulk laxative as ordered. Monitor for fecal impaction.
Bowel incontinence related to lack of sphincter control	Patient will use bowel training program. Continence will be achieved within 1 mo.	Institute bowel training program. Provide toileting opportunity after each meal. Provide privacy and comfort for attempts at defecation. Adjust diet to provide optimal fiber in diet. Keep patient clean, dry, and odor free.
Ineffective coping related to inability to handle excessive stress	Patient will identify desired ways of coping within 3 wk. Patient will learn new coping techniques within 2 mo.	Assist to identify present coping mechanisms. Assist to identify stressors. Instruct in ways to develop more effective coping mechanisms, such as relaxation techniques, alterations in perspective, exercise, or imagery. Refer for counseling as needed.

swallowing and are afraid of choking are afraid to eat alone, but are embarrassed when eating with others. It is essential to explore each patient's causes of anorexia and feelings about eating.

Food from home often is a welcome addition to institutional meals. The person bringing it will need to be advised of any restrictions on the patient's dietary intake and the importance of adherence.

 Assignment Considerations

Oral Rehydration for the Elderly

Institutionalized elderly patients are at high risk for dehydration. Instruct the UAP to directly offer small amounts of fluid, especially water, to patients throughout the day (unless contraindicated) and to assist by opening containers and positioning fluids within reach. A variety of fluids, such as juice, milk, or low-sodium liquids, should be available. Coffee, tea, and soda should be limited because of the diuretic effects (Pinto, 2008).

Nausea and Vomiting

Persistent nausea and vomiting interferes with eating and hinders nutrition. Nausea and vomiting may be related to illness, anesthesia, pain, effects of cancer treatment, or stress. Transient nausea is not treated, but when the disorder persists, medication with antiemetics, GI tube feedings, and administration of intravenous fluids are necessary. Nursing interventions are discussed in Chapter 3.

 Assignment Considerations

Smells Exacerbate Nausea

When caring for patients who are prone to nausea, all health care personnel should be instructed to avoid using heavy perfume. Some very sensitive patients may even be affected by the fragrance from common products such as laundry detergent, lotions, hair products, soaps, or makeup.

 Complementary and Alternative Therapies

Ginger for Nausea

Ginger has been used for centuries in Asia to combat nausea and vomiting, motion sickness, and dyspepsia. It is available candied in capsules, fluid extract, and tablets, and tincture or as fresh gingerroot that can be grated and used to make tea. Ginger may decrease the action of histamine (H_2)-receptor antagonists and proton pump inhibitors and may increase absorption of medications taken orally. Ginger may decrease the effect of antidiabetic medications. It should not be used during pregnancy or lactation.

 Clinical Cues

A quick and temporary measure that relieves nausea is to have your patient sniff a fresh alcohol prep pad.

Accumulation of Flatus (Gas)

Surgical intervention, mechanical obstruction, and accidental injury to the intestinal tract can cause disturbances in the passage of material. Whenever ingested material cannot pass through the intestinal tract as it should, the material accumulates in the stomach and the intestines. Pressure and distention occur when peristalsis is decreased or the flow of chyme is inhibited by an obstruction. Flatus (gas) is formed by the action of digestive juices and bacteria on the ingested material, resulting in bloating.

Nursing Management. Assisting the patient to ambulate has traditionally been the nursing intervention for sluggish peristalsis or bloating. This works for some patients, but others continue to have discomfort. If the physician will permit it, a slight Trendelenburg's position can be useful in speeding the expulsion of gas. Placing the buttocks and legs higher than the trunk and head causes gas to rise toward the rectum, making it easier to expel flatus. For patients who do not have abdominal incisions, massaging the abdomen gently is helpful. Work up the right side, across, and down over the left colon to move gas toward the rectum. Use both hands, placing the left hand behind the right after moving the gas along the bowel before lifting the right hand. This helps prevent gas from moving backward. Advise the patient to avoid chilled or hot drinks as these may create more gas. Antiflatulent medications that contain simethicone, such as Phazyme, are helpful if the patient is not NPO. The physician may order the insertion of a rectal tube or a rectal suppository to help the patient move the gas out of the intestine.

 Patient Teaching

Exercise to Reduce Gas and Bloating

Teach the patient experiencing bloating and excessive gas the following exercise unless contraindicated:
- Lie on your back with your legs extended and a pillow under your knees.
- Slowly raise your right leg, bend the knee, and bring the leg down toward the abdomen.
- Hold this position for a count of 10, then slowly lower your leg back down to the bed.
- Take three slow deep breaths and repeat the exercise with the left leg.
- When you feel the need to expel gas, do so; do not hold back.
- Repeat the exercise three or four times with each leg. Perform the exercise several times a day with rest periods between the exercise periods.

 Think Critically

Can you teach a patient three ways to prevent the occurrence of excessive gas postoperatively?

Constipation

When constipation occurs, the stool is hard, dry, and difficult to pass. There may be a bloated feeling, and defecation may be painful. Consistency of stool is greatly influenced by the type of food eaten and the quantity of liquid consumed. A diet low in fiber or inadequate fluid intake predisposes to constipation. Physical inactivity, ignoring the gastrocolic reflex, stress, and some neurologic disorders affecting the nerves in the intestinal tract also may contribute to constipation. Opioid medications can also contribute to constipation by slowing peristalsis. A new drug, methylnaltrexone bromide (Relistor), is available for patients with advanced illness who are receiving opiates for palliative care and who are not responding to laxatives.

Besides not passing stool regularly, signs and symptoms of constipation include hypoactive bowel sounds, abdominal distention, a firm abdomen, and abdominal discomfort or pain.

 Elder Care Points

Constipation is a problem among many people over age 60. Decreased GI motility, lack of exercise, limited fluid intake, and constipating medications taken for various conditions all contribute. In the very elderly, difficulty getting to the bathroom and suppression of the defecation urge may also contribute to the problem. Reliance on laxatives is common among the elderly, and is to be discouraged. Counsel individual patients about ways to increase dietary fiber and encourage fluid intake of at least 2500 mL/day, if not contraindicated by the presence of cardiac or renal disease.

Nursing Management. The first step is to identify the cause of constipation. Initial treatment may include a rectal suppository or enema to induce evacuation, or the administration of a laxative. A stool softener may be prescribed. Fiber and liquids are increased in the diet. If this does not resolve the problem, the patient is placed on one of the bulk-forming laxatives to be used daily, such as Metamucil. If the patient has become impacted with stool, digital extraction may be needed. The patient may be medicated with a mild analgesic 30 to 60 minutes before impaction removal to decrease the discomfort of the procedure and an oil retention enema usually is given. Then the nurse applies a lubricant, such as K-Y jelly or the anesthetic lubricant lidocaine (Xylocaine) jelly, into the rectum and around the anus and, using a gloved finger, breaks up and removes the feces.

Counsel the patient to add lots of raw fruits and vegetables to the diet, to eat more whole-grain cereals and breads, add bran to the diet, and drink lots of fluids. Fruit juices are particularly helpful as they contain fructose, which is a natural laxative. Help the patient to design an acceptable exercise program, such as walking, bicycling, running, swimming, or active sports participation. Advise her to heed the urge to defecate without delay.

? Think Critically

Can you list six foods high in fiber that a patient might add to the diet to combat constipation?

Diarrhea

The frequent passage of liquid or semiliquid stool is called *diarrhea.* It occurs with a variety of illnesses, food poisoning, excessive stress, and inflammation of the bowel. Mild diarrhea is not treated. If diarrhea persists for more than 24 to 48 hours or the number of stools is so excessive that great quantities of fluid are lost, treatment should begin. Signs and symptoms include multiple liquid or semiliquid bowel movements, hyperactive bowel sounds, and abdominal cramping.

Antidiarrheal agents such as diphenoxylate hydrochloride (Lomotil), loperamide hydrochloride (Imodium), tincture of opium (paregoric), or a combination product, such as Kaopectate, are administered (see Table 30-1). If the diarrhea is severe, nothing is given by mouth until it subsides. If diarrhea is moderate, only clear liquids are permitted by mouth. Severe, long-term diarrhea may require the use of total parenteral nutrition. When diarrhea is caused by infection, stool cultures and antibiotics may be necessary. As the condition improves, the diet is advanced.

 Complementary and Alternative Therapies

Probiotics for Infectious Diarrhea

When probiotics ("friendly" bacteria that are normally present in the intestinal tract) are used in conjunction with rehydration therapy, risk for diarrhea and duration of diarrhea are reduced (Yantis, 2009).

 Nutrition Considerations

Foods that Thicken Stool

When a patient has severe diarrhea and is allowed to resume solids foods, slowly introduce foods that help to thicken the stool, including applesauce, pretzels, bananas, white rice, white toast, or yogurt.

Nursing Management. For patients with diarrhea, monitor intake and output and assess the amount of fluid lost in the stool, measuring it if needed. Administer ordered medications and replace lost fluids. Monitor the patient for electrolyte imbalances and watch for signs of dehydration, such as decreased skin turgor, thick oral secretions, and decreased urine output. Taking small amounts of an electrolyte replacement solution, or Gatorade, helps prevent imbalances. Avoiding coffee or tea helps, as caffeine is a gastric stimulant and increases peristalsis. Thorough hand hygiene is essential when caring for the patient, and Standard Precautions are followed (see Appendix B). When infection is the cause of the diarrhea, follow contact precautions to prevent spread of the infection.

Taking warm sitz baths may relieve soreness and discomfort in the tissues, help cleanse the area, and avoid excessive wiping. Keeping the patient clean and dry is a high priority. Relieving odor in the room may be done with a deodorizing spray and by emptying and cleaning bedpans and commodes quickly.

Clinical Cues

Frequent, loose bowel movements cause rectal irritation. Instruct or assist the patient to apply a lubricant such as A&D ointment, Desitin ointment, or petroleum jelly to protect the skin and promote comfort.

Bowel Training

Severe illness, trauma, neurologic damage, or prolonged bed rest may bring about bowel incontinence. This is very embarrassing for the alert patient. The nurse must make every effort to keep the patient clean and dry. Tracking the time of incontinent movements and offering toileting after each meal may help eliminate the problem. Should incontinence be persistent, the cause should be identified and then a bowel training program instituted. For bowel training, the patient should be in a private environment 20 to 40 minutes after a meal and assume a normal sitting position for defecation if possible, or a side-lying position if bedridden. The nurse or patient performs digital stimulation by gently inserting and rotating a gloved, well-lubricated finger into the rectal sphincter. This action should be done on a regular basis to mimic the patient's normal bowel pattern. A warm drink or prune juice may also help to stimulate the bowels. Consistency and patience are vital to the success of retraining the bowel. In accordance with National Patient Safety Goals, encourage safety and instruct your patient to call for help in getting to and from the toilet. Reassure the patient that calling for help ensures safety and provides an opportunity to observe the progress of the training program.

Get Ready for the NCLEX® Examination!

Key Points

- Peristalsis moves food through the GI tract.
- The process by which the nutrients are used in the body after digestion and absorption is called *metabolism*.
- *Anabolism* is the building of body tissues from the nutrients. *Catabolism* is the breakdown of larger molecules into smaller molecules so that energy is available.
- The gallbladder stores bile and can be removed without harm to the body.
- The pancreas provides enzymes for digestion and insulin, and daily replacement of these substances must occur if the pancreas is removed. The secretion of lipase from the pancreas decreases with age, altering fat digestion.
- Problems of the GI system include infection, inflammation, trauma, and structural defects. Continued irritation and inflammation of the GI mucosa can lead to intestinal bleeding and increased peristalsis with inadequate absorption of nutrients.
- Immunization for hepatitis A and B prevents liver disease. Hepatitis B and C are risk factors for liver cancer.
- Controlling alcohol consumption helps prevent cirrhosis of the liver and pancreatitis.
- If damage to the liver is halted before all tissue is affected, the liver can regenerate.
- Check urine color for darkness (color of tea) and check stool for whitish or clay color; these findings suggest that the bile ducts may be blocked.
- Taste and smell diminish with age, and the gradual loss of these senses may decrease appetite. Poor dentition may make eating difficult for the elderly person. Medications can affect appetite and digestion.
- Ambulation and oral simethicone are helpful in reducing gas.
- Severe diarrhea can cause fluid and electrolyte imbalances and dehydration.
- Increasing fiber, fluids, and exercise helps prevent or relieve constipation.
- Bowel training is designed to mimic and restore the patient's normal bowel pattern.

Additional Learning Resources

SG Go to your Study Guide for additional learning activities to help you master this chapter content.

evolve Go to your Evolve website (http://evolve.elsevier.com/deWit/medsurg) for the following FREE learning resources:
- Animations, audio, and video
- Answers and rationales for questions and activities
- Concept Map Creator
- Glossary with pronunciations in English and Spanish
- Interactive Review Questions and Exercises and more!

 Online Resources
- Standard and Transmission-Based Precautions, www.cdc.gov/hicpac/2007IP/2007ip_part1.html#2
- Cleveland Clinic: Gastrointestinal Disorders, http://my.clevelandclinic.org
- National Digestive Diseases Information Clearinghouse (NDDIC): Constipation, http://digestive.niddk.nih.gov

Review Questions for the NCLEX® Examination

1. The nurse is planning care for several patients who had diagnostic testing. Which patient will require the most time for postprocedural care?
   1. Patient had an ultrasound
   2. Patient had hepatobiliary scintigraphy
   3. Patient had a liver biopsy
   4. Patient had a *Helicobacter pylori* antibody test

2. A decreased secretion of intrinsic factor is a physiologic change associated with the aging process; therefore an elderly patient with decreased intrinsic factor is likely to demonstrate which behavior?
   1. A refusal to eat salty or sweet foods
   2. A change in stools after eating fatty foods
   3. Fatigue and activity intolerance
   4. Difficulties with mastication

3. The nurse is preparing a patient for a gastrointestinal diagnostic procedure. Which nursing intervention would promote the psychological well-being of the patient?
   1. Applying skin barrier ointments to prevent breakdown
   2. Attending to patient's fears and anxiety
   3. Providing oral care
   4. Assessing for dehydration and electrolyte imbalance

4. During abdominal assessment, the nurse auscultates the abdomen before palpation or percussion. What is the most accurate explanation for the nurse's action?
   1. "The sequence prevents abdominal guarding."
   2. "The sequence is necessary to accurately assess the presence of peristalsis."
   3. "The sequence reduces patient anxiety during the examination."
   4. "The sequence is performed to prevent abdominal tenderness."

5. A patient is consuming large quantities of laxative fluid as part of the bowel preparation for a diagnostic procedure. Which side effect is most likely to occur?
   1. Constipation
   2. Rashes
   3. Dehydration
   4. Chest pains

6. A 30-year-old woman is admitted with complaints of severe nausea and vomiting over the past 2 days. On admission she is hypotensive and extremely weak. What is the priority nursing diagnosis?
   1. Ineffective breathing pattern
   2. Activity intolerance
   3. Deficient fluid volume
   4. Decreased cardiac output

7. The nurse emphasizes the importance of eating natural sources of fiber to a patient who has frequent constipation. Which patient statement indicates effective health teaching?
   1. "I will consider eating more white bread."
   2. "Drink fluids only while consuming meals."
   3. "I will add more milk to my morning cereal."
   4. "I will eat more fruits and vegetables."

8. The nurse discusses healthy lifestyle measures with a group of older adults during a senior seminar. What instruction(s) should the nurse include as accurate information? (Select all that apply.)
   1. Consume sufficient fiber.
   2. Eat a normal, well-balanced diet.
   3. Exercise regularly.
   4. Drink at least three glasses of fluids.
   5. Take laxatives regularly.

9. An elderly woman of Puerto Rican descent is admitted for persistent anorexia and dehydration. There are no apparent underlying organic causes for loss of appetite. Which intervention(s) would be culturally appropriate? (Select all that apply.)
   1. Determine food preferences.
   2. Encourage family visits.
   3. Provide small amounts of food and fluid frequently.
   4. Consider parenteral nutrition.
   5. Consult dietitian and speech therapy.

10. A patient with vomiting and diarrhea needs intravenous fluid therapy. The physician orders an infusion of normal saline to infuse 1000 mL over 8 hours. The drip factor is 10 gtt/mL. Calculate the drops per minute to infuse per _____ gravity.

Critical Thinking Activities

Scenario A
Mr. Bruns, 66 years old, was admitted with jaundice, abdominal distention, abdominal pain, and malaise. He is to undergo an ERCP. He is apprehensive and frightened about what may be wrong with him.

1. What is involved in an ERCP procedure?
2. Explain pretest care to help alleviate Mr. Bruns' apprehensions.
3. What is included in the post-test care?
4. What could be possible causes of his jaundice?

Scenario B

Ms. O'Malley is a resident in your extended care facility. She has been losing weight, has no appetite, and is becoming more withdrawn. Her daughter has a new job and is not able to visit as many times a week as she had been.

1. What assessments would you think appropriate for Ms. O'Malley at this time?

2. What nursing interventions could you institute that might improve her nutritional status?

3. What could you do to help her loneliness now that her daughter cannot visit as often?

Scenario C

You are making home visits to an elderly patient to check his blood pressure. During the visit he tells you that he is having trouble with constipation.

1. What questions should you ask to further assess the problem?

2. Why is constipation a common problem for people over age 60?

3. Would you recommend the use of an over-the-counter laxative? Why or why not?

4. What dietary and lifestyle recommendations would you make?

Care of Patients with Disorders of the Upper Gastrointestinal System

Objectives

Theory

1. Discuss obesity and its management, including bariatric surgery.
2. Compare the signs and symptoms of oral, esophageal, and stomach cancer.
3. Illustrate the cause of gastroesophageal reflux disease (GERD).
4. Explain the etiology and prognosis for Barrett's esophagus.
5. Describe the pathophysiology, means of medical diagnosis, and treatment for gastritis.
6. Compare and contrast the treatment and nursing care of the patient with GERD and a patient with a peptic ulcer.
7. Review the difference in the care of the patient with a nasogastric tube for decompression and care of the patient with a feeding tube.

8. Compare the care for a patient receiving total parenteral nutrition with care of the patient receiving enteral feedings.

Clinical Practice

1. Implement a teaching plan for a patient who has GERD.
2. Plan postoperative care for a patient having gastric surgery.
3. Demonstrate proper care of the patient with a Salem sump tube for gastric decompression.
4. Manage a tube feeding for the patient receiving formula via a feeding pump.
5. Review a nursing care plan for the patient with a gastrointestinal disorder.

Key Terms

achlorhydria (ă-chlŏr-HĪ-drē-ă, p. 657)
anastomosis (ă-năs-tŏ-MŌ-sĭs, p. 656)
bariatric (BĀ-rē-ĂT-rĭk, p. 641)
dumping syndrome (DŬM-pĭng SĬN-drŏm p. 642)
dyspepsia (dĭs-PĔP-sē-ă, p. 646)
dysphagia (dĭs-FĀ-jē-ă, p. 643)

Helicobacter pylori (p. 649)
hematemesis (hē-mă-TĔM-ĕ-sĭs, p. 651)
melena (mĕ-LĒ-nă, p. 655)
roux-en-Y (roo-ĕn-WĪ, p. 642)
stomatitis (stō-mă-TĪ-tĭs, p. 643)
vagotomy (vă-GŎT-ŏ-mē, p. 656)

EATING DISORDERS

ANOREXIA NERVOSA

Anorexia nervosa is classified as a psychological disorder (see Chapter 46), but it has serious nutritional consequences. In many contemporary cultures, the emphasis on a slim body has influenced young women's body image. The patient with anorexia nervosa refuses to eat adequate quantities of food and is in danger of literally starving to death. Although it is a psychiatric disorder, the patient may be admitted to the medical floor for treatment of malnutrition by enteral or parenteral therapy. Diagnosis requires extensive interviewing and treatment—including behavior modification and nutrition support—which may take months to years.

BULIMIA NERVOSA

Bulimia nervosa is another psychological disorder covered in Chapter 46. The bulimic patient consumes large quantities of food and then induces vomiting to get rid

of it so that weight is not gained. Laxatives may be taken to purge the system after an eating binge. Some patients with anorexia nervosa also are bulimic. Some individuals practice bulimia occasionally, without harm. When it is practiced frequently, it can lead to severe fluid and electrolyte imbalances, starvation, and death. Treatment of bulimia includes psychotherapy, antidepressant medication, and behavior modification.

OBESITY

Obesity is a worldwide problem, and is particularly prevalent in industrialized nations. Over two thirds of adults in the United States are overweight or obese, and over one third are obese. In the United States, obesity is associated with over 112,000 deaths related to cardiovascular disease, 15,000 deaths due to cancer, and over 35,000 deaths from other causes related to being overweight (Weight-Control Information Network, 2010). Children are showing a trend for increasing obesity. There is an ongoing search to see if there is a genetic predisposition to this disorder. Prevention of obesity and encouraging healthy and nutrition dense foods are goals of *Healthy People 2020.*

Etiology and Pathophysiology

Several factors must interact for obesity to occur, including genetics, a diet of foods high in calories and fat, lack of exercise, and overconsumption of food. Some medications increase appetite. Known contributors to obesity include readily available high-calorie prepackaged and high-fat fast food, plus "supersized" portions available in restaurants.

For some people overeating is a reaction to stress; for others overeating is a substitute for absent pleasures. Some obese people seem to metabolize nutrients differently than others. The way a person develops fat cells and deposits fat is another factor in obesity. Genetic predisposition is most likely a factor since obesity seems to occur among family members.

Signs and Symptoms

A person is considered obese if he weighs more than 20% above the ideal weight for his height, age, and body type. Approximately 3 million Americans are *morbidly obese,* defined as 100% over ideal body weight, or having a body mass index over 40.

Obese patients should be counseled to lose weight in order to avoid developing one or more of the many diseases in which obesity is a contributing factor. Complications of obesity include:

- Diabetes mellitus
- Hypertension
- Hyperlipidemia
- Coronary artery disease
- Obstructive sleep apnea
- Cholelithiasis
- Arthritis with back and/or knee problems
- Increased susceptibility to infectious disease and decreased wound healing.

? Think Critically

You have a friend who is overweight and she asks your opinion about the effectiveness and safety of over-the-counter "diet" pills. How would you respond?

Diagnosis

To determine whether a patient is obese, the following measurements are used:

- Height and weight chart: if more than 20% above ideal body weight for age and body build, the patient is considered obese.
- Measure the waist and then the hip circumference. Calculate the waist-to-hip ratio (waist measurement divided by the hip measurement). If the ratio is more than 1.0 in men or 0.8 in women, it indicates that the person is overweight. This is a more accurate indicator for obesity in the elderly.

- A body mass index (BMI) of more than 30 indicates obesity.

$$BMI = \frac{Weight\ (kg)}{Height\ (m^2)}$$

Thyroid function should be determined to ascertain that hypothyroidism is not a cause of the weight gain.

Treatment

A general health assessment should be conducted before a patient is placed on a weight reduction diet. A physician will usually prescribe a lower-calorie diet and exercise. The patient is taught ways to change thinking about food and weight. Those with a BMI over 40 may have surgery to achieve weight reduction if they meet established criteria. Participation in a support group and behavior modification with some sort of reward for weight loss are part of the total treatment plan. Teaching stress reduction and alternate ways of coping are essential to success. Medications that suppress appetite or block fat absorption may be used on a short-term basis. Sibutramine (Meridia) is the commonly used appetite suppressant. It is a selective serotonin reuptake inhibitor, which enhances the feeling of fullness when eating; sibutramine can be combined with norepinephrine, which increases the metabolic rate, thereby burning more calories. Side effects of sibutramine include dry mouth, insomnia, and constipation. Orlistat (Xenical) inhibits lipase, causing fats to remain partially undigested and unabsorbed. Gastrointestinal side effects of orlistat include diarrhea (sometimes uncontrolled), abdominal cramping, and nausea.

🍂 Elder Care Points

The elderly may become obese due to decreased mobility from arthritis or other joint disorders. Cooking and eating are less appealing if the person is living alone, and snacking on junk food may replace meals. Metabolic rate slows with age, and a decreased calorie intake is needed to maintain a normal weight.

Bariatric Surgery. Bariatric surgery reduces gastric capacity. The patient undergoes extensive counseling and assessment. The patient must agree to modify his lifestyle and follow the stringent regimen required to lose weight and keep weight off. Three common types of bariatric surgery are gastric restrictive, malabsorptive, and gastric restrictive combined with malabsorptive surgery.

Restrictive procedures. *Laparoscopic adjustable gastric banding* is performed by placing an inflatable band around the fundus of the stomach. This procedure may be performed laparoscopically. The band is inflated and deflated via a subcutaneous port to change the size of the stomach as the patient loses weight. For *vertical banded gastroplasty,* the surgeon creates a small stomach pouch by placing a vertical line of staples. A band is placed to provide an outlet to the small intestine (Figure 29-1).

Malabsorptive and combination procedures. The total gastric bypass procedure causes severe nutritional deficiencies and is no longer recommended. The roux-en-Y gastric bypass (RYGB) limits the stomach size, and the duodenum and part of the jejunum are bypassed. This limits the absorption of calories.

> **? Think Critically**
>
> What impact on nutritional status might a roux-en-Y bypass have on an individual? Why? What might be the physical long-term consequences?

Complications. With the RYGB procedure, there is danger of leakage of stomach contents into the abdomen in the early postoperative period. Later, gastric stretching may cause the staple line to break and a leak to occur. Signs and symptoms are tachycardia, dyspnea, or restlessness. An upper gastrointestinal (GI) series or computed tomography scan can diagnose the problem. The band in the vertical banding procedure may erode into the stomach over time and cause leakage. RYGB patients are also at risk for dumping syndrome, which results in nausea, weakness, sweating, and diarrhea. Other complications of major surgery may occur in the respiratory and cardiovascular systems (see Chapter 5 for complications of surgery). There is greater risk of pulmonary dysfunction, thrombus formation, and death, for the obese patient. About a third of patients who undergo bariatric surgery develop gallstones. Urso-deoxycholic acid therapy can be used to treat the gallstones, although poor compliance and cost are issues for this therapy (Patel et al., 2009).

All bariatric surgery patients are at risk of nutritional deficiencies. Those with the RYGB procedure are most likely to develop deficiencies of iron, vitamin B_{12}, calcium, and folate. Supplements must be taken for life.

❖ NURSING MANAGEMENT

▪ Assessment (Data Collection)

Data collection includes establishing whether there is a family history of obesity, determining contributing factors, and obtaining an accurate record of eating patterns for a 7-day period. Physical assessment includes measuring weight and height, calculating BMI, and taking a skinfold thickness measurement. A general health assessment is performed.

▪ Nursing Diagnosis and Planning

Examples of nursing diagnoses relevant to the care of obese patients include:
- Disturbed body image related to excess weight
- Imbalance nutrition more than body requirements related to high fat diet
- Chronic low self-esteem related to excess weight

Goals should be long term, and expected outcomes might include:
- Patient will make positive statements about decreasing body size.

Gastric bypass

Vertical banded gastroplasty

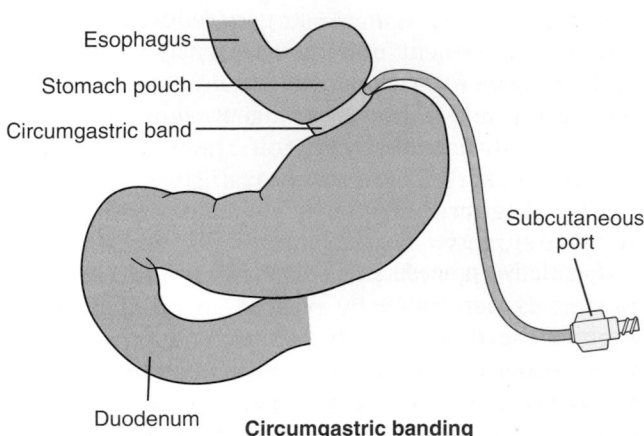

Circumgastric banding

FIGURE 29-1 Bariatric surgical procedures.

- Patient will consume less fatty food and more fruit and vegetables.
- Patient will verbalize feelings of self-worth.

■ Implementation

The diet and exercise plan should be designed according to the patient's lifestyle and preferences. Encourage the patient to keep an eating and exercise diary. Weekly meetings for counseling and evaluation are important to provide guidance. Offer support by being available to talk about the positive aspects and frustrations of staying on the diet. Discourage fad diets and emphasize the importance of a well-balanced, nutritious, low-calorie diet. Commercial programs are available to assist patients with weight reduction. Weight Watchers and TOPS (Take Off Pounds Sensibly) are two commercial programs that have shown good long-term results with maintenance of normal weight.

Preoperative and postoperative care for the bariatric surgery patient depends on the type of surgical procedure performed, but general principles are similar to other types of abdominal or abdominal laparoscopic surgery. Because of the weight and size of the client, lifting apparatus must be available as well as an extra-wide bed and chair. Hospitalization may be for 1 to 5 days depending on the procedure and the patient. If a nasogastric (NG) tube is in place, do not reposition it, as you might disrupt the suture line. Feedings are designed in consultation with a dietitian; you would anticipate feeding progression in the early postoperative period, then onto multiple small meals, a balanced meal plan, and possibly parenteral nutrition (PN) in high-risk patients (National Clearinghouse Guidelines, 2009). For example, feedings begin with 1 ounce of clear liquid at a time, advancing to pureed foods, juice, thinned soups, and milk. The diet is increased in 1-ounce increments taken over 5 minutes until the patient's appetite is satisfied. The diet is maintained for 6 weeks and then progressed to regular foods. Nausea, vomiting, and discomfort may occur, especially if too many liquids are ingested. The patient remains under medical supervision to monitor for vitamin deficiency or malnutrition.

■ Evaluation

The patient's diet and exercise diary should be evaluated each week if possible. Weight is tracked on a graph to show progress in weight loss. If the outcomes are not being met, the plan's interventions must be reconsidered.

UPPER GASTROINTESTINAL DISORDERS

STOMATITIS

Stomatitis is a generalized inflammation of the mucous membranes of the mouth. Causes include trauma from ill-fitting dentures or malocclusions of the teeth, poor oral hygiene, and nutritional deficiencies. Excessive smoking, excessive drinking of alcohol, pathogenic microorganisms, radiation therapy, and drugs (especially those used in chemotherapy for malignancies and anticonvulsants) are other contributors to the problem.

Common symptoms of stomatitis include pain and swelling of the oral mucosa, increased salivation or excessive dryness, severe halitosis, and sometimes fever. Small crater-like aphthous ulcers may appear in the mouth, commonly called "canker sores."

Treatment of stomatitis is chiefly symptomatic, unless a specific infectious causative agent is identified. Nursing measures to control the symptoms of stomatitis—including special mouth care, artificial saliva, and diet—are discussed in Chapter 8.

 Complementary and Alternative Therapies

Lysine for Canker Sores

Many people who develop "canker sores" from food sensitivities or stomach upset often can heal them more quickly by taking the dietary supplement lysine three or four times a day. This often helps cut the time of a "fever blister" on the lips as well (Dugdale, 2009).

DYSPHAGIA

Dysphagia means difficulty in swallowing. It is the most common symptom of disorders of the esophagus and varies from a mild sensation that something is sticking in the throat, to a complete inability to swallow solids or liquids. Tumors, esophageal diverticula, inflammation, or motility disorders from a neurologic disorder may cause swallowing problems. If the patient is experiencing choking or difficulty with swallowing, he is kept on nothing-by-mouth (NPO) status. A modified barium swallow test is ordered to determine the specific cause. Videofluoroscopy is used during the test to visualize the swallowing process.

Treatment and Nursing Management

Have the patient take some "practice swallows" before beginning the meal. Watch to see that the larynx rises with each swallow. Observe the kinds of food the patient can tolerate and the conditions under which difficulties are experienced. Knowing the consistency and temperature of the foods most easily ingested by the patient is helpful. Some patients may strangle on liquids, but will tolerate soft and semisolid foods. Others may have the feeling that high-fiber foods are not moving past a certain point in the esophagus. Measures that may be helpful in relieving dysphagia include instructing the patient to chew the food more thoroughly or to eat semisoft or pureed foods. Drinking liquids throughout the meal may help; however, **liquids will cause many patients to choke. If thin liquids are a problem, adding thickener to liquids makes them easier to swallow.** Sitting upright with the head forward and the neck flexed with the chin slightly tucked aids in swallowing. Head position may be altered, depending on the particular type of problem present. A speech pathologist should be consulted to design the most effective therapy for the patient.

The patient may be a candidate for neuromuscular electrical stimulation (NMES). One type of NMES device stimulates muscle at rest, to compensate for muscle wasting. Another NMES device is used for patients who have swallowing issues related to neurologic disorders such as stroke. Some helpful strategies to improve swallowing include licking lollipops to strengthen tongue movements, practicing vowel sounds to stimulate movement, and sucking or blowing through a straw to strengthen the soft palate (Nazarko, 2010). Meals should be served in a relaxing atmosphere with pleasant surroundings and relief from emotional stress.

Nursing diagnoses for patient with swallowing problems are:

- Impaired swallowing
- Risk for imbalanced nutrition: less than body requirements
- Risk for aspiration

 Elder Care Points

The older patient may have experienced a stroke that has impaired swallowing ability. Swallowing pills is a frequent difficulty for this age group. Instruct the elderly patient to take a drink of water, swallow, place the pill on the back of the tongue, take another drink of water, tuck the chin down slightly and swallow; follow by drinking at least 6 to 8 ounces of water.

Patients with chronic dysphagia are subject to respiratory problems resulting from the aspiration of food into the respiratory tree. Both acute and chronic dysphagia are likely to produce nutritional deficiencies and electrolyte imbalances. If the dysphagia is such that the patient cannot swallow sufficient amounts of food for adequate nutrition, tube feeding may be indicated. This sometimes is necessary when the dysphagia is the result of cerebral damage, as in cerebrovascular accident.

 Clinical Cues

When your patient has a swallowing problem, the oral suction equipment should always be readily available. Aspiration of food or mucus can occur quickly. The patient or family should be taught how to quickly use the oral suction apparatus (Yankauer).

If the patient cannot swallow anything because of a neurologic condition (see Chapters 22 and 24), or if the esophagus is obstructed and cannot be corrected surgically, the patient must have a gastrostomy. An opening in the wall of the stomach is created, and a permanent

feeding tube is sutured in place. Nursing interventions for feeding tubes are discussed later in this chapter.

CANCER OF THE ORAL CAVITY

Etiology, Pathophysiology, and Signs and Symptoms

In May 2010, there were approximately 25,800 new cases of oral cancer in the United States (American Cancer Society, 2010). Although the specific cause is unknown, oral or throat cancer is curable if discovered early. Cell mutation occurs until an area of cells becomes neoplastic. A genetic factor is most likely present. Oral and pharyngeal cancer risks are cigarette smoking, use of smokeless tobacco, pipe smoking, and heavy alcohol use. The human papillomavirus is another risk factor. Leukoplakia, a precancerous lesion, may occur on the tongue or mucosa. Dental examinations should include inspection for this lesion. Sores or discolorations on the lips or in the mouth that do not heal within 2 weeks should be checked by a physician.

Diagnosis and Treatment

Diagnosis is made by physical examination and biopsy. Oral cancer treatment varies depending on the structures involved. Radiation, chemotherapy, and surgery are treatment options. *Mandibulectomy* (removal of the mandible), *hemiglossectomy* (removal of half of the tongue), or *glossectomy* (removal of the tongue) with resection of other parts of the mouth may be necessary. If the cancer has spread to the cervical lymph nodes, radical or modified neck dissection is performed. This surgery involves wide excision of the primary tumor with removal of the regional lymph nodes, the deep cervical lymph nodes, and lymph channels. A tracheostomy accompanies these procedures to protect the airway (see Chapter 14). A drain is placed to prevent fluid accumulation. Tube feedings are used as long as swallowing is difficult.

Nursing Management

Postoperative care includes close monitoring of respiratory status, airway, and oxygenation. Cold packs and elevation of the head are used to prevent excessive swelling in the neck that might compress the airway, circulation, and nerves. Aseptic wound care and tracheostomy care are provided. Nutritional support is an ongoing concern and is very important in the healing process. Many of these patients are malnourished before surgery. See Chapter 8 for the specific care of the cancer patient undergoing radiation and/or chemotherapy.

 Think Critically

You are caring for a young woman who was recently informed that she would need surgery and radiation treatment for oral cancer. What are the implications for her sense of body image and psychological well-being?

CANCER OF THE ESOPHAGUS

Etiology and Pathophysiology

Cigarette smoking is a major cause of esophageal cancer in the United States. When combined with heavy alcohol consumption, the risk for esophageal cancer greatly increases. Both substances are irritants to the mucosa of the esophagus. Cigarettes and smokeless tobacco are responsible for 14,530 deaths from esophageal cancer annually (American Cancer Society, 2009a). The cancer is usually well advanced when discovered. The tumor is either adenocarcinoma or squamous cell cancer.

Gastroesophageal reflux disease (GERD) is a cause of Barrett's esophagus, which is a precancerous condition. One percent of patients with Barrett's esophagus eventually develop esophageal cancer (Mayo Clinic Health Letter, 2010). The cellular changes caused by irritation of the stomach fluids may eventually become malignant.

Signs, Symptoms, and Diagnosis

Signs and symptoms may include progressive dysphagia, a feeling of fullness in the throat, regurgitation of foods, or foul breath. At first the dysphagia only occurs with meat, but then with soft foods and eventually even with liquids. Pain occurs late in the disease and is substernal, epigastric, or in the back and occurs with swallowing. Weight loss is typical. Barium swallow with fluoroscopy may show a narrowed esophagus. Definitive diagnosis is by esophagogastroduodenoscopy (EGD) and biopsy.

 Think Critically

A 76-year-old Chinese man complains of progressive difficulty swallowing and fullness of the throat. When making clinical decisions, what would be the most effective approach for this patient?

Treatment

Care of the patient with Barrett's esophagus is focused on encouraging measures to prevent GERD and on regular checkups. Patients should be encouraged not to use tobacco products and not to indulge in heavy alcohol use.

 Think Critically

If a patient who smokes is awaiting surgery for esophageal cancer, is it appropriate to prevent him from smoking?

An esophagectomy, or removal of most of the esophagus, may be performed if cancer is localized just to the esophagus. Newer forms of treatments may be combined and include radiofrequency ablation (RFA), which uses bursts of radiofrequency energy to burn away abnormal cells; cryotherapy, which freezes abnormal cells and causes sloughing of dead tissues; photodynamic therapy, which uses a medication that causes damaged cells to be sensitive to light; and endoscopic mucosal resection, which is a procedure wherein a saline solution is injected under the abnormal tissue, which makes it easier to suction away (Mayo Clinic Health Letter, 2010). For patients who have advanced-stage cancer, palliative care includes the insertion of expanding metal stents or high-dose intraluminal brachytherapy (radiation source is placed internally near the abnormal tissue) to relieve severe dysphagia (Sreedharan et al., 2009).

Nursing Management

Postoperative care is the same as for any patient having thoracic or abdominal surgery. Maintaining a patent airway is the top priority. Nutrition is initially supplied by parenteral fluids. When bowel sounds return, small amounts of water are given orally every hour. Gradual progression to small, frequent, bland meals is the next step. The patient should be upright when eating to prevent regurgitation. Pain, increased temperature, and dyspnea may indicate leakage of the feeding into the mediastinum. Intolerance of food is evidenced by vomiting and abdominal distention. The patient may need a feeding tube for several weeks or a gastrostomy tube to sustain nutrition.

HIATAL HERNIA (DIAPHRAGMATIC HERNIA)

Etiology and Pathophysiology

Loss of muscle strength and tone, factors that cause increased intra-abdominal pressure (such as obesity or multiple pregnancies), and congenital defects contribute to the formation of a hiatal hernia. Hiatal hernia is the result of a defect in the wall of the diaphragm where the esophagus passes through; this creates protrusion of part of the stomach or the lower part of the esophagus up into the thoracic cavity. Women are more frequently affected with hiatal hernia than are men.

Signs and Symptoms

Signs and symptoms of hiatal hernia include indigestion, belching, and substernal or epigastric pain or feelings of pressure after eating caused by reflux of gastric fluid into the esophagus. The symptoms are more severe when the patient lies down.

Diagnosis and Treatment

Hiatal hernia is diagnosed by an upper GI series. Treatment includes weight reduction, avoidance of tight-fitting clothes around the abdomen, administration of antacids and histamine (H_2)-receptor antagonists, and elevation of the head of the bed on 6- to 8-inch blocks. If esophagitis is present, proton pump inhibitors are used. The patient is instructed not to eat within several hours of going to bed. Intake of alcohol, chocolate, caffeine, and fatty food is limited, and smoking should be avoided. Ingestion of fats relaxes the sphincter, allowing reflux (Pinto & Schub, 2009). Occasionally a patient with reflux esophagitis, which is caused by the hernia, may bleed extensively. If bleeding or discomfort cannot be controlled, surgical correction of the hernia is required.

Nursing Management

The patient with hiatal hernia is taught ways to prevent pain and reflux. If weight is above normal, encourage weight reduction. Remind the patient to stay upright for 2 hours after eating and not to eat for 3 hours before bedtime. Lifting or moving heavy items is to be avoided. If the head of the bed cannot be raised, a wedge pillow should be used to elevate the upper body; this position helps prevent reflux and assists gravity in maintaining the stomach in the abdominal cavity. Prescribed H$_2$-receptor antagonists or proton pump inhibitors should be taken at bedtime to prevent reflux and damage from acid entering the esophagus. The patient should avoid foods that cause bloating, which increases abdominal pressure. Increased abdominal pressure may push the stomach upward through the diaphragmatic defect.

GASTROESOPHAGEAL REFLUX DISEASE

Etiology and Pathophysiology

Gastroesophageal reflux disease (GERD) is a syndrome, not a disease. Ninety percent of patients with GERD have a hiatal hernia. GERD occurs equally in men and women. It is caused by transient relaxation of the lower esophageal sphincter. The relaxation allows fluids or food to reflux into the esophagus from the stomach. Delayed stomach emptying is another factor. Certain foods and medications contribute to this mechanical problem. Being overweight is common among patients with GERD. GERD may contribute to bronchoconstriction and asthma symptoms due to irritation of the upper airway by gastric secretions. About 75% of patients with asthma have GERD (Nazario, 2009).

Signs and Symptoms

Heartburn (dyspepsia) and reflux are the most common symptoms of GERD. Other symptoms may include chest pain, coughing, dysphagia, belching, flatulence, and bloating after eating. Some patients do not experience symptoms; for those who do, the symptoms are aggravated by lying down.

Diagnosis

GERD is diagnosed by EGD and sometimes barium esophagram. Occasionally, other tests such as an esophageal manometry, ambulatory 24-hour pH

monitoring, or radionuclide measurement of gastric emptying are performed. Esophageal manometry measures pressures in the esophagus; pressures will be increased during episodes of reflux. For 24-hour pH monitoring, a tiny tube with a transducer is introduced into the esophagus to take measurements of the esophageal pH.

Treatment and Nursing Management

Diet therapy, lifestyle changes, drug therapy, and education are the mainstays of GERD treatment. The diet should exclude foods that cause sphincter relaxation. Drug therapy may include antacids, H$_2$-receptor antagonists, proton pump inhibitors, and prokinetic drugs (Table 29-1). Check for drug interactions with other drugs the patient is taking. Verify that the patient can afford the drugs prescribed, as some are very expensive.

 Patient Teaching

Measures to Decrease the Symptoms of GERD

DIETARY ALTERATIONS
- Avoid any food in the diet that increases gastric acid and causes pain.
- Avoid high-fat and spicy foods, including garlic.
- Do not eat large meals; instead, eat four to six small meals a day.
- Eat slowly and chew food thoroughly, and avoid using a straw for liquids to decrease belching and reflux.
- Avoid carbonated beverages as they increase bloating.
- Eliminate or limit alcohol, tomato-based products, caffeine, citrus juice, raw onions, chocolate, peppermint, and spearmint from the diet. These foods either relax the esophageal sphincter or increase acid production.

LIFESTYLE ALTERATIONS
- Wait 2 to 3 hours after eating before lying down.
- Do not wear clothes that constrict around the middle of the body.
- If overweight, lose the extra pounds; a 10% weight loss can decrease symptoms considerably.
- Sleep with the head of the bed elevated 4 to 6 inches with blocks or a foam bolster pillow.
- Take medications as directed in relationship to meals and bedtime.
- Stop smoking as it may stimulate gastric acid secretion.
- Participate in regular stress-reducing activities such as exercise, meditation, deep breathing, and laughter.

 Safety Alert

Proton Pump Inhibitors and Cardiac Problems

The Food and Drug Administration (FDA) has issued a warning that long-term use of the proton pump inhibitors esomeprazole (Nexium) or omeprazole (Prilosec) may increase the risk of heart problems. Patients taking these drugs should consult their health care provider.

Table 29-1   Commonly Prescribed Drugs for Upper Gastrointestinal Disorders

CLASSIFICATION*	ACTION	NURSING IMPLICATIONS	PATIENT TEACHING
Antacids			
There are four antacid families consisting of compounds of aluminum, magnesium, calcium, and sodium. Gelusil, Maalox, Mylanta-II, Riopan, Di-Gel, Amphojel, Gaviscon	Neutralize stomach acid	Aluminum hydroxide compounds promote constipation, whereas magnesium hydroxide compounds promote diarrhea. Sodium compounds may adversely affect hypertension and heart failure. All antacids may adversely affect the dissolution and absorption of other drugs. One hour should be allowed between antacid administration and administration of another drug. Magnesium compounds are used cautiously in patients with renal insufficiency.	Antacids for treatment of peptic ulcer should be taken seven times a day: 1 hr and 3 hr after meals, and at bedtime. Separate from other drug administration by 2 hr. Shake liquid preparations well before pouring from container. Chew antacid tablets thoroughly, and follow with a glass of water or milk. Report problems of constipation or diarrhea to the physician. Take even after pain has disappeared; consult physician.
Histamine (H$_2$)-Receptor Antagonist			
Cimetidine (Tagamet) Famotidine (Pepcid) Nizatidine (Axid) Ranitidine (Zantac)	Suppress acid secretion by blocking H$_2$ receptors on parietal cells	Cimetidine may interact with many other drugs; check drug interactions for other drugs patient is receiving. Cimetidine may cause confusion and other CNS effects. Separate administration of these drugs and antacids by 1 hr. Monitor for decreased abdominal pain and ulcer symptoms.	These drugs should be taken with meals and at bedtime. Once-a-day dose should be taken at bedtime. Advise patient to avoid cigarettes, aspirin, and other NSAIDs. Advise to avoid alcohol or only consume it in moderation and only in conjunction with food. Advise to use stress-reduction techniques.
Proton Pump Inhibitors			
Omeprazole (Prilosec) Omeprazole and sodium bicarbonate (Zegerid) Lansoprazole (Prevacid) Dexlansoprazole (Kapidex)	Suppress secretion of gastric acid	May cause headache, nausea, vomiting, or diarrhea. Use is preferably limited to 4-8 wk.	Follow regimen of diet and stress reduction for ulcer healing.
Misoprostol (Cytotec)	Prevents gastric ulcers caused by long-term therapy with NSAIDs	May cause diarrhea or abdominal pain. Not safe during pregnancy.	
Rabeprazole (Aciphex)		Do not crush delayed-release tablets.	This is a slow-release preparation that acts throughout the day. Teach patient to wear sunscreen as drug may cause sun sensitivity.
Pantoprazole (Protonix)		Do not crush tablets.	A slow-release preparation.
Esomeprazole (Nexium)		Do not administer with digoxin, rabeprazole, or iron salts.	May affect absorption of digoxin, rabeprazole, and iron salts.
Miscellaneous			
Sucralfate (Carafate)	Sucralfate provides protective coating barrier over ulcer crater	Monitor for constipation.	Take only as directed. Wait 30 min before taking any other drug.

*Names of generic drugs are listed first, followed by the brand names of drugs in parentheses.

Continued

Table 29-1 **Commonly Prescribed Drugs for Upper Gastrointestinal Disorders—cont'd**

CLASSIFICATION	ACTION	NURSING IMPLICATIONS	PATIENT TEACHING
Antimicrobials			
Clarithromycin (Biaxin)	Suppresses protein synthesis in bacteria Used to kill *Helicobacter pylori*	Assess for drug allergy. Report hematuria or oliguria. Administer every 12 hr to maintain serum levels. Do not crush tablets. Monitor for diarrhea, abdominal pain, or signs of jaundice.	May cause diarrhea, anorexia, or nausea. Must be taken at regular intervals to be effective. Take the entire prescription. Taking acidophilus between doses may alleviate diarrhea. Increase fluid intake if diarrhea occurs.
Amoxicillin (Amoxil)	Causes cell wall of bacteria to swell and burst, preventing replication	Assess for drug sensitivity. Assess for side effects. Monitor renal function. Monitor for blood in stool and abdominal pain.	Take on an empty stomach with a full glass of water. Take at regular intervals around the clock to sustain blood levels. Take entire prescription.
Tetracycline	Bacteriostatic Inhibits protein synthesis in microorganism	Assess for drug sensitivity. Monitor CBC, liver, and kidney functions. Increases effect of warfarin and digoxin. Decreases effect of penicillin and oral contraceptives.	Do not take with dairy products or antacids; separate by 2 hr. Avoid sun exposure. Avoid using Clinistix, Diastix, or Tes-Tape for diabetic urine testing.
Metronidazole (Flagyl)	Kills amebas and *Trichomonas;* degrades DNA in organism	Do not give during second and third trimesters of pregnancy. Increases action of anticoagulants. Decreases action of phenobarbital and phenytoin. May cause toxicity if administered with cimetidine or lithium. Patient should have vision examination before and after therapy. Monitor for neurotoxicity. Discontinue if fever, chills, rash, or itching occurs.	Do not drink alcohol during or for 48 hr after therapy has ended. May cause severe vomiting and prostration. Urine may turn dark brown. Notify physician of numbness or tingling. Dizziness may occur; avoid hazardous activities. May cause dry mouth; chew sugarless gum or sip water frequently.
Antispasmodics			
Dicyclomine hydrochloride (Bentyl, Antispas) Propantheline bromide (Pro-Banthine)	Block acetylcholine, thereby decreasing smooth-muscle spasm and GI motility and inhibiting gastric acid secretion	These drugs interact with many other drugs; check each drug patient is taking for interactions. Most of these drugs are contraindicated in glaucoma, prostatic hypertrophy, myasthenia gravis, and other conditions; consult information on each drug individually. May predispose to drug-induced heat stroke. Monitor vital signs and urine output carefully.	Take 30-60 min before meal. Patient can suck on hard candy to relieve mouth dryness unless contraindicated. Drink 2500-3000 mL of fluid to prevent constipation. Avoid driving and hazardous activities if drug causes dizziness, sleepiness, or blurred vision. Report rash or skin eruption to physician.
Metoclopramide (Reglan)	Hastens gastric emptying and relaxes pyloric and duodenal segments of GI tract	Assess for neurologic or psychotropic side effects such as restlessness, anxiety, ataxia, or hallucinations. Not for long-term use.	Take before meals.

CBC, complete blood count; *CNS,* central nervous system; *GI,* gastrointestinal; *NSAIDs,* nonsteroidal anti-inflammatory drugs.

If these therapies do not control the problem, endoscopic noninvasive therapies often are effective. Laparoscopic surgical fundoplication—wherein the fundus of the stomach is wrapped around the esophagus to create a new valve junction (Figure 29-2)—is effective in 92% of patients (Fisichella & Patti, 2009). This is the same procedure used to correct a hiatal hernia.

? Think Critically

Many patients with GERD and hiatal hernia do not really modify their diet and lifestyle, over the long term; instead they rely on medications, which can be expensive, to decrease their symptoms. What measures could you use to show patients that lifestyle changes may control symptoms without medication?

Complications

Irritation results when stomach contents containing hydrochloric acid, pepsin, and other enzymes are refluxed into the esophagus. Constant irritation may cause cellular changes, such as the precancerous lesions in Barrett's esophagus. Reflux is also a risk factor for aspiration of stomach contents and pneumonitis. Acid reflux into the mouth, over time, may cause dental caries.

GASTROENTERITIS

Gastroenteritis is inflammation of the stomach and small intestine. It is caused by intake of food or water contaminated with a virus, a pathogenic bacteria, or parasites. The Norwalk virus is a common cause, as are *Giardia* and *Shigella*. Signs and symptoms of gastroenteritis include vomiting, diarrhea, abdominal cramping, and distention. Fever, elevated white blood cell count, and blood or mucus in the stool may occur. In healthy adults the disorder is self-limiting and does not require hospitalization. The young child, the elderly, and the chronically ill may need intravenous (IV) therapy to take in enough fluid to compensate for the fluid lost during gastroenteritis.

The gastroenteritis patient should be kept NPO until vomiting has stopped. When tolerated, fluids containing glucose and electrolytes should be started (Pedialyte, Gatorade). If diarrhea continues beyond 3 or 4 days, stool studies for the causative organism should be performed. Therapy to eradicate the causative agent can then be started. Rest is important during the course of the vomiting and diarrhea. After 24 to 48 hours, medication may be prescribed for the vomiting, abdominal cramping, and diarrhea.

🍎 Nutrition Considerations

Dietary Guidelines for the Patient with Vomiting

- Liquid diet for 12 to 24 hours. Frequent, small amounts of clear liquids are best.
- Avoid milk, ice cream, pudding, cheese, yogurt, citrus juice, and cream soups.
- Foods allowed on the liquid diet are electrolyte solutions, carbonated beverages, bouillon, unflavored gelatin, apple juice, peach or pear juice, plain hard candy, sugar, honey, sugar substitutes, and frozen Popsicles.
- When nausea and vomiting stop:
  - Add some of the following foods for the next 12 to 24 hours: soda crackers, toast and jelly without butter, tea, rice, pretzels, bananas, applesauce, cooked cream of wheat or cream of rice, and fruit or vegetable juice (BRATT diet: banana, rice, applesauce, tea, and toast).
  - If above diet is tolerated without further symptoms, add the following foods for the next 12 to 24 hours: potatoes (not fried), soups, soft eggs, custards, puddings, white turkey meat or white chicken meat, and cottage cheese.
  - If no further symptoms occur, resume a regular diet but avoid highly seasoned foods, greasy or fried foods, heavy fatty foods, excessively hot or cold foods, raw vegetables, coffee, colas, and milk products. Avoid those foods for 1 week after symptoms have stopped.

GASTRITIS

Etiology

The main cause of gastritis is *Helicobacter pylori* bacteria. Other contributors to acute gastritis are drinking excessive amounts of alcohol, infection from eating contaminated food, and ingestion of drugs, such as aspirin, ibuprofen, corticosteroids, or nonsteroidal anti-inflammatory drugs (NSAIDs).

Pathophysiology

Gastritis is not a disease; it is an acute or chronic inflammation of the mucous membrane lining the stomach. *Atrophic* gastritis involves all layers of the stomach. It is seen in association with gastric ulcer and malignancies of the stomach. Gastritis associated with uremia is common in the patient with kidney failure. The excessive urea that builds up from the kidney

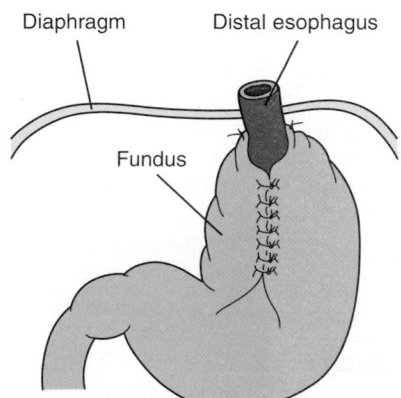

FIGURE 29-2 Nissen fundoplication surgery for hiatal hernia or to treat gastroesophageal reflux disease.

failure causes gastric irritation. Untreated chronic gastritis may progress to ulcer formation and upper GI hemorrhage.

Signs, Symptoms, and Diagnosis

In both acute and chronic gastritis, the main symptoms are anorexia, nausea, vomiting, pain and tenderness in the stomach region, hiccoughs, and sometimes diarrhea. The patient with chronic gastritis may have no symptoms and may suddenly experience massive hemorrhage from the stomach. Diagnosis is by history, physical examination, and endoscopic examination.

Treatment and Nursing Management

Acute gastritis usually is of very short duration. Treatment consists of withholding all foods by mouth and administering drugs that slow down the peristaltic action of the GI tract. If severe dehydration or nausea and vomiting occur, fluids may be given IV. The patient with gastritis must be watched closely for signs of fluid and electrolyte imbalance.

Elder Care Points

If an elderly patient experiences vomiting and is unable to retain fluids for 12 hours, a trip to the emergency department for IV fluids may be needed to prevent severe dehydration.

Chronic gastritis is not as easily treated as acute gastritis. Diet therapy is of primary importance in chronic gastritis because the patient frequently admits to indiscretion in his dietary and drinking habits and finds it difficult to change. The diet for these patients is devoid of spicy or acidic foods. Tact and patience may convince the patient to follow the prescribed diet.

Treatment for chronic gastritis consists of antispasmodics to decrease the pain of stomach spasms, antacids, an H_2-receptor antagonist such as ranitidine to decrease acid secretions and change pH, or a proton pump inhibitor to decrease the secretion of hydrochloric acid. If *H. pylori* is present, antibiotic therapy is administered.

PEPTIC ULCER

Etiology

About 25 million people in the United States have experienced a peptic ulcer. *H.* is rich in an enzyme that may cause corrosion of the upper GI mucosa by damaging its mucous coating, making it more susceptible to damage from gastric acid and pepsinogen. Duodenal ulcers and some prepyloric ulcers are associated with an increased amount or hyperacidity of the gastric juices, and 70% are associated with *H. pylori.* Gastric ulcers, by contrast, are characterized by normal or abnormally low levels of hydrochloric acid, but 90% have been associated with *H. pylori. H. pylori* is also implicated in the development of gastric cancer (Pinto & Schub, 2009).

Elder Care Points

By age 60, approximately 60% of the population in the United States is infected with the *H. pylori* bacterium. However, most people never have symptoms of gastritis, and few develop ulcers.

Both gastric and duodenal ulcers tend to occur in families. Relatives of people with gastric or duodenal ulcers have three times the expected rate for ulcer formation. A genetic link has been found.

Neither hot spicy foods nor caffeine has been proven to be a risk factor for ulcers, but these substances make symptoms worse in many people. Gastric ulcers do occur in those who are poorly nourished because of poverty or because of poor eating habits. Despite the stereotype of the hard-driving executive suffering from an ulcer and ingesting antacid tablets, there is a greater incidence of ulcers in blue-collar workers and among laborers.

Stress does have a bearing on the progression of peptic ulcer. Tension, anxiety, and prolonged stress do alter gastric function. Prolonged physiologic stress produces what is known as a *physiologic stress ulcer,* which is believed to be the result of unrelieved stimulation of the vagus nerves and decreased perfusion to the stomach. A stress ulcer is pathologically and clinically different from a chronic peptic ulcer. It is more acute and more likely to produce hemorrhage. Perforation occurs occasionally, and pain is rare. Stress ulcers are a hazard for patients who are severely ill and in intensive care units for prolonged periods. Patients with multiple trauma, burns, or multisystem disorders are subject to physiologic stress ulcers. Such patients often receive medication to prevent ulcer formation.

Drug-induced ulcers are most often caused by aspirin, NSAIDs, alcohol, and glucocorticoids (Clin-eguide, 2009). Cigarette smoking is known to be a causative factor in peptic ulcer, particularly if over one-half pack a day is smoked (Clini-eguide, 2009).

Safety Alert

Monitor NSAID Use and Acetaminophen

There is an increased risk of peptic ulcer in individuals taking regular doses of over-the-counter (OTC) NSAIDs such as ibuprofen and naproxen. When combined with more than 2 g of acetaminophen per day, the risk increases. Daily doses of acetaminophen over 2 g along with other NSAIDs increase the risk of upper GI bleeding by twofold. Encourage patients who regularly take an NSAID to check the labels on pain, sleep, and cold medications to monitor acetaminophen intake (Kernisan, 2010).

Pathophysiology

Normally, the upper GI mucosa can resist corrosion; all areas exposed to the hydrochloric acid and pepsin in gastric juices have an ample supply of mucous glands that secrete a protective alkaline mucus, but ulcers develop when the mucosa cannot protect itself from corrosive substances, such as gastric acid, pepsinogen, alcohol, bile salts, and irritating food substances. A *peptic ulcer* is an ulceration with loss of tissue of the upper GI tract. The term includes both duodenal and gastric ulcers (Figure 29-3). The most common site for development of a peptic ulcer is in the first few centimeters of the duodenum, just beyond the pyloric muscle.

Signs and Symptoms

Subjective symptoms of uncomplicated ulcer include epigastric pain that might be described as burning, gnawing, cramping, or aching and that usually comes in waves that last several minutes. The daily pattern of pain is associated with the secretion of gastric juices in relation to the presence of food, which can act as a buffer. **For example, with a gastric ulcer the pain is diminished in the morning when secretion is low and after meals when food is in the stomach, and pain is most severe before meals and at bedtime.** Discomfort often appears for several days or weeks and then subsides, only to reappear weeks or months later. Other subjective symptoms include nausea, loss of appetite, and sometimes weight loss. Spontaneous vomiting accompanies duodenal ulcer more often than gastric ulcer.

 Elder Care Points

The elderly patient may not display the typical symptoms. Pain is less typical and may be poorly localized, or it may be described as lower chest discomfort or left-sided pain. Anorexia, weight loss, general weakness, anemia, nausea, and painless vomiting may occur; peptic ulcer is difficult to diagnose in this population.

Gastrointestinal Bleeding. Signs of acute GI bleeding include complaints of weakness and feeling faint, nausea and vomiting, restlessness, thirst, and mental

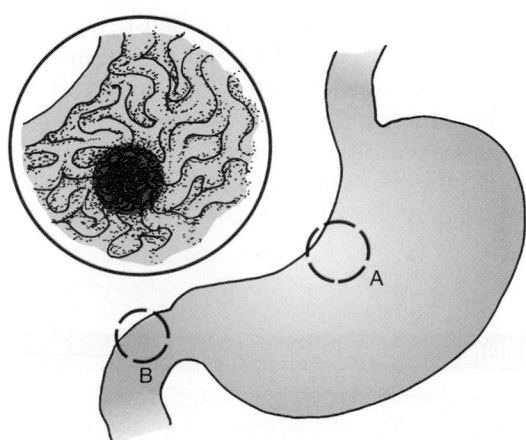

FIGURE 29-3 Peptic ulcers. *A,* Gastric. *B,* Duodenal.

confusion. **Hematemesis** is the vomiting of bright red blood, which indicates an active bleed or blood that has been sitting with gastric juices looks like coffee grounds. Diarrhea, decreased blood pressure, rapid pulse, and other signs of hypovolemic shock may occur. Blood in the GI tract acts as a cathartic and causes diarrhea. If bleeding from the upper GI system is profuse, maroon or bright red blood may appear in stool because of the rapid transit of the blood through the intestinal tract. Black stools almost always indicate the presence of digested blood, which means that the source of bleeding is in the upper GI tract.

 Clinical Cues

Remember that iron salts can cause the stool to be black and that the ingestion of beets can cause the stool to be bright red.

Estimates of blood loss from the GI tract are based in part on blood pressure readings and pulse rates. Blood pressure and pulse rate should be monitored every 15 to 30 minutes when there is evidence of extensive GI hemorrhage. **Changes in the vital signs that signal hypovolemic shock do not appear until after the patient has lost 20% or more of the blood volume.** Central venous pressure readings also are helpful in determining the amount of blood lost, especially in hypertensive patients, whose blood pressure may not reflect hypovolemia.

Additional data useful in determining the status of patients with GI bleeding include hematocrit and hemoglobin levels. These levels can be normal or even slightly elevated at the beginning of a bleeding episode. It takes 4 to 6 hours for the body to shift fluids from other compartments to the intravascular compartment. The shift of fluid changes the ratio of formed elements to fluids in the blood. The white cell count may be elevated in massive GI bleeding, probably because of the body's response to injury or hypovolemia. An elevated level of blood urea nitrogen can indicate digestion of large amounts of blood.

Diagnosis

The technique most commonly used to diagnose peptic ulcer is an upper GI series. Endoscopy can help locate the site of ulceration and bleeding and can differentiate between benign and malignant ulcerations and between the esophageal ulcer and a *diverticulum* (pouching of the intestinal wall).

A gastric analysis to measure the level of hydrochloric acid in gastric juices may be helpful in some cases, but there is significant variation in gastric acid levels among patients with peptic ulcer. Serum tests for *H. pylori* detect antibodies, indicating active or recent infection. The urea breath test involves the measurement of gas released in the breath following ingestion of a radiolabeled urea isotope; when *H. pylori* is present, the test is positive.

 Think Critically

How do the symptoms of a gastric ulcer differ from those of a hiatal hernia?

When the patient is experiencing extensive GI bleeding, the patient's condition is stabilized and diagnostic procedures are done to locate the source of bleeding. These procedures include endoscopic examination of the esophagus, stomach, and small intestine. Barium studies may be ordered.

Treatment

Peptic ulcer is treated conservatively at first, to avoid surgery. Medications to relieve pain from local irritation of the intestinal mucosa include antacids, which reduce the pain of ulcer by neutralizing gastric acid (see Table 29-1).

Treatment of gastric bleeding is begun by inserting a large-bore NG tube and using a normal saline lavage to monitor the quantity of bleeding and evacuate the blood, clots, and stomach contents. This allows the stomach to constrict, halting the blood flow. Antacids are given via the tube to neutralize pepsin and help stop the bleeding. H_2-receptor antagonists or proton pump inhibitors are used to decrease or stop acid secretion (see Table 29-1). Eighty percent of GI bleeding will stop with these treatments.

If there is major blood loss, transfusions of whole blood, packed cells, or fresh frozen plasma may be necessary. Normal saline, Plasmanate (plasma protein fraction), and Ringer's solution may be administered until blood is available. Maintenance of fluid balance is extremely important. Intake and output must be measured and recorded accurately. Oxygen therapy is started to maximize tissue oxygenation.

If the presence of *H. pylori* has been determined, treatment consists of the administration of clarithromycin (Biaxin) plus another antibiotic, an H_2 inhibitor, and a proton pump inhibitor. Sucralfate (Carafate) tablets may be used for short-term (up to 8 weeks) treatment of duodenal ulcer. Sucralfate has negligible acid-neutralizing capacity, as the action of this drug is local. Its benefits probably derive from its adherence to the ulcer site, providing protection from further damage by gastric juices. Misoprostol (Cytotec) is used to replace gastric prostaglandins depleted by NSAID therapy and helps to prevent ulcer formation caused by NSAIDs. Sedatives are sometimes prescribed for the peptic ulcer patient to help reduce anxiety and relieve tension.

! **Safety Alert**

Proton Pump Inhibitor Drug Interactions

Because proton pump inhibitors slow the liver's ability to metabolize and clear some drugs from the bloodstream, they should be used with caution in patients taking diazepam (Valium), phenytoin (Dilantin), and warfarin (Coumadin). Patients taking a proton pump inhibitor along with any of these three drugs should be watched closely for signs of toxicity.

❖ NURSING MANAGEMENT

■ Assessment (Data Collection)

Begin by asking the patient to describe the chief complaint (patient's perception of the main problem).

◎ **Focused Assessment**

Data Collection for Peptic Ulcer

Assess the following areas:
HISTORY
- Pain: characteristics, what affects pain, what relieves it; when pain began
- Nausea or vomiting; presence of "coffee-ground" emesis
- Dark "tarry" stool, or maroon colored stool
- Anorexia, weight loss

PHYSICAL ASSESSMENT
- Vital signs and changes from baseline
- Presence of restlessness, confusion, or thirst
- Skin tone
- Appearance and amount of emesis
- Stool color, characteristics, frequency
- Abdominal tenderness, rigidity, guarding, bloating
- Bowel sounds

LABORATORY DATA
- Complete blood count (CBC)
- Blood urea nitrogen (BUN)

■ Nursing Diagnosis and Planning

Common nursing diagnoses, expected outcomes, and interventions for the patient with a peptic ulcer are found in Nursing Care Plan 29-1. Before a peptic ulcer can be successfully controlled, the patient must understand how and why the ulcer developed in the first place. Once the predisposing factors are understood, it is easier to avoid them. Unless the patient can cooperate fully, there is a strong possibility that ulcers will develop again despite medical or even surgical treatment.

? **Think Critically**

How does reviewing the purpose, schedule, and side effects of medications prescribed for ulcers increase the likelihood of patient compliance?

Nursing Care Plan 29-1 | Care of the Patient with a Bleeding Peptic Ulcer

Scenario

Mr. Lee is a 47-year-old long-distance truck driver admitted to the hospital with a tentative diagnosis of bleeding peptic ulcer. He has had recurrent bouts of epigastric pain that is more pronounced before meals and at bedtime. Mr. Lee states that he eats "whenever I can grab a bite." He eats mostly fried and spicy foods and he smokes two packs of cigarettes a day. He went to the physician because of fatigue and discomfort that seemed to be getting progressively worse in spite of antacid use. He also admits to having some vomiting episodes with blood in the secretions. Mr. Lee is the sole support of his wife and four children and is very concerned about the expense of hospitalization and the time away from work. He is scheduled for an endoscopic examination of the esophagus, stomach, and duodenum.

Problem/Nursing Diagnosis

Worried about costs of hospitalization/Anxiety related to expenses, time off work, and worry about what is wrong with him.

Supporting Assessment Data

Subjective: "I'm the only one working"; expresses worry over hospital expenses; worried about blood in vomitus.
Objective: Self-treated with antacids and continued to work until symptoms progressed.

Goals/Expected Outcomes	Nursing Interventions	Selected Rationale	Evaluation
Patient will verbalize reduction in anxiety before discharge.	Encourage verbalization of concerns and fears.	Verbalizing fears may decrease their intensity.	Verbalizing specific concerns about finances and expresses fear that blood is a sign of serious illness.
Patient will devise plan to cover hospital expenses so as to decrease anxiety.	Advocate for financial consultation regarding hospital expenses.	A plan for meeting financial obligation will somewhat decrease anxiety.	Appointment with social worker to discuss financial situation.
Patient will verbalize understanding of diagnosis and treatment of his condition.	Explain all diagnostic procedures and medications.	Decreases the fear of the unknown and lowers anxiety.	Brochure given about endoscopic procedures and test for *Helicobacter pylori*; reviewed purpose of each medication.
	Assess usual coping techniques and teach new ways to cope as necessary.	Establishes usual coping methods and provides data for other coping methods to be taught.	Uses smoking and television as relaxation.
	Reinforce wife's assurances that they can manage expenses at home.	Reinforcement of information helps patient remember.	Wife says he tends to be a "worry wart"; reinforced information about her ability to cope with expenses.
	Encourage relaxation techniques.	Relaxation techniques help decrease anxious feelings.	Taught relaxation exercise and encouraged to practice it. Continue plan.

Problem/Nursing Diagnosis

Abdominal pain and discomfort/Pain related to irritation and possible ulceration of gastric mucosa.

Supporting Assessment Data

Subjective: Recurrent bouts of epigastric pain more pronounced before meals.
Objective: Epigastric tenderness increases with gentle palpation.

Goals/Expected Outcomes	Nursing Interventions	Selected Rationale	Evaluation
Patient will verbalize relief of pain.	Assess location and severity of pain every shift.	Provides data regarding condition and need for medication.	Pain is epigastric at 3/10; now occurring between meals.
Patient will verbalize ways to prevent gastric pain.	Administer ordered antacids, antispasmodics, and H_2 inhibitors.	Medications neutralize stomach acid or decrease acid production.	Taking medications as ordered.
	Give caffeine-free diet.	Caffeine causes more stomach acid production.	No caffeine drinks; bland diet.

ac, before meals; *BP*, blood pressure; *CBC*, complete blood count; *GI*, gastrointestinal; *Hct*, hematocrit; *Hgb*, hemoglobin; *hs*, at bedtime; *pc*, after meals; *PO*, orally.

Continued

★ Nursing Care Plan 29-1   Care of the Patient with a Bleeding Peptic Ulcer—cont'd

Goals/Expected Outcomes	Nursing Interventions	Selected Rationale	Evaluation
Patient will verbalize ways to prevent gastric pain—cont'd.	Encourage him to quit smoking.	Smoking constricts blood vessels, decreasing perfusion to stomach. Decreased perfusion makes the stomach more susceptible to inflammation.	Encouraged him to quit smoking; said he would think about it. Provided community resource information for stopping smoking.
	Give frequent feedings to neutralize gastric acid.	Keeping food in the stomach helps neutralize acid.	Eating a snack every 2 hr between meals. Continue plan.

Problem/Nursing Diagnosis
Vomiting episodes with blood/Risk for increased bleeding (gastrointestinal) related to irritation of gastric mucosa.

Supporting Assessment Data
Subjective: States has experienced blood-streaked vomitus; history suggestive of peptic ulcer; increasing fatigue.
Objective: Blood-tinged vomitus and blood in stool (positive guaiac test); pale conjunctiva; below-normal Hgb and Hct.

Goals/Expected Outcomes	Nursing Interventions	Selected Rationale	Evaluation
Patient will have no signs of intestinal blood loss by discharge. Hemoglobin and hematocrit will be within normal levels within 30 days.	Monitor CBC count for evidence of continued bleeding. Assess vomitus for blood. Check stool for occult blood as ordered. Monitor vital signs and assess for continued or rapid blood loss as ordered. Teach about foods high in iron (i.e., meat and green leafy vegetables) to correct anemia. Administer iron supplements as ordered.	CBC count may indicate if bleeding is occurring. Blood in vomitus indicates bleeding is still occurring. Blood in stool indicates GI bleeding. Active bleeding will be reflected by vital signs. Eating foods high in iron helps correct anemia. Iron supplementation helps correct anemia.	Hgb 11.9 g/dL and Hct 32. No vomitus this shift. Stool positive for occult blood ×2. Pulse 92 and BP 138/86. Agrees to try and eat more spinach, chard, and lean beef. Iron supplement not ordered yet. Continue plan.

Postprocedure
Mr. Lee's physician found a duodenal ulcer on endoscopic examination. He has prescribed sucralfate (Carafate), 1 g PO qid 1 hr ac and hs; ranitidine (Zantac), 300 mg hs; and Mylanta II, 30 mL 30 min pc, in hopes of healing the ulcer and preventing surgery.

Problem/Nursing Diagnosis
No knowledge of risk factors for peptic ulcer/Deficient knowledge related to factors that contribute to peptic ulcer and information about medications.

Supporting Assessment Data
Subjective: States was unaware that cigarette smoking contributed to ulcers; never has heard of the medications prescribed for him, except for the antacid.

Goals/Expected Outcomes	Nursing Interventions	Selected Rationale	Evaluation
Patient will verbalize factors that contribute to ulcer formation. Patient will attempt to quit smoking within 2 wk.	Instruct in contributing factors of ulcer formation (i.e., explain how the eating behavior of "grab a bite" and eating spicy or fried foods are contributing to ulcer formation).	Understanding how behavior affects health may help the patient to make better choices.	Acknowledged that smoking, his diet, and lifestyle contribute to his ulcer. States that he will quit eating foods that cause pain (i.e., spicy foods); has cut smoking down to ½ pack per day, states he will try to quit; will begin exercise program for stress reduction.

Goals/Expected Outcomes	Nursing Interventions	Selected Rationale	Evaluation
Patient will attempt to quit smoking within 2 wk—cont'd.	Assist him to learn new ways to cope with stress.	Practicing relaxation and deep breathing helps decrease stress.	Taught deep-breathing exercise.
	Discuss smoking cessation strategies (i.e., set a stop date, enlist help of family, use of a prescribed nicotine patch, substituting an activity such as chewing gum).	Nicotine is very addictive and having a formalized plan increases success.	Expresses interest in talking to doctor about getting a prescription for the nicotine patch.
	Discuss ways to manage proper eating when on the road (e.g., packing healthy snacks or choosing baked foods, not fried).	Knowing good food choices for his situation can help him eat properly when on the road.	Discussed food places that have appropriate choices. Wife agrees to pack fruits and whole grain crackers.
Patient will verbalize reason for each medication, dosage schedule, and side effects.	Teach action, dosage, and side effects of sucralfate (Carafate), ranitidine (Zantac), and Mylanta II. Obtain feedback for material taught.	Understanding how to take medications and what to expect, or report, helps with compliance and prevents toxic reactions.	Went over each medication and gave list with dosages. Discussed possible side effects and what to report to the physician.

Critical Thinking Questions
1. How would you interact with this patient to try to help him quit smoking?
2. What does he need to know about taking an antacid if he is taking other medications?
3. Considering he is a truck driver and on the road a lot, what can you do to help him change his diet?

■ Implementation

Blood pressure and pulse rate are measured regularly. Observe skin color, observe for diaphoresis or thirst, and look for other signs of continued blood loss such as restlessness. Watch for impending hypovolemic shock. Measure intake and output and note the character of vomitus, aspirated gastric fluid, and stools. Measure and record the patient's daily weight. Melena stools (black, tarry stools with digested blood) cause an unpleasant odor and the room must be kept as free of odor as possible.

Diet counseling is a top priority once the patient is stable. Currently, most authorities believe that it is best to restrict only those foods that the patient identifies with the onset of symptoms. It is generally agreed that the kind of food is less important than when the food is eaten; therefore the patient is instructed to eat at frequent and regular intervals throughout the day, rather than in two or three large meals. Meals should not be skipped. Alcohol and caffeine should be excluded.

■ Evaluation

The nurse can point out signs of improvement that will help to relieve the patient's anxiety. For example, if an NG tube is being used to lavage and decompress the stomach there will be a decreased showing of hematemesis as the bleeding resolves. **After the bleeding has apparently stopped and the patient's vital signs have stabilized, there must be continuous monitoring for signs of persistent or renewed bleeding.**

Complications

The three major complications of peptic ulcer are hemorrhage, perforation, and obstruction. Hemorrhage occurs when the ulcer erodes vessels, causing bleeding into the stomach. Signs of hemorrhage include the vomiting of blood. If the hemorrhage is unchecked, hypovolemic shock may occur.

Perforation is erosion of the ulcer through all walls of the stomach or intestine. A spilling of the contents of the GI tract into the peritoneal cavity ensues; it constitutes a surgical emergency because of the danger of hemorrhage and peritonitis. **Perforation is characterized by a sudden and severe pain in the upper abdomen that persists and increases in intensity and sometimes is referred to the shoulders.** The abdomen is rigid and boardlike and extremely tender. In a short time the patient shows signs of shock.

Obstruction occurs as a result of scarring and loss of musculature at the pylorus, narrowing the stomach outlet, and is manifested chiefly by persistent vomiting.

Surgical Treatment

Surgical treatment becomes necessary when a chronic ulcer fails to respond to medical treatment; when complications such as perforation, obstruction, or hemorrhage occur; or when malignancy is present.

In *pyloroplasty with truncal or proximal gastric vagotomy*, the pylorus, which has been narrowed by scarring, is widened. The branches of the vagus (tenth cranial) nerve that stimulate acid secretion in the stomach are selectively severed (vagotomy) so that the stomach does not receive impulses from the brain and therefore does not secrete hydrochloric acid. A vagotomy is often done at the same time that a gastric resection is performed.

Subtotal gastrectomy (gastric resection) consists of removing a part of the stomach and then joining the remaining portion to the small intestine by anastomosis. Anastomosis is the joining of two hollow organs by suturing the open ends together so that they become one continuous tube. An *antrectomy*, in which the gastrin-producing portion of the stomach (the antrum) is removed, may be done in conjunction with a truncal vagotomy. When the fundus of the stomach is anastomosed to the duodenum, the procedure is known as a *Billroth I*. In the *Billroth II* procedure, the duodenum is closed and the fundus of the stomach is anastomosed to the jejunum. *Total gastrectomy* is the surgical removal of all of the stomach. The esophagus is anastomosed to the small intestine (Figure 29-4).

Nursing Care of the Patient Undergoing Gastric Surgery

Preoperative care. The diet of the patient is restricted to liquids during the day before surgery. The patient is kept NPO, an NG tube is inserted, and gastric suction is begun to remove all stomach contents before surgery.

The patient receives routine preparations necessary for all major abdominal surgery. These include enemas so that the colon is emptied of fecal material. If the patient has had a barium enema, the nurse should look for and report returns that contain whitish material. This is barium, and it will become hardened if left in the colon, thus presenting the possibility of a fecal impaction later on.

Postoperative care. Care of the patient having gastric surgery is routine, with the following exceptions. After surgery in which part of the stomach has been removed, care must be taken in handling the NG tube to avoid injury to the sutures and to prevent introduction of infectious agents. The surgeon will write specific orders about irrigating fluids and movement of the gastric tube.

After the tube is removed, the patient is given small amounts of liquid to determine tolerance. These liquids are gradually increased. The patient's ability to take them without nausea, vomiting, or abdominal distress is assessed. If the liquids are well tolerated, the patient progresses to small, frequent feedings. Within 6 months, most patients are able to take three regular meals a day. The remaining portion of the stomach stretches to accommodate more and more food. Patients who have

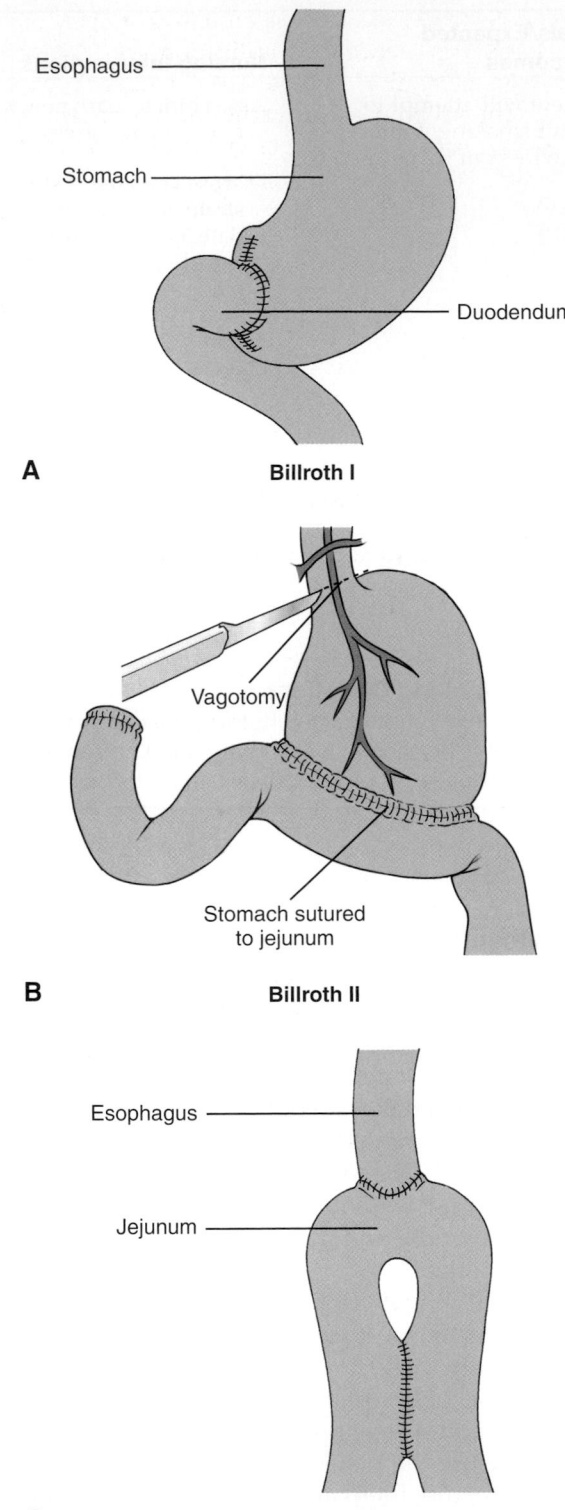

A   **Billroth I**

B   **Billroth II**

C   **Total gastrectomy**

FIGURE 29-4 Stomach surgical procedures. **A,** Billroth I. **B,** Billroth II. **C,** Total gastrectomy.

had a *total* gastrectomy have restricted diets. They are usually restricted to small, frequent feedings of easily digested semisolids for the rest of their lives. Before discharge, the hospital dietitian usually is called to help the patient and his family learn about the special diet needed after undergoing gastric surgery.

Dumping Syndrome. Some patients who have had a gastrectomy experience a complication known as the "dumping syndrome." The patient has nausea, weakness, abdominal pain, and diarrhea and may feel faint and perspire profusely or experience palpitations after eating. These sensations are caused by the rapid passage of large amounts of food and liquid into the jejunum. This occurs because part or all of the stomach and duodenum has been surgically removed. The progress of the ingested foods and fluids is not slowed by passing through the upper portion of the GI tract. When a patient experiences dumping syndrome, instruction is given to avoid eating large meals and to drink a minimum of fluids during the meal. Fluids may be taken in small amounts later, between meals. If sweet foods and liquids seem to aggravate the condition—and they sometimes do—the patient should try to avoid them. It also may be helpful for the patient to lie down flat for 30 minutes after a meal.

GASTRIC CANCER

It is estimated that cancer of the stomach caused 10,620 deaths in 2009 in the United States (National Cancer Institute, 2009). It is usually discovered very late. The 5-year survival rate is 75% if the disease is caught fairly early and only 30% in those with advanced disease. Metastasis to surrounding organs is common.

Etiology

The cause of gastric cancer is unknown, but pernicious anemia and achlorhydria (absence of hydrochloric acid) are often present. It is believed that a diet high in smoked, highly salted, or spiced foods may be a contributor. Food preservatives such as nitrates or nitrites increase the risk. The presence of *H. pylori*—particularly if present from an early age—is a definite factor. Genetic influence plays a role as the risk is increased in family members and in those with blood group A.

Pathophysiology

Gastric cancer grows primarily from the mucous glands. Most tumors arise in the antrum or pyloric area. The lesion begins as an ulcerative crater with an irregular

 Nutrition Considerations

Prevention of Gastric Cancer

Refraining from eating a diet high in smoked and salted foods or pickled vegetables helps prevent gastric cancer. Eating a diet high in fruits and vegetables, particularly those high in beta-carotene and vitamin C, decreases stomach cancer risk. People who eat a lot of red meat each week have double the risk of gastric cancer. Foods such as bacon and many "lunch meats" are high in nitrites, which are carcinogenic. When eating those foods, drinking orange juice reduces the quantity of nitrites. The ascorbic acid in the orange juice counteracts the nitrite concentration.

 Cultural Considerations

Stomach Cancer Incidence

Stomach cancer is almost double in incidence in African American individuals as in non-Hispanic whites. Native Americans and Hispanic Americans are also at an increased risk for stomach cancer. *Helicobacter pylori* is more common in Hispanic and African American individuals. Research with minority populations is underway to determine how *H. pylori* is transmitted in these populations in an effort to decrease stomach cancer incidence.

border and a raised margin. The tumor eventually spreads through the layers of the stomach and spreads to the lymph nodes, the liver, and the ovaries in women.

Signs and Symptoms

Signs and symptoms are similar to those of peptic ulcer, but may be just intermittent abdominal distress. Belching and the use of antacids may relieve the distress. The patient may become pale and weak and complain of fatigue, weakness, dizziness, and sometimes shortness of breath. Anemia is the underlying cause of those symptoms. There is often blood in the stool.

Diagnosis

Diagnosis is by upper GI series and endoscopic examination of the stomach with biopsy. Anemia, verified with a complete blood count, is usually present. Tumor markers such as carcinoembryonic antigen and carbohydrate antigen (CA) 19-9 are useful in determining the degree of invasion of the tumor, and liver metastasis.

Treatment and Nursing Management

Surgical intervention may relieve symptoms such as obstruction, or may debulk the tumor. The same surgical procedures are used as for peptic ulcer. There is only a 40% 5-year cure rate with surgery for gastric cancer. In Japan, laparoscopic surgery for the removal of small tumors is being studied. Adjuvant therapy of radiation and/or chemotherapy may be employed. Radiation has proved to be of value only for palliation. 5-Fluorouracil (5-FU) and cisplatin or 5-FU with epirubicin and cisplatin are the preferred chemotherapy protocols today. Studies are being conducted on the use on directly infusing the chemotherapy into the peritoneal space. A recent study showed that a targeted therapy drug (targets cells that divide rapidly) called trastuzumab (Herceptin) helped patients with metastatic gastric cancer. Other investigational drugs include bortezomib (Velcade), sunitinib (Sutent), and sorafenib (Nexavar) (American Cancer Society, 2009b). Cancer therapy and nursing care are discussed in

Chapter 8. Nursing care after surgery is the same as for the patient who underwent surgery for a peptic ulcer but with excision of involved lymph nodes.

COMMON THERAPIES FOR DISORDERS OF THE GASTROINTESTINAL SYSTEM

GASTROINTESTINAL DECOMPRESSION

Abdominal distention with increased pressure within the abdominal cavity is very uncomfortable. Excess fluids and gases also interfere with ventilation of the lungs and normal function of other nearby organs.

Measures to relieve distention include inserting an NG tube to remove fluids and gas from the stomach. Gastrointestinal tubes vary in length, design, and purpose. The Levin tube and gastric sump tube are shorter because they are intended to reach only as far as the stomach. The Miller-Abbott, Cantor, and Harris tubes are longer tubes that are directed past the stomach and into the small intestine. Intestinal tubes are described in Chapter 30.

🛏 Clinical Cues

NG tube is a generic term that you may see in physicians' orders or in the nurses' or physicians' notes, or you may hear that term in report; however, the purpose of the therapy for the NG tube dictates the type of NG tube. Make sure that you clarify the purpose of the therapy and the type of tube before starting the care of the patient.

Nursing Management

During GI decompression the patient is observed for continuing signs of abdominal distention, which would indicate that excess fluids and gases are not being removed as intended. **Nausea, vomiting, complaints of feeling full or bloated, increasing shortness of breath, and increase in the girth of the abdomen are signs that the stomach and intestines are not being decompressed adequately.**

Applying too much suction can pull the gastric mucosa into the drainage openings, or "eyes," of the tube, causing damage to the mucosa and traumatic ulceration.

📋 Assignment Considerations

Caring for a Patient with a Salem Sump Tube

When assigning assisted ambulation of the patient with a Salem sump tube, remind the CNA or UAP to keep the tube above the level of the stomach to prevent leaking of stomach contents from the pigtail. The main tube should be plugged for ambulation. The assistant can be instructed to reattach the tubing to the wall suction after ambulation is completed, but the nurse is ultimately responsible to follow up and verify that the tube and suction are functioning correctly.

Using a gastric sump tube (Salem, ventral) that has an air vent can help prevent this problem. Sump tubes are usually attached to continuous "low" suction; Levin tubes function best with intermittent suction. **Unless ordered otherwise, use the low setting for suction.** The connecting tubing leading to the suction machine works best if it is kept above the height of entry into the drainage container.

🛏 Clinical Cues

The blue pigtail on the Salem sump tube must be kept above the level of the stomach or it will leak stomach secretions. The pigtail can be cleared by instilling a few milliliters of air, and nothing but air should be instilled through it.

Irrigations with normal saline are usually ordered to keep the tube patent. The amount instilled should be added to the patient's intake count, and the amount of drainage is recorded as output for each shift. If the patient has had surgery on the intestinal tract, the irrigation procedure should be done with aseptic technique rather than clean technique.

The characteristics of the drainage are charted each shift. **If coffee-ground–like material is noticed in the tube, the drainage should be tested for presence of blood** by using a Hemastix strip dipped into the secretions. If blood unexpectedly appears in the drainage, the physician should be notified. Fluid and electrolyte imbalance problems that can be caused by continuous suction and irrigation are discussed in Chapter 3.

An NG tube is uncomfortable for the patient. The naris must be checked for signs of pressure, and the tube may need to be repositioned to relieve the problem. Common complaints are sore throat, dry mouth, earache (from congestion of the eustachian tube), and dry lips and nasal mucosa. Frequent mouth care and application of a lubricant to the lips and nares will help. A room humidifier can also be helpful, but this requires a physician's order. The physician may allow the patient to have limited amounts of ice chips, hard candy, or chewing gum to decrease the problem of dry mouth.

After the tube is removed, the patient is monitored for nausea, vomiting, and abdominal distention. Sometimes it is necessary to insert the tube again.

ENTERAL NUTRITION

If a patient has long-term difficulty taking in food orally, as when in a coma, enteral feeding is indicated. Current practice calls for a nasoduodenal tube, frequently the Dobbhoff or similar weighted-tip tube (Figure 29-5). The tube delivers special-formula liquid feedings into the duodenum.

FIGURE 29-5 Small-bore feeding tube placement.

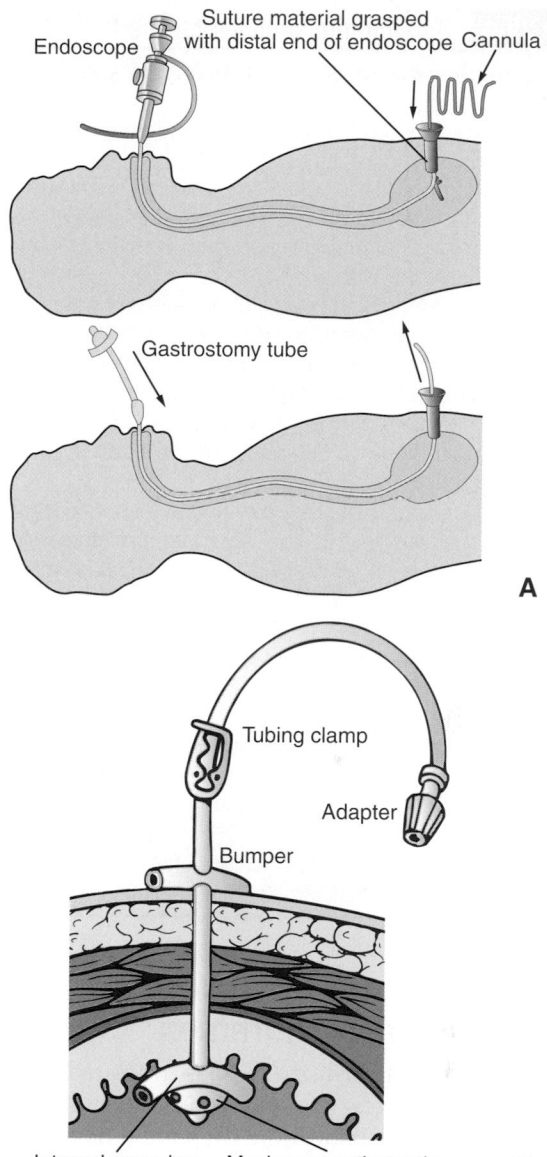

FIGURE 29-6 Percutaneous endoscopic gastrostomy. **A,** Gastrostomy tube placement via percutaneous endoscopy. The gastrostomy tube is inserted through the esophagus into the stomach and pulled through a stab wound made in the abdominal wall. **B,** A retention disk on the inside of the stomach and a bumper disk on the outside secure the tube.

Clinical Cues

When you are working with a Dobbhoff tube always use a large syringe (10 mL or larger) to flush and to give medications because smaller syringes create too much pressure and may cause the tube to rupture.

These tubes are inserted by the physician or a registered nurse, and placement in the duodenum is confirmed by x-ray film before feedings are started. The feedings can be given at specified times throughout the day or on a continuous basis. If continuous tube feedings are ordered, they frequently are administered with a feeding pump.

The patient requiring long-term nutritional support for problems such as inability to swallow may undergo percutaneous endoscopic gastrostomy (PEG). A feeding gastrostomy tube is placed endoscopically through the abdominal wall (Figure 29-6). The patient then receives enteral feedings via the gastrostomy tube. The tube is marked with indelible ink at the point of exit so that correct placement can be checked daily. The area is observed for signs of infection and cleansed daily with soap and water until healing is complete. A 4 × 4 gauze dressing is used over the outside bumper while the area is healing. Box 29-1 presents nursing interventions for the patient receiving tube feedings. **Adding a feeding when there is too much residual from the last feeding may cause regurgitation and aspiration.**

Sometimes the feeding tube is placed in the jejunum via a jejunostomy. If this is the case, the tube is sutured in place, and the spot where the tube enters the abdominal skin is marked. The mark and suture are checked

before beginning a feeding to make certain that the tube has not been dislodged. It is difficult to aspirate anything from a jejunostomy.

Safety Alert

Jejunostomy Tube Displacement

If a jejunostomy tube has moved or the suture is broken, no feeding should be given. Peritonitis may occur if feeding formula spills into the peritoneal cavity. The tube must be replaced by the physician. Always document that placement was checked and whether the suture is intact and the mark is at the skin. If displacement has occurred, document what action was taken.

Box **29-1** Nursing Interventions for the Patient Receiving Enteral (Tube) Feedings

- Be certain tube placement has been checked by x-ray film and is correct.
- Check and record the residual volume every 4 hours or as ordered and record it.
- Verify the drip rate for the feeding on the order sheet.
- Assess the feeding pump to be certain it is set up correctly and that the drip setting is accurate. Be certain the formula being instilled is what was ordered.
- Change the feeding bag and tubing every 24 hours. Change the irrigation set every 24 hours also.
- When continuous feeding is ordered, add only 4 hours of formula to the bag at a time to prevent bacterial growth; a closed system may be used for 24 hours.
- Do not use food dye in the formula as it can cause complications.
- Keep the head of the bed elevated at least 30 degrees during the feeding and for 1 hour after an intermittent or bolus feeding. For continuous feeding, keep the patient in a semi-Fowler's position.
- Monitor laboratory values: blood urea nitrogen, electrolytes, hematocrit, albumin, and glucose.
- Monitor for diarrhea or excessive gas.
- Monitor and record intake and output.
- Monitor and record the patient's weight at least weekly.
- Flush the tube with 30 to 60 mL of water every 4 hours during continuous feeding, and before and after each intermittent feeding.
- Flush with 30 mL of warm water before and after each individual medication; do not mix medications together

or with the feeding formula. Use liquid medications whenever possible.
- If tube becomes clogged, flush with 30 mL of water in a 50-mL piston syringe; use gentle pressure.
- Provide mouth care every 4 hours.
- Clean the nares and around the tube in the naris each shift or twice a day. Inspect the naris for pressure areas.
- Change the tape securing the tube to the nose if it becomes loose or soiled.

FOR GASTROSTOMY TUBE
- Assess the insertion site for signs of infection or excoriation.
- Rotate the tube 360 degrees every day and check for ¼-inch play in and out. If tube cannot be moved, report this to the physician as the retention disk may have become embedded in the tissue.
- Change the dressing once a day, applying a dry sterile dressing.

FOR JEJUNOSTOMY TUBE
- Be certain that the suture holding the tube is in place and that the mark on the tube is at the skin surface before starting or adding to a feeding. If it is not, stop the feeding and notify the physician.
- Do not attempt to aspirate a jejunostomy tube because it will collapse because of a small interior diameter.
- Inspect the insertion site and change the dressing once a day.

TOTAL PARENTERAL NUTRITION

Total parenteral nutrition (TPN) is indicated when the patient cannot ingest or digest foods normally or has a problem with malabsorption. If a patient has continued weight loss and a negative nitrogen balance, TPN is indicated. Conditions that could warrant TPN include severe trauma to the intestinal tract, as with a gunshot wound, and chronic inflammatory conditions. Regional ileitis that prevents absorption of nutrients is an example of an inflammatory condition. Other conditions not related to the intestinal tract but nevertheless capable of seriously interfering with normal nutrition over time include prolonged sepsis, fever, extensive burns, and cancer.

TPN is essentially a form of IV feeding. The amounts and kinds of nutrients needed for long-term nutritional maintenance usually cannot be handled as well by peripheral veins; therefore the nutrient mix is given into a larger central vein such as the superior vena cava. To accomplish this, the physician may choose a direct central line into the vena cava or jugular vein. A peripherally inserted central catheter (PICC) line may be inserted and threaded into the vena cava instead. Lipids may be given via a peripheral vein.

Further information about TPN and the principles for administration are found in Chapter 3.

Clinical Cues

Do **NOT** confuse enteral feedings and TPN feedings. The solutions and routes are not interchangeable. **Infusing an enteral feeding into an IV site can result in death.** First, verify the solution and route. Trace the tube down to the patient's body to ensure that you are using the correct tube.

Care of the patient must be a team effort on the part of physicians, pharmacists, dietitians, and nurses. Nursing care includes assisting with the insertion of the IV central line or PICC line, changing the tubing with each new bag or bottle, changing the dressing, observing the insertion site, and removing the tubing when TPN therapy is discontinued. Day-to-day care includes monitoring vital signs, glucose levels, and fluid and electrolyte balance. The patient is weighed daily and provided frequent mouth care. The rate of TPN is slowly decreased to gradually lower the dextrose load before TPN is discontinued.

Get Ready for the NCLEX® Examination!

Key Points

- A calorie reduction diet combined with exercise and behavior modification are the initial treatments for obesity. Bariatric surgery may be considered for the obese person with a BMI over 40.
- Dysphagia may cause respiratory problems from aspiration.
- Oral cancer and esophageal cancer are associated with alcohol and tobacco use.
- Common symptoms of GERD include dyspepsia and reflux. Diet therapy, lifestyle changes, drug therapy, weight reduction, and education are the mainstays of treatment.
- A peptic ulcer (gastric or duodenal) is ulceration of the upper GI tract. Symptoms include epigastric pain before meals and during the night. Complications include hemorrhage, perforation, and obstruction.
- Monitor vital signs every 15 to 30 minutes when there is evidence of extensive GI hemorrhage. Replacement of blood and fluids may be required.
- Surgical procedures for peptic ulcer include pyloroplasty with vagotomy, subtotal gastrectomy, antrectomy, or total gastrectomy (see Figure 29-4).
- *Helicobacter pylori,* pernicious anemia, and achlorhydria are all implicated in the development of gastric cancer.
- Symptoms of dumping syndrome are nausea, weakness, abdominal pain, diarrhea, faintness, palpitations, and diaphoresis.
- A nasogastric tube (NG) is used for gastric decompression; a nasoduodenal tube is used for enteral feeding. After NG tube removal, the patient is monitored for abdominal distention, nausea, and vomiting.
- When a patient cannot digest foods and liquids normally, total parenteral nutrition (TPN) may be required. The TPN solution must be sterile and administered at the ordered rate into a blood vessel with high-volume blood flow.

Additional Learning Resources

SG Go to your Study Guide for additional learning activities to help you master this chapter content.

⊝volve Go to your Evolve website (http://evolve.elsevier.com/deWit/ medsurg) for the following FREE learning resources:
- Animations, audio, and video
- Answers and rationales for questions and activities
- Concept Map Creator
- Glossary with pronunciations in English and Spanish
- Interactive Review Questions and Exercises and more!

 Online Resources
- Gastric bypass surgery, www.mayoclinic.com/health/gastric-bypass/ MY00825
- Verification of feeding tube placement, www.aacn.org/WD/Practice/ Docs/PracticeAlerts/Verification_of_Feeding_Tube_Placement_ 05-2005.pdf

Review Questions for the NCLEX® Examination

1. A family member tells the nurse, "Dad seems to be having some trouble swallowing lately." What is the nurse's priority action?
   1. Notify the physician.
   2. Consult the speech therapist for advice.
   3. Initiate aspiration precautions.
   4. Observe during "practice swallows."

2. The nurse is supervising a nursing student during the care of a patient with a gastrostomy tube. The nurse should intervene if the student:
   1. aspirates for residual contents before feeding.
   2. flushes the tube after each feeding.
   3. changes the tube and feeding every 4 hours.
   4. cleans and dries the skin around the tube.

3. When screening for the presence of risk factors for oral and pharyngeal cancers, which questions would the nurse ask? *(Select all that apply.)*
   1. How much alcohol do you consume?
   2. Have you had any oral lesions?
   3. Do you have family members who have cancer?
   4. Do you smoke?
   5. Have you been exposed to hepatitis virus?

4. The nurse is reviewing signs and symptoms of esophageal cancer with persons who are at risk. Which statement indicates that the participants have understood the information?
   1. "A feeling of fullness in the throat is an early sign."
   2. "Belching and indigestion are caused by cancerous lesions."
   3. "Common symptoms are halitosis and dryness of the mouth."
   4. "Choking or coughing while swallowing liquids is an early sign."

5. The nurse is taking care of a patient who had a modified radical neck dissection surgery. The patient's spouse asks, "Why do you have to apply cold packs and elevate my husband's head?" Which response is the most appropriate?
   1. "These interventions decrease the need for opiates."
   2. "These interventions reduce neck swelling."
   3. "These interventions promote faster healing."
   4. "These interventions reduce the incidence of postoperative fever."

6. The patient reports a history of gastric ulcer. Which symptom would the nurse most be concerned about?
   1. Epigastric pain that is described as a burning sensation.
   2. Pain is most severe at bedtime.
   3. Reports vomit that "looks like coffee grounds."
   4. Discomfort comes for several days and then subsides.

7. The nurse reinforces diet recommendations to a patient with gastroesophageal reflux disease (GERD). Which patient statement indicates a need for further teaching?
   1. "I should avoid spicy Italian sauces."
   2. "Clothes should be loose around the waist and abdomen."
   3. "I need to wait 30 minutes after eating before lying down."
   4. "I need to consider removing caffeine from my diet."

8. The patient is receiving continuous enteral feedings. Which intervention will address the most common problem associated with the feeding therapy?
   1. Assist the patient to ambulate several times a day.
   2. Assess the skin in the rectal area and apply a barrier cream.
   3. Place an emesis basin and tissues within close proximity.
   4. Frequently offer water, other fluids, or ice chips.

9. While obtaining a clinical history, the patient with a known history of peptic ulcers suddenly complains of a severe upper abdominal pain of increasing intensity that spread to the shoulders. The abdomen has boardlike rigidity. Which sign(s) and/or symptom(s) signal worsening related to the peptic ulcer? *(Select all that apply.)*
   1. Slow, deep respirations
   2. Decreased oxygen saturation
   3. Increased pulse
   4. Hot dry skin
   5. Belching and flatulence
   6. Confusion and restlessness

10. The nurse is caring for a patient who is vomiting blood. The physician orders a normal saline fluid bolus of 500mL to infuse over 30 minutes. What is the correct pump setting in mL/hour?

Critical Thinking Activities

Scenario A
Ms. Sutton, age 52, is experiencing a lot of abdominal discomfort and reflux. She visits her physician, who believes she has GERD. She is 5 feet 3½ inches tall and weighs 158 lb.

1. What measures would be recommended to decrease the symptoms of GERD?
2. What specific instruction would you give Ms. Sutton regarding her diet?
3. Why would losing some weight help her problem?

Scenario B
Mr. Post, age 47, is admitted to the hospital because he has epigastric pain, is vomiting blood, and has a suspected gastric ulcer.

1. What tests might be done to establish a diagnosis for Mr. Post?
2. What kind of information will help Mr. Post avoid difficulty with his diet after he is discharged?
3. What would Mr. Post need to know to keep his ulcer under control and eventually cure it?

Scenario C
The nursing assistant tells you that Mr. Yamamoto had an episode of coughing while he was eating breakfast. You check on the patient and he is not having any respiratory distress, but you notice that there are some food stains on his shirt. He says, "Sometimes water makes me cough." You decide to feed the patient his lunch so that you can observe him eating and inform the physician about your observations.

1. What position will you place him in before feeding?
2. Explain how to observe for problems with swallowing.
3. What dietary modifications can be made for patients that have difficulties with swallowing?

Care of Patients with Disorders of the Lower Gastrointestinal System

Objectives

Theory

1. Compare the etiology and signs and symptoms of various types of hernias.
2. Discuss the characteristics of irritable bowel syndrome.
3. Explain how diverticulitis occurs.
4. Illustrate how the two types of intestinal obstruction occur and the symptoms.
5. Describe the pathophysiology, methods of diagnosis, and treatment for ulcerative colitis and Crohn's disease.
6. Differentiate the signs and symptoms of appendicitis from peritonitis.
7. Plan nursing interventions for the patient having surgery of the lower intestine and rectum.
8. Discuss ways to help the patient psychologically adjust to having an ostomy.

9. Compare the characteristics of hemorrhoids, pilonidal sinus, and anorectal fistula.

Clinical Practice

1. Choose nursing interventions for the patient with inflammatory bowel disease.
2. Assess for the signs and symptoms of appendicitis.
3. Identify types of patients who are at risk for peritonitis.
4. Create a teaching plan for the prevention of colorectal cancer.
5. Write a nursing care plan for the patient with cancer of the colon and intestinal obstruction.
6. Evaluate a nursing care plan for a patient undergoing colostomy, considering the type of stoma and the effluent it produces.
7. Observe the equipment and procedure for changing an ostomy appliance.

Key Terms

anastomosis (ă-năs-tō-MŌ-sĭs, p. 675)
colectomy (kŏ-LĚK-tō-mē, p. 675)
colostomy (kŏ-LŎS-tō-mē, p. 675)
cryotherapy (krī-ō-THĚR-ă-pē, p. 686)
diverticulitis (dī-vĕr-tĭk-ū-LĪ-tĭs, p. 668)
diverticulosis (dī-vĕr-tĭk-ū-LŌ-sĭs, p. 665)
diverticulum (dī-vĕr-TĬK-ū-lŭm, p. 665)
hemicolectomy (hě-mē-kŏ-LĚK-tō-mē, p. 675)
hemorrhoidectomy (HĚM-rŏyd-ĚK-tō-mē, p. 686)
hemorrhoids (HĚM-rŏydz, p. 685)
hernia (HĚR-nē-ă, p. 663)
hernioplasty (hěr-nē-ŏ-PLĂS-tē, p. 664)

herniorrhaphy (hěr-nē-ŎR-ě-fē, p. 664)
ileostomy (ĭl-ē-ŎS-tō-mē, p. 680)
intussusception (ĭn-tŭs-sŭs-SĚP-shŭn, p. 668)
lysed (līzd, p. 669)
mucorrhea (mū-kō-RĒ-ă, p. 665)
paralytic ileus (păr-ă-LĬT-ĭk ĬL-ē-ŭs, p. 669)
peritonitis (pěr-ĭ-tō-NĪ-tĭs, p. 673)
photocoagulation (fō-tō-kō-ăg-ū-LĀ-shŭn, p. 686)
pilonidal (pī-lō-NĪ-dăl, p. 686)
scleropathy (sklěr-ō-pă-thē, p. 686)
steatorrhea (stě-ă-tō-RĒ-ă, p. 674)
volvulus (VŎL-vū-lŭs, p. 668)

DISORDERS OF THE ABDOMEN AND BOWEL

ABDOMINAL AND INGUINAL HERNIA

Etiology and Pathophysiology

If there is a defect in the muscular wall of the abdomen, the intestine may break through the defect. This protrusion is called a hernia or a *rupture.*

The most common locations for a hernia are in areas where the abdominal wall is normally weaker and more likely to allow a segment of intestine to protrude (Figure 30-1). These include the center of the abdomen at the site of the umbilicus and the lower abdomen at the points where the inguinal ring and the femoral

canal begin. The most common contributing factors in the development of a hernia are straining to lift heavy objects, chronic cough, straining to void or pass stool, and ascites. Inguinal hernias are more common in men. A hernia may form at an old abdominal surgical incision.

Hernias are classified as *reducible,* which means the protruding organ can be returned to its proper place by pressing on the organ, and *irreducible or incarcerated,* which means that the protruding part of the organ is tightly wedged outside the cavity and cannot be pushed back through the opening. If the protruding part of the organ is not replaced and its blood supply

663

Direct inguinal hernia   Indirect inguinal hernia

A   Umbilical hernia   Femoral hernia

B

FIGURE 30-1 A, Types of hernias. **B,** Indirect inguinal hernia.

is cut off, the hernia is said to be *strangulated.* An *indirect* hernia protrudes through the inguinal ring. A *direct* hernia protrudes through the posterior inguinal wall.

Signs and Symptoms

If the hernia is not incarcerated, there will just be an abnormal pouching, a "lump" or local swelling out from the abdominal wall or in the groin area (inguinal hernia). When pressure on the abdominal wall is removed by lying down, the swelling disappears. Lifting of heavy objects, coughing, or any activity that puts a strain on the abdominal muscles may force the organ back through the opening, and the swelling reappears.

Some discomfort may accompany the hernia. Pain occurs when the peritoneum becomes irritated or when the hernia is incarcerated or strangulated. The flow of

intestinal contents can be blocked by an incarcerated hernia, and cause symptoms of intestinal obstruction. **This is an emergency because when the blood supply is restricted, part of the intestine may die.**

Treatment

The surgical procedure used in the treatment of a hernia is called a **herniorrhaphy,** which means a surgical repair of a hernia. The defect is closed with sutures. If the area of weakness is very large, a **hernioplasty** is done. In this procedure, some type of strong synthetic material is sewn over the defect to reinforce the area. The procedure is now most often done on an outpatient basis.

Careful discharge instructions are given to the hernia patient to prevent respiratory problems because **the patient should not cough in the immediate post-operative period.** Guidelines on signs and symptoms of complications are sent home with the patient, along with a written list of activities to avoid until healing is complete.

If surgery is not possible because of age or poor surgical risk, the patient may be fitted with an appliance called a *truss,* which simply reinforces the weakened cavity wall and prevents protrusion of the intestines. The truss is put on in the morning before the patient gets out of bed, because the hernia is more likely to be reduced at that time. It is only a symptomatic measure and does not cure the hernia.

Nursing Management

Care after hernia repair is directed at pain control and preventing recurrence of the hernia. The patient is cautioned not to do heavy lifting, pulling, or pushing that increases intra-abdominal pressure. Postoperative care is similar to other surgical patients (see Chapter 5).

? Think Critically

What would you say to a family member who mentions to you that he has a swelling in the groin area and thinks he may have a hernia?

IRRITABLE BOWEL SYNDROME

Irritable bowel syndrome (IBS) is a functional disorder of gastrointestinal motility. In the United States more people suffer with IBS than with diabetes or asthma and IBS is a major reason for missing workdays. In North America, IBS is far more common in women than in men.

Etiology

The cause of IBS is unknown, but it is thought to be due to a hypersensitivity of the bowel wall leading to disruption of the normal function of the intestinal muscles. There is a familial predisposition. Stress, caffeine, and sensitivity to certain foods such as dairy and wheat products seem to trigger IBS in some people.

Pathophysiology

An altered bowel pattern and abdominal pain with bloating are caused by altered motility of the small and large intestines. It is thought that with IBS there is an abnormality of nerve function in the intestine. A chemical mediator, 5-hydroxytryptamine (5-HT) or serotonin, plays a role in bowel motility and visceral sensitivity; 5-HT may be implicated in the pain that occurs with IBS.

Signs and Symptoms

IBS is a group of symptoms that together represent the most common disorder presented by patients who consult gastroenterologists. The three characteristics typical of this disorder are (1) alteration in bowel elimination (either constipation or diarrhea or both); (2) abdominal pain and bloating; and (3) the absence of detectable organic disease. The pattern of bowel dysfunction varies from case to case and each patient seems to have a unique pattern.

Diagnosis

Diagnosis of IBS is based on clinical manifestations and ruling out the presence of organic bowel disease. Diagnostic criteria include:

- Abdominal pain or discomfort that is:
  - Relieved by defecation
  - Associated with a change in stool frequency and/or consistency
- Other symptoms that support the diagnosis:
  - Mucorrhea (mucus in the stool)
  - Abdominal bloating

DIARRHEA OR CONSTIPATION

Treatment and Nursing Management

A good general health assessment is conducted along with a focused assessment. Treatment of IBS is long. Medications are prescribed according to each patient's need. Drugs that have been used include bulk-forming agents, antidiarrheals, antispasmodics, antidepressants, anticholinergics/sedatives, and mild analgesics to relieve discomfort (Table 30-1). A diet high in fiber also may be prescribed. Metamucil or other bulk stool softeners may be recommended.

Gas-forming foods such as legumes and those in the cabbage family should be avoided. Avoiding onions, potatoes, cucumbers, coffee, tea, carbonated beverages, and alcohol can be helpful. In some patients, milk is restricted if they have shown evidence of intolerance to it. Lactase tablets may be used, but these may not help if there is sensitivity to dairy products rather than a lactase deficiency. Wearing loose clothing is more comfortable if bloating or increased abdominal pressure occurs. Give instruction about the medications and diet therapy.

Ineffective coping patterns in response to stress may be present in these patients. Randomized, controlled

Focused Assessment

Data Collection for the Patient with Suspected IBS

For the patient with symptoms suggesting IBS, gather the following data:

HISTORY
- When symptoms first began
- Stool pattern: frequency, character of stool
- Presence of bloating and flatus
- Incidence of pain or cramping; location, duration, character
- Pain that awakens the patient at night
- Precipitating factors for cramping or diarrhea
- Known food intolerances
- Methods of self-treatment
- Known stressors
- Methods of coping with stress

PHYSICAL EXAMINATION
- Presence and character of bowel sounds
- Degree of firmness and tenderness of abdomen
- Location of tenderness
- Appearance of stool

trials have shown cognitive therapy, psychotherapy, and hypnotherapy help to improve overall symptoms (Harvard Women's Health Watch, 2009). Consultation with a psychiatric nursing specialist can help the staff nurse develop more realistic goals and effective nursing interventions to improve the patient's coping skills.

Complementary and Alternative Therapies

Peppermint Oil for the Relief of Abdominal Discomfort

Peppermint oil may provide some temporary relief of abdominal pain for patients with IBS; however, those with gastroesophageal reflux disease (GERD) should avoid this alternative therapy because it can worsen heartburn (Harvard Women's Health Watch, 2009).

Clinical Cues

Having the patient keep a food diary can be very helpful in identifying foods that cause a reaction with bloating and inflammation. If the diary is kept over a period of weeks, a pattern may be established. Food intolerance symptoms may not be evident for up to 4 days after the food is eaten. Sometimes if one food is linked to the symptoms, that food can be simply left out of the diet.

DIVERTICULA

The term **diverticulum** refers to a small, blind pouch resulting from a protrusion of the mucous membranes of a hollow organ through weakened areas of the organ's muscular wall. Diverticula are most prevalent in older individuals and occur most often in the intestinal tract, especially in the esophagus and colon. When diverticula are present, the patient is said to have **diverticulosis.**

Table 30-1 Commonly Prescribed Drugs for Gastrointestinal Disorders

CLASSIFICATION	ACTION	NURSING IMPLICATIONS	PATIENT TEACHING
Antidiarrheals			
Diphenoxylate hydrochloride (Lomotil) Loperamide (Imodium) Opium tincture (Paregoric)	Decrease motility, propulsion, and secretions.	Observe for effectiveness; should be effective within 48 hr. Observe for signs of constipation. Use cautiously in patients with prostatic enlargement as may cause urinary retention. Warn that Pepto-Bismol will make stool black.	Warn that medication will cause dry mouth. Instruct not to take more than recommended dosage as toxicity can occur. With Lomotil, warn not to operate machinery until effect on central nervous system is known. Advise to contact physician if acute diarrhea does not abate within 2 days.
Kaolin-pectin combinations (Kaopectate)	Decrease fluid in stool.		
Bismuth subsalicylate (Pepto-Bismol)	Binds water; coats mucosa, absorbs toxins.		
Antiflatulents			
Simethicone (Phazyme, Mylicon, Di-Gel)	Defoaming action disperses gas.	Warn that the drug does not prevent gas formation, but will decrease bloating and discomfort. Gas is expelled via belching or flatus.	Instruct to chew tablets before swallowing.
Laxatives			
Bulk-forming Methylcellulose (Citrucel) Psyllium (Metamucil, Konsyl)	Act like fiber, absorbing water in the bowel and hastening transit time through the bowel.	None specific; monitor effectiveness.	Instruct to take with an 8-oz glass of water to prevent esophageal or bowel obstruction.
Surfactants Docusate sodium (Surfak, Colace) Docusate potassium (Dialose)	Facilitate absorption of water by stool by decreasing the surface tension. Enhance secretion of fluid and electrolytes in the bowel.	Contraindicated for patients with signs of intestinal obstruction. Act in 24-48 hr. Used to prevent constipation rather than treat it.	Instruct to take with a full glass of water. Not to be used for more than 1 wk without physician's knowledge.
Contact laxatives Bisacodyl (Dulcolax) Phenolphthalein (Feen-a-Mint, Ex-Lax, Modane) *Cascara sagrada* and senna (Senokot, Fletcher's Castoria) Castor oil	Act on intestinal wall to increase secretion of fluid and electrolytes into the intestine.	Most act within 6-12 hr to produce a semi-fluid stool. Bisacodyl is available as a rectal suppository as well as an oral tablet. Phenolphthalein may turn the urine pink. *Cascara sagrada* and senna may cause a brownish yellow or pink tinge to the urine. Castor oil acts within 2-6 hr. Castor oil should not be used routinely to treat constipation. The unpleasant taste of castor oil can be decreased by chilling or pouring over ice or mixing in chilled fruit juice.	Contact laxatives should be used only for occasional treatment of constipation. They are habit forming, decreasing the natural mechanisms for evacuation. Tablets should not be chewed. Take tablets with a full glass of water. Do not exceed recommended dosage. Take bisacodyl 1 hr after taking antacids or milk. Suppository form may cause burning sensation in the rectum.
Drugs for Inflammatory Bowel Disease (IBD)			
Sulfasalazine (Azulfidine) Mesalamine (5-ASA) Olsalazine (Dipentum)	Sulfasalazine is a sulfonamide antibiotic. Mesalamine is the active agent in sulfasalazine.	May cause muscle aches, nausea, fever, or rash. Complete blood counts needed periodically as the drugs can cause agranulocytosis and anemia.	Caution patient to avoid direct sunlight and ultraviolet light to prevent photosensitivity reaction.

5-ASA, 5-aminosalicylic acid; *GI*, gastrointestinal; *IV*, intravenously.

Table 30-1   Commonly Prescribed Drugs for Gastrointestinal Disorders—cont'd

CLASSIFICATION	ACTION	NURSING IMPLICATIONS	PATIENT TEACHING
Drugs for Inflammatory Bowel Disease (IBD)—cont'd			
	Olsalazine contains two molecules of 5-ASA. These drugs reduce inflammation in the bowel by suppressing prostaglandin synthesis and the migration of inflammatory cells into the affected area.	Determine whether allergy to sulfonamides exists before administration.	Advise to use form of contraception other than oral contraceptives as these drugs interfere with their effectiveness. Warn that when used with oral hypoglycemics, an increased hypoglycemic effect may occur. Advise that urine may be tinted orange. GI upset may be minimized by taking drug after meals. Instruct to report rash or sensitivity reaction to physician promptly.
Lubiprostone (Amitiza)	Increases the volume of intestinal fluid, which makes stool easier to pass.	For treating constipation in women over 18 years old. Can cause nausea, diarrhea, and abdominal pain. In rare cases can cause dyspnea.	Teach to take with food and water to decrease side effects. Advise to seek attention immediately if dyspnea occurs.
Infliximab (Remicade)	Monoclonal antibody that neutralizes the activity of tumor necrosis factor–alpha found in Crohn's disease; decreases infiltration of inflammatory cells.	Given IV over at least 2 hr. Dose repeated at 2 wk and then q 6 wk from first dose. Observe for anaphylactic reaction.	May initially cause increased diarrhea. Report nausea, vomiting, abdominal pain, itching, or rash to physician. Need periodic blood counts. Do not breast-feed while taking this drug.
Antispasmodics			
Dicyclomine hydrochloride (Bentyl, Antispas) Propantheline bromide (Pro-Banthine) Oxyphencyclimine hydrochloride (Daricon)	Block acetylcholine, thereby decreasing smooth-muscle spasm and GI motility and inhibiting gastric acid secretion.	These drugs interact with many other drugs; check each drug patient is taking for interactions. Most of these drugs are contraindicated in glaucoma, prostatic hypertrophy, myasthenia gravis, and other conditions; consult information on each drug individually. May predispose to drug-induced heat stroke. Monitor vital signs and urine output carefully.	Take 30-60 min before meal. Patient can suck on hard candy to relieve mouth dryness unless contraindicated. Have patient drink 2500-3000 mL of fluid to prevent constipation. Avoid driving or hazardous activities if drug causes dizziness, sleepiness, or blurred vision. Report rash or skin eruption to physician.
Hyoscyamine (Levsin)	Inhibits action of acetylcholine at postganglionic receptor sites, decreasing spasm and abdominal pain.	May decrease absorption of antacids and antidiarrheals. May increase effects of anticholinergics. May cause urinary retention. Assess for dehydration; encourage adequate fluid intake.	May cause dry mouth. Inform physician of rash, eye pain, difficulty in urinating, or constipation. Avoid hot baths and saunas. May initially cause dizziness or faintness; do not operate machinery until response is known.

Etiology and Pathophysiology

Diverticula tend to develop in people over age 50 who have chronic constipation and/or eat a low-fiber diet. Diverticulitis occurs when the diverticula become inflamed or infected. Waste accumulates in the diverticula and can irritate the mucosal wall. Diverticulitis affects one third of adults over age 60.

Increases in intra-abdominal pressure from constipation and straining to defecate are thought to be factors in the development of colon diverticula. Muscle of the colon hypertrophies, thickens, and becomes rigid. The increased intra-abdominal pressure causes herniation of the mucosa and submucosa through the colon wall. Diverticulitis occurs when food caught in the diverticulum mixes with bacteria. The intestinal wall becomes irritated and infected, and if it is not treated, perforation and peritonitis may occur.

Esophageal diverticula occur when there is herniation of esophageal mucosa and submucosa into surrounding tissue. The disorder is more common in older patients.

Signs, Symptoms, and Diagnosis

A person with diverticulosis may initially be asymptomatic; however symptoms will develop when inflammation or infection occurs because material has lodged in diverticula. For bowel diverticula, there is usually a history of constipation. There may be rectal bleeding. **Diverticulitis of the intestine produces symptoms of diarrhea or constipation, acute severe left lower abdominal pain, fever, and rectal bleeding. The condition may be complicated by intestinal obstruction or by peritonitis if the intestinal wall ruptures.** If bleeding is massive, there will be hypotension and dehydration and eventual shock. Computed tomography with contrast is the preferred diagnostic test. Barium enema and colonoscopy should be avoided in acute cases, due to risk of bowel perforation (Carroll, 2009).

Esophageal diverticula produce complaints of dysphagia, regurgitation, nocturnal cough, and *halitosis* (bad breath). There is a risk of esophageal perforation.

 Think Critically

What is the difference between the signs and symptoms of diverticulitis and those of irritable bowel syndrome?

Treatment and Nursing Management

Diverticulosis often can be managed conservatively. A high-fiber diet, increased fluids and bulk laxatives, or stool softeners to control constipation may be all that are needed.

For diverticulitis, antidiarrheal medication may be prescribed. The role of the LPN/LVN is to reinforce education about the diet, fluid intake, and exercise. Mild pain medication may be used for abdominal discomfort in the ambulatory patient. In acute cases of diverticulitis, parenteral antibiotics, nothing-by-mouth (NPO) status for 2 to 3 days and intravenous (IV) fluids may be necessary. Meperidine (Demerol) may be prescribed for pain, rather than morphine, because morphine increases intraluminal pressure (Carroll, 2009). Recurrent episodes of diverticulitis, or perforation and peritonitis, require surgical removal of the affected part of the colon.

 Safety Alert

Meperidine Toxicity

A metabolite of meperidine (Demerol) is toxic, and the elderly have difficulty metabolizing and eliminating it. The buildup of the toxin in the blood can cause seizures and other mental status changes such as acute confusion. Ask for an alternate analgesic for these patients.

 Nutrition Considerations

Diet for Diverticular Disease

A high-fiber diet is encouraged for the patient with diverticular disease. Eating whole-grain cereals and breads, as well as fruits such as apples, seedless berries, peaches, and pears adds fiber. High-fiber vegetables—squash, broccoli, cabbage, and spinach—and legumes, including dried beans, peas, and lentils, provide bulk that decreases constipation and speeds the transit time in the intestine. Drinking plenty of fluids and water helps regularity. This diet, combined with exercise to prevent constipation, can usually control diverticular disease. Patients who have recurrent diverticulitis are asked to avoid foods with husks, such as peanuts, sunflower seeds, berries with seeds, tomatoes, and popcorn, as a precautionary measure. The husks may get into the diverticulum and irritate it, causing inflammation and eventual diverticulitis.

INTESTINAL OBSTRUCTION

Intestinal obstruction is a sudden or gradual blockage of the intestinal tract that prevents the normal passage of gastrointestinal (GI) contents through the intestines.

Etiology and Pathophysiology

Mechanical obstruction results in blockage of the lumen of the bowel. Examples include tumors, adhesions, strangulated hernia, twisting of the bowel (volvulus), telescoping of one part of the bowel into another (intussusception), gallstones, barium impaction, and intestinal parasites (Figure 30-2). Abdominal adhesions are a common cause of intestinal obstruction. Adhesions form when inflammation from abdominal trauma or surgery has occurred, and fibrous bands of scar tissue hold together two segments of bowel that are normally separated.

Nonmechanical obstruction results from the absence of peristalsis (movement of contents through the bowel stops). Nonmechanical obstructions may

Hernia

Intussusception

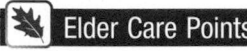

Volvulus

FIGURE 30-2 Mechanical causes of intestinal obstruction.

⚡ Elder Care Points

The elderly are more prone to the occurrence of volvulus and consequent intestinal obstruction, partially because of decreased muscle tone. Suspect this disorder when the elderly patient complains of sudden abdominal pain with vomiting, has abdominal distention with a palpable mass, has increased bowel sounds on auscultation, and exhibits signs of dehydration.

---

occur as a result of paralytic ileus (failure of forward movement of bowel contents) following abdominal surgery, from infection, or as a consequence of hypokalemia. Nonmechanical obstructions may be secondary to intestinal thrombus. Infections can occur in some pelvic inflammatory diseases or peritonitis, in uremia, and in heavy-metal poisoning. All of these conditions can interfere with normal peristaltic action and produce a nonmechanical obstruction.

When obstruction occurs, fluid and gas accumulate in the intestine, increasing intraluminal pressure. Peristaltic waves above the obstruction may occur as the intestine attempts to move material down the tract. These waves may cause severe pain.

Signs and Symptoms
The symptoms of intestinal obstruction vary according to the location of the obstruction. Obstructions occurring high in the intestinal tract are characterized by

sharp, brief pains in the upper abdomen. Frequent bowel sounds are high pitched above the point of obstruction, and bowel sounds are absent below the obstruction. Other symptoms include vomiting, with rapid dehydration and only slight abdominal distention. An acute intestinal obstruction in the upper abdomen can cause respiratory difficulty because of the pressure of the distended abdomen against the diaphragm.

Obstructions of the colon are characterized by a more gradual onset, with marked abdominal distention as the bowel fills, infrequent vomiting (which occurs late in the process if at all), and **pains that last several minutes or longer and correspond to peristaltic waves.** Fecal odor or material in the emesis suggests a complete intestinal obstruction.

Diagnosis and Treatment
Diagnostic x-rays are ordered to locate the obstruction. For some patients, the insertion of an intestinal tube, which is a long tube inserted via the nose (Figure 30-3) relieves the obstruction by decompressing the intestine above the obstruction. Surgery is indicated for obstruction caused by adhesions, volvulus, hernia, or tumor. Adhesions are lysed (broken apart), a volvulus is untwisted, or a colectomy may be necessary if tumor is involved.

Nursing Management
Placing the patient in Fowler's position helps relieve pressure and also aids in removing gas and intestinal contents through the intestinal tube. Fluid and electrolyte status must be monitored closely. Measure

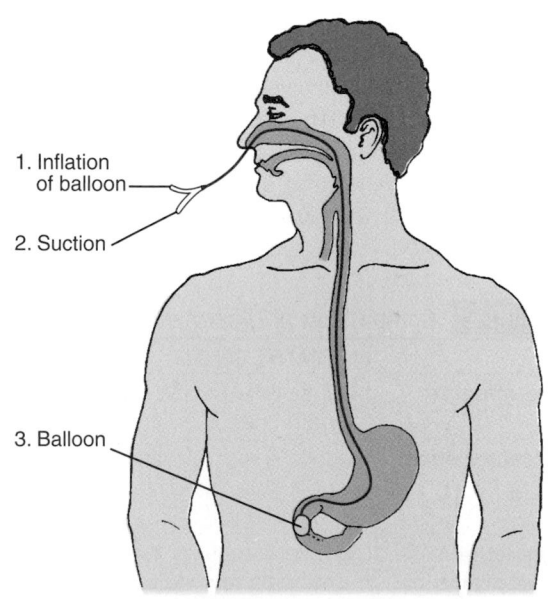

1. Inflation of balloon

2. Suction

3. Balloon

FIGURE 30-3 Miller-Abbott intestinal tube used for decompression. It is advanced through the intestines to the prescribed point. The Miller-Abbott tube has a double lumen and is weighted with tungsten. *(1)* Portion of the metal tip leading to the balloon. *(2)* Portion of the metal tip leading to the lumen that can be suctioned. *(3)* Balloon inflated with air.

abdominal girth every 2 to 4 hours, by placing the tape at the same location on the abdomen each time. Pain control is essential, but worsening pain may signal an unresolved, intestinal obstruction which can lead to rupture of the intestine, peritonitis, shock, and death. If the obstruction cannot be resolved, surgical correction must be done. Postoperative care is the same as for other abdominal surgery patients (see Chapter 5 and Nursing Care Plan 30-1 on pp. 676-678 and 30-2 on Evolve).

BOWEL ISCHEMIA

Bowel ischemia occurs when the blood supply to the bowel is insufficient to support metabolic needs. It can be an acute process with a sudden onset of symptoms, or a chronic condition.

Etiology and Pathophysiology

The problem may involve the arterial or the venous blood supply in the form of emboli, thrombosis, or the gradual narrowing and occlusion of vessels. Ischemia can occur as the result of a bowel obstruction or as the result of hypovolemic shock. Underlying cardiac conditions—such as atrial fibrillation or use of vasoconstrictive drugs—can be contributing factors.

Signs, Symptoms, and Diagnosis

A careful history is necessary, because the symptoms are similar to many other abdominal disorders. The sudden onset of severe abdominal pain signals an acute condition. Nausea, vomiting, diarrhea, and abdominal cramps may also be present. The abdomen is tender to palpation and the patient will exhibit guarding. Bowel sounds will be minimal or absent. The white blood cell count is likely to be elevated. Computed tomography angiography is used to confirm the medical diagnosis.

Treatment and Nursing Management

The patient will be NPO and a nasogastric (NG) tube will be inserted to relieve distention. IV hydration is usually ordered, and a Foley catheter may be used to monitor output in the acute phase. If the damage is not severe, conservative measures such as bowel rest and IV hydration will continue. If damage is severe or if the cause is related to an unresolved anatomical obstruction, the patient may require surgery.

INFLAMMATORY BOWEL DISEASE

Ulcerative Colitis and Crohn's Disease

Inflammatory bowel disease (IBD) commonly starts between ages 15 and 35. There is a growing tendency to include both ulcerative colitis and Crohn's disease under the title of IBD. Ulcerative colitis is an inflammation, with formation of ulcers of the mucosa of the colon. It often is a chronic disease and the patient is usually asymptomatic between acute flare-ups. People with ulcerative colitis have a 40% higher incidence of some types of arthritis. Crohn's disease can involve any part of the GI tract, but most commonly affects the distal ileum and proximal colon.

Etiology

Crohn's disease and ulcerative colitis have a genetic predisposition. Both disorders also have an ethnic correlation as they are more common among the Jewish population. Immunologic activity is thought to be involved as well because anticolon antibodies are often present in the blood. With ulcerative colitis, infections and emotional tension frequently bring about acute attacks.

Pathophysiology

The pathophysiology of IBD is being investigated. It is suspected that ulcerative colitis and Crohn's disease are immunologic responses to the same (as-yet-unknown) etiologic agent. The end result is inflammation of the mucosal lining of the intestinal tract, causing ulceration, edema, bleeding, and fluid and electrolyte loss. Ulcerative colitis and Crohn's disease (regional ileitis) share many of the same characteristics (Table 30-2). One difference is that the inflammatory changes in ulcerative colitis are

Table 30-2 Comparison of Ulcerative Colitis and Crohn's Disease

	ULCERATIVE COLITIS	CROHN'S DISEASE
Area affected	Mucosa only; usually involves rectum and proceeds up the colon	Full thickness of the intestine; most common in small intestine
Characteristics	Mucosa is red, intestinal wall is edematous and friable, bleeding easily; pseudopolyps are present	Edematous bowel wall, inflammatory cells, mucosal ulcerations, granulomas, and "skip" lesions (normal areas)
Signs and symptoms	Diarrhea, frequently bloody; abdominal cramping relieved by defecation; rectal bleeding	Fever, malaise, fatigue, weight loss, intermittent diarrhea, cramping or steady right lower quadrant or periumbilical pain, postprandial bloating
Complications	Massive hemorrhage; hypovolemia, toxic megacolon (rapid dilation of the intestines), cancer of the colon	Fistulas, anal fissures, perianal disease, bowel obstruction or perforation

nonspecific, whereas those in Crohn's disease are granulomatous (a mass of inflamed tissue characterized by the presence of small granules). Patients with long-standing chronic ulcerative colitis are at 10 to 20 times greater risk for developing cancer of the colon than patients with Crohn's disease. The constant inflammation disrupts normal cell function, and cellular mutations may occur. Crohn's disease can affect any area of the intestine, although it more frequently affects the ascending colon and can affect the small intestine (Figure 30-4). Ulcerative colitis most often affects the rectosigmoid and left colon. Changes due to ulcerative colitis tend to be continuous along the affected portion of the bowel, whereas changes due to Crohn's disease are segmental, leaving healthy sections of bowel in between diseased portions ("skip lesions"). With Crohn's disease, radiograph reveals a cobblestone appearance to the mucosa.

Signs and Symptoms

The patient with IBD suffers from attacks of diarrhea that may be bloody and contain mucus; abdominal pain with cramping; malaise; fever; and weight loss. The color of blood in the stool depends on the degree and rapidity of the bleed. Slow bleeding and oozing will show a black, tarry stool. If diarrhea is frequent, the blood may be more reddish. The stool color is also dependent on where in the intestine the bleeding is occurring. Blood tends to be redder when the bleeding location is lower in the intestine. The bouts of IBD symptoms often are precipitated by events that cause undue physical or emotional stress. An acute attack can last for days, weeks, or even months, followed by periods of remission extending from a few weeks to several decades. A few patients experience only one attack, and then remain free of symptoms for the rest of their lives. Others have serious intestinal hemorrhage with fluid and electrolyte imbalances.

⚠ Safety Alert

Opioids and Anticholinergic Medications

If your patient has ulcerative colitis, opioid medications or anticholinergic medications should be avoided if there is fever, leukocytosis, or worsening symptoms because these medications will further reduce the tone of the colon (Beach, 2008).

Diagnosis

Medical diagnosis of IBD usually is based on the patient's medical history and symptoms. Colonoscopy, flexible sigmoidoscopy, mucosal biopsy, barium enema, and stool analysis may be performed to confirm the diagnosis.

Treatment

Treatment for either ulcerative colitis or Crohn's disease varies according to severity of symptoms and whether the condition becomes chronic. Conservative approaches to medical treatment include administration of antidiarrheal drugs, long-term sulfasalazine therapy, and medications to relieve abdominal cramps. The recommended diet consists of low-fat, low-fiber foods that are high in protein and calories. Small frequent feedings are best. Lactose avoidance helps some patients. Corticosteroids are used for moderate to severe cases to decrease the inflammation. During acute attacks, fluid replacement may be necessary. Blood transfusions are given when anemia is present. Oral 5-aminosalicylic acid (5-ASA) derivatives, such as

CROHN'S DISEASE

Skip involvements

ULCERATIVE COLITIS

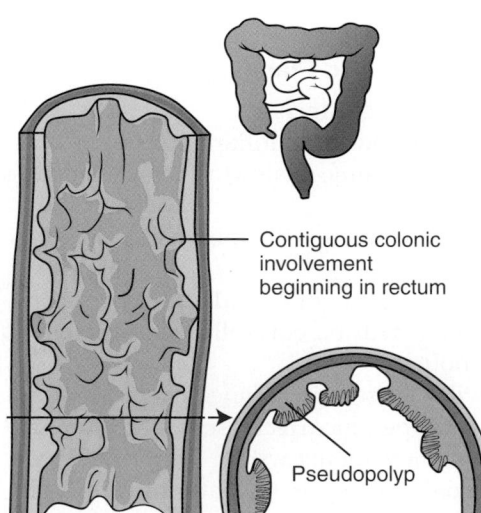

Contiguous colonic involvement beginning in rectum

Pseudopolyp

FIGURE 30-4 Comparison of the distribution of disease and characteristics of lesions of Crohn's disease and ulcerative colitis.

olsalazine sodium (Dipentum), are useful for those patients who cannot tolerate sulfasalazine (see Table 30-1). Budesonide (Entocort) is used to help control disease in the ileum. Patients with advanced disease who are not surgical candidates may be given azathioprine, 6-mercaptopurine, methotrexate, levamisole, or cyclosporine to help control the disease (Tocco, 2009).

Infliximab (Remicade), a monoclonal antibody against tumor necrosis factor, has greater than 80% response rate for Crohn's disease, but only about a 50% success rate with ulcerative colitis. The drug is extremely expensive and is given IV by a set protocol. Certolizumab pegol (Cimzia) is a new drug for patients with moderate to severe Crohn's disease who have not responded to conventional treatments.

Surgical intervention is an alternative treatment for some patients. The surgical procedure usually involves removing the affected portion of the bowel, often by proctocolectomy, and creating an ileostomy. Today a patient with ulcerative colitis may be a candidate for an ileal reservoir (Kock pouch) or an ileoanal anastomosis rather than a standard ileostomy. Both of these procedures allow the patient control over the discharge of wastes from the reservoir, and consequently a collection pouch is not necessary. The patient uses a catheter to empty the reservoir after the Kock procedure. With an ileoanal anastomosis, the patient retains control over the anal sphincter with voluntary defecation. These procedures are not performed often for Crohn's disease because as the disease progresses, the area of the reservoir is involved.

❖ NURSING MANAGEMENT

▪ Assessment (Data Collection)

A complete health assessment is performed with particular attention to pain, nutritional, and fluid and electrolyte status. A thorough abdominal assessment is performed.

▪ Nursing Diagnosis and Planning

Nursing diagnoses might include:
- Pain related to intestinal inflammation
- Deficient fluid volume related to diarrhea fluid loss
- Diarrhea

Other common nursing diagnoses are listed in Table 28-2.

Expected outcomes might include:
- Patient's pain will be controlled with analgesia within 8 hours.
- Patient will regain fluid balance within 24 hours.
- Patient will experience decreased number of diarrhea bowel movements within 24 hours.

Long-term goals are to help the patient adhere to the prescribed regimen, encourage effective coping mechanisms, and participate in prescribed psychotherapy.

▪ Implementation and Evaluation

For an acute attack of IBD, care includes monitoring the number and character of stools, periodic auscultation of bowel sounds, measurement of intake and output, and daily weight measurement. Check for signs of internal bleeding and anemia, and monitor laboratory data for evidence of electrolyte imbalances. Indicators of successful therapy include a decrease in abdominal cramping and discomfort and return of typical bowel pattern.

> **? Think Critically**
>
> Can you describe three key differences between Crohn's disease and ulcerative colitis?

APPENDICITIS

Etiology and Pathophysiology

Appendicitis is an inflammation of the appendix, which is a blind pouch and is therefore easily infected by bacteria passing through the intestinal tract.

Signs, Symptoms, and Diagnosis

Pain in the lower right side, halfway between the umbilicus and the crest of the ileum, at McBurney's point is the best-known symptom of appendicitis. It is usually accompanied by muscle guarding. However, the location of the pain may—and often does—vary among individuals. The patient may rest with the right thigh drawn up. Extending the leg causes pain. **A slight temperature elevation (1° F), nausea and vomiting, and an increase in the white cell count also are characteristic of appendicitis.** Contrast-enhanced computed tomography (CT) scan is the diagnostic test of choice. Ultrasound and perhaps laparoscopy can be used to make the diagnosis if the patient is pregnant (Clin-eguide, 2008).

> **🌿 Elder Care Points**
>
> Peritoneal inflammation does not necessarily cause abdominal rigidity in the elderly patient. These patients often have only diffuse abdominal pain, malaise, and weakness. Confusion may be present and the elderly patient will have an increased risk for falls.

Treatment

Appendicitis is treated by surgically removing the appendix *(appendectomy)*. This procedure may be performed laparoscopically or require an open laparotomy. Patients may be observed for 6 to 10 hours if there is no immediate need for surgery. Before surgery, the patient is NPO. **Under no circumstances should laxatives be given when appendicitis is suspected, because of the increased risk for rupture.**

Cold, Not Heat, for Appendicitis

Never use heat to relieve abdominal pain if appendicitis is suspected. Heat might bring enough blood and fluid to the appendix to cause it to rupture and cause peritonitis. An ice bag may be placed on the abdomen to slow down the inflammation and thus avoid rupture of the swollen and inflamed appendix.

The patient is usually allowed out of bed within several hours of surgery, if there are no complications. The patient undergoing an uncomplicated laparoscopic appendectomy may be discharged the same day after an adequate anesthesia recovery period. The convalescent period is most often uneventful, and the patient may return to her former activities within 1 to 2 weeks. The patient who had an open laparotomy needs 2 to 4 weeks for recovery.

Nursing Management
Assess for nausea, pain level, vital signs, and check the abdomen for rigidity that might indicate a ruptured appendix. A diet history for the previous 24 to 48 hours is obtained to help determine if food poisoning is a cause of the symptoms. Date and character of the last bowel movement and usual bowel pattern are obtained. Common nursing diagnoses are listed in Table 28-2. Preoperatively, pain is the primary nursing diagnosis. Traditionally, the patient is not medicated for pain until the cause of the abdominal pain is diagnosed; the rationale is that analgesia can mask important signs and symptoms. The nurse should initiate nonpharmacologic comfort measures, such as resting quietly (movement tends to aggravate the pain) in a comfortable position. When appendicitis is suspected, obtain an order to apply a cold pack to the area of tenderness. Medication may be given for nausea and vomiting, which will provide symptom relief, and the nurse should advocate for the patient to have pain medication as soon as possible. Postoperatively, pain control and prevention of infection at the surgical site are nursing priorities.

PERITONITIS
Etiology
Peritonitis is an inflammation of the peritoneum. It usually occurs when one of the organs it encloses ruptures or is perforated so that the organ's contents (including bacteria) are spilled into the abdominal cavity. Examples of common causes of peritonitis are ruptured appendix, perforated duodenal or gastric ulcer, ruptured ectopic (tubal) pregnancy, diverticulitis with perforation, and traumatic rupture of the colon, spleen, or liver.

Pathophysiology
As the peritoneum becomes inflamed, there is local redness and swelling of the membrane and production of serous fluid that becomes increasingly purulent as the bacteria multiply. Normal peristaltic action of the intestines slows or ceases and symptoms of intestinal obstruction occur.

Signs and Symptoms
The patient experiences nausea, vomiting, and severe abdominal pain and distention. Fever, chills, tachycardia, and pallor occur, and other symptoms of shock may emerge. **Unless the condition is treated promptly and successfully, peritonitis can be fatal.**

Diagnosis and Treatment
Diagnosis of peritonitis is by history, physical examination, and results of a complete blood count (CBC). A CT scan of the abdomen may be performed to rule out structural problems or tumor. Broad-spectrum antibiotics are given IV and IV fluids and electrolytes are administered to restore a normal balance, and gastric or intestinal decompression is initiated to relieve distention. Surgical procedures needed to repair a ruptured organ are done as soon as the patient's condition will permit. The surgical wound is generally left open after surgery so that healing occurs from the inside out and abscesses do not form.

Nursing Management
Frequent assessment and prompt and accurate reporting of unexpected changes in condition are required. The patient is usually placed in the semi-Fowler's position to facilitate breathing, prevent respiratory complications, and aid in localizing the purulent material in the lower abdomen or pelvis. Vital signs are taken and recorded at least every 1 to 2 hours during the critical stage. If vomiting occurs, the characteristics and amount of vomitus are noted.

A common complication of peritonitis is paralytic ileus. Auscultate at least once a shift for the return of bowel sounds. If the patient passes flatus or feces rectally, this should be recorded on the chart, as it indicates return of peristalsis.

Because of the high fever and toxicity that accompany peritonitis, the patient may be delirious or disoriented and must be protected from self-injury. This includes putting side rails up and having someone at the bedside at all times. The patient should be turned *very gently* and moved in the bed with care because of extreme tenderness in the abdominal region. A high fever and the presence of the gastric tube demand frequent mouth care to protect the lips, prevent halitosis, and cleanse the mouth.

MALABSORPTION
Etiology and Pathophysiology
Many disorders interfere with the normal absorption of nutrients, water, and vitamins from the intestine. Adult celiac disease *(sprue)*, in which the patient cannot properly metabolize gluten (a protein found

in all wheat products, barley, and rye), is one cause. Lactose intolerance is another cause because it results in diarrhea. Pancreatic disease with interference in secretion of pancreatic digestive enzymes also causes malabsorption. Some patients who have undergone chemotherapy for treatment of cancer experience alteration of the intestinal mucosa that causes malabsorption. **Whatever the cause, malabsorption creates a nutritional deficiency.** Pathophysiologically, there is irritation of the intestinal mucosa and consequent diarrhea. Both problems limit the ability of the intestine to absorb nutrients.

 Cultural Considerations

Lactose Intolerance

Lactose intolerance is most common in Native Americans, but it can affect people at any age and any ethnicity. It is caused by lack of the enzyme lactase, which is needed to digest lactose. Assess for bloating, flatulence, cramps, and loose stools or diarrhea after consuming milk or milk products.

Signs, Symptoms, and Diagnosis

A key sign of malabsorption is steatorrhea or passage of stool that is bulky, frothy, and foul smelling and usually floats in the toilet. Other signs and symptoms include weight loss, weakness, and various signs of vitamin deficiency depending on the type of malabsorption the patient is experiencing. Diagnosis is by history, upper and lower GI series, and endoscopy with biopsy. Gluten intolerance is diagnosed by blood tests for gluten antibodies and small bowel biopsy.

 Clinical Cues

If your patient is to undergo testing for gluten intolerance, she must eat wheat and gluten products for 2 weeks before testing; otherwise, the tests will not be accurate.

Treatment and Nursing Management

Treatment is directed at the underlying cause. Pancreatic insufficiency can be treated by administering pancreatic enzymes with meals. Celiac disease is treated by completely omitting gluten from the diet. Nursing management consists of supporting the patient through the diagnostic process and reinforcing teaching about diet and medications. The patient is often required to take supplements of vitamins and minerals as a lifetime therapy.

CANCER OF THE COLON

Cancer of the large intestine, also called colorectal cancer, is the third most common malignancy in both men and women in the United States. Certain forms of colon cancer have been identified as having a genetic link and definitely show a familial tendency for occurrence. Approximately 141,210 colorectal cancer cases were expected to occur in 2011 (American Cancer Society,

2011). Colorectal cancer is one of the most curable of all cancers if it is found in the early stages, and mortality rates have fallen over the last 30 years as detection has become easier. *Healthy People 2020* objectives include the reduction of deaths by colorectal cancer and a decrease in the incidence of invasive colorectal cancer.

 Cultural Considerations

Colorectal Cancer Incidence

Colorectal cancer incidence is highest in African American men and women. Worse yet, mortality rates in African Americans are higher than in the white population. It is not certain whether this is because of access to health care, or is due to other reasons. Always assess an African American over 40 years of age for risk factors and signs and symptoms of colorectal cancer. Encourage annual screening after age 50. High-risk patients need individualized counseling for screening and follow-up (Mayo Clinic, 2009).

Etiology

The cause of colorectal cancer has not been established. The disease mainly occurs in people over age 50, although there is a type that occurs in young people. People most at risk include those with disorders of the intestinal tract, especially ulcerative colitis and familial polyposis. Other risk factors are smoking, alcohol consumption, physical inactivity, obesity, and a diet high in saturated fat and/or red meat, as well as inadequate intake of fruits and vegetables (American Cancer Society, 2011).

 Nutrition Considerations

The Colon and Conjugated Linoleic Acid

In research studies with animals, conjugated linoleic acid (CLA) was found to have a protective effect against inflammation-induced colon cancer. CLA is found in high-fat dairy foods, meats, eggs, and poultry; additional research is ongoing to investigate the applicability to human subjects and risk versus benefit for overweight persons (Evans et al., 2010).

 Health Promotion

Colon Cancer Preventive Measures

Preventive measures include a diet that is high in fiber and low in red meat and animal fat. Nutrients that offer protection against colon cancer are fiber, calcium carbonate, selenium, and vitamin C.

Pathophysiology

The tumor may be polypoid, protruding into the bowel lumen, or it may be annular and extend around the bowel, causing stricture. Most large bowel tumors are adenocarcinomas and are thought to arise from adenomatous polyps that visibly protrude from the mucosal surface of the bowel. The tumor may spread into adjacent structures or via the lymphatics or the bloodstream.

 Complementary and Alternative Therapies

Aspirin, Folic Acid, and Calcium

Recent studies suggest that polyp formation can be reduced by taking a baby aspirin a day and supplementing folic acid and calcium (Wilkes, 2008).

Signs and Symptoms

In the early stages, symptoms are typically mild and vague and depend on the location of the tumor and the function of the affected area. Weight loss may be the first sign. Later signs of colorectal cancer are the result of obstruction of the bowel and extension of the growth to adjacent structures. **Any change in bowel habits, either diarrhea or constipation, could be a sign of colon cancer** (American Cancer Society, 2010a).

Other symptoms include red blood in the stool, black tarry stools, change in stool shape (ribbon-like stool), abdominal distention without weight gain, sensation of incomplete evacuation after a bowel movement, and anemia resulting from intestinal bleeding. Abdominal pain and a sensation of pressure in the lower abdomen or rectum frequently are present. Digital examination may reveal a mass in the anus.

Diagnosis

Screening tests include an annual stool guaiac test or fecal immunochemical test or stool DNA test (frequency for DNA test is undetermined). Beginning at age 50 flexible sigmoidoscopy is recommended every 5 years, colonoscopy every 10 years, double contrast barium x-ray every 5 years, or CT colonography (virtual colonoscopy) every 5 years. Colonoscopy is recommended if any of the screening tests are positive (American Cancer Society, 2010b). If adenomatous polyps are discovered early and removed, colon cancer could be prevented. Tumors of the rectum or lower sigmoid colon are seen by proctosigmoidoscopy. Transrectal ultrasound may be used to determine the extent of a small rectal lesion. Carcinoembryonic antigen is elevated in 70% of patients with colorectal cancer, but since it is nonspecific to this type of cancer, it is mainly used to monitor the effectiveness of treatment.

Treatment

Treatment of colorectal cancer usually involves surgical removal of the affected portion of the intestine. Anastomosis (attachment of one to the other) of the remaining portions is done if the lesion is small and localized (hemicolectomy). A new drug, alvimopan (Entereg), may be used to speed the healing process of the bowel in cases when there is resection and anastomosis. Larger tumors are treated by excising the affected portion of the colon. Occasionally, a surgically created opening on the abdomen (colostomy) is needed to provide for elimination of fecal matter. A permanent colostomy is rarely needed for cancer of the colon. After healing takes place, the colon is reconnected.

Most tumors are resected with an open approach, but laparoscopic surgery is an option for a small, localized tumor. Further treatment depends on the stage of the cancer—whether the tumor is through the bowel mucosa, through the bowel wall, or affecting lymph nodes or has metastasized to other organs.

Colectomy or Hemicolectomy. Colectomy is the removal of the diseased portion of the colon. The remaining ends of the colon are reattached (anastomosed). *Hemicolectomy* is removal of one half of the colon.

Abdominoperineal Resection. Abdominal resection is performed for cancer in the rectum or low sigmoid colon. It is a very extensive surgical procedure in which part of the colon and the entire rectum, anus, and regional lymph nodes are removed. Both an abdominal and a perineal incision are necessary for this procedure. Because of the nature of the surgery, a permanent colostomy is necessary. Because of the high lithotomy position used during surgery, these patients are at increased risk for thrombophlebitis postoperatively.

Adjunctive Treatment. Preoperative, intraoperative, or postoperative radiation and chemotherapy may be given for cancer of the rectum. Use of radiation or chemotherapy for colon cancer depends on the stage of the tumor and the presence of metastasis. When metastasis is present, the patient is usually treated with 5-fluorouracil (5-FU) with or without leucovorin (folinic acid). Oxaliplatin (Eloxatin) is a new drug used with 5-FU and leucovorin for treatment-resistant tumors. Intra-arterial chemotherapy may be directed into the liver if metastasis has occurred. Two other drugs may be used as well. Bevacizumab (Avastin) is an antiangiogenesis medication that reduces blood flow to the growing tumor cells, depriving them of nutrients needed for replication. Cetuximab (Erbitux) and panitumumab (Vectibix) are monoclonal antibodies that bind to protein to slow cell growth. Both are used with other chemotherapy drugs. Irinotecan (Camptosar) is available to treat recurrent colon cancer. Capecitabine (Xeloda) is given orally when the tumor has not penetrated the colon wall.

Nursing Management

An abdominal assessment is performed. Questions are asked regarding bowel pattern and changes, diet pattern, and amounts of red meat and charred or grilled food usually eaten. Determine the amount of alcohol consumption and the degree of cigarette smoking. Assess for a family history of colon cancer. Check diagnostic test results such as the CBC, liver enzymes, and amylase for signs of anemia and possible metastatic involvement of the liver or pancreas.

The patient is likely to be very anxious once a diagnosis of colon cancer has been made. Before surgery, focus on the preoperative care and what the patient needs to be taught. Cover what to expect and provide information about postoperative care. Nursing Care Plan 30-1 describes postoperative care of the patient who has had abdominal surgery with a colectomy.

 Nursing Care Plan 30-1 | **Care of the Patient Undergoing Colectomy for Probable Colon Cancer**

Scenario
Mrs. Simpson, age 58, just returned from surgery and has a dressing over the colectomy site. She has a family history of polyposis of the colon. She had a colectomy because of a malignant lesion in the upper portion of the sigmoid colon. She was NPO even before surgery for a variety of tests. She is experiencing pain and receiving morphine by PCA pump. An NG tube was inserted and attached to suction. She is very frightened, because her father died with colon cancer. She dreads chemotherapy. Mrs. Simpson is a loan officer with a national bank, is very busy, and had put off having a physical exam and sigmoidoscopy until this month, when she noticed some blood in a loose stool. She had experienced some bouts of loose stools but thought these were a result of the stress she was experiencing on her job.

Problem/Nursing Diagnosis
Abdominal pain/Pain related to abdominal surgery.

Supporting Assessment Data
Subjective: "I'm still really hurting."
Objective: Colectomy, abdominal incision with wound drain; pain at 5 on 1-to-10 scale.

Goals/Expected Outcomes	Nursing Interventions	Selected Rationale	Evaluation
Pain will be controlled with analgesia during hospitalization.	Initially assess for pain q 1-2 hr or prn using pain scale and document location and characteristics.	Pain scale use provides more objective measure of pain. Frequency of assessment may be changed to q 3-4 hr as condition improves.	Pain at 2–3 with use of PCA.
	Monitor use of PCA pump.	PCA allows patient better control over pain.	Using PCA appropriately.
Patient will use relaxation techniques to decrease pain before discharge.	Teach relaxation techniques to decrease anxiety.	Relaxation helps decrease pain.	Taught deep-breathing relaxation exercise.
	Provide comfort measures, such as a tidy odor-free room and quiet environment.	Comfort measures help to decrease the subjective experience of pain.	Lights dimmed and linens changed. Patient expresses appreciation. Continue plan.

Problem/Nursing Diagnosis
Ordered NPO/Risk for deficient fluid volume related to NPO status and nasogastric tube.

Supporting Assessment Data
Objective: NPO for 3-5 days; NG tube in place; IV infusing.

Goals/Expected Outcomes	Nursing Interventions	Selected Rationale	Evaluation
Patient will not develop fluid or electrolyte imbalance as evidenced by good skin turgor, moist mucous membranes, and electrolyte studies within normal range.	Assess amount of stomach secretions from NG tube every shift and document.	Volume of stomach drainage must be counted as part of total output.	250 mL light brown fluid drainage this shift.
	Assess for signs of dehydration (i.e., poor skin turgor, decreased amounts, and concentrated urine).	If dehydration persists or worsens, the doctor must be notified so that therapy can be adjusted.	Voiding pale yellow urine; skin dry, but no tenting.
	Maintain IV fluid flow as ordered.	Provides fluid while the patient is NPO	IV flowing at 125 mL/hr.
	Maintain I&O record.	I&O record helps evaluate fluid status.	Intake 1000 mL, output 895 mL this shift.
	Monitor electrolyte laboratory values.	Laboratory values indicate electrolyte imbalances if they occur.	Laboratory specimens to be obtained in A.M. No signs of electrolyte imbalance. Continue plan.

BP, blood pressure; *CBC*, complete blood count; *I&O*, intake and output; *IV*, intravenous; *NG*, nasogastric; *NPO*, nothing by mouth; *P*, pulse; *PCA*, patient-controlled analgesia; *PRN*, as needed; *R*, respirations; *WBC*, white blood cell.

Problem/Nursing Diagnosis

Fresh surgical sites and risk for ileus/Risk for infection related to colectomy and abdominal incision.

Supporting Assessment Data

Objective: Colectomy and abdominal incision with drain.

Goals/Expected Outcomes	Nursing Interventions	Selected Rationale	Evaluation
Patient will not experience wound infection as evidenced by temperature and WBC count within normal range at discharge, wound clean and dry without redness, pain, or purulent drainage.	Assess surgical wounds and adjacent tissues for redness, swelling, warmth, pain, and presence of odors or drainage.	Close observation is necessary to identify the beginning of infection in the early phase.	No redness noted in surrounding tissue. Denies pain or tenderness.
	Track temperature and WBC count.	Changes may indicate beginning infection.	Temp 98.8° F (37.1° C); WBC count 9400/mm^3.
	Reinforce dressings PRN; change q 24 hr or PRN when ordered. Use strict aseptic technique for dressing changes. Clean skin around incision with ordered solution.	Maintaining sterile intact dressing decreases chance of infection.	Incision clean and dry without redness. Sterile dressing changed using sterile technique.
	Maintain patency of drain.	Draining excess fluids from wound site facilitates healing.	Drain in place, small amount of serous fluid noted.
	Monitor temperature and WBC counts.	Rising temperature and WBC counts indicate possible infection.	Temperature 97.8° F (36.6° C); CBC to be drawn in A.M. Continue plan.

Problem/Nursing Diagnosis

Potential for bleeding from surgery/Risk for bleeding related to surgical incision.

Supporting Assessment Data

Objective: Fresh colectomy incision.

Goals/Expected Outcomes	Nursing Interventions	Selected Rationale	Evaluation
Patient will not have excessive blood loss as evidenced by stable vital signs and adequate urine output.	Assess vital signs per postoperative routine: q 30 min for 2 hr; q 1 hr for 2 hr; q 2 hr for 4 hr; then q 4 hr until stable.	Vital signs can indicate hemorrhage.	P 86, R 18, BP 136/84.
	Notify physician for change of mental status, tachycardia with increased respirations or blood pressure 15–20 points below preoperative baseline level; unremitting pain.	Change of mental status is frequently the first sign of decreased cerebral perfusion. Tachycardia with increased respirations and falling blood pressure indicates hemorrhage.	Alert and oriented to person, place, and time. Skin is warm, pink, and dry.
	Monitor hourly urine output; report if <30 mL for 2 consecutive hours.	Decreasing urine output indicates decreased renal perfusion, which can lead to renal failure if prolonged and severe.	Urine output 125 mL over 2 hr.
	Assess dressings for bleeding; check underneath patient.	Postsurgical patients have risk for hemorrhage and blood can pool underneath the patient.	Dressings dry; no drainage under patient.
	Assess abdomen for increasing girth or rigidity.	Increasing abdominal girth or rigidity could signal internal bleeding.	Abdomen not rigid; girth not increasing. Continue plan.

Continued

Nursing Care Plan 30-1 | Care of the Patient Undergoing Colectomy for Probable Colon Cancer—cont'd

Problem/Nursing Diagnosis
Potential for lung problems/Risk for ineffective breathing pattern related to anesthesia, analgesia, and postoperative pain

Supporting Assessment Data
Subjective: "I don't want to cough."
Objective: Underwent general anesthesia; receiving morphine via PCA; shallow breaths.

Goals/Expected Outcomes	Nursing Interventions	Selected Rationale	Evaluation
Patient will not develop atelectasis or pneumonia as evidenced by normal breath sounds in all lobes of lungs.	Assist patient to turn, cough effectively, and deep breathe at least q 2 hr. Monitor for proper use of incentive spirometer. Auscultate lungs every shift.	Coughing and turning assists with lung expansion. Incentive spirometer helps prevent atelectasis. Auscultation tells whether all areas of the lungs are aerating.	Coughing and turning q 2 hr. Decreased breath sounds in bases of lungs. Using incentive spirometer correctly q 2 hr. Decreased breath sounds in bases bilaterally; no adventitious sounds.
	Assist to get out of bed to sit in chair or ambulate as ordered.	Early mobility improves lung function and decreases complications such as pneumonia.	Able to move, stand, pivot, and sit in chair with one-person assist. Continue plan.

Problem/Nursing Diagnosis
Afraid she may have cancer/Anxiety related to fear of cancer, treatment, and possible death.

Supporting Assessment Data
Subjective: Father died of colon cancer; expresses fear of cancer and death; dreads chemotherapy.

Goals/Expected Outcomes	Nursing Interventions	Selected Rationale	Evaluation
Patient will openly discuss fears and concerns with nurse, family, or physician.	Establish trusting relationship with patient by active listening and attentive caring.	A trusting relationship helps patient express feelings.	Not wanting to talk yet; spent quiet time with patient.
	Assess mood, verbal, and nonverbal behaviors that suggest readiness to talk.	Expressions of anxiety and fear will manifest differently for each patient; therefore therapeutic responses are based on assessment of the behavior (i.e., crying, yelling, demanding, rejecting, withdrawn, flat affect, sad expression).	Is withdrawn and quiet; does not wish to discuss situation until pathology report is back. Sat quietly with patient for 15 min.
	Reassure patient that you are available for future discussions.	Patient needs to know that you are willing to return and support her, regardless of how she initially responds to you.	Continue plan.

Critical Thinking Questions
1. Why is it significant that she has familial polyposis?
2. What should other family members be told? What is the nurse's role in disclosing information?
3. Why is a patient such as Mrs. Simpson likely to have IV therapy ordered?

Common nursing diagnoses are located in Table 28-2, but diagnoses specific to cancer (see Chapter 8) are also relevant. Your patient will experience multiple physical and psychological challenges through the diagnosis and treatment process; if interventions are not working, the plan should be changed.

OSTOMY SURGERY AND CARE

In this procedure, an abdominal incision is made, and either the colon (*colostomy*) or the ileum (*ileostomy*) is brought to the outside to drain fecal material.

COLOSTOMY

A colostomy may be required after a colectomy. The colostomy may be permanent or temporary. For a temporary colostomy, the patient will have surgery later for anastomosis of the open ends.

Types of Colostomies

There are three basic types of colostomy surgery for intestinal disorders, and the stomas thus created are called (1) *loop colostomy*; (2) *double-barreled colostomy*; and (3) *single-barreled* or *end colostomy*.

? **Think Critically**

What do you think might be psychological concerns for a person who is to have a colostomy?

Loop Colostomy. During surgery, a loop of the colon is brought through an abdominal incision and onto the surface of the body. Some kind of rod or bridge is placed under the loop to prevent it from slipping back into the abdominal cavity (Figure 30-5). About 2 days later, the surgeon will open the colostomy in surgery or at the patient's bedside. This may be done with an electric cauterizing instrument, a scalpel, or surgical scissors and does not require anesthesia because the bowel has no sensory nerve endings.

Once the surgeon has made the opening in the wall of the intestine, fecal material passes through the opening (stoma) in the loop of the intestine. An appliance for collection of fecal material should be on hand before the intestine is opened so that it can be attached immediately after the stoma has been created. The pouch that collects feces fits over the stoma made by the slit in the loop of intestine. After about 5 to 7 days, the surgeon may remove the bridge if the stoma has adhered to the abdominal wall.

Double-Barreled Colostomy. In a double-barreled colostomy, there are two separate stomas (Figure 30-6). The loop of intestine is completely severed, creating a *proximal stoma* and a *distal stoma*. The proximal stoma

FIGURE 30-5 First stage of loop transverse colostomy. A segment of transverse colon is brought out through the abdominal wall and supported by a bridge. A slit in the bowel allows feces to drain from proximal colon. Support is removed 5 to 7 days after surgery or when the bowel adheres to the abdominal wall.

is the one closer to the small intestine, so fecal material passes through it to the outside. The distal stoma leads to the rectum and should discharge only small amounts of mucus. The distance between the stomas varies; if they are too close together, it is difficult to get a good seal for the collection device around each one. Eventually the colon ends will be reattached.

Single-Barreled or End Colostomy. There is only one stoma in a single-barreled colostomy. It is located on the lower left quadrant of the abdomen and is the proximal end of the sigmoid colon. The end is brought to the abdominal surface, *effaced* (cuffed over itself), and sutured to the skin, making what is called a *surgically mature stoma*. If the colostomy is temporary, the remaining portion of bowel and rectum are left intact. If the colostomy is permanent, an abdominal perineal resection is done to remove the freed bowel, anus, and rectum.

Colostomy Locations

An ascending colostomy is one in which either one end or a loop of a portion of the ascending colon is brought to the surface of the abdomen to form a stoma. The stool from an ascending colostomy is thus watery and unformed.

An ascending colostomy usually is temporary and is done to allow the bowel distal to the ostomy to rest and heal. This is sometimes necessary for the patient with IBD, to reconstruct an intestinal birth defect, or for the patient who has experienced an intestinal tear from trauma. After the rest and healing period, the surgeon

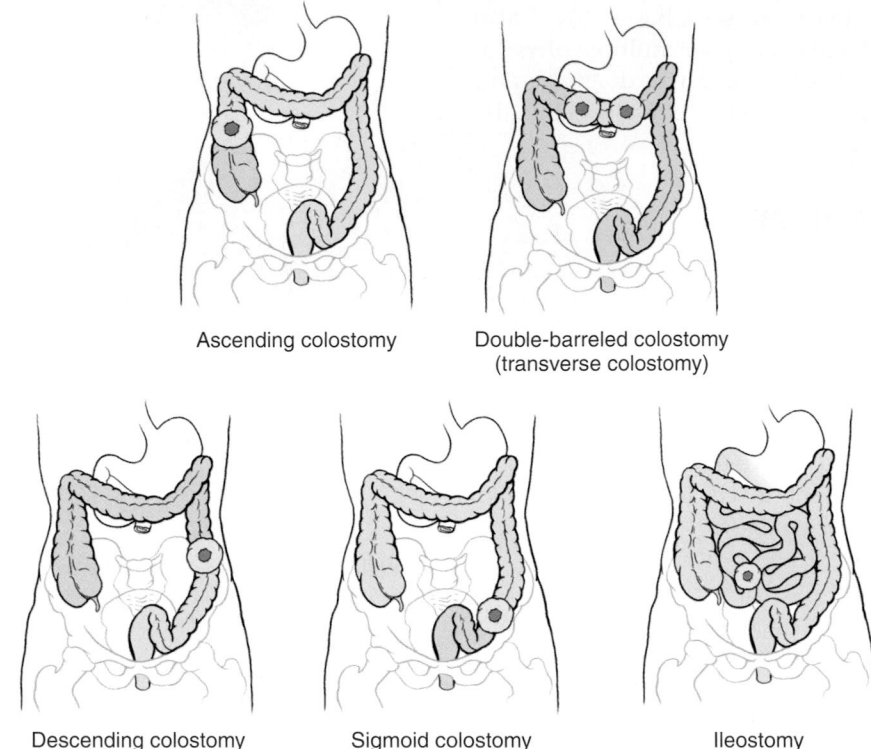

Ascending colostomy

Double-barreled colostomy
(transverse colostomy)

Descending colostomy   Sigmoid colostomy   Ileostomy

FIGURE 30-6 Types of ostomies and intestinal diversions.

will replace and reattach the intestine ends, and fecal material can be defecated normally.

A transverse colostomy is situated toward the middle of the abdomen (location of transverse colon). This kind of colostomy usually is temporary. The stool from a transverse colostomy is semiliquid and is discharged unpredictably.

A sigmoid (descending) colostomy is located on the surface of the lower quadrant of the abdomen (see Figure 30-6). It is the most common type of permanent colostomy and usually is done to treat cancer of the rectum. The stool from a sigmoid colostomy is more solid and well formed and may be discharged no more often than once a day or every 2 days. It is therefore much easier to establish a pattern of evacuation to control the flow of fecal material through a sigmoid colostomy.

ILEOSTOMY

An **ileostomy** is performed to drain fecal material from the ileum. It is indicated when disease, congenital defects, or trauma require bypassing the entire colon. The most common indications for ileostomy are chronic IBD, such as ulcerative colitis and Crohn's disease (regional ileitis), malignancy, and the presence of many polyps in the colon (multiple polyposes). The last disease is hereditary, and the polyps have a high potential for malignancy.

The site for the stoma of an ileostomy must be carefully selected so that it is not near any bony prominences, folds of skin, or scars and is in a place where the patient can see it and care for it (see Figure 30-6). The stool from an ileostomy is liquid, and even though digestion is completed by the time the fecal material reaches the stoma, it still contains digestive enzymes that are highly irritating to the skin.

Surgeons may use other techniques to create an ileostomy. The pouch ileostomy or continent ileostomy frees the ileostomy patient from the need to wear a collection device. A small segment of the ileum is looped back on itself to form a pouch (Kock pouch), and a nipple effect is created (Figure 30-7, *A*). Pressure from the accumulating feces closes the nipple valve, preventing constant drainage through the stoma. The patient empties the pouch every 3 to 4 hours during the day by inserting a catheter into the stoma.

Not every patient can be treated by this surgical technique. It has some disadvantages and must be performed by a surgeon skilled in the procedure. Among those who are not good candidates for a continent ileostomy are patients with chronic inflammatory disease, as the disease tends to recur. Another consideration is the patient's potential for self-care; a catheter must be inserted for periodic drainage of the Kock pouch, and the patient must be able to understand instructions and perform self-care. A third contraindication is related to previous surgery. Patients who have had a conventional ileostomy cannot have a continent ileostomy done if they have less than 29 mm of terminal ileum remaining. This much is needed to construct the nipple valve.

FIGURE 30-7 Ileoanal reservoirs. **A,** Kock pouch. **B,** S-shaped reservoir. **C,** J-shaped reservoir.

The procedure of choice for ulcerative colitis is the creation of a pouch from the terminal ileum; the pouch is sutured directly to the anus. The anal sphincter is left intact and functional. It is a two-stage surgical procedure in which a loop ileostomy is performed and then is closed 3 or 4 months later, when healing is complete. The reservoir may be S-shaped or J-shaped (see Figure 30-7, *B* and *C*). Most patients then have three to eight bowel movements a day. Slight fecal incontinence may be a problem, particularly at night. This procedure is performed only on those patients under age 55 who do not have any anal sphincter deterioration. The mucosa is stripped from the small segment of the rectum that is retained in order to prevent recurrent ulcerative colitis. "Pouchitis" occurs in about 29% of patients and tends to be recurrent. A course of metronidazole (Flagyl) may adequately treat pouchitis. Otherwise, antibiotics and/or steroids are used.

Although not every patient needing an ileostomy can have a continent ileostomy, it is a safe and effective procedure for many. It eliminates the need for an external appliance, is a more natural way to handle waste, greatly reduces fear of embarrassment from leakage of gas and feces, and minimizes periostomal skin problems.

PREOPERATIVE NURSING CARE

Before surgery of the large intestine, fecal material is removed from the colon. To accomplish this, the patient is usually placed on a low-residue diet as early as 7 to 10 days before surgery. The last 24 to 72 hours before surgery, the diet is changed to liquids only. In addition to the dietary preparation, laxatives and enemas are administered to cleanse the lower bowel. Vitamins and minerals may be given to supplement these restricted diets. Antibiotics may be given as prophylaxis against infection of the operative site.

The contents of the stomach are removed by inserting an NG tube and connecting the tube to a suction apparatus the morning of surgery. If it is necessary to remove the contents of the small intestine, a specially designed tube that passes through the stomach and into the duodenum is inserted. This tube is called a Miller-Abbott tube (see Figure 30-3). It is attached to the suction apparatus and given the same care as a gastric tube. The tube is usually left in place after surgery to remove accumulations of mucus and gas that may cause distention and strain on the sutures.

❖ NURSING MANAGEMENT

■ Assessment (Data Collection)

The immediate postoperative care for the intestinal surgery patient is the same as for other patients having major abdominal surgery. Frequent assessment of vital signs, surgical site, and IV site is conducted. Intestinal drainage is assessed for amount and character. The patient is assessed for nausea and treated in the early postoperative period, because vomiting places a strain on suture lines. Intake and output are tracked and fluid balance is assessed. Standard operations on the large intestine are usually of long duration. The prolonged period of anesthesia and exposure of the body, with loss of essential fluids, leaves the patient susceptible to shock. Urine output is assessed frequently, as decreased urine output may be a sign of shock.

Psychosocial assessment postoperatively focuses on the patient's perception of her altered body image; the meaning of the altered body part; her usual and current coping skills, emotional state, support systems, and presurgery lifestyle; and her perception of physical prognosis and its impact on her life.

■ Nursing Diagnosis and Planning

Nursing diagnoses concerning the surgical procedure are similar to abdominal surgery (see Nursing Care Plan 30-1; see also Table 28-2). Nursing Care Plan 30-2 (on Evolve) presents nursing diagnoses and expected outcomes for the patient with an ostomy.

■ Implementation

The gastric or intestinal tube is connected to suction as soon as the patient is returned to her room. The patient is NPO for the first 48 hours after surgery. Peristalsis usually becomes active after this period of time, and the NG tube can be removed. The patient will then be able to take liquids by mouth.

Complementary and Alternative Therapies

Chewing Gum Postoperatively

"Current best evidence suggests that chewing gum should be offered to selected patients with the intent of decreasing postoperative ileus" (Hocevar et al., 2010).

The passing of gas, liquids, or solids through the rectum is an indication of active peristalsis. Observe patients carefully for evidence of the return of peristalsis, and chart it in the nurse's notes. The IV site, fluids, and electrolyte levels are monitored very carefully, as the patient is especially prone to fluid and electrolyte imbalances. Pain assessment is ongoing, and the effectiveness of analgesia should be assessed after administering pain medication.

? Think Critically

How does the effluent from a transverse colostomy, from a sigmoid colostomy, and from an ileostomy differ?

Care of the Stoma

The stoma is inspected for a normal pink or red color, which indicates adequate blood supply. It should look like healthy mucous membrane such as that inside the mouth. Later, the stoma will shrink in size and may be less highly colored. There may be slight bleeding around the stoma and its stem, but any more than slight bleeding should be reported. Most collection devices are transparent, so that checking for color and bleeding does not require removal of the appliance. The skin around the stoma is assessed for irritation or signs of breakdown.

A noticeable lightening or blanching of the stoma may indicate inadequate blood flow through the tissues of the stoma itself. A deepening of color to a purplish hue may indicate obstruction of blood flow to the stoma.

Observe the stoma for signs of edema. In the early postoperative period, the stoma will be slightly edematous and larger than it will be after complete healing has taken place. Stoma edema can be caused by a collection device whose opening is too narrow to accommodate the stoma. The opening of the collection device should be at least ⅛-inch larger than the circumference of the stoma.

Fecal output from the colostomy stoma does not occur for 2 to 4 days, as the patient has been NPO for surgery. If there is a perineal wound, the appearance, amount, and character of drainage are assessed and charted. Carefully inspect for signs of infection. Such a wound may be left open to heal by secondary intention, in which case it may be 3 months before it is completely healed. Initially there will be a drain in the wound. Antibiotic therapy is usually given for a few days postoperatively to prevent infection.

A surgical dressing is never placed over an ileal stoma. If there is a significant decrease in ileal output accompanied by stomach cramping, the ileum may be obstructed. Such symptoms should be reported to the surgeon immediately. If the condition is not relieved, perforation or rupture of the intestine eventually may occur.

Elder Care Points

Elderly patients may require assistance with ostomy care because of poor vision or severe arthritis in the hands. In this case, a family member must be taught the techniques of care. The elderly patient needs easy-to-follow, large-print instructions for care.

Measurement of Intake and Output

Accurate recording of intake and output is especially important in the care of an ostomy patient. Total output of fecal material is calculated every 8 hours. If the stool is liquid, the accuracy of measurement is very important. When the patient's condition is stable, ostomy output is regular, and the patient's nutrition and hydration status are normal, intake and output recording is discontinued.

The ileostomy patient must always be watched for signs of dehydration and fluid imbalance. This is especially important during the immediate postoperative period, but remains a concern as long as the patient has the ileostomy. To prevent dehydration, fluid intake should be sufficient to compensate for the loss of fluid through the feces.

Evacuation and Irrigation

Once the patient is eating again, ileostomy drainage is usually emptied every 2 or 3 hours. The pouch should be emptied when it is half full. The patient sits on the toilet, unclamps the drainage device, and allows the effluent to drain into the bowl. The clamp is then closed, and the outside of the bag is cleansed of any debris. Ileostomies are not usually irrigated unless there is blockage by large particles of undigested food; then irrigation is done by a physician or enterostomal therapist.

A continent ileostomy with a Kock pouch has a drainage tube inserted and attached to suction in the immediate postoperative period to prevent distention and allow the pouch to heal. In about 2 weeks, the patient is taught to insert a catheter into the pouch to drain the contents. As the pouch matures and its capacity increases, the time between drainings will lengthen. The pouch may be irrigated occasionally to remove fecal residue.

A sigmoid colostomy will usually drain formed stool on a relatively regular schedule. Irrigation of the colostomy gives the patient some control over when elimination takes place. The procedure is done daily or every other day at about the same time, and takes close to an hour. A catheter with a cone tip is attached to a bag, which is filled with 500 to 1000 mL of warm (not hot) tap water. The bag is positioned 18 to 20 inches above the height of the stoma. The colostomy appliance is removed and an irrigating sleeve is attached to direct the drainage into the toilet. The cone tip is lubricated and inserted gently into the ostomy stoma, and the water is infused slowly to prevent cramping and distention. The cone tip is removed, and the drainage flows through the sleeve into the toilet. When drainage is complete, the sleeve is removed, skin care is performed, and a clean appliance is secured in place. If the patient is fortunate enough to have a regular evacuation pattern, irrigation is not necessary.

The major reason for irrigating a colostomy is to establish a pattern of predictable bowel movements at the convenience of the colostomate. If the patient prefers not to irrigate, suppositories can be used to stimulate evacuation. The patient does need to wear a drainable pouch if she does not irrigate, as evacuation can be unpredictable.

 Cultural Considerations

Cultural Issues for Ostomy Patients

Be aware that cultural and religious considerations for hygiene and fasting may be important for your ostomy patient. For example, on the Jewish Shabbat, strictly observant practice may prohibit the use of running water or electricity; therefore hygiene must be accomplished before the start of Shabbat. The Muslim patient may observe a strict fasting practice for Ramadan that lasts 28 days, when no food or fluid is consumed between sunrise and sunset. An ileostomy patient could be at risk for dehydration or change of eating patterns could lead to diarrhea or constipation (Black, 2009).

 Assignment Considerations

Ostomy Care

The care of a new postoperative ostomy should not be assigned to unlicensed assistive personnel (UAP) as assessments of the stoma, incision, and skin are essential. When ostomy care for a mature ostomy is assigned to a certified nursing assistant (CNA) or UAP, remind the person to note the color of the stoma and to immediately report if the stoma appearance is not rosy pink or if there is excoriation of the skin. Documenting the appearance of the stoma, the condition of the skin, and the type and amount of effluent is your responsibility regardless of whether the patient or assistive personnel does the actual cleaning and appliance change.

Periostomal Skin Care

Drainage from an ileostomy contains enzymes and bile salts that are highly damaging to the skin. The area of skin around the stoma must be kept clean and protected; fecal material should not be allowed to seep around the opening of the collection device and pool on the skin. In the immediate postoperative period, the pouch should not be changed any more than is necessary to avoid trauma to the skin.

Clinical Cues

Gently placing a cotton tamponade into the stoma opening after removing the appliance will prevent ileostomy contents from getting on the skin and causing irritation.

The two major principles to follow to protect the skin are cleanliness and the provision of a protective barrier to prevent contact between the skin and the discharge from the stoma. If there is a proper seal to prevent seepage of either feces or urine around the stoma, irritation and breakdown of the skin occur much less frequently.

Appliances are generally changed twice a week in order to maintain an effective seal. When the appliance is changed, it should be removed carefully and the skin washed gently with soap and water so that skin is not damaged by vigorous rubbing and scrubbing. The area should be rinsed thoroughly and dried by patting, not rubbing, the skin. In humid weather, a hair dryer on the low setting may be used to dry the skin. Possible causes of skin problems are allergic reactions, yeast infections, or irritation from changing the faceplate too frequently. After cleansing, a protective skin barrier paste—which serves to prevent contact between the skin and the waste being discharged through the stoma—is applied. This may or may not be used for a sigmoid colostomy stoma.

Protective barriers are available in a number of forms and types. The enterostomal therapist or surgeon will indicate which type of barrier is most effective for the individual patient. Should the skin become highly irritated in spite of efforts to protect it, the physician will prescribe topical medications. Fungal infection of the skin sometimes occurs.

Gauze packing of a perineal wound is changed regularly. There initially will be a large amount of serous drainage from the wound.

Elder Care Points

The changes related to aging reduce reaction time and manual dexterity, decrease visual and hearing acuity, and cause memory loss and fatigue. In addition, changes in body contour such as loss of supporting subcutaneous tissues, wrinkling and fragility of skin may result in improper fit of appliances. The elderly patient may have been "educated" about self-care when the ostomy was first established; however, she may have had no follow-up because of transportation issues or because she "didn't want to bother anybody." Nurses should advocate for regular follow-up appointments.

Changing the Collection Device

There are two kinds of pouches or appliances: the temporary/disposable and the permanent/reusable. Both types are either drainable or closed-ended. Each is attached to a faceplate that is secured to the skin around the stoma with a special adhesive. Drainable pouches are used when the flow of waste cannot be regulated and the contents must be emptied frequently (Figure 30-8). Closed-end pouches are used only for security once bowel movements have been regulated. Either new appliance is trimmed to size using a template drawn from the dimensions of the stoma plus ⅛ inch. The appliance should not be constricting to the stoma but must be tight enough so that skin is not exposed to effluent.

Psychosocial Concerns

The ostomy patient will go through the stages of grief and loss (see Chapter 8). Your attitude toward the patient, the stoma, and care has a major impact on the attitude the patient develops about body image changes

FIGURE 30-8 Ostomy collection appliance in place and sealed around the stoma.

and self-care. Disposing of body waste is not a pleasant nursing task, but a matter-of-fact, efficient approach is best when caring for the stoma, the effluent, and the drainage device.

Encourage social interaction, and contact available support groups. **As soon as postoperative pain is well controlled, it is best if the patient can talk with another who has fully adjusted to her ostomy and is living a full and active life.** A series of such visits allows time to formulate and address questions. Such visits do require an order by the physician.

The patient should be guided to express her concerns about the physical and social problems she might encounter as a result of her ostomy. Most patients have concerns about odor, leakage, and noise from the passing of flatus. Nurse and patient should jointly explore changes in lifestyle and realistic alternatives. For example, the colostomy patient might be interested in trying a stoma cap, which is a small flat absorbent device that it placed directly over the stoma. The cap will absorb mucus, but has no capacity to collect stool or fluids; thus irrigation must be done immediately before application. This option might be used for sexual relations or sports (Burch, 2009).

The nurse should indicate that concerns about sexual function are expected. Concerns should be addressed matter-of-factly, and her sexual partner should be included in discussions. The enterostomal therapist is a good resource for specific information and suggestions in this area.

When the patient has prolonged dysfunctional grieving, becomes clinically depressed, or cannot accept her altered body image; referral for professional counseling is appropriate.

Patient Education

After teaching the patient about the physiology of her ostomy and the steps involved in taking care of the stoma and skin, the nurse teaches the patient how to control odor. There will be odor when the drainage pouch is changed or emptied, just as there is with normal bowel movements.

Good basic hygiene is essential. Another measure to control odor is to eliminate from the diet foods known to cause odor or gas. Such foods include eggs, fish, garlic, raw onions, cucumbers, radishes, sauerkraut, corn, broccoli, cabbage, cauliflower, asparagus, dairy products, beans and other legumes, soy, some spices, and chewing gum. Eating too quickly and not chewing food well can cause gas. Carbonated and alcoholic beverages also contribute to the problem.

Gas entering the pouch from the stoma will accumulate there until the pouch is opened and the gas is released. To release gas, open the lower end of the pouch and gently press against its sides. If not released, the gas may cause enough pressure to make the device separate from the stoma. Newer pouches have a charcoal-filtered valve that allows gas to escape. Reusable pouches are washed with soap and water and are rinsed with cool vinegar solution.

The patient with a colostomy will slowly resume a regular diet. All ostomy patients are taught to prevent problems with diarrhea, constipation, and blockage. Dietary guidelines are more important for the ileostomy patient. Blockage of the ileostomy is fairly common.

Patient Teaching

Measures to Prevent Intestinal Blockage for the Ileostomy Patient

Teach the patient the following:
- Eat six small meals a day.
- Eat a soft diet during the healing period.
- Chew food very thoroughly.
- Add other foods to your diet gradually.
- Drink more than 8 cups of fluid per day.
- Avoid the following foods:
  - Dried fruits
  - Corn, including popcorn
  - Nuts
  - Sunflower and other seeds
  - Sausages and foods with casings
  - Apple peel
  - Oranges
  - Pineapple
  - Raw cabbage
  - Celery
  - Chinese vegetables
  - Coconut
  - Mushrooms
- If you experience a blockage in the intestine or of the ostomy:
  - Begin a liquid diet.
  - Cut the opening in your pouch a little larger than normal because the stoma may swell.
  - Take a warm bath to relax the abdominal muscles.
  - Massage the abdomen and area around the stomas as this might increase the pressure behind the blockage and help it to "pop out." Most food blockages occur just below the stoma.
  - Try different body positions, such as a knee-chest position, as it might move the blockage forward.
  - Take oral enzymes to encourage digestion.
- If you are still blocked or have no stomal output for several hours:
  - Call your physician or enterostomal nurse and report the problems.
  - If you cannot reach your physician or the enterostomal nurse, go to the emergency department. Take all of your pouch changing supplies with you.
  - DO *NOT* TRY TO LAVAGE THE ILEOSTOMY.
  - DO *NOT* TAKE A LAXATIVE.
- Other pointers:
  - Ileostomy patients should not take time-release capsules and enteric-coated tablets, as there is not enough time for adequate absorption before the medication is expelled through the stoma.
  - Adequate intake of fluids is important for all ostomy patients, to prevent dehydration and electrolyte imbalance.

Many sources of information are available to the ostomy patient (see Online Resources). These include the local branches of the American Cancer Society, ostomate clubs, enterostomal therapists, and other members of the health care team who have expertise in managing a stoma. Enterostomal therapists are wound care specialists (often with a master's degree, but with certification in wound and ostomy care).

▪ Evaluation

The patient should demonstrate an ability to perform ostomy care and an understanding of how to manage diet and to prevent potential complications such as fluid and electrolyte imbalance, skin breakdown, and blockage of the ostomy. In addition, the patient should demonstrate psychological adjustment to changes in body image. The plan is adjusted if goals are not being met.

ANORECTAL DISORDERS

HEMORRHOIDS

Hemorrhoids are varicosities of the veins of the rectum. They may be *internal* (inside the sphincter muscles of the anus) or *external* (outside the sphincter muscles) (Figure 30-9).

Etiology and Pathophysiology

Venous congestion from interference with venous return from the hemorrhoidal vessels leads to the development of hemorrhoids. Constipation, prolonged standing or sitting, and pregnancy are predisposing causes of hemorrhoids. The habit of sitting on the toilet and straining at the stool for long periods is one of the primary factors responsible for many cases of hemorrhoids. Enlargement of the prostate, uterine fibroids, and rectal tumors are other contributing factors. Chronic liver disease with portal hypertension is another cause.

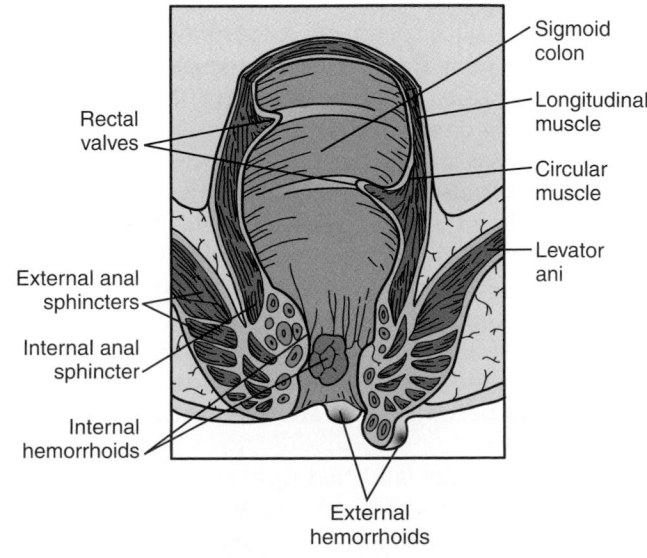

FIGURE 30-9 Hemorrhoids.

Signs, Symptoms, and Diagnosis

Local pain and itching are the most common symptoms of hemorrhoids. Bleeding from the rectum at the time of defecation may also occur. Hemorrhoidal blood is usually bright to dark red. External hemorrhoids are less likely to bleed, but they are more evident, because they appear as tumor-like projections around the rectum. Diagnosis is by physical examination.

Treatment

The symptoms of hemorrhoids may be relieved by correcting constipation, local applications of heat or cold, and sitz baths. The use of ointments that contain a local anesthetic helps relieve the itching and pain. Hydrocortisone ointment and suppositories help decrease the swelling. The patient also should be instructed to wash the anal region with warm water and soap after each bowel movement to prevent infection at the breaks in the mucosa.

Hemorrhoids can be treated by scleropathy (injection of a solution that causes the vessel to dry up and disintegrate). Cryotherapy (freezing) and photocoagulation (burning) are other options. Hemorrhoidectomy using a laser or standard surgical procedure may be performed. Another treatment method is rubber band ligation, in which a rubber band is slipped around the hemorrhoidal vessel, cutting off the blood supply. This causes the hemorrhoid to shrivel and disintegrate. All of these methods are most often done as outpatient treatments. Hemorrhoidectomy may occasionally be done as an inpatient procedure.

Nursing Management

Preoperatively, instruct the patient on rectal hygiene and the use of hydrocortisone suppositories or cream, and sitz baths to decrease swelling. Teach the patient ways to avoid constipation and to promote regular bowel evacuation.

After surgery, the patient receives a prescription for analgesics. A rubber or air-filled ring may be used while the patient is lying down to decrease pain and pressure from the rectal area. Sitz baths are usually ordered twice a day and cold or warm compresses are a comfort measure. Mild, wet dressings that are commercially prepared (Tucks) also may be used on the surgical site. These dressings have a glycerin base and contain a mild astringent that reduces swelling and relieves pain.

Bowel movements after a hemorrhoidectomy will cause some pain, and the usual procedure is to administer a stool softener to make defecation less traumatic. The patient and family should be warned that the patient may become faint, and someone should stay close by.

A high-fiber diet is started right away, as it is best if formed stool is passed regularly. A sitz bath after each bowel movement will offer relief and also cleanses the affected area, keeping it free from irritation. The patient should continue to sit in a tub of warm water after bowel movements until healing is complete.

PILONIDAL SINUS (PILONIDAL CYST)

Etiology and Pathophysiology

The word pilonidal means "having a nest of hair." A pilonidal sinus is a lesion located in the cleft of the buttocks at the sacrococcygeal region. It is sometimes called a *pilonidal cyst*, but it is believed to be a subcutaneous canal (sinus) with one or more openings into the skin (rather than a true cyst or fluid-filled sac). The condition occurs when the stiff hairs in the sacrococcygeal region irritate and eventually penetrate the soft skin in the cleft of the buttocks. Factors that can lead to development of such a sinus include local injury, improper cleaning of the area, and obesity. People who have more than the usual amount of body hair are particularly susceptible.

Signs, Symptoms, and Diagnosis

A pilonidal sinus may cause no trouble until it becomes infected, and then the patient experiences pain in the area, with swelling and a purulent drainage. Diagnosis is by history and examination.

Treatment and Nursing Management

When symptoms are severe or persistent, the area must be incised surgically and the connecting canals opened and drained. Hairs and necrotic tissue must be removed so the area can heal. This is usually done as an outpatient surgical procedure. A drain is left in the cavity so that healing will occur from the inside to the outside.

Postoperative care includes changing of dressings and measures to avoid contamination of the wound. A stool softener and an oil retention enema usually are given before the first bowel movement to avoid strain on the sutures. Antibiotics may be given to control infection.

ANORECTAL ABSCESS AND FISTULA

Etiology and Pathophysiology

An abscess may form where there has been irritation with breaks in the skin or mucosa. Localized infection with a collection of pus forms an anorectal abscess. Tears in the mucosa of the rectum from hard, constipated stools may predispose to abscess and fistula formation. A fistula is a chronic granulomatous tract that travels in a line from the anal canal to the skin outside the anus, or from an anorectal abscess to the anal canal or the area around the anus.

Signs, Symptoms, and Diagnosis

A discharge of pus from the fistula opening may be the first sign of an abscess or fistula. Both abscess and fistula are painful and sitting or coughing aggravates the pain. If a fistula is accompanied by diarrhea, Crohn's disease is suspected because 50% of Crohn's patients develop a rectal fistula. Diagnosis is by history and physical examination.

Treatment and Nursing Management

Antibiotics may be administered to decrease the infection. Medication for pain is prescribed. Incision and drainage of an abscess may be necessary. A fistula usually requires surgical excision and repair. Nursing management involves teaching measures to prevent further incidence of constipation and infection, and rectal hygiene measures. Sitz baths are used to decrease inflammation. Education about pain medication and antibiotic regimens is provided.

COMMUNITY CARE

Nurses in the community should teach self-care and habits that promote healthy function of the GI system.

A healthy diet with appropriate quantities of fiber and fluid, counseling regarding exercise programs, and teaching about the warning signs of colon cancer are all appropriate nursing interventions, to be used whenever possible. Nurses should be a role model for a healthy diet and exercise program to maintain weight within normal limits.

Nurses who work in long-term care facilities and in home settings must be vigilant to spot problems of the GI system. Monitoring nutritional and bowel status is standard practice for every patient. On a continuing basis it is important to assess bowel changes that might indicate colon cancer. Remember that patients who are under care for other disorders still need to have regular cancer screenings.

Get Ready for the NCLEX® Examination!

Key Points

- A hernia can become incarcerated, trapping intestine and cutting off its blood supply and causing intestinal obstruction.
- Diverticulitis produces diarrhea or constipation, left lower abdominal pain, fever, and rectal bleeding. Treatment of diverticulitis includes antibiotics, NPO or a liquid diet, IV hydration, and surgical hemicolectomy.
- A high-fiber diet and lots of fluid are prescribed for the patient with diverticular disease.
- Mechanical bowel obstruction is mainly caused by adhesions, volvulus, intussusception, and strangulated hernia. Nonmechanical bowel obstruction may be a result of paralytic ileus following surgery, hypokalemia, infection, uremia, or heavy-metal poisoning.
- Inflammatory bowel disease (IBD) includes ulcerative colitis and Crohn's disease. An altered bowel pattern, abdominal pain with bloating, and diarrhea or constipation are typical. Problems include ulceration, edema, bleeding, and fluid and electrolyte loss. Drug therapy includes antidiarrheals, sulfasalazine, drugs to relieve abdominal cramping, and corticosteroids.
- Surgery for ulcerative colitis usually involves a proctocolectomy with ileostomy, a Kock pouch creation, or an ileoanal reservoir.
- Appendicitis (inflammation of the appendix) classically causes right lower quadrant pain accompanied by muscle guarding. Nausea and vomiting, a slight temperature elevation, and an increase in the white blood cell count may also occur.
- Peritonitis is an inflammation of the peritoneum. Serous fluid is purulent and normal peristaltic action slows or ceases.
- Malabsorption in adults is usually from sprue or lactose intolerance, radiation therapy, or chemotherapy. Malabsorption can also occur with IBD or diarrhea when transit through the intestines is too rapid.
- Ulcerative colitis, familial polyposis, smoking, alcohol consumption, obesity, physical inactivity, and a diet high in saturated fat or red meat are risk factors for colon cancer.
- Cancer treatment depends on tumor stage and may include surgery, chemotherapy, and radiation. Abdominoperineal resection is done for rectal cancer and may include a colostomy.
- An ileostomy drains fecal material from the ileum and is usually performed for IBD problems. Fluid and electrolyte monitoring is crucial when there is an ileostomy.
- The stoma should be a normal pink or red color. Protective powders and skin paste and a proper fit of the appliance will help to protect the skin. The opening should be cut ⅛-inch larger than the stoma.
- Hemorrhoids are caused by straining at stool for long periods while sitting on the toilet, prolonged standing, prolonged sitting, or pregnancy.
- Anorectal abscess or fistula may be treated with antibiotics, incision and drainage or surgery. Nursing measures include teaching to prevent further constipation and infection.

Additional Learning Resources

SG Go to your Study Guide for additional learning activities to help you master this chapter content.

evolve Go to your Evolve website (http://evolve.elsevier.com/deWit/medsurg) for the following FREE learning resources:
- Animations, audio, and video
- Answers and rationales for questions and activities
- Concept Map Creator
- Glossary with pronunciations in English and Spanish
- Interactive Review Questions and Exercises and more!

 Online Resources
- United Ostomy Association, www.uoaa.org
- Wound Ostomy and Continence Nurses Society, www.wocn.org

Review Questions for the NCLEX® Examination

1. The nurse encourages a patient with irritable bowel syndrome to keep a food diary. What is the best nursing response to the patient regarding the importance of keeping the diary?
   1. "The diary will monitor caloric intake."
   2. "The diary will help identify foods that cause bloating."
   3. "The diary will determine food preferences."
   4. "The diary will reinforce the need for better food choices."

2. A 68-year-old patient complains of mild left lower abdominal pain that is accompanied by frequent diarrhea, fever, and rectal bleeding. Which treatment measure should the nurse anticipate?
   1. Administration of a bulk-forming stool softener
   2. Increasing fluid intake
   3. Encouraging solid foods
   4. Increasing physical activity

3. The patient has a PRN order for loperamide (Imodium). The nurse would administer this medication if the patient says:
   1. "My stomach pain is keeping me awake at night."
   2. "I haven't had a bowel movement for 5 days."
   3. "I had seven liquid stools in the past 2 hours."
   4. "I feel very bloated and I frequently belch."

4. During a home visit, the nurse provides verbal instructions to a patient with a possible blockage of the ostomy. What would be an appropriate instruction for the nurse to give?
   1. Massage the stoma.
   2. Try different body positions.
   3. Take a cold bath.
   4. Begin a high-fiber diet.

5. The nurse is caring for a patient who is postoperative following an ileostomy. Which order should the nurse question?
   1. Strict I&O for 8 hours
   2. NPO
   3. NG tube to low wall suction
   4. Occlusive dressing over stoma

6. In caring for an ostomate, which statement is true regarding medication administration?
   1. Time-release capsules can be given to patients with an ileostomy.
   2. Enteric-coated tablets are adequately absorbed by patients with ileostomy.
   3. Glycerin suppositories are readily evacuated in the distal colostomy stoma.
   4. An antiemetic suppository can be effectively absorbed when inserted in the distal colostomy stoma.

7. The patient has a new colostomy. Which behavior is an early sign of acceptance in the change of body image?
   1. Patient allows the nurse to empty the colostomy bag.
   2. Patient refuses to look at the ostomy site.
   3. Patient holds and examines a new appliance bag.
   4. Patient continues to ask for bedpan to have a bowel movement.

8. The patient develops a paralytic ileus as a complication of peritonitis. Which patient comment suggests a return of peristalsis?
   1. "I feel thirsty; may I have some water?"
   2. "I would like to try and walk to the toilet."
   3. "When will I be allowed to have solid food?"
   4. "I am sorry to pass gas while you are here."

9. What would be included in the recommended diet for patients with inflammatory bowel disease? (Select all that apply.)
   1. Low fat
   2. High fiber
   3. High protein
   4. Low calorie
   5. Lactose avoidance

10. The nurse admits a 23-year-old patient with possible appendicitis. The nurse anticipates which sign(s) and/or symptom(s)? (Select all that apply.)
    1. Increased red cell count
    2. Abdominal tenderness
    3. Anorexia and vomiting
    4. Mild fever
    5. Dark black stools

Critical Thinking Activities

Scenario A
Mrs. Blein, age 29, has had frequent bouts of diarrhea associated with physical and emotional stress since her early teens. She is admitted to the hospital with a diagnosis of possible ulcerative colitis. Her admitting physician, a gastroenterologist, feels certain that she has ulcerative colitis and that she will benefit from an ileostomy, as previous efforts on the part of several other physicians have brought no lasting relief from Mrs. Blein's symptoms. She is admitted to the hospital to establish a definitive diagnosis. Mrs. Blein is 40 pounds underweight and is suffering from severe diarrhea and fluid deficit.

1. What questions would be relevant when taking Mrs. Blein's nursing history?

2. What should be included on Mrs. Blein's nursing care plan regarding observations, measurements, and nursing interventions?

3. Discuss some benefits of an ileostomy over the alternative of continued bouts of severe diarrhea.

Scenario B
Mr. Huang, age 52, was found to have occult blood in his stool when he underwent a physical examination for a new insurance policy. Fiberoptic flexible sigmoidoscopy revealed a small lesion in the sigmoid colon; the biopsy result was positive for malignancy. He is scheduled for a hemicolectomy.

1. What are the probable postoperative nursing diagnoses that should be on Mr. Huang's care plan?

2. What are the psychosocial concerns that need to be addressed for this patient? What would be appropriate nursing interventions?

3. What further treatment will be necessary for Mr. Huang?

Scenario C

Mr. Frick has a history of diverticulitis. He reports that he has intermittent diarrhea and left lower abdominal discomfort. He is admitted to the hospital for symptoms of nausea, vomiting, and severe abdominal pain and distention. Mr. Frick is diagnosed with peritonitis.

1. What signs or symptoms should you observe for that may signal worsening of his condition?

2. What medical orders do you anticipate that the physician will order to treat Mr. Frick's peritonitis?

3. Discuss general nursing interventions that would be appropriate for Mr. Frick.

Objectives

Theory

1. Explain the plan of care for the patient with cholelithiasis.
2. Describe treatment for the patient with cholecystitis.
3. List the ways in which the various types of hepatitis can be transmitted.
4. Identify signs and symptoms of the various types of hepatitis.
5. Devise appropriate nursing interventions for the patient with cirrhosis and ascites.
6. Indicate potential causes of liver failure.
7. Differentiate the signs and symptoms of acute and chronic liver failure.
8. Discuss the ethical issues associated with liver transplantation.
9. Devise a nursing care plan for the patient with cancer of the liver.
10. Prepare a plan for adequate pain control for the patient with pancreatitis.
11. Compare the treatment options for cancer of the pancreas.

Clinical Practice

1. Perform preoperative teaching for a patient who is to undergo laparoscopic cholecystectomy.
2. Review a nursing care plan, including psychosocial concerns, for the patient who has hepatitis with jaundice.
3. Implement a discharge teaching plan for the patient who has been in the hospital with a flare-up of chronic pancreatitis.

Key Terms

ascites (ă-SĪ-tēz, p. 701)
asterixis (ăs-tĕr-ĬK-sĭs, p. 707)
biliary colic (BĬL-ē-ăr-ē kō-LĬC, p. 691)
caput medusa (KĂP-ĕt mĕ-DŪ-să, p. 701)
cholecystectomy (kō-lĕ-sĭs-TĔK-tō-mē, p. 692)
cholecystitis (kō-lĕ-sĭs-TĪ-tĭs, p. 691)
choledocholithiasis (kō-lĕd-ō-kō-lĭ-THĪ-ă-sĭs, p. 690)
cholelithiasis (kō-lĕ-lĭ-THĪ-ă-sĭs, p. 690)
cirrhosis (sĭr-RŌ-sĭs, p. 701)
encephalopathy (ĕn-sĕf-ă-LŎP-ă-thē, p. 698)
esophageal varices (ĕ-sŏf-ă-JĒ-ăl VĂR-ĭ-sēz, p. 704)

fetor hepaticus (hĕ-PĂ-tĭ-kŭs, p. 707)
hematemesis (hē-mă-TĔM-ĕ-sĭs, p. 704)
hepatitis (hĕ-pă-TĪ-tĭs, p. 694)
icterus (ĬK-tĕr-ŭs, p. 702)
jaundice (JĂWN-dĭs, p. 691)
palmar erythema (ĕr-ĭ-THĒ-mă, p. 701)
paracentesis (păr-ă-sĕn-TĒ-sĭs, p. 702)
prodromal stage (prō-DRŌ-măl, p. 699)
pruritus (prū-RĪ-tŭs, p. 701)
pseudocyst (sū-dō-sĭst, p. 709)
spider angiomas (SPĪ-dĕr ăn-jē-Ō-măz, p. 701)

DISORDERS OF THE GALLBLADDER

CHOLELITHIASIS AND CHOLECYSTITIS

Etiology

Cholelithiasis is the presence of gallstones within the gallbladder or in the biliary tract. The stones may vary in size, from very small "gravel" to stones as large as golf balls. Tiny stones pass into the bile ducts, where they become lodged and obstruct bile flow (Figure 31-1). When stones lodge in the common bile duct, the patient has choledocholithiasis. Cholelithiasis is more likely to occur in people with a sedentary lifestyle, a familial tendency, diabetes mellitus, and obesity. Cholesterol-lowering drugs increase the amount of cholesterol secreted in bile. This cholesterol secretion can increase the risk of gallstones.

 Cultural Considerations

Ethnic Predisposition to Gallstones

Native Americans are genetically more prone to develop gallbladder stones than any other group. Hispanic Americans have the next highest propensity to develop gallstones. Teaching dietary changes to decrease the amount of cholesterol and total fat in the diet may be an effective means of decreasing the incidence of gallstones in these populations (National Digestive Diseases Information Clearinghouse, 2007).

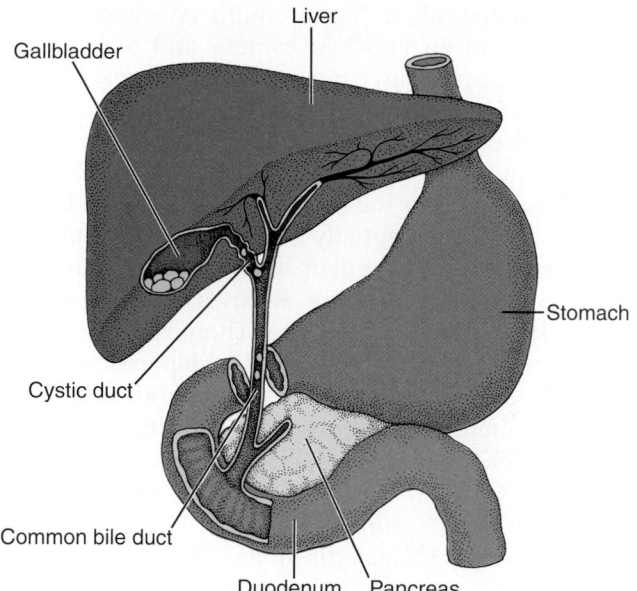

FIGURE 31-1 Gallstones within the gallbladder with obstruction of the common bile and cystic ducts.

Hemolytic disease, extensive resection of the bowel to treat Crohn's disease, bariatric surgery, or rapid weight loss, multiple pregnancies and use of oral contraceptives or hormone replacement therapy also increase the risk for gallstones.

Cholecystitis is an inflammation of the gallbladder and is associated with gallstones in 90% to 95% of occurrences. Other causes include obstructive tumors of the biliary tract and severely stressful situations such as cardiac surgery, severe burns, or multiple trauma.

Pathophysiology

Cholelithiasis (gallstones) develops when the balance between cholesterol, bile salts, and calcium in the bile is altered to the point that these substances precipitate. When cholesterol precipitates, the nucleus of a stone can be formed. The stone grows as layers of cholesterol, calcium, or pigment accumulate over the nucleus. Immobility, pregnancy, and obstructive lesions decrease bile flow. Stasis of bile leads to changes in chemical composition and stone formation. The formation of stones within the gallbladder can cause

irritation and areas of inflammation in the gallbladder wall (cholecystitis). Infection can occur from organisms such as *Escherichia coli*. The organisms enter the gallbladder through the sphincter of Oddi from adjacent structures.

Signs and Symptoms

Symptoms depend on the degree of obstruction to bile flow and extent of inflammation of the gallbladder. The absence of bile in the intestine results in clay-colored stools that float as a result of undigested fat content. If a duct is obstructed by a stone, obstruction of bile flow by stones in the cystic or common bile duct causes strong muscle contractions that attempt to move the stones along; severe pain may be triggered by a fatty meal. Nausea and vomiting, fever, and leukocytosis occur with cholecystitis. Pain may be referred to the right clavicle, scapula, or shoulder. As bile backs up into the liver and blood, jaundice (yellow tint to skin and sclera) occurs. If obstruction is unrelieved, inflammation occurs, and can progress to liver damage.

The symptom most often present in an acute flare-up of chronic cholecystitis is unbearable upper right quadrant pain (biliary colic). The pain sometimes is referred to the back at the level of the shoulder blades. Attacks can occur as frequently as daily or may not appear but once every year or so. Vomiting may accompany acute flare-ups, along with chills and fever. If the inflammation is not corrected or if there is an infection, the gallbladder can become filled with pus and rupture. Rupture spills gallbladder contents into the abdominal cavity and causes peritonitis.

Chronic cholecystitis causes milder symptoms between acute attacks. Symptoms are indigestion after eating fatty foods, flatulence, nausea after eating, and some discomfort in the right upper quadrant. Table 31-1 compares signs and symptoms of gallbladder disorders.

? Think Critically

What questions would you ask when assessing a patient who might have cholecystitis?

Table 31-1 Comparison of Gallbladder Disorders

SIGN/SYMPTOM	CHOLELITHIASIS	ACUTE CHOLECYSTITIS	CHRONIC CHOLECYSTITIS
Pain/biliary colic	Sudden onset, acute	Waves of pain lasting 2-6 hr	Intermittent during the year; pain often referred to back at shoulder blade
Nausea, vomiting	Often present	Frequent	During acute attack
Indigestion and flatulence	—	—	Frequent complaint
Low-grade fever	Present	Present, often with chills	Present
Jaundice	If duct is obstructed	May be present	May be present during attack

Cholelithiasis should be considered in any elderly patient with abdominal pain when another cause cannot be found. Symptoms may be atypical and the presenting symptom of cholecystitis in this age group may be low-grade fever rather than pain.

Diagnosis

Gallstones usually can be diagnosed with ultrasonography or computed tomography (CT) of the gallbladder and biliary tract. Endoscopic retrograde cholangiopancreatography (ERCP) may be done to detect common duct stones. Cholescintigraphy (hepatoiminodiacetic acid [HIDA] scan) diagnoses abnormal contraction of the gallbladder or obstruction. Liver function tests are helpful to diagnose gallbladder and biliary tract disease. Alanine aminotransferase (ALT) and aspartate aminotransferase (AST) will be slightly elevated. If there is common duct obstruction, gamma-glutamyl transpeptidase is elevated. In biliary obstruction, both direct bilirubin and alkaline phosphatase levels are elevated.

The diagnosis of cholecystitis is aided by indicators of infection, such as elevated white blood cell count and sedimentation rate.

Treatment

First, a low-fat diet, loss of excessive body weight, and restriction of alcohol intake are recommended and meals are spaced so that no large amounts of food are put into the intestinal tract at any one time. This avoids overstimulation of gallbladder activity. If the patient does not respond to this therapy or if bile obstruction occurs, correction of the obstructed biliary tract is indicated. Antibiotics are usually only given if peritonitis is present. Fluids are administered and electrolytes are rebalanced.

Postcholecystectomy Diet

If obesity is present, a reduced calorie, low-fat diet may be prescribed for the first 4 to 6 weeks after surgery. Foods to be avoided include whole milk, cream, butter, cheese made from whole milk, ice cream, nuts, fried foods, rich pastries, and gravies. Small frequent meals are helpful. Keeping a record of foods eaten and symptom occurrence will indicate other foods that may be a problem for a particular patient.

If stones may be in the common bile duct, it is explored either before or during surgery. Sometimes small stones may be removed during ERCP, in which the common duct can be visualized. The surgical procedure of choice is cholecystectomy (gallbladder removal). Laparoscopic cholecystectomy is the most common surgical procedure used. Four small incisions are made in the abdomen; abdominal muscles are not cut, and the patient experiences less pain and a quicker recovery than with an "open" cholecystectomy. A laparoscope with an attached camera and a dissecting laser are used along with grasping forceps. Carbon dioxide (CO_2) is instilled into the abdominal cavity to aid visualization. The gallbladder is removed through the incision at the umbilicus. The patient will have dressings over the four small incisions on the abdomen. There is essentially no difference in complications or outcomes for either open cholecystectomy or the laparoscopic procedure. Recovery time is shorter for the laparoscopic procedure (Thomas, 2009).

The nurse should monitor the laparoscopic patient closely for internal bleeding and watch for signs of increasing abdominal rigidity and pain, and for changes in vital signs. Sometimes the retained CO_2 used during a laparoscopic procedure causes "free air" pain. Early and frequent ambulation helps the CO_2 gas dissipate. The patient is discharged after recovering from the anesthesia, or 1 day postoperatively, depending on his age and condition, and must have careful discharge teaching about signs of complications.

Postoperative Laparoscopic Cholecystectomy

Teach the patient to:
- Remove the bandages from the puncture sites the day after surgery and shower.
- Report the following signs and symptoms if they occur:
  - Redness
  - Swelling
  - Bile-colored drainage or pus from any surgical site
  - Severe abdominal pain
  - Nausea, vomiting, chills, or fever
  - Light-colored stool, dark urine, or yellow tint to the eyes or skin as these signs may indicate obstruction to the flow of bile
- Resume normal activities gradually.
- Expect that return to work is probable at 1 week postsurgery.
- Stick to a low-fat diet for several weeks, slowly introducing fattier foods to determine if they cause unpleasant symptoms.

With an open abdominal cholecystectomy, a 2- to 4-day stay in the hospital is usual and there is about a 6-week recovery period. Residual stones can lodge in the common duct after cholecystectomy. ERCP is usually used to remove residual stones.

Oral dissolution therapy is available and works best on small cholesterol stones. Ursodiol (Actigall) and chenodiol (Chenix) are prescribed for 6 months to 2 years to dissolve stones.

An experimental procedure called *contact dissolution therapy* involves injecting a drug, methyl *tert*-butyl ether, into the gallbladder to dissolve stones in 1 to 3 days. It can cause irritation and complications. It is being tested on patients with small stones

(National Digestive Diseases Information Clearinghouse, 2007).

Lithotripsy, or "shock wave" therapy, is occasionally used for gallstones. The procedure involves using sound waves directed through the body to break up the stones. The procedure takes 1 to 1½ hours, and the debris is then carried by the bile into the intestine. To be a candidate for this procedure, there must be no more than three cholesterol gallstones, each smaller than 1½ inches, and the patient must not be obese.

Nursing Management

Preoperative Care. Preoperatively, the gallstone patient may have a nasogastric tube to relieve nausea and vomiting. An analgesic may be ordered to decrease pain, and antiemetics are given for nausea.

> **Clinical Cues**
>
> In the recent past, morphine was not used because it was thought to cause spasm of the sphincter of Oddi; however, this is not supported by research (Carroll, 2009).

Intravenous (IV) fluids are begun to prevent dehydration. Coagulation times are monitored if jaundice is present, and vitamin K, if needed, is administered before surgery to improve clotting ability of the blood. The patient scheduled for gallstone surgery has needs similar to those of any patient having abdominal surgery. Teaching is adapted for the standard procedure or the laparoscopic procedure (see Chapters 4 and 5).

Postoperative Care. The patient is placed in the semi-Fowler's position after he recovers from anesthesia. This position is more comfortable and decreases strain on the sutures. The patient will also be able to take deep breaths and cough more easily in this position.

A patient who has had "open" gallbladder surgery needs proper care of the drains or tubes that may be in place after the surgery. In many cases, the surgery was performed to relieve an obstruction to the flow of bile through the bile ducts or to drain purulent material to the outside. The drainage is absorbed by the dressings over the surgical wound. Dressings must be changed often and should be checked frequently for signs of fresh bleeding. The drain is left in as long as necessary and is then removed by the surgeon.

When an obstruction of the common bile duct has occurred because of stones or tumors, the surgeon may insert a small T-shaped tube (T-tube) directly into the common bile duct during an "open" cholecystectomy (Figure 31-2). This tube must be kept open at all times and is connected to a bedside drainage bag. The length of time the T-tube is left in place varies according to the condition of the patient. Only a small amount of bile will be going to the duodenum. No tension should be put on tubes or drains that have been

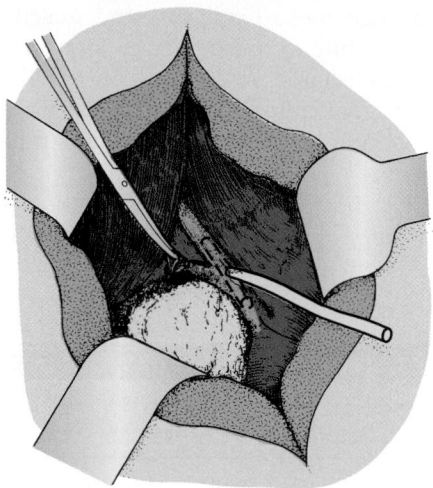

FIGURE 31-2 T-tube inserted into the common bile duct and sutured in place.

inserted in the surgical wound. Dressings must be changed carefully because **T-tubes are sutured in place, and if they are accidentally pulled out, the patient must be returned to the operating room and the incision reopened to replace the tube.**

Montgomery straps are best for holding the dressings in place. The patient should be prepared to expect a greenish yellow discharge (bile) on the dressings. The drainage bag is emptied when the dressing is changed. The patient often goes home with the T-tube in place.

> **Patient Teaching**
>
> ### Caring for a T-Tube
>
> *Teach the patient to:*
> - Wear loose-fitting, older clothes.
> - Coil the drainage tubing and secure it to the abdomen with tape.
> - Take showers rather than baths.
> - Avoid heavy lifting and strenuous activity.
> - Carefully change the dressing every day, cleansing the skin around the tube.
> - Inspect for signs of infection: redness, swelling, warmth, pain, or pus.
> - Take your temperature every day and report to surgeon if greater than 100° F (37° C).
> - Empty the drainage bag at the same time each day.
> - Note the amount, color, and odor of the drainage.
> - Report any change in drainage, abdominal pain, nausea, or vomiting to your surgeon.
> - Return to the surgeon for your follow-up checkup.

The nurse must carefully observe the color of the patient's stools because a return of the normal brown colored stool is an indication that bile is flowing and entering the small intestine. If the bile duct is obstructed, there will be signs of jaundice and stool will be light in color.

The "open" cholecystectomy patient is reluctant to deep-breathe and cough because of pain in the operative area. Encourage these exercises, and auscultate lung sounds every shift to discover any signs of extra secretions or atelectasis. A patient-controlled analgesia (PCA) pump will help the patient to cooperate with turning, coughing, and ambulating and thus prevent complications.

No specific diet is recommended for the patient who has had surgery of the gallbladder, although it is wise to avoid excessive amounts of fatty foods.

 Think Critically

Can you outline the points to be covered for teaching the patient who is about to undergo a cholecystectomy?

Complications

Constant irritation of the gallbladder may contribute to cancer of the gallbladder. Inflammation and infection produce purulent material and a fistula may form. Necrosis, gangrene, and rupture of the gallbladder causing peritonitis may occur. Choledocholithiasis may cause inflammation of the common duct and obstruct the pancreatic duct. This can lead to pancreatitis.

DISORDERS OF THE LIVER

The liver becomes inflamed when injured by trauma, toxins, or tumor invasion. Disruption of the normal functions of the liver occurs depending on how much of the liver tissue is affected. Chronic inflammation causes fibrosis of the liver cells and abnormal function.

HEPATITIS

Etiology and Pathophysiology

There are five types of viral hepatitis (Table 31-2) that cause physical problems. A sixth hepatitis virus, hepatitis G, does not seem to cause the symptoms of hepatitis. Liver cells are damaged either by direct action of the virus on hepatocytes or by cell-mediated immune responses to the virus. Hepatitis viruses cause extensive inflammation of the liver tissue. Liver cell damage results in necrosis of hepatic cells. The Kupffer cells proliferate and enlarge. Bile flow may be interrupted because of the inflammation. With severe inflammation, fibrous scar tissue may form in the liver. Scar tissue often obstructs normal blood and bile flow, causing further damage from ischemia.

Liver cells do have the capacity to regenerate and resume their normal appearance. The cells can function as long as there are no complications.

Hepatitis A and hepatitis E viruses are transmitted primarily by the oral-fecal route. They are responsible for the epidemic forms of viral hepatitis. Hepatitis A virus can be transmitted by food handlers to customers or by mollusk shellfish from contaminated waters. Hepatitis E virus infection is primarily seen in less developed countries. It is transmitted through fecal contamination of water.

Hepatitis B, C, and D viruses may cause chronic inflammation and necrosis of the tissue. A carrier state of hepatitis B, C, or D may occur and asymptomatic individuals can transmit infection to others. **Hepatitis B and C viruses are transmitted by parenteral routes and sexually as they are present in semen, vaginal secretions, and saliva of carriers. Sexual partners of patients who are carriers of hepatitis B or C virus are at high risk for contracting the virus.** Hepatitis D virus coexists with hepatitis B or C virus, and is transmitted in the same ways.

Hepatitis C virus has been the main cause of post-transfusion hepatitis because before 1992 donor blood could not be screened for this type of hepatitis. The number of transfusion-related cases was reduced after screening was implemented. **Intravenous drug use is currently a major cause of hepatitis C infection; therefore users are a target group for screening and counseling. The virus can also be transmitted by straws used to snort cocaine.** Hepatitis B and C viruses can be transmitted from mother to infant. Both can occur in hemodialysis patients. **Hepatitis B and C are the most serious forms of hepatitis, often progressing to chronic hepatitis, cirrhosis, liver cancer, and death.**

 Cultural Considerations

HBV Among Asian Americans

One of 10 foreign-born Asian Americans has chronic HBV infection; in other words, the rate is 100 times greater than that of the non-Asian population (Mosby's Nursing Consult, 2008).

Elder Care Points

Elderly patients who have had several major surgeries and blood transfusions before 1992 are at higher risk for hepatitis B and C. These patients may be carriers of these viruses.

Signs and Symptoms

The clinical signs and symptoms of hepatitis A tend to have an acute onset, whereas in hepatitis B, hepatitis C, and hepatitis D the onset is slower and more insidious. There are three phases of hepatitis A. The first, the *preicteric* phase, precedes jaundice and lasts 1 to 21 days. When symptoms do occur, they may be vague and nonspecific manifestations (see Table 31-2.) The patient might think he has a mild case of influenza because the symptoms are so similar.

The *icteric* phase, characterized by jaundice, lasts 2 to 4 weeks. Urine becomes dark and stools may become light if bile flow is obstructed. Pruritus may occur from the bile pigment deposited in the skin. The liver becomes tender and enlarged.

Table 31-2   Comparison of Hepatitis-Causing Viruses

HEPATITIS A VIRUS (HAV)	HEPATITIS B VIRUS (HBV)	HEPATITIS C VIRUS (HCV)	HEPATITIS D VIRUS (HDV)	HEPATITIS E VIRUS (HEV)
Transmission Mode				
Fecal-to-oral route; poor sanitation and contaminated water and shellfish; often from infected food	Sexual contact, blood and body fluid contact; perinatal from mother to infant	Contact with blood and body fluids, sexual contact with carrier, contact with contaminated surgical, tattooing, and piercing equipment	Blood and body fluid contact; accompanies hepatitis B; close personal contact	Fecal-to-oral route; contaminated water or food
Incubation Period				
15-60 days (average 30 days)	6 wk-6 mo (average 12-14 wk)	6-7 wk	Same as hepatitis B, which precedes it. Chronic carriers of hepatitis B are at risk throughout their carrier state	14-60 days (average 40 days)
Infective Period				
Most infectious 2 wk before onset of symptoms; not likely to be infectious after first week following onset of jaundice	Begins before symptoms appear and persists for 4-6 mo after acute illness; persists for lifetime of chronic carriers	Begins 1-2 wk before symptoms appear; continues throughout life for chronic carriers	Blood is potentially infectious in active hepatitis B infection; may still be present in blood of chronic hepatitis B carriers even though undetectable	
Signs and Symptoms				
Acute onset *First phase (preicteric):* Malaise, fever, loss of appetite, nausea, fatigue, joint aching, skin rash, and upper abdominal discomfort May develop jaundice; malaise and fatigue	Slow onset May be asymptomatic	Slow onset May be asymptomatic until liver damage has occurred	Slow onset May be asymptomatic	Abdominal pain, anorexia, dark urine, fever, hepatomegaly, jaundice, malaise, nausea and vomiting

The *posticteric* phase begins when jaundice is disappearing. Convalescence may take 2 to 4 months. Major complaints are malaise and fatigue. Liver enlargement may continue, but if the spleen was enlarged, it returns to normal in this phase.

For chronic hepatitis B and C, patients are likely to be asymptomatic or have symptoms of chronic liver disease. Acute hepatitis B and C patients could also be asymptomatic. Symptoms include fatigue, nausea, vomiting, poor appetite, right upper quadrant pain, dark urine, and light-colored stools.

Hepatitis D sometimes causes massive destruction of liver cells, liver failure, and death. Hepatitis B and D become chronic in 2% to 10% of infected patients. The patient is then a constant carrier of the virus. There are no currently known signs and symptoms of hepatitis G.

 Clinical Cues

We often assume that liver disorders are associated with jaundice; however, be aware that viral hepatitis without jaundice (anicteric hepatitis) is two to three times more common than viral hepatitis with jaundice.

Diagnosis

Hepatitis is diagnosed by history, physical examination, and laboratory testing. Serologic assays or enzyme immunoassays (EIAs) detect specific antibodies to the various types of hepatitis. Molecular assays can detect viral nucleic acid. These assays do not measure the severity of disease or indicate prognosis. The genotype assay can be used to predict the response to and duration of therapy. Chronic hepatitis is determined by liver biopsy. Elevations in liver function tests (LFTs) are

Table 31-3	Laboratory Test Findings in Acute Viral Hepatitis	
TEST	**ABNORMAL FINDINGS**	
Aspartate aminotransferase (AST)	Elevated in preicteric phase up to 20 times normal; decreases as jaundice subsides	
Alanine aminotransferase (ALT)	Elevated in preicteric phase; ALT/AST ratio is greater than 1; decreases as jaundice subsides.	
Gamma-glutamyl transpeptidase (GGT)	Elevated	
Bilirubin	Elevated unconjugated (direct) bilirubin	
Alkaline phosphatase	Some elevation	
Serum albumin	Normal or decreased	
Serum bilirubin (total)	Elevated to about 8-15 mg/dL (137-257 μmol/L)	
Prothrombin time	Prolonged	

expected findings (Table 31-3). Abnormalities in the white blood cell count, platelets, alkaline phosphatase, albumin, and prothrombin time may also occur depending on the severity of the disease.

Treatment

There is no specific treatment for acute viral hepatitis. Hepatitis A is treated by rest and avoidance of any substances, including alcohol, which can cause liver damage. These measures help the liver to regenerate. A well-balanced diet helps liver cells to heal. Four to six small meals a day are tolerated more readily than three larger ones. Sucking on hard candy is recommended and adds to caloric intake. Nausea may be treated with dimenhydrinate (Dramamine) or trimethobenzamide (Tigan). Phenothiazines are not used because of their hepatotoxic effects. People who have been exposed to the patient should be notified so they can receive prophylaxis.

For hepatitis B, drug therapy is used to decrease the viral load, thereby decreasing the disease progression (Table 31-4). In 2008 the Food and Drug

Table 31-4	Selected Drugs Commonly Prescribed for Disorders of the Liver		
CLASSIFICATION	**ACTION**	**NURSING IMPLICATIONS**	**PATIENT TEACHING**
Diuretic			
Potassium-Sparing Diuretics			
Spironolactone (Aldactone) Amiloride (Midamor) Triamterene (Dyrenium)	Blocks action of aldosterone in the distal nephron, preventing sodium uptake in exchange for potassium secretion. Potassium is "spared" (not secreted) and sodium is excreted. These drugs cause little diuresis.	It is not necessary to supplement potassium for patients taking this type of diuretic alone. Monitor potassium levels.	Avoid foods high in potassium content: bananas, oranges, salt substitutes, dried apricots, and dates.
Loop Diuretic			
Furosemide (Lasix)	Blocks reabsorption of sodium and chloride in the loop of Henle, promoting water secretion. Promotes powerful diuresis.	Give early in the morning. Monitor potassium levels and supplement. potassium as needed Monitor for hypokalemia, I&O. Weigh patient daily. Assess for hearing loss. Monitor for postural hypotension.	Warn that the drug will cause the need to empty the bladder frequently. Caution regarding dizziness when changing positions.
Laxative: Ammonia Detoxicant			
Lactulose (Cephulac)	Prevents absorption of ammonia in the colon; increases water in the stool.	Assess stool amount and color. Monitor serum ammonia level, electrolytes, and I&O. Assess perineal skin frequently for excoriation from diarrhea.	Advise that this drug is intended to cause bowel evacuation and diarrhea is likely.

BP, blood pressure; *GI*, gastrointestinal; *HBV*, hepatitis B virus; *HCV*, hepatitis C virus; *I&O*, intake and output; *INR*, international normalized ratio.

Table 31-4 Selected Drugs Commonly Prescribed for Disorders of the Liver—cont'd

CLASSIFICATION	ACTION	NURSING IMPLICATIONS	PATIENT TEACHING
Antibiotic			
Neomycin (Mycifradin)	Decreases protein synthesis in bacterial cells, causing bacterial death. This prevents the breakdown of protein in the GI tract and helps prevent formation of ammonia.	Monitor renal function and hearing. Observe for dehydration.	Explain the purpose of this drug.
Vasoconstrictor			
Vasopressin (Pitressin)	Causes vasoconstriction; stops bleeding of esophageal varices.	Monitor BP and I&O as may cause water retention.	Explain the purpose of the drug.
Vitamins			
Thiamine (vitamin B$_1$)	Corrects vitamin B$_1$ deficiency that occurs from excessive alcohol use.	Assess thiamine levels.	Explain purpose of the drug.
Vitamin K (AquaMEPHYTON)	Needed for hepatic formation of coagulation factors II, VII, IX, and X.	Monitor prothrombin time and INR.	Explain injection may cause discomfort.
Antiretrovirals			
Lamivudine (Epivir)	Inhibits replication of HBV.	Monitor blood count, viral load, liver functions, amylase, lipase, and triglycerides. Watch for signs of lactic acidosis.	GI complaints and insomnia resolve after 3-4 wk. Drug is not a cure, but will help control symptoms. Notify physician of swollen lymph nodes, fever, malaise, and sore throat. May still pass virus on to others; maintain precautions.
Ribavirin (Rebetol)	Inhibits viral protein synthesis.	Ribavirin is used together with interferon alfa-2b to treat chronic HCV.	Drug may cause fainting or dizziness.
Adefovir dipivoxil (Hepsera)	Prevents DNA replication.	Monitor respiratory status; assess for skin rash.	Report any difficulty breathing or itching, swelling, or redness of the eyes.
Entecavir (Baraclude)	Prevents viral replication.	Monitor renal function.	May cause weakness.
Telbivudine (Tyzeka)	Prevents viral replication.	Monitor renal function and electrolytes.	May cause lactic acidosis and myopathy.
Tenofovir (Viread)	Prevents viral replication.	Monitor renal function and electrolytes.	May cause lactic acidosis and severe hepatomegaly.
Immunomodulator			
Peginterferon alfa-2b (PEG-Intron)	Inhibits viral replication and increases phagocytic action of macrophages, augmenting specific cytotoxicity of lymphocytes.	Perform baseline assessments. Monitor for signs of depression; offer emotional support. Monitor for abdominal pain and bloody diarrhea. Monitor viral load.	Maintain hydration and avoid alcohol. May experience flulike symptoms.
Antimetabolites Neoplastic Metabolites			
5-Fluorouracil (5-FU) and floxuridine (FUDR)	Antimetabolite that acts during cellular metabolism to prevent cellular division.	Perform baseline assessments with attention to temperature. Monitor blood count.	Avoid crowds and exposure to infection. Promptly report fever, diarrhea, vomiting, bleeding, bruising, or redness and burning of the palms of hands or soles of feet.

Administration (FDA) approved a once-daily tablet, tenofovir disoproxil fumarate (Viread), for the treatment of chronic hepatitis B. It works by blocking an enzyme required for replication of the virus. The most common side effect is nausea. Chronic hepatitis C virus treatment is also aimed at reducing the viral load. Treatment is supportive to enhance the patient's natural defenses and promote healing of the liver. Hydration, sufficient rest, and adequate nutrition are the goals. Medication for nausea may be prescribed to encourage adequate nutrition. Vaccines are available to provide active immunity against hepatitis A and B. The vaccine for hepatitis A is administered in two doses, 6 months apart, for lifetime immunity (Dentinger, 2009). The vaccine for hepatitis B produces immunity in about 95% of vaccinated individuals (Degli-Esposti, 2010) and is administered in three or four doses for probable lifetime immunity (MMWR Quick Guide, 2010).

Passive immunity to type A hepatitis can be conferred by the administration of immune globulin (IG). IG is also recommended for those who have been exposed to persons infected with hepatitis B virus who have not been immunized against this virus. There is no protective vaccine for hepatitis C virus.

 Health Promotion

Healthy People 2020 Goal for Hepatitis B

Hepatitis is an occupational hazard for all people who have direct contact with patients or surgical and diagnostic equipment. Standard Precautions must be observed at all times. All health care personnel should be immunized with the hepatitis B vaccine. These practices will help meet the *Healthy People 2020* goal of reducing hepatitis B and the National Patient Safety Goal to reduce the risk of health care–associated infections.

❖ NURSING MANAGEMENT

■ Assessment (Data Collection)

Data collection for a patient with hepatitis should include a nursing history of any previous contacts and whether the contacts have been notified and immunized. By law, viral hepatitis must be reported to the state department of public health. **Because the liver detoxifies many chemicals and metabolizes certain drugs, a complete list of recently taken or current medications is essential. It may be necessary to discontinue some drugs that are particularly toxic to the liver** (see Box 28-1).

Assess for problems related to silent gastrointestinal (GI) bleeding, respiratory distress, and neurologic dysfunction. Mental confusion and coma associated with hepatic encephalopathy occurs from circulating toxins due to liver failure. Encephalopathy is degeneration or disease of the brain.

 Focused Assessment

Data Collection for the Patient with a Liver Disorder

HEALTH HISTORY
- Have you ever had a parasitic infection?
- Do you have a history of cancer?
- How much alcohol do you drink?
- Do you have a history of hepatitis?
- Have you been exposed to hepatitis?
- What drugs do you take?
- Have you been exposed to pesticides or industrial chemicals? Which ones?
- Has your appetite decreased? Have you had nausea or vomiting?
- Are you more fatigued than usual?
- Have you noticed any fever?
- Have you noticed dark-colored urine?
- Have you had any light or clay-colored stools?
- Have you had excessive gas?
- Have you been bruising easily?
- Has your skin been itchy or made you feel uncomfortable?
- Has your abdomen increased in girth lately?
- Do you have abdominal pain? Where? Can you describe it?
- Have you gained weight recently?

PHYSICAL ASSESSMENT
- Inspect the skin for signs of jaundice, scratch marks, and general condition.
- Inspect the sclera and mucous membranes of the mouth for signs of jaundice.
- Gently palpate the abdomen for masses and for liver enlargement.
- Auscultate bowel sounds.
- Measure abdominal girth for a baseline.
- Inspect extremities for signs of edema.
- Check liver function test values and urinalysis for bilirubin presence.

■ Nursing Diagnosis and Planning

Nursing diagnoses specific to hepatitis infection might include:
- Imbalanced nutrition: less than body requirements related to anorexia, nausea, and vomiting
- Fatigue related to disease process and malaise
- Pain related to inflamed liver and pruritus
- Deficient knowledge related to disease process and self-care needed
- Deficient diversional activity
- Disturbed body image related to yellow discoloration of skin

Expected outcomes might be:
- Patient will maintain body weight within normal limits during illness.
- Patient will verbalize lessened fatigue after rest periods each day.
- Patient will verbalize a decrease in pain after pain medication and comfort measures.
- Patient will verbalize knowledge of disease process and self-care within 2 days.
- Patient will engage in appropriate diversional activities during convalescence.
- Patient will list personal strengths that compensate for altered appearance.

Elder Care Points

The elderly patient is at higher risk for drug-induced hepatitis if he has chronic conditions that require the administration of various drugs that can cause liver damage over a long period of time. With liver inflammation, the liver will not function well and drug dosages will need to be lowered; otherwise drug toxicity may occur.

■ **Implementation and Evaluation**

Nursing interventions include reviewing trends of serum liver enzyme levels and serum bilirubin values. Preventing the spread of infection is a major concern when caring for patients with viral hepatitis. The patient and family will need to be instructed regarding special precautions to prevent the spread of the infection, such as proper handling of body secretions, proper hand hygiene, and limiting contact with others.

Sedatives must be given with caution because a diseased liver cannot detoxify them very well. Alcohol is particularly damaging to the liver and should be avoided for 4 months following recovery from hepatitis.

The convalescence of the hepatitis patient is slow and long. A nutritious diet with supplements is prescribed. A variety of diversional activities that are not physically taxing should be planned, such as a new hobby or learning a new skill, handheld computer games, Internet access, puzzle books, and DVDs. Visitors can play cards or board games with the patient. Nursing interventions for selected nursing diagnoses relevant to the patient with hepatitis are found in Table 31-5 and Table 28-2.

 Complementary and Alternative Therapies

Promoting Good Liver Function

Several supplements are known to be beneficial to promoting good liver function. *N*-acetylcysteine (NAC), glutathione (GSH), choline, methionine, milk thistle, carnitine, and antioxidants are helpful. NAC promotes detoxification pathways; choline helps prevent deposition of fat in the liver. Carnitine allows fats to be used as energy and alleviates deposition of fat in the liver and elsewhere in the body. The physician should always be consulted before taking supplements.

Prevention

Transmission Precautions. Both feces and blood of patients with hepatitis A contain virus during the prodromal stage (infected but asymptomatic) and early symptomatic stage. When hepatitis is suspected, adherence to Standard Precautions is essential; patient and family must use precautions at home.

Hepatitis B and D viruses are rarely transmitted by the fecal-oral route, but it is strongly recommended to

 Home Care Considerations

Preventing the Spread of Hepatitis Virus

HEPATITIS A
- Notify close contacts so they can obtain immune globulin protection and hepatitis A vaccine.
- Practice extremely good hygiene, washing with warm water and soap (liquid soap is best).
- Wash hands after using the toilet and before eating and after changing diapers.
- Avoid preparing food during the infectious period.
- Use separate bath and hand towels from other members of the family.
- Avoid sharing toothbrushes.
- Use gloves to disinfect the bathroom fixtures with a 10:1 bleach solution.
- Refrain from sexual contact until the physician states that the infectious period is over.

HEPATITIS B OR C
- Avoid sexual contact until there is no chance of transmission of the virus.
- Advise close contacts to obtain hepatitis B vaccine as indicated.
- Avoid sharing razors or toothbrushes because of the chance of blood transmission.

 Safety Alert

Hepatitis C

Hepatitis C virus (HCV) is transmitted by blood and saliva. Standard Precautions and careful handling of all body fluids are recommended. The first line of defense is scrupulous hand hygiene. Wear gloves when handling plasma-containing body fluids and use extreme caution when handling used needles, syringes, and IV tubing. Needle sticks, open wounds, and the mucous membranes of the eyes, nose, and mouth can serve as portals of entry. Dentists, physicians, nurses, and other health care workers must be informed of a patient's carrier status.

be very careful when disposing of a patient's stool. Standard Precautions guidelines must be carefully followed for handling, sterilizing, and disposing of equipment contaminated with blood. Hepatitis viruses are transmitted by sexual contact, and homosexual men in particular are at risk.

When a patient with viral hepatitis has been admitted to the hospital, the infection control officer must be notified as soon as possible. It is important to familiarize yourself with the hospital's policies and procedures, so that protection for others and follow-up for the infected patient is not overlooked. Infection with hepatitis A in a person who handles food on the job must be reported promptly. The Centers for Disease Control and Prevention (CDC) has published guidelines for the care of patients hospitalized with hepatitis. These same guidelines can be modified for home care to prevent the spread of the infection.

Table 31-5   Common Nursing Diagnoses, Expected Outcomes, and Nursing Interventions for Patients with Hepatitis

NURSING DIAGNOSIS	EXPECTED OUTCOMES	NURSING INTERVENTIONS
Deficient fluid volume related to nausea and vomiting	Patient will cease vomiting within 24 hr. Patient will establish fluid balance within 48 hr as evidenced by moist mucous membranes and good skin turgor.	Administer antiemetics as ordered. Monitor IV infusion site and fluid rate. Encourage clear oral fluids if ordered and tolerated. Monitor electrolyte levels for imbalances. Monitor I&O Provide mouth care q 2 hr while awake.
Imbalanced nutrition: less than body requirements related to nausea, vomiting, and improper diet	Patient will ingest a 1200-calorie diet per day within 7 days after subsidence of acute vomiting. Patient will maintain present weight.	Keep door of room closed to keep odors out. Offer mouth care before meal time. Provide 6 small meals a day plus small, high-calorie snacks between meals. Weigh q 3 days and record. Keep hard candy at bedside for snacking.
Impaired comfort related to jaundice and bile pigments in skin causing itching	Patient will verbalize that itching is decreased.	Assist to bathe with tepid water three times a day. Apply lotion q 2 hr. Provide diversional activities. Teach relaxation techniques.
Deficient knowledge related to ways in which HBV is transmitted, impact of hepatitis on the body, self-care measures, and measures to prevent transmission to others	Patient will verbalize ways HBV is transmitted, impact on body, self-care measures, and measures to prevent transmission to others before discharge.	Teach ways in which HBV is transmitted: parenteral routes, sexual contact, contact with blood and body fluids. Give explanation in understandable terms of what HBV does to the body. Reinforce teaching regarding self-care measures: hygiene, diet, rest, follow-up. Teach importance of not sharing personal articles (especially razor, toothbrush, etc.) with others. Instruct to inform health care workers of the presence of the virus until tests for it are negative. Inform that sexual partner(s) will need injection of special immune globulin for protection and then immunization.
Body image disturbance related to yellow skin color from jaundice	Patient will demonstrate acceptance of present body image by allowing visitors within 3 days.	Assure that jaundice is not permanent. Allow to ventilate feelings about the illness and present appearance. Encourage verbalization of positive aspects about self. Increase fluid intake to help flush bilirubin from blood during recovery.
Fatigue related to vague flulike symptoms	Patient will verbalize less fatigue before discharge.	Assess current level of energy. Assist with ADLs as needed. Suggest that visitors come when energy level is higher. Cluster care and allow for periods of rest. Help identify activities that require more energy and help patient prioritize accordingly.

HBV, hepatitis B virus; *I&O,* intake and output; *IV,* intravenous.

Complementary and Alternative Therapies

Vitamin E and Nonalcoholic Steatohepatitis

Nonalcoholic steatohepatitis (NASH) is a chronic liver disease that resembles alcoholic liver disease and can result in cirrhosis, liver cancer, or death. In a recent study, patients with NASH were given pioglitazone (Actos), which is a diabetic drug, and vitamin E. Although Actos caused undesirable weight gain, there was improvement in liver inflammation and liver enzymes. Patients taking high doses of vitamin E should be monitored by a physician and may need a biopsy to assess response to treatment (NIH News Release, 2010).

Complications

A small percentage of patients with hepatitis can develop massive necrosis of liver cells that results in acute liver failure. *Acute liver failure* is the preferred term according to the American Association for the Study of Liver Diseases. *Fulminant hepatitis* or *necrosis* and *fulminant hepatic failure* are older terms. The only hope for recovery is a liver transplant; without transplant, death occurs in about 75% of these cases. Symptoms of liver diseases include mental confusion, disorientation, and drowsiness, which indicate hepatic encephalopathy. Ascites (abnormal accumulation of serous fluid within the peritoneal cavity) and edema accompany liver failure.

CIRRHOSIS

Etiology

There were 27,555 deaths attributed to chronic liver disease and cirrhosis in 2006 (CDC, 2010). Excessive alcohol ingestion is the leading cause of the cases of cirrhosis in the United States and hepatitis B or C is the second cause (Allegretti, 2009). *Postnecrotic cirrhosis* is caused by viral hepatitis, toxic substances, parasites, or infection. There are three other types of cirrhosis. *Laënnec's cirrhosis,* or *portal cirrhosis,* results from alcoholism. The first change caused by excessive alcohol ingestion is the deposition of fat in the liver cells. This is reversible if alcohol consumption is halted; otherwise, widespread scar formation occurs. *Biliary cirrhosis* is from chronic biliary obstruction and infection. *Cardiac cirrhosis* results from long-standing, severe right-sided heart failure in patients with cor pulmonale.

Cultural Considerations

Liver-Related Deaths

Death related to liver disease is not among the top 10 causes of death for the general population; however for the American Indian and Alaska Native population, chronic liver disease and cirrhosis rank fifth as a cause of death, and for the Hispanic population liver disease is the sixth leading cause of death (Heron, 2010).

Pathophysiology

Cirrhosis is a progressive, chronic disease of the liver. Normal hepatic structures are destroyed and replaced with necrotic tissue. Fibrous bands of connective tissue develop in the organ, which eventually constrict and partition the liver tissue into irregular nodules. If this process is halted before too much liver tissue is damaged, the liver tissue will regenerate. Late cirrhosis is considered irreversible.

When liver cells begin to degenerate, the blood vessels within the liver also fail to function. This causes an obstruction to the flow of blood through the portal circulatory system, causing portal systemic hypertension. There is altered vessel permeability and fluid leakage into the abdomen, resulting in ascites. As pressure increases in the hepatic veins, there is a shift of protein-rich plasma filtrate into the lymphatic ducts. If the pressure is high enough in the ducts, the excess fluid will ooze from the surface of the liver into the peritoneal cavity. The fluid has a high colloidal pressure because of its high protein content and is not readily reabsorbed. Fluid accumulates in the cavity, causing increased abdominal girth and weight gain. Secondarily, the damaged liver's inability to synthesize albumin and the osmotic pressure within the blood vessels falls, allowing fluid to be pulled out into the tissues. The third mechanism contributing to ascites and edema is excess circulating aldosterone, which is not properly metabolized by the damaged liver. The excess aldosterone causes sodium and water retention (Concept Map 31-1).

Signs and Symptoms

Cirrhosis usually progresses without symptoms until severe liver damage is present. Subjective symptoms of liver cirrhosis include fatigue, weakness, headache, anorexia, indigestion, abdominal pain, nausea, and vomiting. Fluid retention in the right hemithorax or ascites can limit expansion of the chest and cause dyspnea. Objective symptoms of liver cirrhosis include excessive gas, skin rashes, and fever. Leg and foot edema and palmar erythema (redness of the palms that blanches with pressure) occur. Sometimes bluish varicose veins, called caput medusa, radiating from the umbilicus (indicating portal hypertension) are seen. Bleeding and bruising because of deficiencies in vitamin K, thrombin, or prothrombin interfere with clot formation. The liver often is enlarged and "knobby" and is palpable below the level of the right rib cage. Abdominal distention is present. The spleen also enlarges. Skin lesions, jaundice, pruritus, bleeding disorders, endocrine disorders, and peripheral neuropathy occur in late disease. Spider angiomas may appear on the face, neck, upper trunk, and arms.

Urine may become dark and foamy, and stools turn clay colored, which indicates that bile is not reaching the intestine. Jaundice occurs either because the liver cannot metabolize bilirubin or because bile flow is

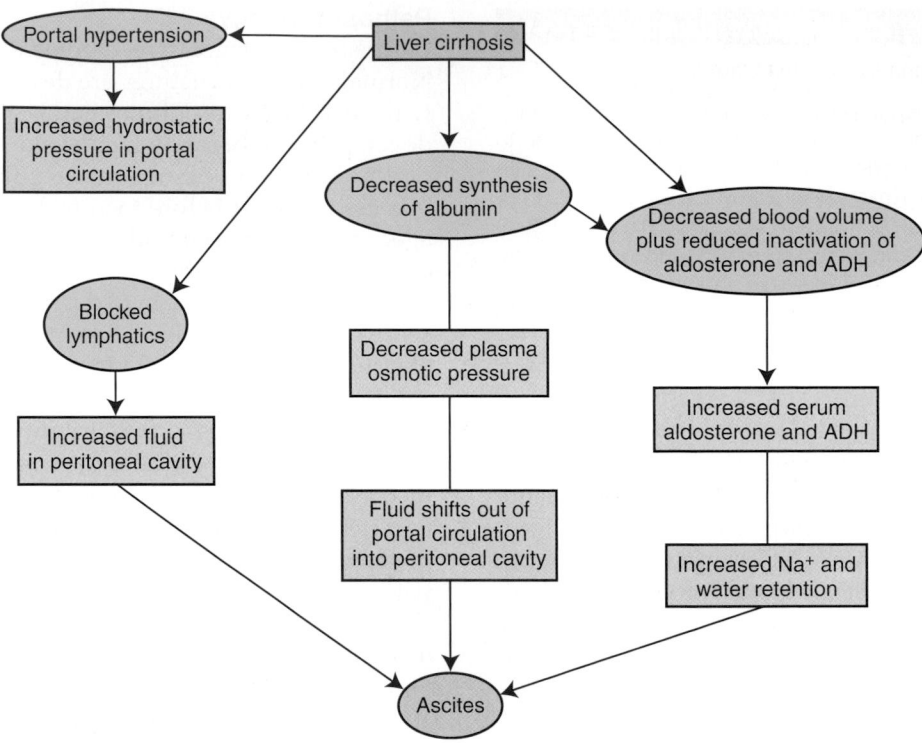

CONCEPT MAP 31-1 Relationship of systemic portal hypertension and ascites in liver cirrhosis.

obstructed. Excessively high levels of bile pigment *(bilirubin)* are present in the blood. The pigment is deposited in the skin, mucous membranes, and body fluids, causing a change in color ranging from pale yellow to golden orange. The first signs of jaundice are usually seen in the sclera of the eye (icterus), which takes on a yellow tint. Jaundice is not always a sign of liver damage. In *hemolytic jaundice,* there may be an increased level of bilirubin as a result of excessive destruction of red blood cells, with resultant release of the pigment into the bloodstream. Figure 31-3 shows the all the signs and symptoms of cirrhosis. **Elevations in liver enzymes usually do not occur until 65% of liver function is gone.** The patient is likely to delay seeking medical attention until symptoms are pronounced.

Think Critically

Can you list the ways in which you would collect data when checking a patient for signs of jaundice?

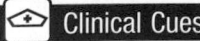
Clinical Cues

In people with dark skin, jaundice is best detected by checking the buccal mucosa, hard palate, palms, soles of the feet, sclera, and conjunctiva.

Diagnosis

A definitive diagnosis of cirrhosis of the liver is made by liver biopsy. Laboratory testing may show a low albumin level and elevated prothrombin time, as well as elevated AST, ALT, ammonia level, and lactate dehydrogenase values. CT and liver scan can help determine the size of the liver and presence of any masses, and outline the hepatic blood flow and any obstruction to it. Magnetic resonance cholangiopancreatography—similar to ERCP but without the use of contrast media—may be performed.

Treatment

Treatment is aimed at stopping the liver damage, restoring the liver's functions and management of symptoms. **Medical treatment of ascites includes restriction of fluid and sodium intake and administration of diuretics.** Abdominal paracentesis can be performed to remove accumulated fluid; however, this a temporary measure that poses problems of rapid fluid shift, loss of protein, and the potential for introducing infectious organisms into the peritoneum. In years past, peritoneal-venous shunt (LeVeen or Denver shunt) involving the shunting of ascitic fluid into the venous system was used. Currently, a transjugular intrahepatic portosystemic shunt (TIPS) may be used to decrease pressure between portal and hepatic veins in the liver and decompress the varices. A catheter is inserted into the jugular vein and threaded through the superior and inferior venae cavae to the hepatic vein and then directed to the portal vein. Stents are placed that extend into both veins.

Safety Alert
Liver Inflammation

Patients with liver inflammation or cirrhosis should avoid taking large doses of vitamins and minerals. Vitamin A, iron, and copper can worsen the liver damage.

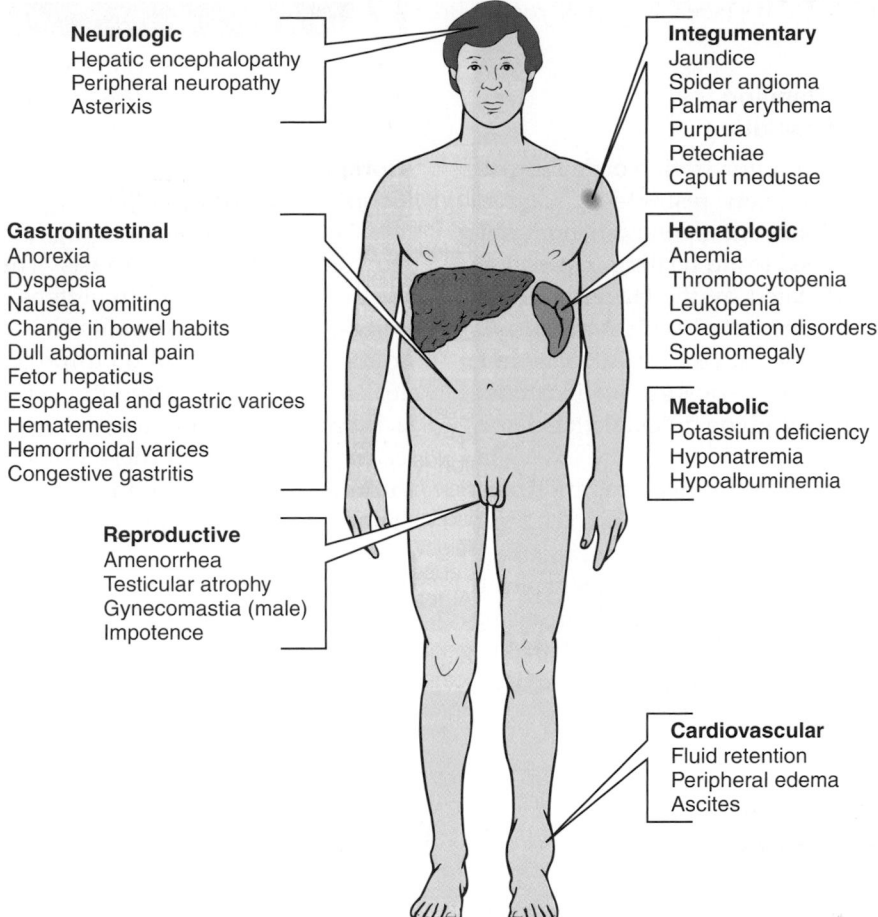

Neurologic
Hepatic encephalopathy
Peripheral neuropathy
Asterixis

Integumentary
Jaundice
Spider angioma
Palmar erythema
Purpura
Petechiae
Caput medusae

Gastrointestinal
Anorexia
Dyspepsia
Nausea, vomiting
Change in bowel habits
Dull abdominal pain
Fetor hepaticus
Esophageal and gastric varices
Hematemesis
Hemorrhoidal varices
Congestive gastritis

Hematologic
Anemia
Thrombocytopenia
Leukopenia
Coagulation disorders
Splenomegaly

Metabolic
Potassium deficiency
Hyponatremia
Hypoalbuminemia

Reproductive
Amenorrhea
Testicular atrophy
Gynecomastia (male)
Impotence

Cardiovascular
Fluid retention
Peripheral edema
Ascites

FIGURE 31-3 The many signs and symptoms of cirrhosis.

Traditionally, limitation of dietary protein intake was prescribed; however, this approach is being challenged and the current recommendation is to manage encephalopathy with medications rather than to restrict protein. Vegetable proteins are preferred because they do not contribute to encephalopathy (Mehta & Rothstein, 2009).

Thiamine and multiple vitamins are given to counteract vitamin deficiency. Neomycin is occasionally given orally or by enema to decrease the colonic bacteria that break down protein. This treatment lowers the formation of ammonia. The bowel is cleansed by enemas to decrease ammonia production further. Lactulose, an exchange resin, is given orally or by a feeding tube to induce diarrhea and prevent diffusion of ammonia out of the intestinal tract. Kidney failure sometimes accompanies liver failure (hepatorenal syndrome).

Cholesterol-binding medications such as cholestyramine (Questran), colestipol (Colestid), and colesevelam (Welchol) may be given to relieve pruritus from bile pigment deposits in the skin.

A relatively new therapy, albumin dialysis has been used to "bridge" the patient who is waiting for a liver transplant or to support function while acute failure is resolving. Theoretically, the albumin binds the toxins, cleanses the blood, and stops the inflammatory process. The therapy has improved level of consciousness related to encephalopathy and reduced mortality rates for chronic liver failure patients who experience an acute episode. It is an expensive therapy that requires specialized equipment and extensive training. Additional research is needed to identify adverse effects and to compare different systems (McCready, 2009).

❖ NURSING MANAGEMENT

■ Assessment (Data Collection)

A thorough assessment to identify specific patient care problems related to abnormal liver function is performed (see Focused Assessment on p. 698). Assess for safety issues related to change in mental status. The patient may have bleeding signs. Pay extra attention to ammonia levels, albumin, AST, ALT, and prothrombin time (PT) results. Increase in ascites is determined by measuring and recording abdominal girth each day. Daily weights should also be initiated if fluid retention is observed. If alcoholism is an issue for your patient, be vigilant for signs of withdrawal, which may occur 6 to 12 hours after the last drink and can continue for 3 to 5 days (see Chapter 47 for additional information).

■ Nursing Diagnosis, Planning, Implementation, and Evaluation

The intake of alcohol and administration of drugs toxic to the liver must be completely restricted. Sedatives and opiates are either avoided or given with great caution. Rest may be prescribed to aid healing. The degree of rest and activity is dictated by the stage of illness. Nutritional deficiencies are treated with supplements and diet. The patient is at great risk for infection and should be protected from exposure to infectious agents; antibiotics should be given quickly when infection occurs.

Nursing diagnoses, expected outcomes, and interventions for the patient with cirrhosis are listed in Nursing Care Plan 31-1 (see also Table 31-5). Stabilization of fluid balance, normalization of vital signs, and progress toward baseline mental status and increasing ability to perform activities of daily living (ADLs) independently are indicators that the expected outcomes are being met; if not, new interventions are chosen for the plan.

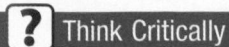 **Think Critically**

Can you identify signs and symptoms that you might find when assessing a patient with advanced cirrhosis of the liver?

Complications

Esophageal Varices. Bleeding from esophageal varices (dilated, distorted, engorged blood veins) is a major complication of cirrhosis. They are the result of portal congestion and hypertension. In advanced cirrhosis, blood that normally flows from the intestines to the portal vein and on through the liver is shunted to other veins, including the veins of the upper stomach and lower esophagus. The added load of blood causes congestion of these veins. When the vein walls rupture, massive bleeding occurs. Another factor in hemorrhage is that the liver is no longer able to make vitamin K, which is an essential component of clotting factors. Varices may rupture and produce hematemesis (vomiting of bright red blood) from increased blood pressure, coughing, vomiting, or mechanical irritation from poorly chewed food. For cirrhosis patients with bleeding esophageal varices, 30% to 60% die within 6 weeks of the first bleed.

 Nursing Care Plan 31-1 | **Care of the Patient with Cirrhosis of the Liver**

Scenario

A 62-year-old man with a 25-year history of alcoholism is admitted with progressive alcoholic cirrhosis. His complaints include thirst, extreme fatigue, a swollen abdomen, edema of the feet and ankles, jaundice, itching, nausea and indigestion, drowsiness, and slight confusion. Esophageal varices are present. All his liver function test results as well as his ammonia level show elevation, and his PT and INR are prolonged. His hematocrit, hemoglobin, and serum albumin levels are low.

Problem/Nursing Diagnosis

Actual (or potential for) difficulty breathing/Impaired gas exchange related to fluid accumulation in the chest (hydrothorax) or abdomen (ascites).

Supporting Assessment Data

Subjective: "I feel like I can't get my breath."
Objective: Shallow rapid breathing, RR 28-32/min; pauses to catch breath after slight exertion of moving in bed.

Goals/Expected Outcomes	Nursing Interventions	Selected Rationale	Evaluation
Patient will maintain adequate oxygenation as evidenced by respiratory rate of 12-24/min and oxygen saturation of <90%.	Assess rate, rhythm, and quality of respirations and do pulse oximeter readings at baseline and after interventions.	Changes in respiratory pattern or pulse oximeter suggest worsening, stabilization, or improvement.	Breathing is shallow and rapid if lying in supine position. If assisted to a sitting position, experiences temporary subjective relief. Pulse oximeter 93% when coached to inhale deeply.
	Place in semi-Fowler's position and observe for relief.	Raising head of bed (HOB) usually alleviates dyspnea, but ascites or hydrothorax may restrict chest expansion.	Relief obtained with HOB at 30 degrees.
	Auscultate lung fields at the beginning of the shift and as required (PRN) for worsening.	Compare findings to your initial assessment to discover changes.	Diminished in the bases bilaterally, with fine crackles.

ADLs, activities of daily living; *BP,* blood pressure; *I&O,* intake and output; *INR,* international normalized ratio; *PT,* prothrombin time; *R,* respirations.

Goals/Expected Outcomes	Nursing Interventions	Selected Rationale	Evaluation
	Administer oxygen as ordered.	Oxygen is generally ordered if saturation falls below 90% (physician may set the parameter higher).	Currently, pulse oximeter shows 93% when awake; however, level drops to 90% when asleep.
	Encourage use of incentive spirometer and teach deep breathing and coughing.	Chest expansion may be limited; therefore patient must be encouraged to make an extra effort to prevent pneumonia and atelectasis.	Willing to try spirometer, but needs continuous reminding. Family members able to help by encouraging him.

Problem/Nursing Diagnosis
Potential for bleeding from esophageal varices/Risk for bleeding related to esophageal varices and decreased clotting factors.

Supporting Assessment Data
Subjective: "Thirsty."
Objective: Elevated liver function test results; cirrhosis, spider angiomas, jaundice, ascites, and prolonged PT.

Goals/Expected Outcomes	Nursing Interventions	Selected Rationale	Evaluation
Patient will not experience life-threatening hemorrhage while hospitalized.	Monitor stool and emesis for blood and other bleeding signs.	Alerts to bleeding.	No signs of bleeding.
	Feed only soft foods.	Prevents mechanical irritation of esophagus.	Eating soft foods; favors puddings and cooked cereals.
	Give vitamin K as ordered.	Vitamin K is needed for synthesis of clotting factors.	Vitamin K administered.
	Monitor vital signs q 2-4 hr as ordered.	Vital sign changes, restlessness, and confusion may indicate bleeding.	BP 120/80, pulse 87/min, R 24/min; is anxious.
	Observe for increasing restlessness and confusion that might indicate hypoxia secondary to bleeding.		Alert and oriented to person and place.
	Monitor PT and INR.	Prolonged clotting times contributes to rapid blood loss.	Laboratory test results pending. Continue plan.

Problem/Nursing Diagnosis
Confusion and drowsiness/Acute confusion related to increased ammonia level caused by liver failure.

Supporting Assessment Data
Subjective: Confused as to month.
Objective: Elevated serum ammonia and drowsiness.

Goals/Expected Outcomes	Nursing Interventions	Selected Rationale	Evaluation
Serum ammonia levels will not increase further during hospitalization.	Neomycin enemas as ordered.	Neomycin kills intestinal bacteria that help digest protein and produce ammonia.	Administered neomycin enema.
Serum ammonia levels will return to normal within 2 mo.	Administer lactulose as ordered.	Lactulose decreases absorption of ammonia.	Lactulose administered; diarrhea occurring. A&D ointment applied to anal area after bowel movements.
	Monitor serum ammonia levels.	Assists in determining likelihood of coma.	Lab work to be drawn in A.M. Continue plan.

Continued

Problem/Nursing Diagnosis
Unfamiliar environment and confused/Risk for injury related to confusion, drowsiness, and weakness.

Supporting Assessment Data
Subjective: "This room looks strange. I can't find the toilet."
Objective: Elevated serum ammonia and slight confusion.

Goals/Expected Outcomes

Goals/Expected Outcomes	Nursing Interventions	Selected Rationale	Evaluation
Patient will not experience injury while hospitalized.	Monitor mental status q 4 hr.	Determines worsening of disorientation.	Oriented to person and place, can recall month with repeated coaching.
	Call bell within reach, bed at lowest level.	Prevents injury from accidental fall from bed.	Bed down, call bell within reach.
	Offer frequent assistance with toileting and other needs (i.e., hygiene, fluids).	Decreases incidents of wandering or falls if trying to meet own needs.	Offered toileting and mouth care q 2-3 hr. No injury sustained. Continue plan.

Problem/Nursing Diagnosis
Cannot perform ADLs/Self-care deficit related to fatigue, drowsiness, and ascites.

Supporting Assessment Data
Subjective: "I'm so sleepy and weak."
Objective: Cannot perform ADLs; very drowsy, ascites present.

Goals/Expected Outcomes

Goals/Expected Outcomes	Nursing Interventions	Selected Rationale	Evaluation
Patient will be able to assist with ADLs within 2 wk.	Bathe with tepid water and apply emollients to decrease itching every shift.	Keeps patient clean and dry, decreases itching.	Baths and emollients have decreased itching slightly.
Patient will be able to perform ADLs independently within 1 mo.	Offer mouth care q 2 hr.	Mouth care improves appetite.	Mouth care given q 2 hr.
	Assist with meal trays.	May lack fine motor coordination to open packages.	Set up meal tray.
	Assist with toileting.	Prevents falls and aids with elimination.	Assisted with toileting. Continue plan.

Problem/Nursing Diagnosis
Fluid retention/Fluid volume excess related to ascites and peripheral edema from portal hypertension.

Supporting Assessment Data
Objective: Ascites, edema of feet and ankles, 6-lb weight gain in 2 days.

Goals/Expected Outcomes

Goals/Expected Outcomes	Nursing Interventions	Selected Rationale	Evaluation
Patient will have no further increase in ascites this week.	Measure abdominal girth every shift.	Determines whether ascites is increasing or decreasing.	Abdominal girth down ⅛ inch.
Patient will return to normal fluid balance within 2 wk.	Administer diuretics as ordered and monitor I&O.	Diuretics remove excess fluid from the body. I&O tracks fluid removal.	Diuretic administered. Intake 400 mL; output 670 mL.
	Weigh daily and record.	Daily weight indicates whether diuretic therapy is effective.	Weight down 1.5 lb.
	Turn at least q 1-2 hr. Provide good skin care.	Turning and skin care prevent pressure sores.	Turned q 2 hr; skin care provided; no reddened or excoriated areas over pressure points. Continue plan.

Critical Thinking Questions
1. Can you describe the correct way to measure abdominal girth?
2. Why is good skin care even more important when a patient has edema and ascites?
3. How high would a PT or INR level have to climb before you would report it to the physician immediately?
4. Why would it be important to monitor this patient for symptoms of alcohol withdrawal?

Treatment options are to put pressure via balloon tamponade with a Blakemore-Sengstaken tube (Figure 31-4), administration of parenteral vasopressors such as vasopressin (Pitressin) to lower portal pressure, injection scleropathy or ligation of the bleeding vessels, embolization of the left gastric vein, or emergency portacaval shunt surgery. Other vasoconstrictors such as terlipressin (Glypressin), somatostatin (Zecnil), and octreotide (Sandostatin) are used to reduce portal blood flow. Nitroglycerin is given to reduce vascular resistance in the liver without interfering with peripheral circulation. A beta blocker may be given to lower blood pressure. The patient is given vitamin K by injection to help rectify clotting factor deficiencies. The treatment of hemorrhage of the upper GI tract is discussed in Chapter 29.

Encephalopathy. Portal systemic encephalopathy is another dangerous complication of cirrhosis. Encephalopathy in this instance is directly related to liver failure and is attributed to the buildup of ammonia and gamma-aminobutyric acid. Symptoms such as delirium, convulsions, asterixis (flapping tremors) and coma occur. Asterixis is observed by having the patient hold out the arms and hands and watching for rapid flexing and extension movements of the hands. There

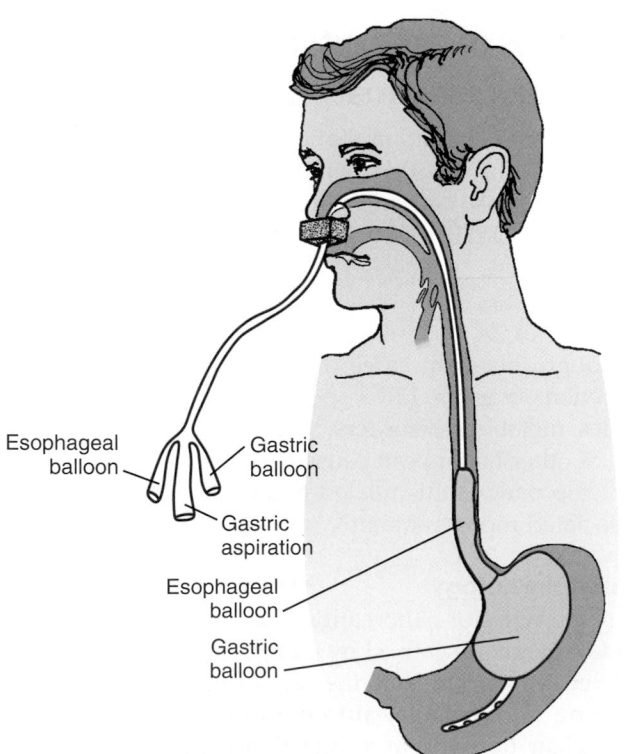

Esophageal balloon
Gastric balloon
Gastric aspiration
Esophageal balloon
Gastric balloon

If the bleeding site is in the esophagus, as from esophageal varices, the esophageal balloon is inflated. If the bleeding site is in the stomach, the gastric balloon is inflated. Inflation of the balloon creates pressure against bleeding vessels.

FIGURE 31-4 Blakemore-Sengstaken tube.

may be rhythmic movements of the legs with dorsiflexion of the foot and rhythmic movements in the face with strong eyelid closure. Fetor hepaticus (breath with a sweet, fecal odor) occurs as liver failure progresses.

LIVER TRANSPLANTATION

Liver transplantation is considered for patients with progressive and advanced liver disease that does not respond to treatment. It is most commonly done for nonalcoholic cirrhosis, chronic active hepatitis, sclerosing cholangitis, metabolic disorders, and biliary atresia in children. Some recovered alcoholics with cirrhosis are candidates. From 70% to 80% of liver transplantation patients survive at least 3 years with good quality of life. Many transplant recipients develop cirrhosis by the fifth year. Organ transplantation, tissue matching, and measures to prevent organ rejection are discussed in Chapter 12. If the patient has encephalopathy preoperatively, an epidural sensor is placed to monitor intracranial pressure (ICP). Every attempt is made to keep ICP within normal limits, as increased ICP levels are correlated with decreased survival rates after transplantation.

🔲 Legal and Ethical Considerations

Liver Transplantation

Available cadaver organs are in short supply. There is controversy about how available organs that fit a patient's genotype should be allotted. Should a person closest to the geographic location of the suitable cadaver liver receive it? Should the person who has been on the transplant list the longest be the recipient? Should the person who is closest to death be given the liver? Should the person whose liver was destroyed by alcohol or from recreational drug use be in line before the person with a metabolic or viral disease that caused end-stage cirrhosis? Should the recipient's age be a factor in the decision? These are examples of questions that enter into the liver transplantation decision.

Nursing Management

After surgery a T-tube and Jackson-Pratt drains will be in place. The patient must take cyclosporine for life to prevent rejection of the new liver. Other immunosuppressants such as azathioprine (Imuran), corticosteroids, tacrolimus (Prograf), monoclonal antibody OKT3, and interleukin-2 receptor antagonists such as basiliximab (Simulect) and daclizumab (Zenapax) may also be added. Strict infection control and prevention is necessary and the patient is monitored closely for signs of hemorrhage or hypovolemia. Measures are instituted to prevent pneumonia, atelectasis, and pleural effusions. Liver functions, serum potassium, serum glucose, and coagulation factors are monitored closely. Right quadrant or flank pain, increasing jaundice, fever, and changes in stool and urine color may indicate organ rejection. Close medical supervision is necessary after discharge.

CANCER OF THE LIVER

Etiology

Primary cancer of the liver is rare in the United States, but is a common malignancy in Africa and Asia and is caused by a parasite called the liver fluke. Liver cancer may be triggered by aflatoxin, a mold that grows on spoiled peanuts, corn, and grains. Metastatic liver cancer is much more prevalent than primary liver cancer, but the end result is the same. Cirrhosis and hepatitis B or hepatitis C increase the risk. Three times as many men as women develop liver cancer.

Pathophysiology

There are two types of primary liver cancer: (1) hepatoma, which arises from the hepatocytes, and (2) cholangiocarcinoma, or bile duct cancer. Benign tumors also occur in the liver. Hepatoma usually develops in people who have cirrhosis. A rare disorder called *hemochromatosis,* which causes deposits of iron in the body, predisposes to the development of hepatoma. Cholangiocarcinoma's cause is unknown, but it occurs more frequently in people with inflammation of the bowel, such as ulcerative colitis.

Pathophysiologically, there is irritation and inflammation with disruption of the structure of normal liver cells. The cancer spreads throughout the organ and invades the portal vein and lymphatics. It may metastasize to the lungs, brain, kidneys, and spleen.

Signs, Symptoms, and Diagnosis

Symptoms may include right upper quadrant pain, fatigue, anorexia, weight loss, weakness, or fever plus signs of poor liver function. Pain may radiate to the back. Because symptoms often are vague, diagnosis of liver cancer occurs late and death may occur within 6 to 18 months.

Diagnostic tests are used to determine the presence of tumor and the stage of the cancer and to find areas of metastasis. Fine-needle biopsy or brush biopsy during ERCP gives a definitive diagnosis.

Treatment and Nursing Management

If no distant spread is found and there is no lymph node involvement, surgical resection may be attempted. If the tumor is primary and has not metastasized, liver transplantation is an option. Treatment is combined radiation and chemotherapy that is infused intravenously or directly into the hepatic circulation. Commonly used agents are 5-fluorouracil (5-FU), floxuridine (FUDR), doxorubicin, and methotrexate. Chemoembolization, wherein an oily substance called lipiodol is added to the drugs given intra-arterially, makes the chemotherapy more effective. The treatment may induce toxic hepatitis, which subsides after the end of therapy. A new drug, sorafenib (Nexavar), has improved the survival of patients with advanced cancer. Other drugs that inhibit tumor growth by interfering with the blood supply that feeds the tumor are being tested in combination with sorafenib and include bevacizumab (Avastin), erlotinib (Tarceva), and sunitinib (Sutent) (NCL Cancer Bulletin, 2007).

Tumor ablation is used for tumors less than 5 cm in diameter. Ethanol or acetic acid is injected through the skin into the tumor. The liquid destroys the cancer cells. The procedure is carried out in the radiology department with the use of ultrasound.

Laser or radiofrequency ablation that causes heat to destroy cancer cells is performed with a local anesthetic. This procedure is used for cholangiocarcinoma. Cryotherapy may be used during surgery; a probe deposits liquid nitrogen to the tumor site and destroys cancer cells.

Radioimmunotherapy is experimental and uses a radioactive isotope that attaches to a radiolabeled antibody against a protein found in liver tumors. It is given intravenously, concentrates in the liver, and irradiates the tumor internally. The side effects of thrombocytopenia and neutropenia occur 4 to 6 weeks after treatment.

Nursing care includes assessing for signs and symptoms of liver failure and blockage in the common bile duct. Additional care is directed at the associated problems, such as ascites and encephalopathy. Surgical care is provided as for other abdominal surgery patients (see Chapter 5). Care of the cancer patient undergoing chemotherapy and radiation is located in Chapter 8.

DISORDERS OF THE PANCREAS

ACUTE PANCREATITIS

Pancreatitis is an inflammation of the pancreas. It may be acute or chronic. Pancreatitis frequently accompanies obstruction of the pancreatic duct from gallstones or from the backflow of bile into the pancreatic duct.

Etiology

Most cases of pancreatitis are related to alcoholism, although there are cases due to biliary disease. Viral infections, trauma, ERCP, penetrating ulcers, drug toxicities, metabolic disorders, scorpion stings, and a variety of other factors can cause pancreatitis. Men tend to develop pancreatitis related to alcohol. In women, it is associated more frequently with gallstones.

Pathophysiology

In some types of pancreatitis, the severe inflammation and damage are caused by escape of pancreatic digestive enzymes. The enzymes act directly on the tissue, causing hemorrhage, autodigestion, and necrosis. It is unclear how the autodigestion is activated. Reflux of bile and duodenal contents into the pancreatic duct is a possible mechanism. A gallstone stuck in the ampulla of Vater can cause edema of the sphincter of Oddi, which might permit reflux of duodenal contents. Alcohol can cause spasm of the sphincter of

Oddi, blocking secretion through the pancreatic ducts. This may lead to activation of the pancreatic enzymes within the pancreas.

Pancreatic abscess or pseudocysts may develop. An abscess may form from the purulent liquefaction of the necrotic pancreatic tissue. A pseudocyst is a sac-like structure that forms on or around the pancreas. It may contain several liters of enzymatic pancreatic exudates. If a pseudocyst ruptures, it may cause hemorrhage. Shock may occur, as well as other life-threatening complications (Concept Map 31-2).

Signs and Symptoms
Pancreatitis causes abdominal pain that is usually acute, but this can vary among individuals. The pain is steady and is localized to the epigastrium or left upper quadrant. As it progresses, it spreads and radiates to the back and flank. Sitting and leaning forward may ease the pain. The severity of the pain may slowly decrease after 24 hours. **Eating makes the pain worse.** Nausea, vomiting, sweating, jaundice, and weakness often accompany pain.

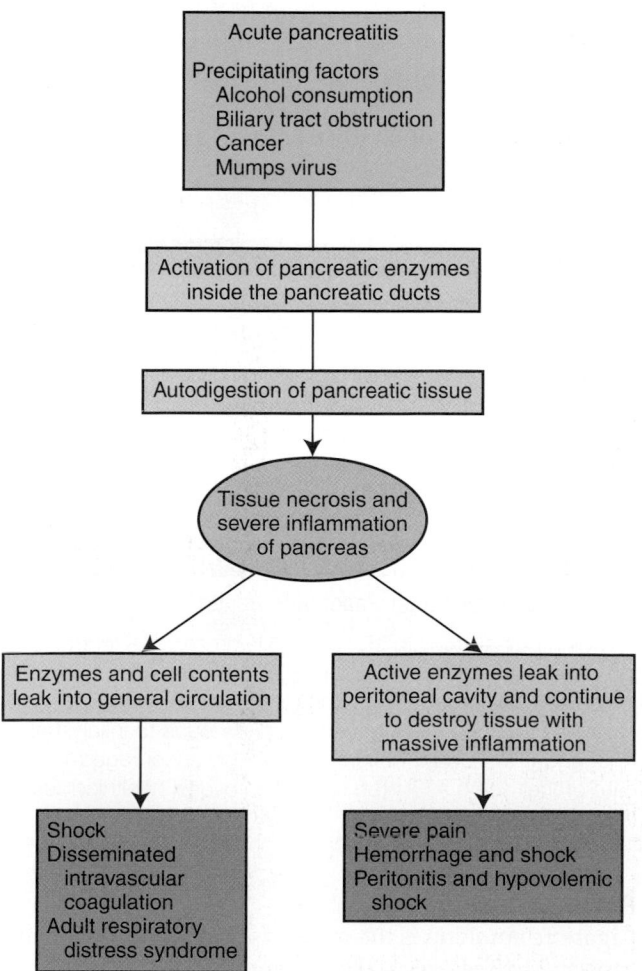

CONCEPT MAP 31-2 Pathophysiology of acute pancreatitis.

 Clinical Cues

The patient with acute pancreatitis may curl up in a tight fetal position (knee-chest) because this opens up the retroperitoneal space and decreases pain. Assuming a supine position for a procedure or assessment, is likely to increase the pain; therefore acknowledge the patient's discomfort and help him to resume the position of greatest comfort when the procedure is over.

Examination of the abdomen will reveal tenderness and guarding. If peritonitis is present, there will be distention and rigidity. Bowel sounds may be reduced or absent. A pseudocyst can be palpated as an epigastric mass in about 50% of cases. If retroperitoneal bleeding is present, there may be bruising in the flanks or a bluish discoloration around the umbilicus. There may be signs and symptoms of respiratory distress (secondary to atelectasis, pleural effusion, or respiratory distress syndrome) such as shock, tachycardia, leukocytosis, and fever. Serum amylase may be two times normal and will remain elevated for 72 hours. Serum lipase remains elevated for several days. If biliary obstruction is involved, mild jaundice may be present. Laboratory values will indicate hypoglycemia, hypocalcemia, and hypokalemia.

Diagnosis
Diagnosis is based on the symptoms, risk factors, and results of tests performed to rule out other disorders. An abdominal sonogram, CT scan, and serum and urine amylase studies are usually ordered.

Treatment and Nursing Management
Vital signs are taken frequently, urinary output is monitored, and the patient is monitored for signs of shock. Observe for signs of restlessness, use of accessory muscles for breathing, irritability, confusion, or dyspnea, which indicate respiratory distress, and administer oxygen as ordered. Pain evaluation and control are primary nursing responsibilities. Monitor laboratory values and note changes. Monitor administration of fluids and observe for electrolyte imbalances. The patient is allowed nothing by mouth during the acute phase to prevent stimulation of the pancreas and further aggravation of the inflammation. Nasogastric intubation with suction may be employed to empty the stomach and duodenum. IV fluids are given until the edema of the pancreas and the pancreatic duct has subsided. If the patient is receiving total parenteral nutrition (TPN), blood glucose needs to be checked regularly, and insulin may be necessary. Most patients with acute pancreatitis recover after receiving this type of treatment.

Assess for tolerance of the diet as the patient slowly resumes bland, soft foods. Pancreatic enzymes are given supplementally when an oral diet is resumed. If abscess or pseudocyst are present, they will be surgically

drained. Intravenous meperidine or morphine via PCA pump may be needed to control pain. Histamine (H_2)-receptor antagonists or a proton pump inhibitor may be given to decrease the hydrochloric acid secretion that stimulates pancreatic activity. Administration of antispasmodics such as dicyclomine (Bentyl) or propantheline bromide (Pro-Banthine) is helpful.

  Clinical Cues

When a powdered form of pancreatic enzymes must be taken, it should be mixed in nonprotein food, such as applesauce. Care must be taken not to let any of the medication remain on the lips or skin as it will cause irritation.

Think Critically

Your patient with acute pancreatitis has a nasogastric tube in place. The patient says, "I want this tube taken out, and I want to eat." What will you say to the patient?

CHRONIC PANCREATITIS

Etiology and Pathophysiology
Chronic pancreatitis is most frequently seen in men who have been drinking alcohol for many years. Repeated bouts of inflammation cause progressive fibrosis of the gland, stricture of the ducts, and eventual calcification.

Signs and Symptoms
Abdominal pain is the major symptom. There may be periods of acute pain, but chronic pain at intervals of months or years is more common. Other symptoms are related to pancreatic insufficiency as less and less pancreatic tissue is functional. Malabsorption with weight loss and steatorrhea, constipation, mild jaundice with dark urine, and diabetes mellitus develop.

Diagnosis
Determination of bicarbonate concentration and output in the duodenum after stimulation with secretin is the definitive test for chronic pancreatitis. Other helpful diagnostic tests are fecal fat determination, fasting blood glucose, arteriography, and radiographic examinations of the pancreas. Pancreatic cancer or another liver disorder can produce the same results on these tests. The differential diagnosis is difficult. Serum amylase and lipase may be elevated slightly or not at all. There may be increases in serum bilirubin and alkaline phosphatase. Leukocytosis and an elevated sedimentation rate are present.

Treatment and Nursing Management
Treatment during an acute episode of chronic pancreatitis is the same as for acute pancreatitis.

After the acute attack has resolved, rest is essential even if the patient does not feel ill. Help your patient by reinforcing information about the disease process and the therapeutic regimen, which will include prescribed pancreatic enzymes to be taken with low-fat meals. Long-term pain control presents problems. The patient is switched to non-narcotic pain medications to try to prevent addiction, but these are often insufficient for pain control. Complications such as diabetes mellitus must be addressed and diet requirements and medications should be reviewed with the patient. Chronic pancreatitis interferes with the patient's usual lifestyle and often is accompanied by depression, so your patient should be periodically assessed for signs of depression and appropriate referrals should be made. **A major nursing action is to be supportive of efforts to abstain from alcohol.** Table 31-6 presents nursing diagnoses and specific interventions appropriate for patients with pancreatitis.

CANCER OF THE PANCREAS

Etiology
The cause of pancreatic cancer is unknown. There were approximately 42,470 new cases of cancer of the pancreas and 35,240 deaths in the United States in 2009. It is more common in men than in women and occurs more often in the over-55 age group. Diets high in red meats and fats may increase the risk. Cancer of the pancreas is often fatal within 1 year. It is usually in a very advanced state when discovered, as the patient is asymptomatic in the early stages.

Cultural Considerations

Pancreatic Cancer Deaths

More African American men die from pancreatic cancer than do men from any other ethnic group (American Cancer Society, 2010). Alcohol use and abuse is a major factor. Working with community leaders to discourage the immoderate use of alcohol might decrease the problem.

Complementary and Alternative Therapies

Healthy Gums for Better Pancreatic Health

In a longitudinal study, men had a 64% greater risk for developing pancreatic cancer if they had gum inflammation and tooth loss. Gum inflammation has been linked to coronary artery disease and the theory is that gum disease leads to inflammation throughout the body. Patients should be encouraged to take care of their teeth as a step toward an overall healthier lifestyle (Lichtenfeld, 2007).

Pathophysiology
Cigarette smoking is the major risk factor for pancreatic cancer; 2 to 3 of every 10 cases are linked to tobacco use. Adenocarcinoma arising from the epithelial cells in the

Table 31-6	Common Nursing Diagnoses, Expected Outcomes, and Nursing Interventions for Patients with Disorders of the Pancreas	
NURSING DIAGNOSIS	**EXPECTED OUTCOMES**	**NURSING INTERVENTIONS**
Acute pain related to pancreatic inflammation	Patient's pain level will decrease per pain scale within 1 hr of instituting nursing measures. Patient will state that pain is controlled within 8 hr.	Medicate with analgesic as ordered. Instruct in use of PCA pump if ordered. Encourage relaxation techniques to decrease discomfort. Assess q 2 hr for adequate pain relief. Administer adjunctive medications as ordered. Assist into knee-chest position for comfort. Maintain NPO status and NG tube for decompression as ordered and explain how these two therapies decrease the pain.
Risk for ineffective breathing pattern related to irritation or pressure to diaphragm from ascites or pancreatic abscess/pseudocyst	Patient will maintain adequate oxygen levels as evidenced by oxygen saturation within normal limits.	Observe for signs of respiratory distress. Auscultate lungs for crackles or abnormal lung sounds. Monitor oxygen saturation with pulse oximeter. Administer supplemental oxygen as ordered. Encourage use of incentive spirometer as ordered. Place in semi-Fowler's position as tolerated to promote better lung expansion.
Risk for bleeding related to potential autodigestion or rupture of abscess resulting in circulatory collapse	Patient will not experience shock symptoms while hospitalized.	Monitor laboratory values for liver enzymes, ammonia, albumin, sodium, potassium, calcium, and magnesium daily. Observe for subtle changes in mental status. Monitor vital signs closely. Observe stool for signs of bleeding. Monitor urine output. Report frank bleeding promptly.
Deficient knowledge related to pancreatitis and its treatment and prevention of recurrence	Patient will verbalize understanding of disease process within 2 wk. Patient will verbalize understanding of treatment regimen within 1 wk. Patient will verbalize ways to prevent recurrence of pancreatitis before discharge.	Instruct in patient-specific causes (i.e., alcohol, ulcer, gallstones) and disease process (i.e., eating triggers digestive enzymes which act directly on the tissues). Explain all aspects of treatment (e.g., NPO and NG decompression decrease the release of enzymes therefore pain is decreased) and reason for each medication (e.g., dicyclomine decreases GI tract spasms). Teach ways to prevent recurrence of pancreatitis (i.e., abstain from alcohol).
Fear related to possibility of disability or death	Patient will verbalize that fear has decreased before discharge.	Establish trusting relationship by attentive, caring attitude. Encourage verbalization of fears; actively listen. Encourage contact with minister, hospital chaplain, or spiritual advisor. Point out any encouraging signs of improvement.

GI, gastrointestinal; *NG*, nasogastric; *NPO*, nothing by mouth; *PCA*, patient-controlled analgesia.

ducts is the most common form of pancreatic neoplasm. Tumor in the head of the pancreas obstructs biliary and pancreatic flow. Cancer in the body and tail of the pancreas usually remains asymptomatic until it is well advanced and invades the liver, stomach, lymph nodes, or posterior abdominal wall and nerves. Metastasis occurs early. Biliary obstruction usually causes liver failure.

 Health Promotion

Smoking Cessation

Most people are aware of the relationship between smoking and lung cancer; however, it is also necessary to tactfully point out the effects on other vital organs, such as the pancreas. Provide referral to community resources for smoking cessation and written materials with options on how to quit.

Signs and Symptoms

Epigastric pain and weight loss are the main symptoms of pancreatic cancer. Anorexia and vomiting may occur, and the patient may develop a dislike for red meat. When the disease is advanced, jaundice appears along with dark urine and clay-colored stools. There is glucose intolerance. There is a high incidence of clot formation with pancreatic cancer.

! **Safety Alert**

Deep Vein Thrombosis

Because of the increased risk of clot formation in patients with pancreatic cancer, it is important to assess for signs and symptoms of deep vein thrombosis (DVT): pain, heat, or swelling in the calves. One leg may be swollen; measure the calf and ankle and compare to the other leg. Check for signs of pulmonary embolus as well: restlessness, apprehension, chest pain, and shortness of breath. Should these signs and symptoms occur, report them to the physician immediately. Joint Commission National Quality Core Measures require rigorous prevention of DVT for all patients.

Diagnosis

Diagnosis is made by ultrasonography, imaging techniques, and fine-needle biopsy. Elevated carcinoembryonic antigen levels occur 80% to 90% of the time when pancreatic cancer is present. However, serum beta-human chorionic gonadotropin and carbohydrate antigen (CA) 72-4 are the strongest indicators of pancreatic cancer. The tumor markers CA 19-9 and CA 242 are used to monitor for potential spread or recurrence.

Treatment

High doses of opioid analgesics are usually required to keep the patient comfortable. Drug dependency should not be a concern. Treating or preventing malnutrition is a major goal. Enteral feedings may need to be given into the jejunum (jejunostomy). TPN may be needed to provide adequate nutrition (see Chapters 3 and 29).

Surgical treatment is appropriate for resectable tumor in about 15% to 20% of patients but has not been highly successful in curing the disease. It provides a 5-year survival rate of less than 5%. Surgery is used mainly to relieve symptoms of obstructive jaundice, severe pain, or other complications. A Whipple procedure, or radical pancreaticoduodenectomy, may be done for cancer of the head of the pancreas. The head of the pancreas, the gallbladder, the duodenum, part of the jejunum, and all or part of the stomach are removed. The spleen may also be removed. The remaining structures are anastomosed to the jejunum. Another option is total pancreatectomy. The patient will usually go to the surgical critical care unit after surgery. Nursing care is the same as for any abdominal surgery, but there are many complications that can occur; vigilance is essential. The patient will need enteral feedings, perhaps for life. A stent may be placed in the pancreatic duct to promote exit of pancreatic secretions and enzymes.

Other treatments include radiofrequency ablation and microwave therapy, which use heat to destroy tissue, and cryosurgery, which uses cold. Embolization therapy can be used to cut off the blood supply to the tumor. Cyberknife treatment—an image-guided radiosurgery that helps target pancreatic tumor without disrupting other tissue—is an option. Intensive external beam radiation therapy may offer pain relief, alleviate duct obstruction, and improve food absorption. Radioactive iodine (^{125}I) seeds may be implanted in combination with systemic or intra-arterial administration of floxuridine.

Gemcitabine (Gemzar) and 5-FU are common for treatment of nonresectable or metastatic tumors (American Cancer Society, 2010). Outcomes for advanced cases are better when erlotinib is added. A combination of drugs has proven most effective, and other commonly used drugs include irinotecan (Camptosar), docetaxel (Taxotere), capecitabine (Xeloda), oxaliplatin (Eloxatin), and cisplatin (Platinol). Other drugs that may be used include the targeted-therapy drug sunitinib, which blocks the growth signal. Octreotide or lanreotide suppresses the hormone release from the tumor. Pasireotide is a new drug that is currently under study. In animal studies, a TAK-1 inhibitor pill or tigatuzumab was combined with gemcitabine, and the outcomes showed promise in the future treatment of advanced pancreatic cancer (Laino, 2009; Science Daily, 2009).

Nursing Management

Nursing care is geared toward managing the severe pain and managing the side effects of treatment. Postoperatively, observe for hyperglycemia, hemorrhage, bowel obstruction or paralytic ileus, wound infection, and intra-abdominal abscess. Monitor the NG tube for clear, colorless, bile-tinged drainage or frank blood with an increase in output, as this may indicate leakage at an anastomosis site. Provide care for the postoperative patient with abdominal surgery (see Chapter 5). Chapter 8 contains information on care of the cancer patient undergoing chemotherapy or radiation.

COMMUNITY CARE

Nurses in the community should promote immunization against hepatitis B virus in all persons at risk. Teenagers and adults should be counseled about the possibility of transmission of hepatitis B virus by sexual contact and advised of measures for protection. The hepatitis A vaccine should be recommended for those traveling in areas where this disorder is prevalent and for those at risk of liver problems. Nurses should be aware of policies and procedures for reporting new cases of hepatitis to local health departments. All health care workers should be tested for the presence of hepatitis C virus.

Nurses in extended care facilities should be alert to signs of jaundice in patients. Dark-colored urine is frequently an early sign of a problem. Cancer and gallstones are both more prevalent in the elderly, and when abdominal pain occurs these disorders must be considered. Home care nurses must be particularly alert to the possibility of liver or pancreatic problems due to medications the patient is taking. Encourage regular laboratory work as recommended when the patient is taking a drug known to be potentially damaging to the liver.

Get Ready for the NCLEX® Examination!

Key Points

- Factors that are associated with cholelithiasis and cholecystitis include hemolytic disease, surgical treatment of Crohn's, rapid-weight-loss diets or starvation, multiple pregnancies or hormonal replacement therapy, major trauma, burns, and cardiac surgery.
- Signs and symptoms of acute cholecystitis include acute pain, fever, anorexia, nausea and vomiting, dehydration, and mild jaundice.
- Typical symptoms of chronic cholecystitis are indigestion, flatulence, nausea after eating fatty foods, and intermittent pain referred to the back.
- There are five main types of hepatitis: A, B, C, D, and E (see Table 31-2). Hepatitis is treated by rest, a nutritious low-fat diet, and avoidance of substances that are harmful to the liver (see Box 28-1).
- Signs and symptoms of liver disorders are fatigue, weakness, anorexia, abdominal pain, nausea and vomiting, skin rashes, itching, fever, dark urine, light-colored stools, peripheral edema, bruising, and jaundice.
- Chronic inflammation causes fibrosis and cirrhosis of the liver cells. Diagnosis of cirrhosis includes liver biopsy, liver function tests, prothrombin time, and albumin levels.
- Bleeding esophageal varices and hepatic encephalopathy are complications of cirrhosis.
- Chemotherapy, radiation, and ablation therapies are used for treatment of liver cancer.
- In acute pancreatitis, inflammation and damage are caused by escape of pancreatic digestive enzymes, causing hemorrhage, autodigestion, and necrosis. Symptoms include acute, steady pain in the epigastrium or left upper quadrant. Serum lipase and amylase are elevated. Treatment consists of pain control, reduction of pancreatic secretions, restoration of fluid and electrolyte balance, and treatment for complications such as shock or diabetes.
- Chronic pancreatitis is related to alcoholism. Long-term pain control is an issue.
- Signs and symptoms of pancreatic cancer are weight loss, anorexia, vomiting, and signs of pancreatic dysfunction. Not smoking cuts the incidence of pancreatic cancer by 50%.
- Treatment of pancreatic cancer includes pain management, and chemotherapy and radiation, which may improve food absorption, relieve pain, and alleviate duct obstruction.

Additional Learning Resources

SG Go to your Study Guide for additional learning activities to help you master this chapter content.

 Go to your Evolve website (http://evolve.elsevier.com/deWit/medsurg) for the following FREE learning resources:
- Animations, audio, and video
- Answers and rationales for questions and activities
- Concept Map Creator
- Glossary with pronunciations in English and Spanish
- Interactive Review Questions and Exercises and more!

Online Resources
- Recommended Adult Immunization Schedule, www.cdc.gov/mmwr/PDF/wk/mm5901-Immunization.pdf

Review Questions for the NCLEX® Examination

1. Before being discharged to home, the patient with gallbladder disease is given instructions regarding the care of the drain and the T-tube. Which patient statement indicates a need for further teaching?
   1. "I must empty the bag the same time each day."
   2. "Loose-fitting clothes must be worn."
   3. "I would have yellowish skin discoloration the rest of my life."
   4. "Passing brown stools indicates return to normal function."

2. If the patient has a history of chronic cholecystitis, which comment is cause for greatest concern?
   1. "I have back pain at the level of the shoulder blade."
   2. "I had nausea after eating a hamburger and fries."
   3. "I have generalized abdominal pain and fever."
   4. "I have discomfort in the right upper part of my abdomen."

3. The nurse is caring for a 57-year-old patient with ascites due to liver insufficiency. The nurse anticipates that the physician will use which therapeutic regimen to reduce portal hypertension?
   1. Vascular shunting of the portal venous systems
   2. Repeated abdominal paracentesis
   3. Diet restrictions and nutrient supplementation
   4. Fluid replacement therapy

4. The patient with high levels of serum ammonia asks, "Why do I have to continue taking lactulose?" What is the best response?
   1. "It destroys ammonia-producing bacteria in the intestines."
   2. "It reduces intestinal absorption of ammonia."
   3. "It corrects vitamin B_1 deficiency."
   4. "It is used in preparation for a diagnostic test."

5. The nurse is caring for a patient who underwent a recent liver transplantation. The nurse reinforces the teaching related to self-care. Which patient statement indicates a need for further instructions?
   1. "I need to report any kind of pain associated with fever and changes in stool color."
   2. "I should expect continued jaundice of the skin and dark yellow colored urine."
   3. "Strict hand hygiene is critical in changing dressings."
   4. "I will need to take these medications for the rest of my life."

6. The nurse is caring for a patient who underwent radical pancreaticoduodenectomy. Which postoperative complication would be the most likely to occur and cause the greatest concern?
   1. Hypoglycemia
   2. Adhesions
   3. Hemorrhage
   4. Anorexia

7. Which statement by the patient indicates a need for further instructions regarding preventing the spread of hepatitis A?
   1. "Bleach solutions must be used to clean the bathroom."
   2. "Somebody else should be doing the cooking right now."
   3. "I can share bath and hand towels with the rest of the family."
   4. "Good hand hygiene prevents the likelihood of passing the virus."

8. A patient has cirrhosis of the liver and ascites. The nurse should question which order?
   1. Bed rest with bathroom privileges
   2. Discontinue furosemide (Lasix) 80 mg
   3. Give 2-g sodium diet
   4. Fluid restriction 1500 mL/24 hr

9. The patient with acute pancreatitis has a bluish discoloration around the umbilicus. What is the significance of this finding?
   1. Associated with respiratory distress
   2. Indicative of infection
   3. Related to biliary obstruction
   4. Suggestive of internal bleeding

10. One goal of nursing care for a patient during the acute phase of pancreatitis is reduction of pain. Which nursing interventions help alleviate pain? *(Select all that apply.)*
    1. Reinforce use of the PCA pump.
    2. Maintain intravenous fluids as ordered.
    3. Provide a bland diet with additional fluids.
    4. Administer dicyclomine (Bentyl).
    5. Give pancreatic enzymes.
    6. Place the patient in a supine position.

Critical Thinking Activities

Scenario A

Mr. Moser is admitted to the hospital with a diagnosis of cirrhosis of the liver. He is 59 years old and has been hospitalized several times for his condition. He suffers from shortness of breath as a result of a swollen and enlarged abdomen, is anemic because of minimal but constant esophageal bleeding, and appears jaundiced. He has severe abrasions on his arms, legs, and abdomen from repeated scratching to relieve his pruritus. Mr. Moser is very depressed and will not converse with you when you enter his room with his breakfast tray the first morning you are assigned to his care. He refuses to eat and indicates his attitude by pushing the tray away and turning on his side, face to the wall.

1. What nursing measures might help relieve some of Mr. Moser's problems?

2. Why do you think he is mentally depressed?

3. How would you go about helping him emotionally?

4. What special observations must you make while caring for Mr. Moser?

5. How would you explain a paracentesis to Mr. Moser if one were ordered for him?

Scenario B

Mrs. Lincoln, age 46, is admitted to the hospital for a laparoscopic cholecystectomy. She is extremely obese and enjoys eating rich, fatty foods, even though she knows this will add to her obesity and precipitate attacks of cholecystitis. You are assigned to care for Mrs. Lincoln when she returns from surgery.

1. How will you position this patient?

2. What would you need to assess to determine whether complications are occurring?

3. What would you need to teach the patient and family before discharge?

4. What problems might occur after discharge? What should be the diet for Mrs. Lincoln?

5. How soon will Mrs. Lincoln probably be able to resume most of her usual activities?

Scenario C

You are working in an employee health clinic and taking a health history from Mr. Austin, who is 52 years old. He reports that he has chronic pancreatitis.

1. What physical signs and symptoms should you ask about?

2. What questions should you ask about diet and lifestyle?

Objectives

Theory

1. Recall the normal anatomy of the musculoskeletal system.
2. Describe how the musculoskeletal system provides the function of motion.
3. Explain how the musculoskeletal system provides protection for the body.
4. Identify the steps included in a nursing assessment of the musculoskeletal system.
5. Discuss the following diagnostic tests: bone scan, arthroscopy, electromyography.
6. List ways in which the elderly can increase musculoskeletal strength and protect bones.

Clinical Practice

1. Gather positioning aids and place them correctly for the patient who has sustained trauma to the left knee.
2. Institute measures to reduce the chance of contracture for patients with musculoskeletal injuries.
3. Assist patients with musculoskeletal injuries with active or passive range of motion.
4. Provide care for a patient who has undergone an arthroscopy.
5. Teach a patient to properly use crutches.
6. Teach an elderly patient with a mobility problem about ways to prevent a fall at home.

Key Terms

ankylosis (ăng-kĭ-LŌ-sĭs, p. 728)
cartilage (KĂR-tĭ-lăzh, p. 716)
contractures (kŏn-TRĂK-chŭrz, p. 727)
crepitation (KRĔP-ĭ-tā-shŭn, p. 718)
isometric exercises (ī-sō-MĔT-rĭk, p. 728)

kyphosis (kī-PHŌ-sĭs, p. 724)
ligaments (LĬG-ă-mĕntz, p. 716)
orthopedic (ŏr-thō-PĒ-dĭk, p. 719)
ossification (ŏs-ĭ-fĭ-KĀ-shŭn, p. 718)
tendons (TĔN-dŏnz, p. 716)

OVERVIEW OF ANATOMY AND PHYSIOLOGY OF THE MUSCULOSKELETAL SYSTEM

WHAT ARE THE STRUCTURES OF THE MUSCULOSKELETAL SYSTEM?

- The musculoskeletal system consists of the bones, joints, cartilage, ligaments, tendons, and muscles.
- There are two distinct groups of bone cells; those that are transformed into mature cells and those bone cells which form cartilage first, and then are gradually replaced by mature bone cells as the person grows older.
- A total of 206 bones make up the human skeleton (Figure 32-1).
- Bone is either compact or spongy. Spongy bone contains red bone marrow (Figure 32-2).
- Bones are classified as long, short, flat, or irregular.
- Each bone has markings on its surface that make it unique (Table 32-1).

- The haversian system is a canal system that runs through the bone and contains the blood and lymph vessels.
- A joint is the articulation point between two or more bones of the skeleton. There are immovable, slightly movable, and freely movable joints.
- Ligaments join the bones of a joint together.
- Tendons are connective tissues that provide joint movement.
- Cartilage is a type of connective tissue in which fibers and cells are embedded in a semisolid gel material. Cartilage acts as a cushion. The meniscus in the knee joint is a type of cartilage.
- A bursa is a fluid-filled sac that provides cushioning at friction points in a freely movable joint.
- Skeletal muscle is made up of hundreds of muscle fibers bundled together surrounded by a connective tissue sheath.
- Fascia is a connective tissue that surrounds and separates the muscles.

Skull

Clavicle

Sternum

Ribs

Ilium

Pubis

Scapula

Humerus

Radius

Ulna

Carpals

Metacarpals

Phalanges

Femur

Patella

Tibia

Fibula

Tarsals

Metatarsals

Phalanges

VERTEBRAL COLUMN
Cervical vertebrae

Thoracic vertebrae

Lumbar vertebrae

Sacrum

Coccyx

Ischium

FIGURE 32-1 Major bones of the human skeleton.

- The muscle coverings contain blood vessels and nerves.
- Muscle has properties that allow it to be electrically excited, cause it to contract, extend, or stretch, and provide elasticity.
- Skeletal muscles are attached to bones by tendons.

WHAT ARE THE FUNCTIONS OF THE BONES?

- Bones provide shape to the body.
- The skeleton provides a rigid framework that supports the internal organs and the skin.
- The skeleton protects the internal organs of the body.
- The skeleton provides attachments for tendons and ligaments and contributes to movement of the body.
- The red bone marrow in the spongy bones forms red blood cells, white blood cells, and platelets.
- The bones store and release minerals, such as calcium and phosphorus.
- The blood and lymph vessels in the canals transport nutrients to the bone cells and remove wastes.
- Bone is maintained by remodeling: existing bone is resorbed into the body and new bone is built by osteoblasts to replace it.

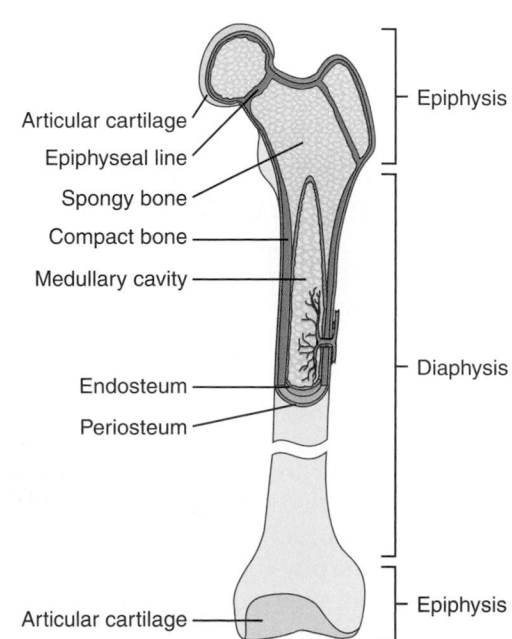

Articular cartilage

Epiphyseal line

Spongy bone

Compact bone

Medullary cavity

Endosteum

Periosteum

Articular cartilage

Epiphysis

Diaphysis

Epiphysis

FIGURE 32-2 General features of long bones.

Table 32-1	Terms Related to Bone Markings	
TERM	**DESCRIPTION**	**EXAMPLES**
Projections for Articulation		
Condyle (KŎN-dīl)	Smooth, rounded articular surface	Occipital condyle on the occipital bone; lateral and medial condyles on the femur
Facet (FĂS-ĕt)	Smooth, nearly flat articular surface	Facets on thoracic vertebrae for articulation with ribs
Head (HĔD)	Enlarged, often rounded, end of bone	Head of the humerus; head of the femur
Projections for Muscle Attachment		
Crest (KRĔST)	Narrow ridge of bone	Iliac crest on the ilium
Epicondyle (ĕ-pǐh-KŎN-dīl)	Bony bulge adjacent to or above a condyle	Lateral and medial epicondyles of the femur
Process (PRĂH-sĕs)	Any projection on a bone; often pointed and sharp	Styloid process on the temporal bone
Spine (SPĪN)	Sharp, slender projection	Spine of the scapula
Trochanter (trō-KĂN-tŭr)	Large, blunt, irregularly shaped projection	Greater and lesser trochanters on the femur
Tubercle (TŪ-bŭr-kŭl)	Small, rounded, knoblike projection	Greater tubercle of the humerus
Tuberosity (tū-bŭr-ĂS-ĭ-tē)	Similar to a tubercle but usually larger	Tibial tuberosity on the tibia
Depressions, Openings, and Cavities		
Fissure (FĬSH-ŭr)	Narrow cleft or slit; usually for passage of blood vessels and nerves	Superior orbital fissure
Foramen (fō-RĀ-mĕn)	Opening through a bone; usually for passage of blood vessels and nerves	Foramen magnum in the occipital bone
Fossa (FĂW-să)	A smooth, shallow depression	Mandibular fossa on the temporal bone; olecranon fossa on the humerus
Fovea (FŌH-vē-ă)	A small pit or depression	Fovea capitis femoris on the head of the femur
Meatus (mē-ĀT-ŭs)	A tubelike passageway; tunnel	External auditory meatus in the temporal bone
Sinus (SĪ-nŭs)	A cavity or hollow space in a bone	Frontal sinus in the frontal bone

From Applegate, E.J. (2010). *The Anatomy and Physiology Learning System* (4th ed.). Philadelphia: Saunders.

WHAT ARE THE FUNCTIONS OF THE MUSCLES?

- Contraction of skeletal muscles is produced by synchronized contraction of many muscle fibers.
- Skeletal muscles contract, thereby providing movement and joint stability, maintaining posture, and producing body heat.
- By shortening and stretching, opposing muscle groups provide movement of the joints.

WHAT CHANGES OCCUR IN THE MUSCULOSKELETAL SYSTEM WITH AGING?

- Ossification, or replacement of cartilage by more solid bony tissue, is not completed throughout the body until age 20 to 25.
- Bone density decreases because of the resorption of minerals.
- The loss of bone mass, or osteoporosis, occurs with aging and is more severe in women.
- The bones of elderly people are brittle and less compact; thus they break easily.
- When a fracture occurs, elderly bones do not heal readily because the physiologic exchange of minerals has decreased with advancing age, making the process of repair much slower.
- Thinning of the intervertebral cartilage and collapse of the vertebra result in *kyphosis* (dowager's hump).

This is partially responsible for the decrease in height in the elderly.
- Joint cartilage thins and erodes from years of use and results in stiffness and crepitation (a grating sound) of the joints.
- Joint motion may decrease, limiting mobility; swelling may occur.
- Ligaments become calcified and lose their elasticity.
- The elderly have a decrease in muscle mass; cells decrease in number and the muscles atrophy. Consequently the elderly have less strength and endurance than younger people.
- Tendons shrink and become sclerotic, slowing muscle movement.
- Muscle cramping, especially at night, increases because of impaired circulation and accumulation of metabolic wastes.

MUSCULOSKELETAL DISORDERS

CAUSES

Disease, trauma, malnutrition, and aging all contribute to musculoskeletal problems. Trauma may cause bruising, strain, sprain, or fracture. Poor nutrition may deprive the body of sufficient calcium and phosphorus to build strong bones. Inadequate protein intake can cause muscle wasting. Malignant tumors place a large nutritional demand on the body, and nutritional imbalances may occur that cause muscle wasting. Tumor may invade bone as either a primary or metastatic cancer. The decrease in estrogen production after menopause in women is thought to be a contributing factor to the occurrence of osteoporosis.

PREVENTION

Preservation of motion and mobility are important to prevent long-term orthopedic (refers to the function and structure of the musculoskeletal system) disability. Weight training and exercise throughout life is needed to maintain bone mass and can decrease the incidence of osteoporosis and increase muscle strength, mass, agility, balance, and coordination, thereby preventing falls and consequent fractures. One of the proposed *Healthy People 2020* objectives is to reduce hospitalizations related to osteoporosis-related hip fractures. For the older adult, maintenance of an exercise diary or personal interviews following workouts helped to increase adherence to recommended weight training and exercise programs (Yeom et al., 2009).

 Complementary and Alternative Therapies

Benefits of Tai Chi

Research in older community–dwelling adults has shown that tai chi has beneficial effects for increasing mobility, strength, balance, and flexibility (Yeom et al., 2009).

Learning to lift and move objects correctly by using large muscle groups can help prevent muscle strain and sprains. Using seat belts when riding in an automobile can reduce the incidence of trauma to bone and muscle during accidents. Wearing bicycle, motorcycle, and other sports helmets will reduce the incidence of skull fractures. Consuming recommended amounts of calcium throughout the life span, obtaining sufficient vitamin D from sunshine, and maintaining adequate protein intake all help build healthy bone and muscle (Kalro, 2009). Refraining from using steroids on a long-term basis can help prevent osteoporosis and fractures. In a study of retired National Football League players, steroid use

 Nutrition Considerations

Nutrition for Bone Growth and Density

Adequate amounts of calcium and phosphorus are essential for bone growth and density. Although green vegetables are a source of calcium, that calcium is not readily absorbed. Dairy products such as cheese, yogurt, and milk are better choices. Nondairy sources of calcium include canned sardines or salmon, tofu, figs, and dried apricots (Phillips, 2009). Magnesium and vitamin K are required for healthy bones as well. These are provided by a healthy diet containing meat and green vegetables, such as spinach.

was linked to musculoskeletal disorders, particular joint health, and to the development of osteoarthritis, physical inactivity, depression, obesity, and diabetes (Brockenbrough, 2009).

 Health Promotion

Smoking and Musculoskeletal Health

Smoking has a significant impact on the bones and joints in that it:
- Increases the risk of developing osteoporosis
- Increases the risk of a hip fracture as you age
- Increases your risk of developing exercise-related injuries
- Has a detrimental effect on fracture and wound healing
- Has a detrimental effect on athletic performance
- Is associated with low back pain and rheumatoid arthritis.

Data from American Association of Orthopedic Surgeons, 2010.

 Think Critically

What could you do now to promote healthy bones during your elderly years?

Diagnostic Tests and Procedures

Specific diagnostic tests of the musculoskeletal system are listed in Table 32-2. Blood counts, blood cultures, and various tests for problems of the immune system may also be performed to detect rheumatoid arthritis or other connective tissue diseases. Other tests include an erythrocyte sedimentation rate (ESR), serum protein electrophoresis, and tests to determine the levels of serum complement and immunoglobulins (see Chapter 10).

 Clinical Cues

Diagnostic tests for musculoskeletal disorders (and other disorders) often use contrast media or radiation. Before diagnostic testing, all patients should be assessed for allergies, and women of childbearing age may need (or want) a pregnancy test.

Range-of-motion (ROM) testing involves both active and passive maneuvers. In active testing, the part being measured must be moved by the patient herself. In passive testing, the evaluator moves the body part while the patient is relaxed.

The measurement of ROM in a joint is called *goniometry* (Figure 32-3 on p. 723). One system of measurement that is commonly used is based on a full circle of 360 degrees. Each joint is evaluated in terms of the number of degrees it can be moved from the 0-degree position.

Muscle strength can be measured on the basis of the ability of a muscle to move the part to which it is attached, working against the force of gravity. A grading system is used, ranging from grade 5 (normal strength) to grade 0 (complete paralysis).

Text continued on p. 723

Table 32-2 Diagnostic Tests for Musculoskeletal Disorders

TEST	PURPOSE	DESCRIPTION	NURSING IMPLICATIONS
Calcium	To measure calcium in the blood	Used to assess calcium availability and metabolism. Calcium is needed for bone formation.	No fasting is required. Test requires 7 mL of venous blood in a red-top tube. Check for interfering factors before the sample is drawn.
Phosphate (phosphorus)	To measure phosphate in the blood	Helps assess phosphorus level in the body. Phosphorus is needed for bone formation.	Should be a fasting specimen. Requires 5-10 mL of venous blood in a red-top tube. Take to laboratory immediately.
Alkaline phosphatase (ALP)	To detect bone disorders Isoenzymes are isolated to distinguish bone from liver, or biliary tract disorders	Helpful in determining if primary or metastatic cancer is present.	Fasting may be required for isoenzyme tests. Requires 7-10 mL of blood in a red-top tube.
Aldolase	To determine extent of muscular trauma and detects polymyositis	Enzyme test using blood.	A fasting state provides more accurate results. Requires 7-10 mL of venous blood in a red-top tube.
Creatine phosphokinase (CPK), creatine kinase (CK)	CPK-MM isoenzymes are used to test for skeletal muscle damage from trauma or disease, such as myositis	Enzyme test using blood.	IM injections will interfere with the test result. Record time and date of venipuncture on the laboratory slip.
Uric acid	To detect abnormally high levels of uric acid in the blood, which is a sign of gout	Collect 5-10 mL of blood in a clot (red-top) tube. *Normal range:* Female: 2.8-6.8 mg/dL Male: 3.5-7.8 mg/dL	No food or fluid restrictions.
Rheumatoid factor	To detect antibodies, indicating possible rheumatoid arthritis, lupus, or scleroderma	Collect 5-10 mL of blood in a clot (red-top) tube Adult: <1:120 titer >1:160 indicates rheumatoid arthritis	No food or fluid restrictions.
Antinuclear antibodies (ANA)	To assess tissue antigen antibodies; useful for diagnosis of rheumatoid arthritis, lupus erythematosus, and other connective tissue disorders	Collect 2-5 mL of blood in a clot (red-top) tube. Check drugs patient is receiving for interference with this test. *Normal finding:* negative	No food or drink restrictions.
X-ray films of the bones or joints	To detect fracture, avulsion, joint damage	No preparation necessary. Part to be x-rayed is positioned by technician and x-ray films are taken.	Explain the purpose, procedure, and possible sensations Assess for pregnancy before testing.
Tomography and xerography	To produce radiographic planes or slices; highlights contrast between structures	Specialized equipment is used; xerography uses a higher amount of radiation than normal x-ray examinations.	Explain that the tomography procedure takes longer, as the machine takes a series of views.
Computed tomography (CT)	To detect musculoskeletal problems, especially of the spine and skull	A special machine is used and the patient is placed on a hard table; the procedure takes 30-60 min. Contrast material may or may not be used. Some patients experience claustrophobia from being encased by the machine. A computer enhances the radiographic findings.	Explain that lying perfectly still is required; the part under study is enclosed in the machine; there is a clicking sound as the machine rotates to take the next view. Assess for allergies to contrast media.

CPK-MM, creatinine phosphokinase isoenzyme; *IM,* intramuscular.

Table 32-2   **Diagnostic Tests for Musculoskeletal Disorders—cont'd**

TEST	PURPOSE	DESCRIPTION	NURSING IMPLICATIONS
Magnetic resonance imaging (MRI)	To diagnose musculoskeletal disorders	Often preferred over bone scan. Magnetic fields and radio waves are used to visualize tissue densities by the density of hydrogen ions. Computer enhancement depicts normal and abnormal tissue.	Instruct patient that there must be no metal on the body and no metal implants because of the strong magnetic fields used. The patient will need to lie still for 15-60 min. Older machines totally encase the patient; newer ones are more open.
Dual energy x-ray absorptiometry (DEXA)	To measure bone density of spine, hip, femur, or forearm To monitor changes in bone density and to diagnose metabolic bone disease	Uses minimal radiation exposure. Patient will lie supine on the imaging table with the legs supported. The scintillator camera is passed over the patient and projected onto a computer screen.	Height and weight will be measured. Instruct patient to remove all metallic objects. Test takes about 30 min.
Bone scan	To detect tumor, metastatic growths, bone injury, or degenerative bone disease; can detect problems earlier than x-ray films	An IV injection or oral dose of a radioisotope is given, and after an interval time for the substance to be taken up by the bone, the area is scanned by scintillation camera.	Explain the purpose and procedure. Check for allergies and pregnancy. Patient will be asked to lie quietly for 30-60 min during the scanning. All metal should be removed from the area to be scanned. Explain that the dose of radiation the patient will receive is lower than usual with radiographs. Assure patient that she will not be "radioactive." The isotope is eliminated from the body in 6-24 hr.
Gallium/thallium scans	To detect bone problems, especially tumor invasion	The radioisotope gallium citrate (GA-70) or thallium-201 is administered before the scan; a bone scan is then performed.	The addition of the radioisotope helps locate areas of rapid bone growth activity that might indicate tumor. Explain that the radioisotope is administered 1-2 days before scanning. The procedure takes 30-60 min, during which lying still is required; sedation may be given.
Arthrography (arthrogram)	To provide radiographic pictures of a joint showing the outline of the joint cavity and soft tissue structures not visible on routine x-ray films	A contrast agent, air, or both are aseptically injected into the joint after the area is anesthetized. Fluid may first be aspirated from the joint space. The joint is manipulated to disperse the contrast agent. X-ray films are taken with the joint held in various positions.	Informed consent is often required. Explain that a needle will be inserted into the joint space after the area is anesthetized. There will be feelings of pressure and some discomfort. Administer an analgesic after the procedure, if needed. Observe for swelling; apply ice as ordered.

Continued

Table **32-2** **Diagnostic Tests for Musculoskeletal Disorders—cont'd**

TEST	PURPOSE	DESCRIPTION	NURSING IMPLICATIONS
Arthrography—cont'd			Advise patient that crackling sounds may be heard or felt in the joint after the test and usually disappear in a day or two. Instruct patient to report any increasing pain or swelling to the physician.
Arthroscopy	To inspect the interior aspect of a joint, usually a knee, with a fiberoptic endoscope to diagnose problems of the patella, meniscus, and synovium; also used to evaluate the progress of arthritis or effectiveness of treatment	After injection of local anesthesia, an incision is made and the arthroscope is introduced into the interior of the joint; instruments for tissue biopsy or surgical procedure may be passed through the arthroscope.	Explain the purpose and procedure. A preprocedure sedative may be administered. When the patient has recovered from any sedation, she is allowed to walk but should not overuse or strain the joint for a few days. The area is observed for bleeding or swelling; ice packs may be used in the immediate postprocedure period, especially if biopsy or surgery was performed. Assessment for swelling, circulation, and sensation is done periodically to detect any complications.
Arthrocentesis	To extract synovial fluid for analysis or to reduce swelling	A needle is inserted into the joint space and synovial fluid is aspirated. Synovial fluid analysis may detect cells indicating infection, inflammation, rheumatoid arthritis, or lupus erythematosus. Corticosteroid may be injected after aspiration of fluid. If a large amount of fluid is aspirated, the joint is immobilized with an elastic bandage. Ice packs are applied to relieve pain and reduce swelling.	Explain the procedure. Have ice packs ready to apply afterward; wrap with elastic bandage if ordered and show patient how to do this; it should be worn for 2-3 days. Instruct patient not to overuse the joint until pain and swelling have subsided. Administer ordered analgesics if needed after corticosteroid injection, as this can be painful.
Culture of synovial fluid	To determine organism responsible for infection	Explain purpose and procedure. See that specimen of fluid is transported to laboratory immediately.	Synovial fluid is aspirated and sent for culture and sensitivity to determine appropriate antibiotic for therapy. Results take 48-72 hr to determine.
Biopsy	Bone biopsy done to detect tumor cells Muscle biopsy done to obtain tissue for cellular analysis, which is helpful in differential diagnosis of several muscle disorders	Under local anesthesia, a piece of bone or muscle is excised and sent for pathologic analysis.	Offer emotional support during the procedures Afterward, medicate for discomfort as needed, apply ice packs to decrease swelling, observe for bleeding; perform circulation and sensation checks distal to the area biopsied.

Table 32-2 Diagnostic Tests for Musculoskeletal Disorders—cont'd

TEST	PURPOSE	DESCRIPTION	NURSING IMPLICATIONS
Electromyelography (EMG)	To detect abnormal nerve transmission to the muscle and abnormal muscle function; determines rehabilitation progress	Needle electrodes are inserted in affected muscles, and, as the muscles are stimulated, the electrical impulses generated by the muscle contractions are amplified and displayed on an oscilloscope; tracings also are made on graph paper.	Obtain a signed consent form. Caffeine-containing drinks and smoking are restricted 3 hr before the test. Muscle relaxants, anticholinergics, and cholinergic drugs should be withheld before the test; check with the physician. Explain to patient that there may be slight discomfort when the electrodes are inserted; explain that she will be asked to relax and contract her muscles. The test usually takes about an hour. If serum enzyme tests are ordered, draw the blood before the EMG.

FIGURE 32-3 Measurement of joint motion with a goniometer.

Other techniques used to evaluate musculoskeletal function include inspection, palpation, and tests for stability of a joint under stress.

❖ NURSING MANAGEMENT

■ Assessment (Data Collection)

History Taking

When reviewing the patient's past history the nurse should keep in mind the significance of disorders that primarily affect other systems but secondarily affect the bones and muscles. For example, sickle cell disease and hemophilia can cause bleeding into the joints and muscles, and psoriasis is sometimes the first sign of psoriatic arthritis, which is an inflammatory condition that affects the spine and the peripheral joints (Habif, 2009). Nutritional deficiencies can affect the mineral composition of bone and muscle, making them more susceptible to trauma and loss of function.

Family history also can be significant, as there are some bone and muscle disorders that are either inherited or have a familial tendency. For example, about 30% of those who have psoriatic arthritis have a family history of psoriasis (Chandran, 2010).

◎ Focused Assessment

Data Collection for the Musculoskeletal System

- Can you tell me what you see as your current problem?
- When is the pain the worst? What seems to bring it on? What relieves it?
- Do you have any pain in your wrists, elbows, knees, hips, or feet?
- Have you experienced any sensory changes? When were they first noticed, and what did they feel like?
- Have you noticed any changes of sensation in your hands, feet, or elsewhere?
- Do you have any joints that are stiff, swollen, or painful?
- Do you have any restriction of movement in any joint?
- Do you have trouble sleeping because of muscle or joint pain?
- Do you have any joint deformity? Bunion? Hammer toe? Deformed knuckle?
- Have you ever suffered an injury to a bone?
- Have you ever experienced a severe muscle strain or muscle problem?
- Is there a history of osteoporosis or arthritis in your family?
- Do you have diabetes, sickle cell disease, psoriasis, systemic lupus erythematosus, or any other chronic metabolic disease?
- Are you taking any steroid medications regularly?
- Do you find that your fatigue level has increased?
- Do you have any problems with bathing, dressing, grooming, toileting, eating, ambulation, or going on social outings?
- Can you easily arise from a seated position?
- Do you have difficulty opening containers?

Continued

Focused Assessment

Data Collection for the Musculoskeletal System—cont'd

- What do you eat or drink that contains calcium? How much of it do you eat or drink?
- What is your daily (weekly) sunshine exposure? Do you take a vitamin D supplement?
- Do you use any alternative therapies or any other type of self-care measures? Are those self-care measures helping?
- Tell me about your work; do you lift, pull, or push? Are you sitting for prolonged periods or doing repetitive motions?
- Does your home have stairs or other features that are causing problems for you?
- Are you able to independently do home maintenance tasks (e.g., mow the lawn)?
- Is the environment you are in most of the day a comfortable temperature for you?
- What type of physical activities or recreational exercise do you routinely do (e.g., sports, gardening)? How often do you participate in these activities?

Physical Assessment

Observe the patient for signs of joint pain, such as limping, poor posture, awkward gait, difficulty in arising or walking, and wincing on movement. Much can be learned about the musculoskeletal system by just watching the patient, noting problems of movement, and changes in facial expression as the routines of bathing and grooming occur. If the patient is admitted with a fracture, obtain a history of the precipitating event so that an assessment can be made of other areas that may have been injured. Sometimes it is necessary to consult family members or someone who lives with the patient about the patient's true ability to perform the activities of daily living (ADLs). **A self-care deficit is one of the primary problems for patients who suffer a problem of immobility.**

 Focused Assessment

Physical Assessment of the Musculoskeletal System

Note the following points:
- *Posture:* Is there evidence of **kyphosis,** such as a rounded upper back, which is called a dowager's hump? Are the knuckles swollen or deformed, indicating arthritis?
- *Gait:* Steady and even? Awkward?
- *Balance:* Able to sit, stand, and walk with a good center of balance?
- *Mobility:* Is any supportive device being used, such as a cane, brace, splint, or elastic bandage?
- *Range of motion:* Able to move neck, shoulders, arms, legs with full range of motion?
- *Strength:* Grips in hands and push-pull in arms equal bilaterally? Straight-leg raising against resistance equal bilaterally?
- *Spine:* Any tenderness of the vertebrae on palpation?
- *Appearance of joints:* Redness, deformity, or loss of motion in elbows, hands, knees, ankles, and feet?
- *Skeletal muscle appearance in arms and legs:* Any degree of atrophy?
- *Ability to perform ADLs:* Independent or needs assistance to dress, bathe, toilet, eat?

 Elder Care Points

Approximately 30% to 40% of inpatient safety incidents are related to falls, and elderly patients are particularly vulnerable because of changes related to aging such as decreased strength, unsteady balance, loss of endurance, slow reflexes, gait disturbances and increased postural sway, and chronic diseases such as arthritis. Conduct a fall risk assessment (see Box 9-4) and initiate fall precautions (Rutledge & Schub, 2010).

 Nutrition Considerations

Vitamin D Associated with Decreased Risk for Falls

In a Cochrane review of 41 trials that included 25,422 subjects, higher vitamin D level was associated with a lowered risk for falls among elderly nursing home residents (Cameron et al., 2010).

 Think Critically

How would you gather data about an elderly patient's ability to perform self-care activities at home before she is discharged? After a hip replacement, can you trust a statement of "I can shop, cook, clean, and do everything I need to do by myself"? If you cannot trust the statement, why not?

■ Nursing Diagnosis and Planning

Caring for immobile patients requires careful planning. Making beds for the bed-confined orthopedic patient is best done by two people. Bathing and grooming are more time consuming when the patient has a limb immobilized or has some other orthopedic device. **Planning for toileting needs at regular intervals is important for the well-being of the patient who is unable to get out of bed herself.** Neglecting such needs may cause incontinence and the time-consuming task of changing the bed and cleaning up the patient; incontinence is also demoralizing for the patient and increases the risk of tissue breakdown from the moisture and irritation of urine or feces. Repositioning the patient at 2-hour intervals needs to be included in the daily work plan to prevent pressure ulcers.

Common nursing diagnoses and example outcomes and interventions for patients with musculoskeletal problems are shown in Table 32-3. Several other secondary nursing diagnoses may be appropriate for patients who are highly immobile. Constipation, impaired tissue integrity, social isolation, risk for injury, and other problems caused by immobility may occur (see Chapter 9).

Interventions and outcomes are designed in collaboration with the patient and other members of the health care team. **The physical therapist and occupational therapist are especially important and act as resources for the patient and the nurse.**

Table 32-3 Common Nursing Diagnoses, Expected Outcomes, and Interventions for Patients with Musculoskeletal System Disorders

NURSING DIAGNOSIS	GOALS/EXPECTED OUTCOMES	NURSING INTERVENTIONS
Impaired physical mobility related to immobilization, loss of limb, stiffness, pain, weakness, or inability to bear weight	ROM of unaffected joints will be maintained. No signs of joint contractures at discharge.	Active ROM at least tid for all unaffected joints while on bed rest. Passive ROM on affected joints as ordered. Ensure that joints are in correct alignment when at rest and after turning. Maintain body in proper alignment. Assess immobilizer for correct fit and positioning every shift; assess for signs of complications due to pressure or pins. Supervise exercise to prepare muscles for ambulation. Instruct in use of ambulatory devices as appropriate; supervise practice; assess for proper "fit" of device. Encourage use of prosthesis for ambulation; assist with practice. Assess for signs of complications in stump and assess that prosthesis is attached correctly. Maintain abduction pillow between legs if one is ordered.
Activity intolerance related to stiffness, pain, impaired mobility, fatigue	Patient will space activities and rest to conserve energy. Patient will use assistive devices to conserve energy.	Determine factors that increase fatigue. Space activities with rest periods throughout the day. Assist to set goals for slow, steady increase in exercise and activity during periods of remission of arthritis symptoms. Perform exercises after heat treatments to decrease discomfort; apply in safe manner. Apply cold as needed after exercise for discomfort. Administer medications to decrease inflammation and pain, allowing greater level of activity. Advise of assistive devices that might make ADLs easier and conserve energy. Assist in obtaining needed devices. Supervise practice with assistive device.
Pain related to injury, surgery, or joint disorder	Pain will be controlled as evidenced by patient verbalization. Pain will be decreased with medication.	Assess for factors contributing to pain level such as increased pressure, infection, positioning, or swelling. Assess pain in systematic, objective manner and track course of pain and effectiveness of pain control (see Chapter 7). Instruct in relaxation, distraction, and imagery techniques to decrease pain. Instruct in use of various heat and cold treatments to decrease pain. Administer analgesic, inflammatory, and steroid medications, as ordered, to decrease pain. Instruct in use and side effects of each drug. Assist to an anatomically correct position to enhance circulation and alignment. Advise of alternative methods of pain control, such as transcutaneous electrical nerve stimulation (TENS). Monitor patient-controlled analgesia (PCA) use for effectiveness of pain control.

ADLs, activities of daily living; *ROM,* range of motion; *tid,* three times a day.

Continued

Table 32-3	Common Nursing Diagnoses, Expected Outcomes, and Interventions for Patients with Musculoskeletal System Disorders—cont'd	
NURSING DIAGNOSIS	**GOALS/EXPECTED OUTCOMES**	**NURSING INTERVENTIONS**
Risk for infection related to trauma or surgical incision	No signs of infection, as evidenced by normal white blood cell (WBC) count and normal temperature; wounds clean and dry.	Follow Standard Precautions and strict Contact Precautions when performing patient care, and use strict aseptic technique for wound or pin care. Assess for signs of infection every shift; assess wound for redness, swelling, and tenderness. Administer prophylactic antibiotics, as ordered. Assess temperature trends and trend of WBC values for signs of infection. Assess patient for subjective signs of malaise. Sniff around cast for signs of foul odor indicating infection.
Risk for ineffective tissue perfusion related to swelling and pressure	No evidence of seriously decreased circulation distal to site of trauma. No evidence of nerve compression from swelling.	Perform neurovascular assessment q 1 hr for 8 hr, then q 2 hr for 48 hr. Question patient regarding sensation distal to site of trauma or surgery. Apply cold to area of injury or surgery, as ordered, to reduce swelling; elevate extremity to slightly above heart level. Immediately report signs of compartment syndrome (i.e., severe, unrelenting pain, numbness) to physician and obtain order for measures to relieve pressure.
Self-care deficit in bathing, grooming, toileting, feeding related to immobilization	Patient will receive assistance for all ADLs, as needed.	Assess degree of inability to perform various self-care activities. Formulate plan to assist patient with ADLs. Answer calls for assistance with toileting promptly; do not leave on bedpan longer than necessary. Open food containers and cut food as needed for self-feeding with one hand. Do not serve extremely hot liquids to patients who have difficulty with coordination or with holding drinking containers or to immobilized patients. Provide assistive devices and help patient to be as self-sufficient as possible without incurring undue fatigue when performing ADLs. Caution patients about change in body's center of gravity when a limb is casted or amputated.
Disturbed body image related to change in appearance and/or loss of mobility or function	Patient will begin adaptation to change in appearance or loss as evidenced by verbalization of feelings of self-worth; maintenance of relationships with significant others; active interest in personal appearance; willingness to resume usual roles and participate in social activities; making plans to adapt lifestyle to meet restrictions imposed by loss.	Assess degree of body image disturbance, noting verbal or nonverbal clues to negative response to changes. Assist to verbalize feelings about effect of loss on usual roles and lifestyle. Be present and supportive during initial dressing changes on stump after amputation. Assist patient to identify strengths and abilities and positive coping mechanisms. Clarify misconceptions about limitations on mobility and activity. Promote activities that require patient to confront the body changes that have occurred, such as bathing, ADLs, or dressing changes. Demonstrate acceptance of patient and encourage significant others to do the same with touch and affection. Encourage as much independence as possible; allow to do things for self.

Table 32-3	Common Nursing Diagnoses, Expected Outcomes, and Interventions for Patients with Musculoskeletal System Disorders—cont'd	
NURSING DIAGNOSIS	**GOALS/EXPECTED OUTCOMES**	**NURSING INTERVENTIONS**
Disturbed body image related to change in appearance and/or loss of mobility or function—cont'd		Assist patient to explore viable options for changes in lifestyle and career. Refer for vocational retraining if needed. Encourage maximum participation in planning of care and self-care to provide a sense of control over life. Encourage participation in social activities and in a support group. Refer for psychological counseling if adaptation does not occur within 6 mo and patient is depressed or in denial.
Impaired home maintenance related to immobility or self-care deficits	Patient will obtain needed assistance with home maintenance.	Assess degree of self-sufficiency and ability to perform ADLs before discharge. Contact social worker for coordination of home care if needed. Obtain bathing and homemaker assistance as needed. Assess continued need for in-home services weekly. Instruct in home adaptations that could aid in efforts at self-care, such as grab bars in bathroom, alterations in counter spaces for food preparation, transportation options for grocery shopping and appointments, or assistive devices for self-feeding and grooming. Assess degree of assistance family members can provide for patient in home environment. Determine safety of home environment for patient.
Risk for disuse syndrome related to immobility or trauma	Patient will not suffer permanent joint deformity or muscle atrophy.	Position joints as ordered; keep rest of body in correct alignment. Begin exercise of affected joint as soon as physician orders. Encourage active exercise of unaffected joints tid. Perform passive ROM as ordered tid. Assist with use of CPM machine, as ordered. Medicate regularly for pain while CPM machine is in use. Use heat and cold treatments before and after exercising stiff or deformed joints. Assess joints for contractures and muscles for atrophy q 24 hr. Encourage participation in ADLs to exercise joints.

CPM, continuous passive motion.

■ Implementation

Lifting and Turning the Patient

When working with the orthopedic patient, all movements must be *gentle* and *firm*. When moving or turning the patient, **obtain sufficient help from adequately trained personnel.** Each person involved, including the patient, should understand exactly what is happening and how the move will be accomplished. If the patient can help without damaging the diseased joint or limb, she should be encouraged to do so. If she is not able to help, explain the procedure to her and instruct her to relax completely during the procedure. Many

times the patient is afraid that moving and turning will cause pain. Explaining the long-term benefits, such as preserving skin integrity and decreasing respiratory problems will increase cooperation.

Interventions to Prevent Disability

The formation of contractures (shortening of skeletal muscle tissue causing deformity), loss of muscle tone, and fixation of joints can be prevented in most cases by consistent nursing intervention. The major components of the intervention are gradual mobilization, an exercise program, proper positioning, and instruction of the patient and family. **Within a matter of a few** days, the structures of immobilized muscles and joints begin to undergo changes. If no effort is made to prevent these changes, the patient will become permanently disabled. The pathologic changes most commonly associated with lack of motion include:

- Contractures
- Loss of muscle tone
- Ankylosis (permanent fixation of a joint)

Preventing Contractures. Joint motion is the result of a shortening and stretching of opposing muscles. For example, when the flexor muscles of the leg contract and shorten, the opposing extensor muscles relax and tighten. When skeletal muscles are not regularly stretched and contracted to their normal limits, they attempt to adapt themselves to this limited use by becoming shorter and less elastic. **An "adaptive shortening,"** or *contracture,* **begins to form within 3 to 7 days after immobilization of a body part,** and the process usually is complete in 6 to 8 weeks. This means that planning and implementing nursing measures must begin immediately to prevent permanent and crippling disability. The most frequent contractures occurring in patients immobilized for long periods are "footdrop," knee and hip flexion contractures, "wrist drop," and contractures of the fingers and arms (Figure 32-4).

Loss of Muscle Tone. *Muscle tone* is defined as the readiness of the muscle to go to work—to contract and relax as needed. If a muscle is not regularly stimulated to action or if it is stretched beyond its normal limits for an extended time, it will lose its ability to contract and relax. For example, in footdrop, the calf muscles are shortened while the opposing flexor muscles

are stretched. The result is loss of muscle tone and inability to produce motion. Performing ROM exercises helps prevent this.

Preventing Ankylosis. Ankylosis is the result of injury or disease in which the tissues of the joint are replaced by a bony overgrowth that completely obliterates the joint. Proper positioning and movement of the joint passively can help prevent this. Sometimes it is extremely difficult to prevent this process (as, for example, in some types of arthritis). In these cases, the physician may brace the joint in the position that will be most useful to the patient, even though there is no motion in the joint.

Gradual Mobilization. The first step of progressive mobilization is assessing the patient's ability to move her limbs, turn herself in bed, transfer herself from bed to chair and back again, and stand and walk. These measurable signs of independent movement represent various stages to which the patient can gradually progress. According to the Joint Commission's National Patient Safety Goals, it is a nursing responsibility to recognize that these patients are at risk for falls while they are learning to regain their mobility.

> **Clinical Cues**
>
> The physician's orders should include level of activity (i.e., bedrest, out of bed to chair, physical therapy to evaluate ambulation); however, if this order is not included—or if your assessment finds that the patient either cannot accomplish the orders, or has already surpassed the ordered level of activity—notify the physician so that he can reevaluate the patient's abilities and update the orders.

Setting goals for progressive mobilization must take into account the pathologic condition causing immobility, any contraindications to movement of a body part, and the ability of the patient to understand and take part in carrying out the rehabilitation activities. In some cases, passive exercises and positioning may be necessary until the patient is able to carry out exercises and positioning on her own. If the patient is to be cared for by family members once back at home, it is essential that they be included in planning and setting goals of intervention to prevent disability and promote mobilization.

Exercise. ROM exercises, both passive and active, are planned and carried out as soon as feasible after immobilization occurs as a result of disease, injury, or surgery. The exercises are done to maintain functional connective tissue within the joint and thereby ensure that every joint retains its function and mobility. **ROM exercises should be done three or four times a day.** Other kinds of exercises are planned according to each patient's needs and the amount of motion allowed by the physician. **Isometric exercises** involve generating tension

A. Footdrop, resulting from improper support of the feet while patient is confined to bed.

B. Wrist drop, resulting from improper support of the hand.

C. Flexion contracture of knee and hip force this patient to walk on tiptoe on the affected side. If both legs are involved, walking is impossible.

FIGURE 32-4 Joint contractures.

between two opposing sets of muscles, for example, trying to flex the lower arm while using the opposite hand to try to extend it.

Safety Alert

Caution with Isometric Exercises

Isometric exercise may be contraindicated in patients with hypertension, increased intracranial pressure, or congestive heart failure, as there is a significant increase in blood pressure and heart rate during the exercise.

Health Promotion

Gentle Stretch for Upper Back

Patients who are kyphotic (or those who hunch over their books while studying!) can develop discomfort and tension in the upper mid-back. Encourage periodic and conscientious attempts to sit upright with the shoulders pulled back. Another exercise is to stand in a corner; place palms on the opposing walls and gently lean into the corner. This may feel uncomfortable at first, so encourage the person to go slow.

Patients suffering from intense joint pain as a result of rheumatoid arthritis will need proper timing of exercises to follow administration of analgesic and anti-inflammatory drugs. If possible, the schedule for drug administration should be adjusted so that the patient receives her first dose of medication in the morning 30 to 60 minutes *before* she begins her exercises.

Sometimes after joint surgery, especially after a total knee replacement, the surgeon will order attachment of an apparatus to the affected limb that provides continuous passive motion (CPM) of the joint within set limits. The apparatus is driven by a motor and requires no effort on the part of the patient or nurse to move the limb (Figure 32-5). It usually is left on all day and is discontinued at night while the patient sleeps. When this type of apparatus is used, the nursing care plan should

FIGURE 32-5 Continuous passive motion machine encourages joint mobility.

include specific instructions regarding its proper application and setting and regular assessment of adequacy of pain medication.

Exercises to recondition muscles for ambulation after injury or immobilization include quadriceps setting and gluteal setting.

Patient Teaching

Quadriceps and Gluteal Muscle Exercises

QUADRICEPS SETTING
- Instruct the patient to straighten the leg out while lying down and tense the leg muscles, straightening the knee, while raising the heel slightly.
- The contraction is held for a count of 5 and released for a count of 5.
- The exercise is done on each leg 10 to 15 times hourly while the patient is awake.
- Commercial breaks on television are a good reminder to do this.

GLUTEAL SETTING
- Instruct the patient to contract the buttocks and pinch them together for a count of 4, then relax for a count of 5.
- Repeat 10 to 15 times hourly.

Positioning. Even though nurses turn a patient, change her body position, and get her up in a chair to prevent pressure ulcers, circulatory stasis, and respiratory and urinary complications, nurses may not realize that changing body position does not necessarily guarantee freedom from orthopedic deformities. **It also is necessary to change joint positions.**

Assessing a patient's need for proper positioning should include watching for early signs of muscle tightness and resistance to joint motion. This can be done during routine ROM exercises and could signal the need for positioning a body part so that the joint is extended and muscles are stretched to their normal capacity.

Patients with flaccid paralysis are not necessarily positioned in the same way as those with spastic paralysis. For example, a footboard is appropriate for proper positioning of the feet to prevent footdrop in a patient with flaccid paralysis. In contrast, putting the soles of the feet of a patient with spastic paralysis in contact with a footboard could trigger muscle contraction and aggravate the spasticity. Using a bed cradle to relieve pressure of the bedclothes can help prevent footdrop in these patients.

Special Beds. A type of bed that often is used for patients in cervical traction is the Roto-Rest bed (see Figure 23-12). This bed very slowly turns the patient about 300 times a day. It provides passive exercise and stimulates peristalsis without risk of injury to the patient. The bed has many other advantages, including several hatches that provide the nurse access to all of the common pressure points on the patient. There is a hatch for bowel and bladder care so that a bedpan can be

FIGURE 32-6 FluidAir bed.

FIGURE 32-7 Wrist splint.

of place, and not cause increased pain (Figure 32-7). If in doubt about how a particular splint is to be applied, seek help from an experienced nurse or the physical therapist.

? Think Critically

You are working in a long-term care facility. Your patient is in a coma because of a head injury that occurred 3 months ago, but her husband visits every day. How could the husband participate to prevent contractures?

placed without moving the patient. The back side of the patient can be bathed through the various hatches also. Once the nurse is familiar with the bed, it greatly simplifies care of the immobilized patient.

The FluidAir bed also is used for various types of immobilized patients. It is an air-fluidized bed and is very helpful in preventing pressure sores (Figure 32-6).

Use of Slings and Splints. A sling used to support the wrist or elbow should support both joints of the arm. The sling should be positioned so that the fastening at the neck area does not rub the neck or press on a neck vessel. When a splint is applied to an extremity, it should support the joint that is to be immobilized, fit properly without impeding circulation or slipping out

Teaching Ambulation with Assistive Devices

For the convalescent patient or for one who may always need support while walking, crutches can mean the difference between freedom to move about and confinement to one location. Before attempting to walk with crutches, the patient should be instructed in their use and manipulation so that she can handle them safely and effectively.

Patient Teaching

Crutch Gaits

GAIT	SEQUENCE	PATTERN
Four-point gait	1. Advance left crutch. 2. Advance right foot. 3. Advance right crutch. 4. Advance left foot. Advantages: most stable crutch gait. Requirements: partial weight bearing on both legs.	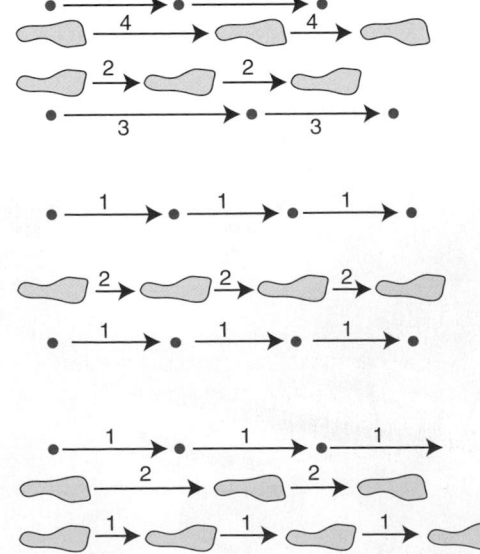
Three-point gait	1. Advance both crutches forward with the affected leg and shift weight to crutches. 2. Advance unaffected leg and shift weight onto it. Advantages: allows the affected leg to be partially or completely free of weight bearing. Requirements: full weight bearing on one leg, balance, and upper body strength.	
Two-point gait	1. Advance left crutch and right foot. 2. Advance right crutch and left foot. Advantages: faster version of the four-point gait, more normal walking pattern (arms and legs moving in opposition). Requirements: partial weight bearing on both legs, balance.	

The type of crutch to be used will depend on the extent of disability or paralysis and the patient's ability to bear weight and maintain balance. If the crutches are too short or too long, the patient will have problems with moving and shifting her weight. When walking, the patient should straighten the elbow and the wrist during weight bearing. The muscles of the arms, shoulders, back, and chest are all used in the manipulation of crutches. Because this is true, many physical therapists start the patient on special exercises to strengthen these muscles several weeks before the patient begins to use the crutches.

 Safety Alert

Crutch Safety

Crutches should be about 16 inches (40 cm) shorter than the patient's height. When in the standing position with axillary crutches, the axillary bar should be two finger breadths below the axilla. The elbow should be flexed at a 30-degree angle when the palms of the hands rest on the handgrip. It is important that the patient not rest her body at the axilla on the top of the crutch; body weight should be borne by the arms on the hand rests of the crutches. If crutches are too long, pressure on the axilla will occur and can cause nerve damage.

To measure for crutches: the patient stands with shoes on the feet and positions the crutch tips at a point 4 to 6 inches (10 to 15 cm) to the side and 4 to 6 inches in front of the feet.

Although the physical therapist supervises the preparation and instruction of the patient before she starts to use crutches and then evaluates her ability to use them correctly, you will sometimes be responsible for assisting a patient with crutch walking while she is in the hospital.

When teaching a patient to ambulate with a cane, be certain that the cane has an intact rubber tip. The cane is the right length if the handgrip is at hip level and the elbow is bent at a 30-degree angle when weight is placed on the cane. **It should be used on the good side unless the physician orders otherwise.** The tip of the cane should be placed 6 to 10 inches (15 to 25 cm) to the side and 6 inches (15 cm) in front of the near foot when walking. The patient should look straight ahead, rather than down, when ambulating. **The cane is advanced at the same time as the affected leg.** The good leg is advanced first when going upstairs and the good leg leads going downstairs.

Walker height is correct when the person's elbow is bent at a 15- to 30-degree angle while standing upright and grasping the handgrips. The walker is lifted or rolled on its wheels slightly in front of the patient while leaning the body slightly forward. A step or two is taken into the walker, and then it is lifted and placed in front of the person again.

 Patient Teaching

Special Maneuvers on Crutches

MANEUVER	SEQUENCE
Walking up stairs	1. Stand at the foot of the stairs with weight on the good leg and crutches.
	2. Put weight on the crutch handles and then lift the good leg up onto the first step of the stairs.
	3. Put weight on the good leg and lift the injured leg and crutches up to that step.
	4. Repeat for each step.
Walking down stairs	1. Stand at the top of the stairs with weight on the good leg and crutches.
	2. Shift weight completely onto the good leg and put the crutches down on the next step.
	3. Put weight on the crutch handles and transfer the injured leg down on the step with the crutches.
	4. Bring the good leg down to that step.
	5. Repeat for each stair step.
Sitting down	1. Crutch-walk to the chair.
	2. Turn around slowly so that the back is to the chair and the backs of the legs touch the seat of the chair.
	3. Transfer both crutches to the side with the injured leg and grasp both handgrips with that one hand.
	4. As weight is supported on the crutches and the good leg, reach back with the free hand and grasp the arm of the chair.
	5. Lower slowly onto the chair seat, using the support of both the crutches and chair.
	6. Sit back in the chair and elevate the leg.
	7. Keep the knee slightly flexed when elevated, because too much extension can decrease the circulation.
	8. To get up, bring both crutches along the side of the injured leg and grasp the handgrip firmly. Make sure the crutch tips are firmly on the floor. Place the other hand on the arm of the chair and push up.
	9. After becoming upright, transfer one crutch to the other hand for walking.

 Elder Care Points

Many elderly patients are hospitalized with injuries they sustain from inability to maneuver crutches, cane, or walker. It is essential that elderly patients be taught proper methods of using assistive devices and that they receive supervised practice before they are discharged.

Psychosocial Care

Unfortunately, many orthopedic conditions require prolonged periods of confinement to bed or, at best, immobilization of a part of the body and restricted physical activities. This leads to frustration and a feeling of hopelessness and despair on the part of the patient. When the patient is young and unaccustomed to depending on others for personal care, a reaction of anger and bitterness may occur. If the patient is a wage earner or a member of the family on whom others are dependent, there is the additional burden of financial and role problems (see Chapter 9).

■ Evaluation

Determining the effectiveness of interventions to treat pain is based mainly on subjective information given by the patient, but the nurse should also be alert to nuances of body language. Observation of the patient's ability to accomplish ADLs gives clues to improvement in mobility and activity tolerance.

Diagnostic test data from radiographs and laboratory reports are used to determine the effectiveness of treatments. For example, radiographs show whether fractures are healing, whereas laboratory reports help to determine how well rheumatoid arthritis is controlled.

Get Ready for the NCLEX® Examination!

Key Points

- The main functions of the musculoskeletal system are motion, support, and protection.
- Exercise and weight training throughout life can decrease musculoskeletal problems late in life.
- Using safety equipment for sports, exercise, when driving, and at work is very important to preventing trauma to the musculoskeletal system.
- Self-care deficit and impaired physical mobility are primary problems for patients with musculoskeletal injuries or disorders.
- Physical and occupational therapists are part of the collaborative team for musculoskeletal care and rehabilitation.
- Contractures can permanently impair the patient's ability to perform ADLs. Positioning must be performed correctly and ROM exercises should be done three or four times a day to promote function and preserve movement.
- The nurse assists with supervising and teaching ambulation with assistive devices.

Additional Learning Resources

SG Go to your Study Guide for additional learning activities to help you master this chapter content.

 Go to your Evolve website (http://evolve.elsevier.com/deWit/medsurg) for the following FREE learning resources:
- Animations, audio, and video
- Answers and rationales for questions and activities
- Concept Map Creator
- Glossary with pronunciations in English and Spanish
- Interactive Review Questions and Exercises and more!

Online Resources
- Arthritis Foundation, www.arthritis.org/index.php
- Back Injury Prevention Guide, www.dir.ca.gov/dosh/dosh_publications/backinj.pdf
- National Association of Orthopaedic Nurses, www.orthonurse.org/ResearchandPractice/ClinicalPractice/tabid/223/Default.aspx

Review Questions for the NCLEX® Examination

1. What action should the nurse perform for the postprocedural care of a patient who just had an arthrocentesis?
   1. Follow up on the results of the serum enzymes that were drawn before the test.
   2. Prepare an ice pack and obtain an elastic bandage.
   3. Check vital signs and pulse every 15 minutes for the first hour.
   4. Encourage the patient to take fluids to flush out the isotope.

2. The nurse is working on a busy orthopedic floor. Which task(s) can be assigned to the UAP? *(Select all that apply.)*
   1. Assist an elderly patient who has an arm sling to perform ADLs.
   2. Report the presence of contractures on a bedridden patient.
   3. Supervise a patient who is learning to use crutches.
   4. Escort a patient in a wheelchair to the radiology department.
   5. Perform passive ROM on a patient who needs a bed bath.
   6. Instruct a patient to reapply a prescribed wrist splint.

3. The nurse evaluates the patient's ability to use the cane. Which action indicates proper use of the cane?
   1. The cane is advanced at the same time as the good leg.
   2. The handgrip is at the hip level.
   3. The cane is used on the affected side.
   4. The patient looks down while ambulating.

4. The nurse is caring for several patients that need diagnostic testing for musculoskeletal disorders. Which patient should not be offered any coffee on the morning of the test?
   1. Patient needs to have a blood sample taken to measure calcium level.

2. Patient needs to have an radiographic examination of the left lower leg with a cast in place.
3. Patient needs to have a bone scan to check for degenerative disease.
4. Patient needs an electromyogram to determine abnormal muscle function.

5. A 50-year-old man complains of joint pains, difficulty rising, and limping. He has poor posture and uncoordinated gait. What is the priority nursing diagnosis?
    1. Self-care deficit
    2. Impaired physical mobility
    3. Ineffective coping
    4. Arthritis

6. The patient reports a grating sound while moving her joints. What is a likely cause of the sound?
    1. Rupture of ligaments and tendons
    2. Rubbing of eroded cartilage
    3. Recently had arthrography
    4. Presence of inflammation

7. The nurse is taking care of an elderly patient with severe degenerative arthritis. What is the initial nursing intervention to accomplish progressive mobilization?
    1. Assist with transfers from bed to chair
    2. Encourage frequent ambulation
    3. Determine ROM of all extremities
    4. Reposition frequently

8. The nurse recruits the assistance of adequately trained personnel to turn an immobile patient. To prevent injury to the patient and the nursing staff, which measure should be taken before repositioning the patient?
    1. Encourage movement of all joints.
    2. Explain the details of the move.
    3. Discourage patient participation.
    4. Medicate patient for anxiety.

9. To manage joint discomfort associated with movement among patients with severe rheumatoid arthritis, the nurse should:
    1. encourage deep-breathing exercises.
    2. administer pain medications immediately after exercise.
    3. schedule pain medication administration before ambulation.
    4. provide a continuous infusion of pain medications.

10. The nurse assesses the condition of a splint applied to the right arm. Which clinical finding is cause for the greatest concern?
    1. Warm skin
    2. Redness of skin
    3. Itching
    4. Palpable distal pulses

Critical Thinking Activities

Scenario A
Miss Simpson has had trouble with her left knee for several years. She is scheduled for an arthroscopy and asks you about the procedure.

1. How would you describe the procedure to her?
2. What is the aftercare for this procedure?
3. How long is she likely to be immobile after the procedure?

Scenario B
Ms. Jackson has been experiencing muscle weakness in her right leg for a few weeks. Her health care provider has scheduled her for an electromyogram (EMG). She asks you about this procedure.

1. Is an informed consent needed for an EMG?
2. How would you describe the test to Ms. Jackson?
3. What care is needed after the procedure?

Scenario C
Ms. White, age 67, sustained a fracture of the right humerus when she fell this morning. A cast has been applied.

1. What would you tell her she needs to do at home to keep her joints mobile?
2. What should she do to protect the muscle mass?
3. What nutritional teaching would you provide?

Scenario D
You are caring for Mr. Moran, a 40-year-old self-employed carpenter. He is a large man with a heavy full leg cast. He is having a lot of pain and expresses fear that moving will increase the pain.

1. Discuss some important considerations in turning, moving, bathing, and toileting for Mr. Moran.
2. What is the psychosocial care for a patient such as Mr. Moran who is immobile?

Objectives

Theory

1. Compare the assessment findings of a connective tissue injury with those of a fracture.
2. Explain the rationale for the "do's and don'ts" of cast care.
3. Outline the potential complications related to fractures.
4. Discuss the pathophysiology and implications of the 6Ps.
5. Compare the preoperative and postoperative care of a patient with a total knee replacement with that of a patient with a total hip replacement.
6. Identify the special problems of patients with arthritis and specific nursing interventions that can be helpful.
7. Explain the process by which osteoporosis occurs, ways to slow the process, and how the disorder is treated.

8. Plan important postoperative observations and nursing interventions in the care of the patient who has undergone an amputation.

Clinical Practice

1. Assess a patient who has a connective tissue injury.
2. Provide pin care for a patient with external fixation.
3. Teach the patient going home with a cast about proper care of the cast and extremity.
4. Observe a physical therapist who is teaching quadriceps exercise and then assist the patient to practice.
5. Assess the skin of a patient who has a prosthetic device on an amputated limb.

Key Terms

arthroplasty (ĂR-thrō-plăs-tē, p. 749)
bivalved (p. 742)
compartment syndrome (p. 741)
dislocation (p. 735)
fasciotomy (p. 742)
fracture (FRĂK-shŭr, p. 736)
nonunion (p. 741)

orthoses (ŏr-thō-sēz, p. 749)
osteogenesis (ŏs-tē-ō-JĔN-ĕ-sĭs, p. 741)
osteomyelitis (p. 741)
osteopenia (ŏs-tē-ō-PĒ-nē-ă, p. 755)
osteoporosis (p. 736)
sprain (p. 734)
subluxation (sŭb-lŭk-SĀ-shŭn, p. 735)

CONNECTIVE TISSUE DISORDERS

SPRAIN

Etiology and Pathophysiology

A sprain is a partial or complete tearing of the ligaments that hold various bones together to form a joint. A sprain occurs when a joint is forced or twisted, during trauma, past its normal range of motion. The ankle, knee, and wrist are most commonly sprained.

Signs, Symptoms, and Diagnosis

- *Grade I* (mild): Tenderness at site; minimal swelling and loss of function; no abnormal motion.
- *Grade II* (moderate): More severe pain, especially with weight bearing; swelling and bleeding into joint; some loss of function.
- *Grade III* (severe, complete tearing of fibers): Pain may be less severe, but swelling, loss of function, and bleeding into joint are more marked.

Diagnosis is by physical and radiographic examination to rule out a fracture or other pathology.

Treatment and Nursing Management

RICE is the acronym used for treatment of sprains: *rest, ice, compression,* and *elevation.* Apply ice immediately after injury and for 24 to 72 hours. Apply the ice bag for 10 to 20 minutes every 1 to 2 hours during the day. Wrap the injured part snugly with an elastic bandage, being careful not to cut off circulation, and elevate. These measures can help minimize swelling and pain and stabilize the joint in proper alignment. The goal of treatment is to protect the ligament until it heals by scarring. Ligaments do not "grow" back together. Air casts, braces, or supports are used only until a joint has been strengthened. If a joint is immobilized too long and muscles are not exercised, muscle atrophy—which begins in a matter of days—can cause permanent disability. In some cases, surgical repair may be necessary. Grade III sprains often require a cast. Patients with Grade II or Grade III sprains need to rest the joint; crutches are needed for a lower extremity sprain. Nonsteroidal anti-inflammatory drugs (NSAIDs) should be prescribed on an around-the-clock basis for the first couple of days to decrease swelling.

STRAIN
Etiology and Pathophysiology
A strain is a pulling or tearing of a muscle, a tendon, or both. A strain occurs by trauma, overuse, or overextension of a joint. The most common muscle strain occurs in the back muscles. (Back problems are discussed in Chapter 23, because they often have a neurologic component.) Muscle strains do occur in other skeletal muscles. The most common sites are the hamstrings, quadriceps, and calf muscles.

 Complementary and Alternative Therapies

Soothing Sore Muscles

Arnica applied topically as an essential oil is supposed to soothe sore tired muscles after a long day's work. Valerian or kava brewed as a tea is also said to relax muscles. A little a honey or apple juice will make the teas more palatable (Blakley, 2009).

 Think Critically

How would you assess for a circulation problem or nerve injury after an ankle sprain or strain?

Signs, Symptoms, and Diagnosis
A history of overexertion or the presence of soft-tissue swelling and pain may indicate a strain has occurred. Bleeding (ecchymosis, hemorrhagic area) will be present if muscle is torn.

Treatment and Nursing Management
Ice and compression should be immediately applied and the part should be rested. The patient is taught to use ice for only 20 minutes per hour. When compression is used, the distal parts of the extremity must be checked for sensation and adequate circulation. Heat can be applied after 48 hours. Anti-inflammatory medications are used for discomfort and, when spasm is present, a muscle relaxant may be prescribed. Time is the greatest healer. The patient is cautioned against reinjury and is taught proper ways to lift and move. Surgical repair may be necessary.

DISLOCATION
Etiology and Pathophysiology
A dislocation is the stretching and tearing of ligaments around a joint with complete displacement of a bone. Subluxation is a partial dislocation. This occurs from trauma. The most common sites are the shoulder, knee, ankle, and temporomandibular joint.

Signs, Symptoms, and Diagnosis
Dislocation often includes a history of an outside force pushing from a certain direction, severe pain aggravated by motion of the joint, muscle spasm, or abnormal appearance of a joint. A radiograph will reveal displacement of bone.

Treatment and Nursing Management
Reduction of displacement under anesthesia, or manual reduction, is necessary. Sometimes spontaneous reduction can be achieved. The goal is to stabilize the joint after reduction and then to rehabilitate to minimize muscular atrophy and strengthen the joint. The nurse should assess for adequate perfusion and movement of the affected part and distal to it; determine if swelling is present and assess the degree of pain. Nursing management is aimed mainly at encouraging rest of the affected part, and pain control. Heat or cold applications may be ordered.

ROTATOR CUFF TEAR
Rotator cuff injury usually results from repetitive activity, such as throwing or making overhead motions with the arm. The rotator cuff is composed of four muscles. If the rotator cuff is torn, there is pain and the patient cannot perform abduction and external rotation of the injured shoulder. Treatment consists of rest, sling support for the shoulder, and NSAIDs for the discomfort. Some physicians treat with injections of steroids or an anti-inflammatory drug. When the acute episode is over, gentle, progressive exercise is prescribed. Heat is recommended before exercising the joint. If the tear will not heal, surgical repair is indicated.

ANTERIOR CRUCIATE LIGAMENT INJURY
Most anterior cruciate ligament (ACL) injuries of the knee occur from athletic activities, but falls and motor vehicle accidents also may cause such injury. Hyperextension, internal rotation, extremes of external rotation, and deceleration are involved. The ligament may be torn from the femur or tibia. Often a loud "pop" can be heard at the time of injury. There is swelling in the hours following the injury and the knee feels unstable and can "give way." Full extension of the leg is difficult. Diagnosis is by physical examination, radiography, or magnetic resonance imaging (MRI) scan. Arthroscopy is performed, at which time repair may be done.

After injury, the knee is immobilized and measures are instituted to reduce swelling and pain. After repair, continuous passive motion (CPM) may be ordered to promote full mobility. A long leg brace with fixed knee flexion may be used as well. Isometric exercises are prescribed in the recovery period, including quadriceps setting (see Patient Teaching box on p. 729), bent-knee leg exercises, and foot exercises.

MENISCAL INJURY

The meniscus is the shock absorber of the knee and lies on top of the tibia between the tibia and the femur. A meniscus tear may accompany an ACL injury. This type of injury often results from fixed-foot rotation in weight bearing with the knee flexed, during sports activities, such as football or skiing. After the injury, mild swelling occurs and there is joint pain. Popping, slipping, catching, or buckling of the knee can occur. Diagnosis is by physical examination to elicit a "click" and localized pain with particular movements of the joint. MRI is the most specific diagnostic test for a meniscal injury. Surgery for repair is done arthroscopically. Postoperatively, pain management is a priority. An exercise program is prescribed for muscle strengthening during recovery.

ACHILLES TENDON RUPTURE

The Achilles tendon attaches to the calcaneus (heel bone). When overstretched, it can rupture. Sports injuries or a fall from a height are the usual mechanisms of injury. Arthritis, diabetes, and taking some antibiotics can predispose to Achilles tendon rupture. Injury most often occurs with bursts of jumping, pivoting, and running, such as occur in tennis, basketball, handball, and badminton. Symptoms are sudden pain at the back of the ankle or calf. There may be a loud "pop" or "snap" sound. A depression can be felt or seen 2 inches above the calcaneus. Pain, swelling, and stiffness follow and then bruising and weakness. There will be an inability to point the toes or stand on tiptoe. Diagnosis is by examination and squeezing the calf muscles while the patient is lying prone. The toes should point downward; if they do not, there is most likely an Achilles tendon injury.

Treatment may be by splinting, casting, or a combination of splinting or casting with surgery. Recovery takes 6 to 8 weeks and is followed by a period of physical therapy.

BURSITIS

Bursitis is an inflammation of the bursae, the saclike structures that line freely movable joints. It occurs from injury or overuse and often appears when a person has engaged in an unaccustomed activity, such as shoulder bursitis after digging up the garden plot in the spring. Bursitis may occur in any heavily used joint, but it most commonly occurs in the elbow, shoulder, or knee. Symptoms are localized tenderness, mild to moderate aching pain, localized to the joint, and exacerbated by activity of the joint. Swelling may be present. Diagnosis is by history of injury and physical examination. Treatment is to rest the joint by altering aggravating activity and using anti-inflammatory agents, ice, massage, and a compression wrap if there is soft-tissue swelling. If these measures—plus time—do not relieve the symptoms, an injection of cortisone into the bursa is administered.

BUNION (HALLUX VALGUS)

A bunion, the most common foot problem, is a painful swelling of the bursa that occurs when the great toe deviates laterally at the metatarsophalangeal joint. It may be hereditary, or it may occur from ill-fitting shoes. Bunions are more common in females than in males. Wearing open-toed shoes of soft leather or athletic shoes that are wider in the toe area helps reduce pain. Metatarsal pads can relieve some of the pressure. Corticosteroid injections are given in the joint if active bursitis is present. Analgesics are used for discomfort. Bone realignment of the big toe with removal of bony overgrowth is performed when walking becomes too painful. Hammertoes are often fixed at the same time.

CARPAL TUNNEL SYNDROME

Etiology, Pathophysiology, Signs, and Symptoms

Carpal tunnel syndrome is a nerve problem that occurs when the median nerve is compressed as it passes through the carpal tunnel in the wrist. It produces pain, numbness, and tingling of the hand, particularly at night. Repetitive movements of the hands and wrists, particularly with constant flexion of the wrist, are contributing causes. Such movement occurs in certain types of factory work and in computer keyboarding. Sometimes there is no known cause.

Diagnosis, Treatment, and Nursing Management

Diagnosis is by physical examination, a compression test, and possibly electromyography to rule out other causes of symptoms. Treatment by rest, splinting, changing the angle of the wrist during repetitive movements, or steroid injection may solve the problem. If the symptoms are of long duration, muscle atrophy occurs, or if sensory loss in the fingers and hands is progressive, surgery is indicated. Surgical decompression of the medial nerve by transection of the carpal ligament is performed, usually as an outpatient procedure.

Postoperatively, blood flow must be assessed hourly by checking color, warmth of the fingertips, and capillary refill. After anesthesia has worn off, sensation of the fingers is assessed. The wrist is immobilized in a splint and the arm is elevated on pillows to reduce edema. The patient is warned to avoid heavy gripping and pinching for up to 6 weeks.

FRACTURES

Etiology and Pathophysiology

A fracture is a break or interruption in the continuity of a bone. Fractures occur mostly from trauma but can occur due to a pathologic process in which bone has degenerated, such as in osteoporosis (metabolic bone disorder that causes a decrease in bone mass) or another metabolic problem. The *mechanism of injury*, or how the injury occurred, can provide clues about the type of fracture. For example, if a patient reports punching a wall or another solid surface, the fifth metacarpal frequently breaks and the patient sustains a "boxer's fracture." Mechanism of injury is also important to help you predict the injury to the neighboring tissues (see Chapter 45). Damage varies according to the type of fracture, but there is always some degree of tissue destruction, interference with the blood supply, and disturbance of muscle activity at the site of injury.

 Safety Alert

Proton Pump Inhibitors and Fracture Risk

In May 2010, the Food and Drug Administration (FDA) issued a warning that proton pump inhibitors (PPIs), including over-the-counter products, increase the risk for fracture of the hip, wrist, and spine. In epidemiologic studies, the risk was highest for people over 50 who had used PPIs for more than a year (Ault, 2010).

Signs, Symptoms, and Diagnosis

A fracture may cause minimal to severe pain depending on the type of fracture, the bone(s) involved, and the amount of displacement. Swelling usually occurs and there may be bleeding into the tissues. Other symptoms of a fracture include pain, tenderness, deformity of the bone, ecchymoses, crepitation with any movement, and loss of function. Box 33-1 presents the most common types of fractures. Figure 33-1 illustrates the characteristics of a variety of fractures. Diagnosis is by physical and radiographic examination.

Elder Care Points

The elderly person is more at risk of sustaining a fracture because of decreased reaction time, failing vision, lessened agility, alterations in balance, and decreased muscle tone, all of which predispose to falls. Nurses should assess for fall risk and initiate fall precautions as needed.

Treatment

The emergency treatment and nursing care of fractures consists of preventing shock and hemorrhage and the immediate immobilization of the part to avoid

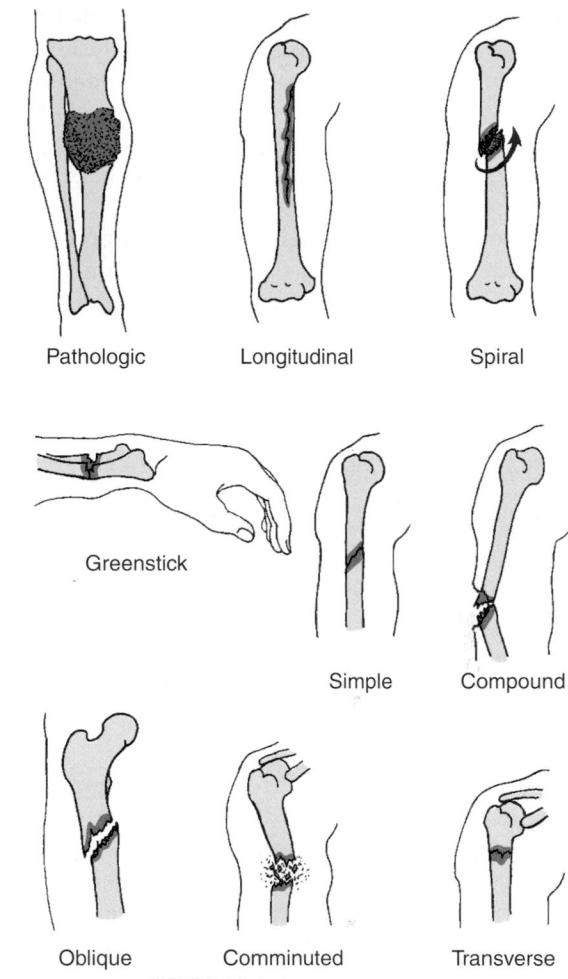
FIGURE 33-1 Types of fractures.

unnecessary damage to the soft tissue adjacent to the fracture. An inexperienced person should never attempt to straighten or set a broken bone. The injured part should be immobilized in the position in which it is found at the time of injury: "splint it as it lies." The limb should be supported firmly so that it will not be jarred when the victim is being moved. If available, ice in a plastic bag can be applied to the fracture area to help minimize swelling.

In the emergency department or clinic, the patient will be examined by a health care provider, and a radiograph will be ordered if fracture is suspected. After a radiograph of the injured part has been made and the type of fracture and extent of damage have been established, the health care provider will decide which method to use in reducing the fracture and providing immobilization. Surgery may be necessary to realign the bones and to reduce the fracture. If the skin was broken when the fracture occurred, tetanus immunization is given. Prophylactic antibiotics are usually administered when a compound fracture has occurred.

The primary aim in the treatment of fractures is to establish a sturdy union between the broken ends so

Box 33-1	Types of Fractures

- *Complete fracture* is when a bone breaks into two parts that are completely separated.
- An *incomplete fracture* is when a bone breaks into two parts that are not completely separated.
- A *comminuted fracture* is one in which the bone is broken and shattered into more than two fragments.
- A *closed (simple) fracture* is one in which there is no break in the skin.
- An *open (compound) fracture* is one in which there is a break in the skin through which the fragments of broken bone protrude.
- A *greenstick fracture*, common in children, is one in which the bone is partially bent and partially broken.

that the bone can be restored to continuity. The healing and repair of a fracture begin immediately after the bone is broken, and proceed through five stages:

1. Blood oozes from the torn blood vessels in the area of the fracture; the blood clots, and begins to form a hematoma between the two broken ends of bone (1 to 3 days).
2. Other tissue cells enter the clot, and granulation tissue is formed. This tissue is interlaced with capillaries, and it gradually becomes firm and forms a bridge between the two ends of broken bone (3 days to 2 weeks).
3. Young bone cells enter the area and form a tissue called "callus." At this stage, the ends of the broken bone are beginning to "knit" together (2 to 6 weeks).
4. The immature bone cells are gradually replaced by mature bone cells (ossification), and the tissue takes on the characteristics of typical bone structure (3 weeks to 6 months).
5. Bone is resorbed and deposited, depending on the lines of stress. The medullary canal is reconstructed during consolidation and remodeling (6 weeks to 1 year).

To facilitate the process of repair and ensure proper healing of the bone without deformity or loss of function, the surgeon must bring the two broken ends together in proper alignment and then immobilize the affected part until healing is complete. The procedure for bringing the two fragments of bone into proper alignment is called *reduction of the fracture.*

Reduction, Surgery, and Stabilization. There are two methods to reduce a fracture: closed reduction and open reduction. In *closed reduction,* the bone is manipulated into alignment; no surgical incision is made. A general anesthetic may be given before the fracture is reduced. An *open reduction* is done after a surgical incision is made through the skin and down to the bone at the site of the fracture. In cases of open (compound) fractures and comminuted fractures, an open reduction is necessary so that the area can be adequately cleansed and bone fragments removed.

There are four methods of stabilizing a fracture after it has been reduced:

- Internal fixation
- External fixation
- Casts, splints, braces
- Traction

Internal Fixation. When a fracture cannot be properly reduced by either open or closed reduction and it is impossible to guarantee adequate union of the bone fragments, the surgeon must perform *internal fixation* of the bone. This means that pins, nails, screws, or metal plates must be used to stabilize the position of the two broken ends. Internal fixation is particularly necessary to treat

A. Tension band wiring technique using Kirschner wires for fracture of a phalanx.

B. Compression plate to the lateral aspect of the femur.

C. Sliding hip screw.

FIGURE 33-2 Examples of internal fixation.

fractures in elderly patients whose bones are brittle and may not heal properly (Figure 33-2).

One of the most common internal fixation procedures is performed on a fractured hip: open reduction and internal fixation (ORIF). An incision is made, the fracture is realigned, and the bone is secured with pins, screws, nails, or plates. A drain will be in place until there is scant drainage (i.e., less than 30 mL/24 hours). If a prosthesis is implanted, there will be more blood loss and the patient may receive autotransfusion of salvaged blood after surgery. Administration of intravenous (IV) antibiotics to reduce the risk of infection is standard. Care includes maintaining good alignment of the affected leg, preventing complications of immobility, and keeping the patient comfortable with pain control measures.

External Fixation. *External fixation* of fractures involves the use of a device composed of a sturdy external frame to which are attached pins that have been placed into the bone fragments. Figure 33-3 shows a fixator that is applied by inserting heavy pins on either side of the fracture and then reducing the fracture by tightening nuts attached to the connecting rods.

External fixation is commonly used for fractures of an extremity or of the pelvis. Indications include:

- Massive open fractures with extensive soft-tissue damage.
- Infected fractures that do not heal properly.
- Multiple trauma with one or more fractures and other injuries, such as burns, chest injury, or head injury.

FIGURE 33-3 External fixation.

External fixation has the advantage of allowing more freedom of movement than traction and usually is more comfortable. With good stability the patient may be able to get out of bed, although he must be assisted and advised not to bear weight on the affected limb. Physical therapy exercises will help the patient avoid many of the problems of immobility, and an occupational therapist can suggest ways to cope with activities of daily living (ADLs). Particularly if the fixator must remain in place for months or years, your patient is likely to have problems with self-image and may feel embarrassed or frustrated about being out in public with an apparatus that is large and bulky.

Casts. Casts are used for stabilizing a fracture after a closed reduction. A cast is rigid and immobilizes the injured body part. The newer fiberglass and polyester-cotton knit casts are light weight, dry quickly, and can bear weight within 30 minutes of application (Figure 33-4). They are less bulky, do not crumble easily, and are less likely to be damaged by wetting. However, synthetic casts cost three to seven times more than plaster casts. They are less easily molded to a body part than are plaster casts, and synthetic casts are not suitable for immobilizing the fragments of severely displaced bones or for stabilizing serious fractures. Their rough exterior surfaces can damage the skin and tend to snag clothing and other soft materials. Synthetic casts are used mostly for upper-extremity fractures. Some physicians still use plaster of Paris casts for lower extremities because plaster casts can bear more weight and last longer with weight bearing. The newly applied plaster cast usually is not dry for about 48 hours. A dry plaster cast is white, has a shiny surface, and will resound when tapped. A wet plaster cast is grayish and dull in appearance and will give a dull thud when tapped. The edges of plaster casts tend to crumble, with bits of plaster dropping down inside the cast and causing the patient discomfort and skin irritation. This can be avoided by covering the rims of the cast with stockinette or applying tape in a "petal" fashion.

There are *long-leg* or and *short-leg* casts, depending on how much leg they cover. A walking *cast shoe* is a canvas sandal with a thick sole that fits over the bottom of the leg cast; this shoe can be used once the patient is allowed to bear weight. When an arm cast is applied, a sling is often used to support the arm and provide extremity elevation. A *spica* cast covers the trunk of the body and one or two extremities. There are long-leg and short-leg spicas that cover one or both legs, and shoulder spicas that include the trunk and one arm.

Braces and Splints. Braces provide support for fractures that have been reduced. The advantage of a brace is that it can be easily removed for assessment and care of the skin, and then reapplied. Examples include a commercial fracture boot to support the distal tibia, ankle, and foot (Figure 33-5). A hinged brace is used for the elbow and knee, which allows for early motion of the joint. An adjustable dial allows for variations in flexion and extension during recovery. A knee immobilizer prevents motion, and provides compression to reduce

FIGURE 33-4 Synthetic limb cast.

FIGURE 33-5 Walking boot.

pain and swelling. Plaster of Paris can be used to create a "backslab" or splint (a slab of plaster that provides support, but does not completely surround the injury). The slab is useful in the early phase because of the swelling that occurs after the injury (Bakody, 2009).

Clinical Cues

Before cast application (especially plaster of Paris), advise the patient that he will feel warmth as the cast sets and dries. Never put a fresh cast on plastic because the heat generated may burn the skin since it cannot dissipate. Also, never cover a fresh plaster cast with a blanket because air circulation speeds drying.

Traction. Traction is the application of a mechanical pull to a part of the body for the purpose of extending and holding that part in a certain position during immobilization. The two general types of traction are *skeletal traction* and *skin traction*. In skeletal traction, the surgeon inserts pins, wires, or tongs directly through the bone at a point distal to the fracture so that the force of pull from the weights is exerted directly on the bone. Skeletal traction uses 10 lb or more of weight and the body acts as the countertraction. With skin traction, a bandage (such as moleskin, or a foam traction boot) is applied to the limb below the site of fracture, and then pull is exerted on the limb. No more than 7 to 10 lb of weight is used for skin traction. Traction may be continuous (as in the alignment and resultant immobility of fractured bones), or it may be intermittent (as in traction on the spinal column to relieve the symptoms of a slipped disk or muscle spasms).

Traction was used more commonly in the past. Current applications of traction are reflected in a small study of severely injured patients, in which the advantages of skeletal traction over external fixation were identified: skeletal traction is simple, takes minutes to apply, is inexpensive, and involves no need for anesthesia. The authors concluded that skeletal traction was a good temporary measure unless the patient was undergoing anesthesia for other reasons (Scannell, 2010).

Figure 33-6 illustrates some of the different types of traction:

- *Buck's extension* is a simple skin traction that is used to treat muscle spasms from fractures of the hip or femur, preoperatively, and for dislocation of the hip.
- *Russell's traction* uses a knee sling to provide support of the affected leg. It is commonly used to treat fractures of the hip or end of the femur.
- *Cervical traction* can be provided through the use of tongs inserted into the skull, the use of a halo device (see Chapter 23), or a head halter.
- *Pelvic traction* with a pelvic belt or sling, although rarely used, may be indicated for pelvic fractures and other pelvic injuries.
- *Balanced suspension with the Thomas splint and Pearson attachment* is used to treat fractures of the femur and pelvis. The Thomas splint supports the thigh and knee and provides countertraction. The Pearson attachment supports the lower leg, although it has generally been replaced with the use of external fixation.

Buck's traction

Russell's traction

Head halter traction

Pelvic traction

Balanced suspension traction

FIGURE 33-6 Examples of common types of traction.

Complications of Fractures

The sooner a fracture is fixed, the less likely the chance for complications. Healing of a fracture can be impeded by improper alignment and inadequate immobilization. Continued twisting, shearing, and abnormal stresses prohibit a strong, bony union. Inadequate levels of serum calcium and phosphorus, vitamin deficiency, and generalized atherosclerosis—which deprives the healing site of adequate blood supply—also can complicate a fracture by delaying healing.

Infection. Infection of the tissue at the fracture site is probably the most serious impediment to healing. Open comminuted fractures, especially, should be taken to surgery within 6 hours to decrease the chance of infection. Typically cefazolin is administered within 1 hour of incision, and three doses are given postoperatively. If the wound is grossly contaminated, additional antibiotics will be ordered. It is important to monitor the patient's temperature and white blood cell (WBC) count for elevations and to monitor the appearance of the area carefully for redness, swelling, heat, or purulent drainage.

Osteomyelitis. Osteomyelitis is a bacterial infection of the bone. The causative organism is most often *Staphylococcus aureus,* which enters the bloodstream from a distant focus of infection, such as a boil or furuncle, or from an open wound, as in an open (compound) fracture. It is usually found in the tibia or fibula, in vertebrae, or at the site of a prosthesis. Osteomyelitis has a sudden onset with severe pain and marked tenderness at the site, high fever with chills, swelling of adjacent soft parts, headache, and malaise. Diagnosis of osteomyelitis is made on the basis of:

- Laboratory findings indicating an acute infection, for example, high sedimentation rate and WBC count
- Radiographs, which may show bone destruction 7 to 10 days after onset of the disease
- History of injury to the part, open fracture, boils, furuncles, or other infections
- Biopsy, in which the bone sample exhibits signs of necrosis

The earlier osteomyelitis is diagnosed and treated, the better the prognosis. Antibiotics are prescribed for 4 to 6 weeks, and the abscess is incised and drained. Dead bone and debris are debrided from the site. The affected limb is immobilized for complete rest. Sometimes amputation is the only cure (see Chapter 6 for care related to infection).

Nonunion. Nonunion (failure to heal) of a fracture can be treated by an electrical bone growth–stimulating device, which uses electrical coils or electrodes to induce weak electrical current in the bone to stimulate healing properties. Examples include an external electromagnetic device, a percutaneous stimulator with electrodes placed at the fracture site, or an implanted direct current stimulator whose current stimulates osteogenesis (growth of bone cells). Use of such devices can prevent further surgery and bone grafting. This treatment is based on the fact that bone has inherent electrical properties used in healing.

Fat Embolism. Fat embolism is a rare but serious complication of a fracture of a bone that has an abundance of marrow fat (e.g., the long bones, pelvis, and ribs). In the early postinjury period, patients with multiple fractures resulting from severe trauma are at risk for this complication. To form an embolism, the fat globules must be large enough or sufficient in number to partially or completely occlude a blood vessel. Rupture of small venules in the area permit entrance of fat globules into the circulation. Signs and symptoms of fat embolism include a change in mental status, respiratory distress, tachypnea, crackles and wheezes on auscultating the lungs, rapid pulse, fever, and petechiae (a fine red rash over the chest, neck, upper arms, or abdomen). Stay with the patient; put him in a high Fowler's position, use a non-rebreather mask to give high-flow oxygen, and establish a peripheral IV line. Summon the physician immediately as there is about an 80% mortality rate from this complication. Anticipate hydration with IV fluids and correction of acidosis. Intubation and mechanical ventilation may also be needed if oxygen levels cannot be maintained with supplemental oxygen.

 Elder Care Points

The elderly patient with a fractured hip is at high risk for fat embolism. Be especially vigilant and assess for this complication.

Venous Thrombosis. The veins of the pelvis and lower extremities are very vulnerable to thrombus formation after fracture, especially hip fracture. Immobility, traction, and casts may contribute to venous stasis. The Joint Commission's National Quality Core Measures call for aggressive prevention of thrombus formation. Compression stockings, sequential compression devices, and range-of-motion (ROM) exercises on the unaffected lower extremities are used to help prevent the problem. To meet National Patient Safety Goals, nurses must be vigilant for the adverse affects of prophylactic anticoagulant drugs that may be ordered, such as aspirin, warfarin, or low-molecular-weight heparin. Fondaparinux (Arixtra), a new class of antithrombotic drug inhibiting factor X_a, a blood clotting component, may be administered along with warfarin sodium.

Compartment Syndrome. Compartment syndrome is a restriction of blood flow that occurs in one or more muscle compartments of the extremities. Compartment syndrome is caused by external or internal pressure and seriously restricts circulation to the area. External pressure can occur from dressings or casts that are too tight. Internal pressure occurs from excessive IV fluid infusion, inflammation, and edema (a shifting of fluid from the vascular spaces to the intracellular spaces). The increased fluid puts pressure on the tissues, nerves, and blood vessels, thereby decreasing blood flow.

> **⌂ Clinical Cues**
>
> Elevation is the key to preventing compartment syndrome; toes and fingers should be higher than the trunk.

The main sign of compartment syndrome is severe, unrelenting pain that is out of proportion to the injury and unrelieved by narcotics. Assess for the six *P*s: pain, pallor, paresthesia, pulselessness, paralysis, and poikilothermia (cold to the touch) (Wright, 2009).

Recognition and immediate notification of the physician can prevent permanent loss of function. If a cast is in place, the cast can be bivalved (split through all layers of the material). Dressings will be cut or replaced. Surgical fasciotomy (linear incisions in the fascia down the extremity) may be necessary to relieve the pressure on the nerves and blood vessels if other measures do not relieve the problem. Figure 33-7 shows the fascial compartments of the calf and forearm.

❖ NURSING MANAGEMENT

■ Assessment (Data Collection)

Initial Assessment (Pretreatment)

Ask the patient to describe the mechanism of injury. Physical assessment of a suspected fracture includes noting pain, swelling, and discoloration, and deformity

in the contour of the bone. With a possible extremity fracture, pulses should be bilaterally checked and compared. Nerve damage in a fractured leg is assessed by having the patient flex and extend his foot. Next obscure the patient's view and touch a toe with a sharp and then a dull object (e.g., the wooden end and then the cotton-tip end of an applicator, respectively); then ask him to identify which toe was touched and to discriminate sharp and dull touch. For checking nerve damage in the arm, have the patient wave his hand, grip your hand, and use the cotton-tip applicator (as above) on the fingers.

> **! Safety Alert**
>
> In-depth assessment and history must be delayed if a broken bone has pierced the skin and the bleeding is severe. Apply direct pressure over the wound. (Observe for shock and treat if necessary.) Avoid introducing infectious agents into the wound and cover the open area with a sterile dressing (clean dressing if sterile supplies are not available).

> **⌂ Clinical Cues**
>
> In cases of fracture, assessment (six *P*s) of extremities should be done bilaterally. Also remember to ask if the patient is left- or right-hand dominant; dominance can account for a weaker grip, but also if the dominant hand is injured it will affect performance of ADLs.

Pain is not always present when a fracture has occurred. Numbness and tingling can also accompany a fracture. **If there is some question as to whether a bone has been broken, it is best to treat the injury**

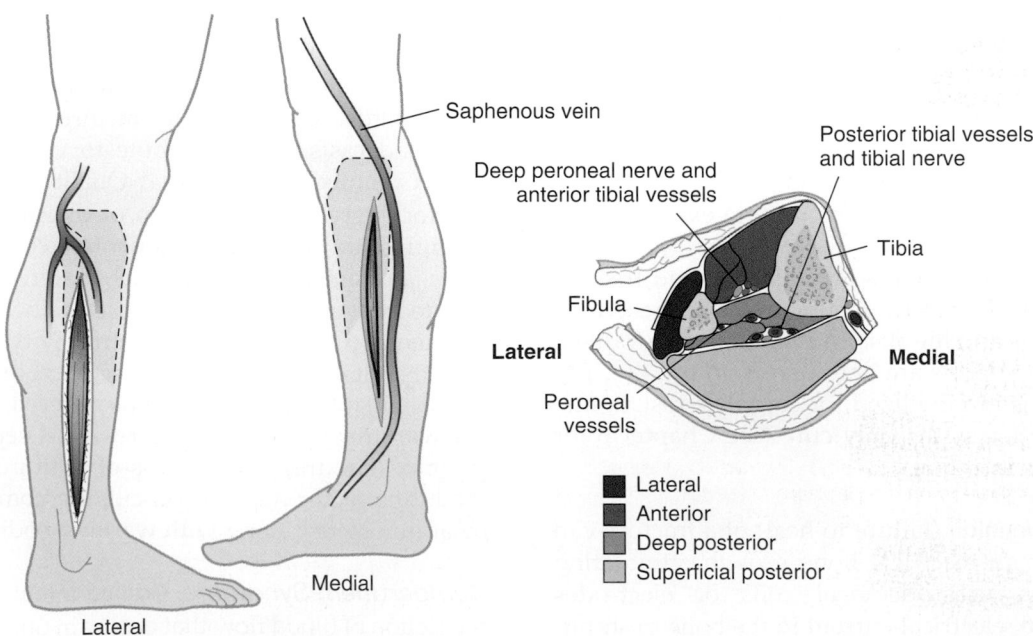

FIGURE 33-7 Fascial compartments of the calf and forearm.

as if it is a fracture. To prevent further trauma and pain, splint the area without moving or manipulating bone. Apply an ice pack, if available, and notify the physician of your findings.

 Think Critically

If you are in the park and you observe a child fall from a tree and obviously suffer a broken forearm, what would you do to assist?

Daily Assessment (Posttreatment)

Attention to pain control is important, especially when the patient is adjusting to fixation devices or a new cast. **If elevating the limb or giving prescribed pain medication does not relieve the patient's complaints within 30 minutes, notify the physician.**

 Focused Assessment

Physical Assessment of Neurovascular Status

Assessment should be performed at least once at the beginning of each shift to establish a baseline for any patient who has suffered a musculoskeletal injury and then performed as required. When a fracture is fresh, this assessment should be performed every 2 to 4 hours.

- *Skin color:* Is the skin pale (decreased blood), blue (decreased oxygenation), bruised (bleeding into surrounding tissues), or red (possible infection)?
- *Skin temperature:* Is the skin increasingly hot to the touch (infection) or cool (decreased blood flow)? Use the back of your hand to do the assessment.
- *Pulses:* Are pulses distal to the injury present and equal bilaterally?
- *Movement:* Can the patient actively move the affected area or the area distal to the injury? If active movement is not possible, passively move the area distal to the injury. How much discomfort is felt with movement?
- *Sensation:* Is numbness or tingling present (paresthesia)? Obscure the patient's view and gently touch a distal area with a paper clip. What and where does the patient feel?
- *Pain:* Where is the pain? What is the nature and intensity? Is pain increasing?
- *Capillary refill:* Does blanching occur when a nail bed distal to the injury is pressed? Assess by pushing on a nail bed, let up, and count the time it takes for color to return. Usual color should return in 3 to 5 seconds.

A thorough assessment of a patient in a cast should include the following:

- Listen to the patient's complaints. If the patient complains of numbness, a tingling sensation, increased pain with motion of the fingers or toes, or sharp localized pain, any of these symptoms could be caused by pressure from a tight cast. Notify the physician if the patient states that he can feel the bone fragments grating against each other (crepitation).
- Check frequently to see whether the cast is properly supported or if there is undue pressure on any underlying part of the body. A sharp, localized, burning pain could mean the beginning of a pressure sore. This should be reported so that the surgeon or orthopedic technician can cut a "window" in the cast to relieve pressure.
- Sniff at the edges of the cast to detect foul odors that are suggestive of infection.

Every immobilized patient should be routinely assessed for the various problems of immobility: skin breakdown, urinary tract infection, constipation, atelectasis, or deep vein thrombosis (DVT). Adequate nutrition and fluids are needed to promote healing and prevent the problems of immobility.

 Nutrition Considerations

Nutrition for Immobile Musculoskeletal Patients

Protein is essential to healing and the diet should be calculated to provide 1 g/kg of body weight. Vitamins D, B, and C and calcium are included in well-balanced meals to ensure optimal soft tissue and bone healing; 500 mg of vitamin C will also help acidify the urine and prevent calcium precipitation that could form kidney stones. Fluid intake of 2000 to 3000 mL/day helps prevent bladder infection, kidney stones, and constipation. A high-fiber diet with lots of vegetables and fruits promotes good bowel function and decreases the chance of constipation. The patient in a hip spica cast or body jacket should receive six small meals a day to avoid abdominal distention and cramping.

 Think Critically

During your neurovascular assessment, you note some decreased sensation and tingling in the fingers of the patient with a lower arm cast. What would you do?

▪ Nursing Diagnosis and Planning

Nursing diagnoses for patients with fractures usually include:

- Pain related to disruption of bone and tissue
- Impaired physical mobility related to disruption of bone
- Self-care deficit related to inability to use an extremity
- Risk for infection related to open fracture

▪ Implementation

Traction devices must be assessed to see that they are in correct position and that the weights are hanging free. The patient's body position should be assessed for proper alignment. Box 33-2 presents points of care.

In caring for the patient with external fixation, for 48 to 72 hours after surgery, the drainage from pin sites may be heavy. Meticulous cleaning of pin sites should be done daily with a 2 mg/mL chlorhexidine solution. The goal is to reduce serosanguineous drainage and crusting that would support infection; also assess for pin loosening (National Guideline Clearinghouse, 2009). Your patient will appreciate a well-organized nurse with a gentle touch, who remembers to premedicate 30 minutes before wound/pin care. For a body part with external pins, daily showering is somewhat

Box 33-2 Points of Care for the Patient in Traction

- Keep the patient in the center of the bed in a supine position.
- Keep the body part in traction in a straight line with the trunk. Misalignment causes pain.
- Be sure the weights are hanging free. If the weights are resting on or against any support, such as the foot of the bed or the floor, the purpose of the traction is defeated. Be careful not to bump against the weights when walking around the foot of the bed. This can be painful to the patient and may cause damage to the healing bone. It is not necessary to lift the weights when pulling the patient up in bed. The amount of pull on the limb will remain the same as long as the weights are hanging free. Also check that the ropes run over the midline of the pulley without interference. Keep knots away from the pulleys, and arrange bedding so that it does not interfere with the ropes and pulleys.
- Check the position of the patient, making sure his body weight is counteracting the pull of the weights. Should the patient slip down in bed so that his feet are resting against the footboard, there will be a loss of force exerted on the limb.
- Observe all bony prominences for signs of impaired circulation and pressure or tissue necrosis.
- To prevent pressure sores, be sure slings and ropes are not pressing against or cutting into an area of the extremity.
- When a patient has skeletal traction, observe the sites of entry of pins, tongs, etc. for signs of infection.
- Devise a systematic routine for observing the patient and the apparatus at specified times during the day so that no aspect of the assessment will be overlooked.

controversial because the water may wash away the protective residual of the chlorhexidine and dressings would need to be changed after every shower (daily dressing changes are of no benefit in preventing infection). Weekly showering may be preferred (Santy et al., 2009).

When the patient is transferred from stretcher to bed, there must be sufficient help available; casts or external fixation devices can be significantly heavy. Pillows for support should be placed on the bed *before* moving the patient onto them. Pillows are used to support the curves of large casts so that the weight of the body will not crack or flatten the cast. The patient in a body cast or spica is more comfortable if pillows are not put under his head and shoulders because the pillows push the chest and abdomen against the front of the cast, causing an uncomfortable crushing sensation and dyspnea. **Hardware of an external fixation device or brace bars between the legs of a cast are never to be used as handles for lifting and turning the patient.** Braces and fixation devices can be displaced if excessive force is applied.

It is important to clarify with the physician how much weight the patient can bear on the affected extremity. Some fractures should have no weight placed on the affected side, whereas other patients will be encouraged to move about without any restrictions.

Care of a Patient with Cast

While the cast plaster is damp (grayish dull appearance), its shape can be changed by careless handling or improper support. Use the palms of the hands or the flat surface of the extended fingers when moving a wet plaster cast because fingertips can sink into the damp plaster and make impressions through the cast that will rub against the tissue under the cast. These can lead to pressure sores. A plaster cast generates heat as it dries; assess the patient's subjective sensation of heat and pain because burns can occur. **During the first 24 to 48 hours after any cast has been applied to an extremity, the extremity should be elevated to minimize swelling.**

The cast should be inspected every day for problems such as flattened areas, soft spots, cracking, and crumbling. The skin around the edges of the cast should receive special attention, including massage with lotion and close observation for signs of pressure or breaks in the skin. Patients must be instructed not to use sharp objects such as pencils or rulers to scratch under the cast. These can tear the skin, leaving an open break for the entrance of bacteria. To relieve itching, use a 60-mL plunger syringe and forcefully direct air under the cast. At home, the patient can use a hair dryer on the coolest setting to blow air into the cast.

A plaster cast will disintegrate if it becomes wet, so the patient will need assistance with bathing. Patients may have permission to shower with a synthetic cast; a plastic covering is secured over the cast and taped to the skin. Instruct the patient to avoid putting the casted area directly under the stream of water.

Depending on the injury or the type of cast, traction, or fixation device, moving or turning the patient for adequate back care may not be allowed or possible. Obtain an order for an overhead trapeze bar so that the patient can lift himself to enable back care to be given and the bottom sheet changed or tightened. Instruct the patient to lift himself straight up so that the amount of pull exerted on the limb in traction will not be altered. This same maneuver can be used when the patient is placed on a bedpan. A small "fracture" bedpan should be used and the lower back supported by a small pillow or folded blanket. When a bedpan is used by the patient in a spica, there is the possibility of a backward flow of urine under the cast unless the head of the bed is slightly elevated. Because the patient cannot bend at the hips to sit up on the pan, the head of the bed should be elevated (on blocks or other device) and the lumbar area of the cast supported to prevent cracking.

When a cast is removed, the underlying skin is usually dry and scaly. Overenthusiastic scrubbing of the area must be avoided to prevent damage to the deeper layers of skin, especially because the cast is frequently reapplied after the physician does the examination. Nursing interventions for selected problems are summarized in Table 32-3.

 Clinical Cues

Ice bags can be used to help control swelling. However, because the weight of an ice bag could make an indentation in a wet plaster cast, the ice bags should be only about half full, and they should be laid against the cast and propped in position, rather than set on top of it.

 Think Critically

Your patient has an arm cast in place and is complaining of severe itching inside the cast. What could you do to help relieve the problem?

■ **Evaluation**

Your patient's pain should be under control and he should be progressing toward independently accomplishing ADLs at his baseline level. There should be no problems associated with immobility (i.e., skin breakdown or constipation, atelectasis, or DVT) or complications (i.e., infection, compartment syndrome). If the goals are not being met, the plan should be revised.

INFLAMMATORY DISORDERS OF THE MUSCULOSKELETAL SYSTEM

LYME DISEASE

Lyme arthritis occurs from a systemic infection caused by the spirochete *Borrelia burgdorferi*. The spirochete is transmitted by the bite of a deer tick. Most cases of this disease are in the New England and mid-Atlantic states, the upper Midwest, and Northern California and Oregon. The disease begins with flu-like symptoms and a "bull's-eye" rash with pain and stiffness in the joints and muscles. Doxycycline, cefuroxime, or amoxicillin taken for 10 to 21 days can prevent the disease's progression. If untreated, 2 to 12 weeks later, stage II begins with carditis and nervous system disorders such as meningitis, peripheral neuritis, or a facial paralysis similar to Bell's palsy. IV antibiotics are the treatment at this point. If undiagnosed and untreated, later chronic complications may occur. The patient may experience fatigue, cognition problems, and arthralgias. In some instances the only sign of Lyme disease is arthritis. Lyme arthritis can cause permanent damage to the nervous system and to the joints.

OSTEOARTHRITIS

Etiology and Pathophysiology

The word *arthritis*, translated literally, means inflammation of a joint. **Osteoarthritis** is a noninflammatory degenerative joint disease that can affect any weight-bearing joint. The exact cause is not known, but risk factors include heredity, aging, female gender, obesity, previous joint injury, and recreational or occupational usage of joints (Lucas, 2009). People with osteoarthritis seem to produce less collagen to strengthen cartilage and cover and protect joints in the body. With time and use, joints become thickened and withstand weight bearing poorly, with consequent damage to cartilage. The synovial cells then release enzymes that cause further cartilage degeneration.

 Health Promotion

Healthy People 2020 Goals Related to Arthritis

The objectives aimed at reducing the disability caused by arthritis include:

- Reducing the mean level of joint pain, activity limitations, care limitations, effect on employment, and the proportion of those who find it "very difficult" to perform specific joint-related activities.
- Increasing health care provider counseling for weight and physical activity; the proportion of those seeing a health care provider for joint symptoms and effective evidence-based arthritis education as an integral part of the managing condition.

Signs, Symptoms, and Diagnosis

Osteoarthritis occurs asymmetrically and typically affects only one or two joints. The chief symptoms are aching pain with joint movement and stiffness, with limitation of mobility. Joints may be deformed and nodules may be present.

Treatment

Treatment consists of pain management, strengthening and aerobic exercise, weight reduction if the patient is overweight, and maintenance of joint function. Salicylates, acetaminophen, or NSAIDs may be used. Acetaminophen in doses of 1000 mg, up to 4000 mg/day, is the standard for the patient with mild to moderate joint pain.

‼ **Safety Alert**

Acetaminophen Usage

All other medications and over-the-counter drugs should be checked for acetaminophen so that overdose does not occur. Taking more of this drug than recommended (no more than 4000 mg/day) can cause irreversible liver damage. The drug should not be taken when drinking alcohol. For the elderly person, the lowest effective dose should be used. Encourage an adequate intake of water, at least 2000 mL, each day to promote excretion of the drug via the kidneys.

Elder Care Points

NSAIDs are not recommended for all elderly persons because of side effects and interactions with other drugs that elderly patients may be taking. NSAIDs decrease effectiveness of the angiotensin-converting enzyme (ACE) inhibitors used for hypertension and heart failure, and NSAIDs increase the effects of anticoagulants.

Corticosteroid injection into the arthritic joint is performed if oral medication does not control the problem. Exercises for joint mobility are encouraged. Surgery or joint replacement may be done to relieve severe pain and improve mobility. The hip and knee are the most common sites for joint replacement.

Complementary and Alternative Therapies

Therapies for Pain Relief

Yoga and massage can help to control and relieve the pain of osteoarthritis. In a Cochrane review, authors concluded that acupuncture can have some small and beneficial effects for reducing pain and improving function in patients with peripheral joint arthritis; however, expectations or the placebo effect may be contributing to these outcomes (Manheimer et al., 2004). Capsaicin cream, or ointment made from cayenne red pepper, blocks pain locally when applied topically to the inflamed joint. It can be used four times a day. It is available over the counter or by prescription. In a research study, Shimoda and colleagues (2010) found that red ginger has anti-inflammatory properties that relieve arthritis pain.

Complementary and Alternative Therapies

Glucosamine and Chondroitin

Glucosamine and chondroitin have been shown in a research study to decrease the pain of osteoarthritis and to contribute to the synthesis of new cartilage. This substance may slow or halt the progression of osteoarthritis. Patients may try 1500 mg of glucosamine sulfate per day as a trial dose (Anderson, 2010).

Injections of hyaluronic acid (HA) (Orthovisc, Synvisc, Supartz, and Hyalgan) into the joint can act as a lubricant and decrease pain and improve function. The intra-articular injections are given once a week for 3 to 5 weeks and may be repeated in 6 months.

A new treatment for knee cartilage injury is the injection of autologous chondrocytes. Healthy articular cartilage cells are removed from the patient and sent to a special laboratory where they are grown for 3 to 4 weeks and then reimplanted. Patients use crutches for 6 to 8 weeks after the surgery. The procedure is successful in about 85% of all cases. It works best in patients younger than age 50 with injury to a small focal area of cartilage (Cluett, 2010).

Nursing Management

Nursing interventions for osteoarthritis include teaching the patient to balance exercise and rest. Gentle exercise is very important in maintaining joint mobility. Walking, knitting, and swimming all help improve mobility and decrease pain. The patient should avoid placing stress on affected joints. Suggest the use of assistive devices to open containers and perform other household functions.

Instruct for moist heat application, and encourage the patient to maintain weight within normal limits. Weight reduction decreases joint stress. Imagery, relaxation, and diversion are helpful to reduce pain. Quadriceps strengthening exercises may relieve pain and disability of the knee (see Patient Teaching on p. 729).

Think Critically

Where would you suggest a patient look for assistive devices available to those with arthritis?

RHEUMATOID ARTHRITIS

Etiology and Pathophysiology

Rheumatoid arthritis (RA) is an inflammatory disease of the joints. It can occur at any age, but is more common among older women. The cause is not known, but hormonal, environmental, genetic, or infectious agents may trigger an underlying autoimmune reaction. An abnormal immune response causes an inflammatory reaction of the synovial membrane. Vasodilation, increased permeability, and the formation of exudate cause red, swollen joints. Rheumatoid factor (RF), which is an antibody against immunoglobulin G, appears in the blood and synovial fluid in most patients.

There are remissions and exacerbations of the disease. As the disease progresses, pannus is formed. *Pannus* is granulation tissue derived from the synovium that spreads over the articular cartilage. Pannus releases enzymes and inflammatory mediators that destroy cartilage. The cartilage becomes eroded and the pannus cuts off nutrition to the cartilage. Over time, the pannus between the bone ends becomes fibrotic, causing ankylosis. Joint fixation and deformity become apparent. Along with these changes, exacerbations cause more damage and there is atrophy of muscles around the joint. Tendons and ligaments stretch and the joint becomes unstable. Muscle spasm draws the bones out of normal alignment. Contractures and deformity occur. Mobility becomes impaired if the knees or ankles are affected. Subcutaneous nodules may form and nodules may occur in the pleura, heart valves, or eyes.

Signs, Symptoms, and Diagnosis

The signs and symptoms of RA are joint pain, warmth, edema, limitation of motion, and multiple joint stiffness in the morning lasting more than 1 hour. The joints of the hands, wrists, and feet are most commonly affected by RA, and involvement is usually bilateral. Subcutaneous nodules may appear over bony prominences. Systemic symptoms of low-grade fever, anorexia with weight loss, malaise, and an iron deficiency anemia resistant to iron therapy may also be present. Joint deformity and consequent dysfunction can occur.

Table 33-1	Comparison of Rheumatoid Arthritis and Osteoarthritis	
CHARACTERISTIC	**RHEUMATOID ARTHRITIS**	**OSTEOARTHRITIS**
Definition	A systemic disease, but pathologic changes and disability result from chronic inflammation of the joints	A progressive degenerative joint disease
Pathology	Chronic inflammation of synovial membranes and formation of chronic granulation tissue (pannus) in the joint; pannus capable of eroding cartilage in joints and spreading to bone, ligaments, and tendons	Microscopic changes in the cartilage in the joint; eventually there is loss of cartilage, bony enlargement, and malalignment of joints
Etiology	Unknown; evidence that the pathologic changes are immunologic	Unknown; may be caused by "wear and tear" of aging
Rheumatoid factors (autoantibodies)	Usually present	Usually absent
Age at onset	30-40 yr	50-60 yr; rarely before age 40
Weight	Normal or underweight	Usually overweight
General state of health	Usually anemic, "chronically ill," with low-grade fever and slight leukocytosis	Well nourished
Appearance of joints	*Early:* Soft-tissue swelling *Late:* Ankylosis, extreme deformity Joint involvement usually symmetrical and generalized	*Early:* Slight joint enlargement *Late:* Enlargement more pronounced, slight limitation of motion Joints usually involved are single-sided and weight-bearing: spine, hips, knees
Muscles	Pronounced muscular atrophy, particularly in later stages	Usually not affected
Other	Morning stiffness; pain on motion; swelling and tenderness of joints; subcutaneous nodules; typical rheumatoid changes seen on radiograph	Stiffness, relieved by moderate motion; joint malalignment; symptoms increase in cold, wet weather

RA pain or immobility of joints interferes with self-care activities necessary to lead an independent lifestyle. Maintaining mobility and controlling pain with the least amount of side effects are the goals for the elderly patient. Table 33-1 presents a comparison of osteoarthritis and rheumatoid arthritis.

According to the American College of Rheumatology, diagnosis is by history of morning stiffness that lasts more than 1 hour, or arthritis pain in three or more joints that lasts more than 6 weeks (Neal-Boylan, 2009). Blood tests for RF, C-reactive protein, and erythrocyte sedimentation rate are ordered. Radiographs confirm the cartilage destruction and bone deformities.

Treatment
Treatment is aimed at relieving pain, minimizing joint destruction, promoting joint function, and preserving ability to perform self-care (Table 33-2). Rest and exercise, medication, immobilization with splints and use of other supportive devices during periods of severe inflammation, and hot and cold treatments are standard treatments. Surgical joint repair or replacement can be done to reduce pain and improve mobility.

NSAIDs (e.g., ibuprofen) are the first-line agents used for arthritis pain. Other medications include salicylates, corticosteroids, antimalarial drugs, methotrexate, gold compounds, sulfasalazine, D-penicillamine, and disease-modifying antirheumatic drugs (DMARDs). Tumor necrosis factor (TNF) inhibitors are a newer type of medication. Systemic corticosteroids have a profound anti-inflammatory effect on arthritis. They were once thought to be "miracle drugs" to treat arthritis; however, their anti-inflammatory action tends to diminish over time, thus requiring higher doses to obtain the same results. Long-term steroid therapy increases the risk for diabetes mellitus, osteoporosis, hypertension, acne, cataracts, and weight gain; therefore long-term oral steroid preparations are reserved for patients who cannot find relief from other drugs. DMARDs provide periods of remission, but they also have some serious side effects. Patients should be tested for tuberculosis (TB) before being started on TNF inhibitors because these drugs may exacerbate TB.

Complementary and Alternative Therapies

Help Patients to Evaluate the Safety of Complementary and Alternative Therapies

Callahan and colleagues (2009) conducted a cross-sectional study of 2141 arthritis patients and found that almost every subject had tried various forms of complementary and alternative medicine (CAM). Patients were most satisfied with dietary, spiritual, and mind-body therapies. Patients with arthritis are particularly vulnerable to "miracle cures" or outright quackery; therefore it is the responsibility of all health care professionals to initiate a dialogue about CAM or other methods that the patient is using in order to evaluate the safety and to incorporate these self-care methods into the overall plan of care.

Table 33-2 **Drugs Used to Treat Rheumatoid Arthritis**

CLASSIFICATION	ACTION/EFFECTS	EXAMPLES	NURSING IMPLICATIONS
Nonsteroidal anti-inflammatory drugs (NSAIDs)	Reduce inflammation and pain	Aspirin, ibuprofen (Advil, Motrin), naproxen sodium (Aleve), COX-2 inhibitors (Celebrex)	May take 2 wk to obtain results; give with food or a full glass of water, but some are best taken 30 min before a meal or 2 hr afterward. May cause GI irritation. Monitor hematologic, renal, liver, auditory, ophthalmic functions, weight gain, and peripheral edema. Teach patient to report heartburn, dyspepsia, nausea, vomiting, diarrhea, or abdominal pain. Teach to avoid alcohol because of increased risk of GI irritation. Dosage in elderly may need to be reduced by half.
Corticosteroids	Reduce inflammation, decrease pain by suppressing the immune system	Prednisone, methylprednisolone (Medrol)	Usually rapid action. Instruct to take daily dose between 6 and 8 A.M. when natural steroids are released. Instruct not to stop taking this drug abruptly. Taper dosage downward as soon as symptoms improve. Monitor elderly closely for fluid retention, elevated blood pressure, and peripheral edema. Handle patients gently to prevent bruising; avoid using tape on skin. May cause osteoporosis, Cushing syndrome, mood changes, weight gain, cataracts, onset of diabetes, muscle weakness, and increased risk of infection.
Disease-modifying antirheumatic drugs (DMARDs)	Reduce inflammation and pain, suppress the immune system, and prevent joint and cartilage destruction	Hydroxychloroquine (Plaquenil), sulfasalazine (Azulfidine), gold salts (Ridaura), D-penicillamine (Cuprimine, Depen), methotrexate (Rheumatrex), azathioprine (Imuran), leflunomide (Arava), others	Plaquenil takes 6 mo to be effective; others take 1-6 mo. May cause rash, diarrhea, and retinal problems. Instruct that frequent eye examinations are necessary. Most of the drugs can cause GI symptoms and blood dyscrasias; monitor blood counts. Gold salts can cause liver toxicity; monitor liver functions. Methotrexate can cause pulmonary, renal, and liver toxicity. Imuran and leflunomide may cause birth defects or fetal death. Alcohol use increases chance of hepatic toxicity. Monitor blood and urine weekly. Check specific nursing implications for each drug.
Biologic therapies (Classifications include tumor necrosis factor inhibitors, interleukin antagonists, selective costimulation modulators or targeted B-cell therapy)	Reduce inflammation by blocking the inflammatory response	Etanercept (Enbrel), infliximab (Remicade), anakinra (Kineret), adalimumab (Humira), abatacept (Orencia) Tocilizumab (Actemra) Denosumab (Prolia)	1-2 wk for onset of action. Increased risk of serious infection and blood dyscrasias; monitor blood counts, temperature, and for malaise closely. May cause demyelinating disorders. Given IV or by subcutaneous injection; may cause injection site reaction. Do not immunize with live virus vaccines. Test for tuberculosis before starting these medications.

Clinical Cues

Monitor patients taking NSAIDs for gastrointestinal (GI) intolerance. Assess liver, kidney, and central nervous system function frequently. Watch for signs of blood dyscrasias and check for tinnitus and hearing loss regularly. The side effects of NSAIDs can be serious and sometimes permanent. If early signs of toxicity appear, they should be reported promptly to the physician.

The injection of steroids directly into a joint (intra-articular administration) has been used successfully in treating painful flare-ups, shortening the period of inflammation, and relieving pain and other symptoms. When intra-articular steroid therapy is used, it is recommended that not more than two or three doses be injected into any joint within 1 year's time.

Elder Care Points

Elderly arthritis patients must be taught to watch for side effects and promptly report to the physician or nurse. Dizziness, which predisposes to falls, can occur with analgesics for arthritis pain, particularly if the medication contains codeine. Advise patients to arise slowly, hold on to furniture until steady, use assistive devices, and to wait for dizziness to pass before walking.

Surgical Intervention and Orthopedic Devices. Casts or braces and splints (orthoses) sometimes are used to immobilize an affected part so that it can rest during an active phase of the arthritic disease. Devices that immobilize the affected joint should allow for motion of adjacent muscles, thereby improving muscle strength and permitting more independence on the part of the patient. Braces also work to prevent deformities by maintaining optimal functional position of the joints.

In the past, surgical intervention for arthritis was reserved for patients who already had suffered severe joint deformity and loss of motion. Currently, the trend is to use surgery in the early stages of arthritis to prevent, or at least modify, deformities and mechanical abnormalities. One such surgical procedure is *synovectomy*, which is the excision of the synovial membrane of a joint. The goal of synovectomy is to interrupt the destructive inflammatory process that eventually leads to ankylosis and invasion of surrounding cartilage and bone tissues. For younger patients with osteoarthritis, *osteotomy* may be an option. In this procedure a wedge of bone is removed to allow for realignment. Tendon reconstruction is performed most frequently on the hand to restore function.

Joint Replacement. An arthroplasty (joint replacement) may be done for a knee, shoulder, elbow, finger, ankle, or hip. The hip and knee are the most frequently replaced joints. Noncemented press-fit prostheses are often used now for young, heavier, and very active patients. The cement used for bone prostheses has a life span of about 10 years.

Total hip replacement. The primary purpose of total hip replacement (THR) is to relieve chronic pain. Hip replacement for osteoarthritis can be performed with minimally invasive surgery and shorter hospital stay for some patients. A hip joint may be replaced with either a low-friction polyurethane socket for the acetabulum with a metallic replacement for the head of the femur or with synthetic materials combined with a porous bone implant (Figure 33-8). The porous bone implant requires 6 weeks of healing, and cemented prostheses patients refrain from full weight bearing for 4 to 6 weeks. For some patients, full weight bearing is avoided for 3 to 6 months. Crutches or a walker are used for ambulation, depending on the ability of the patient. The greatest dangers to successful replacement are infection and failure to function. Possible

FIGURE 33-8 Hip replacement prosthesis.

dislocation is also an issue; this can occur if the hip is internally rotated.

Another procedure is hip resurfacing surgery. This is a bone-conserving hip procedure that can be done to help with pain, improve ambulation, and restore joint function. The procedure involves placing a metal cap over the end of the femur without extensive resecting of the bone. A metal cup is placed in the hip socket and the capped end rotates in the cup (Amanatullah et al., 2010). The advantage of this procedure is that the patient is better prepared for more extensive surgery in the future.

Preoperative care. Preoperatively, the hip replacement patient is given specific instructions about the kind of surgery to be performed, the prosthesis to be used, the postsurgical procedures, and what is expected of him to help achieve the goals of rehabilitation. He is given instructions in postoperative exercises and in the use of ambulation equipment, such as a walker, crutches, or canes. The patient may wish to donate some blood several weeks before surgery in case a blood transfusion becomes necessary after surgery.

A surgical bacteriostatic scrub solution is usually prescribed for use during the daily shower for several days before hip replacement to lessen the chance of infection. Tell the patient that he will be placed in an orthopedic bed with an overhead trapeze bar attached after surgery. He may be transported to and from the operating room on the bed if he is hospitalized before surgery. Show the patient the triangular abductor pillow and explain the between-the-legs position and turning postoperatively (see Chapter 5).

Postoperative care. A blood salvage unit may be in place to collect blood drainage that is then filtered and returned to the patient. There is usually a drain at the surgical hip replacement site with a suction device attached to it. IV fluids will be administered. A Foley catheter will usually be in place. Immediately after surgery, nursing intervention includes all the measures

FIGURE 33-9 Abduction wedge in place to prevent dislocation of hip prosthesis.

required to avoid respiratory and circulatory complications. However, extreme care must be exercised in positioning and repositioning the patient. To prevent dislocation, an abduction wedge or pillow may be secured between the legs (usually in the operating room) and is left in place when the patient is in bed until the surgeon requests its removal (Figure 33-9). The wedge is positioned with the narrower end between the thighs, and the straps should not go over an incision, bony prominence, or drain.

⚠️ Safety Alert

Precautions with Hip Abductor Wedge

Circulation should be checked after each application of the wedge to be certain that the straps are not too tight. Skin should be assessed every shift on the surface of the legs with particular attention to areas over bony prominences.

DVT is a possible complication of joint replacement. Low-molecular-weight heparin, enoxaparin (Lovenox), dalteparin (Fragmin), or tinzaparin (Innohep) can be administered to prevent this problem. It works more quickly than sodium heparin and causes less incidence of hemorrhage because it does not prevent platelets from aggregating at bleeding injury sites. Daily coagulation studies are not needed with this drug as its anticoagulant action is very predictable and stable. It is usually given in a 30-mg dose by subcutaneous injection into the abdomen twice a day.

In most cases the hip replacement patient is allowed to stand at the bedside on the first postoperative day, supported by a walker and two persons. Weight bearing on the operated joint is sometimes allowed, but there should be a specific written order from the physician. The patient will need instruction in transferring himself from bed to chair, wheelchair, and toilet. Whenever he sits, the chair seat should

be raised so that the hips are not flexed beyond a 90-degree angle. In addition to these instructions, the patient may be referred for outpatient or in-home physical therapy. Nursing interventions for selected problems of a patient with total hip replacement (THR) are summarized in Nursing Care Plan 33-1 (see also Nursing Care Plan 5-1). The rehabilitation team includes the patient, family, surgeon, nurse, physical therapist, and occupational therapist.

👥 Patient Teaching

Total Hip Replacement Discharge Teaching

Before he is discharged, the patient who has undergone hip surgery should be given instructions so he can care for himself at home. These include:
- It is all right to lie on your operated side.
- For 3 months you should not cross your legs.
- You should put a pillow between your legs when you roll over on your abdomen or lie on your side in bed.
- It is all right to bend your hip, but not beyond a right (90-degree) angle (demonstrate); avoid sitting in low chairs.
- Continue your daily exercise program at home in the same way you did the exercises at the hospital.

Total knee replacement. Chronic, uncontrollable pain is the main indication for knee arthroplasty. Part or all of the knee joint may be replaced. For the best postoperative result, emphasis is placed on exercise. A continuous passive motion (CPM) machine may be used soon after surgery (see Figure 32-5). To tolerate the exercise, the patient must be well medicated for pain. Within 2 to 5 days, quadriceps-strengthening exercises and straight-leg raising are started. Quadriceps exercise is accomplished by lying supine, straightening the legs, and pushing the back of the knees into the bed. Exercises are taught by the physical therapist, and the nurse often assists the patient in performing them. The arthroplasty patient then progresses to ambulation with a walker or crutches. Other preoperative and postoperative care is similar to that of the patient undergoing any major surgery. After early release from the hospital, the patient continues physical therapy in the outpatient setting.

❖ NURSING MANAGEMENT

■ Assessment (Data Collection)

The RA patient lives every day with pain, limited motion, and the chronic and incurable nature of arthritis; therefore you must carefully seek in-depth information about the patient's social history, his personal and family health history, current general health status, ability to do the things he wants to do, and his experience of pain and how he has been dealing with it.

☆ Nursing Care Plan 33-1 | Care of the Patient after a Total Hip Replacement

Scenario

Miko Yoshima, an 85-year-old woman, has just undergone a total hip replacement for a hip joint damaged by osteoarthritis. She normally lives alone, but has relatives within a 30-minute driving distance. She had been actively gardening and taking care of herself until pain severely limited her mobility over the last few months. (This care plan is specific to problems of hip replacement. All usual care for a postoperative patient should also be included [wound care, respiratory care, monitoring for complications, etc.].)

Problem/Nursing Diagnosis

Restricted from weight bearing/Impaired physical mobility related to pain and activity restrictions after hip replacement.

Supporting Assessment Data

Subjective: "I'm quite uncomfortable."
Objective: Orders for non–weight bearing and up in chair tid; abduction wedge in place when in bed.

Goals/Expected Outcomes	Nursing Interventions	Selected Rationale	Evaluation
Patient will regain sufficient mobility to care for self at home within 3 mo.	Teach use of walker. Encourage ROM and exercises to improve muscle strength and joint flexibility.	Proper use of walker will help prevent falls and injury. ROM helps prevent joint problems in unaffected joints. Exercises decrease muscle atrophy and help strengthen muscles for ambulation.	PT will instruct in use of walker tomorrow. Assisted to perform ROM on shoulders, upper extremities, and other leg. Encouraged ankle rotations and foot exercises on affected leg with supervision.

Problem/Nursing Diagnosis

Incisional pain and joint stiffness/Acute pain related to surgical incision and rehabilitation therapy.

Supporting Assessment Data

Subjective: "My pain is at a 6 on a scale of 1 to 10."
Objective: Face appears pinched and patient is not moving in bed at all.

Goals/Expected Outcomes	Nursing Interventions	Selected Rationale	Evaluation
Patient will experience pain control with patient-controlled analgesia (PCA) pump within 1 hr.	Reinforce instructions on PCA use.	Knowledge of how to use pump provides medication for pain control.	Reinforced instructions; encouraging PCA use as needed.
Patient will have adequate pain control on oral analgesia before discharge.	Assess for pain when vital signs are taken.	Constant monitoring for pain can indicate need for more medication to keep pain from escalating.	Pain level between 2 and 6/10.
	Administer medication bolus per orders PRN.	Administering a bolus of pain medication can stop pain from increasing.	Bolus administered for pain level of 6/10.
	Monitor for excessive sedation, respiratory depression, decreased level of consciousness (LOC), and confusion.	Excessive sedation, respiratory depression, decreased LOC, and confusion can indicate medication toxicity and danger for the patient.	No signs of problems of toxicity or central nervous system (CNS) depression.
	Provide comfort measures: keep linens smooth and clean, reposition q 2 hr and PRN, keep environment quiet and orderly.	Comfort measures and warmth help decrease pain perception.	Provided comfort measures. Replaced warm blankets q 2 hr, as needed.
	Keep warm with added warmed blankets. Put on socks if feet are cold.		Socks with slip-resistant soles applied.

PRN, as needed; *ROM,* range of motion.

Continued

Nursing Care Plan 33-1   Care of the Patient after a Total Hip Replacement—cont'd

Problem/Nursing Diagnosis
Not familiar with needed self-care/Knowledge deficit related to precautions necessary after total hip surgery to prevent dislocation of operative hip.

Supporting Assessment Data
Subjective: "No one I know has had this surgery."

Goals/Expected Outcome	Nursing Interventions	Selected Rationale	Evaluation
Patient will verbalize movement restrictions to prevent hip dislocation within 24 hr.	Explain positional restrictions: no flexion of the hip past 90 degrees, no internal rotation, no adduction of the affected leg.	Flexion, internal rotation, or adduction of the leg may cause hip dislocation. Knowledge is necessary to comply with instructions.	Explained position restrictions.
	Advise not to cross the legs or to bend over from the hips to tie shoes or pick up something off the floor.	These maneuvers cause internal rotation and more than 90 degrees of flexion.	Advised about additional restrictions after discharge. Written instructions given.
	Instruct to only use a raised toilet seat for toileting.	Normal-height toilet seat may cause too much flexion.	States has raised toilet seat at home. Knows to use handicapped toilet stalls when out in public.
	Advise to report pain in hip, buttock, or thigh or continued limp.	Pain or continued limp may indicate dislocation.	Verbalizes understanding of symptoms to report.

Problem/Nursing Diagnosis
Potential for clot formation/Risk for ineffective tissue perfusion.

Supporting Assessment Data
Objective: Decreased mobility and total hip replacement.

Goals/Expected Outcome	Nursing Interventions	Selected Rationale	Evaluation
Patient will not experience deep vein thrombosis before discharge.	Encourage foot and calf exercises q 2 hr.	Encourages circulation and helps prevent clot formation.	Performing exercises q 2 hr while awake.
	Assist and encourage in prescribed physical therapy.		Working with PT.
	Administer low-molecular-weight heparin injections as ordered.	Decreases ability of blood to clot.	Heparin injections administered into abdomen as ordered.
	Assess for signs of thrombus formation, checking calf for warmth, swelling, and pain on foot dorsiflexion.	Finding a thrombus early aids in preventing further extension of clot and preventing embolus.	No redness, swelling, warmth, or pain in affected leg's calf.
	Monitor INR (1.5-2.0 for DVT prophylaxis).	INR indicates potential for blood clotting and thrombus formation.	INR (1.5) within desired limits.

Critical Thinking Questions
1. Besides venous thrombosis, what other complications might occur in this patient?
2. If the patient is anxious about discharge, what could you specifically do to help dispel her anxiety?

DVT, deep vein thrombosis; *INR*, international normalized ratio; *PT*, physical therapist; *tid*, three times a day.

Focused Assessment

Data Collection for the Patient with Rheumatoid Arthritis

During history taking, ask about:
- Pain pattern and pain medication use; other coping methods
- Degree of stiffness and duration after arising
- Family history of rheumatoid arthritis or immune disorders
- Diagnosis with accompanying disorders, such as interstitial lung disease, pericarditis, eye problems, and vasculitis
- Smoking history
- Fatigue level and degree of malaise and methods of coping
- Presence of fever
- Exercise pattern
- Ability to perform ADLs; ability to work; ability for home maintenance
- Adaptive equipment in use
- Usual roles at work, home, and community and social involvement
- Joint deformity or swelling of joints
- Symmetrical involvement from one side of the body to the other
- Pain and degree of limitation with joint movement

■ Nursing Diagnosis and Planning

Nursing diagnoses for arthritis depend on the degree of disability the disease is causing. Common nursing diagnoses might include:
- Chronic pain related to inflamed joints
- Impaired physical mobility related to pain, stiffness, and joint deformity
- Disturbed body image related to joint deformities

Expected outcomes for the above nursing diagnoses of arthritis and subsequent surgical or nonsurgical interventions might be:
- Patient's pain will be controlled with medications, heat, and exercise within 2 weeks.
- Patient's mobility will improve with the use of assistive devices and physical therapy within 3 weeks.
- Patient will demonstrate acceptance of self and appearance by wearing attractive clothing.

Plan for extra time for your patient with arthritis to perform self-care and to ambulate. Allow sufficient time; rushing the patient causes frustration and embarrassment. Even simple procedures will probably take longer, because the patient may not be able to move and turn as easily as a person without arthritis.

■ Implementation and Evaluation

Nursing interventions for arthritis are aimed at providing a balance of rest and exercise, freedom from pain, minimizing emotional stress, preventing or correcting deformities, and maintaining or restoring function so that the patient can enjoy as much independence and mobility as possible.

Rest and Exercise

The purpose of rest is to allow the body's natural defenses and healing powers to overcome the inflammatory process of arthritis. The more inflamed a joint is,

the more rest is needed; this includes rest of the joint and the whole body. Fatigue is a common problem with arthritis and usually requires that the patient has rest periods during the day before he becomes too fatigued or exhausted. During periods of acute exacerbation of arthritis symptoms, the patient may need continuous bed rest. When the patient is lying down, he should maintain good body position and avoid pillows and other devices that support joints in a position of flexion. A firm mattress is recommended, with only one pillow under the head and neck.

It is necessary, however, even in the acute phase of arthritis, to balance rest with exercise. The patient should sit to do tasks whenever possible. Activities should be paced and interspersed with rest. The exercise program is prescribed on the basis of assessment of each patient's status, the severity of inflammation, the particular joints affected by arthritis, and the patient's tolerance for activity. Because anemia and other blood disorders can accompany arthritis, the fatigue experienced by a patient may be somewhat alleviated by correcting underlying blood disorders.

Enlist the patient's cooperation to increase compliance with exercises that must be continued at home. Teach the patient how to perform specific exercises so that they do not increase his pain. Each exercise should be done 3 to 10 times for each joint, with the lower number used on days when pain or fatigue is increased. When joints are inflamed, exercises should not be done. In many instances, doing the exercises in the right way can diminish discomfort. If pain persists for hours after exercises have been done, the patient's status should be reassessed and the exercise program revised. Precautions to avoid joint injury are always necessary for routine physical activities at home, general exercise, or a prescribed exercise program at home.

Patient Teaching

Instructions for Joint Protection

- Always stop an exercise at the point of real pain. Some discomfort can be expected, but it should be minimal. If your joints are still hurting 1 or 2 hours after exercise, you have done too much.
- Always use your biggest muscles and strongest joints. For example, push doors open with your arm instead of your hand; carry a shoulder bag instead of a hand purse.
- Try to do only those jobs that will allow you to stop and rest if you need to when pain develops. Conserve your energy for the things you really want to do.
- Exercise in a way that does not put strain on the joints. Exercising in water decreases joint strain.
- Slow down and move slowly and smoothly. Avoid rapid, jerky movements. Use the palms of the hands rather than the fingers to push up from a bed or chair when arising.
- Turn doorknobs counterclockwise to prevent extensive twisting of the elbow.

Continued

Patient Teaching

Instructions for Joint Protection—cont'd

- Do not lift weights. Pick up heavier items with two hands.
- Let swollen, red, hot, and painful joints rest as much as possible. Do not use them any more than absolutely necessary.
- Change your body position frequently, alternating standing, sitting, and lying down.
- Set your own limits and compete with yourself, not with anyone else.
- Use assistive/adaptive devices, such as Velcro closures and built-up utensil handles to protect joints of the hands. Use a long-handled hair brush.

Applications of Heat and Cold

Either hot or cold may be suitable for treating arthritic joints, depending on the patient's preference and the effectiveness of each. The purpose of either hot or cold applications is to minimize pain, increase the joint's ROM, and improve exercise performance. In general, heat is better for subacute or chronic joint inflammation and cold is more effective in the acute phase when joints are hot, red, and obviously inflamed.

Various forms of heat therapy can be used, including moist or dry heat and superficial or deep heat. For dry heat, a therapeutic infrared lamp is convenient and inexpensive for home use. For treatment of the hands, paraffin baths are effective. Wet heat can be applied by hot tub baths with the water temperature not exceeding 102° F (39° C) or by means of a towel dipped in hot water, wrung out, and applied to the joint. Whirlpool baths promote relaxation and motion with minimal pain, especially when prolonged treatment is indicated. However, immersing the whole body in warm water can cause physiologic changes in respiration and pulse rate and may be contraindicated in debilitated or elderly patients. The patient will need specific instructions on how to avoid injury to the skin and other hazards.

 Safety Alert

Caution with Heat Application

Patients who have decreased sensation in a body part must be very careful when applying heat or they may experience burns. Teach the family and patient to test the degree of heat being applied and to check the area after 5 minutes to make certain that burning is not occurring. A cloth should always be placed between the heat device and the skin.

 Think Critically

If a patient asks about using a heating pad on the joint, what instructions would you give?

 Patient Teaching

Safe Application of Heat and Cold

HEAT
- Recommended for chronic or subacute inflammation.
- Heat should be used for 20 to 30 minutes at a time; repeat the application every 1 to 2 hours while awake.
- Use a shower massager for massage pulsation. Regulate water by turning on cold and adding hot water to desired temperature *before* entering the shower. Use a shower stool if balance is poor or fatigue is likely.
- Use a pad between the heat source and the skin to prevent burning.
- Use the type of heating pad that provides moist heat; it will penetrate best. Do not sleep on the heating pad. Use the low settings because heating pads often cause burns when turned up too high or used for too long.
- Reusable heat packs mold well to body parts because they are pliable. Follow directions explicitly, and test temperature by feel of pack on skin before applying to area in need. Use a light pad or thin dishtowel between pack and skin. Heat in microwave oven. Reheat as needed.
- Heat-producing ointments and gels containing menthol, camphor, capsaicin, or papain (extract from red peppers) may be applied to the sore muscle or joint as long as they do not produce skin irritation. Covering the area after application with plastic wrap helps hold the heat in longer. Wash hands thoroughly after application to prevent eye irritation.

COLD
- Recommended for acute phase of inflammation or acute pain.
- Do not apply to one area for more than 10 to 20 minutes at a time; apply no more than once an hour.
- Discontinue when numbness occurs.
- Not recommended for patients with impaired circulation.
- Ice water bath is useful for hand or foot. Extremity can be exercised during treatment.
- Ice pack can be made by partially filling double plastic bag with ice. Zip-type closures work best. May use thin pad or dishtowel between pack and skin.
- Commercial cold packs mold to body part better than ice bag. Does not stay cold very long. Often takes two of these to finish 10- to 20-minute treatment. Commercial cold pack can be refrozen in the freezer. Disposable chemical packs that are activated when needed are also available.
- Freeze ice in paper cup; peel back part of cup to use so that cup provides a handgrip. Wear rubber glove or use pad to protect hand from ice. Rub ice over body part until skin feels numb, but no longer than 10 to 15 minutes at a time.
- Dry skin well after treatment.

Diet

No special diet will cure or relieve arthritis, in spite of many fraudulent claims to the contrary. However, some patients find that eliminating foods from the "nightshade" family, such as tomatoes, decreases their joint pain. The patient should eat an average, well-balanced diet with no excess or limitations in amount or types of foods. Explain that obesity can put additional stress on the weight-bearing joints and aggravate the arthritic condition; then help the patient review strategies for weight control.

Psychosocial Care

As deformities occur, self-esteem can be affected. Encourage verbalization of feelings. Express acceptance of the patient's appearance. Suggest clothing options that may minimize visible changes. A support group sometimes helps to reframe the disease's effects on the body. Encourage the arthritis patient to gain as much control over the disease as possible with appropriate coping mechanisms, pacing, exercise, and medication.

Resources for Patient and Family Education

The Arthritis Foundation provides some excellent printed material written with the layperson in mind. Another source of information is the Arthritis Information Clearinghouse at the National Institute of Medicine (see Online Resources).

GOUT

Etiology and Pathophysiology

Gout is arthritis of a joint caused by high serum levels of uric acid. Uric acid crystals precipitate from the body fluids and settle in joints and connective tissue. Gout affects men more than women and generally occurs during middle age. It is more common among populations that consume a high-protein diet. Two factors seem to be implicated: (1) a genetic increase in purine metabolism leading to overproduction or retention of uric acid; and (2) consumption of a high-purine diet. Excessive alcohol consumption causes an increased production of keto acids that inhibit uric acid excretion, causing hyperuricemia. Deposits of urate crystals occur in joints and subcutaneous tissues. The big toe is the most common site, but many other joints can be affected. Diuretic therapy sometimes causes a secondary gout because the loss of fluid increases the serum uric acid level in the body. Certain drug therapies interfere with uric acid excretion and can cause a secondary gout.

Signs and Symptoms

Typical signs and symptoms are elevated serum uric acid and tight, reddened skin over an inflamed, edematous joint, accompanied by elevated temperature and extreme pain in the joint.

Diagnosis, Treatment, and Nursing Management

History and physical examination are usually sufficient to diagnose gout, but a blood sample to check serum uric acid level is usually ordered to confirm the diagnosis. Treatment during acute attacks consists of administration of NSAIDs for 2 to 5 days for the pain. Colchicine given orally may bring dramatic pain relief within 24 to 48 hours. Allopurinol (Zyloprim) or probenecid (Benemid) may be prescribed to prevent further attacks. In February 2009 the FDA approved febuxostat (Uloric), which is the first new gout medication to be approved since the 1960s. Teach your patient about gout medication side effects and dosage.

Advise that dietary management includes weight control and restriction of high-purine foods, such as anchovies, sardines, sweetbreads, liver, red meat, kidney, and meat extracts. Alcohol should be restricted. Remind patients who take allopurinol that periodic liver function testing is needed because this drug can cause liver failure. Teach the patient that a fluid intake of 2000 to 3000 mL per day is needed to protect the kidneys from urate crystal deposit and to prevent kidney stones.

 Elder Care Points

Elderly patients with decreased creatinine clearance should not take allopurinol. When the patient has both hypertension and gout, losartan (Cozaar) may be a good choice for therapy. Losartan promotes urate diuresis.

OSTEOPOROSIS

Etiology and Pathophysiology

Osteoporosis makes the person more susceptible to fractures because of the decrease in bone mass. Fragility fractures are often *atraumatic* (occur without trauma.) Starting at age 35, most women lose bone mass at a rate of 1% a year; after menopause, loss of bone mass accelerates to 2% a year. In the United States, 44 million people have osteoporosis and another 34 million have osteopenia (low bone mass) (Qaseem et al., 2008). There is a hereditary tendency for osteoporosis. Risk factors for osteoporosis include age, chronic disease (e.g., liver, lung, kidney), medications (e.g., steroids, anticonvulsants, anticoagulants, proton pump inhibitors, selective serotonin inhibitors), long-term calcium deficiency, vitamin D deficiency, smoking, excessive caffeine or alcohol intake, and sedentary lifestyle. Eating disorders and inflammatory bowel disease lead to osteoporosis because these disorders and disease interfere with nutrition and absorption. The risk of osteoporosis increases considerably in women after menopause because estrogen production is reduced.

 Elder Care Points

Public awareness of osteoporosis for older women has increased, in large part, because the pharmaceutical industry has marketed drugs for prevention of osteoporosis and fragility fractures (Napoli, 2009). However, elderly men have hormone changes around age 70; this increases their risk for osteoporosis. The American College of Physicians recommends that older men should be assessed for risk factors and undergo diagnostic testing (Brown, 2009).

Signs and Symptoms

Osteoporosis is a silent disease and there are no early signs or symptoms. Once the patient has developed osteoporosis, height loss, kyphosis (excessive curvature of the spine), and back pain may occur. Compression fractures of the spine may cause debilitating pain.

Often osteoporosis is diagnosed after the patient sustains a fracture from little or no known trauma.

 Elder Care Points

Patients over age 60 who sustain a nontrauma osteoporotic fracture have an increased risk for death within 5 to 10 years after the fracture event. For elderly women, there may be some underlying risk for fracture and death. For men, there appears to be some connection to the fracture event itself. Additional research is needed to clarify risk factors (Bliuc et al., 2009).

Diagnosis

On radiographs the bone of the patient with osteoporosis appears porous. Dual-energy x-ray absorptiometry (DEXA) is used to assess loss of bone density. DEXA is reported as a T score.

- *Normal bone density:* T score of greater than 1 standard deviation from a healthy young adult
- *Osteopenia:* T score of 1.5 to 2.0 standard deviations below a healthy young adult
- *Osteoporosis:* T score of 2.5 to 3.0 standard deviations below a healthy young adult

Treatment

Treatment is aimed at stopping loss of bone density, increasing bone formation, and preventing fractures. Adequate dietary or supplemental calcium and vitamin D in combination with weight-bearing exercise are standard treatments and estrogen replacement therapy for postmenopausal women may also be used. For premenopausal women, 1000 mg of calcium is recommended and 1500 mg after menopause.

 Nutrition Considerations

Nutrition for Bone Growth and Density

Adequate amounts of calcium and phosphorus are essential for bone growth and density. Although green vegetables are a source of calcium, that calcium is not readily absorbed. Dairy products such as cheese, yogurt, and milk are better choices. Canned sardines or salmon also provide good amounts of calcium. Calcium supplementation is not recommended for the healing of fractures. It has proven not to be readily absorbed and tends to cause kidney stones.

Calcium supplements, if required, should be taken in divided doses during the day. Exposure to sufficient sunlight or vitamin D supplementation is necessary for the proper absorption and metabolism of the calcium. Current guidelines recommend 800 to 1000 units of vitamin D per day, with up to 1400 units during the winter months (Kalro, 2009). Vitamin K is important to bone health as well, and most people obtain vitamin K by eating greens. Daily weight-bearing exercise can decrease the chance of developing osteoporosis. Walking down stairs seems to be especially helpful, but walking for 30 minutes three times a week is sufficient.

Salicylates and NSAIDs are prescribed to control back pain. A back brace may be ordered for the patient who has suffered vertebral compression fractures. The bisphosphonates (i.e., Fosamax or Boniva; Box 33-3), which are cousins to a bone resorption–inhibiting substance found naturally in the body, and hormone therapy are prescribed in addition to calcium and vitamin D supplements for those with osteoporosis. Other classes of medications include parathyroid hormone, bone formation agents, and selective receptor modulators. Miacalcin or Fortical nasal spray, which contains calcitonin, slows the rate

Box 33-3 **Drugs Used for the Treatment of Osteoporosis**

HORMONES
- Estrogen (women)
- Raloxifene (Evista) (selective estrogen receptor modulator)
- Testosterone (men)
- Calcitonin (Miacalcin) (synthetic hormone)
- Teriparatide (Forteo) (synthetic hormone)

BISPHOSPHONATES
- Alendronate (Fosamax)
- Risedronate (Actonel)
- Ibandronate (Boniva)
- Etidronate (Didronel)
- Pamidronate (Aredia)

General Nursing Implications for Bisphosphonates
- Monitor bone density test results.
- Must take regularly (weekly or monthly).
- Observe for hypercalcemia (paresthesias, twitching, colic, or laryngospasm).
- Take with 8 oz of plain water in A.M. 30 to 60 minutes before eating, drinking, or taking any other medication that day (timing depends on the particular drug).
- Swallow the tablet whole. Do not suck or chew on it.
- Store medication in a cool location out of sunlight.
- Remain upright for 30 to 60 minutes after dose to prevent esophageal irritation (timing depends on the drug). Do not eat or drink anything during these 30 minutes to an hour.
- If dose is missed, skip the dose; do not take it later in the day. For the weekly dose medication, take it the next morning after your scheduled dose. Skip the dose if it has been 2 days since it was supposed to be taken and just resume the original schedule. If taking Boniva, take it the next morning after you remember you forgot to take it. Do not take two tablets in any 1 week; wait at least 7 days to take the next dose and then resume your original schedule.
- Take calcium and vitamin D supplements as recommended by the health care provider.
- Perform weight-bearing exercise to increase bone density.
- Advise health care provider if pregnant or planning a pregnancy.

of bone loss. It is an alternative treatment for postmenopausal osteoporosis in women who cannot take estrogens. The spray is used with adequate calcium and vitamin D supplementation.

A clinical trial by the National Cancer Institute (2009) is evaluating zoledronic acid (Zometa) for prevention of osteoporosis and long bone fractures in patients with prostate cancer who are receiving radiation and hormonal therapy.

⚠ Safety Alert

Caution with Bisphosphonate Drugs

There have been some instances of jawbone necrosis in patients who have been taking bisphosphonate drugs. There was also some concern that bisphosphonates increased the risk of femur fracture. Esophageal irritation or erosion can occur if the patient does not remain in an upright position for 1 hour after taking a bisphosphonate drug. The FDA announced in March 2010 that patients should continue to take prescribed bisphosphonates (Lowes, 2010). Patients should be reminded that adverse side effects are varied and any new onset of unusual signs or symptoms should be reported to the physician. These drugs should be stopped after 5 years.

Treatment of Vertebral Fracture. Vertebral compression fractures commonly occur in patients with osteoporosis. These are often treated with pain medication, activity limitation, physical therapy, and bracing. There are two new minimally invasive spine procedures, for those who do not respond to the conservative therapies. *Vertebroplasty* involves the percutaneous injection of polymethylmethacrylate (PMMA), a cement, directly into an osteoporotic spinal area under fluoroscopy. This stabilizes the bone and helps reduce or eliminate pain. *Kyphoplasty* consists of the percutaneous insertion of an inflatable device into the fractured vertebral body under fluoroscopy. The device is inflated, elevating the end plates and restoring the vertebral body toward its original height. Thick PMMA is then injected under low pressure into the cavity. The device is deflated and removed. This provides pain relief and reduces kyphosis (Clin-eguide, 2007).

❖ NURSING MANAGEMENT

■ Assessment (Data Collection)

Assessment for risk factors for osteoporosis should be performed with every general health assessment. Data are gathered about family history of osteoporosis, use of steroid medication, diet, exercise pattern throughout life, and history of smoking and alcohol intake.

■ Nursing Diagnosis and Planning

The main nursing diagnosis is Risk for injury related to possible fracture from thinning of the bone. The expected outcome would be Patient will not experience a fracture during his lifetime.

■ Implementation and Evaluation

Nursing care is focused on promoting screening for osteoporosis, teaching about the benefits of a healthy lifestyle, the need for sufficient intake of calcium and vitamin D, and weight-bearing exercise. Educating about the harmful effects of smoking and excessive alcohol intake is also important. For the patient with osteoporosis, teach about the medications prescribed for the disorder and their side effects, and measures to halt or reverse the disease process.

PAGET'S DISEASE

Paget's disease, more common in men, is a problem of abnormal bone resorption followed by replacement of normal marrow with fibrous connective tissue. The abnormal bone is weak and prone to fractures. The cause of Paget's disease is unknown, although it does occur in clusters in some families. Often the disease is found at the time a fracture occurs as radiographs reveal the abnormality of the bone. Diagnosis is by radiograph and laboratory testing. A 24-hour urine collection for hydroxyproline, which indicates osteoclastic activity, may be performed. Serum alkaline phosphatase is elevated if the disease is active. The main problem is pain. Miacalcin or a bisphosphonate may be given to slow bone resorption. Orthopedic care is given for fractures and necessary joint replacements. A firm mattress, wearing a corset or light brace to relieve back pain, and proper body mechanics are essential. The patient should avoid lifting or twisting.

BONE TUMORS

Etiology and Pathophysiology

Bone is subject to both benign and malignant tumors. Tumors arise from several different types of tissue, including cartilage (chondromas), bone (osteomas), and fibrous tissue (fibromas). Benign tumors often are found on radiograph or at the time of fracture.

Malignant bone tumors are either primary or secondary to metastatic disease. Diagnosing and treating cancer in other parts of the body early can prevent the occurrence of metastases to the bone. Primary malignant bone tumors are most often seen in people 10 to 25 years of age. The most common type is osteosarcoma or osteogenic sarcoma. It grows rapidly and metastasizes. More than half the cases affect the knee area. However, the distal femur, humerus, and proximal tibia are other frequent sites of occurrence. Osteosarcoma may occur in men older than age 60 as a complication of Paget's disease. Other types of primary malignant tumors include Ewing's sarcoma, chondrosarcoma, and fibrosarcoma.

Signs, Symptoms, and Diagnosis

Signs and symptoms of malignant bone tumor include pain, warmth, and swelling. Metastatic bone tumors greatly outnumber primary bone malignancies. Malignancies of the prostate, kidney, thyroid, breast, and

👥 Patient Teaching

Stump and Prosthesis Care

The nurse should instruct the patient in stump care as follows:

- Inspect the stump daily for redness, blistering, or abrasions.
- Use a mirror to examine all sides and aspects of the stump.
- Perform meticulous daily stump hygiene. Wash the stump with a mild soap, and then carefully rinse and dry it. Apply nothing to the stump after it is bathed. Alcohol dries and cracks the skin, whereas oils and creams soften the skin too much for safe prosthesis use.
- Wear woolen stump socks over the stump for cleanliness and comfort. To maintain the size and shape of woolen socks, wash them gently in cool water with mild soap and dry flat on a towel.
- Replace, do not mend, torn socks; mending creates wrinkles that irritate the skin.
- Put on the prosthesis immediately when arising and keep it on all day (once the wound has healed completely) to reduce stump swelling.
- Continue prescribed exercises to prevent weakness.
- Lay prone with hip extension for 30 minutes three or four times a day.
- For lower extremity, replace shoes before wear becomes extreme as gait may be altered.

The nurse should instruct the patient in prosthesis care as follows:

- Remove sweat and dirt from the prosthesis socket daily by wiping the inside of the socket with a damp, soapy cloth. To remove the soap, use a clean, damp cloth. Dry the prosthesis socket thoroughly.
- Never attempt to adjust or mechanically alter the prosthesis. If problems develop, consult the prosthetist.
- Schedule a yearly appointment with the prosthetist.

Adapted from Lewis, S.M., Heitkemper, M.M., Dirksen, S.R., et al. (2010). *Medical-Surgical Nursing: Assessment and Management of Clinical Problems* (8th ed.). St. Louis: Mosby.

FIGURE 33-11 C-leg prosthesis in action.

patient can do for himself and on what strengths he has in his favor. You can be of real assistance to the amputee by helping the patient find short-range goals that can be accomplished without great difficulty and that indicate progress toward independence. For example, you can guide him toward devising ways in which personal needs such as bathing and grooming can be met. Later, give encouragement to sit up, exercise the other limbs, and assist with changing of the dressing. Finally, set a goal for wearing the prosthesis successfully and walking without assistance (Figure 33-11) (see Chapter 9).

COMMUNITY CARE

Rehabilitation programs for amputees, arthritis patients, and others with musculoskeletal disorders exist in most large cities and are being introduced into more communities through agencies such as the YMCA. The Arthritis Foundation has been instrumental in working with the YMCAs to bring programs for exercise to local neighborhoods.

Outpatient rehabilitation programs through clinics work with patients who are regaining mobility and the ability to perform ADLs with a prosthesis. Rehabilitation is moving to a program "without walls," indicating a shift from an inpatient institute to rehabilitation in the home and community.

Home care nurses are particularly instrumental in preventing musculoskeletal injury in home care patients. The premises of the elderly patient are surveyed and recommendations are made to make it safer for the patient. Flat, nonglare surfaces for walking, well-lit walkways, absence of loose rugs, installation of grab bars in showers and bathrooms, and use of communication systems to summon help are some of the measures instituted to protect the elderly patient.

When a home care patient is on crutches, the nurse should assess the patient's ability to go up and down stairs and to sit down and arise from the sitting position safely. Patient Teaching on p. 730 presents the steps for performing these maneuvers correctly. Home care nurses must assess the capability and safety of elderly patients who are newly using assistive devices for ambulation and determine whether alterations in pathways in the home need to be made. Scatter rugs should be removed, and furniture may need to be rearranged to offer a path wide enough to allow the patient to move from one area to another.

Long-term care facility nurses survey patient units and group spaces daily to check for obstacles to ambulation and potential safety hazards. Slowly, our communities are becoming easier to navigate for the elderly, and public places are becoming more accessible for the handicapped and safer for the frail elderly.

Get Ready for the NCLEX® Examination!

Key Points

- Sprains are usually treated with rest, ice, compression, and elevation (RICE).
- Bursitis occurs from injury or overuse.
- Carpal tunnel syndrome causes numbness, tingling, and pain in the hand.
- Fractures occur from trauma or metabolic disease. Assessment includes noting pain, swelling, discoloration, and deformity in the contour of the bone. Complications include infection, osteomyelitis, fat embolism, venous thrombosis, and compartment syndrome.
- Compartment syndrome is an emergency situation. Signs and symptoms include edema, pallor, tingling, paresthesia, numbness, weak pulse, cyanosis, paresis, and severe pain.
- Osteoarthritis occurs asymmetrically and typically affects only one or two joints. Treatment consists of pain management, weight control, exercise, and maintenance of joint function.
- Rheumatoid arthritis is an inflammatory disease of the joints. Symptoms include joint pain, warmth, edema, limitation of motion, and joint stiffness and systemic symptoms. Treatment includes relieving pain, minimizing joint destruction, promoting joint function, and preserving the ability to perform self-care functions. Medications, rest, exercise, and applications of heat and cold are mainstays of treatment.
- Postoperative care after joint replacement is very important to prevent pain, prevent infection, prevent dislocation, and promote mobilization.
- DVT is a common complication of hip and knee joint replacement.
- Gout is caused by high serum levels of uric acid. Symptoms of gout are tight, reddened skin over an inflamed, edematous joint accompanied by elevated temperature and extreme pain in the joint.
- Calcium deficiency and estrogen depletion predispose to the development of osteoporosis, which increases susceptibility to fractures. Treatment includes calcium, vitamin D supplements, bisphosphonates, and other hormonal medications (see Box 33-3).
- The most common primary bone tumor is osteogenic sarcoma.
- Eighty percent of amputations involve lower extremities. Hemorrhage and infection are complications of amputation. Proper stump care is essential to the success of rehabilitation.

Additional Learning Resources

 SG Go to your Study Guide for additional learning activities to help you master this chapter content.

evolve Go to your Evolve website (http://evolve.elsevier.com/deWit/medsurg) for the following FREE learning resources:
- Animations, audio, and video
- Answers and rationales for questions and activities
- Concept Map Creator
- Glossary with pronunciations in English and Spanish
- Interactive Review Questions and Exercises and more!

Online Resources
- Arthritis Foundation, www.arthritis.org
- National Institute of Arthritis and Musculoskeletal and Skin Diseases, www.niams.nih.gov
- National Osteoporosis Foundation, www.nof.org

Review Questions for the NCLEX® Examination

1. After sustaining a rotator cuff tear, the patient's arm is placed in a sling. The patient is instructed to rest and to take ibuprofen (Motrin) for pain. Which patient statement indicates a need for further teaching?

   1. "I will have less stomach upset if I take the pills with food."
   2. "I will not be able to play tennis for a while."
   3. "I need to rest in bed for the next 2 days."
   4. "The sling must be worn most of the time."

2. The nurse is assuming immediate postoperative care of a 23-year-old patient who had carpal tunnel repair. On receiving the patient, what is the priority nursing assessment?

   1. Sensation in the fingertips
   2. Color, warmth, and capillary refill
   3. Condition of the dressing
   4. Range of motion

3. A nurse responds to a roadside emergency and finds a middle-aged man with pain and tenderness over the left leg. The nurse notes a closed bone deformity with inability to move the leg. While waiting for the paramedics, what is the most important nursing action?

   1. Immobilization of the leg
   2. Realigning the bones
   3. Applying warm packs
   4. Elevating the extremity

4. En route to an emergency surgery for open reduction and internal fixation of a fractured femur, the patient signs the surgical consent. During the final surgical team check for the correct surgical site, the patient asks, "What does open reduction and internal fixation of the femur mean?" What is the appropriate nursing action?

1. Answer the patient's question and proceed as planned.
2. Have the surgeon discuss the procedure with the patient.
3. Administer antibiotics and pain medications.
4. Postpone the surgical procedure.

5. The nurse has just received shift report on four assigned orthopedic patients. Which patient should the nurse check on first?

1. A young trauma patient with a below-the-knee amputation is having phantom pain.
2. An elderly woman with a total hip replacement needs assistance with the bedpan.
3. A woman with an external fixation device has a fever and foul odor at pin sites.
4. A man with a full leg cast reports persistent pain despite elevation and pain medication.

6. A patient with a plaster cast of the right arm complains of itching underneath the cast. What should the nurse do to alleviate the symptom?

1. Encourage deep breaths.
2. Insert a cotton-tip applicator under the cast.
3. Forcefully inject 50 mL of air underneath the cast.
4. Administer pain medications.

7. The nurse hears crackles and wheezes in an elderly patient who was admitted for multiple bone fractures. The patient appears apprehensive with an oxygen saturation of 84% on 3 L/min nasal cannula. What is the priority action?

1. Put the patient in a supine position.
2. Deliver breaths with an Ambu bag.
3. Change to a non-rebreather mask.
4. Administer intravenous fluid bolus.

8. The nurse is assisting an elderly patient who has rheumatoid arthritis. The nurse would intervene to teach the patient about joint protection if the patient:

1. turned the doorknob counterclockwise.
2. used the palms of the hands to push off from the bed.
3. lifted a heavy object with the dominant hand.
4. pushed the door open with the arm.

9. A young patient returns from the operating room after a below-the-knee amputation and is alert and quiet. The stump is elevated with a dressing dry and intact. What is the priority nursing diagnosis for this patient?

1. Disturbed body image
2. Risk for bleeding
3. Impaired mobility
4. Knowledge deficit

10. A 24-year-old woman limps into the emergency department after twisting her ankle during a soccer game. On examination, there is local swelling and difficulty maintaining balance. What immediate therapeutic measure(s) should the nurse provide? *(Select all that apply.)*

1. Application of elastic bandage
2. Warm compress
3. Elevation of the ankle
4. Ankle rest and limited weight bearing
5. Apply a topical anesthetic

Critical Thinking Activities

Scenario A
Mrs. Wilson, age 38, has been admitted to the hospital with a diagnosis of fracture of the right tibia. You have been told that when the patient returns from surgery, she will have an external fixation device in place.

1. How would you perform a neurovascular assessment?

2. How can you support the affected extremity?

3. What can you do to decrease swelling?

4. List the observations you must make while the fixator is on Mrs. Wilson's leg.

5. What complications might occur?

Scenario B
Mrs. Cox, age 50, is a moderately obese woman who comes to the orthopedic clinic for treatment of arthritis of the knees and ankles. She has great difficulty walking and would use a wheelchair if she could afford one. Her daughter states that she is becoming more and more inactive and—though her mother says she does not want to become an invalid—she refuses to move about and do things for herself. Mrs. Cox lives alone and prefers not to live with her daughter because the grandchildren make her nervous. In fact, she prefers to be left alone because she feels that she cannot be of use to anyone. Her daughter feels that her mother could find many useful things to do in her neighborhood if she would only try.

1. How does obesity interact with arthritis in causing immobility?

2. What medications might decrease Mrs. Cox's pain?

3. What sort of exercise would be best for this patient?

4. How could you make Mrs. Cox feel more useful and motivate her to move about and get out of the house more?

Scenario C

Mr. Oliver is a 78-year-old who is discharged home after a total hip replacement. You are assigned as his home care nurse to do wound care, assess for complications, and monitor rehabilitation.

1. What teaching for self-care would you reinforce for Mr. Oliver on your first visit?

2. How would you determine whether the home environment is safe for Mr. Oliver?

3. Mr. Oliver is very depressed because he feels he will no longer be able to get out to go fishing and visit with his friends. How would you approach the psychosocial aspects of his care?

Scenario D

During your daily run, you step on an irregular surface and twist your ankle. At home, you notice tenderness at the site, minimal swelling, and loss of function but no abnormal motion.

1. What first aid will you perform?

2. How will you know if you have a sprain or a fracture?

Objectives

Theory

1. Review the anatomy and physiology of the urinary system.
2. State causes of urologic problems and disorders.
3. Discuss ways in which the nurse can help patients to prevent or cope with urologic disorders.
4. Outline the psychosocial impact of urinary incontinence.

Clinical Practice

1. Identify nursing responsibilities in the preprocedure and postprocedure care of patients undergoing urologic diagnostic studies.

2. Perform initial and ongoing nursing assessment of a patient's urologic status.
3. List five nursing responsibilities related to the care of a patient with an indwelling catheter.
4. Write a nursing care plan for a patient with urinary incontinence.

Key Terms

anuria (ă-NŪ-rē-ă, p. 775)
blood urea nitrogen (BUN) (blŭd ū-RĒ-ă NĬ-trō-jěn, p. 767)
creatinine (krē-ĂT-ĭ-nēn, p. 765)
dysuria (dĭs-Ū-rē-ă, p. 775)
hematuria (hē-măt-Ū-rē-ă, p. 773)
micturition (mĭk-tū-RĬSH-ŭn, p. 766)
nephrotoxic (něf-rō-TŎK-sĭk, p. 768)
nocturia (nŏct-Ū-rē-ă, p. 775)
oliguria (ŏl-ĭ-GŪ-rē-ă, p. 775)

polyuria (pŏl-ē-Ū-rē-ă, p. 775)
proteinuria (prō-tēn-YŬR-ē-ă, p. 773)
residual urine (rě-ZĬ-dū-ăl Ū-rĭn, p. 775)
urinary frequency (Ū-rĭ-năr-ē, p. 775)
urinary hesitancy (p. 775)
urinary incontinence (Ū-rĭ-năr-ē ĭn-KŎN-tĭ-něns, p. 766)
urinary retention (Ū-rĭ-năr-ē rē-TĚN-shŭn, p. 775)
voiding (VŎYD-ĭng, p. 766)

OVERVIEW OF ANATOMY AND PHYSIOLOGY OF THE UROLOGIC SYSTEM

WHAT ARE THE STRUCTURES OF THE UROLOGIC SYSTEM AND HOW DO THEY INTERRELATE?

- The kidneys, ureters, urinary bladder, and urethra are the structures of the urinary system (Figure 34-1).
- The kidneys are bean-shaped organs positioned on either side of the vertebral column at the level of the first lumbar vertebra. The left kidney is slightly higher than the right.
- The kidney consists of the cortex, the outer layer, the medulla, and the renal pelvis; the cortex contains blood vessels and nephrons; the medulla contains the collecting tubules; and the renal pelvis gathers the urine and directs it to the bladder (Figure 34-2).
- The nephron is the functional unit of the kidney (1 million nephrons in a kidney).

- The nephron consists of the glomerulus, which is a network of capillaries encased in a thin-walled sac called *Bowman's capsule*, and the tubular system.
- The tubular system of the nephron consists of the proximal convoluted tubule, the loop of Henle, the distal convoluted tubule, and the collecting duct (Figure 34-3). Urine is carried by the ureters from the kidney to the bladder through peristaltic action.
- The bladder, a hollow muscular organ, serves as a reservoir for urine; the inner lining of the bladder is a mucous membrane.
- The urine passes from the bladder down the urethra, which is approximately 3 to 5 cm long in women and 20 cm in men.
- The internal, involuntary, urethral sphincter is controlled by the detrusor muscle that is in the wall of the bladder.

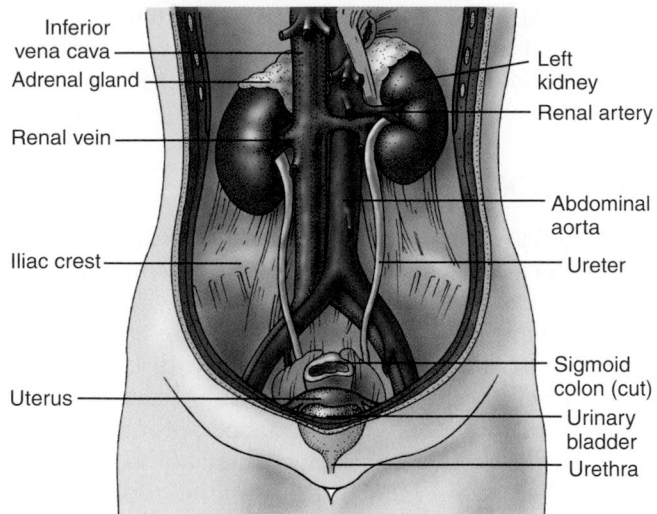

FIGURE 34-1 Structures of the urinary system.

FIGURE 34-2 Structures of the kidney.

FIGURE 34-3 The nephron.

- The external urethral sphincter voluntarily controls release of urine to the outside.
- Blood is brought to the kidney by the renal arteries that branch off the aorta. Blood is returned by veins to the inferior vena cava.

WHAT ARE THE FUNCTIONS OF THE KIDNEYS?

- The kidneys regulate serum electrolytes, by filtration and reabsorption (Table 34-1).
- The kidneys eliminate metabolic wastes, by filtration; they filter about one fourth of the body's blood at any one time.
- Each nephron filters blood plasma through the semipermeable glomerular membrane.
- Glomerular filtration rate (GFR) is the amount of blood filtered by the glomeruli in a given time (GFR: about 125 mL/min).
- The kidneys regulate fluid volume by filtration, reabsorption, and excretion.

- Most of the water and some of the electrolytes are reabsorbed into the bloodstream in the descending and distal convoluted tubules.
- The kidneys assist in maintaining acid-base balance by secreting hydrogen ions into the urine.
- Unwanted substances: urea, **creatinine** (waste products of protein metabolism and skeletal muscle contraction, respectively), and uric acid are retained in the tubules along with some water.
- Approximately 200 L of liquid are filtered in a 24-hour period; 1.5 to 2 L are excreted as urine.
- The kidneys regulate blood pressure by secreting the enzyme renin.
- The kidneys increase red blood cell production by secreting erythropoietin.
- The kidneys metabolize vitamin D into an active form.

WHAT ARE THE FUNCTIONS OF THE URETERS, BLADDER, AND URETHRA?

- Each ureter is a small tube about 25 cm long; it carries urine from the renal pelvis to the bladder.
- The bladder holds the urine; capacity varies from about 1000 to 1800 mL.

Table 34-1	Hormones and Metabolic Actions Associated with Kidney Function

HORMONES	ACTION
Circulating in the Blood to Influence Urine Volume and Concentration	
Aldosterone	Increases the reabsorption of sodium
Antidiuretic hormone (ADH)	Increases permeability in the tubules and reabsorption of water
Atrial natriuretic hormone	Increases the secretion of sodium
Produced by the Kidney	
Erythropoietin	Stimulates the bone marrow to increase red blood cell (RBC) production; increased production of erythropoietin is triggered by a demand for oxygen or when RBC level falls below normal
Calcitriol (active vitamin D)	Increases absorption of calcium and phosphorus
Renin	Assists in the regulation of blood pressure
Affecting Kidney Function	
Parathyroid hormone	Works in conjunction with calcitriol to increase absorption of calcium and phosphorus
Cortisol	Promotes sodium and water retention

- A feeling of bladder fullness and an initial signal to void (empty the bladder) occurs when the bladder contains 150 to 200 mL of urine.
- The micturition (voiding) reflex is then initiated and transmitted to the bladder. Urine then passes from the bladder through the urethra during urination (voiding).
- The flow of urine is controlled by the internal urethral sphincter and the external urethral sphincter.

WHAT CHANGES OCCUR WITH AGING?

- Kidney function begins to lessen after age 45, and renal blood flow and GFR gradually decrease to about half the rate of a young adult by age 65.
- In the male, the prostate gland hypertrophies with age and can cause varying degrees of obstruction to the normal flow of urine.
- Secretion of renin, aldosterone, and vitamin D activation are decreased.
- Degenerative changes in the bladder muscles may lead to residual urine (incomplete emptying of urine) and urinary incontinence (involuntary passing of urine).
- Bladder capacity decreases, to as little as 200 mL and frequent emptying is needed.
- A decreased ability to concentrate urine leads to nocturia (urination during the night).

- Lowered estrogen levels in women result in tissue atrophy in the urethra, vagina, and trigone of the bladder (triangular portion at the base of the bladder), which predisposes to infection and incontinence.

THE UROLOGIC SYSTEM

The kidneys and urinary tract function to maintain the proper balance of fluids, minerals, and organic substances necessary for life. Problems in the heart, lungs, or circulatory system can arise from kidney disorders or kidney failure. Likewise, generalized diseases, such as atherosclerosis, other circulatory impairments, infections, or disturbances in the metabolic processes, may seriously impair the proper functioning of the kidneys.

DISORDERS OF THE UROLOGIC SYSTEM
Causes
In the high volume of blood that is filtered by the kidney, there are some bacteria. These bacteria can colonize the kidney, causing an infection. Also, bacteria can easily enter the urinary tract through the urethra, and then the infection may spread up into the kidneys.

When an immune reaction occurs in the body, the glomeruli that filter the blood are exposed to antibodies and antigen–antibody complexes contained in that blood. These antibodies and antigen–antibody complexes can cause an autoimmune inflammatory reaction known as *glomerulonephritis* that damages the semipermeable glomerular membrane and interferes with normal kidney function.

Once urine is formed, the urinary system must be patent and unobstructed for urine to be excreted. Tumors may form in the bladder, ureters, or kidney and interfere with normal function by altering cell structure or impeding urine flow. Stones in the kidney or ureters may obstruct the flow of urine. In older men, an enlarged prostate may inhibit flow of urine through the urethra.

Tubular necrosis can be caused by lack of oxygen or bacterial or chemical destruction of cells, which affect the functional ability of the nephron and decreases kidney function. Many drugs can be toxic to the kidney, and heavy metals such as mercury can cause considerable damage.

Hypertension is a major cause of end-stage kidney disease; conversely, renal disorders can also cause secondary hypertension. Because so much of the kidney's function is directly related to the capillaries and arterioles, any disorder, such as atherosclerosis and diabetes mellitus, that systemically affects the blood vessels can affect the kidneys. When these vessels become *sclerosed* (hardened), blood flow through the kidney is decreased; kidney function diminishes and eventually this leads to chronic renal failure. Reduced blood circulation related to decreased volume (e.g., hypovolemic shock) or decreased cardiac output (e.g., cardiogenic shock) puts the patient at risk for acute renal failure (ARF).

Patient Teaching
Kidney Health and Healthy Blood Vessels

If your patients have hypertension or diabetes mellitus, design a teaching session that will help them recognize that the atherosclerotic changes that occur in the blood vessels also cause decreased blood flow to the kidneys and eventually reduce kidney function. In accordance with the *Healthy People 2020* goals, emphasize that compliance with the treatment plan for hypertension or diabetes mellitus helps to prevent kidney problems that will occur later in life.

Prevention
One of the best ways to prevent disorders of the urologic system is to drink plenty of water. A minimum fluid intake of 2000 to 2500 mL/day is recommended to initiate good flow through the system.

Health Promotion
Bladder Health

Promote bladder and urinary tract health by encouraging patients to empty the bladder sooner, rather than waiting to urinate. Emptying the bladder prevents urinary stasis and prolonged exposure of waste toxins on the bladder wall, which may contribute to cancer of the bladder. Delayed voiding also causes the bladder wall to stretch beyond normal capacity, and places undue strain on the sphincters. Both can contribute to urinary incontinence later in life.

Controlling blood pressure and maintaining a normal serum glucose level can support healthy blood vessels. A good blood supply promotes good kidney function.

Carefully monitoring for adverse drug effects and avoiding the use of chemicals known to be harmful to the kidney help preserve optimal kidney function. Box 34-1 gives examples of substances that are toxic to the kidney. When drugs that can be harmful to the kidney—such as sulfa compounds—are prescribed, increasing the fluid intake to 3000 to 3500 mL/day reduces the risk of kidney dysfunction. (Increasing fluid intake must be carefully considered when the patient has other conditions, such as congestive heart failure or cirrhosis of the liver.)

Patient Teaching
Over-the-Counter Drugs

Teach your patients to avoid routine use of over-the-counter drugs, such as nonsteroidal anti-inflammatory drugs and acetaminophen, to decrease the possibility of hepatic or renal dysfunction through unnecessary exposure to chemicals. This is in accordance with National Patient Safety Goals—to actively involve patients in their own care to ensure safety.

Think Critically

What changes could you make in your dietary habits or lifestyle that might help to prevent urologic problems?

Box 34-1 **Examples of Substances that Are Potentially Nephrotoxic**

- Anti-infectives
  - Aminoglycosides (gentamicin, streptomycin)
  - Sulfonamides (trimethoprim-sulfamethoxazole)
  - Antifungals (amphotericin B)
  - Antitubercular (rifampin)
  - Cephalosporins (cefaclor)
  - Tetracyclines (doxycycline)
  - Miscellaneous (e.g., vancomycin)
- ACE inhibitors (captopril)
- Antineoplastic agents (cisplatin)
- Immunosuppressants (cyclosporine)
- NSAIDs (salicylates, ibuprofen, indomethacin)
- Other drugs (acetaminophen, furosemide, phenazopyridine HCl)
- Contrast media dye (Gastrografin)
- Anesthetics (halothane)
- Heavy metals (lithium, gold salts, lead)
- Industrial (carbon tetrachloride for cleaning)
- Environmental (pesticides, snake venom)

Diagnostic Tests and Procedures

Patients experiencing problems with the urinary system undergo urine tests, such as a urinalysis, and culture and sensitivity, and general diagnostic tests, such as a complete blood count (CBC), **blood urea nitrogen (BUN)**, serum creatinine, and creatinine clearance. Urea is produced when protein breaks down; it then combines with ammonia and is carried by the bloodstream to the kidneys for excretion. Creatinine is a by-product of skeletal muscle contraction. BUN and serum creatinine are interpreted together and laboratory values should be obtained before the use of radiologic contrast dyes. Creatinine clearance (CC) is a good measure of GFR. Cystatin C is a relatively new test used to evaluate GFR. Cystatin C is a low-molecular-weight proteinase inhibitor that is produced at a constant rate and filtered out by the glomerulus. With impaired kidney function cystatin C levels will rise. Normal value is 0.70 to 0.85 mg/mL (depending on age). This diagnostic test shows promise of being a better indicator of GFR than creatinine clearance; however, its usefulness is currently somewhat controversial (National Kidney Foundation, 2010).

Clinical Cues

Blood urea nitrogen (BUN) level and serum creatinine are the two most common tests used to screen for kidney problems. The normal adult range for BUN is 10 to 20 mg/dL. Serum creatinine: 0.6 to 1.2 mg/dL for adult males and 0.5 to 1.1 mg/dL for adult females. An increase in BUN or serum creatinine can be a signal of decreased kidney function.

Radiologic procedures range from a single view of the kidneys, ureters, and bladder (KUB) to interventional radiology, such as balloon angioplasty.

FIGURE 34-4 Renal biopsy. A needle is inserted through the skin to obtain a tissue sample.

A KUB is used to locate stones and detect structural abnormalities. Angioplasty is used to open blocked vessels and increase blood flow to the organs. Urodynamic tests, such as cystometrography, are used to measure flow volume and muscle function. Biopsies of the kidney or bladder are done in combination with radiologic examinations to locate lesions (Figure 34-4).

 Patient Teaching

Renal Biopsy

Teaching points for patients having a renal biopsy:
- *Explain purpose:* To diagnosis the cause of kidney disease, to detect cancer, or to evaluate kidney transplant rejection.
- *Explain procedure:* Local anesthetic is given. Needle is inserted through skin into the kidney to obtain a small sample under fluoroscopy. Total procedure time is 10 minutes.
- *Explain preparation:* Nothing by mouth (NPO) for 6 to 8 hours before procedure and blood tests will be done before procedure (e.g., hemoglobin and hematocrit, prothrombin time, partial thromboplastin time).
- *Explain postprocedure care:* Must lie on back for 6 to 24 hours (time varies according to facility protocols and physician orders), avoid activities that increase abdominal pressure (e.g., sneezing, laughing), expect that urine will have blood for first 24 hours. Drink 3000 mL of fluid to flush urinary system (unless otherwise contraindicated).
- *Give home care instructions:* Avoid strenuous activity (heavy lifting or contact sports) for 2 weeks. Report bleeding (e.g., bright red or with clots) immediately. Report fever, malaise, or dysuria.

From Pagana, K.D., & Pagana, T.J. (2011). *Mosby's Diagnostic and Laboratory Test Reference* (10th ed.). St. Louis: Mosby.

General nursing responsibilities for diagnostic testing include assessing for allergies to contrast media and possibility of pregnancy, explaining procedures, assisting with specimen collection, reinforcing any dietary and fluid restrictions, and assisting with special preparations, such as bowel evacuation. In addition, Table 34-2 lists common diagnostic tests and procedures, along with nursing implications.

 Think Critically

What is the rationale of having the patient use the clean-catch method, rather than just simply voiding into a collection container?

 Elder Care Points

The aged kidney has less ability to concentrate the urine. This predisposes the patient to dehydration when fluid intake is restricted for diagnostic tests. The contrast agents used for radiographic tests, in conjunction with dehydration, can cause acute renal failure in the elderly patient. The nurse should carefully rehydrate the elderly patient by encouraging several ounces of oral fluid (preferable to intravenous [IV] administration, if possible) every 1 to 2 hours and monitoring vital signs, urinary output, lung sounds, and respiratory effort to prevent fluid overload.

 Clinical Cues

A 24-hour urine collection is usually started in the morning. Have the patient void and discard the urine, note the time on the laboratory slip and in the nurses' notes, and then put each successive voiding into the collection container. At the time when the test is to end, have the patient void, and add this last urine to the collection bottle. Check with the laboratory as to whether the container must be kept on ice during the collection period. Place a sign on the patient's door and over the toilet stating "24-hour urine test in progress" so that everyone will save the urine properly.

❖ NURSING MANAGEMENT

■ Assessment (Data Collection)

History and Present Illness

At the time of admission the nurse should obtain a personal history of illness or injury to any system and previous disorders of the urinary tract, such as frequent urinary tract infections (UTIs) or problems that required surgery. A family history of diabetes, cardiovascular disease, or kidney stones is relevant to an assessment of kidney function.

 Clinical Cues

If the patient appears hesitant to disclose illicit drug use, use a matter-of-fact approach and explain that the information is important because of potential drug-drug interactions and adverse effects on organs such as the kidneys, heart, or liver.

Many substances can be toxic to the kidney (**nephrotoxic**); collect patient history that includes use of prescription or over-the-counter drugs or illicit substances and any occupational exposure to hazardous materials. The complete drug history should be communicated to all health care professionals and conveyed if transferred to another facility; on discharge,

Text continued on p. 773

Table 34-2   Diagnostic Tests for Urologic Disorders

TEST	PURPOSE	DESCRIPTION	NURSING IMPLICATIONS
Urine			
Urinalysis	To detect bacteria, blood, casts, and other abnormalities of the urine	Normal urine is clear, straw to dark amber in color, has a pH of 4.5-6.0, a specific gravity of 1.010-1.030, and is negative for protein, glucose, ketones, and bilirubin. It should have only a rare RBC, no more than 0-4 white blood cells (WBCs), and an occasional cast.	Obtain a fresh 10-mL morning specimen. Send specimen to laboratory immediately. If vaginal bleeding is reported, physician may order a catheterized specimen.
Urine culture and sensitivity (C&S)	To verify UTI and to determine the specific infectious organism and the sensitivity to specific antibiotics	Normally, urine is sterile in the bladder. Several drops of urine are placed in a culture medium. After incubation (several days), the colonies are counted. If >100,000 organisms per milliliter are counted, there is a UTI. *Sensitivity test:* bacteria are exposed to various anti-infectives to see which is most effective in killing the organism.	Instruct patient to perform the *clean-catch* method for specimen collection. A sterile specimen can also be obtained via urinary catheterization. Send specimen to laboratory immediately to prevent change in pH, which can affect bacterial growth.
Urine osmolality	To determine whether the kidneys can concentrate urine; reflects hydration status	Increases in osmolality (i.e., dehydration, azotemia, chronic renal disease). Decreases in osmolality (i.e., low-salt diet, excessive water intake, diabetes insipidus). Normal findings for fasting specimen >850 mOsm/kg.	Give a high-protein diet for 3 days before the urine collection. Restrict foods and fluids for 8-12 hr before obtaining fasting specimen. To collect a fasting urine specimen, have the patient empty bladder at 6 A.M., discard, then collect specimen at 8 A.M. Label as *a fasting specimen* and send to laboratory.
Uric acid	To check for renal failure, gout, kidney stones	Uric acid is an end product of protein metabolism. Level is elevated in renal failure. Normal findings 250-750 mg/24 hr (normal diet).	Take a diet history; specifically ask about purine-rich foods (e.g., liver, beef kidneys, or sardines). Patient needs to fast the night before specimen collection. Instruct on a 24-hr urine collection. (Serum uric acid may be ordered.)
Creatinine clearance	To determine how well kidneys can excrete creatinine	Elevated serum creatinine with decreased urine creatinine indicates decreased kidney function. Normal creatinine clearance is 15-25 mg/kg body weight in 24 hr.	Collect a 24-hr urine specimen. A 5-mL venous blood sample is collected sometime during the 24-hr collection period. Instruct patient to avoid rigorous exercise (according to laboratory protocol: avoid cooked meat, tea, coffee, or drugs) during the collection period.

RBC, red blood cell; *UTI,* urinary tract infection.

Continued

Table **34-2** Diagnostic Tests for Urologic Disorders—cont'd

TEST	PURPOSE	DESCRIPTION	NURSING IMPLICATIONS
Blood			
Blood urea nitrogen (BUN)	To evaluate kidney function and hydration status	High BUN levels can indicate poor kidney function, dehydration, or increased breakdown of body protein (i.e., severe burns or excessive exercise). Lower BUN levels are found in severe liver damage, excessive hydration, and protein deficiency. Normal BUN levels average 7-20 mg/dL (depending on sex and age).	No fasting or patient preparation is required. Take a drug history, as many drugs can alter results. (Record drugs on laboratory slip as appropriate.) Requires 5 mL of venous blood. When drawing specimen, make sure it is not hemolyzed.
Serum creatinine	To evaluate kidney dysfunction when there are a large number of nonfunctional nephrons	Creatinine is a waste product of skeletal muscle activity. It is produced in fairly constant amounts and is excreted through the kidneys. Normal serum creatinine is 0.8-1.2 mg/dL (depending on gender).	Meats, tea, or coffee may be restricted 6 hr before the test. Cephalosporins may be stopped before the test. Record baseline height and weight. Instruct patient to avoid strenuous exercise before test. Requires 5-10 mL venous blood; may include a 24-hr urine collection.
Cystatin C	To detect renal disease in early stage	Cystatin C in the blood binds to specific anti-cystatin C antibody, causing agglutination.	No special preparation needed. Requires a blood draw of 3 mL in lavender-top tube.
Radiology Studies			
Kidneys, ureters, bladder (KUB)	To visualize the urinary structures or radiopaque stones	Single radiographic view of the lower abdomen done without contrast medium.	Patient needs an x-ray gown that has no radiopaque fasteners. Test for pregnancy before any radiologic study.
Intravenous pyelogram (IVP)	To visualize the kidneys, ureters, and bladder To detect obstructions related to stones or tumors	An iodine-based dye is given via IV injection, then radiographs are taken at timed intervals, showing the flow of the dye through the renal system.	Check for allergy to iodine-based dye, verify BUN and creatinine results; inform physician. Bowel prep and NPO may be required. Patient may feel a hot flush or nausea when dye is injected. Postprocedure, encourage PO fluids for rehydration.
Retrograde pyelogram	To visualize the kidneys, ureters, and bladder	During cystoscopy: catheters are threaded into the ureters to inject the dye backward into the kidneys.	Check for allergy to iodine-based dye, verify BUN and creatinine results; inform physician. Bowel prep and NPO may be required.
Cystogram	To visualize the contour of the bladder	Radiographs are taken before and after sodium iodide is instilled into the bladder through a urethral catheter.	Check for allergies to iodine-based dyes. Give a clear liquid breakfast on the day of test. A Foley catheter is usually inserted before the procedure. Patient's bladder may feel very full during the examination, but bladder is drained after the radiographs are taken. Postprocedure, encourage PO fluids for flushing.

NPO, nothing by mouth; *PO*, by mouth, orally.

Table **34-2**	Diagnostic Tests for Urologic Disorders—cont'd		
TEST	**PURPOSE**	**DESCRIPTION**	**NURSING IMPLICATIONS**
Magnetic resonance imaging (MRI)	To detect trauma or tumors in soft tissues	Noninvasive imaging uses a powerful magnetic field to scan radiowave frequencies and form 3D images. Can be done without contrast.	Considered relatively safe. Metal objects are forbidden during the procedure. Pacemakers and implants are contraindicated.
Computed tomography (CT) scan	To determine presence of a cyst, tumor, or renal calculi	A combination of radiologic and computer techniques yields cross-sectional information and indicates the density of tissues.	Contrast medium may or may not be given; check for allergy to iodine. Patient may need to be NPO before examination. Procedure lasts about 30 min; patient must remain quiet and cooperative.
Renal ultrasonography	To show size, shape, and location of kidneys, ureters, bladder; and obstructions to flow	A handheld transducer is passed over the skin and high-frequency sound waves create visual images of the structures.	Patient may be asked to drink fluid to fill bladder before sonogram; other laboratories may require NPO for 8-12 hr before the procedure. Test takes approximately 30 min.
Renal angiography	To assess renal arterial system function and identifies areas of obstruction to blood flow	Under local anesthesia, a catheter is threaded through the femoral artery and up the aorta to the renal artery, and a contrast agent is injected. Fluoroscopy is conducted during the injection to observe for filling of blood vessels. Angiography is performed to detect complications in a transplanted kidney, to evaluate a mass, or to check the extent of kidney trauma.	Requires a signed permission form. Check for allergy to iodine-based dye. A bowel prep or NPO for 6-8 hr may be ordered. Postprocedure care includes direct pressure applied to the puncture site for 20 min, followed by a pressure dressing and additional mechanical pressure. Patient remains flat in bed for 4-12+ hr. Vital signs, popliteal and pedal pulses are checked every 15 min for the first hour and q 2-4 hr, as ordered, for signs of bleeding or shock.
Radionuclide renal scan	To detect perfusion and function; can detect abnormal areas of kidney tissue (e.g., tumors or cysts)	A radioisotope is injected into the blood and a scintillation scanner is passed over the area of the kidney. This yields a pattern of isotope uptake. Procedure may take from 1-4 hr to complete.	Explain that low-dose radiation is used and is quickly eliminated from the body, and that the procedure is not painful, but she must lie very still. There are no dietary restrictions, but the patient should drink 2-3 glasses of water before the test.
Endoscopy			
Cystoscopy	To examine the interior of the bladder	Under short-acting or local anesthesia, a cystoscope is passed up the urethra into the bladder. The scope can be guided into a ureter to extract a stone or to biopsy lesions in the bladder.	Requires a signed permission form. Patient is usually NPO for several hours before the procedure. Give preoperative medication, as ordered. Postprocedure: burning, frequency, and pink-tinged urine may occur. Frank bleeding should be reported. Warm sitz baths and mild analgesics are given for voiding discomfort.

Continued

Table **34-2** Diagnostic Tests for Urologic Disorders—cont'd

TEST	PURPOSE	DESCRIPTION	NURSING IMPLICATIONS
Urodynamics			
Cystometrography (CMG)	To measure bladder capacity, pressures, and sensations	A urinary catheter is inserted and attached to a cystometer. Fluid is instilled and the patient reports when the need to void is first noted, then mild urgency, and finally when bladder feels very full. Readings of bladder capacity and pressure are recorded and plotted.	Sterile technique must be used for catheter insertion and bladder fluid instillation. The patient is monitored for signs of postprocedure infection.
Urethral pressure study	To determine urethral pressure needed to maintain urinary continence	A catheter with pressure-sensing capabilities is inserted into the bladder. As the catheter is withdrawn, the varying pressures of the smooth muscle of the urethra are recorded.	Sterile technique must be used for catheter insertion. The patient is monitored for signs of postprocedure infection.
Electromyography of the perineal muscles	To evaluate the quality of the voluntary muscles used in voiding	Electrodes are placed either in the rectum or the urethra to measure contraction and relaxation of the muscles involved in voiding.	Inform the patient that there is mild discomfort during electrode placement and nerve conduction testing. Analgesics may be given before or after the procedure to relieve discomfort.
Miscellaneous			
Bladder scan	Noninvasive method to measure postvoid residual volume or urinary retention	Portable handheld scanner uses ultrasound to create an image and calculate bladder volume. Can be done at the bedside.	Clean the probe. Palpate for the symphysis pubis and apply gel about 1 inch above. Ensure that the probe makes good contact with the gel-covered skin. Point the probe toward the coccyx. Press the scan button for the bladder volume readout.
Renal biopsy	To obtain tissue specimen to determine cause of renal disease, to check for malignancy, or to evaluate extent of transplant rejection	The patient is placed in the prone position, with a pillow under the abdomen at kidney level. A local anesthetic is given. IVP or ultrasound is used to identify the position for biopsy needle insertion into the lower lobe of the kidney below the 12th rib. The patient must hold breath while the needle is inserted and withdrawn. A tissue sample is extracted and sent to the laboratory.	Requires a signed permission form. Urinalysis, CBC, and coagulation studies should be completed. Patient may be NPO for 6-8 hr before the procedure. Postprocedure, a pressure dressing is applied, and the patient remains prone for 30-60 min and on bed rest for 6-24 hr (time varies according to protocol). Vital signs are taken q 5-15 min for 1 hr and PRN until stable. Report signs of hemorrhage, back pain, shoulder ache, dysuria, or infection. Give 3000 mL of fluid unless contraindicated.

CBC, complete blood count; *PRN,* as needed.

the patient should receive a copy of the information in accordance with National Patient Safety Goals. Collect information about changes in urinary output, including amount and character of urine, pain or discomfort in either the bladder or the kidney region, and abnormal patterns of voiding.

 Focused Assessment

Data Collection for the Urinary System

Ask the following questions when assessing the patient with a urologic problem:
- Do you or your family have a history of hypertension, cardiovascular disease, diabetes, kidney stones, frequent urinary tract infections, or other kidney problems?
- Have you ever had genital herpes or another sexually transmissible infection?
- Do you have any pain when urinating? Any abdominal or flank pain?
- Do you have any difficulty in starting the stream of urine?
- Do you feel as though you empty your bladder completely when you urinate?
- Have you noticed any change in the appearance or smell of your urine?
- Have you needed to empty your bladder more frequently than usual?
- Have you been experiencing any urgency, accompanied by dribbling or leaking urine?
- How many times do you need to get up at night to urinate? (Once a night is average.)
- Have you had any episodes of urinary incontinence?
- Have you ever noticed blood in your urine (other than when menstruating [for women])?
- Do you have any problem with sexual dysfunction?
- Are you experiencing excessive fatigue?
- Have you noticed any itching of the skin?
- How much fluid do you drink in a day?

Physical examination should include the following:
- Inspect the abdomen for any visible abnormalities.
- Palpate all four quadrants for areas of tenderness.
- Palpate above the pubic bone for evidence of bladder distention.
- Inspect genitals as appropriate (e.g., reports of bleeding, discharge, presence of or recent discontinuation of indwelling catheter).
- Examine the urine for color, clarity, volume, and smell.

Clinical Cues

Collecting information about sexual health, sexually transmissible infections, and other genital and reproductive disorders, is important as these may be a source of infection or blockage. You may find that it will be easier for you and the patient to talk about these issues toward the end of the interview, after a sense of rapport has been established.

Physical Assessment

Perform a general physical assessment, including a complete set of vital signs and a baseline weight. Observe for signs of generalized or facial edema. Gently palpate the abdomen and the bladder for distention or tenderness. Visually inspect the external genitalia, particularly if there are complaints of pain, discharge, bleeding, prolapse, or if there is an indwelling or recently removed catheter.

Ongoing Assessment

Nursing responsibilities in the daily assessment of urinary function include (1) measuring intake and output; (2) evaluating abnormal flow of urine; (3) noting the character of urine (i.e., color, odor, clarity); (4) noticing changes in the pattern of voiding; and (5) assessing pain and discomfort. Documentation includes objective observations of amount and characteristics of urine and the patient's subjective reports of pain, discomfort, and abnormalities.

Characteristics of Urine. The color of urine can give helpful information about the status of the patient and the functioning of the kidneys. Table 34-3 lists color variations in urine and the significance of abnormal coloration.

Another characteristic that should be noted is *odor*. Normal urine develops an ammonia-like odor after it has stood for a length of time, but this odor should not be present in freshly voided urine. A foul smell may indicate infection. Acetone in the urine, which occurs during metabolic acidosis, causes it to have a sweet, fruity odor.

Hematuria means blood in the urine. Microscopic hematuria occurs when blood in the urine is not visible to the naked eye. Gross hematuria is a sign of bleeding from some point in the urinary tract. Red blood in the urine is not easily missed, but if the blood has been in the bladder or kidney for a long time, it will deteriorate and cause the urine to be a smoky gray or dark brown. If the blood is noticed as soon as voiding starts, it is likely that the blood is from somewhere in the urethra. If it is noticed at the end of urination, the site probably is near the neck of the bladder. Bleeding throughout voiding indicates that the blood is coming from a site above the neck of the bladder, because the blood has been well mixed with the urine in the bladder.

Proteinuria is the abnormal presence of protein in the urine. Proteins are too large to pass through the structure of the glomerular membrane; therefore presence of protein is suggestive of damage to the membrane that occurs in renal disease, such as nephrotic syndrome or glomerulonephritis. Proteinuria is also seen in other conditions such as preeclampsia, multiple myeloma, and diabetes mellitus (Pagana & Pagana, 2009). Specialized assays are required to detect *microalbuminuria* (presence of albumin in the urine) which is suggestive of *early* kidney disease. This test could be considered essential for those at high risk for renal disease, such as persons with diabetes or hypertension.

Pneumaturia means gas in the urine. This can occur if there is a fistula (abnormal passage) between the bladder and the bowel or vagina.

Table 34-3 | **Common Causes of Variations in Color of Urine**

COLOR	MEDICATION	OTHER CAUSES
Colorless or pale yellow	Diuretics	Dilute urine due to diabetes insipidus, diabetes mellitus, overhydration, chronic renal disease, nervousness, alcohol
Bright yellow	Riboflavin (multiple vitamins)	None
Dark amber to orange	Phenazopyridine HCl (Pyridium) Nitrofurantoin (Macrodantin) Sulfasalazine (Azulfidine) Thiamine (multiple vitamins)	Concentrated urine due to dehydration or increased metabolic state (e.g., fever) Urobilinogen (a by-product of bilirubin normally excreted through stool and urine) Bilirubin (a component of bile normally metabolized and excreted via stool and urine) Foods: excessive carrots
Pink to red	Phenothiazines (e.g., Compazine) Docusate calcium (Surfak) Phenolphthalein (Doxidan) (in alkaline urine) Phenytoin (Dilantin) Rifampin Cascara (in alkaline urine) Senna (Senokot)	Fresh red blood cells Menstrual contamination Myoglobin (a by-product of excessive exercise or skeletal tissue damage) Porphyrin (porphyria is a hereditary metabolic disorder) Foods: beets, blackberries, red food dyes
Brown	Cascara (in acid urine) Metronidazole (Flagyl) (if left standing) Phenothiazines (e.g., Compazine)	Extremely concentrated urine due to dehydration or increased metabolic state Red blood cells (old blood) Bilirubin Urobilinogen Myoglobin Porphyrin
Blue or green	Triamterene (Dyrenium) Amitriptyline (Elavil) Methylene blue	Bilirubin Biliverdin (a blue-green pigment that occurs in bile) Pseudomonas infection
Dark brown to black	Nitrofurantoin (Macrodantin) Iron preparations (if left standing) Levodopa (if left standing) Methocarbamol (if left standing) Quinine Senna (X-Prep, Senokot) Methyldopa (Aldomet)	Melanotic tumors Addison's disease Porphyrin Red blood cells (old blood)

Changes in Voiding Pattern. Ask about or observe urinary frequency during the day and night. Other alterations include the size and force of the urinary stream, feeling of fullness even after voiding, and change in the amount urinated each time. Increased frequency can be a manifestation of some abnormality in the urinary drainage system, particularly in the bladder and urethra. The frequency with which a person feels the urge to urinate can be related to psychological as well as physiologic factors. Excitement, anxiety, and fear can produce increased frequency of urination. Caffeine and other diuretics found in foods and drinks and an increased intake of fluid can increase the number of times a person must urinate. Pathologic conditions that can cause increased frequency include inflammation of the bladder (cystitis) or urethra (urethritis).

 Patient Teaching

Urgency is also symptomatic of inflammation. *Urgency* refers to an almost uncontrollable desire to void. Incontinence sometimes occurs because the patient is not able to get to a toilet quickly enough after the urge to urinate occurs. Box 34-2 includes terminology related to changes in urine output and flow.

Pain and Discomfort. In general, the locations in which the patient with a urinary problem is most likely to experience discomfort are either the bladder area or the region over the kidney.

Bladder pain can be due to the stretching of an overfull bladder. Assessment of the size and location of the bladder is indicated when a patient reports pain in the bladder region. Normally the bladder cannot be felt. If a smooth, rounded mass is felt on palpation in the area

Box 34-2   Terminology Related to Urine Output and Flow

- **Anuria:** Absence of urine. This rarely occurs but may be associated with acute renal failure.
- **Oliguria:** Diminished or abnormally decreased flow of urine; may be due to dehydration, renal failure, or obstruction.
- **Polyuria:** Abnormally high and dilute urine output; the result of excessive solutes and increased excretion of water. Possible causes include hypercalcemia, diabetes insipidus, uncontrolled diabetes mellitus, and increased fluid intake.
- **Nocturia:** Urination that occurs during the night; may be related to the decreased ability of the aging kidney to concentrate urine.
- **Urinary frequency:** Voiding more often than every 2 hours. This can be due to inflammation, decreased bladder capacity, psychological disorders, pregnancy, or increased fluid intake.
- **Urinary hesitancy:** A delay in starting the stream of urine; may be related to partial obstruction.
- **Urinary retention:** Retaining or holding urine in the bladder; various causes including neurologic, psychological, medication, obstruction, or anesthesia.
- **Residual urine:** That which is left in the bladder after voiding; related to poor muscle tone or partial obstruction.

above the pubic bone, the bladder is distended. Bladder pain also can be caused by spasms of the bladder musculature as it attempts to empty itself of clots, bits of tissue, and other cellular debris. This can occur postoperatively or when there is moderate to severe inflammation and bleeding in the urinary tract. Relief sometimes can be obtained by irrigating the bladder to remove the clots and debris.

Flank (side and back area of the body below the ribs and above the hips) pain can also be due to obstruction and distention; in this case the affected organs are the ureters and kidney pelvis. Spasmodic peristaltic contractions along the ureter can be caused by stones, clots, a tumor, inflammatory swelling, or any other condition that prevents the flow of urine from the kidney to the bladder. When evaluating flank pain, note the location and assess for radiation of pain from the kidney or ureter to the genitalia and thigh.

Another kind of discomfort may be painful urination, or dysuria. Dysuria usually is caused by inflammation in either the bladder or the urethra. It often is described as burning and can range from mild to severe. The nurse should also ask the patient when the pain occurs and if it is felt immediately before, during, or after voiding.

 Think Critically

What characteristics of a fresh urine specimen might indicate an infection? Why should UTIs be treated promptly?

■ Nursing Diagnosis

Nursing diagnoses frequently associated with urologic problems and disturbances in urinary flow include the following:

- Impaired urinary elimination related to inflammation
- Urinary retention related to removal of indwelling catheter
- Excess fluid volume related to inability of kidneys to produce urine
- Pain related to ureteral spasm, bladder spasm, or inflammation
- Fatigue related to accumulation of waste products
- Deficient knowledge related to prevention of UTI
- Fear related to cause of hematuria or possibility of malignancy
- Disturbed body image related to urinary diversion

■ Planning

Expected outcomes for the above nursing diagnoses might be:

- Patient will void spontaneously, with decreased symptoms (e.g., urgency, dysuria, hematuria) within 48 hours after starting antibiotics.
- Patient will spontaneously void and empty bladder within 6 hours (maximum 8) after catheter removal.
- Patient will have no signs of fluid volume overload (e.g., weight gain, edema, or crackles in lungs) within 2 days.
- Patient will report bladder pain level less than 3/10 during this shift.
- Patient will have adequate energy to independently perform activities of daily living (ADLs) before discharge.
- Patient will identify four or five ways to prevent recurrent UTIs before leaving the clinic today.
- Patient will verbalize concerns or fears about signs and symptoms (e.g., hematuria) during this shift.
- Patient will demonstrate acceptance of stoma as evidenced by looking at stoma and handling ostomy equipment within 1 week.

Planning care of the patient with a disorder of the urologic system involves considering the effect of the disorder on the other body systems. **Fatigue and irritability are common when kidney function is impaired because of the buildup of waste products in the body and their effect on body cells.** In addition, the nurse should educate the patient and the family to maximize participation in treatment goals and prevent complications. General nursing goals for addressing urologic disorders include:

- Absence of infection
- Absence of pain
- Restoration of normal urinary output
- Return to normal fluid balance

- Assimilation of knowledge for appropriate self-care
- Promoting resolution of body image disturbance
- Prevention of complications

■ Implementation

Caring for patients with urologic problems includes monitoring intake and output, body weight, and signs of edema. Monitoring the drug combinations for potential nephrotoxicity and for possible urinary retention is also very important.

The nurse must use strict aseptic technique when catheterizing patients, emptying drainage bags, handling drainage tubes and stents, and when performing peritoneal dialysis or hemodialysis.

The catheter should be fastened to the upper leg with tape or a catheter strap. Long-term catheter use in the male requires that the tube be secured to the abdomen (Figure 34-5). Connecting tubing should be positioned so that there is no pulling on the catheter when the patient turns, moves in bed, or arises to ambulate; this prevents pulling on the balloon that holds the catheter in place, which would cause tissue irritation and predispose to infection. Irrigation of the bladder is not recommended unless there is an obstruction. If irrigation is needed, it should be done using a closed-system technique to prevent infection (Gould et al., 2009). See Table 35-3 for common urinary catheters and tubes used for urologic disorders. Box 34-3 reviews principles of catheter care.

⚖️ Legal and Ethical Considerations

Urinary Catheters

Urinary catheters are the most common cause of health care–associated infection. In 2008, Medicare stopped paying the estimated $451 million for this complication (Chettle, 2008). Alternatives to catheterization should always be considered to prevent infection, and the care should be carefully documented. In accordance with the 2010 National Patient Safety Goals, when a patient dies of a health care–associated infection, the death is investigated to determine how the infection developed and contributed to the death of the patient. The purpose of the investigation is to prevent future incidents.

| Box **34-3** | Principles of Urinary Catheter and Tube Care |

- Use aseptic technique and gentle handling when caring for any urinary drainage tube.
- Insert urethral catheters using sterile technique.
- Never open a urinary drainage system unless there is no alternative (e.g., the drainage bag must be changed for some reason).
- Empty the drainage bag by opening the drainage port at the bottom of the bag; use aseptic technique and do not allow the drainage tube to touch the collection container. After reclamping the tube, wipe away residual urine from the tube with an antiseptic swab before securing it.
- Use patient's individual collection container for draining the urine storage bag.
- Observe all tubes and level of drainage in the collection bag each time the patient is seen.
- Keep the drainage bag below the level of the catheter or insertion site (indwelling catheter drainage bags should have a backflow valve, but keeping the bag lower prevents backflow). If the bag must be raised above the insertion site, clamp off the tube briefly while repositioning the patient.
- Perform perineal care at least twice daily, cleaning the urinary meatus and catheter with soap and water; rinse well, just as the area would be cleansed if the patient were bathing normally (see agency's policy).
- Keep an intake and output record to help monitor kidney function.
- Encourage fluids to 3000 mL/day unless contraindicated.
- When irrigating, use the correct amount of sterile solution (according to agency policy, or the amount of solution that may be determined by physician's order for nephrostomy tubes, ureteral tubes, or catheters).
- Use a steady, gentle stream to irrigate. Avoid exerting pressure that may traumatize or cause discomfort.
- Do not pull back forcefully on an irrigating syringe attached to a urinary catheter or tube as this creates negative pressure that may damage delicate tissues or collapse the tube.
- When discontinuing an indwelling catheter, never cut the catheter. Use a syringe to deflate the balloon.

FIGURE 34-5 Catheter tubing attached to a collection bag with catheter secured to the abdomen for the male and the thigh for the female.

> **⬧ Clinical Cues**
>
> You can collect a urine specimen from a new drainage bag immediately after the catheter is inserted. If the catheter has been in place for several hours or days, you should not take the specimen from the drainage bag because the urine specimen must be fresh. The tube must temporarily be clamped and the specimen must be drawn from the upper port. Do not forget to unclamp the tube after you have obtained the specimen.

Measuring Intake and Output

The quantity of fluids entering the body, by whatever route, has a direct bearing on fluid balance (see Chapter 3). Patients with urologic disorders are very likely to suffer fluid imbalances, and therefore their intake and output should be measured and the totals recorded every 8 hours during hospitalization or acute illness. In critically ill patients, the urinary output is often measured hourly. **Urine output should be at least 30 mL/hr. For total output, measure all urine excreted, drainage from all tubes, any emesis, and watery stools.** An estimate of the amount of fluid lost through perspiration should also be considered, if perspiration is excessive (e.g., sweating with fever). Any fluid used to irrigate catheters and tubing must be measured and the amount should be added to the total intake and subsequent output.

■ Evaluation

The nurse compares intake and output data over time to determine clinical improvement or the presence of problems. The frequency of comparison will be hour-to-hour for critical patients or over a period of days for patients with chronic conditions. Laboratory data, such as BUN, creatinine, potassium, and urinalysis results, provide further information to evaluate the effectiveness of treatment. A decrease in subjective symptoms, such as flank pain or dysuria, also indicates resolution of the problem.

COMMON UROLOGIC PROBLEMS

URINARY INCONTINENCE

Etiology

In the United States, more than $26 billion a year is spent on incontinence; the problem affects 16.9% of women and 16% of men. Worldwide estimates are 17%. Among institutionalized persons, over 50% are incontinent (Pavlovich-Danis, 2009). Likewise, those who are incontinent appear to be more likely to be institutionalized. Women who have had several children may have anatomical changes that make incontinence more likely. Men may experience the problem because of an enlarged prostate. Other contributing factors include spinal cord injury, neurologic

disorder (e.g., dementia), or functional disorder (e.g., difficulty manipulating clothing fasteners).

When incontinence is occurring, the first step is to identify factors that may be contributing to the patient's incontinence. Immobility, UTI, atrophic urethritis or vaginitis associated with menopause, stool impaction, prostate surgery, delirium or confusion, endocrine problems, and various types of medication, such as alpha-adrenergic agents, beta-adrenergic agonists, and calcium channel blockers, may contribute to the problem of incontinence. Obesity also is a factor, as it causes increased pressure on the bladder.

Pathophysiology

Urine flow out of the bladder is controlled by two circular muscles called *sphincters*. The internal sphincter lies close to the lowermost part of the bladder, and the external sphincter surrounds the urethra. Many factors can cause loss of sphincter control. Unconsciousness, UTI, paralysis, interference with nerve transmission to and from the brain, and loss of muscle tone of the bladder and sphincters are some of the conditions that frequently cause patients to become incontinent.

Signs and Symptoms

There are several types of incontinence: urge, stress, mixed, overflow, functional, or incontinence due to neurologic dysfunction. *Urge incontinence* is the involuntary loss of urine when there is a strong urge to urinate (urinary urgency). *Stress incontinence* occurs when the urethral sphincter fails and there is an increase in intra-abdominal pressure, caused by such things as sneezing, laughing, coughing, or aerobic exercise. *Mixed incontinence* is a combination of different types, such as stress and urge incontinence. *Overflow incontinence* occurs when there is poor contractility of the detrusor muscle or obstruction of the urethra, as in prostate hypertrophy in the male or genital prolapse in the female. *Functional incontinence* is caused by cognitive inability to recognize the urge to urinate or self-care deficit caused by extreme depression. Inability to reach the bathroom due to restraints, side rails, or an out-of-reach walker can also result in functional incontinence. *Neurologic incontinence* is caused by disorders of the neurologic system (e.g., multiple sclerosis or spinal cord injury).

Diagnosis

Diagnosis of incontinence is based on a careful history, and the patient must be able to report symptoms accurately (Table 34-4). The patient may be asked to keep a bladder diary. Routine urinalysis is also performed. When conservative measures do not improve continence, the physician may choose to evaluate the condition with a series of diagnostic tests, including measuring the postvoid residual, stress testing, urodynamic studies, cystogram, or cystoscopy.

Table 34-4 Common Nursing Diagnosis, Expected Outcomes, and Interventions for Patients with Incontinence

NURSING DIAGNOSIS	EXPECTED OUTCOMES	INTERVENTIONS
Functional urinary incontinence related to decreased muscular strength and fine motor coordination	Patient will be able to physically get to the toilet (or commode chair) and accomplish toileting (i.e., undo clothing and sit on toilet) with assistance during this shift.	Assess abilities to stand, walk, and sit. Instruct patient to call for help when needing to go to the toilet. Offer assistance q 2-4 hr. Obtain bedside commode as needed. Suggest clothing with elastic waistband or Velcro fasteners to eliminate zippers and buttons. Encourage independence, as appropriate (consider strength and motor ability).
Stress urinary incontinence related to weak pelvic muscles	Patient will increase control over incontinence within 8-12 wk.	Assess pattern of incontinence and identify actions associated with incontinence (e.g., laughing, coughing) Teach Kegel exercises. Teach to avoid bladder irritants such as coffee, nicotine. Refer to nutritionist for weight loss diet if overweight. Discuss use of incontinence pads or undergarments. Supply information about vaginal cone therapy.
Urge urinary incontinence related to bladder spasms	Patient will experience urge to void and be able to get to the toilet in time to prevent loss of urine.	Instruct patient to keep a voiding diary, or observe for incontinence if unable to self-report. Help patient establish a voiding schedule (e.g., q 3-4 hr). Give antispasmodic medications (e.g., tolterodine) as ordered. Teach patient about side effects of medication (e.g., possible urinary retention).
Self-care deficit, toileting related to impaired cognition	Patient will participate in a routine toileting schedule during hospitalization.	Assess cognitive deficits related to toileting (e.g., unable to remember to go to toilet; senses urge to go, but cannot find the toilet). Observe for odors, stains, or wetness on clothing and linens. Assist (or remind) patient to go to the toilet q 2-3 hr. Provide visual cues to prompt toileting (e.g., commode chair at bedside, large arrows pointing toward bathroom, picture of toilet on the bathroom door). Give positive feedback for efforts.
Risk for impaired skin integrity related to moisture and irritation of urine on skin	Patient's skin will remain dry and intact without breakdown during hospitalization.	Assess for patterns of urinary incontinence (e.g., if patient cannot self-report, check q 2-3 hr). Give fluids primarily during the day and space fluids (e.g., q 2-3 hr) for predictability of voiding. Provide (or assist) with skin care (e.g., clean with mild soap and warm water; use skin barrier creams). Consult with enterostomal therapist (ET nurse) as needed (skin breakdown is progressive).

Table 34-4	Common Nursing Diagnosis, Expected Outcomes, and Interventions for Patients with Incontinence—cont'd	

NURSING DIAGNOSIS	EXPECTED OUTCOMES	INTERVENTIONS
Risk for impaired skin integrity related to moisture and irritation of urine on skin—cont'd		Turn q 2 hr if patient is bedridden or immobile. Ensure adequate nutrition for healing and skin integrity (e.g., high-quality proteins).
Sleep deprivation related to nocturia	Patient will rest and sleep at least 6 consecutive hr each night during hospitalization.	Assess for medication (e.g., calcium channel blockers) side effects that may be contributing to incontinence. Teach patients to avoid taking fluids in late evening hours. Assist (or instruct patient) to ambulate for at least 10 min 1–2 hr before bedtime, then instruct to void before going to bed. Use incontinence pads or undergarments for women and condom catheters for men during the night.
Deficient knowledge related to management of incontinence	Patient will verbalize two or three methods to manage incontinence before leaving the clinic today.	Teach patient about medication side effects (e.g., if on estrogen, patient should report vaginal bleeding or signs of deep vein thrombosis, calf pain, or swelling). Teach Kegel exercises; reinforce that results may take up to 3 mo. Teach bladder training; remind that accidents are expected during training period.
Social isolation related to embarrassment	Patient will maintain usual social contact with friends and family.	Encourage verbalization of feelings (e.g., shame or embarrassment). Assist patient to identify times, settings, and activities when incontinence may occur (e.g., during exercise). Help patient make a plan to deal with incontinence during social occasions (e.g., use of incontinence briefs, mapping out toilet locations, planning fluid intake around social occasions). Refer to support groups.

Treatment

Evidence-based practice indicates that stress incontinence that occurs with exercise, laughing, or coughing may be corrected by exercises to strengthen the pelvic floor muscles (Geriatric Medicine, 2009).

Vaginal weight training with a set of five small, cone-shaped weights that are used along with pelvic muscle exercise is another therapeutic option for incontinence. The lightest cone, which has a string attached, is inserted into the vagina and held in place by muscle tightening for 15 minutes twice a day. When there is no problem holding this cone in place, the next heaviest cone is used. This continues until the heaviest cone can be held in place for the 15-minute period. Maintaining normal weight and using topical estrogen therapy after menopause also decreases the incidence of this disorder.

Various medications, such as phenylpropanolamine, pseudoephedrine, propantheline (Pro-Banthine), oxybutynin (Ditropan), tolterodine (Detrol), dicyclomine hydrochloride (Bentyl), imipramine (Tofranil), doxepin (Sinequan), and other tricyclic antidepressants, have been found to be helpful in treating incontinence. Recently approved drugs for overactive bladder (OAB) include darifenacin (Enablex), oxybutynin, transdermal patch (Oxytrol), solifenacin (Vesicare), trospium (Sanctura), and fesoterodine (Toviaz). Other medications that show promise, but are not yet approved by the Food and Drug Administration, include botulinum toxin A (Botox), tramadol (Ultram), baclofen (Lioresal), duloxetine (Cymbalta), and gabapentin (Neurontin). Table 34-5 provides additional information about selected drugs for urinary incontinence.

Patient Teaching

Kegel Exercises

- To locate the correct muscle, stop the flow of urine while urinating on the toilet by tightening the anus as if preventing a bowel movement.
- Practice for several days each time you urinate. Then begin the exercise program.
- While lying down, slowly count 1-2-3 while tightening the pelvic muscles.
- Release pelvic muscles slowly to the count 1-2-3. Do this 15 times.
- While sitting, repeat the above sequence 15 times: tightening pelvic muscles while counting 1-2-3, and then slowly releasing to the count 1-2-3.
- Stand and repeat the sequence 15 times: tighten to the count 1-2-3, and slowly release to the count 1-2-3.
- Do the pelvic muscle exercises once a day. If you can do them twice each day, improvement in continence will occur more quickly.
- Improvement may be noted in 6 to 8 weeks, but may take as long as 3 months.

Further treatment options for urinary incontinence include biofeedback therapy or an implanted electrical stimulation device called InterStim (Pavlovich-Danis, 2009). A clamp-type device across the penile urethra can be used for men or occlusive devices can be inserted into the vagina or urethra for women; patients or caregivers must be able to apply and remove these devices to prevent tissue damage. Periurethral bulking is a procedure done under local anesthesia in which collagen is injected into the urethra to increase resistance.

 Complementary and Alternative Therapies

Transvaginal Electrical Stimulation

In transvaginal electrical stimulation (TES), the nerves and muscles of the pelvic floor are stimulated by an electrically charged probe. In a small study of TES, women had fewer incontinence episodes and had significant improvements in libido and sexual satisfaction (Katz, 2009).

Surgeries to Correct Incontinence. A variety of procedures may be performed to correct the anatomical position of the bladder, such as bladder neck suspension. These surgeries are most often performed to correct urinary incontinence in women. The *retropubic suspension* (Marshall-Marchetti-Krantz) procedure is performed to correct a cystocele (prolapse of the bladder into the vagina) and urinary incontinence. A low abdominal incision is made and the urethral position is elevated in relation to the bladder. Urethral and suprapubic catheters are in place for several days postoperatively. In the *needle bladder neck suspension* (Pereyra or Stamey) procedure, a vaginal approach is combined with a small suprapubic skin incision to elevate the urethral position in relation to the bladder. Direct visualization of the operative area is not possible

Table 34-5 **Selected Drugs for Urinary Incontinence and Retention**

CLASSIFICATION	ACTION	NURSING IMPLICATIONS	PATIENT TEACHING
Urinary antispasmodics, antimuscarinics Oxybutynin (Ditropan), solifenacin (Vesicare), tolterodine (Detrol), trospium (Sanctura), fesoterodine (Toviaz)	Used to relieve spasms of the bladder; treats overactive bladder and incontinence	Give mouth care, as needed. Monitor I&O. Auscultate bowel sounds. Side effects include dry mouth, increased heart rate, dizziness, abdominal distention, and constipation.	Take fiber foods and fluids to prevent constipation. Do not drive if dizzy or drowsy. Use ice chips or hard candy for dry mouth. May need eyedrops to moisten dry eyes.
Bladder stimulant Bethanechol (Urecholine)	Used to treat urinary retention	Monitor for orthostatic hypotension and bradycardia. Give 1-2 hr after meals or with food for GI complaints. May cause diarrhea, cramping, or increased salivation.	Immediately report severe dizziness or difficulty breathing. Rise slowly from a lying to standing position.
Medication for benign prostatic hypertrophy Tamsulosin (Flomax)	Relieves symptoms of urinary retention associated with obstruction from an enlarged prostate	May cause orthostatic hypotension. Side effects include back pain, chest pain, cough, diarrhea, nausea, dizziness, headache, weakness.	May take 6 mo for symptom relief. Do not crush, chew, or open the capsule. Immediately report a prolonged erection.

GI, gastrointestinal; *I&O,* intake and output.

with this procedure, and it tends to result in more complications than the retropubic suspension. However, the success rate for preventing incontinence is higher. An *artificial sphincter implant* is used more frequently to correct incontinence in males than for females. A mechanical device is placed around the urethra to open and close it.

In a large clinical study, the Stress Incontinence Surgical Treatment Efficacy Trial (SISTEr), the sling procedure was a successful option for women with stress incontinence; 86% of women were generally satisfied with the outcomes (Albo et al., 2007). In the sling procedure a portion of the woman's own tissue is used to reconstruct additional support for the urethra. Following the sling procedure, the nurse should monitor for urinary tract infection and difficulty voiding.

When these measures do not solve the problem, incontinence is managed by intermittent catheterization, indwelling urethral catheterization, suprapubic catheter, external collection system (such as condom catheters), protective pads and garments, or pelvic organ support devices.

 Clinical Cues

Your patient may develop leaking around the suprapubic catheter. If leaking persists and urine is continuously leaking onto the skin, this could mean that the tube is too small. If the tube has been there a long time, the tissue contours may have changed since the initial insertion. Notify the RN or physician for evaluation.

Nursing Management

Use a gentle and matter-of-fact approach when taking an incontinence history. Evidence-based practice supports the use of protocols or guidelines for screening for urinary incontinence (Dowling-Castronovo & Specht, 2009). The patient may be embarrassed by the symptoms, but it is likely that she will welcome the help and suggestions. Observe the clothing for stains and odors and perform a general physical assessment that includes palpation of the bladder. Inspect the genitalia if there is reason to suspect a prolapse, or if there is a catheter present or recently removed.

 Elder Care Points

Assess elderly patients for gross motor strength, fine motor dexterity, and ability to balance and independently ambulate. The elderly patient may be having trouble walking to the bathroom or sitting on or rising from the toilet seat. In addition, clothing fasteners may be problematic.

 Focused Assessment

Assessment for Urinary Incontinence

- What kinds of problems are you having with your bladder?
- Are you having trouble holding your urine (water)?
- When did the urine leakage problem start?
- How often do you accidentally leak urine?
- Are you accidentally soiling your clothing or bed linens?
- When do the accidental leaks occur? Does it happen during the day or the night? Both?
- How often do you wear a pad or other protective device?
- What activities or situations are associated with leakage? For example, does laughing, coughing, sneezing, or exercising cause leakage?
- Are you having difficulty getting to the bathroom in time?
- Are there things about your house that are preventing you from getting to the bathroom in time? For example, do you have to climb stairs or walk a long distance?
- Do you have (or need) assistive devices (e.g., handrails) in the bathroom?

When incontinence is not remedied by correcting an underlying cause, the nurse attempts to help the patient by setting up a voiding and fluid schedule. Assess when the patient is experiencing incontinence. Evidence-based practice suggests that a voiding diary is a useful tool for patients who can self-report (Dowling-Castronovo & Specht, 2009). Box 34-4 provides guidelines for establishing a toileting schedule.

Toileting assistance can be offered at set times just before incontinence usually occurs. Getting the patient on a voiding schedule takes a great deal of patience and persistence on the part of the nurse and the patient. Accidents will happen during the retraining period, and patients need to be assured that this is expected. (See Chapter 23 for care of patients with incontinence related to spinal cord injury.)

Box 34-4	Assisting Patients to Establish a Toileting Schedule

- Assess pattern of incontinence or instruct patient to keep a voiding diary.
- Assist (or remind) patient to go to the toilet at set times (just before the time when incontinence usually occurs).
- Space fluid intake and give the majority of fluids during the day.
- Discourage intake of bladder stimulants, such as alcohol and caffeine.
- Help the patient ambulate for at least 10 minutes an hour or two before bedtime because activity helps to mobilize fluid.
- Apply a condom catheter for males and moisture-proof pants or incontinence pads for women, at night; it is not practical to continue a voiding schedule (every 3 to 4 hours) at night.
- Give positive reinforcement for any small successes.

Assignment Considerations
Bladder Training

In planning and implementing a bladder training program for your confused patient, who is unable to self-report, there are several ways the nursing assistant (NA) can provide valuable help. Ask the NA to record and report any fluids that are offered and consumed and the number of times that clothes, wet bed linens, or incontinence pads need to be changed. Once the schedule is established, direct the NA to help the patient follow the schedule by assisting her to the toilet at the designated times.

Patients may experience transient incontinence or urinary retention after removal of an indwelling catheter that has been in place for several days. Usually the catheter is clamped for intervals and then opened to drainage before it is removed to help rebuild bladder muscle tone. After this has been done for 12 to 24 hours, the catheter is removed. The patient should then be instructed to void every hour to prevent incontinence. **Any bleeding, dribbling, or incontinence of urine or inability to void within 4 to 6 hours (maximum of 8) after removal of the catheter should be reported to the physician.** It takes time to retrain the bladder to hold greater capacity. Gradually the interval between voidings is lengthened to 2, 3, or 4 hours.

Health Promotion
Drinks and Substances to Avoid

Advise patients that avoiding caffeine, alcohol, carbonated beverages, and aspartame may help bladder control. These substances may stimulate or irritate the bladder.

URINARY RETENTION

Urinary retention is retaining or holding urine in the bladder. It can be acute after a surgical procedure, after removal of an indwelling catheter, or with certain medications (e.g., atropine); it may be a chronic condition related to anxiety, neurologic disorders, or obstruction of urine flow through the urethra, as in

enlargement of the prostate gland. A straight catheter is used for a single "in-and-out" catheterization for temporary inability to empty the bladder. Also, patients who have permanent paralysis may use intermittent catheterization to empty the bladder.

Urinary retention will not cause the bladder to rupture, but urine will begin to dribble out of the urethra. Retention of urine stretches the bladder walls, causing extreme discomfort. Assess the degree of bladder distention using gentle palpation before and after intervention. Assist the patient by providing privacy and adequate time for voiding efforts. A caffeinated drink, followed by a warm bath, may help. Instruct to double void: void, sit on the toilet for several minutes, and void again. Schedule a trip to the toilet every 3 to 4 hours. Obtain an order for catheterization if other measures do not relieve the problem. A medication for urinary retention is bethanechol (Urecholine). Examples of medications that relieve the symptoms produced by benign prostatic hypertrophy (enlarged prostate gland) include tamsulosin (Flomax), doxazosin (Cardura), and finasteride (Proscar) (see Table 34-5).

Poor bladder tone or partial obstruction of the urethra can result in dribbling of urine or passing only the overflow, leaving the bladder partially full. During bladder retraining, residual urine can be measured by having the patient void as much urine as possible and then immediately inserting a catheter or performing a bladder scan (see Table 34-2). One hundred milliliters is considered a normal amount of residual urine. Any amount over this can become stagnant and concentrated over time, predisposing the patient to bladder infection and the formation of stones.

Think Critically

The physician ordered removal of an indwelling catheter. Three hours later the patient complains of bladder fullness with inability to void. What should you do?

Get Ready for the NCLEX® Examination!

Key Points

- The urologic system is responsible for maintaining proper balance of the fluids, minerals, and organic substances necessary for life.
- The nephron is the functional unit of the kidney. It consists of the glomerulus, which is a network of capillaries encased in a thin-walled sac called *Bowman's capsule*, and the tubular system.
- Kidney function, GFR, bladder capacity, ability to concentrate urine and secrete renin, and aldosterone all decrease with aging.
- Infection, immunologic disorders, metabolic disorders such as diabetes mellitus, and reduced blood flow secondary to shock or atherosclerosis can result in kidney damage.
- Stones, an enlarged prostate, or tumors may obstruct the flow of urine.

- Tubular necrosis affects the functional ability of the kidney. It can result from lack of oxygen or bacterial or chemical destruction of the nephron.
- Hypertension is a major cause of end-stage kidney disease; conversely, renal disorders can also cause secondary hypertension.
- To promote healthy kidneys, advise patients to drink plenty of water, to empty the bladder at regular intervals, to obtain prompt treatment for bladder infection, to practice good hygiene, to maintain normal serum glucose, and to take blood pressure medication as prescribed.
- BUN and serum creatinine are the most common screening tests for kidney function.
- Monitor intake and output, weight, and signs of edema; monitor drugs for nephrotoxic effects.
- Nursing measures for incontinence include assisting in determining and correcting underlying cause, establishing a voiding and fluid schedule, coaching Kegel exercises, giving medications for incontinence as ordered, and advising to decrease bladder irritants.
- Nursing measures for urinary retention include assessing for bladder distention, providing privacy, instructing to double void, and obtaining an order for catheterization as needed.

Additional Learning Resources

SG Go to your Study Guide for additional learning activities to help you master this chapter content.

evolve Go to your Evolve website (http://evolve.elsevier.com/deWit/medsurg) for the following FREE learning resources:
- Animations, audio, and video
- Answers and rationales for questions and activities
- Concept Map Creator
- Glossary with pronunciations in English and Spanish
- Interactive Review Questions and Exercises and more!

 Online Resources
- Urinary Incontinence, www.mayoclinic.com/health/urinary-incontinence/DS00404
- Urinary Catheters, www.nlm.nih.gov/medlineplus/ency/article/003981.htm

Review Questions for the NCLEX® Examination

1. The nurse is trying to console an elderly patient who is embarrassed about wetting the bed. Which patient comment is consistent with functional incontinence?
   1. "I knew that I needed to go, but I couldn't get out of bed by myself."
   2. "Every time I laugh, cough, or sneeze I pass a little bit of urine."
   3. "When I need to pee, I really have to go right away!"
   4. "My doctor says that my enlarged prostate is causing the problem."

2. What information would the nurse give to a community group about prevention of urologic problems?
   1. Taking an ACE inhibitor, such as captopril, could potentially damage the kidneys.
   2. Drinking several glasses of fluid a day helps to preserve kidney function.
   3. Emptying the bladder decreases prolonged exposure to toxins.
   4. Eating spinach, chocolate, or strawberries causes kidney stones.

3. The night shift nurse is planning care for four patients. Which patient is most likely to have nocturia related to a decreased ability to concentrate urine?
   1. Patient with a high BUN
   2. A pregnant patient
   3. An elderly patient
   4. Patient who had a bladder scan

4. When starting a 24-hour urine collection, what is essential in order to ensure correct results?
   1. Include the first void of the 24-hour period.
   2. Record the time of initial void as the start time of the test.
   3. Discard the last void of the 24-hour period.
   4. Encourage fluid intake before starting the test.

5. Which action by a nursing assistant indicates inadequate knowledge regarding indwelling catheter care?
   1. Keeping the drainage bag below the level of the insertion site
   2. Using aseptic technique to empty the drainage bag
   3. Placing the drainage bag on the bed when repositioning the patient
   4. Performing the perineal care at least twice daily

6. In determining the specific type of urinary incontinence, what is an appropriate assessment question?
   1. "Do you have any difficulty in starting the stream of urine?"
   2. "Do you feel pain when you urinate?"
   3. "Have you needed to empty the bladder more frequently than usual?"
   4. "Have you been experiencing any urgency, accompanied by dribbling or leaking urine?"

7. What is the first action that the nurse should take to assist a patient to develop a toileting schedule?
   1. Encourage use of condom catheters or incontinence pads.
   2. Assess pattern of incontinence.
   3. Schedule trips to the bathroom.
   4. Provide positive reinforcement for small successes.

8. A patient is scheduled to have a renal biopsy. What is included in the preoperative care for this patient? *(Select all that apply.)*

   1. Administer bowel preparation.
   2. Report abnormal coagulation studies.
   3. Enforce nothing by mouth (NPO) for 6 to 8 hours before the procedure.
   4. Check for allergy to contrast media.
   5. Insert indwelling urinary catheter.

9. Which nursing intervention(s) would be appropriate for a patient with stress incontinence? *(Select all that apply.)*

   1. Instruct patient to keep a voiding diary.
   2. Teach patient Kegel exercises.
   3. Offer patient assistance every 3 to 4 hours.
   4. Obtain bedside commode as needed.
   5. Teach patient to avoid bladder irritants, such as coffee and nicotine.

10. _____ is a by-product of skeletal muscle contraction.

Critical Thinking Activities

Scenario A

Mr. Jones, 65 years old, has a history of difficulty passing urine. The physician orders placement of a retention catheter. You attempt to insert a 14-Fr Foley catheter but you meet resistance and the catheter will not pass. The patient reports an uncomfortable sensation in his genital area during the attempt.

1. What is your initial action?

2. Based on your knowledge of pathophysiology, what would you suspect is preventing the passage of the catheter?

3. Once the catheter has been successfully inserted, explain why it is important to keep the drainage bag below the level of the bladder.

4. How would you perform daily catheter care for Mr. Jones?

5. Discuss four or five general principles that you will use while caring for Mr. Jones' catheter.

6. Which tasks would be appropriate to delegate to a nursing assistant (NA)? Select all that apply and give a rationale.

   a. Gathering the equipment for the catheterization procedure
   b. Inserting the Foley catheter
   c. Emptying the drainage bag at the end of the shift
   d. Checking the urinary meatus for complaints of bleeding

Scenario B

A 56-year-old woman, Mrs. Russlyn reports that she has been leaking a little urine occasionally. She makes a joke about hesitating to laugh or sneeze in public.

1. What type of incontinence is associated with dribbling urine when laughing, coughing, or sneezing?

2. What questions will you ask to collect additional data about Mrs. Russlyn's incontinence?

3. What kinds of treatment options are likely to be recommended for Mrs. Russlyn?

Scenario C

You are working in a long-term care facility and caring for Ms. Lilley, an 85-year-old with Alzheimer's disease. She has developed urinary incontinence.

1. What factors might be contributing to your patient's incontinence?

2. Explain how to develop a toileting and fluid intake schedule for Ms. Lilley.

Care of Patients with Disorders of the Urinary System

Objectives

Theory

1. Describe the signs and symptoms of selected urologic inflammatory disorders (e.g., cystitis, urethritis, and pyelonephritis) and nursing interventions for these patients.
2. Discuss nursing management for patients with acute or chronic glomerulonephritis.
3. Analyze types of patient conditions that create a risk for acute renal failure.
4. Compare the needs of patients on long-term hemodialysis with patients who use peritoneal dialysis.
5. Identify the benefits and special problems associated with kidney transplantation.

Clinical Practice

1. Describe the postoperative nursing care of patients having surgery of the kidney.
2. List specific nursing responsibilities in the care of patients with kidney stones.
3. Provide postoperative nursing care of patients having surgery for urinary diversion.
4. Perform interventions to increase patient compliance in the treatment of chronic kidney failure.
5. Devise a nursing care plan for the home care patient with renal failure.

Key Terms

acute renal failure (ă-KŪT, pp. 794, 798)
anuria (ă-NŪ-rē-ă, p. 789)
azotemia (ă-zō-TĒ-mē-ă, p. 802)
chronic renal failure (CRF) (KRŎN-ĭk, p. 801)
cystitis (sĭs-TĪ-tĭs, p. 785)
end-stage renal disease (ESRD) (p. 798)
glomerulonephritis (glō-měr-ū-lō-ně-FRĪ-tĭs, p. 789)
hemodialysis (hē-mō-dī-ĂL-ĭ-sĭs, p. 800)
hydronephrosis (hī-drō-ně-FRŌ-sĭs, p. 790)
lithiasis (p. 791)
lithotripsy (LĬTH-ō-trĭp-sē, p. 793)

nephrectomy (něf-RĚK-tō-mē, p. 790)
nephrostomy (ně-FRŎS-tō-mē, p. 790)
nephrotic syndrome (něf-RĚ-tĭk, p. 790)
oliguria (ŏl-ĭ-GŪ-rē-ă, p. 789)
peritoneal dialysis (pě-rĭ-tō-NĒ-ăl dī-ĂL-ĭ-sĭs, p. 800)
pyelonephritis (pī-ă-lō-ně-FRĪ-tĭs, p. 788)
renal stenosis (stě-NŌ-sĭs, p. 791)
uremia (ū-RĒ-mē-ă, p. 802)
uremic syndrome (p. 802)
urethritis (ū-rě-THRĪ-tĭs, p. 785)
urinary diversion (ūr-ĭ-NĂ-rē dĭ-VĚR-shŭn, p. 796)

The kidneys play a role in maintaining fluid balance, regulating the electrochemical composition of body fluids, providing protection against acid-base imbalance, forming red blood cells, regulating calcium levels, and eliminating waste products. The kidneys also help to control blood pressure, in conjunction with the endocrine system. Circulatory disorders, metabolic disorders such as diabetes mellitus, immunologic disorders, obstruction, bacterial infections, or toxic substances can all cause kidney dysfunction.

INFLAMMATORY DISORDERS OF THE URINARY TRACT

CYSTITIS

Etiology and Pathophysiology

Cystitis is an inflammation of the urinary bladder. It is one of the most common urinary tract infections (UTIs) in women because the female urethra is shorter and the urinary meatus is exposed to contamination from the vagina and anus. The *Escherichia coli* bacterium normally resides in the intestinal tract as a nonpathogenic microorganism and it accounts for about 80% of all UTIs in females.

Cystitis and urethritis (inflammation of the urethra) are often seen in women after they have become sexually active. *Honeymoon cystitis* is a term you may hear; in this case, bacteria have entered the urethra by way of friction during intercourse. In older women, the incidence of cystitis and urethritis increases with age as the decreased muscle tone in the urinary tract prevents complete emptying of the bladder. Urine that sits in the bladder (urinary stasis) provides a good medium for bacterial growth. The estrogen depletion that occurs with aging results in structural atrophy and urinary dysfunction.

In addition, many elderly people purposely restrict fluid intake to decrease the incidence of incontinence.

Elder Care Points

In elderly women, the urethra sometimes becomes displaced and opens into the vaginal outlet; this increases the risk for infection. This structural change occurs because of decreased muscle tone and atrophy of surrounding tissues.

Others restrict fluids to help control heart failure, renal failure, or other disorders that cause fluid retention. Restricting fluid intake decreases urine flow and makes the person more susceptible to urinary tract infection.

Signs, Symptoms, and Diagnosis

The most common symptoms of cystitis are painful urination, frequent and urgent urination, and low back pain. The urinary meatus may appear swollen and inflamed. Cystitis has a tendency to recur, producing less-acute symptoms such as fatigue, anorexia, and a constant feeling of pressure in the bladder region

Elder Care Points

Confusion may be one of the first signs of cystitis or UTI in older adults. If a patient who is normally alert becomes confused, assess the urine for cloudiness, foul odor, or hematuria (blood in the urine), and check for signs of infection (fever, increased white blood cell [WBC] count).

between flare-ups. The urine may appear cloudy or even bloody and have a foul smell. Urinalysis and urine cultures are used to establish a definite diagnosis and to identify the specific causative organism.

Treatment and Nursing Management

Treatment and nursing care of cystitis and urethritis (see description of urethritis on p. 788) are similar. First, specimens are collected for tests to identify the causative organism: urinalysis, urine culture and sensitivity, smear and Gram stain, or culture of the discharge. Specific antibiotics, such as trimethoprim-sulfamethoxazole (Bactrim), are used to combat infection and are combined with urinary analgesics such as phenazopyridine (Pyridium) to relieve discomfort.

Postmenopausal women may benefit from topical estrogen. Table 35-1 shows the most commonly used drugs and nursing implications. The patient is encouraged to drink large amounts of fluids (8 to 12 large 8-oz glasses unless contraindicated) to flush the bladder and to continue the habit once the acute symptoms subside. Evidence-based practice indicates that cranberry-based products, which alter urine pH, also have been used to prevent or treat urinary tract infections (Guay, 2009). Measures to relieve the discomfort include sitz baths and hot water bottles on the back or directly over the bladder region.

Table 35-1 Drugs Used for Urinary Tract Infections

CLASSIFICATION	ACTION	NURSING IMPLICATIONS	PATIENT TEACHING
Sulfonamides			
Trimethoprim-sulfamethoxazole (Bactrim, Septra) Sulfisoxazole (Gantrisin) Sulfamethoxazole (Gantanol)	Active against gram-negative and gram-positive organisms	Assess for allergies to sulfonamides. Record I&O. Fluid intake is a minimum of 3000 mL daily. Monitor laboratory results and symptoms related to anemia, blood dyscrasias, and renal dysfunction. (e.g., hemoglobin, hematocrit, WBCs, BUN). Sulfonamides can potentiate oral anticoagulants, methotrexate, and sulfonylureas (e.g., Glucotrol).	Drink at least 12 large glasses of water each day to prevent crystallization of urine. Immediately report rash, abdominal pain, blood in urine, confusion, difficulty breathing, or fever. Repeat urinalysis after course of medication.
Fluoroquinolones			
Ciprofloxacin (Cipro) Levofloxacin (Levaquin) Newer agents Moxifloxacin (Avelox) Trovafloxacin (Trovan)	Bactericidal Considered second-line drugs; are used as alternatives to other antibiotics	Can be taken with or without food. If antacids are ordered, wait 2 hr after giving Cipro. Monitor WBCs for decreased leukocytes. Can potentiate warfarin and increase theophylline levels. Use cautiously in those patients with history of seizure disorder or alcoholism.	Take all of medication. Drink at least 8 full glasses of water/day to prevent crystalluria.

Table 35-1 Drugs Used for Urinary Tract Infections—cont'd

CLASSIFICATION	ACTION	NURSING IMPLICATIONS	PATIENT TEACHING
Cephalosporins			
First generation Cefazolin (Ancef)	Bactericidal; used to treat infections that do not respond to other, less expensive drugs	Use cautiously in those with allergy to penicillin. *Candida* (yeast) vaginitis is a common side effect.	Can cause dizziness or light-headedness.
Third generation Ceftazidime (Fortaz) Cefixime (Suprax)		May interfere with vitamin K metabolism; therefore may reduce prothrombin levels.	Immediately report rash, restlessness, gastrointestinal symptoms, confusion, or irregular heartbeat.
Fourth generation Cefepime (Maxipime)		Monitor I&O, BUN, serum creatinine.	Avoid alcohol.
Aminoglycosides			
Tobramycin Gentamicin	Effective against resistant infections; use cautiously, as they are nephrotoxic, ototoxic, and can cause agranulocytosis and thrombocytopenia	Monitor BUN, electrolyte, and creatinine levels. Elderly persons are especially vulnerable to problems with hearing, balance, and kidney dysfunction caused by aminoglycosides.	Use sunscreen and avoid direct exposure to sunlight. Report nausea, vomiting, tremors, or tinnitus. Take extra fluid unless contraindicated.
Penicillins			
Extended spectrum Carbenicillin (Geocillin) Ticarcillin/clavulanic acid (Timentin) Piperacillin tazobactam (Zosyn)	Bacteriostatic and bactericidal	Carbenicillin PO only. Ticarcillin/clavulanic acid IV only. Watch for signs of hypersensitivity (e.g., rash, itching, difficulty breathing). Do not give to patients with known allergy to penicillin. May decrease effectiveness of oral contraceptives and warfarin.	Take full course of prescribed medication. Take with water 1-2 hr after meals to increase absorption. Immediately report abdominal pain, decreased urine, watery or bloody diarrhea.
Miscellaneous Urinary Antibiotics			
Nitrofurantoin (Macrodantin, Furadantin)	Wide range of antibacterial action against gram-negative and gram-positive organisms; especially *Escherichia coli*	Monitor I&O. Liquid form can stain teeth; rinse mouth after administration.	Tints urine brown. Take with food and increase fluids. Can cause drowsiness; therefore avoid driving. Report numbness or tingling.
Fosfomycin tromethamine (Monurol)	Effective against most gram-negative and gram-positive organisms	Single-dose treatment. Not for use in children less than 12 yr old.	Can cause headaches and diarrhea.
Doripenem (Doribax) for complicated UTIs, including pyelonephritis	For serious infections caused by gram-positive and gram-negative bacteria	Injection only. Can reduce valproic acid levels to a subtherapeutic level, so level should be monitored.	The most common side effects include headache, nausea, diarrhea, rash, and phlebitis.
Urinary Analgesics			
Phenazopyridine (Pyridium)	Has analgesic effect on urinary mucosa	Is nephrotoxic, hepatotoxic, and can cause gastrointestinal disturbance and anemia.	Colors urine orange and can stain fabric. Discontinue if sclera becomes yellow. Maximum 2 days' use.

BUN, blood urea nitrogen; *I&O,* intake and output; *UTIs,* urinary tract infections; *WBCs,* white blood cells.

FIGURE 35-1 A, A renal staghorn calculus. The renal pelvis is filled and resembles the horn of a stag ("S" on the figure marks the calculus). **B,** Staghorn calculus as seen on an intravenous pyelogram.

Table 35-2 Risk Factors and Treatments for Renal Stones

STONE TYPE	RISK FACTORS	INTERVENTIONS
Calcium oxalate (most common type)	An increased intake of protein, sodium; inadequate fluid intake, prolonged immobility	Increase fluid intake. Medications to bind oxalate (cholestyramine) or calcium (e.g., cellulose phosphate). Diuretics (e.g., hydrochlorothiazide) to encourage flushing. Avoid oxalate sources such as spinach, chard, parsley, peanuts, chocolate, and strawberries.
Calcium phosphate	An increased intake of protein, sodium; inadequate fluid intake, primary hyperparathyroidism	Limit intake of foods high in protein and sodium. Treat underlying hyperparathyroidism.
Uric acid	Excess dietary purine (e.g., organ meats, gravies, red wines, and sardines) Gout (primary or secondary)	Decrease intake of purine sources. Alkalinize urine with potassium citrate or lemonade. Administer allopurinol for gout (decreases production of uric acid).
Struvite (more common in women)	Urinary tract infections	Administer antibiotics for infection and acetohydroxamic acid (inhibits the chemical action of bacteria that contributes to struvite stone formation), as ordered.
Cystine	Hereditary cystine crystal formation	Encourage oral fluids, up to 3 L/day. Medications to prevent crystallization (e.g., tiopronin). Alkalinize urine with potassium citrate or lemonade.

condition removes the cause of the stones. Risk factors for kidney stone formation include:

- Male gender
- A family history of renal stones
- History of intestinal bypass surgery for obesity (these patients have an increased absorption of oxalate from foods)
- Immobility for any reason, which contributes to urinary stasis and calcium loss from bones
- History of recurrent urinary tract infections

Prevention

A continuous flow of dilute urine flushes the tract and removes substances that could form stones. **Ideally, the adult must put out at least 3500 mL of urine every 24 hours to prevent stone formation; likewise, preventing urinary infections and maintaining adequate drainage through tubes and catheters is also necessary.** In those cases in which the urine pH is crucial to stone formation, changing the urine pH can prevent or reduce the incidence of renal calculi. Ascorbic acid or dietary modifications (e.g., cranberry juice or prunes) can be used to acidify urine.

Signs and Symptoms

Some renal stones do not cause noticeable symptoms and can be passed without the person being aware of them. Others may lodge in the renal pelvis and cause symptoms only after the destruction of kidney cells.

The kidney stones that cause severe pain are those that are small enough to move along the ureter with the urine. As the stone rolls along, sharp little spikes scrape the ureteral lining, causing excruciating pain and bleeding. Pain is typically felt in the flank over the affected kidney and ureter, and radiates downward toward the genitalia and inner thigh. Nausea and vomiting often occur because of the severity of the pain. **Moving stones can get trapped along the ureter, causing obstruction of flow and swelling of the ureter.**

 Think Critically

A colleague tells you that your patient is seeking narcotics and is "faking" kidney stone pain and intentionally introducing blood into his urine sample. How would you respond to this?

Diagnosis

Diagnostic tests include urinalysis and a kidney, ureters, bladder (KUB) study to locate stones that are radiopaque (materials such as metal will appear as a white area on the radiograph) and an intravenous pyelogram (IVP) will show a gap (nonradiopaque stone) in the stream of dye being excreted in the urine. Further studies of the blood and urine might be done to determine the levels of substances, such as calcium, uric acid, and cystine that can contribute to stone formation.

Treatment

At first, the physician may try to flush the stone out by increasing the patient's intravenous (IV) fluids or oral fluid intake and managing pain by prescribing opioid analgesics or nonsteroidal anti-inflammatory drugs (NSAIDs) and antispasmodics, such as propantheline bromide (Pro-Banthine) or oxybutynin chloride (Ditropan). If there is pus in the urine, an antibiotic is prescribed to deal with infection.

Some stones can be flushed by irrigation through a ureteral catheter or percutaneous nephrostomy tube or crushed by ultrasound. Usually, a stent will be placed in the ureter to allow the stone fragments to pass more freely. Extracorporeal shock wave lithotripsy (ESWL) has largely replaced surgery for renal stones. For this treatment the patient is placed in a water bath; newer machines use a water-filled mat. Shock waves are generated, pass through the water, bounce off a reflector, and break the stone. Sedation is used to help the patient remain calm and still during the 30- to 45-minute procedure. After the procedure, the patient may experience cramping pain and is given pain medications (e.g., hydrocodone-acetaminophen [Vicodin]) if this occurs. A fluid intake of 3000 to 4000 mL is necessary to help wash the stone fragments from the kidney. The fragments travel in the urine down the ureter and into the bladder for excretion. Early ambulation helps mobilize the fluid and the stone fragments so that they can be eliminated in the urine. Refinements of this treatment are ongoing, with the goal being to break up stones effectively while minimizing the cost and discomfort for the patient.

 Think Critically

Based on your knowledge of anatomy and physiology, what is the difference between a *urethral* catheter and a *ureteral* catheter? (Note the spelling difference!) Why is it important to know the difference between these two catheter sites?

Adjunctive therapy for ESWL includes corticosteroids and calcium channel blockers and alpha antagonists (e.g., tamsulosin), which increase the rate of stone passage. Percussion, diuresis, and inversion (PDI) therapy is used after ESWL. In this procedure, diuresis is promoted and the patient is placed in a prone, reverse Trendelenburg's position and massaged or percussed to encourage stone movement.

When the stone is not passed spontaneously, cystoscopy or surgical intervention is necessary. Nephrolithotomy (incision into the kidney to remove a stone) or pyelonephrolithotomy (surgical removal of a stone from the renal pelvis) can be performed for large stones that will not pass. These procedures may be done percutaneously or with an open procedure. A special forceps is introduced through the nephroscope to retrieve the stone. A nephrostomy tube is inserted as the scope is removed and this remains in place for 1 to 5 days. A fluid intake of 3000 to 4000 mL/day is required to flush any residual stone fragments out of the kidney. The patient is monitored for infection, hemorrhage, and leakage of fluid into the retroperitoneal cavity. When a stone cannot be retrieved by percutaneous procedure, an open procedure is used. If a stone is lodged in a ureter and will not descend after fluid increases, a ureterolithotomy (surgical removal of a stone from a ureter) is performed.

If the stone is 5 mm or greater, the patient could also receive a ureteral stent (usually a soft flexible silicone tube), which is inserted through a cystoscope or nephrostomy tube, or during surgery. The purpose of a ureteral stent is to maintain the patency of the ureter to allow stones to pass through. Stents are not visible on the outside of the body. They are usually removed in 4 to 6 weeks in an outpatient setting. Nursing interventions include monitoring for infection, bleeding, urine output, and pain. Once stones have been removed, chemical analyses of the urine, blood, and the stone itself are necessary to plan effective preventive measures. Table 35-3 provides additional information about common catheters and tubes used for urologic disorders.

Nursing Management

During initial assessment of a patient with kidney stones, the patient may have extreme pain, so use concise questions to gather information about pain,

Table 35-3	Common Catheters and Tubes Used for Urologic Disorders
TYPE	**PURPOSE**
Urethral catheter	Drains urine from the bladder.
Foley catheter	Indwelling catheter for continuous urine drainage from the bladder.
Suprapubic catheter	Continuous drainage of urine from the bladder; inserted in suprapubic area of abdomen through abdominal and bladder wall.
Ureteral catheter	Drains urine directly from the ureter or kidney.
Ureteral stent	Tube placed in ureter to hold it open during healing; not visible on the outside of the body.
Nephrostomy tube	Placed into the pelvis of the kidney to provide drainage of urine directly from the kidney.

changes in urinary output, and characteristics of the urine. Asking family about risk factors and history may be appropriate.

Attempts are made to have the patient pass the stone spontaneously, and all urine is strained to recover the stone or fragments for analysis. This is accomplished by having the patient void into a urinal or collection device and then pouring the collected urine through a fine mesh filter. Fluids are encouraged during this time to facilitate flushing of the stone.

UROLOGIC SYSTEM TRAUMA

TRAUMA TO KIDNEYS AND URETERS
Etiology and Pathophysiology
Accidental injury to the kidneys, ureters, bladder, or urethra should always be considered whenever there has been trauma to the abdominal cavity, lower back, or thoracic cage. Injury to the kidneys is usually caused by blunt trauma that is sustained during a motor vehicle, sports, or occupational accident. Damage can occur as a result of a direct blow, laceration from an adjacent rib or vertebra fracture, or from sudden deceleration, which shears and tears the body tissue. Ureteral injuries are mostly associated with penetrating trauma; the right side is three times more likely than the left side to be involved. Trauma to the urinary system can range from minor contusion to severe hemorrhage that leads to hypovolemic shock.

Signs, Symptoms, and Diagnosis
Signs and symptoms characteristic of trauma to the kidneys include massive hemorrhage, hematuria, abdominal or flank pain, and possibly an enlarged mass in the kidney area. Diagnostic tests include serial urinalyses, hemoglobin and hematocrit tests, and measurements of electrolytes. Rising BUN and serum creatinine levels indicate diminishing renal function. Radiologic studies (KUB, IVP, or CT scan) can demonstrate the extent of damage to the urinary system. MRI or angiography is used in high-risk cases or if CT scan is indeterminate. Hourly measurements of urinary output and observation of the characteristics of the urine can help determine the type and extent of injury.

Clinical Cues
When your patient sustains significant trauma to skeletal muscle tissue, he may develop rhabdomyolysis. Damaged muscles release myoglobin into the bloodstream, and these large muscle proteins can cause **acute renal failure** (sudden loss of kidney function); however, the condition is reversible. Be alert for brown or tea-colored urine after trauma, strenuous exercise, or extensive burns, and report your findings to the physician.

Treatment
Bleeding in the kidney is often self-limiting. Lacerations and contusions without interruption of urinary function usually can be treated conservatively by bed rest. For this reason, the nephrologist may advocate a period of watchful waiting to see whether the kidney can be saved. If the kidney is severely damaged, the patient may undergo a nephrectomy. The remaining kidney then enlarges and is usually able to carry on the work formerly done by two kidneys.

Nursing Management
Preoperative Nursing Care. Patients with kidney trauma are likely to have damage to the colon, spleen, or pancreas. A comprehensive plan for dealing with problems associated with multiple trauma is usually necessary. Preoperatively, the patient is monitored closely for signs of hypovolemic shock, cardiovascular changes, urinary output, and size of the flank hematoma. Grey Turner sign is bruising over the flank or lower back and suggests retroperitoneal bleeding. For most trauma patients, a urethral catheter is inserted into the bladder. An indwelling catheter allows for close observation of urinary output—for example, critically ill patients may need hourly urine output measurements, and a drainage bag with a urometer should replace the standard drainage bag.

Postoperative Nursing Care. Postoperative nursing care for nephrectomy or nephrostomy is described on p. 791.

TRAUMA TO THE BLADDER
Etiology and Pathophysiology
Any violent blow or crushing injury to the lower abdomen may result in rupture or perforation of the bladder wall, with resulting leakage of the urine into

the pelvic tissues or peritoneal cavity. This results in severe inflammation (peritonitis). Bladder trauma is more likely to occur if the bladder is full at the time of an accident, rather than if it is empty.

Signs and Symptoms
Early symptoms of bladder injury are painful hematuria or inability to void, marked tenderness and spasm in the suprapubic area, or the development of a large mass in that area.

 Clinical Cues

In cases of pelvic or perineal trauma, bleeding at the urethral meatus, inability to void, or a distended bladder may indicate a urethral tear. Notify the physician before inserting a catheter, because catheter insertion can increase the damage by extending the tear.

Diagnosis and Treatment
Diagnosis is based on presence of gross hematuria, suprapubic pain, and difficulty voiding. Retrograde or CT cystography is obtained if bladder injuries are suspected. If the bladder has ruptured or is perforated, treatment consists of a suprapubic cystostomy to drain blood and urine.

Nursing Management
Care of the patient demands meticulous attention to drains and dressings to avoid infection and maintain good drainage. Cold applications to the surgical site both before and after surgery may be ordered. You should observe the patient carefully for postoperative shock and massive hemorrhage. Any mass formation in the suprapubic area before or after surgery, or any change in vital signs, should be reported immediately.

UROLOGIC SYSTEM CANCERS

CANCER OF THE BLADDER

Etiology and Pathophysiology
Approximately 70,980 new cases of bladder cancer were diagnosed in 2009 and resulted in 14,330 deaths (American Cancer Society, 2009). This cancer occurs more often in men (ages 60 to 80) than in women. **Smokers have double the risk of developing this cancer.** People living in urban areas or with occupational exposure to nitrates, dyes, rubber, or leather processing (i.e., painters, hairdressers, or textile workers) are at higher risk. The bladder wall is exposed to these carcinogenic chemicals in the urine. Tumors of the bladder usually start in the superficial transitional cell layer and are considered to be papillomas (benign tumors on the epithelial tissue). Bladder tumors are removed—even though they are papillomas—because there is a high risk for invasion into the deeper tissues, and metastasis.

Signs, Symptoms, and Diagnosis
The main symptom of a bladder tumor is hematuria. Frequency, urgency, or dysuria also may be present. Diagnosis is confirmed by IVP and by examining the bladder wall with a cystoscope and biopsy of the tumor.

 Complementary and Alternative Therapies
Healthy Bladder

Smoking cessation and including vegetables such as cabbage or broccoli in the diet contribute to a healthy bladder and a decreased risk of bladder cancer (Pizzorno et al., 2008).

Treatment
Treatment for bladder cancer is surgery, either alone or in combination with chemotherapy or radiation. The type of surgical treatment depends on the clinical stage of the tumor. Every effort is made to preserve the bladder if the tumor is confined to the mucosa or submucosa. In this case, a partial cystectomy or transurethral resection of the bladder tumor (TURB, TURBT) is performed and followed by intravesical chemotherapy (i.e., cisplatin [Platinol], doxorubicin [Adriamycin]) or bacille Calmette-Guérin (BCG) instillations (Intravesical, TheraCys). BCG was originally used as a vaccine against tuberculosis. It has helped patients with bladder carcinoma in situ (site of origin) by reducing tumor recurrence and by eliminating residual malignant cells after surgery. The solution is instilled into the bladder via a urinary catheter. The catheter is clamped for 2 hours and the patient's position is changed every 15 to 30 minutes. Treatments are continued weekly for 6 weeks with possible maintenance doses. Advise your patient that BCG intravesical therapy is likely to cause future tuberculin skin tests to show false positive.

 Clinical Cues

In addition to using Universal Precautions, when disposing of the urine after a BCG treatment, the toilet should be disinfected with bleach for 6 hours after disposing of the waste.

Photodynamic therapy can be used for superficial tumors. In this therapy, a solution of light-sensitive molecules is injected IV. These molecules adhere to cancer cells longer than to normal cells. A cystoscope with a red laser light can then be used to activate the photosensitizers that destroy tumor cells.

Surgeries for Urinary Diversion. Bladder surgery may be minor, such as removing polyps from the bladder interior using a cystoscope, or major, such as cystectomy (removal of the bladder) for bladder cancer. Following cystectomy, there is always the danger of hemorrhage and infection. There are also problems in devising a satisfactory arrangement for urine collection. When the bladder is surgically removed, the surgeon performs a **urinary diversion** to handle the excretion of urine and creates an artificial opening (stoma) on the skin surface. Diversions also can be performed for neurogenic bladder, congenital anomalies, strictures, or trauma. There are several ways in which urinary diversion can be accomplished (Figure 35-2), including ileal conduit or ileal loop, cutaneous ureterostomy, vesicostomy, ureterosigmoidostomy or sigmoid conduit, and ileal reservoir (i.e., Kock, Indiana, Mainz, or Florida pouch). The difference

in these various procedures is the segment of bowel that is used.

Cutaneous ureterostomy and vesicotomy. Ureterostomy is a surgical incision into the ureter that diverts the flow of urine. In a cutaneous ureterostomy, the surgeon detaches one or both ureters from the bladder and brings them to the surface of the body, usually in the region of the flank. The patient may have one or two stomas. If the patient has a cutaneous ureterostomy with two stomas (one from each ureter), the flow

Ureterostomies divert urine directly to the skin surface through a ureteral skin opening (stoma). After ureterostomy, the client must wear a pouch.

Cutaneous
ureterostomy

Cutaneous
ureteroureterostomy

Bilateral cutaneous
ureterostomy

Conduits collect urine in a portion of the intestine, which is then opened onto the skin surface as a stoma. After the creation of a conduit, the client must wear a pouch.

Ileal (Bricker's) conduit

Colon conduit

Ileal reservoirs divert urine into a surgically created pouch, or pocket, that functions as a bladder. The stoma is continent, and the client removes urine by regular self-catheterization.

Continent internal
ileal reservoir
(Kock pouch)

Sigmoidostomies divert urine to the large intestine, so no stoma is required. The client excretes urine with bowel movements, and bowel incontinence may result.

Ureterosigmoidostomy

Ureteroiliosigmoidostomy

FIGURE 35-2 Surgeries for urinary diversion.

of urine, from each stoma, must be measured. Any tubing leading from the ureterostomy should be kept open so that urine can flow freely. The tube is checked frequently for signs of obstruction by mucus or blood clots. A vesicotomy is an incision into the bladder just above the pubic area. After incising the bladder, the surgeon moves it forward and sutures the cut edges to the skin, forming a stoma.

Ileal conduit. An ileal conduit is also called *urinary ileostomy and ileal loop* or *Bricker's procedure.* A portion of the ileum is used as a tube or conduit through which urine flows to the outside. The section of ileum is separated from the intestinal tract. Urine does *not* flow through it to the intestines, as when the ureters are sutured to the sigmoid. The two open ends of the intestines where the section of ileum was removed are rejoined by anastomosis (operative union of structures). The surgeon cuts out a portion of the ileum, leaving nerve and blood supply intact so that it remains a viable tissue. The "borrowed" section of ileum is sutured together at one end to form a pouch, and the other end is brought outside to form a stoma. The ureters are attached to the ileal conduit so that urine can flow through the conduit to the outside.

Ureterosigmoidostomy or sigmoid conduit. A sigmoid or colonic conduit is similar to an ileal conduit, the difference being that a portion of the sigmoid colon is used to form the conduit. The ureters are implanted in the conduit.

Ileal reservoir (Kock pouch). This procedure creates a continent ileal reservoir. The ureters are implanted into a segment of ileum that has been isolated. Special nipple valves connect the pouch to the exterior of the skin. The pouch can then be catheterized via the nipple valve by the patient, providing continence with no exterior collection device. The distal nipple valve is brought flush to the skin on the right side of the abdomen, forming a stoma. The patient is continent of urine, but needs to catheterize the pouch several times a day to empty the urine. An adhesive bandage or gauze pad over the stoma will absorb the secreted mucus. Daily irrigation of the pouch is performed to remove the threads of mucus in the urine that are secreted by the mucous membrane of the ileal or colonic segment of the conduit. Whitish crystals or encrustations in or near the stoma indicate alkaline urine; this should be reported so that treatment can be prescribed to prevent stone formation.

Indiana pouch. This type of pouch is constructed from portions of the ileum and cecum, and the ileocecal valve provides a means of continence. It is larger than the Kock pouch and spherical in shape with lower internal pressure that helps prevent incontinence. The ureters are tunneled into the pouch wall to help prevent reflux into the kidneys. The pouch is emptied via self-catheterization of the nipple valve in the same manner as the Kock pouch.

Clinical Cues

There are significant differences in the irrigation of tubes, drains, and stomas for the urinary system, so make sure to **clarify orders!** For example, the Indiana pouch may be irrigated one to four times a day with 30 to 60 mL of normal saline (size and maturity of the pouch will vary) (United Ostomy Association, 2010), whereas ureteral stents or ureteral catheters are usually not irrigated. If the physician does order irrigation of a stent or ureteral catheter, the amounts of sterile normal saline are much smaller (3 and 10 mL).

Orthotic bladder substitutes. Bladder substitutes or neobladders can be created using a portion of the patient's own intestine; they are more commonly used for male patients with cancer of the bladder, when the sphincter is intact and there is no cancer in the urethra or bladder neck. The advantage is normal micturition. Examples include hemi-Kock, Studer, and ileal W-neobladder.

Nursing Management
Postoperative Nursing Care. Following surgery, observe for pain, abdominal rigidity, fever, and bleeding. Assess the amount and characteristics of the urine and mucus and record accurate output of urine every hour for the first 24 hours and then every 4 to 8 hours. **Regardless of which surgical procedure the patient has had, the urine should never stop flowing.**

The urine should initially be light red or pink and progress to clear within 3 days or less. Bright red bleeding or clots should be reported immediately. The stoma should be pink or red. A pale, dark, or dusky stoma suggests decreased blood flow, which should be reported immediately. Skin irritation and breakdown can be a problem, and every effort is made to keep urine from touching the skin when the patient has an external stoma. A well-fitted and properly adhering collection appliance is essential. A thin gauze roll or tampon is placed into the stoma during appliance changing and cleaning, to prevent leakage of urine onto the skin. For a permanent ostomy, the bag can be used for 3 to 7 days. The bag should be emptied when it becomes one third to half full, to prevent the weight of the urine from pulling the bag loose. At night the bag can be connected to a larger urine container. The bag should be changed in the morning because there is less urine flow. The area around the stoma is washed with a solution of 1:1 vinegar and warm water to remove any crystals. If no crystals are present, warm, soapy water may be used. The area is thoroughly rinsed and patted dry with a towel before a new bag is attached, because any remaining moisture may interfere with the seal of the new appliance. A bath or shower may be taken with the bag on or off.

Most appliances contain an odor barrier; however, odor may be a problem because of poor hygiene, alkaline urine, and normal breakdown of urine when it is exposed to air, and the ingestion of certain foods, such as asparagus. Dilute urine is also less odorous and this is accomplished by increasing fluid intake. Reusable appliances must be washed with soap and water and soaked in dilute white vinegar solution or a commercial deodorizing product for 20 to 30 minutes. The pouch is then rinsed and allowed to dry. Deodorant tablets may be placed in the appliance to decrease odor.

 Complementary and Alternative Therapies

Reduce Odor of Urine

For the patient with a urinary diversion, a diet that includes whole grains, nuts, plums, prunes, and cranberry juice will help to acidify the urine and decrease odors.

Psychological care of the patient facing malignancy and an operation that will radically change his body image should be a primary nursing concern, and there are always sexual concerns when a urinary diversion is performed. Some of the more radical procedures will produce impotence in the male. You must encourage the patient and spouse to talk about fears and concerns and provide emotional support. Help the patient and family to identify appropriate community resources and make referrals as needed for specialized counseling.

CANCER OF THE KIDNEY

Etiology and Pathophysiology

Cancer of the kidney is relatively uncommon; however, these tumors are extremely difficult to treat in the later stages. Neoplasms of the kidney occur in men (ages 50 to 70) twice as often as in women. Risk factors include smoking and exposure to lead or phosphate.

The tumors usually begin growing in the renal cortex. They can become very large, but they are well defined and press into the renal structures rather than invade the tissue. The blood vessels also can become constricted by the tumor growth.

Signs, Symptoms, and Diagnosis

The principal symptoms of malignant tumors of the kidney are hematuria, palpable abdominal or flank mass, and flank pain (although pain and a mass may not be present in the early stages). Other symptoms that may occur are fever, fatigue, weight loss, decreased appetite, and hypertension. Renal angiogram, arteriogram, CT, MRI, or ultrasound may be performed to determine whether the symptoms are being caused by a cyst (nonmalignant) or by a tumor.

Treatment and Nursing Management

The only treatment that has any success is surgical removal of the affected kidney (nephrectomy) before metastasis has occurred. Unfortunately, the patient usually does not have severe symptoms until metastases have occurred. Chemotherapy with a variety of drug regimens is used for metastatic cancer (see Chapter 8). Immunotherapy may be used for recurrent tumors.

Sunitinib (Sutent) and sorafenib tosylate (Nexavar) are drugs for advanced kidney cancer. They act to deprive the tumor cells of blood and nutrients. Temsirolimus (Torisel) and newly approved everolimus (Afinitor) inhibit tumor cell growth and proliferation; these drugs are available to patients who failed to respond to sunitinib or sorafenib. Another recently approved drug, pazopanib (Votrient), interferes with the growth of new blood vessels that would supply the tumor.

Nursing care of the patient is the same as that for patients after nephrectomy (see Chapter 8 for care of patients with cancer).

RENAL FAILURE

Renal failure is the inability of the kidneys to maintain normal function. Renal failure is classified as acute or chronic. The final stage of chronic and irreversible renal failure is called **end-stage renal disease (ESRD)**.

ACUTE RENAL FAILURE

Etiology

Acute renal failure (ARF) occurs suddenly as a result of physical injury, infection, inflammation, or damage from toxic chemicals. Nephrotoxic agents are those that are poisonous to kidney cells and include many drugs, iodine substances used as radiographic contrast media, heavy metals, snake venom, or exposure to industrial chemicals. These toxins may inflict damage on the renal tubules, causing acute tubular necrosis (ATN) and loss of function. They can also indirectly harm the tubules by causing severe constriction of blood vessels that serve the kidney, producing renal ischemia. ATN is responsible for 90% of acute renal failure. Other causes of renal ischemia include circulatory collapse, severe dehydration, and prolonged hypotension in compromised surgical or trauma patients.

Pathophysiology

The pathophysiology of ARF is not well understood. One theory is that cellular or protein debris in the tubules blocks the flow of urine and filtration stops. Another theory is that decreased blood flow results in oxygen deprivation, which causes cellular death and tubular necrosis.

There are three types of acute renal failure, depending on the cause. *Prerenal ARF* is caused by decreased blood flow, such as in hypovolemic shock, or decreased cardiac output, as in cardiogenic shock. *Intrarenal ARF* occurs from glomerular damage, ATN caused by ischemia or toxins, or vascular disease that affects the vessels in the kidney. *Postrenal ARF* is caused by obstruction in the ureters, bladder, or urethra—for example, an enlarged prostate—which causes eventual backup of urine into the kidney, which in turn leads to tissue damage. ARF is potentially reversible, especially if identified early; the patient often regains kidney function. Concept Map 35-1 shows the pathophysiology of renal failure.

? Think Critically

During your clinical experience, which of your patients may have been at risk for ARF? What factors placed these patients at risk?

The course of acute tubular necrosis is divided into three phases: oliguric/nonoliguric, diuretic, and recovery phases. In the oliguric/nonoliguric phase, the patient puts out either a great deal of or very little urine. Oliguria is a urine output of 100 to 400 mL in 24 hours. This phase usually occurs immediately or within 1 week after an ischemic event and lasts for an average of 10 to 14 days; however, it can go on for weeks to months, and prolonged oliguria worsens

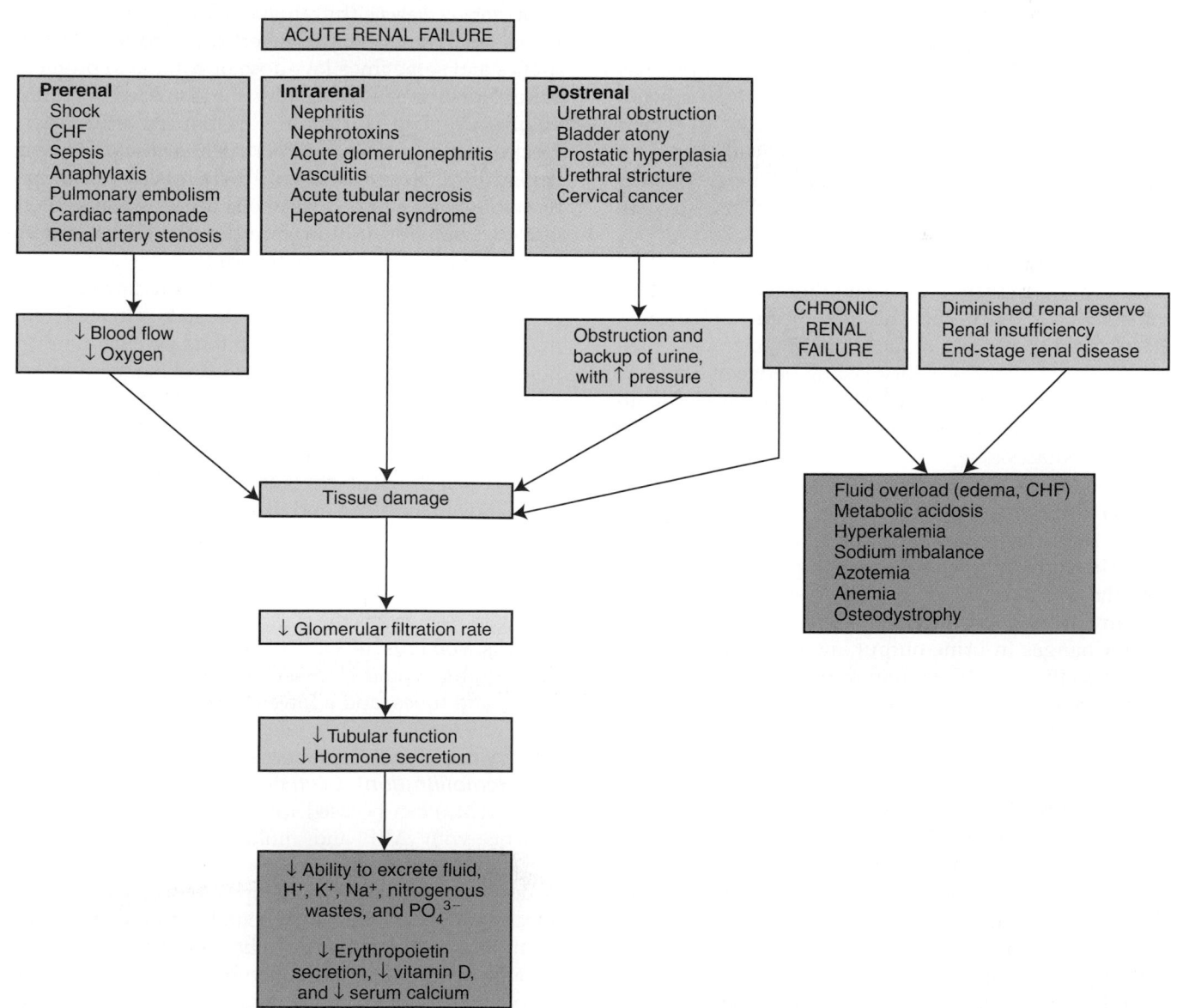

CONCEPT MAP 35-1 Pathophysiology of renal failure.

the prognosis. BUN and creatinine levels rise. When this occurs, there may be volume overload, which can precipitate heart failure, multiple electrolyte imbalances, metabolic acidosis, catabolism (destructive breakdown of body tissue), and end-stage renal failure (ESRF); dialysis is needed.

 Elder Care Points

Because of the overall decreased kidney function related to aging, your elderly patient may be experiencing oliguria even though urine volumes are as high as 600 to 700 mL/day.

Nonoliguric ATN is often due to nephrotoxic agents. Urine output is greater, but the kidneys cannot eliminate waste products efficiently, and BUN and creatinine levels rise and electrolyte imbalances occur. Dialysis is needed less often or for shorter periods, and the prognosis is better than for oliguric failure.

The diuretic phase only occurs if dialysis has not been started early and extracellular fluid volume has built up. In this phase, the kidney is unable to concentrate urine, and output can be between 1000 and 2000 mL/day. With this increased output, there is a danger of dehydration, hyponatremia, and hypokalemia. Approximately 25% of deaths related to ARF occur during this phase.

The recovery phase begins as the kidney function begins to normalize. The concentration of urine, urine output, and electrolyte balance begin to recover. There are 1 to 2 weeks of rapid improvement and then a period of slower recovery lasting between 3 and 12 months. About one third of ARF patients are left with residual renal insufficiency, and about 5% must continue dialysis.

Signs and Symptoms

Renal failure will have an impact on the entire body, and the signs and symptoms will vary according to the phase and response to treatment. Carefully observe for any of the following:

- Changes in urine output and urine results (e.g., specific gravity, proteinuria)
- Electrolyte imbalances (e.g., hyponatremia, hyperkalemia, hypocalcemia)
- Fluid imbalance (e.g., hypotension, hypertension, edema, pulmonary edema)
- Acid-base imbalance (e.g., metabolic acidosis)
- Gastrointestinal effects (e.g., nausea, vomiting, anorexia, constipation)
- Mental status changes (e.g., lethargy, memory impairment)
- Anemia and platelet dysfunction (e.g., fatigue, bleeding signs, and bruising)
- Impaired wound healing and susceptibility to infection (e.g., elevated WBC)

Diagnosis

Diagnostic testing includes urinalysis, creatinine, BUN, CBC, electrolytes, and arterial blood gases. In addition, radiologic studies (such as ultrasound, IVP, CT, or MRI) can be performed if an obstruction is suspected. A renal biopsy may be obtained to assist in determining etiology or to evaluate the extent of kidney damage.

Treatment

Treatment of ARF is aimed toward correcting the underlying cause and preventing or controlling complications and maintaining a tolerable internal environment until the kidneys are able to recover and resume their normal functions. Symptomatic treatment includes correction of fluid and electrolyte balances, management of anemia and hypertension, and cleansing the blood and tissues of waste products with hemodialysis (filtration of blood across a semipermeable membrane) or peritoneal dialysis (filtration of blood across the peritoneal membrane). Volume overload is treated with diuretics and sometimes low-dose dopamine to promote better kidney perfusion. Dialysis is also used to reduce volume overload if it cannot be reduced with drugs. Electrolyte imbalances (hyperkalemia, hypocalcemia, hyperphosphatemia, and mild hypermagnesemia) are monitored and treated. Metabolic acidosis, if severe, is treated with IV sodium bicarbonate. Dialysis with buffer in the dialysate may be used.

Other problems include malnutrition, anemia, and potential for infection. The catabolic state is treated with nutritional management through total parenteral nutrition (TPN). Potassium, phosphate, and magnesium are omitted from the solution while the patient is oliguric. Anemia occurs because the kidney cannot produce normal amounts of erythropoietin. The life span of red blood cells is shortened because of both the toxic wastes circulating in the blood and the hemodilution from fluid overload. To treat this anemia, the physician may order epoetin alfa (Epogen), a synthetic substance that stimulates red blood cell production. Infection frequently occurs with ARF and is the leading cause of death in these patients. You must be vigilant in monitoring for signs of infection that could be associated with IV access sites, drains and tubes, and a lowered immunity state.

Continuous Renal Replacement Therapies (Continuous Hemofiltration). *Continuous renal replacement therapies* (CRRTs) can be used for intensive care unit (ICU) patients with ARF and multisystem organ involvement or for those who are hemodynamically unstable. A double-lumen catheter is typically inserted into the subclavian or internal jugular vein. The blood is removed from the arterial lumen of the catheter and passed through a semipermeable membrane and returned to the venous lumen of the catheter (Dirkes & Hodge, 2008). This method filters out wastes much more slowly than hemodialysis but does not cause such rapid fluid and electrolyte shifts. Continuous arteriovenous hemofiltration (CAVH) uses the patient's own blood pressure to pump the blood. Continuous arteriovenous hemodialysis (CAVHD) combines hemodialysis and hemofiltration, thus removing waste and fluid. Continuous venovenous hemofiltration (CVVH) and continuous venovenous hemodiafiltration (CVVHDF) are both controlled by a pump (Clin-eguide, 2009). Slow continuous ultrafiltration (SCUF) is primarily used for fluid removal, such as for patients with pulmonary edema (Dirkes & Hodge, 2008).

❖ NURSING MANAGEMENT
■ Assessment (Data Collection)

When taking a patient's history, include questions that relate to fluid imbalance (e.g., changes in voiding patterns, weight gain, vomiting, or edema) and potential risk factors (e.g., patient or family history of renal disease or hypertension, recent surgery, trauma, or anesthesia, exposure to nephrotoxic substances and any medications). The patient should also be encouraged to describe specific symptoms (e.g., fatigue, lethargy, weakness, or pain).

All patients need a complete head-to-toe assessment and complete vital signs at the beginning of every shift. Acutely ill patients who are at risk for ARF need frequent reassessment for signs of fluid retention (e.g., skin turgor, edema, lungs sounds, weight, and strict intake and output) and for imbalances in electrolytes (e.g., change of mental status or cardiac dysrhythmias).

■ Nursing Diagnosis and Planning

Examples of nursing diagnoses frequently associated with ARF include:
- Excess fluid volume related to decreased kidney function
- Imbalanced nutrition: less than body requirements, related to nausea and loss of appetite
- Activity intolerance related to metabolic changes
- Risk for infection related to indwelling urinary catheter

Examples of expected outcomes include:
- Patient will have no signs of fluid overload (e.g., weight gain, edema, crackles in lungs, decreased urinary output) for the next 2 hours.
- Patient will receive sufficient calories (based on dietitian's calculation) to prevent catabolism (destructive breakdown of body tissue) during this shift.
- Patient will maintain bed rest and participate in activities of daily living (ADLs) as much as possible (e.g., brushes own teeth) during this shift.
- Patient will not have any signs or symptoms of infection (e.g., fever, cloudy urine) during hospitalization.

■ Implementation

Carefully monitor for signs of fluid imbalance. This includes physical assessment of edema, daily weights, and lung sounds. Strict measurement of intake and output (I&O) is essential. In the acute phase, hourly measurements of urine output are necessary.

Equipment, such as IV control pumps, should be used for accurate and safe delivery of IV fluids. In intensive care settings, arterial or central venous monitoring provides additional information about fluid status. Electrolytes should be monitored and may manifest as changes in the patient's mental status or cardiac dysrhythmias. The patient may be too ill to eat and may require TPN or enteral feedings. Even if the patient is unable to eat, make efforts to reduce noxious stimuli that exacerbate nausea, and administer antiemetics. Provide assistance with ADLs as needed during the acute phase, and progressively provide opportunities for the patient to participate, once fatigue resolves. To prevent infection, you should be vigilant for signs and symptoms of infection. Perform hand hygiene frequently and encourage others to do so. Surgical aseptic technique should be used for procedures such as Foley catheter insertion and central line dressing changes. You can help the patient and the family cope with the stress of this serious condition by allowing them to express concerns and fears, by providing accurate information about ARF, and by making appropriate referrals.

■ Evaluation

Evaluation of outcomes for acutely ill patients must occur frequently, because the plan of care may need frequent revision. For example, **if there are sudden changes or if the hourly urine output drops below 30 mL/hr, the physician must be immediately notified.** The patient should be assessed for signs of worsening, such as shortness of breath and lung crackles associated with pulmonary edema, or decreased cardiac output associated with heart failure. The patient must be transferred from a general medical-surgical unit to the ICU if the condition becomes unstable.

CHRONIC RENAL FAILURE
Etiology

Chronic renal failure (CRF) is a progressive loss of kidney function that develops over the course of many months or years. CRF is caused by destruction of the nephrons. All the causes of ARF may also cause CRF. Hypertension, diabetes mellitus, sickle cell disease, glomerulonephritis, nephrotic syndrome, lupus erythematosus, heart failure, and cirrhosis of the liver may also contribute to CRF.

The most common causes of CRF are glomerulonephritis and nephrosclerosis. **The primary causes of nephrosclerosis are hypertension and atherosclerotic disease of the small arteries in the kidneys.** As the blood supply decreases, the kidney cells degenerate and lose their ability to function, resulting in ESRD.

Diabetes Mellitus

Diabetic nephropathy (kidney disease and dysfunction secondary to diabetes mellitus) is the most common cause of death in patients with diabetes mellitus. In keeping with the *Healthy People 2020* goal, "to reduce kidney failure due to diabetes," help your patients to understand the interrelationship between diabetes and kidney health. For example, you could say, "Mr. Smith, with your hypertension, when your blood sugar goes up, protein starts to leak into your urine. This causes an increased pressure in the kidney vessels, which eventually leads to kidney damage."

Nephrosclerosis is classified as benign or malignant, depending on the severity of the disease and the speed with which hypertensive and atherosclerotic changes occur. The symptoms of nephrosclerosis are similar to those of chronic glomerulonephritis and renal failure. Treatment is the control of hypertension.

Pathophysiology

In the early stages of the disease, renal function can be adequate, but the waste products will begin to accumulate in the plasma. The patient does not experience symptoms until about 65% of the kidney tissue is damaged. As the disease progresses, nitrogenous waste products, such as urea nitrogen and creatinine, build up to higher levels in the blood. In the final or end stage of renal failure, 90% or more of kidney function is lost. Azotemia is the accumulation of nitrogenous products, which is signaled by an increase in BUN and serum creatinine. The patient may experience nausea and vomiting and changes in mental awareness and levels of consciousness. **The kidney is not able to excrete potassium; therefore be alert for high levels of serum potassium (5 to 7 mEq/L), which can adversely affect the heart, causing dysrhythmia and cardiac arrest.**

There are three stages of CRF. In stage 1 there is diminished renal reserve but no accumulation of metabolic wastes. The healthier kidney works harder. Urine concentration is decreased and polyuria and nocturia occur. Stage 2 is renal insufficiency and is signaled by a rise in circulating metabolic wastes; therefore BUN and serum creatinine levels begin to rise. The glomerular filtration rate falls and oliguria and edema occur. Stage 3 is ESRD. Circulating metabolic wastes accumulate in the blood, homeostasis cannot be maintained, electrolyte and fluid imbalances are serious, and dialysis or kidney transplant is necessary to maintain life.

Signs and Symptoms

The symptoms of CRF do not appear early in the disease. A high-normal elevation of BUN is an early warning sign, and the patient is likely to be asymptomatic. **One of the earliest signs of renal impairment is the inability of the kidneys to concentrate urine. This produces polyuria and very dilute urine and the patient may report nocturia.** Renal insufficiency, which occurs before renal failure, can produce occasional headaches and fatigue, but these symptoms usually either go unnoticed or unreported by the patient. At this point, the kidney function is about 20% to 40% of normal. When symptoms do become apparent, kidney function can be as little as 5% to 10% of normal. As renal insufficiency progresses, the kidneys may not be able to produce much urine at all. This causes oliguria and eventually anuria.

Uremia or uremic syndrome includes the clinical signs and symptoms that affect the entire body during ESRD. Uremia signs generally appear when BUN concentration passes 100 mg/dL. The presence of uremic signs is the absolute indicator for initiating dialysis and the goal is to maintain BUN below 100 mg/dL and to keep creatinine below 8 mg/dL.

The skin becomes dry, scaly, and a pallid yellowish gray. Pruritus (severe itching) occurs. Uremic frost (a late sign) appears as evaporated sweat leaves urea crystals on the eyebrows, face, axilla, and groin. Calcium is not absorbed from the intestinal tract, and this leads to the loss of calcium from the body and a corresponding drop in serum calcium. If the hypocalcemia is not corrected, the patient will eventually suffer from muscle cramps, twitching, and possibly seizures. As kidney cells cease to function, they are progressively less able to secrete phosphorus in the urine. An elevated serum phosphate level (hyperphosphatemia) serves to exaggerate the problem of inadequate calcium absorption; phosphate binds with calcium, decreasing its absorption from the intestinal tract. The patient is hypertensive from fluid overload and body weight increases. Pulmonary edema and heart failure may occur. Metabolic changes occur, including triglyceride elevation and carbohydrate intolerance. Dietary protein is restricted in an attempt to decrease the waste products that the kidney can no longer handle; therefore serum protein decreases. Anemia is present due to decreased production of erythropoietin. Anorexia, nausea, and vomiting occur because of gastrointestinal mucosa irritation from waste products circulating in the blood. Constipation often occurs from drug therapy and fluid restriction. Complaints about restless leg syndrome are frequent, and the leg discomfort may interfere with sleep. When circulating wastes are increased, the nervous system cells become irritated and the patient can become irritable and short-tempered. Figure 35-3 shows the manifestations of uremia.

Diagnosis

Creatinine is a stable by-product of skeletal muscle activity, which is excreted completely by the kidneys; therefore creatinine clearance (CC) is a good measure

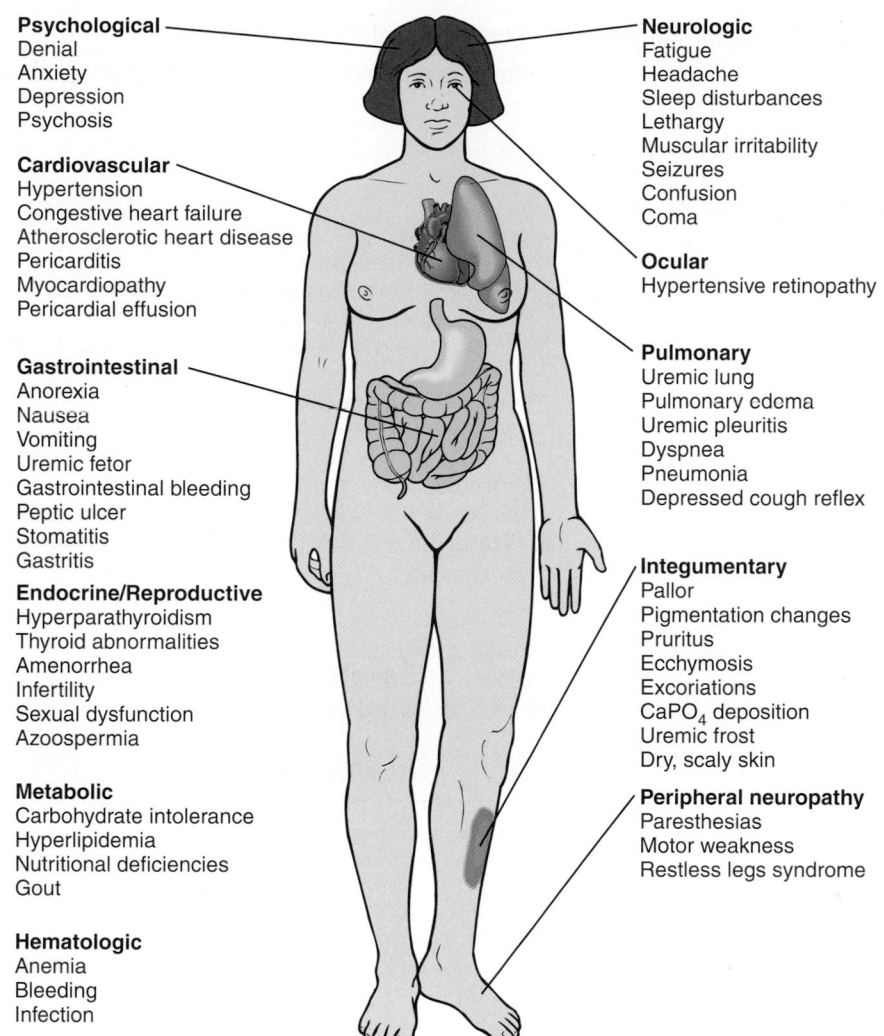

Psychological
Denial
Anxiety
Depression
Psychosis

Cardiovascular
Hypertension
Congestive heart failure
Atherosclerotic heart disease
Pericarditis
Myocardiopathy
Pericardial effusion

Gastrointestinal
Anorexia
Nausea
Vomiting
Uremic fetor
Gastrointestinal bleeding
Peptic ulcer
Stomatitis
Gastritis

Endocrine/Reproductive
Hyperparathyroidism
Thyroid abnormalities
Amenorrhea
Infertility
Sexual dysfunction
Azoospermia

Metabolic
Carbohydrate intolerance
Hyperlipidemia
Nutritional deficiencies
Gout

Hematologic
Anemia
Bleeding
Infection

Neurologic
Fatigue
Headache
Sleep disturbances
Lethargy
Muscular irritability
Seizures
Confusion
Coma

Ocular
Hypertensive retinopathy

Pulmonary
Uremic lung
Pulmonary edema
Uremic pleuritis
Dyspnea
Pneumonia
Depressed cough reflex

Integumentary
Pallor
Pigmentation changes
Pruritus
Ecchymosis
Excoriations
$CaPO_4$ deposition
Uremic frost
Dry, scaly skin

Peripheral neuropathy
Paresthesias
Motor weakness
Restless legs syndrome

FIGURE 35-3 Systemic effects of uremia.

of GFR. CC depends on the amount of blood passing through the kidney; narrowing of the renal arterioles, shock, or dehydration decreases the volume that is available to the kidney for filtration. CC is also affected by the functional abilities of the glomeruli. Urine is collected for a 24-hour period. Urinalysis with culture and sensitivity, hematocrit, and hemoglobin provide additional information. A renal ultrasound, renal scan, CT scan, and renal biopsy are additional diagnostic tests.

Treatment and Nursing Management

Medical treatment and nursing intervention include measures to correct fluid and electrolyte imbalance and acid-base imbalance whenever possible. Decreasing protein in the diet of patients with beginning renal insufficiency may help slow the disease process. A variety of drugs, such as antacids, antihypertensives, antilipemics, epoetin alfa therapy, and vitamin and mineral supplements, are used to counteract the fluid and electrolyte imbalances, treat metabolic acidosis, and control the complications (Table 35-4). Diuretics are used while there is some remaining

kidney function (renal insufficiency) but are not useful during ESRD. In a recent study, a combination of benazepril/amlodipine (Lotrel) showed promise in slowing the progression of chronic kidney disease; however, additional research is needed to verify the results (Napoli, 2010). Inotropic agents, such as digitalis or dobutamine, are used in severe cases of heart failure. Antiseizure medications, such as phenytoin (Dilantin) or diazepam (Valium), also may be needed because uremic toxins can irritate the nervous system. Dialysis and kidney transplant are two major alternatives that offer hope to the patient with ESRD.

Renal Dialysis. Dialysis is indicated for acute renal failure or for renal insufficiency when diet, medications, and fluid restriction have failed. It may also be used for patients with ESRD, drug overdose, hyperkalemia, fluid overload, or metabolic acidosis (Neligan, 2011). Hemodialysis and peritoneal dialysis rely on diffusion to remove waste elements normally excreted in the urine. The principle of *diffusion* states that solute molecules that are in constant motion tend to pass through a

Table 35-4 Common Drugs for Patients with Chronic Renal Disease

CLASSIFICATION	ACTION	NURSING IMPLICATIONS	PATIENT TEACHING
Diuretics			
Furosemide (Lasix)	Promotes urine flow; rids body of excess fluid; used in early stages of chronic renal failure	Potentially nephrotoxic and ototoxic. Strict I&O. Monitor laboratory values for blood dyscrasias. Side effects: vomiting, headache, constipation, and dizziness.	Report fever, sore throat, bleeding, bruising, difficulty swallowing, rash, or change in hearing.
Antihypertensives			
ACE inhibitors Enalapril (Vasotec)	Reduces angiotensin II and aldosterone, which decreases peripheral resistance and sodium reabsorption	Monitor for hypotension, blood dyscrasias, signs of infection, or bruising. African Americans have a higher incidence of angioedema (facial swelling, hoarseness), which can be fatal.	Immediately report cough, difficulty breathing, rash, tremors, blood in stool, or bleeding after brushing teeth. Report persistent dizziness or numbness and tingling.
Vitamins			
Calcitriol (Rocaltrol)	Active form of vitamin D	Monitor serum calcium; normal level 8.4-10.6 mEq/L. Monitor for hypocalcemia.	Report signs of hypocalcemia (e.g., twitching of mouth, numbness of fingers, laryngeal spasm, carpopedal spasm).
Folic acid and vitamin B_{12}	For red blood cell formation	Give with food to promote absorption. Side effects not expected.	Store in dry, light-protected container.
Minerals			
Iron (ferrous sulfate)	Used to treat anemia	Give with water or juice to promote absorption. Do not give with milk products.	Take with food if gastric distress occurs. Sit upright for 30 min after taking. Stool may turn black; this is a harmless side effect.
Ferumoxytol (Feraheme)	Treats iron deficiency anemia of CRF	Administer by IV injection.	The most common adverse reactions include diarrhea, nausea, dizziness, hypotension, constipation, and peripheral edema.
Calcium Supplements			
Calcium carbonate	Prevents problems of calcium loss	Monitor serum calcium. Monitor ECG changes for potential dysrhythmias.	Constipation is a common side effect. Nausea, vomiting, drowsiness, or headache may occur.
Calcium acetate (also binds phosphate)	Give with meals to bind phosphate		
Hematopoietic Growth Factors			
Epoetin alfa (Epogen) Darbepoetin (Aranesp)	Treatment of anemia; promotes red blood cell formation	Can cause hypertension; monitor blood pressure. May need increased doses of heparin. Subcutaneous route is preferred.	Report nausea, vomiting, edema, fatigue, or chest pain.
Resins			
Sodium polystyrene (Kayexalate)	Treatment of hyperkalemia	Can be given mixed with food or in an enema. Monitor electrolytes. Side effects: nausea, vomiting, constipation, and anorexia.	Report any muscle weakness, irregular heartbeat, or stomach pain.

ACE, angiotensin-converting enzyme; *ECG*, electrocardiogram; *I&O*, intake and output.

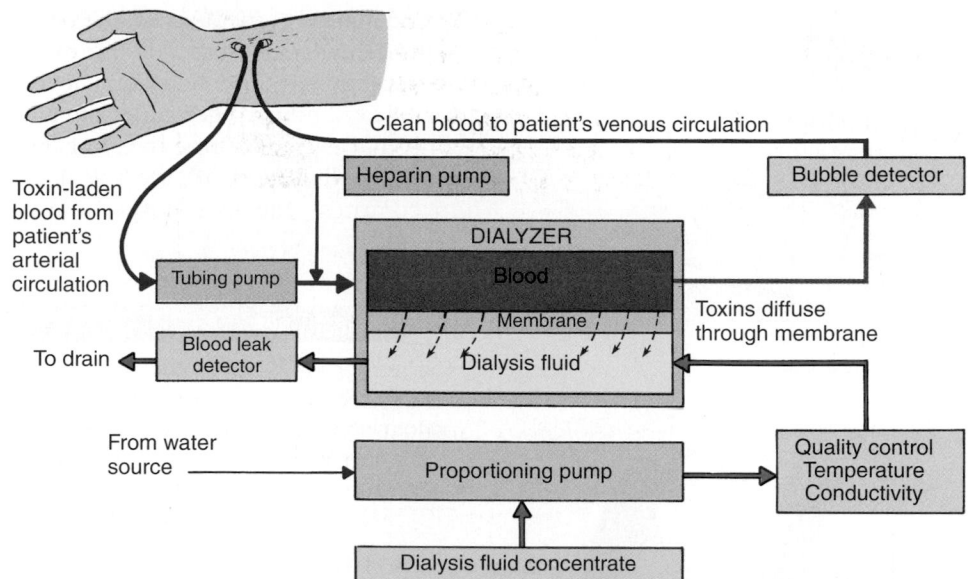

FIGURE 35-4 Schematic of hemodialysis system.

semipermeable membrane from the side of higher concentration to the side of lower concentration.

Hemodialysis. During hemodialysis, blood moves from the arterial circulation through a dialysate bath and back to the venous circulation. A dialysis membrane separates the blood from the dialyzing solution. The molecules of waste pass through this membrane out of the blood and into the dialyzing solution until the two solutions are equal in concentration (Figure 35-4).

A temporary access for hemodialysis can be achieved by inserting a jugular or femoral vein dialysis catheter. The jugular site has a low incidence of thrombosis; it can be used for 1 to 3 weeks and is preferred over the femoral site. Only trained dialysis staff should use these temporary access sites for medication administration or blood draws.

Two kinds of internal access are used for ongoing hemodialysis. An arteriovenous fistula (AVF) is formed by joining an artery and a vein together (Figure 35-5, A). The vein is made into a large superficial vein with an arterial supply that is easily accessible by venipuncture. Most often the radial or brachial artery is joined to the cephalic vein in the arm. A period of 6 to 8 weeks after surgery is needed for the vessel walls to become thickened and usable for the repeated insertion of the hemodialysis needles. Although the AVF has fewer complications and better patency, it requires relatively healthy blood vessels; therefore patients with diabetes, prolonged IV drug use, or peripheral vascular disease may need an alternative access site.

The arteriovenous (AV) access is accomplished by connecting an artery and a vein with a graft of a piece of synthetic material. The hemodialysis needles are then placed directly into the graft (Figure 35-5, B).

Clinical Cues

To assess for a bruit, gently auscultate the shunt with your stethoscope. You should hear an intermittent soft swishing sound that will correlate with the rhythm of your patient's pulse.

Medications frequently prescribed for the dialysis patient include multivitamins, antacids, iron and calcium supplements, antihypertensives (especially angiotensin-converting enzyme [ACE] inhibitors), epoetin alfa, phosphate binders, and possibly anticonvulsants. Darbepoetin (Aranesp) is a newer and longer-acting form of erythropoietin therapy (see Table 35-4).

Complications. The problems that a patient on hemodialysis may experience include fluid overload, electrolyte imbalance, alterations in blood components leading to anemia, and platelet abnormalities that produce bleeding tendencies. Patients can experience dialysis disequilibrium syndrome. This may occur because of rapid decrease in volume and is more likely after the first several treatments. Observe the patient for changes in mental status, headache, vomiting, or seizures. Be alert for cardiac dysrhythmias, signs of air emboli, or hemorrhage. Other major problems are systemic infections or localized infections at the access site.

Hepatitis C and acquired immunodeficiency syndrome (AIDS) are dangers because of blood access and risk of contamination. Patients who had multiple blood transfusions during the early to mid-1980s may have been exposed to the human immunodeficiency virus (HIV). (Hepatitis B is also possible but less of a problem due to vaccination, antibody testing, and strict body fluid precautions. Patients and dialysis staff should receive hepatitis B vaccine.)

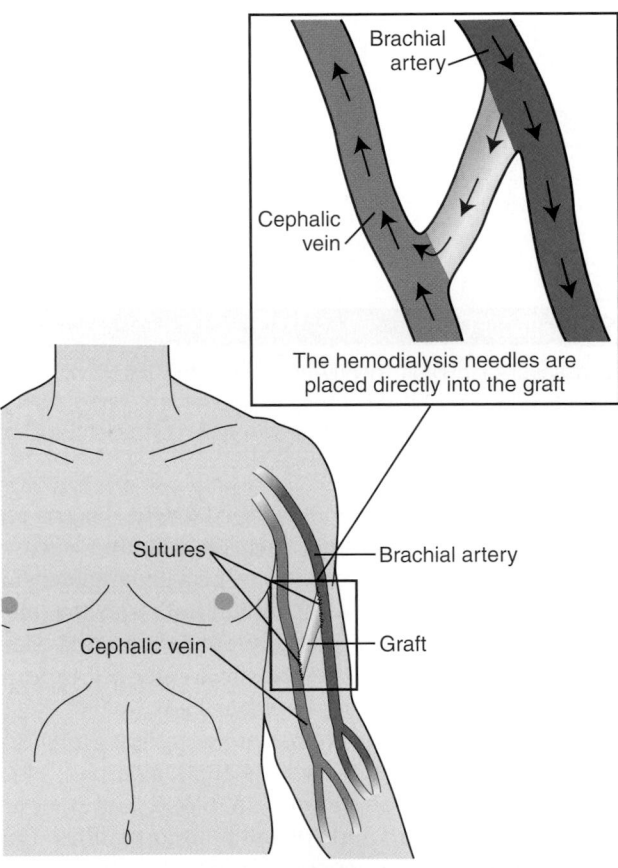

FIGURE 35-5 A, Arteriovenous fistula. **B,** Vascular graft access for long-term hemodialysis.

Nursing management. When caring for the hospitalized patient who has an arteriovenous graft or an AV fistula, it is important to check the site and protect it from injury. The site should be observed at least four times a day for signs indicating clotting or infection, and the peripheral circulation distal to the graft should also be checked (capillary refill and color of nail beds). Palpate for a thrill (vibration in the vessel), by gently laying your fingers on the enlarged vessel. You should be able to feel a buzz or vibration. A *bruit* (soft swishing sound) should be clearly heard on auscultation and the rhythm of the

sound should coincide with the patient's pulse. When a graft has been inserted, the extremity is elevated postoperatively and kept at a level above the heart for 24 to 72 hours. Thereafter, the patient should sleep with that extremity free (i.e., not on the side with the arm tucked underneath the body). Care is taken never to compress the extremity containing the vascular access.

Clinical Cues

The arm or leg in which the arteriovenous shunt has been created should never be used for checking blood pressure or performing venipuncture (peripheral IV lines or blood draws). Post a sign above the bed to alert other members of the health care team.

Antihypertensive drugs are not given the morning of dialysis, as they can cause severe hypotension during the treatment. Nitroglycerin (NTG) patches, digitalis, and anticoagulants also are held. You should also consult with the dialysis nurse to coordinate the timing of medications. Before the patient goes to dialysis, do a physical assessment, check for bruit and thrill at the access site, and obtain a complete set of vital signs and a weight. These measurements will be compared with post-treatment results.

The patient undergoing hemodialysis will have considerable fluid volume shifts that affect homeostasis. You will need to plan to assess this patient more frequently in the hours after dialysis treatment is completed. Postdialysis nursing care includes monitoring the access site for bleeding for 1 hour after the treatment. Assess the patient for signs of confusion or disorientation, hypotension, nausea or vomiting, headache, dizziness, or muscle cramps. Monitor and compare vital signs to pretreatment values and continue assessment of the access site for patency and signs of infection. **Invasive procedures are postponed for 4 to 6 hours after dialysis because the clotting time is extended from the heparin used during dialysis, and prolonged bleeding could occur.**

The scheduling of hemodialysis sessions varies from patient to patient, but treatments usually are done two or three times a week. Stable patients can be treated on an outpatient basis at a dialysis center.

Peritoneal dialysis. Peritoneal dialysis is an alternative procedure that can be used instead of hemodialysis to remove waste products or toxins that have accumulated as a result of ARF or CRF. During peritoneal dialysis, dialyzing fluid which is equal in osmolarity and similar in composition to normal body fluid, is introduced into the peritoneal cavity via a Tenckhoff catheter by gravity or pump (Figure 35-6). Medications such as heparin, insulin, potassium, or antibiotics may be added to the

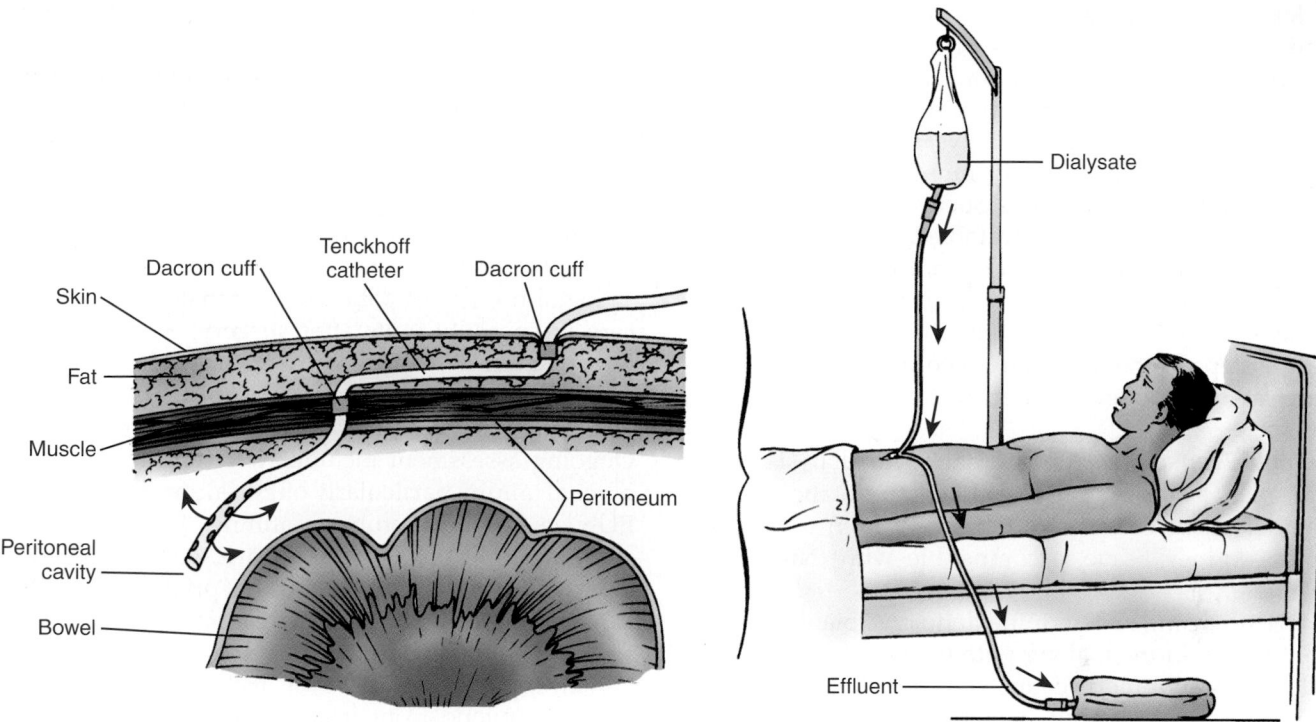

FIGURE 35-6 Peritoneal dialysis through an abdominal catheter.

solution. The solution is left in the peritoneal cavity for a specified time (dwell time) until the concentration of the solutions on either side of the peritoneal membrane is equalized.

After the fluid is infused, the patient can move about during the dwell time. At the end of the dwell time, the dialysate solution containing waste products is drained from the abdominal cavity. The drainage should be colorless or straw-colored unless the catheter was recently inserted, in which case the drainage may be bloody for the first several treatments.

Peritoneal dialysis has several advantages: (1) treatment can be started more quickly than hemodialysis, (2) anticoagulants are not necessary, (3) maturation of the access and canalization of blood vessels is not required, (4) there is less stress on the cardiovascular system because fluid exchanges occur more slowly, and (5) some patients with renal failure fare better on a gentler therapy. Peritoneal dialysis cannot be done when there is severe trauma to the abdomen, after multiple abdominal surgeries, if there are adhesions in the abdominal cavity, or if the patient has a severe coagulation defect, paralytic ileus, or diffuse peritonitis.

There are several types of peritoneal dialysis. The basic principles are the same, but the dwell times, schedule of frequency, and use of a control pump versus gravity flow will vary. The first type is *continuous ambulatory peritoneal dialysis* (CAPD). The CAPD process goes on 24 hours a day, 7 days a week. As a self-dialysis method, CAPD may be the easiest for the patient, and it requires no machinery. For CAPD,

the bag of dialyzing solution is suspended above the level of the abdomen and tubing is attached to the permanently implanted peritoneal dialysis catheter. The clamp on the CAPD tubing is opened and the dialysate solution is allowed to run into the abdomen by gravity flow. After the dwell time (4 to 8 hours), the fluid is drained. A second type is called *nocturnal intermittent dialysis*, which is accomplished either with or without use of a control pump and is performed three to five times per week for 10 to 12 hours at night. This allows the patient to be free between treatment times. A third type, *continuous cycling peritoneal dialysis*, combines CAPD with nocturnal intermittent dialysis for home use. An automated cycling machine allows the patient to do three exchanges at night while sleeping, then during the day there is one exchange, but the dwell time lasts all day long. The last type, *automated peritoneal dialysis*, is regulated by machinery and can be used in acute care settings, in clinics, and at home during the night.

Complications. Potential complications of peritoneal dialysis include peritonitis, leakage, obstruction or other problems with the catheter, respiratory problems, and fluid overload or hypertriglyceridemia (disturbance of lipid metabolism).

? Think Critically

What signs and symptoms might indicate that your peritoneal dialysis patient has peritonitis?

Nursing management. Nursing care for the patient undergoing peritoneal dialysis includes obtaining the patient's weight before and after the treatment; maintaining careful I&O records; maintaining strict aseptic technique in handling the dialysate bags, peritoneal catheter, and all equipment; monitoring vital signs; observing for complications such as peritonitis; and keeping the patient as comfortable as possible. The dialysate solution should be at room temperature and must be instilled slowly. In accordance with National Patient Safety Goals, the patient and family are taught all the steps of the procedure before discharge, to ensure safety and prevent infection.

Kidney Transplant. An alternative to dialysis is to transplant a kidney from a blood relative of the patient, another tissue-compatible donor, or from a cadaver whose kidney tissue is compatible with that of the recipient.

Tissue typing to determine donor-recipient compatibility is performed, along with extensive psychological assessment and counseling for both the live donor and the recipient. Transplant candidates must be free from medical problems that might increase the risks of the procedure or jeopardize the success of the transplant. Malignancy, IV drug abuse, severe obesity, active vasculitis, and severe psychosocial problems eliminate some candidates.

Legal and Ethical Considerations

Organ Donation

Medicare, Medicaid, and the Joint Commission mandate that the local organ procurement organization (OPO) must be notified about brain death of a patient so that a well-trained representative of the OPO can evaluate the suitability of the potential donor and approach the family in a timely manner. Currently, research is being conducted to determine if emphasizing the benefits of donation, such as the desire to help others and save lives, will increase the family's willingness to consent as compared to the traditional neutral approach where the requestor gives information and support and acts as a grief counselor (Emergency Nurses' Association, 2009).

A significant factor in transplant therapy is the shortage of organs. In the United States, more than 100,000 persons are currently on the waiting list, which changes hourly. Stable patients who are waiting for a transplant must live close to a transplant center and be ready immediately when an organ becomes available. Hypertension is brought under the best possible control, any infection is treated, and the patient is dialyzed immediately before transplantation. One of the *Healthy People 2020* goals is to increase the proportion of patients who receive a kidney transplant within 3 years after being put on the waiting list.

There are three types of immunosuppressive drugs to prevent organ rejection: (1) cytokine inhibitors

(e.g., cyclosporine [Sandimmune], tacrolimus [Prograf]); (2) antiproliferative agents (e.g., azathioprine [Imuran]); and (3) antibodies (e.g., muromonab-CD3 [Orthoclone OKT3]). A recently approved drug is everolimus (Zortress), which inhibits the growth of cells that would ordinarily contribute to rejection of the transplanted kidney (Clin-eguide, 2010). Long-term problems for transplant patients are increased susceptibility to infection and a higher risk of malignancy.

Renal transplant patients are transferred to critical care or specialty units after surgery, where they are closely monitored for signs of rejection: fever, increased blood pressure, and pain over the iliac fossa where the new kidney was placed (Figure 35-7). Ongoing assessment includes watching for the signs of renal failure, particularly oliguria, anuria, and rising BUN levels and serum creatinine. Protection from sources of infection is a top priority. Once the new kidney is functioning properly, the primary physician may lift any previous dietary restrictions.

Renal failure and dialysis are very expensive for the patient and family. However, lack of funds does not exclude anyone from needed care. Since July 1973, an amendment to the Social Security Act allows Medicare to pay for most of the cost of treating ESRD, including dialysis and renal transplant. Medical expenses continue after transplant, as the drugs needed to prevent rejection are very expensive.

❖ NURSING MANAGEMENT

■ Assessment (Data Collection)

The assessment findings will vary because of the slow but progressive development of kidney failure and the effect that kidney disease has on other body systems. Take a past medical history that includes medication, previous illness and surgeries, family history of illness, and a report of current complaints and concerns.

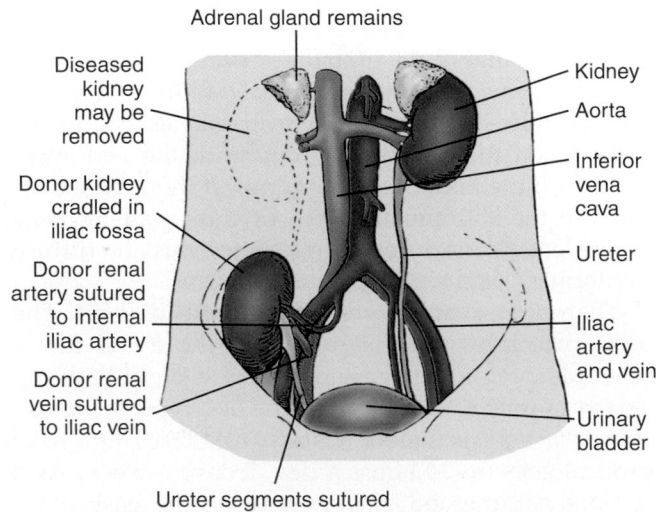

FIGURE 35-7 Placement of transplanted kidney.

Perform a general head-to-toe assessment including complete vital signs and a baseline weight. Observe for changes and symptoms that include:

- Neurologic changes (e.g., lethargy, irritability)
- Cardiovascular abnormalities (e.g., dysrhythmias or hypertension)
- Respiratory abnormalities (e.g., shortness of breath or fluid in lungs)
- Gastrointestinal distress (e.g., nausea, vomiting, constipation)
- Musculoskeletal discomfort (e.g., muscle cramps, twitching, or restless legs syndrome)
- Skin changes (e.g., itching, uremic frost)

Monitor BUN, serum creatinine, electrolytes, and urinalysis. As the disease progresses, assess for impaired urine concentration, decreased output, and anemia.

⬆ Clinical Cues

Although it is common to weigh patients in the morning with the same scale and the same amount of clothing, use your clinical judgment to initiate weights more frequently than once per day if needed. Watch for signs of fluid overload (e.g., facial or peripheral edema, shortness of breath, or crackles in lungs). One kilogram or 2.2 lb of weight gain is equal to approximately 1 L of fluid.

In addition, you should assess patients for sexual difficulties or concerns. Patients may experience medication side effects, such as impotence. Weight gain, peripheral edema, or presence of a shunt may alter body image or feelings of attractiveness. Fatigue caused by anemia or hormonal imbalance can result in decreased libido (sexual desire). Partners may fear that the patient is too ill to participate in sex or that the hemodialysis shunt will be damaged.

⬆ Clinical Cues

Help your patient to verbalize concerns about sexual problems by using a matter-of-fact approach (e.g., "Mr. Smith, have you or your partner noticed any changes in your sexual relations since you started your new medication?"). It is possible that you may not be able to directly solve the problem, but giving the patient the opportunity to talk about it is helpful. In addition, once you have assessed the problem, you can refer the patient to the appropriate resource if the problem is beyond your expertise (e.g., the physician may be able to change medication or the family may need psychological counseling).

■ Nursing Diagnosis

Patients with renal disease will have problems related to anemia, bleeding tendency, susceptibility to infection, nausea, vomiting, anorexia, gastrointestinal bleeding, and fluid overload that exacerbates conditions such as congestive heart failure. Examples of nursing diagnoses frequently associated with chronic renal disease and dialysis include:

- Imbalanced nutrition: less than body requirements related to dietary restrictions and loss of appetite
- Fatigue related to anemia
- Risk for infection related to invasive procedures (e.g., dialysis shunt)
- Acute confusion related to accumulation of toxins
- Sexual dysfunction related to stress and medication side effects

Examples of expected outcomes include:

- Patient will eat at least 50% of all meals during this shift.
- Patient will have adequate energy to independently perform ADLs before discharge.
- Patient will not have any signs or symptoms of infection (e.g., fever, redness, or swelling at shunt site) during hospitalization.
- Patient will demonstrate ability to make safe judgments (e.g., calls for help as needed) and orientation to person, place, and time before discharge.
- Patient will verbalize concerns or fears about sexual dysfunction.

■ Planning

In planning care for the patient with chronic renal disease, consider the stress of prolonged intensive treatment, the frustrations of dealing with an incurable illness, rigid dietary restrictions, fatigue, malaise, occasional limited mobility, and possibly sexual difficulties, all of which take their toll on both the patient and his relatives. Consider the family's needs as well as the patient's when planning nursing intervention.

General nursing goals for care of patients with chronic renal disease include:

- Positive adaptation to therapeutic regimen (i.e., dietary and fluid modifications, dialysis)
- Maintaining fluid and electrolyte balance
- Prevention of complications
- Ensuring knowledge for appropriate self-care
- Assisting with resolution of body image disturbance
- Prevention of caregiver role strain and family dysfunction related to chronic illness

❓ Think Critically

What kinds of behaviors would suggest caregiver role strain for the spouse of a patient who has CRF?

■ Implementation

Daily weight, measurement of I&O, determining the pattern of urination, and restricting fluid as ordered per physician (guidelines: intake 500 to 700 mL plus output from previous 24 hours) are essential to the well-being of the patient with renal damage. In addition to these basic procedures, there should be

THERE ARE TWO DIFFERENT TYPES OF PROTEIN

One is called animal or high-biological protein, which contains ALL essential amino acids

The other type is vegetable or low-biological protein, which contains SOME amino acids

THE HEMODIALYSIS AND THE PERITONEAL MEMBRANE ARE NOT SELECTIVE, WHICH MEANS THAT VITAL AMINO ACIDS AND VITAMINS AS WELL AS UNWANTED WASTES ARE REMOVED

If you are on HEMODIALYSIS, you should aim for **1.2 g of protein per kg of body weight;** e.g., if you weigh 65 kg (143 lb), your protein intake should be about 78 g/day

If you are on PERITONEAL DIALYSIS, you should aim for **1.3 g of protein per kg of body weight;** e.g., if you weigh 70 kg (154 lb), your protein intake should be about 91 g/day

EXAMPLES OF PROTEIN SOURCES

3.5 oz of extra-lean ground beef has 24 g of protein, whereas ribeye has 28 g of protein

Half of a chicken breast (3.5 oz) has 29 g of protein, turkey white meat (3.5 oz) has 30 g of protein

One can of Ensure has 13 g of protein, whereas 1 scoop of Promod has 5 g, and one egg has 6 g of protein

15 large cooked shrimp have 17 g of protein; a 3 oz can of white tuna in water has 22 g of protein

One cup of milk has 8 g of protein, whereas ½ cup of regular tofu has 10 g, and one slice of white bread has 2 g of protein

One cup of cooked corn, peas, potato, pasta, or rice has about 4 g of protein

FIGURE 35-8 Tips for protein intake.

ongoing monitoring of electrolytes, BUN, and creatinine. Hyperkalemia is present, and there is a sodium imbalance. Hypocalcemia and hyperphosphatemia occur (see Chapter 3).

Because of the buildup of nitrogenous wastes from protein metabolism, restriction of protein intake is necessary; only high-quality protein foods (e.g., meat and eggs) are encouraged (Figure 35-8). Potassium is also restricted. Sodium intake often is restricted, especially if the patient is hypertensive. Previously, aluminum carbonate (Basaljel) was used as a phosphate binder; however, concern over elevated aluminum levels has prompted the use of calcium carbonate, which acts as a phosphate binder and a calcium supplement. The complexity of diet restrictions and modifications makes understanding and compliance very difficult for the patient and the family (Table 35-5).

The nurse must assess the patient's health status and learning needs throughout the illness and provide information to manage symptoms and prevent further damage whenever possible. The expertise of other professionals, especially nutritionists, is needed to help accomplish the goals of (1) minimizing uremic toxicity; (2) maintaining acceptable electrolyte levels; (3) controlling hypertension; (4) providing sufficient calories; and (5) maintaining good nutritional status.

Encourage communication between patient and spouse to express feelings about changes in sexual activity, role reversal, and family responsibilities. Kidney-failure patients often have self-care deficits that affect self-esteem and create an increased caregiver burden. Encourage the family to achieve a balance between supporting the patient and allowing as much independence as possible.

Table 35-5 Dietary Restrictions for the Patient with Renal Failure

DIETARY COMPONENT	WITH CHRONIC UREMIA	WITH HEMODIALYSIS	WITH PERITONEAL DIALYSIS
Protein	0.55-0.60 g/kg/day	1-1.5 g/kg/day	1.2-1.5 g/kg/day
Fluid	Depends on urinary output, but may be as high as 1500-3000 mL/day	500-700 mL/day plus amount of urinary output	Restriction based on fluid weight gain and blood pressure
Potassium	60–70 mEq/day	70 mEq/day	Usually no restriction
Sodium	1-3 g/day	2-4 g/day	Restriction based on fluid weight gain and blood pressure
Phosphorus	700 mg/day	700 mg/day	800 mg/day

From Ignatavicius, D.D., & Workman, M.L. (2010). *Medical-Surgical Nursing: Patient Centered Collaborative Care* (6th ed.). St. Louis: Saunders, p. 1617.

Communication

Noncompliant Hemodialysis Patient

John is a 48-year-old man who has end-stage renal disease and is on hemodialysis twice a week. He has not been compliant with his diet and fluid restrictions and has been increased to three dialysis treatments a week. He gained 5 lb over the weekend.

- *Nurse:* "John, I see that you gained five pounds since Friday. Tell me about your weekend."
- *John:* "I never have any fun or do normal things with my friends, so I went fishing with some buddies and we drank a lot of beer. We barbecued fish and some sausage. It was a real feast!"
- *Nurse:* "How are you feeling today?"
- *John:* "I feel rotten. I don't have any energy, and my thinking is slow. My legs are really swollen, and I'm having trouble breathing."
- *Nurse:* "Do you think that might have something to do with the beer and food?"
- *John:* "I suppose it does, but can't a guy have a little fun?"
- *Nurse:* "John, I am concerned. You know that fluid and waste overload puts your whole body out of balance and causes damage in other organs. It's especially hard on the heart."
- *John:* "Yeah, I know you've told me. It's just so hard. You don't understand what it is like."
- *Nurse:* "You are right. I don't have kidney disease, or the strict diet and fluid restrictions. I think it would be very difficult, but I would want to take care of myself for my family and friends."
- *John:* "Well, you know that my wife left me, and I don't see much of the kids, but I sure do enjoy my granddaughter. I really enjoy my times with the guys at the Lodge, too."
- *Nurse:* "Do you have any friends who are in a similar situation who you can talk to?"
- *John:* "No, none of my friends has kidney disease."
- *Nurse:* "There is a young man who comes here for dialysis treatments who is always talking about fishing. Maybe the two of you could give each other some encouragement and support."
- *John:* "Well, don't know; I don't make new friends very easily."
- *Nurse:* "He will be here on Wednesday. How about if we schedule your treatment for the same time? Perhaps you could get acquainted."
- *John:* "O.K. That seems fine."
- *Nurse:* "Next week we can talk again to see how you are doing with your diet, fluid restrictions, and medication schedule."
- *John:* "Thanks. I will try to do better this week."

 Clinical Cues

If your patient is somewhat resistant to listening to the nutritionist, support the diet teaching by showing enthusiasm and providing openings for the nutritionist to give the information. For example, the nurse says, "I'd be interested in hearing about the list of quality protein foods. This sample menu looks pretty good. Do you have more examples we could look at?"

▪ Evaluation

For chronic renal failure, perform and compare data for daily physical assessments, weights, I&O, and laboratory reports. Monitor trends over a period of days to determine clinical improvement or the presence of problems. Daily fluctuations in subjective symptoms, such as fatigue or discomfort, along with ambivalent feelings toward the therapeutic regimen, are expected; however, if symptoms are prolonged or ongoing, the care plan should be revised. Nursing Care Plan 35-1 includes nursing diagnoses, interventions, and outcomes that are commonly used for patients with renal insufficiency and failure.

? **Think Critically**

Your CRF patient is withdrawn and sullen at times, and is sharp and demanding at other times. How will you respond to this? How will you help the family deal with this behavior?

COMMUNITY CARE

A major function of nurses in the community is to assist hypertensive and diabetic patients to achieve good control of their disease to help prevent damage to the kidneys. One of the *Healthy People 2020* goals is to reduce the rate of new cases of ESRD. All nurses can promote healthy kidney function by encouraging the intake of more water and prompt recognition and treatment of urinary tract infections. In addition, nurses can participate in community education to increase awareness of organ donation programs.

Nurses in outpatient clinics assist with urologic procedures, such as cystoscopy and removal or destruction of renal stones. Clinic nurses will also have opportunities to teach patients how to manage problems of incontinence.

Home care nurses are constantly on the alert for signs of ARF or CRF among their patients. Many illnesses, and the variety of drugs that patients receive, may cause kidney damage. Many home care patients have indwelling catheters that must be periodically replaced with new ones. Home health nurses also identify problems of incontinence, and have the advantage of being able to see the environmental and social factors that must be addressed.

Nurses in long-term care facilities deal with a variety of urinary problems. Bladder training for incontinence is a prime consideration. Monitoring for drug toxicities in this population is imperative, as drugs are not excreted quickly and polypharmacy can have additive effects. Keeping residents dry and odor free is very important for physical and psychological reasons. Monitoring for urinary retention or obstruction to the flow of urine is another priority in the elderly population.

Nurses who work in dialysis centers are often the primary nurses for patients in renal failure. These nurses must constantly assess patients for complications, watch for medication-related problems, and continue to reinforce diet and lifestyle modifications. Considerable psychosocial support and counseling may be necessary, as dialysis patients often experience depression, hopelessness, sexual problems, role changes, and relationship problems.

⬥ Nursing Care Plan 35-1 | Care of the Patient with Chronic Renal Failure

Scenario

Mrs. Stevens, age 54, has had hypertension since her early twenties. She was diagnosed with chronic renal failure several years ago. Now, she reports headaches, fatigue, and nausea. States, "I have to sleep with three pillows and I am just exhausted." She feels that "her doctor is keeping something from her" and she is withdrawn and sullen. Tearfully, she reports, "The renal diet is so complex and my husband and son cannot manage the cooking and shopping." Her nephrologist conducted a series of diagnostic tests and recommended hemodialysis and eventual kidney transplant when an organ is available. Laboratory results include hematocrit 25%; hemoglobin 9 g/100 mL, BUN 48 mg/dL, creatinine 3 mg/dL, admission weight: 137 lb ("normal weight around 130 lb"), 3+ pitting edema, bilateral feet and ankles.

Problem/Nursing Diagnosis

Tired and exhausted/Activity intolerance related to anemia.

Supporting Assessment Data

Subjective: "I am just exhausted."
Objective: Hematocrit 25%; hemoglobin 9 g/100 mL, appears tired.

Goals/Expected Outcomes	Nursing Interventions	Selected Rationale	Evaluation
Patient will identify her activity limits for this shift.	Monitor for signs of weakness or increasing fatigue.	These signs and symptoms can signal a potential decreased RBC count and impaired oxygen-carrying capacity.	Able to independently perform basic hygienic needs this morning.
	Check vital signs for changes when activities appear stressful or overtaxing.	Marked increase in pulse or respiratory rate during routine ADLs suggests activity intolerance.	Reported feelings of fatigue and mild dyspnea after walking to the nurses' station. Vital signs at that time were BP 145/90, P 120, R 32/min. Repeat vitals after 30 min of rest: BP 140/80, P 85, R 20/min.
	Have patient use rating scale (scale 1/10) for different types of activities, such as walking to the bathroom or climbing the stairs.	The exertional scale (1/10) allows the patient (and the nurse) to rate and monitor performance and alter activities accordingly.	Ambulating in the hall was "too much" and reported an exertion level of 6/10.
	Adjust activities to allow for periods of rest.	Adequate rest facilitates recovery; activities can be increased or decreased according to the patient's level of tolerance.	Patient was assisted back to her room. Rested for 3 hr.
	Help visitors and patient to discuss what time of day and type of activities will fit the patient's current energy level (e.g., son could visit on Saturday morning and read a book with the patient).	Visitors need specific instructions to prevent overstimulating (or avoiding) the patient.	Patient's family agrees to come in midmorning hours and limit stay to 1 hr.
By discharge, patient will be able to perform ADLs independently without distress.	Assist with ADLs as required and keep personal articles within reach.	Patient's ability to do ADLs will wax and wane. Items close by and assistance as needed will help to conserve energy.	Able to independently comb hair and apply makeup when personal items are within easy reach.

ADLs, activities of daily living; *BP*, blood pressure; *CRF*, chronic renal failure; *I&O*, intake and output; *P*, pulse; *R*, respirations; *RBC*, red blood cell.

Goals/Expected Outcomes	Nursing Interventions	Selected Rationale	Evaluation
Patient will demonstrate increased hematocrit value: 30% and increased hemoglobin 11 g/100 mL.	Monitor for decreased hematocrit and hemoglobin values.	Normal range for hematocrit 37%-47% (female). Normal range for hemoglobin 12–16 g/dL (female).	7:00 A.M. Hematocrit: 24%; hemoglobin: 9 g/100 mL.
	Give epoetin and monitor for side effects (e.g., increased BP, dyspnea, chest pain, seizures, headaches, calf pain). Give iron, multivitamins, and folic acid as ordered. Instruct about foods that supply iron (e.g., lean meat and vegetables) and folic acid (e.g., whole wheat bread).	Nutritional supplements and epoetin are given to help the body with RBC production.	Epoetin given subcutaneously, as ordered. No adverse effects noted.
	Monitor infusions of packed red blood cells, as ordered.	Transfusions may be needed if anemia is severe.	No transfusion ordered at this time. Outcomes partially met. Continue plan.

Problem/Nursing Diagnosis
Believes that information is being withheld and feels that family cannot manage shopping and cooking/Powerlessness related to perceived lack of information and stress of chronic illness.

Supporting Assessment Data
Subjective: "Doctor is keeping something from me."
Objective: Appears withdrawn, sullen, and tearful.

Goals/Expected Outcomes	Nursing Interventions	Selected Rationale	Evaluation
Patient will express feelings associated with chronic illness during this shift.	Encourage expression of feelings (e.g., frustration, anger).	Expression of feelings and beliefs allows the patient and the nurse to clarify how the situation affects behavior and decision making. Taking the time to listen also builds trust and rapport.	Patient stated that she was discouraged and depressed about her illness. Expresses anger toward her physician, because she thinks, "he is not telling the whole story."
	Encourage expression of beliefs about illness and outcomes.	Patient may experience strong feelings and may or may not be able to identify the source. You may not be able to correct all situations, but just talking about the frustration will help some patients.	She "hates the idea of dialysis" and feels like it is "controlling her life."
	Observe for factors contributing to feelings (e.g., lack of information, loss of social roles) and correct if possible. Assist patient to identify factors that can and cannot be controlled.	Identifying factors that cannot be controlled allows the patient to realistically work on achievable goals.	Patient identified that knowing more about dialysis would be helpful.
Patient will participate in planning care and daily goals within 2-3 days.	Provide opportunities for patient to participate in activities that will increase sense of accomplishment (e.g., phoning for an appointment with social services).	A sense of accomplishment empowers the patient to act positively in own behalf.	Assisted patient in making a list of questions for her physician (e.g., "What are the steps for starting hemodialysis? How long can I live on dialysis?").
	Assist patient to identify small, achievable goals and to make realistic plans.	Small goals are more readily accomplished and a feeling of success provides motivation to attempt larger goals.	Patient requested some written information about kidney transplantation and asked to speak to the transplant coordinator.

Continued

Goals/Expected Outcomes	Nursing Interventions	Selected Rationale	Evaluation
Patient will state hopes and plans for the future before discharge.	Emphasize that quality of life can be good for patients on dialysis (e.g., extends time to spend with friends and family).	Emphasizing positive outcomes can create a sense of hope and optimism.	She says that she is not optimistic about getting a donated kidney, but would still like to have the information and the hope that it could happen for her.
	Give positive reinforcement for statements of hope and future planning.	Positive reinforcement encourages repetition of a desirable behavior.	At the end of the shift, patient stated that making the list of questions and talking about her frustrations had helped. Outcomes partially met. Continue with plan.

Problem/Nursing Diagnosis
Renal diet is very complex/Deficient knowledge related to diet and nutrition.

Supporting Assessment Data
Subjective: "The renal diet is so complex and my husband and son cannot manage the cooking and shopping."
Objective: Appears overwhelmed at the amount of information and seems unsure how to use it effectively.

Goals/Expected Outcomes	Nursing Interventions	Selected Rationale	Evaluation
Patient will state willingness to learn about prescribed diet during this shift.	Assess readiness to learn, preferred learning styles, and barriers to learning.	Possible barriers for the patient include being upset, tired, uncomfortable, or anxious about her condition. Learning new information will be difficult under these conditions.	The patient identifies need for herself and her family to learn about her dietary restrictions. Patient also shows interest in attending a group class that will be conducted next month.
	Perform teaching in short sessions.	Complex information is best delivered in manageable pieces.	Limited teaching session to 10 min due to fatigue.
	Use language and terms that patient is able to understand.	Medical jargon and technical terms will not help the patient understand the basic dietary information.	Verbalized understanding of terminology related to health teaching (e.g., restricted protein).
With help, the patient will create a sample diet that is within renal diet parameters within 2-3 days.	Obtain a dietary consultation and reinforce information provided by the nutritional expert.	A renal nutritionist must be consulted to create an individual diet plan based on laboratory values, nutritional requirements, and patient's eating preferences.	Nutritionist came to see the patient and discussed overall nutritional goals and plan. Arrangements have been made with the nutritionist to meet with the family next week.
Patient will apply knowledge about diet and nutrition to reduce nitrogenous waste by-products and solute overload by next outpatient dialysis appointment.	Ensure that the patient has verbal and written instructions.	Written material can be reviewed at a later date and shared with family.	Written information was provided about diet and renal disease.
	Encourage expression of concerns (e.g., cost, preparation, availability of seasonal foods).	Food frequently has a sociocultural base.	Patient is concerned that family will need guidance in shopping.
	Invite the family (especially the person most likely to cook and shop) to attend the teaching sessions.	Costs, food preferences, and family participation should be considered to increase the likelihood of success.	Family will attend teaching session next week.
	Help her review specific information about high-quality proteins (e.g., meat, eggs) and hidden sodium sources (e.g., canned food).	Reviewing information increases retention of new information.	The patient was able to identify high-quality protein foods but continues to be confused about how sodium, phosphorus, and calcium affecting her kidney function. Follow-up teaching sessions will be arranged this week to address the topic. Outcomes partially met. Continue with plan.

Problem/Nursing Diagnosis

Weight gain of 7 lb with pitting edema/Excess fluid volume related to retention of sodium and water from inadequate kidney function.

Supporting Assessment Data

Subjective: "Sleeps with three pillows."

Objective: Admission weight: 137 lb (normal weight around 130 lb), 3+ pitting edema, bilateral feet and ankles.

Goals/Expected Outcomes	Nursing Interventions	Selected Rationale	Evaluation
Patient will have restricted fluid intake (500-700 mL plus output from previous 24 hr) during this shift.	Strict I&O.	Discrepancies in I&O suggest fluid retention and overload.	Fluid intake 1000 mL, output 600 mL.
	Fluid restrictions, as ordered (intake 500-700 mL plus output from previous 24 hr). Assist to establish acceptable schedule for restricted fluids.	Kidneys may produce a small but inadequate output of urine. Limiting fluid prevents overload, whereas spacing fluid throughout the day helps to relieve subjective feelings of thirst.	Patient is aware of and compliant with fluid restrictions.
	Assist with good oral care and discourage mouth breathing; rinse mouth frequently, space fluids throughout the day.	Patient's subjective feeling of moist oral mucous membranes will increase compliance with fluid restrictions.	Subjective relief obtained from frequent, but small quantities of ice chips and periodic mouth care.
	Instruct patient and visitors about fluid restriction.	Visitors may unintentionally offer fluid as a comfort measure if they are uninformed about therapeutic goals.	Patient actively reminds all visitors and staff "not to tempt me."
	Post a sign over the bed to alert visitors and health care team members about fluid restrictions.	Many persons can pass through a patient's room, and all should be aware of precautions to prevent inadvertently offering restricted foods and fluids.	Sign placed above bed for fluid restrictions.
Patient will demonstrate signs of decreased fluid load (e.g., lungs will be clear to auscultation, foot and ankle edema decreased) within 24-48 hr.	Check for signs of fluid overload: edema, crackles in lungs, orthopnea, and changes in mental status.	Peripheral fluid is observed in extremities and face. Edema within body organs (e.g., lungs or brain) manifests as functional impairment.	Fine crackles noted in base of posterior lung fields bilaterally. Reports some mild shortness of breath, especially with exertion or if lying flat in bed. Subjectively feels breathing is okay "when sitting in a chair." Resting pulse oximetry 94%. 3+ pitting edema noted bilaterally in feet.
Patient's weight will return to previous level within 10 days.	Weigh daily (or more frequently if needed) and monitor trends.	An increase in weight is one of the key indicators of fluid imbalance. One kilogram, or 2.2 lb of weight gain, is equal to excess of 1 L of fluid.	Patient's A.M. weight: 137.5 lb.
Patient will demonstrate minimal peripheral edema within 7-10 days.	Administer diuretic (e.g., hydrochlorothiazide) as ordered.	Diuretics can be given in CRF to reduce hypertension and edema; usually discontinued after dialysis is initiated.	Given: hydrochlorothiazide 100 mg. No adverse side effects noted.
	Restrict sodium to 2 g/day, as ordered.	Decreasing solute load decreases fluid retention.	Compliant with 2-g sodium diet. Outcomes partially met. Continue with plan.

Critical Thinking Questions

1. What diagnostic tests do you think the nephrologist would have ordered for Mrs. Stevens?
2. Why might Mrs. Stevens' renal disease not have been diagnosed earlier?
3. If Mrs. Stevens does not agree to hemodialysis, what other alternatives are available to her?
4. What concerns do you anticipate that Mr. Stevens and their son would have?

Get Ready for the NCLEX® Examination!

Key Points

- Teach prevention of infectious disorders, such as cystitis and urethritis (e.g., good hygiene, drinking plenty of water, and seeking prompt treatment for genital discharge or dysuria).
- Symptoms of pyelonephritis include fever, chills, headache, malaise, nausea and vomiting, and pain in the flank radiating to the thigh and genitalia.
- Acute glomerulonephritis is characterized by fever, chills, flank pain, widespread edema, visual disturbances, and significant hypertension; nursing implications include encouraging bed rest, low-protein and low-sodium diet, and administering antihypertensives, corticosteroids, and diuretics as ordered.
- Symptoms of chronic glomerulonephritis include edema, dyspnea, and headache associated with hypertension.
- Hydronephrosis: flow of urine from the kidney is obstructed; kidney dilates and fills with fluid.
- Renal stenosis: renal artery can become blocked or narrowed because of atherosclerosis.
- Renal stones are associated with frequent urinary infections, inadequate fluid intake and concentrated urine, urinary stasis, and urate in the urine.
- Symptoms of trauma to the kidneys, ureters, and bladder may include gross hematuria, pain, or an enlarged mass in renal or bladder area.
- Risk factors for cancer of the bladder: male gender, smoking, and exposure to industrial toxins.
- Symptoms of cancer of the kidney: hematuria and enlargement of affected kidney are major signs.
- ARF: *Prerenal ARF* is caused by decreased blood flow; *intrarenal ARF* occurs from damage in the kidney; *postrenal ARF* is caused by obstruction which causes backup of urine into the kidney.
- ATN can be caused by decreased oxygenation or blood flow, or nephrotoxic substances.
- Three phases of ARF: oliguric/nonoliguric, diuretic, and recovery.
- Nephrosclerosis (hardening of renal arterioles), glomerulonephritis, and diabetic nephropathy are the most common causes of CRF.
- Treatment of CRF: diet management, fluid and electrolyte management, hemodialysis, or peritoneal dialysis and kidney transplant.
- Hemodialysis: use of diffusion to remove waste products normally excreted by the kidneys. Complications include fluid overload, electrolyte imbalance, anemia, platelet abnormalities, and infection.
- Nursing implications for peritoneal dialysis: weigh patient and take vital signs before and after treatment, measure I&O, use strict aseptic technique, and monitor for infection.
- Kidney transplant is another treatment for kidney failure. Signs of organ rejection include elevated blood pressure, fever, pain over transplant area, fatigue, oliguria, and increased BUN and serum creatinine.

Additional Learning Resources

Review Questions for the NCLEX® Examination

1. Which patient statement indicates that she needs additional teaching regarding the discharge instructions for urinary tract infection?
   1. "I will always wipe from back to front after a bowel movement."
   2. "I should avoid wearing tight slacks."
   3. "I won't wash my underclothing with strong detergents."
   4. "I will take a shower instead of a tub bath."

2. A patient with a history of throat infection becomes suddenly ill with fever, chills, flank pain, widespread edema, puffiness about the eyes, visual disturbances, and marked hypertension. The nurse would anticipate which diagnostic test?
   1. Urinalysis
   2. Intravenous pyelogram
   3. Serum amylase
   4. Prothrombin time

3. A 45-year-old man is admitted with a renal calculus. The nurse observes that the patient is stoic and withdrawn, occasionally grimacing, and refuses any type of pain medication. The nursing diagnosis for this patient is *acute pain*. The ultimate goal for this patient is to:
   1. verbalize level of pain.
   2. have a tolerable level of pain.
   3. identify the source of pain.
   4. develop coping strategies.

4. A patient with nephrotic syndrome is admitted with severe generalized edema, ascites, and cloudy urine. The patient is irritable and tired. What is the priority nursing diagnosis?
   1. Risk for infection
   2. Excess fluid volume
   3. Impaired comfort
   4. Fatigue

5. The nurse is assisting in administering bacille Calmette-Guérin (BCG) intravesically to a patient with bladder cancer. Place the steps in the correct order to accomplish this procedure.

   1. Clamp the urethral catheter for 2 hours.
   2. Change position every 15 to 30 minutes.
   3. Aseptically insert a urinary catheter.
   4. Drain urinary bladder.
   5. Instill the BCG fluid.

6. The patient with chronic renal failure (CRF) has a BUN of 120 mg/dL. What is the primary significance of this laboratory value?

   1. It is an expected laboratory result for a patient with CRF.
   2. The value signifies renal insufficiency.
   3. The result in conjunction with uremic signs indicates need for dialysis.
   4. The patient should be referred as a good candidate for peritoneal dialysis.

7. What is included in the nursing care of the patient undergoing peritoneal dialysis? *(Select all that apply.)*

   1. Maintain aseptic technique when accessing a peritoneal catheter.
   2. Instruct the patient to remain supine until the dialysate is drained.
   3. Weigh the patient before and after dialysis.
   4. Monitor vital signs.
   5. Check color and volume of effluent.

8. The nurse is sending the patient to the dialysis clinic. What predialysis nursing intervention should be included? *(Select all that apply.)*

   1. Withholding anticoagulants
   2. Administering antihypertensive
   3. Assessing dialysis access site
   4. Checking vital signs
   5. Monitoring laboratory values

9. While caring for a patient with uremic syndrome, the nurse would anticipate which clinical finding?

   1. Hypercalcemia
   2. Hyperphosphatemia
   3. Polycythemia
   4. Hypokalemia

10. A patient with CRF is on dialysis and waiting for a kidney transplant. The patient says, "I am never going to be at the top of the list for a kidney. I wish I could just die and get it over with." What is the most therapeutic response?

    1. "I am sure you are going to get a kidney. A lot of people donate these days."
    2. "Are you thinking about hurting or killing yourself?"
    3. "I would be discouraged too, but I have never been very good at waiting."
    4. "You seem really down today. What's going on?"

Critical Thinking Activities

Scenario A

Mr. Jakes, 25 years old, complains of sudden onset of fever and chills, flank pain, and "feeling full all over and peeing dark smoke-colored urine." He tells you he had strep throat 2 weeks ago, but is otherwise healthy.

1. Based on Mr. Jakes' history and complaints, what physical assessments should you perform?

2. Why is the history of strep throat 2 weeks ago significant?

3. The physician informs Mr. Jakes that he has glomerulonephritis and prescribes complete bed rest. How long must bed rest continue?

Scenario B

Mr. Mell, a 43-year-old interstate truck driver, complains of severe right lower back pain with nausea, vomiting, and pink-tinged urine. He relates a history of stones and reports, "It always feels like this until the kidney stone passes." The physician orders IV normal saline, morphine, routine laboratory tests to include BUN, creatinine, and an IVP.

1. What are three or four risk factors for kidney stones that might apply to Mr. Mell?

2. His BUN result is 17 mg/dL. What does this result indicate? What is your responsibility in reporting this data?

3. What is the care for Mr. Mell following a lithotripsy?

Scenario C

Mrs. Diaz, 35 years old, has had a nephrostomy for treatment of hydronephrosis due to a renal stone in the pelvis of the kidney. She returns from the surgical unit with a nephrostomy tube, a urethral catheter, and a rubber Penrose drain in place.

1. Explain the purpose of the nephrostomy tube.

2. What is the specific care for these drains and tubes?

chapter

36

The Endocrine System

evolve
http://evolve.elsevier.com/deWit/medsurg

Objectives

Theory

1. Identify the location of each endocrine gland.
2. Diagram the principal actions and target tissues for hormones of the hypothalamus and pituitary, parathyroid, adrenal, and pancreas glands.
3. Summarize the effects of the thyroid hormones.
4. Describe common diagnostic tests for the endocrine system.

Clinical Practice

1. Assess for specific age-related changes of the endocrine system in an elderly patient.
2. Teach patients about the diagnostic tests that might be performed for symptoms of endocrine disorders.
3. Perform a focused assessment on a patient who may have an endocrine disorder.
4. Identify appropriate nursing diagnoses and interventions for problems common to patients with endocrine disorders.

Key Terms

adenohypophysis (ă-DĔN-ŏ-hī-PŎF-ă-sĭs, p. 823)
adrenocorticotropic hormone (ă-DRĔN-ŏ-KŎR-tĭ-kō-TRŌ-pĭk, p. 823)
endocrine (ĔN-dŏ-krĭn, p. 821)
exocrine (Ĕk-sŏ-krĭn, p. 821)
fructosamine assay (p. 827)
glucocorticoids (glū-kō-KŎR-tĭ-kŏydz, p. 821)
glucose tolerance test (p. 827)
hemoglobin A₁c (A1C) (HĒ-mō-glō-bĭn, p. 827)
hormones (HŎR-mōnz, p. 822)
hypersecretion (hī-pĕr-SĔ-KRĒ-shŭn, p. 823)
hyposecretion (hī-pō-SĔ-KRĒ-shŭn, p. 823)

insulin (ĬN-sū-lĭn, p. 822)
mineralocorticoids (mĭn-ĕr-ăl-ō-KŎR-tĭ-kŏydz, p. 821)
negative feedback (p. 823)
parathormone (păr-ă-THŎR-mōn, p. 821)
pressor (p. 821)
target cells (p. 822)
target tissues (p. 822)
thyrocalcitonin (thī-rō-KĂL-sĭ-TŌ-nĭn, p. 819)
thyroid panel (THĪ-rŏyd, p. 827)
thyroxine (THĪ-rŏk-sĭn, p. 819)
triiodothyronine (trī-ī-ō-dō-THĪ-rō-nĕn, p. 819)

OVERVIEW OF ANATOMY AND PHYSIOLOGY OF THE ENDOCRINE SYSTEM

WHAT ARE THE ORGANS AND STRUCTURES OF THE ENDOCRINE SYSTEM?

- The pituitary gland connects to the hypothalamus via the hypophyseal stalk. The pituitary gland has two parts: the anterior pituitary and the posterior pituitary.
- The thyroid gland has two lobes and lies below the larynx over the thyroid cartilage, in front of and on either side of the trachea.
- The parathyroid glands are four to six small glands that are located on the posterior surface of the thyroid gland.

- The adrenal glands are located on the anterior upper surface of each kidney; each is composed of the cortex and medulla.
- The pancreas sits in the upper left aspect of the abdominal cavity. Beta cells, which secrete the hormone insulin, are found in the islets of Langerhans.
- The ovaries are located in the pelvic cavity of the female.
- The testes hang suspended in the scrotum of the male.
- The pineal gland is in the midbrain, in the cranial vault.
- The thymus gland lies at the base of the neck, in the front of the thoracic cavity.

WHAT ARE THE FUNCTIONS OF THE ENDOCRINE SYSTEM?

- Alter chemical reactions and control the rate at which chemical activities take place within cells.
- Change the permeability of cell membranes and select the substances that can be transported across cell membranes.
- Activate a particular mechanism in the cell, such as the system that controls cellular growth and reproduction. The hormones produced by the endocrine system, the target organs on which they act, and the principal actions of each hormone are presented in Table 36-1.

WHAT ARE THE EFFECTS OF THE PITUITARY HORMONES?

- The effects of pituitary hormones when secreted are illustrated in Figure 36-1.

- Any type of dysfunction of the pituitary gland will affect one or more of the hormones, as well as the target organ(s) for the hormone(s).

WHAT ARE THE EFFECTS OF THE THYROID HORMONES?

- The thyroid gland secretes the hormones thyroxine (T$_4$), triiodothyronine (T$_3$), and thyrocalcitonin.
- T$_3$ is the more potent form of thyroid hormone. When T$_3$ is needed, it is converted from the more abundant supply of T$_4$.
- Intake of protein and iodine is needed to synthesize both thyroid hormones.
- Thyroid hormones activate the cellular production of heat; stimulate protein and lipid synthesis, mobilization, and degradation (breakdown); and stimulate the manufacture of coenzymes from vitamins.

Table 36-1   The Principal Endocrine Glands and Their Hormones

GLAND	HORMONE	TARGET TISSUE	PRINCIPAL ACTIONS
Hypothalamus	Releasing and inhibiting hormones	Anterior lobe of pituitary gland	Stimulates or inhibits secretion of specific hormones
Anterior lobe of pituitary	Growth hormone (GH)	Most tissues in the body	Stimulates growth by promoting protein synthesis
	Thyroid-stimulating hormone (TSH)	Thyroid gland	Increases secretion of thyroid hormone; increases the size of the thyroid gland
	Adrenocorticotropic hormone (ACTH)	Adrenal cortex	Increases secretion of adrenocortical hormones, especially glucocorticoids, such as cortisol
	Follicle-stimulating hormone (FSH)	Ovarian follicles in the female; seminiferous tubules in male	Follicle maturation and estrogen secretion in the female; spermatogenesis in the male
	Luteinizing hormone (LH); called interstitial cell–stimulating hormone (ICSH) in males	Ovary in females, testis in males	Ovulation; progesterone production in female; testosterone production in male
	Prolactin	Mammary gland	Stimulates milk production
Posterior lobe of pituitary (storage only: ADH and oxytocin are synthesized in the hypothalamus)	Antidiuretic hormone (ADH)	Kidney	Increases water reabsorption (decreases water lost in urine)
	Oxytocin	Uterus; mammary gland	Increases uterine contractions; stimulates ejection of milk from mammary gland
Thyroid gland	Thyroxine and triiodothyronine	Most body cells	Increases metabolic rate; essential for normal growth and development
	Calcitonin	Primarily bone	Decreases blood calcium by inhibiting bone breakdown and release of calcium; antagonistic to parathyroid hormone
Parathyroid gland	Parathyroid hormone (PTH) or parathormone	Bone, kidney, digestive tract	Increases blood calcium by stimulating bone breakdown and release of calcium; increases calcium absorption in the digestive tract; decreases calcium lost in urine
Adrenal cortex	Mineralocorticoids (aldosterone)	Kidney	Increases sodium reabsorption and potassium excretion in kidney tubules; increases water retention
	Glucocorticoids (cortisol)	Most body tissues	Increases blood glucose levels; inhibits inflammation and immune response

From Applegate, E.J. (2011). *The Anatomy and Physiology Learning System* (4th ed.). Philadelphia: Saunders.

Continued

Table 36-1	The Principal Endocrine Glands and Their Hormones—cont'd		
GLAND	**HORMONE**	**TARGET TISSUE**	**PRINCIPAL ACTIONS**
Adrenal cortex—cont'd	Androgens and estrogens	Most body tissues	Secreted in small amounts; effect is generally masked by the hormones from the ovaries and testes
Adrenal medulla	Epinephrine, norepinephrine	Heart, blood vessels, liver, adipose tissue	Helps cope with stress; increases heart rate and blood pressure; increases blood flow to skeletal muscle; increases blood glucose
Pancreas (islets of Langerhans)	Glucagon	Liver	Increases breakdown of glycogen to increase blood glucose levels
	Insulin	General, but especially liver, skeletal muscle, adipose tissue	Decreases blood glucose levels by facilitating uptake and utilization of glucose by cells; stimulates glucose storage as glycogen and production of adipose tissue
Testes	Testosterone	Most body cells	Maturation and maintenance of male reproductive organs and secondary sex characteristics
Ovaries	Estrogens	Most body cells	Maturation and maintenance of female reproductive organs and secondary sex characteristics; menstrual cycle
	Progesterone	Uterus and breast	Prepares uterus for pregnancy; stimulates development of mammary gland; menstrual cycle
Pineal gland	Melatonin	Hypothalamus	Inhibits gonadotropin-releasing hormone, which consequently inhibits reproductive functions; regulates daily rhythms, such as sleep and wakefulness
Thymus	Thymosin	Tissues involved in immune response	Immune system development and function

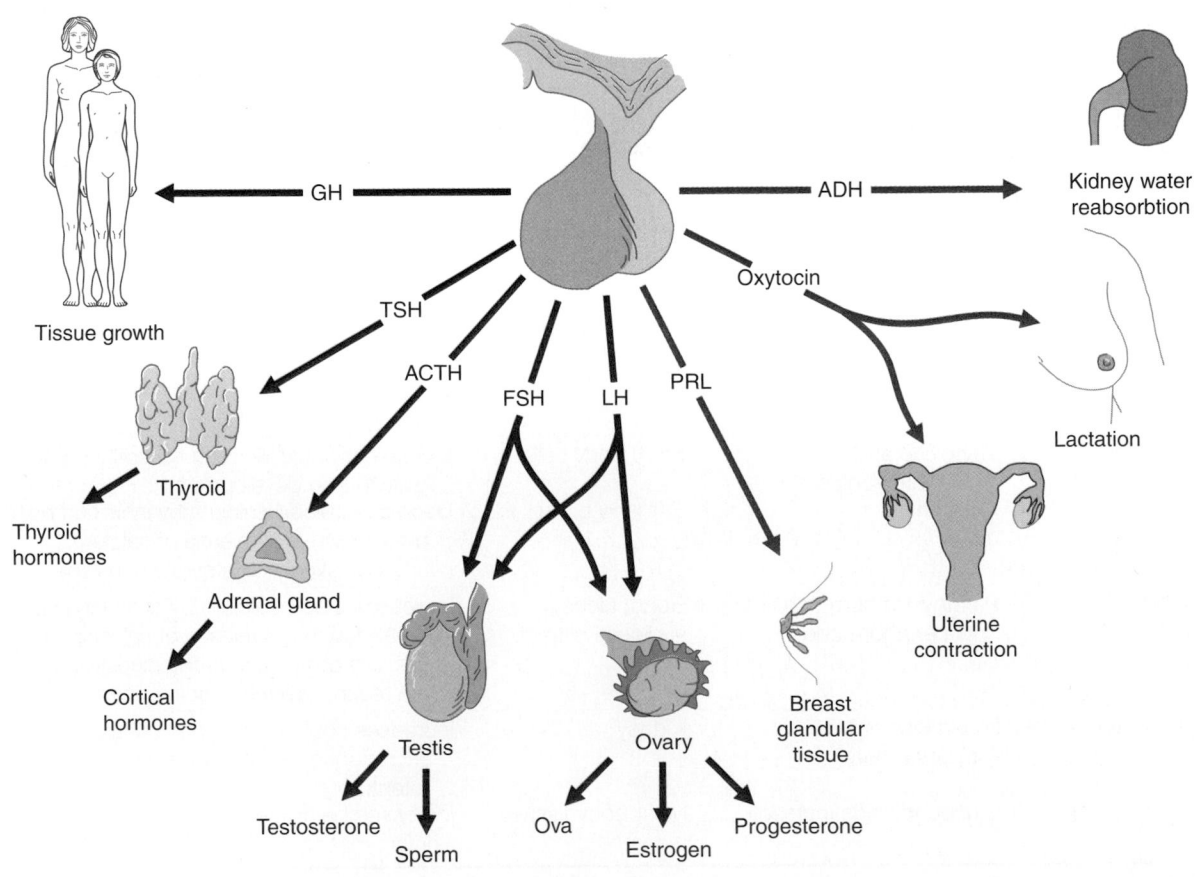

FIGURE 36-1 Effects of hormones from the pituitary gland.

- Thyroid hormones regulate many aspects of carbohydrate metabolism and affect tissue response to epinephrine and norepinephrine.

WHAT ARE THE FUNCTIONS OF THE PARATHYROID GLANDS?

- **Parathormone**, or *parathyroid hormone*, is produced and secreted by the parathyroid glands.
- A low calcium level will stimulate release of parathormone, which increases the plasma level of calcium. A high calcium level will inhibit the release of parathormone.
- Parathormone acts on the renal tubules to increase the excretion of phosphorus in the urine and to stimulate the reabsorption of calcium. Parathormone also acts on bone, causing the release of calcium from the bone into the bloodstream.

 Safety Alert

Parathyroid Deficiency

A deficiency of parathyroid hormone produces muscle cramps, twitching of the muscles, and, in some cases, severe convulsions.

WHAT ARE THE FUNCTIONS OF THE HORMONES SECRETED BY THE ADRENAL GLANDS?

- The adrenal medulla (middle portion) secretes two hormones, epinephrine and norepinephrine, in response to stimulation from the sympathetic nervous system.
- Epinephrine prepares the body to meet stress or emergency situations and prevents hypoglycemia (Figure 36-2). Norepinephrine functions as a **pressor** (causing blood vessel constriction) hormone to maintain blood pressure.
- The hormones secreted by the adrenal cortex are called *adrenal corticosteroids.* (The word *steroid* is sometimes used to designate an adrenal corticosteroid or a synthetic compound with similar properties.)
- The two major types of hormones secreted by the adrenal cortex are the **mineralocorticoids** and the **glucocorticoids** (Figure 36-3).
- The adrenal glands also secrete small amounts of androgenic hormones, which have effects similar to those of the male and female sex hormones.
- The mineralocorticoids affect the electrolytes, particularly sodium, potassium, and chloride. The chief mineralocorticoid is aldosterone, which promotes conservation of water by acting on the kidney to retain sodium in exchange for potassium, which is excreted in the urine.
- Without the mineralocorticoids, a person would die within 3 to 7 days, because these hormones directly control fluid balance, blood volume, cardiac output,

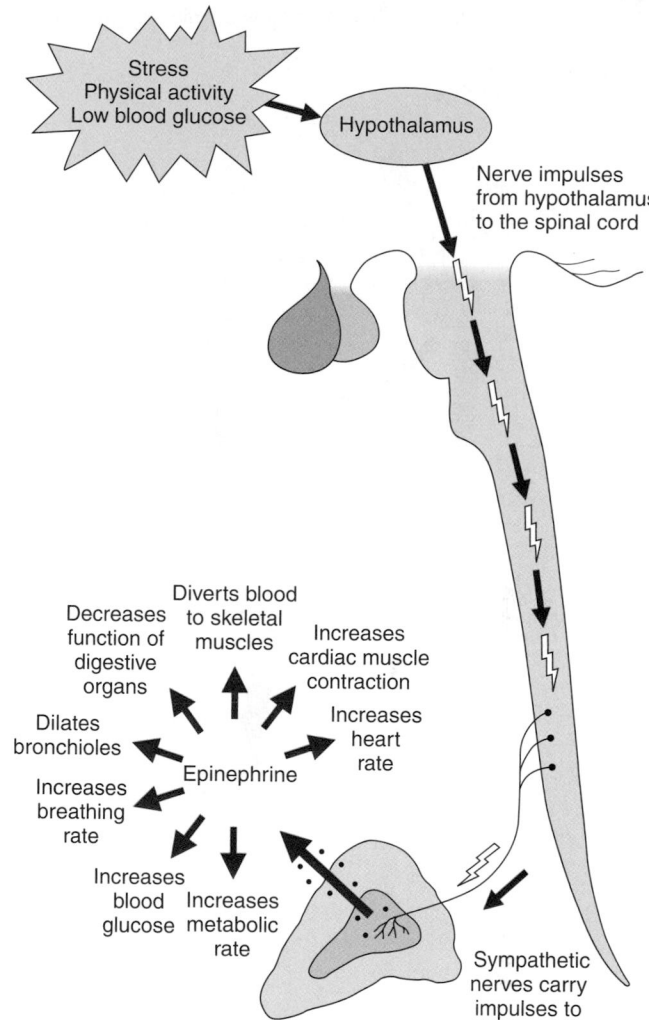

FIGURE 36-2 Effects of epinephrine and control of its secretion.

exchange of nutrients, and wastes in each cell; mineralocorticoids affect all chemical processes and glandular functions within the body.

- The glucocorticoids are essential to the metabolic systems for proper utilization of carbohydrates, proteins, and fats.
- The primary glucocorticoid is cortisol, or hydrocortisone. Cortisol acts to increase glucose levels in the blood. Cortisol also helps counteract the inflammatory response.
- Both aldosterone and cortisol are controlled by adrenocorticotropic hormone (ACTH)–releasing hormone from the hypothalamus and ACTH secreted by the anterior pituitary (see Figure 36-3).

WHAT IS THE HORMONAL FUNCTION OF THE PANCREAS?

- The pancreas is both an **endocrine** (secretes internally) and **exocrine** (secretes outwardly through a duct) gland. Its endocrine function is to produce the hormones insulin and glucagon.

ACTH = Adrenocorticotropic hormone

Stress or low blood glucose

Hypothalamus

Hypothalamus secretes ACTH-releasing hormone

Anterior pituitary secretes ACTH

- ↑ potassium concentration
- ↓ sodium concentration
- ↓ blood pressure/volume

ACTH minor effect

Adrenal cortex secretes cortisol

Adrenal cortex secretes aldosterone

Target tissues
- ↑ blood glucose
- ↑ protein metabolism
- anti-inflammatory

Kidney tubules
- excrete potassium
- reabsorb sodium
- conserve water, reduce urine, increase blood volume

FIGURE 36-3 Regulation of aldosterone and cortisol secretion.

- The beta cells are responsible for producing and secreting insulin. Insulin is needed for the cells of the body to be able to use glucose as fuel (Figures 36-4 and 36-5).

WHAT ARE THE EFFECTS OF AGING ON THE ENDOCRINE SYSTEM?

- The pituitary gland becomes smaller.
- The thyroid becomes more lumpy or nodular; beginning around age 20, metabolism gradually declines.
- Hormones that usually decrease with age include aldosterone, renin, calcitonin, and growth hormone; specific hormones decrease in older women (estrogen and prolactin) and older men (testosterone).
- Hormones that may increase with age include follicle-stimulating hormone (FSH), luteinizing hormone (LH), norepinephrine, and antidiuretic hormone (ADH).
- Hormones that remain unchanged or are only slightly decreased with age include thyroid hormones (T_3 and T_4), cortisol, insulin, epinephrine, parathyroid hormone, and 25-hydroxyvitamin D.
- Blood glucose levels rise with age, with fasting levels climbing about 1 mg/dL for each decade and postprandial levels increasing 6 to 13 mg/dL.

- Although insulin levels remain unchanged with age, decreased glucose tolerance may occur due to changes in the cell receptor sites: the older adult experiences hypoglycemia more quickly than a younger person and may progress to dangerously low levels of blood glucose before signs and symptoms are obvious. This decreased glucose tolerance because of cell receptor change can place the older adult at risk for hyperglycemia and the onset of type 2 diabetes.
- Although thyroid hormone levels may decrease with aging, the body makes up for it by decreasing the rate at which thyroid hormone is broken down; therefore resting levels of thyroid hormone are usually normal in the elderly. Thyroid disorders are, however, twice as common in the older adult. Hypothyroidism is the most common thyroid disorder, especially in older women.
- The amount of hormones secreted by the older adult changes, decreasing the individual's ability to adapt to stress and respond to environmental changes.
- Because of decreasing liver and kidney function in the elderly, hormone replacement therapy must be done very cautiously, to prevent hormone overdosage.

THE ENDOCRINE SYSTEM

The endocrine system regulates metabolism, growth and development, and sexual function and reproductive processes. A primary function of the endocrine system is to synthesize and release hormones directly into the bloodstream and the body fluids. The cells and tissues that are affected by a specific hormone are called its target cells or target tissues.

Some of the endocrine hormones, such as the thyroid hormones, affect practically every cell in the body. Others, such as the sex hormones, exert their special effects on only one kind of organ. Moreover, hormones from one endocrine gland can affect another endocrine gland. The pituitary, for example, secretes several different kinds of hormones that affect other endocrine glands. For this reason, the pituitary gland is often referred to as the "master gland" of the body.

The endocrine system and the nervous system are the two major control systems of the body, and their regulatory functions are interrelated. However, the endocrine system typically controls body processes that occur slowly, such as cell growth, whereas the nervous system controls body processes that occur more rapidly, such as breathing and body movement.

The secretion of a particular hormone normally depends on the need. If an endocrine gland receives a message that its particular hormone is in short supply, it will synthesize and release more of that hormone. If, on the other hand, the hormonal need

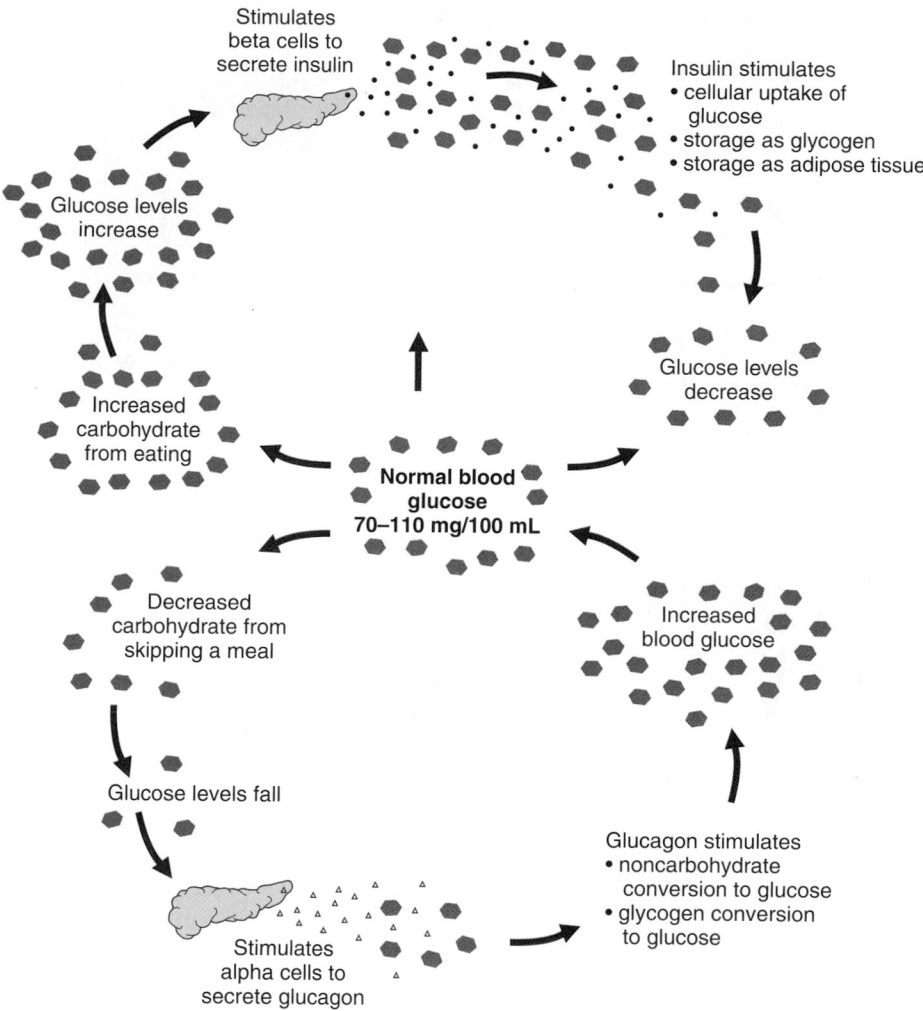

FIGURE 36-4 Effects of insulin and glucagon.

of a target tissue is being satisfied, production or secretion of the hormone will be inhibited—a concept known as negative feedback.

Some glands, such as the adrenal medulla and posterior pituitary, receive their information about hormone levels in the body *directly*, and respond only to stimulation of nerve endings within the glands themselves. However, the posterior pituitary gland *indirectly* receives notice to either release or inhibit hormones: stimulation comes by way of the hypothalamus and the anterior lobe of the pituitary (the adenohypophysis). The hypothalamus contains special nerve endings that produce releasing and inhibiting hormones; these hormones are then absorbed into capillaries of a portal system that transports the hormones to the adenohypophysis (the anterior lobe of the pituitary). Thus the hypothalamus controls the secretion of hormones from the pituitary. The pituitary, in turn, controls the release or inhibition of hormones from other glands. Many of the hormones of the anterior pituitary are "tropic" hormones; that is, they tend to

cause a change in the endocrine gland that is the target of the specific pituitary hormone. An example is adrenocorticotropic hormone (ACTH), which acts on the adrenal cortex. (If you break down this term, you can easily see that the components of *adrenal–cortex–tropic* tell you exactly where or what type of hormone this is and where it comes from.) The major endocrine glands can be found in Figure 36-6; see Table 36-1 for the various tropic hormones and target tissues.

ENDOCRINE SYSTEM DISORDERS

Causes

Endocrine disorders are caused by an imbalance in the production of hormone or by an alteration in the body's ability to use the hormones produced. Dysfunction can occur at any point in the production-secretion-feedback regulation cycle.

Primary endocrine dysfunction means that an endocrine gland is either oversecreting or undersecreting hormone(s)—situations referred to as hypersecretion and hyposecretion, respectively. Tumor or hyperplasia

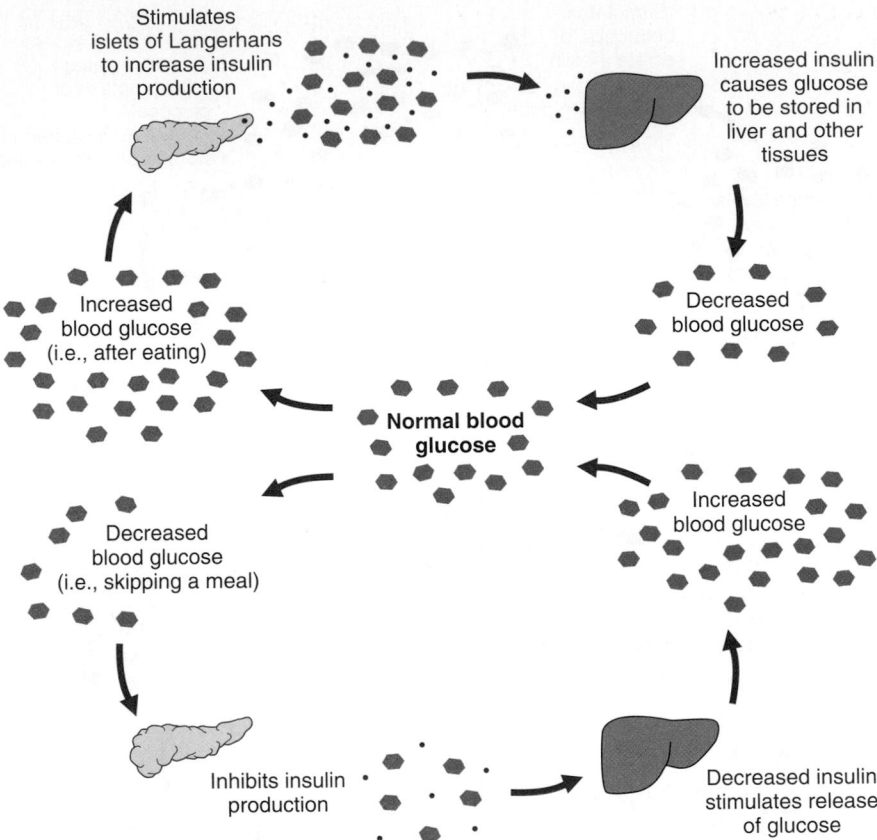

Stimulates islets of Langerhans to increase insulin production

Increased insulin causes glucose to be stored in liver and other tissues

Increased blood glucose (i.e., after eating)

Decreased blood glucose

Normal blood glucose

Increased blood glucose

Decreased blood glucose (i.e., skipping a meal)

Inhibits insulin production

Decreased insulin stimulates release of glucose

FIGURE 36-5 Interaction of blood glucose and insulin.

of the endocrine gland may lead to hypersecretion. Hyposecretion is usually the result of a tumor or an inflammatory process that destroys endocrine glandular tissue or interferes with endocrine function. Infection, mechanical damage, or an autoimmune response may cause such an inflammatory response in a gland.

Secondary endocrine dysfunction occurs from factors outside the gland itself. Medications, trauma, hormone therapy, and other factors may cause secondary dysfunction. Such dysfunction may be temporary or permanent; endocrine function often returns to normal if the cause is corrected (for example, the medication is discontinued).

Prevention

Preventing most endocrine disorders is not possible by lifestyle changes; however, there are some dietary considerations regarding the thyroid gland that may be beneficial.

Pituitary gland

Pineal gland

Parathyroid gland (on posterior surface of thyroid gland)

Thyroid gland

Thymus

Adrenal gland

Pancreas

Ovary (female)

Testis (male)

FIGURE 36-6 Major endocrine glands.

Health Promotion

Preventing Goiter

Goiter, an overgrowth of the thyroid, may be prevented by sufficient intake of iodine. Iodine is available in foods grown near the ocean and in seafood. Iodized salt is the major source for most people.

? Think Critically

Why might a person with an endocrine disorder delay seeking medical care?

Diagnostic Tests and Procedures

Tests of the endocrine system are performed on blood samples, on urine samples, or by scans, ultrasounds, radiographs, or magnetic resonance imaging (MRI). Table 36-2 presents the various tests and procedures and their nursing implications.

Clinical Cues

- Thyroid test results are altered by iodine-based contrast media for radiologic studies.
- Betadine used for skin preparation may also affect thyroid studies.
- Oral contraceptives, aspirin, and other drugs may affect many thyroid tests (Pagana & Pagana, 2012).

Table 36-2 Diagnostic Tests and Procedures of the Endocrine System

TEST	PURPOSE	DESCRIPTION	NURSING IMPLICATIONS
Blood Tests			
Pituitary hormone levels: LH, FSH, GH, ACTH, TSH, prolactin	To detect oversecretion or deficiency of pituitary hormones	Sample of venous blood is drawn; requires at least 1 mL for immunoassay test; check laboratory procedure manual.	Monitor venipuncture site for bleeding; apply bandage or dressing.
Serum T_4 (total thyroxine) *Normal value:* 4.5-11.5 mcg/dL	To assess thyroxine in blood to evaluate thyroid function	Requires a venous blood sample of at least 1 mL.	Aspirin, iodine-containing medications, contrast media, and other drugs may affect result; check with laboratory.
Serum T_3 (total triiodothyronine) *Normal value:* 70-190 ng/dL	Used with T_4 to evaluate thyroid function	Requires a venous blood sample of at least 1 mL.	Same as for serum T_4.
TSH *Normal value:* 1-10 μU/mL	To differentiate between pituitary dysfunction and primary thyroid dysfunction; assist with diagnosis of hypothyroidism	Requires a venous blood sample of at least 1 mL.	Same as for serum T_4.
Antithyroid antibody titer *Normal value:* <1:100	To detect the presence of thyroid antibodies and distinguish between autoimmune disorders and toxic thyroid adenoma	Requires a venous blood sample.	Radioactive iodine will interfere if given within 24 hr of drawing the blood sample.
Calcitonin *Normal value:* <100 pg/mL	Used for differential diagnosis of cancer of the thyroid	Requires a venous blood sample.	If base level is within normal, the pentagastrin stimulation test may be administered by injection to test for calcitonin secretion. Blood samples are then drawn 1½ and 5 min after injection.
Cortisol *Normal value:* 8 AM, 6-23 mcg/dL; 4 PM, 3-15 mcg/dL; 10 PM, <50% of 8 AM value	To assess cortisol production by adrenal glands	Requires sample of venous blood.	Explain that a specimen may be collected two or three times in 24 hr to evaluate circadian effects on cortisol secretion. Keep stress to a minimum. Note time collected on laboratory slip.
Adrenocorticotropic hormone (ACTH) *Normal value:* AM, 20-100 pg/mL; PM, 10-40 pg/mL	To assess ACTH production from pituitary gland	Requires venous blood sample. Place specimen in ice water immediately after drawing.	Prepare ice bath before venipuncture. Note collection time on laboratory slip. Single specimen is best collected in morning.

ACTH, adrenocorticotropic hormone; *ADH,* antidiuretic hormone; *FSH,* follicle-stimulating hormone; *GH,* growth hormone; *IM,* intramuscularly; *IV,* intravenously; *LH,* luteinizing hormone; *NPO,* nothing by mouth; *TSH,* thyroid-stimulating hormone.

Continued

Table 36-2   Diagnostic Tests and Procedures of the Endocrine System—cont'd

TEST	PURPOSE	DESCRIPTION	NURSING IMPLICATIONS
Blood Tests—cont'd			
ACTH stimulation test *Normal value:* after ACTH; serum cortisol >20 mcg/dL	To assess adrenal response to ACTH To detect adrenal cortical insufficiency (Addison's disease)	Baseline venous sample taken for cortisol determination. ACTH is administered IV or IM. Blood sample is withdrawn at 30 and 60 min for further cortisol determinations.	Note time ACTH is administered; note time each specimen is drawn. Instruct patient to avoid strenuous activity on the day before the test. Check with laboratory regarding food restrictions.
Dexamethasone suppression test *Normal value:* after dexamethasone, serum cortisol <5 mcg/dL	To diagnose Cushing syndrome To assess response to dexamethasone	Morning baseline serum cortisol levels are measured. Oral dexamethasone is administered at bedtime. Blood sample is collected the next morning to measure cortisol levels.	Explain the procedure to the patient. Check orders for drugs to be withheld. Both cortisol levels must be drawn at the same time each day. Note time specimens were drawn and patient medications on laboratory slips. Instruct patient to avoid strenuous activity the day before the test.
Thyroid Scans			
Radioactive iodine uptake (RAIU) *Normal values:* <6% uptake in 2 hr; 2%-25% in 6 hr; 15%-45% in 24 hr; 24-hr urine: 40%-80% radioactive iodine excreted in 24 hr	To assess function of thyroid gland To measure the rate of iodine uptake by the thyroid	Trace dose of radioactive iodine (RAI) is given orally. A gamma counter or scintillation counter is placed over the gland to measure the amount of RAI absorbed. Concurrent 24-hr urine specimen may be collected to assess iodine secretion.	Test must not be done during pregnancy or lactation. Explain that the amount of radioactive iodine used is small and will not make the patient "radioactive." Explain the procedure and the time it will take. Instruct how to collect 24-hr urine specimen if required.
Thyroid scan	To determine size, shape, and activity of the thyroid gland To detect hyperactive "hot" spots and hypoactive "cold" spots	After administering RAI, a scintillation camera moves back and forth across the gland to obtain an image of iodine concentration and distribution in the thyroid gland. A computer may provide a three-dimensional image. Often done in conjunction with RAIU.	Same implications as for RAIU. Patient must lie perfectly still during the scanning. Scan takes about 20 min. Rescanning is performed at intervals of 6 and 24 hr after RAI is administered.
Urine Tests			
17-Hydroxycorticosteroids (17-OHCS) *Normal values:* females, 2-8 mg/24 hr; males, 3-9 mg/24 hr	To determine levels of glucocorticoid metabolites	Collect a 24-hr urine specimen in a container with preservative. Medications may interfere; consult with physician and laboratory about medications patient is taking.	Instruct patient in collection procedure. Note start and end time of collection on laboratory slip. Note medications patient is taking on laboratory slip.
17-Ketosteroids (17-KS) *Normal values:* females, 6-15 mg/24 hr; males, 8-22 mg/24 hr; older than age 65, 4-8 mg/24 hr	To determine amount of androgen metabolites in the urine	Collect 24-hr urine specimen. Check with laboratory regarding need to keep specimen chilled.	Same as for 17-hydroxycortico-steroids test.

Table 36-2	Diagnostic Tests and Procedures of the Endocrine System—cont'd		
TEST	**PURPOSE**	**DESCRIPTION**	**NURSING IMPLICATIONS**
Urine Tests—cont'd			
Aldosterone 3-20 mcg/24 hr	To determine urinary aldosterone levels to assist in diagnosis of aldosteronism	Requires 24-hr urine specimen with preservative; specimen must be kept chilled.	Instruct in dietary and medication restrictions. Record diet and medications on laboratory slip.
Fluid deprivation test	To detect diabetes insipidus	While patient is NPO, hourly urine output, specific gravity, osmolality are measured along with body weight and vital signs. Vasopressin is given subcutaneously; hourly measurements are continued for several hours.	Explain the procedure to the patient. Provide urine collection containers. Remind patient to void hourly.
Hypertonic saline test	To stimulate release of ADH to evaluate ADH secretion and detect diabetes insipidus	The patient is loaded with water. An infusion of hypertonic saline is administered. Urine output and urine specific gravity are measured hourly.	Tell patient to produce a urine specimen in the marked container every hour.

Abnormalities in thyroid gland activity (Figure 36-7) are among the most common endocrine disorders. To detect abnormalities, a group of tests—called a **thyroid panel**—is performed. In assessing a patient before administering tests that involve contrast media, the nurse must ask about allergies to iodine or shellfish: an allergy to either of these may indicate that an individual is hypersensitive to contrast media.

Laboratory testing for serum calcium and phosphate levels is usually performed to assess parathyroid function. Adrenal gland function is evaluated by laboratory testing, including electrolyte panels, glucose levels, and hormone levels; a 12-lead electrocardiogram (ECG) may be performed if cardiac dysrhythmias are suspected.

? Think Critically

The physician has ordered laboratory tests to determine if the patient has an endocrine disorder. The patient wants you to tell her the results of the tests. What will you do?

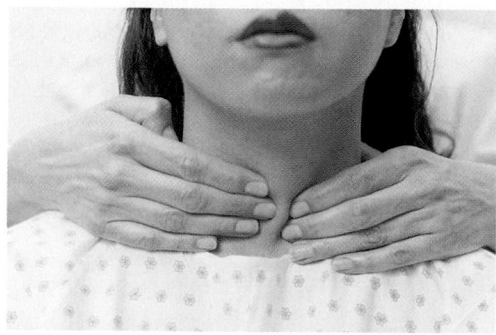

FIGURE 36-7 Posterior palpation of the thyroid gland.

Diagnostic tests for detecting diabetes can be found in Table 36-3. According to 2011 American Diabetic Association guidelines, diagnosis of diabetes mellitus is made using one of four abnormalities:

- Symptoms of diabetes mellitus (see Chapter 38) plus a random glucose level greater than or equal to 200 mg/dL
- A fasting glucose level greater than or equal to 126 mg/dL
- An abnormal A1C hemoglobin level
- A **glucose tolerance test** revealing a postprandial glucose greater than or equal to 200, 2 hours after 75 g of glucose is administered

In a glucose tolerance test, the patient is given a set amount of glucose to evaluate insulin secretion and ability to metabolize glucose.

The **hemoglobin A_{1c} (A1C)** test (formerly called the *glycosylated hemoglobin test*) measures blood glucose over a period of many weeks (Table 36-4). Glucose in the bloodstream attaches itself to the hemoglobin A (red blood cell) molecule and remains there for the life span of the red blood cell. Physicians use A1C test results to prescribe adjustments to a patient's treatment program for managing diabetes. One of the *Healthy People 2020* objectives is to increase the proportion of adults with diabetes who have an A1C test at least twice a year. **Fructosamine assay** is another test to monitor control of glucose over time. The fructosamine assay monitors blood glucose over a shorter time frame than the A1C test, because the assay measures sugar attached to the protein albumin, which has a shorter life span than hemoglobin.

Table 36-3 Diagnostic Tests for Detecting and Monitoring Diabetes Mellitus

TEST	PURPOSE	DESCRIPTION	NURSING IMPLICATIONS
Serum Tests			
Fasting blood glucose *Normal value:* 70-115 mg/dL; elderly: rises 1 mg/dL per decade of age	To determine level of circulating glucose; detect hyperglycemia or hypoglycemia	Requires a fasting venous blood sample.	Explain importance of fasting state to the patient.
2-hr postprandial blood glucose *Normal value:* <126 mg/dL; elderly: rises 5-10 mg/dL with age	To determine need for glucose tolerance test; determine need for change in diabetes therapy	Venous blood sample drawn 2 hr after a meal.	Explain the importance of presenting self for blood sampling exactly 2 hr after finishing a meal.
Glucose tolerance test *Normal values:* Fasting <126 mg/dL; 2 hr, <200 mg/dL	To detect abnormal glucose metabolism; assist in diagnosis of diabetes mellitus	A venous blood sample is drawn after a 10-12 hr fast; patient is given a glucose "load," usually a prepared liquid drink of 300 mL, that contains a specified amount of glucose. Venous blood samples are drawn at 30-min intervals for 2 hr. Phenytoin (Dilantin), birth control pills, diuretics, and glucocorticoids will adversely affect results; consult physician regarding these medications.	Instruct patient to eat a balanced diet with at least 150 g of carbohydrate for 3 days before the test and maintain a normal level of physical activity. Instruct patient to fast for 10-12 hr before beginning the test. Explain that during the test the patient cannot eat, drink, or smoke, and must stay at rest for 2 hr. During the test, instruct patient to report feelings of weakness, dizziness, nervousness, and confusion.
Hemoglobin A$_{1c}$ (A1C) *Normal value:* 3.9%-5.2% (of total hemoglobin)	To determine degree of diabetic control of blood sugar over the preceding 6-8 wk	A sample of venous blood is required. Fasting is not necessary.	Explain to the patient the need for this test to be done periodically to monitor effectiveness of diabetic therapy and determine degree of control over the disease process.
Fructosamine assay *Normal value:* 1.5-2.7 mmol/L	To determine degree of diabetic control of blood sugar over preceding 2-3 wk	A sample of venous blood is required. Fasting is not necessary.	Less influenced by age than A1C.
C-peptide *Normal value:* 0.78-1.89 ng/mL	To evaluate endogenous secretion of insulin when the presence of insulin antibodies interferes with direct assay of insulin	A fasting sample of 1 mL of venous blood is used.	Caution the patient to fast for 8-12 hr before the test. Water is permitted.
Urine Tests			
Ketone bodies	To determine presence of ketones in the urine, which indicates a state of ketoacidosis	A fresh urine sample is tested with a dipstick or with Acetest tablet. Follow instructions on bottle of test material.	Instruct diabetic patient that ketone testing should be done whenever illness has interfered with normal eating and activity for more than 24 hr and whenever signs of hyperglycemia are present.

Table 36-4	Degrees of Control of Blood Glucose Based on Hemoglobin A$_{1c}$ (A1C) Levels	
A1C LEVEL	**RATING**	
4.9%-6.7%	Excellent	
7.6%-8.5%	Good	
9.4%-10.0%	Fair	
12.1%-13.0%	Poor	

❖ NURSING MANAGEMENT

▪ Assessment (Data Collection)

A full physical assessment and history are needed to evaluate the patient who is possibly experiencing an endocrine disorder. The patient's perception of the function of various body systems affected by the endocrine glands is essential.

 Think Critically

Why would it be important to assess the patient's past and current emotional status if you suspect an endocrine disorder?

▪ Nursing Diagnosis

Table 36-5 presents the most common nursing diagnoses, expected outcomes, and nursing interventions for patients with endocrine problems. Additional nursing diagnoses are included in Nursing Care Plans 37-1, 37-2, and 38-1.

 Focused Assessment

Data Collection for the Endocrine System

Ask the following questions:
- Have you gained or lost weight over the past 6 months?
- Has your appetite increased or decreased?
- Have you noticed any changes in thinking? Any difficulty concentrating? Any difficulty with memory?
- Have you become more anxious or nervous? Do you cry a lot?
- Has your personality changed?
- Has your energy level changed?
- Have you experienced muscle cramping or numbness or tingling in your hands and legs?
- Have you been experiencing diarrhea or constipation?
- Have you had more gas or abdominal bloating?
- Have you noticed any facial or ankle swelling?
- Has your voice become huskier?
- Have you been thirstier than usual? Do you urinate more now?
- Have you had heart palpitations? Has your pulse rate changed?
- Has your sleep pattern changed? Do you need more sleep? Are you finding it difficult to sleep?
- *For women:* Have your menstrual periods altered?
- Is there any history in your family of thyroid, pituitary, or adrenal disease, or diabetes?
- Have you noticed a difference in the way you react to the environmental temperature? Are you cold or hot when others are comfortable?
- Have you noticed any changes in the texture or thickness of your hair or eyebrows? What about your fingernails? Are they brittle?
- Has your skin become dry and rough?
- Have you ever had radiation treatments to the head or neck?

▪ Planning

Planning care for a patient with an endocrine problem will depend on what type of problem the patient has. One thing is certain: stress has an effect on the problem.

Table 36-5	Common Nursing Diagnoses, Goals/Expected Outcomes, and Nursing Interventions for Patients with Endocrine Problems	
NURSING DIAGNOSIS*	**GOALS/EXPECTED OUTCOMES**	**NURSING INTERVENTIONS**
Deficient fluid volume related to increased urine output (DI, HyperT, AD)	Patient will display balance between intake and output.	Monitor for dehydration and signs of decreased cardiac output. Measure and record intake and output q 2 hr; maintain ordered IV fluid rate; encourage oral fluid intake.
Constipation related to loss of fluid from intestine, slowed intestinal peristalsis (DI, HypoT, AD)*	Patient will display normal bowel pattern within 2 wk.	Provide high-bulk diet; encourage fluid intake; administer stool softener or laxatives, as ordered. Encourage exercise to promote better bowel function.
Disturbed body image related to changes in physical appearance (PT, HyperT)	Patient will verbalize acceptance of alteration in body appearance within 2 mo.	Allow time for verbalizing feelings. Assist to identify strengths and positive aspects of self and life. Focus on strengths and positive aspects. Give sincere compliments.
Sexual dysfunction related to decreased libido, amenorrhea, or impotence (PT, HyperT)	Patient will acknowledge need for patience until therapy improves the symptoms.	Help patient understand how therapy might help the problem. Assist patient to recognize and maintain personal worth as an individual. Assist to maintain roles within family or living unit. Help significant others understand patient's illness.

AD, Addison's disease; *CS*, Cushing's syndrome; *DI*, diabetes insipidus; *HyperT*, hyperthyroidism; *HypoT*, hypothyroidism; *PT*, pituitary tumors and hypopituitary syndrome.
*Endocrine disorders to which these nursing diagnoses apply are in parentheses.

Continued

Table 36-5   Common Nursing Diagnoses, Goals/Expected Outcomes, and Nursing Interventions for Patients with Endocrine Problems—cont'd

NURSING DIAGNOSIS	GOALS/EXPECTED OUTCOMES	NURSING INTERVENTIONS
Deficient knowledge related to illness and treatment (all endocrine disorders)	Patient will verbalize beginning understanding of concepts taught at end of 2 wk.	Teach patient and significant others about the disease and each aspect of treatment. Provide written instructions regarding medications, their side effects, and what should be reported to the physician. Provide instructions for "sick" days. Alert to signs and symptoms of too much or too little medication. Emphasize the importance of follow-up care. Stress the need for medical-alert tag or bracelet and wallet card.
Imbalanced nutrition: less than body requirements related to anorexia, constipation, increased metabolic rate (PT, HyperT)	Patient will regain and maintain weight within normal limits within 6 mo.	Weigh twice a week. Alter diet as needed to increase fiber and carbohydrate content. Provide small, frequent meals of preferred foods. Provide patient teaching about nutritional requirements.
Fatigue related to weakness, somnolence, lethargy (PT, DI, HypoT, CS)	Patient will verbalize decrease in weakness and fatigue within 1 mo; patient will demonstrate improved energy within 3 mo.	Provide periods of rest. Assist with activities of daily living (ADLs) as needed. Set slower pace for activities. Give patient time to respond to verbal communications. Encourage physical activity to highest level of tolerance.
Risk for injury related to potential increased intracranial pressure (PT), inability to think clearly (HyperT, HypoT), mental and physical sluggishness (HypoT)	Patient will not experience damage from increased intracranial pressure.	Conduct regular checks of neurologic status. Monitor for signs of increased intracranial pressure. Continue hormone replacement therapy as needed to decrease symptoms from tumor or hypofunction.
Readiness for enhanced sleep related to insomnia, hyper-metabolic state (HyperT, CS)	Patient will use relaxation methods to induce sleep.	Assist with rest periods during the day if fatigue is severe. Instruct in relaxation methods to help induce sleep. Provide noise-free, sleep-inducing environment.
Ineffective coping related to emotional lability (HyperT, AD, CS)	Patient will devise plan to cope with mood swings until they resolve.	Encourage verbalization of feelings and concerns. Assure patient that as disease is controlled, moods will be more stable. Help patient identify strengths and focus on them. Teach relaxation techniques to handle stressful times. Explain physiologic causes of changes in mood.
Decreased cardiac output related to fluid depletion (DI, AD), hypometabolic state (HypoT), hypermetabolic state (HyperT)	Patient will be free of signs of heart failure.	Explain to patient how disease process is affecting heart function. Monitor for signs of dysrhythmia and heart failure. Assure that treatment of underlying disease should alleviate heart symptoms.
Risk for infection related to surgical incision (PT, HyperT), anti-inflammatory effect of excess cortisol (CS)	Patient will not develop infection as evidenced by normal temperature, white blood cell (WBC) count within normal range, and absence of visible signs of wound infection.	Maintain strict asepsis for invasive procedures and dressing changes. Monitor temperature, WBC, and subtle signs of infection, as steroids can suppress usual signs. Advise to stay away from individuals who have colds or other infections.
Imbalanced nutrition: more than body requirements related to altered glucose metabolism (CS), hypometabolic state (HypoT)	Patient will regain and maintain weight within normal limits within 3 mo of beginning therapy.	Teach signs and symptoms of hyperglycemia and how to administer ordered insulin; teach regarding correct diet for condition. Assist in designing diet according to food preferences. Teach to balance diet and exercise.

Therefore measures to help the patient decrease stress should be planned. Supplemental hormones, such as corticosteroids, are given in the early morning when such hormones will not interfere with the body's normal release and use of them. General nursing goals for the patient with an endocrine disorder are:

- Prevention of injury
- Maintenance of fluid and electrolyte balance
- Maintenance of hormone balance
- Reduction of stress
- Use of effective coping mechanisms
- Knowledge of self-care
- Tolerance to physical activity
- Promotion of normal bowel function
- Improvement of mental-emotional status
- Integration of body image

■ Implementation

Interventions vary depending on the type of endocrine problem, and are discussed with disorders in Chapters 37 and 38 (see Table 36-5).

■ Evaluation

Evaluation is accomplished by determining whether symptoms are resolving and by laboratory testing to see whether treatment of the endocrine problem is effective. Many of the symptoms of endocrine disorders are subjective, and the nurse must collect reliable data from the patient about symptoms, such as levels of fatigue, feeling cold or hot, and paresthesias. Each patient is questioned about the symptoms and their improvement during the evaluation of care and treatment.

COMMUNITY CARE

Many patients with endocrine disorders are cared for in outpatient settings. Home care nurses often find that the patient with heart disease, neurologic problems, diabetes, or respiratory problems also has a thyroid problem. Careful assessment by the clinic nurse may uncover a developing endocrine problem.

Get Ready for the NCLEX® Examination!

Key Points

- The endocrine system is made up of glands and hormones that regulate metabolism, growth and development, and sexual and reproductive processes.
- The primary regulatory activities of the endocrine system include altering chemical reactions, changing the permeability of the cell membrane, and activating a particular cell mechanism. The secretion of a particular hormone normally depends on the physiologic need for it.
- Any type of dysfunction of the pituitary gland will affect one or more of its numerous hormones, as well as the target organ for that hormone.
- Age-related changes of the endocrine system include decreased size of the pituitary gland, decreased metabolic rate, decreases in some hormone levels, increases in others, and only slight changes in still others.
- Endocrine disorders are caused by an imbalance in the production of hormone or by an alteration in the body's ability to use the hormones produced. Primary endocrine dysfunction consists of either hypersecretion or hyposecretion; secondary endocrine dysfunction occurs from factors outside the gland.
- Endocrine system tests include examination of blood or urine, radiographs, ultrasound, and MRI scans.
- A thyroid panel may be ordered to evaluate thyroid function. Patients with primary hypothyroidism will have low levels of T_3 and T_4 and high levels of thyroid-stimulating hormone (TSH).
- A full physical assessment and history are needed to evaluate the patient with a possible endocrine disorder.
- General goals for the patient with an endocrine disorder include prevention of injury, maintenance of fluid and electrolyte balance, maintenance of hormone balance, reduction of stress, and use of effective coping mechanisms.

Additional Learning Resources

SG Go to your Study Guide for additional learning activities to help you master this chapter content.

evolve Go to your Evolve website (http://evolve.elsevier.com/deWit/ medsurg) for the following FREE learning resources:
- Animations, audio, and video
- Answers and rationales for questions and activities
- Concept Map Creator
- Glossary with pronunciations in English and Spanish
- Interactive Review Questions and Exercises and more!

 Online Resources
- The Hormone Foundation, www.hormone.org
- Common endocrine disorders, www.endocrineweb.com

Review Questions for the NCLEX® Examination

1. The patient is scheduled to have a radioactive iodine uptake (RAIU) thyroid scan. Which statement by the patient indicates a need for additional teaching?

   1. "I am glad I am not pregnant right now, so that I can get this test over with."
   2. "I will remember to save my urine for 24 hours during the test period."
   3. "I hope I can remain calm and still for the test; I'm a little claustrophobic."
   4. "I wanted my little niece to visit me, but I don't want her exposed to the radiation."

2. A patient complains of muscle cramping and twitching. Based on knowledge of the endocrine system, which hormonal deficiency should be evaluated?

   1. Aldosterone
   2. Parathyroid hormone
   3. Estrogen
   4. Melatonin

3. The nurse is taking care of a patient with hyperparathyroidism. Which laboratory results would confirm the diagnosis?

   1. Elevated serum calcium
   2. Increased bone density
   3. Elevated serum phosphate
   4. Increased serum potassium

4. The nurse is caring for several patients who have endocrine problems. For which patient is the nurse most likely to perform a urine dipstick for ketone bodies?

   1. A patient with abnormal thyroid gland activity
   2. A patient with diabetes mellitus
   3. A patient with adrenal cortical insufficiency
   4. A patient with Cushing syndrome

5. A patient is on corticosteroid therapy for an acute exacerbation of a respiratory disease. The initial assessment confirms a nursing diagnosis of *Excess fluid volume*. The underlying etiology for this nursing diagnosis would be:

   1. suppression of normal corticosteroid secretion.
   2. artificial increase in corticosteroids.
   3. increased adrenocorticotropic hormone.
   4. mineralocorticoid insufficiency.

6. The nurse formulates a care plan for a postmenopausal woman who is admitted for hip fracture. Nursing assessments support the nursing diagnosis of Risk for injury. The most likely etiology for the diagnosis would be:

   1. inadequate estrogen secretion.
   2. aldosterone deficiency.
   3. progesterone deficiency.
   4. inadequate parathormone secretion.

7. The older adult can have physiologic increases in circulating antidiuretic hormone (ADH). Based on knowledge of the function of antidiuretic hormone, which condition should the nurse monitor for?

   1. Dehydration
   2. Fluid overload
   3. Increased pulse
   4. Increased urine output

8. A patient is admitted with hyperthyroidism. The initial assessments suggest the nursing diagnosis of Imbalanced nutrition: less than body requirements. An appropriate expected outcome would be:

   1. patient will identify causes of weight loss.
   2. patient will maintain weight.
   3. patient will have a balanced intake and output.
   4. patient will tolerate activities of daily living.

9. The nurse is caring for a patient who had part of the thyroid gland removed. Based on knowledge of anatomy and physiology, which abnormal laboratory value is of particular concern for this patient?

   1. Blood glucose of 150 mg/dL
   2. Serum sodium of 149 mEq/L
   3. Serum calcium of 7 mg/dL
   4. Hemoglobin of 10 g/dL

10. The nurse prepares a patient for a glucose tolerance test. Which instructions must be included? *(Select all that apply.)*

    1. "Eat a balanced diet."
    2. "Maintain a normal level of activity."
    3. "Fast for 24 hours before the test."
    4. "No eating, drinking, or smoking during the test."
    5. "Report dizziness, nervousness, weakness, and confusion."

Critical Thinking Activities

Scenario A

Mrs. Kovash, a 64-year-old widow, comes to the endocrine clinic to be evaluated at the request of her nurse practitioner. She complains that in the past year she has "slowed down" considerably. She states, "I guess I'm just getting old." The nurse practitioner suspects that it may not be simply aging, since Mrs. Kovash has always lived a healthy and active lifestyle.

1. What type of examinations would you expect the health care provider to perform?

2. What would you teach Mrs. Kovash regarding what to expect from the laboratory blood tests?

3. What questions would you ask the patient before tests for evaluation of thyroid function?

Scenario B

The physician tells you that the patient has a new-onset deficiency of antidiuretic hormone. You anticipate that the patient is likely to have dehydration, urinary frequency, constipation, fatigue, and knowledge deficit.

1. Use your knowledge of the endocrine system and explain to the patient why he is dehydrated and constipated.

2. What interventions could you use to address the patient's fatigue?

3. The physician orders intravenous fluid therapy, but the patient is reluctant to get "stuck with a needle." What patient teaching can you provide to help the patient understand the need for this therapy?

Objectives

Theory

1. Give examples of four major problems associated with hyposecretion of pituitary hormones and identify three nursing interventions appropriate for each problem.
2. Outline three nursing interventions appropriate for each problem of hypopituitarism.
3. Plan appropriate nursing assessments and interventions for the patient who might experience complications of a thyroidectomy.
4. Compare and contrast the symptoms of hypoparathyroidism with hyperparathyroidism.
5. Identify six signs and symptoms of adrenocortical insufficiency (Addison's disease).
6. Summarize four major causes of Cushing syndrome.

Clinical Practice

1. From an appropriate list of nursing diagnoses, provide nursing care for a patient with a pituitary disorder.
2. Select appropriate nursing interventions for a patient with adrenal insufficiency.
3. Implement patient teaching for the patient with hypothyroidism.
4. Plan postoperative assessment and nursing care for a patient who has had a hypophysectomy.
5. Evaluate the nursing care of a patient who has had a thyroidectomy.
6. Identify nursing diagnoses and appropriate interventions for a patient with diabetes insipidus.
7. Assist with development of a teaching plan for the patient taking a corticosteroid.

Key Terms

ablation therapy (ăb-LĀ-shŭn THĔR-ă-pē, p. 840)
acromegaly (ăk-rō-MĔG-ă-lē, p. 834)
addisonian crisis (p. 848)
anosmia (ăn-ŎS-mē-ă, p. 835)
apathetic thyrotoxicosis (ă-pă-THĔ-tĭk thī-rō-tŏk-sĭ-KŌ-sĭs, p. 839)
autoimmune thyroiditis (p. 845)
benign pituitary adenoma (bĕ-NĪN pĭ-TŪ-ĭ-tĕr-ē ă-dĕ-NŌ-mă, p. 834)
catecholamines (kăt-ĕ-KŌL-ă-mēnz, p. 847)
Chvostek sign (p. 845)
Cushing syndrome (p. 852)
diabetes insipidus (DI) (p. 835)
diuresis (dī-ŭr-RĒ-sĭs, p. 836)

exophthalmos (ĕk-sŏf-THĂL-mŏs, p. 839)
gigantism (jī-GĂN-tĭzm, p. 834)
Hashimoto's thyroiditis (p. 845)
hyponatremia (hī-pō-nă-TRĒ-mē-ă, p. 838)
hypothyroidism (p. 840)
lability (p. 852)
myxedema coma (p. 845)
Sheehan syndrome (SHĒ-hăn SĬN-drōm, p. 835)
syndrome of inappropriate antidiuretic hormone (SIADH) (p. 837)
tetany (TĔT-ă-nē, p. 841)
thyroid crisis (THĪ-royd krī-sĭs, p. 840)
thyroid storm (TS) (THĪ-royd, p. 843)
Trousseau sign (p. 845)

DISORDERS OF THE PITUITARY GLAND

Many syndromes can occur as a result of a pituitary disorder. Among the more common disorders of the pituitary are:

- Pituitary tumors
- Hypofunction of the pituitary gland
- Diabetes insipidus (DI)
- Syndrome of inappropriate antidiuretic hormone (SIADH) secretion

PITUITARY TUMORS

Tumors of the pituitary gland account for about 10% of all intracranial tumors. Local symptoms are more likely to occur when the tumor is large and creates pressure within the brain. Smaller tumors, as well as the larger ones, can cause various systemic symptoms and endocrine dysfunctions, depending on whether they stimulate or inhibit the secretion of particular hormones.

Etiology and Pathophysiology

A tumor of the pituitary is usually a benign pituitary adenoma. This tumor secretes growth hormone (GH), leading to continued growth of bones and soft tissues. There is increased pressure within the *optic chiasm* (the part of the brain where the optic nerve fibers cross), which, if not relieved, will destroy the optic nerve. It also antagonizes (acts against) the effect of the hormone insulin, resulting in an increase in blood glucose and *glucose intolerance* (see Chapter 38).

Signs and Symptoms

Local symptoms of pituitary adenoma include headache from the pressure of the tumor, and visual disturbance—with possible blindness—from pressure within the optic chiasm. Systemic symptoms may be vague, and progress very slowly. Personality changes, weakness, fatigue, and vague abdominal pain can be present for years before the condition is diagnosed correctly.

The excessive secretion of growth hormone caused by pituitary adenoma results in gigantism in children, leading to excessively tall stature, as the bone growth plates have not yet closed. In adults the result is acromegaly, and the adult's facial features change: the lips thicken, the nose enlarges, and the forehead develops a bulge (Figure 37-1). Also, the adult's hands and feet become enlarged; the first sign may be that the patient's shoes no longer fit. Muscle weakness may occur with acromegaly, and osteoporosis and joint pain are common.

Diagnosis

Diagnosis of a pituitary tumor begins with a complete history and physical examination. Magnetic resonance imaging (MRI) and high-resolution computed tomography (CT) with contrast media may be used to identify, localize, and determine the extent of the tumor. A thorough ophthalmologic examination will be performed to evaluate pressure on the optic chiasm or optic nerves.

Treatment

In some cases the physician may choose to treat the pituitary tumor conservatively with hormone therapy designed to reduce levels of growth hormone. If the tumor continues to grow or presents serious hormonal imbalances, it may be treated surgically or by irradiation. Some specialists prefer to remove the pituitary tumor surgically and then apply radiation to the site to be sure that all tumor cells have been destroyed. *Hypophysectomy*, or removal of the pituitary gland, is the surgical procedure, most often done microsurgically. The usual approach is transsphenoidal via the nose (Figure 37-2).

Nursing Management

After the surgery, the patient is kept in a semi-Fowler's position. The nurse must closely monitor vital signs and the patient's neurologic status. It is important to note and communicate promptly any change in vision, mental status, level of consciousness, or strength. The nurse must also monitor for any complications, such as diabetes insipidus (see p. 835). A nasal drip pad is in place and is changed as needed. Because nasal packing will be in place for 2 to 3 days, the patient must breathe through the mouth. After surgery it is important that the patient not brush his teeth, cough, sneeze, blow

FIGURE 37-1 The progression of acromegaly.

FIGURE 37-2 Transsphenoidal surgical approach for hypophysectomy.

his nose, or bend forward, as these may interfere with the healing process. The nurse assists the patient with mouth rinses and encourages hourly deep-breathing exercises to prevent pulmonary problems.

> **! Safety Alert**
>
> **Coughing**
>
> Coughing after a transsphenoidal hypophysectomy may lead to a cerebrospinal fluid leak.

HYPOFUNCTION OF THE PITUITARY GLAND

Hypofunction of the pituitary gland is a rare disorder characterized by a decrease in the level of one or more of the pituitary hormones.

Etiology and Pathophysiology

The most common cause of pituitary hypofunction is a tumor. Other causes include autoimmune disorders, infections, or destruction of the pituitary. A rare but serious postpartum complication, Sheehan syndrome, involves infarction of the gland secondary to postpartum hemorrhage.

The most common pituitary hormone deficiency involves a decrease in the amount of GH and gonadotropins. This decrease results in metabolic problems and sexual dysfunction. Decrease in GH will lead to short stature in children; in adults it leads to an increase in bone breakdown, resulting in increased bone fragility and risk for osteoporosis. The decrease in gonadotropins may lead to testicular failure in a man and, ultimately, sterility. Ovarian failure, amenorrhea, and infertility occur with decreased gonadotropins in women.

Signs and Symptoms

Signs and symptoms of pituitary hypofunction depend on the cause of pituitary failure and the hormones involved. If the disorder is related to a tumor, the patient may experience headaches, visual changes, anosmia (loss of the sense of smell), or seizures. Other signs and symptoms depend on the hormones decreased, and are outlined in Table 37-1.

Diagnosis

Diagnosis of pituitary gland hypofunction is made by history, physical examination, and diagnostic studies. Laboratory blood tests are performed to measure levels of pituitary hormones. MRI and CT are used to determine the presence or absence of a pituitary tumor.

Treatment and Nursing Management

The mainstay of treatment for hypofunction of the pituitary gland is lifelong replacement of the hormone(s) affected. Somatropin, via subcutaneous injection, is used to replace GH. The patient experiences a feeling of increased energy and well-being, although there are side effects, such as edema, joint pain, and headache. Gonadal hormone therapy is usually offered, including testosterone for men and estrogen/progesterone for women, although associated risks may outweigh the benefits for some patients. If the disorder is caused by a tumor, surgery or radiation for tumor removal is usually performed, followed by hormone therapy.

Nursing management involves recognizing the signs and symptoms of hypofunction of the pituitary. Teach the patient about lifelong hormone replacement therapy, including method and frequency of hormone replacements, side effects, and follow-up.

DIABETES INSIPIDUS

Etiology and Pathophysiology

Diabetes insipidus (DI) is characterized by the production of copious amounts (usually more than 2.5 L/day) of dilute urine. DI results from decreased production of antidiuretic hormone (ADH), which regulates reabsorption of water in the kidney tubules. When ADH is not present in a sufficient amount, the water remains in the tubule and is excreted as urine (Concept Map 37-1). The following are three primary mechanisms of DI:

1. Central DI, associated with brain tumors, head injury, neurosurgery, or central nervous system (CNS) infections
2. Nephrogenic DI, caused by drug therapy (lithium) or kidney disease
3. Dipsogenic DI, caused by excessive water intake (sometimes associated with schizophrenia)

HORMONE DIMINISHED	ASSOCIATED CLINICAL MANIFESTATIONS
Growth hormone (GH)	Decreased muscle mass, reduced strength, pathologic fractures
Follicle-stimulating hormone (FSH), luteinizing hormone (LH)	*Women:* Menstrual irregularities, diminished libido, decreased breast size *Men:* Testicular atrophy, diminished spermatogenesis, loss of libido, impotence, decreased facial hair, decreased muscle mass
Adrenocorticotropic hormone (ACTH), cortisol	Weakness, fatigue, headache, dry/pale skin, diminished axillary and pubic hair, postural hypotension, fasting hypoglycemia, decreased tolerance for stress, susceptibility to infection
Thyroid hormone	Similar to hypothyroidism, although milder: cold intolerance, constipation, fatigue, lethargy, weight gain

Table 37-1 Decreased Hormones in Pituitary Hypofunction and Associated Clinical Manifestations

Adapted from Lewis, S.L., Heitkemper, M.M., Dirksen, S.R., et al. (2011). *Medical-Surgical Nursing: Assessment and Management of Clinical Problems* (8th ed.). St. Louis: Mosby.

Signs and Symptoms

The patient experiences profound diuresis (production of a large amount of urine), often as much as 15 to 20 L in every 24-hour period. Other signs and symptoms include thirst, weakness, and fatigue, often from *nocturia* (urination at night). The patient will exhibit signs of deficient fluid volume, such as tachycardia, hypotension, weight loss, constipation, and poor skin turgor. If untreated, the patient will demonstrate signs of shock and CNS manifestations progressing from irritability to eventual coma, resulting from hypernatremia and severe dehydration.

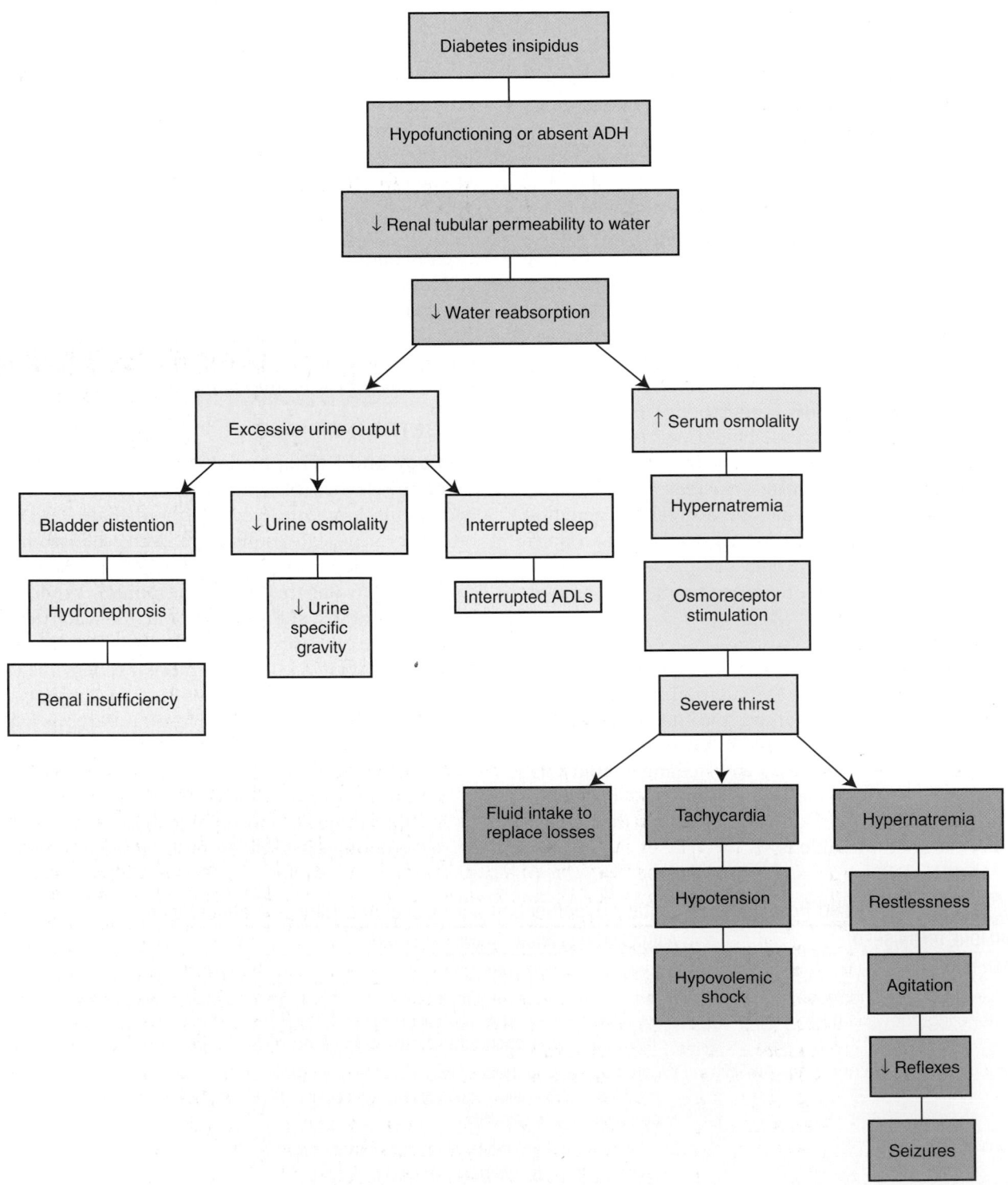

CONCEPT MAP 37-1 Pathophysiology of diabetes insipidus.

Diagnosis

To diagnose DI a complete history is obtained, and a physical examination and laboratory tests are performed, including urine and plasma osmolality, and urine specific gravity. A water deprivation test is done to confirm a suspected case of central DI.

Treatment and Nursing Management

Replacement of fluid and electrolytes, along with hormone therapy, represents the basis of treatment of DI. In central DI, the hormone of choice to replace insufficient ADH is desmopressin acetate (DDAVP), available orally, intravenously, or nasally. Other hormone medication choices exist, such as vasopressin (Pitressin) via nasal inhalation or by injection. For fluid replacement, hypertonic saline is used, titrated to match the patient's urinary output.

Nursing management focuses on early detection, maintenance of fluid and electrolyte balance, and patient education. Baseline vital signs and weight are important to accurately document and monitor throughout therapy. Strict (hourly) intake and output are essential to correct fluid losses and to titrate hypertonic saline infusion.

SYNDROME OF INAPPROPRIATE ANTIDIURETIC HORMONE

Etiology and Pathophysiology

Syndrome of inappropriate antidiuretic hormone (SIADH) is the opposite of DI. Excessive amounts of ADH are produced, resulting in fluid retention (Concept Map 37-2). Numerous factors can cause SIADH, including malignancies and tumors pressing on the pituitary.

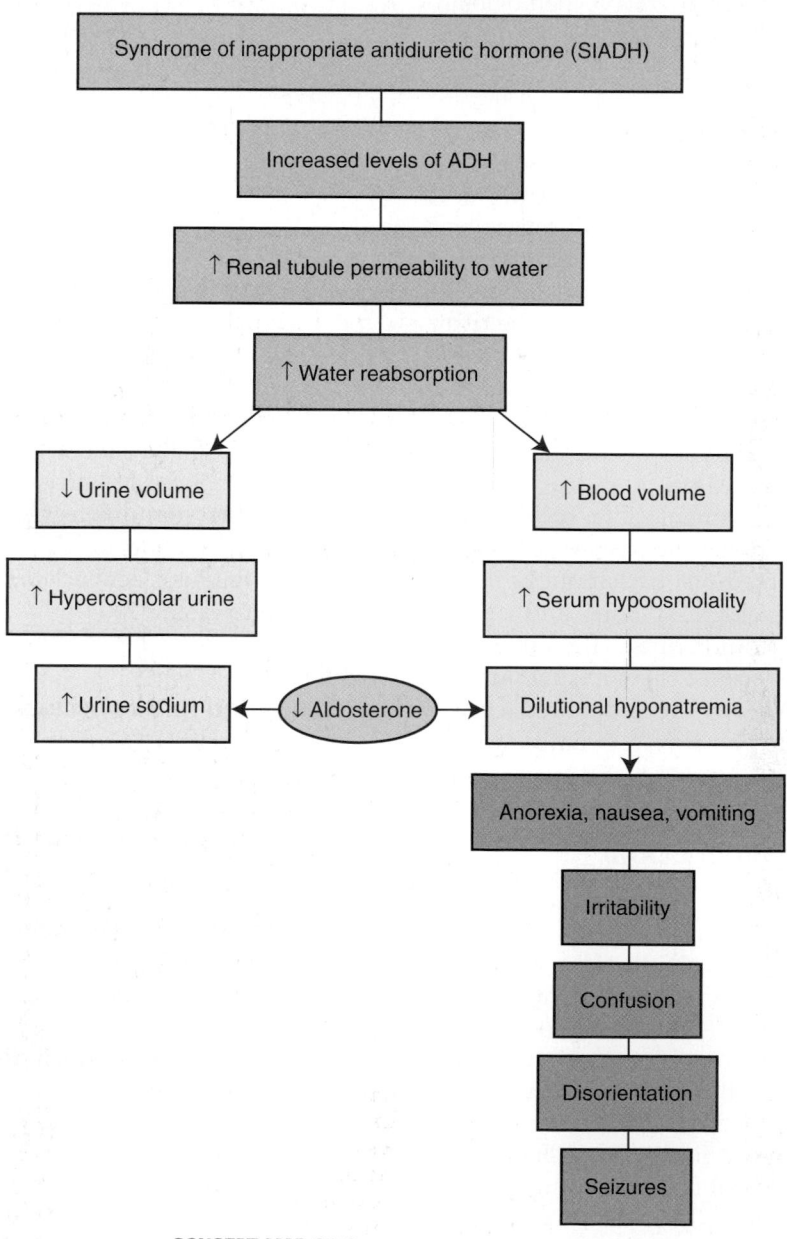

CONCEPT MAP 37-2 Pathophysiology of SIADH.

Signs and Symptoms

Signs and symptoms of SIADH include confusion, seizure, and loss of consciousness accompanied by weight gain and edema. **Hyponatremia** from fluid excess is present with serum sodium often less than 120 mEq/L. As a result of the hyponatremia, the patient will experience muscle cramps and weakness. Urine output will be diminished.

Diagnosis

SIADH is diagnosed by performing urine and serum osmolality tests simultaneously. Results will demonstrate a decreased serum osmolality (less than 280 mOsm/kg) and elevated urine osmolality (more than 100 mmol/kg), which indicates the inappropriate excretion of concentrated urine in the presence of a dilute serum. Other laboratory tests to support the diagnosis include a decrease in blood urea nitrogen (BUN), hemoglobin, hematocrit, and creatinine clearance, and elevated urine sodium.

Treatment and Nursing Management

Treatment of SIADH is aimed at correcting the underlying cause, restricting fluids to 500 to 1000 mL/day, and administering sodium chloride, diuretics, and demeclocycline (a tetracycline) to increase excretion of water. In 2009 the U.S. Food and Drug Administration (FDA) approved tolvaptan (Samsca) for the treatment of hyponatremia in SIADH. Tolvaptan improves serum sodium levels within 8 hours; however, there is a danger of overcorrection and sodium levels need to be closely monitored. Hypertonic enemas may be prescribed to draw out excess water.

Thorough nursing assessment/data collection is essential to monitor treatment and prevent complications of SIADH. The nurse must closely focus on the cardiovascular and neurologic systems and remain alert to the possibility of fluid shifts. The nurse must promptly notify the physician of any change in level of consciousness. Electrolytes are monitored closely (as often as several times per day), and daily weights are measured.

DISORDERS OF THE THYROID GLAND

Abnormalities in thyroid gland activity and resultant changes in the levels of thyroid hormones are among the most common disorders affecting the endocrine system. The thyroid gland secretes the hormones thyroxine (T_4), triiodothyronine (T_3), and thyrocalcitonin (see Chapter 36). The secretion of thyroid hormones is regulated by the hypothalamic-pituitary-thyroid control system (Concept Map 37-3). In other words, all three organs are involved in the closed-loop negative feedback system. Internal conditions, such as low thyroid and norepinephrine (NE) serum levels, can activate the hypothalamus, as can external conditions,

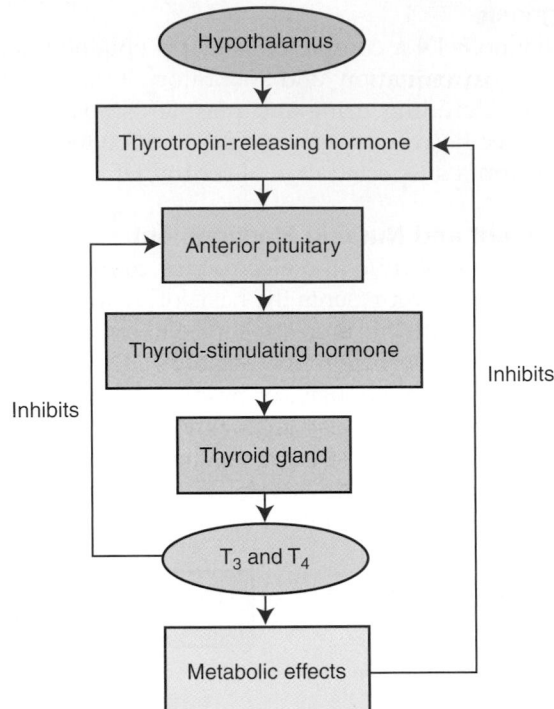

CONCEPT MAP 37-3 Regulation of thyroid hormone secretion by negative feedback control.

such as cold. In response to feedback received by the hypothalamus, thyrotropin-releasing hormone (TRH) is secreted. TRH acts on the pituitary gland, bringing about its release of thyroid-stimulating hormone (TSH). The TSH then acts on the thyroid cells, causing them to release thyroid hormones. When sufficient heat has been produced by increased metabolic activities (if cold was the stimulus), or when there are sufficient levels of thyroid hormone in the body fluids (if a deficit was the stimulus), feedback to the hypothalamus causes it to stop releasing TRH.

GOITER

Etiology and Pathophysiology

The person with a goiter has a greatly enlarged thyroid gland (Figure 37-3). The serum levels of the thyroid hormones may or may not be within normal limits. One type of goiter is caused by a deficiency of iodine in the diet. Iodine deficiency can be prevented by increasing iodine intake—for example, by using iodized salt. Although the administration of iodine will not cure goiter, it will stop the continued enlargement of the gland.

Signs, Symptoms, and Diagnosis

Because there may be no systemic symptoms or changes in the metabolic rate of a person with simple goiter, the first sign that is usually noticed is an enlargement in the front of the neck. Later, if the gland continues to grow bigger, it presses against the esophagus and causes some difficulty in swallowing. The

FIGURE 37-3 Goiter.

goiter also can press against the trachea and interfere with normal breathing. The diagnosis of goiter is established by history and physical examination. Goiter can be associated with increased, normal, or decreased hormone production.

Treatment

If goiter resulting from iodine deficiency is treated early, the growth of the gland can be arrested, and in some cases the enlargement will eventually disappear. Medications prescribed include preparations containing elemental iodine (the iodide ion). A very large goiter that continues to grow and produces local symptoms of pressure—or one that presents the possibility of developing into a malignant growth or a toxic goiter—is surgically removed in a procedure similar to the one sometimes done for hyperthyroidism.

Nursing Management

Iodine preparations should be given well diluted and administered through a straw, as they can stain the teeth. Adverse effects of iodine preparations can include gastrointestinal upset, metallic taste, skin rashes, allergic reactions, and epigastric pain.

HYPERTHYROIDISM

Etiology and Pathophysiology

Patients at greatest risk for hyperthyroidism are adult women between 30 and 50 years of age. *Primary* hyperthyroidism is the result of an abnormality of function involving the thyroid gland itself, and causes excessive circulation of thyroid T_4 and T_3 hormones. However, it is possible that only the T_3 level will be above normal if the patient has Graves' disease, toxic adenoma of the thyroid, or toxic nodular goiter.

High serum levels of T_4 can be caused by either overactivity of the thyroid gland or by excessive doses of T_4 given in replacement therapy. Primary hyperthyroidism is more common in women 30 to 50 years of

age. *Secondary* hyperthyroidism usually is the result of an abnormality in another gland, such as the pituitary gland, that could produce too much TSH and therefore overstimulate the thyroid gland.

Primary hyperthyroidism is also known as Graves' disease or toxic goiter. Medications containing iodine, such as amiodarone (an antidysrhythmic heart medication) can predispose to hyperthyroidism. In addition, it has been discovered recently that women who smoke have nearly twice the risk of developing hyperthyroidism when compared with nonsmokers.

Signs and Symptoms

The earliest symptoms of hyperthyroidism may be weight loss (in spite of a good appetite) and nervousness. Symptoms can vary from mild to severe, and may include weakness, insomnia, tremulousness, agitation, tachycardia, palpitations, exertional dyspnea, ankle edema, difficulty concentrating, diarrhea, increased thirst and urination, decreased libido, scanty menstruation, and infertility. The condition sometimes is not diagnosed in its early stages because of the vagueness of the symptoms. In some cases hyperthyroidism is misdiagnosed as a cardiovascular disease, as symptoms are similar.

 Elder Care Points

The older adult with hyperthyroidism may exhibit milder signs and symptoms or he may exhibit an *atypical presentation,* such as shortness of breath, palpitations, or chest pain. In the older adult, **apathetic thyrotoxicosis,** or simply fatigue and slowing down, can be the only presentation.

If hyperthyroidism is not diagnosed correctly and continues untreated for any length of time, the patient can develop true organic heart disease and may experience myocardial infarction.

The symptoms manifested by a hyperthyroid patient are the result of an accelerated metabolic rate and a speeding up of all physiologic processes. Emotional upheaval occurs as a result of the action of thyroid hormones on the nervous system. The patient often reports episodes of emotional extremes with uncontrollable crying and depression followed by intense physical activity and euphoria. The patient with hyperthyroidism also exhibits an enlarged thyroid gland (toxic goiter) and abnormal protrusion of the eyeballs, or **exophthalmos** (Figure 37-4).

Diagnosis

Medical diagnosis is based on clinical manifestations of hyperthyroidism and the results of laboratory tests for thyroid hormone levels. One indicator of hyperthyroidism is assessment of the heart rate while the patient is sleeping. A rate that is consistently above 80 could signify a toxic state resulting from excessive levels of

FIGURE 37-4 Exophthalmos of Graves' disease.

therapy with radioactive iodine alone, the patient will require adjunctive therapy in the form of potassium iodide and antithyroid drugs.

Antithyroid drugs are prescribed as the initial treatment of hyperthyroidism in children, young adults, and pregnant women. Methimazole (Tapazole) is the main drug used. The patient must take the antithyroid drug at the prescribed time and strictly according to schedule. Iodine preparations such as propylthiouracil (PTU) and potassium iodide (SSKI) have only a temporary effect.

! Safety Alert

PTU Can Cause Liver Failure

In 2009 the FDA issued a safety alert for PTU. Patients should be closely monitored for liver failure, especially for the first 6 months after starting therapy. PTU is not a first-line drug and is used only for patients with allergy or intolerance to methimazole (Osterwell, 2009).

Iodine preparations also may be given for a period of 10 to 14 days before surgery of the thyroid to reduce the vascularity of the gland, minimizing the danger of releasing large amounts of thyroid hormone into the bloodstream during surgery, and to decrease the risk of hemorrhage.

THYROIDECTOMY

Patients who do not respond well to antithyroid drug therapy, who are unable to take radioactive iodine, or who have greatly enlarged thyroid glands are candidates for a subtotal thyroidectomy. Patients with thyroid malignancy undergo a total thyroidectomy. In the subtotal procedure, two thirds of the glandular mass is removed. The remaining portion of the gland is left intact so production and release of thyroid hormones can continue. For most patients, however, surgery is a treatment of last resort, as the potential complications of hemorrhage, hypoparathyroidism, and vocal cord paralysis can be emotionally devastating. Many patients will be rendered hypothyroidic because of surgery or radiation therapy that alters thyroid function. It is then necessary to manage their illness with long-term thyroid replacement therapy.

Because many of the signs and symptoms of hyperthyroidism mimic those of cardiac disease, the nurse caring for the older adult must be alert to the possibility that such signs may be indicative of an endocrine, rather than a cardiac, disorder. Physical and mental rest is extremely important, because physical stress and emotional upset can stimulate greater activity in the thyroid gland. Adequate rest is essential to conserve strength, but it is difficult for a person with hyperthyroidism to relax and get sufficient rest.

The diet of the patient with hyperthyroidism should be sufficiently high in calories to meet metabolic

Treatment and Nursing Management

Hyperthyroidism may be treated medically by administering radioactive iodine and antithyroid drugs, mild sedatives, and beta-adrenergic blocking agents to control tremor, temperature elevation, restlessness, and tachycardia. Radioactive iodine (^{131}I), also known as ablation therapy, is the definitive treatment for hyperthyroidism. It is contraindicated in pregnant and nursing women, as it can disable the infant's thyroid gland. The main disadvantage of ablation therapy is the possibility of hypothyroidism (deficient activity of the thyroid gland) caused by "overeffective" treatment. The hypothyroidism can occur immediately after treatment or long after it is completed; thus the patient must have ongoing follow-up.

Dosage depends on the size of the gland and the thyroid's sensitivity to radiation. Patients receiving small doses can be given the drug orally for several doses on an outpatient basis. Larger doses require isolation of the patient for 8 days, which is the *half-life* (the time required for half the nuclei to undergo radioactive decay) of ^{131}I.

Because the iodine circulates in the blood and is excreted by the kidneys, precautions must be taken when handling needles, syringes, and other equipment likely to be contaminated with blood, and bedpans, urinals, and specimen bottles likely to be contaminated by urine.

All patients receiving radioactive iodine must be observed for signs of thyroid crisis resulting from radiation-induced thyroiditis (discussed later). If hyperthyroidism is not controlled within several months of needs. This will vary from person to person, but continued loss of weight is an indication that more high-calorie foods are needed. It may be necessary to refer the patient to a dietitian, who can work out a satisfactory diet that helps maintain normal body weight.

Patients who are being treated medically for hyperthyroidism must understand that they have an illness that requires ongoing medication and frequent monitoring to assess the effectiveness of treatment. Sometimes it is difficult for the patient's family to accept and deal with the emotional outbursts and mood changes that are present when the disease is not under control. Once hormone levels return to the normal range, the mental and physical symptoms should subside.

Nursing interventions for selected problems of patients with hyperthyroidism are summarized in Nursing Care Plan 37-1.

Preoperative Nursing Care

Preoperative care is similar to any major surgery. If the patient appears nervous, tense, and apprehensive, this should be reported to the surgeon. These symptoms may indicate improper control of the thyroid gland and may predispose the patient to the postoperative complication of "thyroid crisis" (see the following section).

Postoperative Nursing Care

The patient is placed in the Fowler's position (sitting upright to at least 90 degrees) to facilitate breathing and reduce swelling of the operative area. The head may be supported with sandbags on either side to relieve tension on the sutures.

The vital signs are checked continuously in the immediate postoperative period, progressing to hourly once the patient is considered to be stable. The patient is watched closely for signs of bleeding and swelling at the operative area. Any rise in temperature, pulse, or respiration rate should be reported immediately, as it may indicate a high level of thyroxine in the bloodstream. External swelling may cause constriction of the bandage around the neck.

Difficulty in swallowing or breathing also should be reported immediately, as it may indicate internal edema and pressure on the esophagus and trachea.

In many hospitals, a tracheostomy set is kept at the bedside of the postoperative thyroidectomy patient in case severe respiratory complications develop. Other symptoms to be reported are persistent hoarseness or loss of the voice, as they may indicate damage to the vocal cords. Tetany (muscular twitching and spasms) and thyroid crisis are other possible complications. These are rare, but when they do occur, the nurse

---

★ **Nursing Care Plan 37-1**   **Care of the Patient with Hyperthyroidism**

Scenario
Mrs. Jackson, age 35, has been having symptoms of hyperthyroidism. She complains of feeling "hot and soaked with perspiration all the time." She is 25 lb underweight, even though she reports a "ravenous" appetite. Her vital signs are P 110, bounding; RR 30 and somewhat irregular; BP 170/90. She had a physical examination at her physician's office and her serum calcium level was 11.5 mg/dL. She was admitted for control of hypercalcemia and for more diagnostic tests. Mrs. Jackson is very apprehensive, agitated, and irritable.

Problem/Nursing Diagnosis
Apprehensive, agitated, and irritable/Anxiety related to excess circulating thyroid hormone as evidenced by nervousness and agitation.

Supporting Assessment Data
Subjective: "I don't understand what is happening to me. I feel so nervous all of the time."
Objective: Wringing her hands, eyes darting around the room, fidgeting in bed.

Goals/Expected Outcomes	Nursing Interventions	Selected Rationale	Evaluation
Patient will verbalize reduction of anxiety and agitation within 3 days of receiving prescribed medication.	Keep environmental stimuli at a minimum.	Excessive stimuli can worsen anxiety and agitation.	Patient exhibits decrease in agitated behavior.
	No visitors other than family as requested by patient. Approach in a calm and unhurried manner.	Calm approach can lessen patient anxiety.	Patient states that she feels "less anxious."
	Provide 30-min rest periods before lunch, in afternoon, and after supper.	Rest can promote sense of calmness.	Took a nap before lunch.
	Administer antianxiety medications as ordered.		Goal met.

BP, blood pressure; *P*, pulse; *RR*, respiratory rate; *T*, temperature.

Continued

Problem/Nursing Diagnosis
Does not understand what is happening/Deficient knowledge related to lack of information about disease and treatment.

Supporting Assessment Data
Subjective: States that she does not know anything about hyperthyroidism or its treatment.

Goals/Expected Outcomes	Nursing Interventions	Selected Rationale	Evaluation
Patient will verbalize basic understanding of disease and treatment before discharge.	Explain disease process; reinforce information about diagnostic tests and what to expect for each one.	Basic information about disease increases compliance and contributes to long-term self-management.	Patient verbalized basic understanding of hyperthyroidism.
	Stress importance of compliance and keeping appointments with physician.	Treatment of hyperthyroidism is lifelong.	Patient verbalized the importance of long-term follow-up.
	Encourage questions and help the patient to make a list. Reinforce options, as explained by the physician, for treatment.	Making lists is a self-management strategy that the patient can continue to use when talking to doctor or others.	Patient verbalized correct rationale for treatment plan, but decided to ask doctor about options. Continue plan.

Problem/Nursing Diagnosis
Considerable weight loss/Imbalanced nutrition: less than body requirements related to increased metabolic rate.

Supporting Assessment Data
Objective: Lost 25 lb over past 6 months, although appetite has increased considerably.

Goals/Expected Outcomes	Nursing Interventions	Selected Rationale	Evaluation
Patient will gain 2 lb/wk when thyroid production is under control.	Weigh weekly; encourage high-calorie between-meal snacks (e.g., peanut better, dried fruits). Increase caloric intake to 3000 calories per day. Try to accommodate food preferences.	Weekly weight is more reflective of true weight trends (daily weight tends to reflect water gains/losses). High-calorie snacks can be helpful in "sneaking in" extra calories.	Patient demonstrated 4-lb weight gain in 10 days but remains less than ideal body weight. Eating peanut butter and wheat toast as a snack. Continue plan.

Problem/Nursing Diagnosis
Potential for heart damage/Risk for injury (cardiac muscle) related to excess circulating thyroid hormone and excess serum calcium.

Supporting Assessment Data
Objective: Thyroid levels: T_3, 230 mg/dL; T_4, 16 mcg/dL; calcium, 16 mg/dL.

Goals/Expected Outcomes	Nursing Interventions	Selected Rationale	Evaluation
Patient will develop no permanent cardiac problems.	Check vital signs q 4 hr.	Increases in pulse and blood pressure may indicate thyrotoxicosis.	Patient's vital signs are BP 130/80, P 85, RR 28, T 100.6° F.
	Assess cardiac function each shift and watch for symptoms of thyrotoxicosis, such as increased pulse, dyspnea, edema, and rising blood pressure; report as needed	Hyperdynamic vital signs can be taxing on the heart and must be monitored closely.	Patient denies dyspnea.
Patient will have controlled thyroid production within 2 wk.	Medicate with calcium channel blocker as ordered; observe for side effects.	Beta-adrenergic–blocking agents decrease sympathetic tone and decrease stimulation of the heart.	No peripheral edema present.
Patient will have normal serum calcium by discharge.	Give medication to decrease calcium levels (diuretic) and monitor electrolyte levels.		Patient's calcium level is 9.0 mg/dL; AM thyroid levels are pending. Continue plan.

Problem/Nursing Diagnosis

Very moody/Ineffective coping related to labile moods.

Supporting Assessment Data

Subjective: States she has been "very moody"; family says that she keeps changing her mind about things.

Goals/Expected Outcomes	Nursing Interventions	Selected Rationale	Evaluation
Patient will return to her baseline emotional stability when thyroid production returns to normal.	Assure her that mood swings are manifestations of her thyroid disorder.	Knowledge that emotional lability is disease related can lower anxiety.	The frequency of emotional episodes has decreased to approximately once per week.
	Help patient to identify signals of mood change and suggest alternative coping strategies.	Early recognition of mood change allows patient to actively control behavior (e.g., feels irritable, so goes to a quiet corner to be alone).	Reports irritation whenever roommate turns on television; has asked the roommate to adjust the sound.
	Establish trusting relationship; be accepting of behavior; spend uninterrupted time with her each shift; display acceptance of her and her behavior.	Acceptance of behavior and spending time with patient increases trust and self-esteem.	Spent 15 min with the patient. She apologized for being "moody." Reassured that this moodiness will pass after the condition is stabilized.

Critical Thinking Questions

1. Considering Mrs. Jackson's nervousness and agitation, how would you proceed to implement a teaching session about her hyperthyroidism?
2. What specific nutritional suggestions might you offer Mrs. Jackson to help her gain weight?

must be alert for the beginning signs and immediately report observations.

Tetany actually results from injury to, or accidental removal of, the parathyroid glands. Parathyroid hormone is important in regulating body calcium and phosphorus levels, and a deficiency of parathyroid hormone produces muscle cramps, twitching of the muscles, and, in some cases, severe convulsions (see Chapter 36). These symptoms represent a medical emergency and must be reported to the physician at once. Treatment consists of intravenous (IV) administration of calcium gluconate during the emergency stage and subsequent maintenance doses of parathyroid hormone to maintain calcium and phosphorus balance in the body.

Thyroid storm (TS), also known as *thyroid crisis* or *thyrotoxicosis*, is another complication following a thyroidectomy. In the postoperative setting, the condition is caused by a sudden increase in the output of thyroxine caused by manipulation of the thyroid as it is being removed. Another cause of TS may be improper reduction of thyroid medication before surgery.

In a patient with hyperthyroidism, TS also can be triggered by other factors unrelated to surgery (Box 37-1); TS can also be caused by a patient with hypothyroidism who consumes an overdose of levothyroxine.

The symptoms of TS are produced by a sudden and extreme elevation of all body processes. The temperature may rise to 106° F (41.1° C) or more, the pulse increases to as much as 200 beats per minute, respirations become rapid, and the patient exhibits marked apprehension and restlessness. Unless the condition is relieved, the patient quickly passes from delirium to coma to death from heart failure.

Assignment Considerations
Changes in Vital Signs

Remind the UAP to report any sudden changes in vital signs (give specific parameters) or behavior (give examples) in the patient with thyroid disorders.

Treatment of thyroid crisis must begin immediately after the first symptoms are noticed, rather than waiting for laboratory confirmation. Measures are taken to reduce the temperature, cardiac drugs are given to slow the heart rate, and sedatives, such as a barbiturate, are given to reduce restlessness and anxiety.

Box 37-1	Common Causes of Thyroid Storm

- Administration of drugs or dyes containing iodine
- Childbirth (immediately postpartum)
- Congestive heart failure
- Diabetic ketoacidosis
- Inadequate hormone replacement
- Infection
- Pulmonary embolism
- Severe emotional distress
- Stroke
- Trauma or surgery

Safety Alert

Reducing Fever During Thyroid Storm

Aspirin should never be given to patients during thyroid storm, because it increases serum levels of T_3 and T_4. Acetaminophen is the safer choice (Holcomb, 2009).

 Think Critically

What specific assessments would you perform on the patient who returned from having a thyroidectomy 4 hours ago?

HYPOTHYROIDISM

Etiology and Pathophysiology

Hypothyroidism (*hypo-* meaning "under") can be caused by inflammation of the thyroid gland (thyroiditis), iodine deficiency, decreased TSH secretion, hypothalamus dysfunction, atrophy of the thyroid gland, or by treatment of hyperthyroidism (*hyper-* meaning "over") that results in destroying too many thyroid cells and a resultant deficit of thyroid hormone. Genetic defects can cause congenital hypothyroidism, called *cretinism.* Cretinism is caused by a severe lack of thyroid hormone during fetal life and infancy and is characterized by growth failure. Underactivity of the thyroid gland can also be caused by a pituitary or hypothalamus dysfunction that causes inadequate stimulation of the thyroid, inducing secondary hypothyroidism.

Signs and Symptoms

Children with hypothyroidism have delayed physical and mental growth and become very sluggish within a few weeks after birth. Adults who have *myxedema* (very low thyroid production) have a decrease in appetite but an increase in weight because of a slow metabolic rate. Other signs are bagginess under the eyes and swelling of the face. There is a tendency for patients with hypothyroidism to be lethargic and to sleep for abnormally long periods during the day and night. The speech may be slurred, and the individual will appear sluggish in both mental and physical activities. Other signs and symptoms of hypothyroidism are cold intolerance, constipation and abdominal distention, flatulence, impaired memory, depression, husky voice, thinning eyebrows, hair loss, brittle nails, easy bruising, fatigue, muscle cramps, numbness and tingling, dry skin, and nonpitting edema. Gastrointestinal symptoms are the result of decreased peristaltic activity and can lead to paralytic ileus if untreated.

 Elder Care Points

Elderly patients who exhibit lethargy, slow thought processes, and lack of enthusiasm could be demonstrating signs of hypothyroidism rather than a brain disorder such as dementia. Hypothyroidism is particularly common in older women.

Diagnosis and Treatment

Medical diagnosis is based on clinical signs and symptoms and laboratory testing of serum levels of thyroid hormones and TSH. Hypothyroidism can be treated effectively with replacement of thyroid hormones. The dosage is gradually increased until a proper level has been reached, and then a delicate balance must be maintained so that the patient does not suffer from either hypothyroidism or hyperthyroidism. The results of treatment of hypothyroidism are striking, and most patients show a remarkable abatement of their symptoms. The nurse may not see many cases of hypothyroidism in the hospital because treatment usually does not require hospitalization.

Nursing Management

These patients have very rough and dry skin, and they will need massage with lotions and creams to prevent cracking and peeling of the skin. Provisions for extra warmth must also be made for those who have an increased sensitivity to cold. It is important that the patient receive thyroid medication every day.

 Patient Teaching

Self-Care Management of Hypothyroidism

- Take levothyroxine on an empty stomach, as many medications and foods, especially those rich in iron, fiber, calcium, or soy, will interfere with absorption.
- Take levothyroxine at the same time each day; morning is usually recommended.
- It may take 6 to 8 weeks to feel benefit or improvement of symptoms.
- Levothyroxine is lifelong therapy; it should never be stopped by anyone except the practitioner who prescribed it.
- Contact your health care provider if you experience unusual bleeding, bruising, chest pain, palpitations, sweating, nervousness, or shortness of breath.
- Report signs and symptoms of myxedema coma (i.e., dizziness, respiratory distress, low blood sugar, or hypothermia) and hyperthyroidism (i.e., weakness, palpitation, agitation, increased urination, thirst, diarrhea, insomnia).

 Safety Alert

Thyroid Medications

In accordance with the Joint Commission's National Patient Safety Goals, nurses should increase awareness of look-alike, sound-alike products and help patients to recognize the exact name and purpose of their medications. Thyroid medications should not be changed by the patient to the cheapest generic brand, as even slight variations in the level of hormone can be dangerous. Prescription should be labeled "NO substitutions."

The nurse must avoid rushing these patients or giving them the impression of being annoyed by their sluggishness. Forgetfulness, inability to express oneself verbally, and physical inertia are mannerisms that are a direct result of the thyroid deficiency, and the nurse must recognize them as unavoidable as long as the condition is uncontrolled.

MYXEDEMA COMA

Although rare, myxedema coma is life threatening. It can be precipitated by abrupt withdrawal of thyroid therapy, acute illness, anesthesia, use of sedatives or narcotics, surgery, or hypothermia in the hypothyroid patient. Signs and symptoms are loss of consciousness along with hypotension, hypothermia, respiratory failure, hyponatremia, and hypoglycemia. Treatment is administration of levothyroxine sodium IV, fluid replacement, maintenance of an airway and respiration, IV glucose administration, corticosteroids, and provision of warmth.

THYROIDITIS
Etiology and Pathophysiology

Thyroiditis is an inflammation of the thyroid gland. There are three types: acute, such as infection related; subacute, for example, related to upper respiratory viral infection; or chronic, the most common type. Autoimmune thyroiditis, also known as Hashimoto's thyroiditis, is a chronic form that usually affects women between 30 and 50 years of age. Here the body produces antibodies against the thyroid, which in turn destroy the gland. The reasons behind autoimmune thyroiditis are not fully understood; however, there seems to be a genetic predisposition, and it is more prevalent in people with other autoimmune disorders, such as rheumatoid arthritis.

Signs, Symptoms, and Diagnosis

The patient will experience a painless enlargement of the thyroid gland and may have dysphagia caused by the inflammation. Diagnosis is based on laboratory tests, including serum thyroid hormone levels, TSH levels, and radioactive iodine uptake. Needle biopsy of the gland may be performed.

Treatment and Nursing Management

The treatment is thyroid hormone to prevent hypothyroidism and suppress TSH secretion. Thyroid function in this disorder is usually normal or low, rather than increased (as in acute thyroiditis). Left untreated, eventually hypothyroidism will develop. The goal of therapy is to decrease the size of the thyroid and prevent hypothyroidism. Surgery to remove part of the gland may be considered. Nursing management focuses on patient teaching and providing for comfort.

THYROID CANCER
Etiology and Pathophysiology

The incidence of thyroid cancer has become more common in recent years. The most common form of thyroid cancer is papillary carcinoma, which occurs most often in younger women. This cancer is characterized by a slowly growing tumor that can be present for years before it is diagnosed. The cause of thyroid cancer is unknown.

 Cultural Considerations

Thyroid Cancer and Equal Access Health Care

In a study of 4625 patients, Brown and colleagues (2010) found that in an equal access health care system, black and white patients have similar thyroid cancer presentation, similar treatment, and similar survival rates.

Signs and Symptoms

The first sign of thyroid cancer may be a nodule found on a routine physical examination. Only 5% to 10% of nodules are found to be cancerous. Other signs and symptoms of thyroid cancer, such as fatigue, depression, and weight changes, can be easily missed or attributed to other causes.

Diagnosis

The diagnosis of thyroid cancer is made by examination and diagnostic tests. An ultrasound examination is used to assess thyroid size and to locate any nodules. Iodine uptake studies may be used to check for nodules also. *Fine-needle aspiration* is the definitive test, in which a specimen of tissue is taken and analyzed.

Treatment and Nursing Management

The treatment for thyroid cancer is thyroidectomy. In some cases, radioactive iodine (ablation) therapy may be used in lieu of surgery to disable the gland (see p. 838). In 2011, the FDA approved vandetanib, which inhibits tumor growth in symptomatic medullary thyroid cancer (Khatta, 2011).

DISORDERS OF THE PARATHYROID GLANDS

HYPOPARATHYROIDISM
Etiology and Pathophysiology

Hypoparathyroidism is most often caused by atrophy or traumatic injury to the parathyroid glands. **This can occur as a result of accidental removal or destruction of parathyroid tissue during a thyroidectomy,** irradiation of the thyroids, neck trauma, or from idiopathic (having no known cause) atrophy of the glands. A deficiency of parathormone will result in a drop in serum calcium levels and an increase in phosphorus levels.

Signs and Symptoms

Signs and symptoms of hypocalcemia include mild tingling, numbness, muscle cramps, and mental changes, such as irritability. Chvostek sign manifests as muscle irritability when the facial nerve is gently tapped. Trousseau sign manifests as a carpal spasm, elicited by inflating a blood pressure cuff above the systolic blood pressure. Tetany is a serious sign resulting from a lowered serum calcium level. In tetany, muscular twitching and spasms occur because of extreme irritability of neuromuscular tissue. If calcium levels continue to fall, the patient will suffer from convulsions, cardiac dysrhythmias, and spasms of the larynx.

Diagnosis

Medical diagnosis of hypoparathyroidism is established by clinical signs and laboratory data. An electroencephalogram (EEG) may demonstrate abnormalities which return to normal when the calcium level is corrected. A CT scan may reveal brain calcifications if the hypocalcemia is chronic. Changes in bone integrity may be seen on radiograph. Other laboratory tests that confirm the diagnosis include serum calcium, phosphate, magnesium, vitamin D, parathyroid hormone assay, and urine cyclic adenosine monophosphate (cAMP).

Treatment and Nursing Management

Acute hypoparathyroidism with tetany is treated with IV calcium gluconate to raise serum calcium levels to normal range. Oral or parenteral administration of calcium salts is used in the acute phase. In chronic hypoparathyroidism, treatment is aimed at restoring and maintaining normal calcium levels in the blood. This can be accomplished by parathormone replacement therapy, administration of vitamin D in massive doses to enhance absorption of calcium from the small intestine, and oral administration of calcium salts. Nursing care revolves around electrolyte replacement and patient teaching. The nurse must remind the patient that therapy for hypoparathyroidism is lifelong, and advise the patient to wear a medical-alert bracelet.

Nutrition Considerations

Dairy Products Are High in Phosphorus

The nurse should teach the patient with hypoparathyroidism to eat foods high in calcium but low in phosphorus. Milk, yogurt, and processed cheeses are high in phosphorus; therefore are not advised.

Box 37-2	Causes of Hyperparathyroidism

- Parathyroid tumor (benign or malignant)
- Congenital enlargement
- Neck trauma or irradiation
- Vitamin D deficiency
- Chronic renal failure with hypocalcemia
- Lung, kidney, or GI tract cancers

Adapted from Ignatavicius, D.D. & Workman, M.L. (2010). *Medical-Surgical Nursing: Critical Thinking for Collaborative Care* (6th ed.). Philadelphia: Saunders.

HYPERPARATHYROIDISM (VON RECKLINGHAUSEN'S DISEASE)

Etiology and Pathophysiology

Hyperparathyroidism is a common endocrine disorder that occurs most often in postmenopausal women. Excessive synthesis and secretion of parathormone can occur, most often as a result of benign enlargement of the parathyroid glands (adenoma) or hyperplasia of two or more glands. Hypercalcemia (calcium level above 10.5 mg/dL) occurs with hyperactivity of the parathyroid glands. Other causes of hyperparathyroidism are outlined in Box 37-2.

Signs and Symptoms

More than 50% of patients with hyperparathyroidism are asymptomatic (Ferri, 2010). Signs and symptoms of hyperparathyroidism may be mild or severe and include dehydration, confusion, lethargy, arrhythmias, anorexia, nausea, vomiting, weight loss, constipation, thirst, frequent urination, and hypertension. If hypercalcemia exists, there may be skeletal changes, including thinning of the bone and bone cysts. A bone fracture often causes the patient to seek medical attention. The signs of hypercalcemia are manifested in virtually every major system in the body. Hyperparathyroidism and hypoparathyroidism are compared in Table 37-2.

Diagnosis

Laboratory testing for persistent elevated serum calcium and low phosphate levels helps confirm the diagnosis. Serum parathyroid hormone is the best test for the initial confirmation. Serum albumin is also measured because serum calcium needs to be corrected for low albumin levels. Dual-energy x-ray absorptiometry (DEXA) to evaluate osteopenia or a bone survey for bone resorption may also be ordered (see Table 32-2).

Table 37-2	Comparison of Hyperparathyroidism and Hypoparathyroidism	
	HYPERPARATHYROIDISM	**HYPOPARATHYROIDISM**
Serum calcium levels	Increased	Decreased
Serum phosphate levels	Decreased	Increased
Bone resorption	Increased	Decreased
Calcium and phosphate in urine	Increased	Decreased
Neuromuscular irritability	Decreased	Increased (may progress to tetany)

Treatment

The treatment of hyperparathyroidism will depend on the severity of the symptoms produced by hypercalcemia and hypophosphatemia. Infusions of isotonic sodium chloride and administration of diuretic agents promotes excretion of excess calcium in the urine; phosphate therapy is given to correct the deficit; administration of mithramycin binds calcium and enhances secretion from the body; and administration of calcitonin decreases the rate of skeletal calcium release.

 Safety Alert

Caution with Diuretics

Thiazide diuretics should not be used for patients with hyperparathyroidism, because they potentiate hypercalcemia (Ferri, 2010).

Surgical removal of a major portion of the parathyroids (subtotal parathyroidectomy) is recommended for patients who have severe systemic disorders associated with excessively high levels of parathormone. In a large cohort study, patients who had this surgery had a lower incidence of fractures and gastric ulcers compared to patients who did not have surgery (Ferri, 2010). The remaining parathyroid tissue will continue to function and prevent the problem of hypoparathyroidism.

Nursing Management

Nursing management for patients on diuretic therapy includes accurate measuring of intake and output (every 2 to 4 hours), daily weight, monitoring of serum electrolytes, ongoing assessment for electrolyte imbalance, and appropriate nursing intervention. The patient may be placed on continuous cardiac monitoring, depending on the degree of the electrolyte imbalances.

DISORDERS OF THE ADRENAL GLANDS

PHEOCHROMOCYTOMA

Etiology and Pathophysiology

Pheochromocytoma is a rare tumor of the adrenal medulla that secretes catecholamines (epinephrine and norepinephrine). It often causes severe hypertension and if left untreated it can lead to death.

Signs, Symptoms, and Diagnosis

Signs and symptoms of pheochromocytoma are related to excess catecholamine release. Signs include tachycardia and severe hypertension (as high as 250/150 mm Hg) that can be intermittent or persistent. Profuse diaphoresis, severe headache, and palpitations are known as the "classic triad"; however, the classic triad has been challenged, because symptoms do not occur in every case (Cook, 2009).

Pheochromocytoma is diagnosed by measurement of serum catecholamines and 24-hour urine measurement of catecholamine metabolites. CT and MRI may be used to locate the tumor.

Treatment and Nursing Management

Treatment is surgical removal (often laparoscopically) of the tumor (adrenalectomy). Before surgery, the patient may be in hypertensive crisis and require close monitoring of vital signs and administration of antihypertensive medications, such as prazosin (Minipress). The patient should be monitored for signs of orthostatic hypotension related to medication therapy.

ADRENOCORTICAL INSUFFICIENCY (ADDISON'S DISEASE)

Etiology and Pathophysiology

Addison's disease is characterized by decreased function of the adrenal cortex resulting in a deficit of all three hormones secreted by the adrenal cortex. The major problems are related to insufficiencies of the mineralocorticoids and the glucocorticoids. The insufficiency of the androgenic hormones can be compensated for by the ovaries and testes.

Insufficient production of the adrenocortical hormones can result from a disorder affecting the adrenal cortex itself (primary insufficiency) or from a disorder affecting the pituitary gland that stimulates adrenal secretion (secondary insufficiency). Disorders causing a primary insufficiency include idiopathic atrophy, inflammation, infection, and nonsecreting tumors of the adrenal cortex. Secondary insufficiency occurs when the pituitary gland fails to secrete adrenocorticotropic hormone (ACTH) because the gland is underfunctioning or was surgically removed (hypophysectomy), because of certain pituitary tumors, or after abrupt withdrawal of steroid therapy.

 Think Critically

What signs and symptoms might you see in a patient who is developing Addison's disease after stopping steroid therapy?

Signs and Symptoms

In the early stages of Addison's disease, the clinical manifestations may be so vague as to be annoying to the patient but not serious enough to consult a physician. Hence it is easily missed or misdiagnosed. Later, as the hormone insufficiency worsens, there are severe symptoms associated with fluid and electrolyte imbalance and hypoglycemia. Considering the functions of the mineralocorticoids, a major problem is depletion of sodium (hyponatremia), which in turn causes depletion of extracellular fluid and potassium retention (hyperkalemia). The patient experiences generalized malaise and muscle weakness, muscle pain, orthostatic hypotension, and vulnerability to cardiac dysrhythmias.

Insufficiency of the glucocorticoids affects blood glucose levels and causes symptoms of hypoglycemia.

There is also decreased secretion of gastrointestinal enzymes, which results in anorexia, nausea and vomiting, flatulence, and diarrhea. These symptoms, as well as anxiety, depression, and loss of mental acuity, are thought to be related to absence of the peaks of cortisol output that normally occur every 24 hours.

Diagnosis

Diagnosis of Addison's disease is made by examining blood and urine electrolytes. An ACTH stimulation test can determine if the problem lies in the adrenal gland or in the pituitary. CT and MRI scans may be used to locate tumor, calcification, or gland enlargement. Abnormal serum electrolyte levels (hyponatremia and hyperkalemia), decreased glucose tolerance, elevated white blood cell count (leukocytosis), and abnormally low levels of free cortisol are among the criteria used to diagnose Addison's disease (Clineguide, 2009).

Treatment

Replacement therapy providing the missing hormones usually brings about a rapid recovery, but the patient must continue taking the hormones as lifelong therapy.

Nursing Management

Nursing management of the patient with Addison's disease includes:

- Intensive care and support during addisonian crisis when the patient is in a critical condition and in danger of death from fluid volume depletion, hypotension and shock, and impairment of cardiac function.
- Prevention of problems related to fatigue and orthostatic hypotension.
- Alleviation of gastrointestinal problems.
- Instruction of self-care.

Two important nursing measures are to provide both regular feedings throughout the day and adequate rest. The patient may feel well in the morning but may become progressively weaker and fatigued as the day goes on. If fasting is necessary for diagnostic studies or surgery, the patient with Addison's disease probably will need IV glucose to avoid developing profound hypoglycemia. Maintenance doses of glucocorticoids are especially important whenever fasting is required.

Gastrointestinal problems bring on the possibility of imbalanced nutrition, less than body requirements, related to anorexia, nausea and vomiting, and diarrhea. Specific fluid and electrolyte imbalances are covered in more depth in Chapter 3. Stress—even relatively mild physical or emotional stress—can quickly bring on an addisonian crisis for a patient with Addison's disease. The patient must avoid undue physical stress whenever possible, and must learn effective coping mechanisms to deal with emotional stress (Nursing Care Plan 37-2).

 Patient Teaching

Managing Addison's Disease

Teach the patient about the signs and symptoms of inadequate or excessive steroid levels, the importance of prompt reporting, and the following points:

- The nature of the illness and what can be done to control it.
- The purpose of each medication and the side effects to be reported.
- The importance of taking the medication every day and of never stopping corticosteroids suddenly; they need to be tapered off slowly.
- Signs and symptoms to report to the physician immediately (worsening weakness, hypotension, confusion, infection).
- The importance of contacting the physician so that medication dosage can be adjusted to combat the effects of stress.
- Diet adjustments to provide food throughout the day and a bedtime snack.
- The importance of following the prescribed diet to avoid gastrointestinal problems.
- Planned rest periods during the day and sufficient sleep at night, as well as avoidance of physical stress.
- The need for a medical-alert tag or bracelet stating Addison's disease and that the patient is on steroid therapy.

 Think Critically

What specific interventions for a patient with Addison's disease would you use to help teach the patient to decrease stress or to cope with stress?

ACUTE ADRENAL INSUFFICIENCY OR ADRENAL CRISIS

The presence of cortisol in the body allows the blood vessels to function properly in response to epinephrine and other catecholamines by constricting. Conditions that decrease the amount of circulating cortisol interfere with the ability of the blood vessels to constrict. Patients with Addison's disease have a decrease or absence of adrenal cortical secretions, primarily cortisol. Since cortisol is released in response to ACTH from the pituitary gland, abnormalities in ACTH release can also cause a reduction in circulating cortisol. Physical stress from the flu or other infection, or from surgery, can send the patient with Addison's disease into addisonian crisis. Another situation that can cause symptoms of acute lack of cortisol results from prescribed treatment. Steroids are given to treat many autoimmune diseases, and the body becomes dependent on this outside source of cortisol. If administration of the medication is stopped abruptly, acute cortisol insufficiency will occur.

Decreased levels of cortisol result in decreased sensitivity of the blood vessels to sympathetic stimulation. It is the sympathetic stimulation that maintains vascular tone. Lack of vascular tone causes vasodilation, producing hypotension. Cortisol helps maintain blood pressure (BP) and cardiovascular function, so the acute lack of it will decrease BP and produce typical signs and symptoms of shock.

Text continued on p. 852

Scenario

Mr. Cox, age 49, is admitted with a tentative diagnosis of adrenocortical insufficiency (Addison's disease). He has recently experienced weight loss, weakness, poor coordination, vomiting, changes in skin coloration, and loss of body hair. During initial assessment, Mr. Cox is found to be very irritable and easily upset by the questions. His vital signs are BP 90/50, P 70 and slightly irregular, RR 16 and deep. He reports that he feels pretty good when he awakens in the morning but quickly becomes tired and his muscles begin to ache. He is concerned about his weight loss and change in appearance and also has noticed that he has been unable to "think straight." Admission laboratory data: blood glucose, 50 mg/dL; sodium, 90 mEq/L; potassium, 5.6 mEq/L; white blood cell count (WBC), 12,000/mm^3.

Problem/Nursing Diagnosis

Hypotensive/Fluid volume deficit related to low sodium.

Supporting Assessment Data

Subjective: Feels very tired, weak, and uncoordinated.
Objective: BP 90/50.

Goals/Expected Outcomes	Nursing Interventions	Selected Rationale	Evaluation
Patient's BP and pulse will be within 10% of his normal baseline.	Obtain vital signs at the beginning of the shift and as required.	Nursing judgment will dictate the frequency of vital signs; unstable patients may need q 15 min.	BP continues between 90/50 and 100/60. Physician notified. Will repeat BP in 1 hr.
	Monitor for signs of dehydration (i.e., thirst, dry mucous membranes).	Subjective and objective signs and symptoms of dehydration may occur before BP drops.	Reports thirst and dry sensation in mouth. Oral care given. Willing to take ice chips with subjective relief.
	Administer IV and oral fluids as ordered.	Fluid replacement will correct hypovolemia	IV infusing at 125 mL/hr. Oral fluid offered, but refused because of nausea; physician contacted for antiemetic order.
	Initiate I&O and track pattern over several days.	I&O should be balanced; however, in a hypovolemic state, output is likely to be less than input as the fluid balance recovers.	Intake for end of shift 1000 mL of IV fluid and 2000 mL of oral fluid; output 1000 mL of urine and 500 mL of emesis.

Problem/Nursing Diagnosis

Hyponatremia and hypoglycemia/Electrolyte imbalance related to insufficient production of mineralocorticoids.

Supporting Assessment Data

Objective: Blood glucose, 50 mg/dL; sodium, 90 mEq/L; potassium, 5.6 mEq/L.
Subjective: Reports fatigue, weakness, mental acuity changes.

Goals/Expected Outcomes	Nursing Interventions	Selected Rationale	Evaluation
Patient will have a stable glucose 70-100 mg/dL.	Observe for signs of hypoglycemia (i.e., shakiness, hunger, mental confusion) and report promptly.	Hypoglycemia can be a warning sign of impending addisonian crisis; brain tissue is very sensitive to low glucose levels.	Patient's blood glucose level is 110 mg/dL.
Patient will have normal serum sodium and potassium within 24 hr.	Check to see that meals are served on time; provide snacks as needed.	Intake of nutritious foods is important to maintain adequate glucose and sodium levels.	Patient knows signs/symptoms of hypoglycemia. No problems noted at this time.
	Monitor serum sodium and potassium. Watch for signs of hyponatremia (i.e., lethargy, muscle cramps or weakness, headache) or hyperkalemia (i.e., weakness, cardiac dysrhythmias).	Identifying problems with electrolytes in the early phase and acting quickly to restore balance prevents complications.	Physician aware of admission laboratory values and patient condition. Phone order obtained to start an IV with normal saline at 125 mL/hr. Physician will reevaluate patient within the hour.

Continued

Nursing Care Plan 37-2 | **Care of the Patient with Adrenocortical Insufficiency (Addison's Disease)—cont'd**

Problem/Nursing Diagnosis
Has adrenocortical insufficiency/Risk for infection related to decreased immune state.

Supporting Assessment Data
Objective: WBC, 12,000/mm^3.

Goals/Expected Outcomes	Nursing Interventions	Selected Rationale	Evaluation
Patient will not develop an infection during hospitalization.	Observe for signs of infection (fever, malaise, elevated WBC).	Identifying the early signs of infection can prevent complications.	WBC continues slightly elevated 12,500/mm^3, temperature 100.2° F (37.8° C). Physician aware.
	Monitor vital signs, lung fields, and venipuncture sites each shift.	Vital signs and lung sounds should be compared to baseline for changes.	BP 95/62, P 74, RR 16; lungs clear to auscultation. IV site intact, no redness, swelling or complaints of discomfort.
	Protect from exposure to infection (i.e., hand hygiene, advise visitors to check with nurse before entering room).	Decreasing opportunities for transmission is one method of controlling infection.	Sign posted on door instructing all persons to wash hands and to see nurse before entering the room.

Problem/Nursing Diagnosis
Difficulty thinking and remembering/Ineffective coping related to excess cortisol and moods swings.

Supporting Assessment Data
Subjective: "Unable to think straight."
Objective: Very irritable and impatient; serum cortisol results pending.

Goals/Expected Outcomes	Nursing Interventions	Selected Rationale	Evaluation
Patient will develop effective coping mechanisms; patient will use relaxation techniques before discharge.	Teach relaxation techniques and supervise practice; work with patient on other ways to decrease stress in daily life.	Effective coping skills are an important determination of how successfully a patient will manage a long-term illness.	Patient practicing relaxation exercise. Verbalized three methods (listening to music, writing in a journal, talking to brother) to decrease stress.
	Help patient to identify sources of stress and set priorities.	Identifying and prioritizing stressors helps patient to make a plan; indicates what type of resources are needed.	Identified job deadlines and financial concerns as major stressors. Decided to call his boss. Financial representative will come to see patient.
	Encourage verbalization of fears and concerns.	Verbalization of fears and concerns can be cathartic; identifies need for psychiatric referral.	Verbalized that chronic disease would "ruin everything." Agrees to talk to a mental health counselor.
	Discuss alterations in body image and changes that can be expected with therapy.	Anticipatory discussions provide time and opportunity to develop coping strategies.	Sees self as an active person who likes sports and social outings; discussed how the disease affects his self-image and ways that he can continue to participate. Continue plan.

Problem/Nursing Diagnosis

Unfamiliar with Addison's disease/Deficient knowledge related to illness, medications, and necessary changes in lifestyle.

Supporting Assessment Data

Subjective: States that he knows nothing about Addison's disease, its diagnosis, or treatment; unfamiliar with corticosteroid therapy.

Goals/Expected Outcomes	Nursing Interventions	Selected Rationale	Evaluation
Patient will verbalize understanding of medications and dosage schedule before discharge.	Answer questions and discuss medication purpose, side effects, and dose.	Medication compliance is key for treating the disease and preventing complications.	Patient verbalized dosing schedule and the basic action of each medication. Wants a repeat teaching session about side effects.
Patient will verbalize plans for obtaining adequate rest before discharge.	Help him develop a balanced schedule that allows for periods of rest, work, social interaction, and recreation.	Once hormone levels are normalized, the patient with Addison's can expect to resume normal activities, as long as rest periods are integrated into the schedule.	Patient described his intention to integrate rest with desired activities.
	Provide written instructions for symptoms of insufficient corticosteroid medication and those of excess medication.	Written instructions increase the retention of vital information. Patient must be able to self-identify and report problems.	Patient verbalized three signs and symptoms of insufficient hormone (weakness, fatigue, diarrhea) or excessive hormone (hunger, thirst, and increased urination).
	Instruct him to report either set of symptoms to the physician promptly so medication can be adjusted.	Patient must know when to contact physician so that problems can be prevented.	States that he is happy to know that medication adjustment can be done to address stress and symptoms before things get out of control.
	Instruct to report periods of extra stress (minor illness, such as a cold, an emotional upset, or unusual physiologic or psychological stress) so that medication can be adjusted.	Patient must be aware that stress will have greater impact on his life because of Addison's disease.	Tells family to help him recognize minor physical or emotional stresses that he may overlook because those things are "part of my normal crazy life."
	Instruct him to wear a form of medical-alert identification with data concerning steroid therapy.	Medical-alert identification provides lifesaving information if he is ever unable to give health history.	States that he is a little embarrassed to wear jewelry that "publically announces my problem," but agrees to seriously consider it.

Critical Thinking Questions

1. In implementing the patient teaching plan for Mr. Cox, when would you perform your patient teaching, and why?
2. Mr. Cox has put together a proposed activity schedule for after he is discharged from the hospital. He lives in a rural community and must go to the post office to get his mail each day. He asks if you would mind looking at the schedule and giving him feedback on it. The schedule reads: *8 AM breakfast, 9 AM walk dog, 10 AM gardening, 11 AM walk to post office/get mail, 12 PM lunch, 1 PM nap, 2 PM watch television, 3 PM daughter over for visit.* What if any suggestions would you give Mr. Cox, and why?

BP, blood pressure; *I&O,* intake and output; *IV,* intravenous; *P,* pulse; *RR,* respiratory rate.

Treatment

The nurse must closely monitor vital signs, blood glucose, and potassium levels. Adrenal crisis requires immediate fluid replacement therapy, in order to prevent irreversible shock. Intravenous hydrocortisone is given along with sodium, fluids, pressors, and dextrose until blood pressure becomes stable. The hydrocortisone is then tapered off slowly. Hyperkalemia must also be addressed with insulin, Kayexalate and loop diuretics, and by monitoring arrhythmias and the patient's intake and output. Hypoglycemia is treated with IV glucose and with glucagon as needed; blood glucose is monitored every hour.

EXCESS ADRENOCORTICAL HORMONE (CUSHING SYNDROME)

Etiology and Pathophysiology

Cushing syndrome is a rare disorder. The symptoms typical of Cushing syndrome are manifestations of excess levels of the hormones from the adrenal cortex. The condition can be caused by:

- Excessive secretion of ACTH by the pituitary, which may result from faulty release of corticotropin-releasing factor (CRF) from the hypothalamus.
- A secreting tumor of the adrenal cortex.
- Ectopic production of ACTH by tumors outside the pituitary, such as lung cancer.
- Iatrogenic Cushing syndrome from prolonged use of steroid therapy.

Signs and Symptoms

Signs and symptoms presented by the patient with Cushing syndrome are caused by excessive levels of this hormone (Figure 37-5). They include painful fatty swellings in the intrascapular space (buffalo hump) and facial area (moon face), an enlarged abdomen with thin extremities, bruising following even minor traumas, impotence, amenorrhea, hypertension, and weakness due to abnormal protein catabolism with loss of muscle mass.

Unusual growth of body hair (hirsutism) can occur in women with Cushing syndrome, and streaked purple markings in the abdominal area can occur due to collections of body fat. Patients with Cushing syndrome who have a familial predisposition to diabetes mellitus frequently develop type 1 diabetes from the anti-insulin, diabetogenic properties of cortisol.

Diagnosis

The diagnosis of Cushing syndrome is established by laboratory findings indicating consistently high levels of free plasma cortisol rather than the usual 24-hour fluctuations. A 24-hour urine test should be performed. If cortisol is elevated, a dexamethasone suppression test should be ordered: for the test, the patient is given a steroid at night, and blood and urine cortisol levels are then measured in the morning.

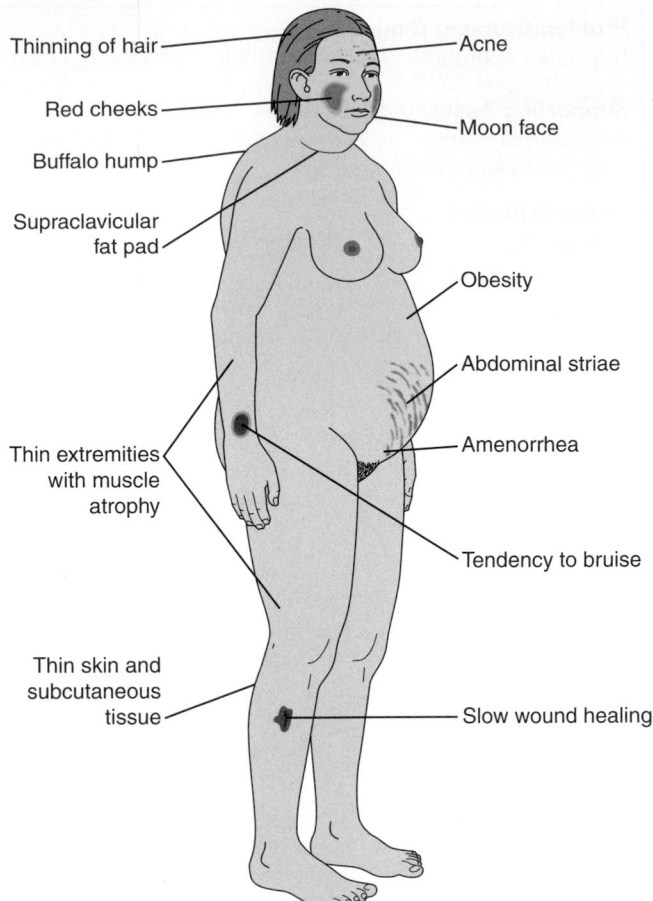

FIGURE 37-5 Common characteristics of Cushing syndrome.

Treatment

Pituitary Cushing syndrome can be treated by microsurgery on the pituitary gland. In some instances the disorder can be prevented by using steroids cautiously. Steroid administration is normally restricted to the Cushing syndrome patient who does not respond to other forms of therapy. If Cushing syndrome is arising from an adrenal tumor, adrenalectomy is indicated. In this instance, replacement of glucocorticoids is necessary (Box 37-3).

Clinical Cues

Secondary Cushing syndrome produced by long-term cortisone therapy is often reversible, if the medication is tapered off and stopped. However, most people taking cortisone are taking it for other health disorders and cannot manage without it. No one should take steroids for a condition other than the specific health disorder for which steroids are prescribed.

Nursing Management

The nursing care of the patient with Cushing syndrome is primarily concerned with helping the patient cope with the many systemic problems presented by the disorder. The nurse must assist the patient with psychosocial concerns presented by emotional lability

Box 37-3 General Nursing Implications for the Administration of Corticosteroids

When giving a corticosteroid drug:
- Question the patient about history of peptic ulcer, glaucoma, cataracts, diabetes, or psychiatric problems (these conditions may contraindicate the use of steroids).
- Take an extensive drug history and seek specific drug information; many medications interact with steroids.
- Take baseline vital signs and particularly note blood pressure before the start of therapy; steroids may elevate the blood pressure.
- Assess for signs of infection before starting the therapy as steroids may mask the signs and symptoms of infection.
- Check dosage very carefully and administer only the amount ordered. Spread topical ointment or cream very sparingly.
- Never stop steroid therapy abruptly; such abrupt withdrawal may cause death in the patient who has been on long-term therapy.
- Advise that increased stress, such as infection or surgery, may cause acute adrenal insufficiency.
- Give a daily dose in the morning.
- When not contraindicated, give a diet low in sodium and high in potassium.
- Give oral doses with food to decrease gastrointestinal irritation.

Regarding possible side/adverse effects of the drug:
- Assess for side effects when patient has been on glucocorticoid therapy for more than 10 days.
- Monitor the older adult for signs of osteoporosis. Give vitamin D and recommend weight-bearing exercise to prevent osteoporosis.
- Assess for changes in muscle strength.
- Watch for signs of depression in patients on high-dose steroid therapy.
- Monitor for signs of hypokalemia, such as nausea, muscle weakness, abdominal distention, and irregular heart rate.
- Monitor blood sugar of diabetic patients closely as glucocorticoids may cause hyperglycemia.
- Check blood pressure regularly during therapy to monitor for hypertension.
- Observe stool for signs of gastrointestinal bleeding.
- Monitor weight, as steroids may cause increased appetite and weight gain.

- Instruct to report slow healing of wounds to the physician.
- Advise patients on long-term steroid therapy that they should have regular checkups for glaucoma and cataracts.

The nurse should teach the patient to:
- Take oral doses in the morning with food.
- Not discontinue the drug abruptly but taper down the dosage before stopping it, and only with the approval of the practitioner who prescribed it.
- Be aware that increased hunger and overconsumption could cause weight gain.
- Watch for signs of hypokalemia, such as muscle weakness, fatigue, anorexia, and irregular heartbeat.
- Take the drug only as prescribed.
- Eat foods such as fresh and dried fruits, juices, potatoes, meats, and nuts that are high in potassium.
- Report signs of Cushing syndrome, such as moon-shaped face, puffy eyelids, edema in the feet, increased bruising, dizziness, bleeding, and menstrual irregularity.
- Carry a medical-alert card and wear a bracelet stating patient is on steroid therapy when on long-term steroids.
- Avoid people with infections and stay away from crowds, especially during cold and flu season.
- Advise all other physicians and dentists about steroid therapy.
- Be aware that more insulin may be needed if diabetic.
- Be aware that antibody response from immunization while taking steroids may be reduced; do not take a live-virus vaccine.
- Use aspirin and other NSAIDs cautiously as they will increase the risk of gastrointestinal bleeding when taken during steroid therapy.
- Be aware that steroids decrease the effect of barbiturates, phenytoin, and rifampin and that the doses of these drugs may need to be increased.
- Have clotting time monitored closely when taking an anticoagulant at the same time as the steroid.
- Be aware that taking steroids along with potassium-wasting diuretics may cause hypokalemia; increase potassium intake in diet.

NSAIDs, nonsteroidal anti-inflammatory drugs.

and by depression, when these occur. The patient needs assurance that the symptoms will improve, with proper treatment.

COMMUNITY CARE

Nurses in long-term care facilities must be on the alert for signs of thyroid dysfunction, especially among their elderly female patients. The nurse often is the one to notice subtle changes in the patient that have occurred over many months.

Nurses can be instrumental in preventing secondary Cushing syndrome by cautioning patients to seek means of treatment other than long-term steroid therapy for arthritis or allergies. The nurse must teach patients receiving a new prescription for steroids that this medication must be tapered, never stopped abruptly.

Get Ready for the NCLEX® Examination!

Key Points

- A pituitary tumor secretes growth hormone and antagonizes the effect of insulin. Treatment consists of hormone therapy or surgery.
- Hypofunction of an endocrine gland typically mandates lifelong hormone therapy.
- Hypofunction of the pituitary gland is characterized by a decrease in pituitary hormones and metabolic and sexual dysfunction.
- DI can occur as a result of decreased production of ADH, and can lead to hypernatremia, dehydration, and coma. Replacement of fluid, electrolytes, and hormones is required.
- In SIADH, excessive amounts of ADH are produced, resulting in fluid retention. Treatment includes correcting the underlying cause, restricting fluids, and administering medications. Monitor the cardiovascular and neurologic systems, electrolytes, and weight.
- Signs and symptoms of hyperthyroidism are the result of an accelerated metabolic rate, although the older adult may have milder or opposite symptoms. Ablation therapy is usually the definitive treatment. Thyroidectomy is a treatment of last resort.
- Hypothyroidism causes a decrease in appetite and an increase in weight. Myxedema coma can be precipitated by abrupt withdrawal of thyroid therapy, acute illness, or other stressors.
- The most common type of thyroiditis is autoimmune or Hashimoto's. Treatment includes thyroid hormones or surgery.
- Thyroid cancer occurs most often in younger women. Treatment includes ablation therapy, thyroidectomy, or both.
- Hypoparathyroidism can occur from removal or destruction of parathyroid tissue. Treatment includes administration of calcium, hormone replacement, and vitamin D.
- Hyperparathyroidism is characterized by excessive synthesis and secretion of parathormone. Therapies include infusions of sodium chloride with diuretics, phosphate, mithramycin, and calcitonin; subtotal parathyroidectomy may be done. Nursing care includes monitoring intake and output (I&O), weight, and electrolytes.
- Pheochromocytoma is a potentially fatal adrenal medulla tumor; treatment is surgical removal of the tumor.
- In Addison's disease, there is decreased function of the adrenal cortex and a deficit of all hormones. Symptoms include severe fluid and electrolyte imbalances and hypoglycemia.
- Cushing syndrome involves excess levels of adrenal cortex hormones; it may be treated surgically.

Additional Learning Resources

SG Go to your Study Guide for additional learning activities to help you master this chapter content.

 Go to your Evolve website (http://evolve.elsevier.com/deWit/medsurg) for the following FREE learning resources:
- Animations, audio, and video
- Answers and rationales for questions and activities
- Concept Map Creator
- Glossary with pronunciations in English and Spanish
- Interactive Review Questions and Exercises and more!

Online Resources
- Pituitary Disorders Education and Support, www.pituitarydisorder.net
- American Thyroid Association, www.thyroid.org
- Cushing's Support and Research Foundation, www.csrf.net
- Cushing's Help Organization, www.cushings-help.com
- National Adrenal Disorders Foundation, www.nadf.us
- MedicAlert Foundation, www.medicalert.org

Review Questions for the NCLEX® Examination

1. A 50-year-old man outputs 15 L of urine within a 24-hour period. He has poor skin turgor with low blood pressure and increased heart rate. The nurse would plan to administer which medication?

   1. Furosemide (Lasix)
   2. Desmopressin acetate (DDAVP)
   3. Regular insulin
   4. Spironolactone (Aldactone)

2. A 45-year-old man has muscle cramps and weakness. He is weak and confused. Serum sodium is 115 mEq/L. The nurse should report the condition and obtain an order to:

   1. give hypertonic enema.
   2. encourage fluid intake.
   3. infuse hypotonic intravenous fluids.
   4. administer vasopressin.

3. A 35-year-old woman reports episodes of emotional extremes with uncontrollable crying and depression followed by intense physical activity and euphoria. She complains of drying of the eyes and difficulty swallowing. Her symptoms confirm a nursing diagnosis of Ineffective coping. What is an etiology for this diagnosis?

   1. Parathyroid hormone deficiency
   2. Excessive thyroid hormone secretion
   3. Deficient estrogen production
   4. Growth hormone deficiency

4. A patient received large doses of radioactive iodine (^{131}I) for hyperthyroidism. Which nursing intervention(s) should be included? *(Select all that apply.)*
   1. Monitor vital signs.
   2. Restrict fluids.
   3. Encourage low-fat, high-fiber diet.
   4. Properly handle contaminated materials.
   5. Encourage physical activity.

5. The nurse is caring for a post-thyroidectomy patient. What should the nurse monitor for? *(Select all that apply.)*
   1. Bleeding and swelling
   2. Hypothermia
   3. Increase in pulse
   4. Difficulty swallowing
   5. Difficulty breathing

6. A post-thyroidectomy patient complains of severe muscle cramping followed by muscle twitching and convulsions. What is an appropriate nursing action?
   1. Prepare for intubation.
   2. Obtain calcium gluconate.
   3. Force fluids.
   4. Administer antibiotics.

7. The nurse is reviewing the medications that each of her patients will receive during the shift. Which patient is likely to receive levothyroxine?
   1. Patient who has von Recklinghausen's disease
   2. Patient who has hypothyroidism
   3. Patient who has hyponatremia
   4. Patient who has Graves' disease

8. A 25-year-old woman complains of amenorrhea with weakness, easy bruising, and painful, fatty swelling on the back. Which assessment question would be most appropriate to ask this patient?
   1. Have you been taking steroid therapy for a prolonged period?
   2. Have you been taking any medications that contain iodine?
   3. Have you been taking lithium for several years?
   4. Have you had a recent pregnancy with postpartum bleeding complications?

9. The nurse provides patient instructions regarding taking iodine preparations. It is important for the nurse to include which instruction(s)? *(Select all that apply.)*
   1. "Dilute the preparations well."
   2. "Use a straw to prevent staining of the teeth."
   3. "Watch for easy bruising."
   4. "Report severe epigastric pain."
   5. "Anticipate a metallic taste."

10. The nurse is caring for a patient with adrenocortical insufficiency (Addison's disease). Which set of laboratory values would be the primary interest for this patient?

1. Serum sodium, white blood cell count, and blood glucose
2. Serum calcium, serum phosphate, and vitamin D level
3. Urine osmolality, plasma osmolality, and urine specific gravity
4. Serum T_4, serum T_3, and thyroid-stimulating hormone

Critical Thinking Activities

Scenario A
Mrs. Timms has a tentative diagnosis of hyperthyroidism. She is 45 years old, 5 feet 7 inches tall, and weighs 102 lb.

1. What subjective and objective signs and symptoms would you expect Mrs. Timms to present during nursing assessment?

2. How would you go about preparing Mrs. Timms for diagnostic laboratory tests for thyroid function?

3. If Mrs. Timms' physician decided to treat her condition with large doses of radioactive iodine, what special nursing care will she require?

4. What other forms of therapy are used to treat hyperthyroidism?

Scenario B
Mr. Lau, age 37, is receiving adrenocorticoid hormones as replacement therapy for Addison's disease.

1. What kinds of problems does insufficiency of the adrenal cortex hormones bring about?

2. What should be included in your instructions to Mr. Lau to help him manage his illness?

Scenario C
Mrs. Josten, age 48, is hospitalized for a cholecystectomy. She has Cushing syndrome, as well as gallbladder disease. She is 35 lb overweight and depressed.

1. What kinds of problems is Mrs. Josten likely to have as a result of her Cushing syndrome?

2. What would be your concerns in the immediate postoperative period?

3. What would you want to include in your discharge teaching plan?

Scenario D
A patient complains of fatigue, constipation, cold intolerance, flatulence, hair loss, and dry skin. You suspect that the patient may have a thyroid problem.

1. What other questions could you ask this patient?

2. What laboratory tests is the physician likely to order and what are the normal values for those tests?

3. The patient is prescribed levothyroxine. What teaching points should you share about the medication?

Objectives

Theory

1. Compare and contrast the two major types of diabetes mellitus.
2. Analyze the four kinds of factors that influence the development of diabetes mellitus.
3. Review the signs and symptoms of an insulin reaction (hypoglycemia) and discuss appropriate nursing interventions.
4. Summarize the acute and long-term complications and results of poorly controlled diabetes mellitus.
5. Identify sources of support and information for people with diabetes and their families.

Clinical Practice

1. Teach a newly diagnosed person with diabetes about the disease, treatment, and self-care.
2. Perform a focused nursing assessment/gather data for the management of type 1 and type 2 diabetes mellitus.
3. Interpret laboratory tests used in the diagnosis and management of diabetes mellitus.
4. Assess for/gather data related to signs and symptoms that might indicate that the patient with diabetes is in early ketoacidosis.
5. Teach a patient how to recognize and self-treat hypoglycemia.

Key Terms

basal insulin (p. 863)
bolus dose (p. 863)
correction dose (p. 863)
diabetic nephropathy (p. 860)
diabetic neuropathy (p. 876)
endogenous (ĕn-DŎJ-ĕn-ŭs, p. 857)
exogenous (ĕks-ŎJ-ĕn-ŭs, p. 857)
gastroparesis (găs-trō-pă-RĒ-sĭs, p. 876)
glucometer (p. 867)
glycemic control (glī-SĒ-mĭk, p. 859)
glycosuria (glī-cōs-Ū-rē-ă, p. 859)

hyperglycemia (hī-pĕr-glī-SĒ-mē-ă, p. 859)
incretin mimetics (p. 866)
insulin resistance (p. 857)
insulin-to-carbohydrate ratios (p. 860)
ketoacidosis (kē-tō-ă-sĭ-DŌ-sĭs, p. 857)
medical nutrition therapy (MNT) (p. 860)
metabolic syndrome (p. 875)
neuroglycopenia (nū-rō-GLĪ-kŏ-PĒ-nē-ă, p. 876)
polydipsia (pŏl-ē-DĬP-sē-ă, p. 859)
polyphagia (pŏl-ē-FĀ-jă, p. 859)
polyuria (pŏl-ē-Ū-rē-ă, p. 859)

DIABETES MELLITUS AND HYPOGLYCEMIA

DIABETES MELLITUS

Diabetes mellitus is a disturbance in metabolism and use of glucose that is secondary to a malfunction of the beta cells of the pancreas. Beta cells are responsible for making insulin. Because insulin is involved in the metabolism of carbohydrates, proteins, and fats, diabetes mellitus is not limited to a disturbance of glucose homeostasis; however, intolerance to glucose is an underlying issue, regardless of the type of diabetes.

Diabetes mellitus, the most common form of diabetes, is a deficiency of the pancreatic hormone insulin, which results in the body's failure to metabolize sugars and starch. Sugars accumulate in the blood and urine, and the by-products of alternative fat metabolism

disturb the acid-base balance of the blood, causing a risk of convulsions and coma.

 Nutrition Considerations

Brown Rice and Whole Grains

In a recent study, Sun and colleagues (2010) found that substituting brown rice and whole grains for white rice was associated with a lower risk for developing diabetes.

Types of Diabetes Mellitus

Nearly 23.6 million Americans (approximately 8% of the population) have diabetes mellitus, and millions more have diabetes and do not know it. The cost of treating diabetes in the United States is approximately $132 billion a year (Luger & Chabanuk, 2009).

Table 38-1   Clinical Categories of Diabetes Mellitus and Characteristics

TYPE (FORMER NAMES)	CHARACTERISTICS
Type 1 (insulin dependent; IDDM; juvenile diabetes; juvenile-onset)	Little or no endogenous insulin produced. New patients can be any age but usually are young. Patient must receive exogenous insulin and follow prescribed diet and exercise program. Renal, cardiovascular, retinal, and neurologic complications likely if disease is not kept under tight control.
Type 2 (non–insulin-dependent; NIDDM; adult-onset diabetes; maturity-onset diabetes)	Rarely develop ketosis; may develop hyperglycemic, hyperosmolar nonketotic syndrome (HHNS). Patients vary in need for exogenous insulin. New patients are usually over 30 and most are obese. Disorder often responds to diet and exercise.
Latent autoimmune diabetes (LADA) (slow onset type 1 diabetes or type 1.5 diabetes; type 1 diabetes, according to the World Health Organization)	Usually not overweight, have no signs of metabolic syndrome, and may have a history of autoimmune disease. Demonstrate rapid failure of oral hypoglycemic drugs. Insulin should be started within 1 year of diagnosis.
Prediabetes (impaired glucose tolerance and impaired fasting glucose)	Glucose levels higher than normal but lower than those with diabetes. Are at high risk for atherosclerotic disease and cardiovascular problems. Progression to diabetes is not inevitable. Weight loss and increased physical activity can delay or prevent diabetes and return blood glucose levels to normal.
Gestational diabetes	Occurs only during pregnancy. After pregnancy, women with gestational diabetes have 20%-50% chance of developing diabetes within 5-10 years.
Statistical risk of diabetes	Those who have had impaired glucose tolerance in the past but have normal glucose tolerance now; prediabetes; latent diabetes; subclinical diabetes. Those who are predisposed to diabetes because of family history, age, race, or obesity.

Table 38-1 summarizes the major characteristics of various forms of diabetes mellitus. Type 1 diabetes—formerly known as insulin-dependent diabetes mellitus (IDDM)—accounts for about 5% to 10% of all cases. Type 1 diabetes occurs when the body's immune system destroys beta cells. There is no known way to prevent type 1 diabetes. Persons who have type 1 diabetes require injections of exogenous (from outside the body) insulin to maintain life, because they produce little or no endogenous (inside the body) insulin on their own. In general, persons with type 1 diabetes are more prone to a serious complication, *ketosis,* associated with an excess production of ketone bodies, leading to ketoacidosis (metabolic acidosis). Moreover, type 1 diabetes is more likely to appear early in life. In fact, type 1 diabetes was formerly called *juvenile diabetes* or *ketosis-prone diabetes* because of its typical early onset and potential for ketoacidosis.

Type 2 diabetes—formerly called non–insulin-dependent diabetes mellitus (NIDDM)—makes up 90% to 95% of all known cases of diabetes. Type 2 diabetes is believed to begin with insulin resistance, which is a situation whereby insulin interaction with glucose becomes less efficient, and therefore fat metabolism is abnormal. As the need for insulin rises, the pancreas gradually loses the ability to produce it. Type 2 diabetes has a tendency to develop later in life than does type 1, and patients with type 2 rarely develop diabetic ketoacidosis. Box 38-1 lists the signs and symptoms of type 1 and type 2 diabetes. Factors associated with development of type 2 diabetes are listed in Box 38-2.

 Cultural Considerations

Ethnicity and Type 2 Diabetes

Although rare, type 2 diabetes is being diagnosed more frequently in children and adolescents, particularly in American Indians, African Americans, and Hispanic/Latino Americans.

Box 38-1   Symptoms of Type 1 and Type 2 Diabetes

TYPE 1
- Very thirsty (polydipsia)
- Frequent urination (polyuria)
- Extremely hungry (polyphagia)
- Rapid loss of weight
- Irritability
- Weakness and fatigue
- Nausea and vomiting

TYPE 2
- May experience polydipsia, polyuria, and polyphagia
- More commonly experience excessive weight gain
- Family history of diabetes mellitus
- Poor healing of scratches, abrasions, and wounds
- Blurred vision
- Itching
- Drowsiness
- Increased fatigue
- Tingling or numbness in the feet

Factors Associated with Development of Type 2 Diabetes

- Older age
- Obesity
- Family history of type 2 diabetes
- History of gestational diabetes
- Impaired glucose metabolism
- Physical inactivity
- Race/ethnicity (African Americans, Hispanic/Latino Americans, American Indians, some Asian Americans, Native Hawaiian/Pacific Islanders)

Data from U.S. Department of Health and Human Services, Centers for Disease Control and Prevention. (2010). *National Diabetes Fact Sheet: General Information and National Estimates on Diabetes in the United States.* Atlanta, Ga.: USDHHS.

Latent autoimmune diabetes (LADA) is a type 1 diabetes, according to the World Health Organization. Other names for this condition are "slow onset type 1 diabetes" or "type 1.5 diabetes." It is believed that the presence of islet cell antibodies in the blood (which are not present in healthy individuals) will eventually destroy the beta cells, and insulin production will cease. Patients with LADA are usually not overweight, have no signs of metabolic syndrome, and may have a history of personal or familial autoimmune disease. The diagnosis is based on three criteria: (1) onset after age 30, (2) islet cell antibodies circulating in the blood, and (3) insulin is not required sooner than 6 months after diagnosis. Patients can be misdiagnosed as type 2 diabetes, and rapid failure of oral hypoglycemic drugs suggests LADA. Evidenced-based management suggests that metformin can be used in the early phase and insulin should be started within 1 year of diagnosis; both may offer some protective effects against the destruction of the beta cells, whereas sulfonylureas may hasten destruction of beta cells and therefore are not recommended (Kapustin, 2008).

Gestational diabetes may occur as a result of the stress of pregnancy. It may be treated with diet, oral hypoglycemia agents, or insulin. After delivery, the condition must be reevaluated; approximately 5% to 10% of women with gestational diabetes go on to be diagnosed with type 2 diabetes after delivery. The baby also carries an increased risk of type 2 diabetes later in life.

Etiology and Pathophysiology

At least four sets of factors influence the development of diabetes mellitus: genetic, metabolic, microbiological, and immunologic. In a recent study funded by the National Institutes of Health (2010) scientists used computer analysis to evaluate 226 environmental factors affecting diabetes. They found that a pesticide derivative (PCB) was strongly associated with developing diabetes, and that the nutrient beta-carotene served a protective role.

Genetic factors are included in the etiology of diabetes because diabetes tends to run in families. It is known that the risk of having some form of diabetes increases in proportion to the number of relatives who are affected, the genetic closeness of the relatives, and the severity of their disease.

Metabolic factors involved in the etiology of diabetes are many and complex. Emotional or physical stress can unmask an inherited predisposition to the disease, probably as a result of glucogenesis induced by increased production of hormones from the adrenal cortex (especially the glucocorticoids). Perhaps even more significant than metabolic factors is the association of type 2 diabetes and obesity. About 80% of type 2 diabetes patients are obese (greater than 20% above their ideal body weight), and there is a higher incidence of type 2 diabetes in persons who lead a sedentary life and eat a high-calorie diet. **With weight reduction and increased physical activity, blood glucose can be restored to normal levels and maintained there—hence the importance of diet and exercise in the management of type 2 diabetes.** In type 2 diabetes there also seems to be a relationship to aging and a reduction in the function of the pancreatic beta cells and how they synthesize insulin.

Think Critically

What is one way in which you or your family members might decrease the risk of type 2 diabetes in later life?

Some forms of type 1 diabetes may be related to the viral destruction of beta cells. There are known cases in which children developed type 1 diabetes after having had a recent viral infection. The mumps or coxsackie virus is thought to be the trigger. Evidence that supports viruses as causative factors include:

- Both type 1 and viral infections tend to have sudden onsets.
- Seasonal fluctuations in the onset of type 1 diabetes—late autumn and early spring—correspond with the times of the year when "flu" and other viral illnesses are most common.
- Viral infections can and often do attack the pancreas; many viral infections are characterized by inflammation of the pancreatic beta cells.

Signs, Symptoms, and Diagnosis

The American Diabetes Association (ADA) recommends screening all adults, especially if overweight, for type 2 diabetes starting at age 45, to be repeated every 3 years: either hemoglobin A_{1c} (A1C or HbA_{1c}), fasting plasma glucose (FPG), or 2-hour 75-g oral glucose tolerance test (OGTT) are appropriate screening methods. The ADA recommends that screening begin at an earlier age, and at more frequent intervals, if the person has one or more risk factors associated with type 2 diabetes (ADA, 2009).

In addition to laboratory tests (see Chapter 36), the health care provider depends on clinical signs and symptoms of diabetes mellitus to establish a diagnosis. The classic symptoms of diabetes mellitus, regardless of type, are related to an elevated blood glucose level, or **hyperglycemia.** Hyperglycemia increases the concentration of the intravascular fluid, raising its osmotic pressure and pulling water from the cells and interstitial fluid into the blood. This causes cellular dehydration and the loss of glucose **(glycosuria),** electrolytes, and water in the urine. Cellular dehydration causes thirst and a resultant increased intake of water **(polydipsia)** and diuresis with increased urination **(polyuria).** Hunger **(polyphagia)** is the result of the body's effort to increase its supply of energy foods, even though the intake of more carbohydrates does not meet the energy needs of the cells.

Clinical Cues

Classic signs and symptoms of diabetes mellitus are polydipsia, polyuria, and polyphagia.

Fatigue and muscular weakness occur because the glucose needed for energy is not metabolized properly. Weight loss in patients with type 1 diabetes occurs for two reasons: (1) the loss of body fluid; and (2) in the absence of sufficient insulin, the body begins to metabolize its own proteins and stored fat. The oxidation of fats is incomplete and fatty acids are converted into ketone bodies: beta-hydroxybutyric acid, acetoacetic acid, and acetone. When the kidney is unable to handle accumulated ketones in the blood, ketosis occurs. The overwhelming presence of the strong organic acids in the blood lowers the pH and leads to a severe and potentially fatal acidosis. The metabolism of body protein when insulin is not available causes an elevated blood urea nitrogen (BUN) level. This is because the nitrogen component of protein is discarded when the body metabolizes its own protein to obtain the glucose it needs.

People with diabetes are prone to infection, delayed healing, and vascular diseases. Poor control of diabetes makes the person prone to develop an infection. The propensity for infection is thought to be partly a result of decreased normal function of leukocytes and abnormal phagocyte function. Another contributing factor to infection and delayed healing probably is decreased blood supply to the tissues because of atherosclerotic changes in the blood vessels. An impaired blood supply means a deficit in the protective cells brought by the blood to a site of injury.

It is believed that the neurologic, vascular, and metabolic complications of diabetes predispose the person to infections by allowing organisms to enter tissues that are normally better defended and less accessible. For example, a neurogenic bladder predisposes the patient to stagnant urine and accumulations of bacteria, and a leg ulcer resulting from peripheral vascular disease is without the protection of the skin as a barrier to organisms.

? Think Critically

If a friend complains of thirst, fatigue, and frequent urination, what questions would you ask? What would you suggest this person do?

Management of Diabetes

There is no cure for diabetes mellitus; the goal is to maintain blood glucose and lipid levels within normal limits and to control these factors to prevent complications. Studies have demonstrated that there are benefits of tight **glycemic control** (control of glucose in the blood) for people with both type 1 and type 2 diabetes. Patients attempting tight control follow an intensive therapy plan of blood glucose testing and insulin injections, three or more times a day, or they use an insulin pump. There are some risks associated with perfect control of blood glucose levels, and "tight control" is not indicated for every patient. The most serious control issue is hypoglycemia, or insulin reaction. In a recent study (Finfer & Delaney, 2008), tight glucose control was associated with increased mortality rate in critically ill patients. American Diabetes Association guidelines now recommend glucose targets of 140 to 180 mg/dL for critical patients. For the noncritically ill, premeal target is 140 mg/dL or less and random readings should be 180 mg/dL or less. The health care provider will adjust these parameters for the individual patient.

Research has demonstrated that lowering A1C levels to 7% is associated with decreased microvascular complications (eye, kidney, and nerve diseases) of diabetes. If the patient is elderly and very frail or if the life expectancy is short, the American Geriatrics Association recommends an A1C of 8% (Lee, 2009).

The protocol for control of diabetes mellitus is highly individualized and depends on the type of diabetes a person has, age, general state of health, ability to follow the prescribed regimen, and acceptance of responsibility for managing illness, along with a host of other factors.

The overall goal of diabetes management is achieved when fasting blood glucose stays within normal limits, A1C tests show that blood glucose has stayed within normal limits from one testing period to the next, the patient's weight is normal, blood lipids remain within normal limits, and the patient has a sense of health and well-being.

Elder Care Points

Older adults experience hypoglycemia more quickly than do younger people, and the elderly are more prone to hypoglycemic episodes. The older adult may progress to dangerously low levels of blood glucose before signs and symptoms are obvious. Severe hypoglycemia in the older adult can precipitate myocardial infarction, angina, stroke, or seizures. For this reason, "tight" control may not be the best thing for the older adult.

Diet. **Diet is the cornerstone of diabetic treatment.** Weight gain is common in persons with type 2 diabetes, because of high caloric intake and decreased availability of endogenous insulin to fully use ingested food. Weight gain can make a patient with type 2 diabetes more insulin resistant. In many cases, people with type 2 diabetes can control their blood glucose by reducing caloric intake and increasing physical exercise. There is no such thing as a "typical" person with diabetes, and because diabetes is an unstable and changing process, each patient's needs will change from time to time. A person can eat the "perfect" breakfast 3 days in a row, which results in a "perfect" postprandial (after-meal) blood glucose value, only to eat the very same breakfast the next day and have a high blood glucose measurement. This can be frustrating for the patient. The strategies that are effective in managing diabetes can be altered by many factors (e.g., stress, illness, activity, health beliefs), and the strategies that are effective for one person with diabetes may not be effective for someone else.

Medical nutrition therapy (MNT) is now recommended for all persons with either type 1 or type 2 diabetes. A registered dietitian (RD) or a certified diabetes educator (CDE) performs an in-depth assessment of type of diabetes, height-to-weight ratio, usual dietary intake, food preferences, exercise level, and daily schedule. A range of interventions are considered when designing a plan that is individualized for the patient. These interventions include: reduced energy and fat intake, carbohydrate counting, simplified meal plans, healthy food choices, individualized meal planning strategies, exchange lists, insulin-to-carbohydrate ratios (adjusting insulin doses to match carbohydrate intake), physical activity, and behavioral strategies (American Dietetic Association, 2009). In general, MNT is geared toward providing adequate nutrition with sufficient calories to maintain normal body weight and control of cholesterol, and to adjust the intake of food so that blood glucose is kept within safe limits.

Meal plans generally include a consistent carbohydrate intake, with 45 to 60 g of carbohydrate per meal (ADA, 2009). If the patient chooses to eat sweets, 10% to 35% of total intake does not have a negative effect, but sweets would count as carbohydrates. Proteins should make up 15% to 20%; for patients with diabetic nephropathy (kidney disease secondary to high blood glucose level), protein intake of 1 g/kg of body weight is recommended. Meals should include 14 g of fiber per 1000 kilocalories, which is the recommendation for the general public. Reduction of saturated fats, *trans* fats, and dietary cholesterol also improves cardiovascular outcomes (American Dietetic Association, 2009).

 Clinical Cues

Emphasis should be placed on the positive aspects of the diet—on the foods allowed rather than those that are forbidden. A patient should not be made to feel guilty about having difficulty staying on the diet or the times when she "cheats" and eats foods that are not allowed.

Cultural preferences must be considered when devising meal plans. One of the most effective means of helping a person with diabetes follow the prescribed diet is by teaching about food values and how they affect diabetes. Initially, three or four teaching sessions performed by the RD or CDE lasting 45 to 90 minutes are recommended, with annual follow-up as a minimum. The ADA and the American Dietetic Association have worked together to devise simplified methods of calculating a diabetic diet and planning meals for a person with diabetes. Organizations such as the ADA and the Joslin Diabetes Center, affiliated with Harvard Medical School, have instructive material (see Online Resources on p. 877).

 Elder Care Points

Weight loss is seldom a goal for the older person with type 2 diabetes unless weight is more than 1½ times normal for height and frame. Older adults are more susceptible to nutritional deficiencies from teeth problems, illness, and decreased appetite. Diet is frequently managed by reducing concentrated sugars and by adhering to a meal schedule.

 Think Critically

How would you obtain accurate data about what your patient with diabetes is eating each day?

Exercise. Physical exercise is an important part of managing diabetes. Muscular activity improves glucose utilization for energy and improves circulation. In addition to lowering blood glucose levels by "burning up" the glucose, exercise makes the insulin receptors on cells more sensitive to the hormone, and thus improves utilization of the available glucose. Because diabetic control also considers blood lipid levels, exercise contributes to that control by reducing triglyceride levels and increasing high-density lipoprotein (HDL) levels.

The exercise program should be designed for the individual patient. The plan should consider the age and overall physical condition of the patient, ability to carry out the exercises regularly, and how well controlled the diabetes is. For some patients a brisk walk of 1 or 2 miles daily is as much exercise as they can tolerate. Others may be able to perform more strenuous exercises, but they must be cautioned against extremes, especially if they are taking insulin. Exercise can rapidly lower blood glucose levels and cause serious hypoglycemia.

All exercise programs should begin with milder forms of exercise and gradually increase until the patient's level of tolerance or the desired therapeutic effect is reached. A program should not be started until the blood glucose is under control. The exercise program should be planned so that the exercises are performed at the same time every day, preferably after a meal, when the blood glucose is highest. Blood glucose should be checked before beginning to exercise. The patient is encouraged to wear a medical-alert bracelet (Figure 38-1) and to exercise with a friend who knows the signs and symptoms of hypoglycemia and how to treat it.

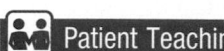

Patient Teaching

Home Treatment for Hypoglycemia

Patients should always have an emergency supply for treating glucose. When signs of hypoglycemia are present and the patient is able to swallow, give one of the following:

- ½ cup of juice
- 1 cup of 2% or skim milk
- ½ cup of regular soda (not sugar-free)
- 6 or 7 hard candies, such as Life Savers (not sugar-free)
- 1 small box of raisins (2 tablespoons)
- Three glucose tablets
- 1 tablespoon of honey
- 1 tablespoon of sugar
- 5 small cubes of sugar
- 1 small tube of cake icing (2 oz)
- 1 small tube of glucose gel
- Follow up with a longer-acting source, such as crackers and cheese or a meat sandwich.

If the patient is unable to swallow (groggy or unconscious):

- Turn the patient onto the side.
- Administer 1 mg of glucagon by injection after mixing the solution in the bottle until it is clear. Call 911 if unable to give injection.
- Feed the patient as soon as she is awake and able to swallow. Give a fast-acting source of sugar (see above list) and a longer-acting source, such as crackers and cheese or a meat sandwich.
- If the patient does not awaken within 15 minutes, give another dose of glucagon and inform a health care provider of the situation immediately.
- If a health care provider cannot be contacted, call 911 or the local emergency service.

FIGURE 38-1 Medical-alert bracelets.

Clinical Cues

Patients should be advised to check with their health care provider before starting an exercise program. Certain activities may be ill advised if there are complications. For example, patients with neuropathy, retinopathy, or renal insufficiency may be unable to safely balance, see, or perform rigorous or strenuous activities.

Elder Care Points

Physical limitations may discourage older adults with diabetes from exercising. The older patient with diabetes is at risk of developing hypoglycemia up to 24 hours after exercising if the exercise is too strenuous. Walking, swimming, or stationary bicycle riding are considered to be among the safest activities for this group. Exercise should begin slowly and build up to 30 to 45 minutes, three or four times a week. The gradual increase helps prevent hypoglycemia, stress fractures, and cardiovascular complications.

Increasing Food Intake During Exercise. During moderate exercise (such as brisk walking, bowling, or vacuuming) 5 g of simple carbohydrate should be consumed at the end of 30 minutes and at 30-minute intervals during the continued activity. (A food example with 5 g of simple carbohydrate is 1 tsp honey.) Jogging, swimming, or scrubbing floors should be preceded by consumption of 15 to 20 g of complex carbohydrate plus protein 15 to 30 minutes before beginning the exercise, and then, if the activity continues for more than 30 minutes, 10 g of simple carbohydrate should be taken every 30 minutes. Vigorous exercise (such as fast jogging, skiing, or playing tennis) requires intake of 30 to 40 g of complex carbohydrate plus protein 15 to 30 minutes ahead of time and then 10 to 20 g of simple carbohydrate intake every 30 minutes after the first half-hour.

Performing exercise when insulin or an oral antidiabetic agent is at its peak of action can bring on an acute hypoglycemic reaction. Eating a piece of fruit before even light exercise, if done between meals, also can help prevent hypoglycemia in people with type 1 diabetes. Once a patient begins to follow a regular exercise program, the insulin dosage and diet may need to be revised. In general, the patient may need to take less insulin and to increase caloric intake with regular exercise. Keeping a daily record of exercise, along with weight, insulin dosage, and blood glucose levels, can help motivate the patient to continue exercise.

Health Promotion

Insulin and Exercise

Advise patients to avoid injecting insulin into an area that will soon receive extra exercise (e.g., the leg). The abdomen is a good site for insulin injection as absorption is steady, rapid, and not affected by exercise.

Oral Hypoglycemic Agents. Oral hypoglycemic agents (OHAs) or antidiabetic agents may be prescribed for patients with type 2 diabetes to manage their blood glucose levels. These medications are not a form of oral insulin; pharmacologically, they are from completely different classes of medications. There are now six major categories of OHAs that act in different ways to help achieve blood glucose control. Information about these medications can be found in Table 38-2.

Table 38-2   Oral Hypoglycemic Agents

GENERIC NAME (BRAND NAME)	MAIN SITE OF ACTION	HOW THEY CONTROL BLOOD GLUCOSE	OTHER CONSIDERATIONS
Biguanides			
Metformin (Glucophage) Also available in combination with other OHAs: with sulfonylurea agents (Glucovance and Metaglip), thiazolidinediones (Avandamet), and DPP-4 inhibitors (Janumet)	Liver	Keep liver from releasing excessive insulin; make muscle cells more sensitive to insulin	Do not cause hypoglycemia or hyperinsulinemia Do not lead to weight gain Contraindicated in renal failure, liver disease, and acidosis
Alpha-Glucosidase Inhibitors			
Acarbose (Precose) Miglitol (Glyset)	Intestine	Reduce demand for insulin by slowing absorption of complex carbohydrates, resulting in less of a blood glucose "spike"	Contraindicated in people with inflammatory bowel disease or other intestinal diseases
Thiazolidinediones			
Pioglitazone (Actos) Rosiglitazone (Avandia)	Muscle cells	Make muscle cells more sensitive to insulin; decrease liver production of glucose	Contraindicated in people with congestive heart failure Actos and Avandia have black box warning for cardiac risk
Sulfonylureas (Long-Acting)			
Glimepiride (Amaryl) Glipizide (Glucotrol) Glyburide (DiaBeta, Micronase, Glynase PresTab)	Pancreas	Stimulate pancreas to secrete more insulin	Quick action can cause hypoglycemia Contraindicated in advanced kidney or liver disease, or for those with sulfa allergies
Nonsulfonylurea Insulin Glinides			
Nateglinide (Starlix) Repaglinide (Prandin)	Pancreas	Stimulate insulin secretion, but shorter acting than sulfonylureas	Must be taken immediately before eating Lower risk of hypoglycemia than sulfonylureas
DPP-4 Inhibitors			
Sitagliptin (Januvia) Saxagliptin (Onglyza)	Endocrine system	Enhance a natural body system called the incretin system, which helps regulate glucose by affecting alpha and beta cells in the pancreas	May cause delayed gastric emptying (can affect absorption of other medications) Reduced dosage may be required in patient with renal impairment, as medication is excreted via the kidneys
Dopamine Agonist			
Bromocriptine mesylate (Cycloset)	Brain	Increasing dopamine activity improves metabolism problems related to diabetes and A1C levels	Can cause nausea, vomiting, dizziness, and headaches

Safety Alert

Sulfa Drug Allergy

Because the sulfonylureas are from the same family of drugs as the sulfonamide antibiotics, they must be given with caution to persons known to have an allergy to sulfa drugs.

Patients receiving OHAs should know that these medications do not eliminate the need for following their diet and exercise program. Some may be under the impression that if they go off their diet and indulge themselves, they can just take more pills to compensate. Others who have been on a diet and exercise program for a time and then have an OHA prescribed for them think it is acceptable to stop planning their meals and exercising regularly. All OHAs are capable of producing gastric irritation, nausea, vomiting, and diarrhea. Liver damage with jaundice, bone marrow depression, and allergic skin reactions may result in some patients.

Clinical Cues

Metformin is the preferred drug for type 2 diabetes, so many of your patients will be taking this OHA. Metformin should be held before surgery or a procedure requiring contrast media and for 48 hours afterward until renal function is verified.

Insulin Therapy. Insulin therapy can be prescribed for patients with either type 1 or type 2 diabetes. The goal of insulin therapy is to closely mimic basal insulin, which is the amount of insulin that would normally be produced by the pancreas throughout the day to maintain a healthy blood sugar level between meals. The pancreas also produces extra insulin after meals (*postprandial*). The health care provider can use a variety of rapid-acting, short-acting, intermediate-acting, and long-acting insulins that best suit the individual patient (Table 38-3). A single daily injection of intermediate- or long-acting insulin, or a combination insulin (such as Humulin 70/30 that combines short- and intermediate-acting insulins), can be used for some patients. The multiple daily injection (MDI) regimen is more often prescribed and offers the advantage of being more physiologically appropriate. MDI combines short- and intermediate-acting insulins, injected two or more times a day. The patient could also be placed on an intensified regimen. This regimen relies on the patient's ability to accurately perform blood glucose monitoring. The basal dose, again, would be intermediate- or long-acting insulin. A bolus dose, or correction dose, of short- or rapid-acting insulin is used to manage elevations in blood glucose and bring the next blood glucose measurement into range.

Table 38-3 Common Types of Insulins: Onset, Peak, and Duration of Action

PREPARATION	BRAND NAME	ONSET (HR)	PEAK (HR)	DURATION (HR)
Rapid Acting				
Insulin aspart injection	NovoLog	0.25	1-3	3-5
Insulin lispro injection	Humalog	0.25	0.5-1.5	5
Insulin glulisine injection	Apidra	0.3	0.5-1.5	3-4
Short Acting				
Regular human insulin injection	Humulin R	0.5	2-4	5-7
	Novolin R	0.5	2.5-5	8
Buffered regular human insulin injection	Velosulin BR	0.5	1-3	8
Intermediate Acting				
Isophane insulin NPH	Humulin N	1.5	4-12	16-24+
	Novolin N			
	ReliOn N	1.5	4-12	24
Insulin zinc suspension (Lente)	Novolin L	1	6-8	5.7-24
Insulin detemir injection	Levemir	1	6-8	5.7-24
Long Acting				
Insulin glargine injection	Lantus	2-4	None	24
Combination Insulin				
70% Insulin aspart protamine suspension/ 30% insulin aspart injection	NovoLog Mix 70/30	0.25	1-4	24
75% Insulin lispro protamine suspension/ 25% insulin lispro injection	Humalog Mix 75/25	0.25	1-2	24
70% Human insulin isophane suspension (NPH)/30% human insulin injection (regular)	Humulin 70/30 Novolin 70/30 ReliOn 70/30	0.5	2-12	24
50% Human insulin isophane suspension (NPH)/50% human insulin injection (regular)	Humulin 50/50 Novolin 50/50	0.5	3-5	24

Adapted from Ignatavicius, D.D., & Workman, M.L. (2010). *Medical-Surgical Nursing: Critical Thinking for Collaborative Care* (6th ed.). Philadelphia: Saunders.

Clinical Cues

You are likely to hear and see the term *sliding scale*. This concept has been used for years, so many health care providers, nurses, patients, and hospital systems may continue to use this term; however, the sliding scale method has been deemed ineffective because hypoglycemic events are common.

Clinical Cues

If regular insulin and longer-acting insulin are to be mixed in one syringe, the regular insulin is drawn up first to prevent any contamination of the regular bottle of insulin with the longer-acting variety. "Clear to cloudy" is an easy way to remember which insulin to draw up first. The clear (regular) insulin is drawn up first, followed by the cloudy (longer-acting) insulin. **Remember, every insulin dose must be verified by another nurse as it is drawn up, every time.** This habit will also help you meet the National Patient Safety Goal to increase the safety of administering medications.

Insulin cannot be taken orally or given via a feeding tube, because it is destroyed by gastric juices. Insulin pens, filled with insulin, are another alternative to the traditional syringe-and-needle apparatus. The patient selects the correct dose on a dial, and the insulin is delivered by a small needle at the end of the pen.

Safety Alert

Insulin Pen Injectors

Patients must be careful when dialing the dose of insulin into a pen injector. If performed incorrectly, the numbers of the dosage will be transposed (e.g., 52 units instead of 25 units.) This could potentially happen if the pen is held in the left hand, or if the number scale is held upside down.

Safety Alert

Read the Labels on Prefilled Pens

In 2009 the Food and Drug Administration (FDA) approved Aprida SoloStar prefilled insulin pens. This pen contains a rapid-acting insulin analogue. Lantus SoloStar, from the same company, also comes in insulin pen form; however, Lantus is a long-acting insulin. During comparative studies, users were able to differentiate the two pens; however, patients should be advised to carefully check the labels before injection. The nurse must also continue to have another nurse double-check the insulin type and dose when using prefilled pens.

Injectable insulin continues to be the most common delivery method, so it is critical that nurses be educated in all aspects of injectable insulin therapy. Insulin injections are rotated within one body area to enhance absorption. Patients are given charts showing the places on the arms, legs, buttocks, and abdomen

Front   Back

FIGURE 38-2 Rotation sites for injection of insulin.

where insulin can be injected (Figure 38-2). They are then encouraged to keep a daily record of injection sites to help remember which sites have been used and to avoid the problem of altered or erratic absorption.

Patient Teaching

Guidelines for Subcutaneous Insulin Injection

- Wash your hands thoroughly.
- Check the type of insulin and expiration date on the bottle label.
- Check that the syringe type is correct (e.g., U100 for U100 insulin).
- Roll the bottle of insulin between the palms of your hands to mix it gently.
- Cleanse the top of the rubber stopper with an alcohol swab.
- Remove the needle cover and pull the plunger back to a point equal to the desired amount of insulin you will draw up; place the needle into the bottle above the surface of insulin and inject the air (this prevents bubbles).
- Turn the bottle and syringe upside down, holding them with one hand; with the bevel of the needle well into the insulin, slowly draw up the correct amount of insulin.
- Remove air bubbles in the syringe by tapping on the barrel of the syringe, reinjecting into the bottle, and then redrawing up the correct dosage of insulin without bubbles.
- Remove the needle from the bottle; select a site for injection that has not been used in the past month.
- Clean the site with an alcohol swab; pinch up the area of skin and insert the needle all the way at a 90-degree angle; inject the insulin.
- Pull the needle straight out quickly. Blot the site with the alcohol swab; do not rub the site.
- Do not recap the needle; dispose of the syringe and needle in a puncture-proof container.

Insulin requirements change as metabolic needs are altered by diet, exercise, age, and even changes in seasons. In the summer, for example, many people are outdoors and exercising more than during the winter months. Also, as a person grows older, the level of physical activity may decrease. Insulin requirements also are altered when the patient has an infection or illness or is under added stress.

 Clinical Cues

Some patients are able to use the insulin-to-carbohydrate ratio. The patient must receive extensive MNT and be taught to interpret blood glucose patterns, to count carbohydrates, and to calculate bolus doses based on carbohydrate intake. One unit of insulin will cover 15 g carbohydrate for most patients (weight and insulin sensitivity must also be considered). See Table 38-4 for an example of lunch calculation. Contact the diabetic educator for assistance if you identify a patient who could use this type of management system.

 Think Critically

How would a patient know that her insulin requirement has changed?

Table 38-4	Example of Carbohydrate Counting for Lunch	
FOOD SOURCE		**GRAMS OF CARBOHYDRATES**
2 oz tuna, canned in water		0
1 hamburger bun		30
15 fat-free Pringles		15
1 tablespoon reduced-fat mayonnaise		0
1 tomato and 1 lettuce slice		0
1 medium dill pickle		0
Sugar-free pudding made with fat-free milk		15
	Total:	**60**
	Insulin (1:15 ratio):	**4**

Modified from Ignatavicius DD, & Workman ML. (2010). *Medical-Surgical Nursing Patient-Centered Collaborative Care* (6th ed.). St. Louis: Saunders, p. 1495.

Insulin Pump. An alternative to insulin therapy by daily injections is the insulin pump. These pumps can deliver a continuous infusion of insulin through an automated system composed of a battery-driven electronic "brain," an electric motor and drive mechanisms, and a syringe (Figure 38-3). The syringe is attached to plastic tubing and a subcutaneous needle, which is inserted into the abdomen or thigh. Pumps are helpful in managing diabetes because they allow for improved blood glucose control; people using pumps tend to have fewer episodes and less severe hypoglycemia when compared with MDIs.

The pump continuously delivers basal insulin to maintain blood sugar levels between meals and can be programmed to administer a bolus dose for meals of elevated blood sugar levels. Current models do not yet have a mechanism by which the pump can sense the body's ever-changing needs for insulin *and* take corrective action; however, there is an insulin pump with real-time continuous blood glucose monitoring, which allows the patient to take immediate corrective action based on blood glucose (Miller, D.K., 2009). Today's pumps internally record and manage data, such as blood glucose values, insulin delivered, and carbohydrate consumption.

At present, insulin pumps are recommended only for a select few patients who are willing and able to monitor their blood glucose frequently during the day, and who can understand the principles of basal-bolus insulin and carbohydrate counting.

 Clinical Cues

The insulin pump will have to be disconnected for certain diagnostic tests, such as magnetic resonance imaging. Most patients can safely be without the pump for an hour, but blood glucose should be checked before disconnecting and after reconnecting (Miller, D. K. 2009).

Only 4 buttons mean you can do all functions in just a few steps

Tactile side buttons allow discreet bolus programming, even through clothing

IR communication supports wireless data transfer

ACCU-CHEK Spirit

Automatic alerts for low insulin, low battery, etc., help ensure uninterrupted therapy

Rubber end caps help absorb the knocks, drops and bumps of everyday life

Backlight allows operation in any lighting situation

Intuitive text icons like [STOP] and [i] simplify programming—scroll forward and backward quickly and easily

315-unit insulin cartridge means fewer fills and changes—it's the largest of all pump brands

FIGURE 38-3 Insulin pump.

Table 38-5 Injectable Hypoglycemic Agents

GENERIC NAME (BRAND NAME)	MAIN SITE OF ACTION	HOW THEY CONTROL BLOOD GLUCOSE	OTHER CONSIDERATIONS
Incretin Mimetic			
Exenatide (Byetta)	Subcutaneous	Mimics the action of incretins Stimulates insulin secretion, suppresses glucagon release, delays gastric emptying	Administer before breakfast or dinner (not lunch) to avoid severe hypoglycemia Give 1 hr after oral hypoglycemic agents
Synthetic Hormone			
Pramlintide (Symlin)	Subcutaneous	Synthetic form of the hormone amylin Slows gastric emptying, suppresses glucagon release, suppresses glucose production by the liver, decreases appetite	Black box warning: potential to cause severe hypoglycemia; patients started on this medication should have their rapid-acting insulin dosage cut in half Pramlintide cannot be mixed with insulin and must be administered as a separate injection
Human Glucagon–like Peptide-1 Analogue			
Liraglutide (Victoza)	Subcutaneous	Stimulates the release of insulin when blood glucose levels are elevated	Not a first-line treatment, but may be used in type 2 diabetics as an adjunct to diet, exercise, and oral hypoglycemic agents

From Fonseca, V.A. & Kulkarni, K.D. (2008). Management of type 2 diabetes: Oral agents, insulin, and injectables. *J Am Diet Assoc 108*(4), Suppl 1. Mosby's Nursing Consult. (2010). FDA approves injectable Victoza for type 2 diabetes. Drug Information FDA approvals. Retrieved from www.nursingconsult.

Other Injectable Agents. Historically, insulin was the only injectable medication for the management of diabetes; however, new injectable agents have been introduced. One new category of medications is called incretin mimetics because they mimic the action of *incretins*, which are hormones released from the intestine; they lower postprandial blood glucose levels in a number of ways (Table 38-5). Other injectable medications to treat diabetes are synthetic hormones, such as pramlintide. Although these medications are administered subcutaneously, none of these new medications should ever be mixed in the same syringe with insulin, and the patient must be monitored carefully for hypoglycemia.

⚠ Safety Alert

Pramlintide

The medication pramlintide (Symlin) carries with it an FDA *black box warning* (a type of warning sometimes carried on prescription medications indicating the potential for serious adverse effects). This medication has the potential to cause severe hypoglycemia within 3 hours of administration. It is critically important that the nurse observe the patient closely for any signs or symptoms of hypoglycemia.

Preoperative and Postoperative Insulin Management. The emotional and physical stress of surgery can increase the blood glucose level and alter the amounts of medication needed for glycemic control. Patients with type 2 diabetes may be taken off OHAs up to 48 hours before surgery and started on insulin by injection to achieve adequate control of their diabetes during this stressful period. The patient should be reassured that the diabetes is not worse, and that the insulin injections are only a temporary measure. A patient with type 2 diabetes will have bolus or correction dose orders along with the usual insulin order. Blood sugar determinations are done more frequently.

For all diabetic patients, intravenous fluids are begun as soon as the patient is ordered "nothing by mouth" (NPO) and are continued until the patient is eating again after surgery. During surgery, an insulin infusion of regular or short-acting insulin may be used, usually mixed in 5% dextrose or 0.9% NaCl solution, depending on hospital policy. Blood glucose is monitored closely during surgery and every 2 to 4 hours postoperatively; urine is checked for ketones when glucose levels are high.

⌂ Clinical Cues

Be especially alert for signs of hypoglycemia in patients who are receiving an insulin infusion. Blood glucose is monitored hourly. The rate of infusion is adjusted according to an algorithm.

Islet Cell Transplantation. An experimental procedure for treatment of type 1 diabetes is transplantation of insulin-producing islet cells. The procedure is controversial. Ethical issues include (1) two to four donor pancreases are needed for the required number of islet cells, (2) about a third of recipients will develop antibodies that would prohibit any future whole-pancreas transplant attempts, and (3) lifetime immunosuppressive medications are highly nephrotoxic. The option may be discussed with patients who have very unstable metabolic control and have frequent life-threatening hypoglycemic episodes (Ruggenenti et al., 2008).

❖ NURSING MANAGEMENT

■ Assessment (Data Collection)

The nurse should assess every patient for signs and symptoms of potential diabetes mellitus. Assess the skin for signs of poor wound healing or areas of infection. The feet should be inspected for signs of tight-fitting shoes and beginning sores. The patient should be weighed to determine whether weight is within normal limits.

 Focused Assessment

Data Collection for Diabetes

The following questions should be asked to establish a database that indicates the patient may have diabetes, has poorly controlled diabetes, or has no signs of diabetes:

- Has anyone in your family ever been told he or she has diabetes? What about your parents and grandparents?
- Have you had any recent weight loss or weight gain?
- Have you become increasingly hungry over the past few months?
- Has your thirst increased? Are you drinking more fluids than you used to?
- Do you have to urinate (go to the toilet) more than you used to?
- Have you noticed that you are more tired than you were 6 months ago?
- Do you have any trouble with scratches and wounds healing?
- Do small scratches or abrasions become easily infected?
- Have you noticed any numbness or tingling or "funny" sensations in your hands, legs, or feet?
- Is constipation becoming a problem?
- Are you having any sexual difficulties? Any impotence (men)? Any frequent vaginal infections (women)?

If the patient is known to have diabetes, ask these questions also:

- Do you feel that you can easily and correctly perform your blood glucose determinations? (Check the patient's performance using her own machine.)
- How do you calibrate your blood glucose monitor?
- Are you having any trouble sticking to your dietary plan?
- How are you planning your meals?
- Are you taking your insulin/oral medication regularly?
- Are you having any problems in relation to the medication?
- Are you keeping records of your blood glucose readings and your insulin injections? (Check records, if available.)
- Are you seeing your primary health care provider at regular intervals?
- Are you having your eyes examined regularly?
- Are you visiting the dentist regularly?

For the patient newly diagnosed with diabetes, the nurse must assess whether the patient is a good candidate for using a **glucometer** (blood glucose–monitoring machine) (Figure 38-4). The patient must have adequate peripheral circulation to easily obtain a drop of blood for the test. Manual dexterity is needed to perform the fingerstick to obtain a large enough drop of blood, to place the drop on the right spot, and to correctly read the meter. Patients with arthritis or visual impairment may have difficulty with these steps. The patient must be able to time the test,

FIGURE 38-4 Blood glucose monitor.

remember the correct sequence of the steps, and remember to do it at the designated times. Determining whether the patient can cope with learning the procedure and whether there is willingness to fit it into the daily routine are other assessment factors. Periodic assessment of glucose monitoring techniques, medication administration, and compliance with treatment regimen are essential. There is a new device available that offers continuous blood glucose monitoring. This device consists of a sensor that is surgically inserted under the skin, a radiofrequency transmitter, and a monitor. Blood glucose readings are taken every 5 minutes; the device displays the readings when a button is pushed. It also signals a result that is too high or too low, alerting the patient to view the blood glucose value and to take corrective action (Medtronic MiniMed, 2010).

■ Nursing Diagnosis

The following nursing diagnoses are common for patients with diabetes mellitus:

- Imbalanced nutrition: less than (or more than) body requirements related to alterations in insulin availability or utilization
- Deficient knowledge related to newly diagnosed disease process, possible complications, and self-care needs
- Risk for infection related to elevated blood glucose level
- Ineffective coping related to denial of need for effective self-care
- Disturbed sensory perception related to effect of elevated blood glucose on vascular and nervous systems

- Risk for injury related to severe decrease in tissue perfusion in feet
- Pain related to nerve damage secondary to peripheral vascular disease

There are many other nursing diagnoses related to the various complications that the patient with diabetes may develop over the years. Nursing care plans must be carefully individualized to the particular problems and needs of each patient (Nursing Care Plan 38-1).

■ Planning

Always check the calibration of the glucometer before use. You should know the schedule for meal tray delivery and plan glucose testing and insulin injections for appropriate times throughout the day. Fingersticks for blood glucose testing should be performed 30 minutes before breakfast. If an hour has elapsed without insulin being given after the reading was obtained, the test must be repeated before insulin administration.

When a patient is NPO for tests or procedures, monitor for signs of hypoglycemia and obtain the patient's food tray immediately when the patient returns from testing. The insulin dose should be adjusted according to health care provider order during the NPO period; insulin should not be withheld. Assessment for hyperglycemia must be planned for times during the shift when the patient is undergoing the added stress of illness or surgery.

To avoid delays, make certain that the patient's insulin, appropriate syringes, or oral medication are on the unit ahead of scheduled medication time. Examples of expected outcomes for the patient with diabetes mellitus include:

- Patient will attain a body weight within normal limits within 6 months.
- Patient will demonstrate knowledge of disease process, possible complications, and self-care methods.
- Patient will constantly monitor for signs of infection.
- Patient will develop coping methods to perform self-care.
- Patient will verbalize ways to preserve and protect vision.

✳ Nursing Care Plan 38-1   Care of the Patient with Diabetes Mellitus

Scenario
Mr. Blackburn, age 49, is 5 ft 7 in tall and weighs 350 lb. He was admitted to the hospital for surgical repair of a hernia. During the preoperative evaluation, his blood glucose value was 420 mg/dL. On further examination by the health care provider, Mr. Blackburn reported symptoms of extreme thirst, hunger, and excessive urination. Surgery was rescheduled; further workup confirmed the suspected diagnosis of type 2 diabetes mellitus. Mr. Blackburn was extremely upset at learning the diagnosis and not being able to have his surgery. His response to the diagnosis was to ask the surgeon if he could be prescribed "some pills" and "get on with it."

Problem/Nursing Diagnosis
Extremely overweight/Imbalanced nutrition: more than body requirements related to alteration in glucose utilization by cells.

Supporting Assessment Data
Objective: Blood glucose 420 mg/dL; weighs 350 pounds.

Goals/Expected Outcomes	Nursing Interventions	Selected Rationale	Evaluation
Patient will develop meal plan that will assist in maintaining ideal body weight and blood sugar within normal limits.	Perform dietary assessment (i.e., typical intake, nutritional knowledge, cultural preferences).	Patient's current diet and general knowledge of nutrition and cultural preferences can be considered and modified.	Normally eats a lot of fast foods, but likes fruits and vegetables and would like to improve diet.
Patient will demonstrate knowledge of correct meal planning within 3 mo.	Instruct in diabetic meal planning and carbohydrate counting.	The relationship of meal planning to control of chronic disease is new information.	States that he "doesn't get it" when asked about meal planning and carbohydrate counting.
	Assist with construction of an acceptable meal plan for attaining desired weight and to normalize serum glucose levels.	Any meal plan must be individualized for weight goals, lifestyle, and food preferences.	Able to correctly identify appropriate portion sizes of sample menu.
Hemoglobin A$_{1C}$ and fructosamine assay levels will show compliance with dietary plan within 6 mo.	Reinforce health care provider's instructions to follow up for repeat laboratory tests and for additional dietary education.	Long-term goal is to achieve: Normal value (A1C): 3.9%-5.2% (of total hemoglobin) Fructosamine assay: Normal value: 1.5-2.7 mmol/L	A1C and fructosamine assay level and reassessment of dietary success to be done at follow-up. Continue plan.

Problem/Nursing Diagnosis

Has no knowledge about diabetes/Deficient knowledge related to disease process, possible complications, and self-care.

Supporting Assessment Data

Subjective: Patient asks health care provider if he could be prescribed "some pills" and "get on with it."

Goals/Expected Outcomes	Nursing Interventions	Selected Rationale	Evaluation
Patient will verbalize basic knowledge about disease process within 1 mo.	Instruct patient about the disease process of diabetes using a variety of teaching methodologies based on the content and learning style.	Varied methods that target the patient's learning style increase retention of information (i.e., written material, demonstrations, videos).	Patient verbalized basic knowledge of disease process.
Patient will verbalize ways to prevent the complications of diabetes within 3 mo.	Instruct regarding the potential complications of diabetes and how to decrease the risk of complications.	Knowledge empowers patient to achieve self-care and to take preventive measures.	Patient states, "I need to lose weight." Patient acknowledges complications of diabetes but states he needs more information.
	Instruct in oral medication or insulin administration.	Long-term self-management of medication is essential.	Very resistant to the idea of insulin injections, but shows interest in learning about oral medications.
Patient will demonstrate proper foot care within 1 mo.	Instruct in proper foot care techniques (i.e., daily inspection, cleaning, foot attire).	Poor circulation and peripheral neuropathy can lead to infection or amputation.	Demonstrates proper foot care.
	Seek feedback regarding material taught by verbalization and demonstration of skills.	Provides opportunity for reinforcement, or praise. Reteaching or redesign of materials might be necessary.	Expresses appreciation of time spent in teaching him about various topics; requests written information about foot care and medication side effects.

Problem/Nursing Diagnosis

Recently diagnosed with type 2 diabetes mellitus/Risk for unstable glucose level.

Supporting Assessment Data

Objective: Admitting blood glucose 420 mg/dL.

Goals/Expected Outcomes	Nursing Interventions	Selected Rationale	Evaluation
Patient will have a premeal blood glucose of 70-140 mg/dL while in the hospital.	Monitor the blood sugar before meals and at bedtime or as ordered.	Illness and stress will affect blood sugar level and patient is newly diagnosed, so response to therapy must be closely monitored.	Blood glucose 230 mg/dL at 6:00 AM. Health care provider aware and order for correction dose of insulin obtained.
	Monitor for signs of hypoglycemia (i.e., hunger, sweating, confusion) and hyperglycemia (i.e., increased urination, thirst, rapid breathing).	Hypoglycemia must be treated immediately because brain cells need a continuous source of glucose. Hyperglycemia can cause long-term damage, but can also be life threatening if ketoacidosis occurs.	Does not exhibit any signs of hypoglycemia (i.e., weakness, anxiety, palpitations) or hyperglycemia (i.e., nausea, acetone breath, or dry mucous membranes). "Feels pretty good considering."
Patient will demonstrate blood glucose levels within acceptable limits within 1 mo.	Instruct in glucose monitoring technique appropriate to patient.	Proper instruction, including return demonstration, is important in ascertaining correct fingerstick values.	Able to perform fingerstick and check value. "I'm good with gadgets."
	Instruct to record blood glucose findings after testing.	Keeping a daily record is important in monitoring day-to-day fluctuations in blood glucose.	Likes to keep records. "It's good to have the data right where I can see it." Continue plan.

Continued

Nursing Care Plan 38-1   Care of the Patient with Diabetes Mellitus—cont'd

Problem/Nursing Diagnosis
Feels loss of control/Situational low self-esteem related to diagnosis of chronic disease requiring lifestyle changes or insulin injections for survival.

Supporting Assessment Data
Objective: Patient with newly diagnosed diabetes.

Goals/Expected Outcomes	Nursing Interventions	Selected Rationale	Evaluation
Patient will verbalize own strengths within 1 mo.	Encourage verbalization of feelings related to diagnosis of diabetes and need for lifestyle changes. Allow expression of frustrations.	Verbalization of feelings is an important first step toward identifying one's own strengths. Frustration is a normal human response to a real or perceived threat.	Initially, very quiet, appears withdrawn and angry after health care provider informs of new diagnosis of diabetes mellitus. "I guess I am taking out my frustrations on you and the doctor." Reassured that frustration is normal.
Patient will express that control over the disease and life is possible.	Encourage exploration of strengths and positive measures of self-worth (i.e., roles, accomplishments). Explain how control over disease and life is possible.	Remembering past achievements can help patients realize their strengths. After feelings are expressed, patient will be more receptive to information. Knowledge and tools can help him achieve control.	States, "I am a hard worker. I own my own business—I can certainly learn to manage this too." "I think I am beginning to understand. Balancing food intake and insulin is like balancing a spreadsheet of expenditures at my business."
	Praise efforts at learning and practice of self-care techniques.	Positive reinforcement is a powerful tool for helping a patient accomplish acceptance of a situation.	Goal met/reevaluate as needed.

Critical Thinking Questions
1. The RN has planned the first teaching session for Mr. Blackburn, which you are to help implement. The topics planned for today include meal planning, short-term complications of diabetes, long-term complications of diabetes, foot care, and actions/side-effects/interactions of oral hypoglycemia agents. When the RN asks for your collaboration on the plan, what would you recommend?
2. Mr. Blackburn has visitors coming to see him. You greet them in the hallway, and notice they are carrying bags from Krispy Kreme and Baskin Robbins. How would you respond to this situation?

- Patient will demonstrate methods to prevent injury to feet.
- Patient will verbalize that pain is within acceptable limits after medication and nonpharmaceutical measures are administered.

■ Implementation

Intervention is geared toward assisting the patient with self-care, performing blood glucose determinations, administering medication when the patient is ill and cannot self-administer, observing for signs and symptoms of complications, assessing learning needs, and carrying out a teaching plan as indicated. Be sure to encourage others involved in your patient's care to be alert for signs and symptoms.

 Assignment Considerations

Observations

Remind the UAP to report any breaks in the skin observed while giving physical care to the patient with diabetes. Report excessive urination or changes in vital signs, such as increasingly rapid respirations.

Monitor the trend of blood glucose, A1C, and fructosamine assay readings over time, rather than focus only on the current reading. Assess how well the patient is eating and taking fluids. Intake and output recordings are appropriate if the patient is ill or having surgery. Any type of stress can alter the control of the patient's diabetes. Electrolytes also should be monitored, with particular attention to potassium levels, which can shift suddenly when insulin is insufficient.

Every patient on insulin should be monitored for hypoglycemia after insulin injections. After injection of each type of insulin, you must know when hypoglycemia might occur, and you should assess the patient at that time. Patients are taught to report signs of hypoglycemia promptly, to avoid a crisis.

Monitoring for signs of ketoacidosis also is essential. Some of the earliest symptoms may be polyuria, fatigue, anorexia, abdominal pain, and a "fruity" smell to the breath. Look for beginning signs of dehydration with decreased tissue turgor, sunken eyeballs, and dry mucous membranes (Table 38-6). Report such findings to the health care provider promptly.

Patient Education

The patient must be able to self-manage diet, medication, and progress. In addition, adjustments in lifestyle, recreational choices, and self-image will probably need to be made. The patient must be taught the correct steps for blood glucose monitoring (see Figure 38-4).

Noncompliance can be devastating to the patient's welfare and can mean the difference between leading a nearly normal life or becoming an invalid; eventually, noncompliance may mean the difference between life and death for the person with diabetes. Many hospitals and clinics have developed standardized teaching programs for diabetes education because the task of diabetic teaching is very challenging and complex (Figure 38-5).

Table 38-6	Comparison of Hypoglycemia and Ketoacidosis	
HYPOGLYCEMIA	**KETOACIDOSIS**
Etiology	
Overdosage of insulin	Failure to take insulin
Skipped or delayed meal	Illness or infection
Unplanned strenuous exercise	Overeating or too many carbohydrates
	Severe stress (surgery, trauma, emotional upset)
Symptoms	
Headache	Increased thirst (polydipsia)
Weakness	Increased urination (polyuria)
Hunger (polyphagia)	Acetone breath odor ("fruity")
Pallor	Dry mucous membranes and sunken eyeballs (dehydration)
Irritability	Nausea and vomiting
Lack of muscle coordination	Deep respirations (Kussmaul's respirations)
Apprehension	Abdominal pain and rigidity
Shakiness	Paresthesias, weakness, paralysis
Diaphoresis with cool, clammy skin	Hypotension
Blurred vision	Minimal urine output (oliguria) or none (anuria) (late sign)
Rapid heartbeat	Stupor or coma (late sign)
Confusion	
Coma (late)	
Treatment	
If patient can swallow, give 3 glucose tablets or equivalent glucose gel, 6 oz of juice, 6 oz regular cola, 8 oz of 2% or skim milk, or 6 to 8 Life Savers	IV fluid and insulin with correction of electrolyte imbalances
If patient cannot swallow, administer glucagon by IV push	Severe cases are hospitalized for stabilization
If at the hospital: give $D_{50}W$ solution	
Prevention	
Eat meals 4-5 hr apart, plus prescribed snacks	Take correct dose of insulin
Take correct dose of insulin	Consult health care provider when ill (even for minor illnesses)
Test blood glucose level regularly and more frequently during illness	Follow diet; do not overeat and do not overload with carbohydrates
Eat extra food when exercising more than usual	

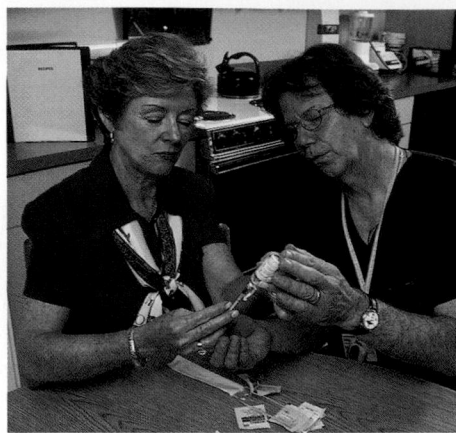

FIGURE 38-5 Nurse teaching patient with diabetes.

Major topics covered in a standardized program usually include:

- Pathophysiology of diabetes mellitus, including functions of the pancreas and contributing or precipitating factors in the development of diabetes
- How to manage a diet program
- Blood glucose monitoring at home
- Foot care
- Urine testing when blood glucose level is over 240 mg/dL to check for acetone
- Identification tag, identification card, and medical information (see Figure 38-1)
- Information on what to do on "sick" days, especially when nauseated or vomiting and unable to maintain diet
- Community resources and help groups available to patient with diabetes and family
- Travel tips
- Devices that make insulin administration easier (especially for the elderly, visually impaired, or patients with arthritis)

 Patient Teaching

What to Do on Sick Days

A bad cold, flu, or minor gastrointestinal upset can create problems for diabetic patients.

MEDICATION

- Take insulin as prescribed. Adjust the dosage as directed, depending on blood glucose readings.
- If taking an oral hypoglycemic, take usual dose. Do not increase the dose unless ordered to do so by the health care provider. If vomiting and unable to take medication by mouth, the health care provider may temporarily order insulin.

DIET

- Eat a normal diet on schedule.
- If nausea and vomiting occur, replace carbohydrate solid foods in the normal diet with liquids that contain sugar (fruit juice, regular soft drinks, or Jell-O).
- Take at least 1 cup of water or calorie-free, caffeine-free liquid each hour. If nauseated, take small sips to help avoid vomiting.

MONITORING

- Test blood glucose at least every 4 hours and record result. If severely ill, check blood glucose every 2 hours.
- Test urine for ketones if blood sugar level is over 240 mg/dL.

NOTIFYING THE HEALTH CARE PROVIDER

- Call the health care provider right away for vomiting or abdominal pain or a temperature above 100.2° F (38.8° C).
- Notify the health care provider if blood glucose is above 200 mg/dL or if urine test shows ketones in the urine.
- Report to the health care provider if blood glucose level that was above 200 mg/dL does not come down with an additional dose of insulin.
- If unable to reach the health care provider, go to the hospital emergency department.

 Patient Teaching

Instructions for Traveling

- Carry extra medication or insulin in case a bottle gets lost or broken. Keep a 48-hour supply of pills, insulin, and syringes in a purse, briefcase, or carry-on luggage, along with the blood glucose–monitoring device.
- Wear a Medic-Alert bracelet or tag, and carry a medical information card in a purse or wallet.
- Carry an emergency supply of fast-acting sugar at all times in case of a hypoglycemic episode. Also carry longer-acting foods, such as peanut butter and crackers.
- Plan ahead at least 2 days for replenishing supplies for blood glucose monitoring, insulin, and syringes in case the correct items are hard to find in a foreign city. (It is best to take supplies for the entire trip.)
- If ill, seek medical attention immediately before a dangerous condition occurs.
- Stick to prescribed meal plans as much as possible, substituting available foods according to food group classification.
- Obtain sufficient rest and avoid stressful situations as much as possible to prevent stress-induced hyperglycemia.
- It is best to travel with someone who is familiar with diabetes and treatment. It is best to advise the airline or ship personnel about the diabetes.
- Obtain the usual amount of exercise or adjust food and medication accordingly.
- Drink a glass of water every 2 hours to prevent dehydration.
- Check blood glucose level frequently.
- Obtain a letter from the health care provider about the diabetes, as well as extra prescriptions for medications.
- Protect insulin from temperature extremes.
- Eat something at least every 4 hours.
- Call airlines and ship companies ahead of departure to request diabetic meals.
- Before departure, research food substitutions, so that personal meal plans are consistent.
- Remember time zones: going westward lengthens the day; take more insulin. Going eastward shortens the day; take less insulin.

Patient Teaching

Working with the Older Adult Who Has Diabetes

- Assess hearing and vision and use aids and adequate lighting.
- Set a time for the teaching session that is agreeable to the patient.
- Arrange a quiet, nondistracting environment for the session.
- Be certain that the patient is comfortable before beginning.
- Keep the sessions short—no more than 15 to 20 minutes at a time.
- Limit information to a few major concepts per session.
- Go slowly and seek feedback that the patient has understood each point when finished presenting it.
- Allow time for the patient to jot down important points.
- Repeat key concepts frequently; if the patient does not understand, try rephrasing the concept.
- Use bold-type printed materials with a white or yellow background.
- Leave printed materials that are illustrated with simple drawings and that are not crowded with text.
- Printed materials should be written at a fifth- to tenth-grade reading level depending on the patient.
- If the patient becomes frustrated or distracted, stop the session and reschedule it.
- Summarize what has been taught and what has been learned at the end of the session.

The patient and significant others, staff nurses, health care providers, diabetic specialist, nurse educator, dietitian, podiatrist, and periodontist are all involved in the educational process. Because of frequent updates and changes in diabetes management, all persons responsible for the care of diabetic patients should read and continue to study and learn about the current protocols.

■ Evaluation

For a patient with diabetes, the learning that has taken place and compliance with the treatment regimen are the essential components. Monitor A1C and fructosamine assay levels to determine the degree of control of blood glucose. Question the patient about exercise and diet and give feedback. Observe demonstrations of learned skills for insulin injection, proper foot care, dietary planning, and glucose monitoring. If the expected outcomes are not being met, the nursing care plan must be revised. Collaboration with the health care provider and dietitian are necessary to design or redesign a plan that is effective.

Complications

In general, people with diabetes are susceptible to two types of complications: short-term (acute) problems and long-term problems.

Short-Term Problems. Acute complications arise when the blood glucose suddenly becomes either too high (hyperglycemia) or too low (hypoglycemia) (see Table 38-6).

 Safety Alert

Hyperglycemia or Hypoglycemia

When there is doubt as to whether the patient is suffering from hyperglycemia or hypoglycemia, treatment is begun for hypoglycemia until a blood glucose determination is obtained to prevent brain damage from extremely low cerebral glucose levels.

When a patient is admitted to the hospital with hyperglycemia, decisions about the proper modes of therapy are based on whether the patient has type 1 or type 2 diabetes and the presence of objective and subjective symptoms. Type 1 diabetes is more likely to be complicated by ketoacidosis, whereas type 2 diabetic patients may suffer hyperglycemic hyperosmolar nonketotic syndrome (HHNS; HHNC, HNKC, and HHNK are also common abbreviations).

Diabetic ketoacidosis. Diabetic ketoacidosis (DKA) is a serious condition caused by incomplete metabolism of fats due to an absence or insufficient supply of insulin. When insulin is not present in adequate amounts to meet metabolic needs, the body breaks down protein and fat for energy. This produces an abundance of the by-products of fat metabolism, which are potent organic acids called *ketones.* In an attempt to rid itself of excess ketones, the body excretes some via the lungs. This produces a characteristic fruity odor to the breath. Acetone, a ketone body, is excreted in the urine, causing acetonuria or ketonuria. As the kidney excretes excess glucose and ketones, it also eliminates large quantities of water and electrolytes. These pathologic changes are responsible for metabolic acidosis, dehydration, and electrolyte imbalances.

Signs and symptoms of DKA can be life threatening and are listed in Table 38-6. Intravenous (IV) fluids are administered first, then electrolyte imbalances are addressed in conjunction with an insulin drip. Electrolytes, especially potassium, and serum glucose are monitored closely. **The goals of treatment are to restore the normal pH of the blood and other body fluids, correct the fluid and electrolyte imbalance, lower the blood glucose level gradually, and provide life-support measures as necessary if the patient is comatose.** Infection is the most frequent cause of DKA; however, other causes include poor compliance with the prescribed regimen of diet and insulin therapy and insulin pump failure. After the patient is stabilized, the underlying cause must be determined and treatment or corrective measures implemented.

Clinical Cues

If you suspect a patient is in DKA, immediately ensure that there is at least one patent IV access and anticipate an order for IV therapy.

Hyperglycemic hyperosmolar nonketotic syndrome.
Hyperglycemic hyperosmolar nonketotic syndrome (HHNS) occurs in people with type 2 diabetes who experience high blood glucose levels because of illness or added stress, such as infection. Glucose levels between 600 and 1000 mg/dL are not unusual; in some cases the blood glucose can reach well over 1000 mg/dL. The extremely high level of glucose in the blood causes severe dehydration and circulating fluid volume depletion. Blood osmolality is considerably elevated (greater than 350 mOsm/kg). HHNS is different from DKA because a small amount of circulating insulin remains available, resulting in the absence of ketosis and acidosis. Because ketosis and acidosis are absent, the gastrointestinal symptoms do not occur and the patient does not seek early medical care in the course of illness. The patient's mental state may progress from confusion to complete coma. Also—in contrast to DKA—the HHNS patient may suffer generalized or focal seizures.

Elder Care Points

Older adults are at greater risk for HHNS, as they become dehydrated more quickly than do younger patients. HHNS may be the first indicator that the patient has diabetes. HHNS most frequently occurs after a febrile illness or gastrointestinal flu, during which the patient has stopped eating properly and possibly has discontinued oral hypoglycemic agents.

Things that may precipitate HHNS in a person with type 2 diabetes are (1) medications, such as steroids, thiazides, phenytoin, and beta blockers; (2) acute illnesses, such as infection, myocardial infarction, and trauma; (3) chronic illnesses, such as cerebrovascular accident, and psychiatric illnesses, such as dementia; and (4) treatments, such as total parenteral nutrition and peritoneal dialysis.

Treatment of HHNS focuses on fluid replacement and correction of electrolyte imbalances. Because fluid replacement will initially be rapid, cardiovascular status and lung sounds must be assessed frequently. Small amounts of insulin may be used until the patient is stabilized. Blood glucose and intake and output must be monitored closely. The underlying illness that triggered the HHNS must be identified and treated. HHNS can be fatal, and mortality risk is directly correlated with higher elevations of blood glucose and the resultant severity of dehydration.

Rebound hyperglycemia. Rebound hyperglycemia, also known as the *Somogyi effect*, follows a period of hypoglycemia, often during sleep. When hypoglycemia occurs, the body secretes glucagon, epinephrine, growth hormone, and cortisol to counteract the effects of low blood sugar. The patient may report nightmares and night sweats along with morning elevated serum glucose; if the patient increases the insulin dose, it worsens the problem.

The Somogyi effect is diagnosed by checking blood sugars during the night; once verified, the usual treatment is to lower the insulin dosage or move the time of the intermediate-acting insulin to bedtime. Changing or increasing the bedtime snack also helps.

The *dawn phenomenon* is characterized by elevated blood glucose in the morning. The dawn phenomenon is caused by release of growth hormone, glucagons, and epinephrine during the night, as part of the body's natural circadian rhythm. These hormones act to raise the body's blood sugar. The dawn phenomenon is the reason why most people with diabetes do not tolerate carbohydrates well in the morning. The treatment is an intermediate-acting insulin at night.

Hypoglycemia. The word *hypoglycemia* means low blood glucose. Hypoglycemia is a common complication of type 1 diabetes mellitus. Most often it is a response to either too large a dose of insulin or too much exercise in relation to the amount of food eaten. People with diabetes must be taught to monitor for the signs and symptoms of hypoglycemia: tremulousness, hunger, headache, pallor, sweating, palpitations, blurred vision, and weakness. Symptoms may progress to confusion and loss of consciousness. Individual reactions vary considerably. Some patients are alert with a glucose level of 40 mg/dL, whereas others at this level are comatose.

Treatment depends on the degree of hypoglycemia and level of consciousness. If the patient is alert enough to tolerate oral intake safely, glucose levels of 40 to 60 mg/dL respond to ingestion of food such as milk, crackers, or juice. Glucose levels of 20 to 40 mg/dL respond best to concentrated sugars, such as honey, table sugar, or juice. Patients must be taught how to self-treat hypoglycemia (see Patient Teaching on p. 861). In the hospital, if the person is experiencing seizures or is not alert enough to tolerate oral intake safely or has a very low blood sugar, a solution of 50% glucose is given IV. When an IV access cannot be established, 1 mg of glucagon is administered intramuscularly. The injection is repeated in 15 minutes if symptoms are not resolved.

Long-Term Problems. The long-term consequences of diabetes mellitus are chiefly the result of damage to the large and small blood vessels. Elevated blood glucose levels over a period of years seriously damage blood vessels and the organs they serve. Diabetes is the seventh leading cause of death in the United States for all age groups (Centers for Disease Control and Prevention, 2010). In addition, cardiovascular disease and other causes of death often can be attributed to diabetes.

Patients who have had diabetes for more than 10 years are likely to develop one or more of the complications of the disease. The less closely the blood glucose has been controlled, the more likely the development of cardiovascular, eye, and renal complications. **Improperly treated or untreated diabetes is the leading cause of new blindness, renal failure leading to dialysis, and nontraumatic lower limb amputations.** Although not every person with diabetes will suffer from long-term complications, many will be hospitalized for one reason or another in some later stage of the disease.

Cardiovascular disease. Thickening of the vessels, chiefly the *basement membrane* (thin layer of connective tissue under the epithelium), occurs when blood glucose is elevated over a long period. The vessels of the retina, renal glomeruli, peripheral nerves, muscles, and skin are affected. Larger vessels also are affected, predisposing the patient to atherosclerosis and vascular occlusion. Two out of three people with diabetes die prematurely from heart attack or stroke. In compliance with the Joint Commission Core Measures, aggressive measures should be taken to prevent stroke in patients at risk. This includes considering the use of statins and giving education about how to prevent stroke and recognize symptoms.

Metabolic syndrome. Metabolic syndrome (formerly known as *insulin resistance syndrome*) is the term used to describe a condition whereby a patient has insulin resistance, hypertension, and increased very-low-density lipoprotein (VLDL) and decreased HDL cholesterol concentrations. Metabolic syndrome is induced by poor diet and obesity, which in turn lead to higher levels of circulating insulin. This hyperinsulinemia contributes to vascular damage and stimulates other hormones that cause vasoconstriction and hypertension. Diabetes mellitus and metabolic syndrome create an increased risk of cardiovascular disease (see Chapter 18 for additional information).

A healthy diet that is low in saturated fats, high in fiber, limited in carbohydrates, and contains 15% protein is the primary intervention. Moderate exercise for at least 30 minutes a day or vigorous exercise for 20 minutes three times a week and resistance training are also recommended.

Health Promotion

Skip the Diet Soda

Recent studies have shown that drinking even one diet soda a day is associated with an increased risk of weight gain, impaired glucose control, and metabolic syndrome, as well as a 67% increased risk for diabetes. It is hypothesized that artificial sweeteners may actually increase the desire for high-calorie foods or interfere with the body's ability to estimate need for more food.

Nephropathy. Diabetic nephropathy occurs directly from changes in the renal blood circulation. Factors that influence whether a person with diabetes will develop kidney disease include genetics, blood glucose level, and blood pressure. After years of having

to filter too much blood with elevated blood glucose, the filtering mechanism of the kidney begins to fail, allowing large particles that normally would have been filtered out (such as protein) to exit through the urine. In the early phase, microalbuminuria, there are small amounts of protein in the urine. If nothing is done to prevent further damage, microalbuminuria progresses to a later phase, macroalbuminuria, with large amounts of protein in the urine. Finally, the patient enters end-stage renal disease, and requires either a kidney transplant or hemodialysis to perform the filtering for the kidneys.

Nephropathy can be prevented by keeping tight control of blood glucose. Research has demonstrated that tight blood glucose control reduces the risk of developing microalbuminuria, may prevent people with microalbuminuria from progressing to macroalbuminuria, and can even reverse microalbuminuria.

Peripheral vascular disease. Gangrene, which often leads to amputation, is far more common in people with diabetes. More than 60% of nontraumatic amputations occur among people with diabetes. Vascular changes frequently cause very poor circulation in the feet and lower extremities. Healing of wounds in these areas is difficult because of poor blood supply. Since the diabetic's increased levels of glucose in the blood provide a good medium for bacterial growth, it is harder to eradicate infection. Learning and practicing excellent foot care are essential to prevent

 Patient Teaching

Foot Care

- Inspect each foot daily for cuts, cracks, blisters, abrasions, or discoloration of the toes; report any abnormality to the health care provider. Use a mirror if unable to bend to see the bottom of the foot. Be certain to check between the toes.
- Wash the feet in warm (not hot) water, using mild soap; do not soak the feet as this can cause cracking of the skin.
- Thoroughly dry the feet after washing, paying special attention to drying between the toes. Rub in a nonscented, nonmedicated cream if the skin is dry; do not put the cream between the toes.
- Cut the nails straight across; have corns, calluses, and ingrown nails managed by a podiatrist. Smooth the nails with an emery board after cutting to prevent cuts on the legs from rough nails while sleeping.
- Wear a clean pair of cotton socks each day.
- Wear properly fitted shoes with a firm sole that do not pinch or bind the foot; never walk barefoot.
- Break in new shoes gradually.
- Never wear open sandals or sandals with straps between the toes.
- Use socks and blankets to warm the feet; do not use a heating pad or hot water bottle near them.
- Test the temperature of bath water with wrist or forearm before stepping into the tub or shower.
- Elevate the feet whenever possible to improve circulation.

amputation. Aggressive screening and early intervention could prevent at least 50% of amputations (Bonham, 2007).

Retinopathy. Visual impairment and blindness are common sequelae of diabetes mellitus. The three most common visual problems are diabetic retinopathy, cataracts, and glaucoma. Retinal damage, which can cause visual impairment and blindness, occurs in most people with diabetes within 10 years of diagnosis. Changes in the retinal vessels lead to hemorrhages and to retinal detachment. Recent surgical techniques using photocoagulation of destructive lesions of the retina with laser beams offer hope for preserving sight by preventing progress of diabetic retinopathy. Tight glucose control, frequent eye examinations, and treatment can help preserve vision.

Diabetic neuropathy. Approximately 60% to 70% of people with diabetes have mild to severe neuropathy. Pathologic changes in the nervous system cause deterioration, with symptoms such as paresthesia, numbness, and loss of function. Diabetic neuropathy primarily affects the peripheral nerves, causing sexual impotence in the male, constipation, neurogenic bladder, and pain or anesthesia (lack of feeling) in the lower extremities. It is for this reason that foot care and daily inspection of the feet are so important. Because the patient often cannot feel cuts, blisters, or abrasions on the foot, there is great danger that a neglected sore might become infected. Although it may be mild at the beginning, eventually partial or almost total anesthesia of the affected part creates a potential for serious injury without awareness. In contrast, some patients experience debilitating pain and hyperesthesia; some lose deep-tendon reflexes. Other problems related to diabetic neuropathies are the result of autonomic nervous system involvement. These include orthostatic hypotension, delayed gastric emptying or gastroparesis, diarrhea or constipation, and asymptomatic retention of urine in the bladder.

 Complementary and Alternative Therapies

Acupuncture for Neuropathy

"Acupuncture has shown some benefit in managing the pain associated with diabetic neuropathy" (Moquin et al., 2009, p. 201).

HYPOGLYCEMIA

Etiology and Pathophysiology

The organs involved in meeting the challenge of carbohydrate ingestion include the intestines, liver, and pancreas (specifically, the beta cells that produce insulin). Thus any condition affecting these organs and their systems can lead to hypoglycemia. Examples other than diabetes mellitus include gastrectomy and surgical bypass procedures. These types of surgery provide more rapid access of glucose to the absorptive sites in the small bowel. Tumors of the pancreas (insulinomas), liver disease, and disorders of the adrenal cortex and pituitary gland can also produce abnormally low blood glucose levels. People who abuse alcohol and other substances are also prone to hypoglycemia.

Functional hypoglycemia, for which there is no known cause, may be a very early indicator of diabetes mellitus. In fact, studies have shown that almost one third of the people who have functional hypoglycemia may eventually develop diabetes if the hypoglycemia is not effectively controlled.

Signs and Symptoms

Signs and symptoms of hypoglycemia include rapid heartbeat, tremulousness, weakness, anxiety, nervousness, and hunger. Symptoms can occur rather suddenly, within 4 hours after a meal is eaten. Some physiologic symptoms may be mistaken for indications of a psychiatric illness. These symptoms include irritability, personality change, temper tantrums, and other psychoneurotic manifestations.

Diagnosis and Treatment

Diagnosis of hypoglycemia is done with measurement of blood sugar values. The patient's insulin levels and C-peptide levels can also be measured. The diagnosis may be made using a glucose tolerance test or a medically supervised fast. Computed tomography (CT) scan, ultrasound, and other diagnostics may be used if an insulinoma (insulin-secreting tumor) is suspected.

Hypoglycemia is treated by modifying eating patterns. Smaller and more frequent meals that are relatively free of simple sugars are recommended. The diet should be high in proteins and low in carbohydrates, and carbohydrates should be complex ones, such as those found in fruits, vegetables, and whole grains. Refined sugar and white flour are omitted. Cases in which gastric surgery and intestinal bypass are believed to be the cause of hypoglycemia may be treated with drugs that reduce intestinal motility.

Complications

Untreated fasting hypoglycemia can lead to severe neuroglycopenia (shortage of glucose in the brain) and possibly death.

Nursing Management

In addition to information about the patient's physical and mental symptoms, assessment should include a detailed history of eating habits. Does the patient eat regularly? How often during each day? What kinds of foods constitute a typical meal? Does she crave sweets? Have there been episodes of weakness, sweating, visual disturbances, and confusion or inability to concentrate? If these symptoms have occurred, when are they most noticeable (i.e., in a fed or fasting state)? Nursing interventions for patients with hypoglycemia include explaining the nature of the disorder and the need for diagnostic testing, objective observation and reporting of symptoms, and reinforcement of dietary instruction and restrictions.

COMMUNITY CARE

One major objective of *Healthy People 2020* is to "increase the proportion of persons with diabetes who receive formal diabetes education." Nurses play a crucial role in home care, and in teaching the elderly population who have diabetes. If nurses could follow the progress of these patients over the years with good assessments and implement ongoing patient education programs, the incidence of complications could certainly be decreased.

Long-term care nurses must be alert to the signs of diabetes. When a resident does not properly recover from a viral illness, in-depth assessment for signs of diabetes is proactive. Home care and clinic nurses must be persistent in assessing compliance with diabetic regimens and must also be instrumental in teaching the public about the signs and symptoms of diabetes and self-care to prevent complications (see Online Resources). At present, diabetes is costing the United States more than $132 billion a year in health care expenditures. This is an area where nurses can be instrumental in cutting health care costs.

Get Ready for the NCLEX® Examination!

Key Points

- Diabetes mellitus involves a disturbance in glucose metabolism. Type 1 diabetes usually appears at a young age, and the patient requires insulin for life. Type 2 diabetes usually develops later in life, but is now being diagnosed more frequently in younger people. Gestational diabetes may occur in pregnancy. Patients with LADA may be initially misdiagnosed with type 2 diabetes; recommendations are to start insulin within 1 year of diagnosis.
- The goal in diabetes is to maintain blood glucose and lipid levels within normal limits to prevent complications.
- The cornerstone of therapy for people with diabetes is diet and exercise. Insulin must be taken for type 1 diabetes; OHAs (and insulin) may be prescribed for type 2.
- The diet plan provides optimal nutrition and calories to maintain normal body weight and allows adjustments to food intake to keep blood glucose within safe limits.
- The emotional and physical stress of surgery and illness can increase the blood glucose level and alter the amounts of medication needed.
- Basal insulin is the amount of insulin that would normally be produced by the pancreas throughout the day.
- A bolus or "correction" dose of short- or rapid-acting insulin is used to manage elevations in blood glucose and bring the next blood glucose into range.
- DKA is a serious condition caused by incomplete metabolism of fats due to the absence of insulin marked by metabolic acidosis, dehydration, and electrolyte imbalances.
- HHNS occurs in people with type 2 diabetes because of illness or stress. Glucose levels are often between 600 and 1000 mg/dL, leading to severe dehydration.

- Hypoglycemia is often a response to either too much insulin or too much exercise. Monitor for hypoglycemia after insulin injections.
- If there is doubt whether the patient is suffering from hyperglycemia or hypoglycemia, treat for hypoglycemia until you obtain a blood glucose level.
- The long-term consequences of diabetes mellitus result from damage to large and small blood vessels. Cardiovascular disease, nephropathy, peripheral vascular disease, retinopathy, and neuropathy can all be reduced by strict blood glucose control.

Additional Learning Resources

SG Go to your Study Guide for additional learning activities to help you master this chapter content.

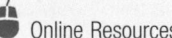 Go to your Evolve website (http://evolve.elsevier.com/deWit/medsurg) for the following FREE learning resources:
- Animations, audio, and video
- Answers and rationales for questions and activities
- Concept Map Creator
- Glossary with pronunciations in English and Spanish
- Interactive Review Questions and Exercises and more!

Online Resources
- American Diabetes Association, www.diabetes.org
- American Dietetic Association, www.eatright.org
- *Diabetes Forecast* magazine, http://forecast.diabetes.org
- Joslin Diabetes Center, www.joslin.org
- National Guideline Clearinghouse http://guideline.gov/content.aspx?f=rss&id=34168

Review Questions for the NCLEX® Examination

1. A 30-year-old woman is admitted for urinary tract infection. A urinalysis reveals presence of ketones, glucose, and nitrates. Which question would the nurse ask to further assess possible diabetes mellitus?
   1. "Have you noticed an extra roundness to your face?"
   2. "Have you had more gas or abdominal bloating?"
   3. "Have you been thirstier than usual? Do you find you urinate more now?"
   4. "Have you experienced any pain or discomfort with urination?"

2. Which teaching technique(s) would be most useful for the older diabetic patient? (Select all that apply.)
   1. Set a time for the teaching session that is agreeable to the patient.
   2. Invite the patient to join a teaching session for new diabetic patients.
   3. Allow time for the patient to jot down important points.
   4. Use bold-type printed materials with a white type on a dark blue or black background.
   5. Keep the sessions at a limit of 1 to 2 hours and give frequent breaks.
   6. Teach all necessary information in one session.
   7. Repeat key concepts frequently; if the patient does not understand, try rephrasing the concept.

3. A patient newly diagnosed with diabetes is given diet instructions. What should the nurse do to effectively motivate the patient to comply with dietary recommendations? (Select all that apply.)
   1. Emphasize good food choices.
   2. Apply diet prescriptions to patient-preferred foods.
   3. Instill guilt to self-regulate when "cheating" occurs.
   4. Focus on the benefits of diet compliance.
   5. Involve meal preparers in diet teaching.

4. A 50-year-old woman was recently diagnosed with type 2 diabetes mellitus and desires to start a healthy lifestyle to control her disease. What is the initial recommendation that the nurse should make?
   1. Encourage brisk walking.
   2. Lose 10 to 15 pounds.
   3. Ensure adequate glucose control.
   4. Develop an exercise schedule.

5. The nurse is supervising a nursing student who is performing foot care for a diabetic patient. The nurse would intervene if the student:
   1. inspects the feet for cuts, cracks, blisters, abrasions, or discolorations.
   2. washes the feet in warm water using a mild soap and dries between each toe.
   3. applies a pair of clean white socks after bathing.
   4. places a protective cover between a heating pad and feet and uses the lowest setting.

6. A patient who works as a personal trainer is diagnosed with insulin-dependent diabetes. What should the nurse teach regarding self-administration of regular insulin?
   1. If you have a strenuous workout, skip your insulin for the day.
   2. Inject the insulin before moderate exercise.
   3. Exercise during the insulin peak of action.
   4. Use the abdomen as an insulin injection site.

7. The home health nurse is visiting an elderly patient who has successfully managed her type 2 diabetes for years. During the visit, the nurse notes that the patient has severe arthritis, poor vision, and several dry, red areas on the lower extremities. What is the priority nursing diagnosis?
   1. Risk for noncompliance related to social circumstances
   2. Risk for ineffective self-health management related to aging
   3. Risk for infection related to poor peripheral perfusion
   4. Risk for disturbed sensory perception related to degenerative changes

8. The nursing assistant informs the nurse that the diabetic patient's blood glucose reading is 750 mg/dL. What is the nurse's priority action?
   1. Immediately notify the RN and the health care provider.
   2. Assess the patient for responsiveness and ketoacidosis.
   3. Check the record to verify if the patient has type 1 or type 2 diabetes.
   4. Ensure that there is at least one patent IV access.

9. The nursing assistant tells you that a known diabetic patient has a blood glucose level of 60 mg/dL. What symptoms would the nurse be most likely to observe with this glucose level?
   1. Confusion, tremulousness, pallor, sweating, and weakness
   2. Dry, flushed skin and mild irritability
   3. Deep, rapid breathing and abdominal pain
   4. Incoherent moaning, combativeness, and seizure activity

10. During a routine checkup, the health care provider tells the diabetic patient that tests results reveal microalbuminuria. Which long-term complication is specific to this test result?
    1. Metabolic syndrome
    2. Nephropathy
    3. Retinopathy
    4. Peripheral vascular disease

Critical Thinking Activities

Scenario A

Mrs. Lopez is 42 years old and has had type 2 diabetes mellitus for the past 10 years. She is admitted to the hospital for treatment of an infection of the great toe on her left foot, which is the result of improper care of an ingrown toenail. She is 45 lb overweight and admits to frequent binges of eating foods not on her diet. She does not exercise regularly because she says the housework she does gives her enough exercise. When asked about the OHA and diet that have been prescribed for her, she tells you that she only takes her medicine and follows her diet "most of the time."

1. Describe the essential components of a teaching plan for Mrs. Lopez to help her manage her illness better. Why is foot care an important part of this plan?

2. What could you suggest to Mrs. Lopez to help her lose weight?

3. What do you think might motivate Mrs. Lopez to accept more responsibility for managing her illness?

4. What laboratory testing would be recommended to track Mrs. Lopez's compliance with her treatment regimen?

Scenario B

Mr. Tobin is a 22-year-old construction worker who has recently experienced fatigue, excessive thirst and urination, and weight loss. A routine urinalysis revealed glycosuria and a trace of acetone. His health care provider has arranged for Mr. Tobin to have additional diagnostic testing to determine if he has diabetes mellitus.

1. If Mr. Tobin is found to have type 1 diabetes mellitus, what kind of information will he need to manage his illness?

2. How would you explain the importance of good or tight control of his blood glucose levels to Mr. Tobin?

3. What criteria could be used to determine whether his diabetes is under control?

Scenario C

Mr. Smith is 76 years old and has recently been diagnosed with type 2 diabetes mellitus. It has been difficult to control his blood sugar and his health care provider has added insulin to his treatment regimen. Mr. Smith was issued a glucometer by the hospital but says that the test strips are too expensive for him to buy very often. Mr. Smith lives alone, cooks for himself, and likes a glass of wine with dinner. Other than an occasional fishing trip, he does not exercise regularly.

1. How would you approach a teaching program for this patient?

2. What resources could you suggest that might assist him to purchase the test strips for the glucometer?

3. How can a glass of wine be incorporated into an acceptable meal plan for a patient with diabetes?

4. What sort of exercise program could you recommend to this patient?

Scenario D

You are making a home visit to a patient who normally administers her own insulin. On arrival you notice that she has tremulousness, is pale and sweating, and she seems more irritable and distractible than usual. She reports taking her insulin, but she is unable to tell you when she took it, or exactly how much she injected. She thinks her last food was during supper, last night, but she is unsure.

1. You check her blood glucose level with her home device and get a reading of 55 mg/dL. What does this value indicate?

2. Based on your assessment of the patient's symptoms and the blood glucose level, what is your next nursing action?

3. How will you determine that it is safe to leave the patient?

chapter

39

Care of Women with Reproductive Disorders

evolve

http://evolve.elsevier.com/deWit/medsurg

Objectives

Theory

1. Identify the female reproductive organs and their role in the overall health of the individual.
2. Describe normal physiology and age-related changes in the female reproductive system.
3. Discuss common menstrual disorders and their nursing interventions.
4. Explore methods of contraception.
5. Review causes and treatment of infertility.
6. List changes associated with menopause, its treatment options, and appropriate nursing interventions.
7. Explain the screening procedures recommended for maintaining reproductive health.

8. Compare and contrast benign and malignant disorders of the female reproductive system.
9. Understand the role of robotic gynecologic surgery as an alternative to open surgery.
10. Discuss the nurse's role during screening procedures, data collection, and education of women concerning reproductive health.

Clinical Practice

1. Teach techniques of breast self-examination and vulvar self-examination to a patient.
2. Plan the nursing care of a woman with a reproductive disorder.
3. Describe the causes of and interventions for common disorders of the female reproductive tract.

Key Terms

amenorrhea (ă-měn-ŏ-RĒ-ă, p. 904)
anovulation (ăn-ŎV-ū-LĀ-shŭn, p. 905)
climacteric (klī-MĂK-těr-ĭk, p. 882)
cystocele (SĬS-tō-sēl, p. 903)
dowager's hump (p. 891)
dysmenorrhea (dĭs-měn-ō-RĒ-ă, p. 902)
dyspareunia (dĭs-pă-RŪ-nē-ă, p. 890)
effleurage (ĕf-lū-RĂZH, p. 902)
endometriosis (ĕn-dō-mē-trē-Ō-sĭs, p. 906)
enterocele (ĕn-TĚR-ō-sēl, p. 903)
fibroids (FĪ-broydz, p. 905)
hirsutism (HĚR-sūt-ĭszm, p. 904)
hysterectomy (hĭs-těr-ĔK-tō-mē, p. 903)
lymphedema (lĭm-fĕ-DĒ-mă, p. 913)
menarche (mĕ-NĂR-kē, p. 882)

menopause (MĚN-ō-păwz, p. 882)
menorrhagia (měn-ō-RĀ-jă, p. 904)
menses (měn-sēz, p. 882)
menstruation (měn-strū-Ā-shŭn, p. 882)
metrorrhagia (mĕ-trō-RĀ-jă, p. 904)
mittelschmerz (MĬT-ĕl-shmārts, p. 883)
myomectomy (mī-ō-MĚK-tŏ-mē, p. 905)
oligomenorrhea (ŏl-ĭ-gō-měn-ŏ-RĒ-ă, p. 904)
polycystic ovarian syndrome (pŏ-lē-SĬS-tĭk, p. 904)
prolapse (PRŌ-lăps, p. 882)
pruritus (prū-RĪ-tŭs, p. 890)
rectocele (RĚK-tō-sēl, p. 903)
sentinel node biopsy (SĚN-tĭ-nĕl nōd BĪ-ŏp-sē, p. 911)
stress incontinence (STRĚS ĭn-KŎN-tĭ-nĕns, p. 903)

OVERVIEW OF ANATOMY AND PHYSIOLOGY OF THE FEMALE REPRODUCTIVE SYSTEM

WHAT ARE THE PRIMARY EXTERNAL STRUCTURES OF THE FEMALE REPRODUCTIVE SYSTEM?

The *vulva,* or *pudendum,* is the name given to the external female genitalia. It is made up of the following structures:

- The *mons pubis* is a rounded mound of fatty tissue that protects the symphysis pubis. The mons pubis is covered with pubic hair.
- The *labia majora* are two elongated, raised folds of pigmented skin that enclose the vulvar cleft. The pubic hair extends along these folds.
- The *labia minora* are soft folds of skin within the labia majora. They are soft, shiny, and made up of fat tissue and glands, and have no hair follicles.
- The *clitoris* is located at the top of the vulvar cleft, above the urethral opening. It is made up primarily of erectile tissue and is highly sensitive to touch. It is a primary source of pleasurable sensation during sexual activity.
- The *urethral meatus,* or external opening of the urethra of the urinary bladder, is located below the clitoris within the folds of the labia minora.
- The *vaginal vestibule* is situated below the urethral meatus within the labia minora and is the entrance to the vagina.
- The *perineum* is the flat muscular surface lying between the vagina and the anus.

WHAT ARE THE PRIMARY INTERNAL STRUCTURES OF THE FEMALE REPRODUCTIVE SYSTEM?

- The *vagina* is a muscular tube lined with membranous tissue with transverse ridges called rugae. It connects the external and internal female sexual organs (Figure 39-1).
- The *uterus* (womb) is a hollow pear-shaped organ with a thick muscular wall. It lies at the upper end of the vagina. It is capable of expanding to many times its normal size to accommodate a growing fetus. The lower opening of the uterus is the *cervix,* which dilates during labor to allow for delivery of the infant.
- There are two *fallopian tubes* that branch outward from the right and left side at the top of the uterus. They form the pathway for the *ovum* (egg) from the ovary to the uterus.
- There are two *ovaries,* one located near the end of each fallopian tube. These almond-shaped glands excrete estrogen and progesterone into the bloodstream. At birth, the ovaries contain all the eggs (*oocytes*— primitive ova or eggs) the woman will ever produce, approximately 400,000 in each ovary, most of which will never mature for possible fertilization.
- The *bony pelvis,* located at the base of the body between the hips, supports the pelvic organs, including the growing uterus during pregnancy. Uterine support is assisted by the *pelvic floor,* a collection of strong muscles and supportive tissues that brace the pelvis and provide both support and protection for the pelvic organs.

FIGURE 39-1 Female reproductive organs.

WHAT ARE THE ACCESSORY ORGANS OF THE FEMALE REPRODUCTIVE SYSTEM?

The breasts, or *mammary glands,* located on the upper chest, are the accessory organs. They are composed of fibrous, adipose, and glandular tissue, and are responsible for *lactation* (milk production), which provides nourishment for the infant.

WHAT ARE THE PHASES OF THE FEMALE REPRODUCTIVE CYCLE DURING THE CHILDBEARING YEARS?

The *ovarian cycle* has two phases:
1. *Follicular phase*—the first 14 days of a 28-day cycle. *Follicle-stimulating hormone (FSH)* and *luteinizing hormone (LH)* stimulate the maturing of immature ova in preparation for fertilization. Estrogen peaks when the ovum is released *(ovulation)* about 14 days before the next menstrual period. The ovum lives up to 24 hours after fertilization.
2. *Luteal phase*—the 15th to 28th days of the cycle. LH and progesterone are the primary hormones in this phase. The blood supply to the uterus increases in preparation for possible implantation of a fertilized ovum. If fertilization and implantation do not occur, the lining of the uterus will degrade and be shed during menstruation, and the cycle begins again.

The *menstrual cycle* has four phases that are described in Box 39-1.

Box 39-1   Stages of the Menstrual Cycle

FIRST TO FIFTH DAYS
Stage I: Menstrual Stage (Dismantling Stage)
1. Endometrium sloughs away as menstrual flow begins.
2. Progesterone and estrogen are no longer secreted.
3. New follicle starts to mature.

SIXTH TO FOURTEENTH DAYS
Stage II: Growth and Repair (Estrogen or Proliferative Stage)
1. Follicle grows and egg matures.
2. Endometrium returns to normal state and then begins to thicken in response to estrogen.
Stage III
Ovulation occurs 14 days before menses, regardless of length of menstrual cycle. It takes place when follicle ruptures and releases egg. If pregnancy does not occur, the corpus luteum deteriorates, estrogen and progesterone decline, and the thickened tissue on the endometrium of the uterus is sloughed off and is discharged via the vagina as a menstrual "period."

FIFTEENTH TO TWENTY-EIGHTH DAYS
Stage IV: Secretory Stage (Postovulatory or Progesterone Stage)
1. Corpus luteum secretes progesterone.
2. Endometrium continues to thicken in response to estrogen and progesterone. Prepares to receive fertilized ovum.

WHEN DOES SEXUAL DEVELOPMENT OCCUR IN THE FETUS?

During the first weeks of pregnancy, the male and female sexual organs are undifferentiated. After the 7th week, rapid changes occur. By the 12th week the external genitalia are formed and fully differentiated as male or female, as dictated by the union on the XX or XY chromosomes at conception. The internal structures also are forming during this period.

WHAT CHANGES TAKE PLACE AS GIRLS MATURE INTO WOMEN AND BECOME CAPABLE OF REPRODUCTION?

The period of sexual maturation is called *puberty.* It usually occurs between ages 9 and 17 years for girls, with the average onset being 12 years of age. It involves a period of accelerated growth, then the hips begin to widen and the breasts begin to develop. Axillary and pubic hair appears. Puberty is completed by the onset of the menstrual cycle, or **menses.** The beginning of menstruation is called **menarche. Menstruation** (shedding of the uterine lining) will continue at intervals of approximately 4 weeks throughout the childbearing years except when pregnancy occurs.

WHAT CHANGES TAKE PLACE AS A WOMAN ENTERS MENOPAUSE?

Toward the end of the childbearing years, women enter the phase known as the **climacteric.** The menses become irregular in both pattern and flow and eventually cease altogether. **Menopause** has occurred when the menses have completely ceased for at least 12 months.

WHAT CHANGES OCCUR WITH AGING?

After menopause, some atrophy of the female organs, loss of elasticity, dryness of the vaginal membranes, and reduction of bone mass occur because of the decrease in estrogen levels. Loss of natural tissue elasticity may allow internal organs to sag, or **prolapse,** into the vagina.

Reproductive health can be disrupted by a variety of disorders, such as infertility, spontaneous abortion, premature labor, infection, and the growth of abnormal tissue, including cancerous and noncancerous tumors. As the childbearing years draw to a close, hormone production slows until the reproductive cycle ceases altogether. Nursing care of patients with diseases of the female reproductive system is further complicated by the emotional effects of such disorders. The reproductive organs represent the biologic aspect of sexual identity, and women may feel their personal identity is threatened by disorders of this system.

THE FEMALE REPRODUCTIVE SYSTEM

MENSTRUATION

During the first year following menarche, the menstrual cycle may be somewhat irregular, but by the second year a regular cycle of approximately 28 days is normally established.

Attitudes and ideas regarding menstruation are formed early. They are based on the thoughts and beliefs expressed by other women and on personal experience. Incorrect perceptions about this normal process may increase physical discomfort or cause the young woman unnecessary embarrassment or fear. It is important that the nurse understand her own attitudes about sexuality and the reproductive process, before attempting to provide information to women about these sensitive issues. The nurse should encourage a healthy view of menarche as a natural physiologic process marking reproductive maturity.

Normal Menstrual Bleeding

Menstrual blood consists of shed endometrial tissue, blood, mucus, and vaginal and cervical cells. Shedding of the uterine lining occurs during the menstrual cycle at intervals of approximately 4 weeks, and produces bleeding. Menstrual bleeding occurs about 14 days after ovulation and lasts between 2 and 8 days. The amount of actual blood loss is only 40 to 80 mL. Blood flow may be heavy at first, but gradually reduces to spotting. The color may change from bright red to brown and the blood may have a musty odor. Once a menstrual pattern is established, a change from this pattern is reason to consult a health care provider. The length of the menstrual cycle can be influenced by stress, drugs, nutrition, or illness. Women should be encouraged to keep a calendar of their individual menstrual cycle to determine regularity and to recognize deviations. Mild cramping may occur, and some mood swings may be associated with the hormonal changes. Mittelschmerz is a sharp pain in the right or left lower quadrant, sometimes felt at the midcycle around the time of ovulation; the pain may last a few hours. Some women are sensitive to this phenomenon, and others never experience it.

Normal Vaginal Discharge

The vagina is a warm, moist, dark vault in which microorganisms can flourish. Normal vaginal secretions contain cervical mucus, endometrial fluid, exudate from Bartholin's glands and Skene's ducts, and products of normal flora. An increase in secretions normally occurs during pregnancy and at the midpoint of the menstrual cycle when ovulation occurs, and a decrease in secretions normally occurs after menopause. The main line of defense against infection is lactic acid, which causes an acidic pH. Any change in this pH can result in infection.

Normal vaginal discharge has an off-white color and is without odor. If the vaginal discharge develops an odor, changes color or consistency, or causes irritation or burning of the vaginal mucosa, a health care provider should be consulted.

NORMAL BREASTS

Breasts are made of adipose tissue, milk-producing glands called lobules, ducts, and fibrous tissue that rest on the chest muscle. They may not be completely symmetrical (one may be slightly larger than the other) and may feel a bit lumpy and tender, especially during the middle of the menstrual cycle. Age, pregnancy, medication, and diet can affect the way the breasts feel. As the woman ages, the denseness and adipose tissue content decreases. Birth control pills, hormone replacement therapy, and pregnancy may cause the breasts to increase in size.

CONTRACEPTION AND FERTILITY

Many women start sexual relationships and risk pregnancy before they are ready to have children. Other women give birth, and do not wish to bear more children. For these groups of women, information concerning techniques of contraception is essential to prevent unwanted, unintended pregnancies. Many sexually active women of childbearing age are concerned about regulating, planning, or preventing pregnancy. With the assistance of a health care provider, they can select the birth control method best suited to their physical health, sexual activity, desire to have children at a future date, cultural and religious beliefs about family regulation, and lifestyle.

Contraceptive Options

Women should make an informed decision concerning methods of reliable birth control, and nurses are responsible for providing comprehensive education concerning the advantages, limitations, and side effects of the various contraceptive drugs and devices (Table 39-1). Some methods of birth control provide protection against sexually transmitted infections (STIs), but some do not. Newer contraceptive regimens reduce the hormone-free interval, thereby decreasing the occurrence of menstrual periods. The best contraceptive methods for young adults are abstinence, the use of planned contraception, the correct use of condoms to prevent STIs (Figure 39-2), and lifestyle counseling.

Oral Contraceptives

Oral contraceptives (OCs) are the most popular method of reversible hormonal contraception. OCs are effective if used properly, and offer noncontraceptive benefits—relief from breast tenderness, bloating, and premenstrual syndrome (PMS) symptoms—but OCs have contraindications and cautions for use (Samra-

Text continued on p. 887

Table 39-1   Methods of Contraception

HOW METHOD WORKS	SIDE EFFECTS/PRECAUTIONS	DEGREE OF EFFECTIVENESS
Abstinence		
Sexual contact avoided.	Reliable method of preventing pregnancy and STIs.	100%
Fertility Awareness Methods		
Basal body temperature (BBT) BBT is measured and charted daily on awakening. Coitus is avoided on the day of temperature rise and for 3 subsequent days.	Temperature must be taken before any activity, or it will rise above its basal level. The special thermometer should be kept at bedside.	80%-90% for all fertility awareness methods if done correctly
Calendar or rhythm method Woman charts her monthly menstrual cycle on a calendar and avoids intercourse during fertile period.	Not effective for woman with irregular menstrual cycles. Several months of charting are necessary to establish clear pattern of menstrual cycle.	Fertility awareness methods that monitor multiple parameters (e.g., symptothermal method) may be more effective, but most important aspect of success is faithful adherence to the method; also, the woman must feel comfortable enough with her body to make the necessary observations each month
Ovulation or Billings method Cervical mucus changes are assessed. During ovulation, mucus is clear with high stretchability ("egg white" consistency). Degree of stretch is tested by pinching a small amount of cervical mucus between the thumb and forefinger and stretching it between them (called *spinnbarkeit*). During ovulation, mucus smeared on a glass slide will dry into a "fern" pattern.	Woman must feel very comfortable with her body and confident in her ability to detect and assess changes.	
Symptothermal method Variety of parameters are recorded, including cervical mucus changes, BBT pattern, *mittelschmerz* (brief sharp abdominal pain that may occur with ovulation), increased libido (sexual drive).	More effective for women with regular menstrual cycles. Requires significant accurate record keeping.	
Chemical predictor test A test kit that contains a chemically treated strip that will turn color when estrogen or luteal hormone levels are present in urine.	Increase in hormone levels occurs 12-24 hr before ovulation.	
Mechanical or Barrier Contraception		
Intrauterine device (IUD) A small, sterile, flexible plastic device that is inserted by a physician into the uterus. Can be a copper device (ParaGard) or a device containing the hormone levonorgestrel (Mirena). Can provide 5 yr of protection.	May increase menstrual flow or cause cramping or low back pain. Increased incidence of PID in women with multiple sex partners, women whose partners have multiple partners, and women with previous incidence of PID. Patient must check placement by feeling for string once each month.	Up to 99% effective; must be removed by health care provider

Data from Hacker, N., Gambone, J., & Habel, C./ (2010). *Essentials of Obstetrics and Gynecology,* 5th Ed., Philadelphia: Saunders., Hatcher, R., Trussell, A., Nelson, W., et al. (2007). *Contraceptive Technology* (19th ed.). New York: Ardent Media; Yranski, P., & Gamache, M. (2009). New options for barrier contraceptives, *JOGNN* 37 (3):384-389; Fischer, M. (2009). Implanon: a new contraceptive implant, *JOGNN* 34(3):361-368; Fontenot, H., & Harris, A. (2009). Latest advances in hormonal contraception, *JOGNN* 34(3):369-371; Fantasia, H. (2009). Options for intrauterine contraception, *JOGNN* 34(3):375-379; and Theroux, R. (2009). Hysteroscopic approach to sterilization, *JOGNN* 34(3):356-360.
FDA, Food and Drug Administration; *GI,* gastrointestinal; *PID,* pelvic inflammatory disease; *STIs,* sexually transmitted infections.

Table 39-1	Methods of Contraception—cont'd		
HOW METHOD WORKS		**SIDE EFFECTS/PRECAUTIONS**	**DEGREE OF EFFECTIVENESS**
Mechanical or Barrier Contraception—cont'd			
Male condom A sheath commonly made of latex that is placed over the erect penis before intercourse. Oil-based lubricants such as petroleum jelly can cause latex to break down and reduce effectiveness. Some condoms, made of polyurethane, are compatible with oil-based lubricants.		Inexpensive, readily available, easy to use correctly. *Precautions:* (1) leave space at tip for semen to collect rather than being forced upward out of the condom; (2) store in a cool place, and not for excessively long, to avoid breakage due to aging of the latex or heat damage; (3) handle carefully to avoid spilling semen and possibly introducing it into the vagina.	88%-98% if used properly; use of spermicide increases effectiveness to 98%-99%
Lea's Shield A one-size reusable silicone barrier that is held in place by the vaginal walls. Used with a spermicide and inserted before each intercourse act. Lea's Shield is a one-size prescription and is nonhormonal.		Effectiveness enhanced with use of spermicide. Provides STI protection. Should not be left in place for more than 48 hours or used during menstruation. Woman should urinate before and after insertion.	84%-90%
Female condom Sheath with retaining ring that is placed in the vagina before intercourse. Open end with large entrance ring extends outside the vagina. Can be inserted up to 8 hr before intercourse.		The penis must remain inside the sheath, not between the sheath and the vaginal wall. Acceptance of the method has been slow as it is more expensive and more difficult and time-consuming to place properly than the male condom. Effectiveness enhanced with use of spermicide. Provides protection against STIs.	79%-90%; most failures occur when the penis is withdrawn too far and reenters the vagina beside rather than within the condom
Diaphragm A latex or rubber dome-shaped cup that fits snugly over the cervix. Spermicide is applied to the cervical side of the diaphragm and it is inserted into the vagina so the fitted ring holds it securely in place at the top of the vagina to wall off the cervix. The spermicide enhances effectiveness, should there be a leak around the edge or tear in the diaphragm.		A diaphragm must be fitted professionally and should be refitted annually or with a gain or loss of 7-10 lb, and particularly after pregnancy.	82%-94%
Cervical cap Cervical cap fits over the cervix. Filled with spermicidal jelly and applied over the cervix. Fem Cap is prescription fitted to each woman.		Can be in place up to 48 hr before sexual intercourse. Similar to diaphragm. It is recommended that women void before and after insertion and after intercourse. Should not be used during menstruation.	82%-94%
Vaginal sponge A nonprescription soft polyurethane sponge traps and absorbs semen and has spermicidal properties.		Sponge is moistened with 2 tablespoons of water and squeezed before insertion. Must remain in place 6 hours after intercourse. Prolonged use can increase risk for toxic shock syndrome.	82%-94%

Continued

Table 39-1   Methods of Contraception—cont'd

HOW METHOD WORKS	SIDE EFFECTS/PRECAUTIONS	DEGREE OF EFFECTIVENESS
Spermicidal Methods		
Gels, foams, creams Work by killing sperm within the vagina. Must be applied before intercourse.	Available without prescription. More effective when used as an adjunct to condoms, diaphragms, and caps.	Foam alone, 79%-90%; creams and gels alone, 79%
Hormonal Methods		
Oral contraceptives (OCs) "The pill" contains a combination of synthetic estrogen and progestin, hormones that prevent ovulation and thicken cervical mucus, making it difficult for sperm to travel upward (also true for injectable and timed-release hormonal methods). Traditionally based on a 28-day cycle with 7 hormone-free days that result in monthly menstruation. *Seasonale* is an OC that reduces menstrual periods to 4 times a year. *Lybrel* is an OC that is taken 365 days a year and suspends menstruation indefinitely (FDA approved in 2007).	Prescription required. Must be taken faithfully to be effective. *Precautions:* Not recommended for women older than 35 who smoke, or women with a history of heart or liver disease, breast or uterine cancer, blood clots or venous inflammation, or unexplained vaginal bleeding. At least three regular ovulatory cycles should be evidenced before adolescents start OC use. May cause nausea.	97%-99.9%
"Minipill" Contains a small dose of progesterone and no estrogen. Causes endometrium to be hostile to implantation.		97%-99.9%
Low-dose regimens *Mircette* uses low-dose estrogen for 5 of the 7 traditionally "hormone-free" days, resulting in shorter, lighter menses. *Loestrin 24 Fe* provides 24 days of combined hormones with a 4-day hormone-free interval. *Yasmin* is similar to Loestrin, but has been shown to relieve symptoms of premenstrual dysphoric syndrome. Both approved in 2006.	There is evidence of increased risk of venous thromboembolism in users of OC's containing drosperinone or levonorgestrel (Parken, et al. 2011).	97%-99.9%
Injectable contraceptives (Depo-Provera) Synthetic timed-release progesterone is injected q 12 wk, preventing ovulation.	Injections given in clinic or office. Must be repeated q 12 wk to remain effective. *Precautions:* See oral contraceptives.	99.7%
Sustained-release implants Implanon, a thin, flexible rod containing synthetic hormone, is placed under the skin of the forearm in a minor surgical procedure (replaces Norplant). Effective for 3 yr (FDA approval in 2006).	Small incision required to place and to remove. Less popular now that injection is available. *Precautions:* See oral contraceptives.	98.4%-99.4%
Emergency contraception Taken orally the day following unprotected intercourse, it induces menses and prevents implantation in the uterus.	Not to be used as a routine form of contraception. Women receiving the "morning-after" pill should also get assistance in choosing an effective, ongoing method of contraception.	97%-99.9%

Table 39-1	Methods of Contraception—cont'd		
HOW METHOD WORKS	**SIDE EFFECTS/PRECAUTIONS**	**DEGREE OF EFFECTIVENESS**	
Hormonal Methods—cont'd			
Vaginal ring			
The NuvaRing (etonogestrel and ethinyl estradiol) is a flexible silicone ring inserted into vagina for 3 wk and removed for 1 wk to allow for menstruation.	Leukorrhea and vaginal infection are possible side effects. Other side effects similar to OCs but fewer GI problems since it does not pass through GI tract.	97%-99.9%	
Skin patch			
A transdermal skin patch containing norelgestromin and ethinyl estradiol applied to dry skin of back, buttocks, upper arm, or torso. Replaced each week for 3 wk. Not applied 4th wk to allow for menstruation.	The FDA is investigating evidence that a higher level of estrogen is absorbed during sunbathing or while in saunas, giving rise to increased risk for complications (symptoms similar to OCs). Risk of thromboembolus may be higher than with OCs.	97%-99.9% (may not be effective in obese women: >200 lb [90 kg])	
Delayed menstruation			
Seasonale is an OC that delays menstruation so that the woman experiences four menstrual periods a year. *Seasonique* is an OC that provides 84 days of combined hormones followed by a week of low-dose estrogen rather than a hormone-free interval. The four menstrual periods a year are lighter and with less discomfort.	A popular choice. Requires follow-up research concerning long-term effects.	97%-99.9%	
Permanent Contraception			
Tubal ligation (female) (Surgical or nonsurgical hysteroscopic technique)			
Fallopian tubes are surgically cut or tied to prevent sperm from reaching ovum. Nonsurgical transcervical insertion of an Essure microchip into each fallopian tube causes local inflammation and closure of fallopian tubes.	Sterilization procedures are considered permanent, as reversal may not be effective.	100%	
Vasectomy (male)			
The vas deferens (sperm ducts) are cut and tied to prevent sperm from entering ejaculatory fluid.	Use another form of birth control until two sperm analyses are negative.	100%	

Latif, 2011) (Figure 39-3). The nurse should counsel the woman concerning options, and collect data that can determine which contraceptive choice is best for her. The health care provider assists the woman in making the final choice. Traditional OC regimens are based on a 28-day cycle with a 7-day hormone-free interval that allows for menstruation and gonadotropin levels to rise and for ovarian follicular growth to occur. When the OC cycle is not resumed *on schedule,* the risk of unplanned pregnancy occurs. Newer OCs reduce the hormone-free interval, thereby reducing menstrual discomforts and decreasing risk of contraceptive failure (Borgelt-Hansen, 2011). Seasonale is a popular oral contraceptive that provides delayed menstruation, so that a woman has only four menstrual periods a year (Drug.com, 2011). Another regimen (Lybrel) was approved by the Food and Drug Administration (FDA) in 2007; the regimen involves low-dose combined hormones for 365 days per year without a hormone-free interval, allowing a woman to postpone menstruation indefinitely. The first "four-phasic" OC, estradiol valerate and dienogest (Natazia), was approved in 2010. Natazia provides four dosage combinations of progestin and estrogen hormones during each 28-day cycle.

Clinical Cues

It is important to tell patients that birth control pills and most other birth control methods are not 100% effective in preventing conception. Abstinence is the only 100% effective method to prevent pregnancy.

Emergency Contraception

Known as the "morning-after" pill, emergency contraception is indicated after unprotected intercourse. It is not meant to be used on a regular basis, but was

HOW TO USE A MALE CONDOM

1. Apply condom before any contact with vagina because sperm are present in secretions *before* ejaculation.

2. Squeeze air from the tip of condom, and hold it while unrolling condom over erect penis. Leave a half-inch space at tip.

3. Use water-soluble lubricants, if needed.

4. To remove condom, hold it at the base of penis to prevent spillage as you withdraw from the vagina.

5. Dispose and use a new one each time. Be sure to check expiration date on condoms.

Squeeze air from tip of condom

Hold condom at base of the penis to prevent spillage

A

HOW TO USE A DIAPHRAGM

1. The diaphragm can be inserted up to 4 hours before intercourse. Apply spermicide on the rim and inside the center of diaphragm.

2. Compress diaphragm using thumb and finger of one hand, and use other hand to spread the labia.

3. While squatting (or placing one foot on a chair), insert into vagina with spermicide toward cervix. Direct diaphragm inward and downward behind and below cervix.

4. Tuck the front rim of diaphragm into the pubic bone, and feel cervix through the center of diaphragm.

5. Leave in place at least 6 hours after intercourse.

6. To remove, assume squatting position and bear down. Hook a finger over top rim, and pull diaphragm down and out.

7. Wash diaphragm with mild soap and dry after each use. Dust with cornstarch, if needed, and inspect occasionally for small holes.

B

Begin to insert diaphragm into vagina with spermicide toward cervix

Tuck diaphragm behind the pubic bone

FIGURE 39-2 Proper application of **(A)** a condom, and **(B)** a diaphragm.

developed to decrease the number of unwanted pregnancies and elective abortions. Emergency contraception prevents pregnancy in one of three ways: by preventing ovulation or fertilization, slowing transport of the sperm and egg, or altering the uterine lining to prevent implantation. "Plan B one-step" is one tablet of levonorgestrel only, taken within 72 hours of unprotected sex; the tablet was approved in July 2009 and is available without prescription to women over 17 years

FIGURE 39-3 Contraceptives.

of age. Next Choice, a generic version of the original two-pill plan B contraception, is available by prescription to those age 17 or younger. Ulipristol acetate (Ella) is a one-pill emergency contraceptive that is approved for use for up to 5 days after unprotected sex (Fine, 2010). The American College of Obstetricians and Gynecologists (ACOG) stated in July 2009 that emergency contraception is safe for women of all ages (ACOG, 2009a).

Legal and Ethical Considerations
The "Morning-After" Pill

Although the "morning-after" contraceptive pill can be sold over the counter in most states, there has been considerable unwillingness by certain pharmacists to provide it. The pharmacists claim that dispensing the pill is against their religious principles. It may not be ethical for pharmacists to withhold the medication from a woman because of the pharmacists' personal beliefs.

The woman is advised to take an antiemetic before each dose of emergency contraception to minimize nausea and vomiting. Since emergency contraception is not effective if the woman is already pregnant, failure to menstruate by 21 days after initiation of emergency contraception requires evaluation for pregnancy. There is no evidence that emergency contraception causes abortion, ectopic pregnancy, or fetal anomalies if taken when the woman is already pregnant (Fontenot & Harris, 2008).

A copper intrauterine device (IUD) can be inserted up to 7 days after unprotected sexual intercourse to prevent implantation of the zygote in women who prefer long-term contraception. A woman who seeks emergency contraception should be educated concerning methods of birth control and prevention of STIs.

Infertility
Many women dream of having children but find difficulty in conceiving. For these women, preconception guidance and infertility treatments may be helpful.

Preconception guidance involves gathering data concerning the woman and her partner in order to provide information necessary to make an informed, individualized decision concerning conception or fertility assistance. Screening for genetic disorders may be required.

 ## Cultural Considerations

Fertility

Symbols and rites that celebrate fertility are practiced by many cultures. In the United States, throwing rice at the bride and groom is a wish for family growth. Distributing candy or cigars in celebration of a birth is also common in the United States. In some countries, rubbing the swollen abdomen of a statue of a fertility goddess is a popular practice for women seeking to conceive.

Primary infertility is the inability of the couple to conceive a child after at least 1 year of active, unprotected sexual relations without using contraceptives. *Secondary infertility* is the inability to conceive after having once conceived, or the inability to maintain a pregnancy long enough to deliver a viable infant. Approximately 10% to 20% of American couples have infertility, and today more couples are seeking medical intervention. Infertility services also assist women who wish to have a child without a male partner.

The ability to conceive depends primarily on both partners having normal reproductive physiology, physiologically and psychologically sensitive interaction, and proper timing of intercourse. Factors in the male that contribute to infertility include problems with the sperm, abnormal ejaculation, abnormal erections, and abnormal seminal fluid. Chapter 40 presents a discussion of problems in the male reproductive system. Factors contributing to infertility in a woman include:

- Problems with ovulation
- An abnormality in the pathway between the cervix and fallopian tube
- An abnormality in the endometrium of the uterus, or malformation of the uterus
- Tumors in the reproductive tract
- Vaginal or cervical environment that is inhospitable to sperm motility or viability.

Repeated pregnancy loss can be caused by:

- An abnormality in fetal chromosomes that result in spontaneous abortion
- Abnormalities of the cervix or uterus
- Disorders of the endocrine or immune system
- Infections
- Environmental factors, such as toxic agents

Preconception counseling helps the couple evaluate problems or risks related to conception.

 ## Communication

Emotional Impact of Infertility

The emotional impact of infertility is intense. Some couples become almost desperate to conceive. The nurse should be alert to evidence that psychological intervention may be needed to assist the couple to deal with the stress of their situation. Indications that a referral may be needed may include, but are not limited to, inability to focus on anything other than the desire to have a child, and tension in the relationship of the couple, including blaming each other.

There are many causes of infertility; some involve a problem in the woman, and some in the man. Diagnosis includes a detailed health history and laboratory tests such as serum prolactin levels and other endocrine evaluations, semen analysis, sperm antibody agglutination studies, and chromosome studies. Tests for tubal patency and other possible abnormalities in both the male and female reproductive tract may also be needed.

Nursing Management. Interventions the nurse can discuss with the patient regarding infertility may include nonmedical actions such as:

- Using water-soluble lubricants during intercourse, because these do not have spermicidal properties.
- Recommending that the male partner avoid environments that cause high scrotal temperatures, such as saunas, or using a laptop computer on the lap for long periods, since these can reduce sperm production, as well as the life span of the sperm.
- Using condoms when the woman has an elevated antisperm antibody level. After several months, condoms can be removed during the woman's fertile period.
- Referring the couple for stress management, nutrition counseling, and lifestyle analysis.

Interventions for infertility can also involve medical therapy such as the use of drugs that stimulate ovulation. Drugs to treat thyroid or adrenal problems in the man may enhance spermatogenesis.

 ## Complementary and Alternative Therapies

Herbal Products and Fertility

Since there is widespread use of complementary and alternative medicines (CAMs) such as herbs and oils, women should be instructed that use of herbs and oils such as licorice root, wormwood, fennel, ephedra, goldenseal, flaxseed, pennyroyal, cascara, sage, and periwinkle should be avoided while trying to conceive and carry a pregnancy (Breslin and Lucas, 2003). Herbal products that may be used to promote fertility include nettle leaves, dong quai, and red clover flowers. Vitamin E, calcium, and magnesium supplements have also been used. There is currently no scientific evidence that these herbal products are effective.

Assisted Reproduction. Assisted reproductive therapies (ARTs) (Box 39-2) are available, but are associated with many ethical and legal issues such as the risk for having a multifetal pregnancy, freezing embryos for later use, and the use of a surrogate mother. Micromanipulation allows the removal of a single cell from an embryo for genetic analysis. Defective genes can be replaced. Success rates of ARTs vary, and the procedure is usually expensive and rarely is covered by health insurance. Donor eggs or donor sperm can be used, making future legal challenges for custody a possibility.

MENOPAUSE

Menopause is defined by the World Health Organization as the cessation of menses for 12 consecutive months due to a decrease in estrogen production. The *perimenopausal period* or *climacteric* is the time around the actual cessation of the menstrual cycle. Signs and symptoms of the climacteric and menopause include hot flashes (a sensation of warmth), hot flushes (a visible redness and moistness of the skin), and night sweats due to vasomotor instability resulting from low estrogen levels. These symptoms usually decrease as the woman's body adjusts to the lower level of estrogen. Changes in the menstrual flow and menstrual irregularity require the woman to "be prepared" for an unexpected menstrual period. The aging process—as well as the decrease in estrogen levels—can cause thinning of the vaginal walls *(atrophy)*, dryness, and itching of the vagina (pruritus). These changes may result in painful sexual relations (dyspareunia) and can also lead to increased susceptibility to infections because the vaginal pH increases.

The psychological response to menopause represents a change that can challenge a woman's coping skills and may require family support to help the woman maintain a sense of purpose in life. Other women feel a sense of freedom from the need for contraception or medication for cramping.

Elder Care Points

The significant reduction in estrogen after menopause (about 80% less than during the reproductive years) causes a decrease in natural vaginal lubrication. Women may be prescribed vaginal creams containing estrogen to restore moisture and elasticity to vaginal tissues. Vaginal estrogen (Estring), which contains slow-release, low-dose estrogen, may be used in place of cream. Women should be cautioned not to use estrogen cream as a lubricant for sexual intercourse as their partner may absorb the estrogen. Nonmedicated lubricants should be used for this purpose, if necessary. Studies have shown that the estrogen contained in some vaginal creams can be systemically absorbed and therefore should be used with caution (Bachman, 2009).

Western culture values youth and beauty; therefore some women may see the onset of menopause as a loss of attractiveness, and the first step toward old age. Other cultural groups value the wisdom gained from life's experiences, and for women in these cultures the onset of menopause may carry less negative psychological impact. Nurses must understand the perceptions of the woman and the family before designing and implementing a teaching plan to address this "change in life."

Health Risks of Menopause

The major health problems that occur at or after menopause include the development of osteoporosis and coronary heart disease.

Osteoporosis. Osteoporosis is a decrease in bone mass that raises the risk for bone fractures. The decrease in estrogen during menopause slows bone growth; therefore bone deteriorates and thins before new bone growth occurs. Estrogen also enables vitamin D to assist in calcium absorption in the intestine, and a decrease in estrogen is associated with a decrease in calcium, which is essential to healthy bone tissue. Box 39-3 provides a list of some lifestyle activities that may increase the risk of developing osteoporosis. A new drug, denosumab (Xgeva, Prolia), developed for women who have osteoporosis and are at risk for facture was approved by

---

Box 39-2	Some Assisted Reproductive Therapies (ARTs)

- **In vitro fertilization (IVF-ET):** Woman's eggs are collected from the ovary, fertilized in the laboratory, and transferred into the uterus at the embryo stage of development.
- **Zygote intrafallopian transfer (ZIFT):** After in vitro fertilization, the ovum is placed into the fallopian tube at the zygote stage of development.
- **Therapeutic donor insemination (TDI):** A donor's sperm inseminates the woman.
- **Intracytoplasmic sperm injection:** Injection of one live sperm directly into the mature egg.
- **Surrogate mother:** The surrogate mother can be inseminated with the partner's sperm or an egg, fertilized by the partner's sperm in vitro. The egg is transferred to the uterus of the surrogate mother; she becomes a gestational carrier.

ET, embryo transfer.

Box 39-3	Lifestyle Activities that Increase Risk of Osteoporosis

- *Inadequate lifetime intake of calcium and vitamin D:* prevents reaching peak bone mass by age 30
- *Smoking:* Decreases estrogen production
- *Excess alcohol intake:* Interferes with calcium absorption and depresses new bone growth
- *Excess caffeine, cola, or soft drink intake:* Results in imbalanced calcium and phosphorus or demineralizes bone

the FDA in 2010 and is often prescribed with vitamin D and calcium supplements. Women are then monitored for low calcium levels and jaw osteonecrosis. The use of nitroglycerin ointment to increase bone density is currently under study (Khosla, 2011).

⬥ Elder Care Points

Older women who are on long-term estrogen replacement therapy are at increased risk for endometrial cancer, as well as the possibility of breast cancer, and it is particularly important that these women have annual pelvic examinations and perform breast self-examination regularly.

The first signs of osteoporosis are loss of height, back pain, and the development of a so-called **dowager's hump** in which vertebrae fail to support the upper body in an upright position (Figure 39-4). The ACOG Women's Health Care Physicians recommend bone density screening for menopausal women.

Coronary Heart Disease. The decrease in hormones in postmenopausal women causes an increased risk for coronary heart disease due to changes in lipid metabolism and a rise in total cholesterol. Diet and exercise can have a positive effect in minimizing the effects of these risks. See Chapters 20 and 21 for details concerning cardiovascular diseases.

5' 6"
5' 2"

| Years past menopause | 5 | 10 | 15 |

FIGURE 39-4 Osteoporosis. With progression of osteoporosis, the vertebral column collapses, causing loss of height and back pain. *Dowager's hump* is the term used for this curvature of the back.

Treatment Options During Menopause

Hormone Therapy. In the past, hormone (estrogen) replacement therapy (HRT) was the cornerstone of interventions to reduce the discomforts of menopause (hot flashes and vaginal atrophy) and protect women from developing coronary heart disease and osteoporosis. Research offers evidence that HRT can increase the risk of blood clots, stroke, heart attack, and breast cancer. The ACOG recommends careful selection of patients for HRT, and detailed education concerning risks of therapy. Current guidelines state that hormone therapy should be used by well-informed and well-monitored patients and for menopausal symptoms only, at the lowest effective dose (Prentice, 2009).

Bioidentical hormones. Bioidentical hormones such as oral estradiol, estradiol transdermal patches, or oral micronized progesterone (Prometrium) are clinically synthesized from steroidal molecules taken from wild yam or soy, but have chemical structures identical to hormones produced in the human body. They differ from "natural hormones" such as conjugated equine hormone (Premarin), which comes from the urine of pregnant mares and has a chemical structure different from the human. Progesterone is a bioidentical hormone that has a different chemical structure than progestins such as synthetically produced medroxyprogesterone (Provera). Both synthetic and bioidentical hormones interact with the same estrogen and progesterone receptors on target cells, but their physiologic side effects maybe different.

Bioidentical hormones that are made (compounded) by individual pharmacies are not FDA regulated or approved and may not be monitored for consistency and purity (Borsage & Freeman, 2009). Nurses should be alert to research findings that involve "hormone therapy" and should inquire if the hormones researched are bioidentical or synthetic (Weil, 2009).

Alternative Therapies. Some CAM therapies have been helpful in relieving specific discomforts of menopause. Homeopathy, acupuncture, and certain herbs may offer relief, but each may have contraindications as well. Herbal therapy has not been fully researched or regulated, and some side effects or interactions with food or drugs are possible. Phytoestrogens, soy products, and vitamins B, C, and E have also been helpful in relieving menopausal discomforts.

Health Promotion

Using CAM Therapies for Menopause

Women should be encouraged to consult with a health care provider before using CAM therapies such as soy isoflavones, black cohosh, or other herbs. For some women these substances may be contraindicated. Certain herbs may interact with other medications the patient is taking.

Nutrition Considerations

Managing Menopause

When phytoestrogens are recommended by the health care provider, teaching about these substances should be provided. Phytoestrogens are found in foods such as wild yams, cherries, dandelion greens, alfalfa sprouts, and black beans. Food sources of soy include tofu, soy milk, and roasted soy nuts.

Medications such as alendronate (Fosamax) can be prescribed for women with osteoporosis, but side effects should be explained carefully. After taking Fosamax, the woman must be able to remain upright for at least 30 minutes. Diet, exercise, and support groups are very effective in helping to manage menopause. When hot flashes significantly affect a woman's quality of life, nonhormonal medication may be recommended. Studies have shown that medications such as venlafaxine (Effexor) and clonidine (Catapres), soy isoflavones, and CAM therapies such as black cohosh (*Cimicifuga racemosa*) may offer relief of hot flash symptoms (NCAM, 2011).

HEALTH PROMOTION AND DISEASE PREVENTION

Women's health care can be defined as the promotion of the physical, psychological, and spiritual well-being of women. In the twenty-first century, women are increasingly economically independent and empowered to make health care decisions. Health care education of the adolescent includes information concerning puberty, menstruation, and sexuality. A teen needs information concerning safe sex, contraceptives, and choices concerning high-risk behaviors. Adult women require information concerning Papanicolaou (Pap) smears, breast self-examination, nutrition, exercise, and lifestyle management. Perinatal education is important. Older women require information regarding menopause, long-term illness, and disabilities that affect health care needs. Today many older women live alone with below-poverty-level income and are without caregivers or easy access to health care. The nurse must have an understanding of these needs and of the normal physiologic changes of each age group in order to devise a plan of care to maintain health or treat illness.

It is of utmost importance that women of all ages be knowledgeable about the function of their bodies, health care needs, and signs and symptoms of wellness, as well as those of illness. Young women often first enter the health care system for a Pap smear or for contraceptive advice. Support, reassurance, and understanding of cultural and personal needs are the primary responsibilities of the nurse during this first contact. A complete history, physical examination, age-appropriate screening tests with clear interpretations, referrals, and education concerning nutrition, lifestyle, and health care to meet individual needs are essential responsibilities of the nurse and the health care team.

Health Screening and Assessments

Health screening is a form of preventive care. *Primary prevention* is designed to decrease the probability of becoming ill (for example, by maintaining a health or nutrition history, and by providing immunizations). *Secondary prevention* is designed to focus on detection of specific at-risk diseases so that early treatment may be given (such as annual mammograms). *Tertiary prevention* minimizes the impact of an already-diagnosed condition.

All adult women may be at risk for obesity, high cholesterol, high blood pressure, osteoporosis, and dental disease. Pregnant women or women planning pregnancy may be at risk for a folic acid deficiency that could result in a neural tube defect in the developing fetus; therefore prenatal vitamins, including folic acid supplements, may be prescribed.

Health screening begins with the woman's visit to her health care provider. It is your responsibility to introduce yourself, ask pertinent questions, and document all information gathered. The data collected identify the patient and summarize her personal health history, the community in which she lives, and her available support system. Some information concerning the woman's culture, lifestyle, and usual coping mechanisms will enable the design of an individualized plan of care. All data collection should include information regarding use of nonprescription as well as prescription medications and CAM therapy.

Breast Self-Examination. Breast self-examination (BSE) should be done monthly, about 1 week after menstruation begins, or on a specific date each month after menopause. The nurse plays a major role in teaching and encouraging women to perform BSE to detect breast lumps and thickened areas. Figure 39-5 illustrates the steps in the procedure. In addition, the American Cancer Society has videotapes available that demonstrate BSE.

New tests that may replace current mammography for breast cancer are currently being researched; these include the cone-beam breast computed tomography scan. The scanner merges 300 x-ray scans taken in 10 seconds into three-dimensional images. The breast is not compressed for the test. Ultrasound elastography has been supersensitive in identifying 100% of malignant tumors during trials, and the technique may replace breast biopsy.

 Clinical Cues

If the health care provider has recommended that a woman have a mammogram and the woman does not want to because she has previously experienced a fair amount of discomfort during the procedure, suggest that she take some acetaminophen an hour before the scheduled test, unless contraindicated. Also compare the benefits of discovering breast cancer early with the few minutes of breast discomfort from the compression by the machine.

1. POSITIONS

Visual Inspection: Standing in each position, look for changes in contour and shape of the breasts, color and texture of the skin and nipple and evidence of discharge from the nipples.

Arms raised above head

Hands on hips

Bending forward

Arms relaxed at side

Palpation: Flat and Side-Lying: Use your left hand to palpate the right breast, while holding your right arm at a right angle to the rib cage, with the elbow bent. Repeat the procedure on the other side. The side-lying position allows a woman, especially one with large breasts, to most effectively examine the outer half of the breast. A woman with small breasts may need only the flat position.

Side-lying Position: Lie on the opposite side of the breast to be examined. Rotate the shoulder (on the same side as the breast to be examined) back to the flat surface.

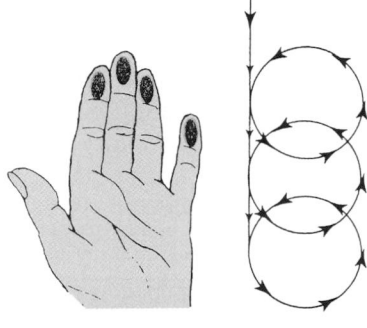

Flat Position: Lie flat on your back with a pillow or folded towel under the shoulder of the breast to be examined.

2. PERIMETER

The examination area is bounded by a line that extends down from the middle of the armpit to just beneath the breast, continues across the underside of the breast to the middle of the breast bone, then moves up to and along the collarbone and back to the middle of the armpit. Most breast cancers occur in the upper outer area of the breast (shaded area).

3. PALPATION WITH PADS OF FINGERS

Use the pads of three or four fingers to examine every inch of your breast tissue. Move your fingers in circles about the size of a dime.

Do not lift your fingers from your breast between palpations. You can use powder or lotion to help your fingers glide from one spot to the next.

4. PRESSURE

Use varying levels of pressure for each palpation, from light to deep, to examine the full thickness of your breast tissue. Using pressure will not injure the breast.

5. PATTERN OF SEARCH

Vertical Strip:

Using the following search pattern to examine all of your breast tissue, palpate carefully beneath the nipple. Any incision should also be carefully examined from end to end. Women who have had any breast surgery should examine the entire area and the incision.

Start in the armpit, proceed downward to the lower boundary. Move a finger's width toward the middle and continue palpating upward until you reach the collar bone. Repeat this until you have covered all the breast tissue. Make at least six strips before the nipple and four strips after the nipple. You may need between 10 and 16 strips.

Nipple Discharge:

Squeeze your nipples to check for discharge. Many women have a normal discharge.

Axillary Examination:

Examine the breast tissue that extends into your armpit while your arm is relaxed at your side.

6. PRACTICE WITH FEEDBACK

It is important that you perform breast self-examination (BSE) while your instructor watches to be sure you are doing it correctly. Practice your skills until you feel comfortable and confident.

FIGURE 39-5 Recommended breast self-examination procedure.

Vulvar Self-Examination. Many women are unaware of the importance of vulvar self-examination (VSE). Although serious lesions in this area are less common than in the breast, early detection allows for rapid and often minimally invasive treatment. Delay in detection of vulvar lesions can lead to severe surgical disfigurement, and even death. Just like BSE, VSE should be performed monthly. It usually is done in a sitting position. One hand is used to hold a mirror, the other to separate the labia and expose the area surrounding the vagina. Using both touch (to palpate for lumps or thickening beneath the skin) and visualization, the self-examination begins at the top of the mons pubis and works downward to the clitoris, the labia majora, labia minora, the perineum, and finally the area around the anus. The woman should note any changes and report them to her health care provider. These include new moles, warts, or growths; new areas of pigmentation—especially white, red, or dark skin areas; ulcers or sores; and areas of continuing pain, inflammation, or itching. Most of these findings will not be malignancies and will require little, if any, treatment. Treatment of malignancies that have been detected early often is relatively easy and can avoid deformative surgeries such as *vulvectomy* (excision of the vulva) and prevent *metastasis* (spread of a malignancy to other areas of the body).

Diagnostic Tests

The nurse often is asked to assist with various diagnostic tests. Providing the woman with a clear explanation of what will be done and what she can do to minimize discomfort is essential. Consent may be required with certain procedures, and the nurse is responsible for ensuring that the health care provider has obtained an informed consent. All questions should be answered clearly and accurately before the procedure has started. Table 39-2 describes common gynecologic diagnostic tests.

Pelvic Examination. The nurse assembles the equipment and directs the woman to take deep breaths and relax all muscles during exhalation (Box 39-4). The woman can be instructed to bear down as the speculum is being inserted. The speculum is gently placed into the vagina by the health care provider. The blades are then opened to view the cervix. Specimens may be collected for laboratory examination. A Pap smear may be obtained to determine the presence of abnormal cells. After the examination, the nurse can assist the woman to a sitting, then a standing position. Disposable tissues may be provided to wipe lubricant from the perineum. The patient usually dresses and then speaks with the health care provider. Teaching may include the purpose of the tests performed, the need for routine checkups, and the need for Pap smears from the age the woman becomes sexually active (or from ages 20 to 40) and every 1 to 3 years thereafter.

Clinical Cues

Talking to the patient and holding her hand, if possible, during the pelvic examination aids with distraction and enhances relaxation.

Elder Care Points

Women of advanced years may feel that they no longer need regular mammograms and Pap smears, particularly if they are not sexually active. They need to be aware that the incidence of breast and endometrial cancers increases with age and that annual screening becomes more, not less, important.

❖ NURSING MANAGEMENT

■ Assessment (Data Collection)

The nurse is responsible for collecting essential data regarding the patient's reproductive history and gynecologic concerns. This can be difficult for both the patient and the nurse, as it involves discussing intimate aspects of the patient's body and personal life. The nurse should also record information on the cultural beliefs and attitudes regarding sexuality and sexual identity, reproduction, and body image, as these all affect the assessment process.

Cultural Considerations

Culture and Women's Health

Cultural considerations can be particularly significant in the care of women's health. Cultural views regarding sexuality, reproduction, and the role of women in society will have a direct bearing on the type of care sought and the amount and type of information the woman is willing and able to provide. The nurse must not pass judgment based on her own cultural bias, but must be culturally sensitive and supportive to the needs of women from diverse cultural backgrounds.

■ Nursing Diagnosis

Nursing diagnoses commonly associated with gynecologic disorders include:
- Activity intolerance related to anemia from excessive blood loss, weakness, or disabling discomfort
- Excess fluid volume related to premenstrual fluid retention
- Impaired skin integrity related to pruritus, genital lesions, and vaginal discharge
- Pain related to menstrual cycle, decreased vaginal lubrication, or vaginal irritation

- Sexual dysfunction related to dyspareunia (painful intercourse) or emotional issues
- Ineffective coping related to negative attitude about human sexuality or menstruation
- Disturbed body image related to surgery, fear of mutilating surgery, and loss of femininity

- Deficient knowledge about practices of personal feminine hygiene, normal anatomy, and physiology of the female reproductive organs, or safe methods of contraception
- Situational low self-esteem related to sterility, menopause, and surgery on a reproductive organ

Table 39-2   Common Gynecologic Diagnostic Tests and Diagnostic Procedures

PURPOSE	DESCRIPTION	NURSING IMPLICATIONS
Pelvic Examination		
Visual inspection of the external genitalia, vagina, and cervix to obtain specimens such as a Pap smear.	*Equipment:* Gloves, vaginal speculum, lubricant, light, table with stirrups. *Process:* Inspection via the vaginal speculum; manual palpation through abdominal wall, vaginally, and rectally of internal organs.	Some discomfort during examination (decreased or eliminated if the patient remains fully relaxed). Nurse to ensure that patient is appropriately draped and correctly positioned in the stirrups. Examination time is usually 5-10 min.
Pap Smear, Thin Prep		
To obtain samples of cells and fluids for pathology/cytology studies.	*Equipment:* Sterile specimen collection equipment. *Process:* Exudate, mucus, and cells obtained from surface with sterile swab or scraping tool and placed on laboratory slide or into preservative solution for pathology evaluation.	Cultures and smears of the cervix may cause mild bleeding and cramping.
Endometrial Biopsy		
Postmenopausal bleeding, menstrual difficulties, infertility workup.	*Equipment:* Same as pelvic examination plus suction biopsy apparatus. *Process:* A suction biopsy of the endometrium is performed via the cervical opening.	Severe cramping may occur during procedure. Patient is usually premedicated. Normally some vaginal bleeding follows; flow should not be heavy.
Colposcopy		
Endoscopic examination of the vagina and cervix to evaluate abnormal cells and lesions, particularly after a positive Pap smear.	*Equipment:* Same as pelvic examination plus colposcope. *Process:* Area is visualized through the scope, with photos and possible biopsies of lesions requiring further study.	Patient is positioned as for pelvic examination. Procedure takes a few minutes. Biopsy may cause a small amount of bleeding and minor cramping. No tampons should be used until healing has occurred.
Hysteroscopy		
Endoscopic examination of the interior of the uterus; may also involve procedures such as biopsy or removal of fibroids, adhesions, and septums. Endometrial laser ablation (destruction of areas within uterine lining) may also be performed.	*Process:* Hysteroscope is inserted vaginally, usually under local anesthesia. May also be done in combination with laparoscopy.	Occasional injury to cervix or uterine wall. If endometrial ablation is done, the woman will have difficulty becoming pregnant as the lining destruction is permanent.
Dilation and Evacuation (D&E)		
To detect cause of excessive bleeding; to remove hypertrophied uterine lining, retained placenta, or tissue remaining from incomplete abortion.	*Equipment:* Done in operating room. *Process:* The cervix is dilated and the interior of the uterus is cleansed by scraping, suction, or both.	Mild cramping and bleeding for up to 1 wk. Next period may be either early or late. Complications include uterine perforation, excessive bleeding, infection. Instruct patient to report heavy bleeding, clotting, sharp/severe abdominal pain, abnormal or foul discharge.

Continued

PURPOSE	DESCRIPTION	NURSING IMPLICATIONS
Mammography		
To screen the breasts for abnormal growths, particularly cancer.	*Equipment:* Done in the radiology department with special radiographic equipment. *Process:* A full-field digital mammography machine records images on a computer screen and can computer-enhance questionable images for increased accuracy.	Breast discomfort from compression of the tissue during the test; occasional mild bruising. Instruct patient to wear no deodorant or lotion on the upper body and to wear clothing that allows top to be easily removed.
Hysterosalpingography		
To detect uterine tumors, adhesions, or developmental anomalies; to detect tubal obstruction preventing ova from reaching uterus.	Patient is placed in the lithotomy position on fluoroscopy table with a speculum in the vagina. Contrast media is injected through the cervix. Fluoroscopy is performed and radiographs are taken.	Have patient void before the procedure. Vaginal discharge may occur for 1-2 days post-test and may be bloody. Instruct patient to report fever, pain, or other signs of infection.
Ultrasound (Sonogram)		
Pregnancy: To determine gestation; screen for birth defects or placental abnormalities. *Gynecology:* To determine presence, location, and size of abdominal mass; to determine whether a mass is *cystic* (fluid filled) or solid; locate intrauterine device; monitor ovulation in infertility.	*Equipment:* Ultrasound machine. *Process:* Sound wave transducer emits inaudible sound waves that record interior structures on the ultrasound screen. A videotape is made so results can be restudied and evaluated. A "picture" of the fetus may be provided to the parents.	Some tests require a full bladder, which may be uncomfortable during the test. The nurse should assist the woman to immediately empty her bladder after the examination. Skin should be clean, dry, and free of lotions or powder. During pregnancy, up to two ultrasound examinations may be required. The use of independent three- or four-dimensional ultrasound procedures for purposes of providing mementos to parents is not recommended, as the long-term effects of the extra energy used in these examinations on the fetus has not been researched.
Pelvic/Vaginal Ultrasound		
To detect thickness of uterine lining, size of uterus, presence of fibroids; size of ovaries; and presence of cysts or tumor.	*Process:* Ultrasound transducer is passed over pelvic area or the transducer is inserted into the vagina and guided over areas of the surface.	Advise that there will be minor discomfort if vaginal transducer is used.
Breast Ultrasound		
To differentiate benign tumor from malignant tumor. Useful in women with dense breast tissue and fibrocystic disease.	*Process:* A noninvasive painless procedure.	An ultrasound will not detect microcalcifications that a mammogram can detect.
PET Scan		
To stage breast cancer and detect skeletal lesions.	*Process:* Performed in radiotherapy unit.	
Breast MRI		
Used for women with dense breast tissue.	*Process:* Images are taken with a magnetic resonance image machine.	Premedication to lessen anxiety for women with claustrophobia may be advised. Patient must not wear metal during test.
Breast Biopsy		
To diagnose breast cancer. Usually performed when a suspicious breast lump is detected.	*Process:* A needle aspiration can be done on an outpatient basis under local anesthesia. An incisional biopsy can be done in a same-day surgery setting under local or general anesthesia. All removed tissue or fluid is sent to laboratory for analysis.	Check incision for bleeding. Encourage verbalization of fears. Schedule follow-up appointment for results of laboratory studies.

MRI, magnetic resonance imaging; *Pap,* Papanicolaou; *PET,* positron-emission tomography.

Box 39-4	Preparing the Woman for a Pelvic Examination

- The unit should provide privacy and good lighting.
- Assemble clean gloves and supplies.
- Orient the patient to the equipment and the purpose of the examination.
- Encourage the woman to void because a full bladder will make the examination more uncomfortable.
- Position and drape the patient appropriately.
  - Lithotomy
  - Side-lying
  - Knee-chest
- Stay with the woman, encouraging her with information to promote comfort.

 Focused Assessment

Data Collection for Gynecologic History

Sample questions when collecting data from a patient with a gynecologic problem include:

- How old were you when you began menstruating?
- Are your periods regular? How often do they occur? How long do they last?
- How heavy is your flow? Do you ever pass clots or pieces of tissue? Do you have pain before or during your period?
- Do you have cramps, headaches, or abdominal or back pain at other times of the month?
- Do you have mood swings, depression, or periods of tearfulness associated with your menstrual cycle?
- Are you having any vaginal discharge or itching?
- Do you have bleeding or spotting between your periods?
- Do you have any problems urinating, including burning, pain, or incontinence?
- How many times have you been pregnant?
- Have you had any miscarriages?
- Have you ever had a pelvic infection?
- Do you perform breast and vulvar self-examination?
- When was your last Pap smear?
- When was your last mammogram?
- Are you taking any medications routinely?
- Are you currently using any method of birth control, and if so, which method?
- Do you feel comfortable with your method or have a desire to change methods?
- Do you have any specific concerns or questions that we have not talked about?

Ask questions in a tactful yet matter-of-fact manner, and appreciate that the patient has the right to choose not to answer. A symptom diary can be very helpful. Note patterns of coping and available support persons.

■ Planning

Planning the care of a patient with a gynecologic problem depends on the specific disorder. However, prevention of infection, effective patient education, and emotional support are appropriate goals for the plan of care for all patients with a gynecologic problem. The needs of a patient facing gynecologic surgery would include pain management, education regarding the procedure and follow-up care, infection prevention, and supportive care specific to the procedure. A woman who will lose the ability to bear children because of an early hysterectomy may have very different supportive needs from those of the postmenopausal woman undergoing the same procedure. Surgery for breast cancer brings fears of a major change in body image and the possibility of death if the disease is not controlled. These issues need to be addressed in the plan of care. The plan for the patient with an infection would include scheduling appropriate medication, monitoring for effectiveness of treatment (e.g., decreased fever, swelling, pain resolving), and monitoring for signs of an allergic response to the prescribed antimicrobial agent.

Expected goals or outcomes include:

- Patient uses energy conservation techniques while maintaining activities of daily living.
- Patient maintains adequate fluid volume without excessive fluid retention.
- Skin remains intact with healing of existing wounds.
- Patient verbalizes an acceptable level of pain relief and ability to engage in normal activities.
- Patient expresses satisfaction with physical intimacy patterns and experience.
- Patient develops improved method of communication, problem-solving techniques, and positive attitude to enable effective coping with signs and symptoms.
- Patient evidences enhanced body image and self-esteem with ability to accept altered body part or function.
- Patient demonstrates motivation to learn and verbalizes understanding of female hygiene and safe sex practices.
- Patient recognizes and accepts positive aspects of self.

In the clinic setting, women may be attending for annual visits, reproductive or contraceptive counseling, treatment of infections or STIs, prenatal and postnatal care, and a variety of other reasons. If the facility uses standardized care plans as a reference, they must be adapted to express the needs of the individual patient.

The plan of care must address education, pain management needs, emotional and physical care, family impact, cultural influences, and financial constraints. Specific goals of care for any patient are based on nursing observation and assessment, prescriptions for medication and therapies, the patient's personal desires and goals, and input from other members of the health care team. The patient should agree to the goals, and they must be clearly communicated to other care providers through well-written care plans and documentation. Team conferences should be convened when appropriate. Nursing Care Plan 39-1 presents one example of a nursing care plan for a woman having a hysterectomy.

Nursing Care Plan 39-1   Care of the Patient After Hysterectomy

Scenario
Marilyn Blair, age 52, has just returned to the unit after abdominal hysterectomy for multiple fibroids, metrorrhagia, and greatly increased uterine size that caused abdominal pain. She has an IV infusion of 1000 mL normal saline in the left forearm, an indwelling urinary catheter, an abdominal dressing, and patient-controlled analgesia (PCA) pump containing morphine. Her vital signs are BP, 138/82; P, 86; R, 16; T, 98.2° F (36.8° C).

Problem/Nursing Diagnosis
Pain and discomfort related to surgical incision/Pain related to abdominal surgery.

Supporting Assessment Data
Subjective: Pain at 7/10 on pain scale: "It hurts to turn."
Objective: Abdominal hysterectomy incision.

Goals/Expected Outcomes	Nursing Interventions	Selected Rationale	Evaluation
Pain will be controlled by prescribed analgesia, avoiding episodes of acute pain.	Instruct her in use of PCA pump. Give booster medication as ordered if needed.	When patient feels in control, anxiety is reduced and less pain medication may be required.	Analgesia via PCA pump provides good relief.
	Assess location, type, and quality of pain q 3-4 hr using a pain scale.	Assessing location and quality of pain may alert nurse to developing complications.	Pain at 3-5 on pain scale.
	Assist with repositioning and support with pillows to attain comfort. Provide quiet, darkened atmosphere for rest and sleep.	Changing position prevents stasis of circulation; comfortable, supported position promotes relaxation.	Assisted to reposition q 2 hr. Sleeping long intervals on side with pillow behind back and between knees for comfort.
	Monitor for side effects of analgesics, especially respiratory rate. Administer antiemetic as ordered at first signs of nausea to prevent vomiting and further pain.	Morphine can depress respiratory rate.	Respirations 18. No nausea or emesis.
	Check Foley catheter and tubing for patency frequently to prevent bladder distention.	Bladder distention can increase pain and cause infection due to stasis of urine in bladder.	Bladder not distended, Foley draining clear urine. Continue plan.

Problem/Nursing Diagnosis
Potential for hemorrhage/Potential for deficient fluid volume related to potential hemorrhage.

Supporting Assessment Data
Objective: Abdominal hysterectomy.

Goals/Expected Outcomes	Nursing Interventions	Selected Rationale	Evaluation
Vital signs (VS) will remain stable; no signs of shock or hemorrhage.	Monitor VS frequently per postoperative protocol routine.	A rapid pulse and falling blood pressure can indicate development of shock.	VS are at baseline: BP 118/68; P 84; R 16.
	Check abdominal dressing and beneath patient for signs of bleeding with each set of VS; assess for bleeding from vaginal area.	Gravity can cause fluids to drain to a point beneath the patient.	Abdominal dressing clean and dry; no visible vaginal drainage.
	Assess for signs of intra-abdominal bleeding; such as increasing abdominal girth, decreasing bowel sounds, and increasing abdominal pain and rigidity.	Intra-abdominal bleeding is a complication of abdominal hysterectomy.	Abdomen soft; bowel sounds have returned; no evidence of intra-abdominal bleeding. Continue plan.

Problem/Nursing Diagnosis
Surgical incision causing pain on inspiration/Risk for ineffective breathing pattern related to pain.

Supporting Assessment Data
Subjective: "It hurts to take a deep breath."
Objective: Abdominal hysterectomy.

Goals/Expected Outcomes	Nursing Interventions	Selected Rationale	Evaluation
Patient will have no signs of atelectasis or pneumonia as evidenced by clear breath sounds in all lung fields and afebrile status.	Assist patient to use an incentive spirometer, sit up to deep-breathe and cough q 2 hr while awake; give small pillow and instruct her on how to splint incision before coughing. Enlist aid of family or significant others in reminding patient to deep-breathe. Report adventitious, diminished, or absent breath sounds or crackles.	Cough and deep-breathing exercises can prevent development of atelectasis. Pain can prevent patient from taking deep breaths. Others can provide encouragement and support. Abnormal breath sounds can be sign of developing complications.	Able to deep breathe and cough at 8 and 10 A.M. and 12 and 2 P.M. Sitting on side of bed q 2 hr while awake. Family helping and reminding patient to do breathing exercises. Lung sounds clear bilaterally; all VS are WNL; T, 98.0° F (36.7° C). Continue plan.

Problem/Nursing Diagnosis
Skin disrupted by surgical incision/Risk for infection related to surgery.

Supporting Assessment Data
Objective: Abdominal surgical incision.

Goals/Expected Outcomes	Nursing Interventions	Selected Rationale	Evaluation
Patient will be without signs and symptoms of infection at discharge.	Administer prophylactic antibiotics as ordered. Monitor incision for signs of redness, swelling, purulent drainage, or hardness. Keep dressing clean and dry. Use careful aseptic technique when changing dressings. Monitor WBC count and temperature. Assess vaginal drainage for signs of odor or change in character. Assess abdomen for signs of infection, increasing pain, localized tenderness, swelling, increased erythema (redness) around wound edges, decreased bowel sounds.	Antibiotics kill pathogens. Redness, swelling, drainage, and pain at an incision site may be signs of infection. A wound dressing must be kept clean and dry to prevent contamination that can cause infection. Odor or purulent appearance of vaginal drainage may indicate infection. Tenderness, swelling, increased erythema, and decreased bowel sounds are signs of intra-abdominal infection.	Tolerating prescribed medications. No incisional redness, swelling, hardness, or purulent drainage. Dressing clean and dry. WBC count WNL; afebrile. Vaginal drainage is minimal and without odor. Abdomen soft, active bowel sounds; no signs or symptoms of infection. Continue plan.

Continued

Nursing Care Plan 39-1   Care of the Patient After Hysterectomy—cont'd

Problem/Nursing Diagnosis

Potential for blood clots from inactivity/Risk for injury related to possibility of thrombophlebitis from bed rest and abdominopelvic surgery.

Supporting Assessment Data

Objective: Abdominal hysterectomy and decreased activity level.

Goals/Expected Outcomes	Nursing Interventions	Selected Rationale	Evaluation
Patient will not exhibit signs of thrombophlebitis at time of discharge.	Encourage ambulation as soon as it is ordered; explain benefits of walking. Assist with leg and ankle exercises q 2 hr.	Range-of-motion exercise and early ambulation can prevent the development of thrombus formation. Leg exercises increase circulation and prevent blood pooling.	Leg and ankle exercises q 2 hr while awake, and is tolerating ambulation.
	Monitor SCDs q shift.	SCDs prevent pooling.	SCDs functioning properly.
	Encourage added fluid intake as soon as diet order allows.	Extra liquids keeps blood more fluid and less likely to clot.	Presently NPO with IV fluids.
	Inspect lower legs q shift; check for positive Homans' sign.	A positive Homans' sign may indicate development of thrombophlebitis.	Homans' sign negative. Continue plan.

Problem/Nursing Diagnosis

Worried that she has lost her femininity/Disturbed body image related to removal of uterus.

Supporting Assessment Data

Subjective: "I wonder how this will affect my husband's view of me."
Objective: Abdominal hysterectomy.

Goals/Expected Outcomes	Nursing Interventions	Selected Rationale	Evaluation
Patient will express her concerns over loss of uterus before discharge. Patient will accept new body image within 3 mo as evidenced by lack of depression and reinvestment in usual activities.	Provide openings for conversation regarding patient's concerns over loss of her uterus and its meaning to her. Explore her feelings regarding sexuality after hysterectomy. Encourage expression of positive aspects of having the hysterectomy and how she as a person is unchanged.	Enabling patient to verbalize and express concerns will make it possible to establish a patient-centered plan of care and teaching.	Patient is able to begin discussion about her concerns; will continue tomorrow. Continue plan.

Critical Thinking Questions

1. Following an abdominal hysterectomy, this 52-year-old woman appears depressed and states she is worried her marital relations will "never be the same." What is the best response of the nurse?
2. Aside from an abdominal hysterectomy, what other options for the treatment of uterine fibroids are available?

BP, blood pressure; *IV*, intravenous; *NPO*, nothing by mouth; *P*, pulse; *R*, respirations; *SCD*, sequential compression device; *T*, temperature; *VS*, vital signs; *WBC*, white blood cell; *WNL*, within normal limits.

■ Implementation

The patient's needs must always be addressed when implementing various aspects of the plan of care. Table 39-3 on p. 901 contains detailed information on various types of surgical procedures that are used for different gynecologic problems. Education must be done in a manner appropriate to the patient's knowledge base and her ability to learn new information. Patient teaching should form an important aspect of each nursing contact.

■ Evaluation

Any nursing intervention requires evaluation of its effectiveness. This can be accomplished by asking the following questions: How effective were pain control measures? How is the patient tolerating the change

Table 39-3	Gynecologic Surgical Procedures	
REASONS FOR PERFORMING	**DESCRIPTION**	**NURSING CARE AND TEACHING POINTS**
Dilation and Evacuation (D&E)		
Excessive vaginal bleeding; incomplete abortion; removal of placental fragments; therapeutic abortion.	Scraping away the inner lining of the uterus (endometrium) via the cervix.	Observe for excessive bleeding postoperatively.
Conization or Conical Excision		
To remove abnormal or early cancerous tissue; biopsy.	Removal of cone of tissue with scalpel or electrical cutting wire.	Office procedure. May cause some bleeding.
Fistulectomy		
Presence of rectovaginal fistula (channel between rectum and vagina) or urethrovaginal fistula (channel between bladder and vagina).	Surgical excision of the fistula and repair of the tissue to prevent passage of urine or feces into the vagina.	Observe for excessive bleeding or for vaginal fecal drainage postoperatively.
Hysterectomy		
Prolapse of pelvic organs; pain associated with pelvic congestion; endometriosis; excessive/debilitating uterine bleeding; fibroids; noninvasive uterine or cervical cancer.	Removal of entire uterus, vaginally or abdominally.	Observe for excessive bleeding; paralytic ileus can occur. Ends childbearing if premenopausal, which may have profound emotional impact.
Panhysterectomy		
Cancer; pain associated with pelvic inflammatory disease; recurrent ovarian cysts.	Removal of entire uterus, fallopian tubes, and ovaries.	See hysterectomy. Removal of ovaries induces menopause in premenopausal women.
Radical Hysterectomy		
Invasive cancer.	Removal of uterus, tubes, ovaries, upper third of vagina, and lymph nodes.	See hysterectomy and panhysterectomy. Vaginal alteration may affect ability to have sexual intercourse. Possible lymphedema due to removal of nodes.
Anterior and Posterior Colporrhaphy		
Presence of prolapse of bladder and rectum into the vagina; may accompany a uterine prolapse.	Repair of the anterior and posterior wall of the vagina.	Observe for excessive bleeding.
Salpingectomy		
Tubal pregnancy; tumor; traumatic injury.	Removal of a fallopian tube.	Will not cause infertility if other tube/ovary is intact.
Oophorectomy		
Tumor; cystic disease; endometriosis; traumatic injury; severe hormonal disorder.	Removal of an ovary.	See salpingectomy. Only a portion of one ovary is necessary to provide normal hormonal balance before menopause.
Vulvectomy/Endoscopic Laparoscopy		
Malignancy.	Radical vulvectomy: surgical excision of the labia, clitoris, perineal structures, femoral and inguinal lymphatic tissues.	Major disfigurement; extreme supportive measures, including professional counseling, often required.

in diet or new therapy? Have there been any adverse reactions to medications or treatments? A decision to continue the plan of care or revise the plan of care is the outcome of evaluation.

DISORDERS OF THE FEMALE REPRODUCTIVE SYSTEM

MENSTRUAL DYSFUNCTIONS

Premenstrual Syndrome

Premenstrual syndrome (PMS), also known as *ovarian cycle syndrome,* is the presence of physical, psychological, or behavioral symptoms that regularly recur within the luteal phase of the menstrual cycle and significantly disappear during the remainder of the cycle. These signs and symptoms—which occur between ovulation and menstruation—include weight gain, bloating, irritability, changes in eating patterns, fatigue, mood swings, and a fear of losing control of emotions. Management includes lifestyle modifications, diet high in B vitamins, and exercise changes; stress management; and avoidance of fatigue (ACOG, 2008).

Premenstrual Dysphoric Disorder

Premenstrual dysphoric disorder is a more severe form of PMS and is described officially in the *Diagnostic and Statistical Manual of Mental Disorders,* fourth edition, text revision (DSM-IV-TR), a classification of disorders that is published by the American Psychological Association. Premenstrual dysphoric disorder is thought to be a decreased ability to cope with normal stressors, rather than being an appearance of new stressors. Functional changes such as depression and impaired concentration may interfere with the normal lifestyle or work responsibilities.

Strategies for self-care may include exercising to manage stress, changing patterns of lifestyle, and maintaining a healthy diet. Consumption of refined sugar, salt, red meat, alcohol, and caffeinated beverages should be limited. Dietary supplements in the form of calcium, magnesium, and vitamin B_6 may be helpful. Exercise may increase beta-endorphin levels, which results in relief of depression and mood elevation. Peer support groups can also be helpful. Psychological counseling and prescribed medications such as diuretics or nonsteroidal anti-inflammatory medications (such as ibuprofen) may provide relief. Fluoxetine (Sarafem, a selective serotonin reuptake inhibitor), Zoloft, and Paxil have been approved by the FDA for the management of menstrual disorders. An oral contraceptive with drosperinone (YAZ) 3 mg and ethyl estradiol 20 mg has been found to be effective in treatment of premenstrual dysphoric syndrome (Htay, 2011).

Dysmenorrhea

Dysmenorrhea is painful menstruation; it is a common gynecologic complaint. There are two classifications of dysmenorrhea.

Primary Dysmenorrhea. Primary dysmenorrhea usually occurs 6 to 12 months after the menarche (when the process of ovulation becomes established and regular menstruation occurs). Primary dysmenorrhea is thought to be due to the release of high levels of prostaglandins in the first 2 days of menstruation, causing uterine contractions and vasoconstriction that result in abdominal cramps. Backache, weakness, decreased appetite, and central nervous system symptoms such as dizziness, headache, and poor concentration may also occur but rarely last longer than 48 hours, which coincides with the decrease in prostaglandin levels.

The most important management of dysmenorrhea is to promote an attitude of positive sexuality and self-worth. Correction of myths and misinformation is essential, and management is related to the woman's individual responses.

A heating pad promotes vasodilation, and often relieves cramps. Back massage and soft rhythmic massage of the abdomen (effleurage) can also relieve discomfort. Exercises such as the *pelvic rock* relieve discomfort by releasing endorphins, suppressing prostaglandins, and shunting the blood flow away from the pelvic organs, which results in less pelvic congestion. The pelvic rock is accomplished while in the hands-and-knees position, alternating arching the back and constricting abdominal and gluteal muscles while exhaling, and then hollowing the back and relaxing the muscles while inhaling. Several CAM therapies can also be helpful, such as aromatherapy and meditation. A balanced low-fat diet with foods that are natural diuretics (such as cranberry juice, asparagus, and watermelon) may decrease edema-related symptoms. Medications such as nonsteroidal anti-inflammatories are prostaglandin inhibitors, and may relieve many discomforts. Health care providers may prescribe an OC, which provides relief from menstrual discomfort, such as heavy menstrual bleeding, along with advantages of contraceptive protection. Many herbal preparations and over-the-counter CAM medications are available for self-treatment. The nurse should be aware of side effects and interactions of CAM therapies with prescribed drugs.

? Think Critically

Why should the nurse ask the patient about over-the-counter medications and herbal remedies she is taking, and document their use?

Secondary Dysmenorrhea. Secondary dysmenorrhea occurs usually after 25 years of age and is caused by pelvic pathology such as endometriosis, pelvic inflammatory disease, uterine polyps, or fibroids. Pain associated with secondary dysmenorrhea is characterized by a dull, lower abdominal pain that radiates to the back or thighs. The pain may occur before the menstrual period, and may last throughout the days of menstrual flow. Management involves treating the cause of the pelvic pathology. Temporary relief may be obtained with the same therapies used for primary dysmenorrhea (Table 39-4).

PELVIC RELAXATION SYNDROME

When the muscles, ligaments, and fascia that support the pelvic floor weaken, the pelvic organs may descend toward the vaginal orifice. The descent of pelvic organs may affect the bladder (cystocele), rectum (rectocele), bowel (enterocele), or uterus (uterine prolapse).

Etiology and Pathophysiology

Because the lack of estrogen results in weakening of tissue structures, pelvic relaxation syndrome may occur as women age. The bladder protrudes through the vaginal wall, forming a cystocele, or into the rectum, forming a rectocele. Our increasing life span results in these problems occurring more commonly. Heavy lifting, constipation, and obesity contribute to the weakening of the pelvic floor muscles and tissues. Pelvic surgery and the strain of vaginal childbirth may also contribute to the development of pelvic relaxation syndrome.

Signs and Symptoms

Symptoms relate to the specific organs involved. In a cystocele, urinary frequency or incontinence is most common. A rectocele may result in constipation, soiling, or painful defecation. A uterine prolapse may result in dyspareunia. The uterus may protrude from the vaginal orifice. The woman often complains of general symptoms that include a sense of fullness in the pelvis and backache. Stress incontinence (loss of small amount of urine during coughing, sneezing, or lifting objects) may occur.

Diagnosis

Diagnosis is confirmed by history and physical examination. Obtain an obstetric history concerning the number of vaginal deliveries and the size of the infants, which may have contributed to the problem. A history of stress incontinence or constipation may indicate how the problem may interfere with activities of daily living. A computed tomography scan may be required if other pelvic pathology is suspected. The patient and the health care provider determine if a nonsurgical or surgical approach to management is most appropriate.

Treatment and Nursing Management

Nonsurgical Management. *Nonsurgical* management includes teaching the woman how to perform Kegel exercises in order to strengthen the pubococcygeal muscles that support the pelvic floor (see Chapter 34). Lifestyle changes include increasing fluid intake and a high-fiber diet to avoid constipation, avoiding heavy lifting, and maintaining an optimum weight. Hormone therapy may be prescribed. A *pessary* (a hard rubber or plastic ring) can be fitted into the vagina by the health care provider to provide support to the pelvic structures.

Complementary and Alternative Therapies

Biofeedback and Transcutaneous Electrical Nerve Stimulation

Biofeedback and transcutaneous electrical nerve stimulation (TENS) may be offered by a licensed provider to help strengthen the pelvic floor muscles.

Surgical Management. The procedure to repair a cystocele or rectocele is called an anteroposterior repair *(colporrhaphy)*. A hysterectomy (removal of the uterus) may be indicated. The management of stress

Table 39-4   Medications Used to Relieve Dysmenorrhea

MEDICATION	SIDE EFFECTS	NURSING IMPLICATIONS
Nonsteroidal anti-inflammatory drugs (NSAIDs) (Ibuprofen, Motrin, Naproxen)	Nausea, dyspepsia, itching, rash	Contraindicated in hemophilia, bleeding ulcers, bleeding disorders. Do not take with aspirin. (Check labels on cold/allergy medications that may contain NSAIDs.) Take around the clock when menses start to treat discomforts. Take with meals. Avoid alcohol.
Mefenamic acid (potent prostaglandin synthesis inhibitor) (COX-2 inhibitors)	Diarrhea, nausea, abdominal distention	Contraindicated in hemophilia, bleeding ulcers, bleeding disorders. Used for women who cannot tolerate NSAIDs.
Oral contraceptives	Women who smoke should not use hormone therapy. Risks and benefits should be discussed with health care provider.	Used with caution in women with blood clotting disorders, cardiovascular disorders, or cancer.
Levonorgestrel-releasing intrauterine system (LNG-IUS)	Requires invasive application and medical follow-up	Can be used in combination with contraceptive therapy.

incontinence includes minimally invasive surgery performed under local anesthesia, called a tension-free vaginal tape (TVT) sling procedure, wherein a transvaginal mesh sling is inserted to support the urethra. This procedure is contraindicated in women who plan to become pregnant or have a urinary tract infection or a blood-clotting problem (Altman, 2011). Postoperatively, the nurse must monitor bowel and bladder patency. Residual urine may be measured after voiding via ultrasound or catheterization. Routine postoperative pain management is provided. See Chapter 35 for treatments for urinary incontinence.

POLYCYSTIC OVARIAN SYNDROME

Polycystic ovarian syndrome is a congenital condition in which many cysts develop on one or both ovaries and produce excess estrogen. High levels of testosterone and luteinizing hormone (LH) and low levels of follicle-stimulating hormone (FSH) occur. Signs and symptoms include irregular menstruation, infertility, hyperinsulinemia, and glucose tolerance problems. Excessive hair on the body (hirsutism) is common.

Treatment of polycystic ovarian syndrome involves use of OCs to inhibit LH and testosterone production. Surgical removal of the cysts may be indicated. If pregnancy is desired, ovulation-stimulating medications are prescribed. The nurse should advise the patient concerning the importance of follow-up care to monitor the progress of this condition.

DYSFUNCTIONAL UTERINE BLEEDING

Dysfunctional uterine bleeding is uterine bleeding that occurs at times other than the normal menstrual cycle, or abnormal bleeding during menstruation. Uterine bleeding may be considered abnormal if the interval between menstruations is less than 21 days or more than 45 days, the duration of menstrual flow is more than 7 days, or the amount of blood loss exceeds 80 mL.

Oligomenorrhea (decreased menstruation) usually refers to menstrual periods that occur at an interval of 45 days or longer. The cause often involves a problem with the hypothalamus, the pituitary gland, or ovarian function. Hormone therapy is the treatment of choice, and the woman should be educated concerning advantages and disadvantages of hormone therapy. The use of OCs can decrease menstrual flow. Structural abnormalities can cause obstructions or destruction of the endometrium, resulting in oligomenorrhea. The woman should be taught to keep close records of her menstrual cycle and associated symptoms.

Amenorrhea means absent menstruation. *Primary amenorrhea* refers to women who have not had a normal onset of menstrual periods (they never started to menstruate). *Secondary amenorrhea* applies to women who began normal menses that later ceased. Some causes can include anatomical defects such as *imperforate* (closed) hymen, an endocrine dysfunction affecting female hormones, chronic disease, extreme weight loss or obesity, emotional disturbances, drug side effect, excessive exercise, or poor nutrition. Amenorrhea occurs with pregnancy, but that is a normal occurrence. Goals of treatment include progression of normal pubertal development; prevention of complications such as osteoporosis, endometrial hyperplasia, or heart disease; and promotion of fertility.

Metrorrhagia is bleeding between menstrual periods. Occasionally, a brief episode of "spotting" occurs 14 days before the expected menstrual period (corresponding to the time of ovulation). This is known as "mittle staining" and is considered normal. Women who take OCs or have IUDs may have bleeding between menstrual periods, which is termed *breakthrough bleeding*. The problem is usually resolved by adjusting medication or dosage. Causes of abnormal metrorrhagia include leiomyomas, uterine polyps, trauma, foreign body, malignancy, infection, or an interrupted pregnancy. The treatment depends on the cause. Nursing responsibilities include providing reassurance, support, and education.

Menorrhagia is excessive menstrual bleeding or extended duration of the menstrual period. There are many causes, including hormone imbalances, malignancies, fibroids, infections, and the use of some drugs. One cause of heavy menstrual bleeding is von Willebrand's disease, which is caused by a chromosome factor VIII dysfunction. Symptoms often include frequent nosebleeds and delayed postpartum hemorrhage. Blood tests should be taken during menstruation for accurate diagnosis (James, 2009). Treatment of menorrhagia depends on the cause. The hemoglobin and hematocrit should always be assessed to determine the seriousness of the blood loss. In 2010 the FDA approved a nonhormonal treatment of menorrhagia with the drug tranexamic acid (Lysteda). This oral medication works by reducing clot breakdown in the uterus. Lysteda should not be used with oral contraceptives, as the risk for thrombus formation or strokes increase with the combination (FDA, 2010). Nursing interventions include education concerning follow-up care, an iron-rich diet to combat anemia, and information concerning treatment options.

ABNORMAL UTERINE BLEEDING

Abnormal uterine bleeding is defined as uterine bleeding not related to the menstrual period. It is often caused by anovulation and a failure of hormonal changes during the menstrual cycle. Abnormal uterine bleeding most often occurs at the beginning (menarche) or end (menopause) of the reproductive years. Bleeding due to continuous estrogen production can also occur due to thyroid dysfunction, polycystic ovarian disease, infection, trauma, or neoplasm. Use of some herbal products that promote estrogen activity can also cause dysfunctional or abnormal uterine bleeding.

 Elder Care Points

Vaginal bleeding in elderly women is a possible warning sign of cervical or uterine cancer. An immediate pelvic examination to determine and treat the cause of such bleeding is advised. The incidence of these cancers increases with age.

Monitoring the hemoglobin and hematocrit is essential, and hospitalization may be required if the hemoglobin falls below 8 g/100 mL. Severe bleeding may be treated with intravenous conjugated estrogens (Premarin) until bleeding stops or slows significantly. A dilation and evacuation (formerly known as a dilation and curettage) and endometrial biopsy may be required. The woman may be given oral contraceptives for 3 to 6 months, after which the bleeding pattern will be reassessed.

Persistent anovulation (failure to ovulate) with continuous estrogen stimulation of the endometrium can cause abnormal tissue changes in the uterus. Nursing interventions include educating the patient concerning the use of unsupervised CAM therapies and proper use of OCs, providing support during treatments, and ensuring that the patient is aware of treatment options.

LEIOMYOMA

Commonly known as uterine fibroids, leiomyomas are benign tumors of the uterine muscle. Ovarian hormones influence growth of leiomyomas, and they are common in women taking birth control pills. Leiomyomas spontaneously shrink during and after menopause. Common symptoms include backache, a sense of lower abdominal pressure, constipation, urinary frequency or incontinence, and abnormal uterine bleeding. A pelvic examination and ultrasound may help confirm the diagnosis.

Medical management of leiomyomas depends on the size and location of the fibroids, the symptoms experienced, the desire for future pregnancies, and how near the woman is to natural menopause. In mild cases, monitoring and supportive care to relieve symptoms are indicated. Nonsteroidal anti-inflammatory drugs or OCs may be prescribed. In severe cases, leuprolide (Lupron) or nafarelin (Synarel)—gonadotropin-releasing hormone (GnRH) agonists that shrink the fibroids—and other hormones may be prescribed to suppress estrogen. These drugs may cause menopausal symptoms and bone demineralization, and their use is limited to a 6-month period to reduce the fibroids and prepare for surgery.

Uterine artery embolization involves the injection of special pellets into selected blood vessels that supply the fibroid, resulting in shrinkage of the fibroid. It is performed under conscious sedation by an interventional radiologist (a physician who is a radiologist and specializes in invasive procedures not requiring general anesthesia). Cramping, nausea, fever, and malaise (postembolic syndrome) may occur postoperatively as the fibroid degenerates. Postoperative pain may require an overnight hospitalization and treatment with fentanyl or hydromorphone (Dilaudid) by patient-controlled analgesia. Maintenance of hydration and ambulation to prevent complications are encouraged postoperatively. After 6 weeks, magnetic resonance imaging (MRI) confirms the effectiveness of the procedure. Postoperative teaching includes avoiding the use of anticoagulant drugs, including aspirin; avoiding douches, sexual intercourse, and the use of tampons for 4 weeks postoperatively; monitoring urine output; preventing constipation; and returning for follow-up care.

Myomectomy is the removal of the tumor from the uterine wall and can be accomplished by use of an endoscope via an abdominal incision *(laparoscopy)* or vaginally *(hysteroscopy)*. It is performed in the proliferative phase of the menstrual cycle and does minimal damage to the uterine lining, allowing for positive pregnancy outcomes in the future. Fibroids can eventually return. *Hysteroscopic endometrial ablation* involves resection of submucosal fibroids followed by scraping and burning of tissue. This procedure significantly reduces future fertility. *Laser cauterization* of the fibroids can also be done laparoscopically or vaginally but may scar the uterine wall and prevent future pregnancies. *Magnetic resonance–guided focused ultrasound surgery (MRgFUS)* is a safe way to significantly reduce symptoms of premenopausal uterine fibroids with a rapid return to quality of life (Stewart et al., 2006 and Hacker, 2010).

A hysterectomy may be performed if the woman does not wish future pregnancies. A laparoscopic supracervical hysterectomy preserves the cervix and is less invasive, with fewer complications (Hacker, 2010). However, for benign disease, the vaginal route for hysterectomy is preferred (ACOG, 2009b). Currently in the United States, approximately 22% of hysterectomies are performed vaginally, 12% laparoscopically and 66% abdominally (Clinical Insights, 2010). Of the 600,000 hysterectomies performed within the United States each year, approximately 40% are for fibroids, 17% are for endometriosis, and 14% treat vaginal prolapse (Clinical Insights, 2010). The postoperative teaching plan should include information concerning advantages and disadvantages of hormone therapy, comfort measures for pain relief, and when to resume normal activities. The use of lubricants for vaginal intercourse and a plan for follow-up care should also be provided. Danger signs to report to the health care provider include bleeding and abnormal vaginal discharge.

ENDOMETRIOSIS

Endometriosis is a common disorder in which endometrial tissue (the inner lining of the uterus) is found outside the uterus, particularly on the ovaries, in the rectovaginal septum (wall separating the rectum and the vagina), and in the pelvis and abdomen. It usually undergoes the same changes as the normal endometrium during the menstrual cycle and may bleed at the time of menses, which can cause irritation, pain, and the formation of adhesions. Other symptoms may include excessive menstrual flow, bleeding between periods, painful bowel movements, and painful coitus.

Continuous hormonal contraceptive therapy and drugs such as medroxyprogesterone acetate (Depo-Provera) or norethindrone (Ortho Micronor) suppress growth of the endometrial tissue. Danazol (Cyclomen, Danocrine) and GnRH agonists such as leuprolide or nafarelin create a "pseudomenopause" by interfering with hormones that stimulate ovulation and menstruation. Menopausal symptoms such as hot flashes, decreased *libido* (sexual drive), and reduced bone density may occur. Continuous hormonal contraceptive treatment may be continued for 3 to 6 months. Surgical treatment may include a laparoscopy to remove adhesions or laser evaporation of the uterine tissue.

If the woman does not desire children in the future, a complete hysterectomy and removal of all endometrial lesions is the treatment of choice. Treatment for menopausal symptoms may be needed postoperatively.

Robotic Gynecologic Surgery

Robotic surgery is surgery performed by a surgeon's medical manipulation of robotic "hands" and electronic monitors. Robotic surgery has benefits such as shorter operative time, shorter hospitalization, and more sophisticated surgery. Limitations include increased hospital cost, which must be weighed against the shorter hospital stay. Robotic surgery is not indicated for very short procedures such as endoscopic sterilization. A vaginal hysterectomy is preferred over an open hysterectomy or robotic procedure because of the lower morbidity rates of vaginal approach over any other type. Urogynecologic reconstructive surgery and fistula repair is best accomplished by robotic approach. The application of robotic surgery to treatment of gynecologic cancers is promising. Robotic surgery may be preferred over minilaparotomy for tubal anastomosis or reproductive endocrinology (Akl and Magrina, 2009).

INFLAMMATIONS OF THE LOWER GENITAL TRACT

Etiology and Pathophysiology

Inflammations or infections of the vulva, vagina, or cervix most often occur when the acid environment of the vaginal secretions changes, enabling the survival of pathogenic organisms. The acid environment of the vaginal vault is maintained by estrogen levels and by the presence of *Lactobacillus*. Risk factors that alter the bacterial flora and pH environment within the vagina include aging; poor nutrition; the use of medications such as steroids, OCs, or antibiotics; and douching.

Organisms can also gain entrance to the vagina through contaminated hands, clothing, loss of skin integrity due to trauma or surgery, or sexual intercourse. Vulvar infections typically occur as a result of skin trauma caused by itching and scratching. Although *Candida albicans* is present in low levels in the vaginal area, a change in vaginal pH can lead to an overgrowth, resulting in vulvovaginitis (Table 39-5).

Signs, Symptoms, and Diagnosis

A history and physical examination usually reveal the nature of the problem. Often lesions may be present, and *dysuria* (painful urination) often occurs because the acidic urine comes into contact with open lesions. An abnormal vaginal discharge may occur that often causes *pruritus* (itching discomfort). Women with cervicitis may experience bloody spotting after intercourse.

The diagnosis of the specific condition may be accomplished by culturing vaginal discharge or lesions, blood tests for specific infections, or a colposcopy or biopsy of the lesion. Drug therapy is based on the diagnosis.

Treatment and Nursing Management

You can teach the woman about the risks and prevention of genital infections, as well as the treatment protocol for the specific infection. Infections of the lower genital tract are typically treated with local creams, vaginal suppositories, or systemic antimicrobials. Hand hygiene, wearing loose cotton underwear, and the use of intermittent warm, local, moist heat provide comfort and decrease irritation. Genital infections can cause the woman embarrassment, may lower self-image, and may negatively affect relationships. Providing psychological support is very important. Since many organisms that cause lower genital tract infections are spread by sexual intercourse, prompt treatment is essential in order to prevent the spread of infection to the upper genital tract. The importance of recognizing symptoms and seeking medical care should be stressed. A nonjudgmental attitude of the nurse will empower the woman to ask questions and seek advice. The nurse ensures that the woman fully understands directions for taking medication or applying creams, and visual aids should be used whenever possible to ensure clarity of directions. Infections of the lower genital tract that are also STIs, such as pelvic inflammatory disease, are discussed in Chapter 41.

TOXIC SHOCK SYNDROME

Toxic shock syndrome (TSS) is a rare and potentially fatal disorder caused by strains of *Staphylococcus aureus* that produce toxins that cause shock, coagulation

Table 39-5	Comparisons of Two Types of Common Vaginal Infections	
	BACTERIAL VAGINOSIS	**YEAST INFECTION**
Primary causative organism(s)	*Gardnerella* (most common).	*Candida* (formerly called *Monilia*).
Onset	May be asymptomatic.	Abrupt; preceding menstruation.
Odor	Fishy, most noticeable after intercourse.	None or mild "musty" odor.
Itching	Usually none (does not invade vaginal wall).	Severe; most prominent symptom.
Discharge	Thin, gray, may be frothy.	Thick, white, "cottage cheese" when colonization is heavy.
Sexually transmitted	Possibly; 70% of women have this organism present in vaginal flora.	Possibly. Associated with high estrogen levels; diabetes mellitus; tight underclothing that increases warmth and moisture.
Vulvar signs	Absent.	Redness; excoriation from scratching; may have edema of labia.
Vaginal signs	Vaginal pH above 4.6. Little redness; discharge adherent to vaginal wall, normal cervix.	Normal cervix, no discharge. Lesions and edema from scratching.
Treatment	Metronidazole orally, sometimes vaginally; clindamycin in second trimester if pregnant (associated with adverse pregnancy outcomes).	Miconazole, clotrimazole, or nystatin vaginally as directed. Oral treatment: fluconazole (Diflucan) 150-mg single dose. Nonprescription treatment is available.

defects, and tissue damage if they enter the bloodstream. It is associated with the trapping of bacteria within the reproductive tract for a prolonged time. Risk factors include the prolonged use of high-absorbency tampons, cervical caps, or diaphragms. Symptoms of TSS include:
- Sudden spiking fever
- Flulike symptoms
- Hypotension
- Generalized rash resembling a sunburn
- Peeling skin on the palms or soles

Treatment includes hospitalization and intensive care with supportive treatments and intravenous antimicrobials. The nurse plays an important role in preventing TSS by teaching the woman hand hygiene when inserting tampons, and the importance of changing tampons every 4 hours. Tampons should not be used when sleeping as they will likely remain in place longer than 4 hours. Diaphragms and cervical caps should not be left in place for a prolonged time or be used during menstruation.

CANCER OF THE REPRODUCTIVE TRACT

Vulvar Cancer

Vulvar intraepithelial neoplasia (VIN) refers to the growth of abnormal tissue on the vulva that may be precancerous. Cancer of the vulva is rare, and occurs most commonly in elderly women. Symptoms include red, brown, or white patches on the skin of the vulva. Treatment includes surgical removal of the pathologic tissue. Some strains of VIN are associated with the human papillomavirus (HPV). The incorporation of the HPV vaccine (Gardasil) into the standard immunization regimen for all girls will further reduce the incidence of this condition.

Cancer of the Cervix

Cervical cancer is the second leading cause of death in women 20 to 29 years of age (Klisc & Kaplan, 2009). Risk factors for cervical cancer include multiple sex partners, sexual intercourse with uncircumcised males, starting intercourse at a young age (younger than 20 years of age), multiple pregnancies, obesity, and history of HPV infection or an STI. The HPV vaccine given to girls at or before puberty may prevent the type of HPV infection that causes cervical cancer. Regular pelvic examinations and Pap smears may enable early diagnosis and provide opportunity for early and more successful intervention. ACOG recommends that cervical cancer screening should begin at age 21 and be repeated every 2 years between ages 21 and 29 in asymptomatic women. Women with three consecutive negative screenings at age 30 should have repeated testing every 3 years until age 65, when testing of asymptomatic women is no longer necessary. Women with cervical pathology or cancer should be screened annually for 20 years after treatment (ACOG, 2009c).

Treatment of cervical cancer may include cryosurgery, electrosurgical incision, or surgical conization of the cervix. Advanced cervical cancer may require a hysterectomy with bilateral salpingo-oophorectomy (removal of the uterus, including the fallopian tubes and ovaries) followed by radiation and chemotherapy. See Chapter 8 for discussion of care of a patient receiving radiation or chemotherapy.

Cancer of the Uterus

The most common malignant tumor of the female reproductive tract is endometrial cancer. It is a slow-growing cancer that most often occurs after menopause. The treatment of choice is a hysterectomy with bilateral salpingo-oophorectomy. Treatment is often complicated by the fact that many women with cancer of the uterus may be elderly, or have chronic conditions such as diabetes. Surgery is often followed by radiation and chemotherapy. Chemotherapy agents used are doxorubicin (Adriamycin), cisplatin (Platinol), 5-fluorouracil (5-FU), carboplatin (Paraplatin), and paclitaxel (Taxol). See Chapter 8 for discussion concerning care of the patient receiving chemotherapy and radiation therapy.

Cancer of the Ovary

Approximately 70% of ovarian tumors are benign. Ovarian cancer is known as a "silent cancer" because signs and symptoms are often nonspecific or vague, such as fatigue or abdominal distention with no detectable precancerous changes in the ovary.

 Health Promotion

Symptoms of Ovarian Cancer

The American Cancer Society lists warning signs of ovarian cancer as:
- Abdominal pain
- Feeling full quickly when eating
- Feeling a frequent or urgent need to urinate
- Increased abdominal girth

An important risk factor for the development of ovarian cancer is having a sister or mother with the disease, or inheriting the *BRCA1* or *BRCA2* gene, which is also associated with breast cancer. Exposure to talc powder, fertility drugs, obesity, pelvic irradiation, or mumps has also been linked to the development of ovarian cancer. Women on hormone therapy should be informed concerning the risks for ovarian cancer (Morch, 2009). Factors that may prevent ovarian cancer include one or more term pregnancies, breast-feeding, bilateral tubal ligation, prophylactic oophorectomy, and the use of OCs (American Cancer Society, 2011). Ovarian cancer is classified according to the type of tissue within the ovary that is involved. Diagnosis is often made during a routine pelvic examination. An ovarian cancer tumor marker (CA-125; assessed by a blood test) combined with pelvic ultrasound can detect ovarian cancer, but not at an early stage. Researchers at Yale Medical School have a new test under development and trials that could detect ovarian cancer in the early stages. However, at this date, the CA-125 test is not covered as a routine screening by most insurance companies. Once diagnosis is established, a *panhysterectomy* (removal of the uterus, the fallopian tubes, and the ovaries) is followed by chemotherapy and radiation. Newer drugs have improved the survival rate to 50%. Cisplatin and carboplatin are used for stage III and stage IV disease. Altretamine (Hexalen) is used

for recurrent ovarian cancer. Paclitaxel and topotecan (Hycamtin) are used to treat metastatic ovarian cancer. See Chapter 8 concerning care of the patient with cancer.

DISORDERS OF THE BREAST

Although the breast is not a reproductive organ, it is affected by hormonal changes that occur during the menstrual cycle and during and after pregnancy.

BENIGN DISORDERS OF THE BREAST

Fibroadenoma

Fibroadenomas are commonly found in the teenager and young adult. Fibroadenomas are firm, rubbery, mobile nodules of fibrous and glandular tissue that may or may not be tender on palpation. They usually occur in the upper outer quadrant of the breast and do not change during the menstrual cycle. A fine-needle aspiration or biopsy may be performed to determine the presence of cancerous cells.

Fibrocystic Breast Changes

Fibrocystic breast changes (FBCs) were formerly called *fibrocystic breast disorder*. This condition is common during the reproductive years. It is a palpable thickening of portions of the breast tissue associated with pain and tenderness. Multiple smooth, well-delineated cysts may form that are most painful during the premenstrual phase of the menstrual cycle. The "lumps" make BSE more difficult and are a frequent source of anxiety. Women with FBCs can learn to recognize the size and shape of their normal lumps and should report any change in these findings to their health care provider. Treatment of fibrocystic changes is conservative and based on supportive care. Vitamin E supplements, the elimination of caffeine and alcohol, reduction of fat in the diet, and the use of nonsteroidal anti-inflammatory drugs such as ibuprofen help control discomfort found with FBCs. Wearing a supportive bra and the use of heat are also helpful.

 Complementary and Alternative Therapies

CAM Therapy for FBCs

Relaxation techniques and herbal therapy with angelica, lady's mantle, or evening primrose oil are helpful in FBCs.

Intraductal Papilloma

Intraductal papilloma is the development of small elevations in the epithelium of the ducts of the breasts under the areola. The ducts erode, causing a serosanguineous discharge from the nipple. Treatment includes excision of the mass and analysis of the discharge to determine if cancer cells are present.

The nurse should clarify and reinforce the explanations of diagnostic procedures to be performed, and recognize the anxiety and apprehension that the woman feels, until the final diagnosis is confirmed. The woman should be encouraged to express her concerns, and supportive care should be provided.

BREAST CANCER

The United States has a high breast cancer rate, with approximately 230,480 women and 2140 men diagnosed with breast cancer in 2007. The breast cancer rate for white women is higher than the rates for African American or Asian American women (Kerlikowski, 2009). The increased incidence of breast cancer may be due to the advanced technology that can detect cancer at an earlier stage. Although the risk of developing breast cancer increases with the woman's age, many other factors contribute to the risk (Box 39-5). Breast cancer is identified according to the structure affected, and is staged according to the size and degree of invasiveness (Table 39-6).

| Box 39-5 | Risk Factors for Breast Cancer* |

- Family history of relative with breast cancer
- Early menarche, late menopause
- Late first pregnancy or no children
- Abnormal cells in previous breast biopsy
- Obesity
- Environmental exposure to hormone-modulating chemicals such as pesticides and polycyclic aromatic hydrocarbons found in meat barbequed or grilled at high temperatures
- Inherited *BRCA1* or *BRCA2* gene

*Note that the specific cause of breast cancer has not been established. It is most likely due to genetic factors combined with environmental factors resulting in a cumulative risk level. The first four risk factors are included on the National Cancer Institute (NCI) risk assessment tool available at www.cancer.org.

Etiology and Pathophysiology

The development of breast cancer is thought to be related to the hormones estrogen and progesterone. For example, women who start to menstruate at an early age (early menarche) or who experience late menopause are exposed to more estrogen spikes during

| Table 39-6 | Stages of Breast Cancer |

CANCER STAGE	LOCATION	DESCRIPTION	5-YEAR SURVIVAL RATE
Stage 0	Carcinoma in situ	Lobular carcinoma in situ (LCIS)—cancer cells in lining of a lobule. Ductal carcinoma in situ (DCIS)—cancer cells in lining of a duct.	100%
Stage I	Early stage of invasive cancer	Tumor is <2 cm in diameter. Cancer cells have not spread beyond the breast.	100%
Stage II	Invasive	Any one of the following: • Tumor is <2 cm across. Cancer has spread to lymph nodes under the arm. • Tumor is between 2 and 5 cm. Cancer may have spread to lymph nodes under the arm. • Tumor is >5 cm. Cancer has not spread to lymph nodes under arm.	92%-81%
Stage III	Locally advanced	Large tumor, but cancer has **not** spread beyond the breast and nearby lymph nodes.	
Stage IIIA		Any one of the following: • Tumor is <5 cm. Cancer has spread to underarm lymph nodes attached to each other or to other structures. • Tumor is >5 cm. Cancer has spread to underarm lymph nodes.	67%
Stage IIIB		Any one of the following: • Tumor has grown into chest wall or skin of the breast. • Cancer has spread to lymph nodes behind the breastbone. *Inflammatory breast cancer* is a rare type of Stage IIIB wherein breast looks red and swollen because cancer cells block the lymph vessels in the skin of the breast.	54%
Stage IIIC		Any size tumor that has: • Spread to lymph nodes behind the breastbone and under the arm. • Spread to lymph nodes under or above the collarbone.	This was defined only a few years ago, hence survival rate not yet available
Stage IV	Distant metastatic	Distant metastatic cancer. Cancer has spread to other parts of the body.	20%

From National Cancer Institute: Cancer Information Service at www.cancer.gov and *Breast Cancer Facts & Figures: 2009-2010,* (retrieved from www.cancer.org, June 2011).

monthly ovulation, whereas women who have had multiple pregnancies have fewer monthly ovulating cycles and hormonal spikes.

Recently, the genes *BRCA1* and *BRCA2* were identified as genes involved in the inherited form of breast cancer. Not all women who carry these genes will develop breast cancer, and some women who do not carry these genes will still develop breast cancer. A small percentage (5% to 10%) of newly diagnosed breast cancer is the inherited type, but 80% of the women with this gene develop breast cancer (Kerlikowski, 2009). Genetic testing for this gene is available.

Legal and Ethical Considerations

BRCA1 and *BRCA2* Genes

If all women are tested for the presence of the *BRCA1* or *BRCA2* gene, the ethical problem is the action to take if the gene is present. Should the young woman have a prophylactic mastectomy? Should the woman be given prophylactic treatment with tamoxifen? Does the knowledge of the potential risk for cancer produce anxiety that may result in life changes that can have a negative outcome? Would there be health insurance implications?

In 2009 the U.S. Preventive Services Task Force did not recommend that routine genetic testing be done. *BRCA* testing costs about $2975 per test and is not usually covered by insurance. Significant risk factors that may warrant genetic counseling or *BRCA* testing include:

- In women of Ashkenazi Jewish descent:
  - A first-degree relative with breast/ovarian cancer
  - Two second-degree relatives on same side of family
- In women of non–Ashkenazi Jewish descent:
  - Two first-degree relatives with breast cancer, with one younger than age 50
  - Three first- or second-degree relatives with breast cancer
  - A first-degree relative with bilateral breast cancer
  - A history of breast cancer in a male relative

Signs, Symptoms, and Diagnosis

Although 90% of breast lumps are detected by the woman during a BSE, most early breast cancer can be detected by mammography (radiographic examination of the breast) before it can be clinically palpated. A nipple discharge or change in the skin pattern such as "dimpled skin" on the breast may also be a sign of breast cancer. Any unilateral breast change should be immediately reported to a health care provider. Even a short delay in diagnosis can result in invasion of surrounding tissue and metastasis to other the parts of the body. Refer to Table 39-2 for details on the role of ultrasound or MRI diagnostic tests in confirming diagnosis.

Prevention

A healthy lifestyle that includes exercise and a diet rich in antioxidants and phytoestrogens—such as vegetables, fruits, whole grains, and soy products—may protect against the development of many cancers. Monthly BSE (see Figure 39-5) and regular scheduled mammograms between ages 50 and 74 have been recommended by the ACOG, but research concerning a needs-based or individual-risk screening plan is ongoing (Kerlikowski, 2009). At present, the drug tamoxifen is used to prevent recurrent breast cancer; however, tamoxifen is not used as a general prophylactic measure in women with risk factors because of potential side effects such as increased bone pain, photosensitivity, headache, and increased risk for pulmonary embolism or uterine malignancies. The drug raloxifene (Evista) is FDA approved for the prevention of osteoporosis in postmenopausal women, and may play a significant role in breast cancer prevention. Raloxifene tends to cause more dangerous side effects than tamoxifen such as thromboembolism and stroke. Aromatase inhibitors such as exemestane may be more effective than tamoxifen and have fewer side effects (Liu, 2011).

Some women who have known genetic *BRCA1* or *BRCA2* predispositions have elected to have prophylactic bilateral mastectomies. The psychological implications and effect on self-image should be carefully measured against the preventive benefits. The decision is between the woman and her health care provider.

Treatment

Treatment options are based on the type of breast cancer, stage of the disease, patient's age, physical and menopausal status, and other health factors that may affect the woman's ability to undergo the specific treatment. In general, the primary treatment is usually surgical removal of the tumor and varying amounts of surrounding tissue. The types of surgery include:

- *Lumpectomy* (removal of tumor only).
- Partial or *segmental mastectomy* (removal of tumor and a portion of the surrounding breast tissue and axillary lymph nodes).
- Simple or *total mastectomy* (removal of entire breast and axillary lymph nodes).
- *Modified radical mastectomy* (removal of breast, axillary lymph nodes, and lining over the chest wall muscles).
- *Radical mastectomy* (removal of breast, axillary lymph nodes, and chest wall muscles under the breast). Radical mastectomy was once common, but high success rates with a reduction in disfigurement are now made possible by using appropriate staging of the disease when making treatment decisions.

A suggested nursing care plan for a woman undergoing a lumpectomy in a same-day surgery unit is presented in Nursing Care Plan 39-2. If there is concern

Nursing Care Plan 39-2   Care of the Patient After Breast Lumpectomy

Scenario

A 24-year-old woman is ready for discharge from the same-day surgery unit after undergoing a breast lumpectomy for a suspicious breast lesion. She expresses concern about the amount of scar tissue that will form and that her breasts may no longer be the same size after the lumpectomy.

Problem/Nursing Diagnosis

Worry about abnormal breast appearance/Anxiety and disturbed body image related to asymmetrical breasts and scar tissue as a result of undergoing a breast lumpectomy.

Supporting Assessment Data

Subjective: Concern about scar tissue and that breasts will no longer be the same size.
Objective: Lumpectomy.

Goals/Expected Outcomes	Nursing Interventions	Selected Rationale	Evaluation
Patient will use positive coping strategies to adjust to changes in body image as evidenced by use of support system and available resources.	Assess for previous problem with self-esteem.	Previous coping strategies can be revealed by discussing previous experiences.	Patient discussed previous experiences and recognizes the stages of loss she experienced.
	Assess for signs of anxiety or inability to focus.	Anxiety can be an expected result of a diagnosis that may involve a possible cancer.	Patient expressed understanding of prognosis as explained by physician.
	Encourage verbalization of feelings.	Verbalization can reduce anxiety and focus on the problem of altered body image.	Patient expressed her concerns about scar tissue and alteration in breast symmetry.
	Involve family and multidisciplinary health care team in offering support.	Providing patient with broad support base and resources assists in adjustment.	Patient expressed understanding of healing process and resources available for assistance after discharge.
	Provide accurate information concerning prognosis.	Provides an opportunity to correct misinformation.	Patient expressed understanding of need for follow-up care.
	Encourage her to help care for wound.	Looking at and touching wound indicates readiness to participate in self-care to achieve optimum wound healing.	Patient states will actively participate in wound dressing changes.

Critical Thinking Questions

1. What factors influence a woman's perception of the importance of body image?
2. What other problems or issues might there be for a woman sent home the same day after a breast lumpectomy?

---

that cancer cells have invaded the lymph nodes, an axillary node dissection may be done during breast surgery, in which the lymph nodes under the affected arm are removed and sent to the laboratory. This procedure may result in swelling of the affected arm. Sentinel node biopsy is popular, wherein one node is removed and, if laboratory results show no evidence of cancer, the remaining nodes are left intact.

Tamoxifen (Nolvadex) blocks estrogen by binding with the estrogen receptors. This drug is usually prescribed for 5 years. Nausea and anorexia may occur, and cholesterol and triglyceride levels should be monitored. Approximately 25% of women have a type of breast cancer tumor that manifests the human epidermal growth factor receptor-2 protein (*HER2*-positive breast cancer). Studies have shown that the monoclonal antibody trastuzumab (Herceptin) added to chemotherapy is very effective at reducing the risk of tumor recurrence (Kelanu, 2010). The woman should be monitored for cardiovascular side effects of this drug.

Research is ongoing concerning the customizing of treatment options for women with breast cancer. The National Institutes of Health and the National Cancer Institute (NCI) are researching a treatment trial called TAILORx (Trial Assigning Individual Options for Treatment). Women are assigned to treatment regimens based on genetic findings. The results of these trials may enable a change from standardized treatment to customized treatment protocols (Kerlikowski, 2009).

Radiation therapy often is done following lumpectomy or segmented mastectomy, to destroy micrometastases and decrease cancer recurrence rates. Radiation therapy options include whole-breast radiotherapy using external beam radiation weekly for 7 weeks; intensity-modulated radiation therapy (IMRT), which minimizes damage to surrounding tissue; accelerated partial breast irradiation (APBI), using a balloon catheter in the local tumor site; interstitial brachytherapy, with pellets inserted around the tumor site (Figure 39-6); or external beam radiation (EBRT) after healing occurs. Chemotherapy also may be considered as part of treatment, in combination with surgery and radiation. Aromatase inhibitors such as anastrozole (Arimidex) or letrozole (Femara) or exemestane (Aromasin) reduce the risk of recurrence by inhibiting the enzyme aromatase, which results in decreased estrogen production. Exemestane has been shown to lower the risk of breast cancer by 65% in postmenopausal women at high risk of breast cancer with less side effects than tamoxifen (Liu, et al., 2011). Aromatase inhibitors are not used in premenopausal women with functioning ovaries. An estrogen receptor agonist such as fulvestrant (Faslodex) binds with estrogen receptors, and can be used when tamoxifen fails. Ovarian ablation is the surgical removal or irradiation of the ovary to stop estrogen production. The use of goserelin (Zoladex) may be an alternative to chemotherapy. See Chapter 8 concerning care of the patient receiving chemotherapy or radiation therapy.

 Safety Alert

Aromatase Inhibitors

Skin moisturizers and some vaginal creams that contain estrogens—used on a regular basis—can be dangerous to women with estrogen-receptor–positive cancer, especially if they are taking aromatase inhibitors (Olson et al., 2009).

Breast Reconstructive Surgery

Plastic surgery of the breast may be done to reduce breast size (reduction mammoplasty), enlarge breast size (augmentation mammoplasty), or reconstruct (reconstruction mammoplasty) the breast after breast cancer surgery.

Reduction Mammoplasty. Problems related to an excessively large breast include back and shoulder pain, pressure on nerves from brassiere straps, inability to buy clothing that fits, and psychological problems related to fear of ridicule or unwelcome sexual advances.

A mammogram may be necessary before surgery in women older than 40 years of age. The amount and degree of scarring should be discussed with the woman, as the scar is determined by the technique of surgery. Although data suggest that breast reduction surgery does not interfere with successful breast-feeding, it is possible milk production may be affected (Spector & BFAR, 2011). Decreased nipple sensation or loss of part of the areola may also be a side effect of surgery that the woman should be aware of, preoperatively. Information concerning successful breast-feeding after breast reduction surgery may be obtained from the La Leche League International.

Augmentation Mammoplasty. Breast augmentation is usually initiated by the patient who wishes to improve self-image and attain a sense of increased femininity. Breast augmentation can be accomplished by insertion of a saline implant under the pectoralis muscle.

Reconstructive Mammoplasty. Reconstructive mammoplasty creates a new breast when the natural tissue has been removed during mastectomy. A nipple/areola reconstruction provides a more natural appearance. Saline implants can be used or skin and tissue may be taken from other parts of the body (autologous reconstruction), and tattooing of the nipple area provides natural-looking coloring.

Step 1: During the lumpectomy or shortly thereafter, a deflated balloon is placed inside the cavity created by removal of the tumor.

Step 2: Patient returns to clinic for 1 to 5 days of outpatient treatment, where a radioactive seed is inserted through a catheter into the balloon twice a day for 10 minutes each time. The seed targets radiation to the area where tumors are more likely to recur, while minimizing exposure to healthy tissue.

Step 3: The balloon is deflated and the catheter is removed. No source of radiation remains in the patient's body between treatments or after the final procedure.

FIGURE 39-6 Brachytherapy.

Nursing Management for Breast Cancer Surgery

Preoperative Care. Most women need extensive education before breast surgery. Many surgeons now provide educational programs for their patients, but it is important for the nurse to determine whether the patient did, in fact, receive adequate information and if she has a good understanding of what was taught. Women often are particularly concerned about the change in their appearance following breast surgery. It can be helpful to talk with a Reach to Recovery volunteer, or to a nurse with extensive professional or personal knowledge. Teaching points will vary depending on the amount of tissue to be surgically removed and whether or not a prosthesis will be implanted either during the initial surgery or at a later date (Figure 39-7).

Postoperative Care. Postoperative care will include pain management, observation for signs of infection, and continued supportive and educational measures. Because breast tissue is highly vascular, bleeding may be a problem. Surgical dressings should be observed frequently during the first 48 hours following the procedure.

Body image and disfigurement issues, as well as the focus in our society on the breast as a marker of femininity or sexual attractiveness, make treatment for breast cancer a highly emotionally charged experience. Women require ongoing supportive care, and most will benefit greatly from participating in a support group and from visits by American Cancer Society Reach to Recovery volunteers. These women have all undergone treatment for breast cancer and have been trained to do peer counseling.

Collaborative Care. Collaborative care is essential to reduce anxiety and stress in the breast surgery patient. Emotional support and accurate information are essential. The woman and her partner may differ in how much information they want to discuss. Issues concerning self-image and loss of control should be addressed.

Complications

Lymphedema. Lymphedema is swelling of the arm that sometimes occurs after breast cancer surgery due to the damage to, and resulting congestion of, the lymphatic tract. Lymphedema can also be idiopathic, or of unknown origin; it can also be a congenital problem. Lymphedema occurs within 5 years of treatment in about 42% of women who undergo breast node biopsy or cancer surgery (Fu et al., 2009). Lymphedema can become a chronic condition. The use of sentinel node biopsy—with removal of additional lymph nodes only if the sentinel lymph node is positive for cancer—has reduced the occurrence of lymphedema because the less aggressive the surgery, the less damage to the lymph tissue and therefore the less chance of developing lymphedema. Nursing interventions to help reduce the risk of lymphedema during the postoperative care from breast node biopsy or breast cancer surgery include the following.

FIGURE 39-7   Reconstructive breast surgery. **A,** Appearance of the chest following bilateral mastectomy. **B,** Postoperative breast reconstruction before nipple reconstruction. **C,** Postoperative breast reconstruction after nipple and areolar reconstruction.

- Do not assess blood pressure in the affected arm.
- Do not give injections or do venipuncture in the affected arm.
- Provide meticulous skin care.
- Teach the patient to wear gloves in the kitchen and when gardening to prevent skin irritation or injury.
- Teach the patient to avoid heavy lifting.
- Wear a compression garment during strenuous activities.
- Elevate and exercise the arm daily.

The nurse should review exercises that may be helpful (Figure 39-8). Discharge teaching should focus on the need for follow-up care, exercises to improve range of motion, prevention of infection, side effects of medical therapy, and community resources available.

Lymphedema clinics are available in some states. The standard of care is complex physical therapy, which involves techniques that provide lymphatic drainage, specialized pressure bandaging, application

FRONT WALL CLIMBING
Patient stands facing the wall, elbows slightly bent. Palms are placed at shoulder level and fingers are flexed and unflexed as hands "walk" up the wall as high as possible. Hands are then walked back down to shoulder level. Patient moves toward wall as fingers climb higher and then away from wall as fingers move downward.

SIDE WALL CLIMBING
With operative side to wall, arm is extended until fingers touch wall. Patient moves toward the wall as fingers climb higher until body touches it. Maneuver is reversed as fingers climb back down wall.

ROPE TURNING
One end of rope is tied to door knob. Patient holds other end of rope and swings it in a circular motion, being sure entire arm and not the wrist is in motion.

YARDSTICK OR BROOM LIFT
Holding a yardstick or broom handle with both hands, the back is placed against a wall. Arms are extended straight downward and, with elbows straight, the stick is raised by the straightened arms until knuckles touch the wall over the head.

FIGURE 39-8 Postmastectomy exercises.

of a compression garment, exercising, and skin care (Fu et al., 2009).

The diagnosis and treatment of breast cancer in women can be a direct threat to the sense of femininity and body image. Anxiety, denial, anger, and depression are common reactions. Many women fear that after treatment for breast cancer they will no longer be attractive to their peers. A combination of peer support and psychotherapeutic, spiritual, and educational guidance can help women cope with the diagnosis and treatment. Nurses play a key role in education and referral.

HOME CARE

Home health nursing is a standard of care in the United States. Hospital stays are becoming progressively shorter, and women frequently go home very quickly after illness, surgery, or childbirth. Intravenous antibiotic therapy is increasingly frequent in home settings, as many health problems are being treated outside the hospital setting.

Many women recover at home following surgical procedures. Home health nursing responsibilities include pain management, observation of the surgical site for signs of infection (redness, swelling, pain, presence of exudate, foul odor, fever), or reopening of the surgical wound because of trauma or poor healing response. If the procedure involves the pelvic reproductive organs, the nurse must also assess the amount and duration of bleeding, any increase in the volume of flow, and any change (e.g., purulence or foul odor) that indicates the presence of infection.

The majority of patient teaching is often the responsibility of the home health nurse. Even conscientious teaching by the hospital nurse frequently needs extensive follow-up: the patient's learning ability may be impaired by immediate concerns such as acute pain, recovery from anesthesia, or emotional stresses associated with the diagnosis and its impact on daily living.

Patient Teaching

Teaching the Older Adult

Advanced age can inhibit the ability of the woman to learn at a time when information concerning comfort and health is vital. In any teaching plan, you should:

- Promote readiness and motivation to learn. The woman must sense that the information applies to her and is important.
- Provide brochures; reliable sources confer credibility of information.
- Include the woman's experiences and interests; personalizing teaching makes it more meaningful.
- Ask questions to confirm understanding.
- Provide socialization and opportunity to share. Use group sessions when possible.
- Provide short teaching sessions.
- Face the patient, and talk loudly and clearly.
- Use a quiet, adequately lit environment.

The home health nurse must be prepared to give accurate, detailed information as part of home care. The nurse also should assess the patient's need for more general education regarding reproductive health, such as regular BSE and VSE, Pap smears, and need for information regarding contraception or STIs.

The home health nurse must be able to function independently; she needs to communicate with the other members of the care team by phone, written documentation, and group conferences. The nurse also is often the primary source of information about appropriate support groups and informational programs that could assist the patient and her family.

COMMUNITY CARE

Community care can take many forms. In the area of general reproductive health, low-cost women's health care clinics and organizations such as Planned Parenthood offer pregnancy testing, counseling and instruction on contraception and prevention of STIs, programs concerning BSE and VSE, and screening procedures such as pelvic examinations and mammograms. Instruction and low-cost screening may also be made available by local chapters of organizations such as the American Cancer Society. These outreach programs make information and services available to all women at a reasonable cost. Such programs assist in the prevention and early detection of disease, reducing the long-term effects of potentially serious illness and the cost of intrusive health care.

Community care also takes the form of educational public service announcements on radio and television and in newspapers and magazines. These give the public valuable information on sexual health and disease prevention and treatment.

School nurses can and should play a major role in reproductive education and health maintenance. Drugs, alcohol, and early sexual activity are major health care concerns for our adolescents. The school nurse is in a position to become a trusted source of accurate, nonjudgmental information for young people, who are often confused and may lack education in the realities of reproductive health.

In recent years, a variety of programs have been developed for women at risk for serious diseases of the breast or reproductive organs. Such programs are sponsored by national organizations such as the American Cancer Society or by local groups or health care providers. These programs provide education and offer support groups for women undergoing treatment for breast or uterine cancer, infertility, fetal loss, and other serious health concerns. The nurse can assist in referring women to these community programs, or may volunteer herself as a group facilitator or resource person.

Get Ready for the NCLEX® Examination!

Key Points

- Women should keep a calendar of their individual menstrual cycles to determine regularity and recognize deviations from their normal cycle.
- Premenstrual syndrome (PMS), also known as ovarian cycle syndrome, is the presence of physical, psychological, or behavioral symptoms that regularly occur in the luteal phase of the menstrual cycle.
- Premenstrual dysphoric disorder is a more severe type of PMS described officially in the DSM-IV-TR, a classification of disorders published by the American Psychological Association.
- Personal contraceptive techniques include fertility awareness methods, the basal body temperature (BBT) method, calendar and rhythm methods, the ovulation or Billings method, and the symptothermal method.
- Mechanical contraception includes the use of the male condom, female condom, diaphragm, spermicides, cervical cap, and intrauterine device (IUD).
- Hormonal contraception methods include the use of oral contraceptives (OCs), injectable contraceptives, transcutaneous patches, intrauterine and vaginal inserts, and sustained-release implants.
- Permanent contraception includes tubal ligation (female) and vasectomy (male).
- Emergency contraception may be indicated after unprotected intercourse, but is not meant for regular use.
- Menopause is described as cessation of menses for a 12-month period due to decreased estrogen production. The perimenopausal period or climacteric is the period around the actual cessation of the menstrual period. Common symptoms include irregular menstruation, hot flashes or hot flushes, fatigue, insomnia, emotional swings, depression, back pain, headache, irritability, and decreased libido.
- A decrease in estrogen can increase the risk for the development of osteoporosis and increased blood cholesterol levels.
- Osteoporosis is a decrease in bone mass that increases the risk for bone fractures.
- Breast self-examination (BSE) should be done monthly 1 week after menstruation begins, or on a specific date each month after menopause.
- Risk factors for cancer of the cervix include multiple sex partners, early sexual activity, multiple pregnancies, infection with HPV, and smoking.
- Leiomyomas (fibroids) of the uterus are common among women between 25 and 40 years of age, and may cause vaginal bleeding between menstrual periods.
- Endometriosis is a condition in which endometrial tissue is found outside the uterus.
- Pelvic relaxation syndrome can affect the bladder (cystocele), the rectum (rectocele), or the uterus (uterine prolapse).
- Exercise to restore arm function is very important following mastectomy.
- Disorders of the female reproductive system often affect the woman's self-image.
- Specific genes have been identified that can predict the risk of specific types of breast cancer.
- Screening measures such as mammography, BSE, VSE, and Pap smears allow early detection and treatment of cancer of the reproductive tract.
- Modern technology can assist the woman who has fertility problems.
- The nurse must understand the perceptions of the woman and family before designing a teaching plan.

Additional Learning Resources

SG Go to your Study Guide for additional learning activities to help you master this chapter content.

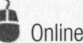 **evolve** Go to your Evolve website (http://evolve.elsevier.com/deWit/medsurg) for the following FREE learning resources:
- Animations, audio, and video
- Answers and rationales for questions and activities
- Concept Map Creator
- Glossary with pronunciations in English and Spanish
- Interactive Review Questions and Exercises and more!

Online Resources
- Breast cancer information, www.breastcancer.org
- National Cancer Institute, www.cancer.gov
- Uterine fibroids, www.emedicinehealth.com/uterine_fibroids/article_em.htm
- National Lymphedema Network, www.lymphnet.org
- North American Menopause Society, www.menopause.org

Review Questions for the NCLEX® Examination

1. A female patient complains of irritability, fatigue, mood swings, and fear of losing control during the days before menstruation. The initial assessment suggests a nursing diagnosis of ineffective coping related to cyclic hormonal changes. Which instruction would likely promote patient coping?

   1. "Avoid calcium-containing foods."
   2. "Exercise regularly."
   3. "Have occasional alcohol."
   4. "Consider a sodium-rich diet."

2. A 44-year-old patient complains of irregular menses with hot flashes. She is informed that she is approaching the climacteric period. Her nurse finds the patient withdrawn and crying. An appropriate statement by the nurse would be:

   1. "It is not the end of the world."
   2. "You seem upset. I am here to listen."
   3. "Everything will be all right."
   4. "Aging is not for the faint of heart."

3. The nurse instructs a premenopausal female patient on how to perform breast self-examinations. Which patient statement indicates understanding?
   1. "I examine my breast about 1 week after menses."
   2. "I can use my thumbs to palpate for lumps and nodules."
   3. "I should pay special attention to the area between the breast and underarm."
   4. "I do not have to see the physician for clinical breast examinations."

4. The nurse is discussing various methods of contraception with a woman. When discussing mechanical methods of contraception that do not provide any protection from STIs, the nurse would specifically include the:
   1. symptothermal method.
   2. Billings method.
   3. use of water soluble lubricants during sexual activity.
   4. use of IUDs.
   5. use of oral contraceptives.

5. The nurse empowers a patient who had a right radical mastectomy by providing specific instructions regarding postoperative care of the surgical site and surgical complications. Which patient statement would indicate a need for more teaching?
   1. "Blood pressures cannot be taken on the right arm."
   2. "I can resume intense weight training immediately after discharge."
   3. "No injections must be given in the right arm."
   4. "When gardening, I need to wear gloves."

6. A 44-year-old patient who had a right radical mastectomy expresses concerns regarding her physical appearance. Further assessment indicates a nursing diagnosis of disturbed body image. An important goal for this patient would be to:
   1. participate in activities of daily living.
   2. demonstrate acceptance of change in appearance.
   3. perform aseptic wound care.
   4. state signs and symptoms of infection.

7. Abnormal bleeding between menstrual periods that is associated with uterine polyps, leiomyomas, trauma, and foreign body is referred to as:
   1. metrorrhagia.
   2. menorrhagia.
   3. oligomenorrhea.
   4. pseudomenopause.

8. Which nursing intervention(s) would help relieve symptoms of dysmenorrhea? (Select all that apply.)
   1. Pelvic rocking exercises
   2. Cold compresses
   3. Effleurage
   4. Low-fat diet
   5. Nonsteroidal anti-inflammatory medications

9. The nurse is discussing healthy lifestyle activities with a woman. Which statement(s) by the woman indicate(s) a need for follow-up teaching? (Select all that apply.)
   1. "I will use herbals such as angelica or evening primrose oil during menstruation to decrease breast tenderness."
   2. "I will focus on drinking caffeine-free colas to keep my fluid intake adequate."
   3. "I will douche regularly with an alkaline solution to maintain vaginal health."
   4. "I will wear form-fitting, nylon clothing and underwear for warmth and to prevent infections."
   5. "As I approach menopause, I will eat wild yams, cherries, and alfalfa sprouts as a source of phytoestrogens."

10. The nurse is taking the gynecologic history of a postmenopausal Mexican American patient. Which technique(s) would help develop rapport with the patient? (Select all that apply.)
    1. Establish direct eye contact.
    2. Involve family members.
    3. Touch the patient.
    4. Use a polite tone of voice.
    5. Respect privacy.

Critical Thinking Activities

Scenario A
Mrs. Long is a 45-year-old college instructor, married, with two teenage children. She found a lump during breast self-examination that was diagnosed as malignant. Mrs. Long does not want to have the radical mastectomy recommended by her surgeon.

1. What are some possible reasons for Mrs. Long's hesitation about having a radical mastectomy?
2. What alternative surgical procedures are available to Mrs. Long?
3. What types of resources are available to help Mrs. Long make this decision?

Scenario B
A young, newly married woman tells the clinic nurse that she wants to delay pregnancy until she graduates from school, but does not want to take pills or use any intrusive method such as an IUD.

1. How would you counsel her?
2. What evidence-based information should you provide?

Objectives

Theory

1. Understand the effects of aging on the male reproductive system.
2. Summarize the medical and nursing management of erectile dysfunction.
3. Describe factors involved in fertility, infertility, and contraception in the male patient.
4. Discuss the most common diagnostic tests and examinations of the male reproductive system.
5. Describe the assessment of the male reproductive system.
6. Outline the pathophysiology and manifestations of common disorders of the male reproductive tract.
7. Evaluate the plan of care for a patient with a disorder of the male reproductive tract.
8. Identify the psychological and emotional impact of disorders of the male reproductive tract.
9. Understand the role of drug therapy in disorders of the male reproductive tract.

10. Compare and contrast four types of surgical treatments for benign prostatic hyperplasia (BPH).
11. Diagram the preoperative and postoperative nursing care of a patient with BPH.
12. Discuss inflammations of the male reproductive system and their treatments.
13. Illustrate the patient teaching involved for early detection of testicular and prostate tumors.
14. Describe the nursing care of a patient with prostate cancer.

Clinical Practice

1. Teach a patient about the procedure for a prostate biopsy.
2. Outline a nursing care plan for a patient with prostate cancer.
3. Devise a teaching plan for testicular examination for young adult men.
4. Prepare materials describing treatment to a patient experiencing erectile dysfunction.

Key Terms

androgens (ĂN-drō-jĕnz, p. 919)
azotemia (ă-zō-TĒ-mē-ă, p. 927)
cremasteric reflex (p. 926)
ejaculation (ē-jăk-ū-LĀ-shŭn, p. 919)
erectile dysfunction (ED) (p. 923)
erection (ĕ-RĔK-shŭn, p. 919)
gonads (GŌ-năds, p. 918)
gynecomastia (jīn-ĕ-kō-MĂS-tĭ-ă, p. 928)
impotence (ĬM-pō-tĕnz, p. 923)
infertility (ĭn-fĕr-TĬL-ĭ-tē, p. 924)
libido (lĭ-BĒ-dō, p. 920)
orchiectomy (ŏr-kē-ĔK-tō-mē, p. 933)

premature ejaculation (p. 924)
priapism (PRĪ-ă-pĭz-ĕm, p. 924)
PSA velocity (p. 934)
prostate-specific antigen (PSA) (prŏs-tāt, p. 922)
retrograde ejaculation (p. 924)
rugae (RŪ-jē, p. 919)
semen (SĒ-mĕn, p. 919)
spermatogenesis (p. 919)
tamponade (tăm-pŏn-ĀD, p. 929)
urodynamics (ū-rō-dī-NĂM-ĭks, p. 927)
vasectomy (vă-SĔK-tō-mē, p. 920)

Many diseases and disorders, and many medications, can affect the male reproductive system. The urinary system and reproductive system are so closely linked in the male that a disorder in one system often affects the other. Assessment of the reproductive system is an essential part of any comprehensive health history. The nurse needs to be comfortable with his or her own sexuality and knowledgeable about the male reproductive system to be helpful to the patient.

OVERVIEW OF ANATOMY AND PHYSIOLOGY OF THE MALE REPRODUCTIVE SYSTEM

WHAT ARE THE STRUCTURES OF THE MALE REPRODUCTIVE SYSTEM?

- The male gonads (sex glands) are the testes; they are oval shaped and are encased in the scrotum along with the epididymis, seminal vesicles, and vas deferens (Figure 40-1).

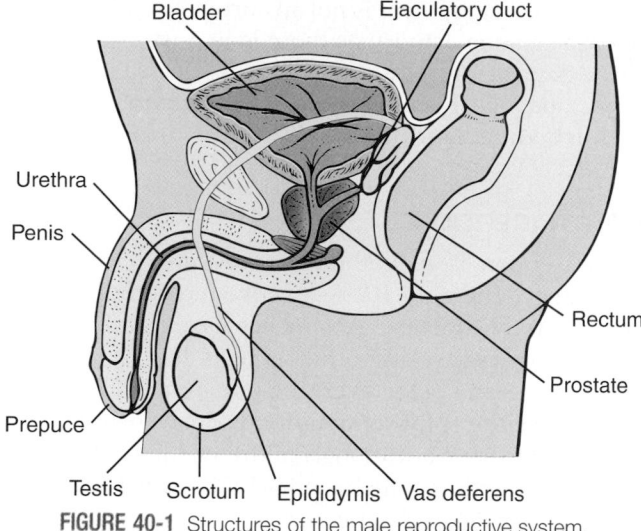

FIGURE 40-1 Structures of the male reproductive system.

- The scrotum is covered with wrinkled skin (rugae) and is very sensitive to temperature, pressure, touch, and pain.
- The penis is a cylindrical, erectile organ that hangs in front of the scrotum. It contains three columns of erectile tissue that can cause it to extend and enlarge in circumference, becoming stiff. The penis is covered with skin and includes a foreskin (unless circumcision has been performed). The scrotum and penis make up the external genitalia of the male.
- The prostate gland is shaped like a walnut, encircles the urethra, and is located below and to the rear of the bladder.
- The bulbourethral (Cowper's) glands are small pea-sized glands located in the urethral sphincter, posterior to the urethra.

WHAT ARE THE FUNCTIONS OF THE ORGANS OF THE MALE REPRODUCTIVE SYSTEM?

- The scrotum—a thin-walled, muscular sac—holds the testes, the epididymis, and the vas deferens. The scrotum hangs from the pubic bone, and suspends the testes outside the body where they remain several degrees cooler than the body; the cooler temperature is needed for the production of viable sperm.
- The spermatic cord attaches the testes to the body. It contains the blood vessels and nerves that supply the testes.
- The seminiferous tubules within the testes produce sperm (spermatogenesis). These tubules collect and transport the sperm to the epididymis. Testosterone also is produced in the testes.
- The epididymis is a long tube (almost 6 m) that conducts sperm from the testes to the vas deferens. Immature sperm mature as they travel through this tube. Mature sperm are stored in the lower portion of the epididymis.

- The vas deferens is a muscular tube that connects to the epididymis. It stores sperm and then carries it to the ejaculatory duct by peristaltic movements.
- The prostatic section of the urethra receives the sperm and carries it to the penile portion of the urethra for ejaculation. Secretions from the seminal vesicles and ducts of the prostate gland are mixed with the sperm in an alkaline solution that assists in neutralizing the acidity of the vaginal tract.
- The seminal vesicles produce a fluid that is thick and contains fructose to nourish the sperm and provide energy. The fluid also contains prostaglandins, which contribute to the motility of the sperm. This fluid mixes with the sperm to form seminal fluid, or semen. The average volume of semen ejaculated is 2.5 to 4 mL, but may vary from 1 to 10 mL.
- The prostate gland produces thin, milky, and alkaline secretions that contribute to the seminal fluid and enhance the motility of the sperm.
- The bulbourethral glands secrete an alkaline mucus-like fluid in response to sexual stimulation.
- These secretions of the bulbourethral glands neutralize the acid of residual urine in the urethra and provide some lubrication at the tip of the penis for intercourse.
- The penis is flaccid until sexual arousal causes the arterioles to the erectile tissue to dilate and the veins to constrict, engorging the penis with blood until it is enlarged and rigid. This is an erection. Erections are stimulated by anticipation, memory, visual sensations, or touch on the glans penis and skin of the genital area. If stimulation continues, ejaculation will occur. This is the forceful expulsion of semen from the urethra. Thoughts, emotions, some medications, or medical disorders can sometimes inhibit erection. The penis transfers semen to the vagina of the female. It also carries urine through the urethra to be excreted.

HOW IS SPERM PRODUCTION CONTROLLED?

- The hypothalamus, the anterior pituitary, and the testes secrete hormones that control male reproduction.
- The hypothalamus secretes gonadotropin-releasing hormone (GnRH) in response to an unknown stimulus.
- GnRH stimulates the anterior pituitary to release luteinizing hormone (LH) and follicle-stimulating hormone (FSH). LH stimulates the testes to produce testosterone. FSH binds with cells in the seminiferous tubules, making them respond to testosterone. Testosterone and FSH stimulate the formation of sperm (spermatogenesis).
- The male sex hormones are called androgens.
- At puberty, testosterone levels rise and cause maturation of the male reproductive organs. Sperm take 70 days to mature and are constantly being produced once puberty has occurred.

- Normal sperm count is 100 million/mL. Sterility occurs when the sperm count, for one reason or other, drops to less than 20 million/mL.

WHAT CHANGES OCCUR WITH AGING?

- The scrotum becomes more pendulous and there are fewer rugae.
- Prostate enlargement may occur with risk of urethral obstruction.
- Plasma testosterone and progesterone levels decrease.
- There is decreased sperm production, but fertility remains intact. Ejaculate volume decreases.
- After age 60, the cycle of sexual response lengthens. Arousal takes longer and more direct penile stimulation may be needed; the firmness of the erection may be decreased.
- Sexual activity in the older man is closely related to his sexual activity in earlier years.
- Vascular problems are the major causes of impotence.
- Certain medical disorders, or the use of various medications in the older man, may have side effects that can have an impact on sexual function.

THE MALE REPRODUCTIVE SYSTEM

The male reproductive organs are shared with the urinary tract, and disorders in functioning of one system often affect the other. For this reason, a male patient who has a disorder or dysfunction of the reproductive tract is often treated by a urologist.

FERTILITY

If the anatomy and physiology of the male reproductive tract are intact, sexual function is influenced by the functioning of the hypothalamus, pituitary, and testes; the metabolism and transport of sex hormones (such as GnRH and others); and the cognitive and sensory centers in the brain. A sexual desire (libido, the ability to respond to sexual stimulation with a penile erection) and the ejaculation of semen containing live sperm are necessary for fertility. Both the parasympathetic and sympathetic nervous systems influence the normal sexual response cycle.

Elder Care Points

The decrease in testosterone with age decreases muscle strength, bone mass, libido, and erectile function, and affects the psychological sense of well-being. Testosterone replacement therapy is thought to decrease visceral fat and improve bone density and muscle strength, libido, and energy, but may not improve erectile function of the penis. There is no evidence that DHEA supplements, available over the counter, benefit the older man. Studies are ongoing concerning the benefits of testosterone therapy in the elderly.

As a man ages, there is not an abrupt cessation of gonadal hormone activity as there is in a woman. In the man, there is a gradual decrease in testosterone and other anabolic hormones, such as growth hormone and dehydroepiandrosterone (DHEA).

CONTRACEPTION

Contraception is a method of preventing unwanted pregnancy. The only 100% effective method of contraception is abstinence. Abstinence is encouraged for adolescents and young adults and is taught in many school programs. However, the nurse must be able to provide contraceptive options for the many couples that prefer not to have additional children added to the family. Contraception is the responsibility of *both* the male and the female. Female contraception is discussed in Table 39-1.

Reversible Contraception

Reversible contraception involves the use of spermicidal creams, gels, or foams applied before intercourse to kill sperm in the vagina. These are more effective if used in conjunction with a condom. A male condom is an effective reversible contraceptive technique if it is applied and used properly. The condom sheath is typically made of latex. Proper application includes timing of application and removal, and providing a space at the tip for semen to collect. Oil-based lubricants such as petroleum jelly can cause latex to deteriorate, so these lubricants reduce reliability of latex condoms. Condoms made of polyurethane are compatible with oil-based lubricants. Latex condoms provide some protection against sexually transmitted infections (STIs).

Permanent Contraception: Vasectomy

Sterilization of the male by vasectomy is a popular method of permanent contraception. The term **vasectomy** refers to a surgical procedure performed on the vas deferens for the purpose of interrupting the continuity of this duct, which conveys the sperm at the time of ejaculation. This is considered a permanent procedure, but occasionally a vasectomy can be successfully reversed by vasovasotomy (microsurgery) at a later time if a man's life circumstances change.

A vasectomy is done on an outpatient basis in a clinic or physician's office, with a local anesthetic. An incision is made into the scrotal sac on each side, and the vas is lifted out. A segment of the vas is cut out, the ends are bound, and the incision is closed.

Instruct the patient to use ice applications and acetaminophen or ibuprofen for scrotal pain and swelling the first 12 to 24 hours postoperatively. The patient should wear jockey shorts or a scrotal support for comfort. Sexual intercourse may be resumed in about 1 week or whenever the patient finds it comfortable. Two negative sperm counts are needed after vasectomy before the patient is infertile and some form of contraception should be used until then.

Since seminal fluid is manufactured in seminal vesicles and the prostate gland, there is no decrease in semen ejaculation following a vasectomy. However, the semen does not contain sperm. After vasectomy, the sperm cells produced by the vas deferens are reabsorbed by the body. Vasectomy has no effect on libido or sexual performance, and provides no protection from STIs. Some patients consider storing fertile sperm in a sperm bank before a vasectomy. Since reversal of a vasectomy may or may not be successful, using frozen sperm at a later date to father a child remains an option.

 Clinical Cues

After the vasectomy, instruct the patient to use another method of birth control until sperm counts are negative, because active sperm are still present in the vas. Another sperm count should be done 1 year later to verify that the vas deferens is not intact.

❖ **NURSING MANAGEMENT**

■ **Assessment (Data Collection)**

Because certain kinds of male reproductive disorders predominate in certain age groups, the age of the patient is relevant to nursing assessment. In men over age 50, the assessment is directed more toward detecting prostate problems, whereas younger men are carefully assessed for STIs and testicular cancer.

It may be awkward for the new nurse to obtain a sexual and reproductive history, but with experience in interviewing male patients of all ages, she will soon become more comfortable and adept at obtaining necessary data. Because questions about urinary problems are usually less sensitive than those dealing with sexual dysfunction, it is best to begin with questions of this kind and then lead into more sensitive ones.

Open-ended questions that start out with "Tell me about..." or "When did you first notice..." give the patient room to discuss only those things he is comfortable talking about. It also is helpful to relate his problem to the inconvenience it has caused in his daily life. For example, tenderness and discomfort in the scrotal area could make sitting at a desk or walking very difficult and interfere with getting assigned work done. Frequent urination can cause distracting and sometimes embarrassing interruptions in his work schedule or recreational activities.

Good communication depends on the sender and receiver of messages using mutually understood language. Many people do not know the medical names of their sex organs. If the nurse suspects that the patient does not understand what particular part of the body she is talking about, or if the nurse herself is not familiar with the term the patient is using, it is important to phrase questions differently or ask for clarification from the patient.

 Focused Assessment

Data Collection for the Male Reproductive System

Ask the following questions:
• Have you noticed any changes in patterns of urination; any differences in the stream of urine?
• Do you ever have any discharge coming from the penis?
• Have you felt any masses or bumps in the scrotum or groin?
• Do you have any tenderness or pain in the scrotum or penis?
• Do you have any rectal or perineal pain?
• Do you perform regular testicular examinations?
• Have you had past infections of the reproductive system?
• What drugs do you take regularly?
• Do you have difficulty obtaining or maintaining an erection?

 Health Promotion

Health Screening and Assessments

Regular self-evaluation of the testes is encouraged, such as testicular self-examination for early detection of cancer. The nurse can encourage the patient to perform self-examination and teach proper techniques and follow-up care (Figure 40-2). (Privacy should be provided during examination and obtaining specimens.)

? **Think Critically**

Can you think of five relatives or friends for whom you could provide information on testicular self-examination? How would you approach them on this subject?

■ **Diagnostic Tests**

Tests for general state of health, such as complete blood cell count, urinalysis, chemistry profile, and thyroid tests, are done initially for problems concerning the male reproductive tract. Serum acid phosphatase is usually elevated in the patient with prostate cancer. Serum alkaline phosphatase is elevated if malignancy of the prostate has metastasized to the bone. A kidney-ureters-bladder (KUB) x-ray, an intravenous pyelogram, and cystoscopy with uroflowmetry studies also

FIGURE 40-2 Testicular self-examination.

may be done (see Chapter 34 for more information on these tests). Blood tests are done to detect specific UTIs.

Tumor protein marker studies are performed for patients with testicular cancer for follow-up to determine the success of treatment or recurrence of the disease. The primary tumor markers are alpha-fetoprotein (AFP) and the beta subunit of human chorionic gonadotropin (beta-hCG). A prostate-specific antigen (PSA) test detects levels of a glycoprotein produced by the prostate that is elevated in prostate cancer. Diagnostic tests that relate to the male reproductive organs are summarized in Table 40-1.

 Think Critically

How would you begin your assessment interview with a 52-year-old man? Would you have any difficulty asking the questions necessary to obtain a good reproductive organ history and information about present problems?

■ Nursing Diagnosis

Nursing diagnoses commonly used for problems of the male reproductive system may include:

- Urinary retention related to urinary obstruction
- Anxiety related to inability to empty bladder completely or dribbling
- Pain related to pressure of pelvic mass or distended bladder; surgical incisions; or bladder spasms
- Sexual dysfunction related to inability to achieve erection
- Ineffective sexuality pattern related to decreased libido
- Disturbed body image related to changes in sexual function
- Potential fluid volume excess related to bladder irrigation.
- Risk for infection related to stasis of urine

Table 40-1   Diagnostic Tests for the Male Reproductive System

TEST	COMMENTS
Digital rectal examination	A lubricated, gloved finger is inserted into the rectum to evaluate the consistency and size of the prostate and detect any nodules.
Semen analysis	Through masturbation, the patient provides a specimen of semen, which is analyzed for volume and for sperm content and motility.
Testicular self-examination (TSE)	Monthly self-examination is encouraged (see Figure 40-2).
Prostate-specific antigen (PSA) level	A sample of blood is examined for the level of glycoprotein produced only by the prostate. An elevated level is found in benign prostatic hyperplasia, and levels above 10 mg/mL may be indicative of prostate cancer. However, abnormal levels do not indicate a positive diagnosis. The American Cancer Society recommends annual digital rectal examinations and PSA levels for men over 45 yr of age or young men with high-risk factors.
Transrectal ultrasound	Recommended when PSA and/or digital rectal examination results are abnormal. May also be used to guide needle biopsies of the prostate.
Urography	Radiologically detects changes caused by ureter abnormalities and follows urine excretion pathway.
Uroflowmetry	Measures the volume of urine expelled from the bladder per second. Detects outflow tract obstruction. Patient voids into a urine flowmeter. Privacy is provided.
Prostate tissue analysis (biopsy)	Specimens of prostate tissue or fluids can be obtained by perineal or transrectal needle aspiration. If procedure is outpatient based, the patient is taught to report hematuria or change in urine flow after the procedure.
Cystoscopy	A lighted instrument is inserted through the urethra into the bladder. Used to detect prostate hypertrophy and bladder tumors. This is done as a sterile procedure.
Urethral smears	Used for laboratory microscopy study to identify pathogens. Prostate massage increases secretions in the urethra. A sterile swab is inserted into the urethra to obtain the specimen. Often used to diagnose some sexually transmitted infections.
Endocrine Studies	
Luteinizing hormone (LH) level	LH secreted by the pituitary stimulates Leydig cells in the testes to produce testosterone. High levels may indicate testicular failure.
Prolactin level	Prolactin, a hormone secreted by the pituitary, potentiates testosterone production.
Follicle-stimulating hormone (FSH) level	FSH is secreted by the anterior pituitary gland and stimulates the Sertoli cells in the seminiferous tubules to complete formation of mature sperm. Increased FSH levels indicate decreased spermatogenesis.
Testosterone level	Testosterone is secreted by the Leydig cells of the testes. High levels may indicate a testicular tumor. Low levels may occur in the aging man. Because testosterone levels are highest in the morning and lowest in the evening, it is important to obtain a morning sample.

Additional nursing diagnoses may be appropriate for the patient undergoing surgery or for one who has cancer (see Chapters 4, 5, and 8).

■ Planning

Expected outcomes are written for individual patients based on the nursing diagnoses chosen. Interventions are planned to help the patient meet the expected outcomes. The nurse plans her interaction with the patient based on his age, educational level, degree of comfort in discussing reproductive problems, and culture.

Expected outcomes for the patient with problems of the male reproductive system are:
- Patient will have normal urinary flow without obstruction.
- Patient will have normal urinary elimination after surgery.
- Patient will have bladder spasms controlled with medication.
- Pain will be resolved after surgical recovery.
- Patient will have intact self-esteem 3 months after surgery.
- Patient will explore avenues for achieving sexual satisfaction.
- Patient will focus on positive traits and capabilities to increase a positive body image.
- Patient will not experience a fluid imbalance. Patient will not experience any infection from stasis of urine or from surgery.

■ Implementation

Nursing actions for selected problems of the male reproductive system are found within the sections on specific disease that follow. Privacy should always be provided when assessing the genitals, performing catheter care, or doing dressing changes. There are wide variances in the degree of modesty in men. The female nurse must be especially cautious and display a matter-of-fact, respectful manner when providing care. Sensitivity to embarrassment is necessary. Rather than stating "Don't worry; I'm used to this," it might be better to state, "I understand that this may be embarrassing for you; I will try to be as quick about it as I can."

Some patients express inappropriate comments when they feel that their sexuality is threatened. A male patient with sexual dysfunction, or one about to undergo surgery that may affect his sexuality, might make sexual comments or advances to a female nurse; she should be tactful and matter-of-fact in setting limits on such behavior, without taking the patient's inappropriateness personally.

■ Evaluation

Evaluation assesses how effective the nursing actions are in helping the patient achieve the expected outcomes. If the actions and treatments are not achieving the desired effect, a revision in the plan of care is necessary.

DISORDERS OF THE MALE REPRODUCTIVE SYSTEM

ERECTILE DYSFUNCTION

Erectile dysfunction (ED), also known as impotence, is the inability to achieve or maintain an erection that is firm enough for sexual intercourse more than 25% of the time. Impotence can also involve ejaculation problems. Erectile dysfunction has both psychological and organic causes.

🔼 Clinical Cues

Sexual Activity Among Elderly Men

Cultural factors can affect erectile function in the older man. Some cultures may frown on sexual activity among elders, and some elderly men may not seek guidance for erectile dysfunction.

Factors that interfere with the mechanisms of penile erection will cause erectile dysfunction. Any condition that impairs the blood supply to the penis, impairs pathology of the nervous system or hormonal supply, or impairs psychosocial responses can interrupt the process of penile erection. Anxiety and depression can affect achieving or maintaining an erection. Organic causes can include diabetes mellitus and other endocrine disorders, disorders of the urinary tract, neurologic disorders, and chronic illness (such as sickle cell anemia, hypertension, cardiovascular disease, liver disease, and cancer). Medications and drug and alcohol abuse can interfere with sexual performance. Some antihypertensive drugs, diuretics, tranquilizers, and medications used to prevent gastroesophageal reflux disease (GERD) can cause sexual problems. Antiparkinson medications can enhance sexual desire but not the ability to perform (Wold, 2008).

A complete history and physical examination is needed to rule out any physical illness that may affect sexual performance. Sleep laboratories can monitor nighttime penile erections to detect organic causes of impotence. A Doppler probe can measure arterial flow in the penis essential for erections, and nerve conduction tests can rule out neurologic pathology related to impotence. Review the patient's medications for side effects affecting erectile function and conduct a complete psychological evaluation for psychological causes of impotence before devising an individualized treatment plan. Studies have shown that among patients who seek help for ED, nearly 30% have undiagnosed hypertension, 15% have diabetes mellitus, and 5% have significant coronary artery disease (Jackson et al., 2006).

Treatment

Medical treatment depends on the cause of ED. Medical conditions are treated, the medications prescribed are reviewed and adjusted, hormone therapy may be prescribed for hypothalamic-pituitary disorders, and vascular surgery may be indicated for penile blood flow obstruction.

The primary intervention for ED is modifying reversible causes of the problem. Drug therapy includes phosphodiesterase (PDE-5) inhibitors, taken an hour before sexual activity. These drugs should not be taken with nitrate-based drugs used for heart problems, as a serious drop in blood pressure can occur from the combination. If these methods fail to resolve ED, surgical interventions include inserting a penile implant that can be rigid or flexible. One type of implant includes a pump, inflatable cylinders, and a reservoir for emptying after erection. The erection produced is usually firm enough to enable intercourse (Figure 40-3). Complications of oral therapy include priapism, a persistent abnormal erection that can develop into a urologic emergency. Treatment options are presented in Table 40-2.

The nurse must be aware of relationship problems within the family unit. Asking open-ended questions concerning sexual function or problems can provide information that will be helpful to the plan of care. Referral to a sex therapist may be indicated to help the patient integrate his sexual belief, practices, and abilities into a healthy lifestyle. Community support groups for patients with ED and their partners may be available, such as Impotence Anonymous (I-Anon).

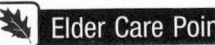

Elder Care Points

The elderly man who has been consistently participating in intercourse throughout the years has the best chance of maintaining this capability. When abstinence has occurred over a considerable time, ED may become a problem. With patience and treatment, this problem may be overcome. The man can reproduce as long as he can participate in intercourse.

EJACULATION DISORDERS

Spinal cord injuries, neurologic disorders such as multiple sclerosis, diabetes mellitus, urologic surgery, or the side effects of various medications can cause problems with ejaculation. Premature ejaculation is the most common ejaculation problem in men and it occurs when the ejaculation reflex is not controlled and the release of semen occurs before release is desired. Chemical, vibratory, and electrical stimulation can be used to treat premature ejaculation.

Retrograde ejaculation occurs when the semen travels toward the bladder rather than exiting the penis. Determining the physical and psychological factors causing the retrograde problem is the priority for selecting appropriate treatment and planning care. Retrograde ejaculation may occur after prostatectomy.

If fertilization is desired, men with retrograde ejaculation may have sperm harvested from their urine for artificial insemination. When spinal injury is the problem, an electro-ejaculation device inserted into the rectum stimulates the prostate and enables sperm collection for artificial insemination.

INFERTILITY

Infertility is defined as failure of a couple to achieve a pregnancy after at least 1 year of frequent, unprotected intercourse. Approximately 25% to 30% of infertility causes may be due to male factors.

Hypothalamic-pituitary disorders and ED contribute to infertility, but testicular disorders are the most frequent organic cause of male infertility. Drugs, infections, systemic disease, and congenital disorders can cause testicular failure.

A semen analysis with sperm count and activity is performed. Laboratory tests performed include FSH, LH, and testosterone levels to determine if hormone therapy is indicated. A postejaculation urine specimen may be examined to diagnose retrograde ejaculation of semen into the bladder. An ultrasound of the seminal vesicles may reveal dilated vesicles and obstruction of the vas deferens near the ejaculatory duct. Surgical resection of the ejaculatory duct may be indicated. A fine-needle aspiration or biopsy of the testicles may reveal pathology that can be treated. Discussion

Flaccid · Erect

INFLATABLE PENILE IMPLANT

Flaccid · Erect

FLEXIBLE ROD PENILE IMPLANT

FIGURE 40-3 Penile implants.

Table 40-2 Treatment Options for Erectile Dysfunction

OPTION	COMMENT
Medications Taken About 1 Hour Before Intercourse	

PDE-5 Inhibitors
  Sildenafil (Viagra)
  Vardenafil (Levitra): rapid onset
  Tadalafil (Cialis): longer lasting
	Side effects can include headache, dyspepsia and nasal congestion. Contraindicated in patients taking nitrates and patients with hypertension or retinopathy. Usually taken ½ to 4 hr before sexual stimulation. Viagra can cause color vision disturbances and should not be taken more than once per day.

Yohimbine	Useful if organic disease is cause of ED.
Trazodone	Has sedation as side effect.
Intraurethral prostaglandin E_1 suppository (alprostadil)	Works locally on corpora cavernosa as a vasodilator.
Intracavernosal injections of vasodilating drugs	Currently replaced by oral sildenafil therapy. May cause priapism.

Vasoactive drugs
  Papaverine gel
  Alprostadil (Caverject)
  Phentolamine (Vasomax)
	Can be administered by topical gel, local self-injection, or insertion of medication pellet (alprostadil) into the urethra. Side effects can include pain, fibrotic nodules, and hypotension.

Complementary and Alternative Therapies	
Siberian ginseng *Ginkgo biloba* Acupuncture Aromatherapy Sandalwood Rose Jasmine Ylang ylang oil Imagery Biofeedback Relaxation	Thought to increase penile blood flow, but research-based evidence is lacking. These therapies may be used in conjunction with other options. Research-based evidence of effectiveness is lacking but research is ongoing.
Other	
Sexual therapy	The psychosocial factors that may be causing ED are discussed with a qualified sexual therapist. Counseling should include the partner.
Penile implants	Can be semi-rigid rod or an inflatable prosthesis.
Negative pressure (vacuum constrictive devices)	Used to induce erection by suction. A band is placed at base of penis to maintain erection. May be cumbersome to use. Injury can occur if constriction band is left in place longer than 1 hr.

ED, erectile dysfunction.

with both partners concerning technique and timing of intercourse is indicated.

Pathology may be corrected with medications, hormone therapy, or surgery. In vitro fertilization, or intracytoplasmic sperm injection (ICSI) after sperm extraction, is often successful in treating male infertility.

The environment should be evaluated for toxins such as pesticides, lead, mercury, or radiation exposure—all of which can affect fertility. Occupational influences on fertility include exposure to heavy metals, solvents, fumes, or polycyclic aromatic hydrocarbons (DeFleurian, 2009). The patient seeking fertility should be instructed to avoid excessive heat around the scrotal area, which could decrease sperm development. Hot tubs, using a laptop on the lap, and tight underwear should be avoided. Stress reduction techniques, information concerning timing and technique of intercourse, optimum nutrition, and health practices should be reviewed with both partners. When infertility is attributable to the man, his self-image may be affected; therefore diplomatic, caring, and considerate family interactions are essential.

HYDROCELE

There is normally a small quantity of fluid in the space between the testis and tunica vaginalis within the scrotum (Figure 40-4). A larger-than-normal amount of fluid accumulating in this space is known as *hydrocele*. The fluid accumulation may be caused by infection, such as epididymitis or orchitis, or accumulation may occur after trauma; hydrocele involves interference with lymphatic drainage of the scrotum. Many times the cause is unknown. Hydrocele causes enlargement of the scrotum and usually is painless, but the weight and added bulk of the fluid can cause discomfort.

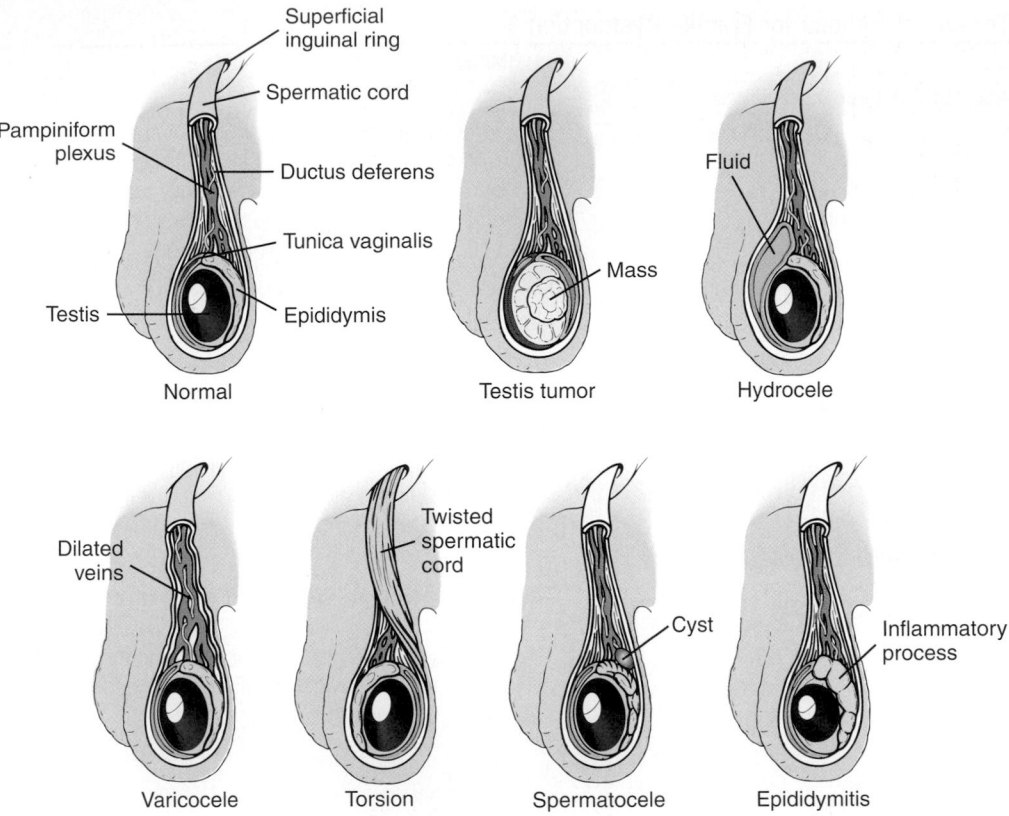

Superficial
inguinal ring

Spermatic cord

Pampiniform
plexus

Ductus deferens

Tunica vaginalis

Testis

Epididymis

Normal

Mass

Testis tumor

Fluid

Hydrocele

Dilated
veins

Varicocele

Twisted
spermatic
cord

Torsion

Cyst

Spermatocele

Inflammatory
process

Epididymitis

FIGURE 40-4 Scrotal masses.

Treatment, when indicated, is aspiration or surgical incision and drainage of the sac. A pressure dressing and a drain are left in place postoperatively. The patient will need to wear an athletic support for several weeks.

VARICOCELE

Dilation and clumping of the tributary vessels of the spermatic vein cause the painful swelling called *varicocele* (see Figure 40-4). Varicocele usually occurs on the left side of the scrotum, due to retrograde blood flow from the left renal vein. The discomfort is rarely enough to warrant surgery. If infertility has been a problem, surgical correction via injection of a sclerosing agent or ligation of the spermatic vein may improve the infertility problem.

Nursing measures to help the patient cope with fatigue, weakness, and fever are appropriate, because these problems often are associated with urogenital infections and surgical procedures. Fluid intake should be increased to help prevent fluid deficit, reduce fever, increase urinary flow, and remove debris and bacteria. The patient is advised to wear scrotal support after any intervention.

TESTICULAR TORSION

Testicular torsion is a twisting of the testes and spermatic cord (see Figure 40-4). It is commonly caused by elevated hormone levels in young adult men but can also

be the result of scrotal trauma. Signs include sudden acute scrotal pain and an absence of the **cremasteric reflex** (retraction of the testicles when the inner thigh is stroked). Nausea and vomiting may also occur. A Doppler ultrasound scan may reveal diminished blood flow and confirm the diagnosis. To avoid testicular ischemia and necrosis, emergency surgery secures the testicle within the scrotum or possibly removes the testicle. The nurse provides routine postoperative wound care, with emphasis on providing support and relieving anxieties concerning the patient's sexual self-image and future sexual performance.

PRIAPISM

Priapism is a prolonged penile erection resulting in a large, hard, and painful penis, unrelated to sexual desire or activity. The cause can be neurologic, vascular, or the result of medications such as those designed to increase sexual performance. The most common disease that causes priapism is sickle cell disease, which causes a local accumulation of erythrocytes that result in engorgement of the corporal bodies. Circulation to the penis may be compromised, and voiding may be impaired while the penis remains erect, so prompt treatment is essential.

Treatment can be conservative, to promote dilation of vessels and relief of pressure. Sedation, bed rest, warm baths or enemas, and urinary catheterization may be prescribed. Aspiration of the corpora cavernosa with a large-bore needle or a shunting procedure to divert blood may be necessary to prevent ischemia of the penis. The nurse should provide supportive care to the patient, who not only may be in pain, but may be embarrassed by the loss of erectile control and fearful of the effect of this condition on future sexuality.

PEYRONIE'S DISEASE

Peyronie's disease is a condition in which a plaque of nonelastic fibrous tissue develops in the tunica portion of the dorsal corpus cavernosa of the penis. The loss of elasticity in that section of the penis results in the inability to have a uniform erection of the penis. The penis will curve upward when erection occurs. Inability to penetrate the vagina may result, and the erection may become painful as well as embarrassing.

Treatment may include conservative measures such as local injections to dissolve the plaque. The size of the lesion and the level of erectile dysfunction may indicate a need for surgical intervention.

BENIGN PROSTATIC HYPERPLASIA

Etiology and Pathophysiology

Enlargement of the prostate, also known as benign prostatic hyperplasia (BPH), occurs when the prostate gland enlarges and extends into the bladder neck, causing obstruction of urine flow. An enlargement of the prostate often begins to develop before age 30. Fifty percent of men show evidence of enlargement by age 60, and 80% of men in their eighth decade develop BPH (American Urological Association, 2010).

Signs and Symptoms

BPH produces no symptoms until the growth becomes large enough to press against the urethra (Figure 40-5). Then the patient begins to experience difficulty in urinating, evidenced by a decrease in the caliber of the stream of urine, hesitancy, and dribbling after voiding. There may be frequency, nocturia, and urgency due to irritation of the distended bladder wall. In the later stages there may be complete obstruction of the urinary flow. Retention of urine (urinary stasis) is defined as more than 60 mL of residual urine after a void. Urinary tract infections can result from urinary stasis, as the retained urine acts as a medium for organism growth. Gradual dilation of the ureter *(hydroureter)* and kidneys *(hydronephrosis)* can occur. Nitrogen products can accumulate in the blood (azotemia) and cause renal failure if the urinary obstruction is not relieved. The American Urological Association has developed a tool to assess symptoms related to urinary obstruction, which aids in clarifying the severity of the problem. The tool gives a numerical score to the severity of each symptom of urinary retention. The total numerical score is used to determine appropriate treatment options.

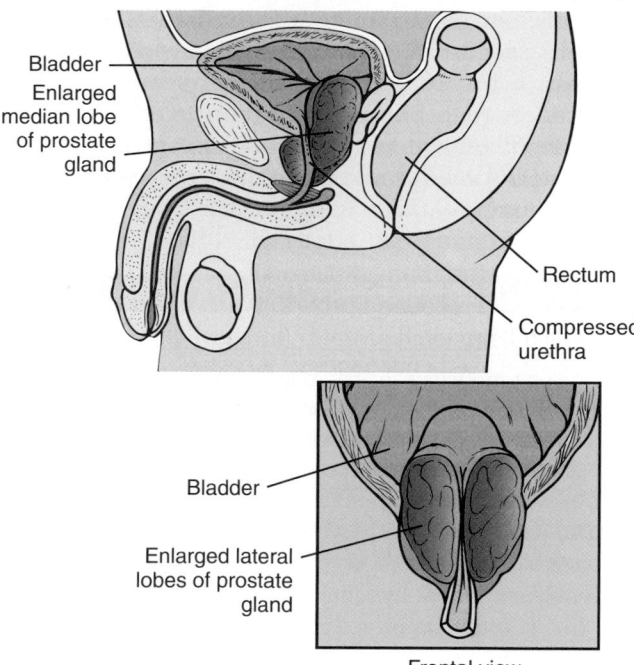

FIGURE 40-5 Benign prostatic hyperplasia.

Diagnosis

A digital rectal examination will reveal an enlarged prostate. The "gold standard" test for bladder outlet obstruction is increased bladder pressure relative to urinary flow. Pressure flow studies can be performed (urodynamics). A postvoiding ultrasound or catheterization to determine residual urine volume is also a helpful diagnostic aid. A transrectal ultrasound differentiates BPH from prostate cancer, and a serum creatinine level can rule out renal insufficiency.

Treatment

If the patient cannot void, an immediate catheterization will relieve the emergency problem, and follow-up care concerning the cause and severity of the prostate enlargement will then be carried out.

Drug Therapy. Drug therapy includes:
- *Alpha-adrenergic blockers,* which promote relaxation of smooth muscle and reduce blood pressure. Side effects of doxazosin (Cardura), terazosin (Hytrin), tamsulosin (Flomax), and alfuzosin (Uroxatral) include dizziness and orthostatic hypotension. These drugs offer prompt relief but may not reduce the prostate size. A new drug, silodosin, has recently been approved by the Food and Drug Administration (FDA) (Hussar, 2010).
- *5-Alpha-reductase inhibitors* (ARIs) are steroids and may take several months to work. Antiandrogen agents such as finasteride (Proscar) and dutasteride (Avodart) can decrease prostate size by reduced dihydrotestosterone (DHT) production.

Side effects include decreased libido and increased breast size (gynecomastia). Finasteride has been approved for use to prevent prostate cancer in select patients (Barnett et al., 2009). The FDA has approved the use of tamsulosin and dutasteride in combination; the use of silodosin in combination with dutasteride or finasteride is still under study (Hussar, 2010).

 Safety Alert

5-ARIs and Cancer

The 5-alpha reductase inhibitors (5-ARIs) now have a warning issued by the FDA that individuals taking these drugs may be at an increased risk for developing high-grade prostate cancer (FDA, 2011).

Herbal Therapy. Plant extracts such as saw palmetto (*Serenoa repens*) are thought to relieve symptoms and increase urine flow in some patients, although research has not proven its effectiveness. Side effects may include an increase in blood pressure and gastrointestinal disturbances. Saw palmetto should not be taken if the patient is receiving hormone replacement therapy. Research concerning the role of complementary and alternative medicine therapies in the treatment of BPH is ongoing.

 Complementary and Alternative Therapy

Antioxidants for BPH

Pumpkin seeds are also thought to decrease prostate size, and antioxidants such as pomegranate juice may be helpful in BPH (Pavlorich-Danis, 2007).

Surgery. Indications for surgical intervention include hematuria, urinary retention, bladder stones, and urinary tract infections. Balloon dilation, transurethral incision of the prostate, laser resection, and microwave thermotherapy are newer surgical treatment options. The nurse should review the surgical options that were presented by the health care provider to ensure that the patient has a clear understanding of treatment options (Table 40-3).

Serum PSA is a protein-specific antigen that is produced by the prostate tissue and is elevated in BPH, cancer of the prostate, prostatitis, and after prostate biopsy. Interpretation of PSA levels should take into consideration any diagnostic procedures involving the prostate gland. An elevated PSA is therefore not *always* indicative of cancer. The value of routine PSA screening is currently under question.

[?] Think Critically

A patient has been experiencing increasing difficulty in emptying his bladder; he is diagnosed with BPH. His physician has recommended prostate surgery, but he is reluctant to have surgery. What other options are available to this patient that might prevent further organ damage?

Nursing Management

Preoperative Care. Urinary drainage is accomplished by insertion of a catheter using sterile technique. If the obstruction is severe, a urologist may insert a special rigid catheter. A high fluid intake is encouraged, and antibiotics are routinely prescribed. The nurse should interview the patient to assess the understanding of the procedure to be performed and the impact on his lifestyle, self-image, and sexual function.

Preoperative teaching includes deep-breathing exercises, range-of-motion leg exercises, the general preoperative and postoperative routine, and explanation of care for the incision, catheters, irrigation system, and drains (see Chapters 4 and 5).

Postoperative Care. The postoperative nursing care of the patient varies according to the type of prostate surgery performed (Figure 40-6). The general principles of postoperative nursing care that apply to all patients having major surgery are necessary for the patient undergoing a prostatectomy. Potential postoperative complications are bleeding, urinary incontinence, and bladder spasms. Because hemorrhage always is a danger, vital signs are taken per agency protocol, then every 4 hours. The patient is monitored for pallor and rising pulse, which, along with blood pressure changes, may indicate excessive bleeding and shock. A high-fiber diet and a stool softener may be prescribed to prevent straining, which increases intra-abdominal pressure and can cause further bleeding.

Patients with suprapubic prostatectomy and transurethral resection of the prostate (TURP) will return from surgery with a three-way urethral catheter connected to continuous bladder irrigation with sterile normal saline (Figure 40-7). Blood-tinged urine is usual for the first few days following the surgery. To decrease clot formation, the bladder irrigation flow rate is adjusted to keep the urine diluted to a reddish pink, clearing to a pink tinge within 48 hours. Some pieces of tissue and small clots may be seen in the drainage. Additional intermittent irrigation with 20 to 30 mL of normal saline may be needed to clear the catheter of obstruction (Nursing Care Plan 40-1). Hemorrhage is a possible complication and occurs most frequently in the first 24 hours. Strict sterile technique must be used when irrigating the bladder, and the catheter should be connected to a closed drainage system to prevent infection.

 Clinical Cues

When caring for a bladder irrigation system:
- Use sterile normal saline unless otherwise ordered.
- Monitor rate of irrigation.
- Monitor and record intake and output.
- Record the amount of irrigation fluid instilled and the amount returned. The difference equals the urine output.
- Check drainage tubes for kinks and clots.
- Observe for signs of bladder spasms and medicate promptly as needed.

Table 40-3	Surgical Interventions for Male Urogenital Problems
TREATMENT	COMMENTS
Minimally Invasive Treatment (Day Surgery)	
Transurethral microwave thermotherapy (TUMT)	Heats and coagulates prostate tissue via a transurethral probe. A urinary catheter may be left in place for 1 wk after treatment to facilitate passing of necrotic tissue and prevent urinary retention. Antibiotics, analgesics, and bladder antispasmodics are prescribed after the procedure.
Transurethral needle ablation (TUNA)	Places radiofrequency needles directly into the prostate to coagulate specific tissue areas. Hematuria may occur for 1 wk after this procedure.
High-intensity focused ultrasound (HIFU)	High-intensity, low-frequency ultrasound waves destroy prostate tissue. Has been found effective in treatment of BPH, but continued research concerning aftereffects are ongoing.
Surgery	
Open prostatectomy Suprapubic prostatectomy Retropubic prostatectomy	Involves an external abdominal incision that allows complete visualization of prostate tissue. Suprapubic enters via the bladder and retropubic does not enter the bladder. There is risk for infection and erectile dysfunction, postoperative pain, and a longer recovery period.
Perineal prostatectomy	The removal of the prostate via an incision in the perineum has high risk for postoperative wound contamination, incontinence, and impotence.
Transurethral resection of the prostate (TURP)	TURP is the "gold standard" of treatment for BPH and is performed under spinal anesthesia. A resectoscope is inserted into the urethra to excise and cauterize obstructive prostate tissue. A large three-way catheter is inserted to provide hemostasis and allow urinary drainage. May be performed as day surgery at many facilities.
Transurethral incision of the prostate (TUIP)	The TUIP incises the prostate. May be performed as day surgery at many facilities.
Laser prostatectomy	A modified TURP; uses a laser beam to destroy prostate tissue. Minimal postoperative bleeding occurs, but a catheter may be required for 1 wk postoperatively to prevent urinary retention due to edema.
Transurethral electrovaporization of the prostate (TUVP)	Electrosurgical vaporization and desiccation destroy prostate tissue. Complications include hematuria and retrograde ejaculation.
Transurethral photoselective vaporization of prostate (PVP)	Uses a green light laser beam to coagulate prostate tissue.
Urethral stent	A metallic stent is placed in the urethra to hold the urethra open. This is usually a temporary measure as displacement is common.
Laparoscopic radical prostatectomy	Provides better visualization and less postoperative complications and has a shorter hospital stay.

Persistent bleeding turning the urine darker than cherry red or bright red, or viscous drainage with many clots, should be reported immediately to the surgeon. Traction may be applied to the catheter to supply pressure (tamponade) to prevent excessive bleeding. The surgeon does this by pulling against the balloon and then taping the catheter to the thigh or abdomen. This pressure may cause the patient to have a sensation of a continuous need to void. The nurse checks frequently to see that the catheter and tubing are not kinked and that outflow is appropriate. Irrigation is continued for 2 to 3 days. The patient may have some urinary frequency and burning after catheter use is discontinued. Some blood in the urine is not unusual for several more days.

The patient who has had a suprapubic prostatectomy will have a suprapubic catheter in addition to a urethral catheter. Each catheter is attached to a separate sterile drainage system. After the urethral catheter is removed (sometime after the third day), the suprapubic catheter is clamped, and the patient attempts to void. Residual urine is measured afterward by unclamping the suprapubic catheter. When there is no more than 60 mL of residual urine after voiding, the suprapubic catheter is removed. Dribbling of urine often occurs after prostatectomy due to decreased sphincter tone, but usually stops within about 6 months. Patients who experience incontinence are taught perineal muscle strengthening (Kegel) exercises for this problem and are given instruction in bladder training (see Chapters 34 and 35). Teaching begins 24 to 48 hours after surgery. Kegel exercises and coping strategies should be taught to enable early return to a normal lifestyle.

When the urethral or suprapubic catheter is removed, the patient must be carefully monitored for ability to void. Intake and output are tracked closely. Any difficulty in voiding within 6 hours after removal must be reported to the surgeon promptly, as a distended bladder may cause bleeding.

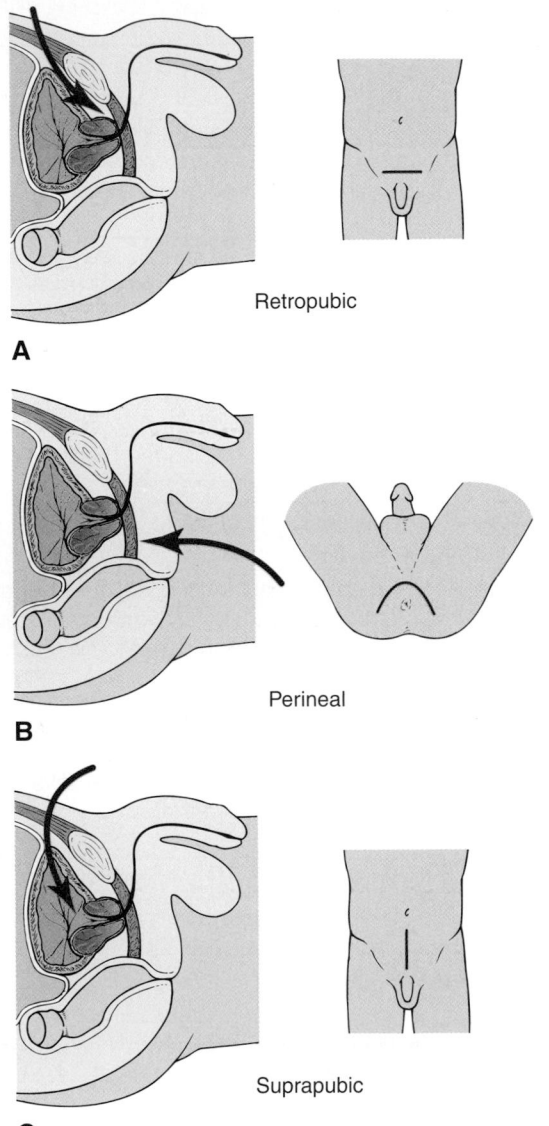

FIGURE 40-6 Three approaches to perform a prostatectomy. **A,** Retropubic approach involves a midline abdominal incision. **B,** Perineal approach involves an incision between the scrotum and anus. **C,** Suprapubic approach involves an abdominal incision.

Retropubic

A

Perineal

B

Suprapubic

C

FIGURE 40-7 Continuous bladder irrigation (CBI) system.

The nurse monitors the incisional dressings and changes them as often as necessary to keep the patient dry and comfortable. Urine is very irritating to the skin, and any area that is exposed to urine drainage is thoroughly cleansed before a new dressing is applied.

Prophylactic antimicrobials and analgesics are administered in the early postoperative period. Bladder spasms often are a problem for the post-TURP and post–suprapubic prostatectomy patient. Before giving medication, the nurse checks to see that the tubing is not kinked and the catheter is draining well, as obstruction can cause bladder spasm. Abdominal distention may be a sign of catheter obstruction as well. The patient who has had a radical procedure may have a patient-controlled analgesia pump to control pain.

Clinical Cues

Belladonna and opium (B&O) rectal suppositories are effective for bladder spasms if they are given when the spasms first begin. Relaxation techniques and an anticholinergic drug, such as oxybutynin (Ditropan), may be used to help relieve bladder spasms.

Discharge teaching includes care of the catheter, management of incontinence, maintaining hydration, preventing constipation, observing for signs of infection, and management of anxiety related to impaired sexual function and self-image (see Patient Teaching on p. 935). *Retrograde ejaculation* (semen discharged into the bladder) may cause the urine to appear cloudy. Frequent planned urination and avoidance of irritating foods such as citrus, caffeine-containing products, and alcohol should be initiated. The patient should be taught to monitor output and contact the health care provider if unable to void. BPH can recur, so annual digital rectal examinations should be continued (see Nursing Care Plan 40-1).

Nursing Care Plan 40-1   **Care of the Patient After Prostatectomy**

Scenario

A 65-year-old man is admitted to the postoperative unit after a prostatectomy. His vital signs are stable, and a bladder irrigation system is set up at the bedside. The patient is awake and oriented, and the physician's orders include diet as tolerated.

Problem/Nursing Diagnosis

Prostatectomy/Risk of deficient fluid volume secondary to postoperative hemorrhage and limited fluid intake.

Supporting Assessment Data

Objective: Transurethral prostatectomy.

Goals/Expected Outcomes	Nursing Interventions	Selected Rationale	Evaluation
Patient evidences normal fluid volume and stable vital signs.	Monitor vital signs.	A change in vital signs can indicate fluid deficit.	Vital signs stable.
	Monitor intake and output.	Encouraging oral fluids as tolerated and recording amount and type of output enable identification of fluid volume status.	Intake >3500 mL; output >3200 mL. Taking sufficient oral fluids.
Patient evidences clear to pink urinary drainage with no clots.	Perform closed bladder irrigation as prescribed.	Irrigation removes accumulating clots that can obstruct urine outflow and precipitate further hemorrhage.	Irrigation outflow pink with few clots.
	Administer IV fluids as prescribed.	IV therapy can help maintain fluid balance.	IV infusion at 150 mL/hr.

Problem/Nursing Diagnosis

Does not know anything about wound care/Deficient knowledge related to lack of knowledge regarding self-care after discharge.

Supporting Assessment Data

Subjective: "No, I've never had to do any wound care before. What do I have to do?"

Goals/Expected Outcomes	Nursing Interventions	Selected Rationale	Evaluation
Patient will list signs of infection, explain need for increased fluid intake, demonstrate care of wounds, dressings, and catheter, and follow medication regimen.	Instruct to report signs of infection: fever, chills, malaise, increased pain, purulent drainage, excessive swelling.	Finding infection early means early treatment.	Able to provide accurate feedback of all instructions.
	Instruct to avoid heavy lifting, driving, and sexual activity until permitted by urologist.	Heavy lifting or sexual activity may cause disruption of tissue and bleeding.	States he understands and will comply with restrictions.
	Instruct to report new onset of burning on urination or cloudy urine.	Burning on urination or cloudy urine may indicate bladder infection.	No burning on urination; no cloudy urine.
	Explain what each medication is for and when and how to take it.	Helps with compliance with medication regimen.	States understands when and how to take the medications.
	Provide written information about signs and symptoms of urethral stricture or infection and instruct to report these.	Written instructions can be reviewed at home and help to get quick attention for problems.	Given written instructions regarding complications and what to report to surgeon.

Continued

⭐ **Nursing Care Plan 40-1** | **Care of the Patient After Prostatectomy—cont'd**

Problem/Nursing Diagnosis

Worried about being able to achieve an erection/Risk for sexual dysfunction related to inability to achieve erection.

Supporting Assessment Data

Subjective data: "Do you think my wife will leave me if I can no longer have an erection to meet her sexual needs?"
Objective data: Prostatectomy 6/25.

Goals/Expected Outcomes	Nursing Interventions	Selected Rationale	Evaluation
Patient will discuss concerns before discharge.	Encourage verbalization of problems and concerns.	Verbalization of concerns helps with identifying solutions.	Verbalizes concern about the possibility of not being able to obtain an erection.
	Provide information on alternative ways to achieve erection.	Gives the patient useful information in case of need.	Provided with information about the alternate ways to achieve erection.
Patient will discuss concerns with his spouse before discharge.	Counsel in other ways to achieve intimacy. Include spouse or significant other in discussions. Assist to make plan to meet sexual needs.	Addressing individual needs of patient encourages learning and retention. Provides tools to cope with sexual problems.	Agrees to include spouse in discussions regarding his sexual concerns.

Critical Thinking Questions

1. What are the priority nursing interventions if the nurse notices that the urinary outflow is less than the irrigation input after bladder irrigation?
2. Why is it important to attend to complaints of pain from bladder spasms as soon as possible? What is the medication generally used for this type of pain?

IV, intravenous.

INFLAMMATIONS AND INFECTIONS OF THE MALE REPRODUCTIVE TRACT

Many of the inflammations and infections affecting the male reproductive system are similar to those of the female reproductive system in cause and effect. For example, urethritis in the male and female can be caused by common pyogenic and colonic bacteria and by *Neisseria gonorrhoeae.* The male also can be infected with *Trichomonas vaginalis* or *Chlamydia,* which are transmitted by sexual contact. There always is the possibility that the sexual partners will reinfect one another, until both are treated simultaneously.

Nonspecific genitourinary infections in the male—including nongonococcal urethritis (NGU)—may be caused by various organisms, but these infections present substantially the same clinical picture. Among the symptoms of nonspecific urethritis are mucopurulent discharge from the urethra, painful urination of varying degrees of severity, and the occasional appearance of blood in the urine. A microscopic examination of a smear from urethral secretions may not show any specific organisms, but there may be an excessive number of white cells.

Epididymitis

Epididymitis is an inflammation of the epididymis and may result from an infection of the prostate or urinary tract infection. The patient with epididymitis complains of groin pain plus swelling and pain in the scrotum. In men younger than 35, the major cause of epididymitis is *Chlamydia trachomatis,* a sexually transmitted organism. Symptoms include scrotal pain, swelling, induration of the epididymis, and eventual edema of the scrotal wall. The adjacent testicle may become involved. The urine may contain pus (pyuria), and chills and fever may follow. Antibiotics, ice packs, analgesics, sitz baths, and elevation of the scrotum are the prescribed treatment protocol. A local anesthetic may be injected into the spermatic cord to manage pain.

Orchitis

Orchitis is inflammation of the testicle and may affect one or both testes. It may be caused by local or systemic infection (viral or bacterial) or by trauma. Bilateral orchitis is serious and often causes sterility. *Mumps orchitis* occurs in about 20% of adult men who contract mumps. Gamma globulin usually is given to lessen the possibility or severity of mumps orchitis. The symptoms and treatment parallel those of epididymitis.

Prostatitis

Prostatitis is an inflammation of the prostate that occurs from an infectious agent or other causes. The National Institutes of Health (NIH) classification (Goldman et al., 2007) system includes:

- *Type I: Acute bacterial prostatitis* with recovery of bacteria from fluid and signs of illness such as fever

- *Type II: Chronic bacterial prostatitis* with recovery of bacteria from fluid and no signs of systemic illness
- *Type III: Nonbacterial prostatitis/chronic pelvic pain syndrome:* recovery of leukocytes; microscopic purulence of prostate fluid is present but few or no bacteria are recovered
- *Type IV: Asymptomatic inflammatory prostatitis (prostatodynia):* no bacteria or leukocytes in prostate fluid but persistent symptoms of prostate discomfort, including poor urinary flow, frequency, and dysuria

Symptoms include recurrent urinary infection, pelvic pain, and sexual dysfunction and are often mistaken for BPH. Since blood PSA levels are often elevated in prostatitis, misdiagnosis of prostate cancer can occur. Prostate massage, useful for diagnosis, presents a risk for bacteremia. The various types of prostatitis can be diagnosed with a segmented culture of the initial stream urine, midstream urine, prostate fluid before and after massage, and postmassage urine specimen. Treatment includes bed rest, analgesia, bladder sedatives, sitz baths, and stool softeners to avoid straining. Antibiotics may be prescribed according to culture and sensitivity laboratory findings.

Antibiotics diffuse poorly into the prostatic fluid, so chronic prostatitis is often treated with alpha-adrenergic blockers (tamsulosin); fluoroquinolones may be prescribed. The patient is taught to recognize symptoms of urinary tract infection and to reduce retention of prostatic fluid by ejaculation. The patient should be taught to avoid foods that increase prostatic secretions such as alcohol, chocolate, tea, and spices. Follow-up care to detect reinfection is essential.

CANCER OF THE MALE REPRODUCTIVE TRACT
Cancer of the Penis
Cancer of the penis is rare, occurring mostly in males with human papillomavirus infections or males who were not circumcised.

Cultural Considerations
Incidence and Mortality Rate of Penile Cancer

Penile cancer is very rare in the United States. Testicular cancer is more common in whites; prostate cancer occurs most frequently, and has a high mortality rate, among African American men.

A nontender nodule may appear on the penis, and biopsy will show a squamous cell–type carcinoma. Laser resection of the lesion is the treatment of choice unless the cancer has spread. Radical resection of the penis followed by radiation and chemotherapy may be required. The shaft of the resected penis can respond to sexual stimulation and enable orgasm and ejaculation. After a total removal of the penis (penectomy) the patient may experience orgasm via stimulation of the scrotum and perineal area.

Testicular Cancer
Testicular cancer occurs most commonly in men ages 15 to 40 and is the leading cause of cancer death in men 25 to 35 years of age. Studies have identified a gene mutation that may predispose a man to develop a type of familial testicular cancer (American Cancer Society, 2011). The 5-year survival rate for testicular cancer is greater than 95% (American Cancer Society, 2011).

Men most at risk for testicular cancer are those who have had an undescended or partially descended testicle. Men who were exposed to diethylstilbestrol (DES) in utero also may be at high risk for testicular cancer, but evidenced-based research is lacking. All males between ages 15 and 40 should practice testicular self-examination on a monthly basis. Cancer symptoms appear slowly and involve painless enlargement of the testes, backache, and weight loss.

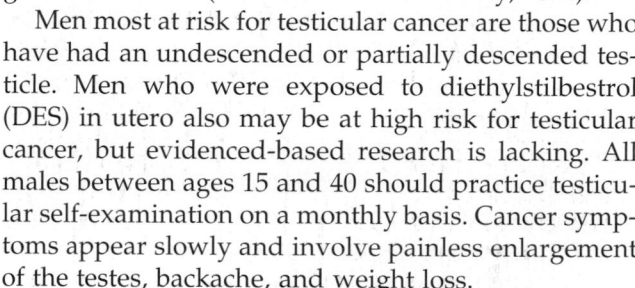

Health Promotion
Testicular Self-Examination

- Should be performed monthly.
- Perform after bathing when scrotal skin is relaxed.
- Roll each testicle between thumb and fingers.
- Report lumps to health care provider.

If a mass is found and thought to be malignant, diagnostic tests for tumor marker proteins such as elevated levels of AFP, beta-HCG, alkaline phosphatase, and lactate dehydrogenase are obtained to confirm diagnosis. Computed tomography (CT) scans and/or ultrasound should be performed to detect sites of testicular mass. Testicular cancer spreads rapidly via lymph and blood vessels. A microscopic tissue analysis is performed *after* surgical removal of the mass, for definitive diagnosis.

There are three stages for classifying the malignancy of testicular cancer. In *stage I*, the tumor is confined to the affected testis. In *stage II*, malignant cells have spread to the regional lymph nodes, usually on the same side as the affected testis. In *stage III*, there is metastasis to other organs, such as the lungs and liver.

If the testicular tumor is limited to the scrotal sac and there is no metastasis, a laparoscopic surgical removal of the testis (orchiectomy) may be all that is necessary to cure the patient of his disease. A gel prosthesis can be implanted. Care is taken to preserve the nerves associated with ejaculation. The nursing care focuses on teaching and providing psychological support. Ice bags and scrotal support provide comfort, and the importance of follow-up care is stressed. Removal of only one testis will not affect the patient's ability to produce the male hormone testosterone or render him impotent, as there remains another testis to carry on adequate testicular function.

Further treatment for stage II testicular cancer may include radiation. Chemotherapy is reserved for advanced stages of cancer and may results in a high percentage of complete remission. See Chapter 8 for a detailed discussion of radiation and chemotherapy in the care of cancer patients.

Some men view an orchiectomy as a loss of manhood. The nurse can be instrumental in assisting the patient to accept the procedure. Time for questions and discussion of concerns should be provided for the patient and his sexual partner. Sperm banking before surgery is an option for the young patient who may face chemotherapy. Continued follow-up care is essential.

Prostate Cancer

Carcinoma of the prostate is the second most common cause of cancer deaths in men (following lung cancer). The American Cancer Society predicted approximately 240,080 new cases for 2011 in the United States with 23,720 men dying of prostate cancer (American Cancer Society, 2011). Carcinoma of the prostate is usually a slow-growing cancer that is dependent on the hormone androgen. Some studies have identified an association of the prostate cancer antigen gene *(PCA3)* which can be measured via urinary assay as a significant risk factor. Studies are in progress to determine the effect of finasteride, beta-carotene, and beta-blocker drugs on prevention of prostate cancer (Smeltzer et al., 2010). The drug dutasteride (Avodart) is currently under study for use in men with BPH to boost the predictive power of PSA and, possibly, more effectively prevent prostate cancer or enable earlier intervention for prostate cancer.

Clinical Symptoms and Screening. If prostate cancer is detected early, the possibility of cure is high. Early detection by digital rectal examination can reveal a hardened lobe of prostate early in the course of the disease. Routine PSA screening of young healthy men is not recommended by the American Cancer Society; screening every 4 years, beginning at age 45, to 75 is recommended by the United States Preventive Task Force and National Comprehensive Cancer Network (Porche, 2011; Daskwich, 2011). Men with prostate cancer often exhibit some sexual dysfunction.

[?] Think Critically

What sort of psychological care would the patient undergoing a prostatic biopsy need from the nurse? What might be some of the patient's concerns?

An elevated PSA (about 4 ng/mL) screening test may indicate prostate pathology, but is not diagnostic for prostate cancer. The **PSA velocity** is a trend in PSA levels over time that may indicate a need for further tests to diagnose prostate cancer. A transrectal ultrasound may be done, and bones may be scanned to detect metastasis. A ProstaScint scan can detect prostate cancer cells when the PSA levels are low. A urine test to detect prostate cancer, Progensa (PCA-3) assay is closely related to biopsy outcomes. Transrectal, transurethral, and transperineal prostate biopsy and tissue analyses determine the severity or extent of prostate cancer.

Treatment and Nursing Care. Since prostate cancer is relatively slow growing, conservative treatment may involve monitoring and follow-up care. Annual digital rectal examinations are done, and PSA levels are monitored in high-risk patients. When surgical therapy is indicated, a laparoscopic radical prostatectomy is considered the most effective treatment for long-term survival before metastasis occurs. Other treatment options are listed in Table 40-4. A new drug, denosumab, is awaiting FDA approval for treatment of bone loss (osteoporosis) in men who have had androgen deprivation therapy for prostate cancer (Smith, 2009).

A multidisciplinary approach integrates surgery, radiation, and androgen restriction. Following surgery, PSA levels are monitored, and a decrease may indicate treatment success. In the early stages, radiation therapy may be the treatment of choice. Gamma teletherapy (external) and brachytherapy (internal) are used for cancer of the prostate and provide greater preservation of sexual ability.

Chapter 8 presents a detailed discussion concerning care of the cancer patient receiving radiation and chemotherapy. Hormonal therapy is designed to suppress androgen stimulation of the prostate by decreasing plasma testosterone. Removal of the testes may be done to result in prostate atrophy. A luteinizing hormone–releasing hormone (LHRH) agonist such as leuprolide, goserelin, or androgen agents such as flutamide (Eulexin) suppress androgen and may be used in combination with radiation therapy. The nurse should provide a sensitive, caring approach to the patient and family to help them cope with the diagnosis and make informed choices. Preoperative care involves restoration of urinary drainage, prevention of urinary tract infection, and understanding the options for treatment and their impact on sexual function. Complications of surgery may include bleeding, catheter obstruction, and sexual dysfunction. Impotence or retrograde ejaculation may occur. Options to enable erections and improve sexual function via prosthetic devices or medication should be discussed with the patient. The nursing care of a patient with a prostatectomy includes reducing anxiety, relieving discomfort, maintaining fluid balance, monitoring for bleeding or infection, catheter care, and teaching the patient self-care and the need for continued follow-up care.

Table 40-4 Treatment Options for Prostate Cancer

TREATMENT	COMMENTS
Radical prostatectomy	The prostate gland, seminal vesicles, and portions of the neck of the bladder are removed. ED and incontinence are two long-term complications. A laparoscopic approach provides fewer complications and shorter hospital stay. Robotic prostatectomy reduces risk of incontinence and impotence.
Cryosurgery	A freezing technique destroys prostate tissue. Complications include urethral damage, ED, and incontinence.
Radiation therapy	May be prescribed when the patient is not a candidate for surgery or may be offered in combination with surgery and hormone therapy.
External beam radiation	Most popular form of radiation therapy, given weekly on an outpatient basis for 2 mo. Side effects can include skin irritation, GI cramping and bleeding, ED, and bone marrow suppression. Cure rates for patients with localized cancer are comparable to radical prostatectomy.
Brachytherapy	The implantation of radioactive seeds into the prostate gland. It may be offered in combination with external beam irradiation.
Hormone therapy	Designed to reduce androgens. Leuprolide (Lupron, Viadur), goserelin (Zoladex), and triptorelin (Trelstar) are common drugs used; produces a chemical castration.
Chemotherapy	Used for hormone-resistant cancer or late-stage cancer. The prostate has limited response to chemotherapy.
Bisphosphonates	Reduce bone complications in advanced stages of prostate cancer. Drugs may include zoledronic acid (Zometa), risedronate (Actonel), etidronate (Didronel), or alendronate (Fosamax).

ED, erectile dysfunction; *GI*, gastrointestinal.

Elder Care Points

For the older adult undergoing chemotherapy or radiation therapy:
- Monitor for infections.
- Promote assisted ambulation.
- Institute fall precautions.
- Encourage use of incentive spirometer.
- Minimize pain.
- Reorient to environment as needed.

COMMUNITY CARE

Nurses in the community can be instrumental in teaching and promoting testicular self-examination in men between ages 15 and 40. Encouraging all men over 50 to have an annual digital rectal examination and PSA test may help reduce the death rate from prostate cancer through earlier detection and treatment.

Each nurse should be sufficiently knowledgeable about BPH and prostate cancer to direct patients toward treatment options and reliable information.

Nurses in long-term care facilities must be watchful for urinary obstruction in elderly male residents. Alert men should be questioned regularly about problems with urination; men with cognitive impairment who do not have a normal urinary stream should be placed on intake and output recording to detect any problems with urinary obstruction. Palpation just above the symphysis pubis may reveal a distended bladder.

All nurses can be instrumental in teaching perineal muscle (Kegel) exercises to decrease the incidence of incontinence. Incontinence is one of the prime causes of

Patient Teaching

Discharge Instructions for the Patient with a Prostatectomy

The patient is instructed regarding the following points:
- Drink 12 to 14 glasses of water during the day to keep the urine flowing freely.
- Do not lift any object weighing more than 8 lb.
- For 2 to 3 weeks following surgery (depending on physician's instructions), avoid strenuous activities.
- If blood is noticed in the urine, lie down and rest; drink more fluids and call the surgeon if the bleeding continues.
- Depending on the type of employment, it may be possible to return to work within 2 to 4 weeks. Consult the surgeon.
- Keep the catheter clean; cleanse the catheter and around the meatus daily with soap and water and rinse thoroughly.
- Report any cloudiness or foul smell in the urine.
- Report signs of infection such as fever, chills, or purulent wound drainage.
- After catheter removal, dribbling of urine may occur for up to 6 months. The problem usually will resolve. Perineal strengthening exercises help.
- After healing is complete, report any changes in the force or size of the urine stream to the surgeon.
- Report for annual checkups to detect recurrence of tissue growth or the development of prostate cancer.

loss of self-esteem in older adults, and can be corrected in many cases. Correcting incontinence also greatly decreases the nursing care time that needs to be spent with the patient, thereby cutting health care costs.

Home care nurses supervise or assist with dressing changes for the patient who has radical surgery, monitor side effects and complications in patients undergoing radiation, teach self-care, and provide psychosocial support for patients with prostate cancer and sexual dysfunction. Collaboration with the physician, social worker, and community agencies can provide avenues of help for these patients.

Nurses in the community can assist patients who are suffering from erectile dysfunction by including assessment for this problem when working with male patients. Knowledge about treatment options, a matter-of-fact optimistic attitude, and a comfortable manner when speaking about this topic can provide hope and guidance. Sometimes this problem is brought to light when speaking with the spouse of the older patient. Many times a satisfying sexual life can be reinstituted for these couples, providing added fulfillment and joy in the later years.

Get Ready for the NCLEX® Examination!

Key Points

- Anxiety, depression, various medications and certain diseases can contribute to erectile dysfunction.
- Complications of treatment for erectile dysfunction can include priapism, which requires prompt intervention.
- Testicular cancer occurs most commonly in men ages 15 to 40 years, and the 5-year survival rate is 95%.
- Nurses can be instrumental in teaching and promoting use of monthly testicular self-examination and monitoring for prostate cancer by digital rectal examination and PSA testing.
- Serum PSA levels become elevated when prostate disease is present (such as BPH or prostatitis) and therefore may not be a reliable marker indicating cancer.
- The medical treatment of BPH involves medications that relax the bladder and urethra (alpha blockers) and reduce prostate tissue through reduced DHT production (5-alpha reductase inhibitors).
- Indications for surgical intervention for BPH include urinary retention, gross hematuria, bladder stones, and urinary tract infections.
- Nursing care is planned based on the patient's age, educational level, degree of comfort in discussing reproductive problems, and culture.
- Patient education concerning disorders of the reproductive tract should include information about the impact on sexual activity.
- Elderly patients who have consistently participated in intercourse through the years have the best chance of maintaining this capability into old age.
- Nurses in long-term care facilities must watch for signs of urinary obstruction in elderly men.

Additional Learning Resources

SG Go to your Study Guide for additional learning activities to help you master this chapter content.

evolve Go to your Evolve website (http://evolve.elsevier.com/deWit/medsurg) for the following FREE learning resources:
- Animations, audio, and video
- Answers and rationales for questions and activities
- Concept Map Creator
- Glossary with pronunciations in English and Spanish
- Interactive Review Questions and Exercises and more!

 Online Resources
- Agency for Healthcare Research and Quality, www.ahrq.gov

Review Questions for the NCLEX® Examination

1. A 22-year-old man complains of sudden acute scrotal pain. Initial examination reveals absence of the cremasteric reflex. Doppler ultrasound reveals a diminished blood flow. This condition would most likely be:
   1. varicocele.
   2. testicular torsion.
   3. hydrocele.
   4. priapism.

2. The physician prescribes finasteride (Proscar) to a patient with benign prostatic hyperplasia. The nurse must discuss which anticipated side effect of the medication?
   1. Increased libido
   2. Increased ejaculate volume
   3. Erectile dysfunction
   4. Increased PSA levels

3. A patient is discharged after having a vasectomy. Which statement by the patient would indicate a need for further teaching?
   1. "I don't want any more children."
   2. "Now I can go home and have sex without fear of impregnating my wife."
   3. "There is a possibility that this procedure can be reversed in the future."
   4. "I should use ice packs to the scrotum after surgery to reduce swelling."

4. The nurse is taking care of a 40-year-old Hispanic man who had a bilateral orchiectomy. Clinical interviews with the patient confirm mounting concerns regarding his "manhood." The nurse would effectively approach the patient's disturbance in body image by:
   1. establishing eye contact.
   2. demonstrating sensitivity to nonverbal cues.
   3. asking specific questions.
   4. involving nonessential members of the family.

5. A patient who had transurethral resection of the prostate (TURP) complains of increasing bladder spasms. An appropriate initial nursing action would be to:

1. medicate with a belladonna and opium suppository.
2. check the urinary catheter tubing for kinks and obstruction.
3. teach relaxation exercises.
4. encourage use of patient-controlled analgesia.

6. A 25-year-old African American man was hospitalized for a prolonged penile erection unrelated to sexual desire or activity. A likely cause would be:

1. diabetes mellitus.
2. sickle cell disease.
3. hemophilia.
4. urinary infection.

7. A postprostatectomy patient expresses concerns regarding his ability to have intimate relations with his wife. The nurse identifies a nursing diagnosis of risk for sexual dysfunction. Priority nursing interventions would be geared toward which of the following nursing goals?

1. Identify signs and symptoms of infection.
2. Facilitate verbalization of personal concerns with his partner.
3. Demonstrate good aseptic wound care.
4. Facilitate development of alternative coping strategies.

8. A 65-year-old man complains of difficulty urinating, described as decreased caliber of the urine stream. He also has accompanying hesitancy, dribbling, and urgency. A digital rectal examination reveals an enlarged prostate. Which nursing intervention(s) would be appropriate? *(Select all that apply.)*

1. Teach to decrease caffeine and artificial sweeteners.
2. Teach to limit spicy foods and alcohol intake.
3. Apply a condom catheter.
4. Restrict fluid intake.
5. Plan a timed voiding schedule.

9. A patient states, "The doctor says I have a hydrocele." How should the nurse explain a hydrocele? *(Select all that apply.)*

1. "A fluid collection within the scrotum that can be drained."
2. "Sometimes caused by an infection of the testis that causes inflammation."

3. "An inflammation of the testes and scrotum from an illness such as mumps."
4. "Possibly from an injury with inflammation."

10. The loss of elasticity in a section of the penis that results in the inability to have a uniform erection is referred to as _____.

Critical Thinking Activities

Scenario A
Your brother, who is 20 years old, tells you of a friend who has just learned that he has testicular cancer and is scheduled for surgery tomorrow. Your brother is concerned about the effect the surgery will have on his friend's "manhood." He also says that, if ever he has that kind of cancer, he "doesn't want to know about it, and certainly wouldn't allow surgery."

1. What information could you give your brother about testicular cancer and self-examination of the testes?

2. How could you explain that removal of a testis does not render a man less masculine?

Scenario B
Mr. Watts, age 67, has been admitted to the hospital to undergo a transurethral resection of the prostate. He is assigned to your care on his second postoperative day. Mr. Watts seems disoriented and restless, and when you begin to give him his bath, he tells you that his bladder is full and he needs to urinate. You check the catheter and find that it apparently is not draining as it should.

1. What would you tell Mr. Watts about his need to void?

2. What would you do about the catheter, which seems to be obstructed?

3. What observations should you make while caring for this patient?

4. What special precautions should be taken for his safety?

Objectives

Theory

1. State the signs and symptoms of common sexually transmitted infections (STIs).
2. Discuss the danger of contracting human papillomavirus (HPV) and preventive measures.
3. Explain the procedure for the various tests for STIs.
4. Describe the treatment of common STIs, their prevention, and the resources available to those who need information about STIs.
5. Compare the symptoms of gonorrhea in male and female patients.
6. List the ways in which human immunodeficiency virus (HIV) is transmitted.

7. Identify the three stages of syphilis and discuss prevention, treatment, and complications.
8. Discuss the nurse's role in preventing, identifying, reporting, and treating common STIs.

Clinical Practice

1. Devise a teaching plan for the patient who has experienced a first incidence of genital herpes.
2. Instruct a female patient on ways to prevent contracting or transmitting HIV.
3. Teach a female patient and a male patient ways to prevent STIs.

Key Terms

agglutination (ă-GLŪ-tĭ-NĀ-shŭn, p. 941)
bacterial vaginosis (băk-TĔ-rē-ăl vă-jĭ-NŌ-sĭs, p. 939)
chancre (SHĂNG-kĕr, p. 947)
gram negative (p. 941)
gram positive (p. 941)
oophoritis (oof-ō-RĪ-tĭs, p. 939)

pelvic inflammatory disease (PID) (PĔL-vĭk ĭn-FLĂ-mă-tŏ-rē dĭ-ZĒZ, p. 939)
peritonitis (pĕr-ĭ-tō-NĪ-tĭs, p. 939)
salpingitis (săl-pĭn-GĪ-tĭs, p. 939)
sexually transmitted infection (STI) (p. 938)

The term **sexually transmitted infection (STI)** refers to those particular infections spread by intimate physical contact. Modes of transmission include sexual intercourse and contact with the genitals (sexual organs), rectum, or mouth. STIs can also be transmitted via blood contact, and can be transmitted to the fetus via the placenta or to the newborn during the birth process.

The incidence of STIs continues to rise throughout the world. Although all sexually active people must be considered potentially at risk, people with multiple sexual partners are at very high risk for contracting an STI. The largest population groups affected by STIs are adolescents and young adults (Centers for Disease Control and Prevention, 2011). Teens are engaging in sexual practices at an earlier age and have an opportunity for multiple partners. They are often unaware of signs and symptoms of STIs and are reluctant or unable to access confidential health care. Inflamed tissue and open lesions associated with STIs increase the risk of developing human immunodeficiency virus (HIV) infection, which can result in acquired immunodeficiency

syndrome (AIDS). AIDS is an STI for which there is currently no cure (see Chapter 11). The risks of STIs do not disappear with age. Over 10% of HIV cases occur in patients older than 50 years (Wold, 2012). Safe sex practices are essential at all ages.

 Think Critically

What safe sex practices can help prevent the spread of STIs?

STIs have a major impact on reproduction and general health. Because STIs are communicable, these infections are of concern both to the patient and to the general public health. One of the goals of *Healthy People 2020* is to increase efforts to "promote responsible sexual behaviors, strengthen community capacity and increase access to quality services to prevent STIs and their complications." Another *Healthy People 2020* objective is to "prevent HIV infection and its related illness and death." The progress in reaching these national objectives is monitored by the U.S. Department of Health and Human Services.

COMMON INFECTIONS OF THE FEMALE REPRODUCTIVE TRACT

PELVIC INFLAMMATORY DISEASE

Pelvic inflammatory disease (PID) refers to any inflammation in the pelvic cavity. If the infection is located in the fallopian tubes, it is called salpingitis. Infection of the ovary is called oophoritis; involvement of the pelvic peritoneum is called pelvic peritonitis. The organisms causing the infection are usually introduced from the outside, traveling through the uterus to infect pelvic organs. Therefore PID is much more common in sexually active women, particularly women with multiple sexual partners. Most of these infections are commonly caused by two sexually transmitted organisms, *Neisseria gonorrhoeae* and *Chlamydia trachomatis,* and the most common complication is infertility due to fallopian tube damage. However, PID can also be the result of an infection following pelvic surgery or childbirth and is not *always* an STI.

Symptoms of acute PID include severe abdominal and pelvic pain and fever, frequently accompanied by a foul-smelling purulent vaginal discharge, and the woman appears acutely ill. Chronic PID usually causes backache, a feeling of pelvic heaviness, and disturbances in menstruation. However, mild cases may produce no symptoms but still cause significant reproductive damage. Acute PID usually is treated with intravenous antimicrobials, symptom relief, and patient support and teaching. See Chapter 39 for other common inflammations and infections of the female reproductive tract.

CANDIDIASIS

Candidiasis (moniliasis) is a yeast infection, and although it is not considered a sexually transmitted infection, recurrent infections increase the risk for STIs in sexually active women. Candidiasis is caused by a change in the vaginal pH, which allows the yeast-like fungus *(Candida albicans)* to grow. The pH of the vagina can be altered by diabetes mellitus, oral contraceptives, some systemic antibiotic use, or the frequent douches often practiced by sexually active women. Symptoms of candidiasis include itching, burning on urination, and a white, cheese-like discharge. Treatment includes vaginal miconazole or clotrimazole for 3 to 7 days or oral fluconazole in a single dose.

BACTERIAL VAGINOSIS

Bacterial vaginosis occurs when normal lactobacillus in the vagina is replaced by *Mycoplasma hominis* or anaerobic bacteria. Bacterial vaginosis is associated with minor vaginal tissue trauma often caused by frequent sexual activity or douching. Symptoms include a grayish-white discharge that has a fishy odor. Although not considered an STI, this condition can increase the risk for STIs and does have serious consequences if it

occurs during pregnancy. Treatment includes metronidazole or clindamycin (see Chapter 39 for other common inflammations or infections of the female reproductive tract).

RISK FACTORS FOR TRANSMISSION OF SEXUALLY TRANSMITTED INFECTIONS

Although men and women are equally susceptible to STIs, **women are diagnosed with STIs at a much higher rate than men.** Biologically, young, sexually active women have a large proportion of columnar epithelium lining the cervix and a vaginal pH that can be altered by frequent douching. An alteration of vaginal pH can place the woman at higher risk for an STI. During and after the sexual act, male secretions and semen are in contact with female mucous membranes for a period of time longer than female secretions are in contact with male mucous membranes. Therefore women have an increased risk for STI.

 Cultural Considerations

Media Effects on STIs

Custom and culture can also affect the development of STIs. STI rates increase in societies in which the media (television, magazines, movies, and Internet chat rooms) focus on sexuality and premarital sexual experiences of people with varying behaviors and values, including greater sexual freedom.

The mucus plug in the cervix of women (that protects the upper genital tract) becomes more permeable around the menstrual period, which can result in an increased risk for infections in the upper genital tract, such as pelvic inflammatory disease (PID).

Contraceptive choice may influence a woman's increased risk of STIs because the use of oral contraceptives alters the cervical secretions, resulting in a more alkaline environment in the vagina and thus a more favorable setting for growth of organisms that cause STIs. The use of long-acting oral contraceptives may reduce the use of condoms, thus increasing the risk of exposure to STIs in both partners.

Cultural Considerations

Contraception Choices

In societies or cultures in which women are passive, they may not insist on condom protection before intercourse. The condom offers protection from STIs, but the man often decides whether or not it is to be used.

Women may not seek medical care as quickly as men for symptoms of an STI. Often a vaginal discharge is considered a normal variance and health care may not be sought until the infection spreads and symptoms of PID occur. In men, urinary tract infections associated with sexual activity may be the first sign of an STI. Men may seek earlier health care intervention because the signs and symptoms are obvious and distressing. STIs can have long-term effects in the form of sterility, complicated pregnancy, or neonatal infection. Health care screening services and easy access to health care are important in preventing the spread of STIs.

PREVENTION OF HUMAN PAPILLOMAVIRUS

The Advisory Committee on Immunization Practices of the Centers for Disease Control and Prevention (CDC) has recommended routine human papillomavirus (HPV) vaccinations for all girls and women 9 to 26 years old. Gardasil provides protection against strains 6 and 11 that cause genital warts, and against 16 and 18 (the cancer-causing HPV strains). Gardasil can be given to girls as young as 9 years of age, and to women up to 45 years of age. Three doses are required. (The second dose is given 2 months after the first, and the third dose is given 6 months later.) Although the vaccine is effective in preventing genital warts and precancerous lesions of the cervix, it does not protect against other HPV infections, so recommendations for routine cervical cancer screening are still valid. A second HPV vaccine was approved in 2009 by the Food and Drug Administration (FDA) for prevention of infection from HPV strains 16 and 18. According to 2009 guidelines, HPV protection is for both boys and girls and remains effective for approximately 6 years (CDC, 2011).

LESIONS OF SEXUALLY TRANSMITTED INFECTIONS

In men, the lesions related to STIs may appear under the prepuce, on the head or body of the penis, or on the scrotum, perianal area, rectum, or inner thighs. In women, lesions of STIs can appear on the vulva, vagina, cervix, perianal area, or inner thighs. Lesions around the mouth can occur in cases of oral sexual practices. Lesions can also be found far from the genital area. For example, lesions of syphilis include a classic rash on the palms of the hands and soles of the feet. Lesions of *Neisseria gonorrhoeae* may spread and cause pustules on the extremities as part of an "arthritis-dermatitis" syndrome. Examples of common organisms involved in STIs are listed in Box 41-1.

REPORTING SEXUALLY TRANSMITTED INFECTIONS

STIs must be reported to the local public health agency in accordance with state and local statutory requirements. The CDC and local health authorities establish these regulations and provide regular updates and reporting forms to health care providers for monitored infections. Syphilis, gonorrhea, chlamydia, chancroid, lymphogranuloma venereum, hepatitis B, PID, HIV infection, and AIDS are reportable diseases in all parts of

Box 41-1	Causes of Sexually Transmitted Infections

BACTERIA
- *Neisseria gonorrhoeae*
- *Chlamydia trachomatis*
- *Treponema pallidum* (syphilis)
- *Haemophilus ducreyi* (chancroid)
- *Mycoplasma hominis*

VIRUSES
- Human herpesvirus 2 (herpes simplex virus type 2)
- Hepatitis B virus
- Human immunodeficiency virus (HIV)
- Human papillomavirus (HPV)

YEASTS AND FUNGI
- *Candida albicans*
- *Candida glabrata*
- *Candida tropicalis*

PARASITE
- *Trichomonas vaginalis* (trichomoniasis)

Data from www.cdc.gov/std/trichomoniasis/default.htm.

the United States, according to the public health guidelines from the CDC. The requirements for reporting other STIs differ by state, and clinicians must be familiar with state and local reporting requirements. This tracking information is used to determine community resource needs and is evaluated in terms of the national goals of *Healthy People 2020*.

TRANSMISSION OF SEXUALLY TRANSMITTED INFECTIONS

STIs are primarily passed through some type of intimate contact, either genital to genital, mouth to genital, or genital to rectum. They occur in both heterosexual and homosexual relationships. Some infections, such as HIV or hepatitis B or C, also may be passed through blood contact, by the sharing of contaminated needles, or—though rarely—through transfusion with contaminated blood. Accidental transmission to medical personnel may occur via needle or sharps injuries or by direct exposure to open wounds or body fluids.

Blood-borne infections may be transmitted to the fetus before birth. The newborn is at risk for contracting any STI that may reside in the vagina at the time of birth. Depending on the organism, such exposure can lead to a variety of serious problems for the infant, including pneumonia and blindness.

? Think Critically

What are the four major modes of transmission for STIs?

In many states screening for some STIs—particularly for syphilis—is required for a marriage license. However, it is expensive to screen for all STIs. The greatest hope for controlling STIs is public awareness and willingness to take responsibility for prevention, and for treatment should infection occur.

COMMON DIAGNOSTIC TESTS

Table 41-1 lists the more common STIs and contains information about modes of transmission, diagnoses, symptoms, treatments, and nursing responsibilities.

A variety of tests are used to detect STIs. Noninvasive diagnostic techniques have been developed that use urine samples. *Smears* and *cultures* may be taken directly from the site (e.g., vaginal, cervical, or urethral swabs). In some instances, organisms also can be cultured from the blood. *Biopsies* are microscopic tissue examinations performed on a sample taken from the affected area and are usually done to differentiate between benign and malignant tissues, but can also provide a differential diagnosis in diseases that have specific cellular changes or organisms present.

Numerous types of blood tests can help detect STIs. They look for specific antibodies formed by the presence of certain microorganisms, or for the effects of antigens (substances in the bloodstream that stimulate the production of antibodies). Such effects include the tendency for agglutination—the clumping together of cells in a variety of characteristic patterns.

Staining procedures differentiate organisms by using dyes that have been found to stain some bacteria in specific ways. An example of this would be a Gram stain, in which bacteria are first stained with crystal violet, then treated with a strong iodine solution, decolorized with ethanol or ethanol acetone, and then counterstained with contrasting dye. Those retaining the initial stain are considered gram positive; those losing the stain but accepting the counterstain are considered gram negative. Current development of noninvasive testing and screening procedures using urine samples will increase public acceptance of mass screening. See Chapter 6 for further discussion on testing for infectious agents.

❖ NURSING MANAGEMENT

Identifying microorganisms is a complex procedure. When collecting or assisting in the collection of specimens, the nurse has several specific responsibilities to ensure that the samples will allow accurate studies to be performed. These include:

- Ensure that appropriate laboratory request slips have been prepared according to the health care provider's specific orders. If antimicrobials have been started, note this on the laboratory slip.
- Check the laboratory manual for any specific restrictions or preparations for the tests ordered.
- Urethral swabs should not be done within 1 hour of the last void as organisms will have been flushed away.

- Female patients should not douche before vaginal cultures or smears.
- Some tests will give a false-positive reading if the patient is on specific medications or has other types of infection present. Check the patient's history.
- Antimicrobials may cause cultures to be negative even though the drug or the dose may not be sufficient to cure the infection. Document the medication history.
- Stool present in the rectum can prevent good rectal swabs from being obtained.
- Cultures and smears usually are obtained with a *sterile* swab and sent to the laboratory.
- Prepare the patient. (See information on preparing the patient for a pelvic examination in Chapter 39.)
- Explain what tests have been ordered and any specific home preparation. Answer all questions.
- Provide appropriate draping and privacy, and remain with the patient during the procedure.
- Provide emotional support as needed.
- Make sure that specimens are appropriately labeled and delivered to the laboratory with the corresponding laboratory slips.

■ Assessment (Data Collection)

Screening for potential STIs or risk for acquiring such an infection should be part of any patient history data collection. However, it often is difficult to get accurate information. Patients may not disclose symptoms such as inflammation, rash, or discharge if they fear it is related to sexual activity. Adolescents may fear parental disapproval, rejection, or disciplinary action if they admit to being sexually active, and so may hide symptoms. Fear of finding a serious disorder such as HIV also may make the patient reluctant to cooperate with data collection.

 Communication

Gathering Information

When someone is diagnosed with an STI, the public health department is responsible for collecting the names of sexual partners so that they can be contacted and treated. Many people do not wish to give out this information. Professionals who deal with these issues regularly, such as public health nurses, often have special training in obtaining an appropriate history.

Obtaining a history on a patient seeking treatment for an STI requires tact and sensitivity. Such a history involves very intimate questions and may involve a variety of cultural and personal issues. The nurse must maintain an open and nonjudgmental attitude.

Text continued on p. 948

Table 41-1   Common Sexually Transmitted Infections

INFECTION	MODES OF TRANSMISSION	SYMPTOMS	MEDICAL DIAGNOSIS	MEDICAL TREATMENT	NURSING INTERVENTIONS
Chlamydia trachomatis 	Direct sexual contact. May be transmitted to the newborn during vaginal delivery. Most common STI in the United States.	*Male* Often asymptomatic. Dysuria frequency of urination, watery, mucus-like discharge. Causes about half the cases of epididymitis and nongonococcal urethritis. *Female* Approximately 75% have no symptoms. Yellow vaginal discharge, urinary frequency, dysuria. May have unusual odor after intercourse. Can result in PID, ectopic pregnancy, and sterility. *Neonate* Exposure can cause eye infections and pneumonia.	By cervical culture, DNA probe, enzyme immunoassay, ELISA, or nucleic acid amplification. *Screening protocol* Test women ages 15-25 via low vaginal swab (SOLVS) or first void urine (SVU). Test men seen in GU clinic via urine sample. TMA, SDA, or PCR test and test for gonorrhea as well.	A 7-day course of antibiotics such as doxycycline (Vibramycin), ofloxacin (Floxin), or levofloxacin (Levaquin); ciprofloxacin. A single dose of azithromycin (1 g PO) for patients with compliance problem. Erythromycin for pregnant women.	*Education* Encourage patients to seek attention for any unusual vaginal or penile discharge. Partner(s) must be treated concurrently. Condom use for prevention of future infection, with abstinence until course of treatment completed. Must complete antibiotics to ensure effective treatment and prevent development of PID. CDC recommends screening all pregnant women and sexually active young women.
Human papillomavirus (HPV) Condylomata acuminata (venereal warts) caused by HPV	Spread during sexual contact. Highly contagious. Can be transmitted to newborn during vaginal delivery.	Warts are flat or raised, rough, cauliflower-like growths on the vulva, penis, perianal area, vaginal or rectal walls, or cervix. The flat variety is more likely to lead to tissue changes that contribute to cervical or penile cancer. *Neonate* Laryngeal papillomas.	Biopsy, colposcopy, anoscopy, Pap smear.	Freezing, laser therapy, surgical removal, cryotherapy. Topical podophyllin, imiquimod, and podofilox are alternative treatments for external warts. Topical TCA or interferon is used for difficult cases. Some lesions can cause cancer.	*Education* Teach about mode of infection and use of condoms to prevent spread. Regular Pap smears due to risk of cervical cancer. Two vaccines are available and are recommended for all women ages 9-45. Should remain supine for 15 min after vaccination as fainting may occur (Munoz, 2009).

Genital herpes	Caused by herpes simplex virus (HSV) types 1 and 2. Highly contagious, spread by direct contact; not limited to sexual contact. Self-inoculation also possible, for example, from lip ulcer (fever blister) to genitals. Invades nerve cells located near the site of infection. Lies dormant, flare-ups erratic and unpredictable. Some patients have frequent recurrence, others rarely or none. Neonate may be infected during delivery if mother has active disease (more common if initial episode occurs during pregnancy).	*Primary* Fever, headache, malaise, myalgia, burning genital pain, dysuria (female), painful intercourse. Vesicles in genital area that ulcerate, crust over, and resolve spontaneously in about 2 wk. *Secondary* Burning genital pain, possible numbness and tingling 24 hr before lesions appear, vesicles. *Male* Lesions may appear on glans penis, shaft of penis, prepuce, scrotal sac, inner thighs. *Female* Vulva, vaginal surface, buttocks, cervix. Cervical lesions may be superficial with diffuse inflammation, or a single, large, necrotic ulcer. Primary infection during pregnancy associated with high risk of premature labor and spontaneous abortion. *Neonate* Local infections of eyes, skin, or mucous membranes to severe disseminated infection that can be lethal may occur.	Lesions usually easily identified by experienced clinician. Can be confirmed by viral cultures of fluid from vesicles.	No known cure. Treatment with acyclovir, valacyclovir, or famciclovir may reduce symptoms and accelerate healing. For individuals with frequent recurrence, continuous treatment may reduce frequency. Viral shedding may continue after lesions are healed.	Keep lesions clean and dry to prevent secondary infection. Increased fluids will dilute urine for greater comfort. Topical anesthetics and oral analgesics may help manage pain. Strict gloving and observation of Contact Precautions are necessary. *Education* Use of condoms with spermicide to help prevent spread, avoidance of sex if lesions present; scrupulous hand hygiene. If patient becomes pregnant while disease is active, infant will be delivered by cesarean section to protect it from exposure.

AIDS, acquired immunodeficiency syndrome; *ARC,* AIDS-related complex; *CD4,* T helper cell; *CDC,* Centers for Disease Control and Prevention; *CNS,* central nervous system; *DNA,* deoxyribonucleic acid; *ELISA,* enzyme-linked immunosorbent assay; *FDA,* Food and Drug Administration; *FTA-Abs,* fluorescent treponemal antibody absorption; *HBIG,* hepatitis B immune globulin; *HBsAg,* hepatitis B surface antigen; *IM,* intramuscular; *Pap,* Papanicolaou; *PID,* Pelvic Inflammatory Disease; *PO,* oral; *RPR,* rapid plasma reagin; *STI,* sexually transmitted infection; *TCA,* trichloroacetic acid; *VDRL,* Venereal Disease Research Laboratory.
*2008 Centers for Disease Control and Prevention Treatment Guidelines.

Continued

Table 41-1 Common Sexually Transmitted Infections—cont'd

INFECTION	MODES OF TRANSMISSION	SYMPTOMS	MEDICAL DIAGNOSIS	MEDICAL TREATMENT	NURSING INTERVENTIONS
Gonorrhea (GC)	Easily transmitted by direct sexual contact. Transmitted to the newborn during vaginal delivery if mother has active disease. Autoinoculation via fingers to eye possible. Occasionally becomes blood-borne.	Incubation: 2-6 days after exposure. May be asymptomatic. *Male* Dysuria with frequency; scant to copious purulent discharge from penis, unilateral testicular pain. If untreated may develop urethral stricture, epididymitis and can cause sterility. *Female* Vaginal discharge, burning on urination. Untreated, results in PID. May involve rectum, eyes, oropharynx. *Neonate* Due to exposure at birth to mother's vaginal secretions, is at risk for ophthalmia neonatorum, which can cause blindness, and other infections within 2-5 days after birth. *Children* Infection in children over 1 yr of age is likely due to sexual abuse.	Confirmed by presence of the causative organism, *Neisseria gonorrhoeae*, in vaginal or urethral smear, rectal or pharyngeal culture. Nucleic amplification test using urine sample is accurate.	A single dose of ceftriaxone IM is treatment of choice.* Cefixime tablets are awaiting FDA approval. Hospitalize if PID or severe illness occurs. Empirical treatment for chlamydia is recommended by CDC.	Observation of Standard Contact Precautions and frequent hand hygiene. *Education* Teach about prevention, treatment, and importance of completing treatment, naming all contacts for treatment and having follow-up cultures to ensure that treatment has been effective. Encourage safer sex practices to prevent reinfection. Be sure patient understands how to take prescribed medication. Teach CDC recommendations for sexually active patients to be screened for GC infection.

STI	Etiology/Transmission and Manifestations	Diagnosis	Treatment	Prevention/Education
Hepatitis B	Caused by hepatitis B virus (HBV). Transmission via sexual contact, blood contact, and to the fetus via the placenta in an infected mother. May have anorexia, malaise, vomiting, abdominal pain, dark urine, jaundice, skin rashes, arthralgias, arthritis. Acute infection may be asymptomatic. Infection may be persistent and result in a chronic carrier state and may develop chronic active hepatitis, cirrhosis, hepatocellular carcinoma, hepatic failure, and death. Infants born infected are at high risk for chronic hepatitis B infection.	Serologic testing for HBV infection gives definitive diagnosis.	No specific therapy is available. HBIG is given prophylactically following known exposure. Hepatitis B vaccine (Hep B) is recommended for people at risk for exposure, including health care workers. Hep B vaccine is currently given as part of normal childhood immunizations with a three-dose regimen beginning at birth. Postexposure interval before vaccination administration should not exceed 7 days for needle-stick exposure and 14 days for sexual exposure.	Appropriate handling of all blood or body fluids to prevent transmission of infection. Prevention of needle-stick injuries. *Education* Universal vaccination of newborns with single-antigen Hep B vaccine before discharge; routine screening of all women for HBsAg. Final dose of three-dose regimen should be given between 6-12 mo of age for infants from Alaska, Pacific Islands, Africa, and other endemic areas.

Continued

AIDS, acquired immunodeficiency syndrome; *ARC*, AIDS-related complex; *CD4*, T helper cell; *CDC*, Centers for Disease Control and Prevention; *CNS*, central nervous system; *DNA*, deoxyribonucleic acid; *ELISA*, enzyme-linked immunosorbent assay; *FDA*, Food and Drug Administration; *FTA-Abs*, fluorescent treponemal antibody absorption; *HBIG*, hepatitis B immune globulin; *HBsAg*, hepatitis B surface antigen; *IM*, intramuscular; *Pap*, Papanicolaou; *PID*, Pelvic Inflammatory Disease; *PO*, oral; *RPR*, rapid plasma reagin; *STI*, sexually transmitted infection; *TCA*, trichloroacetic acid; *VDRL*, Venereal Disease Research Laboratory.
*2008 Centers for Disease Control and Prevention Treatment Guidelines.

Table 41-1   Common Sexually Transmitted Infections—cont'd

INFECTION	MODES OF TRANSMISSION	SYMPTOMS	MEDICAL DIAGNOSIS	MEDICAL TREATMENT	NURSING INTERVENTIONS
Human immunodeficiency virus (HIV), AIDS, ARC	HIV is transmitted by intimate contact with body secretions of an infected person or exposure to infected blood or by perinatal transmission from mother to newborn.	Initially, flulike symptoms several weeks after HIV exposure. Antibodies appear in blood a few months to 1 yr later. A latent period follows with gradual reduction in CD4 cells. CD4 cell decline results in reduced immune function, resulting in opportunistic infections, such as Kaposi sarcoma, *Pneumocystis jiroveci* (formerly *Pneumocystis carinii*) pneumonia, and oral candidiasis. CD4 count below 200/mm^3 is diagnostic of AIDS.	Diagnosis of HIV infection based on reactive enzyme immunoassay (EIA) confirmed by a more specific assay (e.g., Western blot or immunofluorescent assay).The ELISA and HIV-RNA tests are recommended by the CDC (Swan, 2009), AIDS and ARC may be diagnosed based on laboratory results and/or specific diagnostic criteria. The FDA has approved a rapid test for HIV screening that provides results in less than 1 hr. A positive rapid HIV test requires further testing for confirmation.*	Currently there is no cure. Drug regimens interrupt reproduction of viruses. There are five major classes of antiretroviral drugs that are tailored to individual patient needs. Raltegravir is the first HIV integrase inhibitor and is used for initial antiretroviral therapy (Lennox, 2009). Postexposure prophylaxis (PEP) treatment should start within 72 hr of exposure (Kurtyka, 2010).	Nurses should assess patients for individual risk factors and recommend HIV testing as many patients are unaware of their status. Patients who are HIV positive or who have been diagnosed with AIDS or ARC should receive specific professionally trained counseling on lifestyle practices, treatment protocols, and follow-up procedures. Provide support and information to improve general health. Safe sexual practices should be used to prevent spread. Avoid breastfeeding. Cesarean birth if pregnant.

			Screening / Laboratory	Antibiotics	Education
Syphilis	Direct body contact; organism (*Treponema pallidum*, a spirochete) requires warm, wet environment to survive; can be destroyed with plain soap and water. Can penetrate intact mucous membrane. Placental transmission to fetus in about 50% of women with active disease during pregnancy.	Syphilis has three stages. *Primary* (after 3-wk incubation period) **Chancre** (hard, painless sore) on the mucous membrane of the mouth or genitals, often unnoticed in women. Chancre teeming with spirochetes, very contagious at this stage. Spirochetes enter bloodstream 3-7 days after infection and begin to multiply rapidly (bacteremia). Symptoms disappear within 3-8 wk. *Secondary* (6 wk later) Symptoms vary. May have generalized skin rash. Serology test is positive. Symptoms may disappear as the disease enters latent period. *Tertiary* (late: 1-20 yr after infection) Spirochetes have had access to all body tissues. "Gumma," a soft encapsulated tumor, appears on any organ, causing symptoms (including neurologic). *Congenital* Stillbirth, CNS damage.	*Screening* VDRL and RPR tests, performed on blood or spinal fluid if neurosyphilis is suspected. May be negative in primary, but always positive in secondary and tertiary phases. *Confirmation:* Dark-field microscopy of scrapings from chancre. FTA-Abs blood test. Tests for other STIs should also be done.	*Antibiotics* Single-dose benzathine penicillin G or adequate blood levels of penicillin given over an 8- to 14-day period, or ceftriaxone 1 g IM for 14 days.	*Education* Caution patients not to ingest alcohol for 24 hr before VDRL or RPR (may cause false-positive result). Remember that chancre is highly infectious (gloved contact only). Encourage naming of contacts so everyone can be treated. Encourage condom use to prevent reinfection. Explain importance of follow-up (usually 3- and 6-mo VDRL) to ensure treatment has been effective. Follow-up usually at 1, 2, 3, 6, 9, and 12 mo for HIV-positive individuals.
Trichomoniasis	Sexually transmitted.	Pruritus; frothy gray-green vaginal discharge; dysuria.	*Laboratory* Laboratory observation of protozoa; ulceration on cervix or vaginal wall.	Metronidazole (Flagyl), single 2 g dose for woman and partner.	*Education* Educate concerning safe sex practices and importance of seeking early care for symptoms.

AIDS, acquired immunodeficiency syndrome; *ARC*, AIDS-related complex; *CD4*, T helper cell; *CDC*, Centers for Disease Control and Prevention; *CNS*, central nervous system; *DNA*, deoxyribonucleic acid; *ELISA*, enzyme-linked immunosorbent assay; *FDA*, Food and Drug Administration; *FTA-Abs*, fluorescent treponemal antibody absorption; *HBIG*, hepatitis B immune globulin; *HBsAg*, hepatitis B surface antigen; *IM*, intramuscular; *Pap*, Papanicolaou; *PID*, Pelvic Inflammatory Disease; *PO*, oral; *RPR*, rapid plasma reagin; *STI*, sexually transmitted infection; *TCA*, trichloroacetic acid; *VDRL*, Venereal Disease Research Laboratory.
*2008 Centers for Disease Control and Prevention Treatment Guidelines.

Focused Assessment

Data Collection for STIs

The following questions are asked when assessing the patient with or at risk for an STI:

- Are you currently sexually active?
- At what age did you become sexually active?
- Do you currently have more than one sexual partner?
- Have you had other partners in the past?
- If yes to either of the last two questions: Do you understand the risks associated with having multiple sexual partners?
- If a sexually active female: Are you having regular gynecologic examinations with Papanicolaou (Pap) smears? If yes, when was your last examination?
- If a sexually active female: Are you currently pregnant or trying to become pregnant?
- Are you checked at least annually for STIs even if you do not have symptoms?
- If currently in a nonmonogamous relationship: Are you using condoms to help prevent STIs?
- Have you ever had an STI? If yes, ask for specific information (what, when, how treated; was follow-up done?).
- Do you have symptoms or reasons to believe you might have an STI now? If yes, ask for specific information (symptoms, duration; partner[s] symptomatic?).

Think Critically

What factors make it difficult to take an accurate history or provide education for a patient with an STI?

Physical examination for STIs involves exposure of the most private parts of the anatomy. Such an examination is usually performed by both a health care provider and a nurse, particularly when there are gender differences between the medical personnel and the patient. It is the nurse's responsibility to provide appropriate draping and to give the patient privacy when he or she is undressing for the examination.

Patients may request that a family member be allowed to remain with them, and they have this right. The nurse should escort such individuals into the room and have them sit or stand by the patient in a manner that allows them to provide support. The nurse also should make sure that any required equipment, supplies, specimen containers, and laboratory slips are ready in the examination room.

■ Nursing Diagnosis

Nursing diagnoses for the patient who has an STI may include:

- Deficient knowledge related to modes of transmission, signs and symptoms, and treatment
- Pain related to inflammation
- Anxiety related to intimate examination and personal information required
- Fear of being HIV positive
- Noncompliance related to repeated infection with STIs and refusal to use condoms

■ Planning

Expected outcomes for the patient with an STI may include:

- Patient will verbalize knowledge of self-care to prevent recurrence or other STI.
- Patient will be free of pain after treatment.
- Patient will cope adequately with history taking and physical examination.
- Patient will have decreased fear of HIV diagnosis after examination and treatment.
- Patient will comply with safer sex practices.
- Patient will comply with treatment requirements.

In addition to managing the treatment protocol and any pain related to an STI, patient education and emotional support are primary aspects of planning for patients with or at risk for STIs. Education in this area often is hampered by the patient's reluctance to discuss sexual issues. This may result from cultural views or more personal feelings. Patients of all ages may wish to protect themselves or their partners from possible condemnation or embarrassment through disclosure of sensitive information. The nurse must maintain a nonjudgmental attitude and give assurance that information will be kept confidential within the health care system.

When planning education, consider the patient's existing knowledge and ability to understand information provided. Select appropriate teaching aids, such as pictures, pamphlets, and three-dimensional models, to assist in the education of the patient.

Emotional support is another important aspect of care for the patient with an STI. Allow time in the teaching plan for listening to the patient's concerns and for answering questions. Be prepared with information on support groups, counseling services, and informational programs that may be of assistance. In the case of serious infections, such as HIV, support programs and professional counseling are of particular importance to the patient.

■ Implementation

Symptom Relief

STIs carry a variety of symptoms, some of which may cause mild discomfort or significant pain. Review Chapter 7 on pain management techniques and Table 41-1 for specific nursing interventions. Nursing Care Plan 41-1 gives specific nursing interventions for a patient with chlamydia.

Prevention of Spread

The spread of STIs is a major health concern in the United States. People often become sexually active at a young age, and it is not uncommon for individuals to have had a variety of sexual partners over the years. Strategies for prevention and control of STIs are given in Box 41-2.

⭐ Nursing Care Plan 41-1 | Care of the Patient with Chlamydia

Scenario
A 21-year-old woman is admitted to the clinic and diagnosed with a chlamydia infection.

Problem/Nursing Diagnosis
Does not know what chlamydia is/Deficient knowledge related to new diagnosis of chlamydia infection.

Supporting Assessment Data
Subjective: "What is chlamydia?"
Objective: Positive test for chlamydia.

Goals/Expected Outcomes	Nursing Interventions	Selected Rationale	Evaluation
Patient will verbalize understanding of disease prevention, transmission, and treatment protocols.	Assess readiness to learn about chlamydia.	Readiness to learn is essential for successful learning to occur.	Patient asking questions about her diagnosis.
	Determine knowledge base concerning chlamydia.	Learning plan should build on existing knowledge.	Patient discussing her understanding.
	Identify barriers to learning.	Language barriers, cultural beliefs, and embarrassment can alter learning effectiveness.	Patient speaks fluent English and is willing to discuss illness.
	Teach the medication regimen.	Compliance with medication regimen is essential for successful treatment.	Patient verbalizes understanding of when and how to take medication.
	Review safer sex practices.	Safer sex practices can prevent exchange of body fluids and minimize risk of STI transmission.	Patient demonstrates understanding of safer sex practices.
	Schedule follow-up appointments.	Follow-up testing is an essential part of confirming successful treatment of chlamydia.	Patient promises to return for follow-up care.

Problem/Nursing Diagnosis
Vaginal discharge/Impaired tissue integrity related to testing positive for chlamydia.

Supporting Assessment Data
Subjective: "I've had a small amount of vaginal discharge."
Objective: Chlamydia test positive.

Goals/Expected Outcomes	Nursing Interventions	Selected Rationale	Evaluation
Patient will evidence signs of successful treatment of chlamydia as evidenced by absence of symptoms and completion of medication regimen.	Assess for signs and symptoms of chlamydia such as vaginal discharge and dysuria.	Absence of symptoms may indicate successful treatment.	Patient does not evidence continued signs of the disease.
	Assess for risk factors for reactivation of disease.	Minimizing risk factors can prevent reinfection.	Patient states she is now in a monogamous relationship.
	Encourage woman to identify partners to enable treatment.	Treating sexual partners can minimize risk for reinfection and spread of infection.	Patient has contacted other partners, who have come in for examination.
	Teach safer sex practices and risk for recurrence.	Use of safer sex practices can minimize reinfection.	Patient evidences understanding of safer sex practices.

Critical Thinking Question
1. What are the long-term problems associated with untreated chlamydia?

Box 41-2   Prevention of STIs

The prevention and control of STIs are based on the following major strategies:

- Early education of adolescents concerning abstinence programs and safer sex practices.
- Education and counseling of people at risk on ways to avoid STIs through changes in sexual behaviors.
- Identification of asymptomatically infected people and of symptomatic people unlikely to seek diagnostic and treatment services.
- Effective diagnosis and treatment of infected people.
- Evaluation, treatment, and counseling of sex partners of people who are infected with an STI.
- Pre-exposure vaccination of patients at risk for vaccine-preventable STIs such as hepatitis B and HPV.
- Follow-up of patients at risk or under treatment to ensure compliance.

HPV, human papillomavirus; *STIs*, sexually transmitted infections.
Adapted from www.cdc.gov/std/hpv/default.htm.

 Health Promotion

Preventing STIs

Although the only absolute prevention is abstinence, certain behaviors significantly reduce the risk of contracting an STI. These behaviors include using condoms with a spermicide containing nonoxynol-9, which acts as a barrier and has viricidal and bactericidal action; limiting sexual contacts, preferably to one partner; and avoiding sexual contact if a partner is known to be infected or if lesions are observed in the genital, perianal, or oral regions. If the patient or the sexual partner is an intravenous (IV) drug user, education regarding nonsharing of needles is important.

▪ Evaluation

Initially, each patient teaching contact should be evaluated for effectiveness by reviewing information discussed to determine whether learning has occurred. Over time, evaluate whether the patient is following the recommendations. Follow-up cultures that are negative are a good indicator that treatments were followed as prescribed. During the follow-up interview, the nurse can inquire about use of safer sex practices and evaluate retention of information previously taught.

COMMUNITY CARE

Most communities have clinics, often through the public health system, that provide screening and treatment for STIs. These may be low cost or no cost, and they provide a valuable service by assisting the community to control the spread of STIs.

Patient education is an important service provided by community clinics. The health department and organizations such as Planned Parenthood are just two of the community agencies that routinely provide pamphlets, posters, and classes on preventing and treating STIs. Confidential screening and education on safer sexual practices are important services provided by these clinics. Public service announcements, such as the television spots on HIV/AIDS awareness, are another source of public education. In many areas, information and education are made available through schools and colleges and are directed both at students and their families and at the general community.

Get Ready for the NCLEX® Examination!

Key Points

- STIs are primarily passed through intimate contact with body fluids. Needle sticks or blood transfusions with contaminated blood can also spread STIs. An STI can also be transmitted to the newborn during the birth process.
- One objective of *Healthy People 2020* is to "prevent HIV infection and its related illness and death."
- STIs can be caused by bacteria, viruses, or protozoa.
- Contraceptive choice influences a woman's risk for STIs.
- A properly used condom offers protection from the transmission of STIs.
- STIs can cause sterility, complicate pregnancy, or cause neonatal infection.
- Many STIs are reportable to the public health department.
- Awareness of symptoms of STIs can aid in early diagnosis, treatment, and education of patients.
- Nursing responsibilities include helping to identify, screen, and educate patients at risk for STIs.
- PID is an inflammation of the pelvic cavity often caused by STIs and can cause sterility.

- Candidiasis is a yeast infection caused by a change in vaginal pH that can be the result of frequent douching, use of oral contraceptives, or systemic antibiotic therapy.
- Bacterial vaginosis occurs when normal lactobacillus in the vagina is replaced by pathogenic organisms, and it increases the risk for STIs.
- Education concerning safer sex practices can prevent STIs.

Additional Learning Resources

SG Go to your Study Guide for additional learning activities to help you master this chapter content.

evolve Go to your Evolve website (http://evolve.elsevier.com/deWit/medsurg) for the following FREE learning resources:
- Animations, audio, and video
- Answers and rationales for questions and activities
- Concept Map Creator
- Glossary with pronunciations in English and Spanish
- Interactive Review Questions and Exercises and more!

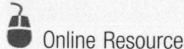
Online Resources
- STI information, www.cdc.gov/std; www.womenshealth.gov
- Kids' Health, www.kidshealth.org

Review Questions for the NCLEX® Examination

1. Changes in the vaginal pH predispose the woman to develop various forms of infections. Which product decreases vaginal resistance to infections?
   1. Vaginal douche
   2. Tampons
   3. Latex condoms
   4. Spermicidal agents

2. The nurse is taking the clinical history of an adolescent with a tentative diagnosis of gonococcal urethritis. Initial assessment confirms a nursing diagnosis of fear. A likely etiology for the diagnosis would be:
   1. potential death.
   2. parental disapproval.
   3. disfigurement.
   4. loss of reproductive function.

3. The nurse is teaching a patient about her diagnosis of genital herpes. Which statement made by the patient indicates that further teaching is necessary?
   1. "Once my lesions are healed I am no longer communicable."
   2. "Primary lesions will resolve in about 2 weeks."
   3. "This infection can spread to other parts of my body."
   4. "A cesarean section may be necessary if the infection is active during pregnancy."

4. While inserting an indwelling urinary catheter, the nurse finds raised, rough, cauliflower-like growths on the vulva and vaginal walls. A likely causative agent would be:
   1. herpes simplex virus.
   2. human papillomavirus.
   3. Treponema pallidum.
   2. Neisseria gonorrhoeae.

5. Which statement is true regarding the venereal disease research laboratory (VDRL) test?
   1. VDRL tests are used for screening and diagnosis.
   2. False-negative reactions are associated with malaria, leprosy, and viral pneumonia.
   3. The VDRL values increase quantitatively after completion of therapy.
   4. False-negative reactions are associated with alcohol consumption.

6. The nurse is counseling a patient concerning the importance of early detection and treatment of sexually transmitted infections. Which serious complication(s) result(s) from STIs? (Select all that apply.)
   1. Sterility
   2. Pregnancy complications
   3. Stroke
   4. Neonatal infections

7. The nurse talks with the parents of a 9-year-old girl regarding the human papillomavirus (HPV) vaccinations. The information session must include which statement(s)? (Select all that apply.)
   1. The vaccine is a one-dose immunization.
   2. The vaccine prevents genital warts.
   3. The vaccine prevents some precancerous lesions of the cervix.
   4. The vaccine protects against some other full-blown HPV infections.
   5. The vaccine eliminates the need for routine cervical cancer screening.

8. An important nursing responsibility is the reporting of certain sexually transmitted infections to the CDC and local health authorities. Which infection(s) should the nurse prepare to report? (Select all that apply.)
   1. Gonorrhea
   2. Syphilis
   3. Bacterial vaginosis
   4. Candidiasis
   5. Chlamydia

9. The nurse is assessing the patient for clinical signs and symptoms of syphilis. What are the classic manifestations of syphilis? (Select all that apply.)
   1. An open ulcer on the genitals
   2. A red rash on the palms of the hands
   3. A cough and fever
   4. A red rash on the soles of the feet

10. A neonate is at risk for _____ when exposed to a birth canal infected with Neisseria gonorrhoeae.

Critical Thinking Activities

Scenario A
A friend confides that she has a rash in her genital area that occurred after she began having sex with her latest boyfriend. She is afraid she may have syphilis or genital herpes and does not know what to do.

1. What would you say to convince her that she needs to see an experienced clinician for diagnosis and treatment?

2. Where can she go if she does not want to see her regular health care provider?

Scenario B
A patient confides in you that he has three girlfriends, all of whom are taking oral contraceptives, so he sees no reason to use condoms.

1. What could you tell him about the importance of using condoms and his risky behavior?

chapter

42

The Integumentary System

ℯvolve

http://evolve.elsevier.com/deWit/medsurg

Objectives

Theory

1. Review the structure and functions of the skin.
2. Compare and contrast the various causes of integumentary disorders.
3. Analyze important factors in the prevention of skin disease.
4. Plan specific measures to prevent skin tears.
5. Interpret laboratory and diagnostic test results for skin disorders.
6. State nursing responsibilities in the diagnosis of skin disorders.
7. Write outcome objectives for a patient with a nursing diagnosis of Impaired skin integrity.

Clinical Practice

1. Teach three patients to perform a self-assessment of the skin.
2. Analyze the changes that have occurred with aging that affect the skin barrier for one of your elderly patients.
3. Perform a focused integumentary assessment on a patient.
4. Provide skin care for an elderly patient with dry skin.
5. Implement a teaching plan appropriate for adolescents and young adults for the prevention of skin cancer.

Key Terms

biopsy (BĪ-ŏp-sē, p. 957)
erythrasma (ĕ-rĭth-RĂZ-mă, p. 957)
exudate (ĔKS-ū-dāt, p. 957)
keloid (KĒ-loid, p. 958)
keratoses (kĕr-ă-TŌ-sēs, p. 958)
macule (MĂK-ūl, p. 959)
papule (PĂP-ūl, p. 959)

plaque (plăk, p. 959)
pustule (PŬS-tūl, p. 959)
senile lentigines (SĒ-nĭl lĕn-TĬJ-ĭ-nēz, p. 954)
senile purpura (SĒ-nĭl PŬR-pū-ră, p. 960)
vesicle (VĔS-ĭ-kŭl, p. 959)
wheal (WĒL, p. 959)

OVERVIEW OF ANATOMY AND PHYSIOLOGY OF THE INTEGUMENTARY SYSTEM

WHAT IS THE STRUCTURE OF THE SKIN, HAIR, AND NAILS?

- The skin consists of two layers of tissue, the epidermis and the dermis (Figure 42-1).
- The skin is attached to underlying structures by subcutaneous tissue.
- The epidermis consists of squamous epithelium and contains no blood vessels; cells receive nutrients by diffusion from vessels in the underlying tissue.
- Cell growth occurs from the bottom of the epidermis and pushes cells above to the surface, where they eventually die and slough off or are washed off. This layer is called the *stratum corneum.*
- The bottom layer of the epidermis contains melanocytes that contribute color to the skin.

- The dermis, also called the corium, is thicker than the epidermis and consists of dense connective tissue.
- The dermis contains both elastic and collagenous fibers that give it strength and elasticity.
- The dermis contains blood vessels and nerves as well as the base of hair follicles, glands, and nails that are derived from the epidermis.
- A hair consists of a shaft and a root made up of dead keratinized epithelial cells.
- The hair root is below the surface of the epidermis and is enclosed in a hair follicle that is embedded in the dermis.
- Fibroblasts that produce new cells to heal the skin are contained in the dermis.
- Glands contained in the skin are *sebaceous* (sweat producing) or *ceruminous* (wax producing).
- Nails are dead stratum corneum with a very hard type of keratin.

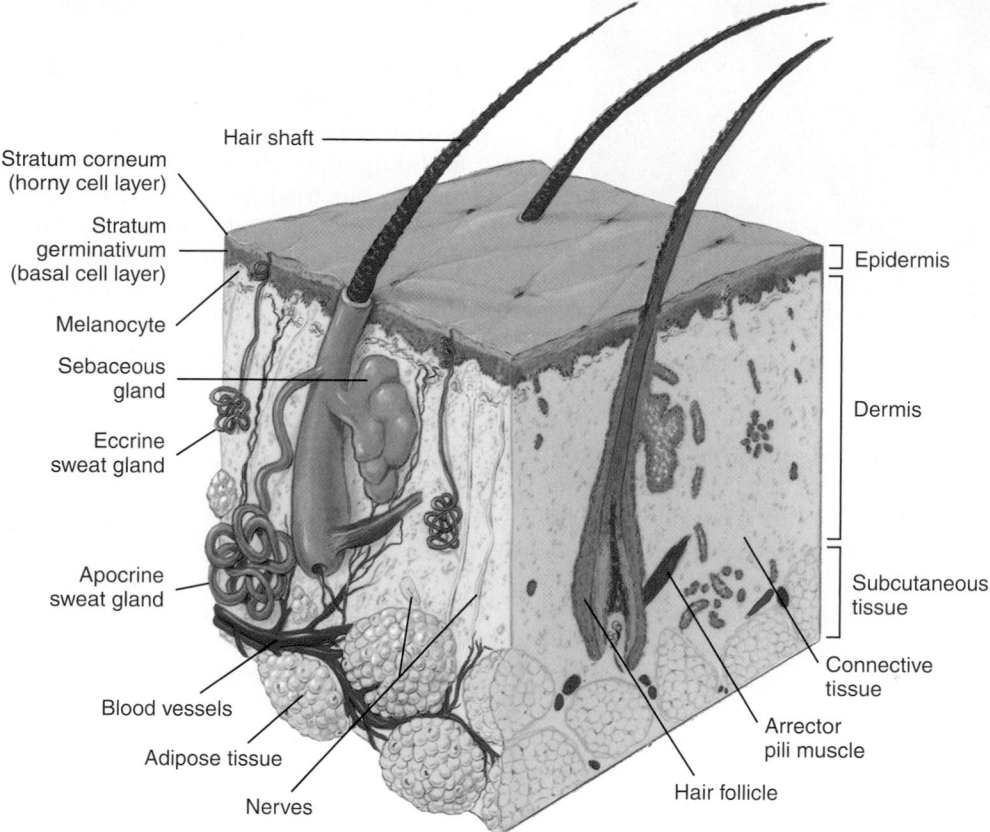

FIGURE 42-1 Structure of the skin.

WHAT ARE THE FUNCTIONS OF THE SKIN AND ITS STRUCTURES?

- The skin acts as a protective covering over the entire surface of the body.
- The keratin in the skin makes it waterproof, preventing water loss from the underlying tissues and too much water absorption during swimming and bathing.
- Skin provides a barrier to bacteria and other invading organisms.
- Skin protects underlying tissues from thermal, chemical, and mechanical injury.
- The skin helps regulate body temperature by dilating and constricting blood vessels and by activating or inactivating sweat glands.
- When the skin is exposed to ultraviolet light, molecules in the cells convert the rays to vitamin D.
- Melanin pigment absorbs light and acts to protect tissue from ultraviolet light.
- The nerve receptors in the dermis transmit feelings of heat, cold, pain, touch, and pressure.
- Hair follicles contained in the skin produce hair.
- Sebaceous glands secrete sebum that functions to keep hair and skin soft and pliable. Sebum also inhibits bacterial growth on the surface of the skin and, because of its oily nature, helps prevent water loss from the skin.

- Sweat glands act to excrete water and salt when the body temperature increases; sweat evaporates, producing a cooling effect.
- Sweat glands in the axillae and external genitalia secrete fatty acids and proteins as well as water and salts. They become active at puberty and are stimulated by the nervous system in response to sexual arousal, emotional stress, and pain.
- Hair color is produced by melanocytes in the skin and depends on the type of melanin produced.
- The shape of the hair shaft determines whether hair is straight or curly.
- Hair assists the body to retain heat.
- Nails cover the distal ends of the fingers and toes.
- Each nail has a free edge, a nail body, and a nail root that is covered by skin.
- The cuticle of each nail is a fold of stratum corneum.

WHAT CHANGES OCCUR IN THE SKIN AND ITS STRUCTURES WITH AGING?

- The number of elastic fibers decreases and adipose tissue diminishes in the dermis and subcutaneous layers, causing skin to wrinkle and sag.
- Loss of collagen fibers in the dermis makes the skin increasingly fragile and slower to heal.
- The skin becomes thinner and more transparent.
- Reduced sebaceous gland activity causes dry skin that may itch.

FIGURE 42-2 Senile lentigines (age spots or liver spots).

- Thinned skin and decreased sebaceous gland activity reduce temperature control and lead to an intolerance of cold and a susceptibility to heat exhaustion.
- A reduction in melanocyte activity increases risk of sunburn and skin cancer.
- The number of hair follicles decreases and the growth rate of hair declines; the hair thins.
- A decrease in the numbers of melanocytes at the hair follicle causes gradual loss of hair color.
- Nail growth decreases, longitudinal ridges appear, and the nails thicken; nails become more susceptible to fungal infections.
- Some areas of melanocytes increase in production, producing brown "age spots" or "liver spots," properly named senile lentigines (Figure 42-2).

THE INTEGUMENTARY SYSTEM

The skin is the first line of defense against invasion by pathogenic bacteria living in the environment. When an area of the skin is destroyed by disease or trauma, its protective functions are immediately impaired. This impairment makes the body susceptible to infection. If very large areas of skin are destroyed, as in an extensive burn, fluid and electrolyte balance is disturbed. Protein and body heat are lost from burned areas. Skin diseases are common; they are often difficult to diagnose and cure and tend to recur. The physical effects of skin diseases are not often serious. However, when the disorder renders the patient unattractive, there is a psychological impact that threatens self-image and damages self-esteem. The skin also reflects systemic diseases.

DISORDERS OF THE INTEGUMENTARY SYSTEM
Causes

More than 3000 disorders of the skin have been officially named, and many more are not included in any official nomenclature. The majority of the recognized and named skin disorders arise from some pathology in the skin itself. The remainders are manifestations of some systemic disease. Skin disorders may occur from immunologic and inflammatory disorders, proliferative

and neoplastic disorders, metabolic and endocrine disorders, and nutritional problems. Physical, chemical, and microbiologic factors also can damage the skin.

Many patients with dermatologic disease are not hospitalized and are seen only in physicians' offices and outpatient clinics. Others do not seek medical attention but treat their skin disorder themselves with home remedies and over-the-counter drugs. In some cases self-care measures are successful, but they also have the potential for aggravating the condition or only temporarily relieving more severe symptoms. This can lead to delay in treatment and allows the disease to progress to a chronic and sometimes untreatable state.

Prevention
Hygiene. The ritual of the daily bath is almost an obsession with the average American. Traditionally, plenty of soap, hot water, and friction were considered a necessity for cleanliness; however, many facilities have adopted disposable cleaning cloths to replace the individual bathing basin. In a recent study, Johnson and colleagues (2009) cultured bath basins and cleaning sponges and found bacteria growing in 98% of the samples, including *Staphylococcus aureus* (23%), vancomycin-resistant enterococci (13%), and methicillin-resistant *S. aureus* (8%). Soap and water continues to have a place in hygiene, but beyond infection control, the astute nurse will assess for and consider skin type. Blondes and redheads with a fair complexion usually have very delicate skin that requires special care to prevent drying and irritation. If the skin appears dry and scaly, frequent bathing with soap and hot water only aggravates the condition. Oils and creams are available that cleanse the skin quite effectively and help replace the natural oils at the same time. On the other hand, people with dark hair usually have skin that is oilier and less susceptible to excessive drying and irritation. The person with oily skin will need to clean the skin frequently with a liberal amount of soap and water and there will be less need to apply additional oils to the skin.

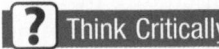
? Think Critically

You assist an elderly patient with a bath and notice that he has very dry skin. What interventions would you use?

Clinical Cues

Remember to dry areas where two skin surfaces touch, such as the axilla and under the breasts.

Diet. Even borderline deficiencies of vitamins and minerals will cause the skin to take on a sallow and dull appearance. Severe nutritional deficiencies lead to skin breakdown and the development of sores and ulcers. Dehydration causes loss of skin turgor and predisposes to pressure ulcers. People can be so concerned about their physical appearance that they refuse to eat properly for fear of gaining weight; however a well balanced diet will enhance appearance.

Age. Young people are not the only ones who should be concerned with the care of their skin. As we grow older, our skin undergoes certain changes that easily lead to irritation and breakdown if proper care is not given. The oil and sweat glands become less active, and the skin has a tendency to become dry and scaly. It also loses some of its tone, becoming less elastic and more fragile. Frequent cleansing of the skin becomes unnecessary as the skin ages, and alcohol and other drying agents must be used sparingly, if at all. Assist older patients to establish a regular routine of massaging oil, cream, or oily lotion into the skin.

 Elder Care Points

The elderly patient who has dry skin does not need a full bath every day; cleansing of the axillae and genital-rectal area between bathing days should be sufficient. Elderly patients should use a mild lotion-based soap or body wash for bathing. After showering or bathing, a lotion or cream that helps seal in moisture should be applied while the skin is still damp. Moisturizing lotion or cream should be reapplied at bedtime.

Environment. Several environmental factors can have a direct effect on the health of the skin. These include prolonged exposure to chemicals, excessive drying from repeated immersions in water, very cold temperatures, and prolonged exposure to sunlight. Some of these are occupational hazards. A change of jobs may be necessary to eliminate contact with a factor that is causing a skin disorder. One of the *Healthy People 2020* objectives is to reduce occupational skin diseases or disorders among full-time workers.

Overexposure to the ultraviolet rays of the sun can seriously and permanently damage the superficial and deeper layers of the skin. The damage results in severe wrinkling and furrowing, as well as loss of elasticity, and the skin assumes a tissue-paper transparency. In addition to the potential for premature aging and degenerative changes, solar damage also can result in malignant changes. Ultraviolet rays from the sun have long been known to be carcinogenic. This is especially true for fair-skinned people who have subjected their skin to prolonged exposure to sunshine. Although sunburns are particularly harmful, it is the normal daily exposure of unprotected fair skin to sun that causes long-term damage.

 Health Promotion

Sun Exposure Precautions

Health teaching to inform the public about the dangers of solar ultraviolet radiation should include the following information:

- Although fair-skinned people who freckle easily are more likely to suffer sun-damaged skin, people of all complexions and races can and do burn if exposed to sufficient sunlight.
- Although a good tan might be considered by many to be desirable, dermatologists say that there is no such thing as a "healthy tan." Tanning causes damage to the skin. If one insists on lying out in the sun, the initial exposure should be slow and gradual, and an adequate sunscreen with a sun protection factor (SPF) of at least 30, as well as ultraviolet A (UVA) and ultraviolet B (UVB) protection, should always be used. Too much sun too soon only leads to blistering and peeling.
- Select a sunscreen preparation on the basis of skin type and ability to tan, as well as its active ingredients and the amount of time to be spent in the sun. Remember that the sunscreen can be washed off by water or perspiration or rubbed off on sand and towels and must be periodically reapplied. Apply sunscreen liberally 15 to 30 minutes before sun exposure (American Academy of Dermatology, 2010). Reapply every 2 hours.
- Avoid exposure to the sun during the time its rays are most hazardous; that is, between 10 A.M. and 2 P.M. standard time or 11 A.M. and 3 P.M. during daylight saving time. Local radio and television stations often give information about current weather conditions and the chances for being burned by the sun at particular times during each day.
- You can be sunburned on a cloudy or overcast day.
- Light, loosely woven clothing will not give adequate protection from the sun's rays.
- Remember that snow, water, and sand can reflect the sun's rays and increase the intensity of exposure.
- Do not try to gauge how much you are being burned while in the sun. It may be 6 to 8 hours before a painful burn becomes obvious.
- Wear sunglasses and a hat when you go out in the sun, and, when possible, wear protective clothing.
- **Never use a tanning booth;** there is an eightfold increased risk to develop melanoma for persons under age 36 (Strayer & Schub, 2009).

 Complementary and Alternative Therapies

Ultraviolet Radiation Protection

An oral form of fern plant extract may help protect the skin from ultraviolet (UV) radiation. The fern extract is from *Polypodium leucotornos* and is a natural antioxidant with tumor inhibition properties. Initial studies showed that volunteer subjects could tolerate threefold to sevenfold longer sun exposure time. A 2004 study showed a microscopic decrease in sunburned cells and less infiltration of mast cells, which typically respond in allergic disorders (Fox, 2009).

Clinical Cues

It is estimated that 90% of persons between 50 and 71 are not getting adequate vitamin D. During spring, summer, and autumn, 5 to 15 minutes of sun exposure without sunscreen twice per week to the face, arms, hands, and back is sufficient for adequate vitamin D production (Kalro, 2009).

 Think Critically

You are talking to a young man who works as a ski instructor. He is fair-skinned and says that "on really sunny days, my hat is in my pocket and I never use sunscreen." Discuss some issues related to this man's integumentary health.

INTEGRITY OF SKIN

Good nursing care includes protection of the skin and prevention of skin tears. A skin tear is a potentially preventable, traumatic wound that occurs primarily on the extremities of older adults because of age and debility. The wound occurs as a result of careless handling, friction alone or shearing and friction forces that separate the epidermis from the dermis or separate both structures from the underlying tissue. More than 1.5 million skin tear injuries occur each year among institutionalized adults in health care facilities; 80% occur on upper extremities, 50% have no apparent cause, 25% are wheelchair injuries, and 25% are caused by simply bumping into objects (Miner et al., 2009). The epidermis thins and becomes less elastic with age, making it susceptible to tearing with little trauma. Those individuals who require total care are at the highest risk. Risk factors for skin tears, other than age over 65, are presented in Box 42-1.

The Payne-Martin classification system (Ayello & Sibbald, 2008) classifies skin tears as:

- *Category I:* A skin tear without tissue loss
- *Category II:* A skin tear with partial tissue loss
- *Category III:* A skin tear with complete tissue loss in which the epidermal flap is missing

Nursing Management

Rigorous nursing care (Box 42-2) to prevent skin tears is obviously preferable to treating skin tears that could have been avoided. However when a skin tear is discovered, steps for its management are:

- Gently cleanse the skin tear with saline.
- Allow the area to air-dry, or pat dry gently and carefully.
- If the skin tear flap has dried, remove it using scissors and sterile technique.
- If the skin tear flap is viable, gently roll the flap back into place using a moistened cotton-tipped applicator.

Box 42-1 Risk Factors for Skin Tears in the Elderly

Assess the patient for the following factors:
- Dry skin with dehydration
- Areas of ecchymoses
- Presence of friction, shearing, or pressure from bed or chair
- Impaired sensory perception
- Impaired mobility
- Taking multiple medications
- Prolonged use of corticosteroids
- Presence of renal disease, congestive heart failure, or stroke impairment
- Incorrect removal of adhesive dressings
- Rough handling when being bathed, dressed, transferred, or repositioned

Box 42-2 Measures to Prevent Skin Tears and Protect Fragile Skin

- Have patients wear long sleeves and long pants to protect the extremities, or protect the fragile skin on extremities with stockinettes.
- Provide adequate lighting to reduce the risk of bumping into furniture or equipment.
- Maintain the patient's nutrition and hydration; offer fluids between meals.
- Lubricate the skin with cream or lotion twice a day, paying special attention to the arms and legs.
- Use an emollient soap for bathing, and do not use soap every day on extremities if no soiling has occurred.
- Use a lift sheet to move and turn patients.
- Avoid wearing rings or bracelets that could snag the skin.
- Use transfer techniques that prevent friction or shear.
- Pad bed rails, wheelchair arms, leg supports, or other equipment where the patient might bump an extremity.
- Support dangling arms and legs with pillows or blankets.
- Use nonadherent dressings on fragile skin. Use gauze wraps or stockinettes to secure dressing. If tape must be used, use a paper or nonallergenic tape and apply it without tension.
- Mark the dressing with an arrow showing the direction it should be removed.
- Remove tape and dressing with extreme caution:
  - Use a solvent or saline to loosen the adhesive bond.
  - Slowly peel tape away from anchored skin (stabilize skin).
- If a thin hydrocolloid or solid wafer skin barrier is used as a protective barrier between the skin and the dressing, allow it to fall off naturally.

- If bleeding has stopped, silicone-coated net dressings are preferred; Steri-Strips or petroleum-based protective ointments are also used. Cyanoacrylate skin protectants are in a liquid form; when applied, a barrier is created to protect damaged skin. The substance does not need to be removed because it will shed in approximately 1 week (Fleck & Kesselman, 2009).

- If bleeding continues, dress with alginate and a secondary dressing.
- Manage the same as a skin graft. The flap should not be disturbed for about 5 days to allow the skin flap to readhere.
- Assess and measure the size of the skin tear.
- Document assessment and treatment.

Bolhuis (2008) recommends that a skin tear protocol is essential to ensure that adequate attention is given to the wound. The dressing should (1) continuously cleanse the wound, (2) conform to the wound, (3) absorb exudates, and (4) keep the wound bed moist and reduce pain and discomfort. The wound must be watched for signs of infection. Extra padding for the involved extremity will help to prevent additional injuries.

Clinical Cues

According to the Wound, Ostomy, and Continence Nurses Society, transparent adhesive dressings are no longer recommended for covering skin tears (Miner et al., 2009).

Diagnostic Tests and Procedures

Skin Biopsy. Removing a sample of tissue (biopsy) from a skin lesion usually is performed with a local anesthetic. It can be done by shaving a top layer off a lesion that rises above the skin line *(shave biopsy),* by removing a core from the center of the lesion *(punch biopsy),* or by excising the entire lesion *(excisional biopsy).*

Skin biopsy is used to differentiate benign from malignant lesions and to help identify the causative organism in bacterial and fungal infections. No special patient preparation is necessary beyond a simple explanation of the procedure and its purpose. If a local anesthetic is to be used, the patient is asked about any personal or family history of allergies. After the procedure, the patient is given instructions for the care of the biopsy site. Usually the bandage is changed daily. The site may or may not be treated with a topical antibiotic solution or ointment. Sutures from an excisional biopsy will need to be removed in 10 to 14 days.

Culture and Sensitivity Tests. When a bacterial, viral, or fungal infection of the skin is suspected, culture and sensitivity tests can be used to identify the causative organism and the drug most appropriate for treating the specific infection. A sampling of exudate (drainage) is taken from the lesion and sent to the laboratory for culturing. Once the organism has been cultured, colonies can be tested for sensitivity to certain anti-infective agents. Care must be taken when handling the specimen and its container to avoid contaminating people who will later be handling the specimen.

Safety Alert

Skin Drainage or Weeping

Whenever there is a question of a pathogenic process, weeping or drainage from skin lesions, or the suspicion of scabies, Standard Precautions should be employed when touching the patient's skin to prevent self-contamination or transmission of an organism.

Microscopic Tests. Various stains and solutions are used to prepare skin, hair, scales, or nail material for study. These tests can identify fungal, bacterial, and viral organisms. To check for organism infestations, scrapings are suspended in mineral oil and examined under the microscope.

Special Light Inspection. Inspection of the skin is one of the principal means by which skin lesions are diagnosed. To facilitate the diagnosis of certain kinds of skin disorders, special lights may be used by the examiner. A *cold light* is one in which the light is transmitted through a quartz or plastic structure to dissipate the heat. Because there is no danger of burning the skin, the cold light can be applied directly to the skin to illuminate its layers for visualization of malignant changes.

A *Wood's light* is a specially designed ultraviolet light. The nickel oxide filter holds back all but a few violet rays of the visible spectrum. This special light is especially useful to diagnose fungal infections of the scalp and chronic bacterial infection of the major folds of the skin (erythrasma). Under a Wood's light, fungal lesions and erythrasma are fluorescent. Erythrasma usually is seen on the inner thighs, scrotum, and axilla, under the breasts, and in the area between the toes.

Diascopy. Diascopy uses a glass slide or lens pressed down over the area to be examined, blanching the skin and thereby reducing the erythema caused by increasing blood flow to the area. The shape of the underlying lesion is then revealed.

Skin Patch Testing. When a rash is suspected to be of an allergic nature, patch testing is used to identify the responsible allergen. Test chemicals or substances are introduced to unaffected skin, usually on the forearm or back, by superficial scratches or pricks. If a localized reaction producing a wheal (smooth, slightly elevated area that is pale or reddened) occurs, the test is positive. Patch tests are sometimes evaluated at a later time.

Nursing Care for Diagnostic Tests. Check to see that the patient has signed an informed consent, if one is needed, for biopsies. Reinforce what the physician has told the patient about the procedure and assess if the patient understands or has additional questions.

Check for allergies to the anesthetic or skin prep solution. Properly label any specimens and send them to the laboratory. Apply a dressing and give both verbal and written postoperative instructions to the patient. Tell the patient approximately when the results will be back and that the patient will be notified. Advise if a follow-up visit is necessary.

❖ NURSING MANAGEMENT

■ Assessment (Data Collection)

History Taking

Diagnosing skin disorders requires a thorough history to identify factors that predispose a patient to skin disease or factors that cause some type of skin disease.

 Focused Assessment

Data Collection for Skin Disorders

The following questions should be asked when seeking data on a skin disorder:

- When did the rash or lesion first appear?
- Can you think of any event or different food you ate or substance you were using just before it appeared?
- What is your usual dietary pattern? What do you eat and drink?
- Have you noticed if anything makes it worse?
- What seems to make it better?
- Have you been using any chemicals lately for household cleaning or in pursuit of your hobbies?
- Have you been out in the country or the woods lately?
- Have you been traveling? Did you visit a tropical area?
- Have you had any recent exposure to animals?
- What drugs are you taking? Do you take any over-the-counter medications?
- Have you ever had a drug reaction?
- Have you ever had radiation therapy?
- Do you have a history of any skin disorders in your family?
- Does anyone in the family currently have similar symptoms, such as a rash?
- Do you have any allergies?
- Are you experiencing itching? Pain? Fever?
- Have you had any gastrointestinal problems that began about the same time that the rash or lesion appeared? What about a runny or stuffed-up nose? Cough?
- Has the skin condition had an impact on your social life or work?

Scabies, lice, and other parasites can be transmitted through close personal contact with infected persons at work, recreation, home, or school. It is important to know if exposure has occurred, so that others can be notified and treated.

Many drugs can produce skin eruptions in certain individuals. Drug allergy or reaction can produce lesions and rashes that imitate those found in a long list of diseases, including measles, chickenpox, fungal infections, skin cancers, and psoriasis.

Itching and pain are the most common complaints. If the patient has recently been exposed to severe cold, her skin may be drier than usual and she may complain of severe itching *(winter itch)*. If the disorder is caused by an allergy, the patient also may complain of shortness of breath, cough, or some gastrointestinal symptoms. The patient also may be able to relate what other factors, such as stress or excitement, could be related to the appearance of the skin lesions.

Physical Assessment

A thorough inspection of the skin under good lighting is essential. Provide privacy and have the room at a moderate temperature so that the patient does not become chilled. Dress the patient in a gown that allows access to all areas of the skin.

 Cultural Considerations

Coin Rubbing

Coin rubbing is a Southeast Asia folk remedy that is intended to draw the illness out of the body. An oiled coin is rubbed over the skin surface and creates bruiselike marks or patterns of red lines or welts on the skin. The redness is interpreted as a sign that the remedy is bringing the illness to the surface (D'Avanzo, 2008).

Seborrheic **keratoses** are common in the elderly. They appear as wartlike, greasy lesions on the trunk, arms, scalp, and sometimes the face. They are not a cause for concern.

Darkly pigmented people will have areas that are darker than other parts of the skin. This is due to hormonal influences. The darker areas are the nipples, areola, scrotum, and labia minora. This is true among both African Americans and Asians. When the skin of a darkly pigmented person is damaged, scar tissue may hypertrophy, forming a **keloid** (a thick ridge of scar tissue that stands up from the surrounding skin) (Figure 42-3).

The hair of African Americans differs in texture. It varies from being long and straight to being short, thick, and tightly curled. It is very dry and fragile and requires daily grooming with oil. If an African American child suffers from malnutrition, sometimes the hair will turn a coppery red. Asians tend to have straight hair.

FIGURE 42-3 A keloid scar.

Clinical Cues

When trying to differentiate between a macule and a papule, shine a flashlight at a right angle to the lesion. A papule will cast a shadow. If there is no shadow the lesion is a macule. To determine whether there is fluid in a lesion, place the tip of a penlight against the side of the lesion. If the light illuminates it with a red glow, it is fluid filled. If there is no light illumination, the lesion is solid.

 Clinical Cues

Pallor in a dark-skinned person presents as an ashen-gray tone to the skin. In a brown-skinned person, pallor gives the skin a yellow-brown color.

The skin should be lightly palpated to detect changes in texture and surface elevations. Palpation also is used to detect pain, areas of increased warmth, and tenderness. When checking the temperature of the skin, the back of the hand should be used. Skin turgor is assessed by lifting a fold of skin on the forearm, chest, or abdomen between two fingers and seeing how fast it falls back into place.

◎ **Focused Assessment**

Physical Assessment of Skin

Perform physical examination of the entire skin surface. Proceed from head to toe. Compare from one side of the body to the other. Use the metric system when measuring lesions; document all findings. Check the patient for:

- General appearance of skin surface: texture, elasticity, thickness
- Condition of areas between skinfolds
- Type of lesions and distribution, size, and appearance; photograph or measure and document measurements
- Appearance of skin adjacent to lesions; note whether reddened areas blanch when mild pressure is applied
- Localized or generalized skin edema
- Characteristics of secretions: color, viscosity, amount
- Odor: description of odor; strong or faint; source—local or generalized
- Temperature changes: location of hot spots or cold areas of the skin
- Check the back and the soles of the feet, including between the toes
- Observe patient for scratching, rubbing, or picking at lesions
- Observe for scratching of the scalp or pubic areas
- Inspect the hair for texture, brittleness, thinning, and cleanliness
- Inspect the nails for chipping, splitting, discoloration, and ragged or inflamed cuticles

Table 42-1 shows characteristics of various types of skin lesions. As you are performing your assessment you can simultaneously be teaching the patient about self-examination of the skin.

Table 42-1	Types of Skin Lesions
LESION	**DESCRIPTION**
Macule	Circumscribed, flat area with a change in skin color; <1 cm in diameter *Examples:* Freckles, petechiae, measles, flat mole (nevus)
Papule	Elevated, solid lesion; <1 cm in diameter *Examples:* Wart (verruca), elevated moles
Vesicle	Circumscribed, superficial collection of serous fluid; <1 cm in diameter *Examples:* Varicella (chickenpox), herpes zoster (shingles), second-degree burn
Plaque	Circumscribed, elevated superficial, solid lesion; >1 cm in diameter *Examples:* Psoriasis, seborrheic and actinic keratoses
Wheal	Firm, edematous, irregularly shaped area; diameter variable *Examples:* Insect bite, urticaria
Pustule	Elevated, superficial lesion filled with purulent fluid *Examples:* Acne, impetigo

From Lewis, S.L., Heitkemper, M.M., Dirksen, S.R., et al. (2011). *Medical-Surgical Nursing: Assessment and Management of Clinical Problems* (8th ed.). St. Louis: Mosby.

Patient Teaching

Self-Assessment of the Skin

Teach the patient that the skin should be examined every few months. For back or other areas, suggest that a family member or close friend examine that area of skin. If any changes have occurred, consult physician right away. Advise that warts, moles, or discolorations of the skin should be checked each month for:

- Darkening or spreading of color or increasing unevenness of color
- Increase in size or diameter
- Change in shape; that is, has the lesion become elevated, or have its formerly regular edges become irregular?
- Redness or swelling of surrounding skin, or any other noticeable change around the lesion
- Itching, tenderness, or other change in sensation
- Crusting, scaling, oozing, ulceration, or other change in the surface of the lesion
- When assessing for melanoma, check for the ABCDs: A = asymmetrical, B = irregular border, C = color, D = diameter change greater than ¼ inch

Elder Care Points

When checking skin turgor on an elderly patient, test the upper chest because the skin of the arms and hands of the elderly has often lost elasticity and is not a reliable index. Gently pinch a small amount of skin and lift up and let go. Note the time it takes for the skin to move back to its normal position. If the skin stays "tented" or takes more than 8 to 10 seconds to return to normal position, the patient is dehydrated. Elderly patients bruise more easily as the skin becomes thinner and collagen is lost. Patches of **senile purpura,** deep red areas, may occur even from minor injuries.

Assessing the Skin for Signs of Breakdown

Skin should be thoroughly assessed when the patient is admitted to your facility. Skin assessment is performed every shift on immobile patients, noting the condition of skin over bony prominences. Findings must be accurately documented.

Legal and Ethical Considerations

Skin Lesion Documentation

All data gathered when assessing the skin and any lesions should be accurately documented as to location, size, appearance, and characteristics. Measure lesions using a ruler device and note the measurements in the chart. For pressure ulcers, many facilities take photos and enter those in the chart so that healing progress can be demonstrated.

Once every 24 hours, usually during the bath, the skin is totally assessed. When a reddened area is found, it is checked for blanching by pressing gently in the center of the area to see if it turns from red to white or to a paler color on darker skin. **Blanching** usually indicates that the redness is temporary and will resolve when pressure on the area is relieved. (See Chapter 43 for additional information pressure ulcers.)

Assignment Considerations

Observation While Bathing

Unlicensed assistive personnel are generally assisting with hygiene, and the nurse should give specific instructions to report reddening, bruising, breaks in the skin, or new lesions. **Remember that total skin assessment cannot be delegated; this is the nurse's responsibility.**

■ Nursing Diagnosis and Planning

Nursing diagnoses are based on the analysis of the data gathered from assessment. Diagnoses commonly associated with skin disorders are presented in Table 42-2. Nursing goals for patients with skin disorders are to:

- Restore the skin to normal
- Decrease pain and itching
- Protect the skin from further damage
- Prevent infection
- Prevent scarring as much as possible

Planning of the daily work schedule should include consideration of time necessary for dressing changes, soaks, special baths, and other skin treatments.

■ Implementation

Some general rules when caring for patients with a skin disease may be helpful as a guide until specific orders are obtained:

- Bathing with soap is usually contraindicated in all inflammatory conditions of the skin.
- Dressings covering the skin lesions that have been applied by a physician should not be removed when the patient is admitted unless there are specific orders to do so.
- Do not attempt to remove scales, crusts, or other exudates on the skin lesions until the physician has had an opportunity to examine the patient.
- Observe the skin very carefully at the time of the patient's admission, and record observations on the chart or report them to the nurse in charge.
- Avoid excessive handling or rubbing of the skin against the sheets and bedclothes when changing the bed.
- Lotions or other skin products should not be used on the skin unless the physician has approved their use.

Once the physician has determined the type of lesions present, specific treatments will be ordered to relieve the patient's symptoms and promote healing. The two most commonly used treatments are special dermatologic baths and wet compresses or dressings. In addition, lotions, salves, or ointments may be applied locally at frequent intervals.

Table 42-2 Common Nursing Diagnoses, Expected Outcomes, and Nursing Interventions for Patients with Skin Disorders

NURSING DIAGNOSIS	GOALS/EXPECTED OUTCOMES	NURSING INTERVENTIONS
Impaired skin integrity related to injury and treatment; excoriation or scaling; infectious process	Patient's skin will be intact within 2 wk (4 mo for burns). Number of lesions will decrease within 2 mo. Patient will exhibit no signs of infection within 3 mo.	Cleanse skin and apply topical medications as prescribed. Monitor for signs of adverse reaction to topical medication. Preserve integrity of grafted areas with aseptic dressing technique and splinting. Apply light treatments as prescribed.
Pain related to itching, soreness, or tenderness of lesions, exposure of denuded skin to air, or involvement of nerve tissue	Patient's pain will be controlled by medication and relaxation or distraction techniques.	Apply topical medication as ordered. Administer analgesia as ordered and as required (PRN). Provide medicated baths as prescribed. Teach relaxation techniques. Provide distraction activities.
Chronic low self-esteem related to disrupted skin surface and lesions	Patient will show increase in self-esteem by socializing with others within 3 wk.	Suggest ways to cover lesions. Help patient list positive aspects and achievements. Encourage socialization with others. Show acceptance and matter-of-fact attitude when dealing with patient's lesions.
Risk for infection related to loss of intact skin barrier	Patient will not experience skin infection before lesions are healed.	Cleanse skin carefully and gently. Use aseptic technique when attending to lesions. Apply ordered topical medication. Encourage patient to keep hands off affected skin areas. Encourage hand hygiene for patient.
Anxiety related to chronic, recurring nature of skin disorder; reaction to diagnosis of cancer; slow healing	Patient will verbalize feelings within 3 wk. Patient will explore options for treatment of cancer. Patient will identify short-term and long-term goals that realistically match the slow healing process.	Provide atmosphere of acceptance. Allow patient time to verbalize feelings. Assist to recognize positive coping techniques by looking at ways patient has coped with anxiety in the past. Provide information on treatment and prognosis for skin malignancy.
Deficient knowledge related to cause and treatment of skin disorder	Patient will verbalize knowledge of factors related to appearance of skin disorder. Patient will verbalize knowledge of treatment for disorder. Patient will demonstrate self-care techniques.	Explain the etiology of the skin disorder and measures to prevent possible recurrence, if any. Instruct in various methods of treatment. Teach the side effects of medications. Instruct in self-care techniques for medication application, dressing changes, and so on. Obtain feedback of information and skills taught.
Sleep deprivation related to itching or pain	Patient will obtain at least 7 hr of rest per day.	Administer medication to relieve itching. Keep environment cool to decrease itching sensation. Caution patient to take cool or tepid baths or showers to decrease itching. Caution not to scratch lesions as this often makes itching worse. Suggest ways to use distraction (e.g., card or game playing, intense concentration on learning something, or reading an absorbing book) to decrease focus on itching. Administer hypnotic as ordered.

Continued

Table 42-2	Common Nursing Diagnoses, Expected Outcomes, and Nursing Interventions for Patients with Skin Disorders—cont'd	
NURSING DIAGNOSIS	**GOALS/EXPECTED OUTCOMES**	**NURSING INTERVENTIONS**
Sleep deprivation related to itching or pain—cont'd		Administer analgesics as ordered. Encourage use of meditation, relaxation, or imagery techniques to decrease pain. Provide restful, quiet environment. Use massage as appropriate to promote relaxation and sleep. Allow usual bedtime rituals that help patient induce sleep.
Social isolation related to long treatment process; disfigurement	Patient will maintain social contact with family and friends. Patient will reintegrate into community within 3-24 mo.	Encourage family and friends to send cards, call, and visit. Encourage patient to continue dialogue with family and friends. Refer to psychologist or social worker for grief work and reintegration of new body image. Refer to support group for expression of feelings and realization patient is not alone with such problems. Encourage return to employment or job training. Encourage return to church or community activities.

Although the vast majority of skin diseases are *not* contagious, nurses should be careful to observe rules of cleanliness and Standard Precautions when caring for any patient with a skin eruption. **Special care is needed to avoid spreading infection from the fluid in all pustules and in the vesicles of fever blisters and cold sores.**

Giving Medicated Baths

Among the agents that may be added to the bath water are sodium bicarbonate, sodium chloride, cornstarch, oatmeal, medicated tars, oils, potassium permanganate, and special bath preparations.

 Safety Alert

Prevent Falls

A nonslip bath mat should be used in the tub when giving medicated baths. The substances used for the bath can make the tub very slippery. Showers should have nonslip mats in them as well, especially when showering an elderly person.

Patient Teaching

Easy Cleanup After an Oatmeal Bath

Put dry, uncooked oatmeal into an old nylon stocking to make an oatmeal sachet. Place the sachet in the tub and squeeze it repeatedly. After the bath is finished, discard the sachet.

During the bath, the patient must be protected from chilling, because the bath usually lasts from 30 minutes to an hour, and most patients with skin diseases have a lowered resistance to cold. **When the patient is removed from the tub, the skin is dried by patting rather than by rubbing.** If medication is to be applied locally, it should be put on as soon as the bath is completed in order to keep *pruritus* (itching) at a minimum. **Medication is applied in a thin layer unless otherwise ordered.**

The medicated bath has a very soothing and relaxing effect on the patient and also helps relieve the itching and burning commonly associated with skin diseases. The nurse should encourage the patient to rest in bed and perhaps to take a short nap after each bath.

Laundry Requirements

The bed linens and gowns used for patients with severe skin diseases may need special laundering to eliminate all traces of soap. If the patient is to be cared for at home, vinegar may be added to the rinse water to neutralize the soap. One tablespoon of vinegar is used for each quart of water. Only detergent without perfume or other additives should be used. Dryer sheets should not be used as they contain chemicals that often cause skin problems. Residue from dryer sheets can remain in the dryer and affect laundry that has been washed separately for the sensitive-skinned person. New clothes should be washed before wearing when skin sensitivity is a problem. Washing removes chemical fabric finish products.

Application of Wet Compresses or Dressings

Wet dressings may be applied to the skin in various ways. The two general types used are *open dressings* and *closed dressings*. Open compresses must be changed repeatedly and are never allowed to dry. They usually need to be remoistened every 20 to 30 minutes. The solution used should be at room temperature or warmer. This type of dressing is used when the dermatologist wishes to have air circulating to the skin lesions. Closed dressings are thoroughly soaked with the prescribed solution and wrapped with an airtight, waterproof material. It is recommended that you obtain specific instructions from the dermatologist before applying wet dressings to any skin lesions.

 Clinical Cues

When changing wet dressings, inspect the skin adjacent to the wound for signs of maceration from the moisture; this condition could cause the wound to enlarge.

Application of Topical Therapy

Many skin lesions are treated by directly applying medications to the surface of the affected area. This method is called *topical therapy*. Lotion, cream, ointment, powder, or gel may be used. The physician prescribes the kind of medication to be used and the way in which the drug is to be applied. Patients with skin conditions do not always consult a physician and sometimes choose to treat themselves at home. All patients should be instructed in the proper application of topical medications (Box 42-3). Occlusive dressings must not be applied over the area after application of the medication unless ordered by the health care provider (see Table 42-2 and Chapter 43).

 Think Critically

If a patient has an order for a topical cream to be applied to an area of rash on the right upper thigh, how would you apply this cream?

■ Evaluation

Evaluation of treatment and nursing interventions for skin disorders is based on improved appearance of the skin, absence of signs of infection, relief from itching and pain, and signs of healing. Many skin disorders are slow to respond to treatment, and patience is required on the part of the patient and the nurse. Even a

---

Box 42-3   Guidelines for Applying Topical Medications*

POWDERS
- Dry the area thoroughly before applying powder to prevent caking.
- Do not apply to raw and denuded areas.
- Some powders, such as cornstarch, can actually serve as culture media for the growth of bacteria.

OINTMENT
- Use only a small amount and gently massage into the skin until a thin film covers the area. An exception is when ointment is used as an occlusive dressing, as for a burn.
- Ointments tend to leave a greasy feeling to the skin. They are best for chronic lesions, because they help the skin retain moisture and natural oils.
- Avoid putting ointment on areas where the skin is creased and overlaps itself.

GELS
- A gel is a semisolid mixture that tends to liquefy when applied to the skin. It is absorbed into the skin and dries quickly, leaving a thin, nonocclusive film.
- If applied to abraded or sensitive areas, alcohol in the base can cause a burning or stinging sensation.

LOTIONS
- These are actually powders suspended in water; they will leave a residue once the liquid evaporates from the skin. This residue should be washed off before a fresh dose is applied.
- Be sure powder is uniformly dispersed in solution before applying, then use a firm stroke to distribute the medication evenly. Do not "dab" on lotions, as this can be irritating to the skin.

ALL TYPES
- Always apply topical medications sparingly and in a thin film that extends beyond the affected area about ¼ inch. Thick layers of topical medications are wasteful, and some of these drugs, such as corticosteroids, are very expensive.
- Too much of some topical medications (e.g., antifungal agents) can chemically irritate the skin and delay healing. Thick layers also tend to soften the skin too much.
- If the skin condition appears to be getting worse after a topical agent is applied, or if the patient develops eczema, suspect an allergic contact dermatitis caused by the drug.

*Allergies must be assessed before applying a topical medication.

minor fungal skin infection may take from 7 to 14 days to clear with topical medication. A fungal infection of a nail may take up to a year to clear. A major part of evaluation is to determine that treatment is not aggravating the condition.

Get Ready for the NCLEX® Examination!

Key Points

- The skin is essential for the maintenance of life; it is the first line of defense against pathogenic organisms. Skin has two layers, the epidermis and the dermis. New cells to heal the skin are contained in the dermis.
- Factors in the prevention of skin disorders include cleanliness, appropriate diet, proper skin care, limiting exposure to the sun and careful handling of fragile skin.
- With age the skin becomes thinner and more fragile, less elastic, and drier.
- Fragile skin requires special attention: protective clothing (such as long sleeves), lubrication with creams or lotions, bed transfer techniques that prevent shear, padded side rails and assistive devices, use of nonadherent tape, and use of solvent to loosen dressings and to peel slowly.
- Several types of diagnostic measures are used: biopsy, culture, microscopic examination of scrapings or tissue, special light inspection, diascopy, and skin patch testing.
- A thorough health history is key in the diagnosis of skin disorders (see Focused Assessment on p. 959).
- Teach self-examination of the skin, including the ABCDs: A = asymmetrical; B = irregular border; C = color change; D = diameter greater than ¼ inch (see Patient Teaching on p. 960).
- Standard precautions are used when touching patients with weeping lesions or when drainage is present.
- Treatments for skin disorders include medicated baths, special laundry precautions, application of compresses or dressings, and topical therapy.
- Systemic therapy may be used for some fungal infections and for serious bacterial infections.

Additional Learning Resources

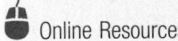 **SG** Go to your Study Guide for additional learning activities to help you master this chapter content.

evolve Go to your Evolve website (http://evolve.elsevier.com/deWit/medsurg) for the following FREE learning resources:
- Animations, audio, and video
- Answers and rationales for questions and activities
- Concept Map Creator
- Glossary with pronunciations in English and Spanish
- Interactive Review Questions and Exercises and more!

Online Resources
- American Cancer Society, www.cancer.org
- Agency for Healthcare Research and Quality, www.guideline.gov

Review Questions for the NCLEX® Examination

1. What physiologic changes in aging predispose the older adult to skin breakdown? *(Select all that apply.)*
   1. Skin becomes thicker
   2. Loss of collagen
   3. Increased elastic fibers
   4. Decreased adipose tissues
   5. Reduced sebaceous gland activity

2. The nurse notes that the elderly patient has "liver spots" on the hands and forearms. What is the significance of this finding?
   1. This a typical condition for aged skin because of concentrated, increased melanocyte production.
   2. The spot is a sign of potential liver problems and the finding should be reported to the physician.
   3. The liver spot is a premalignant lesion that is common in the elderly; teach the patient how to monitor for changes.
   4. The appearance of the liver spot indicates that there is dryness; gently cleanse the skin and apply cream.

3. A patient with a suspicious skin lesion is scheduled for a punch skin biopsy. What is the most accurate explanation that the nurse would give about the procedure?
   1. "It is shaving a top layer off a lesion that rises above the skin line."
   2. "It is removing a core from the center of the lesion."
   3. "It is removing the entire lesion."
   4. "It is aspirating a tissue sample."

4. The nurse reads in the patient's record that the physician observed "circumscribed, superficial vesicles with a collection of serous fluid." The nurse anticipates that the physician will make which recommendation for the patient?
   1. A prescription for a topical application for acne
   2. Isolation precautions for herpes zoster
   3. Over-the-counter antihistamine for an insect bite
   4. Patient education to self-monitor the wart

5. The nurse needs to apply a dressing to a patient who has fragile skin. Which intervention would the nurse use to protect the patient from skin tears?
   1. Ask the physician to give specific orders for wound care.
   2. Gently clean and apply a sterile transparent dressing.
   3. Tape the dressing with paper tape and avoid tension.
   4. Allow any tape and gauze dressing materials to fall off naturally.

6. A nurse is observing a nursing assistant provide skin care to an older adult patient. Which action by the nursing assistant indicates a need for further training?
   1. Using soap and hot water every day to clean the patient's body
   2. Alerting the nurse about a wet dressing
   3. Reporting redness and blanching over the sacral area
   4. Applying lotion while the skin is still damp

7. The nurse is supervising a new graduate nurse (GN) who is examining a new patient with skin lesions. The nurse would intervene if the GN:
   1. gently handles the patient's extremities to avoid skin tears.
   2. observes the condition of the skin and measures the size of the lesions.
   3. removes the scales and crusts from the lesions to clean the skin.
   4. assesses for and documents any home remedies that the patient has tried.

8. The nurse is giving instructions to a caregiver regarding the proper application of skin ointment. Which statement by the caregiver indicates a need for additional teaching?
   1. "I should use the ointment sparingly."
   2. "I will gently massage in a thin film."
   3. "I must avoid creased areas."
   4. "I should apply a thick layer to the area."

9. The nurse reminds teenagers regarding the importance of protecting the skin from ultraviolet rays. What information should the nurse include? *(Select all that apply.)*
   1. Use a sunscreen with a sun protection factor (SPF) of at least 30.
   2. Apply sunscreen thinly.
   3. Wear light, loosely worn clothing.
   4. Gauge exposure while in the sun.
   5. Wear sunglasses and a hat.

10. The patient has a rash of unknown origin. Which assessment question(s) would help determine the underlying cause of the lesion? *(Select all that apply.)*
    1. "When did the rash or lesion first appear?"
    2. "Can you think of any event or different food you ate or substance you were using just before it appeared?"
    3. "What drugs are you taking? Do you take any over-the-counter medications?"
    4. "Have you ever had radiation therapy?"
    5. "Do you have a history of any skin disorders in your family?"

Critical Thinking Activities

Scenario A
You have been asked to give a presentation to a ninth-grade class on skin care and prevention of skin cancer.

1. What specific information would you include on the subject of general skin care?
2. What would you say about lying out in the sun?
3. What information would you give regarding the use of tanning booths?
4. What would you say about protection when out in the sun?

Scenario B
Mrs. Hess, an 83-year-old resident of a long-term care facility, has very dry skin. She asks you to look at spots on her hand that are brown and "ugly."

1. What could this lesion on Mrs. Hess' hand be?
2. What would you tell her?
3. Mrs. Hess asks you why she bruises so easily. She says she hates these reddish purple areas she gets on her arms and legs. What would you answer?
4. What nursing measures should be instituted for skin care for Mrs. Hess' dry skin?

Scenario C
You and a home health aide have been assigned to care for an elderly woman in the patient's home for several days. The patient has a noncontagious itchy rash, and the physician has suggested using oatmeal as a soothing bath and topical application of lotion and has ordered daily assessments to monitor the patient's condition. In addition, the patient's daughter has asked that the linens be washed on a daily basis.

1. Discuss which tasks you (the nurse) should perform.
2. Which tasks can be delegated or assigned to the home health aide? What specific instructions should be given to the home health aide about assigned duties?
3. During one of the home visits the daughter asks the nurse to look at a mole on her own back. "I can't see it very well, and of course my mother is not able to help me either." What would you do and say in this situation?

Objectives

Theory

1. Describe the etiology of dermatitis.
2. Plan psychosocial interventions for the patient who has psoriasis.
3. Compare and contrast the treatment of fungal skin or nail disorders to the treatment of bacterial skin disorders.
4. List the main nursing care points for patients with herpes virus infections.
5. Discuss the types of acne and their treatment.
6. Compare the characteristics of the various types of skin cancer.
7. Analyze the important points of caring for an immobile patient to prevent pressure ulcers.
8. Prepare care plan interventions for each stage of a pressure ulcer.
9. Summarize important assessment points for the patient who has sustained a burn.

10. Evaluate the nurse's role in emergency burn care.
11. Evaluate the psychosocial needs and interventions for burn patients.
12. Describe the process of rehabilitation for the patient with a major burn.

Clinical Practice

1. Teach a family about care for the patient and home when scabies is present.
2. Assess the skin of family members for signs of skin cancer.
3. Provide care for a patient with a stage III or stage IV pressure ulcer.
4. Apply Standard Precautions and sterile technique for the care of a burn.
5. Visit a burn intensive care unit and observe the wound care of a patient who is in the acute stage of a major burn.

Key Terms

allograft (ĂL-ō-grăft, p. 986)
autograft (ĂW-tō-grăft, p. 986)
autoinoculation (ăw-tō-ĭn-Ŏ-kū-LĀ-shŭn, p. 970)
biologic dressings (bī-ō-LŎJ-ĭk, p. 986)
biosynthetic (bī-ō-SĬN-thĕt-ĭk, p. 986)
carbuncles (KĂR-bŭn-kŭlz, p. 970)
cellulitis (p. 970)
Curling's ulcer (p. 982)
dermabrasion (dĕrm-ă-BRĀ-zhŭn, p. 968)
dermatophytosis (DĔR-mă-tō-fī-TŌ-sĭs, p. 972)

eschar (ĔS-kăr, p. 980)
escharotomy (ĔS-kă-RŎ-tŏ-mē, p. 986)
furuncles (fyū-RŬN-kŭlz, p. 970)
mycoses (mī-KŌ-sēz, p. 972)
onychomycosis (ŏn-ĭ-kō-mī-KŌ-sĭs, p. 972)
purulent (PŬ-rū-lĕnt, p. 981)
serosanguineous (SĔR-ō-săng-GWĬN-ē-ŭs, p. 981)
shearing action (p. 977)
tinea pedis (TĬN-ē-ă pē-dĭs, p. 973)
xenograft (ZĒ-nō-grăft, p. 986)

INFLAMMATORY INFECTIONS

Many skin diseases result from infection with bacteria, viruses, or fungi or from infestation with parasites. Diseases of this kind require special precautions to avoid spreading the infectious organism or the parasite. Hand hygiene is a first-line measure in the prevention of health care–associated infections and is mandated as one of the Joint Commission's National Patient Safety Goals. The Center for Infectious Diseases, a division of the Centers for Disease Control and Prevention, recommends that Contact Isolation, as well as Standard Precautions, be implemented for a number of these diseases (Box 43-1). There are skin infections that are not

necessarily contagious; however, it can be difficult to quickly determine if the condition that you are observing is a contagious type. Therefore isolate, perform hand hygiene, and use Standard Precautions (see Appendix B) if there is any doubt.

DERMATITIS

Dermatitis is not contagious unless a secondary infection has occurred in the lesions.

Etiology, Pathophysiology, Signs, and Symptoms

Contact dermatitis is a delayed allergic response involving cell-mediated immunity. On contact with the skin, the allergen is bound to a carrier protein and forms a

| Box **43-1** | Review of Contact Isolation Requirements |

Specifications for Contact Isolation are as follows:

- A private room is indicated. In general, patients infected with the same type of organism may share a room.
- Gloves are worn when entering the room. Change gloves after contact with infective material, such as wound drainage or feces, and before treating a different location on the body. Perform hand hygiene before donning clean gloves.
- Remove gloves when leaving the room, and perform hand hygiene using an antimicrobial agent.
- Gowns are indicated if soiling is likely, particularly if there is drainage from an uncovered wound or the patient is incontinent.
- Articles contaminated with infective material should be discarded in a biohazard waste receptacle or bagged and labeled before being sent for decontamination and reprocessing.
- Patient care equipment should be used only for the one patient and should be left in the room until no longer needed.
- Skin disorders that require Contact Isolation include:
  - Diphtheria, cutaneous
  - Furunculosis, group A *Streptococcus*
  - Herpes simplex, disseminated, severe primary, or neonatal
  - Herpes zoster (varicella-zoster)
  - Varicella (chickenpox)
  - Impetigo
  - Infection or colonization by bacteria with multiple drug resistance (any site)
  - Pediculosis
  - Scabies
  - Skin wound or burn infection, major (draining and not covered by dressing, or dressing does not adequately contain purulent material), including those infected with *Staphylococcus aureus*
  - Vaccinia (generalized and progressive eczema vaccinatum)

sensitizing antigen. T cells become sensitized to the antigen. Local skin irritation is evident within a few hours or days after exposure to an antigen. Erythema and swelling, pruritus, and the appearance of vesicular lesions follow. Many chemicals, cosmetics, soaps, latex, and poison ivy or oak can cause such a reaction.

Atopic dermatitis affects about 10% of the population and is more common in infancy and childhood, but does affect some adults. It results from a complex activation process that involves mast cells, T lymphocytes, Langerhans cells, monocytes, B cells that produce immunoglobulin E, and other inflammatory cells that release histamine, lymphokines, and other inflammatory mediators. Atopic dermatitis seem's to have a genetic, allergic association, as it is more prevalent in families.

Stasis dermatitis generally occurs on the legs as a result of venous stasis and edema and is seen in conjunction with varicosities, phlebitis, and vascular trauma. Erythema and pruritus occur first, and then there is scaling, development of petechiae, and *hyperpigmentation* (excessive pigmentation). Lesions may become ulcerated, particularly around the ankles and tibia.

Seborrheic dermatitis is a common inflammation involving the scalp, eyebrows, eyelids, ear canals, nasolabial folds, axillae, chest, and back. It is most common on the scalp. The cause is unknown. Lesions appear as scaly, white or yellowish plaques with mild pruritus.

Diagnosis and Treatment

Diagnosis of dermatitis is done by inspection and by compiling a complete history, looking for possible exposure to causative substances.

In general, treatment is aimed at avoidance of the contact irritant or allergen, good skin lubrication, preservation of skin moisture, and control of inflammation and itching. Topical agents are often used. Corticosteroids may be used topically, or sometimes orally or by injection to intervene in a severe episode of dermatitis (see Box 37-3 for nursing implications).

Nursing Management

Teach patients to avoid contact irritants and to properly care for their skin. Instruct them in the proper way to apply topical agents. Caution any patient who is experiencing pruritus to avoid becoming hot and to bathe in tepid water. The skin should be patted rather than rubbed dry.

ACNE

Etiology, Pathophysiology, Signs, and Symptoms

Acne is a disorder of the skin characterized by papules and pustules over the face, back, and shoulders. Some types of acne are related to cosmetics or to chemicals in the environment. For example, occupational acne is due to prolonged contact with oils and tars.

There are many kinds of acne, but the two major types are *acne rosacea* and *acne vulgaris*. Acne rosacea usually begins between ages 30 and 50. It is characterized by erythema (redness), papules, pustules, and telangiectases. It occurs on the face over the cheeks and bridge of the nose. *Comedos* (dilated hair follicles filled with skin debris, bacteria, and sebum) do not occur. Factors that cause facial flushing precipitate worsening. Tea, coffee, alcohol (especially wine), caffeine-containing foods, spicy foods, sunlight, and emotional stress cause flare-ups.

Acne vulgaris is more common than acne rosacea. Factors that contribute to the development of acne include hereditary disposition, increased androgen levels, and premenstrual hormonal fluctuations. Use of heavy creams, use of certain drugs, and exposure to increased heat also contribute to the disorder. Acne vulgaris typically begins in early puberty, continues through the teens, and then begins to subside. Occasionally it persists, or it can recur several years later. The onset of acne vulgaris in adolescents is related to increased release of sex hormones, which stimulate activity of the sebaceous glands, causing increased production of sebum. Ducts leading from the sebaceous glands become plugged with sebum. It is not known why in some persons the ducts from these glands become plugged, but the increased production of sebum triggers the formation of blackheads and whiteheads. The color of blackheads is the result of particles of melanin, the skin's own pigment, combined with sebum and keratin. Accumulations of sebum, skin particles, and dead skin cells can cause an inflammatory reaction. Bacterial infection leads to the formation of pustules. An extensive inflammation can lead to the formation of cysts, with swelling above and below the surface of the skin.

There are many misconceptions about acne vulgaris and its treatment. It is not a contagious disease. It is not due to uncleanliness or poor personal hygiene. Diet can contribute to the formation of lesions, but generally there is little or no relationship between the intake of certain foods and the appearance of the lesions of acne. Typically, chocolate, colas, and fried foods do not need to be eliminated from the diet in an effort to prevent or cure acne. A well-balanced diet is all that is recommended in the management of acne.

Diagnosis and Treatment

Diagnosis is by history and physical examination. Acne rosacea is treated by avoiding the triggers for flare-ups and with topical antibiotics, metronidazole (MetroGel), and retinoids. Sometimes oral antibiotics are prescribed.

Mild, noninflammatory cases of acne vulgaris respond well to efforts to remove blackheads and whiteheads by promoting dryness and peeling of the top layer of skin. The medication is applied directly on the skin. Nonprescription drugs, such as lotions, creams, and gels that contain sulfur, benzoyl peroxide, and sulfur combined with resorcinol, usually are effective for noninflammatory acne.

Among the topical medications, retinoic acid (tretinoin [Retin-A]) is the best agent for *papular* and *pustular* acne problems. It should be used once or twice a day. Benzoyl peroxide is the most frequently used topical agent for acne and is available both by prescription and over the counter. A newer drug, azelaic acid (Azelex), is available and is applied topically twice a day. The U.S. Food and Drug Administration (FDA) (Drugs.com, 2010) approved Veltin Gel, a water-based topical agent for the treatment of acne vulgaris in patients 12 years and older.

Antibiotics such as tetracycline and erythromycin also are sometimes prescribed topically and orally for cystic acne to inhibit the growth of bacteria in the plugged ducts.

Isotretinoin (13-*cis*-retinoic acid) given to treat cystic acne has been especially effective in controlling cases that are resistant to other forms of treatment. The drug is marketed under the trade name Accutane. An FDA-restricted program, iPledge, is intended to prevent fetal exposure: all distributors, prescribers, and pharmacies are required to register, and patients must be eligible and meet monthly requirements (Hartner, 2007). Accutane is taken by mouth daily for 2 to 4 months and inhibits activity of the sebaceous glands. Its effects are sustained for months to years after it has been discontinued. Almost all patients experience some adverse reaction to this drug. **Accutane is used only for severe cystic acne that is resistant to all other treatment. There are serious adverse side effects, including organ damage and mental problems.** Laboratory testing includes hemoglobin, hematocrit, glucose, triglycerides, uric acid, alkaline phosphatase, and liver enzymes.

If the patient has deep scarring and pitting as a result of cystic acne, appearance can be improved by dermabrasion. This dermatologic procedure involves mechanically scraping away the outer layers of skin and smoothing out its surface by applying motor-driven wire brushes or diamond wheels. Chemical dermabrasion is done by applying phenol or trichloroacetic acid to remove the scars.

Nursing Management

Teach the patient about the nature of the particular skin disease and give support while he is trying to cope with its physiologic and psychosocial effects. Acne can be particularly distressing to adolescents, who are often deeply concerned about their appearance and acceptance by their peers.

The face should be washed gently with a mild soap. Scrubbing the skin and using a harsh soap is damaging and contributes to inflammation. Special medicated soaps do not seem to be any better than a mild face soap. If the hair is oily, it should be shampooed frequently and kept off the face.

It is not a good idea to squeeze pimples and pustules. This can press the sebum and accumulated material more firmly in the clogged duct, increase the chance of inflammation, and spread an infection to other parts of the skin and body. Blackheads and whiteheads are best removed by applying a prescription medication that causes peeling of the skin. The hands should be kept off of the face.

Because the management of acne can go on for years and requires periodic evaluation by a dermatologist, patients and their families will need continued support and encouragement to follow the prescribed regimen. They will need to know the expected results of prescribed medications, any adverse reactions that might occur, and symptoms that should be reported immediately.

Think Critically

What skin care measures would you recommend to a young teenager who is just beginning to experience face blemishes such as blackheads or whiteheads? The kids at school are calling him "scab face."

PSORIASIS

Etiology, Pathophysiology, Signs, and Symptoms

Psoriasis is a noncontagious, chronic, and recurring skin disorder that typically appears as inflamed, edematous skin lesions covered with adherent silvery white scales (Figure 43-1). These scales are the result of an abnormally rapid rate of proliferation of skin cells. When the scales are removed, there is pinpoint bleeding. The plaques most often appear on the skin of the elbows, knees, and base of the spine. It also may affect the scalp, in which case it can be confused with *seborrheic dermatitis*. When the fingernails are involved, there can be pitting of the surface of the nails. The palms and soles also can be affected, making it difficult for the patient to carry out activities of daily living (ADLs).

In some cases the skin eruptions of psoriasis are accompanied by inflammation of the joints, especially those of the fingers and toes. This is called *psoriatic arthritis*. Psoriasis affects about 2% of the U.S. population. There is a genetic predisposition for the disease. It is likely that an immunologic event triggers the disorder as the first lesion commonly appears after an upper respiratory infection. T cells are mistakenly activated and they trigger immune responses that speed up the growth cycle of skin cells. Kimball and colleagues (2010) found that patients with moderate to severe psoriasis had a higher incidence of cardiac disease and risk for stroke.

Diagnosis and Treatment

Diagnosis is by history, physical examination, and ruling out other skin disorders. Each case of psoriasis is treated individually. The disease is unpredictable, tends to go into remission spontaneously, and sometimes will clear up temporarily with or without treatment.

FIGURE 43-1 Psoriasis lesion on the hand.

Mild cases usually respond to steroid creams (triamcinolone acetonide [Kenalog]), but there is a possibility that eventually the disease will become resistant to steroids. Sunlight in moderate doses can help, because the ultraviolet (UV) rays slow down the rate at which epithelial cells are produced. Extremes of UV radiation can have the opposite effect, resulting in an aggravation of the condition. Calcipotriene (Dovonex), a vitamin D analogue cream, helps to regulate skin cell production, decreasing the incidence of psoriasis plaques.

Tar preparations also act to impede the proliferation of skin cells and have long been used to heal psoriasis lesions. They may be administered in the form of baths, topical applications, or shampoos. Combinations of artificial UV radiation and a coal tar product often are prescribed for severe cases. This usually requires hospitalization so that the dosage of each component of therapy can be measured precisely. A form of therapy called PUVA combines application of one of a class of drugs called psoralens, which penetrates the skin, with exposure to ultraviolet light type A (UVA).

Antimetabolites have been used to treat severe psoriasis, helping to control the disorder by their antiproliferative action. Methotrexate is the most commonly used antimetabolite for this purpose. Acitretin (Soriatane) or cyclosporine is sometimes used. Brimhall and colleagues (2008) performed a systematic review of the new biologic agents for psoriasis and found a rank order efficacy for infliximab, etanercept, efalizumab, and alefacept. The review also disclosed an increase of previously unreported adverse advents. Ustekinumab (Stelara) was approved by the FDA in 2009; it targets proteins that are believed to have a role in the development of psoriasis.

Nursing Management

Patients with psoriasis will need instruction about the nature of their disease, the purpose of the prescribed treatment, and information about ways to avoid aggravating it. **The skin should be kept as moist and pliable as possible. Humidifiers to increase moisture in the environment are sometimes helpful.** Lubricating lotions and creams should be approved by the dermatologist before they are applied.

Minor scratches and abrasions and bacterial infections can trigger the formation of lesions at a new site. **Because any irritation or break in the skin seems to stimulate the growth of psoriatic plaques in a person susceptible to psoriasis, the patient should be cautioned to avoid injury of any kind.** This includes hangnails, damaged cuticles, blisters from poorly fitting shoes, scratches from pets, and potentially harmful agents in the environment such as radiation and chemicals.

STEVENS-JOHNSON SYNDROME

Stevens-Johnson syndrome (SJS) is an allergic reaction with skin manifestations. It is usually triggered by a medication. The signs and symptoms appear within

14 days of starting drug therapy. Offending drugs are the anticonvulsants carbamazepine (Tegretol) and phenytoin (Dilantin), the antimalarial sulfadoxine-pyrimethamine (Fansidar), and the antibiotic sulfamethoxazole-trimethoprim (Bactrim, Septra). However, over-the-counter medications can cause SJS. Lesions that may be mistaken for chickenpox develop on the face, trunk, palms, extensor surfaces of joints, soles of the feet, and dorsum of the hands. The lesions have irregular borders and may have blistered, necrotic centers.

Treatment of SJS is to discontinue the drug and provide supportive care with fluids and nutrition. Wound care is similar to that for a burn. The lesions are painful, and analgesia is provided. Sedatives may be necessary. If not treated early, SJS can cause death.

 Clinical Cues

Assess the skin of every patient daily. If new skin lesions appear, seek an opinion from a physician. Check the medication profile and medication history to see what medications the patient has been receiving. Alert the physician if the patient has been taking a medication known to cause SJS.

BACTERIAL INFECTIONS

Etiology, Pathophysiology, Signs, and Symptoms

Cellulitis is an infection of the dermis and subcutaneous tissue and is generally caused by *Staphylococcus*. It may occur as an extension of a skin wound, as an ulcer, or from furuncles or carbuncles. The area will be erythematous, swollen, and painful. It is treated with systemic antibiotics, and Burow's soaks may be used to relieve pain. Burow's solution is an astringent and topical antiseptic also called aluminum acetate solution.

Furuncles (boils) are inflammations of hair follicles. The organism responsible is usually *Staphylococcus aureus*. Any skin area with hair can be affected. Initially there is a deep, firm, red, painful nodule 1 to 5 cm in diameter. The nodule changes to a large and tender cystic nodule accompanied by cellulitis. The lesion may drain large amounts of pus and necrotic tissue.

Carbuncles are a collection of infected hair follicles and most often occur on the back of the neck, the upper back, and the lateral thighs. It begins as a firm mass and evolves into an erythematous, painful, swollen mass. It may drain through many openings in the mass. Abscesses may develop with fever, chills, and malaise.

Diagnosis, Treatment, and Nursing Management

Diagnosis is by history and examination. Treatment of both furuncles and carbuncles is application of warm compresses to provide comfort, promote localization, and cause spontaneous drainage. Abscess formation requires incision and drainage. Recurrent episodes are treated with systemic antibiotics.

Nursing interventions are aimed at healing the infected areas and preventing recurrence. Rinsing very well after bathing to eliminate soap residue is recommended. The patient is taught to avoid using cosmetic products and over-the-counter topical remedies on the affected areas. A clean washcloth and towel should be used for bathing each day until the carbuncle or furuncle is healed. Linens should be washed in hot soapy water and thoroughly dried before reuse.

VIRAL INFECTIONS

HERPES SIMPLEX

Herpes simplex virus type 2 (HSV-2) is most often associated with genital herpes, whereas herpes simplex virus type 1 (HSV-1) lesions are primarily nongenital (Figure 43-2). Either type can cause lesions in the genital area as well as other regions of the body. **Autoinoculation** of the virus is possible by direct contact, for example, lips to fingers to genitals or lips to fingers to eyes.

 Health Promotion

Preventing Spread of Herpesvirus

Patients with genital herpes need to be aware that the disorder can be transmitted even when no lesions are present. When a person has a "cold sore," the virus can be transferred to others. Contact with the lesion should be avoided. Care should be taken not to share drinking glasses and eating utensils, lipstick, or other items that touch the lesion.

Complementary and Alternative Therapies

Lemon Balm for Cold Sores

Lemon balm in a concentrated cream base has been shown to relieve the symptoms of *herpes labialis* (infection of the lips; commonly known as cold sores or fever blisters) (Yarnell et al., 2009).

Etiology and Pathophysiology

When initial infection occurs, the virus is imbedded in a nerve ganglion that innervates the site of the lesion. Reactivation of the virus causes new lesions to occur at

FIGURE 43-2 Herpes simplex virus lesions.

the same site. The virus travels along the nerve to the site of the original infection. Reactivation is brought about by exposure to ultraviolet light, skin irritation, fever, fatigue, or stress.

Signs and Symptoms

An infection with HSV-1 appears as lesions on the lips and nares that are commonly called cold sores or fever blisters. As with other types of herpesvirus infections, no drug will completely cure the infection.

Diagnosis, Treatment, and Nursing Management

Diagnosis is by physical examination and history. Sometimes topical and oral acyclovir (Zovirax), famciclovir (Famvir), or valacyclovir (Valtrex), available by prescription, hastens healing. The symptoms of itching and burning that accompany oral herpes infection sometimes can be minimized by applying warm compresses to the sores, followed by local application of tincture of benzoin or spirits of camphor to aid drying and facilitate healing. The disease usually is self-limiting, which means that it does not progress and will subside on its own, but it can recur. Contagion is possible up to 5 days after appearance of the lesion. Docosanol cream (Abreva) sold over the counter is a helpful treatment for this disorder.

Patients should be cautioned to use good personal hygiene to avoid spreading the virus to the eyes and genital area and other body parts. Hand hygiene is a very simple, but essential, part of preventing spread of the virus.

HERPES ZOSTER

Etiology and Pathophysiology

The causative organism for this skin disorder is herpes varicella-zoster. The virus causes chickenpox (varicella), mostly in young children, and shingles (herpes zoster) in all ages. In herpes zoster, the herpesviruses replicate in the peripheral nerve ganglia, where they lie dormant until reactivated by trauma, malignancy, possibly stress, or local radiation (Figure 43-3).

FIGURE 43-3 Herpes zoster (shingles).

Approximately 1 million cases per year occur in the United States, and about 25% of the population will be affected at some point in their lifetime (Centers for Disease Control and Prevention [CDC], 2011). The risk is greater for immunocompromised individuals (those with cancer or HIV/AIDS). A vaccine is available for children to prevent chickenpox.

 Elder Care Points

Approximately 50% of individuals who live past 80 years of age develop shingles. There is a vaccine available (Zostavax) that is about 50% effective in preventing shingles; it appears to be effective in attenuating the disorder if it occurs and is effective for about 6 years (CDC, 2009).

Signs and Symptoms

Herpes zoster begins with vague symptoms of chills and low-grade fever and possibly some gastrointestinal disturbance. There may be only aching or discomfort along the nerve pathway with or without erythema. About 3 to 5 days after onset, small groups of vesicles appear on the skin. They usually are found on the trunk and spread halfway around the body, following the nerve pathways leading from the spinal nerve to the skin.

 Safety Alert

Danger of Herpes Zoster Transmission

No health care worker, or visitor, should be in contact with a patient who has chickenpox or shingles if they have never had the disease. A pregnant woman should not care for a patient with chickenpox or herpes zoster. The virus is highly contagious and can harm a fetus.

The vesicles eventually change from small blisters to scaly lesions and are accompanied by pain and itching. The lesions usually affect only one side of the body or face. The pain of shingles often is quite severe. Pain can persist for several days or weeks after the skin lesions are completely healed. The pain of postherpetic syndrome is not easy to control.

Diagnosis and Treatment

Diagnosis is by history and physical examination. There is no cure for herpes zoster. The condition can persist for months, especially in older and debilitated patients. Herpes infections may be recurrent as immunity does not occur. **The earlier the condition is diagnosed and treatment begins, the better are chances to decrease the amount and duration of the associated pain** (Farage et al., 2009).

Symptomatic treatment usually involves administering an analgesic to relieve pain. Capsaicin, an over-the-counter analgesic that is applied topically five times a day, decreases pain for some patients. A paste made from aspirins and water placed on the lesions decreases pain for others. Antibiotics may be prescribed prophylactically against secondary bacterial infection of the lesions. Most physicians prescribe oral acyclovir (Zovirax), famciclovir (Famvir), or valacyclovir (Valtrex) to diminish the extent or duration of the lesions. Valacyclovir is used only in otherwise healthy patients. Famciclovir (Famvir), if given within the first 2 to 3 days of the outbreak, seems to shorten the duration of the chronic pain that frequently follows shingles. Systemic corticosteroids are often used to decrease pain and in an attempt to prevent postherpetic pain syndrome. Their use is controversial. Tricyclic antidepressants and gabapentin (Neurontin), an anticonvulsant drug, have been used with variable success at controlling pain.

Narcotic analgesics are avoided if possible, because they can lead to addiction when used for an extended time. If the pain persists and is intractable, the physician prescribes a corticosteroid to reduce inflammation. Vidarabine, administered intravenously (IV), is sometimes given to patients who have an immune deficiency. It is usually effective in reducing, if not completely relieving, the pain.

Even though shingles may be difficult to live with while it is running its course, the only lasting complication from the disease is postherpetic neuralgia (unless the virus attacks the eye, in which case it can cause blindness). However, the prognosis is obviously less favorable in patients who have an underlying malignancy or who are immunocompromised.

Nursing Management

Care includes symptomatic relief from the pain and itching and prevention of a secondary bacterial infection.

Complementary and Alternative Therapies

Tai Chi Boosts Immunity to Shingles

Research has shown that Tai Chi resulted in a level of immune response close to that of the varicella vaccine and that Tai Chi boosted the positive effects of the vaccine. The study involved a clinical trial of 112 adults ages 59 to 86 who took part in a 16-week program of Tai Chi (National Institutes of Health, 2007).

Cold compresses, calamine lotion, and diversional activities are sometimes helpful. Rest and adequate nutrition can promote healing and shorten the acute phase of shingles. Teaching imagery, deep muscle relaxation, or use of distraction activities may help decrease pain. Evidence supports initiation of isolation procedures based on symptoms rather than waiting for a confirmed diagnosis. If lesions are disseminated or if the patient is immunocompromised, airborne and Contact Isolation are necessary. If the lesions are localized and the patient is not immunocompromised, Standard Precautions are sufficient. Transmission precaution isolation needed until all the blisters are crusted (Riley, 2008)

FUNGAL INFECTIONS

Fungal infections are called mycoses; systemic fungal infections involving the lungs and other internal organs are called *systemic mycoses*. There are actually two groups of fungi: (1) fungi that are truly pathogenic to humans; and (2) fungi that cause *opportunistic infections* (can cause an infection when the host has an altered immune system).

True pathogenic fungi can cause infection in an otherwise healthy person, but relatively few fungi are able to do this. Fungal infections are rarely fatal if they involve only the superficial tissues of the body. Nevertheless, mycotic skin infections can be exasperating because they are difficult to diagnose and are often resistant to treatment.

The most common types of fungal infections involving the skin are *tinea pedis* (athlete's foot or dermatophytosis), *tinea cruris* (jock itch), *tinea of the scalp* (commonly known as ringworm), and *tinea barbae* (barber's itch). *Moniliasis* (thrush) is a fungal infection that can attack the mucous membranes of the mouth, rectum, and vagina *(candidiasis)*. (This condition is discussed more fully in Chapter 11.)

The skin fungal infections produce itching, some swelling, and a breakdown of tissue. Because fungi thrive in warm, moist places, a tropical climate or other environmental factors that produce prolonged heat and moisture can encourage the development of fungal infections.

The elderly are prone to develop fungal infections of the fingernails or toenails (onychomycosis) (Figure 43-4). Hands and feet should be thoroughly dried after becoming wet, with special attention to drying between the toes after the bath or shower. Nails should be cut straight across without rounding the edges. Wearing clean socks daily helps prevent fungal growth. In the toenails, the condition may become quite painful. Treatment requires oral antifungal medication daily for several months or topical agents daily for a year or more.

Complementary and Alternative Therapies

Treatment of Nail Fungus

Tea tree oil used topically daily on the nail and cuticle has been successfully used for treatment of yeast and fungal infection (Combest, 2007). It must be used regularly to be effective, and may take weeks or months to cure the infection. Another inexpensive treatment that may work with consistent daily use is the topical application of Vicks VapoRub twice a day. This salve contains camphor, menthol, and eucalyptus. It seems to arrest the development of further fungal growth, allowing a fungus-free nail to grow. It takes about 6 months of treatment and is not effective for everyone.

FIGURE 43-4 Onychomycosis (nail fungus).

There are many side effects of the oral antifungal medications. Liver function should be monitored during drug administration. Diagnosis of fungal infections is confirmed by microscopic examination of skin scrapings that have been treated with potassium hydroxide (KOH) solution. Fungal specimens generally show the typical filaments of fungal organisms. Patients should be taught how to prevent recurrence of fungal infections.

Patient Teaching

Preventing Recurrent Fungal Infection

Instruct the patient to do the following:

- Wear shoes that provide ventilation for the feet. Wear cotton socks when rubber-soled shoes or sneakers must be worn.
- Wash and dry the feet at least daily, being careful to completely dry the skin between the toes.
- Sprinkle an antifungal powder on the feet and between the toes if there is a tendency to have athlete's foot. An antifungal spray may be used rather than powder.
- Change hose or socks daily; do not wear them more than one day without washing.
- Change underpants or shorts daily; do not wear them more than one day without washing.
- Use only clean towels, changing them at least every other day.
- Change bed linens at least once a week and wash in hot water.
- Do not use the combs, hairbrushes, or hair clips or ties of others, and do not allow them to use yours.
- Inspect pets regularly for ringworm. Have a veterinarian check the animal if an infection is suspected.

TINEA PEDIS

Tinea pedis (athlete's foot) affects the feet, particularly between the toes. The infection may spread to the entire foot and cause blistering, peeling, cracking, and itching. If it continues unchecked, it can spread to other parts of the body. The condition can be complicated by a severe bacterial infection.

Etiology, Pathophysiology, Signs, and Symptoms

Most cases of tinea pedis are contracted and spread in swimming pools, spas, showers, and other public facilities of this type. *Trichophyton mentagrophytes* and *Trichophyton rubrum* are the usual infecting agents. These organisms may be normal flora that spread easily under conditions of excessive warmth and moisture. The skin between the toes becomes inflamed and develops cracks that become painful fissures. Itching is often present.

Diagnosis and Treatment

Diagnosis is by physical examination. Treatment of tinea pedis consists of keeping the area dry, clean, and exposed to the air and sunlight as much as possible. Clean cotton socks should be worn every day, and the affected areas between the toes should be separated by gauze or cotton. Soaks of Burow's solution help. Various topical antifungals can be prescribed, including ciclopirox (Loprox), miconazole, clotrimazole (Mycelex), econazole (Spectazole), ketoconazole (Nizoral), and naftifine (Naftin). Some medicated powders, such as undecylenic acid–zinc undecylenate work to keep the feet dry and also help control fungal growth. Other treatments are available without prescription. Systemic treatment for stubborn infection includes oral itraconazole (Sporanox) and terbinafine (Lamisil).

Nursing Management

Encourage the patient to keep the feet clean and dry and to wear clean cotton socks every day. Daily application of the topical agent must be done diligently to eradicate the problem. The patient should only use his own towel, and the shower or tub should be thoroughly cleaned and disinfected after bathing to prevent transmission to other family members. Personal footwear should be used in public places, such as the swimming pool and in the showers at fitness centers, and feet should be washed and dried thoroughly after using public facilities.

PARASITIC INFECTIONS

PEDICULOSIS AND SCABIES

Etiology and Pathophysiology

The parasites that cause *pediculosis* and *scabies* are found throughout the world in all types of climates. They can infest anyone. The parasites are particularly troublesome, however, where people live under crowded conditions and are negligent in their personal hygiene. The occurrence of pediculosis and scabies in the United States has recently increased significantly because of the growth of the homeless population and communal living. These parasites are often found among schoolchildren. The parasites are also found in nursing homes, dormitories, and sometimes hospitals.

Three basic types of lice that infest human beings are (1) the head louse, *Pediculus humanis capitis;* (2) the body louse, *Pediculus humanis corporis* (Figure 43-5); and (3) the pubic or crab louse, *Phthirus pubis.* In addition, human beings also may be infested by *Sarcoptes scabiei,* the mange mite that produces scabies. The lice are oval and 2 to 4 mm long. All types are acquired by contact with infested people or their clothing, bed linen, and bedding. Pets have also been known to carry lice and the scabies mite.

Signs and Symptoms

The most prevalent symptom of louse infestation is severe itching. The resultant scratching can lead to excoriation of the skin and secondary infection causing impetigo, furunculosis, and cellulitis. Systemic infections are not commonly associated with louse infestation, but they can and do occur in the forms of glomerulonephritis, septicemia, pneumonia, and cystic abscesses. If the lice infest the eyelids and eyelashes, the eyelids become red and swollen. Swelling may also occur in the lymph glands of the neck of a person heavily infested with head lice. The body louse can transmit typhus fever, trench fever, and some other diseases. Other types of lice are not known to be transmitters of disease.

The scabies mites burrow under the top layers of the skin and live their entire life there. They are more likely to be found in the skin between the fingers and toes, in the groin, and in other areas where there may be folds of skin. Excretions from the mites produce irritation with intense itching and blistering. Secondary infection is not uncommon with scabies, and some deaths have occurred when the scabies infestation has led to pneumonia or septicemia.

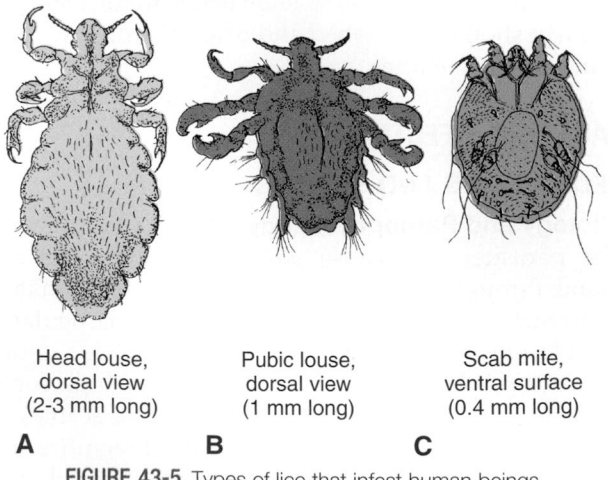

Head louse, dorsal view (2-3 mm long)

A

Pubic louse, dorsal view (1 mm long)

B

Scab mite, ventral surface (0.4 mm long)

C

FIGURE 43-5 Types of lice that infest human beings.

Diagnosis

Diagnosis is by body inspection and by examination of skin scraping of a lesion under the microscope. Lice eggs are deposited at the base of the hair shaft and can be seen on close inspection. Scabies causes curved or linear white or erythematous ridges in the skin that are easily visible.

Treatment

The prescription drugs most commonly used and considered most effective against lice and scabies are permethrin (Nix Elimite), pyrethrins (RID), and malathion (Ovide). These substances must be carefully used and the patient's liver functions monitored as they can be very toxic. They are available as creams, lotions, and shampoos. Lindane has been found to be especially harmful and is no longer recommended. A fine-toothed (nit) comb is then used to remove the nits (eggs) that may have remained on the hair. Benzyl alcohol lotion 5% is effective for head lice. It works by suffocating the lice. The amount required is based on the length of the hair and a second treatment is required in 7 days (Meinking et al., 2010).

Nursing Management

Contact Isolation is recommended. In addition, clothing, bedding, hats, stuffed animals, and other infested articles must be decontaminated to prevent reinfection. Laundering in hot water and machine drying using the hottest cycle is effective. Dry cleaning of nonwashable bed coverings or clothing can be effective. Mattresses, upholstered furniture, carpets, and other articles should be sprayed with a specific disinfectant. All combs and brushes should be soaked in very hot water for more than 5 minutes. For items that cannot be cleaned, such as some stuffed animals, sealing them in plastic bags with the air expelled for 14 days can be effective. You must instruct all family members about the infection and ways to prevent reinfestation.

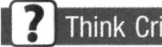 **Think Critically**

How would you approach and instruct the parents of an 8-year-old who has scabies?

NONINFECTIOUS DISORDERS OF SKIN

SKIN CANCER

Skin cancer is often neglected because there is no pain associated with it and patients fear that treatment will involve extensive or disfiguring surgery. More than 2 million cases a year of basal cell and squamous cell cancers occur in the United States. These are highly curable cancers. It is expected that 70,230 persons will have been diagnosed with melanoma, the most serious type of skin cancer, in 2011, and that 8790 deaths from melanoma will occur (American Cancer Society,

2011a). Most melanoma deaths could have been averted through early diagnosis and treatment. Information on Kaposi sarcoma and T-cell lymphoma is located in Chapter 11.

Etiology and Pathophysiology

Several factors predispose an individual to developing skin cancer. Among these are internal changes in the cells that may be due to hereditary factors and external influences such as chronic exposure to ionizing radiation, petrochemicals, or vinyl chloride or to other irritants in the environment. Sunburn as a child is a particular risk factor. Since characteristics are inherited susceptibility to skin cancer tends to run in families. Blue-eyed blondes and redheads seem to be most susceptible, probably because they lack sufficient pigment to protect the skin cells from outside irritants. Those with a white complexion have a 10-fold greater risk of developing melanoma (Strayer & Schub, 2009).

A major cause of skin cancer today is the alteration in the ozone layer of the earth's atmosphere that allows more UV radiation to reach the earth's surface. This type of radiation is inflicting much quicker damage to skin with much less sun exposure than in years past. Another problem is that the quickly proliferating skin cells of the younger generation are even more susceptible to this type of damage, and it is mostly the young who spend large amounts of time in the sun. Nurses should instruct all people about the dangers of sunning without an appropriate protective sunscreen.

[?] Think Critically

You and a girlfriend are going on a beach vacation. She invites you to go to a tanning salon before the trip. "We want to look tan and sexy out there." How will you respond?

Signs, Symptoms, Diagnosis, and Treatment

Signs and symptoms vary according to the type of lesion. Diagnosis is by examination, biopsy, and pathology study. The three main types of skin malignancy are basal cell carcinoma, squamous cell carcinoma, and melanoma. *Basal cell carcinoma* usually appears first as a small, scaly area and tends to become larger as the disease progresses (Figure 43-6). It occurs most often on the face and trunk. As the scales shed, there is a small amount of bleeding and a scab will form. When the scab is shed, the affected area becomes wider, and it is bordered by a waxy, translucent, raised area. **If such a sore has not healed within a month, it may be a basal cell carcinoma.** This spreading may continue very gradually during several months or years. Even though these malignancies do not metastasize, they can invade underlying tissues, and death can result from complications such as infection or hemorrhage from encroaching into a blood vessel. Small lesions

FIGURE 43-6 Basal cell carcinoma.

can be removed under local anesthesia in a doctor's office. Larger lesions respond well to radiation therapy.

Squamous cell carcinoma is caused by sunlight, affects the epidermis, and can become invasive and metastasize to other areas of the body. It appears on the head and neck most frequently. The tumor begins as a small nodule that rapidly becomes ulcerated (Figure 43-7). Treatment must begin early if the condition is to be relieved before the skin cells sustain extensive damage. Surgical procedures involve total removal or destruction of the lesions and the surrounding tissues that have been invaded. Radiation therapy is advised for patients who are poor surgical risks or who are fearful of surgery.

Elder Care Points

Actinic keratoses occur very frequently on the skin of the elderly. They appear on fair-skinned people as a small, scaly, red or grayish papule particularly on areas of skin that are often exposed to the sun. These lesions should be removed as they can evolve into a squamous cell carcinoma that can grow rapidly and metastasize.

Malignant melanoma is the least common form of skin cancer. It arises from pigment-producing cells and varies in its course and prognosis according to

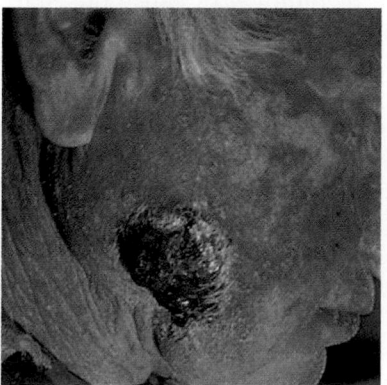
FIGURE 43-7 Squamous cell carcinoma.

FIGURE 43-8 Melanoma.

its type (Figure 43-8). Causative factors are genetic predisposition, solar radiation, and steroid hormone influence. There are several types of melanoma, but the three major kinds of malignant melanoma are superficial spreading, nodular, and lentigo maligna melanoma. In general, the superficial lesions can be cured, but the deeper lesions tend to metastasize more readily through the lymphatic and circulatory systems. Characteristics of the three main types of skin cancer are shown in Table 43-1.

Malignant melanoma always requires surgical removal of the tumor and excision of adjacent tissues and possibly nearby lymphatic structures. Chemotherapy may be employed to destroy tumor cells believed to have migrated beyond the tumor site. Radiation therapy usually is not indicated unless there is extensive metastasis. The radiation does not eliminate the disease, but it can relieve symptoms by reducing tumor size. Interferon alfa-2b has been found to prolong life in patients who have undergone malignant melanoma surgery and are at high risk for systemic recurrence (American Cancer Society, 2011). An oral agent, PLX4032, is being investigated; thus far there has been a 70% response in metastatic melanoma (Wendling, 2009). A new drug combination, may be helpful for patients with metastatic melanoma. The new treatment uses paclitaxel, carboplatin, and sirolimus to overcome chemoresistance (Meier et al., 2009).

The type of removal of cancerous skin tissue will depend on the type of malignant growth present. **In all but the most extensive growths, treatment is relatively simple and completely successful if started early.** Although benign precancerous lesions do not inevitably develop into malignant lesions, the most advisable course of action is to remove them when they are first diagnosed. Removal is performed by surgery, *electrodesiccation* (tissue destruction by heat), *cryosurgery* (tissue destruction by freezing with liquid nitrogen), topical application of 5-fluorouracil (5-FU), interferon therapy, laser therapy, and molecular therapy. Radiation therapy is sometimes used to destroy the cancer.

Table 43-1   Three Major Types of Skin Cancer

TYPE	CHARACTERISTICS
Basal cell carcinoma	Slowly enlarging, firm, scaly papule. Crusted or ulcerated center that may be depressed; has pearly (semitranslucent) raised border. Dilated capillaries around lesion. Accounts for 70% of all skin cancers. Rarely spreads and is easily treated.
Squamous cell carcinoma	Appearance variable. Frequently seen as well-defined, irregularly shaped nodule or plaque. May be elevated, nodular mass, or fungated mass. Varying amounts of scale and crusting. May have ulcerated center. Predominantly on sun-exposed areas: head, neck, hands; 75% occur on the head. Spreads rapidly.
Malignant Melanomas	
Superficial spreading melanoma (SSM)	Appears in a variety of colors: white, red, gray, black, blue over a brown or black background. Has irregular surface and notched border. Small tumor nodules may ulcerate and bleed. Horizontal growth can continue for years. Vertical growth worsens prognosis.
Nodular malignant melanoma (NMM)	Nodule with uniformly grayish black color, resembles a blackberry. May be flesh colored with specks of pigment around base of nodule. Itching, oozing, and bleeding may occur. Prognosis less favorable than superficial type.
Lentigo maligna melanoma (LMM)	Relatively rare. Arises from a lesion that resembles a large flat freckle that is of variable color from tan to black. Has irregularly spaced black nodules on the surface. Often located on the back of the hand, on the face, and under fingernails. Develops very slowly; may ulcerate. Tends to metastasize; prognosis poor.

Nursing Management

While performing daily care of patients, you often are in a position to notice these lesions in their early stages and should do your best to persuade the person with such a lesion to seek prompt medical attention.

Assignment Considerations

Report Different Skin Lesions

When assigning hygiene care to unlicensed assistive personnel, ask them to report any odd-looking lesions they find on the patient's skin. Skin cancers are often discovered on further assessment of suspicious lesions.

Because victims of skin cancer run a high risk of eventually developing another malignancy, either at the original site or elsewhere in the body, they should visit a physician at least once a year after the skin cancer has been cured. Although most skin cancers are easily curable, they should not be considered harmless and something to forget about after treatment (see Chapter 8).

Another nursing function is educating the patient about the type of cancer, and helping to decrease fear. For many people, the diagnosis of "cancer"—even of an easily cured skin lesion—causes a change in body image and, possibly, in self-esteem. You can assist patients to talk about concerns and the future, point to community resources and support groups, and answer questions about treatment.

PRESSURE ULCERS

When a patient is on bed rest, or constantly sitting because of paralysis, pressure against the skin in various areas interferes with circulation. Because cells die very quickly without adequate blood supply, a pressure ulcer can develop. Depending on the patient's general condition, weight, and other factors, skin damage may occur within a few hours to a few days. Areas most prone to pressure ulcer formation are those over bony prominences. When the patient is placed in a position in which the bone is pressing on the skin where the skin is against the bed, the circulation to that area is compromised (Figure 43-9). Shearing action (where superficial layers of tissue are pulled and stretched across deeper layers of tissue) can cause damage to the skin if the patient is slid along the sheets for positioning, rather than lifted.

Risk Factors and Prevention

Every patient needs and deserves good skin assessment, but there are risk factors that make some patients more susceptible to problems, such as confinement, immobility, incontinence, malnutrition, decreased level of consciousness or confusion, obesity, diabetes mellitus, dehydration, edema, excessive sweating, and extreme age. Preventing pressure ulcers is far more desirable, more cost-effective, and less time-consuming than treating them. In fact, the importance of excellent nursing care is now a financial issue because as of 2008, Medicare/Medicaid will no longer reimburse for hospital-acquired pressure ulcers (van Rijswijk &

FIGURE 43-9 Bony prominences most susceptible to skin breakdown depending on position.

Box 43-2 Best Practice for the Prevention of Pressure Ulcers

- Assess the skin of all patients every 8 to 24 hours (interval depends on condition), paying particular attention to the bony prominences (see Figure 43-9).
- Reposition bed rest patients at least every 2 hours; use a written schedule for systematically turning and repositioning each patient.
- Use positioning devices, such as pillows, foam wedges, and padding, for bed rest patients, to keep body prominences from being in direct contact with one another.
- For patients on bed rest who are completely immobile, use devices that totally relieve pressure on the heels, by raising the heels off the bed. Do not use donut-type devices.
- When the side-lying position in bed is used, avoid positioning directly on the trochanter.
- For bed rest patients, maintain the head of the bed at the lowest degree permitted by medical condition. Limit the time the head of the bed is elevated.
- Use lifting devices, such as a trapeze or bed linen, to move rather than drag patients who cannot assist during transfers and position changes.
- For patients with limited mobility, use a pressure-reducing device on the bed, such as a foam, static air, alternating air, gel, or water mattress.
- Minimize skin injury caused by friction and shear forces by proper positioning and correct transferring and turning techniques. Reduce friction injuries by using lubricants, protective films, protective dressings, and protective padding. Use lift devices to reposition patients rather than sliding them on the bedding.
- Skin cleansing should occur at the time of soiling and at routine intervals based on patient need and preference. Avoid hot water, and use a mild cleansing agent that

minimizes irritation and dryness of the skin. Cleanse gently, minimizing the force and friction applied to the skin.
- Keep the environmental humidity above 40% and avoid exposure to cold. Treat dry skin with moisturizers.
- Do not massage bony prominences.
- Minimize skin exposure to moisture due to incontinence, perspiration, or wound drainage. When sources of moisture cannot be controlled, underpads or briefs that absorb moisture and present a quick-drying surface to the skin should be used. Use an incontinence management program for incontinent patients. Check for incontinence at least every 2 hours.
- Correct inadequate dietary intake of protein and calories with nutritional intervention either by oral supplementation or enteral or parenteral feedings.
- For wheelchair-bound patients, use a pressure-reducing device such as those made of foam, gel, air, or a combination of items. Do not use donut-type devices.
- Positioning of wheelchair-bound patients should include consideration of postural alignment, distribution of weight, balance and stability, and pressure relief by device or repositioning.
- Any person at risk for developing a pressure ulcer when sitting in a chair or wheelchair should be repositioned, shifting the points under pressure at least every hour (every 15 minutes is preferable); patients who are able should be taught to shift weight every 15 minutes.
- If a potential for improvement of mobility and activity status exists, institute a rehabilitation program. Maintain current activity and mobility status with a range-of-motion exercise program.

Lyder, 2008). Pressure relief, positioning, padding, use of pressure relief devices, adequate nutrition, and excellent skin care are the hallmarks of pressure ulcer prevention. Box 43-2 presents interventions for preventing pressure ulcers based on the Institute for Clinical Systems Improvement health care protocol.

 Nutrition Considerations

Nutrition and Wound Healing

Ongoing research is being conducted about the optimal amounts; however, increased energy, protein, zinc, and vitamins A, C, and E are shown to reduce pressure ulcers in high-risk patients by 25% (Crowe & Brockbank, 2009).

Signs and Symptoms

Once a patient has developed a pressure ulcer, treatment depends on the stage of the ulcer. Several kinds of preprinted forms can be used to assess the risk of developing pressure ulcers. These assessment tools take into account the general condition of the skin, control of urination and defecation, mobility, mental status, and nutritional status. They provide a more systematic approach to evaluating a patient's potential for pressure

ulcer development. Many agencies use either the Braden scale system (Figure 43-10) or the Norton system for systematic assessment of the skin.

The presence and stage of an ulcer must be documented on admission to any health care facility or service. Classifying an ulceration can also be helpful in evaluating the effectiveness of treatment and progress toward healing and repair. The National Pressure Ulcer Advisory Panel (NPUAP) has updated pressure ulcer definitions for the prediction and prevention of pressure ulcers and a staging system for classification:

- *Suspected deep tissue injury:* Intact skin with a purple or maroon discoloration. Tissue may be firm, boggy, painful, cool, or warm.
- *Stage I:* An area of intact skin that is reddened, deep pink, or mottled that does not blanch (Figure 43-11).
- *Stage II:* Partial-thickness skin loss involving the epidermis and/or dermis. The skin appears blistered or abraded, or has a shallow crater. The area surrounding the damaged skin is reddened and probably will feel hot or warmer than normal (Figure 43-12).

Patient's Name _____		Evaluator's Name _____		Date of Assessment			
SENSORY PRECEPTION Ability to respond meaningfully to pressure-related discomfort	**1. Completely limited:** Unresponsive (does not moan, flinch, or grasp) to painful stimuli, due to diminished level of consciousness or sedation. OR Limited ability to feel pain over most of body surface.	**2. Very Limited:** Responds only to painful stimuli. Cannot communicate discomfort except by moaning or restlessness. OR Has a sensory impairment that limits the ability to feel pain or discomfort over half of body.	**3. Slightly Limited:** Responds to verbal commands, but cannot always communicate discomfort or need to be turned. OR Has some sensory impairment that limits ability to feel pain or discomfort in one or two extremities.	**4. No Impairment:** Responds to verbal commands. Has no sensory deficit which would limit ability to feel or voice pain or discomfort.			
MOISTURE Degree to which skin is exposed to moisture	**1. Constantly Moist:** Skin is kept moist almost constantly by perspiration, urine, etc. Dampness is detected every time patient is moved or turned.	**2. Very Moist:** Skin is often, but now always moist. Linen must be changed at least once a shift.	**3. Occasionally Moist:** Skin is occasionally moist, requiring an extra linen change approximately once a day.	**4. Rarely Moist:** Skin is usually dry, linen only requires changing at routine intervals.			
ACTIVITY Degree of physical activity	**1. Bedfast:** Confined to bed.	**2. Chairfast:** Ability to walk severely limited or non-existent. Cannot bear own weight and/or must be assisted into chair or wheelchair.	**3. Walks Occasionally:** Walks occasionally during day, but for very short distances, with or without assistance. Spends majority of each shift in bed or chair.	**4. Walks Frequently:** Walks outside the room at least twice a day and inside room at least once every 2 hours during waking hours.			
MOBILITY Ability to change and control body position	**1. Completely Immobile:** Does not make even slight changes in body or extremity position without assistance.	**2. Very Limited:** Makes occasional slight changes in body or extremity position but unable to make frequent or significant changes independently.	**3. Slightly Limited:** Makes frequent though slight changes in body or extremity position independently.	**4. No Limitations:** Makes major and frequent changes in position without assistance.			
NUTRITION Usual food intake pattern	**1. Very Poor:** Never eats a complete meal. Rarely eats more than a third of any food offered. Eats two servings or less of protein (meat or dairy products) per day. Takes fluids poorly. Does not take a liquid dietary supplement. OR Is NPO and/or maintained on clear liquids or IVs for more than 5 days.	**2. Probably Inadequate:** Rarely eats a complete meal and generally eats only about half of any food offered. Protein intake includes only three servings of meat or dairy products per day. Occasionally will take a dietary supplement. OR Receives less than optimum amount of liquid diet or tube feeding.	**3. Adequate:** Eats over half of most meals. Eats a total of four servings of protein (meat, dairy products) each day. Occasionally will refuse a meal, but will usually take a supplement if offered. OR Is on a tube feeding or TPN regimen that probably meets most of nutritional needs.	**4. Excellent:** Eats most of every meal. Never refuses a meal. Usually eats a total of four or more servings of meat and dairy products. Occasionally eats between meals. Does not require supplementation.			
FRICTION AND SHEAR	**1. Problem:** Requires moderate to maximum assistance in moving. Complete lifting without sliding against sheets is impossible. Frequently slides down in bed or chair, requiring frequent repositioning with maximum assistance. Spasticity, contractures, or agitation leads to almost constant friction.	**2. Potential Problem:** Moves feebly or requires minimum assistance. During a move, skin probably slides to some extent against sheets, chair, restraints, or other devices. Maintains relatively good position in chair or bed most of the time but occasionally slides down.	**3. No Apparent Problem:** Moves in bed and in chair independently and has sufficient muscle strength to lift up completely during move. Maintains good position in bed or chair at all times.				
				Total Score			

At risk = 15-18; Moderate risk = 13-14; High risk = 10-12; Severe Risk = 9.
Key: IV, intravenously; NPO, nothing by mouth; TPN, total parenteral nutrition.

FIGURE 43-10 Braden scale for predicting pressure sore risk.

FIGURE 43-11 Stage I pressure ulcer.

FIGURE 43-12 Stage II pressure ulcer.

FIGURE 43-13 Stage III pressure ulcer.

- *Stage III:* The skin is ulcerated. There is a crater-like ulcer, and the underlying subcutaneous tissue is involved in the destructive process. The ulcer may or may not be infected. Bacterial infection is almost always present at this stage, however, and accounts for continued erosion of the ulcer and the production of drainage (Figure 43-13).
- *Stage IV:* There is deep ulceration and necrosis involving deeper underlying muscle and possibly bone tissue. The ulcer can be dry, black, and covered with a tough accumulation of necrotic tissue, or it can be made up of wet and oozing dead cells and purulent exudates. Depth can be determined (Figure 43-14).

FIGURE 43-14 Stage IV pressure ulcer.

- *Unstageable:* Full-thickness wounds with eschar and/or tissue that obscures depth determination.

Assignment Considerations

"On-Time"

The On-Time Quality Improvement for Long-Term Care was developed by the Agency for Healthcare Research and Quality. Part of the program includes assessment tools that can be completed by certified nursing assistants. The tool provides information about nutritional status, behavior, incontinence, and contributing factors. Data is then available to physicians, nurses, dieticians, etc. The program fosters teamwork and communication and helps to identify patients that are at risk for pressure ulcers (Hudak et al., 2008).

A new technology called *pressure mapping* may help to identify areas of high pressure. The patient lies (or sits) on a sensor-filled mat and the mat sends data to a computer, which creates a display of color coded images. Red areas indicate higher pressures, and blue or green images suggest lesser pressures. The patient can then be repositioned accordingly. The technology is an adjunct to, not a replacement for, good nursing assessment (Hanson et al., 2009).

Treatment and Nursing Interventions

Débridement. Removal of any eschar (dead, necrotic tissue) has to occur for a pressure ulcer to heal. The exception is a heel ulcer with dry eschar that has no edema, erythema, drainage, or boggy tissue. *Débridement* can be done surgically with forceps and scissors or mechanically. Mechanical débridement is accomplished by whirlpool baths, wet-to-dry saline dressings, dextranomer beads sprinkled over the wound, or other proteolytic enzymes or chemical products that break down the dead tissue and absorb the exudate. When wet-to-dry dressings are used, the patient should be medicated for pain before the dressing is pulled from the wound, as pulling necrotic tissue pulls some viable tissue with it. **This method is not recommended because of the damage that occurs to new granulation tissue.** Carefully read the instructions for whatever product is being used. Surgical débridement may be done in the patient's room, the physician's office, or the surgical suite depending on the depth and extent of the wound. Surgical débridement may require a skin graft to cover the area exposed. Whenever surgical débridement, forceful irrigation, or whirlpool débridement is to occur, be certain to provide sufficient analgesia for the patient, as the procedure is painful.

Cleansing and Dressing. Many hospitals and larger long-term care facilities have a wound care nurse specialist who oversees wound treatment; nurses should consult these specialists for valuable advice about wound cleansing and dressing materials. After sharp débridement with bleeding, clean and dry dressings are used for 8 to 24 hours, then moisture-retaining dressings are applied. Ulcers are cleaned whenever the dressing is changed. Normal saline or other non-toxic solutions, such as Shur-Clens, and light mechanical action with sponges or irrigation equipment is a way of cleansing that prevents disruption of granulation tissue. At least 250 mL of solution and a 30-mL syringe with a small catheter or 18-gauge needle attached is used to irrigate and to reach undermined areas and tunnels. A reddened wound bed requires gentle irrigation with a 30- to 50-mL needleless syringe to prevent damage to newly developing tissue.

Wound dressings are selected according to the characteristics of the wound. Common dressing materials include moisture retentive dressings, hydrogel dressings, hydrocolloid wafers, alginates, biologic dressings, and absorptive dressings. Use hypoallergenic tape when tape is necessary. Choose a dressing that keeps the ulcer moist and the surrounding skin dry. Prevent abscess formation by loosely filling all cavities with dressing material. Pressure must be kept off the wound for it to heal.

Other Treatment Methods. Houghton and colleagues (2010) found that application of electrical stimulation increased the rate of healing of pressure ulcers for community-dwelling spinal cord injury patients. In this study, high-voltage pulsed current was applied to the wound area (stage III or greater). At 3 months, the size of the wounds was reduced and appearance was improved.

In some facilities, vacuum-assisted wound closure is being used. A suction tube covered by a special sponge is sealed into place for 48 hours. Low-negative suction pressure is applied through the tube. This seems to stimulate the formation of granulation tissue. This treatment is used for chronic ulcers (Gestring, 2011).

For an ulcer that will not heal with other methods, hyperbaric oxygen therapy may be prescribed if the equipment is available in the community. The patient is placed in the hyperbaric oxygen chamber for the treatments. Tissue becomes flooded with more oxygen

Table 43-2	Color of Purulent Exudate and Probable Pathogen	
COLOR EXUDATE	**MAY INDICATE**
Beige with a fishy odor	*Proteus*
Brown with a fecal odor	*Bacteroides*
Creamy yellow	*Staphylococcus*
Green-blue with a fruity odor	*Pseudomonas*

than is normally available when breathing atmospheric-pressure air. This is an effective treatment for other difficult-to-heal wounds as well (Hilton, 2009).

Documentation. Pressure ulcers should be measured and documented when they are discovered and at least once a week thereafter. Document the characteristics of the wound and any exudate present. Exudate is usually purulent (containing pus) or serosanguineous (containing serum and blood). Serosanguineous exudate is amber colored and blood tinged. Purulent drainage may be one of several colors (Table 43-2).

All aspects of risk assessment, preventive measures instituted, objective description and measurement of pressure ulcers, treatment, and progress toward healing are documented regularly in the patient's chart. The Pressure Ulcer Scale for Healing (PUSH) tool is a good way to objectively document your findings. Photographs are often taken of the ulcer on discovery and during treatment to document progress.

BURNS

Etiology and Pathophysiology

Burns are injuries to the skin caused by exposure to extreme heat, hot liquids, electrical agents, strong chemicals, or radiation. Inhaling smoke or fumes also causes injury. About 450,000 Americans seek care for burns each year. The majority of burns are relatively minor, but approximately 40,000 patients are hospitalized each year. Fire and burns kill approximately 4000 victims each year in the United States (American Burn Association, 2011). Thirty years ago most patients with burns over 50% of the body did not survive. Today, because of fluid resuscitation, burn wound excision and grafting techniques, new skin coverings, and nutritional supplementation, a patient may survive a 99% burn.

Electrical burns damage tissue deep within the body. The extent of damage is not always visible and the entrance site and exit site may appear small. Cardiac monitoring should be initiated even if the patient does not complain of chest pain.

Chemical burns result from accidents in homes or industry. The severity of the injury depends on the duration of contact and the concentration of the chemical. The amount of tissue exposed to the chemical and the action of the chemical affect severity. Alkalis (e.g., industrial cleaners and fertilizers) cause greater injury and burn by liquefying tissue. Acids damage the tissue by coagulating cells and proteins. Chemicals for swimming pools, rust removers, and bathroom cleaners are acids. Organic compounds damage tissue by their fat solvent action.

Radiation skin injury is most often from therapeutic radiation treatment. In industries in which radioactive isotopes are used, the degree of injury depends on the amount and type of energy deposited over time. See Chapter 8 for care of skin damaged by radiation treatments.

Burns cause an acute inflammatory response (see Chapter 6). Serious burns have local and systemic effects. **All burns should be considered potentially life threatening until they are thoroughly assessed.** When a burn area is large, the inflammatory response can result in a massive shift of water, electrolytes, and protein into the tissues. This causes severe edema. Evaporation from denuded areas is four times that from intact skin. Hyperkalemia occurs when potassium is released from the damaged cells. Hyponatremia is caused by the stress response and potassium shifts. Metabolic acidosis develops. The loss of fluids from the vascular space leads to hypovolemia with low blood pressure and possible hypovolemic shock. There will be an increased hematocrit due to concentration of the blood, which is missing the components that have shifted into the tissues. The increased viscosity of the blood causes slowing of blood flow in the small vessels, which in turn causes tissue hypoxia. There is danger of kidney failure from both the hypovolemia and the cellular debris that the kidneys must clear from the body. Lung tissue injury from inhalation of heat and smoke may cause alveolar edema.

The decreased perfusion to other organs causes changes in the gastric mucosa that impair its integrity. A type of ulcer called Curling's ulcer can occur within 24 hours.

The stress response to the trauma releases catecholamines, aldosterone, cortisol, and antidiuretic hormone. A hypermetabolic state results, and unless nutrition needs can be met, the body falls into negative nitrogen balance. A low-grade fever may develop as core temperature rises.

Signs, Symptoms, and Diagnosis

Burn severity depends on the cause, the temperature and duration of contact, the extent of burned area, and the anatomical site of the burn. Signs and symptoms vary from slight reddening of the skin to full loss of tissue down to bone with black, charred areas. Blisters may form. A dry, scablike crust forms over a superficial burn. Eschar is a hard, leathery layer of dead tissue that results when there has been a full-thickness injury. It is dark brown to black.

Diagnosis of the depth of burn is made based on a classification system.

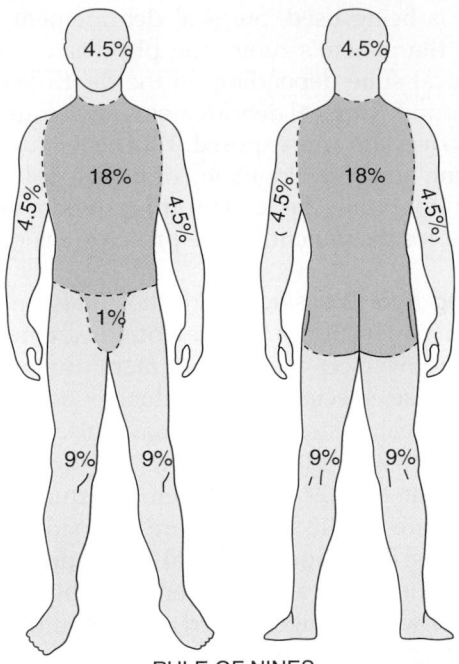

RULE OF NINES

FIGURE 43-15 Chart used for burn area estimate ("rule of nines").

Classification of Burns

The classification of burns is based on the amount of the body surface that has been burned and the depth of the burn. The extent of a burn is roughly calculated outside of the hospital according to the "rule of nines" and is expressed as a percentage of total body surface (Figure 43-15). The figures used in this method are fairly accurate for gross assessment in adults. The Lund-Browder classification or the Berkow chart can be used to compute the depth of the burn as well as the extent of the injury according to relative age, and the total burn estimate is used as the basis for treatment.

The depth of a burn is more difficult to determine, because various graduations of injury are sustained in a major burn. Some small patches may be more deeply burned than the areas adjacent to them. Burn depth originally was classified according to degrees, a first-degree burn being the most superficial and a fourth-degree burn being the deepest.

A more current method to evaluate the depth of burns is based on the layers of skin that have been damaged (Figure 43-16). *Partial-thickness wounds* (Figure 43-17) are those in which the epidermal appendages (sweat and oil glands and hair follicles) are not destroyed and the wound will heal by itself if no further injury occurs from either infection or inappropriate treatment (see Table 5-1 for the phases of wound healing). Grafting may or may not be necessary. *Full-thickness wounds* (Figure 43-18) involve all layers of skin and the destruction of the epidermal appendages. Wounds of this type will require grafting for the wound

		WOUND APPEARANCE	WOUND SENSATION	COURSE OF HEALING
PARTIAL-THICKNESS BURN	1st-degree	Epidermis remains intact and without blisters. Erythema; skin blanches with pressure.	Painful	Discomfort lasts 48-72 hours. Desquamation in 3-7 days
	2nd-degree	Wet, shiny, weeping surface Blisters Wound blanches with pressure.	Painful Very sensitive to touch, air currents	Superficial partial-thickness burn heals in < 21 days. Deep partial-thickness burn requires > 21 days for healing. Healing rates vary with burn depth and presence/absence of infection.
FULL-THICKNESS BURN	3rd-degree	Color variable (i.e., deep red, white, black, brown) Surface dry Thrombosed vessels visible No blanching	Insensate (↓ pinprick sensation)	Autografting required for healing
	4th-degree	Color variable Charring visible in deepest areas Extremity movement limited	Insensate	Amputation of extremities likely Autografting required for healing

Diagram labels: EPIDERMIS, Sweat duct, Capillary, Sebaceous gland, Nerve endings, DERMIS, Hair follicle, Sweat gland, Fat, Blood vessels, Bone

FIGURE 43-16 The tissues involved in burns of various depths.

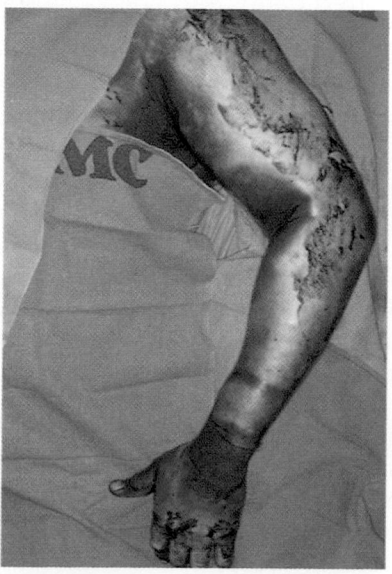

FIGURE 43-17 Partial-thickness burn injury.

FIGURE 43-18 Full-thickness burn injury.

to heal and for optimal function to be restored. Table 43-3 provides a guide for estimating the depth of a burn.

Emergency Treatment
First, all burn patients are treated as trauma patients. Establishment and maintenance of an airway is the first priority. The patient may have other life-threatening injuries besides their burns. Hemorrhage does not usually occur with burns. If a burned patient shows signs of bleeding, he must be checked for some other type of injury, such as a penetrating wound, fracture, or laceration that occurred at the same time that he was burned.

Generally, patients are undressed and covered with a sterile or freshly laundered sheet: however, clothing that is stuck to the burn area is not removed before the patient is in the hospital (Murphy et al., 2009). Rings, bracelets, and watches should be removed from injured extremities to avoid a tourniquet effect when swelling occurs. Do not apply salves or ointments or any greasy substance to a burned area, because the removal of greasy substances is very painful and increases the possibility of infection. Blisters should not be disturbed initially, as they serve as a protective covering over the wound. Box 43-3 outlines first aid for minor burns.

The seriously burned victim is generally given nothing by mouth. Oxygen is administered if pulse oximetry indicates a problem with respiratory function or if inhalation injury is suspected. Assessment for carbon monoxide inhalation includes checking the mucous membranes for a cherry-red color. Intravenous fluid therapy and more extensive medical treatment are

Table 43-3   Classification of Burn Depth

CHARACTERISTIC	SUPERFICIAL BURN	SUPERFICIAL PARTIAL-THICKNESS BURN	DEEP PARTIAL-THICKNESS BURN	FULL-THICKNESS BURN	DEEP FULL-THICKNESS BURN
Color	Pink to red	Pink to red	Red to white	Black, brown, yellow, white, red	Black
Edema	Mild	Mild to moderate	Moderate	Severe	Absent
Pain	Yes	Yes	Yes	Yes and no	Absent
Blisters	No	Yes	Rare	No	No
Eschar	No	No	Yes, soft and dry	Yes, hard and inelastic	Yes, hard and inelastic
Healing time	3-5 days	Approximately 2 wk	2-6 wk	Weeks to months	Weeks to months
Grafts required	No	No	Can be used if healing is prolonged	Yes	Yes
Example	Sunburn, flash burns	Scalds, flames, brief contact with hot objects	Scalds; flames; prolonged contact with hot objects, tar, grease, chemicals	Scalds; flames; prolonged contact with hot objects, tar, grease chemicals, electricity	Flames, electricity, grease, tar, chemicals

From Ignatavicius, D.D., & Workman, M.L. (2010). *Medical-Surgical Nursing: Patient-Centered Collaborative Care* (5th ed.). Philadelphia: Saunders.

Box 43-3   First Aid for Minor Burns

- Run cool water over the burn continuously for 10 to 15 minutes.
- Apply cool compresses if continuous water flow is not available.
- Do not apply ice, ice water, butter, or ointments.
- Do not pop blisters.
- Cover loosely with a sterile gauze bandage.
- Take ibuprofen or acetaminophen for pain.

started as soon as possible. The American Burn Association has identified criteria for minor and major burn injuries. It recommends that all major burn injury patients be treated in a burn center. Every emergency department has guidelines that indicate whether a burn victim needs to be transferred to a burn center.

Emergent Phase of Burns

The emergent phase averages 24 to 48 hours, but may last as long as 3 days. It begins with fluid loss and edema formation and lasts until edema fluid is mobilized and diuresis begins.

The first hour of treatment after burning can be crucial to the eventual outcome of a serious burn. Other life-threatening injuries must be treated first.

If possible, details of the nature of the accident should be obtained so that a more thorough assessment can be made. Knowing the causes of the burn and whether there is any possibility of thermal damage to the respiratory tract, can alert the team to the specific needs of the patient. The depth and extent of the burn area are estimated and multiple IV lines are established. A tetanus toxoid injection is given in the emergency department; it is the only intramuscular injection given initially.

Respiratory Support. There is a potential for respiratory obstruction if upper airway passages have been burned. Swelling will occur, and it will become increasingly difficult for the patient to breathe. Signs of respiratory distress such as increased respiratory rate, use of accessory muscles, nasal flaring, retractions, restlessness, and confusion may occur. Early intubation is recommended for an extensive upper airway injury.

Lower airway injury (damage to lung parenchyma) is caused by breathing in smoke and soot from the fire. This type of injury may also require intubation and ventilation and may be life threatening.

Patients who should be watched closely for signs of developing respiratory problems include those who have:

- Burns of the face and neck
- Singed nasal hair or darkened membranes in the nose and mouth
- Smoky-smelling breath
- Dark or black sputum
- Burning sensation in the throat or chest
- A history of having been burned in an enclosed space

Watch for increasing restlessness, coughing, hoarseness, rapid shallow respirations, *stridor* (high-pitched musical sound on inspiration), and falling oxygen

saturation (below 95%). Humidified oxygen is given if the patient is experiencing respiratory distress; intubation and mechanical ventilation may be required. Keep necessary equipment at hand and constantly assess the patient's respiratory effort. Employ the use of an incentive spirometer, coughing, turning, and early ambulation to maintain good respiratory function. Respiratory therapy treatments may be ordered.

Fluid Resuscitation and Prevention of Shock. **A major concern in the care of a burn victim is to prevent shock due to circulatory collapse.** The two most important measures used to relieve profound shock in a burn patient are:

- Replacement of lost fluids and electrolytes (fluid resuscitation)
- Enhancement of tissue perfusion

The loss of fluids and electrolytes results from the sudden capillary leak and shifting of the blood plasma and tissue fluids from their normal site to the area of the burn. This shift occurs in the first 24 to 48 hours after the burn. The fluids are then lost by movement from the vascular space to the interstitial spaces. Fluid resuscitation needs are based on one of several burn formulas. The Parkland formula for fluid resuscitation is:

$$4 \text{ mL Ringer's lactate (RL)} \times \% \text{ burn} \times \text{weight in kg}$$

One-half of the required fluid should be given within 8 hours of the time of the burn. The second half is given over the next 16 hours. After that, fluids are based on specific volume and electrolyte imbalances and response to treatment. **Fluid replacement is calculated from the time of injury, not from the time of arrival at the medical facility.** An important nursing function is to keep IV access sites patent and secured in place, and to see that the fluids are administered at the ordered rates.

🖳 Clinical Cues

In trauma patients, a Foley catheter is inserted to monitor hourly urine output and provide data to determine whether fluid resuscitation is adequate. The minimum urine flow for an adult is 30 mL/hr. To obtain accurate hourly measurements, the standard drainage bag should be changed to a drainage bag that has a urometer.

Unless fluids are replaced immediately, the cardiac output will drop and the resultant profound shock may be fatal to the patient. The patient's vital signs must be checked hourly and recorded accurately. It should be noted that a blood pressure reading taken by cuff from an extremity may not be reliable. An arterial line may be inserted for more accurate monitoring of blood pressure changes. The state of sensorium or level of consciousness is another key observation in the assessment of tissue perfusion. Constantly assess the patient's level of alertness and clarity of thinking. Ask the patient who he is, where he is, his age, what happened, and so on. There are significant dangers to fluid resuscitation; for example, excessive fluid potentiates adult respiratory distress syndrome, and extreme fluid deficit will cause acute renal failure. It is very important to monitor the signs of adequate fluid resuscitation and know when to increase or decrease the fluids based on clinical findings.

After the first 24 hours, 5% dextrose in water (D_5W) is given to maintain a serum sodium level of 135 to 145 mEq/L. Fluid intake and output and daily weights are measured as long as the patient has open wounds. Laboratory data are checked frequently for evidence of either a deficit or surplus of specific electrolytes.

Pain Management. As soon as IV lines are established and fluid resuscitation is begun, pain control can begin. Measures to relieve pain include the administration of morphine or hydromorphone hydrochloride (Dilaudid) IV. Doses of IV morphine may be higher than you are accustomed to seeing: 2 to 4 mg every 5 to 10 minutes is the standard starting dose, and the patient may require a much larger total dose because of the severe pain (Connor-Ballard, 2009a). Fentanyl is another powerful opioid medication that can be combined with a benzodiazepine, such as midazolam, before painful wound care procedures. Ketamine and propofol are anesthetic agents that are used for control of pain during procedures. The massive fluid shifts that occur after a burn injury make absorption from an intramuscular site unpredictable in the first 24 hours after the burn.

For chronic pain, gabapentin and methadone can be prescribed. Nonsteroidal anti-inflammatory drugs (NSAIDs) work to control pain, but may not be used if ongoing grafting is necessary or because of stress ulcers.

Acute Phase of Burns

The acute phase extends from the time of fluid mobilization and diuresis to when the burned area is completely covered by skin grafts or when burns are healed. Goals during this phase include management of pain and anxiety, prevention of wound infection, promotion of nutritional intake, and rehabilitation therapy.

Prevention of Infection. Although wound infection is no longer the major cause of death in burn victims (the main cause of death is pneumonia), its prevention is important to recovery. Today patients are taken to the operating room very early after the burn. Burn eschar is excised away from the wound and the area is covered with a biologic or biosynthetic skin. During the granulation stage of repair, the wound should look slightly pink and somewhat shiny. Healthy granulation tissue does not emit exudates. **A very wet wound that has a foul odor indicates infection.** A greenish blue wound exudate is a sign of *Pseudomonas* infection. Signs of inflammation, such as redness and swelling of the tissues adjacent to the wound, may indicate *cellulitis* (acute inflammation of the subcutaneous tissues). Signs of infection should be reported to the physician. If wound sepsis occurs, IV antibiotics specific to bacteria in the wound are given and topical antibacterial soaks are applied to the wound.

Critically burned patients have a high risk for ventilator-acquired pneumonia. Wahl and colleagues (2010) reported that use of the Joint Commission's Core Measures decreased the complications and the mortality rate associated with catheter-related bloodstream infections and ventilator-acquired pneumonia, although there was no decrease in ventilator, use intensive care unit (ICU), or hospital days. Examples of Core Measures for ICU patients include protocols to prevent deep vein thrombosis, tighter glucose control, head of bed elevated at 30 degrees, and reinforcement of mandatory weaning and spontaneous breathing trials.

Wound Treatment. There are six general principles for the daily care of burn wounds (Demling & Desanti, 2004):

1. Cardiopulmonary status should be monitored during the procedure.
2. Tubes and catheters are a source of infection and must not become wet.
3. Patient must be kept warm; heat lamps or radiant heat shields can be used.
4. Infection must be prevented via use of gowns, gloves, masks, and so on, and cleansing should progress from "cleaner to dirtier" wounds.
5. Analgesia and sedation should be preadministered. Provide adequate stress management.
6. Motion must not be impaired (except for new grafts).

Burn wounds are cleansed using sterile technique at least once daily with diluted chlorhexidine. The goal is to remove excess exudate and drainage and to minimize the danger of infection. Wounds of the face or ears are left undressed. After the wounds are cleaned, a topical ointment such as bacitracin is usually applied every 8 hours to prevent infection and promote healing. Burns on the hands, extremities, or trunk may be cleansed at the bedside, on a shower table in the burn unit treatment room, or in a whirlpool bath. Cleansing is done at least once a day and these wounds are dressed. Dressings are composed of layers of sterile gauze saturated with topical medications, biologic dressings, synthetic dressings, or artificial skin. The wound is then wrapped with stretch gauze, such as Kling, or with elastic mesh webbing. Silver sulfadiazine has long been used for burn care and is still frequently used; however, it is poorly absorbed through eschar and it releases silver for only a few hours. Other, newer silver preparations include hydrogels, ionic silver powder, alginate combinations, and silver site dressings (Fleck & Kesselman, 2009). Table 43-4 lists the most common topical medications and their nursing implications.

Escharotomy. Eschar is a source of infection, and it impairs healing. Removal of eschar and skin grafting are usually done within 1 week after the burn (Figure 43-19). When tissue perfusion or quality of respiration is compromised because of eschar constriction, an **escharotomy** is performed. **An incision into the burn eschar with a scalpel or electrocautery relieves pressure caused by circumferential burns that encircle an extremity or that constrict movement of the chest.** The incisions extend into the subcutaneous tissue. If the pressure is not relieved, arterial blood flow in the extremity will be compromised, possibly causing necrosis; nerve damage from the pressure also may occur. An escharotomy on the chest improves lung expansion and oxygenation. The procedure does not cause discomfort as the nerve endings have been destroyed by the burn. No anesthesia is required.

Be alert for compartment syndrome. This occurs when there is increased pressure within a compartment (e.g., arm, leg) that causes compromise of circulation to the area. Fluid accumulation from edema is the cause in burn patients. Monitor for increasing pain, paleness and tenseness of the tissue, numbness or tingling, discoloration in the distal portion of the extremity, and decreased sensation *(paresthesia)*.

Débridement. *Débridement* involves removing the eschar and necrotic material from underlying tissues. It is usually done in the operating room. Whirlpool tubs are used 3 to 4 days after grafting procedures. Pain medication is given before the bath. Enzyme compounds, such as collagenase (Santyl), containing proteolytic agents may be applied topically to digest necrotic tissue. They are used in conjunction with a Polysporin powder to prevent bacteria from entering the bloodstream from the wound. Surgical débridement and grafting may require IV anesthetic agents, sedation, nitrous oxide, or narcotic analgesia.

Grafting. Surgical removal of eschar and applications of biologic dressings are done within the first week after the burn injury. Biologic dressings are materials obtained from cadavers or from animals. It is most desirable to graft the patient's own skin (autograft), but, when this is not possible, a *homograft* (the skin of another person [allograft], obtained from a cadaver), a heterograft (xenograft, usually obtained from a pig), or artificial (biosynthetic) skin, such as Biobrane, can be used as a temporary measure. Biobrane is a nylon fabric with a silicone film, which allows exudate to pass through. The many synthetic dressings available consist of silicone, plastics, or alginate (brown seaweed combined with other substances) and remain in place

Table 43-4   Topical Medications Commonly Used for Burns

MEDICATION	ACTION	NURSING IMPLICATIONS
Silver sulfadiazine (Silvadene, Flamazine)	Interferes with DNA synthesis by binding to bacterial cell membrane.	Assess for allergy to sulfonamides. Observe for rash, itching, or burning, which may indicate allergic reaction. Observe for leukopenia. Not effective against *Pseudomonas* infections. Cream must be removed and reapplied once or twice per day.
Mafenide acetate (Sulfamylon)	Bacteriostatic agent; effective against both gram-positive and gram-negative organisms.	Assess for allergy to sulfonamides. Observe for signs of allergic reaction. May cause metabolic acidosis; monitor blood gases and electrolyte levels. Application may cause pain for 30-40 min; medicate before applying. Penetrates eschar and is effective against *Pseudomonas*. Very effective for electrical burns.
Silver nitrate	Antimicrobial action.	Dressings must be kept continually wet with 0.5% solution. Stings on application; stains fabric. Monitor electrolyte levels as may cause imbalances. Penetrates wound only 1-2 mm.
Sodium hypochlorite solution (Dakin's)	Bactericidal action; inhibits blood clotting and may dissolve clots.	Observe for signs of irritation. Keep dressings moist with the solution at all times. Helps dry wounds and assists débridement.
Collagenase (Santyl) with polymyxin B (Polysporin) powder	Digests collagen in necrotic tissue; powder prevents infection.	Monitor for wound infection.
Gentamicin sulfate (Garamycin)	Interferes with protein synthesis in bacterial cell.	Monitor for ototoxicity and nephrotoxicity. Use with caution if decreased renal function is present. Monitor creatinine clearance during treatment. Used when there is resistance to other drugs.
Polymyxin B–bacitracin	Wide-spectrum antibiotic action.	May cause itching, burning, and inflammation. Will not penetrate eschar. Must be applied q 2-8 hr.
Nystatin	Interferes with fungal DNA replication.	May cause itching or allergic reaction. Requires long-term use to clear fungal infection.

FIGURE 43-19 Escharotomy of the lower extremity.

for 1 to 14 days. **The patient's own skin is the only permanent graft material.** Some success has been achieved in growing skin cells harvested from the patient in cultures, but this is a slow, expensive process. The epithelial sheets grown are then used for grafting.

When autografting is performed, there is a donor site from which a split-thickness piece of skin has been removed. That piece of skin may be used intact, or it may be cut into a mesh pattern (Figure 43-20). It takes longer for a mesh graft area to heal as the skin cells need to grow into the holes between the links of skin. In 2008 the FDA approved Artiss, which is a fibrin sealant used for adhering skin grafts for burn patients. "Dressings and splints are typically removed on the fourth or fifth day following skin grafting; they may, however, be reapplied for a more lengthy period of time to maintain proper positioning" (American Burn Association White Paper, 2009).

Donor sites may be covered by a film dressing to hasten healing and decrease pain. Often the donor site is more painful than the graft site. Once the donor site has healed completely, skin may be harvested from that site again.

FIGURE 43-20 Typical appearance of meshed autografts. **A,** Appearance during application of meshed autograft. **B,** Appearance of meshed autograft after healing.

Pressure dressings are worn as soon as grafts heal to decrease scarring that can inhibit mobility. The pressure dressing may be an elastic wrap or a custom-fitted, elasticized piece of clothing that provides uniform pressure over the burned area. These pressure dressings must be worn 23 hours a day, every day, until the scar tissue is mature. Scar maturity takes 12 to 24 months. Daily exercise and splint applications are done to prevent contracture formation. After burns are fully healed and the scar tissue has matured, plastic surgery may be performed to try to rebuild lost structures such as the nose or an ear or to enhance appearance.

Complications

When a sizable burn occurs, blood flow is shifted to the brain, heart, and liver because of the fluid shifts that occur. The gastrointestinal tract receives decreased blood and gastric motility is impaired. Monitor peristalsis and be alert to signs of paralytic ileus. Severe abdominal distention may occur. Curling's ulcer may develop, inducing gastrointestinal bleeding. Stools are monitored for signs of occult blood. A histamine (H_2)–receptor antagonist, such as cimetidine (Tagamet), ranitidine (Zantac), famotidine (Pepcid), or nizatidine (Axid), may be administered IV to prevent this complication.

Contractures always are a threat with major burns and sometimes with minor burns. Proper positioning and regular exercise are essential to prevent musculoskeletal deformities following a burn. Painful as the motion of physical therapy exercises may be, the muscles and skin must be exercised and stretched every day if normal motion is to be maintained. Sometimes it is necessary for the patient to continue visiting the physical therapist for several months after discharge from the hospital. Ambulation two or three times a day is begun as soon as the fluid shift has stabilized for patients who have no fractures or serious injuries to the feet or legs.

Rehabilitation Phase of Burns

The patient who has experienced a major burn is transferred to a rehabilitation facility. The rehabilitation phase begins with wound closure and ends when the patient reaches the highest level of function possible. This phase may last for years. Continued physical therapy and psychological care are essential to help the patient achieve his optimal level of function. Some patients must learn to use adaptive devices or alter the way they formerly accomplished tasks.

When the patient is ready to accept some responsibility for self-care, preparation for release from the hospital begins. Teach how to apply topical agents without contaminating the wound and how to change dressings if these are used. A family member, if available, is included in burn care education.

Maturing scars usually appear red, hard, and raised before they eventually begin to fade and soften. Pressure garments and masks help prevent thick and disfiguring scars but are uncomfortable (Figure 43-21). The patient may resist wearing them unless he understands their intended purpose. Your encouragement and reinforcement of the purpose can help.

Reintegration into roles, community activities, and employment takes time. Participation in a support group of burn victims is sometimes helpful. In this way the patient and family realize that they are not alone in their struggles with the many problems that the injury has brought. Assessment of the home environment and family interaction is essential before discharge. Knowing how the patient formerly coped with stressful situations helps professional personnel involved support him. Having friends visit and making short trips out in public is helpful in dealing with the reactions of others to burn scars and disfigurement.

FIGURE 43-21 Pressure garments are individually fitted.

Referral for job retraining may be required if the patient will be unable to return to a former occupation because of residual physical deficits. See Chapter 9 for rehabilitation goals and principles.

❖ NURSING MANAGEMENT

Care of the burn patient is interdisciplinary and includes the services of the physician, surgeon, nurses, dietitian, respiratory therapist, physical therapist, occupational therapist, psychologist or psychiatrist, and social worker. Other health professionals are added to the team as needed. Collaborative planning meetings are scheduled at least once a week initially. Input for the plan of care is contributed by all members of the team.

■ Assessment (Data Collection)

A thorough assessment of all body systems and psychological response is performed on admission and continues throughout because of the potential for complications. The patient's vital signs and pain level must be checked and recorded at regular intervals. The condition of the wounds also should be assessed systematically to determine whether healing is taking place as it should and infection is being avoided. Wounds are carefully assessed at each dressing change. Signs that indicate infection include:
- Strong odor
- Color change to dark red or brown
- Redness around edges extending to nonburned skin
- Texture change
- Exudate and purulent drainage
- Sloughing of graft

Such signs should be reported as culture or biopsy is needed.

? Think Critically

? Think Critically

What would you do if, when taking vital signs, you find that the pulse on the burned arm is weaker than that on the other, non-burned extremity?

■ Nursing Diagnosis

Care of the burn patient is extremely complex and you should anticipate that multiple nursing diagnoses will apply. The plan of care must be frequently revised and updated. Nursing diagnoses commonly used for burn patients are included in Nursing Care Plan 43-1. Additional diagnoses include:
- Imbalanced nutrition: less than body requirements related to increased caloric demands and inability to orally ingest sufficient calories
- Anxiety related to pain, guilt associated with injury, financial concerns, appearance, treatment, and prognosis
- Disturbed body image related to disfigurement secondary to burn injury
- Ineffective coping related to alteration in roles
- Compromised family coping related to care and support of burn victim
- Deficient knowledge related to home care

■ Planning

Examples of appropriate expected outcomes are written for the individual patient, such as:
- Patient will regain nutritional balance.
- Patient will decrease anxiety.
- Patient will integrate the altered body image.
- Patient will develop new coping mechanisms.
- Family will develop ways to cope with caring for patient at home.
- Patient and family will learn to provide good care at home.

■ Implementation

Managing Pain

The nurse must use gentleness and care in handling the patient as she turns him or administers treatments. This reduces the amount of pain; also, the less the patient is handled, the less danger there is of contaminating the wounds. **Despite advances in burn care, research studies show that pain continues to be undertreated and even experienced clinicians tend to overestimate the efficacy of opioids.** In one study, 74% of patients reported procedural pain at 7 on a scale of 1 to 10 at least once during burn care (Connor-Ballard, 2009b). Morphine or hydromorphone hydrochloride (Dilaudid) should be administered via a patient-controlled analgesia pump when possible. Boluses are necessary before treatments or surgical procedures and at bedtime. Sedatives such as lorazepam (Ativan), midazolam (Versed), and haloperidol (Haldol) should be used along with analgesia.

★ Nursing Care Plan 43-1   Care of the Patient with a Burn

Scenario

Mr. Young, age 33, sustained partial- and full-thickness burns over both arms when a container of gasoline he was carrying ignited. He also suffered superficial partial-thickness burns on his hands and face. In the emergency department, his wounds were cleaned and a topical agent was applied; no dressings were applied. IV lines were established, and fluids were administered to avoid potential fluid and electrolyte imbalance. He received morphine for pain and on admission to the unit was fairly comfortable, conscious, and oriented. He is in the emergent phase.

Problem/Nursing Diagnosis

*Superficial partial- and full-thickness burns on the arms, hands, and face/*Deficient fluid volume related to fluid shift and loss of fluids via open wounds.

Supporting Assessment Data

Objective: Partial-thickness burns over hands and face with full-thickness burns on arms; burn areas becoming edematous.

Goals/Expected Outcomes	Nursing Interventions	Selected Rationale	Evaluation
Patient will have adequate circulating blood volume as evidenced by blood pressure (BP), pulse, and urine output.	Monitor vital signs q 2 hr.	Falling BP and rising pulse can indicate hypovolemia.	BP 120/80. Pulse 78/min. Respirations 24/min. Temperature 98.6° F (37° C).
	Monitor urine output, report drop below 0.5 mL/kg/hr.	Urine output may also indicate hypovolemia as kidneys will be less perfused.	Urine output at 45 mL/hr.
	Monitor laboratory values for electrolyte imbalances.		Potassium is 4.5 mEq/L. Sodium is 140 mEq/L.
	Maintain IV fluids on schedule.	Adequate fluid resuscitation prevents hypovolemia.	IV fluids on schedule. Continue plan.

Problem/Nursing Diagnosis

*Open wounds with dead tissue/*Risk for infection related to burn damage to skin.

Supporting Assessment Data

Objective: Skin on face, hands, and arms damaged by burns.

Goals/Expected Outcomes	Nursing Interventions	Selected Rationale	Evaluation
Patient will not experience infection of burn wounds as evidenced by normal vital signs and normalization of WBC count.	Assess for medication allergy.	Medication ordered may be contraindicated.	No allergies to medication.
	Use strict aseptic technique for wound care.	Infection is the greatest cause of burn wound depth.	Strict aseptic technique provided to wounds.
	Do not submerge catheters or insertion sites during cleansing.	Invasive catheters are potential portals of infection.	Peripheral IV catheter and site covered with plastic for cleaning process.
	Assign private room and use Contact Isolation Precautions. Use Standard Precautions, including hand hygiene.	Major burns generally require Contact Isolation Precautions (follow facility procedures). Hand hygiene is a first-line measure to prevent infection.	Contact Isolation Precautions initiated. Isolation supplies gathered and placed outside the door. Sign posted for isolation procedures and instructing visitors to see the nurse before entering.
	Apply topical silver sulfadiazine as ordered to wounds tid.	Suppresses bacterial growth and promotes healing.	Wounds cleansed, silver sulfadiazine applied, and wounds redressed.
	Monitor WBC count for signs of infection; assess and cleanse wounds tid.	Cleansing wounds helps prevent infection and promotes healing.	Results for WBC count pending. No signs of wound infection.
	Encourage adequate nutrition.	High caloric intake with sufficient vitamins and minerals is needed for healing.	Not taking food as yet. Continue plan.

ADLs, activities of daily living; *IV,* intravenous; *PT,* physical therapy; *WBC,* white blood cell.

Problem/Nursing Diagnosis
Extensive burns and painful care procedures/Pain related to burn wounds and cleansing procedures.

Supporting Assessment Data
Subjective: States is in constant pain at an 8-10 level.
Objective: Grimacing and holding body rigid.

Goals/Expected Outcomes	Nursing Interventions	Selected Rationale	Evaluation
Patient's pain will be controlled to tolerable levels with analgesia.	Assess for quality, location, and intensity of pain. Assess patient's "acceptable" level.	Pain is subjective and patient must report own experience. "Acceptable" level reflects the patient's expectations and tolerance.	Reports pain at 4/10 currently; medicated 3 hours ago. Acceptable level is 4/10, but requests additional medication before dressing change.
	Assess for and control noxious social or environmental stimuli.	Perception of pain is affected by various noxious stimuli, such as loud noise, visitors, dirty sheets, bad odors.	Reports that visitors are laughing loudly in the stairwell; would like to have door closed.
	Administer IV analgesia as ordered, giving boluses as appropriate before procedures and at bedtime.	IV narcotic analgesia is best for burn pain control initially.	Bolus given for pain of 4 before dressing change.
Patient's pain will be controlled with oral medication before discharge.	Teach relaxation and imagery techniques to assist with pain control.	Relaxation and imagery techniques have proven helpful in pain control.	Began instruction on relaxation technique.
	Supply diversionary activities to diminish pain awareness.	TV, card games, visitors, computer games, and reading help divert attention from pain.	Is watching TV; not ready for greater activity yet. Continue plan.

Problem/Nursing Diagnosis
Cannot use hands and arms/Self-care deficit: hygiene, feeding, toileting, and grooming related to inability to use hands and arms.

Supporting Assessment Data
Objective: Burns on hands and arms being treated and grafted; unable to use hands and arms for self-care activities.

Goals/Expected Outcomes	Nursing Interventions	Selected Rationale	Evaluation
Patient will assist with self-care activities within 3 mo.	Assist with hygiene, toileting, grooming, and feeding as needed.	Assistance as needed must be provided to prevent infection and increase well-being.	Requires full assistance with ADLs today.
	Allow him to make decisions as much as possible to lessen feelings of helplessness.	Participation in care decreases feelings of dependency and increases feelings of control.	Choosing time for bath. Unable to use hands and arms at this time.
	Allow him to do as much as he is able to do.	Gradual resumption of activities can occur with encouragement and time.	"At least I can walk to the bathroom by myself." Continue plan.

Continued

Nursing Care Plan 43-1   **Care of the Patient with a Burn—cont'd**

Problem/Nursing Diagnosis

*Fears he will not be able to work at job and support family/*Situational low self-esteem related to burned hands and worries about role in family as "bread winner."

Supporting Assessment Data

Subjective: "With my hands and arms burned, I won't be able to work anymore. I'm not much of a man anymore if I can't take care of my family."

Objective: Unable to use hands and arms because of burns.

Goals/Expected Outcomes	Nursing Interventions	Selected Rationale	Evaluation
Patient will verbalize frustrations and concerns before discharge.	Establish trusting relationship, actively listen to concerns and frustrations.	A trusting relationship helps him to freely verbalize concerns and facilitates acceptance of treatment plan.	Expressed concerns about helplessness.
	Help him establish his active role in recovery of use of hands and arms.	Collaboration helps improve his self-esteem.	States wants to recover self-sufficiency.
	Allow him to do whatever ADLs are possible for him.	Performing self-care helps increase self-esteem.	Unable to perform any arm or hand movements yet.
	Praise him for his efforts with PT exercises and use of splints.	Praise encourages his actions.	Passive PT thus far.
	Help him establish small, accomplishable goals on a weekly basis.	Accomplishing small goals increases self-esteem.	Is thinking about goals for next week.
	Review past successes in overcoming obstacles.	Reflecting on past strengths helps patient to envision transferring success to current challenges.	Recalls having a broken arm as a child and remembers learning to adapt and function with a cast in place.
Patient will discuss possible job retraining if needed.	Refer for job retraining if needed.		Need for job retraining unknown at this time. Continue plan.

Critical Thinking Questions

1. With partial-thickness burns on his hands, do you think Mr. Young will be able to use his hands as a mechanic again?
2. Since he had burns on his face, what specific assessments should be made to see whether there has been an inhalation injury?
3. Will he probably need skin grafting? If so, where? Is it likely that autografts could be used?

Pain often continues even after the wound appears to have healed completely. Exercises to prevent contractures can cause pain because they stretch the skin while it is very tender. Splints to prevent musculoskeletal complications can also cause discomfort. Analgesics will allow the patient to get sufficient rest, but they should be given judiciously as the pain becomes less acute. If a patient begins to depend too much on one kind of analgesic, alternative drugs can be given.

 Complementary and Alternative Therapies

Helping Patients to Cope with Pain

Proper body positioning, distraction therapy, music, television, games, and virtual reality technologies may help burn patients to cope with pain. These adjunctive interventions do not replace medication or attentive nursing care (Arnstein, 2010).

Preventing Infection

An aseptic environment is needed for burn care. Standard Precautions are used for all burn care, and protective isolation techniques are used. Those in attendance usually wear sterile caps, gowns, shoe covers, and gloves while caring for the patient. Contact Isolation measures are used for infected wounds. Gloves are worn for all contact with open wounds, and are changed when handling wounds on different areas of the patient's body and between handling soiled and sterile dressings. **Patient care items are not shared, and great attention is paid to maintaining asepsis for all patient care.** Bed linen is changed daily and whenever soiled, and a bed cradle or some other device is used to support the weight of the top covers to keep them off the burned areas.

Managing Itch

Administer antihistamines proactively before itching becomes intense (American Burn Association White Paper, 2009). Nonpharmacologic measures to reduce itching, such as relaxation techniques, meditation, guided imagery, and music therapy, are used along with medication. Therapeutic touch may prove helpful. Acupressure and acupuncture may assist with pain and itch relief.

Nutritional Support

Enteral feedings are started shortly after the fluid resuscitation is completed for a major burn victim. The patient with large burns often develops paralytic ileus as a response to the trauma. The stomach stops working when this occurs, and a nasogastric tube must be inserted and attached to intermittent suction. Bowel sounds should return 48 to 72 hours later, and then intake may begin with high-protein, high-calorie drinks if tolerated.

A diet high in protein and calories is necessary for healing. The patient has increased metabolic needs directly proportional to the size of the burn area. Nutritional needs may be increased 50% to 150% above normal and caloric requirements may be as high as 5000 calories per day. Caloric needs are calculated to include the patient's weight, age, and percentage of burn over total body surface (Chan & Chan, 2009). Only high-calorie liquids are given to drink. Free water intake is restricted. Dietary supplements include vitamins, especially vitamins A, C, and D. Minerals such as zinc and copper are supplied because deficiencies are seen in burn patients. Consultation with a nutritionist is essential because of the dietary issues that can occur for burn patients. There appears to be a maximum glucose load, and high carbohydrate intake can lead to hyperglycemia, dehydration, and respiratory problems. Excessive lipid intake has been associated with impaired wound healing, and ability to tolerate protein is related to renal function and fluid balance (Chan & Chan, 2009).

 Complementary and Alternative Therapies

Helping Burn Patients to Relax

In a small pilot study, Klein and Hoffman (2010) found that relaxation and visual image techniques lowered hypermetabolic states for burn patients.

Psychosocial Support

Burn patients may face loss of mobility and independence, or disfigurement involving the face or other parts of the body usually visible to others. Many will experience post-traumatic stress syndrome and others may feel guilt, anger, or depression. Strive to develop an attitude of acceptance of the patient, a calm approach to dressing changes and discussions of scar formation, and an optimistic emphasis on what the patient can do and will be able to do in the future. When a patient has difficulty coping with the physical and psychosocial effects of a severe burn, effective nursing intervention can help the patient deal with his fears, anxieties, and sense of loss. Assist the patient through the grief process. Encourage the patient to relate what is experienced and his feelings about what has happened or is happening. Also encourage him to ask questions and to verbalize his concerns about the care and the treatment plan. The nurse can reinforce the patient's self-esteem by emphasizing the strengths the nurse has noticed when the patient was coping with pain, inconvenience, or some other unpleasant situation. Involving the patient in performing self-care as much as possible and giving some sense of control over the situation are helpful.

The patient's body image may have been severely disrupted. Assist the patient to grieve over the loss and integrate the present body image. If the burns were caused by a suicide attempt or a risky behavior, psychiatric therapy will probably be necessary to deal with feelings of guilt. A psychiatric clinical nurse specialist should be consulted to help the staff and the patient work through the complex psychological issues (Klein, 2009). Referrals to a psychologist, psychiatrist, social worker, or religious leader may also be necessary.

 Clinical Cues

Noise, lights, or certain people—visitors or staff—may be very irritating to the patient; these factors usually can be adjusted. If the patient is unhappy about being isolated, bringing in a television, radio, computer games, and books may help.

Patient-Family Education

The patient and family are taught about daily skin and wound care before discharge. They must be familiar with dressing instructions, lubrication of grafts, and donor site care. Moisturizing with an alcohol-free skin moisturizer is necessary at least three times a day. Pressure dressings or garments must be worn for 23 hours daily. Direct sunlight should be completely avoided for 1 year after injury because of increased sensitivity to ultraviolet rays.

Medication dosages, precautions, and potential side effect information are sent home with the patient. Nutritional needs and particular diet recommendations are discussed. Adequate protein and calories are very important to full recovery. Referral is made to support groups or peers and counseling as needed for readjustment to life after the burn incident. The need for follow-up care is stressed, and appointment dates and times are established. See Nursing Care Plan 43-1 for interventions for selected problems in a burn patient.

Evaluation

Although the physician chooses the type of medication to be applied topically or administered systemically for pain, infection, and wound healing, the nurses are responsible for continued assessment of the burn wounds to evaluate the effectiveness of the prescribed treatments. The nurse should perform a systematic and ongoing assessment of scar tissue formation and evaluate if the patient is making an adjustment to the fact that burn scars may take as long as 12 to 24 months to mature completely. If outcomes are not being met, interventions are changed.

COMMUNITY CARE

Nurses in the community can do much to educate the public about the dangers of unprotected sun exposure and the signs of skin cancer. Nurses vigilantly assess changes in skin lesions that may indicate cancer. Skin self-screening is taught at every opportunity.

School nurses perform assessments for signs of lice and scabies. They teach families how to deal with these problems and how to prevent their spread.

One of the objectives for *Healthy People 2020* is to reduce the number of hospitalizations for older adults that result because of pressure ulcers; therefore nurses employed outside the hospital setting are tasked with the challenge of prevention. Long-term care nurses must promote good skin integrity in all residents, handling the elderly with special care so as not to tear the skin. Patients who are immobile are turned diligently to prevent pressure ulcers, and skin is inspected regularly. Home care nurses can encourage elderly patients to use skin emollients to moisten and protect the skin.

Teaching fire safety to children and parents and to workers in various occupational settings helps to decrease fire injury. Home care nurses must continually assess patient homes for fire dangers and reinforce teaching to prevent home fires.

Get Ready for the NCLEX® Examination!

Key Points

- Dermatitis causes erythema and itching; a thorough history is necessary to locate the offending agent. Teach to avoid causative factors and how to apply topical medications.
- Acne often occurs at puberty; there is an accumulation of sebum and dead skin cells, which causes an inflammatory reaction. Drying agents that cause peeling work best to rid the skin of blackheads and whiteheads.
- There is a genetic predisposition to psoriasis, which appears as inflamed, edematous skin lesions with adherent silvery white scales. It can be controlled, but not cured.
- Stevens-Johnson syndrome is a potentially life-threatening allergic reaction usually triggered by medication.
- Hospitalized patients with bacterial skin infections require contact isolation.
- Viral skin disorders are caused by herpesviruses.
- Herpes zoster lesions follow nerve pathways; it is a very painful condition, and postherpetic neuralgia can occur. Anyone who has not previously had chickenpox or the immunization should not care for a patient with herpes zoster.
- Fungi prefer warm, moist places; for example, tinea pedis is one of the most common fungal infections and occurs on the feet.
- Treatment of pediculosis and scabies requires treating both the patient and objects that may harbor the parasites.
- Exposure to ultraviolet radiation (sunlight) is a major cause of skin cancer. Encourage use of a hat and sunglasses, and sunscreen with UVB protection and a sun protection factor (SPF) of 30.

- Skin cancer has increased in incidence, but is highly curable if treated in the early stages. All patients should be screened for skin cancer lesions and taught prevention measures and self-screening.
- Basal cell, squamous cell, and melanoma are the usual carcinomas arising from the epidermis.
- Actinic keratoses are a premalignant lesion common on the skin of older adults.
- If squamous cell carcinoma is not treated early, it can become invasive and metastasize.
- Melanoma is the most aggressive of the skin cancers and needs to be treated early to prevent metastasis.
- Pressure ulcers are a potential problem for all immobile patients. Assessment includes risk factors and staging. Pressure ulcers should be measured and documented on discovery and then measured and documented regularly to show progress in healing. Treatment depends on the stage and location.
- Burns are caused by extreme heat, hot liquids, electrical agents, strong chemicals, or radiation. Treatment is based on classification.
- Burn care is divided into phases: emergency care, emergent care, acute care, and rehabilitation. Pain control is a major concern in every phase.
- Burn patients must be assessed for signs of respiratory problems. Suspect an inhalation injury if there are burns on the face or neck, singed nasal hair, darkened membranes in nose or mouth, or a history of burn in a small space.
- With a major burn, fluid shifts can cause hypovolemic shock. Early fluid resuscitation is essential to prevent death.

- Burn care is aseptic. Eschar must be removed and wounds must be débrided. Débridement can be very painful, but is essential for healing and prevention of infection. Contracture prevention begins at the time of admission; special splints and positioning are used to preserve anatomical alignment.
- Early grafting with biologic or synthetic substances helps burn wounds heal more quickly. When skin grafts are healed, pressure dressings or garments are used to prevent excessive scarring.
- Burn patients can have problems with body image and also experience grief, loss, anger, or depression.

Additional Learning Resources

SG Go to your Study Guide for additional learning activities to help you master this chapter content.

e**volve** Go to your Evolve website (http://evolve.elsevier.com/deWit/ medsurg) for the following FREE learning resources:
- Animations, audio, and video
- Answers and rationales for questions and activities
- Concept Map Creator
- Glossary with pronunciations in English and Spanish
- Interactive Review Questions and Exercises and more!

 Online Resources
- Acne and Rosacea, www.acnesociety.org
- American Burn Association, www.ameriburn.org
- American Cancer Society, www.cancer.org
- American Melanoma Foundation, www.melanomafoundation.org
- Melanoma Education Foundation, www.skincheck.com
- National Cancer Institute, www.cancer.gov
- National Pressure Ulcer Advisory Panel, www.npuap.org

Review Questions for the NCLEX® Examination

1. In managing dermatitis, the nurse provides which instruction(s)? *(Select all that apply.)*

    1. Avoid the irritant or allergen.
    2. Provide adequate skin lubrication.
    3. Wash skin frequently with germicidal soaps.
    4. Maintain skin moisture.
    5. Apply steroid-based preparations.

2. A teenager is diagnosed with acne vulgaris. What information should be included in the patient education regarding acne vulgaris? *(Select all that apply.)*

    1. Acne vulgaris results from accumulations of sebum in occluded sebaceous glands.
    2. Acne vulgaris is caused by increased levels of androgens and fluctuating premenstrual hormones.
    3. Application of heavy creams and heat exposure contribute to the development of acne.
    4. Alcohol, caffeine-containing foods, spicy foods, sunlight, and emotional stress cause flare-ups.
    5. These lesions are not a sign of uncleanliness.

3. A male patient has inflamed, edematous skin of the elbows and knees accompanied by swelling of the joints of the fingers and toes. On examination, the skin is covered with adherent silvery white scales. Which question would provide more information regarding the patient's condition?

    1. "What do you do for a living?"
    2. "How much do you smoke?"
    3. "Have you had an upper respiratory tract infection recently?"
    4. "Have you recently changed your laundry detergent?"

4. A patient has skin lesions on the face, trunk, palms, extensor surfaces of joints, soles of the feet, and dorsum of the hands. On inspection, the lesions have irregular borders and blistered, necrotic centers. The physician makes the medical diagnosis of Stevens-Johnson syndrome. What is the priority nursing diagnosis for this patient?

    1. Disturbed body image
    2. Self-care deficit
    3. Risk for infection
    4. Acute pain

5. The nurse is developing a plan of care for a wheelchair-bound patient. To prevent development of pressure ulcers, which nursing interventions must be implemented? *(Select all that apply.)*

    1. Maintain postural alignment.
    2. Use pressure-relieving devices.
    3. Teach to shift weight every 15 minutes.
    4. Use donut-type devices.
    5. Reposition in the chair every hour.

6. The nurse notes a reddened area on the patient's sacral area and checks for blanching. What is the best rationale that supports this nursing action?

    1. Blanching suggests that the redness is probably temporary and will resolve when the pressure to the area is relieved.
    2. Checking for blanching is part of the daily routine for assessing any patient who is at risk for pressure ulcers.
    3. Evidence of blanching indicates that the patient is at high risk for a pressure ulcer according to the Braden scale.
    4. Occurrence of blanching indicates that the redness is associated with a localized skin infection.

7. The nurse is caring for a 50-kg burn victim who has a calculated 30% burned total body surface area. According to the Parkland formula, what is the rate of infusion for lactated Ringer's solution during the first 8 hours?

    1. 38 mL/hr
    2. 188 mL/hr
    3. 250 mL/hr
    4. 375 mL/hr

8. While performing the initial assessment, the patient with extensive burn injuries suddenly develops increasing hoarseness and stridor. Pulse oximetry is 86%. What is the priority nursing action?

   1. Encourage the patient to take deep breaths.
   2. Provide humidified oxygen.
   3. Administer respiratory treatments.
   4. Suction respiratory secretions.

9. A school-age girl with evidence of severe itching in the scalp is checked for pediculosis. The nursing diagnosis of *Deficient knowledge* related to unfamiliarity with managing the disease is identified for the child and the parent. What instructions would the nurse include? *(Select all that apply.)*

   1. "Machine wash clothes and bedding using the cold cycle."
   2. "Share combs and hairbrushes with family members, but not with friends."
   3. "Soak all combs and brushes in very hot water for more than 5 minutes."
   4. "Seal items that cannot be washed in air-expelled plastic bags for 14 days."
   5. "Reinfestation is unlikely if all family members are treated."

10. Place the patients in order from 1 to 4 (1 being the highest risk, 4 having the lowest risk) for their risk for developing a pressure ulcer based on the Braden scale.

    1. _____Elderly patient who is NPO for procedure; able to independently ambulate and accomplish ADLs
    2. _____Patient who is paraplegic, well nourished, with strong upper body strength to self-transfer to wheelchair
    3. _____Thin elderly patient who walks occasionally, but has limited mobility and cognitive impairments; reluctant to eat
    4. _____Patient who is comatose and unresponsive after a near-drowning accident; receives enteral feedings and is incontinent

Critical Thinking Activities

Scenario A

Mrs. Nash, age 32, has been assigned as your patient on the evening shift. She has severe dermatitis, which is probably allergic in origin. Her physician has ordered a topical lotion, dermatologic baths twice a day, and an antihistamine to relieve itching.

1. What kinds of data would you include in your ongoing assessment of Mrs. Nash's skin disorder?

2. What nursing care problems is Mrs. Nash likely to present?

3. What objectives and nursing measures to meet them would you include in Mrs. Nash's nursing care plan?

4. What would you teach Mrs. Nash about the application of topical agents when she returns home?

Scenario B

Ms. Moore, age 22, was badly burned when her clothing caught fire while she was grilling hamburgers on her patio. She has partial-thickness and full-thickness burns over her abdomen and down the front of both upper legs.

1. What is the priority of care after assessment when Ms. Moore reaches the emergency department?

2. What nursing measures should be taken to prevent infection of her burns?

3. What nursing measures would be included in the patient's nursing care plan to ensure that she did not suffer from an undetected fluid and electrolyte imbalance?

4. How is Ms. Moore's pain treated? Why?

5. List some specific things you and the other nurses could do to help her handle her sense of loss and altered self-image as a result of the appearance of the burns and scars.

Scenario C

Mrs. Chaco is an elderly patient who was admitted to your unit for dehydration and malnutrition. She responds to verbal commands, but seems somewhat confused by your questions. She will quietly sit in a chair, with some movement of her arms, but makes no attempts to walk or stand. She can feed herself, but her appetite and food and fluid intake are very poor. She has had one episode of incontinence with a scant amount of dark yellow urine.

1. Rate this patient's risk for pressure ulcers using the Braden scale.

2. Discuss interventions that you will use to address her positioning and apparent lack of spontaneous mobility.

3. Discuss interventions that you could use to address her nutritional issues.

4. What instructions will you give to the nursing assistant about cleaning the skin?

Care of Patients During Disasters, Bioterrorism Attacks, and Pandemic Infections

Objectives

Theory

1. Analyze differences between an emergency situation and a disaster.
2. Discuss an emergency preparedness plan for a health care facility.
3. Compare the stages of psychological response that occur with a disaster.
4. Compare and contrast the parameters used in the triage system for victims after a disaster versus the routine triage that occurs in hospital emergency departments.
5. Identify responsibilities and duties of the nurse in the care of disaster victims.
6. Explain safety measures to be employed for a chemical emergency.
7. Demonstrate knowledge of measures to be taken in the event of a nuclear disaster.
8. Explain warning signs that suggest a bioterrorism attack has occurred.
9. Differentiate the signs and symptoms of the various agents that could be used for a terrorist attack.
10. Synthesize the importance of debriefing of health care personnel after a disaster.

Clinical Practice

1. Participate in a disaster drill.
2. Teach a group of adults how to prepare safe water after a disaster has disrupted the water supply.
3. Identify the measures you would take for your own safety when assisting others after a disaster has occurred.

Key Terms

bioterrorism (p. 1010)
debriefing (p. 1016)
decontamination (dē-kŏn-tăm-ĭ-NĀ-shŭn, p. 1009)
disaster (p. 997)

mass casualty (p. 999)
pandemic (p. 1015)
surge capacity (p. 1000)
triage (TRĒ-ăhzh, p. 999)

DISASTER PREPAREDNESS AND RESPONSE

An extraordinary event, such as a multivictim incident involving an explosion or a train crash, requires a rapid and skilled response to manage the wounded. There may be walking wounded, critically wounded, and fatally wounded victims. This type of event usually can be handled by the community's emergency medical services and the hospital emergency departments.

A disaster **exists when the number of casualties exceeds the resource capabilities of the area;** thus the community's existing emergency resources may be overwhelmed. Natural disasters include epidemics, earthquakes, explosions, hurricanes, tornadoes, fires, and floods. Intentional terrorist attacks or accidental man-made disasters may result from transportation incidents or events involving chemical, biologic, or nuclear materials. A disaster causes mass casualties, psychological as well as physical trauma, and permanent changes within the community.

The governmental agencies for disaster planning are the Department of Homeland Security, the Office of Domestic Preparedness, and the U.S. Public Health Service. The American Red Cross is a voluntary organization that traditionally provides the basic essentials of shelter, food, and first aid during a natural disaster (Figure 44-1). In most communities, the local Office of Emergency Services (OES), the Red Cross, and the Salvation Army work together to formulate disaster plans. They coordinate their services with each other and with other agencies in planning for essential services, such as shelter, transportation, communication, and welfare. The Centers for Disease Control and Prevention (CDC) has a website with information on all types of disasters, weather events, and mass casualty events.

Special courses in civil defense and disaster nursing are usually offered by the OES, the Red Cross, and professional organizations. These courses help nurses and

FIGURE 44-1 September 19, 2005. A Red Cross volunteer checks on a resident affected by the extreme heat in Algiers, Louisiana, after Hurricane Katrina. © American Red Cross.

volunteer workers to understand the function and co-ordination of agencies involved in a particular type of disaster. To increase availability of volunteer health care professionals, registries such as the Emergency Systems for Advance Registration of Volunteer Health Professionals (ESAR-VHP) have been designed to pro-actively verify credentials, provide disaster response training, and coordinate deployment of professionals in conjunction with local, state, and national response plans. Such programs are intended to avoid the chaos of disaster and the underutilization of skilled volun-teers (Peterson, 2006).

? Think Critically

Consider your current level of nursing knowledge and your personal circumstance at home to include your family, pets, and any preparations that you have (or have not!) made for a disaster event. What would be your reaction if your instructor called you and asked you to help because of a local environmental disaster?

Whether the disaster is natural or related to war, it will involve physical injuries, loss of property, and interruption of the normal activities of daily living. People often will need food, clothing, shelter, medical and nursing or hospital care, and other basic necessi-ties of life.

Disaster supplies, with all the recommended items, should be prepared by every household.

Every family should have a contact person out of the geographic area where extended family members can call to receive information about the welfare of their relatives. Communication into and out of the disaster region is often cut off. Each member of a family living together should know whom they are to call if sepa-rated from one another.

🏃 Health Promotion

Preparing Disaster Supplies

Community members should be encouraged to prepare for a disaster. Preparations should include a minimum of 3 days' supplies. At a minimum, have the basic supplies listed below. Keep supplies in a kit that you can use at home or take with you in case you must evacuate.

- Water in plastic containers (1 gallon per person per day). Change the supply every 6 months.
- Nonperishable food that requires no refrigeration, prepara-tion, or cooking and little water, including:
  - Ready-to-eat canned meats, fruits, and vegetables
  - Canned juices, milk, and ready-to-eat soups
  - Sugar, salt, pepper
  - Peanut butter, jelly, crackers, granola bars, trail mix
  - Foods for infants or elderly on special diets
  - Hard candy, instant coffee, tea bags, cookies in tins
- Disposable dishes and eating utensils, or camping or military "mess kit"
- Flashlight
- Battery-operated or hand-crank radio (NOAA Weather Ra-dio, if possible)
- Extra batteries
- First aid kit containing an assortment of bandages, scissors, tweezers, needle, antiseptic, thermometer, and moistened towelettes
- Supply of essential prescription medications
- Nonprescription drugs: pain reliever, antacid, vitamins, laxa-tive, anti-inflammatory agents
- Sanitation and personal hygiene items (e.g., hand sanitizer, soap, disinfectant wipes)
- Copies of personal documents (medication list and pertinent medical information, proof of address, deed/lease to home, passport(s), birth certificate(s), insurance policies, copies of insurance cards and official identification)
- Cell phone with chargers
- Family and emergency contact information
- Extra cash or traveler's checks
- Emergency blanket
- Map(s) of the area
  Consider the needs of all family members and add supplies to your kit:
- Medical supplies (hearing aids with extra batteries, glasses, contact lenses, syringes, cane)
- Baby supplies (bottles, formula, baby food, diapers)
- Games and activities for children
- Pet food, water, and medications
- Two-way radios
- Extra set of car keys and house keys
- Manual can opener
  Additional supplies to keep at home or in your kit, based on the types of disasters common to your area:
- Whistle
- N-95 or surgical masks
- Matches in waterproof container
- Rain gear
- Towels
- Work gloves, disposable gloves
- Tools/supplies for securing your home: shut-off wrench to turn off household gas and water, multipurpose tool, utility knife, pliers, scissors

- Type ABC fire extinguisher: ordinary combustibles (type A), flammable liquids (type B), and electrical equipment (type C)
- Jacket, hat, change of clothes, sturdy shoes
- Tube tent and blanket or sleeping bag
- Plastic sheeting and duct tape
- Household liquid bleach
- Entertainment items
- Paper and pencil
- Aluminum foil
- Signal flare

Some agencies advocate keeping a 3- to 6-week supply of food and water on hand. Food items should be used and replaced every 6 months to maintain freshness.

Data from American Red Cross (2010). *Be Red Cross ready.* Available at www.redcross.org/www-files/Documents/pdf/Preparedness/checklists/Be_Red_Cross_Ready.pdf.

Most people know about these recommendations, but few are truly prepared. In fact, one of the barriers of disaster preparedness, at all levels, is an underlying belief that "it probably won't affect me" (Legg, 2009). At the system level, disaster events are viewed as "low risk" with "high impact" (Ahmad, 2009); thus administrators may be reluctant to divert time, money, and attention to disaster preparedness when health care systems are strained by the daily workload. All nurses must encourage people in the community to prepare. You should *proactively* (take it upon yourself to) seek out disaster training at your work setting and advocate for sufficient emergency supplies and support.

 Think Critically

You have just started your new nursing job. During your orientation and preceptorship you do not receive any training about the hospital's disaster plan or what your role would be as a staff nurse. What should you do?

COMMUNITY PREPAREDNESS

The law enforcement agency, the city or county emergency management department, and the state public health department are responsible for coordinating efforts to assist people when a disaster happens. The American Red Cross may disperse personnel and supplies to assist with essential needs and medical care. If the state requests assistance, Homeland Security determines if the Federal Emergency Management Agency (FEMA) is to be called. If so, FEMA brings personnel and aid to the area. If a disaster is of major proportions, a Disaster Medical Assistance Team (DMAT) may be activated at the state or federal level. These units bring medical, paraprofessional, and support personnel along with medical equipment and supplies to sustain an operation for a minimum of 72 hours. The team provides triage (sorting out of casualties by priority of need for treatment), evacuation,

primary health care, and assistance to local health care facilities that are overwhelmed. The emergency management team sets up a communications system, and the emergency medical services (EMS) personnel at the scene notify the emergency departments at the hospitals of the situation. With pagers, telephone trees, and instant computer alert messages, essential personnel are notified of a disaster or mass casualty (many-victims incident).

Community residents are instructed about what to do in the event that an earthquake, wildfire, hurricane, tornado, or flood occurs in their area.

 Safety Alert

Fire

In the event of a wildfire, if told to evacuate, leave quickly. If at home and the smoke detector goes off, do not wait to dress or gather belongings—get out of the dwelling. If fire or smoke is evident, drop to the floor and crawl to the exit. Cover your mouth and nose with a moistened cloth if smoke is present. Feel any door before opening it. If it is hot, find another way out. If clothes catch on fire, drop to the ground and roll to suffocate the fire. Keep rolling until flames are out.

 Safety Alert

Earthquake

If an earthquake strikes and you are indoors, stay there. Get under a desk or table, or stand in a corner or door frame. Cover your head with your arms. If outdoors, get into an open area away from trees, buildings, walls, and power lines. If driving, pull over to the side of the road and stop away from trees, buildings, and power lines. Stay inside the vehicle. If you are in a crowded public place, do not rush for the doors. Move away from display shelves containing objects that could fall and large-pane windows. If you are in a high-rise building, stay away from windows and outside walls. Avoid using the elevators. Get under a table or desk. After the shaking has stopped, assist those injured, applying first aid as needed. Do not use the telephone unless there is a life-threatening injury or fire. If uninjured, check for gas leaks. If you find any, turn off the utility at once. Turn off water if water pipes are broken. Turn on the portable radio for instructions and news reports.

Safety Alert

Tornado, Hurricane, and Flood

Choose ahead of time where you could go if evacuation is necessary. Evacuate when you are told to do so. Listen to a National Oceanic and Atmospheric Administration (NOAA) Weather Radio or local radio or television stations for evacuation instructions. Keep a road map handy because you may have to take unfamiliar routes. Take these items with you:
- Prescription medications and medical supplies, glasses, hearing aid, and other assistive devices
- Bedding and clothing, including sleeping bags and pillows

Continued

Safety Alert

Tornado, Hurricane, and Flood—cont'd

- Bottled water, battery-operated radio and extra batteries, first aid kit, and flashlight
- Maps and documents, such as driver's license, Social Security card, proof of residence, insurance policies, wills, deeds, birth and marriage certificates, and tax records, if they are readily available within the home

Patient Teaching

Preparing for a Hurricane

People living in a hurricane-prone area should be taught to prepare a disaster kit and keep it refreshed every 6 months.
When a hurricane "watch" is issued:
- Bring inside any outdoor furniture, trash cans, potted plants, toys, and the like that could be picked up by the wind.
- Protect the windows with hurricane shutters or ½-inch outdoor plywood boards.
- Fill your car's gas tank.
- Have cash on hand.
- Check batteries and stock up on canned food, first aid supplies, drinking water, and medications.
- Do not stay in a mobile home.
When a hurricane "warning" is issued:
- If not advised to evacuate, stay inside and away from windows.
- Be aware that the calm "eye" of the storm is deceptive. The worst winds will blow from the opposite direction once the "eye" passes over.
- Be alert for flying debris. Stay in a room, bathroom, or closet with no windows.
After the hurricane passes:
- Stay away from floodwaters once the hurricane is past. Do not drive through flowing water. If the water is rising, go to higher ground immediately.
- Do not let children play in the floodwater.
- Stay away from standing water as there may be a downed power line touching it.
- Use tap water for drinking and cooking only when local officials say it is safe.

Adapted from National Oceanic and Atmospheric Administration. *Hurricanes: Unleashing Nature's Fury.* Available at www.weather.gov/om/brochures/hurr.pdf.

If advised to evacuate the area, residents should gather essential belongings, medications, pets, and keepsakes and leave immediately. If tornado sirens are sounded, people should take refuge in a basement or in an inner room without windows, such as a closet or a bathroom, to avoid flying debris. Getting into the bathtub and covering oneself with cushions or a mattress can also protect a person from flying debris. If outside, it is best to lie in a culvert or ditch below ground level.

HOSPITAL PREPAREDNESS

The Joint Commission requires that hospitals have an emergency preparedness plan in place. There are guidelines for emergency preparedness by type of facility. Emergency department physicians undergo formal training for disaster events. Emergency department nurses are encouraged to obtain certification in emergency preparedness. Health care systems must self-evaluate surge capacity, which is defined as the maximum services that a facility can offer when every resource is mobilized (Barishansky & Langan, 2009); therefore the emergency plan should be tested with drills at least twice a year.

The emergency preparedness plan will identify who will be in charge and the chain of command for the facility. The designated communications officer is responsible for internal communication, such as keeping the staff informed, and for external communication, such as contacting other agencies for help, or reporting data about infection or chemical contamination that could have widespread effects (Rebmann, 2009). There will be a hospital incident commander (physician or administrator) who assumes responsibility for launching the emergency preparedness plan. This person's role as commander is to view the entire situation, to bring in needed human and supply resources, and facilitate the flow of patients through the system. Usual hospital routine will be altered to accommodate care for high numbers of patients. Departmental roles will be changed. Physical therapy and other departments may close down usual operations and become the minor treatment area for the nonurgent patients. The concept of "reverse triage" or sending relatively stable patients home can be used to free up beds. Using an evidence-based computer model, researchers determined that any patient who had a 12% or less risk for an adverse event within the next 4 days could be discharged under disaster circumstances (Kelen et al., 2009).

A medical command physician will focus on determining the number, acuity, and medical needs of the casualties arriving from the scene of the disaster. This person will organize the emergency health care team response to the injured or ill patients. Specialists trained for the particular type of disaster will be called in to help as the need is foreseen. Decisions will be made about who is to be evacuated to a facility with a higher level of care.

A triage officer, usually a physician, with the assistance of triage nurses, will rapidly evaluate each patient at the hospital and send the patient to the appropriate area for immediate or eventual treatment. The emergency department supervisor or charge nurse collaborates with the medical command physician and triage officer to organize nursing and ancillary personnel to meet patient needs. A telephone tree will be activated to call in off-duty staff. In addition to these personnel, there will be a supply officer, communications officer, infection control officer, and public information officer. The public information officer will manage the media. Hospital staff, at all levels, will be called on to assist with whatever care is needed. Long-term care facilities may need to evacuate residents, or they may need to take in people from other facilities or the community.

 Think Critically

If a disaster occurred in your community and you were not injured, where would you call, or go, to see how you could help?

PSYCHOLOGICAL RESPONSES TO DISASTER

Any intense event results in an emotional response. Natural disasters or massive injuries from a man-made event have both physical and emotional effects. The phrase "they are in shock" is used to explain the emotional state of the victims following one of these events. Although emotions can trigger physical signs and symptoms, the condition is usually not life threatening unless the individual affected has a preexisting condition that puts her at risk.

Signs and symptoms of emotional shock include headaches, nausea, and chest pain. Preexisting medical conditions may worsen due to the stress. Remaining calm and seeing to immediate physical needs can reassure the victim that someone is in charge that has control over the situation. Severe emotional trauma, such as post-traumatic stress disorder, may take years of therapy to process.

Following a major disaster, psychological events occur in stages (Crisis Management Consultants, 2010):

- *Impact stage.* Survivors are stunned, apathetic, and disorganized. For several hours after the initial event, they may have difficulty following directions and will need strong support and firm guidance.
- *Heroic stage.* Individuals want to be helpful, and may minimize or ignore their own injuries and demonstrate rescue behavior that is risky to self.
- *Honeymoon stage.* Survivors are grateful that they are still alive. There is a strong sense of brotherhood and community spirit.
- *Disillusionment stage.* Reality of loss occurs. Ongoing physical and emotional fatigue can result in

substance abuse and discouragement. Survivors feel abandoned and ignored by the larger community because of the gap between resources and need.

- *Reconstruction stage.* This stage may continue for years as people rebuild lives and even begin to see the crisis, in retrospect, as a growth and opportunity period.

TRIAGE

After a disaster, care of victims is prioritized according to a triage system that is different from regular emergency department triage (Table 44-1). Those victims with life-threatening conditions and a good chance of survival are cared for first. **When there are more victims of a disaster than medical personnel to treat them, those who are likely to survive are treated first; these patients are given red, yellow, or green tags (some classification systems may also include a white tag). The mortally wounded and those who are not expected to survive are attended later, and these patients are issued a black tag** (Figure 44-2). The choice of issuing tags is difficult for most nurses, but in a disaster, the good of many must prevail over benefit to the few.

Even though triage may have been done in the field, triage is performed again at the emergency care facility. Green-tagged patients usually comprise the greatest number in large-scale disasters. Patients need to be managed until they are able to be treated. If not managed, patients can become a health hazard by walking around with infection, radioactivity, or chemical contamination. A special bracelet with a disaster number may be applied to tagged patients.

 Think Critically

Are you and your family prepared for a disaster? Do you have a disaster kit on hand? If you have children, do you have measures in place for their care by others if you are unable to reach them? Is there an out-of-state contact person for family to call and inform of their status?

Table 44-1 **Disaster Triage System**

CLASSIFICATION	TRIAGE TAG	TYPICAL CONDITIONS	TREATMENT
Class I: Emergent	Red tag	Immediate threat to life, such as airway compromise or hemorrhagic shock	Immediate
Class II: Urgent	Yellow tag	Major injuries, open fractures, large wounds	Within 30 min to 2 hr
Class III: Nonurgent	Green tag	"Walking wounded" (closed fractures, sprains, strains, contusions)	Wait for more than 2 hr
Class IV: Minor	White tag	Minor injuries not requiring physician care (abrasion, bruises)	Dismiss
Class V: Dead or expected to die	Black tag	Dead, or imminently dying with little chance of survival	None

Stoppler, M.C. (2007). Medical triage: code tags and triage terminology. *Medicinenet.com*. Available at *www.medicinenet.com/script/main/art.asp?articlekey=79529*.

FIGURE 44-2 Example of triage tags.

Nursing Roles and Responsibilities During Disaster

Your basic nursing skills will serve you well if you are called on to work under disaster conditions; for example, you could be asked to:

- Perform emergency nursing measures.
- Evaluate the environmental and physical risks and shortages (e.g., no electrical power).
- Know measures for prevention and control of environmental health hazards (e.g., hand hygiene and food and water safety.)

Other responsibilities require specialized knowledge that is not part of a nurse's routine daily job. You must study this material now and review it periodically before a disaster happens.

- Be prepared for self-survival (i.e., stock your own household with emergency supplies).
- Know the disaster plan for your workplace and identify your duties accordingly.
- Know the meaning of warning signals of disaster and the action to be taken.
- Know measures for protection against radioactive, chemical, or biologic contamination.
- Know the community disaster plans and community health resources.
- Know and interpret community resources for citizen preparedness, such as first aid and medical self-help courses.

During emergency care, you will perform needed procedures such as inserting catheters, nasogastric tubes, and possibly intravenous (IV) lines and drawing blood. In many types of disasters outside the hospital you may need to improvise because of lack of equipment. Basic principles of nursing apply in a disaster, but adaptation to "crisis standards" is necessary if there is a disparity between need and availability of equipment, supplies, or personnel. You may be called on to exercise leadership and judgment in determining the condition of each victim, using supplies and equipment, and detecting changes in the environment that might be hazardous. Performing nursing procedures in a disaster situation demands skill and judgment to provide for the good of the greatest number of people. You may be asked to help cook, serve food, pass out water, or do whatever else is a priority need at the time. Proactive development and understanding of crisis standards, to include an ethics committee, is recommended (Rebmann, 2009).

The U.S. Department of Health and Human Services recommends that nurses be skilled in the following areas if they are to be involved in providing health care during a disaster:

- Participating in planning and providing care for large groups of people under extreme duress in various types of disaster situations
- Developing and revising nursing procedures aimed at providing comfort and safety during and after a disaster
- Knowing your own limitations and seeking help as needed

Observing, recording, and reporting information about patients to appropriate authorities must be done in an organized manner. General physical and mental conditions of patients and signs and symptoms that may indicate change in condition must be quickly identified. During a disaster, preventing the spread of infection is a primary nursing concern. Table 44-2 identifies the communicable diseases that can become epidemic after a disaster. Infection control is a top priority when large groups of people are together in a shelter because the incidence of communicable disease is much greater. Although the National Patient Safety Goal is intended for the prevention of health care–related infections under normal circumstances, hand hygiene has an even greater potential as a basic infection control measure to protect large groups of people that may gather together after a disaster.

The emotional and physical comfort and safety of large numbers of disaster victims must be attended to with limited supplies, equipment, utilities, and personnel. You must understand the emotional stress caused by: fear, problems of displacement and separation of families, personal and material losses, crowded living conditions, increasing anxiety, and continuing danger. You will need to help people of different cultural backgrounds and religious beliefs accept and adapt to temporary living conditions in crowded and often adverse

situations (Legg, 2009). Encourage people to verbalize their concerns and fears. **In a disaster situation, the nurse should provide basic instructions about appropriate self-care within the current environment and encourage people to provide for their own needs.**

Care of Special Populations

Ideally, there should be a community database that includes the needs of vulnerable groups (elderly, disabled, and immunocompromised persons) that require special assistance, because a delay can result in death. Loss of electrical power is a serious issue for those who require oxygen or other life-sustaining mechanical equipment (Drill, 2009). The elderly may be without their prescriptions for chronic or other serious health conditions. Eyeglasses or hearing aids may be lost, and many elderly cannot see or hear well without these aids. Developmental concerns should be considered; for example, infants need diapers, formula, bottles, and powdered milk. Infants are especially vulnerable to diarrhea and dehydration related to contaminated water sources.

The disabled may need a means of mobility if they are separated from their belongings. They may need assistance with bathing, eating, and general activities of daily living. Immunocompromised people need special attention and care to prevent infection when in large crowds. You can direct people to where they can obtain assistance, or you may obtain needed items for them.

Water and Food Safety

Disruption or contamination of the water supply is probable when a disaster occurs. Floodwater or storm water should not be used to wash dishes, brush teeth, wash and prepare food, wash hands, make ice, or make baby formula. People have to be taught how to purify water.

 Health Promotion

Preparing Safe Water

When the normal water supply is disrupted, water may be purified by:

- Bringing it to a rolling boil for 3 to 5 minutes. Let the water cool before drinking.
- Adding household liquid bleach containing 5.25% sodium hypochlorite. Add 16 drops of bleach to a gallon of water and let stand for 30 minutes.
- Distilling the water. To distill, fill a large pot halfway with water. Tie a cup securely to the handle on the pot's lid so that the cup will hang right side up when the lid is upside down. Set the lid upside down on the top of the pot so that the cup hangs down into the pot below the lid (the cup should not dangle in the water). Boil the water for 20 minutes. The water that drips from the lid into the cup is distilled. This method frees water of microbes that may remain after bleach treatment.

Data from United States Environmental Protection Agency (EPA). (2011). *Ground water and drinking water.* Retrieved from http://safewater.supportportal.com/ics/support/default.asp?deptID=23015; American Red Cross. (2009). Be Red Cross ready–*Get a kit. Make a plan. Be informed.* (Brochure). Washington, D.C.; Federal Emergency Management Agency (FEMA) and American Red Cross (2004). *Food and water in an emergency.* (Brochure). Jessup, MD.

Table 44-2 Communicable Diseases with Epidemic Potential (All Except Tetanus) in Natural Disasters

DISEASE	TRANSMISSION	AGENT	CLINICAL FEATURES	INCUBATION PERIOD	DIAGNOSIS	TREATMENT	PREVENTION/CONTROL
Waterborne							
Cholera	Fecal/oral, contaminated water or food	Vibrio cholerae serogroups O1 or O139	Profuse watery diarrhea, vomiting	2 hr-5 days	Direct microscopic observation of V. cholerae in stool	Intensive rehydration therapy; antimicrobials based on sensitivity testing	Hand hygiene, proper handling of water/food and sewage disposal
Leptospirosis	Fecal/oral, contaminated water	Leptospira species	Sudden-onset fever, headache, chills, vomiting, severe myalgia	2-28 days	Leptospira-specific IgM serologic assay	Penicillin, amoxicillin, doxycycline, erythromycin, cephalosporins	Avoid entering contaminated water; safe water source
Hepatitis	Fecal/oral, contaminated water or food	Hepatitis A and E viruses	Jaundice, abdominal pain, nausea, diarrhea, fever, fatigue, and loss of appetite	15-50 days	Serologic assay detecting anti-HAV or anti-HEV IgM antibodies	Supportive care; hospitalization and barrier nursing for severe cases; close monitoring of pregnant women	Hand hygiene, proper handling of water/food and sewage disposal; hepatitis A vaccine
Bacillary dysentery	Fecal/oral, contaminated water or food	Shigella dysenteriae type 1	Malaise, fever, vomiting, blood and mucus in stool	12-96 hr	Suspect if bloody diarrhea; confirmation requires isolation of organism from stool	Nalidixic acid, ampicillin; hospitalization of seriously ill or malnourished; rehydration	Hand hygiene, proper handling of water/food and sewage disposal
Typhoid fever	Fecal/oral, contaminated water or food	Salmonella typhi	Sustained fever, headache, constipation	1-3 days	Culture from blood, bone marrow, bowel fluids; rapid antibody tests	Ampicillin, co-trimoxazole, ciprofloxacin	Hand hygiene, proper handling of water/food and sewage disposal; mass vaccination in some settings
Acute Respiratory							
Pneumonia	Person to person by airborne respiratory droplets	Streptococcus pneumoniae, Haemophilus influenzae, or viral	Cough, difficulty breathing, rapid breathing	1-3 days	Clinical presentation; culture respiratory secretions	Co-trimoxazole, chloramphenicol, ampicillin	Isolation; proper nutrition; if cause is Streptococcus, polyvalent vaccine to high-risk populations
Direct Contact							
Measles	Person to person by airborne respiratory droplets	Measles virus (Morbillivirus)	Rash, high fever, cough, runny nose, red and watery eyes; serious postmeasles complications (5%-10% of cases)—diarrhea, pneumonia, croup	10-12 days	Generally made by clinical observation	Supportive care; proper nutrition and hydration; vitamin A; control fever; antimicrobials in complicated cases with pneumonia, dysentery; treat conjunctivitis, keratitis	Rapid mass vaccination within 72 hr of initial case report (priority to high-risk groups if limited supply); vitamin A in children 6 mo–5 yr of age to prevent complications and reduce mortality risk

Disease	Transmission/Source	Causative Agent	Signs and Symptoms	Incubation	Diagnosis	Treatment	Prevention
Bacterial meningitis (meningococcal meningitis)	Person to person by airborne respiratory droplets	Neisseria meningitides serogroups A, C, W135	Sudden-onset fever, rash, neck stiffness; altered consciousness; bulging fontanel in patients less than one year	10-12 days	Examination of CSF—elevated WBC count, protein; gram-negative diplococci	Penicillin, chloramphenicol, ampicillin, ceftriaxone, cefotaxime, co-trimoxazole; supportive therapy; diazepam for seizures	Rapid mass vaccination
Wound-Related							
Tetanus	Soil	Clostridium tetani	Difficulty swallowing, lockjaw, muscle rigidity, spasms	2-10 days	Entirely clinical	Tetanus immune globulin	Thorough wound cleansing, tetanus vaccine
Vector-Borne							
Malaria	Mosquito (Anopheles species)	Plasmodium falciparum, P. vivax	Fever, chills, sweats, head and body aches, nausea and vomiting	7-30 days	Parasites on blood smear observed using a microscope; rapid diagnostic assays if available	Chloroquine, sulfadoxine-pyrimethamine	Mosquito control; insecticide-treated nets, bedding, clothing
Dengue fever	Mosquito (Aedes aegypti)	Dengue virus-1, -2, -3, -4 (Flavivirus)	Sudden-onset severe flulike illness, high fever, severe headache, pain behind the eyes, and rash	4-7 days	Serum antibody testing with ELISA or rapid dot-blot technique	Intensive supportive therapy	Mosquito control; insecticide-treated nets, bedding, clothing
Japanese encephalitis	Mosquito (Culex species)	Japanese encephalitis virus (Flavivirus)	Quick-onset, headache, high fever, neck stiffness, stupor, disorientation, tremors	5-15 days	Serologic assay for JE virus IgM-specific antibodies in CSF or blood (acute phase)	Intensive supportive therapy	Mosquito control, isolation of cases, mass vaccination
Yellow fever	Mosquito (Aedes, Haemagogus)	Yellow fever virus (Flavivirus)	Fever, backache, headache, nausea, vomiting; toxic phase—jaundice, abdominal pain, kidney failure	3-6 days	Serologic assay for yellow fever virus antibodies	Intensive supportive therapy	Mosquito control, isolation of cases, mass vaccination

CSF, cerebrospinal fluid; ELISA, enzyme-linked immunosorbent assay; HAV, hepatitis A virus; HEV, hepato-encephalomyelitis virus; IgM, immunoglobulin M; JE, Japanese encephalitis; WBC, white blood cell.
From Waring, S.C., & Brown, B.J. (2005). The threat of communicable diseases following natural disaster: A public health response. Disaster Management and Response, 3(2), 44-45.
Copyright © 2005 with permission from the Emergency Nurses Association.

Box 44-1	Keeping Food Safe to Eat

Perishable foods should not be held above 40° F (4.4° C) for more than 2 hours. A refrigerator will ordinarily keep food chilled to below 40° F for 2 to 4 hours. It is wise to have a quick-response digital thermometer on hand. If a power outage occurs, do the following:

- Keep the refrigerator and freezer doors closed. A freezer that is half full will keep food safe for up to 24 hours; a full freezer will keep food safe for 48 hours.
- If it appears that the outage will be for more than 2 to 4 hours, pack refrigerated milk, dairy products, mayonnaise, meats, fish, poultry, eggs, gravy, stuffing, and leftovers into coolers and surround them with ice.
- When uncertain as to how long the power has been out, check the internal temperature of foods in your refrigerator with the quick-response thermometer. If the internal temperature is above 40° F, throw the food away.
- Throw away food that may have come into contact with flood or storm water.
- Throw away food that has an unusual odor, color, or texture.
- Food containers with screw-on caps, snap-on lids, crimped caps (beer bottles), twist-off caps, and snap-open caps, as well as home-canned foods, should be discarded if they have come into contact with floodwater because they cannot be disinfected.
- If cans have come into contact with floodwater or storm water, remove the labels and wash them with hot soapy water or dip them in a solution of 1 cup of bleach in 5 gallons of clean water. Relabel the cans with a marker.

Data from American Red Cross (2011). Food safety. Retrieved from www.redcross.org/portal/site/en/menuitem.d229a5f06620c6052b1ecfbf43181aa0/?vgnextoid=74f561150e8ae110VgnVCM10000089f0870aRCRD&vgnextchannel=74e51a53f1c37110VgnVCM1000003481a10aRCRD; American Red Cross (2009). Be Red Cross ready–Get a kit. Make a plan. Be informed. (Brochure. Washington, D.C.; and Federal Emergency Management Agency (FEMA) and American Red Cross (2004). *Food and water in an emergency.* (Brochure). Jessup, MD.

Healthy People 2020 objectives include improved food and water safety; during a disaster, special attention is required to safeguard food and water supplies. If there is a power outage, and people can stay in their homes, they will need to know how to keep their food supply safe to eat (CDC, 2011) (Box 44-1).

Nursing Management in the Reconstruction Stage

Working toward restoring community and family life after the disaster—according to available resources—involves the nurse and other members of the health care team. Individual self-help and work therapy are encouraged, as are activities of daily living, with adaptations designed to attain and maintain a clean and healthy environment. Existing community facilities and resources must be used as much as possible for continued patient care.

You can promote the effectiveness of the health service agency in disaster preparedness by knowing and interpreting the agency's disaster plan. Understand the relationship among the agency plan, the local government plan, and the community agencies' plans. Trying to maintain and restore community health by controlling environmental health hazards is an important responsibility for every nurse.

PREPARING FOR CHEMICAL, NUCLEAR, OR BIOLOGIC DISASTERS

CHEMICAL DISASTER

A chemical emergency can occur from a transportation accident, or an explosion at a chemical plant. Chemical agents such as the Sarin gas used in the Tokyo subway attack can also be used by terrorists. Awareness of a chemical attack or accident is difficult because most chemical agents vaporize quickly from their liquid form. A lesson learned during the Sarin attack is that chemical agents are difficult to identify and front-line staff are not always informed. At 8:28 A.M. the first victims began to arrive at the hospital and at 9:40 A.M. an expert in Sarin began treating patients with Sarin antidote, but police analysis of the chemical was not available until 11:00 A.M., and emergency staff members got that information by watching the television news (Powers, 2009).

Many chemical agents give off no odor or have a familiar odor such as that of onion, garlic, or almonds. Indications that a chemical attack has occurred might include (Peterman, 2010):

- Foglike or low-lying cloud suddenly appearing in the atmosphere
- Many dead birds, domestic animals, or insects within a particular area
- Many dead, dying, or sick people in an area or downwind from a suspicious cloud or fog
- An atypical, unexplained odor for the location

Chemical agents (Table 44-3) that might be used in a terrorist attack include pulmonary/choking agents, blood agents, vesicant (blistering) agents, and nerve agents (Science & Technology Review, 2010). Currently, Homeland Security considers cyanide (blood agent) to be one of the most likely substances to be used in an attack. Cyanide is plentiful and readily available, requires no special scientific or technical knowledge, is rapidly lethal, and treatment requires a large amount of a specific antidote (Emergency Nurses Association [ENA], 2010).

The public should be informed of what to do in the event of a chemical disaster.

Table 44-3 Chemical Agent Symptoms and Care

CLINICAL PRESENTATION	DECONTAMINATION PROCEDURES	TREATMENT
Vesicant Agents (e.g., phosgene, mustard, lewisite)		
Ocular: Eyelid swelling and inflammation, severe pain, conjunctivitis, and keratitis. *Dermal:* Pain, erythema, blisters, and burning followed by necrosis. *Respiratory:* Immediate upper airway irritation; burning of mucous membranes, laryngitis, shortness of breath, productive cough; inhalation and systemic absorption may cause pulmonary edema and death. *Gastrointestinal:* Nausea and vomiting, diarrhea, and abdominal pain. *Cardiovascular:* High-dose of lewisite exposure may cause capillary permeability and subsequent intravascular fluid loss, hypovolemia, and organ congestion. *Renal:* High levels of lewisite may cause renal failure caused by hypotension. *Hepatic:* High levels of lewisite may cause hepatic necrosis and hypoperfusion.	Decontamination for eyes must begin immediately by flushing eyes with water 5-10 min and skin to minimize tissue damage. Decontaminate before bringing into health care facility. Negative-pressure room if available. All clothing is removed and skin washed with soap and water. If showers are available, showering with water alone is adequate. Place contaminated clothing and personal belongings in biohazard bag. Contain decontamination runoff. Patients whose clothing or skin is contaminated can contaminate health care providers by direct contact or through off-gassing vapor.	*For phosgene:* Restrict fluids. Obtain chest radiographs and blood gases. Oxygen/PEEP. *For mustard:* Possible tracheostomy. Establish IV: Do not push fluids as with thermal burns. Drain vesicles and large blisters and irrigate with topical antibiotics. Antibiotic eye ointment. Morphine as needed (PRN). *For lewisite:* Treat affected skin with British anti-lewisite (BAL) ointment, if available. Treat affected eyes with BAL ointment, if available. Treat pulmonary symptoms. BAL deep IM; repeat q 4 hr × 3. Morphine PRN. Severe poisoning: shorten interval for BAL injections to q 2 hr.
Nerve Agents (e.g., Sarin)		
Respiratory: Bronchial constriction and spasm; severe respiratory distress or apnea; miosis; rhinorrhea. *Gastrointestinal:* Do not induce emesis.	Decontaminate before bringing into health care facility. Negative-pressure room. Contain decontamination runoff. Patients whose clothing or skin is contaminated with liquid or solid nerve agents can contaminate health care providers by direct contact or through off-gassing vapor. If exposed to liquid nerve agent, irrigate eyes 5-10 min with water or saline within minutes of exposure to limit injury. If exposed to liquid nerve agent, cut and remove all clothing and wash skin immediately with soap and water. If shower is not available, wash with 0.5% bleach solution. If exposed to vapor only, remove outer clothing and wash exposed skin with soap and water or 0.5% bleach solution. Place contaminated clothing and personal belongings in biohazard bags.	*Nerve agent protocol:* Intubate and ventilate as needed. Mark 1 antidote kits. Atropine. Pralidoxime chloride (2-PAM C1). Diazepam for seizures. Reevaluate q 3-5 min for worsening.
Blood Agents (e.g., cyanide)		
Dermal: Possible cherry red color to skin. *Respiratory:* Respiratory distress secondary to cellular hypoxia, tachypnea, dyspnea, bradypnea, apnea.	Decontaminate before bringing into health care facility. Negative-pressure room. Contain decontamination runoff.	*For cyanide:* Administer cyanide poisoning kit for significant cyanide toxicity and persistent high anion gap metabolic acidosis.

PEEP, positive end-expiratory pressure.

Continued

Table 44-3	Chemical Agent Symptoms and Care—cont'd	
CLINICAL PRESENTATION	**DECONTAMINATION PROCEDURES**	**TREATMENT**
Blood Agents—cont'd		
Cardiovascular: Dysrhythmias caused by acidosis. *Neurologic:* Syncope, seizures, lethargy, confusion, coma.	Patients whose clothing or skin is contaminated with cyanide can contaminate health care providers by direct contact or through off-gassing vapor. Patients exposed only to vapor require no decontamination. Avoid dermal contact with gastric contents that may contain ingested cyanide-containing materials. Remove contaminated clothing and wash with soap and water.	Amyl nitrite, sodium nitrite, sodium thiosulfate. Hydroxocobalamin. Sodium bicarbonate for acidosis.
Pulmonary/Choking Agents (e.g., chlorine)		
Acute exposure to gas can cause immediate coughing, eye and nose irritation, tearing. *Dermal:* Skin irritation, burning pain, inflammation, and blisters. Treat as thermal burns. Liquefied, compressed chlorine can cause frostbite. Treat by rewarming affected areas in a water bath of 102°-108° F (38.8°-42.2° C) for 20-30 min. Continue until flushing has returned to affected area. *Ocular:* Do not irrigate frostbitten eyes; if exposed to vapor, irrigate for at least 15 min; check for corneal damage. *Respiratory:* Airway constriction, pulmonary edema and hemoptysis may occur.	Health care providers are at minimal risk of secondary contamination from patients who have been exposed to chlorine gas. Remove contaminated clothing and wash with soap and water. Flush exposed skin and hair with plain water for 2-3 min; then wash twice with soap and water. Clothing or skin soaked with industrial strength bleach or similar solutions may be corrosive to personnel and may release chlorine gas.	*For chlorine:* Dyspnea. Oxygen by mask. Chest radiograph. Bronchodilators. Give supportive therapy and treat other problems.

! Safety Alert

Chemical Disaster

When a chemical disaster has occurred in your neighborhood, you should do the following unless you are told to evacuate immediately:

- Close all windows and doors to the dwelling.
- Turn off all fans, heaters, and air conditioning systems.
- Close the fireplace damper.
- Wet some towels and jam them in the cracks under the doors. Use plastic garbage bags or plastic sheeting and duct tape to cover doors, windows and skylights, electrical outlets, exhaust fans or vents, window air conditioners, and heat registers.
- Go to an above-ground room with the fewest windows and doors.
- Take your emergency kit and a portable radio with you.
- Stay inside until you are told all is safe or you are asked to evacuate.

Chemicals are dispersed as a gas or liquid or are aerosolized and may contaminate skin, clothing, and any object they touch. The vapor from a liquid or solid toxic chemical also is harmful. Those exposed to toxic chemicals should be decontaminated in the field before transport to a medical facility. Decontamination is usually done with running water and scrubbing. If not done in the field, decontamination should be done outside the medical facility.

The Tokyo Sarin attack highlights the importance of decontamination to protect staff and preserve the hospital environment: 110 staff members developed signs and symptoms of Sarin exposure; in a makeshift overflow area, 38 of 83 workers (45.8%) were exposed (Powers, 2009). In a small study, Brinker and colleagues (2009) found that emergency physicians and anesthetists had familiarity with personal protection equipment (PPE) for airborne diseases such as severe acute respiratory syndrome (SARS), but their knowledge of self-protection for chemical agents was lacking. Chemical warfare agents can produce immediate respiratory distress if inhaled; therefore respirator masks are essential. This research points out a need for ongoing staff education.

Patient Teaching

Removal and Disposal of Contaminated Clothing

If you are in an area where a chemical spill has occurred and the liquid or solid comes into contact with your clothing, you will need to (1) remove and bag contaminated clothing and (2) decontaminate your skin. Chemicals will penetrate the clothing and contaminate the skin. If the exposure to a chemical was by vapor (gas), you will only need to remove your clothing and the source of the toxic vapor. Perform the following steps:

- Quickly take off clothing that has a chemical on it. Any clothing that has to be pulled over the head should be cut off instead of pulling it over the head.
- When helping others remove clothing, be careful not to touch any contaminated areas. Remove clothing as quickly as possible.
- As quickly as possible, wash any chemicals from your skin with large amounts of soap and water. If the eyes are burning, rinse with plain water for 10 to 15 minutes.
- If contact lenses are worn, remove them and place with the contaminated clothing.
- After washing yourself, carefully place all contaminated clothing and contact lenses into a plastic bag. Avoid touching contaminated areas; use tongs, a stick, or a tool to place the clothing in the bag. Place the implement within the bag as well when finished using it.
- Thoroughly wash eyeglasses worn at time of chemical contamination before wearing again. Wash hands thoroughly again after cleaning glasses.
- Carefully seal the bag and place it within another plastic bag and seal the outer one.
- Dress in clothing that has not been contaminated (i.e., clothes that have been in the closet or dresser drawers).
- When health department or emergency personnel arrive, have them handle the bags and arrange for disposal.

Adapted from FEMA (2010). After a chemical attack. Available at: www.fema.gov/hazard/terrorism/chem/chem_after.shtm.

Depending on the chemical agent, there may be an antidote that can be used (see Table 44-3). Each hospital should have a set of protocols in place. Symptomatic supportive care is supplied with oxygen, IV fluids, and comfort measures.

NUCLEAR DISASTER

A nuclear disaster may be the result of an accident at a nuclear power plant, a disruption of a nuclear power plant by terrorists, or a nuclear or "dirty bomb" (one containing radioactive substances). The amount of damage to each person depends on the type of radiation, the dose received, the length of time of exposure, and the route of the exposure. **Time, distance, and shielding are key to the quantity of radiation an individual will receive.** The shorter the time of exposure, the farther away from the radiation source, and whether or not the person was shielded by materials that are impermeable to radiation are details pertinent to radiation risk (ENA, 2010) (see Chapter 8). Some types of radiation produce particles and other types produce rays. Particles will adhere to airborne dust particles, may be inhaled, and will settle on clothes, crops, water supplies, and other surfaces.

Decontamination is done with showering and scrubbing the skin to remove particles. Radiation exposure to rays does not require decontamination, although rays can cause serious health effects or death, as they do internal damage to tissues. However, if the exposure is from a terrorist attack, it would not be immediately known if the exposure to radiation was in the form of particles or rays. Therefore everyone exposed, or suspected of being exposed, will need to be decontaminated. Personnel performing triage and decontamination must be protected from radioactive particulates and contaminated dust (Figure 44-3).

Usually, specially trained units supply personnel to handle decontamination. Minimal protective equipment includes protective gear for clothes and shoes (Tyvek suit), double gloves (one under clothing and taped to the skin, and one over the clothing cuffs), and a high-efficiency particulate air (HEPA) respirator mask with a full facepiece. If no such mask is available, a fit-tested N-95 respirator mask such as used for tuberculosis precautions is better than no mask. Radiation detection badges are worn underneath the protective clothing. After disposing of the protective garb in specially marked biohazard containers, each person will be assessed to make certain radiation contamination has been eliminated (Radiation Emergency Medical Management, 2010b).

Exposure to high doses of radiation rays that penetrate the body even for a few minutes may result in acute radiation sickness syndrome. Three subsyndromes may be seen, depending on the dose of radiation received: bone marrow syndrome, gastrointestinal syndrome, and cardiovascular/central nervous system syndrome. Bone marrow tissue is affected first; then with increased dosage, the gastrointestinal lining is affected. The person who receives a high enough

FIGURE 44-3 Assisting a victim of a radioactive event to a decontamination showering area during a drill.

dose of radiation to cause cardiovascular/central nervous system syndrome will experience effects on the bone marrow and gastrointestinal system as well. The effects of radiation are progressive as the dosage increases. Signs and symptoms may include nausea, vomiting, diarrhea, leukopenia, signs of bleeding or hemorrhage, lethargy, confusion, ataxia, convulsions, hair loss, and respiratory complications with fever and pneumonia (Table 44-4). Treatment of life-threatening injuries takes precedence over the radiologic damage (ENA, 2010).

Once injuries are managed and decontamination is complete, nursing care is supportive, with strict infection control procedures in place. Maintaining an accurate record of the onset and duration of the clinical symptoms is essential for the physician to decide on treatment strategies. Record hair loss, inflamed mucosa, and locations of erythema hourly and, if possible, record skin symptoms with a camera. Serial blood counts will be performed. Nausea is treated with antiemetics. Blood problems may be treated with blood component transfusions.

When the radiation exposure has been in the form of particulates that have entered the body, treatment depends on the type of radiologic substance. The four types of agents used to reduce the radiation damage by reducing exposure to the radiologic substance are chelating agents, isotope-specific blocking agents, excretion agents, and diluting agents.

Chelating agents bind with the radioactive material and allow it to be excreted without being absorbed into the tissues. Radioactive iodine exposure is treated with potassium iodide, an isotope-specific blocking agent, to prevent the thyroid cancer this type of radiation causes. Excretion agents are used when radioactive material has been ingested; these reduce the time the radiologic material is in the gastrointestinal tract. Diluting agents reduce the concentration of the radioactive material. Water is the best example of a diluting agent. Special precautions need to be used when administering a mobilizing or diluting agent as the fluids produced could be radiologically contaminated (Radiation Emergency Medical Management, 2010a).

BIOLOGIC DISASTER

Bioterrorism involves the deliberate release of microorganisms or toxins derived from living organisms that cause disease or death to humans or animals or plants

Table 44-4	Acute Radiation Syndrome			
SIGNS AND SYMPTOMS*	**TIME OF ONSET***	**DURATION**	**TREATMENT**	
Initial or Prodromal (Dose Dependent)				
Nausea, vomiting, diarrhea Progressive cognitive impairment at high doses	Minutes to days after exposure	May last for several days	Serial CBC obtained every 2-3 hr for 8-12 hr; then every 4-6 hr for 2-3 days. Record all symptoms and time of onset (vomiting is correlated with prognosis). Fluids and antiemetics. Chelating, blocking, excretion, or diluting agents.	
Latent				
Feels and appears relatively healthy	Hours to weeks after prodromal phase		Patient education about significance of latent stage, need for infection control, and possible progression to phase of manifest illness. Continue to monitor for symptoms and CBC.	
"Manifest Illness" (Obvious Illness)				
Signs and symptoms leukopenia purpura, hemorrhage Pneumonia Hair loss Diarrhea, fever, electrolyte disturbance Convulsions, ataxia, tremor, lethargy	Hours-weeks	Hours to months	Supportive and symptomatic treatment. Isolation for leukopenia as needed. Possible stem cell replacement.	
Recovery or Death				
Death	Days to year Death may occur within 1-2 days at >3000 rads; death occurs 3 wk-6 mo at >200-600 rads		Educate those who recover about increased future risk for cancers and advise to have frequent health checkups.	

From ENA. (2010). *Sheehy's Emergency Nursing: Principles and Practice* (6th ed.). St. Louis: Mosby.
CBC, complete blood count; *rads*, unit of absorbed radiation dose.
*Progression through phases and symptoms depends on the dose and type of radiation received.
From ENA. (2010). *Sheehy's Emergency Nursing: Principles and Practice* (6th ed.). St. Louis: Mosby.

on which we depend for food. There are 180 potential pathogens that could be used (Ahmad, 2009); however, anthrax, plague, smallpox, botulism, viral hemorrhagic fevers, and tularemia are category A because they pose a threat to national security (Peterman, 2010). These organisms cause a high death rate and public panic and fear is likely to accompany any breakout. Relative to nuclear or explosive materials, pathogens are easily disguised and transported. In fact, the scenario of "suicide coughers" is considered a public health nightmare (Bhardwaj et al., 2009).

Biologic Agents

Biologic agents (Table 44-5) are divided into three groups (Centers for Disease Control and Prevention [CDC], 2010; Peterman, 2010):

- *Category A agents:* Easily disseminated, and some may be transmitted from person to person as well. These could cause mass casualties and require a well-organized and extensive health care system response for management.
- *Category B agents:* Delivered through water and food sources. These produce moderate amounts of illness and low death rates. Public health department action is needed for management. Examples are Q fever, brucellosis, glanders, ricin toxin, epsilon toxin of *Clostridium perfringens,* and *Staphylococcus aureus* enterotoxin B.
- *Category C:* Agents that have not been weaponized as yet, but have the potential for high morbidity

and mortality. These agents are plentiful and easy to produce and disseminate. Examples include *Hantavirus,* tick-borne encephalitis, yellow fever, and multidrug-resistant tuberculosis.

Symptoms from exposure to a biologic agent are not immediate. There are various incubation periods. So, unless someone knows that she has been exposed to a strange powder or substance, decontamination does not take place. Nurses particularly need basic knowledge about the category A agents because they are easily disseminated and spread from person to person.

Anthrax. Anthrax is a category A agent caused by the gram-positive bacteria *Bacillus anthracis,* which forms spores. It is primarily a disease of sheep and cows. Animal vaccination programs have controlled naturally occurring anthrax in the United States. There are three forms of the disease: cutaneous, gastrointestinal, and inhalational. Aerosolized inhalable anthrax is most likely to be used for a terrorist attack. The greatest chance of inhaling the spores after aerosolization is during the first day after the event, before the particles hit the ground. Symptoms in those who have inhaled the spores will resemble a nonspecific influenza at first. A rapid downhill progression is then seen with respiratory failure, shock, and possibly death over a 2- to 5-day period. Features that differentiate anthrax illness from flu are shortness of breath, a nonproductive cough, chest discomfort, myalgia, and fatigue. The lack of a sore throat and rhinorrhea and the appearance of

Table 44-5 Category A Agents of Bioterrorism

PATHOGEN AND DESCRIPTION	CLINICAL MANIFESTATIONS	TRANSMISSIBILITY	TREATMENT
Anthrax (Bacillus anthracis)			
Inhalational			
Bacterial spores multiply in the alveoli Toxins cause hemorrhage and destruction of lung tissue High mortality rate	Incubation period: 1-2 days to 6 wk Abrupt onset Dyspnea, diaphoresis, fever, cough, chest pain, septicemia, shock, meningitis, respiratory failure, widened mediastinum (seen on chest radiograph)	No person-to-person spread Found in nature and most commonly infects wild and domestic hoofed animals Spread through direct contact with bacteria and its spores Spores are dormant, encapsulated bacteria that become active when they enter a living host	Antibiotics prevent systemic manifestations Effective only if treated early Ciprofloxacin (Cipro) is the treatment of choice Penicillin Doxycycline Postexposure prophylaxis for 30 days (if vaccine not available) Vaccine has limited availability
Cutaneous			
95% of anthrax infections Least lethal form Toxins destroy surrounding tissue	Incubation period: up to 12 days Small papule resembles an insect bite Advances to a depressed, black ulcer Swollen lymph nodes in adjacent areas Edema	Spores enter skin through cuts or abrasions Handling of contaminated animal skin products	

From Lewis, S.L., Heitkemper, M.M., Dirksen, S.R., et al. (2011). *Medical-Surgical Nursing: Assessment and Management of Clinical Problems* (8th ed.). St. Louis: Mosby.
Continued

Table 44-5   Category A Agents of Bioterrorism—cont'd

PATHOGEN AND DESCRIPTION	CLINICAL MANIFESTATIONS	TRANSMISSIBILITY	TREATMENT
Anthrax (Bacillus anthracis)—cont'd			
Gastrointestinal			
Intestinal lesions in ileum or cecum Acute inflammation of intestines	Nausea, vomiting, anorexia, hematemesis, diarrhea, abdominal pain, ascites, sepsis	Ingestion of contaminated, undercooked meat	
Botulism (Clostridium botulinum)			
Spore-forming anaerobe Found in soil Seven different toxins Lethal bacterial neurotoxin	Incubation period: 12-72 hr Abdominal cramps, diarrhea, nausea, vomiting, cranial nerve palsies (diplopia, dysarthria, dysphonia, dysphagia), skeletal muscle paralysis, respiratory failure	Spread through air or food No person-to-person spread Improperly canned foods Contaminated water Contaminated wound	Induce vomiting Enemas Antitoxin Mechanical ventilation Penicillin No vaccine available Toxin can be inactivated by heating food or drink to 185° F (85° C) for at least 5 min
Plague (Yersinia pestis)			

Bacteria found in rodents and fleas
Forms
  Bubonic (most common)
  Pneumonic
  Septicemic (most deadly)
	Incubation period: 2-4 days
	Hemoptysis, cough, high fever, chills, myalgia, headache, respiratory failure, lymph node swelling
		Direct person-to-person spread
		Transmitted through flea bites
		Ingestion of contaminated meat
			Antibiotics only effective if administered immediately
			Drug of choice: streptomycin or gentamicin
			Vaccine under development
			Hospitalization
			Isolation for containment

Smallpox			
Variola Major and Minor Viruses			
United States ended routine vaccination in 1971 Global eradication declared in 1980	Incubation period: 7-17 days Sudden onset of symptoms Fever, headache, myalgia, malaise, back pain Lesions progress from macules to papules to pustular vesicles	Highly contagious Direct person-to-person spread Transmitted in airborne droplets Transmitted by handling contaminated materials (i.e., linens)	No known cure Cidofovir (Vistide) under testing Isolation for containment Vaccine available for those exposed Vaccinia immune globulin (VIG) available
Tularemia (Francisella tularensis)			
Bacterial infectious disease of animals Mortality rate about 35% without treatment	Incubation period: 3-10 days Sudden onset Fever, swollen lymph nodes, fatigue, sore throat, weight loss, pneumonia, pleural effusion, ulcerated sore from tick bite	No person-to-person spread Aerosol or intradermal route Spread by rabbits and ticks Contaminated food, air, water	Gentamicin treatment of choice Streptomycin, doxycycline, and ciprofloxacin are alternatives Vaccine in developmental stage
Hemorrhagic Fever			
Caused by several viruses, including Marburg, Lassa, Junin, and Ebola Ebola virus is life threatening	Fever, conjunctivitis, headache, malaise, prostration, hemorrhage of tissues and organs, nausea, vomiting, hypotension, organ failure	Carried by rodents and mosquitoes Direct person-to-person spread by body fluids Virus can be aerosolized	No intramuscular injections No antiplatelet drugs Isolation for containment Ribavirin (Virazole) effective in some cases No known treatment available

nausea and vomiting may occur with flu as well. Treatment is with ciprofloxacin (Cipro) or doxycycline (Vibramycin) for 14 days. Antibiotics are adjusted after culture and sensitivity results are known. Treatment continues for 60 days if infection is proven as the disease can continue to develop from germinating spores up to that time. Otherwise prophylaxis lasts for 10 to 14 days when cultures are completed and results obtained. Other care is supportive for respiration, fluid and electrolyte balance, and comfort. Extended precautions are not necessary as anthrax is not transmissible from person to person. There is a vaccine, but it is currently only available to persons with a high occupational risk for anthrax (Mosby's Nursing Consult, 2010) (see Online Resources).

Botulism. Botulism is a category A agent caused by the botulinum toxins produced by *Clostridium botulinum*. There are three forms of botulism: food-borne, wound, and inhalational. Foods can become contaminated with botulism spores when canned or processed under conditions favorable for toxin production (e.g., insufficient heat). Botulism is not contagious and the organism is destroyed by chlorine in water supplies or by boiling foods for 10 minutes (Mosby's Nursing Consult, 2010). Organisms are naturally present in the soil and can cause wound infection. Inhalational botulism does not occur naturally and would most likely indicate a terrorist attack.

Double vision, drooping eyelids, and difficulty swallowing and speaking may be the early symptoms of botulism. A triad of symptoms is classic for the disorder:

- Symmetrical descending flaccid paralysis progressing to respiratory weakness
- Absence of fever
- Alertness and orientation without sensory deficits

Respiratory support may require intubation and mechanical ventilation. If a large number of persons are infected, the community health care resources would be taxed to provide adequate care for all. Treatment is with botulinum antitoxin if the toxin type is A or B. The CDC and public health departments stock these antitoxins. Early treatment is required as the antitoxin does not reverse the muscular paralysis that has already occurred. The adult antitoxin costs about $25,000. Supportive therapy may be needed for several weeks until new synapses can grow to replace those damaged by the toxins (see Online Resources).

Plague. Plague is a category A agent caused by a gram-negative bacillus, *Yersinia pestis*. The bubonic form starts as a skin infection and spreads to the lymph nodes; it is naturally transmitted by infected fleas that bite rodents or people. Pneumonic plague is the most likely type to be spread by a terrorist attack with aerosolized plague organisms. Fortunately, plague bacilli are killed by sunlight and remain viable in aerosolized form for only about an hour after release. Clinical signs are an abrupt onset of pneumonia with bloody sputum *(hemoptysis)* that follows a rapidly progressive course. Disseminated intravascular coagulation (DIC) can develop leading to multiorgan system failure. Death is likely within 24 hours of infection if treatment is not started.

Gentamicin (Garamycin) is the drug of first choice for this organism. Ciprofloxacin and doxycycline are used to treat pneumonic plague and are given for 7 to 10 days. If treated early, the infection is usually not fatal. Plague can be transmitted from person to person, and respiratory droplet precautions along with Standard Precautions are necessary until 48 hours after treatment has been initiated. Researchers are currently working on a vaccine (Mosby's Nursing Consult, 2010).

Smallpox. Smallpox is caused by variola virus. It is communicable, has no known effective treatment, and has a high mortality rate. The disease was declared eradicated worldwide in 1980, but laboratory strains of the virus still exist. Because it is so lethal and highly contagious, it is listed as a category A agent.

Smallpox has an average incubation period of 12 to 14 days. Symptoms begin with fever for 1 to 4 days and then a rash occurs. High fever may be accompanied by headache, backache, malaise, vomiting, and delirium. The rash contains firm, deep-seated vesicles or pustules all in the same stage of development on any one area of the body (Figure 44-4). The rash starts on the buccal and pharyngeal mucosa, spreads to the face, hands, and forearms, and then spreads to the rest of the body over several days. A cough may develop. Lesions progress from macules to papules to vesicles to pustules to scabs, with each stage lasting 1 or 2 days. It must be differentiated from chickenpox. With chickenpox, the lesions appear before illness symptoms and are usually concentrated on the trunk. Chickenpox lesions are usually more superficial and are "flimsy," rather

FIGURE 44-4 Face lesions on a boy with smallpox.

than firm as in smallpox. Chickenpox lesions do not usually occur on the palms and the soles of the feet; smallpox lesions do occur in those areas (Figure 44-5). Chickenpox lesions are often in various stages within the same area of the body, whereas smallpox lesions are all in the same stage within a body area.

Smallpox is communicable from the onset of rash until all scabs have separated from the skin. Patients should be treated with strict Airborne Infection Isolation and Contact Precautions, and be placed in a negative-pressure room with an HEPA-filtered exhaust system. All linens and gowns *must* be incinerated to prevent spread of the disease.

Although there is no treatment for smallpox, receiving the smallpox vaccine within 4 days of exposure can reduce the severity of the disease. The vaccine is not available in large amounts, and for that reason isolation and quarantine of infected patients will be the most likely course of action. Smallpox vaccine has significant possible side effects. If health care workers are to be vaccinated, you will receive all the necessary information about the vaccine and how to take care of the vaccination site. Medical management is supportive, with antimicrobial drug treatment for secondary infection of lesion sites, fluid and electrolyte replacement, and nutritional therapy. Those vaccinated

FIGURE 44-5 Comparison of smallpox and chickenpox lesions. **A,** Smallpox. **B,** Chickenpox.

against smallpox before 1972 have no immunity now. The vaccine provides immunity for only 3 to 5 years, but those who had multiple vaccinations may have some residual immunity.

[?] Think Critically

Can you explain to someone how to distinguish smallpox lesions from those of chickenpox?

Tularemia. Tularemia is a category A agent caused by a gram-negative coccobacillus, *Francisella tularensis*. It is a vector-borne illness that is transmitted by an infected tick, mosquito, or deer fly bite, by direct exposure to contaminated animal tissues and fluids, or by ingestion of contaminated food or water. A variety of small mammals are natural reservoirs of the organism. It is seen throughout the United States except in Hawaii. If aerosolized, it could be inhaled, and this is the most likely form for a terrorist attack. The disease is not spread by person-to-person contact.

Tularemia occurs in three different forms: cutaneous, pneumonic, and typhoidal. The pneumonic form is the one most likely to occur in a terrorist attack. The pneumonia caused by the inhaled form is difficult to differentiate from other pneumonias. Symptoms include abrupt onset of fever, chills, headache, muscle aches, nonproductive cough, and sore throat. Laboratory testing can establish the correct diagnosis.

Treatment or prophylaxis is with streptomycin and gentamicin, the drugs of first choice. Doxycycline, chloramphenicol (Chloromycetin), and ciprofloxacin may also be used. The course of treatment should extend through 10 to 14 days depending on the drug used. Tularemia is fatal if not treated with the proper antibiotics. Standard Precautions are used, but the inhalational form is not transmitted by person-to-person contact and no other extended precautions are necessary. A vaccine for protection from tularemia is under review by the U.S. Food and Drug Administration.

Viral Hemorrhagic Fevers. The hemorrhagic fevers are a group of illnesses caused by four families of viruses: arenaviruses, filoviruses, flaviviruses, and bunyaviruses. The viruses, which are within the category A agents, cause Ebola, Marburg, and Lassa hemorrhagic fevers. Junin, Machupo, Guanarito, and Sabia hemorrhagic fevers occur more frequently in the Southern Hemisphere. There are no vaccines available for these diseases. These occur in different geographic parts of the world. Reservoirs for the viruses are rodents and arthropods. Human infection usually occurs by being bitten by an infected arthropod, by contact with infected animal carcasses, or by inhaling aerosolized rodent excreta. Once contracted, the virus can be transmitted from person to person by blood and body fluids. Contact and Airborne Infection Isolation Precautions are necessary. Only special biosafety laboratories can test for the viral hemorrhagic fevers. Such tests are performed at the CDC. It is thought that an aerosolized form of Ebola or Marburg virus might be used for a terrorist attack. Travelers from a region experiencing an outbreak could also carry the virus into other countries (CDC, 2011).

The incubation period is from 2 to 42 days, depending on the virus, and there is a prodromal syndrome lasting less than a week. Signs and symptoms are marked fever, fatigue, dizziness, muscle aches, and loss of strength. Symptoms may progress to abdominal pain, nonbloody diarrhea, weakness, and exhaustion. Later bleeding begins, starting with bleeding under the skin and petechiae and progressing to spontaneous bleeding and DIC. Many body systems are affected. Hypotension, conjunctivitis, pharyngitis, plus skin rash may reflect increasing capillary permeability. Shock, nervous system malfunction, seizures, delirium, and coma may occur. Mortality rates can be very high with Ebola, but are not always so with the other viruses.

There is no specific treatment for these hemorrhagic fevers; treatment is supportive. The antiviral ribavirin may be useful in treating Lassa fever. Contact and Airborne Expanded Precautions are essential. Double gloves, impermeable gowns, leg and shoe coverings, face shields, eye protection, and an N-95 mask are required for patient contact. A negative-pressure room is desirable.

Prevention measures include use of insect repellant, bed nets, window screens, and proper clothing, and the eradication of rodents from living spaces. Mosquito abatement is performed in areas of outbreak, when possible. All linens and gowns used for patient care must be incinerated.

PANDEMIC INFLUENZA INFECTION

Pandemic infection is an international outbreak of disease. Experts at the CDC indicate that an influenza epidemic is a naturally occurring event that eventually is going to happen (Chappell & Bridges, 2009). Most of us have had firsthand experience with the flu, but the H1N1 (swine) flu episode in 2009 heightened our awareness of how readily a disease moves back and forth across international borders. The SARS outbreak in China made health care professionals feel particularly vulnerable to airborne respiratory infections (see Chapter 15).

A report from the state of New York suggests that equipment and staffing issues may exist if H5N1 (avian flu) occurs. The population of New York is 19 million, and there are 3981 intensive care (ICU) beds; 15% of H5N1 victims will require ICU care. There are 6100 ventilators, and 85% of those ventilators are in use at any one time; three times as many ventilators would be needed for pandemic flu. Most of the deaths

(70%) related to flu will occur in the hospital. Furthermore, by 2025 there will be a nationwide shortage of 500,000 nurses (Donnellan, 2009). Equipment and staffing issues are likely to be much worse for areas in the world with limited resources.

Preparations for pandemic flu include teaching people to be prepared to stay at home for at least 2 weeks. Nurses also need to reassure people that basic measures for prevention of respiratory infection can be effective. These include healthy lifestyle to support the immune system, hand hygiene, covering the mouth during coughing or sneezing, disposing of tissues, and staying away from public places if at all possible (Donnellan, 2009).

Nurse's Role in Preparedness and Response

In addition to learning about hospital protocols, community resources, and specific knowledge related to disaster care, you should explore your feelings about professional participation in a disaster event. Under normal circumstances, such as caring for HIV/AIDS patients, a nurse's duty to care is high, because the risk of harm to self is low; however, when the danger to the nurse is unclear or apparent—such as in the SARS outbreak—the nurse could decide that preservation of self is reasonable (Twedell, 2009). In a small study of nurses' intention to respond to a biological disaster, those with dependent children and more nursing experience were less likely to respond. Nurses said they were more likely to respond if the cause of the disease was known and treatable and if personal protection equipment was available. Also, those with emergency or disaster experience were more likely to respond (Grimes & Mendias, 2010). Arming yourself with knowledge, preparing your own household, and having ethical discussions with colleagues will help you in your decision-making process.

The nurse's role during a bioterrorism event includes:

- Recognizing clusters of cases or unusual cases suggestive of a biologic event
- Promptly evaluating and assisting with medical management
- Promptly communicating with the local public health department and infection control department
- Working closely with law enforcement, emergency management, public health, and other government agencies

Recognizing a Bioterrorism Event. Many of the likely bioterrorism agents do not produce symptoms right away. Certain signs or events may present a warning that a bioterrorism attack has occurred. Some of the signs include (Peterman, 2010):

- Rapidly progressing flulike illness, particularly in the young and among those previously healthy

- Rapidly progressive respiratory illness, especially in young, previously healthy people
- Unusual or extensive rashes, especially if preceded by flulike symptoms
- Flaccid muscle paralysis
- Severe bleeding disorders
- A large group of patients with food-borne illness
- Sudden death of many animals in the community

Nursing Management. When such patterns are discovered, implement the hospital and community response plan. **Strictly adhere to infection control procedures and policies.**

If your assessment has aroused suspicion of a biological event, ask these questions:

- Was there a sudden onset of severe respiratory or gastrointestinal problems?
- Has the illness progressed rapidly?
- Has the patient been healthy otherwise?
- Are the patient's family, friends, or colleagues ill?

If the answers indicate that an infectious agent is present, immediately take the following steps:

- Notify your supervisor and the infection control department of the situation.
- Put a surgical mask on any patient who is coughing.
- Pay strict attention to Standard Precautions and hand hygiene, and encourage the patient and family to do the same.
- Wear an N-95 or P-100 respirator mask (one certified by the Occupational Safety and Health Administration [OSHA]).
- If indicated, isolate the patient in a negative-pressure room; obtain specimens for laboratory testing.
- Use all recommended personal protective equipment whenever caring for the patient, and pay strict attention to Standard and Expanded Precautions.

When a known terrorist airborne event has occurred and victims are triaged to the hospitals and to emergency field medical units, victims will need to be decontaminated before being brought into the medical facility. Outside shower areas will be set up to accomplish the decontamination. Whether the agent used in the attack is biologic or nuclear, the outside of the body must be thoroughly scrubbed. Personnel in biohazard suits handle this task (Figure 44-6). Clothing must be removed and sealed in plastic biohazard bags to prevent contamination of others. The skin should be scrubbed in every area with warm soapy water for at least 30 seconds. The hair should be soaped and shampooed several times.

FIGURE 44-6 Personnel wearing biohazard suits perform a decontamination scrub during a hospital bioterrorism drill.

In a crisis situation, give firm directions with a kindly tone. Let people know what will happen next. Active listening and assisting with problem solving provide needed psychosocial support. If a family has been separated, help locate children and other family members. Direct people to available support services to meet physical and psychological needs.

Debriefing. Critical incident stress debriefing (CISD) teams provide sessions for small groups of personnel to help with effective coping strategies. After the turmoil and the emotional impact of the disaster, including its aftermath, personnel may find it difficult to return to their normal routine. Without intervention, some may develop post-traumatic stress disorder (see Chapter 46). There is strict confidentiality and unconditional acceptance of any information shared during the sessions. Participants are encouraged to bond by talking about where they were and what they were doing when they first heard about the disaster, and to describe what they saw, heard, or smelled during the event; they are asked to share how they felt during the event, discuss how they feel now, and encouraged to describe physical symptoms that have occurred since the incident. Facilitators reassure that strong reactions are normal, and they offer coping strategies. These coping strategies may include avoiding use of alcohol or drugs, eating a well-balanced diet, watching for obsessing or fixation, taking time off from work, socializing with friends and co-workers, and getting help if necessary.

Get Ready for the NCLEX® Examination!

Key Points

- A disaster exists when the number of casualties exceeds the resource capabilities of the area.
- Nurses should be proactive in being familiar with the facility's disaster plan, in encouraging people to stock a disaster kit at home, and teaching the public about what to do when a disaster occurs (see Health Promotion on p. 998).
- A chain of command is set in place when a disaster occurs, and it must be followed to ensure that appropriate notification and information is provided to the Office of Emergency Services.
- The stages of psychological response include impact, heroic, honeymoon, disillusionment, and reconstruction.
- Triage for a disaster is based on saving those with life-threatening conditions and a likelihood of survival first.
- Reverse triage can be used to increase surge capacity.
- First aid, safety measures, and prevention and control of health hazards are priorities.
- Special populations such as the elderly, infants, disabled, and immunocompromised individuals need help to stay safe and meet basic life requirements.
- Teach people how to purify water (see Health Promotion on p. 1003).
- Knowledge of food safety when there has been a power outage or a flood is essential (see Box 44-1).
- Warning signs that a bioterrorism event has occurred include rapidly progressing flulike illness, respiratory illness in otherwise healthy young people, unusual rash, paralysis, bleeding disorders, outbreaks of food-borne illness, and sudden death of animals.
- Decontamination of individuals affected by a chemical, radiologic, or bioterrorism event is performed before they are allowed into the health facility.
- Debriefing by a trained team after a disaster helps prevent long-term psychological problems among the personnel involved in caring for people affected by the event.

Additional Learning Resources

SG   Go to your Study Guide for additional learning activities to help you master this chapter content.

 evolve   Go to your Evolve website (http://evolve.elsevier.com/deWit/medsurg) for the following FREE learning resources:
- Animations, audio, and video
- Answers and rationales for questions and activities
- Concept Map Creator
- Glossary with pronunciations in English and Spanish
- Interactive Review Questions and Exercises and more!

Online Resources
- Anthrax, www.bt.cdc.gov/agent/anthrax
- American Red Cross, www.redcross.org
- Botulism, www.bt.cdc.gov/agent/botulism
- Chemical agents, www.bt.cdc.gov/planning/personalcleaningfacts.asp
- Safety Kits, www.ready.gov/build-a-kit
- Weather Safety, www.nws.noaa.gov/safety.php/brochures/hurr.pdf

Review Questions for the NCLEX® Examination

1. A large number of patients are arriving at the hospital from the scene of a chemical disaster. What is the nurse's priority action?
   1. Take vital signs to determine which patients are in distress.
   2. Call poison control for assistance in determining antidotes.
   3. Decontaminate all patients outside the hospital by showering.
   4. Instruct all caregivers to don personal protective equipment.

2. At a disaster scene, the nurse notices that a person has been triaged with a black tag who has respiratory distress and severe total body burns. What should the nurse do?
   1. Immediately obtain a portable oxygen tank and apply an oxygen mask.
   2. Seek out emergency services personnel to transport patient to the hospital.
   3. Try to locate family members so that they can be present when the person dies.
   4. Stay with the person for as long possible to give support and comfort.

3. The nurse is participating in a disaster drill. A mock victim with a green tag asks, "What does this tag mean?" What is the nurse's best response?
   1. "You can go home because you no longer need health management."
   2. "You potentially pose a health hazard so you must sit in the green area."
   3. "You will have to remain in waiting room for approximately 6 hours."
   4. "You will be seen and treated immediately by a physician."

4. While admitting a young, previously healthy patient with a severe respiratory illness, the nurse becomes suspicious of a bioterrorism event. Which question would the nurse ask to confirm the suspicion?
   1. "Have you been washing your hands frequently?"
   2. "Has the illness progressed rapidly?"
   3. "Have you had flulike symptoms?"
   4. "Are you a local resident?"

5. A patient is tentatively diagnosed with chickenpox. During skin assessment, what is the nurse likely to find that confirms the diagnosis?
   1. Skin lesions are firm.
   2. Skin lesions are found on palms and soles.
   3. Skin lesions occur in various stages.
   4. Skin lesions occur with other signs and symptoms.

6. The nurse is teaching a group of people about water and food safety following a disaster. Which comment by an audience member indicates a need for additional teaching?
   1. "Contaminated water should be boiled for at least 20 minutes."
   2. "Sixteen drops of bleach to a gallon of water will purify the water."
   3. "A full freezer will keep food safe for 48 hours."
   4. "Any food that has an unusual odor, color, or texture should be thrown away."

7. Which patient needs to be put immediately into isolation?
   1. Diagnosed case of botulism poisoning
   2. Probable case of inhalational anthrax
   3. Known exposure to a high dose of radiation rays
   4. Suspected smallpox, but probable chickenpox

8. Which behavior by the nurse indicates that there is a need for additional counseling beyond the counseling offered through a critical incident stress debriefing?
   1. Talks openly about the incident, but is not ruminating
   2. Avoids coworkers and friends for a prolonged period
   3. Takes extra vacation time away from the city
   4. Attempts to resume a healthy lifestyle, but is not sleeping well

9. In the event of a hurricane watch, which measure(s) must be done? *(Select all that apply.)*
   1. Bring inside any outdoor furniture, trash cans, potted plants, toys, and the like that could be picked up by the wind.
   2. Fill your car's gas tank and sit in the car until the threat passes.
   3. Have cash on hand.
   4. Check batteries and stock up on canned food, first aid supplies, drinking water, and medications.
   5. Look out the window to watch for the "eye" of the storm.

10. There is a power outage and the IV pumps are no longer functional. The nurse must deliver a fluid bolus of 500 mL over 20 minutes. The drip factor for available IV tubing is 10 gtt/mL. What is the drip rate in drops/minute? _____

Critical Thinking Activities

Scenario A
A hurricane has hit the town in which you live. There is widespread wind damage in much of the town, many streets are flooded, and a lot of people are injured. The power is out and the phones are dead. Your neighbor has a gash in his lower leg and is bleeding.

1. Describe how you would stop the bleeding.

2. How would you transport him to a health care facility? What precautions would you take on the journey?

3. If teenagers want to go out and wade in the floodwater and see if they can rescue stranded people or animals, what would you tell them?

Scenario B
You and several other health professionals have been asked to come and teach a community group about what to do in the event of a disaster or bioterrorism attack.

1. Outline what should be included in the teaching plan.

2. If questions arise about a nuclear disaster, what would you say about measures they could take?

Scenario C
You are working in a busy walk-in clinic. You recognize that emergency departments and clinics are likely to be the first places where infected people will begin to show up if there is a biologic event. You must be vigilant for clusters of cases or unusual cases that may suggest that a bioterrorism event has occurred among the population that serves the clinic.

1. What signs or events would suggest that a bioterrorism event has occurred?

2. What assessment questions would you ask if you suspect a patient has been exposed to a bioterrorism agent?

3. If you determine that an infectious agent is likely, what should you do?

Care of Patients with Trauma or Shock

Objectives

Theory

1. List the basic principles of first aid.
2. Summarize the importance of mechanism of injury and index of suspicion in caring for patients with traumatic injury.
3. State the key components of assessing a trauma patient.
4. Discuss prevention of injuries from extremes of heat and cold.
5. Describe specific interventions in the emergency care of accidental poisoning by ingestion and inhalation.
6. Describe emergency care of victims of insect stings, tick bites, and snakebites.
7. Review the appropriate nursing actions and care needed for the patient who has experienced a respiratory or cardiac arrest.

8. Identify signs and symptoms of shock.
9. Compare and contrast the treatment of cardiogenic, hypovolemic, and neurogenic shock.
10. Evaluate how your personal attitudes, beliefs, and values affect your ability to care for victims of abuse.

Clinical Practice

1. Observe how the triage nurse in the emergency department sets priorities for patient care.
2. Observe how the emergency team works together on a major accident victim.
3. Role play with fellow students, practicing techniques to calm a combative patient.

Key Terms

anaphylaxis (ă-nă-fă-LĂK-sĭs, p. 1031)
angioedema (ăn-jē-Ō-ĕ-DĒ-mă, p. 1036)
automated external defibrillator (AED) (ĂW-tō-mā-tĕd ĕks-tĕr-năl dē-fĭb-rĭ-LĀ-tŏr, p. 1033)
C-A-B (chest compressions, airway, breathing) (p. 1032)
flail chest (p. 1032)
hands-only CPR (p. 1032)
hypovolemia (hī-pō-vō-LĒ-mē-ă, p. 1033)
index of suspicion (p. 1022)
mechanism of injury (p. 1022)

multisystem organ dysfunction syndrome (MODS) (p. 1038)
perfusion (pĕr-FŪ-zhŭn, p. 1033)
poison control center (p. 1029)
push hard, push fast (p. 1033)
shock (shŏk, p. 1033)
systemic inflammatory response syndrome (SIRS) (p. 1038)
triage (TRĒ-ăhzh, p. 1022)
vasoactive (vă-zō-ĂK-tĭv, p. 1036)

PREVENTION OF ACCIDENTS

HOME SAFETY

According to statistics compiled by the National Safety Council (2010), accidents in the home account for one half of all unintentional injury deaths. People under 5 and over 65 years of age are the principal victims of fatal mishaps occurring in the home. The two most dangerous rooms in the house are the kitchen and the bathroom (Box 45-1).

HIGHWAY SAFETY

Motor vehicle accidents are the leading cause of accidental death in the United States. Improper driving, which is responsible for almost 90% of all accidents, can be caused by the influence of alcohol and/or drugs, fatigue, excessive speed, distractions, or emotional instability. Emphasis on using seatbelts, better enforcement of laws against driving drunk, and discouraging use of cell phones have helped to decrease accidents. Improvements in emergency medical services (EMS) and care of accident victims have significantly decreased vehicular deaths.

WATER SAFETY

Water safety rules include selecting safe swimming areas, ensuring supervision of children and adults who are not strong swimmers, diving where the water is sufficiently deep and is free of rocks or obstacles, never swimming alone, and avoiding swimming distances beyond one's ability. **The victim of a diving injury preferably should not be removed from the**

Box 45-1 | Home Safety

KITCHEN
- For a gas, coal, or wood-burning stove have vents or flues; keep windows open a crack. Never light the stove with kerosene or gasoline. Turn off all flames after cooking. Repair any gas leakage.
- Use pot holders. Keep handles of pots and pans turned away from edge of stove.
- Keep matches, sharp instruments, and poisons, such as bleach and household cleansers, out of children's reach. Place child safety locks on storage cabinets.
- Wipe up spills on floor.
- Keep electrical appliances in good working order.
- Place broken glass in a heavy paper sack to prevent cuts through plastic bags.

STORAGE AREAS
- Always keep cellars, attics, and garages neat.
- Clean and disinfect the area where garbage is kept, and dispose of garbage frequently.
- Never place poisonous substances in drinking glasses, cold drink bottles, or other containers that have been used for food or drink.
- Always label poisonous compounds; read labels of poisons and store the containers out of reach.

LIVING ROOM
- Be sure floors are not slippery. Use rubber mats under rugs to prevent slipping.
- Replace frayed or torn carpets.
- Cover electrical sockets.
- Replace frayed electrical cords. Keep electrical cords off floor where people walk.
- Place heaters a safe distance from walls. Use screens around fireplace.

- Pad sharp edges on furniture as necessary.
- Check ashtrays for lit matches or cigarettes when going to bed or leaving the house.

FURNACE
- Have a professional check and maintain the furnace every year, especially for leaks.
- Change filters monthly.

BATHROOM
- Use a rubber mat in the tub.
- Store medicines out of children's reach. Keep all medicines capped and labeled. Throw out old medicines. Keep phone number of poison center close to telephone.
- Be cautious in using appliances plugged into a wall plug near water.
- Keep hot water heater set at 120° F (48.8° C) or lower.

BEDROOM
- Do not smoke in bed.
- Use rubber mats under scatter rugs.

STAIRWAYS
- Cover with carpeting or rubber safety treads.
- Replace torn or frayed carpeting. Keep stairs clear of toys and cleaning equipment.
- Install handrails and proper lighting.
- Use gates at top and bottom for young children and confused elders.

GENERAL AREAS
- Install smoke and carbon monoxide alarms throughout the house.
- Make sure candles are away from flammable materials. Never leave a lit candle unattended.

water until EMS arrives, because of possible neck and spinal cord injury. **The victim is placed on a flat surface and is moved as a unit, taking care to rigidly stabilize the neck.** Venema and colleagues (2010) reviewed 29 rescue reports and concluded that bystander intervention makes a critical difference in the survival of drowning victims. First, the rescuer should call for help. If possible, try to reach the victim without going into deep water. After the rescued person is brought out of the water, he must be given cardiopulmonary resuscitation (CPR) and rescue breathing if he is not breathing and is pulseless. If he is breathing, he should be placed on his side (Figure 45-1) and his head should be turned to one side to prevent aspiration. Near-drowning victims should be transported to a

medical facility. They usually aspirate water, and pulmonary edema may occur. Bacterial or fungal pneumonia may follow aspiration of fresh water. There is danger of delayed cardiac irregularities for any victim who struggled in the water.

FIRST AID AND GOOD SAMARITAN LAWS

First-aid providers must proceed step-by-step. Deliberate action will help to instill confidence in those you are trying to help. Table 45-1 shows guidelines for first aid. Most states have adopted "Good Samaritan" laws that protect medical personnel from liability when rendering emergency medical care for victims of accidental injury. These laws guard against liability for care, as long as medically trained individuals act in good faith and to the best of their ability. Individuals who offer care are held to the standard of care consistent with their level of training. If a nursing assistant stops to provide emergency care, she will be held to a different standard than the physician who stops at the same accident scene. Both are expected to do the best they can in the circumstances. A bad outcome is not proof

FIGURE 45-1 Recovery position.

Table 45-1	General Principles of First Aid
ACTION	**REASONING**
Before attending to the victim or victims of an accident, quickly survey the accident scene to determine whether there are further hazards to yourself and the victims.	Spillage of gasoline after a motor vehicle accident can cause a fire or explosion, or there may be danger to the victim, yourself, and onlookers from oncoming traffic and secondary collisions. In both highway and home accidents, live electrical wires may be in the vicinity. Whenever there is a high risk of death from hazardous conditions in the immediate environment, the victims should be moved at once, regardless of the nature of their injuries. Victims may receive severe burns from lying on a sun-baked street or sidewalk while waiting for the ambulance. Although it may not be safe to move the victim to a shaded area, it is advisable to place clothing, newspaper, or some other protective covering between skin and the hot pavement.
If there are several victims of the accident, make a quick check on each one before beginning treatment.	The most serious and life-threatening injuries must be treated first; those victims who do not seem to be in immediate danger can be attended to by someone else who is capable of watching them and reporting any change in their condition.
Use a calm tone and short sentences to explain what you are doing. You must sound as if you are in control of yourself and the situation.	Giving reassurance to the victim will decrease anxiety and promote cooperation. Using short, simple explanations facilitates understanding during duress. Forcing yourself to remain calm can increase your own ability to function in an emergency situation.
Do not move the victim unless he is in immediate danger or until you have immobilized injured parts.	This is particularly true if spinal injury is suspected. Moving the victim can cause further injury if precautions are not taken.
Do not remove an object that has penetrated a part of the body and is still in place.	A knife, piece of metal, or sliver of wood that is protruding from the chest or abdomen should be left as is until it can be removed in a controlled situation by trained professionals. Removal of the object can cause further damage and make bleeding worse. Bandages are applied around the object to stabilize it and control bleeding as necessary.
Look for a Medic-Alert bracelet or necklace.	If the victim is wearing one or has some other identification showing specific medical needs, bring this to the attention of the ambulance or hospital personnel.
Try to determine the mechanism of injury.	This will give clues about the type of injury sustained and the treatment required. When evaluating the victim, begin at the head and work downward to the toes (see Focused Assessment on p. 1023).
Do not try to give anything by mouth to a person who is unconscious or has a decreased level of consciousness.	Aspiration of the material into the air passage may occur, causing breathing difficulty or complete airway obstruction.
Give an organized and chronological report to the EMS or physician, including details of incident (if you were a witness), assessment of injuries, and care rendered.	Any details of events leading to incident, mechanism of injury, baseline assessment data, and care rendered will be useful in the emergency care at the hospital. Being brief and organized is important because the EMS personnel must simultaneously intervene and take a history if the victim is in critical condition.

of improper care. Even in states in which there are no such protective laws, malpractice suits of this kind very rarely occur.

? Think Critically

You come upon an automobile accident in which several people were involved and stop to render aid. How would you assess the situation for safety for yourself and the victims? How would you act to ensure safety at the scene?

EMERGENCY CARE

The nurse may need to give emergency care in a variety of community, clinic or hospital settings, but emergency nursing is generally associated with care of patients in the emergency department (ED) of a hospital. In a survey of hospital ED directors, 90% said that overcrowding and long wait times are an issue. One of the *Healthy People 2020* objectives is to reduce the proportion of patients that wait beyond the recommended time frame to see an emergency physician. A new Joint Commission's Core Measure holds hospital facilities accountable for the "latest time the patient was receiving care in the ED, under ED services or awaiting transport." An increased number of uninsured patients and downsizing of hospitals contribute to overcrowding, which leads to decreased patient satisfaction, frustration for health care personnel, and increased risk for poor outcomes. In a study of 4574 patients who were admitted for chest pain, the authors concluded that serious complications were three to five times more likely to occur if they were treated in a crowded ED (Pines et al., 2009). Two problems were identified: more than 43% of ED patients are nonurgent, and there are significant transfer delays for those who need to be admitted to an inpatient bed (Olshaker, 2009); thus all health care professionals must work toward educating patients about appropriate use of emergency services and the entire hospital administration and staff must support the timely transfer of ED patients to inpatient beds.

Emergency nurses need excellent assessment and clinical decision-making skills and the ability to prioritize care under stressful conditions. Frequently emergency nurses follow protocols to initiate diagnostic testing or to start therapy, such as oxygen administration or peripheral intravenous access. Clinical decisions, prioritization, and use of protocols are based on (1) events or incidents that preceded the emergency visit, (2) mechanism of injury, and (3) index of suspicion. For example, two patients arrive at the hospital in an unresponsive state. For the first patient, friends report, "She was drinking and taking a lot of drugs for fun and then we found her passed out with vomit on her mouth." For the second patient, bystanders report hearing him complain of chest pain and needing his heart medication and finding him unresponsive in the parking lot. Both patients are unresponsive, but preceding events suggest that the first patient is an overdose with possible aspiration, whereas the second is more likely to have an acute cardiac problem.

Mechanism of injury refers to how the injury occurred; an experienced clinician may use this information to predict damage and complications. For example, toddlers frequently sustain dramatic looking "goose eggs" on the forehead by falling against a coffee table, but these incidents are usually more traumatic for the parents than the child. A high index of suspicion is required to detect problems that are not initially obvious. For example, a patient reports being kicked and punched several times in the abdomen. At first the patient appears to be stable with minor abrasions; however, this patient will require serial abdominal assessments to detect slow hemorrhage or internal tissue damage. Maintaining a *high index of suspicion* is important in a busy emergency setting, because everyone (including the patient) is anxious for discharge or transfer to make room for others in the waiting room.

TRIAGE: INITIAL SURVEY

The process of setting priorities for treatment is known as triage. One of the most common methods for triage of patients uses "ABCDE" as a memory trigger for the sequence of assessment. *A* is airway, *B* is breathing, and *C* is circulation. *D* can mean either the need for defibrillation or, in a trauma setting, assessment of neurologic disability. *E* is exposed: all areas of the body should be exposed so that injuries are not missed underneath clothing.

AIRWAY AND RESPIRATION

A patent airway and oxygenation are priority. A simple way to assess airway is to ask the person to tell you his name and to ask how he is feeling. If the airway is partially obstructed, the voice quality may sound muffled or coarse. With severe shortness of breath, a person cannot complete full sentences. A confused answer suggests possible decreased cerebral perfusion and oxygenation. If the patient is unconscious, look for the rise and fall of the chest.

The most common cause of airway obstruction in the unconscious person is the tongue. The head tilt–chin lift maneuver repositions the trachea and tongue and opens the airway. The jaw-thrust method should be used if a spinal injury is suspected. For this, position yourself at the head of the victim; place your elbows on either side of the head, and place your thumbs on his lower jaw near the corners of the mouth and pointing toward his feet; place your fingertips around the bone of the lower jaw, and lift (Figure 45-2 on p. 1024). (Note: Jaw thrust is no longer taught to the lay rescuer; however, health care professionals must learn this maneuver.)

After ensuring that the airway is patent, take a pulse oximetry reading and apply oxygen as needed and monitor respiratory rate and effort. Emergency equipment for resuscitation and intubation should be checked every day and use of the equipment should be reviewed periodically.

Clinical Cues

During emergency situations, "verbal orders" may appear to be the norm to inexperienced bystanders; however, the health care team members are frequently working off well-established algorithms, such as Advanced Cardiac Life Support (ACLS). Nurses are responsible to seek clarification of orders; even under extreme circumstances, the excuse of misunderstanding a verbal order is not acceptable. The physician is responsible for writing and signing orders as soon as the crisis has passed.

◎ Focused Assessment

Evaluation of Accident and Emergency Patients

AREA OF ASSESSMENT	MODE OF ASSESSMENT	RATIONALE
Primary Survey	ABCDE	A systematic approach is needed for assessment.
A: Airway	Assess for signs of breathing and respiratory distress, gasping, wheezing, *stridor* (high-pitched sound made by partial airway obstruction), choking. Check mouth for easily removable foreign body.	Adequate air exchange is necessary for the body's oxygen needs. The tongue may block the airway in an unconscious patient.
	Do not tilt head and hyperextend neck; immobilize cervical spine as needed for suspected injury.	Any patient with an unknown degree of trauma is at risk for cervical spine injury. Movement may worsen the injury.
B: Breathing	Quickly assess breathing. Watch chest and abdomen for rhythmic rise and fall. Note rate and quality of respirations.	Normal breathing requires no intervention. Abnormal breathing should be further evaluated and assisted as needed.
C: Circulation/ hemorrhage	Feel for pulse in carotid or femoral artery; note rate and quality. Check for bleeding.	Absence of a pulse indicates cardiac arrest or obstructive shock. A rapid bounding pulse may indicate fright or hypovolemia. A rapid thready pulse may indicate further blood loss, leading to shock.
D: Disability or, if nontrauma patient, defibrillation	If nontrauma patient, place defibrillator pads and follow the automatic external defibrillator (AED) instructions.	In the presence of primary cardiac arrest, early defibrillation significantly increases the chance for survival.
	If trauma patient: Note if alert, oriented to time, place, person. Note response to verbal stimuli. Check for Medic-Alert identification. Assess ability to move all extremities.	Additional assessment of trauma patients helps identify injuries.
E: Exposure	Remove clothing to look for injuries that may be covered, especially if the patient is not alert or cannot communicate. Look for life-threatening injuries. Keep patient warm.	The only way to verify if there are other injuries is to look. Protect patient privacy.
Secondary Survey	Head to toe	Initiated after life-threatening injuries are addressed.
Head, face, neck, neurologic status	Look for bleeding, bruising, abrasions. Inspect pupils, assess level of consciousness. Note and record Glasgow Coma Scale score for baseline.	Alterations in level of consciousness can be caused by a variety of conditions such as head trauma, stroke, hypoglycemia, or drug overdose.
	Maintain cervical spine precautions, assess for neck injury.	Neck injuries may be hidden by the cervical collar.
Chest	Listen to breath sounds. Look for equal chest expansion.	Tension pneumothorax can develop after a chest injury.
Abdomen/ genitourinary system	Auscultate for bowel sounds. Palpate for tenderness, guarding, and fullness. Look for bloody urine.	Abdominal trauma can result in ruptured spleen or bladder, or liver damage.
	Note bruising or abrasions, such as Grey Turner's or Cullen's sign.	External trauma may indicate internal damage.
Limbs	Assess adequacy of circulation in all extremities.	Dislocations or fractures can compress nerves and blood vessels.
Log roll	Using at least four people, stabilize the neck and head and gently log roll the victim to assess the back of the head, neck, back, and buttocks.	Bleeding and fractures may obscure additional injuries that are located on the back. In penetrating injuries observe for entrance and exit wounds.

CONTROL OF BLEEDING

Severe bleeding can rapidly lead to irreversible hypovolemic shock. Arterial blood is bright red and gushes in spurts at regular intervals. Blood from a severed or punctured vein leaks slowly and steadily and is dark red. Even major bleeding can usually be stopped by **applying pressure directly** over the wound. When in a health care work setting, Centers for Disease Control and Prevention and Occupational Safety and Health Administration requirements mandate use of personal protective equipment that includes barrier devices such as gloves when in contact with body fluids. In a community setting, adapt available material.

▣ Safety Alert

Protective Gear

In a community setting, personal protective equipment may not be present where needed. If gloves are not available, create a barrier with plastic or multiple layers of cloth. Hands and any other skin in contact with blood should be washed as soon as possible.

Head tilt–chin
lift maneuver

Jaw-thrust
maneuver

FIGURE 45-2 Opening the airway.

The palm of the hand is used, preferably after a clean cloth or sterile dressing has been placed over the open wound. However, if no dressing is available and the blood loss is substantial, contamination of the wound is not as important as controlling the hemorrhage. Once the bleeding has stopped, a compression dressing and bulky bandage are applied and left in place to prevent disturbing clots. If blood soaks through the original dressing, additional dressings are applied over the soaked ones. The wrap should not completely constrict circulation. Elevating and immobilizing the injured part will help to control bleeding.

Clinical Cues

Many patients are on antiplatelet drugs such as aspirin and clopidogrel (Plavix) or anticoagulants such as warfarin (Coumadin) to treat heart and vascular conditions. If there is injury, bleeding will be significant and may be difficult to stop.

If bleeding is copious and cannot be stopped with a pressure bandage and immobilization, the artery leading to the wound can be compressed to decrease or even stop the flow of blood. Pressure points for control of arterial bleeding are shown in Figure 16-3. If compression of the pressure point is successful, the distal pulse will be absent and the victim will notice a tingling and numbness in the area. Compression of pressure points on the neck and head should be avoided unless there is no other choice because of interference of the blood supply to the brain.

NECK AND SPINE INJURIES

Presence of neck or spinal injury should be suspected in any situation in which the individual has sustained multiple injuries, a fall, or is unconscious. **Examples of accidents which would increase index of suspicion for spinal injury include motor vehicle collisions, diving, biking, or any situation in which the neck**

receives significant force. In emergency or accident situations, the rescuer may be distracted by severe bleeding or other life-threatening conditions and thus overlook the possibility of a spinal cord injury.

⚠ Safety Alert

Cervical Spine Immobilization

In any traumatic injury in which there is the potential for spinal injury, victims are treated as spinal cord–injured patients until a spinal injury is ruled out. Cervical spine immobilization is implemented before the person is moved to a stretcher. Improper immobilization of the neck or back may result in permanent damage and paralysis.

If the victim must be moved to safety before EMS arrives, the neck may be immobilized with a coat, or towel, rolled in the shape of a collar. The purpose is to keep the neck as straight as possible, preventing it from flexing or hyperextending. Applying a cervical collar or other commercial device and maintaining traction on the head requires advanced training (Figure 45-3). A cervical collar is not particularly comfortable for the patient and it partially obscures assessment of the neck, jaw, and upper mid-chest but removal of the collar is strictly at the discretion of the physician (see Chapter 23).

CHEST TRAUMA

Thoracic trauma is a major cause of accidental death, exceeding head and facial injuries. There also can be contusion of the myocardium, rupture of the aorta, and tracheobronchial or tracheoabdominal injuries.

Fractured ribs are very painful, as breathing causes movement at the site of injury. The treatment goal is to decrease pain so that the patient can breathe adequately. Intercostal nerve block with local anesthesia may be used to control pain. Narcotic drug therapy is used cautiously since it can depress respirations. **Binding the ribs is no longer recommended**.

When three or more ribs are broken in two or more places, the chest wall becomes unstable. This condition is called *flail chest*, which produces paradoxical respirations. When the patient breathes in, the fractured portion of the chest is drawn inward instead of expanding outward as the rest of the chest does; with exhalation, the flail portion expands outward as the rest of the chest collapses normally. This process interferes with oxygenation, as the lungs cannot expand normally. Emergency treatment consists of turning the patient onto the affected side so that the ground or bed will act as a splint and reduce the pain of breathing. The patient is observed for signs of external and internal bleeding, pneumothorax, and shock.

Once the patient is in an emergency facility, flail chest is treated by intubation and mechanical ventilation while the ribs heal. The patient often has to be given a

SHORT SPINE BOARD

PHILADELPHIA COLLAR

LONG SPINE (FRACTURE) BOARD

Rolled towels or 1 liter bags of IV fluids

FIGURE 45-3 Spinal immobilization.

neuromuscular blocking agent such as pancuronium bromide (Pavulon) to prevent fighting the action of the ventilator. Sedation and pain medication are used to decrease anxiety over being totally paralyzed.

Pneumothorax, Hemothorax, and Tension Pneumothorax

An open, or "sucking," chest wound is one in which pneumothorax (accumulation of air), or hemothorax (accumulation of blood) results from penetration of the pleural cavity. Symptoms of pneumothorax or hemothorax include labored, shallow respirations, lack of movement on one side of the chest when the person inhales and exhales, and chest pain. In the field, emergency medical personnel will cover a sucking chest wound at the end of a forceful expiration with an *occlusive dressing*—that is, one made of plastic wrap, aluminum foil, Vaseline-covered gauze, or any other

material that seals the wound and prohibits the flow of air into the pleural cavity. **One corner of the dressing is left unsealed to allow accumulated air to escape.** The patient should be placed in a semi-Fowler's position if possible. Once the patient is in an emergency facility, treatment includes chest tube insertion with closed system drainage (Chapter 15).

Tension pneumothorax develops when air enters the pleural space on inspiration but remains trapped there rather than being expelled on expiration. It can occur from trauma, mechanical ventilation, or rib fracture during cardiopulmonary resuscitation. The air in the pleural space increases with each breath, and the pressure within the chest builds, which gradually collapses the lung. If unrelieved, this increasing pressure will cause a *mediastinal shift*, resulting in a decrease in cardiac output and blood pressure. Mediastinal shift means that the structures in the mediastinum—the heart, great vessels, trachea, and esophagus—are all shifted to the unaffected side of the chest. The vena cava can become "kinked" and cause cardiac arrest. In this case, a flutter valve needle or Heimlich valve may be used until a chest tube can be placed to remove the air from the pleural cavity.

ABDOMINAL TRAUMA

Penetrating abdominal trauma is usually the result of a knife or gunshot wound. At the scene, external wounds with evisceration can be temporarily covered with a piece of nonadhering material such as plastic wrap or aluminum foil. This will keep the protruding intestinal contents moist and relatively free of contamination. After the occlusive covering is applied, a clean folded towel or sheet is placed over it to retain body heat in the protruding organs. No attempt should be made to replace the abdominal organs through the wound. The victim is transported to a medical facility as quickly as possible.

Particularly with gunshot injuries, exit and entrance wounds are anticipated, thus all clothing must be removed by the EMS and/or ED staff and the anterior and posterior body surfaces must be examined. The amount of surface bleeding may be misleading because the path of a bullet is not necessarily linear. Information about the weapon or the attack, such as the length of the knife, caliber of the gun, or position of the shooter, is invaluable because it helps to predict the degree of damage (Hussey, 2010).

Blunt trauma is less dramatic, but can result from improperly worn seat belts, or physical assault. Rapid changes in speed, crushing, or shearing actions result in hemorrhage and damage to internal organs. The survival rate for blunt trauma is 90% to 95% (Hussey, 2010), but the victim must be observed closely for symptoms of shock, and serial abdominal assessments must be performed. A bluish tinge around the umbilicus may indicate abdominal hemorrhage (Cullen's sign).

Ecchymosis or bruising along the flank is a sign of retroperitoneal bleeding (Grey Turner's sign).

Focused abdominal sonography for trauma (FAST), peritoneal. lavage, or computed tomography may be performed to diagnose intra-abdominal bleeding. Additional diagnostic tests include serial hemoglobin and hematocrit, blood chemistries, and urinalysis. Treatment includes two large-bore intravenous (IV) lines, nasogastric tube, Foley catheter, and type and crossmatch for blood.

Cultural Considerations
Uninsured Trauma Patients More Likely to Die

In a national analysis, young uninsured trauma patients (155,011) were more likely to die than insured patients. Being uninsured was more significant for mortality risk than gender or race. Mechanism of injury (e.g., penetrating trauma versus blunt trauma) or physician bias against the underinsured may have been confounding factors; nevertheless the results of this study strongly suggest the need for policies and interventions to address the needs of this young, vulnerable group (Wendling, 2010).

MULTIPLE TRAUMA

The most common cause of multiple trauma is motor vehicle accidents. Among the elderly, falls are the most common cause. Head injury, fractures, and chest and abdominal injuries are anticipated. Airway management is always the first priority (see Focused Assessment on p. 1023). In head trauma, ventilation and oxygenation may be compromised due to decreased level of consciousness and C-spine precautions must be observed when performing airway interventions. Threats to breathing may include injuries such as pneumothorax, rib fractures, or open chest wounds. The multiple trauma patient has high risk for hypovolemic shock. Tension pneumothorax and cardiac *tamponade* (compression) can also compromise circulation and lead to shock.

Think Critically

What do you have available at home or in your car that could be used to hold pressure on a bleeding wound? Are you prepared to respond to an emergency?

METABOLIC EMERGENCIES

INSULIN REACTION OR SEVERE HYPOGLYCEMIA

Brain cells needs a constant supply of glucose. If glucose levels drop, level of consciousness is altered and blood vessels dilate. The classic clinical picture of a patient who has received too much insulin includes altered level of consciousness; cold, clammy skin; and hypotension, dizziness, and tachycardia. Most, but not all, patients experiencing hypoglycemia have diabetes.

Treatment

First obtain a glucose reading, if at all possible; if glucose monitoring equipment is not available, but you suspect hypoglycemia, initiate treatment without delay. If the patient is awake, give him a glass of milk. Glucose tablets or hard candy may also be used. Alteration in level of consciousness often results in impaired swallowing. Attempts to give glucose by mouth could result in aspiration. If a patient has a decreased level of consciousness, IV glucose may need to be given. If an IV line is not in place, intramuscular glucagon can be given by medical personnel or trained family members. Mental status should improve within minutes of receiving glucose. The patient should be given a protein meal, such as a meat sandwich, as soon as he is alert enough to eat. Follow-up care includes teaching about prevention of hypoglycemic episodes, recognition of the signs and symptoms of hypoglycemia, and emergency treatment.

OTHER METABOLIC EMERGENCIES

Other metabolic emergencies include thyroid storm, addisonian crisis, and diabetic ketoacidosis. See Chapters 37 and 38.

INJURIES CAUSED BY EXTREME HEAT AND COLD
HEATSTROKE

Heatstroke is the result of a serious disturbance of the heat-regulating center in the brain and can be exertional or nonexertional. Exertional heatstroke tends to occur in young, healthy individuals who engage in prolonged physical activity in a hot environment. The very young, very old, chronic invalids, those on medications such as anticholinergics, or those with weight or alcohol problems are at risk for nonexertional heatstroke (National Oceanic and Atmospheric Administration [NOAA], 2009). Normally, the body is able to regulate body temperature even with increased activity or changes in environmental temperatures by increasing perspiration and by using other internal mechanisms. In heatstroke, these mechanisms fail to function properly and the patient's temperature rises, the skin becomes dry and hot, and there may be convulsions and collapse. Alteration in neurologic function is a finding common to both types of heatstroke. Other symptoms include visual disturbances, dizziness, nausea, and a weak, rapid, irregular pulse. The body temperature may go as high as 108° to 110° F (42.2° to 43.3° C). Untreated heatstroke could result in complications or death related to cerebral edema and hemorrhage, dilation of the heart and rupture of the myocardial fibers, disseminated intravascular coagulation, pulmonary edema, and kidney or liver failure (Brege, 2009).

Prevention

In hot weather or if active in warm weather, take precautions. Drink plenty of fluids that are nonalcoholic, noncaffeinated, and low in sugar content (the wrong fluids can increase fluid loss); do not wait until thirsty to drink fluids. Stay indoors and if air conditioning or adequate cooling is not available in the home, go to a public place with air conditioning (NOAA, 2009).

In the heat, wear lightweight, light-colored, loose-fitting clothing. Limit outdoor activities to morning and evening hours, using sun protection such as wide-brimmed hats, sunglasses, and sunscreen. Try to rest often in shaded areas and limit exertion if possible.

Treatment

A person suffering from heatstroke should be placed in the shade and cooled immediately by sprinkling with water and fanning until EMS arrives. Active cooling measures at the hospital include removal of extra clothing or coverings, wiping the skin with cool wet towels or application of ice packs to the groin and axillae, use of a cooling blanket, iced saline lavage, and infusion of cold fluids. Active cooling measures are discontinued when the rectal temperature reaches 102.2° F (39° C); this prevents rebound hypothermia (Brege, 2009).

HYPOTHERMIA

People most at risk for hypothermia are the elderly, very young and thin children, the mentally ill, the homeless, and others unable to alter their ambient environment. Hypothermia is a serious lowering of the total body temperature caused by prolonged exposure to cold. The extremities can withstand lower temperatures (20° to 30° F lower). When the core (central) temperature drops even 2° or 3° F, fatal cardiac dysrhythmias or respiratory failure can occur.

Symptoms of hypothermia range from mild shivering and complaints of feeling cold and loss of coordination to eventual loss of consciousness and a deathlike appearance. In severe hypothermia, the body's protective mechanisms will drastically slow the metabolic processes and require less than half the normal oxygen. Pulse and respiration are barely detected, reflexes are absent, and the person is unconscious.

Prevention

Prevention of hypothermia includes eating high-energy foods, exercising, wearing layers of clothing, and covering the head. From one half to two thirds of the body's heat is lost through the head. Hypothermia in elderly individuals can easily be misdiagnosed because the symptoms resemble those of so many diseases to which the elderly and weak are most susceptible. Mild hypothermia (90° to 95° F [32° to 35° C] body temperature) is usually tolerated fairly well. Moderate hypothermia (84° to 90° F [29° to 32° C] body temperature) results in a mortality rate of about 21%. Severe hypothermia (core temperature below 82° F [28° C]) has an even higher mortality rate.

Most oral clinical thermometers used in hospitals and clinics do not register temperatures below 94° F (34.5° C). In the ED, rectal, bladder, or esophageal probes will be used to monitor true core temperature throughout the warming process.

 Elder Care Points

With aging, the body's ability to withstand the cold is lessened. Older people may also be less active, which generates less body heat. The elderly are at risk for accidental hypothermia after exposure even to mild cold weather or a small drop in temperature (Box 45-2).

Treatment

Once hypothermia is diagnosed, the core must be rewarmed first with continuous monitoring. The goal is to prevent lactic acid or cold blood that has pooled in the extremities from being rapidly shunted to the heart, which can cause ventricular fibrillation. **The heart is extremely sensitive when cold, and the patient must be handled carefully to prevent dysrhythmias.** Rewarming outside a health care facility should be more gradual by wrapping the patient in a blanket or submerging him in a tepid bath.

FROSTBITE

Frostbite is a localized injury to tissue caused by freezing. Exposure of the tissues to extreme cold constricts the blood vessels, damages vessel walls and tissue

---

Box 45-2 **Prevention of Hypothermia in the Elderly**

- Room temperature should not be lower than 65° F (18° C). An indoor thermometer should be kept in the house and checked daily during the cool seasons.
- An energy audit with suggestions from the utility company can prevent heat loss from the home.
- Suggest heating one or two rooms and closing off the other rooms of the house.
- Suggest aids, such as a throw or quilt, extra socks, and warm hats to be worn indoors.
- Recommend wearing several loose layers of clothing to retain body heat.
- Head covering should be worn even while sleeping to prevent heat loss.
- Advise against using fireplaces in extremely cold weather because a substantial amount of heat is lost through the flue.
- Arrange for someone to check in daily with elderly persons who live alone.
- Suggest an early alert system be installed, allowing the individual to call for help by pressing a button, if unable to get to the phone.

cells, and leads to the formation of blood clots. Frostbite occurs most often in the fingers, toes, cheeks, and nose, where exposure usually is greatest and blood supply is most easily hampered. Frostbite can be categorized by four degrees of severity; however a simplified classification divides injury into superficial or deep (Edlich, 2010). The appearance of a first-degree injury (superficial) includes reddened skin, swelling, waxy appearance, hard white plaques, and sensory deficit. Second-degree injury (superficial) also has redness and swelling and formation of blisters filled with clear or milky fluid that form within 24 hours of injury. In third-degree injury (deep), the blisters are blood filled and over several weeks black eschar forms. Fourth-degree injury (deep) involves full-thickness damage affecting muscles, tendons, and bone, resulting in tissue loss.

Prevention

Like hypothermia, frostbite can be prevented by wearing protective clothing and avoiding exposure to extreme cold. Those who are intoxicated or under the influence of drugs may not realize they are suffering from frostbite; likewise, when a person is significantly hypothermic, cognition and judgment are impaired. Friends, families, or bystanders must take the initiative to direct impaired individuals toward shelter and warmth.

Treatment

Once the patient is removed from the cold, the affected area should be warmed by immersion for about 10 minutes in water heated to between 100° and 110° F (38° and 43° C); however, the **rewarming process should not be started if there is a chance of refreezing** (Ferri, 2011). Handle the frostbitten part gently. *Never* rub or massage skin that has been frozen. Rubbing snow or ice on the part is dangerous and can cause further damage to the fragile tissues. Wrap the affected area in bulky clean or sterile bandages, being sure to separate skin areas, as between the fingers. Elevate the affected area. Avoid alcohol or sedatives as they tend to further depress function. A tetanus immunization is given if not up to date. Débridement of dead tissue and skin grafting or amputation will be necessary if the deeper tissues have been destroyed. Extent of tissue injury may be unknown for several months.

Safety Alert

Frostbite

Do not try to hasten the warming process by using water that is hotter than recommended, as this can add to the damage.

POISONING

ACCIDENTAL POISONING

The American Association of Poison Control Centers reported that there were 2,482,041 cases of poisoning in 2007 (Harding, 2010). **Children are the most frequent victims of accidental poisoning.** Aspirin poisoning is a serious issue for children under age 5. Other poisons frequently ingested by children include bleaches, soaps and detergents, insecticides, and vitamin and iron preparations. Most of us recall at least one childhood episode of unsupervised tasting of a plant or wild fruit for fun and adventure; thus children are at risk for ingestion of poisonous mushrooms, plants, or toxic berries. The elderly are also at risk for accidentally taking too much prescribed medication, because of forgetfulness, confusion about dosage or frequency, or inability to read small print on a medication bottle.

Prescription drugs such as narcotic analgesics, antidepressants, antipsychotics, or cardiovascular medications may be used when self-harm or harm to another is the motive. Alcohol and illegal drugs can also be involved during an accidental or suicide attempt.

Prevention

Prevention of accidental poisoning begins with a realization that there are literally thousands of poisonous substances in our environment. Even water is poisonous if you drink too much (Camacho, 2009). Every home has a variety of poisons in the medicine cabinet, under the kitchen sink, or in the laundry room, utility room, and garage. Encourage families to look at their environment through the eyes of their children and elders to discover potential poison sources.

Symptoms

The symptoms of poisoning vary according to the substance ingested and the time that has elapsed since it first entered the body. Poisoning should be suspected if the victim becomes ill very suddenly and there is an open poison or drug container nearby. A peculiar odor to the breath may be present; for example, a garlic smell is associated with organophosphate poisoning. Other symptoms of poisoning include pain or burning sensation in the mouth and throat, an increase or decrease in pulse or respiratory rate, nausea, vomiting, disorientation, visual disturbances, loss of consciousness, or a deep, unnatural sleep.

Treatment

The health care team must first ensure circulation, airway, and breathing. Listen carefully to the patient, family or EMS personnel because they provide invaluable information as to *what* was taken (or inhaled) and *when* the event occurred. Availability of the

Health Promotion

Poison Prevention

- Destroy all medicines that are no longer being used. In some instances, drugs undergo chemical changes with age, and become toxic compounds.
- Store poisons and inedible products separately from edible foods.
- Do not transfer poisonous substances from their original container to an unmarked one. *Never* place a poison in a container (such as a soft drink bottle) that is normally used for edible solids or liquids.
- Never tell children that medicine is candy. Explain that medicine will make the child feel better and that it must be taken only as the doctor has directed.
- Always read the labels of chemical products before using them.

---

container and any of the contents may help in identifying the poison. The poison control center at 1-800-222-1222 is immediately consulted and the caller should be prepared to give patient's age; weight; medical and medication history; allergies; what, when, and why the substance was taken; current signs and symptoms with vital signs and laboratory results and any treatment rendered (Schaeffer & Badillo, 2009). Poison control gives advice about severity of toxicity and treatment options.

Treatment of Ingested Poisons. Remember to ask about first-aid measures that were initiated before arrival at the hospital. Syrup of ipecac is no longer recommended as a home remedy; however, it was recommended for years. If ipecac was given at home, initiate aspiration precautions because vomiting is likely to occur. A sample of vomitus should be saved for analysis and identification.

Treatment in the ED includes activated charcoal to decrease absorption of poison, gastric tube insertion (a sample of stomach contents should be saved for analysis), irrigation to remove stomach contents, sorbitol to enhance bowel excretion, and antidotes that are specific to the poisons. In severe cases, hemodialysis, hemoperfusion, hemofiltration, or exchange transfusion may be performed (Camacho, 2009).

After decontamination, the patient may be admitted to the intensive care unit or a medical unit, or may be observed in the ED. If a suicide attempt underlies the incident, a psychiatric consultation must be obtained before the patient is discharged.

FOOD POISONING

There are 6 to 8 million cases of food poisoning per year in the United States (Ferri, 2011). Decomposing food is not necessarily harmful, but decomposing foods frequently harbor pathogenic organisms and serve as an excellent growth medium. The toxins

of bacteria are usually what cause the illness, although some types of organisms are invasive. *Staphylococcus aureus* frequently grows in creamed foods that have not been refrigerated adequately. In the summertime, during picnic season, custards, cream pies, mayonnaise, and processed foods are common culprits. *Clostridium perfringens* is likely to show up around Thanksgiving or Christmas, when we forget to put the leftover turkey in the refrigerator. *Enterotoxigenic coli* may accompany you home from travel in a foreign country. And in the summer of 2010, we all thought twice about eating eggs because of *Salmonella*. Botulism is usually associated with home canned goods; botulism fatality is related to quantity of toxin.

Prevention

Cleanliness, good personal hygiene, and proper preparation and handling of foods are essential to prevent food poisoning.

Health Promotion

Safe Food Handling Tips from the National Health Institute

- Carefully wash your hands and clean dishes and utensils.
- Use a thermometer when cooking. Cook beef to at least 160° F (71° C), poultry to at least 180° F (82° C), and fish to at least 140° F (60° C).
- Do *not* place cooked meat or fish back onto the same plate or container that held the raw meat, unless the container has been thoroughly washed.
- Promptly refrigerate any food you will not be eating right away. Keep the refrigerator set to around 40° F (4° C) and your freezer at or below 0° F. Do *not* eat meat, poultry, or fish that has been refrigerated uncooked for longer than 1 to 2 days.
- Do *not* use outdated foods, packaged food with a broken seal, or cans that are bulging or have a dent.
- Do *not* use foods that have an unusual odor or a spoiled taste.

Health Promotion

Healthy People 2020 Food Safety

Standards for food handling from farm and field to home or factory are in place to prevent contamination of food with illness-causing organisms. In addition to concerns regarding microorganism contamination, the agencies have also implemented standards for labeling of foods to identify potential allergens. These agencies are tracking instances of illness linked to food consumption to be able to immediately implement changes needed to protect the public.

Symptoms and Treatment

Food poisoning should be suspected when more than one person in a group, family, or community is affected by an acute gastrointestinal disturbance. Symptom onset ranges between 1 and 16 hours, with nausea, vomiting, diarrhea, and abdominal cramps. Food is withheld and rehydration is the primary therapy. Small frequent amounts of oral electrolyte solutions are appropriate if tolerated. Parenteral fluids are given for intractable vomiting and diarrhea or for severe dehydration. Antidiarrheals are usually not given, because the illness is normally self-limiting. Antibiotics are sometimes given. Botulism is treated with an antitoxin (Ferri, 2011).

INHALED POISONS

When a person has inhaled a poisonous substance, call for emergency help. Never attempt to rescue a person without notifying others first. If it is safe to do so, rescue the person from the danger of the gas, fumes, or smoke. Open windows and doors to remove the fumes. Take several deep breaths of fresh air, and then hold your breath as you go in. Hold a wet cloth over your nose and mouth. Do not light a match or use a lighter because some gases can catch fire.

After rescuing the person from danger, loosen clothing from around the neck and chest. Check and monitor the person's pulse, airway, and breathing. If necessary, begin CPR and rescue breathing (see American Heart Association recommendations for rescue breathing and CPR, p. 1032).

Symptoms that may indicate inhaled poison include excessive coughing; shortness of breath, wheezing, and a burning sensation of the nose and throat; pale or bluish color to skin; dizziness, headache, nausea, and vomiting; and chest pain or tightness. Carbon monoxide is the most commonly inhaled poison and results in a **cherry red color of the mucous membranes.** A carboxyhemoglobin level should be obtained and the patient should be treated with 100% oxygen until the carboxyhemoglobin level is less than 10%. In carbon monoxide poisoning, the readings of pulse oximetry and the values of arterial blood gases can appear normal despite significant toxic exposure (Ferri, 2011).

BITES AND STINGS

HUMAN BITES

A human bite is usually superficial; when the teeth sink into the flesh, there is a rectangular pattern of four incisors and triangular marks from the incisors. A common injury occurs when a tooth meets the skin and muscle of a clenched fist. Human bites have a high incidence of infection and require copious irrigation and débridement of devitalized tissue (Habif, 2010).

ANIMAL BITES

Family pets, especially dogs and cats, are the most common source of animal bites. When a wild animal, such as a squirrel or fox, attacks and bites a human being without provocation, one should always suspect rabies as the cause of the animal's unusual behavior.

Treatment

Bite wounds should be rinsed immediately with soap and hot running water for 5 to 10 minutes. The affected area is then treated with antibiotic ointment, covered with a clean bandage, and immobilized. Medical attention includes copious irrigation; suturing is usually done if the wound is on the face or hand. Puncture wounds on the arms or legs are frequently left unsutured and allowed to drain. If the victim has not had a tetanus shot in the past 5 years, a booster will be given.

The possibility of rabies must always be considered in an animal bite. The local animal control agency should be contacted to catch the animal if necessary. If it has been killed, animal control will take the body for examination. If a diagnosis of rabies in the animal has been confirmed or if there is no proof that the animal has been immunized against rabies, the victim is given rabies immune globulin (20 IU/kg infiltrated around the wound and the remainder given intramuscularly) and a series of five intramuscular injections. Antibiotics are given for deep puncture wounds, particularly cat bites (Habif, 2010).

SNAKEBITE

In the United States, 45,000 snakebites occur annually; 8000 are from poisonous snakes, of which less than 1% to 2% are fatal (Ferri, 2011). There are four kinds of poisonous snakes in the United States: copperheads, rattlesnakes, coral snakes, and cottonmouths (or water moccasins). Copperheads, rattlesnakes, and cottonmouths are all called pit vipers because they have pits or depressions behind their nostrils; coral snakes are small snakes with characteristic red, black, and yellow bands. Coral snakes do not have fangs; they inject their venom by a chewing motion.

A venomous snakebite usually can be distinguished by two fang marks (though there may be only one on a small surface, such as the toe or finger), severe pain and swelling in the area, discoloration at the site of injection of venom, nausea and vomiting, respiratory distress, and shock. Nonpoisonous snakebites usually appear as either small scratches or lacerations.

Treatment

Nonpoisonous snakebites are treated as simple wounds and require only a cleansing of the wound with soap and water and the application of a mild antiseptic. First aid for a poisonous snake bite includes washing the wound, lowering the extremity or area and immobilizing it, keeping the victim calm, and seeking medical attention as quickly as possible. In the field, do *not* apply suction, make incisions over the wound, apply ice, or give alcoholic beverages or stimulants.

Once the snakebite victim reaches a hospital or clinic, the wound is débrided and irrigated to remove the venom and damaged tissues. Skin grafting may be required later. The victim is observed for at least

8 hours and given a tetanus immunization, antivenin medications, and other drugs to prevent complications and provide relief. Sheep immunoglobulin–based antivenin is safer and preferred for pit viper bites over horse serum–based antivenin. Antivenin advice is available at 877-377-3784 (Ferri, 2011).

INSECT BITES AND STINGS

Systemic reactions to the bites and stings of insects and bees account for more deaths each year in the United States than do snakebites. A systemic reaction is caused by hypersensitivity to the venom of bees, wasps, hornets, fire ants, or harvester ants. Symptoms of a systemic reaction include hives, swelling, general weakness, tightness in the chest, abdominal cramps, constriction of the throat, loss of consciousness, and possibly death from severe anaphylaxis. When the interval between the sting or bite and the development of symptoms is short, the possibility of death increases. Ice packs may be applied to the area of the bite or sting while medical help is being sought.

The black widow and the brown recluse spiders are the best known spiders that have a potentially serious bite. The symptoms of a black widow spider bite may not be obvious initially; the bite may feel like a pinprick with some slight redness and swelling. Within a few hours intense pain and stiffness will occur. Other symptoms include chills, fever, nausea, and severe abdominal pain. The brown recluse spider bite produces a mild stinging, redness, and pain within several hours. A fluid-filled blister forms at the site of the bite. The tissue sloughs off, leaving a deep, hard-to-heal ulcer.

 Elder Care Points

Anyone over age 65 should seek medical attention if bitten by a brown recluse or black widow spider. The elderly are more at risk for developing complications related to the bite.

Treatment

Treatment for a systemic reaction is to inject aqueous epinephrine (1:1000 solution) in dosages of 0.3 to 0.4 mL for adults and 0.15 to 0.3 mL for children. An antihistamine, such as diphenhydramine (Benadryl), is given. An ice pack may be applied to reduce swelling and relieve pain. Patients who appear to be in shock should be kept warm and should remain lying down with the legs elevated and the head flat. If symptoms persist after 20 minutes and the patient has not yet reached a medical facility, a second injection of epinephrine should be given.

The female worker honeybee injects a venom sac that may remain embedded in the victim's skin. **The "stinger" should be removed as quickly as possible.** Do not use tweezers to remove an insect stinger; this may cause squeezing of the venom sac and worsen the symptoms. Use a credit card or any rigid item with a smooth, flat edge to scrape out the stinger.

An emergency kit that contains drugs, syringe, tourniquet, towelette, and tweezers is available by prescription and is used for treatment of systemic reactions to stings and bites. Individuals with known hypersensitivity to insect and bee venom should carry medical identification and an emergency kit and be thoroughly familiar with its use *before* the need arises. Persons who have systemic reactions or even severe local reactions with swelling beyond two joints should be referred for hyposensitization therapy.

Applying a paste of baking soda and water or household ammonia and a cold compress treats less serious stings of bees, wasps, yellow jackets, and hornets. Meat tenderizer also has been found effective in relieving the symptoms of minor insect sting reactions. Topical cortisone cream can relieve inflammation and itching.

Bites from venomous spiders, scorpions, and other poisonous insects are treated in the same manner as poisonous snakebites. Antivenin specific to the spider, scorpion, or other poisonous creature is available at hospital EDs and clinics that serve rural areas.

Ticks can carry Rocky Mountain spotted fever or Lyme disease. The tick is removed by grasping it as close to the skin as possible with tweezers and pulling it straight out without twisting. Applying turpentine, mineral oil, petroleum jelly, nail polish, or insecticide on the tick is not recommended because the tick may regurgitate stomach contents into the skin (Harvard Women's Health Watch, 2009). After the tick is removed, wash the area with soap and water and apply a mild disinfectant. A physician can be consulted for possible infection or disease symptoms.

ELECTRIC SHOCK AND BURNS

When an electric current passes through the body, it can cause severe damage to the entire body, including cessation of breathing, circulatory failure, and serious burns. The current travels along the path of least resistance, and may be conducted through the heart. The amount of voltage and current involved, the length of time in contact with the electricity source, and the condition of the skin all play a role in how much damage may occur as a result of an electric shock.

Emergency treatment of electric shock involves CPR if breathing has ceased or the heart has stopped, and treatment of burns or other concurrent injuries. The proper procedure for separating a victim from a live conductor of electricity is shown in Figure 45-4. **Remember that water serves as a conductor of electricity, and wet objects can transmit a fatal electric current to a person trying to rescue the victim of electric shock.** All electric shock victims, including those struck by lightning, must be observed for cardiac dysrhythmias after the injury.

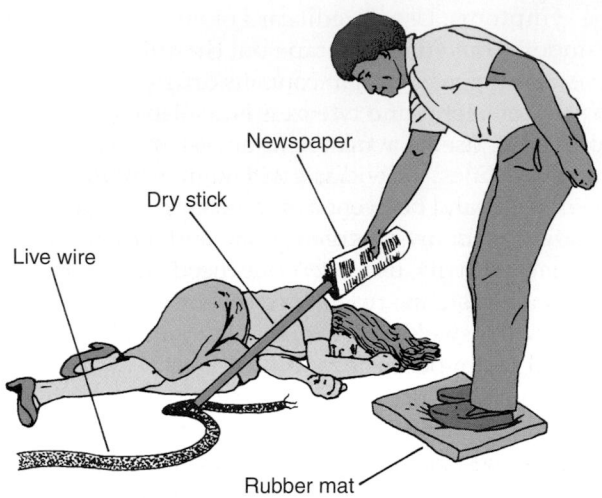

Live wire
Dry stick
Newspaper
Rubber mat

FIGURE 45-4 Separating a victim from a live electrical wire while avoiding similar shock.

Lightning

If outdoors when lightning occurs, avoid water, high ground, open spaces, and metal objects. Do not seek shelter under canopies, small picnic or rain shelters, or trees. If out in the open, do not lie down, but crouch down on the balls of the feet; this minimizes height and body contact with any ground currents. If inside, avoid plumbing fixtures and electrical appliances, including computers and cord phones. If in the car, do not touch surfaces that readily conduct electricity (Hyett, 2009).

CHEMICAL BURNS

Strong chemicals capable of burning the skin and mucous membranes will continue to destroy tissue unless they are diluted and removed immediately. For this reason, any area burned by chemicals must be quickly flushed with large amounts of water (with some exceptions) until all traces of the chemical have been removed; the burned area is then covered with a dressing.

Water is not used for burns caused by dry lime or phenol. Dry lime should be brushed from the skin and clothing unless there is enough water to remove *all* traces of the powder. Small amounts of water will react chemically with the lime to produce a highly *corrosive* (destroys gradually) substance. Phenol (carbolic acid) is not water soluble. The phenol is first removed by alcohol and the burned area is then rinsed with water. **If a corrosive chemical has been ingested, the poison control center should be contacted for instructions and proper dosage of an antidote.** Vomiting should *not* be induced or encouraged. No attempt should be made to neutralize an ingested chemical substance, as this can cause further damage to the esophagus and stomach.

Patients with chemical burns should be transported to a hospital as soon as possible. If possible, the treating physician should be informed about (1) the offending agent, physical form, and concentration; (2) the route and volume of exposure; (3) the timing and extent of irrigation; and (4) any coexisting injuries.

CHOKING EMERGENCIES

Obstructed airway is the sixth leading cause of accidental death. Adults as well as children can become choking victims and need immediate intervention to prevent death from asphyxiation. Both partial and complete airway obstruction should be treated, especially with poor air exchange with the partial obstruction. **If the person is conscious and able to cough or speak, he may not need assistance in expelling the object from his throat.** In this situation, encourage him to cough rigorously and breathe as deeply as he can. His coughing efforts are more effective than outside intervention; stay with him and call for help as needed. When the choking victim cannot speak, cough, or independently expel the foreign object, abdominal thrusts are used to force the object up and out (see Chapter 14).

You are dining in a restaurant and observe someone at another table apparently choking. What steps would you take to assist?

CARDIOPULMONARY RESUSCITATION

Many phenomena cause sudden cessation of breathing and circulation, from electric shock to drowning to cardiac arrest. **CPR is indicated when the person shows (1) absence of response to stimuli, (2) absence of respirations, and (3) absence of a carotid pulse.** When a person stops breathing spontaneously and his heart stops beating, "clinical death" has occurred. Within 4 to 6 minutes, the cells of the brain, which are most sensitive to lack of oxygen, begin to deteriorate. If the oxygen supply is not restored immediately, the patient suffers irreversible brain damage and "biologic death" occurs.

The 2010 American Heart Association Guidelines for *cardiopulmonary resuscitation* (CPR) have been revised according to research and discussion by international experts. For many of us, these changes mean having to let go of the familiar A-B-C (airway, breathing, chest compressions) and adopt the C-A-B (chest compressions, airway, breathing). The new guidelines emphasize the importance of high-quality CPR and recommend hands-only CPR for the lay rescuer. These recommendations are based on research that indicates that the highest survival rates for cardiac arrest among adults occurs for witnessed ventricular tachycardia, where the critical interventions are chest compressions and defibrillation. For the lay rescuer, "look, listen, and feel" and the step of palpating for the pulse have been eliminated completely. Even health care providers should not delay or interrupt chest compressions by more than 10 seconds for pulse checks. The idea of hands-only CPR for lay rescuers is intended to encourage bystanders to intervene only with chest compressions and to **push hard, push fast** at a rate of at least 100 compressions per minute. Beyond the fear of contagion, it was determined that the positioning of the head and delivering the initial breaths was delaying the delivery of chest compressions. In the health care setting, high-quality CPR means that the chest compressions must be delivered with the correct depth and rate with adequate recoil and that any pauses for ventilation, pulse checks, or switching rescuer positions or procedures such as application of equipment or defibrillation must be kept to the absolute minimum.

Health care providers are held to a higher standard of care and intervention must be based on assessment of the patient and tailored to address the most likely cause. For example, if the nurse were to witness a sudden collapse of a patient in the hospital, ventricular fibrillation (VF) with cardiac arrest would be a likely assumption. The sequence would be to establish unresponsiveness, check pulse and respirations in 10 seconds or less, activate the response team, start compressions, defibrillate with the **automated external defibrillator (AED)** as soon as it is available, and ventilate with an Ambu bag. The nurse must adapt and delegate as personnel and equipment arrive at the scene.

In the community, the use of the AED combined with activation of the EMS response system and CPR gives the victim of VF the best chance for survival. AEDs are now located in many public buildings, health clubs, airlines, malls, and sporting venues. As soon as the AED is brought to the scene, the device must be turned on; it will audibly give step-by-step instructions. A single shock is delivered instead of the previously recommended sequential three shocks. When the AED indicates that it is analyzing the rhythm, all CPR and any direct contact with the victim must stop. If the AED identifies a shockable rhythm, it will either automatically charge, or give instructions to charge the device. Once the AED is charged, the instructions will state "stand clear" of the victim. To avoid being shocked, everyone must avoid touching the victim when the charge is delivered.

Table 45-2 presents recent changes to techniques of CPR. For the most up-to-date science, refer to a current CPR handbook. Recertification is generally required every 2 years; however, studies show that skills are not retained for that length of time unless reviewed.

SHOCK

Shock is a condition that starts at the cellular level and gradually spreads to produce clinical signs and symptoms. The hallmark of shock is lack of **perfusion** (blood supply) to tissues, which results in lack of oxygen and nutrients. Conditions of low circulating volume (hypovolemic shock); decreased cardiac output (cardiogenic shock); or maldistribution of volume (neurogenic, anaphylactic, or septic shock) cause decreased perfusion. Perfusion requires adequate blood volume, the blood vessels must be intact, and the pump (the heart) must be working correctly.

SIGNS AND SYMPTOMS

Early recognition and treatment of impending shock results in better outcomes. Typical clinical symptoms of shock reflect lack of oxygen to essential organs. Signs and symptoms reflect decreased cardiac output, such as confusion, restlessness, diaphoresis, rapid thready pulse, increased respiratory rate, cold clammy skin, and diminishing urinary output to less than 20 mL/hr (Figure 45-5). A **change of mental status or an increase in pulse may be the first signs of shock.**

HYPOVOLEMIC SHOCK

Hypovolemic shock is the most common form of shock. A blood loss of even 500 mL in a typical adult may cause hypovolemic shock. Table 45-3 shows the amount of blood loss and consequent clinical manifestations. Any significant loss of fluid volume can result in hypovolemic shock (Concept Map 45-1). Plasma leaking from a burn, severe vomiting and diarrhea, and internal bleeding secondary to pancreatitis are examples of conditions leading to hypovolemia.

 Elder Care Points

The elderly may develop shock with smaller blood loss because of decreased vascular tone and impaired cardiac function.

Treatment

The primary interventions for **hypovolemia** are to stop the fluid loss, if possible, and to replace fluids. **In all situations of hypovolemic shock, volume replacement is essential.** To infuse large volumes of fluid and/or blood products, adequate IV access is extremely important. Two large-bore peripheral IV sites or placement of a central line with multiple lumens are needed (Strickler, 2007). If large volumes of fluid are required for fluid resuscitation, warming of the fluids can help prevent hypothermia. If hemorrhage is present, crystalloids (i.e., normal saline or lactated Ringer's) or colloids (e.g., albumin, or Voluven, approved by the Food and Drug Administration in 2008) will be infused until blood products are available for transfusion. Packed red cells are given to replenish

Table 45-2   CPR for Adults

COMPONENT	ACTION FOR LAY RESCUER	ACTION FOR HEALTH CARE PROVIDER
Recognize symptoms and need for assistance	No breathing or gasping only. You find an unresponsive victim, call for help.	Tailor actions to the situation. If it is likely that the victim has had an airway problem (e.g., drowning), do 2 min of CPR and rescue breathing before leaving the victim to call. The sudden collapse of an adult is likely to be cardiac in origin; call for help, start CPR, and defibrillate as soon as the AED is available.
Pulse check	Lay rescuers are not taught this step.	≤10 sec, carotid.
CPR sequence	C-A-B.	C-A-B.
Compression rate	At least 100/min. Pushing hard, pushing fast, and allowing for the chest to recoil between compressions has been found to be the most effective.	At least 100/min. Pushing hard, pushing fast, and allowing for the chest to recoil between compressions has been found to be the most effective.
Compression depth	At least 2 inches (differs for children and infants).*	At least 2 inches (differs for children and infants).*
Compression interruption	Minimize interruptions in chest compressions.	Limit interruptions to less than 10 sec (i.e., rotating compressors, delivering shock, pulse check). Rescuers should change compressors q 2 min to prevent fatigue and decreased efficiency of compressions.
Airway	Untrained lay rescuers should not delay compressions to perform airway maneuvers.	Head tilt–chin lift; use jaw thrust if cervical injury is suspected.
Compression ratio to rescue breathing (no advanced airway placed)	Compressions only for untrained lay rescuers.	30:2 for one or two health care rescuers.
AED use	Use as soon as possible.	Use as soon as possible. For an out-of-hospital, unwitnessed cardiac arrest, EMS may initiate 1½ to 3 min of CPR before attempting defibrillation.

AED, automated external defibrillator; *CPR,* cardiopulmonary resuscitation; *C-A-B,* chest compressions, airway, breathing.
*Consult a pediatrics text and the American Heart Association guidelines for additional data that is specific to children and infants.

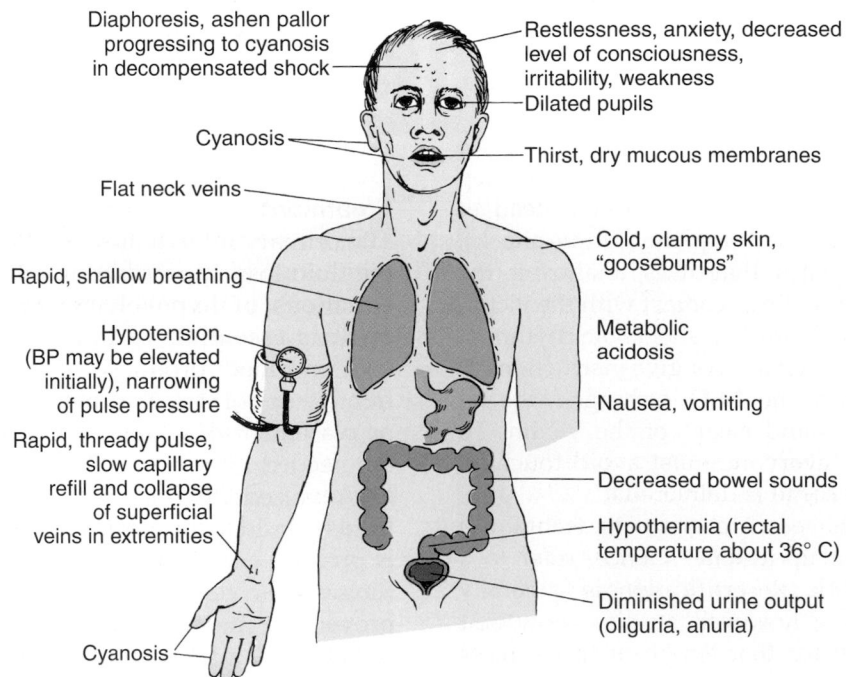

Diaphoresis, ashen pallor progressing to cyanosis in decompensated shock

Cyanosis

Flat neck veins

Rapid, shallow breathing

Hypotension (BP may be elevated initially), narrowing of pulse pressure

Rapid, thready pulse, slow capillary refill and collapse of superficial veins in extremities

Cyanosis

Restlessness, anxiety, decreased level of consciousness, irritability, weakness
Dilated pupils

Thirst, dry mucous membranes

Cold, clammy skin, "goosebumps"

Metabolic acidosis

Nausea, vomiting

Decreased bowel sounds

Hypothermia (rectal temperature about 36° C)

Diminished urine output (oliguria, anuria)

FIGURE 45-5 Clinical signs of shock.

Table 45-3	Clinical Manifestations of Blood Loss
VOLUME LOST	**CLINICAL MANIFESTATIONS**
10%	None
20%	At rest, no signs or symptoms; slight postural hypotension when standing; tachycardia with exercise.
30%	Blood pressure and pulse normal when supine; postural hypotension and tachycardia with exercise.
40%	Below-normal blood pressure, central venous pressure, and cardiac output at rest; rapid, thready pulse and cold, clammy skin.
50%	Shock and potential death.

Adapted from Lewis, S.L., Heitkemper, M.M., Dirksen, S.R., et al. (2010). *Medical-Surgical Nursing: Assessment and Management of Clinical Problems* (8th ed.). St. Louis: Mosby.

CONCEPT MAP 45-1 Hypovolemic shock.

cell volume. Units of packed cells contain citrate as an anticoagulant. If multiple units of blood are rapidly infused, the citrate can bind with ionized calcium, decreasing the amount of circulating calcium. This can depress cardiac function and alter coagulation. If a large volume of blood is lost, clotting factors will also need to be replaced. Fresh frozen plasma is given for replacement of clotting factors.

Checking Blood Products During an Emergency Situation

Resuscitation of a victim in hypovolemic shock is an emergency situation; however, before administering blood there are several safety checks that must be conducted. (1) Match the blood or blood component to the order, (2) match the patient to the blood or blood component, and (3) use a two-person verification process. This verification process is in compliance with National Patient Safety Goals, and avoiding a transfusion reaction in a compromised patient is just good nursing practice.

If fluid loss is from gastrointestinal sources, isotonic solutions will be used to replenish the fluid and electrolytes. Burn patients require replacement of lost plasma, which is rich in protein. Crystalloids containing salt and colloids, such as albumin, will be administered to rehydrate burn victims (see Chapter 43). Monitor vital signs, level of consciousness, and urine output to assess response to therapy.

 Clinical Cues

Oxygen should always be administered to patients in shock or suspected shock.

? **Think Critically**

You are caring for a patient who has vomited large amounts of blood. You expect to see a compensatory increase in pulse, but in fact the pulse rate remains between 50 and 60 beats/min. Why would you want to double-check this patient's medication history?

CARDIOGENIC SHOCK

Cardiogenic shock occurs when the heart is incapable of pumping enough blood to meet the needs of the body (Concept Map 45-2). Myocardial infarction is the primary cause of coronary cardiogenic shock due to direct damage of the heart muscle from a heart attack. Heart muscle can be rendered ineffective as a pump by causes such as cardiomyopathy, valvular dysfunction, or pulmonary edema.

Treatment

In cardiogenic shock, increasing the volume by giving additional fluid will overwhelm an already inefficient pump. Chemical and mechanical treatments are used to support the impaired heart muscle without increasing workload of the heart. Vasopressor agents (e.g., norepinephrine and dopamine), inotropic agents (e.g., dobutamine), or phosphodiesterase inhibitors (e.g., inamrinone) are all used to increase the contractility of cardiac muscle (positive inotropy) (Schub, 2010). However, as the heart works harder, it requires more

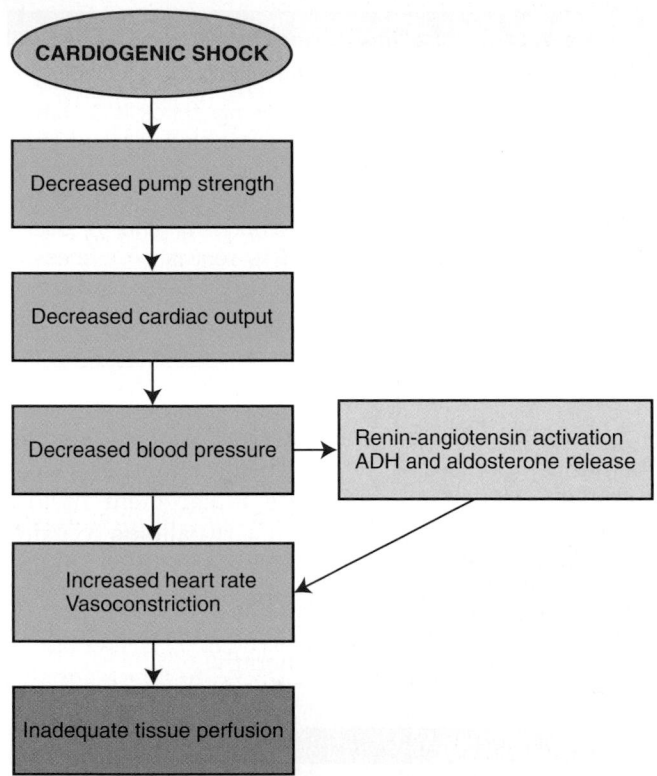

CONCEPT MAP 45-2 Cardiogenic shock.

oxygen. If the heart is already damaged, pushing it to do more will only worsen the inadequate circulation. In conjunction with the positive inotropes, vasodilators (e.g., nitroglycerin) are judiciously used to decrease cardiac workload.

When the heart ejects blood into the systemic circulation, it has to overcome the pressure of the closed aortic valve and the resistance of the peripheral blood vessels. Think of an adjustable nozzle on a hose: as the nozzle opening is enlarged, less pressure is required than if the nozzle is turned to the smallest setting. Similarly, if the blood vessels are dilated, the heart does not have to work as hard to expel the blood. Diminished workload lessens the oxygen demand of the cardiac muscle. Thus, when inadequate circulation is occurring, blood pressure (BP) rises to overcome restricted flow, and vasodilator medications are used to open up blood vessels. When blood vessels dilate, the pressure in the system decreases, which drops BP. Vasodilators must be used cautiously to enhance cardiac performance without compromising BP. The intraaortic balloon pump (IABP) is a mechanical left ventricular assist device that supports cardiac function; IABP is used in critical care units.

OBSTRUCTIVE SHOCK

Tissue perfusion can be impaired when there is a mechanical obstruction to blood flow. In conditions such as pericardial tamponade, tension pneumothorax, or constrictive pericarditis, there is a physical obstruction that prevents adequate filling or emptying of the heart. In conditions such as aortic dissection or massive pulmonary embolus there is a problem in the blood vessels that prevents forward flow of blood.

Treatment
Pericardial tamponade is treated by inserting a needle into the pericardial sac and removing the fluid that is compressing the heart. Tension pneumothorax is also treated by needle decompression. A needle or thoracostomy tube is inserted to release the air trapped in the chest that is putting pressure on the heart. Constrictive pericarditis does not usually have a sudden onset. It is usually a chronic problem with acute episodes. Medical treatment with anti-inflammatory medications may help, but the only definitive treatment is surgery. Aortic dissection is one of many causes of chest pain and diagnosis can be difficult, but the patient must be taken immediately to the operating room for repair of the vessel. Massive pulmonary embolus (PE) is usually fatal. A less severe PE will be treated with heparin to prevent further clot formation. Thrombolytic therapy in PE is controversial.

MALDISTRIBUTION OF FLUIDS (DISTRIBUTIVE SHOCK)

Distributive shock (Concept Map 45-3) involves a maldistribution of the fluid within the vascular system. If the vessels dilate and the volume of fluid stays the same, the pressure decreases (vasogenic shock). "Distributive shock is analogous to turning on all the faucets in a house at once" (Wilmot, 2010). All forms of distributive shock involve vasodilation of blood vessels, resulting in a "relative hypovolemia." There has not been actual volume loss, but physiologically the patient appears to be hypovolemic.

ANAPHYLACTIC SHOCK

Acute allergic reactions can result in life-threatening anaphylactic shock. For the body to produce this hypersensitive reaction, a previous exposure to the antigen must have occurred. In anaphylactic shock, the antigen-antibody reaction that occurs releases vasoactive substances that cause massive vasodilation as well as increased capillary permeability. This combination of factors results in hypotension. These mediators can also cause bronchoconstriction and angioedema of the laryngeal tissue, causing an acute airway emergency. Other signs and symptoms may include skin rash and generalized flushing, headache, or light-headedness.

Treatment
If possible, the antigen should be removed immediately. With a bee sting, prompt removal of the stinger may help. If the anaphylaxis is due to an ingested or

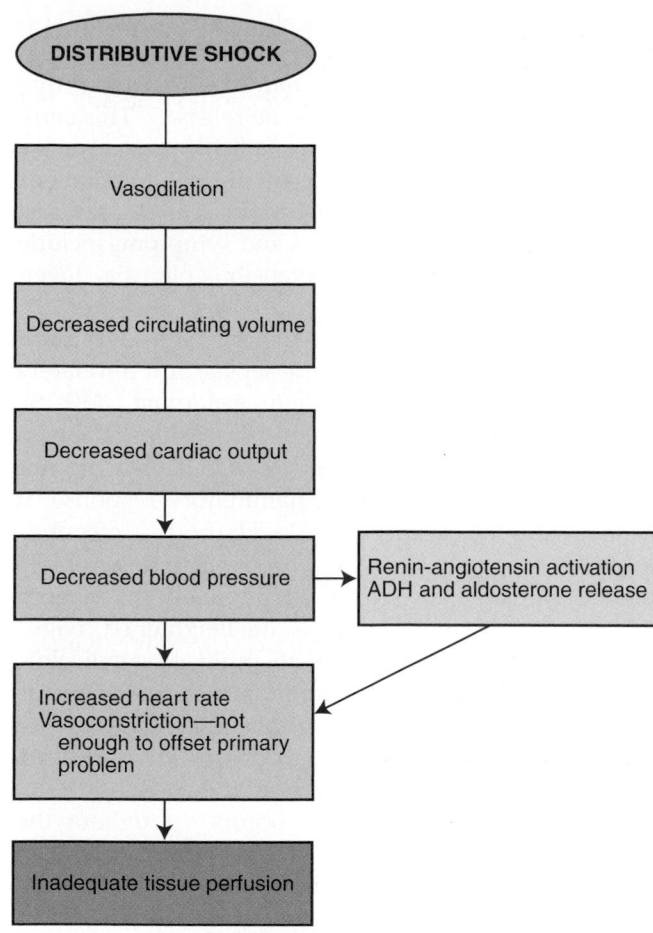

CONCEPT MAP 45-3 Distributive shock.

inhaled substance, removal may not be possible, so treatment begins immediately. Treatment of anaphylactic shock includes airway management, including intubation when necessary, and administration of epinephrine intravenously or—if there is no IV access—intramuscularly. Epinephrine helps maintain BP, counteracts the effects of the released mediators, and inhibits further release of mediators from mast cells and basophils. Bronchodilators may also be administered.

Administration of fluid is also needed. Although the actual circulating volume reduction due to leaking capillaries is not enough to cause hypotension, vasodilation is more than enough to cause a significant drop in BP. An antihistamine such as diphenhydramine (Benadryl) is given; dexamethasone or methylprednisolone is given to reduce inflammatory response. Patients should be monitored for several hours even if response to treatment is good because antihistamines and epinephrine will wear off (Wilmot, 2010).

NEUROGENIC SHOCK

Neurogenic shock, the rarest form of shock, has a triad of symptoms: hypotension, bradycardia, and hypothermia. Spinal injury or anesthesia can cause a blockage in sympathetic outflow from the vasomotor center of the brainstem. Most blood vessels are never completely constricted or completely dilated. This in-between state is known as *vascular tone* and allows for constriction or dilation as necessary. The sympathetic nervous system maintains this state of readiness. When spinal cord injury happens or high levels of spinal anesthesia are administered, the sympathetic impulses regulating the state of the blood vessels are blocked and passive vasodilation occurs. The volume of fluid circulating in the blood vessels is the same, but the space within the blood vessels enlarges. This results in a lower BP leading to hypotension and a shock state. Proper stabilization of spinal injuries can prevent or minimize conditions that lead to neurogenic shock (Tocco, 2009).

Treatment

Treatment includes administering crystalloids to maintain a mean arterial pressure of 85 to 90 mm Hg. Dopamine is given for a combination of hypotension, bradycardia, and decreased cardiac output. Hypothermia is treated with warming blankets and environmental temperature control. Spinal cord injury patients are at high risk for deep vein thrombosis, so you should anticipate orders for heparin prophylaxis, compression stockings, and sequential compression devices for the lower legs (Tocco, 2009).

SEPSIS AND SEPTIC SHOCK

Patients who have delayed seeking treatment for an infection of any kind are at risk for sepsis. An immunocompromised patient with multiple tubes and IV lines is also at risk. In 2001, health care professionals from critical care organizations and societies met at an international conference to update previous definitions of sepsis. The diagnosis of sepsis is based on documented or *suspected* infection and two or more signs of *systemic inflammatory response syndrome* (SIRS). According to the guidelines from the 2001 conference, SIRS occurs when two or more of the following are present (Glow, 2009):

1. Temperature greater than 102.2° F (39° C) or less than 96.8° F (36° C)
2. Heart rate greater than 90 beats/min
3. Respiratory rate greater than 20 breaths/min or $PaCO_2$ less than 32 mm Hg
4. White blood cell count greater than 12,000 cells/mm^3 or less than 4000 cells/mm^3 or greater than 10% bands

Other symptoms of sepsis include altered mental status, significant edema, hyperglycemia, hypotension, hypoxemia, coagulopathy, oliguria, ileus, and decreased capillary refill. During septic shock, the inflammatory process, in addition to causing clotting and activation of the immune system, releases chemicals that cause vasodilation and increased capillary permeability. The vasodilation, as with the other forms of distributive shock, causes BP to fall. The leaking capillaries cause fluid loss, which increases the severity of the hypotension. The infecting organism secretes toxins from the cell wall that also react with the blood vessels and cell membranes, causing further increased capillary permeability and further loss of fluid from the vascular space, cellular injury, and greatly increased cellular metabolic rate.

Bacteria commonly associated with infections lead to sepsis and septic shock. Gram-negative bacteria such as *Pseudomonas aeruginosa, Escherichia coli,* and *Klebsiella pneumoniae,* and gram-positive bacteria such as *Staphylococcus* and *Streptococcus,* are normally present in the environment. Health care–associated infections can lead to sepsis with deadly outcomes. Meticulous care must be taken with IV sites, Foley catheters, and other devices that disrupt the body's protective mechanisms.

Treatment and Nursing Management

In 2003, 11 international organizations launched the "Surviving Sepsis Campaign." Recommendations include initiation of a sepsis resuscitation bundle in the first 6 hours. Early detection of sepsis is a cornerstone to successfully outcomes; thus the importance of good nursing assessment and prompt reporting of findings is underscored. When a patient is at risk for sepsis, monitor for slight changes in condition: warm, dry, flushed skin; full, bounding pulse; normal to high BP; and elevated urine output. The temperature may be normal or slightly elevated. Some patients do experience a high temperature with sepsis; however, the elderly or others may experience hypothermia when septic.

When sepsis is identified, the nurse must be vigilant for signs of septic shock. **Watch the urine output. If it begins to decrease hourly, notify the physician.** Monitor breath sounds for crackles, and check for an increasing heart rate. Assess for increased fatigue, feelings of anxiety, and changes in mental status. Watch for dependent edema. If shock occurs, the skin will become cool and clammy and the peripheral pulses will be weak and thready. BP will fall as hypovolemia becomes more pronounced.

Once sepsis is suspected, appropriate treatment begins immediately. This includes fluid resuscitation with crystalloids or colloids to maintain BP and oxygenation; intubation and mechanical ventilation may be required. Blood cultures are obtained and broad-spectrum antibiotic therapy is started within 1 hour of diagnosis of septic shock. Norepinephrine or dopamine may be ordered to maintain mean arterial pressure greater than 65 mm Hg. Dobutamine or steroid therapy may be used if the BP and cardiac output do not respond to fluid challenge or vasopressors.

SYSTEMIC INFLAMMATORY RESPONSE SYNDROME

The inflammatory response is part of the cascade of events that is part of the body's immune response. Once the threat has been dealt with, feedback mechanisms inhibit the release of the chemicals and the immune system goes back into a state of readiness. In some situations this does not happen, and the substances that cause inflammation continue to be released. This clinical picture is known as systemic inflammatory response syndrome (SIRS). **SIRS can occur under infectious or noninfectious conditions; therefore it may manifest in any type of shock.** The signs and symptoms include tachycardia, tachypnea, hypotension, oliguria, fever, and signs of poor perfusion.

It is thought that SIRS is the first part of a continuum that leads to sepsis, then severe sepsis, and ultimately multisystem organ dysfunction syndrome (MODS). When two or more organ systems show signs of abnormality, the condition is called MODS. When the immune system initiates the inflammatory response, it also initiates the clotting cascade. The body is responding to an unknown threat and prepares to fight off foreign organisms and/or to stop bleeding, so both systems are activated. In sepsis, the heightened coagulant state of the body leads to multiple small clots forming in the microcirculation, which is known as *disseminated intravascular coagulation (DIC).* These small clots clog up the circulation to organs. This clotting leads to organ damage throughout the body.

The extensive clotting that occurs throughout the body in DIC uses up most of the clotting factors in the blood. As a result, bleeding occurs easily. Patients may ooze blood from previously dry wounds, from their gums, and around IV catheters, and may bruise very easily. The clinical sign most noticeable is bleeding from any break in the skin.

If an event occurs that triggers clotting, normally the process to dissolve the clot is also activated. This allows the clot to stop the bleeding and then be reabsorbed when no longer needed, conserving the clotting factors for reuse. One of the substances involved in the breakdown of the clot is activated protein C. Drotrecogin alfa (activated) (Xigris) is given to decrease clotting in the extremely small blood vessels and keep the blood flowing. Although it may seem contradictory to give a medication that will dissolve clots when the patient is bleeding, the clots that have formed in the small blood vessels are harming the patient, as they are keeping the clotting factors from being available in the areas they are needed. Administration of this medication is an attempt to disrupt the abnormal clotting.

The usual clinical progression starts with symptoms indicating SIRS, moving into sepsis, then severe sepsis and MODS complicated by DIC. If this sequence of events continues, mortality rates range from 28% to 80%. The wide range is due to multiple variables such as age, preexisting illnesses, and access to treatment. Early recognition and effective treatment of this cascade of events are the most significant factors in reducing mortality risk.

❖ NURSING MANAGEMENT

The nurse must be vigilant for patients who are at risk for developing shock. For example, postsurgical patients are always at risk for hemorrhage, which could lead to hypovolemic shock or infection, which could lead to sepsis and septic shock. Maintaining adequate fluid volume and BP are key components in adequately managing shock.

■ Assessment (Data Collection)

Ongoing evaluation of the patient's level of consciousness, vital signs (including temperature), skin signs, and urine output are all essential to the recognition and management of shock. Serial assessment data are compared to the previous data and to the baseline assessment. **Watching for changes and trends in physical and laboratory findings is extremely important.** This information must be reported to the physician in order to make treatment decisions. In accordance with National Patient Safety Goals, recognition and response to changes in a patient's condition is particularly applicable to the prognosis of shock. Many hospitals have implemented rapid response teams to help with the assessment and management of patients who are unstable.

■ Nursing Diagnosis, Planning, and Implementation

The primary nursing diagnosis for shock is Ineffective Tissue Perfusion. The planning of care for the patient in shock should include measures to monitor and maintain a patent airway, body temperature, and skin integrity (Nursing Care Plan 45-1).

The treatment goals in shock are to restore circulating volume and to treat the underlying cause, if possible. In most types of shock, BP responds to administration of IV fluids. The exception to this is cardiogenic shock in which the pump cannot manage the fluids that are already present and pump support is needed. If an IV is not in place, volume can be redistributed to the central circulation by laying the patient flat and elevating the legs 10 to 12 inches. Pneumatic "shock trousers" can also be applied to increase the blood pressure, particularly in hypovolemic shock.

■ Evaluation

If interventions are effective, there should be improvement in tissue perfusion. This can be evaluated by looking at BP, urine output, and level of consciousness. These are key indicators of adequacy of blood flow to vital organs. Other indicators to monitor include capillary refill, color and temperature of

---

⭐ Nursing Care Plan 45-1 — Care of the Patient Exhibiting Symptoms of Shock

Scenario
Bob Jones, a 22-year-old, was involved in a motor vehicle accident, and sustained abdominal injury and multiple fractures.

Problem/Nursing Diagnosis
Multiple trauma/Deficient fluid volume related to blood loss.

Supporting Assessment Data
Objective: BP 90/40, P 150, skin pale and clammy.

Goals/Expected Outcomes	Nursing Interventions	Selected Rationale	Evaluation
Patient will have adequate BP to maintain vital organ perfusion.	Monitor vital signs, CVP (when used), urine output, q 5 min to 1 hr as indicated by patient condition.	Maintain a high index of suspicion for hypovolemia and shock. Early detection and treatment of shock prevents complications.	BP is maintained at greater than 90 mm Hg systolic and urine output is ≥30 mL/hr.
	Maintain patent IV sites. Administer fluids as ordered.	Volume replacement is essential and requires adequate access.	IV fluid bolus of 500 mL given. IV fluids infusing at 150 mL/hr via peripheral IV sites in both forearms (total of 300 mL/hr).
	Note quality/strength of peripheral pulses with vital signs.	Weak, thready pulses indicate decreased cardiac output.	Pulses are weak and thready.
	Monitor laboratory and x-ray results.	Evaluate patient's response to therapy.	Laboratory and radiograph results are pending.

BP, blood pressure; *CVP*, central venous pressure; *IV*, intravenous; *P*, pulse.

Continued

Nursing Care Plan 45-1   Care of the Patient Exhibiting Symptoms of Shock—cont'd

Problem/Nursing Diagnosis
Very low blood pressure/Risk for impaired gas exchange related to altered blood flow.

Supporting Assessment Data
Objective: BP 80/40, blood loss secondary to trauma, respiratory rate 32/min.

Goals/Expected Outcomes	Nursing Interventions	Selected Rationale	Evaluation
ABGs, pulse oximetry, and respiratory rate are within patient's normal range.	Maintain patent airway. Elevate head of bed if tolerated by BP and spinal fracture is ruled out.	Enhances lung expansion.	Patient breathing is rapid, but not labored at 32/min. Supine position maintained for BP 90/40.
	Administer oxygen to keep SaO_2 ≥92%. Monitor pulse oximetry.	Maximizes the oxygen-carrying capacity of the available hemoglobin.	SaO_2 is ≥92%. Pulse oximetry reading is 99% on non-rebreather mask.
	Auscultate breath sounds q 2-4 hr.	The patient is at risk for ARDS.	Lung sounds clear or changes are identified and reported promptly.
	Investigate alterations in level of consciousness.	Decreased levels of oxygen can cause alterations in sensorium.	No change in level of consciousness. Is alert, talkative, and seems anxious.

Problem/Nursing Diagnosis
Very anxious about injuries/Patient/family fear due to uncertainty of condition related to presence of a life-threatening situation.

Supporting Assessment Data
Subjective: Patient states that he is scared and wants to know if he will live.

Goals/Expected Outcomes	Nursing Interventions	Selected Rationale	Evaluation
Patient/family will express concerns and fears.	Maintain a calm and reassuring presence.	This will reduce anxiety and the patient's oxygen need.	Patient/family is reassured when the nurse is present.
	Explain activities, medications, treatments, and equipment simply and honestly.	Information facilitates cooperation and increases feelings of control.	The patient/family states that all of their questions were answered.
	Demonstrate concern and respect for patient and family.	Extending an attitude of concern makes it easier for patients/families to discuss concerns.	The patient/family discussed concerns with the health care team.

Critical Thinking Questions
1. What complications is this patient at risk for developing?
2. If this patient were 72 instead of 22 years old, how would that change your care?

ABGs, arterial blood gases; *ARDS*, acute respiratory distress syndrome; *SaO₂*, percentage of hemoglobin saturated with oxygen.

the skin, and the amplitude of pulses in the extremities. With adequate fluid and medication administration, BP should be maintained above 90 mm Hg systolic. This should provide enough blood flow to the kidneys to generate 20 to 30 mL of urine output per hour. If there are no neurologic problems, the patient should return to previous level of consciousness.

PSYCHOLOGICAL AND SOCIAL EMERGENCIES

THE COMBATIVE PATIENT

One half of all health professionals have been verbally assaulted and one quarter have been physically assaulted. Patient factors associated with an increased incidence of attacks on health care personnel include paranoid schizophrenia, personality disorders, dementia, and substance abuse or a history of abuse or

| Box 45-3 | Strategies for Approaching a Combative Patient |

- Offer help on a one-to-one basis. Several people trying to simultaneously talk to or subdue the patient may add to fear and disorientation.
- Establish eye contact.
- Use the person's name frequently.
- Explain who you are and what you are trying to do.
- Express genuine concern about the situation.
- Use a soft voice.
- Make sure the patient can hear and understand what is being said.
- Observe for signs of drug or alcohol use.

| Box 45-4 | Questions to Detect Abuse |

- Have you been hit or hurt in any way in the past year?
- Who injured you? Has it occurred before?
- Are you afraid of anyone?
- Do you feel safe at home?
- Does your partner use drugs or alcohol? How does his or her behavior change after using them?

violence (March & Grose, 2010). Patients who are not diagnosed as mentally ill can also become violent when nurses and other health care personnel fail to respect their rights and needs or when they are feeling threatened. Signs and symptoms that usually precede an attack include increasing agitation or resistance, aggressive behavior, pacing, frowning, hyperalertness, increasing demands, and glaring. Approach in a non-threatening manner, use a calm tone of voice, and remain calm (Box 45-3). Language barriers and hearing difficulties need to be considered as possible contributors to an escalating situation. It may be necessary to help the patient by exerting control. Physical force should be used only after it is apparent that talking with the patient is not effective. One may simply tell the patient to stop screaming, to sit down, or to put down a weapon-like object. If physical restraint becomes necessary, enough people must be available to control the patient (see Chapter 48).

If restraints are used, clearly explain that restraints are not a punishment for wrongdoing, but will help the patient to regain control of himself. The patient should be advised about the duration of restraint and the conditions (i.e., calm behavior, talking rationally) of removal. The Joint Commission and most facilities have standards related to the use of restraints.

DOMESTIC VIOLENCE AND ABUSE

Approximately 2 million injuries and 1000 to 1600 deaths per year are the result of partner violence (Schub & Jaffe, 2010). Although many more women (1 in 5) are battered by their intimate partners, men (1 in 14) sometimes also suffer from battering (Pinto & Grose, 2010). Signs of battering include bruises, swellings, lacerations, fractures, hematomas, blackened eyes, abdominal injuries (especially during pregnancy), burns, and open wounds. Bruises or fractures in various stages of healing and signs of old lacerations and wounds in the presence of new ones indicate a need for a thorough assessment for battering. Often

the victim may explain all of the injuries as the result of logical accidents rather than disclose that battering by an intimate partner has occurred.

Psychologically the person may display signs of depression, low self-esteem, anxiety, and stress. Box 45-4 presents the types of questions that might be asked to elicit more information. Asking these questions after establishing rapport with the patient may encourage honest sharing of thoughts and feelings. Research shows that women actually welcome the opportunity to talk about domestic violence, but health care personnel do not routinely ask unless there is a high index of suspicion. Health care personnel's response to domestic violence is based on subjective evaluation and is affected by education and experience in the area of abuse (Olive, 2007). If battering is revealed, the person is referred to an appropriate shelter and community resources and the incident is reported to the appropriate agency. **Some states have laws requiring health care providers to report domestic violence.**

 Clinical Cues

It is estimated that an abused woman may be beaten as many as 35 times before being able to make the final break with her abuser (Pinto & Grose, 2010). As a nurse, you may feel frustrated, astonished, or helpless as you meet women who repeatedly return to their abusers. Women are likely to think of the safety of their children (Olive, 2007); therefore using discussions about the physical dangers to children and long-term psychological effects may help an abused woman to take action.

Child Abuse

If the child and caregiver make frequent trips to the clinic or ED for unexplained or questionable injuries, abuse could be occurring. Suspicion increases when the mechanism of injury, as reported by the caregiver (or child), does not match the injury pattern. **Child abuse or suspicion of child abuse must be reported by law.**

 Think Critically

A caregiver reports that the child reached for a hot surface; there is a perfectly round burn in the middle of the palmar surface. What might you conclude about the caregiver's explanation?

Elder Abuse

An estimated 1.6 million elderly adults are abused every year, primarily at home by family caregivers (Schub & Grose, 2010). Neglect is the most common form, but also assess for physical, emotional, psychological, or financial abuse. The elderly patient should be assessed for signs of fear, withdrawal, anxiety, or evasiveness. The caregiver should be assessed for a hostile, critical, or unsympathetic attitude. The same signs of physical abuse listed for domestic abuse should be searched for, as well as signs of malnutrition, uncleanness, or severe depression. **The law requires that signs of elder abuse be reported.** Immediate safety must be established; but referrals to support groups, counseling, respite care, Meals on Wheels, and transportation services can alleviate stress for caregivers. Placement in a nursing home or care facility may be the best option (Champion, 2009), although many families will require financial assistance.

Get Ready for the NCLEX® Examination!

Key Points

- Good Samaritan laws protect medical personnel from liability when offering emergency medical care for victims of accidental injury.
- Three elements that emergency nurses use for clinical decisions are (1) events or incidents that preceded the emergency visit, (2) mechanism of injury, and (3) index of suspicion.
- *Triage* is the process of setting priorities for treatment.
- Neck or spinal injury is suspected in multiple injuries, falls, or blunt force impact.
- Flail chest occurs when three or more ribs are broken in two or more places; flail chest compromises respirations, as the chest wall is unstable. Treatment includes intubation and mechanical ventilation.
- Symptoms of pneumothorax or hemothorax include labored, shallow respirations, lack of movement on one side of the chest when the person inhales and exhales and chest pain. Penetrating abdominal trauma is frequently associated with gun or knife wounds. Patients with blunt trauma to the abdomen should have serial assessments to identify slow hemorrhage or occult injury.
- Poison control centers need the following information to assist in diagnosis and treatment: patient's age; weight; medical and medication history; allergies; what, when, and why the substance was taken; current signs and symptoms, with vital signs and laboratory results; and any treatment rendered.
- Clean bite wounds immediately with soap and hot running water for 5 to 10 minutes.
- Chemical burns should be flushed with large amounts of water (with some exceptions) until all traces of the chemical have been removed.
- The new American Heart Association guidelines emphasize C-A-B (chest compressions, airway, breathing) and the importance of high-quality CPR, and recommend hands-only CPR for the lay rescuer.
- Treatment of shock generally includes infusion of large volumes of IV fluid.
- Blood pressure support in cardiogenic shock involves support for the pump (the heart) rather than adding volume.
- Signs and symptoms that usually precede aggression or attack include increasing agitation or resistance, aggressive behavior, pacing, frowning, hyperalertness, increasing demands, or glaring.
- Victims of domestic abuse and violence may be reluctant to voluntarily reveal abuse or identify the abuser.

Additional Learning Resources

SG Go to your Study Guide for additional learning activities to help you master this chapter content.

evolve Go to your Evolve website (http://evolve.elsevier.com/deWit/medsurg) for the following FREE learning resources:
- Animations, audio, and video
- Answers and rationales for questions and activities
- Concept Map Creator
- Glossary with pronunciations in English and Spanish
- Interactive Review Questions and Exercises and more!

Review Questions for the NCLEX® Examination

1. To control a gushing bleed of the lower leg, what should the nurse do initially?
   1. Apply direct pressure to the wound.
   2. Compress the artery above the wound.
   3. Check the circulation to the foot.
   4. Snugly secure a bulky dressing.

2. In the event of any type of poisoning that occurs in the home setting, what is the initial course of action?
   1. Save the poison container and contents.
   2. Save a sample of vomitus for analysis.
   3. Call poison control.
   4. Induce vomiting.

3. A teenager—alert, oriented, and in no apparent distress—is brought to the ED by EMS on a backboard with spine immobilization in place. He reports diving into a lake and bumping his head. Based on the mechanism of injury, which assessment is the nurse most likely to initiate?
   1. Assessment of water safety behavior
   2. Serial abdominal assessments with hematocrit
   3. Frequent vital signs to monitor for shock
   4. Peripheral motion and sensation with mental status checks

4. The nurse makes a home visit to a 70-year-old patient on a cold winter day. On arrival the patient demonstrates excessive coughing, shortness of breath, drowsiness, and confusion. Mucous membranes are cherry red. What is the nurse's first action?

   1. Question the patient about recent food or fluid consumption.
   2. Call for emergency help and open the windows.
   3. Search the house for evidence of poisons and then call poison control.
   4. Locate the source of odors or try to get the patient to walk out of the house.

5. The nurse is talking to a community group about strategies to prevent heat-related illness. What advice is appropriate to give to the group? *(Select all that apply.)*

   1. Drink fluids that are nonalcoholic, noncaffeinated, and low in sugar content.
   2. When you are thirsty, drink fluids and avoid eating salty foods.
   3. Stay indoors with cooling systems.
   4. In the heat, wear lightweight, light-colored, loose-fitting clothing.
   5. Limit outdoor activities to spring or fall when the weather is cooler.
   6. Use sun protection such as wide-brimmed hats, sunglasses, and sunscreen.

6. A family of six people arrives at the ED with similar symptoms of diarrhea, cramps, and nausea and vomiting that started approximately 6 hours after eating a picnic lunch. Which order from the physician should the nurse anticipate?

   1. Administer antidiarrheal medication.
   2. Establish peripheral intravenous access.
   3. Obtain stool specimens for culture and sensitivity.
   4. Give oral rehydration therapy.

7. A patient is brought to the ED with severe gastrointestinal bleeding and hypovolemic shock. What is the priority intervention for this patient?

   1. Insert a nasogastric tube and attach to low wall suction.
   2. Draw a blood sample for a type and crossmatch.
   3. Measure the amount of emesis and check for blood.
   4. Establish two large-bore peripheral IV sites.

8. When taking care of a patient with sepsis, what is the first sign that would signal impending septic shock?

   1. Increasing urine output
   2. Decreasing heart rate
   3. Decreasing blood pressure
   4. Change in mental status

9. A patient is 6 hours postoperative with signs of deficient fluid volume. The physician orders a fluid challenge of 200 mL lactated Ringer's stat over 20 minutes. What would be considered a desirable response to the treatment?

   1. Decrease in blood pressure
   2. Increase in urinary output
   3. Increase in body weight
   4. Increase in pulse rate

10. A patient was bitten by a stray dog and rushed to the emergency department. Which measure must be done first?

   1. Apply antibiotic ointment on affected sites.
   2. Cover with a clean bandage and immobilize.
   3. Rinse wound with soap and hot running water for 5 to 10 minutes.
   4. Give tetanus booster shot if patient has not had one in the past 5 years.

Critical Thinking Activities

Scenario A

While watching a sporting event from the stands, you notice the person sitting in front of you has slumped over. You touch her shoulder and ask if she is all right. There is no response and you see no signs of breathing.

1. What is the most likely explanation for this witnessed event of sudden unconsciousness?

2. What should you do first?

3. An AED is on scene. What is your role in use of this equipment?

4. How do "Good Samaritan Laws" affect you and any interventions that you may perform on this woman?

Scenario B

You are on your way home from work and you see a car hit a teenage boy on a bicycle. You stop to help the bicyclist. He is unconscious, has a large scalp laceration that is bleeding profusely, and has an obviously fractured left leg.

1. If you need to open his airway, what method would you use?

2. What should you do about the scalp laceration and broken leg?

3. What is your legal obligation in this setting?

Scenario C

While working as a student nurse in the hospital's emergency unit, you notice that patients who have been injured or are very ill sometimes become hostile and combative. Some try to assault members of the emergency team and others use abusive and threatening language.

1. Discuss with your classmates some reasons why patients may behave in these ways when they are injured or very ill.

2. What are some ways in which violent patients, who are not mentally ill, can be handled to prevent assault and encourage cooperation with the emergency staff?

3. What resources are available to help manage combative patients?

4. What patient history or information might help to clarify aggressive behavior?

Scenario D

Your 80-year-old male patient admitted yesterday for pneumonia has become confused, hypotensive, oliguric, clammy, and pale.

1. What are the possible explanations for his clinical signs and symptoms?

2. What are your priorities for his care?

3. Discuss what treatment is indicated.

4. How will you know if your treatment has been effective?

Care of Patients with Anxiety, Mood, and Eating Disorders

http://evolve.elsevier.com/deWit/medsurg

Objectives

Theory

1. Analyze the significance of anxiety in the general adult population.
2. Compare and contrast normal anxiety and anxiety disorders.
3. Describe the signs and symptoms and treatment for anxiety disorders.
4. Discuss assessment, nursing diagnoses, and nursing interventions for patients with anxiety disorders.
5. Discuss the variances of normal mood and discuss mood alterations that become debilitating.
6. Discuss assessment, nursing diagnoses, and nursing interventions for patients with bipolar disorder and major depressive disorder.

7. Summarize factors that are essential when assessing a suicidal patient.
8. Analyze the impact of family, peer, and media pressure on patients with eating disorders.
9. Discuss assessment, nursing diagnoses, and nursing interventions for patients with eating disorders.

Clinical Practice

1. Watch the movie *As Good as It Gets* and discuss behaviors that are debilitating for the main character.
2. Implement a teaching plan for a patient with a mood disorder to increase medication compliance.
3. Identify at least six interventions for the nursing diagnosis Risk for self-directed violence related to suicidal ideations.

Key Terms

affect (ĂF-ĕkt, p. 1052)
anorexia nervosa (ăn-ŏ-RĔK-sē-ă nĕr-VŌ-să, p. 1060)
bipolar disorder (bī-PŌ-lăr dĭs-ŎR-dĕr, p. 1051)
bulimia nervosa (bū-LĒ-mē-ă nĕr-VŌ-să, p. 1060)
dual diagnosis (dū-ăl dī-ăg-NŌ-sĭs, p. 1055)
dysthymia (dĭs-THĪ-mē-ă, p. 1051)
electroconvulsive therapy (ECT) (ĕ-LĔK-trō-kŏn-VŬL-sĭv THĔR-ă-pē, p. 1057)
flight of ideas (p. 1051)
generalized anxiety disorder (GAD) (jĕn-ĕr-ăl-ĪZD ăng-ZĪ-ĭ-tē dĭs-ŎR-dĕr, p. 1046)
hypersomnia (hī-pĕr-SŎM-nē-ă, p. 1052)
hypomania (hī-pō-MĂN-ē-ă, p. 1051)

insomnia (ĭn-SŎM-nē-ă, p. 1052)
lanugo (lă-NŪ-gō, p. 1061)
major depressive disorder (MĀ-jŏr dĕ-PRĚ-sĭv dĭs-ŎR-dĕr, p. 1055)
mania (MĀ-nē-ă, p. 1051)
obsessive-compulsive disorder (OCD) (ŏb-SĔS-ĭv cŏm-PŬL-sĭv dĭs-ŎR-dĕr, p. 1047)
phobic disorder (FŌ-bĭk dĭs-ŎR-dĕr, p. 1047)
post-traumatic stress disorder (PTSD) (pōst-trăw-MĂT-ĭk strĕs dĭs-ŎR-dĕr, p. 1047)
pressured speech (p. 1051)
psychomotor retardation (sĭ-kō-MŌ-tĕr rē-tăr-DĀ-shŭn, p. 1055)

ANXIETY AND ANXIETY DISORDERS

Anxiety is considered normal and healthy unless it becomes debilitating and prevents a person from functioning in everyday life. Abnormal or debilitating anxiety is intense and feels life threatening to the individual. One of four people will experience symptoms of an anxiety disorder during his or her lifetime. Elderly people are at high risk for anxiety disorders because of physical illness, psychosocial stress, depression, cognitive impairment, and personal factors related to female gender, lower education, or substance abuse.

Anxiety is often self-limiting and alleviated without specific medical or nursing intervention. However, intervention may be necessary to prevent potential harm toward self or aggression toward others. Nurses can be instrumental in helping a patient recover from a panic level of anxiety. Table 46-1 describes the various levels of anxiety and their nursing management, and Figure 46-1 depicts the relationship among stress, anxiety, and related behaviors. By remaining calm and supportive, the nurse provides a safety net for the patient. Anticipate that panic-level anxiety is challenging and will often require medication. Patients with anxiety need teaching

Table 46-1   **Nursing Management for Levels of Anxiety**

LEVEL OF ANXIETY	ASSESSMENT	NURSING GOAL	NURSING MANAGEMENT
Mild	Increased alertness, motivation, and attentiveness.	To assist patient to tolerate some anxiety.	Help patient identify and describe feelings. Help patient develop the capacity to tolerate mild anxiety, and use it conscientiously and constructively.
Moderate	Perception narrowed, selective inattention, physical discomforts.	To reduce anxiety; long-term goal directed toward helping patient understand cause of anxiety and new ways of controlling it.	Provide outlet for tension such as walking, crying, working at simple, concrete tasks. Encourage patient to discuss feelings.
Severe	Behavior becomes automatic; connections between details are not seen; senses are drastically reduced.	To assist in channeling anxiety.	Recognize own level of anxiety. Link patient's behavior with feelings. Protect defenses and coping mechanisms. Identify and modify anxiety-provoking situations.
Panic	Overwhelmed; inability to function or communicate; possible bodily harm to self and others; loss of rational thought.	To be supportive and protective.	Provide nonstimulating, structured environment. Avoid touching. Stay with patient. Medicate patient with tranquilizers if necessary.

Adapted from Zerwekh, J., & Claborn, J. (2003). *NCLEX-PN: A Study Guide for Practical Nursing.* Dallas: Nursing Education Consultants (p. 112).

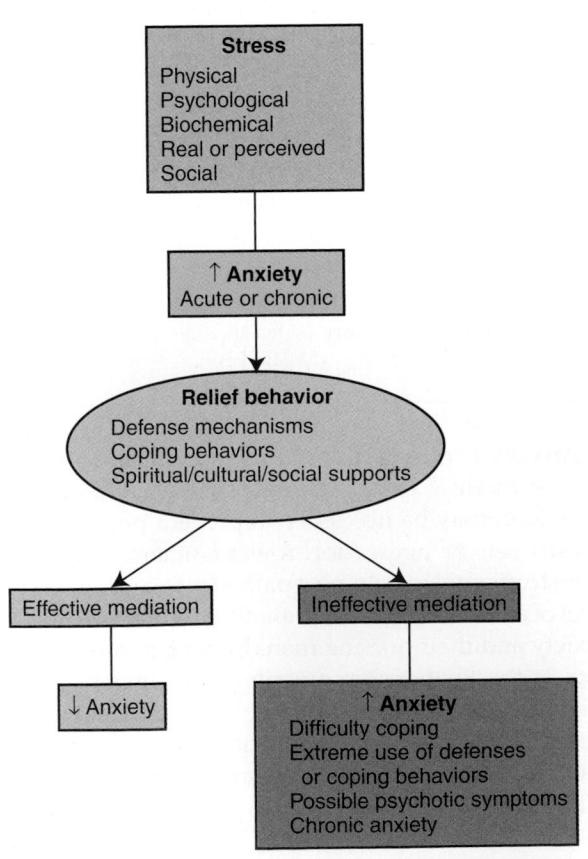

FIGURE 46-1 Stress, anxiety, and behavioral effects.

about how to prevent further attacks. They need to be taught how to relax and should attempt to determine the underlying cause of their anxiety. Anxiety can recur at a greater level of severity; therefore early intervention is important.

? Think Critically

Recall a time when you felt very anxious. What were your feelings and behaviors? What strategies did you use to manage your own anxiety?

GENERALIZED ANXIETY DISORDER

A person who experiences persistent, unrealistic, or excessive worry about two or more life circumstances for 6 months or longer is exhibiting symptoms associated with **generalized anxiety disorder (GAD).** GAD usually develops slowly and is chronic in nature. As a case study, let us consider John Evans. John Evans has GAD. He worries about his work performance, despite good evaluations. John worries that his children are not happy, smart, popular, or excelling, and he worries constantly about their future. John worries about paying the bills, and he worries about the well-being of his elderly parents. There are currently no actual problems, yet despite his wife's support and reassurance, John cannot stop worrying. He experiences the signs and symptoms of excessive physiologic response such as tachycardia, restlessness, sweating, fatigue, muscular tension, and shortness of breath. His cognitive symptoms include difficulty with problem solving and poor concentration. John also demonstrates limited coping skills.

PHOBIC DISORDER

A person with a phobic disorder experiences excessive fear of a situation or object. This fear can lead to avoidance or extreme anxiety that interferes with normal responsibilities and routines. As another case study, let us consider Max Payne. Max has a specific type of phobia known as social anxiety disorder. Max is chronically unable to hold a job; he fears scrutiny of his abilities and is afraid of being embarrassed by coworkers or supervisors. Work settings cause him to feel pressured, overwhelmed, and distressed and he experiences physical symptoms such as trembling, blushing, and nausea. He avoids opportunities by creating a variety of excuses not to pursue them, and this further lowers his self-esteem. He acknowledges that his fears are unreasonable, but he continues to make excuses to avoid professional challenges or situations of occupational risk taking.

OBSESSIVE-COMPULSIVE DISORDER

When a person has an obsessive-compulsive disorder (OCD), she experiences an *obsession*, recurrent or intrusive thoughts that she cannot stop thinking about, and these thoughts create anxiety. A *compulsive act* is an act that the person feels compelled to perform. For example, a person may experience anxiety and so performs repetitive handwashing in an attempt to reduce that anxiety. Time spent in these thoughts and rituals can become overwhelming to the point of interfering with normal life. Consider the case study of Jane Forman, who is constantly thinking about the boyfriend who left her. Jane does not want to think about him; however, she *ruminates* (repeatedly talks or thinks about the same topic) on their relationship. She scrubs and cleans everything that he might have touched. Jane begins to miss work and stops socializing with friends because she cannot stop cleaning. Her compulsive thoughts have led to obsessive behavior, and Jane Forman has an obsessive-compulsive disorder.

POST-TRAUMATIC STRESS DISORDER

Individuals with post-traumatic stress disorder (PTSD) have endured one or more extreme life-threatening events, and the remembrance of these events now produces feelings of intense horror, with recurrent symptoms of anxiety and nightmares or flashbacks.

 Cultural Considerations

PTSD and Immigrant Patients

Patients who have emigrated from war-torn countries such as Vietnam or Afghanistan are at risk for PTSD. Language differences and a reluctance to seek professional help for psychiatric problems are barriers to care.

As a case study, consider Holly Harris, who was a rape victim 2 months ago. In her consciousness Holly frequently relives the traumatic experience, although she tries to avoid thinking or talking about what happened. She feels detached from others and disinterested in her normal activities. She fears she may not ever be able to have loving feelings toward a man and feels bleak about the future in general. She is irritable and has difficulty sleeping and concentrating. She is hypervigilant, yet she startles very easily.

 Cultural Considerations

PTSD and Military Personnel

In studies of war veterans, there was an increased risk for PTSD for those who were young, female, Hispanic, or African American and for those who had more combat experience (Westgard, 2009).

Diagnosis of Anxiety Disorders

To help clinicians define and diagnose behavioral disorders more consistently, the American Psychiatric Association publishes a regularly updated manual that establishes guidelines for how diagnoses are made. The *Diagnostic and Statistical Manual of Mental Disorders,* fourth edition, text revision (DSM-IV-TR) provides a set of diagnostic criteria (specific behaviors) and a specific time frame for each mental health disorder. For example, a patient might feel mildly anxious for 1 or 2 days before surgery, but mild anxiety for a short period before such an event would be considered normal; therefore that patient would not meet the criteria for any of the anxiety disorders. In contrast, a person such as John Evans (described previously) is *dysfunctional* because of **continuous worry for at least 6 months** and his behavior would meet the criteria for GAD.

The DSM-IV-TR also uses a multiaxial approach that further describes health in physical, social, and functional areas:

- Axis I: Major mental health disorder (e.g., major depression)
- Axis II: Personality disorders or mental retardation (e.g., dependent personality)
- Axis III: Physical health disorders (e.g., diabetes mellitus)
- Axis IV: Psychosocial or environmental factors (e.g., death in the family)
- Axis V: Global Assessment of Functioning (GAF)

Scores on Axis V (the GAF) range from 1 to 100 for functioning in daily life. For example, many nursing students would score between 81 and 90 because of mild anxiety before tests, but general satisfaction with life; whereas many people in jail would score below 50 because of a prolonged inability to hold a job, with history of legal problems and social dysfunction.

Treatment of Anxiety Disorders

People with anxiety disorders can be treated with supportive therapy and *anxiolytic* (antianxiety) medications. Supportive therapy may include individual therapy and education about relaxation techniques and stress management. Patients who are anxious need much reassurance, and a nurse who is nonjudgmental will be a good listener. Evidence-based practice indicates that for elderly patients with GAD, cognitive-behavioral therapy (CBT) is the first-line psychotherapy (Box 46-1).

A relatively new short-term therapy for PTSD is eye movement desensitization and reprocessing (EMDR). In EMDR, while the patient thinks about the distressing event, she shifts her gaze from one side to the other. As unpleasant feelings are uncovered, the therapist redirects the eye movements and this helps the patient to release the emotions. In another new therapy for PTSD, the patient wears a headset and is exposed to a virtual reality environment. The clinician controls what the patient hears, sees, and smells, and the patient learns to tolerate anxiety (Helwick, 2010).

Box 46-1	Advanced Practice Psychotherapeutic Interventions

- *Psychodynamic therapy:* Therapist helps the patient to link a past event to current feelings. This insight is thought to help patient modify feelings and behavior.
- *Cognitive-behavioral therapy:* Therapist helps the patient to identify unhealthy thoughts or undesirable responses that occur because of a situation or event and then the patient is assisted to change ways of thinking about an event and therefore to change emotional response and behavior.
- *Motivational interviewing:* Therapist enhances motivation for change by matching the patient's ability to problem solve, with specific strategies. Principles include expressing empathy, developing discrepancy, supporting self-efficacy, and rolling with resistance.
- *Interpersonal therapy:* Therapist helps the patient to identify the problem, then selects a strategy to address the problem. The goal is to eliminate symptoms by improving social relationships.
- *Group therapy:* Therapist leads group sessions of 5 to 10 patients who have similar needs or problems. Patients share feelings, thoughts, ideas, and experiences; they realize, "I am not alone in my experience."
- *Behavioral therapy:* Therapist assists the patient to change behavior, by using rewards, punishment, repetition, imitation, or exposure to stimuli—but understanding of the underlying cause is not essential. There are four types of behavioral therapy: modeling, operant conditioning, systematic desensitization, and aversion therapy.

 Clinical Cues

Your patient may need referral to a stress management class; however, there are a few basic suggestions that you can make to help your patient cope with stress. These suggestions include talking to a friend, listening to music, taking a warm bath or shower, doing a large muscle activity such as walking, or throwing ice cubes against the back fence.

Benzodiazepines are commonly prescribed for anxiety disorders. Drugs from this category are alprazolam (Xanax), chlordiazepoxide (Librium), oxazepam (Serax), lorazepam (Ativan), and diazepam (Valium). Patients taking these drugs must be advised to use medications with caution because *tolerance* (the need for an increased dosage to achieve the desired effect) and physical and psychological dependency can occur.

⚠ Safety Alert

Sensitivity to Benzodiazepines

Elderly patients are very sensitive to benzodiazepines and use is generally restricted during alcohol or sedative withdrawal. Lorazepam (Ativan) and alprazolam (Xanax) can cause confusion, oversedation, or disinhibition (Lyons et al., 2009).

Buspirone (BuSpar), in a class by itself, takes 3 to 4 weeks to reach therapeutic efficacy. The advantage of BuSpar is less sedation with a decreased risk of dependency. Another class of drugs, the selective serotonin reuptake inhibitors (SSRIs), are becoming first-line drugs for anxiety because they have fewer adverse effects. Examples from the SSRI category include citalopram (Celexa) and sertraline (Zoloft). Table 46-2 presents a list of common medications used to treat anxiety.

In a new experimental therapy for anxiety disorders, propranolol was used to decrease the fear associated with a frightening memory. Researchers found that the timing of the drug in relation to the threatening event was the essential element. Other studies suggested that well-timed psychotherapy could potentially be used instead of the drug to accomplish the manipulation of the memory and fear response (Harvard Medical School, 2009).

❖ NURSING MANAGEMENT

■ Assessment (Data Collection)

You should assess the anxiety-prone patient for subjective feelings of fear, apprehension, isolation, or the need for increased space. Assess the patient's ability to concentrate and make rational judgments, and explore the sources of preoccupation and worries. Physical symptoms may include trembling, feeling shaky, increased muscle tension, muscle soreness, easy fatigability, and restlessness. Patients may be hypervigilant, have

Table 46-2 Medications Used to Treat Anxiety

CLASSIFICATION	ACTION	NURSING IMPLICATIONS	PATIENT EDUCATION
Benzodiazepines			
Alprazolam (Xanax) Chlordiazepoxide (Librium) Diazepam (Valium) Lorazepam (Ativan) Oxazepam (Serax)	Has depressant action on the CNS and inhibits stimulation of the brain. Used for anxiety disorders and insomnia.	Watch for signs of orthostatic hypotension. Watch for side effects: palpitations, dry mouth, nausea and vomiting, and occasional nightmares. Elderly patients have significantly increased risk for falls.	Do not take any other CNS depressants, including alcohol. Potentially addictive; use only as prescribed. Can cause drowsiness and lethargy. Do not stop taking these medications abruptly.
Nonbenzodiazepines			
Buspirone (BuSpar)	Interacts with serotonin receptors (see Chapter 49). Used for anxiety and sleep disorders.	Always a scheduled medication, never PRN. May cause headaches, dizziness, or drowsiness, but much less so compared to the benzodiazepines.	Takes 7-10 days for symptoms to subside and several weeks for optimal results. No evidence of tolerance or physical dependence. Do not stop taking this medication abruptly.
Duloxetine (Cymbalta) approved for GAD	Increases activity of serotonin and norepinephrine.	Most common side effects are nausea, dry mouth, sleepiness, and constipation.	Advise that driving or operating machinery could be dangerous.
SSRIs (see Table 46-4)			

CNS, central nervous system; *FDA,* Food and Drug Administration; *GAD,* generalized anxiety disorder; *PRN,* as needed; *SSRIs,* selective serotonin reuptake inhibitors.

difficulty sleeping, and be very irritable. In addition, an autonomic nervous system response can cause an increase in blood pressure, dyspnea, palpitations, dry mouth, dizziness, and nausea.

Cultural Considerations

The Hispanic/Latino Patient

The Hispanic/Latino patient may believe that an emotional trauma will result in a fright sickness called *susto.* Symptoms of *susto* include crying, insomnia, restlessness, nightmares, diarrhea, and fever. Treatment is brushing the body with a rough object. The patient might also believe in *brujeria,* which is a magical or supernatural illness. Symptoms include paranoia, delusions, hallucinations, and being controlled by others. The patient may reject the physician in favor of a *brujo* (witch) for reversal of the spell or hex.

Evidenced-based guidelines suggest that screening tools can be used by *any* health care worker if an elderly patient is showing signs of an anxiety disorder. These assessment tools include the Mini-Mental State Examination (see Chapter 48), Geriatric Anxiety Inventory, Short Anxiety Screening Test, Hospital Anxiety and Depression Scale, and Rating Anxiety in Dementia Scale (Smith & Brighton, 2009). After initial screening, the physician is notified, to determine the diagnosis.

Clinical Cues

When would you give a drug ordered as a short-acting anxiolytic? Observe the patient for signs of anxiety, such as pacing, restlessness, and facial expressions of fear or concern. Assess for feelings of apprehension and the patient's ability to concentrate. For example, "Mrs. Smith, you seem a little restless. Let's sit for a while and you can tell me what is going on." If therapeutic communication is not successful, and the patient shows progressively escalating signs of hostility, trembling, agitation, irritability, or inability to relax and converse, it would be appropriate to offer the medication.

Elder Care Points

Elderly patients frequently have strong spiritual beliefs that assist in coping with stress and illness. Friendships, social contacts, and activities associated with religious organizations also play a large part in positive mental health. Evidence suggests that elderly patients will benefit from tactful assessment and individualized interventions that incorporate personal spiritual beliefs (Phillips et al., 2009).

■ Nursing Diagnosis

Nursing diagnoses for anxiety include:
- Anxiety related to threat to self-concept
- Fear related to threat in the environment

- Impaired social interaction related to extreme anxiety in social situations
- Ineffective coping related to panic attack
- Ineffective role performance related to perceived inability to complete work responsibilities
- Powerlessness related to loss of control when facing a specific phobic object (e.g., a spider)
- Complicated grieving related to multiple loss of fellow soldiers (i.e., war trauma)
- Post-trauma syndrome related to an overwhelming, life-threatening event (e.g., rape)

■ Planning

Expected outcomes are written for the specific individual nursing diagnoses chosen to resolve the patient's problems. For the nursing diagnoses above, example outcomes might include:

- Patient will demonstrate decreased symptoms of anxiety (e.g., pacing, crying) within 3 days.
- Patient will verbalize feelings of safety before discharge.
- Patient will attend group meeting today accompanied by primary nurse.
- Patient will practice three coping strategies to use during a panic attack before discharge.
- Patient will identify three tasks at which she excels at work, during this shift.
- Patient will verbalize increased feelings of control when encountering phobic object within 1 month.
- Patient will express grief and loss related to multiple losses before discharge.
- Patient will experience fewer nightmares related to traumatic event within 3 months.

Planning care for a patient with an anxiety disorder involves promoting a physically and psychologically safe environment. For example, provide a quiet, clean, and noncluttered environment and verbal reassurance ("Mrs. Smith, you are safe here. The staff is here to help you."). Methods to reduce the symptoms of anxiety include therapeutic communication, such as active listening, being physically present, offering emotional reassurance, giving clear and concise instructions, and using pharmacologic methods.

 Complementary and Alternative Therapies

Essential Oils

Essential oils that have a calming and soothing effect include basil, bergamot, chamomile, jasmine, rose, and lavender. These oils can be used in an aromatic bath or as massage oil.

 Complementary and Alternative Therapies

Reduce Stress to Decrease Anxiety

Research has demonstrated that massage reduces cortisol levels with "stress alleviating" effects and increases serotonin and dopamine with "activating" effects. Yoga, exercise, and amino acid therapy also can potentially reduce stress, anxiety, and depression (Wilson, 2009).

 Nutrition Considerations

Promoting Relaxation

Advise your patient that stimulants such as coffee and colas should be avoided to help decrease anxiety and nervousness. Consumption of raw nuts and seeds, whole grains, and fresh fruits and vegetables helps to build the body's reserve and strength. Bananas, rice, milk, and pasta contain tryptophan, which helps to induce relaxation.

As the acute anxiety passes, the focus of care is to help the patient recognize that certain behaviors (such as avoidance) are being overused. The patient is then assisted to develop new methods of coping and to resume participation in family, social, and occupational roles.

 Elder Care Points

The elderly population often expresses somatic complaints rather than openly verbalizing emotional distress. You may observe the anxious elder complaining of an upset stomach, inability to sleep, fatigue, or increased need to urinate. Medications (e.g., sertraline [Zoloft], levothyroxine [Synthroid], theophylline [Slo-Phyllin]) that the elder is taking may increase feelings of anxiety. Certain medical conditions, such as problems with the thyroid gland, problems with the cardiac system, and altered blood sugar, can also mimic anxiety disorders.

■ Implementation

When intervening with a patient who is experiencing extreme levels of anxiety, you must maintain a calm and reassuring attitude. Stay with the patient and attend to physical needs as necessary. Attempt to make the immediate surrounding environment less stimulating. For example, dim the lights, turn off the television or radio, and limit the number of people in the area. Be sure to use clear, simple statements, and repeat them as necessary. When extreme levels of anxiety resolve, use additional interventions to help the patient learn to control her anxiety (see Table 46-1).

 Clinical Cues

Anxiety is contagious and can spread rapidly from person to person until the entire unit is affected; likewise, the nurse is not immune to these feelings. Fortunately, you can use therapeutic communication skills to help the patient de-escalate. Use a calm voice and a relaxed body position, and convey confidence in your own ability to maintain control of your own anxiety. Self-control by the nurse helps the patient to mimic calm behavior and control her anxiety.

When the anxiety is under control, you can assist in helping the patient to use problem-solving strategies. The long process of determining root causes of the anxiety can take years of therapy, but you can make referrals as needed, and provide support.

Evaluation

Ongoing evaluation of patients with anxiety is necessary. Evaluation includes the status of the patient before discharge from the hospital, clinic, or emergency department. Carefully document that outcome criteria were met and symptoms were relieved. **If symptoms are not totally resolved, you should clearly document that the patient's level of anxiety is not a threat to self or others at the time of discharge.** Also include the plan for follow-up care and a plan to obtain emergency care if needed.

MOOD DISORDERS

The incidence of mood disorders is very high. Unfortunately, these disorders are often inaccurately diagnosed and treated. **Dysthymia** refers to a disturbance in mood that may manifest in either depression or elation **(mania).** An individual experiencing clinical depression is more than just sad. Depressed or dysthymic individuals feel a sense of hopelessness and despair that cannot be alleviated by usual means. This hopelessness can lead to thoughts of suicide.

Mania is an elevation in mood that includes increased grandiosity or irritability that is present for at least 1 week. A manic person may exhibit **pressured speech,** which is talking that is loud and rapid and difficult to interrupt; or **flight of ideas,** where the speaker goes from topic to topic with little or no connection. There is an inability to concentrate, a decreased need for sleep or nutrients, and an increase in goal-directed activity, impulsive spending, and hypersexuality. Unstable and frequently changing, or *labile,* behavior is often seen in manic patients; a mood of frivolity and joking can rapidly change to agitation and extreme paranoia. **The agitation and irritability seen in manic patients can often lead to aggressive behavior.** Manic individuals may require hospitalization for an inability to eat or sleep for days that leads to complete physical and mental exhaustion and aggressive behavior. Sometimes individuals will rapidly switch from being extremely depressed to being euphoric and manic. This condition is called *bipolar disorder* and occurs equally in men and women. It often is initially diagnosed in young adults, but it may be diagnosed at any time during the life span.

BIPOLAR DISORDER

Bipolar disorder is suspected when a patient experiences episodes of extreme sadness, hopelessness, and helplessness interspersed with periods of extreme elation and hyperactivity. According to the DSM-IV-TR, two types of bipolar disorder are recognized. Bipolar I disorder is characterized by episodes of major depression with at least one episode of manic or hypomanic behavior. Bipolar II disorder is characterized by one or more depressive episodes with at least one episode of hypomania. **Hypomania** is an inflated or irritable mood for at least 4 days. Patients may display loud, rapid speech, and flight of ideas, decreased need for sleep, distractibility, and an increase in goal-directed activity, but hospitalization is not indicated because it does not involve psychotic behavior.

Treatment

Lithium carbonate is the drug of choice used to stabilize manic behavior. Lithium has a narrow therapeutic range, so serum lithium levels must be determined 8 to 12 hours after the first dose, then two or three times per week for the first month, and then weekly to monthly. See Table 46-3 for nursing implications for lithium. Because it may take 2 to 3 weeks for lithium to become effective, antipsychotics such as chlorpromazine (Thorazine) or haloperidol (Haldol) are given to decrease the initial level of hyperactivity. Anticonvulsant drugs such as divalproex sodium (Depakote) and carbamazepine (Tegretol) are effective in the treatment of mania and quetiapine (Seroquel), which is an atypical antipsychotic (see Box 49-1 and Table 49-2), is also used for mania. Lamotrigine (Lamictal) is effective for the depressive episodes. The Food and Drug Administration (FDA) has approved risperidone (Risperdal Consta) (2008) and ziprasidone

Table 46-3	Nursing Implications for Patients on Lithium			
CLASSIFICATION	ACTION	NURSING IMPLICATIONS	PATIENT TEACHING	
Antimanic	Alters the release, synthesis, and reuptake of neurotransmitters in the brain (i.e., dopamine, norepinephrine, and serotonin) (see Chapter 49). Does not cure bipolar disorder, but helps to decrease the manic behavior.	Takes 7-14 days to reach therapeutic level (1.0-1.5 mEq/L). Blood levels should be drawn 8-12 hr after the first dose, then two or three times/wk for the first mo and then weekly to monthly until a maintenance level is reached. Sodium depletion or dehydration could cause toxicity; therefore monitor fluid intake and dietary sodium. Diuretics should be avoided. Monitor renal and thyroid function periodically.	Normal salt intake. Drink 2500-3000 mL of fluids per day. Take with meals to decrease gastric distress. Avoid caffeinated drinks because of diuretic effects. Immediately report diarrhea, vomiting, tremors, or lack of coordination.	

HCl (Geodon) (2009) for treatment of bipolar disorder. All of these can be used safely in combination with lithium. In addition to stabilizing the patient with medication, it is sometimes necessary to hospitalize patients with manic symptoms, particularly if they are a danger to themselves or others, or are suffering from exhaustion caused by extreme hyperactivity. Recently, Diazgranados and colleagues (2010) used one dose of intravenous ketamine (Ketalar) with treatment-resistant bipolar depression, and subjects showed improvement in 40 minutes.

❖ NURSING MANAGEMENT

■ Assessment (Data Collection)

Assessing for mood disorders involves observing for mood, affect, and physical signs and symptoms. You assess mood by asking the patient questions about feelings and observing facial expressions and verbalizations. **Affect** is a term used to describe a person's external expression of emotion. A person with a flat or blunted affect may report feeling fine, but you notice that her facial expression and overall demeanor convey sadness. The sadness described by depressed individuals is intense and creates feelings of worthlessness and hopelessness. Conversely, the mood of a manic patient is one of grandiosity and general well-being. In the midst of a manic episode, the patient may feel invincible and recklessly engage in extremely dangerous behavior.

Many physical signs and symptoms are classic for mood disorders. An initial question concerns sleep. A depressed patient may report sleeping all of the time **(hypersomnia)** or falling asleep easily, but then waking up after 2 to 3 hours and being unable to get back to sleep **(insomnia)**. Manic patients are unable to sleep, and it is not unusual for them to tell you they have not slept for days.

■ Nursing Diagnosis

Typical nursing diagnoses for mania may include:
- Imbalanced nutrition: less than body requirements related to shortened attention span while trying to eat
- Risk for other-directed or self-directed violence related to labile emotional state
- Sleep deprivation related to hyperactivity
- Impaired verbal communication related to flight of ideas and pressured speech
- Interrupted family processes related to inability to perform child care duties
- Noncompliance related to refusal to take medications during manic phase

■ Planning

For the nursing diagnoses above, example outcomes include:
- Patient will consume at least 1500 calories during a 24-hour period.

- Patient will refrain from hurting self or others during this shift.
- Patient will sleep and rest at least 6 hours within a 24-hour period.
- Patient will demonstrate a decrease in pressured speech and flight of ideas before discharge.
- Patient and family will identify and use substitutes and resources for child care until the patient is able to resume family responsibilities.
- Patient will identify two methods of ensuring medication compliance before discharge.

Planning care for a patient with mania involves promoting safety, adequate nutrition, and sleep. Patients in a manic state can be a source of danger to others on the unit. Manic patients can quickly escalate in behavior from good-natured humor into active aggression. Often it is necessary to assign a nurse or nursing assistant to stay with the patient until the medications have reduced agitation and hyperactivity.

📷 Assignment Considerations

Hygienic Care of Manic Patients

On a medical-surgical unit, the nursing assistants (NAs) are likely to assist patients with hygienic needs in the morning. When caring for a manic patient, inform the NA that the patient may have a shortened attention span and a tendency to be argumentative; therefore the hygienic care may have to be accomplished in small steps over the course of the day, for example, washing hands and face on waking, brushing teeth after breakfast, combing hair midmorning, and talking a shower in the afternoon.

■ Implementation

Nursing interventions for the manic patient include keeping the patient safe, providing a high-calorie intake, administering antimanic medications, and providing for a restful sleep. Manic patients often come into the hospital malnourished. Small, frequent, high-calorie meals and finger foods are often necessary because the manic patient will not sit down long enough to eat. Close observation and documentation of mood, verbalizations, and behavior are very important. It may be necessary to place a manic patient in a quiet area away from others, to decrease environmental stimulation.

When communicating with a manic patient, it is essential that you maintain a calm demeanor. **Until the medications are effective, therapeutic communication consists of setting limits.** When setting limits, it is necessary that you clearly state your initial expectations of the patient's behavior. For example, you might say, "Mr. Smith, I am talking to Ms. Jones right now, so please stop interrupting us and wait for me in the dayroom. I will be with you as soon as we are finished." State the consequences for noncompliance with the request and remember that consistent follow-through on consequences is essential. "If you interrupt us one more time,

I will not help you with your project today and you will have to wait until tomorrow." To avoid being manipulated by the patient, it is important that all staff members be consistent. Sometimes, because of the severity of the mania, the manic patient is unable to comply with simple requests. In these instances, it is necessary to distract or redirect the patient rather than attempt to use reason.

When the patient is stabilized, providing her with information about medications and the rationale for their long-term use is important in order to increase medication compliance. Compliance is important because it is not unusual for the patient to stop taking medications once the manic symptoms subside (Nursing Care Plan 46-1).

 Nursing Care Plan 46-1 | **Care of the Patient with Bipolar Disorder (Manic Phase)**

Scenario

Bobby Holmes, 25 years old, is diagnosed with bipolar disorder. He is currently euphoric, grandiose, loud, and very talkative. Although he can be charming, he is currently argumentative and intrusive and is verbally aggressive toward other patients. He states, "I'm going to get in your face whenever I feel like it!" He is continuously walking around the unit and has trouble sitting still for meals or conversation. He states, "I haven't slept well or eaten much for the past 3 days."

Problem/Nursing Diagnosis

Poor impulse control and argumentative/Risk for other-directed violence related to manic state.

Supporting Assessment Data

Subjective: "I'm going to get in your face whenever I feel like it!"
Objective: Argumentative, intrusive, and verbally aggressive toward others.

Goals/Expected Outcomes	Nursing Interventions	Selected Rationale	Evaluation
Patient and others on unit will remain free from harm during this shift.	Observe patient's behavior frequently (q 15 min).	Changes in behavior can signal impending violence toward self or others.	Patient pacing and talking loudly; checked q 15 min × 3.
	Redirect or distract patient (e.g., walk outside, make bed, talk to nurse).	Helps control impulses and channel excess energy.	Patient easily redirected with verbal suggestions; likes to talk to nursing staff and mental health assistant.
	Move patient away from others as necessary.	Agitated and aggressive behavior is contagious and will escalate in proximity to others.	Patient was verbally directed to go to room. Patient was observed for 1 hr on a 1:1 basis by mental health assistant.
	Administer tranquilizing medications as ordered and monitor effectiveness.	Chemical restraints may be necessary if patient cannot control his behavior.	Administered PO Ativan. Patient continues to be hypervigilant and loud, but able to sit for 5-6 min without pacing, 45 min after given Ativan. Patient and others remain free from harm. Outcome met. Continue plan.

Problem/Nursing Diagnosis

Too agitated to eat/Imbalanced nutrition: less than body requirements, related to inability to sit long enough to eat.

Supporting Assessment Data

Subjective: "I haven't . . . eaten much for the past 3 days."
Objective: Patient observed continuously moving and not eating meals.

Goals/Expected Outcomes	Nursing Interventions	Selected Rationale	Evaluation
Patient will assume regular eating habits within 1 wk.	Weigh daily.	To monitor nutritional status.	Patient's current weight is 160 lb (normal weight is 170 lb).
	Record food intake and calculate calorie counts.	To determine if nutritional intake is adequate.	Patient ate sandwich (300 calories) and glass of milk (120 calories).

CNS, central nervous system; *PO*, oral.

Continued

Goals/Expected Outcomes	Nursing Interventions	Selected Rationale	Evaluation
	Determine food likes and dislikes.	Increases likelihood that he will eat if given favorite food.	Patient will eat any type of food, but needs constant reminders to finish food.
	Offer small, frequent, high-calorie meals and finger foods.	To meet nutritional needs "on the run."	Patient was offered eggs, toast, bacon, and orange juice for breakfast. Patient was able to eat bacon, orange juice, and toast "on the run" but refused eggs.
	Stay with patient during meals.	Provides support and encouragement to eat as much as possible.	Patient able to eat meals, but requires less coaching if given PRN Ativan 30 min before meals.
	Administer vitamin and mineral supplements.	To replace any dietary deficiencies.	Patient agrees to take supplements for duration of hospitalization. Patient eating three meals per day, but requires monitoring and Ativan. Outcome partially met. Continue plan.

Problem/Nursing Diagnosis

Not sleeping × 3 days/Sleep deprivation related to manic activity.

Supporting Assessment Data

Subjective: "I haven't slept well ... for the past 3 days."
Objective: Observed continuously walking.

Goals/Expected Outcomes	Nursing Interventions	Selected Rationale	Evaluation
Patient will return to his normal patterns of rest and sleep within 3 days.	Provide a quiet environment with low stimuli.	Quiet environment is conducive to rest and sleep.	Patient placed in private room; however, quiet environment was not helpful last night.
	Monitor and record sleeping patterns.	To determine if rest is adequate and normal pattern is resuming.	Patient slept 2 hr last night and 6 hr after lunch.
	Before bedtime provide comfort measures such as back rub, warm bath, and relaxing music.	Teaches habits that signal bedtime and helps with relaxation.	Patient having difficulty with sleeping; warm milk offered. Suggested resting in bed even if not sleepy, but patient continued to be restless, rising frequently to come to nurses' station last night.
	Prohibit intake of caffeine foods in the evening hours.	CNS stimulants can cause restlessness.	Patient agrees to stop drinking coffee for duration of hospitalization, "but it won't make any difference."
	Administer sedative medications as ordered.	Potentiates sedation at the biochemical level.	Restoril offered for sleep, but refused. Patient is sleeping 2-3 hr at night, but has not been able to reestablish normal cycle. Outcome partially met. Continue plan.

Critical Thinking Questions

1. How will you respond to Bobby's intrusiveness and constant need for attention?
2. Why is Bobby at risk for injury to himself if he is not hospitalized during the manic phase?

See Evolve for Nursing Care Plans for patients with anxiety, depression, and anorexia nervosa.

■ Evaluation

Ongoing evaluation of patients with bipolar disorder is necessary. You must determine whether the outcome criteria for the patient's physical needs—such as safety, nutrition, and rest—were met. In addition, are the symptoms resolving? Is the patient able to communicate effectively and resume social and occupational roles? Do both the patient and the family have a plan to maintain medication and follow-up appointments?

MAJOR DEPRESSIVE DISORDER

Major depressive disorder is diagnosed when at least five symptoms characteristic of depression have been present for at least 2 weeks. These symptoms include an overwhelming feeling of sadness, inability to feel pleasure or experience interest in daily activities, weight gain or loss not attributed to dieting, sleep disturbances, fatigue or loss of energy, feelings of worthlessness, difficulty in making decisions or concentrating, and suicidal thoughts. The depressed patient often has psychomotor retardation in which speech, movements, and thought processes are slowed. However, it is not uncommon to see agitation and irritability in a depressed person. These symptoms may be *subjective* (described by the patient) or *objective* (observable by others).

Before making a diagnosis of depression, the physician must be certain that there are no medical conditions present that could mimic depression, such as hypothyroidism or chronic fatigue syndrome. In addition, patients who have suffered a stroke or myocardial infarction, have cancer, or are newly diagnosed with a chronic disease such as diabetes all need to be screened for depression, because major illness can lead to depression. Moreover, many classifications of medications may induce a pharmacologic type of depression. Examples are antihypertensives, sedatives, anxiolytics, antipsychotics, steroids, and hormones. In addition, substance abuse—especially of alcohol—often produces symptoms that mimic depressive symptoms. In other cases, drinking large amounts of alcohol will actually cause a person to feel depressed because alcohol is a central nervous system depressant. A diagnosis of alcohol dependence needs to be considered. When a person has an emotional problem such as depression and abuses a substance such as alcohol, she has a dual diagnosis. See Chapter 47 for more on substance abuse.

 Think Critically

How would you differentiate symptoms of depression and hypersomnia from the medication side effects of drowsiness or sedation?

There is increasing evidence that major depressive disorder is caused by a biochemical imbalance. However, most scientists agree that the majority of chronic illnesses result from a combination of heredity and environment. What is not understood is how these elements interact to precipitate an episode of major mental illness. Whereas the signs and symptoms of mild depression usually subside, research findings indicate that an attack of major depression is very likely to recur with even greater severity; therefore, regardless of the cause, symptoms of depression need to be addressed and not ignored.

 Elder Care Points

Although the elderly have many risk factors for depression (such as loss of friends and body changes) that increase with age, symptoms of major depression are not a normal part of the aging process. Research shows that the majority of older adults are not depressed most of the time. Our senior citizens want to enjoy good mental health, but cost and access to mental health services are barriers.

Treatment

Patients who are depressed respond best to a combination of antidepressant medication and psychotherapy.

 Complementary and Alternative Therapies

St. John's Wort

Herbal remedies such as St. John's wort have been used for mild to moderate depression and anxiety; however, patients should be advised that taking monoamine oxidase inhibitors (MAOIs) or SSRIs with St. John's wort can cause adverse drug-herb interactions.

 Complementary and Alternative Therapies

Music Therapy for Depression

Evidenced-based practice suggests that persons with major depression are receptive to music therapy and show improvement in moods (Maratos et al., 2008).

Hospitalization may be necessary if there is a high potential for suicide. Since the 1960s, medications have made a great difference in the lives of people who are depressed. The four main categories of medications used to treat depression are the MAOIs, tricyclic antidepressants, SSRIs, and other chemically unique antidepressants. Tricyclics and MAOIs are very effective in treating depressive symptoms; however, they can cause some serious side effects (Table 46-4).

SSRIs cause fewer side effects and are becoming first-line drugs, but they are very expensive and do not work for every patient. Newer drugs such as mirtazapine (Remeron) and venlafaxine (Effexor) show promise, but there is less research on these chemically unique drugs; therefore SSRIs are preferred. Evidence-based practice indicates that medications should be

Table 46-4 Nursing Implications for Antidepressant Drugs

CLASSIFICATION	ACTION	NURSING IMPLICATIONS	PATIENT TEACHING
Tricyclics			
Amitriptyline (Elavil) Clomipramine (Anafranil) Imipramine (Tofranil) Maprotiline (Ludiomil) Nortriptyline (Pamelor)	Inhibit the reuptake of neurotransmitters (serotonin and norepinephrine) (see Chapter 49). Used to treat major depression.	Watch for side effects: dry mouth, blurred vision, tachycardia, cardiac dysrhythmias, postural hypotension, constipation, urinary retention, and esophageal reflux. Usually taken at bedtime. Monitor patient for suicidal ideation. An overdose of these medications could be fatal.	Mood elevation may take 7-28 days. Full recovery from major depression may take 6-8 wk. Avoid taking alcohol and working around machines and heavy equipment. Drowsiness, dizziness, and hypotension will subside after the first few weeks. Do not stop taking these medications abruptly.
MAO Inhibitors (MAOIs)			
Isocarboxazid (Marplan) Phenelzine (Nardil) Tranylcypromine (Parnate)	Inhibits the MAO enzyme, thereby preventing the breakdown of dopamine, norepinephrine, and serotonin.	Common side effects: weight gain, postural hypotension, edema, change in cardiac rate and rhythm, urinary retention, constipation, insomnia, weakness, and fatigue. Monitor blood pressure very closely during the first few weeks of treatment. Take a medication history to identify use of medications that increase the heart rate, such as ephedrine, stimulants, alcohol, narcotics, TCAs, or antihypertensives; report findings to physician or RN.	Avoid foods high in tyramine, such as aged cheeses; red wine, sherry, and beer; pickled or smoked fish; fermented meats; and artificial sweeteners, because drug-food interactions can cause a life-threatening hypertensive crisis. If the medication is discontinued for any reason, dietary restrictions should continue for at least 14 days. Go to the emergency department immediately for headaches.
Selective Serotonin Reuptake Inhibitors (SSRIs)			
Citalopram (Celexa) Escitalopram (Lexapro) Fluoxetine (Prozac) Paroxetine (Paxil) Sertraline (Zoloft)	Block the reuptake of serotonin. Used for depression, anxiety disorders, and bulimia.	These medications elevate mood faster than the TCAs or MAOIs. They are not as sedating and do not have the anticholinergic side effects of TCAs or MAOIs. Common side effects include nausea, nervousness, insomnia, anxiety, and sexual dysfunction.	Take with food if GI distress occurs. Take drug in the A.M. for optimal effects. Full therapeutic effects may take up to 4 wk. Decreased libido or impotence may occur; check with physician rather than stopping medications abruptly.
Atypical Antidepressants			
Trazodone (Desyrel) (also called Oleptro) Bupropion (Wellbutrin) Nefazodone Mirtazapine (Remeron)	Block the reuptake of norepinephrine, serotonin, and dopamine. Used to treat depression in patients who are not responding to other antidepressants.	Side effects are similar to the SSRIs. Bupropion, in doses >450 mg/day, can cause seizures: assess for history of head trauma or seizure disorder. Nefazodone can cause liver failure. Mirtazapine can cause agranulocytosis.	Immediately contact your doctor if *priapism* (a painful, prolonged erection of the penis) occurs. Immediately contact your physician if seizures occur. Report yellowing of the skin or sclera, anorexia, or malaise. Immediately report sore throat, fever, or other infection signs.

Table 46-4	Nursing Implications for Antidepressant Drugs—cont'd		
CLASSIFICATION	**ACTION**	**NURSING IMPLICATIONS**	**PATIENT TEACHING**
Venlafaxine (Effexor)		Venlafaxine, in doses >300 mg/day, potentiates risk of sustained hypertension; assess for history of hypertension.	Continue taking BP medications as ordered.
Duloxetine Cymbalta		Side effects are similar to the SSRIs.	Monitor for hypoglycemia.
Desvenlafaxine (Pristiq)		Common side effects: dizziness, fatigue, headaches, nausea, dry mouth, diarrhea, constipation, decreased appetite.	Instruct patient and family to report suicidal ideations.

BP, blood pressure; *FDA*, Food and Drug Administration; *GI*, gastrointestinal; *MAO*, monoamine oxidase; *MAOIs*, monoamine oxidase inhibitors; *TCAs*, tricyclic antidepressants.

started at the lowest dose and increased gradually; however, it is also important that the patient receives a sufficient dose for an appropriate length of time. If the patient experiences medication failure, compliance is more difficult to achieve (Costell, 2003).

Safety Alert

Serotonin Syndrome

SSRIs have the potential to cause serotonin syndrome. This is a potential life-threatening condition that could start 30 minutes to 48 hours after taking the medication. Symptoms include change of mental status, increase in pulse and fluctuation in blood pressure, loss of muscular coordination, and hyperthermia. Treatment includes stopping medication, administering intravenous (IV) fluids, and decreasing temperature.

Electroconvulsive therapy (ECT) is the oldest form of brain stimulation therapy used for severe depression. After several regimens of medication are unsuccessful, or if the patient is severely depressed or actively suicidal, ECT is considered. Particularly for older patients, remission rates for ECT treatment range from 70% to 90% (Sherman, 2009), and evidence suggests that ECT is more effective than pharmacology (Kavanagh & McLoughlin, 2009). Basically, ECT consists of electric shock delivered to the brain via electrodes applied to the temples. This shock artificially induces a grand mal seizure lasting 30 to 90 seconds. The patient typically receives 8 to 12 treatments spread over several weeks. ECT is frequently done on an outpatient basis in the early morning.

The potential risks associated with the procedure include increased intracranial pressure, increased blood pressure (especially for those with essential hypertension), and cardiac dysrhythmias. Short-term memory loss, occasional headaches, and confusion are expected but will resolve in minutes to hours after the procedure, and this should be explained to the patient and family before treatment. The patient should take nothing by mouth for 6 to 8 hours before the procedure.

Basic preoperative preparation includes obtaining a signed consent and removing dentures, jewelry, hairpins, contact lenses, and hearing aids. The patient will receive a preoperative medication such as atropine sulfate and a short-acting general anesthetic. After the procedure is completed, vital signs are monitored and the patient is reoriented. Before discharge, the patient is fed and the family is reminded about the expected short-term memory loss.

Newer forms of brain stimulation therapy have shown promise. Repetitive transcranial magnetic stimulation (rTMS) and magnetic seizure therapy (MST) are noninvasive methods; a magnet is placed on the skull and then areas of the brain are stimulated by pulsations. Vagus nerve stimulation (VNS) and deep brain stimulation (DBS) use a surgically implanted pacemaker to stimulate nerve tissue. VNS was approved in 2005 and rTMS was approved in 2008 to treat depression in certain circumstances. MST and DBS are currently considered experimental treatments (National Institute of Mental Health, 2009).

Programs are continuously being developed to improve outcomes for mental health patients. For example, IMPACT (Improving Mood–Promoting Access to Collaborative Treatment) is an evidenced-based intervention for older patients who have major depression. A nurse, social worker, or psychologist and the primary care provider use a collaborative team approach that includes assessment, education about treatments, activities, and the patient's preference for depression treatment, such as antidepressant medications and psychotherapy (SAMHSA's National Registry of Evidenced-Based Programs, 2007).

❖ NURSING MANAGEMENT

▪ Assessment (Data Collection)

You should collect information about feelings of sadness, hopelessness, and a loss of interest in usual activities. In accordance with 2010 National Patient Safety Goals, nurses are responsible for identifying patients at risk for suicide. Assess for changes in ability to fulfill family, social, or occupational obligations. Appetite must be assessed, along with recent weight loss or gain and changes in normal patterns of eating. A person who is depressed may also have many somatic complaints, such as headache, stomachache, dizziness, nausea, indigestion, constipation, and change in sexual responsiveness. The inability to concentrate and indecisiveness are also hallmarks of mood disorders.

■ Nursing Diagnosis

Common nursing diagnoses for patients experiencing depression include:

- Fatigue related to psychomotor retardation
- Hopelessness related to inability to achieve career goals
- Spiritual distress related to questioning the meaning of life
- Complicated grieving related to loss (e.g., divorce)
- Chronic low self-esteem related to past failures
- Self-care deficits for bathing/hygiene, dressing, grooming, feeding related to lack of motivation
- Risk for self-directed or other-directed violence related to repressed anger and grief

■ Planning

For the nursing diagnoses above, example outcomes might include:

- Patient will participate in at least one unit activity today and gradually increase participation as depression and fatigue resolve.
- Patient will identify two short-term goals that would contribute to achieving overall long-term career goals by the end of shift.
- Patient will verbalize renewal of faith in a higher power after two or three visits from hospital clergy.
- Patient will express feelings of loss and sadness about divorce within 1 month.
- Patient will relate at least one "success story" about self every day for 1 week.
- Patient will participate with assistance (e.g., verbal coaching) in activities of daily living (ADLs) (e.g., brush own teeth) for 1 week and gradually increase independent completion of ADLs before discharge.
- Patient will refrain from harming self or others during this shift.

Planning care for a patient with depression involves promoting safety, adequate nutrition, and rest. Initially, the patient may require assistance in performing ADLs until the severe depression subsides. Mental energy and concentration to work on complex psychological issues are not available to a person who is still in the depths of depression. However, as the energy level improves, you need to help the patient begin to set some small goals such as meeting her own hygienic

needs, and gradually work toward the greater goal of reentry into the workforce. It is important to remember that an increased energy level also increases the risk for self-harm.

■ Implementation

The priority nursing intervention for a depressed patient is to protect the patient from acting on impulses to harm herself. Medications to treat an underlying depression often are indicated, and you must help the patient understand that sometimes pharmacologic intervention is necessary to combat depression at the biochemical level; reversing depression is not merely a matter of thinking happy thoughts. Also, comparing the need for medication to that for a condition such as diabetes or a heart problem may help the patient to feel less stigmatized. **Once the antidepressant medications begin to take effect, the risk for self-harm actually increases because the patient now has sufficient energy to complete the act.** Genuine caring and concern and close monitoring are very important.

Depressed patients can be difficult to be with because of their self-defeating thoughts and verbalizations. Set limits on the amount of time spent ruminating in negative thoughts and redirect the patient to discussions of the present reality. For example, focus on the small successes that the patient has achieved during the shift, such as combing her own hair or attending a group session.

⌂ Clinical Cues

When you spend a lot of time caring for a depressed patient, you may find that you feel very tired, subdued, or even mildly depressed. Share this experience with your clinical instructor or a classmate, and remember that in order to give excellent patient care, identifying your feelings and protecting your own mental health are essential.

? Think Critically

What types of goals would be suitable for a 25-year-old female nursing student who is depressed? She is taking Zoloft, an SSRI, and feeling better, but continues to be overwhelmed.

Most depressed people complain of some type of sleep deprivation. You should provide an environment that is conducive to sleep and educate the patient and family about the importance of regular sleep.

■ Evaluation

Daily evaluation of the patient's depression includes determining whether the outcome criteria for the patient's physical needs were met. These include safety and issues related to decreased energy levels, such as helping with ADLs. Also evaluate the patient's ability to participate in social activities and to express feelings. Part of this overall assessment will include determining the effectiveness of medications. Sometimes it takes several different trials of a combination of drugs to achieve the desired effect. In addition, many of the medications take 2 to 4 weeks to become effective, and the initial side effects of drowsiness and nausea may discourage long-term compliance.

SUICIDAL PATIENTS

❖ NURSING MANAGEMENT

■ Assessment (Data Collection)

Risk factors for suicide include family history of suicide, history of a previous attempt, terminal illness, addiction to drugs or alcohol, diagnosis of major depressive disorder or bipolar disorder, and excessive stress. Suicide assessment includes determining the level of risk (low, moderate, or high) for accomplishing the act of suicide, the presence of a distinct plan, and means of acting on the plan. Be caring in your approach; however, do not be afraid to be direct. You cannot cause the patient to commit suicide with your questions. Moreover, the patient is likely to feel relieved that you are not afraid to hear about suicide and that you are capable of dealing with this painful disclosure.

> ### 🔲 Clinical Cues
>
> If you are working on a busy medical-surgical unit and you identify a patient with signs of suicidal thoughts or behaviors, first ensure patient safety, and then immediately report these behaviors to the physician or RN. The patient may need a psychiatric consultation, transfer to a medical-psychiatric unit, or initiation of intensive suicide precautions (i.e., one-on-one observation). These measures are beyond the routine care provided on a medical-surgical unit.
>
> **The probability of a completed suicide attempt increases with male gender, weapon availability (guns or knives), poor support system, social isolation, and the influence of mood-altering chemicals. However, all suicide threats and gestures should be taken seriously.** Patients who are actively suicidal are considered unstable, and if you gather data that support this suspicion, the facts should be immediately reported to the physician or RN.

> ### ◎ Focused Assessment
>
> #### Questions to Ask a Potentially Suicidal Patient
>
> - Are you feeling suicidal?
> - Do you have a plan? How do you plan to take your life?
> - Can you think of any event that may have caused you to feel this way?
> - Do you have a lethal weapon in your possession?
> - Who is a part of your support system?
> - Do you drink or use drugs on a regular basis?
> - Has anyone in your family made a previous suicide attempt?
> - Are you currently taking any antidepressants?
> - Have you experienced a major loss within the last year?
> - What is your history with past close relationships?
> - Have you given away any of your possessions recently?
> - Have you been having difficulty remembering things lately?

> ### ❓ Think Critically
>
> Women are two times more likely to attempt suicide, but men are four times more likely to complete the suicide act. Why might older white men have the highest rate for completed suicide?

■ Nursing Diagnosis

Common nursing diagnoses for patients at risk for suicide include:
- Risk for self-directed violence related to impulsive behavior
- Risk for suicide related to history of previous suicide attempt
- Powerlessness related to history of dependency in relationships
- Hopelessness related to viewing the future as bleak and grim
- Spiritual distress related to loss of belief in God
- Ineffective coping related to overuse of avoidance
- Chronic low self-esteem related to unmet dependency needs

■ Planning

For the nursing diagnoses above, example outcomes might include:
- Patient will refrain from injuring self during this shift.
- Patient will refrain from suicide attempts during this shift and will stop verbalizing suicidal thoughts before discharge.
- Patient will identify three examples of dependency in her relationships and describe how this dependency affects her life during group therapy session.
- Patient will verbalize one or two future events that she could look forward to and enjoy.
- Patient will demonstrate renewal of her usual spiritual activities (e.g., attending church) within 2 months.
- Patient will identify at least two additional coping mechanisms by the end of the week.
- Patient will list at least two ways to meet her own needs during this shift.

Planning care for a patient at risk for suicide involves ensuring a safe environment by determining the level of risk and initiating the appropriate suicide precautions.

> ### ⚖ Legal and Ethical Considerations
>
> #### Safe Environment for a Suicidal Patient
>
> Although patients have the right to bring and keep personal items, you have the legal responsibility for maintaining a safe environment for a suicidal patient. Belts, shoelaces, and even undergarments such as a bra could be used in a self-strangulation attempt and should be taken away as necessary.

As the risk for suicide decreases, the focus of nursing care shifts to assisting the patient to develop alternative methods to cope and solve problems.

■ Implementation

Protecting a suicidal patient from self-harm is a priority nursing intervention. Suicide precautions for a high level of risk consist of placing the patient in a seclusion room with one-to-one (1:1) observation, where one caregiver is assigned to be with the patient continuously. A physician's order is required for 1:1 seclusion; however, a 1:1 measure can be initiated temporarily by the nursing staff, until the physician is notified. The observer may have to remain close enough (arm's length) to immediately intervene if the patient attempts self-harm. As the level of risk decreases, the patient is allowed to have more personal space, for example, 1:1 may continue in the dayroom, but visual contact must be maintained at all times. In addition, all items with a potential for self-harm must be removed, such as sharp or pointed objects, glass objects, or pills. Observe the patient for "cheeking," which is a ploy to avoid taking medication by holding the pill in the cheek pouch rather than swallowing it. Suicidal patients have been known to hoard medication and then use it in an attempt to overdose.

When assessment indicates that the suicide intent is less lethal, it is sufficient to maintain close observation and contract with the patient to refrain from taking action. A no-suicide contract—preferably written—should be initiated and renewed as needed. Active listening and a caring attitude are necessary to build a trusting relationship with a severely depressed, suicidal patient. Even if the patient is unwilling to talk to you, you must indicate to the patient both verbally and nonverbally that you care and are available to listen. Your attention and presence convey your respect, and help the patient to build self-esteem and a sense of self-worth.

■ Evaluation

Unstable, suicidal patients need to be reassessed and evaluated frequently (i.e., every 15 to 30 minutes), and the plan of care should be adjusted accordingly to ensure safety and prevent self-harm. As the patient stabilizes and the level of risk decreases, you will evaluate patient outcomes related to gaining new coping skills, renewing hope and a sense of purpose, improving communication skills to get needs met, and preparing to resume life in a community setting. The status of the patient just before discharge should be carefully documented to reflect the absence of suicidal ideations and a follow-up plan with a specific method to access emergency care if suicidal feelings return. According to the Joint Commission's National Quality Core Measures, when patients are discharged from a facility the plan of care should be communicated to the provider who assumes the care of the patient. This is particularly important for patients who have attempted suicide or expressed suicidal thoughts.

EATING DISORDERS

ANOREXIA NERVOSA

Anorexia nervosa is characterized by the patient's refusal to maintain minimal body weight or eat adequate quantities of food. There is a disturbance in the perception of body shape and size and an extreme fear of becoming fat. The patient strives for perfection and control by controlling caloric intake. These patients may act immaturely and are socially insecure and exhibit fluctuating moods. Intricate food rituals (e.g., shifting food around the plate, collecting recipes, and making elaborate meals for others) develop, and the patient may have superstitions about food (e.g., ice cream goes straight to your hips). Excessive exercise is commonly used as another means of staying thin. In many cultures, the emphasis on a slim body has influenced young women's body image. Anorexia nervosa occurs in about 1 of 100 to 200 females in late adolescence or early adulthood. About 10% of cases occur in males. Anorexia nervosa is a dangerous disorder; 6% to 20% of patients with this diagnosis will die from starvation or suicide. Other psychiatric conditions such as anxiety or depression can accompany anorexia nervosa.

Diagnostic criteria include:
- Refusal to maintain body weight at or above a minimally normal weight for age and height (body weight less than 85% of that expected).
- Intense fear of gaining weight or becoming fat, even though underweight.
- Disturbance in the way in which one's body weight or shape is experienced, or denial of this problem.
- Absence of at least three consecutive menstrual cycles after onset of menstruation in the female.

 Think Critically

How does your own culture influence your body image?

BULIMIA NERVOSA

Patients with bulimia nervosa induce vomiting after consuming large quantities of food. This binge eating occurs in a frenzied state and usually in secrecy; afterward, the patient experiences feelings of shame and self-criticism. Laxatives may be taken to purge the system after the binge. Ninety percent of patients with bulimia are young women. Bulimia and anorexia nervosa can occur simultaneously in some patients, and both conditions are difficult to cure.

TREATMENT OF EATING DISORDERS

The goal of treatment in eating disorders is to restore nutritional health and a normal body weight. If weight is below 75% of ideal body weight and the patient is medically unstable, the first step is hospitalization to correct fluid and electrolyte imbalances and severe weight loss. After the medical condition is stabilized, behavior modification is the focus of treatment. Therapy is long term, requiring 1 to 6 years for reversal of the disorder. Both inpatient treatment and outpatient treatment are required with individual, group, and family therapy. Support groups can provide opportunities for growth and sharing of feelings and information. The long-term goal is for the patient to achieve a sense of self-worth and self-acceptance that is not exclusively based on appearance.

❖ NURSING MANAGEMENT

■ Assessment (Data Collection)

Collect information about compulsive dieting, severe weight loss, or an unrealistic body image. The patient and the family may be in denial. Amenorrhea and electrolyte imbalances occur, and as the disease progresses, a host of other symptoms appear. Problems related to vitamin and nutrient deficiencies occur, including dry skin, constipation, muscle wasting, and facial puffiness. Lanugo (downy hair covering the body) may occur. Cardiac dysrhythmias, hypotension, and hypothermia can be life threatening.

Individuals with bulimia nervosa may maintain a normal weight. Assess for tooth marks on the knuckles from repeated attempts to induce vomiting and dental caries from exposure to stomach acid. Other signs and symptoms include fluid and electrolyte imbalances, complaints of heartburn, vomiting of blood, or constipation due to dehydration.

■ Nursing Diagnosis

Common nursing diagnoses for patients with eating disorders include:

- Imbalanced nutrition: less than body requirements related to refusal to eat and fear of gaining weight
- Risk for electrolyte imbalance related to self-induced vomiting and limited intake
- Disturbed body image related to sociocultural and media influence
- Chronic low self-esteem related to repeated negative feedback from parents
- Ineffective coping related to using maladaptive dietary practices to cope with stress
- Dysfunctional family processes related to the emotional growth and development of the adolescent family member

 Clinical Cues

The patient with an eating disorder is attempting to gain a sense of control by controlling dietary intake; therefore it is important to avoid power struggles over food. Use a matter-of-fact approach and help the patient to experience control in non–food-related areas. For example, "Jane, go ahead and finish your lunch and then you can show me what CDs you decided to take on your school trip."

■ Planning

For the nursing diagnoses above, example outcomes might include:

- Patient will take at least _____ calories per day for 1 week and gradually increase caloric consumption to regain 85% of ideal body weight within _____ months.
- Patient will refrain from self-induced vomiting during this shift.
- Patient will discuss four or five ways in which culture and media are influencing her self-image.
- Patient will identify examples of negative feedback from parents and discuss how that feedback is affecting her during today's group session.
- Patient will identify three alternative coping strategies to replace maladaptive dietary practices before discharge.
- Patient and family will identify three family activities (non–food related and non–exercise related) that provide support to the adolescent (e.g., discussing a homework assignment).

Planning care for a patient with an eating disorder involves ensuring a safe environment and helping to restore weight and correct nutritional deficiencies. As the physical needs are met, the focus of nursing care shifts to assisting the patient to develop a more realistic body image, increase self-esteem, increase feelings of control, and practice new coping skills. *Healthy People 2020* goals include decreasing the proportion of adolescents who use eating behaviors to control weight.

■ Implementation

The initial interventions for eating disorders are targeted toward physical health and safety. Suicide precautions are initiated if necessary, and fluid and electrolyte imbalances are corrected. Nutritional status, weight gain, and behaviors such as excessive exercise or self-induced vomiting are monitored. Use a supportive, nonjudgmental approach to assist the patient in building self-esteem, assertiveness, a realistic body image, and age-appropriate peer relationships. Power struggles and discussions of food should be avoided.

Clinical Cues

Evidence-based practice indicates that patients can learn to interrupt negative thoughts and substitute positive affirmations (Peden et al., 2005). Teach your patients to use a personal positive affirmation statement that can be said out loud on a regular daily basis. You may even want to use a positive affirmation to build your own confidence while you are in nursing school. Wake up every morning and say to your mirror, "I am a good student and I am going to be a great nurse!"

■ **Evaluation**

In the acute phase, patients with eating disorders need evaluation of outcome criteria that ensure safety, nutritional, and electrolyte and fluid balance needs. Changing beliefs about food or body image, building self-esteem, learning new coping skills, and restructuring eating habits may take months or even years; therefore even small gains should be carefully documented. Evaluate the patient's readiness to resume life in a community setting with healthier eating habits and the family's ability to support the patient's efforts.

COMMUNITY CARE

As hospital stays become shorter, many patients with anxiety, mood, or eating disorders will be hospitalized only long enough to stabilize their life-threatening symptoms. They will then be seen in outpatient clinics, in long-term care, at home, or in day hospitals. Medication compliance is a major nursing responsibility. Once a patient feels better and the crisis is over, there may be a tendency to stop taking medications. Regular visits to the clinic or physician and a social support system are essential.

Get Ready for the NCLEX® Examination!

Key Points

- The four levels of anxiety are mild, moderate, severe, and panic.
- Examples of anxiety disorders include generalized anxiety disorder, phobic disorder, obsessive-compulsive disorder, and post-traumatic stress disorder.
- Assess for physical symptoms of anxiety: increased blood pressure, pulse, respirations, and urinary output; dry mouth, nausea, diarrhea, trembling, muscular tension, restlessness, hypervigilance, and insomnia.
- Assess for the psychological symptoms of anxiety: feelings of impending doom, fear, guilt, anger, helplessness, irritability, and low self-esteem.
- Interventions for patients with anxiety disorders include remaining calm, decreasing environmental stimuli, teaching relaxation techniques and stress management, medicating with anxiolytics as necessary, and determining root causes of anxiety as indicated.
- Bipolar disorder is characterized by episodes of extreme sadness, hopelessness, and helplessness alternating with periods of extreme elation and hyperactivity.
- Assess for physical indicators of bipolar disorder: hypersomnia or insomnia, change in appetite, and somatic complaints such as headache, stomachache, dizziness, nausea, indigestion, and change in sexual responsiveness.
- Assess for psychological indicators of bipolar disorder: irritability, grandiosity, delusions, labile emotions, flat affect, sadness, indecisiveness, and inability to concentrate.
- Interventions for patients in the acute manic phase include ensuring the safety of the patient and others, providing a high-calorie diet and finger foods, setting limits on behavior, administering and monitoring the effectiveness of antimanic medications, and encouraging rest and sleep.

- Major depressive disorder is diagnosed when at least five symptoms characteristic of depression have been present for at least 2 weeks.
- Assess for physical indicators of depression: weight loss or weight gain, sleep disturbances, fatigue or loss of energy, and psychomotor retardation.
- Assess for psychological indicators of depression: feelings of sadness, worthlessness, hopelessness, or excessive guilt; inability to feel pleasure or disinterest in daily activities; difficulty in making decisions or concentrating; and recurrent thoughts of death or suicide.
- Interventions for depressed patients include active listening, assessing for suicidal ideations, attending to physical needs, administering and monitoring the effectiveness of antidepressant medications, assisting in setting goals, and educating about medications and ECT.
- Assess for suicide plan, including lethality level and means to act on the plan.
- Interventions for suicidal patients in the acute phase include developing a trusting relationship, one-on-one observation, removing dangerous objects, and initiating a no-suicide contract.
- Anorexia nervosa is the extreme fear of becoming fat, with a disturbance in perception of body size.
- Bulimia nervosa is characterized by the practice of inducing vomiting after binge eating.
- Assess for physical symptoms of an eating disorder: amenorrhea, electrolyte imbalances, dry skin, constipation, muscle wasting, facial puffiness, lanugo, dysrhythmias, hypotension, hypothermia, and dental caries (related to self-induced vomiting).
- Assess for psychological and behavioral symptoms of an eating disorder: denial of problem, compulsive dieting, preoccupation with food, unrealistic body image, low self-esteem, and shame (related to binge eating).

- Interventions for patients with eating disorders include monitoring nutritional intake and weight gain, monitoring behaviors such as excessive exercise and self-induced vomiting, and assisting to build self-esteem and assertiveness.

Additional Learning Resources

SG Go to your Study Guide for additional learning activities to help you master this chapter content.

 evolve Go to your Evolve website (http://evolve.elsevier.com/deWit/medsurg) for the following FREE learning resources:
- Animations, audio, and video
- Answers and rationales for questions and activities
- Concept Map Creator
- Glossary with pronunciations in English and Spanish
- Interactive Review Questions and Exercises and more!

Online Resources
- National Institute of Mental Health, www.nimh.nih.gov/index.shtml
- Depression, www.nlm.nih.gov/medlineplus/depression.html
- Mental Health, www.webmd.com/mental-health/default.htm

Review Questions for the NCLEX® Examination

1. A patient is irritable, pacing, crying, and becoming increasingly more agitated. The physician orders a PRN medication for acute anxiety. What is the most likely medication to be ordered?
   1. Amitriptyline (Elavil)
   2. Buspirone (BuSpar)
   3. Lorazepam (Ativan)
   4. Quetiapine (Seroquel)

2. A 40-year-old man is diagnosed with generalized anxiety disorder. Which behavior would the patient be more likely to display with this diagnosis?
   1. Runs out of the room when he notices a spider in the corner
   2. Continuously checks to see if doors are shut and locked
   3. Has difficulty concentrating and excessively worries about his family
   4. Wakes at night screaming because of recurrent nightmares

3. The nurse determines that there is a need to medicate an elderly patient for anxiety. Which strategy would help the nurse to make this clinical decision?
   1. Listen to verbalization of apprehension.
   2. Be sensitive to somatic complaints.
   3. Initiate therapeutic communication.
   4. Observe for escalation of agitation.

4. The patient is taking lithium. What symptoms are early signs of lithium toxicity?
   1. Hypertension and headache
   2. Diarrhea and slurred speech
   3. Confusion and blurred vision
   4. Convulsion and polyuria

5. A patient is hospitalized for dehydration and weight loss. He is very restless and exhibits flight of ideas with easy distractibility. The nurse identifies the priority nursing diagnosis of Imbalanced nutrition: less than body requirements. Which intervention is most appropriate?
   1. Give three high-calorie meals on a regular schedule.
   2. Offer finger foods, such as a meat and cheese sandwich.
   3. Provide a pleasant, odor-free environment.
   4. Encourage family meals and socialization while eating.

6. The patient is disheveled and disinterested in daily activities such as bathing or hygiene. He reports overwhelming feelings of sadness and loss of energy. The nursing diagnosis of Self-care deficit for bathing and hygiene is identified. Which intervention(s) would be appropriate? *(Select all that apply.)*
   1. Explain the importance of hygiene to health and appearance.
   2. Encourage the patient to "look good and feel good."
   3. Plan extra time to help the patient to complete ADLs related to hygiene.
   4. Instruct the nursing assistant to do partial hygiene.
   5. Encourage some participation and set limits.
   6. Do everything for the patient until he feels better.
   7. Have the same caregiver assist on a daily basis if possible.

7. The nurse is admitting an adolescent with a tentative diagnosis of anorexia nervosa. Which behavior is most likely to characterize this disorder?
   1. Eating in secrecy
   2. Excessive exercise
   3. Suicidal ideations
   4. Difficulty sleeping

8. A male patient demonstrates an overwhelming feeling of worthlessness, difficulty in making decisions or concentrating, and suicidal thoughts. The nurse determines the suicide risk by asking which question(s)? *(Select all that apply.)*
   1. "Are you feeling suicidal?"
   2. "Do you have a plan? How do you plan to take your life?"
   3. "Why do you want to commit suicide?"
   4. "What would you accomplish by killing yourself?"
   5. "Do you drink or use drugs on a regular basis?"
   6. "Have you considered how your family would feel?"
   7. "Have you recently given away any of your belongings?"

9. A patient who is taking a selective serotonin reuptake inhibitor suddenly develops a rapid pulse, fluctuating blood pressure, fever, loss of muscle coordination, and mental status changes. The nurse anticipates that the physician is most likely to order which medical therapy?

   1. Infuse intravenous fluids and administer an antipyretic.
   2. Obtain an ECG and start oxygen per nasal cannula.
   3. Administer an antidote and encourage PO fluids.
   4. Monitor the patient closely and continue the medication.

10. The nurse is caring for an 18-year-old patient who is diagnosed with anorexia nervosa. The nurse identifies Imbalanced nutrition: less than body requirements as a priority nursing diagnosis. What is an appropriate expected outcome?

    1. The patient will be able to eat 35% or more of her meals.
    2. The patient will be able to develop improved eating behaviors.
    3. The patient will be able to verbalize the importance of eating.
    4. The patient will be able to identify barriers to eating.

Critical Thinking Activities

Scenario A

You are working in a clinic, and the mother of an adolescent who was recently diagnosed with cancer becomes hysterical. You briefly assess her and find she is at a panic level of anxiety.

1. Explain why closed questions (questions that can be answered with a yes or no, or with very specific answers) and short simple sentences delivered in a firm, kind tone would be effective while she is at a panic level of anxiety.

2. What signs and behaviors would indicate that your interventions are successfully helping this mother to reduce her anxiety?

Scenario B

You are caring for an elderly couple in their home. The husband suffered a stroke 6 months ago. One day the wife takes you aside and tells you that she is concerned about her husband. She says that he is not sleeping well and that his appetite is poor. On further questioning, you find that he is verbalizing a desire to "end it all."

1. What questions would you ask the husband? What questions would you ask the wife?

2. What type of community supports might be available for this couple?

Scenario C

Bill Jones, a 35-year-old, comes into the emergency department after a high-speed chase with the police. He is using vulgar, profane language and is unable to sit down even for a few minutes. Bill switches rapidly from being fun loving and humorous to angry and aggressive. The psychiatrist tells you that Bill has bipolar disorder and orders a dose of intramuscular Thorazine.

1. How would the team approach Bill to give him the injection?

2. What are the major safety concerns for this patient while he is in the emergency department?

3. What other nursing interventions are necessary at this time?

Scenario D

You are assigned to care for Jaycee, a 17-year-old who has been admitted for treatment of anorexia nervosa. She tells you she would like to delay breakfast to take a walk around the unit. You kindly, but firmly, tell her that she cannot delay breakfast. Later you walk into her room and she is doing jumping jacks; the breakfast is untouched. She tells you she really cannot eat this morning because she feels so fat.

1. How will you respond to Jaycee?

2. What can you do to help her gain a more realistic body image?

Scenario E

You are caring for Mr. Moreno, an elderly patient who suffers major depression. Several regimens of medication were tried without success and the psychiatrist has recommended electroconvulsive therapy (ECT).

1. Give Mr. Moreno and his family a brief explanation of ECT.

2. What are the most common side effects?

3. What are the risks associated with the procedure?

4. Outline the preprocedural and postprocedural care for a patient undergoing ECT.

Care of Patients with Substance Abuse Disorders

Objectives

Theory

1. Summarize the significance of substance use disorders in the general adult population.
2. List the diagnostic criteria included in the medical diagnosis of substance abuse disorder.
3. Identify the physical, behavioral, and psychological indicators of substance use disorder.
4. Discuss the significance of denial and rationalization in substance use disorder.
5. Analyze the effects of substance use disorders on family and friends.
6. Discuss symptoms and complications of withdrawal from alcohol.

7. Identify at least six nursing interventions appropriate for a patient with a substance use disorder.

Clinical Practice

1. Visit a 12-step group and identify the advantages and disadvantages of the program for substance abuse patients.
2. Contribute to a teaching plan for a community presentation on smoking cessation.
3. Review a care plan with at least three nursing diagnoses and five nursing interventions per diagnosis for a patient who is at risk for alcohol withdrawal.
4. Devise a care plan with at least three nursing diagnoses and five nursing interventions per diagnosis for a patient who is taking central nervous system stimulants (e.g., cocaine).

Key Terms

abuse (ăb-ūz, p. 1066)
addiction (ă-DĬK-shŭn, p. 1066)
co-dependency (KŌ-dĭ-PĔN-dĕn-sē, p. 1067)
confabulation (kŏn-făb-ū-LĀ-shŭn, p. 1071)
denial (dĕ-NĪ-ăl, p. 1066)
dependency (dĭ-PĔN-dĕn-sē, p. 1066)
detoxification (dĕ-tŏk-sĭ-fĭ-KĀ-shŭn, p. 1069)
dual diagnosis (p. 1066)
enabling (ĕn-Ā-blĭng, p. 1067)

Korsakoff's syndrome (SĬN-drōm, p. 1071)
psychoactive substances (sī-kō-ĂK-tĭv SŬBZ -tăn-sĕz, p. 1066)
rationalization (ră-shŭn-ăl-ī-ZĀ-shŭn, p. 1066)
substance abuse (SŬBZ-tănz ăb-ŪZ, p. 1065)
substance use disorder (SŬBZ -tănz ūz dĭs-ŌR-dĕr, p. 1065)
tolerance (TŎL-ŭr-ŭns, p. 1066)
Wernicke's encephalopathy (ĕn-sĕf-ă-LŎP-ă-thē, p. 1071)
withdrawal (p. 1068)

SUBSTANCE AND ALCOHOL ABUSE

Substance abuse (excessive use of drugs or alcohol that creates problems) has the potential for causing medical problems and death for the patient, and also causes many emotional and physical problems for family, co-workers, and friends. There are many theories about the cause of substance and alcohol abuse. In 1956 alcoholism was recognized by the American Medical Association as a medical disease rather than a moral weakness. However, change in attitude takes time, and there are still many stigmas associated with alcoholism and the abuse of other substances. Research conducted in the mid-1980s identified a genetic predisposition to alcoholism. Neurobiologic theories suggest that some people are born deficient of endorphins (the brain's own morphine-like substances) or that other people have hormonal influences that make them more susceptible to peer pressure, and so are more likely to abuse substances. Social and psychological theories suggest that users are trying to avoid adult responsibilities and use substances as a dysfunctional coping method. Ongoing research suggests that a variety of factors and circumstances increase the risk for substance abuse: aging (Matthews, 2009), personality disorders (Bates, 2009), male gender (Back et al., 2010), post-traumatic stress disorder (Calhoun et al., 2010), and discrimination against those with lesbian, gay, or bisexual preference (McCabe et al., 2010).

? Think Critically

What personal experiences have you or your family had with substance abuse, and how might such experiences affect your care of the patient who has a substance abuse disorder? Of the patient's family?

A substance use disorder is diagnosed when individuals have problems with alcoholism or substance abuse. This term implies that there is a recognizable

Box **47-1**	Common Terms Used to Describe Substance Use Disorders

- *Abuse:* Use of a psychoactive substance in a nontherapeutic manner or illicit use of prescription drugs.
- *Dependency:* Presence of physical and psychological symptoms of addiction.
- *Psychological dependence:* Craves or feels compelled to take a substance to feel good.
- **Addiction** or physical dependence: Needs the substance to prevent symptoms of withdrawal, not merely to sustain the feeling of euphoria that was present with early use of the drug.
- *Tolerance:* Need for increased amounts of substances to achieve the desired effect.
- *Withdrawal:* Stopping the drug results in a group of symptoms. Withdrawal symptoms are usually the opposite of the symptoms caused by use of the chemical.

set of signs and symptoms related to the ingestion of a psychoactive substance. **Psychoactive substances** are any mind-altering agents capable of changing a person's mood, behavior, cognition, level of consciousness, or perceptions. **Abuse** of substances is considered maladaptive and nontherapeutic, and manifestation of psychological or physical symptoms implies a **dependency** on substances. Box 47-1 lists common terms associated with substance use. The *Diagnostic and Statistical Manual of Mental Disorders,* fourth edition, text revision (DSM-IV-TR) outlines diagnostic criteria. The current definition suggests a substance abuse disorder if, within a 12-month period, the individual repeatedly demonstrates failure to meet usual obligations, creates danger to self or others, has legal problems, or has poor interpersonal relationships because of substance use. As the science of psychiatric diagnosis evolves it is possible that terms such as abuse and dependency will be combined in the general treatment approach of substance use disorder (Bates, 2010).

Dual diagnosis indicates that a patient has been diagnosed with a substance abuse problem and with a mental health disorder.

This chapter addresses some of the more commonly abused substances: alcohol, narcotic analgesics, opiates (e.g., heroin) cocaine, amphetamines (includes methamphetamines), nicotine, cannabis (marijuana), hallucinogens (e.g., lysergic acid diethylamide [LSD]), and inhalants.

> ### ? Think Critically
>
> Treating *dual diagnosis* patients can be challenging and difficult. For example, your patient has schizophrenia and admits to drinking alcohol and using "lots of drugs all of the time." What are the additional challenges to think about when this patient is discharged to a community setting?

SIGNS AND SYMPTOMS

Symptoms of substance abuse vary greatly, depending on the substance and on the duration of use and the tolerance **that has developed.** The patient should be observed for physical, behavioral, and psychological signs (Figure 47-1). Problems with fine motor control may be observed when the individual is trying to perform simple tasks such as walking or eating. Observe the skin for needle tracks, bruises, excessive perspiration, excoriation, or poor condition that suggests malnutrition. Behavioral symptoms (see Figure 47-1) should be compared to baseline; other conditions such as dementia, delirium, and metabolic or psychiatric disorders must be considered if behavioral changes are noted. For psychological symptoms, denial and rationalization are the most common defense mechanisms used by substance abusers. A typical example of denial would be: "I drink a few on the weekend." A classic example of rationalization is, "I just have a few drinks to relax." To be effective in treating these

Behavioral symptoms
Little or no direct eye contact
Disoriented or have a decreased level of consciousness
Slurred speech
Incoherent, or loud and boisterous
Mood varies from complacent to extremely agitated
May have paranoid ideation
Delusions, hallucinations, or illusions could be present

Physical symptoms
Blood pressure, pulse, and respiration may be decreased or increased
Impaired coordination
Unsteady gait
Pupils may be dilated or constricted
Grooming varies: extreme neatness to being unkempt

Substance abuse

Psychological symptoms
Denial
Rationalization

FIGURE 47-1 Signs and symptoms of substance abuse.

Table **47-1**	Common Defense Mechanisms	
DEFENSE MECHANISMS	**CHARACTERISTICS**	**EXAMPLE**
Denial	A simple and primitive defense mechanism. Person ignores reality and absolutely refuses to be swayed by evidence.	An alcoholic states, "I do not have a problem with alcohol. I never drink before 5 P.M."
Rationalization	Justifying a behavior or action by making an excuse or an explanation.	A student states, "I failed the class because the teacher didn't like me."
Displacement	Discharging intense feelings for one person onto another object or person who is less threatening.	A woman has an argument with her coworker and goes home and kicks the dog.
Identification	Modeling behavior after someone else.	A student starts dressing and talking like a popular schoolmate.
Intellectualization	Excessive reasoning and logic to counter emotional distress.	A nursing student is upset by the death of a patient, but talks at length about the equipment on the code cart.
Reaction-formation	An intense feeling that is unknowingly acted out in an opposite manner.	You treat someone whom you unconsciously dislike in an overly friendly manner.
Regression	Returning to an earlier level of behavior when severely threatened.	A 7-year-old child resumes bed-wetting and thumb sucking during the first few days of hospitalization.
Repression	Unconsciously blocking an unwanted thought or memory from open expression.	A student truly does not remember cheating on an important test.
Splitting	Viewing people or situations as all good or all bad.	A patient praises a nurse one day and then hates and scorns her the next day.
Sublimation	Rechanneling an impulse into a more socially desirable acceptable activity.	A student has generalized angry feelings about school so she takes up kickboxing as an after-school sport.

patients, you must remember that substance abusers usually do not seek help voluntarily. Denial and rationalization become entrenched behaviors and are difficult to eradicate. A review of defense mechanisms is presented in Table 47-1.

Legal and Ethical Considerations

Substance Abuse Among Health Care Workers

Those in the health care field are particularly vulnerable to substance abuse because of the availability of drugs and the tendency to care for others while ignoring personal problems. The American Nurses Association estimates that substance abuse among nurses reflects that of the general population at about 10%. In other words, if you work with 10 nurses, potentially one of them will have a substance abuse problem (Copp, 2009). Approximately 40 states have established confidential programs to assist impaired health care professionals to get help for the problem rather than immediately forfeiting their professional license. Signs and symptoms to be aware of among health care workers include frequently calling in sick or always working (to have access to drugs), sloppy patient care, frequently leaving for breaks, offering to give pain medications, and patients complaining of no relief after receiving pain medications (Pinto & Schub, 2009).

EFFECTS OF SUBSTANCE ABUSE ON FAMILY AND FRIENDS

Anyone living in proximity to a substance-dependent person will be affected. People who are abusing substances are unavailable for emotional intimacy because

life becomes centered on the substance of choice rather than on relationships or responsibilities. **Family members experience a multitude of feelings, including anger, rage, embarrassment, guilt, shame, and hopelessness. The family also uses denial and rationalization to cope.**

Two terms commonly associated with the family and friends of a substance abuser are *enabling* and *co-dependency*. **Enabling** is "helping" a person so that consequences from unhealthy behavior are less severe; thus, enabling "helps" the unhealthy behavior to continue.

In maintaining their own denial about the situation, *enablers* cover up for their troubled loved one and attempt to maintain a status quo. Calling in sick for the abuser is one common example of enabling behavior. Enabling keeps the substance-dependent person from facing consequences, and enabling ultimately supports continued denial. Enablers often have a difficult time understanding that their behavior is counterproductive to the health and well-being of the substance abuser and the abuser's family. Self-righteousness is a typical attitude observed in enablers, and it is difficult to confront.

? Think Critically

How might a family enable their loved one? Is enabling ever helpful?

Co-dependency is another behavior that occurs in circumstances of substance abuse. **The *co-dependent***

is any family member or friend who overcompensates and tries to "fix the situation" or to control the substance abuser. For example, a teenage son may repeatedly go to the bar and retrieve his drunk mother when she binges and then assume all household and child care duties until she can function. Because overcompensating does not work, co-dependents feel powerless, and attempt to control even more. A vicious, self-destructive cycle is established that is difficult to break. The overcompensating also keeps the substance abuser from facing reality objectively.

DISORDERS ASSOCIATED WITH SUBSTANCE ABUSE

ALCOHOL ABUSE

Alcohol is a central nervous system (CNS) depressant and is the most commonly abused substance. It is widely available, legally sanctioned, and relatively inexpensive, and abuse of this substance is found at all socioeconomic levels.

Alcoholism is a major health problem and is a factor in many other instances of death and morbidity. Some of the medical conditions include *cirrhosis* (liver damage), cardiomyopathy, gastrointestinal bleeding, pancreatitis, hypertension, stroke, sleep disturbances, malnutrition, peripheral neuropathies, cognitive impairment, *leukopenia* (decreased white blood cells), *thrombocytopenia* (decreased platelets), and chronic infection. Alcohol is also frequently associated with traffic accidents, murder, spousal abuse, child abuse, rape, and suicide. Concurrent abuse of other substances *(polysubstance abuse)* is frequent. Until alcoholism reaches advanced stages, it is often easy to conceal the problem from the general community. Beginning in early 2010, the Joint Commission conducted a pilot phase to develop and refine Core Measures for the assessment and treatment of alcohol use (see Online Resources).

Cultural Considerations

Religion and Alcohol

In a recent study of college students, students who were the least religious were 27 times more likely to be heavy drinkers and 9 times more likely to be moderate drinkers compared to students who had strong religious affiliations and beliefs (Wells, 2010). How does your own cultural and religious background influence your attitudes toward alcohol consumption?

SYMPTOMS OF INTOXICATION AND WITHDRAWAL

A 12-oz bottle of beer, a 6-oz glass of wine, and a 1.5-oz single shot of whiskey contain the same amount of alcohol. It takes approximately 1 hour for the body to metabolize one standard drink. A person is intoxicated when the amount of alcohol ingested creates physical or mental impairment. A number of factors

can affect intoxication, such as the quantity and speed of alcohol ingestion; the history of alcohol use (e.g., heavy drinker, novice drinker, social drinker); general health status; and concurrent use of other drugs or substances that depress the central nervous system. Familiar early symptoms that you may have experienced or observed include: drowsiness, slurred speech, loss of coordination, loss of inhibition, euphoria, and mild impairment of judgment. If drinking continues, motor function worsens, confusion progresses, and increasingly stronger stimuli are required to arouse the drinker. The late signs of excessive ingestion include urinary incontinence, coma, low blood pressure, respiratory depression and possibly death (Cohen, 2011).

Withdrawal occurs when a person who has a physical dependence on alcohol stops drinking. Early symptoms of withdrawal may manifest within 6 to 12 hours after the last drink; these include anxiety, irritability, and agitation. Progressive symptoms include increased blood pressure and pulse, tremors, nausea and vomiting, diaphoresis, delirium tremens ("DTs"), hallucinations, and seizures. Major withdrawal symptoms can occur 2 to 3 days after the last drink and may last 3 to 5 days.

Elder Care Points

The elderly are at great risk for alcohol and substance abuse. Drinking can be an attempt to alleviate depression, pain, or loneliness. The function of vital organs (especially the liver and kidneys) diminishes with age; loss of body mass and decrease in body fluids results in a higher concentration of ingested substances. With damage to the liver and kidneys, the by-products of alcohol are not cleared from the body as efficiently. Organ damage or failure and neuropsychiatric effects can occur (Pinto & Walsh, 2008).

Diagnosis

To establish a diagnosis of alcohol dependence, the following criteria must be met: presence of withdrawal, significant impairment in family relationships and occupational productivity, *blackouts* (a temporary loss of recent memory that occurs while drinking), drinking in spite of serious consequences to health or occupation, and evidence of tolerance.

Making the diagnosis of alcohol dependence is not necessarily difficult. The difficulty lies in getting the patient to admit that there is a problem. Unless there is *self-diagnosis* ("I am an alcoholic"), treatment will be for the benefit of the treatment team and the family, but will not foster long-term recovery for the patient.

? Think Critically

You are caring for a patient with a history of alcohol abuse, who has been admitted for surgery. After a visitor leaves, you notice the smell of alcohol on the patient's breath. How would you handle this situation?

Treatment

At one time it was thought that allowing alcoholics to experience a painful withdrawal would frighten them so much they would never drink again. Today we know that **withdrawal can be life threatening,** especially withdrawal from alcohol and certain anxiolytics, such as benzodiazepines. Withdrawal treatment consists of two phases. Initial priorities focus on detoxifying and stabilizing the patient. Detoxification **refers to the process of ridding the body of the abused substance, without causing harmful ill effects.** Treatment decisions may be based on assessment scales such as the Clinical Institute Withdrawal Scale for Alcohol Revised (CIWA-Ar) (Clin-eguide, 2009a). CIWA-Ar indicates the severity of the withdrawal and suggests whether admission to the hospital is warranted, or if outpatient treatment is adequate. Chlordiazepoxide (Librium), diazepam (Valium), or oxazepam (Serax) is given in titrated doses. Phenytoin (Dilantin) and magnesium sulfate (if magnesium levels are low) may be given to prevent seizures. Promethazine (Phenergan), prochlorperazine (Compazine), ibuprofen (Motrin), or dicyclomine (Bentyl) may be given for the symptoms of nausea, vomiting, pain, or cramps. Intravenous fluids are used to correct dehydration, and a "banana bag," which includes normal saline, magnesium sulfate, folic acid, and multivitamins, may be ordered

(Tierney, 2009). Table 47-2 lists the medications used to treat substance abuse.

Once the patient is stable and able to participate in a treatment program, therapy consists of confronting the patient's denial and encouraging self-diagnosis. Disulfiram (Antabuse) is a drug that causes unpleasant reactions if the patient decides to return to drinking anytime after starting the drug and including 14 days after stopping it. Even small quantities of alcohol that might be inhaled from shaving lotion could trigger serious reactions such as chest pain, nausea and vomiting, hypotension, weakness, blurred vision, and confusion. Naltrexone (ReVia) can be used to block the craving for alcohol and to prevent relapse in the recovery phase; nalmefene (Revex) is similar to naltrexone, but lasts longer and is more potent. An oral form of Revex has been used in research studies, but it is currently only available in parenteral form. Acamprosate (Campral) has been used successfully in Europe and has been approved for use in the United States; patients show significantly higher rates of completing therapy programs on this drug. Vivitrol is a once-monthly injectable form of naltrexone that was approved in 2006.

Group therapy helps break through denial and also gives the patient a new sense of belonging and identity. Behavioral therapy helps with self-discipline and discourages impulsive behavior. Limit setting is one of the

| | Table 47-2 | Drugs Used to Treat Substance Abuse |

CLASSIFICATION	ACTION	NURSING IMPLICATIONS
Drugs Used to Treat Acute Alcohol Withdrawal		
Benzodiazepines Chlordiazepoxide (Librium) Diazepam (Valium) Lorazepam (Ativan) Oxazepam (Serax)	Have depressant action on the CNS and inhibit stimulation of the brain. Used for acute withdrawal and to prevent seizures.	Dilute with normal saline and give IV dose slowly. Watch for phlebitis. Have respiratory resuscitation equipment available. Can cause drowsiness and lethargy. Watch for signs of orthostatic hypotension. May cause paradoxical excitement, especially in the elderly.
Antiseizure Phenytoin (Dilantin)	Suppression of neuronal activity that might cause seizures. Used for all types of seizures except absence seizures. Depresses activity of the CNS.	Give IV bolus dose slowly (50 mg/min). Use IV normal saline, not D₅W. Can cause purple glove syndrome (pain, discoloration, and tissue damage) if given into hand vein. Therapeutic level is 10-20 mcg/mL. Maximum infusion rate is 150 mg/min.
Magnesium sulfate		Give IV infusion over 4 hr. Overdose signs include sedation, confusion, intense thirst, and muscle weakness. IV calcium gluconate is the antidote for magnesium intoxication.
Vitamins Thiamine	Contributes to enzyme production for carbohydrate metabolism. Used to correct thiamine deficiency found among alcoholics.	Assess for symptoms of Wernicke's encephalopathy (confusion, ataxia, memory loss). Dilute IV dose and give slowly.

CNS, central nervous system; *D₅W,* 5% dextrose in water; *IV,* intravenous.

Continued

Table 47-2   Drugs Used to Treat Substance Abuse—cont'd

CLASSIFICATION	ACTION	NURSING IMPLICATIONS
Drugs Used to Discourage Relapse		
Naltrexone (ReVia) (Vivitrol: approved 2006)	Competitively binds to opiate receptors to prevent narcotic's effects. Used for alcohol rehabilitation.	Advise patient about side effects of naltrexone: dizziness, fatigue, headache, nausea, nervousness, sleeplessness, and vomiting. Screen for history of liver problems. Vivitrol is a once-monthly injection. Caution that concurrent use of heroin can cause withdrawal symptoms or even death.
Acamprosate calcium (Campral)		Advise patient about side effects of Campral: diarrhea, fatigue, nausea, and flatulence.
Nalmefene (Revex)	Similar to naltrexone.	Must be administered IM or IV. Side effects include nausea, vomiting, tachycardia, hypertension.
Drugs Used to Treat Heroin Abuse or Discourage Relapse		
Opioid Analgesic Methadone Buprenorphine (Suboxone, Subutex)	Produces mild euphoria; used as a heroin substitute in rehabilitation programs.	Extreme caution with use in elderly or debilitated patients, or patients with renal or hepatic impairment, hypothyroidism, Addison's disease, head injury, urethral stricture, enlarged prostate, or respiratory conditions. Advise patient about side effects of dizziness or drowsiness. Monitor for constipation and encourage fluids and fiber. Methadone tablets should be dissolved in orange juice. Buprenorphine is taken sublingually.
Drug Used to Treat Heroin Overdose		
Narcotic Antagonist Naloxone (Narcan)	Competes with opioid receptors and blocks (or reverses) the action of narcotics. Used for patients who have narcotics overdose.	Abrupt reversal of CNS depression may cause nausea, vomiting, increased pulse and blood pressure. Short half-life; watch for recurrent respiratory depression. May have to give repeated doses q 2-3 min or an IV infusion.
Drugs Used to Treat Nicotine Addiction		
Nicotine polacrilex (Nicorette) Nicotine transdermal (Nicotrol)	Delivers lower doses of nicotine. Used in smoking or tobacco cessation programs.	Apply patch immediately after opening to avoid evaporation. Do not cut or fold patch. Instruct patient to chew gum slowly for about 30 min. Advise patient about gradual withdraw from gum after 3 mo; not recommended for use longer than 6 mo. Advise patient to suck on lozenge until dissolved; no chewing, biting, or swallowing. Do not eat or drink for 15 min after finishing lozenge. Advise patient that patch should not be used longer than 3 mo. If no benefit within 4 wk, unlikely that continued use will produce desired effects; consult health care provider.
Bupropion (Zyban)	Weakly blocks reuptake of serotonin, epinephrine, and dopamine (see Chapters 46 and 49). At lower doses, used in smoking cessation programs; at higher doses is used as an antidepressant.	Advise patient that Zyban may cause insomnia; do not take at bedtime. Do not chew, divide, or crush tablets. Treatment usually lasts 7-12 wk. May not notice therapeutic effect for 1 wk. Avoid alcohol while taking this drug.
Varenicline (Chantix)	Blocks nicotine from binding at the receptor sites.	Teach patient to begin taking Chantix 1 wk before stop date. Side effects include nausea or decreased appetite, headaches, insomnia, or vivid dreams. Use cautiously in renal impairment. May cause suicidal tendency.

IM, intramuscular.

hallmarks of behavioral therapy, and it is essential that all members of the behavioral team participate and completely agree about the limits. Brief intervention therapy at 1-year follow-up has been shown to significantly reduce weekly alcohol intake (McQueen et al., 2009). The acronym FRAMES defines the brief approach: Feedback about personal status, Responsibility to change, Advice for change, Menu for options, Empathy in counseling, and Self-efficacy for changes (Durkin & O'Connor, 2009). In accordance with *Healthy People 2020* the use of evidence-based screening in level 1 and 2 trauma centers is essential and brief intervention therapy should be initiated.

[?] Think Critically

A woman brings her 85-year-old father into the clinic and insists that he be admitted to a detox (detoxification) program. The man tells you, "At my age, with my health problems, my fixed income and everything else I have to worry about, having a drink or two is the least of my problems." Discuss your personal reactions and your professional responsibilities in dealing with this family.

Referral to a 12-step program, such as Alcoholics Anonymous (A.A.), is also integral to most treatment plans. A.A. has been in existence for over 50 years and is the dominant approach to alcoholism rehabilitation in the United States; although there is no "cure" for alcoholism, there is hope for ongoing recovery. Evidence-based practice shows that active participation in A.A. results in decreased alcohol consumption. Physicians and nurses can assist by helping the patient to make the first call for A.A. information, locating local sites, and asking about the meetings (Clin-eguide, 2009a). Box 47-2 lists the 12 steps of A.A.

Complications

A serious effect of chronic alcohol abuse is damage to brain cells. A condition that is reversible with treatment is Wernicke's encephalopathy. This condition precedes Korsakoff's syndrome (substance-induced persisting dementia), which is irreversible. If the individual has a history of alcohol use and displays the symptoms of confusion, ataxia, and significant memory loss, Wernicke's encephalopathy is suspected. Treatment involves giving large doses of thiamine (vitamin B_1) and abstaining from alcohol. Thiamine acts as a nerve insulator in the body and is absent in the diets of most chronic alcoholics.

Clinical Cues

Thiamine should always be given before glucose to prevent triggering Wernicke's (Clin-eguide, 2009a).

The individual with Korsakoff's syndrome has grossly impaired memory and gait disturbance. Confabulation (making up stories) frequently is seen as an

Box 47-2 The Twelve Steps of Alcoholics Anonymous

1. We admitted we were powerless over alcohol—that our lives had become unmanageable.
2. Came to believe that a Power greater than ourselves could restore us to sanity.
3. Made a decision to turn our will and our lives over to the care of God *as we understood Him.*
4. Made a searching and fearless moral inventory of ourselves.
5. Admitted to God, to ourselves, and to another human being the exact nature of our wrongs.
6. Were entirely ready to have God remove all these defects of character.
7. Humbly asked Him to remove our shortcomings.
8. Made a list of all persons we had harmed and became willing to make amends to them all.
9. Made direct amends to such people wherever possible, except when to do so would injure them or others.
10. Continued to take personal inventory and when we were wrong, promptly admitted it.
11. Sought through prayer and meditation to improve our conscious contact with God, *as we understood Him,* praying only for knowledge of His will for us and the power to carry that out.
12. Having had a spiritual awakening as the result of these steps, we tried to carry this message to alcoholics, and to practice these principles in all our affairs.

From Alcoholics Anonymous. (2005). *The Big Book Online* (4th ed.). New York: AA World Services, Inc. (pp. 59–60). The Twelve Steps are reprinted with permission of Alcoholics Anonymous World Services, Inc. (AAWS). Permission to reprint the Twelve Steps does not mean that AAWS has reviewed or approved the contents of this publication, or that AAWS necessarily agrees with the views expressed herein. A.A. is a program of recovery of alcoholism only—use of the Twelve Steps in connection with programs and activities which are patterned after A.A., but which address other problems, or in any other non-A.A. context, does not imply otherwise.

attempt to communicate. A brain scan will show brain atrophy; currently there is no treatment to reverse this condition.

ABUSE OF OTHER CENTRAL NERVOUS SYSTEM DEPRESSANTS

Other CNS depressants subject to abuse and dependence are barbiturates and anxiolytics, including benzodiazepines. It is not uncommon to see these drugs used in conjunction with alcohol, but this practice can be fatal because of the additive effects. Drugs in this category may be purchased illegally, or initially they may be prescribed by a physician for insomnia, or to ease anxiety. There has been an increase in nonmedical use of prescription drugs and in 2008, emergency department visits for misused prescription or over-the-counter drugs matched the number of visits for illicit drugs (*Morbidity and Mortality Weekly Report*, 2010). The increase of abuse of prescription drugs suggests that policy and practice changes are required, such as health provider education, universal use of prescription monitoring programs, routine monitoring of insurance claims information, and increased vigilance for signs of abuse.

Benzodiazepines (e.g., lorazepam [Ativan], oxazepam [Serax], temazepam [Restoril]) have familiar side effects: drowsiness, hypotension, relaxation, and slurred speech. The chronic user may display lack of motivation, memory loss, poor concentration, irritability, aggression, anxiety, and an increased appetite with weight gain. If an individual has been abusing drugs that depress the CNS and goes through withdrawal, symptoms would include an elevation in pulse and blood pressure, nervousness, and heightened anxiety. Flunitrazepam (Rohypnol) is classified as a benzodiazepine and may look like a packaged prescription medication because it is produced and used in Europe and Mexico for insomnia; however, it is illegal in the United States. Rohypnol gained notoriety in the 1990s as the date-rape drug. It produces *anterograde amnesia* (inability to remember events that happened while under the influence of a substance), along with muscle relaxation, drowsiness, and slowed motor performance.

 Elder Care Points

Insomnia is not atypical in the elderly population. Great care must be taken when prescribing sedatives and hypnotics for this group. Decreased liver and renal function can quickly lead to toxicity and dependence. Benzodiazepines, in particular, have a long half-life and are not excreted readily by the body. Therefore patients with poor liver and renal function are subject to a cumulative effect and may experience toxic side effects. Patient education is very important.

Treatment

As with detoxification from alcohol, the benzodiazepine addict may be given a drug from a similar category in titrated doses. The amount depends on the severity of the addiction. With the long half-life of benzodiazepines, the initial symptoms of withdrawal may not appear for 3 to 5 days. Table 47-3 presents the symptoms of intoxication with and withdrawal from CNS depressants. Long-term treatment consists of referral

Table 47-3 | Characteristics of Commonly Abused Substances

SUBSTANCE	USUAL METHODS OF ADMINISTRATION	SYMPTOMS ASSOCIATED WITH USAGE	EFFECTS OF OVERDOSE	WITHDRAWAL SYNDROME
Alcohol	Oral	Drowsiness, ataxia, initial euphoria and aggressive or belligerent behavior, muscular incoordination. At higher alcohol levels, slurred speech, marked ataxia and muscular incoordination, marked cognitive impairment.	Amnesia, tremors, hypothermia, seizures, respiratory failure, coma, death.	Nausea, vomiting, anorexia, agitation, hallucinations, seizures, increased body temperature, increased blood pressure and heart and respiratory rate, possibly death.
Opiates (narcotic analgesics)	Oral, inhalation, IV	Euphoria, drowsiness, decreased respirations, constricted pupils.	Decreased respirations, shallow breathing, clammy skin, seizures, possibly death.	Watery eyes, runny nose, yawning, anorexia, irritability, tremors, panic, cramps, nausea, chills, and sweating.
CNS stimulants (cocaine, amphetamines)	Inhalation, oral, IV, smoked	Increased alertness, excitation, euphoria, increased pulse and blood pressure, insomnia, anorexia.	Agitation, hyperthermia, hallucinations, convulsions, cardiac dysrhythmias, possibly death.	Apathy, long periods of sleep, irritability depression, disorientation.
CNS depressants (anxiolytics and barbiturates)	Oral	Slurred speech, disorientation, drunken behavior without odor of alcohol.	Shallow respiration, clammy skin, dilated pupils, weak and rapid pulse, coma, possibly death.	Anxiety, insomnia, tremors, delirium, convulsions, possibly death.
Cannabis (marijuana)	Inhaled, oral	Euphoria, relaxed inhibitions, increased appetite, disoriented behavior.	Fatigue, paranoia, psychosis.	None.
Hallucinogens (LSD, PCP)	Oral	Illusions, hallucinations, impaired perception.	Effects are increased and intensified, psychosis, flashbacks, possibly death.	None.

CNS, central nervous system; *IV*, intravenous; *LSD*, lysergic acid diethylamide; *PCP*, phencyclidine.

to a 12-step program (i.e., Narcotics Anonymous) and perhaps individual and/or group psychotherapy. Patients need to be taught alternative ways to induce sleep and relieve anxiety.

ABUSE OF OPIATES

Opiate analgesics can also be obtained both legally and illegally. The process of addiction may begin with a prescription drug for severe pain. If these individuals rely totally on narcotics to relieve chronic pain and have a tendency to abuse drugs, addiction may occur. Conversely, if narcotics and a variety of measures are used to alleviate the pain, there may be some increased tolerance and physical dependence. However, tolerance and physical dependence can be treated by slowly decreasing dosages of the opiates. For symptoms of use, withdrawal, and overdose see Table 47-3.

 Complementary and Alternative Therapies

Pain

Assist your patients to explore adjunctive therapies to alleviate pain. These include meditation, visualization, biofeedback, hypnosis, and acupuncture. Aromatherapy with fragrant oils such as jasmine or patchouli can stimulate endorphins (natural pain killers produced by our bodies).

Treatment

The greatest danger with opiates is an overdose which can result in respiratory depression and death. Treatment for an overdose usually consists of administration of a narcotic antagonist, such as naloxone (Narcan).

 Clinical Cues

A dose of IV Narcan can produce dramatic and rapid results. Your lethargic overdosed patient may arouse very suddenly with nausea, vomiting, tachycardia, and an increased blood pressure. **Do *not* assume that the danger is over.** The half-life of Narcan is short, and the opiate action will resume and cause respiratory depression; therefore anticipate that a continuous Narcan infusion may be ordered.

 Clinical Cues

If activated charcoal is ordered as part of the treatment for an overdose of opiates, make sure that the patient is fully alert and able to protect his own airway (Clin-eguide, 2009b).

Withdrawal from opiates is not life threatening, but patients can experience abdominal cramps, irritability, profuse sweating, yawning, muscle aches, fever and chills, and cravings. Treatment involves helping the individual withdraw from the drug. Methadone maintenance programs are successful in helping patients

who have a heroin addiction. Buprenorphine (Suboxone or Subutex) has been approved in the United States for opiate substitute therapy; however, in one survey, 81% of general psychiatrists were reluctant to prescribe buprenorphine. This represents a significant barrier to treatment, considering that current estimates for the United States indicate 1 million heroine users and 3 million addicted to prescription drugs compared to 220,000 slots for methadone clinics (Thomas et al., 2008). See Table 47-2 for nursing implications related to medications to treat opiate overdose and recovery.

If a street drug such as heroin is the substance of choice, rehabilitation is difficult unless the environmental and social factors (e.g., breaking off relationships with friends who abuse substances) are also changed. It is not unusual for an individual addicted to heroin to require up to 2 years in some type of supervised alternative living program. Group, individual, and behavioral therapy and a referral to a 12-step program (i.e., Narcotics Anonymous) are also essential to success. In a systematic review of psychosocial treatments, Cleary and colleagues (2009) found that motivational interviewing combined with cognitive-behavioral therapy reduced substance abuse for the short term and improved mental state (see Box 46-1). In a 5-year study of physicians with substance abuse problems, a zero tolerance approach showed that 72% were successfully abstaining. The program included intensive monitoring and mandatory testing with severe consequences for even a single relapse (Dupont et al., 2009). For convicts in South Dakota and Hawaii, a similar zero tolerance method has also produced remarkable results (Boschert, 2010). Network therapy is an evidence-based program that uses the patient's social network to support abstinence; biweekly meetings and aversive consequences are also part of the therapy (SAMHSA, 2007).

Support groups are useful to any individual who is trying to make a major life change or to someone who has experienced a major life-changing event. Substance abusers who are trying to change to a totally different lifestyle can also benefit from this extra support. The purpose of support groups is to help promote healthy relationships, learn and practice new coping skills, and reduce stress and anxiety. Support groups borrow from the principles of group therapy: universality (we have similar experiences), cohesiveness (we have a feeling of belonging), catharsis (expressing feelings make us feel better), altruism (you help me, I'll help you), information giving (this worked for me, it might help you), improved social skills (you can say this in group, now say it to your family), and intrapersonal learning (Yalom, 2005). Nurses should refer patients and encourage them to use this valuable resource.

ABUSE OF STIMULANTS

The two common categories of CNS stimulants are cocaine and amphetamines. Both categories of drugs have legitimate medical uses, but are also abused. **Amphetamines can cause an increase in pulse rate and blood pressure, general excitation, anorexia, and hyperactive reflexes and can produce life-threatening conditions such as cardiac dysrhythmias, seizures, or hyperthermia.**

Misuse can range from small and infrequent amounts to ingestion of large amounts, which cause prolonged sleeplessness and anorexia. Sleep deprivation of this magnitude can lead to extreme agitation and hostility, as well as a transient psychosis, and can be fatal. People who are withdrawing from stimulants will experience drowsiness, headache, lethargy, nausea, alterations in eating and sleeping patterns, and sometimes cravings.

Methamphetamine, known as "speed," "meth," "crank," or "crystal," is injected or smoked (Figure 47-3). White men ages 20 to 35 have the highest abuse rate for methamphetamines. It is highly addictive, and users end up taking progressively larger doses. "Meth labs" are unfortunately easy to establish in any average household, garage, trailer, or the like, where common household chemicals, brake fluid, antifreeze, batteries, matches, ammonia, or over-the-counter medications (Clark, 2008) are "cooked," creating a harmful residue that lingers on the walls and in the air well after the cooking process is finished. Chronic users may develop toxic psychosis and experience paranoia, hallucinations, and delusions. They are also at risk for *pericarditis* (inflammation of the heart lining).

Cocaine use has increased dramatically. It is highly addictive and can cause death, even in small doses.

FIGURE 47-2 Methamphetamine.

FIGURE 47-3 Crack cocaine.

Cocaine is a short-acting substance and is more commonly used for binges. It produces euphoria, increased energy, and a sense of well-being. The stimulating effects are very fast acting and energizing. However, the effects after the "high" are equally intense, and individuals are subject to severe emotional lows. The powder is either "snorted" (intranasal administration) or dissolved and taken intravenously. "Crack," a purified form of cocaine, is smoked by placing it in a pipe or smoking it with marijuana or tobacco (Figure 47-3). This "freebasing" of cocaine reduces it to its purest form. This is the most dangerous type of administration; it produces an immediate rush and accounts for many overdoses and lethal reactions.

Treatment

Treatment for abuse of CNS stimulants is similar to treatment for alcohol abuse. Initially the treatment protocol is symptom specific and managed by medications. Anxiolytics or antipsychotics may be used for agitation or aggressive behavior, and antidepressants may be used for the depressive symptoms. Experimental studies are being conducted on the use of familiar drugs as potential treatments for cocaine addiction: methylphenidate (Ritalin), amantadine (Symmetrel), fluoxetine (Prozac), propranolol (Inderal), and ondansetron (Zofran). In a recent study, an experimental anti-cocaine vaccine did not produce complete abstinence; however, participants did have better social functioning (Martell et al., 2009). A combination of behavioral and group therapy and referral to a 12-step program have been shown to reduce cocaine use (Clin-eguide, 2009b). These patients must also be taught ways to cope with the psychological craving that often leads to relapse. Two new approaches are currently being studied to address cognitive problems in addictive disorders: computer-assisted cognitive rehabilitation and pharmacologic manipulation of neurotransmitters. This type of adjunctive therapy is important because cognitive impairment has been shown to hinder treatment length and engagement and to cause the therapist to view the patient as unmotivated (Fals-Stewart & Lam, 2010).

ABUSE OF NICOTINE

Nicotine is highly addictive and causes increased respiration, decreased pulmonary function, and a chronic cough. Use of tobacco is related to more than 400,000 deaths per year and contributes to the development of lung cancer and other lung diseases, such as emphysema. Pipe smokers and people who chew tobacco are more prone to oral cancer. Smoking has been implicated in many other health conditions, including heart disease, stroke, many cancers, hypertension, premature wrinkling of the skin, bad breath, and discoloration of the fingernails. In addition, environmental tobacco smoking results in 38,000 deaths each year (Agency for Healthcare Research and Quality [AHRQ], 2009). **Withdrawal symptoms can begin as soon as 24 hours after the cessation of smoking and include irritability, tension, decreased heart rate, and insomnia.** Cigarettes are legal and accessible, and the craving continues long after the patient quits smoking; therefore resumption of the habit is common and many smokers stay in denial about the effects of nicotine.

 Cultural Considerations

New Consumer Markets

There has been a decrease in smoking in the United States in the past 25 years. In 1966 the U.S. Surgeon General's health warnings were placed on all cigarette packages. Since then, similar warnings have been put on other tobacco products. Television and radio advertising for cigarettes was banned in 1971. Education and an increase in cigarette taxes, along with restrictions on smoking in public places, have also contributed to the decrease. Nevertheless, new potential consumer markets are being targeted around the world. For example, cigarette manufacturers have now identified China as a good alternative consumer market, and as a result, many Chinese men and teenagers have developed this high-risk habit.

Treatment

Nicotine replacement therapy (NRT) is available from patches, lozenges, gum, sublingual tablets, inhalant, and nasal spray. Self-help groups, hypnosis, and acupuncture are among the treatments available for nicotine addiction. In 1997 bupropion (Zyban) was approved as a stop-smoking aid in the United States. Varenicline (Chantix) is a new medication that acts to block nicotine from binding at the receptor sites. Cessation smoking programs support the *Healthy People 2020* goals and emphasize the positive effects of quitting, such as better overall health for the individual and the family, an increased sense of smell and taste, and saving money. Evidence-based practice suggests that nursing intervention for smoking cessation increases likelihood of quitting and helps patients succeed (Zarling, 2007). Multicomponent interventions for smoking cessation that include an on-site visit, follow-up phone calls, enhanced education about NRT, and motivational interviewing are effective. The most useful aspects of counseling are helping the patient develop a plan and identifying barriers to quitting. The plan can include setting a stop date, asking friends and family for help, anticipating how to combat cravings, and removing all tobacco products and accessories from the house, car, and workplace. The combination of counseling and medications is more successful than using one without the other (AHRQ, 2009).

 Clinical Cues

The AHRQ (2009) recommends the "five *As*" approach for helping patients to quit using tobacco: (1) *Ask* about tobacco use, (2) *Advise* to quit, (3) *Assess* willingness to quit, (4) *Assist* to quit, and (5) *Arrange* follow-up.

 Legal and Ethical Considerations

Do As I Say, Not As I Do

Evidence suggests that nurses who use tobacco are less effective in helping patients with smoking cessation interventions; possibly they have the same misconceptions and difficulties in quitting that patients have. To be more effective in helping patients to quit, nurses who are using tobacco should actively participate in their own smoking cessation efforts (Zarling, 2007).

ABUSE OF CANNABIS

The leaves and flowering tops of the *Cannabis sativa* (marijuana) plant are dried and loosely rolled in cigarette paper and smoked. It is commonly used as a "gateway substance" (substance that leads the way or opens the gate to more dangerous and serious substance abuse) by teenagers and as a recreational drug by adults. There is active and controversial discussion of legalizing marijuana for medical purposes. The active ingredient in marijuana is effective in controlling nausea in patients who are receiving chemotherapy and helping relieve some types of chronic pain. Some proponents suggest that marijuana lowers intraocular pressure in patients who have glaucoma, but the Glaucoma Research Foundation (2011) advises that marijuana is not as effective as medications that are currently prescribed.

Marijuana is typically smoked, but it can also be ingested. It acts quickly (15 minutes), and the effects last for up to 4 hours. **General effects are a mild euphoria, increased appetite, and increased sensitivity to sound, colors, and other environmental elements. Impaired coordination, mental concentration, and altered judgment are also present.** In large doses, the person may experience psychotic symptoms. Marijuana is thought not to be physically addictive, but it may lead to psychological dependence and a lack of motivation and ambition. There is no particular withdrawal syndrome for cannabis, so treatment must focus on issues related to the general dangers of substance abuse. In addition, patients should be advised that a recent study showed that people who smoked both marijuana and tobacco were 2.5 times more likely to develop lung disease (Tan et al., 2009).

 Think Critically

Substance abuse crosses all ethnic, gender, age, and socioeconomic backgrounds. You have three patients: a homeless elderly Asian American woman, a well-to-do African American teenager, and a middle-aged white man who works as a carpenter. You must assess all three for marijuana (and other substances) use. First, identify your own biases and then describe your approach.

ABUSE OF HALLUCINOGENS AND INHALANTS

Two common drugs that cause hallucinations are lysergic acid diethylamide (LSD) and phencyclidine hydrochloride (PCP, or angel dust). These hallucinogens are thought to be somewhat less physiologically addictive compared to other psychoactive substances; however, there are extremely unpredictable effects. Hallucinogens cause distortion of the senses, an inability to separate fact from fantasy, impaired sense of time, and severely impaired judgment. Users never know whether they will have a good "trip" or a bad one. Uncontrolled *flashbacks* (feelings and sensations associated with use despite being drug free) can occur. This group of drugs is very dangerous because use is known to cause panic, paranoia, and death from extremely impaired judgment.

Inhalants are psychologically and physiologically addictive. Commonly abused inhalants include glue, nail polish remover, aerosol-packaged products (e.g., deodorants), and paint thinner and other types of solvents. Symptoms of use are acute confusion, excitability, and sometimes hallucinations. Prolonged use of inhalants causes permanent damage to all body organs and a psychological dependence. Inhalants are most frequently used by teens and children because they are inexpensive and easily accessible.

 Think Critically

You are caring for a 14-year-old who admits to you that he has been experimenting with glue sniffing. He tells you that he has stopped and he asks you not to share this information with his parents. How will you handle this situation? Who can you consult to clarify your legal and ethical obligations?

Treatment

Medical treatment and intervention for both hallucinogens and inhalants may include provision of safety for the individual who may be experiencing a bad "trip." Emergency measures may be necessary to provide respiratory support for an individual who has impaired gas exchange as a result of inhalants.

❖ NURSING MANAGEMENT
▪ Assessment (Data Collection)

A general physical assessment, including vital signs, is necessary. Any life-threatening physical problems must be quickly identified and treated. For example, patients can and do die from cardiac dysrhythmias associated with stimulant abuse, whereas patients who have overdosed on heroin are at risk for respiratory arrest.

Any patient who enters the health care system should be screened for substance abuse, so that early intervention can prevent the immediate and long-term consequences of substance misuse (Tierney, 2009). Obtain a substance and alcohol history that includes the type of substance used, the amount taken, and the pattern of use. For patients scheduled for surgery, a thorough preoperative history is absolutely essential, because a patient who normally drinks a lot of alcohol can return from surgery to a busy surgical unit and develop symptoms of alcohol withdrawal. An event of this type complicates postoperative recovery and can be fatal.

 Focused Assessment

Data Collection for Substance and Alcohol Use

Ask the following questions during history taking to determine past and present substance and/or alcohol use:

- Have you ever had a drinking or substance abuse problem?*
- When did you last drink or use drugs of any kind?*
- What substances (alcohol, tobacco, or illicit substances) are you currently using?
- What other types of drugs (prescription and nonprescription) do you routinely take?
- How much do you drink or how much do you use?
- How often do you drink or use substances?
- Have you ever tried to cut down or control your substance use or drinking?
- Have you noticed that now it takes more of the substance or drink to get the same effect you got several months ago?
- Have you noticed any withdrawal symptoms?
- Have you ever been treated for liver disease, hepatitis, heart disease, anemia, or overdose?
- Have you had any recent falls, accidents, or injuries?
- Have you ever stopped drinking or using drugs for a period of time?
- Have you ever been in treatment for substance abuse?
- Is there a family history of alcoholism or substance abuse?
- What is your marital status? If married, are you happily married?
- Have you ever been in trouble with the law?
- What is your occupation? Are you experiencing any difficulties at work?

*Direct questioning is found to yield highly sensitive responses, despite the common expectation that alcoholics deny or minimize alcohol usage (Tierney, 2009).

A quick and simple assessment tool for alcohol abuse is the CAGE questionnaire, which includes four questions regarding the patient's feelings about his or her drinking and specific habits. A "yes" answer to two or more of the four questions has a 90% correlation with alcohol abuse (Ewing, 1984). Also, obtain information about past and current function in family, social, and occupational roles. Remember that denial is a primary defense mechanism used in these disorders. Therefore it often is necessary to ask the family to describe their perception of the user's problem and the extent of substance use. At the appropriate time, assess the impact of the user's behavior on the family and explore the presence of co-dependent or enabling behaviors.

■ Nursing Diagnosis

Nursing diagnoses for substance use disorders include:

- Confusion related to excessive or chronic alcohol consumption
- Ineffective denial related to physical and psychological dependence on a substance
- Interrupted family processes related to substance addiction that override family responsibilities
- Risk for injury related to impaired judgment
- Ineffective role performance related to impaired ability to complete assigned work duties
- Noncompliance related to the commitment of abstinence from a substance

Clinical Cues

Patients will enter the health care system with medical complaints or injuries who also have unidentified substance abuse problems. When taking a routine admission history, ask about the use of substances. This information is needed to evaluate drug-drug interactions and any potential toxic effects on the body organs (i.e., heart, kidneys, liver). Use a matter-of-fact tone of voice: "Sir, what kind of prescription, over-the-counter, or illicit (street) drugs do you use? Do you smoke or drink alcohol?" In accordance with National Patient Safety Goals, your findings contribute to a complete list of medications. This medication reconciliation list should be communicated to the health care team within the organization, sent to other facilities if the patient is transferred, and provided to the patient when discharged.

■ Planning

Expected outcomes are written for the specific individual nursing diagnoses chosen to resolve the patient's problems. For the nursing diagnoses above, they might include:

- Patient will demonstrate less confusion after receiving thiamine and abstaining from alcohol before discharge.
- Patient will discuss how reliance on substances is affecting his quality of life during today's group therapy session.
- During weekly sessions with social service counselor, the patient and family will communicate

needs and identify sources of support to sustain the family.
- Patient will remain safe from harm or injury during this shift.
- Patient will resume job duties within _____ months.
- Patient will participate in a 12-step program at least three times per week.

Elder Care Points

When working with elderly patients, be on the alert for substance use disorders; this group is at high risk because of loneliness, multiple losses, and limited resources. Health care providers frequently overlook substance abuse in elderly patients because behaviors may be attributed to aging, depression, or dementia. Stevenson and Masters suggested a "best predictor model" for older women who had a high risk for alcohol abuse (Stevenson & Masters, 2005). They found that scores of 1 or higher on the T-ACE questionnaire (Tolerance, Annoyance, Cut-down, Eye opener; similar to CAGE), regular use of over-the-counter drugs, ingestion of large amounts of coffee, and using alcohol to induce sleep were associated with alcohol abuse.

Collaborative goal setting is very important when working with an individual who is addicted to a substance. In addition to working with the patient, it is necessary that you collaborate with the family. Setting goals with the patient and excluding the family or friends often leads to failure or relapse. Planning care for a patient with a substance use disorder includes promoting physical and psychological safety, providing a safe withdrawal from the substance, and ensuring adequate nutrition and sleep. To prevent relapse, education regarding substance abuse becomes a priority goal. The education may be started in a treatment center, but needs to be continued after discharge for at least 1 year. People who abuse substances need opportunities to learn and practice new coping skills in a supportive environment.

Think Critically

Do you have any bad habits such as smoking, drinking alcohol, or drinking too much coffee? How does your personal behavior affect what you will say to your patients about making changes for a healthier lifestyle?

■ Implementation

Nursing intervention depends on the severity of the substance abuse disorder. Initial interventions for the patient focus on physical recovery. For example, cardiac monitoring, pulse oximetry, IV access, and other emergency measures may be indicated. Potentially fatal effects of drugs and/or alcohol, such as cardiac dysrhythmias, hypotension, and respiratory depression, must receive priority attention. If the patient is intoxicated, orienting to person, place, and time and providing for physical safety are essential. You may need to insist that the patient remains in a protected environment until judgment and coordination return. Ensuring adequate sleep and a balanced diet high in proteins and multivitamins are also part of early intervention.

If the patient is having symptoms of withdrawal, detoxification must be medically managed by giving antianxiety agents, such as chlordiazepoxide (Librium). Close monitoring of vital signs is important because signs of alcohol withdrawal include an increase in blood pressure and heart rate. Preventing the patient from experiencing a seizure or delirium tremens is an essential part of the detoxification process.

Clinical Cues

When monitoring and reporting changes in blood pressure, keep several factors in mind: patient's baseline, trends (if available), and medications (last dose and type). Also assess for accompanying subjective symptoms such as dizziness or light-headedness (hypotension), headache, or blurred vision (hypertension).

Assignment Considerations

One-to-One Observation

Frequently a CNA or UAP is assigned to sit with a patient who needs one-to-one (1:1) observation. Before assigning personnel to this task, clarify with the physician or RN the purpose of 1:1 observation and the stability of the patient. For example, recall that opioid withdrawal is not life threatening, but the restless patient may be temporarily placed on 1:1 observation to prevent *elopement* (leaving) to seek drugs to satisfy the intense craving. It would be appropriate to assign a CNA or UAP to prevent elopement. In contrast, an agitated patient who is withdrawing from alcohol is not physically stable and his care should be managed by an RN.

Once the substance is cleared from the body, nursing intervention is directed toward helping the patient lead a drug-free life. This includes alleviating the symptoms and confronting denial. You must also observe for signs of suicide. Addicted patients often feel they cannot live without the euphoria and consolation of the substance experience.

Patients who are in the early recovery process from substance abuse benefit greatly from therapeutic conversations with the nurse, and a caring, concerned attitude is very important. Studies have shown that two 15-minute monthly meetings and two 5-minute follow-up nurse calls have beneficial effects (Clini-eguide,

2009b). Patients must grieve the loss of the substance, and they also feel guilt and shame for acts that were committed while under the influence. To help the patient "work through" these feelings, you need to be an active listener, offering support and validation as necessary. Mandating a patient to stop is usually not an effective intervention; however, you should support the patient's decision to stop. Assist by reminding him that the physical symptoms of withdrawal will not last forever. The craving will last longer than the withdrawal symptoms, but is manageable if the patient has a strong motivation to change toward a healthy lifestyle. Help your patient to identify ways to cope with the craving. For example, help him to make a list of activities that he could use to distract his attention from the craving, such as calling a friend, taking a brisk walk, cleaning the house, or eating a nutritious snack. Help him identify settings, circumstances, or relationships that were part of his substance abuse pattern, then identify alternative settings and relationships that are now part of his new lifestyle. For example, polysubstance use might routinely occur in a bar or lounge with friends after having a few beers, but is less likely to occur in a movie theater with friends who are having popcorn.

If the patient is addicted to heroin, the recovery process will be lengthy because of the lifestyle changes that are necessary. Typically, with heroin addiction, there have been some illegal actions and maladaptive coping. The patient needs to be educated about the disease process and needs to learn new coping methods (Nursing Care Plan 47-1).

Intervening with the Family

A trusting relationship needs to be developed with the family or they may continue to focus on the patient rather than focus on their own recovery. Families need to learn in what manner they might have been enabling their loved one, and they need time to practice new behaviors that will require the substance abuser to be responsible for himself. Family members should be encouraged to express how the crisis is affecting them. There may be a need to refer families to legal or social services if the person is abusing illegal drugs or if there was an arrest for driving while intoxicated. The family feels shame and guilt and shares the stigma associated with substance abuse. Encourage them to seek support from groups such as Al-Anon or Alateen. Family members may consider substance abuse a moral weakness, rather than a disease. Educating them about the neurobiologic theories may help them to reconsider their attitudes and relieve some guilt. **To be effective in working with substance abusers, nurses must examine their own attitudes and make certain the patients and families are treated with respect.**

Nursing Care Plan 47-1   **Care of the Patient with a Substance Abuse Disorder**

Scenario

Jerry Sanders is a 42-year-old man brought in by his supervisor for admission to a "detox" unit. The supervisor last saw Mr. Sanders drinking about 10 hours ago. He states that Jerry is a good worker but could lose his job. Mr. Sanders jokingly replies, "My boss is a worrier. I'm just a social drinker. My wife and kids know I'm okay." The supervisor states that the wife frequently makes excuses but seems unaware of the problem. Mr. Sanders seems slightly anxious and irritable. He appears thin and malnourished.

Problem/Nursing Diagnosis

Showing early signs of withdrawal/Risk for injury related to effects of substance and complications of withdrawal.

Supporting Assessment Data

Objective: Slightly anxious and irritable; last known drink 10 hours ago.

Goals/Expected Outcomes	Nursing Interventions	Selected Rationale	Evaluation
Patient will remain free from any injury this shift. Patient will withdraw from drugs or alcohol without any undue effects.	Assess for early symptoms of withdrawal (e.g., agitation, irritability, anxiety) and notify physician or RN of first signs.	Early detection of withdrawal allows for prompt intervention to prevent life-threatening complications.	Is anxious and irritable.
	Administer medications (e.g., chlordiazepoxide [Librium]) as prescribed by physician.	Decreases neurologic irritability at the biochemical level.	Thirty minutes after administration of Librium, patient appears more relaxed.
	Remain with patient during times of confusion and disorientation.	Provides support and decreases agitation.	Currently alert and oriented.
	Restrain and/or place in seclusion as ordered if the patient becomes a danger to self or others.	May temporarily be unable to control aggressive or self-harm impulses. May attempt to leave.	Is verbally hostile and denies substance abuse problems, but shows no signs of physical aggression.
	Ensure safe environment (i.e., call bell within reach, bed in lowest position).	Safety is a priority, and patient judgment and coordination may be temporarily impaired.	Did not sustain any injury during the shift. Outcomes met. Continue plan.

Problem/Nursing Diagnosis

Not admitting to problem/Ineffective denial related to minimization of the symptoms of addiction.

Supporting Assessment Data

Subjective: States "My boss is a worrier. I'm just a social drinker."
Objective: Supervisor's report and Mr. Sanders' perception of problem are mismatched.

Goals/Expected Outcomes	Nursing Interventions	Selected Rationale	Evaluation
Patient will acknowledge the abuse of substances and the unhealthy impact on his life.	Approach the patient in a nonjudgmental manner.	Helps to build trust and rapport.	Is agreeable to talking but is unable to disclose feelings.
	Gently confront the denial as you gain the trust of the patient.	Breaking through denial is essential to recovery.	Denial continues.
Patient will openly acknowledge the need for substance abuse treatment.	Help the patient see the need for treatment and abstinence.	May be unaware of or is ignoring the long-term consequences.	Denies need for treatment.
	Inform the patient about the negative aspects of addictive processes.	Helps the patient to make an informed decision.	Verbally acknowledges that substances are harmful for others, "but I don't drink that much."
	Encourage patient to list the harmful effects that he has experienced.	Increases insight and facilitates self-diagnosis.	Denies that substances are harming him.

Continued

Nursing Care Plan 47-1	Care of the Patient with a Substance Abuse Disorder—cont'd

Goals/Expected Outcomes	Nursing Interventions	Selected Rationale	Evaluation
Patient will agree to attend 90 12-step meetings in 90 days.	Encourage attendance at a 12-step program to help break through the denial.	Provides support by others who have experienced the same difficulties.	Agrees to go to a 12-step program, but thinks it is unnecessary. Outcomes not met. Continue plan.

Problem/Nursing Diagnosis

Wife is affected, but is not openly acknowledging problem/Dysfunctional family process: alcoholism related to altered family roles, unexpressed feelings, family history of alcoholism.

Supporting Assessment Data

Subjective: Per supervisor, wife frequently makes excuses but seems unaware of the problem.
Objective: Wife is absent; supervisor is advocating for treatment.

Goals/Expected Outcomes	Nursing Interventions	Selected Rationale	Evaluation
Family will be able to identify and share feelings.	Invite family to participate.	Family may be unaware, or need assistance to break through their denial.	Wife and children did come in to talk with physician and social worker about Mr. Sanders' condition.
	Assess for presence of denial, shame, or guilt.	Feelings of denial, shame, and guilt are expected, but may be repressed.	Family members expressed support for Mr. Sanders, but are unable to disclose personal feelings.
	Encourage expression of genuine feelings.	Opportunity for expression of feelings helps to build trust and rapport.	Trust and rapport are being established, but communication between family members continues to be ineffective.
	Teach how to recognize feelings and safe ways to express them (e.g., "I love you, but I am not going to stay here while you drink").	New communication methods are needed to help the family break old patterns.	Currently family is not openly acknowledging how Mr. Sanders' behavior affects each member, but they agree to attend group therapy.
	Educate the family about the altered roles present in addictive families. (e.g., wife overcompensating for husband).	Family members may be unaware of how the illness is affecting role function.	Family is not identifying dysfunctional roles, but appear open to exploring the family situation.
	Define the term *enabling* for family members.	Identifying and defining enabling helps family to recognize this behavior.	Entire family appears to be in denial at this time; denies enabling behaviors.
	Encourage family members to state at least one time when they engaged in enabling behavior.	Increases insight into own behavior.	
	Offer family members alternative choices to enabling behavior (e.g., telling him that he must call in sick for himself).	Family needs new ways to cope with old problems.	Family open to learning more about disease process and how to cope with Mr. Sanders' behavior.
	Have family members practice and role play alternative responses to enabling behavior.	Practice in a safe environment allows family to test new skills.	Family having difficulty with role play.
Family will agree to attend at least six 12-step meetings.	Encourage family members to attend a 12-step support meeting.	Provides support by sharing with others who are experiencing the same problem.	Family agrees to go to a 12-step group this weekend. Outcomes not met. Continue plan.

Problem/Nursing Diagnosis

Drinking excessive alcohol and not eating enough to meet daily needs/Imbalanced nutrition: less than body requirements related to poor food intake, inadequate absorption of nutrients, poor appetite.

Supporting Assessment Data

Objective: Appears thin and malnourished.

Goals/Expected Outcomes	Nursing Interventions	Selected Rationale	Evaluation
Patient will self-select a nutritious diet.	Assess ability to feed self.	May have impairment in fine motor coordination.	Is able to independently feed self; shows some fine tremors in hands.
Patient will gain 5 lb within 1 mo; signs of peripheral neuropathy (numbness and tingling) will disappear.	Watch for nausea, vomiting, diarrhea. Administer antacids, antiemetics, and IV fluids as ordered.	Alcohol can cause gastritis and alterations in absorption.	Currently no nausea or vomiting.
	Document intake and output and food intake. Weigh patient.	To monitor nutritional status and progress toward goal.	Weighs 140 lb (ideal body weight 165 lb). Finishes food trays.
	Collaborate with patient to determine food preferences.	Increases likelihood of consumption.	Eats all types of food.
	Encourage small, frequent meals, high in proteins with 50% carbohydrates.	Small meals are easier to tolerate, and foods rich in nutrition will replace loss due to poor dietary practices.	States that he sometimes forgets to eat but knows he should gain some weight ("Will try harder").
	Administer multivitamins, especially thiamine (vitamin B_1) and niacin, as ordered.	Patient is at risk for Wernicke's encephalopathy.	Agrees that supplements are a good idea and will continue to take them after discharge.
	Consult nutritionist.	Collaboration with specialist ensures best plan.	Consultation with nutritionist deferred because patient agrees to eat everything on food trays. Outcomes partially met. Continue plan.

Critical Thinking Questions

1. What are some questions that would be appropriate to ask the wife (if she is willing to come in and meet with the healthcare team)?
2. Mr. Sanders is currently far from being ready for self-diagnosis. What are some things that might signal that he is breaking through the denial?

? Think Critically

A patient tells you that he drinks socially, but his wife and children tell you that he drinks to the point of intoxication at least three times a week. What would you say to the family? What would you say to the patient?

■ Evaluation

Recovery from a substance use disorder is a lengthy process. Ridding the body of substances can take weeks, particularly if there is coexisting liver damage. Often the patient is malnourished, physically exhausted, and in poor general health. Return to an optimum healthy state may take 6 months to 1 year. Recovery of psychological or emotional health takes even longer. If the patient started abusing drugs at a very young age, emotional development may have been arrested. Coping mechanisms to deal with anxiety or emotional pain were never properly developed; the individual used the drug(s) instead.

Consequently, nurses working in the hospital may only see early physical recovery. Evaluating overall effectiveness of substance abuse treatment is measured in years rather than weeks. Admitting a patient to a hospital and guiding him safely though detoxification is a very necessary, but small, beginning step in the overall process.

COMMUNITY CARE

Nurses who work in emergency departments and busy outpatient clinics often see individuals who have medical problems related to substance abuse. Often these patients are treated only for their presenting medical problem. In these instances, the medical treatment team is reinforcing the patient's denial system. *Healthy People 2020* goals include a proactive approach to use these incidental contacts to screen for substance abuse and appropriately refer these patients to prevent costly long-term complications.

As is the case with the general patient population, inpatient hospital stays for individuals who are addicted are usually short. If the patient has some type of insurance, it is not unusual for the insurance company to pay only for medical detoxification. Any further treatment that is necessary would be performed on an outpatient basis.

Making a decision to become sober and/or substance free often requires lifestyle changes. Changes of this magnitude are not made overnight. Addicted individuals often need ongoing medical support, as well

Elder Care Points

In dealing with substance abuse issues, elderly patients are likely to prefer home and community settings. Frame questions and substance problems with a linkage to a medical condition, to decrease feelings of stigma. Older patients are likely to have better adherence to treatment plans and less relapse (Matthews, 2009).

as support from the recovery community. Encourage your patients who are attempting recovery to seek out help and make the recovery process a number one priority. As a nurse, you can be instrumental in facilitating public awareness and in educating patients about the responsible use, and ultimate hazards, of mood-altering substances. Nurses should also be politically attuned to and advocate for legislation that regulates product availability and marketing of substances such as tobacco and alcohol.

Get Ready for the NCLEX® Examination!

Key Points

- Substance use disorder is diagnosed when ingestion of psychoactive substances such as alcohol or drugs results in recognizable signs and symptoms.
- Psychoactive substances are mind-altering agents capable of changing or altering a person's mood, behavior, cognition, arousal level, level of consciousness, and perceptions.
- Abuse implies use of a psychoactive substance in a nontherapeutic manner or the illicit use of prescription drugs.
- Dependence implies the presence of physical or psychological symptoms of addiction; when the substance use is stopped, withdrawal symptoms appear.
- Withdrawal symptoms occur when there is an attempt to stop using a substance. Symptoms of withdrawal from CNS depressants include increased blood pressure and pulse, nervousness, and heightened anxiety.
- Symptoms of withdrawal from CNS stimulants include drowsiness, headache, lethargy, nausea, alterations in eating and sleeping patterns, and cravings.
- Medical conditions related to alcohol abuse include liver damage, cardiomyopathy, hypertension, gastrointestinal bleeding, stroke, sleep disturbances, malnutrition, peripheral neuropathies, chronic infection, cognitive impairment, Wernicke's encephalopathy, and Korsakoff's syndrome.
- Assess for physical, psychological, and behavioral symptoms of abuse or withdrawal.
- Take a history from the patient and the family to determine type, amount, and pattern of use.
- General nursing interventions include observing for life-threatening conditions, safely managing detoxification, orienting the patient to reality, providing a balanced diet

high in protein and multivitamins, setting limits, confronting denial, identifying enabling behaviors and teaching new coping mechanisms, and referring the patient to a 12-step program.
- Denial and rationalization are primary defense mechanisms used by the substance abuser and the family. Substance abuse affects family and friends; they may experience anger, rage, guilt, embarrassment, shame, and hopelessness. Enabling behaviors ("helping" a person so that the consequences of his unhealthy behavior are less severe) or co-dependency (family member or friend attempts to control the behaviors of the substance abuser) further inhibit recovery.
- Elderly people may drink to alleviate depression and loneliness. Decreased liver and renal function can quickly lead to toxicity and dependence.

Additional Learning Resources

SG Go to your Study Guide for additional learning activities to help you master this chapter content.

 Go to your Evolve website (http://evolve.elsevier.com/deWit/medsurg) for the following FREE learning resources:
- Animations, audio, and video
- Answers and rationales for questions and activities
- Concept Map Creator
- Glossary with pronunciations in English and Spanish
- Interactive Review Questions and Exercises and more!

Online Resources
- Alcoholics Anonymous, www.aa.org
- The Joint Commission's Core Measures, www.jointcommission.org/performance_measurement.aspx
- Narcotics Anonymous, www.na.org

Review Questions for the NCLEX® Examination

1. The nurse is taking a history on an adolescent who needs emergency surgery. He freely admits to using marijuana, alcohol, cocaine, and hallucinogens. What is the most important question that the nurse should ask this patient?
   1. "Do your parents know that you are using all these drugs?"
   2. "When was the last time you drank or took a substance?"
   3. "How frequently are you using these drugs and alcohol?"
   4. "Have you ever tried to control your substance use?"

2. The patient comes to the emergency department with a history of alcohol abuse. The physician makes the medical diagnosis of Wernicke's encephalopathy and orders large doses of vitamin B_1. Which response indicates that the treatment is working?
   1. No seizure activity
   2. Less confusion and improvement of memory
   3. Decreased urge to drink alcohol
   4. No tremors, nausea, or vomiting

3. When asked regarding alcohol consumption, a patient who reputedly drinks heavily responds, "I really do not have a problem with drinking. I just have a few beers now and then." Which defense mechanism is the patient expressing?
   1. Intellectualization
   2. Sublimation
   3. Displacement
   4. Denial

4. The teenage son of an alcoholic cares for his younger siblings. When asked about his father's whereabouts, the boy often responds, "He is working somewhere and will not be back for a while." What is the priority nursing diagnosis?
   1. Ineffective coping: individual
   2. Dysfunctional family processes: alcoholism
   3. Readiness for enhanced family coping
   4. Readiness for enhanced parenting

5. The wife of a substance abuser demonstrates enabling behavior. Which outcome would be appropriate for the nursing diagnosis of Ineffective denial related to her husband's substance problem?
   1. Wife will identify family behaviors related to substance abuse.
   2. Wife will accept responsibility for her husband's behaviors.
   3. Wife will verbalize ways to enhance her husband's self-esteem.
   4. Wife will list reasons for her husband's substance abuse.

6. A postoperative patient who is a self-confessed drinker is given chlordiazepoxide (Librium) for increased blood pressure, increased pulse, tremors, nausea and vomiting, and diaphoresis. Why did the physician prescribe this medication for the patient?
   1. To prevent postoperative clot formation
   2. To reduce the symptoms of alcohol withdrawal
   3. To control the blood pressure
   4. To relieve postoperative nausea and vomiting

7. A self-confessed alcoholic asks, "What is the purpose of the disulfiram (Antabuse) that has been prescribed by my doctor?" What is the best explanation to give to the patient?
   1. "It blocks the craving for alcohol."
   2. "The medication causes unpleasant symptoms when you drink."
   3. "The medication keeps you from having seizures."
   4. "It controls symptoms of nausea, vomiting, pain, or cramps."

8. The patient's wife indirectly suggests that her husband has a substance abuse problem. Which initial assessment question(s) would the nurse ask the husband? *(Select all that apply.)*
   1. What substances (alcohol, tobacco, or illicit substances) are you currently using?
   2. How often do you drink or use illicit substances?
   3. When did you last drink or use drugs of any kind?
   4. How do you feel about people who abuse substances?
   5. Why does your wife think you have a substance abuse problem?
   6. Is there a family history of alcoholism or substance abuse?

9. The nurse is teaching a community group about substance abuse among children and teens. Which statement by an audience member indicates a need for additional teaching?
   1. "Inhalants are most frequently used by children and teens."
   2. "Marijuana causes mild euphoria, increased appetite, and altered judgment."
   3. "African American teenagers have the highest rate of abuse for methamphetamines."
   4. "Withdrawal from heroin is not life threatening."

10. A patient is in the early recovery process and is attempting to lead a drug-free life. Which intervention is the most appropriate to assist the patient?
    1. Remind the patient of the discomfort and pain that occurred during detoxification.
    2. Tell the patient that there is no need to feel guilty or ashamed.
    3. Help the patient to identify relationships that were part of the substance use pattern.
    4. Advise the patient that stopping forever is the only choice for a drug-free life.

Critical Thinking Activities

Scenario A

Mr. Samm, a 65-year-old white man, is recently widowed and misses his wife very much. He comes to the physician's office and he is stumbling. His speech is slurred, and his breath has an alcohol-like odor. He begins to cry and states he has changed his mind. He does not want to see the physician, but is going to drive home.

1. How will you ensure his safety?

2. What type of assessment will you perform on this patient?

Scenario B

Ms. Brown, age 29, is an ambulatory postoperative patient. She admits to a past history of illicit substance abuse, but claims to be drug free for several months. You notice that she leaves the unit and when she returns her coordination is slightly impaired and she seems inappropriately euphoric and giddy. Shortly thereafter, you observe her hiding a plastic bag; you suspect that she may be taking an illicit substance.

1. How would you handle this situation?

2. What types of documentation should you perform?

Scenario C

Mr. Martinez, a 32-year-old construction worker, was admitted for emergency orthopedic surgery yesterday evening following an on-the-job accident. He begins yelling profanity and is irritable and argumentative. He seems to be having trouble concentrating on your questions. His wife says he forgot to tell the physician that he drinks 12 beers every night.

1. What do you suspect is wrong with Mr. Martinez?

2. What other signs and symptoms would you watch for if you suspect alcohol withdrawal?

3. List the nursing interventions to care for Mr. Martinez during the initial phase of withdrawal.

Scenario D

Ms. Genavarian's father confides that his daughter has a substance abuse problem. He reports that the family has frequent arguments about the issue. Further assessment reveals that Mr. Genavarian believes that the behavior is "just weakness," whereas the daughter and wife maintain that "it's not that big of a deal."

1. Discuss some of the emotional and psychological responses that are common among patients and families when there is a substance abuse problem.

2. What could you say to Mr. Genavarian to help him understand that substance abuse is a medical problem?

3. How could you help Mrs. Genavarian to understand that she may be enabling her daughter's behavior?

Care of Patients with Cognitive Disorders

Objectives

Theory

1. Discuss the incidence and significance of cognitive disorders in the elderly population.
2. Compare and contrast the etiology and symptoms of *delirium* (acute cognitive disorder) and *dementia* (chronic cognitive disorder).
3. Describe the signs and symptoms of Alzheimer's disease in relation to the three stages: (1) preclinical Alzheimer's disease, (2) mild cognitive impairment (MCI) due to Alzheimer's disease, and (3) dementia due to Alzheimer's disease.

4. Choose appropriate nursing interventions for the care of patients with Alzheimer's disease.
5. Identify the assessment skills that are necessary to accurately monitor a cognitive disorder.
6. Identify nursing interventions that can be used to assist the family and friends of patients who have cognitive disorders.

Clinical Practice

1. Devise a care plan with at least six interventions for a patient who is confused and disoriented.
2. Implement a teaching plan for a family member who is caring for an elderly parent with Alzheimer's disease in the family home.

Key Terms

Alzheimer's disease (ĂWLTZ-hī-měrz dĭ-ZĒZ, p. 1085)
biomarker (p. 1088)
cognition (kŏg-NĬ-shŭn, p. 1085)
confabulation (kŏn-fă-bū-LĀ-shŭn, p. 1086)
delirium (dĕ-LĬR-ē-ŭm, p. 1085)
delusion (dĕ-LŪ-shŭn, p. 1086)

dementia (dē-MĚN-shē-ă, p. 1085)
global amnesia (GLŌ-băl ăm-NĒ-zhē-ă, p. 1097)
hallucinations (hă-lū-sĭ-NĀ-shŭnz, p. 1086)
illusions (ĭ-LŪ-shŭnz, p. 1086)
sundowning (SŬN-doun-ĭng, p. 1094)
vascular dementia (VĂS-kū-lăr dē-MĚN-shē-ă, p. 1085)

OVERVIEW OF COGNITIVE DISORDERS

Cognition refers to mental processes of perception, memory, judgment, and reasoning. It includes the ability to perceive and process information. **A *cognitive disorder* is diagnosed when there is a significant change in cognition from a previous level of functioning.** Cognitive disorders greatly affect the quality of life for affected individuals, families, and friends. Although cognitive disorders do occur across the life span, they are often linked to the neurobiologic changes that accompany aging. Cognitive disorders have become increasingly common with the aging of the population. Disorders of cognition include delirium and dementia.

Delirium **(acute confusion) is characterized by a change in overall cognition and level of consciousness over a short time.** Dementia, **on the other hand, is characterized by several cognitive deficits, memory in particular, and tends to be more chronic.** Both conditions are classified according to etiology (cause or origin of disease). Examples of etiologies for delirium are ingestion of a toxic substance or a serious infection. An example of etiology for dementia is multiple small blood clots that cause brain tissue damage (known as vascular dementia). Alzheimer's disease (a degenerative disease of the brain) is another example of dementia, although the exact cause is unknown. The difference between the two conditions is that **delirium is an acute condition that requires immediate treatment and dementia is a chronic condition.** Reversing the symptoms of delirium depends on timely diagnosis and treatment. It also is important to note that **delirium can coexist with dementia.** If delirium is recognized and promptly treated, the patient with preexisting dementia should be restored to a previous level of functioning.

DELIRIUM

Many conditions or physiologic alterations can cause delirium. Some examples are cerebrovascular accident; drug overdose, toxicity, or withdrawal; tumors; systemic infections; fluid and electrolyte imbalances; and malnutrition. The onset of acute delirium is sudden. The patient may be alert or lethargic, depending on the cause of the delirium, or may appear very confused. The attention span changes and overall awareness of the environment is decreased. Orientation is impaired, as are recent and immediate memory. Speech may be incoherent, and overall thinking can be disorganized and distorted. The patient will not be able to communicate her thoughts to you in a meaningful way. In delirium, a patient may experience illusions (misinterpretations of reality). For example, a pen appears to be a knife, or a shadow on the floor appears to be a menacing monster. If your patient appears to be talking to someone who is not there, it is likely that she is experiencing hallucinations (seeing or hearing things that are not there). If she insists that you are an angel of death and destruction, this is an example of a delusion (belief in a false idea).

 Clinical Cues

Haloperidol is the first-line medication for treatment of delirium. It can be given orally, intravenously (IV), or intramuscularly. If the IV route is used, cardiac monitoring should be initiated as arrhythmias can occur (Qaseem et al., 2008).

Problem-solving ability and judgment may be diminished, but not completely absent. Consequently, the patient may not make good decisions, or may become combative or hostile if the nurse or family member attempts to intervene. The general features of delirium are the same for all the causes, and nursing care is basically the same; the main difference is in diagnosis and treatment of the underlying cause.

 Elder Care Points

In hospitalized older adults with preexisting dementia, it is not unusual to see a patient who has been previously conscious and oriented become drowsy, disoriented, combative, and unable to recognize family and friends. The astute nurse suspects delirium or acute confusion. An important evaluation is to note the type and response to medications. Anticholinergic medications have potent central nervous system effects and can cause a sudden episode of confusion. Is the dose too high for age and physiologic functioning? Is there a cumulative effect? Are the medications interacting? Delirium and dementia can coexist, and the acute condition needs to be recognized and treated, not merely dismissed as part of the overall dementia.

 Clinical Cues

Does your patient have depression, dementia, or delirium? A patient with depression can have poor personal hygiene, can have difficulty with concentration, and may be very quiet and withdrawn or very agitated (see Chapter 46). You will have to observe for subtle differences to detect depression, dementia, or delirium. For example, your depressed patient may speak very little, but the speech is generally logical and will contain sad and negative thoughts and feelings of hopelessness. The patient with dementia may confabulate or will have difficulty finding words. The patient with delirium is more likely to be incoherent or loud.

SUBSTANCE-INDUCED DELIRIUM

Substance-induced delirium can be caused by withdrawal from a substance, intoxication with a substance, or side effects from a medication (see Chapter 47). Many classes of medications can produce symptoms of delirium. Some common examples are anesthetics, analgesics, sedative-hypnotics, any products with anticholinergic activity (tricyclic antidepressants, antihistamines, theophylline derivatives, and antipsychotics), and histamine (H_2)-receptor blockers (e.g., famotidine, cimetidine, and ranitidine). Commonly prescribed beta blockers and nonsteroidal anti-inflammatory drugs (NSAIDs) can also cause symptoms of delirium.

Diagnosis and treatment depend on taking a thorough history. If the patient is unable to give you a history, elicit help from the family. It is not unusual for a person to be taking large amounts of over-the-counter medications and forget to mention them because the medications were not prescribed by a physician. Pay attention to drug interactions and incompatibilities, and consult with the pharmacist as needed. Early recognition can facilitate a faster recovery. If the medication accumulates over several days, elimination of the substance from the body takes much longer and places the patient in even greater danger.

 Elder Care Points

Older adults have a high risk for substance-induced delirium because of overall decreased metabolism and reduction in liver and kidney function. A general principle that providers should use in prescribing medications to elders is to give the smallest amount possible and increase the amount only as symptoms indicate. Therefore you must carefully observe and report subtle changes in behavior, vital signs, and laboratory results.

DEMENTIA

There are several different types of dementia, and these conditions are also classified according to the underlying cause. Examples include Alzheimer's disease, frontotemporal lobe dementia, Huntington's disease, Korsakoff's syndrome, vascular dementia, acquired immunodeficiency syndrome (AIDS) dementia complex, and Parkinson's disease. The onset for dementia is slow, and the condition may progress over months to years. The patient is generally alert. Orientation to person, place, and time and recent memory may be impaired. In later stages of dementia, patients lose remote memory as well. You would observe that the patient has difficulty with abstracting thoughts and a poverty of thoughts. Confabulation (making up experiences to fill conversational gaps) and impaired judgment are common. Often, there is a noticeable change in personality. Hallucinations, delusions, and illusions usually are not present. These patients experience fragmented sleep rather than a reversed cycle.

Complementary and Alternative Therapies

Herbs with Sedative Effects

Herbs that have a sedative effect include chamomile, hops, and valerian. These can be used in a tea or taken in capsules. A popular method of promoting sleep is to place a few drops of lavender onto the pillowcase. If your patients are using herbs or alternative therapy, advise them to inform their physician because of potential drug-herb interactions, or for contraindications due to medical conditions.

ALZHEIMER'S DISEASE

Etiology and Pathophysiology

Alzheimer's disease (AD) is the most common degenerative disease of the brain. Approximately 5.4 million Americans have AD (Alzheimer's Association, 2011), and there is no known cause or cure. AD typically affects people over 65 years of age, but can also strike younger people. The 85+ age-group is currently the fastest growing age-group in the United States. It is estimated that 50% of this age-group have AD.

In AD, there is a loss of neurons in the frontal and temporal lobes. The atrophy in these areas accounts for the patient's inability to process and integrate new information and to retrieve memories. Brain biopsies of AD patients have revealed nerve cells that are tangled and twisted and an abnormal buildup of proteins. Production of neurotransmitters (e.g., acetylcholine, serotonin) is relatively decreased for these patients (see Chapter 49). Risk factors for developing Alzheimer's include lack of exercise, lower educational level, depression, chronic kidney disease, obesity in midlife, disadvantaged childhood environment, exposure to metals or toxins, and a previous head injury (Bassil & Grossberg, 2009a).

Health Promotion

Diet and Memory

Studies show that fish and omega-3 polyunsaturated fats, fruits and vegetables, curcumin (curry spice), and a traditional Mediterranean diet may lower the risk for loss of cognitive function and/or Alzheimer's disease. Moderate consumption (250 to 500 mL per day) of wine is also associated with a reduced risk, but the evidence is insufficient to recommend that the nondrinker take up wine consumption (Bassil & Grossberg, 2009a).

Health Promotion

Exercise for the Brain

Longitudinal studies have shown that challenging intellectual activity is associated with a decreased risk for dementia. Reading, writing, debating, learning something new, using your nondominant hand, and playing memory or puzzle games exercise the brain (Bassil & Grossberg, 2009b).

Signs and Symptoms

AD has a slow onset and variable rate of progression. Eventually, it is fatal. According to the Alzheimer's Association (2011), behavioral patterns and symptoms are divided into seven stages: (1) no impairment, (2) very mild cognitive decline, (3) mild cognitive decline, (4) moderate cognitive decline, (5) moderately severe cognitive decline, (6) severe cognitive decline, and (7) very severe cognitive decline. During the first two stages, there will be no symptoms or there will be changes that appear to be due to normal aging. The early signs and symptoms of beginning mental deterioration include forgetfulness, recent memory loss, difficulty learning and remembering, inability to concentrate, and a decline in personal hygiene, appearance, and inhibitions. Later the patient becomes quite confused and unable to make judgments, has difficulty communicating, suffers losses in motor function, and becomes dependent on others. Behavioral manifestations can also be categorized in three stages, mild, moderate and severe (Rohl, 2006 & Hussey, 2011) (Box 48-1).

Box 48-1 | **Behavioral Patterns in Mild, Moderate, and Severe Alzheimer's Disease**

MILD
- Slow, progressive loss of intellectual ability
- Difficulty in learning new things
- Small but noticeable changes in ability to perform at work or socially
- Decline in ability to plan ahead
- Increase in memory loss
- Decreased ability to perform usual ADLs
- Variable mood; depression is common and worsens symptoms
- Noticeable personality change
- Social withdrawal

MODERATE
- Unable to recognize familiar objects and persons
- Needs repeated instructions for simple tasks
- Needs total care—can be very burdensome for the family
- Wanders away
- Incontinent
- Outbursts of anger, hostility, paranoia

SEVERE
- Unable to speak or ambulate
- Profound memory loss
- Difficulty swallowing
- Weight loss
- Bedridden
- Fetal position
- End-stage consequences of poor nutritional state and bedridden status: pressure sores, respiratory failure, contractures, pneumonia

ADLs, activities of daily living.

Patients have a progressive loss of common cognitive functions. You observe that the patient has trouble remembering words *(anomia)* or verbally expressing himself *(aphasia)*, and he is unable to write down his thoughts *(agraphia)* or understand written language *(alexia)*. If he holds a common object such as a spoon, he does not seem to recognize it *(agnosia)*, and he cannot put on his shirt, although he has the strength and motor movement to dress himself *(apraxia:* inability to perform an activity despite motor function). He has difficulty planning ahead and he attends fewer social functions. He also displays some problems with balance and gait. For example, an 85-year-old retired attorney displays the criteria for dementia according to the *Diagnostic and Statistical Manual of Mental Disorders,* fourth edition, text revision (DSM-IV-TR).

Complementary and Alternative Therapies

Pet Therapy

Pet therapy may help patients to improve memory (e.g., calling the therapy dog's name), coordination (e.g., throwing a ball for the dog), object identification (e.g., directing the dog to get the ball), language (e.g., talking to the dog), and attention (e.g., caring for the dog). Research conducted about pet therapy programs demonstrates consistent positive outcomes for both physical responses, such as improvement in vital signs, and psychological parameters, such as a decrease in anxiety, fatigue, depression, and confusion (Coakley & Mahoney, 2009).

Think Critically

It is not uncommon for patients with dementia to act in a sexually inappropriate way because of loss of social reserve. Your elderly male patient is reaching to fondle your breasts when you turn him to do hygienic care and linen changes. How will you handle this?

Diagnosis

In 2011, new criteria and guidelines for the diagnosis of AD were presented as the result of an international collaboration to review the original 1984 criteria and incorporate research findings to improve the diagnostic process. The new guidelines propose three stages: (1) preclinical AD, (2) very mild cognitive impairment (MCI) caused by AD, and (3) dementia caused by AD.

Currently there are no criteria for physicians to use in making the diagnosis of preclinical AD. Future research on preclinical AD is based on the assumption that there are biologic processes that are occurring before the onset of actual symptoms. The proposed research goals for the preclinical stage are to identify biomarkers that will confirm a diagnosis of AD. (A **biomarker** is an objective measure that indicates the presence of disease.)

In making the diagnosis, the physician uses a detailed medical and family history and conducts a thorough physical, neurologic, and functional assessment. The benefits of early diagnosis include being able to include the patient in the planning, to proactively ensure safety, to reduce the family's blaming the patient for behaviors that are part of the disease process, and to counter patient and family denial (Bennett, 2009). Your patient may undergo magnetic resonance imaging (MRI) to rule out pathologic lesions. The diagnostic use of positron emission tomography (PET) and single-photon emission computed tomography (SPECT) are controversial, but are being considered. Apolipoprotein E4 genotyping is used to confirm the diagnosis of late-onset AD. Research for new diagnostic tests for AD will continue. Three new clinical criteria may be predictors for early AD: amyloid protein in the spinal fluid, plus a biomarker with slight cognitive changes, or brain atrophy on imaging (Sullivan, 2010). The DSM-IV-TR provides behavioral criteria for AD.

Treatment

Current medications do not cure AD, but may improve intellectual functioning and slow the progression of the disease (McGuinness et al., 2009) The evidence indicates that the benefit of these drugs is modest (Qaseem et al., 2008). Research is being done on immunotherapies that target the protein that contributes to the formation of the neurofiber tangles (Alzheimer's Association International Conference on Alzheimer's Disease, 2010). Table 48-1 describes medications used to treat cognitive disorders and their nursing implications. Behavioral interventions such as the three *R*s (repeat, reassure, redirect) or the ABCs (antecedents, behaviors, consequences) can be adapted to match the patient's current level of function (Kalapatapu & Neugroschi, 2009). In a recent study (Ancoli-Israel, et al., 2008), patients with AD and obstructive sleep apnea showed improvement in cognition after 6 weeks of continuous positive airway pressure (CPAP) therapy.

❖ NURSING MANAGEMENT

■ Assessment (Data Collection)

You may be the first health care professional who encounters a patient who is in the early stages of AD. Know and be vigilant for the 10 warning signs of AD (Alzheimer's Association, 2010) (Box 48-2). For example, the family may tell you, "We think Dad is having problems with his memory and in completing daily tasks, and we also think he is attempting to hide his forgetfulness because he keeps misplacing things and can't seem to solve ordinary problems. He insists on driving, but we are beginning to question his judgment. He often acts like he is searching for

Table 48-1   Drugs Used to Treat Cognitive Disorders

CLASSIFICATION	ACTION	PATIENT EDUCATION	NURSING IMPLICATIONS
Donepezil (Aricept) Galantamine (Razadyne) Memantine (Namenda) Rivastigmine (Exelon) Transdermal patch has been recently approved	Causes elevated acetylcholine levels in the brain and slows progression of Alzheimer's disease symptoms.	Take with food to decrease GI distress. Slows progression of symptoms, but is not a cure. Take frequent drinks of cool liquids or use sugarless gum or candy for dry mouth. Increase fiber and fluids to prevent constipation. Common side effects (nausea, vomiting, headaches and dizziness, GI bleeding, urinary frequency, anorexia) should be reported to physician.	Be alert for abdominal pain, fatigue, hypotension, and agitation. Monitor CBC, liver, and renal function tests. Signs of overdose include severe nausea and vomiting, bradycardia, hypotension, convulsions, or severe muscle weakness. Rivastigmine patch: first patch should be applied on the day following the last oral dose, then rotate sites, replace every 24 hr.
Tacrine (Cognex)		Immediately report jaundice, nausea and vomiting, or malaise.	Used in the past, but is rarely prescribed now due to liver toxicity. If prescribed, liver function tests should be monitored weekly for 18 wk after starting the medication.

CBC, complete blood count; *GI*, gastrointestinal.

Box 48-2   Ten Warning Signs of Alzheimer's Disease

1. Memory loss that disrupts daily life
2. Challenges in planning or solving problems
3. Difficulty completing familiar tasks at home, at work, or at leisure
4. Confusion with time or place
5. Trouble understanding visual images and spatial relationships
6. New problems with words in speaking or writing
7. Misplacing things with inability to retrace steps
8. Decreased or poor judgment
9. Withdrawal from work or social activities
10. Changes in mood or personality

Alzheimer's Association. (2010). *10 signs of Alzheimer's.* Retrieved from www.alz. org/alzheimers_disease_10_signs_of_alzheimers.asp?type=more_information.

---

the right word. We can't seem to teach him how to position a can to use a can opener. He is even confused about times when we have recently visited him, and he is moody and withdrawn during our regular visits. " Ask the patient and the family questions about memory, ability to perform activities of daily living (ADLs), and any subtle changes in personality. Give specific common examples (e.g., "Does he forget to turn off the stove or to lock the doors?"). Refer this type of patient to the RN or physician because he needs an in-depth assessment and an extensive physical examination. Assessment should include the necessary data to plan measures to protect the patient.

 Clinical Cues

Before you begin to assess your elderly patient, consider the changes that normal healthy older adults might be experiencing because of aging. For example, it is normal to have some decline in memory; however, the healthy older adult should be able to create new memories, act purposefully, and accomplish ADLs independently (Bennett, 2009).

■ **Nursing Diagnosis and Planning**

Nursing diagnoses are identified to maximize safety and to minimize complications due to loss of cognitive function. For example, Risk for injury, Wandering, Confusion, Self-care deficits, and Caregiver role strain are some of the diagnoses that are used for patients with AD. Planning care for a patient with AD is based on the stage of the disease, and the family should be encouraged from the beginning to participate in developing the long-term goals (Nursing Care Plan 48-1). As the disease progresses, the patient will sustain losses in every area of function.

 Clinical Cues

When caring for confused patients, evidenced-based practice supports the need for careful observation and documentation of patterns of behavior. This process, *dementia care mapping,* can be used to improve care (McEvoy, 2004). For example, you observe that your confused patient consistently tries to get out of bed on the right side, despite the fact that the safety devices are on the left and that there is more room on the left side. This suggests that the patient has an automatic habit of getting out on the right side; these data can now be used to adapt the room and increase patient safety.

★ Nursing Care Plan 48-1   Care of the Patient with Alzheimer's Disease

Scenario
Mrs. Jane Best, an 85-year-old with Alzheimer's disease, lives with her daughter. The daughter works full time and occasionally leaves Mrs. Best at a senior citizen day care center where you are working. "Mom is confused and withdrawn most of the time and needs reminders to eat and coaching to go to the bathroom. I really try my best, but Mom can be difficult." The daughter appears tired, but is very patient with her mother. You observe Mrs. Best wandering alone and trying to go outside. You have to redirect her several times, and she mistakes you for her daughter.

Problem/Nursing Diagnosis
Intellectual and memory impairment/Chronic confusion related to cognitive impairment.

Supporting Assessment Data
Subjective: Per daughter, patient is "confused most of the time."
Objective: Mistakes you for her daughter.

Goals/Expected Outcomes	Nursing Interventions	Selected Rationale	Evaluation
Patient will function at an optimal level for the degree of cognitive losses at this time.	Identify yourself.	Patient may not recognize people previously introduced.	Patient repeatedly mistakes nurses for her daughter. Does recognize physician.
Patient will follow concrete instructions.	Speak clearly and calmly and use short phrases and repeat as needed. Face the patient directly when you talk. Use pictures to communicate.	Facilitates communication. Stimulation of two senses (visual and auditory) facilitates understanding.	Speaking slowly and clearly and repeating helps patient to understand. Use of arrows to bathroom also appears helpful.
	Be consistent in approach and assign the same staff and maintain daily structure and routine.	Familiar faces and repetitive patterns decrease confusion.	Patient functions best when AM routine is followed and primary nurse helps her.
	Break down all tasks into simple steps and encourage completion of one step at a time.	Single steps are less complex and easier to achieve.	This AM patient was able to brush own teeth if instructed, step by step.
	Encourage reminiscing about the past.	Remote memory is more likely to be intact than recent memory.	Appears to enjoy talking about "Maggie's cat." Outcomes met. Continue plan.

Problem/Nursing Diagnosis
Unable to independently perform ADLs/Toileting/feeding/self-care deficit related to cognitive and perceptual impairment.

Supporting Assessment Data
Subjective: Per daughter, "needs reminders to eat and coaching to go to the bathroom."
Objective: Needs repetitive verbal prompting.

Goals/Expected Outcomes	Nursing Interventions	Selected Rationale	Evaluation
Patient will perform ADLs independently or with minimal assistance from caregivers.	Assess the patient's ability to perform ADLs independently or with minimal assistance.	Provides baseline for daily planning (abilities may wax and wane).	Is able to physically perform most ADLs, but needs verbal coaching for each step.
	Encourage patient to maintain independence in performing ADLs.	Maintain maximal independence for as long as possible to increase self-esteem and stimulate mental processes.	Daughter reports that "it is really faster just to do everything for her" but acknowledges the benefit of allowing her independence.

ADLs, activities of daily living; *ID*, identification; *NA*, nursing assistant.

Goals/Expected Outcomes	Nursing Interventions	Selected Rationale	Evaluation
Patient will perform ADLs independently or with minimal assistance from caregivers—cont'd	Allow patient to wear own clothes. Use clothing with zippers and Velcro.	Familiar objects decrease confusion. Ease of equipment decreases frustration.	Usually recognizes own clothing, but needs coaching for dressing; can manipulate Velcro fasteners.
	Praise for any and all accomplishments.	Reinforces desired behavior.	Appears to enjoy interaction and feedback.
	Use simple, direct explanations when demonstrating the specific behavior you want the patient to complete.	Verbal and visual cues help to decrease confusion.	Follows instructions, but rarely asks for help.
	Maintain toileting schedule.	Bowel and bladder routine decreases incontinence.	Toileting schedule q 4 hr; patient usually continent.
	Encourage the use of finger foods.	Simplifies eating while maintaining intake.	Eats all food if encouraged. Has difficulty cutting meat with knife and fork. Outcomes met. Continue plan.

Problem/Nursing Diagnosis

Withdrawn/Social isolation related to anxiety and depression, apathy, and confused state.

Supporting Assessment Data

Subjective: Per daughter, confused or withdrawn most of the time.
Objective: Walking alone.

Goals/Expected Outcomes	Nursing Interventions	Selected Rationale	Evaluation
Patient will participate in group activities.	Assess preferred patterns of social activity from earlier years.	Ideally, current socialization should mimic past patterns.	Social contact usually limited to family. Occasionally went to church.
Patient will demonstrate socially acceptable behavior.	Provide group activities that are simple, such as singing or simple crafts.	Simple activities decrease frustration and are a vehicle to interaction.	Appears to enjoy movies and musical groups.
	Stay with the patient during social activities as needed.	Provides support and reassurance.	Does not initiate conversation with others, but will respond if spoken to.
	Do not force a patient who is becoming agitated to participate in any social activity.	Socialization can be stressful, and forcing is counterproductive.	Readily agreed to go to all activities today.
	Gradually increase social interaction with other staff and patients.	Gradual exposure increases comfort level and familiarity.	Will sit with others, but does not initiate any interaction. Will speak to other patients if they speak to her. Outcomes met. Continue plan.

Problem/Nursing Diagnosis

Daughter is the primary caregiver/Risk for caregiver role strain, related to high emotional and physical demands, safety concerns for the relative, and caregiver isolation.

Supporting Assessment Data

Subjective: "I really try my best, but Mom can be difficult."
Objective: Daughter works full time and appears tired, but very patient with her mother.

Goals/Expected Outcomes	Nursing Interventions	Selected Rationale	Evaluation
Caregiver will verbalize ways to perform the caregiver role without becoming exhausted.	Assess caregiver's ability to meet the needs of the patient.	Baseline for planning.	Daughter expresses willingness to care for her mother, but does work full time.
Caregiver will openly express feelings.	Actively listen to caregiver's fears and concerns.	Allowing expression helps to build trust and rapport; also helps speaker and listener to clarify issues.	Fears for mother's safety; is concerned about wandering.

Continued

⊛ Nursing Care Plan 48-1   Care of the Patient with Alzheimer's Disease—cont'd

Goals/Expected Outcomes	Nursing Interventions	Selected Rationale	Evaluation
Caregiver will openly express feelings—cont'd	Educate the caregiver about cognitive disorders and the patient's specific cognitive deficits.	Accurate information allows daughter to have realistic expectations.	Written information given and discussion of cognitive disorders provided for daughter.
	Help caregivers be realistic about the prognosis for their loved one.	Being realistic about prognosis helps the family to begin the process of anticipatory grieving.	Daughter appears unsure about the future, knows that her mother is going to get worse.
	Make caregiver aware of community resources such as respite care.	Community supports are available to provide care, education, support, and advice.	Referred to support group for caregivers of Alzheimer's disease patients.
	Encourage participation in support groups.	Sharing with people who are experiencing similar problems decreases feelings of alienation and allows sharing of information.	
	Support caregiver in taking steps to maintain own health.	Daughter must be healthy to continue supporting her mother.	Daughter discussed respite care and plans to take occasional breaks. Continue plan.

Problem/Nursing Diagnosis
Unfamiliar environment/Wandering related to cognitive impairment and loss of judgment.

Supporting Assessment Data
Subjective: Per daughter, "Mom is confused."
Objective: Wandering by herself and trying to get outside despite repetitive redirection.

Goals/Expected Outcomes	Nursing Interventions	Selected Rationale	Evaluation
Patient will remain within the boundaries of the center (or the family property) unless accompanied by others.	Place in a limited-access unit. Put complex locks on the doors. Allow access to fenced yard.	Securing the environment allows the patient to roam safely, but without restraints.	Patient remained safe in secure unit. Went out to grounds with nursing student in the AM.
	Use identification bracelets or sew ID labels on clothes.	ID methods facilitate location and return if she does get lost.	Discussed sewing labels into clothes with daughter.
	Label all rooms and doors.	Patient may be wandering because she cannot find the bathroom, cafeteria, etc.	Arrows to bathroom appear especially useful.
	Remove visual cues that trigger wandering (e.g., car keys, coat).	Visual cues such as car keys can trigger a past familiar behavior (e.g., driving to work).	Asked for coat, was reassured that it was in the storage closet. Redirected into common area.
	Notify police and neighbors to be on the alert.	Police and neighbors can quickly contact caregiver.	Discussed with daughter about notifying neighbors and police. Outcomes met. Continue plan.

Critical Thinking Questions
1. How would you react if Mrs. Best's daughter complains about the care that Mrs. Best is receiving at the senior center?
2. What interventions could you initiate to protect patients like Mrs. Best from physical injury related to confusion?

■ Implementation and Evaluation

Patients with AD need interventions that enhance memory. For example, put up holiday decorations that are appropriate to the season, or use photos of family and friends to help them reminisce. Reminiscence therapy could also include creating a life-story book that helps the patient to review accomplishments and increase self-esteem (Manepalli et al., 2009). Although safety is a primary concern, restraints are rarely appropriate for these patients; creative interventions that are specific to the individual and family can ensure safety while preserving dignity. For example, one family placed a pleasant musical bell on the front door to prevent the confused elder from leaving the house undetected. Supporting the family will be a priority, particularly if the patient is being cared for at home. Help the family to have realistic expectations and refer them to respite care and support groups. Placing written name tags on commonly used household objects, such as the bathroom door or the patient's room door, seems to help the patient function better within the home setting. Visual cues such as the picture of the toilet on the bathroom door are helpful as the disease progresses.

AD patients may seem to require very infrequent evaluation, because the disease can progress very slowly and obvious changes in behavior or success in meeting goals may seem very gradual. However, vigilant evaluation will help you detect subtle changes in behavior that may signal delirium or progression of the disease. Also, any small successes can and should be shared with the family.

VASCULAR DEMENTIA

Vascular dementia was formerly known as multi-infarct dementia. It is the second most common type of chronic cognitive disorder. *Vascular dementia* **is a broad term used to describe any type of dementia caused by vessel disease.** People who are predisposed to this type of dementia have a history of hypertension, hyperlipidemia, diabetes mellitus, and abuse of nicotine and alcohol.

 Cultural Considerations

Race Factors

African Americans have twice the risk for developing AD and Hispanic Americans have 1.5 times the risk. African Americans are also at greater risk for developing vascular dementia compared to whites. Patients with risk factors for vascular dementia, such as hypertension and diabetes, should be identified and educated to optimize healthy lifestyle practices (Alzheimer's Association, 2010).

Any type of vessel disease in the brain will cause brain damage. Lack of oxygen to the brain tissue because of clots or hemorrhage can cause death of brain tissue in a short time. The parts of the brain originally affected by cell death will be permanently damaged.

The onset can be gradual or abrupt, and the neurologic impairment is localized rather than global. The progression of symptoms is more rapid than in AD. Neurologic deficits are present in whatever part of the brain has been destroyed. **Prompt treatment of hypertension and vascular disease is necessary to prevent long-term complications.**

AIDS DEMENTIA COMPLEX

AIDS dementia complex (ADC) is caused by infection with human immunodeficiency virus (HIV). The central nervous system can be affected, and the patient may also have *peripheral neuropathy* (disturbance in the function of peripheral nerves that results in numbness or muscle weakness). ADC affects cognition, behavior, mood, and motor ability. There is great variability in the manifestation of symptoms. In the beginning, symptoms can be easily mistaken for depression: apathy, loss of interest, difficulty concentrating and slowed thinking, and irritability. Early symptoms may also include unsteady gait and poor hand coordination for things such as writing. In the later stages, the patient can develop bowel and bladder incontinence, confinement to bed, and psychosis or mania. ADC is diagnosed by computed tomography or MRI, spinal tap, and a mental status examination. Treatment includes anti-HIV drugs, and symptoms are treated with antidepressants, antipsychotics, and anxiolytics.

❖ NURSING MANAGEMENT

■ Assessment (Data Collection)

On admission, an extensive mental status examination should be conducted by the physician and the RN to obtain a baseline for the patient's thought content, intellectual functioning, mood, affect, and judgment. After the baseline is established, the Mini-Mental State Examination (MMSE) can be used for ongoing assessment. The MMSE is a popular shortened version of the mental status examination that was developed by Folstein and colleagues in 1975. It can be used for patients who have cognitive disorders or thought disorders to assess orientation, memory, and ability to follow commands. It consists of 11 easily scored items and should take about 5 to 10 minutes to administer. Examples of items would include "What day is it? What city is this? What am I holding (common objects such as a pen or paper clip)?

Differentiating between delirium and dementia is often difficult for the nurse because the patient is not a reliable historian. A mood disorder, such as depression, can further complicate the picture (see Chapter 46). Accurate recognition of these three conditions requires excellent assessment skills. An effective way to assess whether a patient has delirium or dementia is to note function in the following five areas: judgment, affect, memory, cognition, and orientation (JAMCO).

Focused Assessment

Quick Assessment Guide for Delirium and Dementia: JAMCO

*J*udgment: Does patient have insight into her behavior? Is the patient aware of danger or safety issues?

*A*ffect: Is affect blunt, flat, inappropriate, suddenly changed, or variable?

*M*emory: Is memory intact? Does the patient have remote memory, but not recent or immediate? Is memory better during the day?

*C*ognition: Is the patient able to process abstract thoughts? Are thoughts fragmented or disorganized? Does the patient make up answers to questions (confabulate) to hide deficits?

*O*rientation: Is the patient oriented to person, place, and time? Does the patient recognize family and friends?

First, what is the status of the patient's *judgment?* Your patient insists on driving, despite the fact that she has had several minor accidents within the past 2 weeks. This connotes poor judgment, and you must work with the patient and the family to seek alternative transportation.

Assessing and documenting *affect* (emotional or feeling tone) are also important. Has there been a sudden change in mood from the previous assessment? The family will often say that they note a difference in mood when they visit the patient. You should pay attention to what family members tell you and elicit their opinions about the changes that they are seeing in their loved one.

 Clinical Cues

Mood and affect are frequently assessed simultaneously. *Mood* is the current state of emotion that a person is experiencing. *Affect* is the demonstration of emotion, usually by facial expression and body position. Ordinarily, we expect affect and mood to match, so when we are in a "good mood" we would display a cheerful affect. Likewise, depressed people often display a flat or sad affect. In a flat affect, the face is devoid of expression and the patient may appear to have little or no energy for interaction. A sad affect is usually apparent, and the patient may cry, frown, or have a worried, preoccupied expression.

When assessing *memory,* it is important to note recent and remote memory. In some types of dementia, a patient may not be able to remember what was on the breakfast tray, but may be able to talk at great length about events in her younger years. When assessing delirium, you may find that both recent memory (a few hours before) and immediate memory (a few minutes before) are absent.

 Think Critically

Think of one or two ways you can assess immediate, recent, and remote memory. How would you know whether the patient's memory is accurate?

Cognition is the ability to abstract and process information. Obviously, there are links and overlaps to memory and perception when assessing cognition. The family should also be consulted whenever possible for valuable baseline information about the patient's past performance. For example, a patient's son tells you, "My mother was a former math teacher; now she cannot seem to balance her checkbook, and that was something that she could easily do in the past."

Finally, is the patient *oriented* to person, place, and time? Are there times when the patient is disoriented? It is not unusual for a patient to be completely oriented during the daytime hours and become confused and disoriented at night. This phenomenon is known as sundowning and needs to be documented. A dose of trazodone in the afternoon or evening may be ordered to reduce the symptoms associated with sundowning (Kalapatapu & Neugroschi, 2009).

 Complementary and Alternative Therapies

Agitated Patient

Music, recordings of soft ocean sounds, light touch or hand massage (avoid touching if the patient is violent or angry), or aromatherapy may help to calm an agitated patient with sundown syndrome. Having your patient sit by a light box in the early morning may also help, particularly if the patient has depression. These adjunct therapies may decrease need for pharmaceuticals (Nazarko, 2009).

 Think Critically

What implications does sundowning have for planning care and activities for the patient?

A mental status assessment needs to be completed at least once per shift, so that any change can be detected promptly and appropriate interventions taken. This assessment should include orientation to person, place, and time and the other elements of JAMCO. The MMSE can be used at the nurse's discretion to validate mental status changes or according to the agency's policy for long-term care patients. When abrupt changes are noted, the RN and the physician should be notified to perform more detailed assessments.

 Clinical Cues

In cases of delirium or acute confusion, you must assess the patient's medication history, look for any signs of infection, and assess current fluid and electrolyte status. Also, if you have reason to suspect that the patient may have sustained a fall, assess for head trauma.

 Think Critically

How would you approach a pain assessment for a patient with dementia?

■ Nursing Diagnosis

Nursing diagnoses for patients with cognitive disorders include:

- Acute confusion related to delirium induced by infection
- Chronic confusion related to slow progressive memory loss
- Social isolation related to inability to recognize friends and family
- Self-care deficits, bathing/hygiene/eating, related to decreased psychomotor abilities
- Risk for injury related to faulty judgment
- Sleep deprivation related to age-related sleep pattern changes
- Disturbed sensory perception related to hallucinations
- Wandering related to disorientation to time and place
- Risk for caregiver role strain related to prolonged 24-hour responsibility of caregiving

■ Planning

Expected outcomes are written for the specific individual nursing diagnoses chosen to resolve the patient's problems. For the nursing diagnoses above, they might include:

- Patient will demonstrate orientation to person, place, and time within 24 to 48 hours after starting antibiotic therapy.
- Patient will recognize self and primary caregiver (e.g., daughter) during hospital stay.
- Patient will interact with family and friends during weekly visits.
- Patient will perform ADLs with assistance as needed during this shift.
- Patient will be safe and free from harm during this shift.
- Patient will rest and sleep for at least 6 hours every 24-hour period.
- Patient will decrease behaviors that suggest hallucinations (e.g., listening to voices) within 1 week.
- Patient will remain on unit or within fenced grounds during this shift.
- Family will identify signs and symptoms of caregiver role strain during counseling session at the end of the week.

⬦ Clinical Cues

When assisting elderly and confused patients to eat, slowly give one bite of an item, allow adequate time for chewing and swallowing, and then give another bite of a different food item. This varies the taste and texture and enhances the enjoyment of eating. Also remember to include some time for socialization during the meal.

In accordance with National Patient Safety Goals, nurses must identify patients that have safety risks; this includes patients with cognitive disorders. Planning care for a patient with delirium involves accurately assessing the acute condition, stabilizing the patient, reducing environmental stimuli, providing reality orientation, and assisting the physician in determining the cause. Planning care for a patient with dementia frequently involves the caregivers and should be done with long-term goals in mind. Patients in the early stages of AD may be experiencing difficulties with ADLs; however, they may attempt to hide their condition. Forgetting to turn off the stove or to lock the doors is not uncommon. Regardless of the cause, the loss of cognition is devastating, and it is important to maintain the patient's dignity, provide for safety and optimal level of functioning, and promote quality of life.

■ Implementation

Interventions to provide safety and minimize anxiety for patients with dementia and delirium are similar. **However, when caring for a patient whose sudden change in behavior may be due to delirium, time is of the essence.** Assess the patient frequently, document your findings, and be certain the physician is notified. Because the level of consciousness may be clouded, reduce distractions in the environment; for example, having the television on can create background noise that increases confusion (Lyons et al., 2009). It may be necessary to medicate patients with anxiolytics for severe anxiety, or with antipsychotics if the misinterpretation of the environment causes them to be aggressive.

⚠ Safety Alert

Antipsychotic Drugs

Nurses should be aware that atypical antipsychotics such as olanzapine (Zyprexa) and risperidone (Risperdal) are approved for use in schizophrenia, but are not approved for use with older patients who display behavioral changes related to dementia. Clinical trials showed an increased risk of death in this population with use of these drugs (Drugs. com, 2010).

Patients may be able to remember their own name, but may be confused about place and time. A patient who is experiencing acute confusion or delirium will benefit from repeated orientation to person, place, and time. It is not adequate to repeat this information once or twice. It must be repeated frequently and in a calm, soothing manner. Your calm attitude is very important in reducing the anxiety that is inevitably present for the patient. Box 48-3 lists guidelines to conduct reality orientation for confused patients.

Box 48-3 Guidelines for Reality Orientation

WHAT IS REALITY ORIENTATION?

- Reality orientation is a therapeutic program consistently implemented by all nursing staff to orient a patient to person, place, and time. This method includes the use of verbal communication techniques, as well as written signs indicating the current date, month, or room identification. Clocks with large numbers are included to help the patient know the correct time (Manepalli et al., 2009).
- Special group sessions are also used to orient patients. These sessions focus on person, place, and time as well as certain holiday events. These groups improve orientation and provide opportunities for social interaction.

WHEN TO USE REALITY ORIENTATION

- The use of reality orientation is appropriate when a patient is experiencing acute confusion or delirium. A sudden episode of confusion is very frightening, and orienting the patient is a way to allay fear and anxiety.
- Patients experiencing global amnesia do not benefit from repeated verbal reality orientation.
- For patients with dementia, gentle reminders of the day or time need to be repeated often and without the expectation that the patient will remember something that was said 5 minutes ago.
- All aspects of reality orientation are helpful for all patients with cognitive disorders. However, in patients experiencing acute confusion, the ultimate expectation is that the patient will become completely oriented and return to a previous level of functioning. With chronic confusion, the goal is to preserve dignity and maintain optimum function.

EXAMPLES OF WAYS TO IMPLEMENT REALITY ORIENTATION AND REDUCE CONFUSION

- Under no circumstances should nurses ever chastise or become frustrated when a patient cannot remember. This has no therapeutic value.
- Verbalize to patients in a consistent and caring manner who you are, where they are, and the date and time:

"Hi, Mr. Jones. I am your nurse, Betty, at the Davis Nursing Care Center. It is 8 AM on Wednesday, October 25, and it is time for breakfast."
- Look directly at the patient when you are speaking.
- Ask only one question at a time.
- Ask questions that can be answered with a "yes" or "no": "Would you like to eat in the dining room?"
- Eliminate environmental distractions when talking to a patient.
- Break down tasks such as dressing into simple one-step tasks.
- Ask the patient to do only one task at a time.
- Gently touch the patient to convey acceptance.
- If possible, provide caregivers who are familiar to the patient.
- Provide general orientation to the calendar year by using holiday decorations.
- Decrease the noise level in the environment by avoiding paging systems and call lights that ring or buzz.
- Label photos of people familiar to the patient with the names of the people who are in the photos.
- Limit visitors to one or two at a time.
- Place the patient's name in large block letters in his room and on clothing.
- Use symbols rather than words on signs indicating location of dining room or bathroom.
- When misperceptions are present, clarify them for the patient: "No, Mr. Jones, I am not your daughter; I am your nurse, Betty. Your daughter will be here after you eat your lunch."
- When special low-stimulus units designed for patients with chronic confusion are not available, use yellow tape to mark specific boundaries for the patient.
- Give frequent reassurances.
- Keep the patient's room well lit.
- Encourage the use of hearing aids and prescription glasses.
- Have clocks, calendars, and personal items in clear view of the patient.
- Encourage reminiscing about happy times in life.

Assignment Considerations

Reality Orientation

Nursing assistants (NAs) can be instrumental in the ongoing orientation of confused patients. First, identify those patients who would benefit from reality orientation. Then give the NA specific instructions about how to orient to person, place, and time (e.g., "Hi, Mrs. Collins. I am Judy, the nursing assistant at Sunshine Care Center. It is 8 A.M. on Tuesday, June 28, 2010. It's a nice warm summer day today."). Instruct the NA in how to use visual cues to orient patients (e.g., "Mrs. Collins, this calendar will help you remember the day, month, and year.").

Legal and Ethical Considerations

Use of Restraints

Remember, having to restrain a patient is considered an unusual circumstance that requires clear documentation and adequate elaboration as to the events leading to the need for restraints, all alternatives tried before restraint, the type of restraint, strict accounting for time in and out of restraints, and the care given to the patient while in restraints. (Do *not* forget to offer and document bathroom breaks, fluid and food, and skin care.)

A patient experiencing acute confusion may become combative, or may attempt to crawl out of bed or remove therapeutic equipment. In 1992 the Food and Drug Administration issued a warning stating that restraints should no longer be considered as first-line management of a patient's behavioral problems.

When using restraints, your patients may be at risk for physical problems such as immobility, strangulation, or asphyxiation, or for psychological issues such as anger, humiliation, loss of autonomy, and decreased functioning. Evidenced-based practice suggests that hourly assessments should include attention to the patient's immediate condition, evaluation of the patient's reaction to the restraints, assessment of medical and behavioral problems, and determination of the need for continuing the restraints (Nadler-Moodie, 2009). It is recommended that institutions have policies and procedures that address the safe and legal use of restraints (Rutledge & March, 2008). In accordance with the Joint Commission's National Quality Core Measures, the total number of hours in restraints or seclusion must be noted with supporting documentation. Box 48-4 presents guidelines on the use of restraints and alternatives to restraints.

An individual with chronic confusion in the late stages of dementia will not benefit from repetitive information. If **global amnesia** (generalized loss of memory) is present, the patient will not be able to remember family, friends, or events, regardless of how many times you repeat the information. Moreover, expecting the patient to remember leads to frustration for you and the patient. Use of pictures or symbols, such as arrows pointing to the bathroom, can facilitate daily tasks and clarify communication. In addition, creative therapies such as video histories, use of familiar songs,

and pet therapy and aromatherapy may enrich the quality of life for these individuals.

 Complementary and Alternative Therapies

Smell

The limbic or "old brain" is associated with the sense of smell. Use of familiar smells reinforces remote memories. For example, the smell of pine or fir can trigger past memories of happy Christmas times spent with family and friends. Aromatherapy can be administered by inhalation, bathing, massage, or topically (Manepalli et al., 2009).

 Complementary and Alternative Therapies

Massage

Massage has been used to reduce agitation in patients with Alzheimer's disease (Manepalli et al., 2009). Additional benefits include meeting the human need for nurturing touch, decreasing mild depression, reducing mental stress, improving circulation, and relieving muscle tension and stiffness.

Box 48-4   Alternatives to and Guidelines for the Use of Restraints

ALTERNATIVES TO RESTRAINTS

Acute Care Settings
- Encourage family members and friends to stay with the patient.
- Assign a nurse or nursing assistant for one-on-one observation.
- Encourage oral feedings instead of intravenous or nasogastric feedings. (Avoid inserting tubes that can be pulled out.)
- Remove catheters and drains as soon as possible.
- Decrease glaring lighting, reduce noise, and minimize stimulation.
- Keep the patient close to the nurse's station.
- Be certain the call button is within easy reach.
- Place the bed in the lowest setting, and use three side rails to keep the patient from rolling out.
- Check on the patient frequently to offer nutrition, fluids, pain relief, and toileting assistance as appropriate.

Long-Term Care Facilities
- Place the mattress on the floor to prevent the patient from falling out of bed.
- Talk to the patient, even when the patient is not responding to you or is responding in an inappropriate way.
- Incorporate relaxation techniques into the care plan, such as back massage and hydrotherapy.
- Use therapeutic communication techniques to encourage the patient to verbalize feelings.
- Encourage ambulation whenever feasible.
- Encourage participation in recreational, physical, and occupational therapy.
- Encourage participation in as many ADLs as possible.
- Initiate diversional activities, such as listening to radio, television, and music.
- Maintain a schedule for toileting.

GUIDELINES FOR THE SAFE USE OF RESTRAINTS
- Use the least restrictive type of restraint that will accomplish the objective.
- Obtain informed consent from the patient or the patient's relatives before using restraints.
- Have an institutional policy on restraints written and available for the patient and family.
- Make certain that all staff have adequate in-service training on the use of restraints.
- Use hand mitts for patients who are receiving IV therapy or have catheters or nasogastric tubes.
- If hand mitts do not work, consider wrist restraints.
- All restraints must have a physician's order.
- Restraints must not be used to punish or control the patient.
- Apply restraints snugly, but ensure that circulation is not impeded.
- Check the area distal to the restraint every 2 hours (or according to the agency policy) for circulation and function.
- Remove the restraints and change the patient's position at least every 2 hours.
- Apply active or passive ROM to the affected joints and muscles.
- Secure restraints to the bed frames, not the side rails.
- Tie restraints with knots that can be quickly released.
- Consider restraints as a temporary solution.
- Clearly document in the patient record the reason for the restraint, the type selected, and the time frame for use.
- Document care given to the patient while in restraints.

ADLs, activities of daily living; *IV,* intravenous; *ROM,* range of motion.

Complementary and Alternative Therapies

Using Mirrors to Stimulate Responses

In a small study of patients with dementia, nurses used mirrors to stimulate and communicate with patients. They found that patients recognized themselves and expressed laughter and enjoyment (Freysteinson, 2009).

? **Think Critically**

Is it always necessary to encourage a patient to see and acknowledge reality? What about elderly patients who have severe dementia and believe they are living in their own homes, even though they are in a nursing home?

Nurses who care for patients with dementia need to be aware of the importance of maintaining the dignity of the patient and family. In the later stages of dementia, there are numerous deficits in self-care, such as grooming and toileting. It is very important to treat both patients and families with respect. **Call the patient by name, provide for privacy, and individualize your care for this patient based on culture and history.** It is well documented in the nursing literature that when patients are seen as people or human beings, nurses are likely to be more compassionate and caring.

 Elder Care Points

When working with the elderly, do not confuse clear and supportive communication with "elderspeak." Elderspeak is a style of speech that includes baby talk, exaggerated tones and slow speed, elevated pitch and volume, and simplified vocabulary. Being overly nurturing ("Come on, sweetie, let's eat now.") or overly controlling ("Sit down and finish your food!") is perceived as patronizing and demeaning, without improving communication.

Assessment of and Interventions for the Family

The family should also be assessed for their knowledge and ability to relate to the illness and care of a family member with dementia. The goal of treatment is preservation of function (Bennett, 2009) and this should be clarified when working with the family. For example, if the patient lives at home, the family will need to realize that **a person with dementia responds much better if there are daily routines and a structured environment.** Assist the family to develop a schedule that includes adequate time for hygiene care, meals, medications, and activities such as walking. Home care nurses are in an excellent position to make suggestions to help the family create a safe environment. For example, potentially hazardous areas can be evaluated and then suggestions made for gates across stairwells, or better lighting in dark hallways.

 Clinical Cues

Evidence-based practice suggests that structured activities, such as "Simple Pleasures" (Buettner et al., 1996), benefit patients and families. In this classic intervention, family members or volunteers are asked to make items such as fleece-covered hot water bottles. Handling the handmade item reduces agitation in the patient with dementia. The family sees the impact of the gift and the family-patient interaction is improved.

If the patient has a tendency to wander or get lost, the family will live in a constant state of hypervigilance to ensure the safety of their loved one. Help family members to recognize potential wandering behaviors: looking for keys, preparing to go to "work," restlessness and pacing, getting lost going to the bathroom or to the bedroom, or performing a task without actually accomplishing anything (e.g., moving dirty dishes from place to place without actually washing them). Nurses can make practical suggestions such as sewing identification labels into clothing, or using a bell that signals when an exit door is opened. Box 48-5 presents additional tips for families.

Families should also be assessed for signs of caregiver role strain (Nguyen, 2009). Observe and assist family members to recognize when they themselves experience denial, irritability, anxiety, sleeplessness, and anger—and note that these signs suggest the illness of the elder is taking its toll on the caregivers. Family members often are exhausted from the daily requirements of round-the-clock care. Evidence suggests that families who receive intensive support and counseling are able to manage the care of the AD patient in the home for longer periods of time (Grossberg et al., 2010).

Encourage caregivers to consider day care or respite care. These options give the family members a much-needed psychological and physical rest. In addition, families should be encouraged to use support groups, such as the Alzheimer's Association (see Online Resources). One of the *Healthy People 2020* objectives is to help family caregivers to access caregiver support services.

? **Think Critically**

How would you help a family member to recognize and acknowledge the need for respite care?

Families also need to be encouraged to talk openly and frankly about quality of life, and about end-of-life issues such as advance directives. Preferably these talks should be completed before the diagnosis of dementia, when the patient still has cognitive functioning. If not, the family caregiver becomes the spokesperson and needs to be encouraged to get a power of attorney and a living will for the patient. Families need considerable support in these matters. Refer to Nursing Care Plan 48-1 for additional nursing management information.

Suggestions for Families Caring for a Person with Alzheimer's Disease

- Make and keep a copy of the daily schedule, and stick to the schedule as closely as possible.
- Establish bedtime rituals.
- Orient the person as necessary to maintain safety and promote maximum functioning.
- Avoid multiple caregivers.
- Simplify the environment to minimize illusions and confusion; keep decorative items to a minimum.
- Keep the environment as quiet as possible.
- Schedule rest breaks throughout the day for yourself and your loved one.
- Change your expectations; forcing thought and interaction causes frustration.
- Offer the person help when needed, and distraction as necessary.
- Always supervise the use of medications.
- Use sense of touch; there is an increased need for touch.

- Always approach the person from the front before touching.
- Use distraction if agitated. Walking, gardening, rocking in a rocking chair, sanding wood, and folding laundry are good examples of distraction.
- Use many of the safeguards for young children, such as storing all cleaning solutions, pesticides, medications, and nonedible items in locked cabinets.
- Put protective caps on all unused electrical outlets.
- Remove all sharp objects.
- Remove all throw rugs, and keep hallways and stairs free of clutter.
- Keep the house well lit.
- Allow smoking only under very close supervision.
- Attach safety grab bars in the bathroom.
- Protect windows and doors with Plexiglas.
- Rather than restrict the person from wandering, provide a safe area in which to wander.

■ **Evaluation**

Because confusion is present in all cognitive disorders, keeping the patient free of injury is of primary importance. Is the patient returning to or moving toward a previous level of cognitive and psychomotor functioning? Has the cause of acute delirium been determined or eliminated? An additional expected outcome, particularly with patients with dementia, is that the family will be able to verbalize the stages of illness and maintain realistic expectations for their loved one.

COMMUNITY CARE

If patients with dementia or delirium are hospitalized, the inpatient stay will typically be for a short time. For a variety of reasons, financial and personal, many families are choosing to keep their elders at home. Nurses who make home visits will often encounter families attempting to care for a relative who is experiencing either of these conditions. Teaching must be done about

the causes and stages of these illnesses. In addition, families are eager for practical knowledge that will make the living arrangement more acceptable (see Box 48-5).

In the later stage of dementia, nursing home placement sometimes is necessary. Many nursing homes have special units set aside for AD patients. In these units, safety precautions are a primary concern. Entrance and exit doors have special codes so that patients cannot wander off the unit. "Wandering pathways" are created using corridors, walkways, or outdoor spaces that allow for walking and roaming with security and safety (Nazarko, 2009). Nurses in these units spend considerable time educating families about the stages of AD and helping families with the inevitable grieving process.

In addition to observing patients with delirium in the acute hospital setting, nurses often interact with these patients in outpatient clinics, emergency departments, or physician's offices. Excellent assessment skills are necessary to prevent any further decline.

Get Ready for the NCLEX® Examination!

Key Points

- Cognition includes the mental processes of perception, memory, judgment, and reasoning.
- Delirium is acute confusion; signs and symptoms may include a shortened attention span, disorientation, impairment in recent and remote memory, incoherent speech, disorganized thinking, and possible presence of delusions, hallucinations, and illusions.
- Dementia is chronic confusion that has slow onset (months to years); signs and symptoms include impairments in memory, poverty of thoughts, difficulties

with abstract thoughts and judgments, confabulation, and changes in personality. In later stages, global amnesia is present. Attention span and alertness are normal, and there are usually no hallucinations, delusions, or illusions.
- Assess *judgment, affect, memory, cognition,* and *orientation* (JAMCO). *Judgment* is the presence of judgment and insight. *Affect* is the demonstration of emotion, and is usually apparent in facial expression or body position. (*Mood* is the current state of emotion that a person is experiencing.) *Memory* is assessed for

impairments in recent, remote, and immediate memory. *Cognition* is the ability to abstract and process information. *Orientation* to person, place, and time should be assessed.

- Alzheimer's disease is the most common degenerative disease of the brain and usually affects people over age 65.
- Vascular dementia describes any type of dementia caused by vessel disease, which causes brain damage. Onset is usually more abrupt, and neurologic impairment is localized rather than global.
- Goals of treatment for cognitive disorders include achieving an optimal level of functioning, ensuring safety, educating caregivers, and preserving the dignity of the patient and family.
- Nursing interventions for AD depend on the stage of illness. General interventions include maintaining a calm and soothing manner, ensuring environmental safety, using appropriate reality orientation, and monitoring the effects of medications.
- Elders are sensitive to the cumulative effects of medications because of decreased metabolic and liver function; the smallest amount of medication possible should be prescribed and doses should be increased only when symptoms indicate the need.
- Families are frequently electing to care for their elders at home; teach the family about cognitive disorders and provide practical knowledge about living arrangements.

Additional Learning Resources

SG Go to your Study Guide for additional learning activities to help you master this chapter content.

evolve Go to your Evolve website (http://evolve.elsevier.com/deWit/ medsurg) for the following FREE learning resources:
- Animations, audio, and video
- Answers and rationales for questions and activities
- Concept Map Creator
- Glossary with pronunciations in English and Spanish
- Interactive Review Questions and Exercises and more!

 Online Resources
- Alzheimer's Association, www.alz.org

Review Questions for the NCLEX® Examination

1. The nurse is reviewing the medications ordered for several patients who have Alzheimer's disease. Which physician's order is the nurse most likely to question?
   1. Memantine (Namenda)
   2. Rivastigmine (Exelon) transdermal patch
   3. Donepezil (Aricept)
   4. Tacrine (Cognex)

2. A nursing student is caring for a patient who has dementia due to Alzheimer's disease. Which action indicates the need for further education and training?
   1. Uses season-appropriate holiday decorations and a calendar with large numbers
   2. Labels family photos with names of family members and discusses photos with patient
   3. Encourages the patient to acknowledge that he is not living in his own home
   4. Helps the patient to perform one task at a time, giving step-by-step instructions

3. The nurse is working in a long-term care facility and notices that one of the residents with chronic dementia is uncharacteristically drowsy and lethargic. What is the most appropriate nursing intervention?
   1. Monitor the patient, but allow her to sleep.
   2. Stimulate her by inviting her to join a social group.
   3. Call the physician to report a change of mental status.
   4. Perform a mental status examination and obtain vital signs.

4. An elderly man with dementia displays a sudden change in behavior with slurred speech and combativeness. He appears to be having hallucinations. What is the priority nursing diagnosis?
   1. Impaired verbal communication
   2. Disturbed sensory perception
   3. Risk for injury
   4. Acute confusion

5. The nurse in an acute medical-surgical unit is caring for a confused, elderly patient who is trying to get out of bed. Which alternative to restraints would be appropriate for the patient and the setting?
   1. Put the patient's mattress on the floor.
   2. Keep the patient close to the nurses' station.
   3. Put four side rails up instead of tying the patient down.
   4. Use hand mitts and a soft vest with Velcro fasteners.

6. A confused elderly man is hospitalized for a recent fall. He is accompanied by a daughter, who cries and says, "I can't take care of him any longer!" Initial assessment confirms a nursing diagnosis of Caregiver role strain. Which nursing intervention(s) would be appropriate? *(Select all that apply.)*
   1. Encourage verbalization of feelings.
   2. Refer to respite care or day care programs.
   3. Tell the daughter to calm down and maintain composure.
   4. Reassure the daughter that everything will be okay.
   5. Encourage admission to a nursing home.
   6. Assess for alternative family support and resources.
   7. Tell the daughter to focus on past happy times with the father.

7. Which measure should the nurse use if the patient has sundowning phenomenon?

   1. Complete complex tasks during the morning.
   2. Keep the patient in a dark, quiet room during the day.
   3. Orient the patient to the time of day at sundown.
   4. Put the patient to bed before sundown.

8. The caregiver of a male patient with Alzheimer's disease is given instructions regarding donepezil (Aricept). Which caregiver statement indicates a need for further instructions?

   1. "I should always give Aricept with food to minimize gastric distress."
   2. "I thought Aricept was rarely used because of liver problems."
   3. "I must increase fiber and fluid in his diet."
   4. "I need to provide frequent sips of cool liquids."

9. The nurse is assessing the dietary preferences of a patient with chronic confusion. Which assessment question would be the most appropriate to use with this patient?

   1. "Do you have cultural preferences with regard to food?
   2. "What would you usually eat during a typical day?"
   3. "Do you prefer water or milk with your meals?"
   4. "What did you think about the dinner that was served last night?"

10. The nurse observes that a patient with dementia cannot put on his shirt, although he has the strength and motor movement to dress himself. Which intervention would be appropriate to accomplish dressing while maximizing the patient's dignity?

    1. Verbally coach the patient using simple directions.
    2. Leave the patient alone and give extra time and privacy.
    3. Have the wife help the patient get dressed.
    4. Give the patient a shirt with Velcro fasteners.

Critical Thinking Activities

Scenario A
Oneida Lampert, 82 years old, has Alzheimer's disease. Her daughter tells you that Mrs. Lampert has "good days and bad days" but seems to be more forgetful and more withdrawn. "Do you have any suggestions for me? I know Mom is going to get worse, but I'd like to care for her at home as long as possible."

1. What are some questions you should ask the daughter?
2. What can you do to help the daughter with the practical issues of caring for Mrs. Lampert at home?

Scenario B
You are caring for Mr. Dixon, who is a 75-year-old patient residing in a nursing home for the past 6 months. Today he becomes uncharacteristically combative when the nurse's aide attempts to give him a bath. You have never observed Mr. Dixon exhibit this type of behavior before.

1. What would your initial nursing interventions be?
2. How might you explain Mr. Dixon's sudden change in behavior?

Scenario C
Jill Botello, a 40-year-old schoolteacher, accompanies her father, Sam Miller, to the physician's office where you are working. Mr. Miller, currently 65 years old, was diagnosed with vascular dementia 2 years ago. His condition is progressively deteriorating, and Ms. Botello tells you that she is fearful that this type of dementia could happen to her.

1. How would you respond to Ms. Botello?
2. What type of preventive education might be helpful for Ms. Botello?

Scenario D
The night shift nurse recommends that you call the physician and obtain an order to restrain Mr. Loncola, who is an elderly patient with dementia. The patient currently has a feeding tube and an IV which he keeps trying to pull out. He is easily agitated and strikes out at caregivers. In addition, he is physically strong enough to get out of bed and has a history of falls.

1. What assessments would you make before calling the physician for the restraint order?
2. What interventions could you try before using restraints?
3. If restraints are ordered, describe what you must document.

Objectives

Theory

1. Discuss the incidence of thought disorders in the general population.
2. Describe the signs and symptoms of schizophrenia.
3. Identify at least four nursing diagnoses and the major nursing interventions that would be appropriate for a patient with a thought disorder.
4. Compare and contrast behaviors for each of the various personality disorders.
5. Choose at least four nursing diagnoses and the major nursing interventions that would be appropriate for a patient with borderline personality disorder.

6. Illustrate how the nurse can identify and modify personal feelings that can occur when caring for a patient with borderline personality disorder.
7. Analyze your personal feelings related to caring for patients with manipulative behaviors.

Clinical Practice

1. Watch the movie *A Beautiful Mind* and develop a teaching plan to help the wife understand the husband's bizarre and erratic behavior.
2. Develop a care plan with at least six nursing interventions for a patient who is paranoid and suspicious.
3. Write a care plan with at least six nursing interventions for a patient who is manipulative.

Key Terms

akathisia (p. 1105)
alogia (p. 1104)
anhedonia (p. 1106)
atypical antipsychotics (ā-tǐ-pǐ-kǎl ǎn-tē-sī-KŎT-ǐks, p. 1106)
avolition (p. 1104)
borderline personality disorder (BPD) (BŎR-děr-līn pěr-sŏ-NĂL-ǐ-tē dǐs-ŎR-děr, p. 1114)
command hallucinations (KŎM-mănd hǎ-lū-sǐ-NĀ-shǔns, p. 1108)
conventional antipsychotics (kŏn-VĔN-shǔn-ǎl ǎn-tē-sī-KŎT-ǐks, p. 1105)
delusions (dě-LŪ-zhǔn, p. 1102)
dystonic reaction (dǐs-TŎN-ǐk rē-ĂK-shǔn, p. 1105)
hallucinations (hǎ-lū-sǐ-NĀ-shǔn, p. 1102)
illusion (ǐ-LŪ-shǔn, p. 1104)

loose associations (p. 1109)
milieu therapy (mēl-yoo THĔR-ǎ-pē, p. 1114)
negative symptoms (NĔG-ǎ-tǐv, p. 1104)
neologisms (NĒ-ō-lō-jǐzm, p. 1109)
oculogyric crisis (p. 1105)
personality disorders (pěr-sŏ-NĂL-ǐ-tē dǐs-ŎR-děrz, p. 1113)
positive symptoms (p. 1103)
psychotherapy (sī-kō-THĔR-ǎ-pē, p. 1114)
psychotic features (sī-kǒ-tǐk, p. 1102)
schizophrenia (skǐt-sō-FRĒ-nē-ǎ, p. 1102)
splitting (p. 1114)
tardive dyskinesia (TĂR-dīv dǐs-kǐ-NĒ-zHē-ǎ, p. 1105)
therapeutic alliance (p. 1110)
thought disorders (p. 1102)
word salad (p. 1109)

OVERVIEW OF THOUGHT DISORDERS

The *Diagnostic and Statistical Manual of Mental Disorders,* fourth edition, text revision (DSM-IV-TR) defines thought disorders by the presence of psychotic symptoms. Schizophrenia is the most common thought disorder. Examples of psychotic features are hallucinations (hearing, seeing, smelling, tasting, or feeling something that is not really there), delusions (false fixed ideas), and disorganized speech and/or behavior.

The incidence of thought disorders is not as high as that of mood disorders, but thought disorders tend to be more chronic and debilitating. It is estimated that 1.1% of the general population is affected with schizophrenia, and in the United States this represents 2.4 million Americans (National Institute of Mental Health, 2010).

NEUROTRANSMITTERS

Many of the medications used to treat mental disorders are thought to affect the activity (production, release, destruction, or blocking [or reuptake] at the receptor site) of neurotransmitters. Neurotransmitters

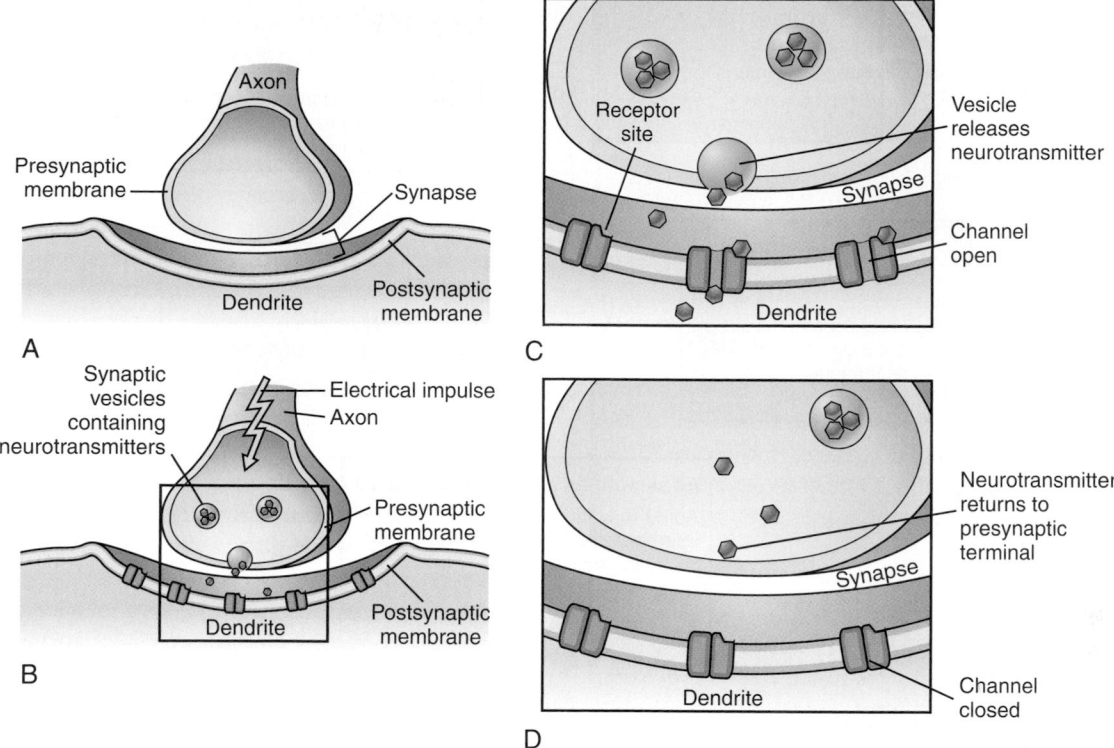

FIGURE 49-1 Neurotransmitters. **A,** Axon with stored neurotransmitters and dendrite with receptor sites. **B** and **C,** Electrical impulse causes release of neurotransmitter. **D,** Receptor sites close and neurotransmitter returns to storage.

are chemical messengers that are produced and stored in the nerve terminal *(axon)* (Figure 49-1). An electrical impulse causes the release of the neurotransmitter, and it then moves into the gap *(synaptic cleft)* between the nerve endings and attaches to receptor sites on the receiving nerve cell *(dendrite)*. This causes a reaction in the dendrite, the receptor sites close, and the neurotransmitter travels back across the gap into storage *(reuptake)*.

Serotonin is a neurotransmitter of the central nervous system. It is important in sleep, pain perception, and emotional states. Lack of serotonin can lead to depression. Norepinephrine and acetylcholine are neurotransmitters of the autonomic nervous system. Norepinephrine plays an important role in the *fight-or-flight reaction* (constriction of the blood vessels, dilation of the pupils, increased heart rate, increased awareness and vigilance). Acetylcholine causes decreased heart rate and force of contraction and plays a role in the sleep-wake cycle. Dopamine is located mostly in the brainstem. It is thought to play a role in controlling complex movements, motivation, and cognition. For patients with schizophrenia, it is thought that there is an imbalance of neurotransmission of dopamine—which may cause hallucinations and delusions— and serotonin, which may contribute to the negative symptoms (Hoban, 2010). Antipsychotic drugs work by blocking dopamine receptors.

SCHIZOPHRENIA

Etiology and Pathophysiology

The exact cause of schizophrenia is unknown; however, current research favors the theory that there is a neurobiologic basis with a genetic component. As with most chronic conditions, an unfavorable social environment contributes to a poor prognosis. Schizophrenia usually develops in late adolescence or the early 20s.

 Complementary and Alternative Therapies

Omega-3 Fatty Acids

In a small study, Amminger and colleagues (2010) found that omega-3 fatty acids were as effective at preventing progression to psychosis as antidepressants, antipsychotics, or cognitive-behavioral therapy; however, more research is needed to substantiate long-term outcomes.

Signs and Symptoms

The signs and symptoms are divided into positive (present) and negative (absent) symptoms (Figure 49-2). Positive symptoms are present in schizophrenic patients, but should not be there. These include the presence of hallucinations, delusions, and disordered thinking or loose associations between thoughts. Voices *(auditory hallucinations)* will tell the person what to do, and delusions develop as the disorder progresses.

Positive symptoms
Hallucinations
Delusions
Disorganized speech
Bizarre behavior

Negative symptoms
Blunted affect
Poverty of thought (alogia)
Loss of motivation (avolition)
Inability to express pleasure or joy (anhedonia)

Cognitive symptoms
Inattention, easily distracted
Impaired memory
Poor problem-solving skills
Poor decision-making skills
Illogical thinking
Impaired judgment

Co-occurring problem
Anxiety
Depression
Substance abuse
Suicidality

All symptoms alter the individual's
Ability to work
Interpersonal relationships
Self-care abilities
Social functioning
Quality of life

FIGURE 49-2 Signs and symptoms of schizophrenia.

Delusions can be either grandiose or persecutory. An individual who believes he is a king is having *delusions of grandeur*. Individuals with *delusions of persecution* believe that they are being persecuted by agencies, by other people, or by supernatural beings. An **illusion** is a misinterpretation of something that really exists. For example, an electrical cord appears to be a snake, or a pencil is misinterpreted to be a knife blade. When *ideas of reference* occur, the individual believes that events or situations are occurring because of—or specifically for—him. A common *idea of reference* is to believe that people on the television are sending special telepathic messages. *Positive symptoms* are much more responsive to medication therapy compared to the *negative symptoms*; however, some patients will tell you that "the voices are always there, but if I take my medications the voices are less intrusive."

? Think Critically

Why might friends and family fail to recognize that there is a problem when schizophrenia first develops in a teenager or young adult? Describe how you might feel, and how it would change your life, if someone you loved developed schizophrenia in early adulthood.

! Safety Alert

Be Cautious, Not Fearful

Nursing students are often afraid to enter a psychiatric unit, because patients with schizophrenia can be bizarre and unpredictable; however, these patients are usually not overly prone to violence. Older men or those with a history of violence, substance abuse, or victimization are more likely to demonstrate violence (Bryan et al., 2009). To protect yourself and others, ask the charge nurse to give advice about potentially violent patients.

Negative symptoms are abilities or personal characteristics that are *absent* or lost to the patient. For example, think of elements of personality that make people motivated, socially outgoing, happy, and active in daily life, and then take away those elements. The results are *negative symptoms*: apathy, social isolation, psychomotor retardation, flat affect (obvious absence of emotional expression), poverty of thoughts **(alogia),** lack of motivation **(avolition),** and inability to experience pleasure or joy **(anhedonia).** These symptoms are notoriously more difficult to treat because the symptoms, in and of themselves, inhibit the individual from seeking help. *Negative symptoms* are also linked to acquisition of important social skills and prognosis (Roberson, 2009). For example, if your teenage patient withdraws because of feelings of persecution, he will miss the important socialization tasks that occur during adolescence, such as exploring identity and preparing to live independently away from his parents.

In addition, these patients also have cognitive impairments that manifest as difficulty with memory, judgment, problem solving, and decision making. Concurrent mental health problems such as anxiety and depression can also occur. Overall there is an impact on the individual's quality of life, and some will have great difficulty functioning in society.

Diagnosis

There are different types of schizophrenia (paranoid, catatonic, disorganized, undifferentiated, and residual), and diagnosis is based on guidelines in the DSM-IV-TR. Table 49-1 provides a description of the different types of schizophrenia.

Table 49-1	Types of Schizophrenia and Associated Behaviors
TYPE	**BEHAVIORS**
Paranoid	Exhibits extreme suspiciousness, delusions of grandeur, and delusions of persecution. Can be hostile and aggressive. Auditory hallucinations are common.
Catatonic	Exhibits a stuporous condition associated with rigidity, unusual posturing, and waxy flexibility (maintains a limb in one position for a long time). Also demonstrates echopraxia (imitating the motions of others) and echolalia (involuntary repetition of words spoken by others). Exhibits unpredictable behavior because behavior is controlled by delusions and hallucinations.
Disorganized	Exhibits flat affect, silliness, and incoherence. Has gross thought disturbances, including word salad and neologisms. Delusions and hallucinations are common.
Undifferentiated	Exhibits symptoms found in more than one type, but does not meet adequate criteria for paranoid, catatonic, or disorganized types.
Residual	Exhibits negative symptoms (i.e., apathy, social isolation, psychomotor retardation, blunted affect, poverty of thoughts, and lack of motivation) of schizophrenia, with no evidence of hallucinations, delusions, or disorganized thoughts.

Treatment

Evidence suggests that early treatment for schizophrenia improves long-term prognosis. Patients who are treated for first episodes generally respond to the therapeutic effects and require lower doses of antipsychotic medications. After starting a medication, the patient should be monitored for 2 to 4 weeks for therapeutic response (American Psychiatric Association, 2004). Antipsychotic medications (neuroleptics) treat the positive symptoms of schizophrenia (Box 49-1). The conventional antipsychotics are very effective in stopping the auditory hallucinations, enabling the patient to connect thoughts in a logical manner, and eliminating the delusional system. They do cause serious and unpleasant side effects, and are becoming less commonly prescribed. However, some patients respond well to these drugs and, particularly for older patients who have taken them for a long time, it is likely that a successful drug regimen will continue.

The side effects for these medications include the familiar anticholinergic effects (i.e., dry mouth, flushing, urinary retention and constipation). In addition, these drugs have *extrapyramidal side effects* (EPSs): dystonia, pseudo-parkinsonism, and akathisia (Figure 49-3). Dystonia or dystonic reaction is an acute muscle contraction, especially of the tongue, face, neck, and back. Oculogyric crisis, a fixed upward gaze or muscle spasm of the eye, can occur. *Pseudo-parkinsonism,* or drug-induced parkinsonism, includes a poor balance, flat affect, slowed movements, tremors, and drooling. Akathisia manifests as motor restlessness (e.g., tapping a foot, rocking, pacing) or apprehension and irritability. Treatment for akathisia, dystonia, or pseudo-parkinsonism is to lower the dosage or change the medication, and to give benztropine (Cogentin) or diphenhydramine (Benadryl).

Tardive dyskinesia is a primary concern because **symptoms are irreversible once they have developed.** Symptoms include tongue protrusion, lip smacking, sucking, chewing, blinking, lateral jaw movements, grimacing, shoulder shrugging, pelvic thrusting, wrist and ankle flexion or rotation, foot tapping and toe movements, and rapid, purposeless, and irregular movements. Movements are often described as writhing and wormlike. Monitor for signs of tardive dyskinesia, particularly in patients who have been taking a conventional antipsychotic medication for longer than 6 to 12 months.

Other adverse effects associated with the use of antipsychotic medications include blurred vision; bone marrow suppression; cardiac dysrhythmias; endocrine changes such as elevation of blood sugar, weight gain, and breast enlargement; and *hepatotoxicity* (liver injury and jaundice). *Neuroleptic malignant syndrome* is a rare reaction; however, it is life threatening, and frequently the patient will be transferred to the intensive care unit. Symptoms include high fever, increased pulse, muscle rigidity, stupor, incontinence, elevated white blood cell count, hyperkalemia, and renal failure.

Box 49-1	Drugs Used to Treat Schizophrenia
CONVENTIONAL DRUGS	**NEWER (ATYPICAL) DRUGS***
Chlorpromazine (Thorazine)	Clozapine (Clozaril)†
Fluphenazine (Prolixin)	Aripiprazole (Abilify)
Haloperidol (Haldol)	Olanzapine (Zyprexa)
Loxapine (Loxitane)	Quetiapine (Seroquel)
Molindone (Moban)	Risperidone (Risperdal)
Perphenazine (Trilafon)	Ziprasidone (Geodon)
Thioridazine (Mellaril)	Paliperidone (Invega)
Thiothixene (Navane)	Iloperidone (Fanapt)
Trifluoperazine (Stelazine)	Asenapine (Saphris)

*These drugs have fewer side effects than the conventional medications.
†First atypical antipsychotic, now rarely prescribed due to potential agranulocytosis. Weekly monitoring of white blood cell count is necessary.

Pseudo-parkinsonism
• Stooped posture
• Shuffling gait
• Rigidity
• Bradykinesia
• Tremors at rest
• Pill-rolling motion of the hand

Acute dystonia
• Facial grimacing
• Involuntary upward eye movement
• Muscle spasms of tongue, face, neck, and back (back muscle spasms cause trunk to arch forward)
• Laryngeal spasms

Akathisia
• Restless
• Trouble standing still
• Paces the floor
• Feet in constant motion, rocking back and forth

Tardive dyskinesia
• Protrusion and rolling the tongue
• Sucking and smacking movements of the lips
• Chewing motion
• Facial dyskinesia
• Involuntary movements of the body and extremities

FIGURE 49-3 Characteristics of pseudo-parkinsonism, acute dystonia, akathisia, and tardive dyskinesia.

Elder Care Points

Elders who are taking antipsychotic medications are at a higher than usual risk for developing serious side effects. Baseline cardiac, renal, hepatic, and hematologic studies need to be done before initiating psychotropic drugs. The beginning dosages should be one half to one third of the normal adult dosage. Elders need to be watched very closely for difficulty swallowing, constipation and fecal impactions, weight gain, memory impairment, and orthostatic hypotension.

Clinical Cues

Clozapine (Clozaril), the first of the atypicals, is significantly more effective than the other atypicals, but is less frequently prescribed because patients can develop *agranulocytosis* (decreased white blood cells). Patients on this drug must have weekly blood tests (Calandra, 2009). The Joint Commission's National Quality Core Measures require that documentation reflects appropriate justification when patients are discharged with prescriptions of multiple antipsychotic medications.

Examples of newer medications—sometimes referred to as **atypical antipsychotics** (see Box 49-1)—have the advantages of fewer side effects, especially tardive dyskinesia, and offer some success with treating the negative symptoms. Olanzapine comes in a quickly dissolving oral form that is a potential alternative to an injection. This form is more expensive; however, it eliminates the risk of needle-stick injury if the patient is combative, and it discourages "cheeking" (attempts to avoid swallowing by holding the pill in the cheek pouch). Aripiprazole (Abilify) is the first in a new class of antipsychotics, the dopamine system stabilizers. The most recently approved medications for schizophrenia include paliperidone (Invega), iloperidone (Fanapt), and asenapine (Saphris). Table 49-2 presents medication side effects and nursing implications for drugs used to treat thought disorders.

For patients with positive symptoms that do not respond to medication, repetitive transcranial magnetic stimulation (rTMS) or electroconvulsive therapy (ECT) may be considered (Matheson et al., 2010) (see Chapter 46 for additional information about ECT and rTMS).

Negative symptoms are treated with a therapeutic environment, including a therapeutic relationship with the nurse, and education regarding basic living skills. **Historically, individuals with schizophrenia were shunned and stigmatized** because of unusual and bizarre behavior. Evidence-based practice indicates that with early intervention these individuals can cope with symptoms and maintain independent and productive lives outside of an institution. Community mental health teams decrease likelihood of relapse (Malone et al., 2009). Programs such as the Program for Assertive Community Treatment (PACT), Assertive Community Treatment (ACT), and Functional Adaptation Skills Training (FAST) include elements of patient and family support, education about disease management, and skills training (American Psychiatric Association, 2004; National Institute of Mental Health, 2007). If left untreated, individuals with schizophrenia are particularly vulnerable to poverty, homelessness, drug abuse, and suicide.

Evidence suggests that cognitive-behavioral therapy (CBT) should be used in conjunction with medication

Table 49-2 Antipsychotic Drugs Used to Treat Thought Disorders and Nursing Implications

COMMON SIDE EFFECTS	NURSING IMPLICATIONS
Anticholinergic Side Effects	
Dry mouth	Provide adequate fluids. Suggest sugarless hard candy or gum and good oral care.
Urinary retention and hesitancy	Monitor voiding and elimination patterns.
Constipation	Administer stool softener. Encourage fluids and fiber foods.
Blurred vision	Remind patient that blurred vision will cease once the body becomes accustomed to the drug.
Photophobia	Remind patient to wear sunglasses when in the sun.
Sexual dysfunction	Remind patient to alert treatment team for sexual difficulties.
Common Extrapyramidal Side Effects	
Pseudo-parkinsonism: Masklike facies, stiff and stooped posture, shuffling gait, drooling, fine tremors, and pill-rolling movement.	May need to switch to a different antipsychotic. Administer anticholinergic medications such as trihexyphenidyl (Artane) or benztropine (Cogentin).
Akathisia: Characterized by pacing and motor restlessness.	Notify physician. Antipsychotic may need to be changed or an anticholinergic added to the drug regimen. Symptoms disappear when the drug is discontinued.
Other Adverse Neuromuscular Effects	
Tardive dyskinesia: Typically manifests after 6–12 mo or more of medication therapy. It is characterized by tongue protrusion, lip smacking, sucking, chewing, blinking, lateral jaw movements, grimacing, shoulder shrugging, pelvic thrusting, wrist and ankle flexion or rotation, foot tapping and toe movements, and rapid, purposeless, and irregular movements.	Prevention by assessment; encourage checkups every 3 mo. Discontinuing the drug does not always relieve the symptoms. No specific treatment other than discontinuing the drug. Give soft foods. Have patient wear soft shoes or slippers.
Neuroleptic malignant syndrome: A rare but potentially fatal reaction to antipsychotic medications. It is characterized by high fever, increased pulse, muscle rigidity, stupor, diaphoresis, hyperkalemia, incontinence, elevated white blood cell count, and renal failure.	Early detection increases survival rate. Stop all medications. Give supportive, symptomatic care. Decrease body temperature. Hydrate (oral and IV). Correct electrolyte imbalance. Medicate for dysrhythmias as ordered. Renal dialysis for renal failure.
Cardiovascular Side Effects	
Orthostatic hypotension Tachycardia Paliperidone (Invega) can cause cardiac dysrhythmias (i.e., QT prolongation)	Check blood pressure and pulse before giving medications. Inform patient to dangle feet before getting out of bed to prevent falls. Inform patient that tolerance will develop in several weeks. Report to physician or RN any history of cardiac disease before starting the medication. Increase fluid intake to expand vascular volume as ordered.
Miscellaneous Side Effects	
Sleepiness and fatigue	Inform patient that tolerance to the dosage will develop in 1-2 wk.
Photosensitivity	Administer medication at bedtime. Avoid direct sunlight. Wear protective clothing and sunscreen when outside.
Weight gain	Monitor food intake.
Hives and contact dermatitis	Notify physician if there is a rash; may need to discontinue or change the drug.

IV, intravenous.

in the treatment of schizophrenia (American Psychiatric Association, 2004). In CBT, the therapist helps the patient to identify stressors, to make plans, and to modify behaviors. For example, the patient is assisted to recognize that hallucinations increase during the late evening hours. The plan might include listening to music and going to bed earlier. If the voices continue or get louder the patient knows to say, "Stop!"

⚖ Legal and Ethical Considerations

Rights of Psychiatric Patients

Psychiatric patients have the right to refuse medication and other therapies. Denial, paranoia, stigmatization, and lack of insight into illness contribute to the decision to refuse. In emergency situations, such as potential harm to self or others, the physician can order administration of involuntary medications. For routine ongoing treatment, the patient must be deemed incompetent and a court order must be obtained if the staff are to override the patient's right to refuse therapy.

⌂ Clinical Cues

Nursing students often have difficulty applying therapeutic communication skills with schizophrenic patients because these patients have trouble answering questions, conversing coherently, or expressing feelings. Remember to offer yourself ("Mr. Elliott, if you would like to talk or walk around the unit, I can spend some time with you today.") and attempt to understand ("Mr. Elliott, I am having a little difficulty understanding what you are saying, but I can tell you are trying to say something important."). Spending even a few seconds with a paranoid schizophrenic patient is therapeutic because your attention builds trust and rapport, and allows the patient to practice social skills. Also remember that the purpose of therapeutic communication is to meet the patient's needs, not to have your questions answered.

❖ NURSING MANAGEMENT

■ Assessment (Data Collection)

When collecting information from patients who have thought disorders, the interview must be brief. Because there is a problem with logical thought processing, it is difficult for the individual to remain focused for very long. Mental status assessment tools, such as the Mini-Mental State Examination (MMSE) (see Chapter 48), are useful in evaluating thinking processes and the ability to abstract information. Assessment of a thought disorder involves observing the person's ability to think in a logical manner and the presence of psychotic features. Assessing the content and themes of hallucinations and delusions is important to ensure safety. For example, the patient may be receiving command hallucinations in which the voices are directing him to harm himself or others. Your patient may be experiencing delusions of persecution and be suspicious of staff and therefore refuse to eat. In addition, you should observe for stressors that seem to trigger or exacerbate disorganized behavior.

Patients with thought disorders may have difficulty verbalizing physical symptoms, and routine physical assessment should be performed to identify or monitor potential health problems. In addition, an initial and ongoing assessment of functionality, including activities of daily living and social skills, should be conducted. For example, the patient may have a disheveled appearance and dress in a bizarre fashion. Clothes may be worn in layers, backward, or inside out and be inappropriate to the season, or the patient may disrobe and stride about naked. One of the nursing goals would be to help the patient recognize and adopt socially appropriate attire.

■ Nursing Diagnosis

Typical nursing diagnoses for thought disorders may include:

- Acute confusion related to extreme anxiety and delusional thoughts
- Disturbed sensory perception (hallucinations) related to biochemical imbalance
- Impaired verbal communication related to disorganized thoughts and loose associations
- Social isolation related to extreme distrust
- Self-care deficit, bathing/dressing/eating, related to cognitive deficits
- Noncompliance related to medication regimen
- Risk for other-directed or self-directed violence related to command hallucinations

■ Planning

Sample outcomes for the nursing diagnoses above might include:

- Patient will verbally acknowledge that delusional thinking and beliefs (e.g., accuses others of being FBI agents) increase during times of intense anxiety.
- Patient will spend decreased time attending to hallucinations (e.g., less time talking to self, less time listening for voices) before discharge.
- Patient will communicate basic needs more clearly within 1 week.
- Patient will attend the community meeting for _____ minutes today.
- Patient will wash his face and hands with supervision this morning.
- Patient will identify three methods that will help him to continue medications (after discharge) at first follow-up appointment.
- Patient will refrain from hurting self or others during this shift.

Clinical Cues

Monitor your own appearance and clothing when you are working with patients who have thought disorders. First, be a role model for clean, matching, and appropriate clothing. Second, avoid flashy and dangling jewelry because patients are easily distracted by such objects. Third, watch what you put around your neck. An agitated patient can grab a long necklace, a scarf, a tie, or a stethoscope during a takedown.

Planning care for a patient with a thought disorder involves promoting safety, monitoring medications intended to relieve agitation or psychosis, and ensuring adequate nutrition and sleep. **Care for these disorders will be long term, with intermittent treatment for acute episodes.** Patients need to be educated about the medications and coping skills necessary to function outside of a hospital setting. It is not unusual for a patient to stop taking medications because the voices returned and told him that all medications are unnecessary or harmful. For patients who are noncompliant with medications, a long-acting injectable form may be prescribed to prevent relapse (American Psychiatric Association, 2004).

 Think Critically

Can you think of some ways that nurses could devise to help individuals with thought disorders comply with the medication regimen?

■ **Implementation**

A priority intervention in working with schizophrenic patients is to administer antipsychotic medications. As with any medication, nursing responsibility includes not only giving the medication, but also monitoring the effectiveness and any adverse effects. Antipsychotics have many serious side effects, some of which can be life threatening.

 Patient Teaching

Antipsychotic Medications

Patients taking antipsychotic medications should be advised not to use alcohol. Combining alcohol and antipsychotic medications may result in impaired judgment, thinking, and coordination. This is due to the additive effect of the central nervous system depression (Drugs.com, 2010).

 Clinical Cues

In accordance with National Patient Safety Goals, there should be at least two identifiers before giving medication or blood products or taking blood samples. When patients are not able to state their correct legal name (because of confusion or psychosis), an alternative method would be to have two health care providers verify the patient's identity.

When dealing with an actively psychotic patient, use a calm and caring approach. Do not touch the patient without warning or permission, especially if he is agitated or paranoid. During active hallucinations, state reality and help the patient return to reality. "Mr. Elliott, you seem to be listening to something. I am not hearing any voices. Come and talk to me." Strategies for helping patients to manage persistent auditory hallucinations include monitoring what triggers the hallucinations, talking with someone, listening to music, watching TV, saying "stop," using earplugs, doing deep breathing or relaxation exercises, and doing a favorite activity.

You may have great difficulty understanding the patient because of neologisms (making up new words), word salad (disorganized mix of words, phrases, and fragments), or loose associations (expression of ideas that do not logically connect).

 Cultural Considerations

Language

During times of stress, it is natural to revert to your first language. If your patient speaks English as a second language, obtain the assistance of a translator to determine if the patient is having disturbances in communication (e.g., the patient's verbalizations might sound like word salad, but are actually a mixture of English and another language). Also, you can be charged with giving substandard care if you fail to call for a translator when the patient is unable to speak or understand English.

Use therapeutic communication and be attentive, respond to the underlying feelings, and gently verbalize concern. "Mr. Elliott, you seem really anxious to tell me something. I am trying to understand."

 Think Critically

You are caring for a patient who does not trust you. How does his distrust affect medication compliance? How will you establish trust and rapport with this patient?

General nursing interventions for the negative symptoms include establishing trust and teaching the patient and family how to manage the signs and symptoms. An attitude of acceptance is necessary to promote trust. Begin by offering yourself and being available to the patient even if he initially rejects your overtures to establish a therapeutic relationship: "I'm here if you want to spend some time talking today." You should model conventional social behaviors such as greeting the patient by name: "Good morning, Mr. Elliott," and making friendly eye contact.

Cultural Considerations

Eye Contact

Lack of direct eye contact does not necessarily signal disinterest or an unwillingness to communicate. Direct eye contact may be considered a sign of disrespect by people from different cultural backgrounds (i.e., Asian, Hispanic/Latino).

Give your patient positive feedback for making attempts to overcome negative symptoms: "You seemed very interested in the group discussion topic today." Do not make promises that you cannot keep, and if you make a promise, be sure to follow through.

Consistently invite your patient to join groups even if he rejects the initial invitations: "Mr. Elliott, we are going to play cards. Would you like to join us?" Acknowledge and thank the patient for his efforts to interact, even if he spends only a few seconds with you: "Thank you for talking to me today." Leave the door open for future interactions: "I understand if you don't want to talk today; maybe we can try tomorrow."

Although these patients may have difficulty sustaining an interaction for even 1 or 2 minutes, your persistent effort builds the therapeutic alliance (relationship between the patient and nurse) and increases the patient's self-esteem.

Complementary and Alternative Therapies

Music Therapy

Music therapy can be used with selected patients to treat positive and negative symptoms of schizophrenia. Participation in music groups increases socialization and stimulates interest. Encourage participants to express how the music makes them feel and to discuss their favorite kinds of music. Focused projects such as a performance event help patients to meet individual goals and experience success.

Administering medications and teaching the patient and family about antipsychotic medications are two additional nursing interventions. In addition, the side effects of the medications must be monitored. Nursing Care Plan 49-1 lists specific nursing diagnoses, expected

Nursing Care Plan 49-1   Care of the Patient with Schizophrenia

Scenario

Jake Green is a 29-year-old man who was diagnosed with schizophrenia 8 years ago. He was taken to the emergency department yesterday after he destroyed his own trailer home. Jake states, "There were demons in the walls." He is disheveled and unkempt and appears paranoid and reluctant to interact with the staff or other patients. He appears to be hearing voices and tells you, "I am Jesus, saving you, saving you; hear the demons. You, all of you are demons, yourselves are demons."

Problem/Nursing Diagnosis

Delusions continue/Acute confusion related to delusional thinking, loosening of associations, or neurobiochemical imbalances.

Supporting Assessment Data

Subjective: States "You, all of you are demons, yourselves are demons."
Objective: Believes he is Jesus and believes others are demons.

Goals/Expected Outcomes	Nursing Interventions	Selected Rationale	Evaluation
Patient will be able to talk for 5 min without discussion of delusions. Patient will be able to distinguish between reality and nonreality before discharge.	Assess the themes of delusions. Assess for situations that trigger anxiety and stress.	Delusional themes suggest fears and safety issues. Anxiety and stress are theorized to increase delusions and disorganized behavior.	Has a belief that he is being persecuted by demons. Currently very anxious and actively delusional; assessment for associated triggers continues. Patient is making continuous reference to demons.
	Reflect the underlying feelings ("It's frightening if you feel someone is trying to hurt you.").	Acknowledging feelings validates the patient's experience without agreeing with the delusional content.	Appears suspicious and fearful.
	State reality as you perceive it ("I believe that the hospital is a safe place.").	Corrects misperceptions without directly arguing against patient's perspective.	Reassured that the hospital is a safe place, but he continues to be fearful.
	Avoid arguing about the patient's delusional system.	Arguing causes patient to verbally defend own beliefs and potentially strengthens the delusional system.	Occasionally, patient appears to recognize certain staff members, but overall is highly delusional.

Goals/Expected Outcomes	Nursing Interventions	Selected Rationale	Evaluation
Patient will be able to distinguish between reality and nonreality before discharge—cont'd.	Redirect discussions to real people and events.	Helps patient to stay focused on reality	Continues unwavering in his beliefs in demons. Does respond when called by name (Jake); however, continues to verbalize the belief that he is Jesus.
	Administer antipsychotic medications as ordered and monitor for effectiveness and side effects.	Counteract psychosis at the biochemical level.	Agrees to take risperidone (Risperdal) if administered by certain nurses. Outcomes not met. Continue plan.

Problem/Nursing Diagnosis
*Not attending to basic ADLs/hygiene/grooming/*Self-care deficit related to cognitive impairment.

Supporting Assessment Data
Objective: Disheveled and unkempt.

Goals/Expected Outcomes	Nursing Interventions	Selected Rationale	Evaluation
Patient will independently perform self-care within 1 wk.	Encourage the patient to independently perform ADLs according to current level of ability.	Performing ADLs helps the patient to focus on real tasks and decreases time spent in delusional thinking.	Is not initiating ADLs, but will perform brief tasks (e.g., washing face) with coaching.
Patient will dress appropriately and maintain appropriate hygiene before discharge.	Make available only the clothes the patient is to wear.	Limiting choices decreases confusion and indirectly suggests appropriate attire.	Is continuously changing clothes unless locked out of room.
	Intervene as necessary if patient is unable to complete daily care.	Initially the patient may not be able to complete ADLs due to impaired thought processes.	Mental health assistant verbally directed patient to shower. Patient became hostile; therefore shower deferred for today. Will try to have his brother assist him tomorrow.
	Offer positive reinforcement for any completed portion of ADLs.	Increases likelihood that desired behavior will be repeated.	Acknowledges feedback by looking up when spoken to.
	Assist the patient to make a structured plan if necessary.	Having a plan provides structure, goals, and ways to achieve goals, which helps the patient to complete tasks.	Verbally advised that shower is deferred for today, but that brother will help tomorrow. Agrees to wash hands and face today. Outcomes not met. Continue plan.

Problem/Nursing Diagnosis
*Hearing voices of demons/*Disturbed sensory perception related to neurobiochemical imbalance and anxiety.

Supporting Assessment Data
Subjective: States, "hear the demons."
Objective: Appears to be hearing voices.

Goals/Expected Outcomes	Nursing Interventions	Selected Rationale	Evaluation
Patient will verbalize three ways to cope with hallucinations this week.	Observe behavior that suggests that hallucination is occurring (e.g., talking to self, listening intently).	Staff can interrupt the hallucination in progress.	Observed in listening position and talking to self. Is actively hallucinating today (more than yesterday), appears upset; reason unclear.
Patient will verbalize a decrease in hallucinations before discharge.	Assess for theme of hallucinations, especially command hallucinations (e.g., voices that say, "Kill others.").	Knowing themes helps to anticipate violent or unexpected behavior.	Hearing command hallucinations ("I have the word, the word to save you.").

ADLs, activities of daily living.

Continued

Nursing Care Plan 49-1   **Care of the Patient with Schizophrenia—cont'd**

Goals/Expected Outcomes	Nursing Interventions	Selected Rationale	Evaluation
Patient will verbalize a decrease in hallucinations before discharge—cont'd.	Redirect when hallucinations occur (e.g., "Talk with me.").	Interrupts hallucination in progress.	Patient does attend to nurse when spoken to; although he appears fearful, he will stay for 10-15 sec if he is given adequate space (e.g., 5 ft).
	Help patient recognize the feelings that are present before the hallucination.	Anxiety, fear, and stress are theorized to exacerbate hallucinations.	Unclear why patient is so agitated today; he is unable to verbalize specific feelings.
	State reality (e.g., "I understand that you hear voices. I do not hear those voices.").	Helps patient to recognize and stay focused on reality.	Patient is actively hallucinating; only able to attend to nurse's voice for a few seconds.
	Teach patient to identify and use strategies to interrupt the hallucinations (e.g., seek out nursing staff, sing, listen to music).	Allows patient to cope with hallucinations. (For some patients, hallucinations never completely resolve.)	Unable to identify or teach alternative coping methods. Appears less agitated if not approached by other patients.
	Administer antipsychotic medications and monitor effectiveness and side effects.	Counteracts psychosis at the biochemical level.	Agrees to take risperidone (Risperdal) if administered by certain nurses. Outcomes not met. Continue plan.

Problem/Nursing Diagnosis
Paranoid and avoiding others/Social isolation related to mistrust, bizarre behavior, or cognitive impairment.

Supporting Assessment Data
Subjective: "...all of you are demons."
Objective: Reluctant to interact with the staff or other patients.

Goals/Expected Outcomes	Nursing Interventions	Selected Rationale	Evaluation
Patient will engage in social interaction with others on the psychiatric unit (meals, outings, groups) within 2 wk.	Convey a warm, accepting attitude.	Builds therapeutic relationship.	Has some trust toward selected nurses.
	Spend some structured time with the patient every day.	Encourages social interaction with a set time and purpose.	Able to tolerate 10-15 sec of contact with nurses. Responds to his own name.
	Determine patient's interests.	Patient more likely to engage if interested in activities.	Family states that Jake is interested in baseball. Does show some interest in watching sports on television.
	Model social interaction and conversation.	Patient may be unaware of how to converse with others.	Is not initiating any conversations. Is able to attend group meeting for less than 1 min.
	Create opportunities for socialization (e.g., card games).	Patient may not know how to independently engage others.	
	Acknowledge and thank patient for any efforts to interact and participate in groups.	More likely to repeat behavior if encouraged and acknowledged.	Unable to participate in any group interaction today.
	Encourage the patient to interact with others, even if only briefly.	Brief contacts allow for gradual trust and familiarity to decrease suspiciousness.	Declined going to group music class this afternoon. Appears more restless and suspicious compared to yesterday. Patient unable to verbalize source of distress, no known event or trigger identified. Will continue to observe. Outcomes not met. Continue plan.

Critical Thinking Questions
1. Why is it important for a patient like Jake to have consistent social support after he is discharged from the hospital?
2. What can nurses do to help decrease the social stigma of chronic mental illnesses such as schizophrenia?

| Box 49-2 | Specific Nursing Interventions for Patients Who Are Angry, Hostile, Aggressive, Manipulative, or Paranoid |

ANGRY, HOSTILE, AND AGGRESSIVE BEHAVIOR
- Continuously assess for nonverbal cues (pacing, fidgeting, and increase in verbalizations) and intervene early.
- Maintain a calm, self-assured attitude, even if you are frightened.
- Listen and acknowledge that you care and want to help.
- Be culturally aware of how your patient is interpreting eye contact.
- Allow the patient to have adequate personal space.
- Encourage the patient to find a quiet, safe place.
- Maintain your own safety—have adequate staff visually present in the background. However, only one person should attempt verbal de-escalation.
- Stand to the side or sideways to present yourself as a smaller target. Your hands should be relaxed at your sides or with the palms turned upward.
- Be aware of the exits and position yourself so that the patient is not blocking the exit.
- Ask for permission before touching. Defer therapeutic touching if the patient is highly agitated.
- Honestly verbalize the patient's options. For example, say, "You can stay in the dayroom if you can remain calm; otherwise it will be necessary for you to go to the quiet (seclusion) room."
- Set a time frame for verbal de-escalation. If progress is made within the time limit, continue. If not, remind the patient of the initial time limit.
- Offer appropriate PRN medications as ordered. If the patient continues to escalate and the behavior becomes aggressive, physical restraints may be necessary.
- Application of physical restraints requires a team approach by trained staff.
- Inform the patient of the staff's intentions and actions. Accurately document the entire episode, including all efforts to use the less restrictive measures before resorting to physical restraints.

MANIPULATIVE BEHAVIOR
- Set clear and realistic limits on specific behaviors.
- Establish realistic and enforceable consequences.
- Make certain that all staff are informed of the limits and are in agreement.
- Specific limits need to be documented in the plan of care/nurses' notes.
- The decision to discontinue limits should be made by the entire staff and should be made only when the patient has demonstrated consistent behavior.
- Be self-aware and establish clear boundaries.

PARANOID BEHAVIOR
- Assign only one or two staff members to the patient.
- Initially make brief contact with the patient, and do not make unnecessary demands.
- Increase credibility by being honest, adhering to a stated schedule, and following through on commitments.
- Do not touch a patient who is paranoid.
- Do not mix medications with food.
- Supply food in commercially wrapped packages if the patient is refusing to eat.

PRN, as needed.

outcomes, and nursing interventions for individuals with thought disorders. Box 49-2 lists additional interventions for patients who are angry, hostile, aggressive, manipulative, or paranoid.

■ Evaluation

To evaluate the effectiveness of nursing interventions, it is necessary to determine expected outcomes and then monitor the patient's progress. **Compliance with antipsychotic medications will decrease hallucinations and delusions (positive symptoms) and improve sleep.** It takes longer to achieve expected outcomes for the negative symptoms of schizophrenia than for the positive symptoms. **Outcomes for the negative symptoms would include a decrease in psychomotor retardation, increase in self-care, improved affect, and an increase in motivation. In addition, the patient would exhibit a trusting attitude toward others and a decrease in social withdrawal.**

OVERVIEW OF PERSONALITY DISORDERS

Personality disorders are enduring patterns of behavior in which there is no loss of contact with reality or impaired cognition. The patient with a personality disorder demonstrates an ongoing, inflexible pattern of behavior that is *very* different from the individual's culture.

Symptoms of personality disorders are usually first observed in late adolescence and early adulthood. Four characteristics of personality disorders are:
1. Inflexible and maladaptive response to life events
2. Serious difficulty in areas of personal and work relationships
3. Tendency to evoke interpersonal conflict
4. Tendency to evoke a negative empathic response from others

An actual diagnosis may not be made until the person reaches the late 20s or 30s; by then the entrenched behaviors are quite evident. It is not uncommon to note failed marriages, poor work histories, and considerable difficulty with interpersonal relationships.

The DSM-IV-TR describes 10 different personality disorders. Depending on the descriptive characteristics, these disorders are clustered into three separate categories. Cluster A includes behaviors that are considered *odd* or *eccentric* (schizotypal, schizoid, and paranoid). Cluster B describes behaviors that are considered *dramatic, emotional,* and *erratic* (antisocial,

Box 49-3   Description of Personality Disorders

CLUSTER A (ODD AND ECCENTRIC)
- *Schizotypal:* Exhibits difficulty with close relationships, distortions in thinking and feeling, and odd or eccentric behavior.
- *Schizoid:* Exhibits withdrawal from social relationships and a restricted affect.
- *Paranoid:* Exhibits distrust and suspiciousness of others and feels that others wish him harm or evil.

CLUSTER B (DRAMATIC, EMOTIONAL, AND ERRATIC)
- *Antisocial:* Exhibits disregard for, and violation of, the rights of others; lacks empathy.
- *Borderline:* Exhibits instability in interpersonal relationships and self-concept, labile emotions, and marked impulsivity.
- *Histrionic:* Exhibits pattern of extreme emotionality and attention-seeking behavior.
- *Narcissistic:* Exhibits grandiose behavior, intense need for admiration, and lack of empathy.

CLUSTER C (ANXIOUS AND FEARFUL)
- *Avoidant:* Exhibits social inhibition, feelings of inadequacy, and fear of rejection.
- *Dependent:* Exhibits behavior that is submissive and clinging; needy.
- *Obsessive-compulsive:* Exhibits behavior that is concerned with excessive orderliness, perfectionism, and need for control.

borderline, histrionic, and narcissistic). Individuals with Cluster C behaviors appear *anxious* and *fearful* (avoidant, dependent, and obsessive-compulsive). A final type of personality disorder is personality disorder NOS (not otherwise specified). Box 49-3 provides a brief description of each of these personality disorders. In this chapter we review borderline personality disorder because it is more commonly diagnosed, and caring for patients with a borderline personality presents many challenges.

BORDERLINE PERSONALITY DISORDER

Borderline personality disorder (BPD) is defined by the DSM-IV-TR as "a pattern of instability in interpersonal relationships, self-image and affect, and marked impulsivity" (American Psychiatric Association, 2007). Individuals with this disorder attach quickly and easily to others and fear *real* or *imagined abandonment.* Emotions and relationships are very intense. In response to potential abandonment from caregivers or significant others, it is not unusual to see *self-mutilating behavior* (e.g., cutting on hands and wrists, cigarette burns) or *suicidal gestures.* Evidence-based practice suggests that the therapeutic goals for patients who self-mutilate include acquiring new coping methods, better impulse and emotional control, and increasing self-awareness (Starr, 2004).

? Think Critically

You are assigned to escort a young female patient to the smoking area. As she is finishing her cigarette, she touches the hot ash to her wrist and sustains a burn before you can stop her. She publicly announces to the staff and the other patients that you were negligent in watching her. How would you handle this?

Splitting, a primitive defense mechanism, involves the initial idealization of a caregiver or friend, followed by a hasty devaluing of that same person. The patient with BPD also may idealize one or two team members and devalue others. For example, the patient may say, "You are the best nurse I have ever had. No one else understands me like you do." When the nurse returns after 2 days off, the patient would say, "I can't believe you didn't call me when you were off. I felt horrible and began cutting on my wrists, and it is your fault." It is very important that the staff decide on an approach to use with a particular patient. To implement the plan properly, all team members must be consistent with the approach.

Impulsivity in at least two of the following areas also is characteristic of BPD: gambling, overeating, spending impulsively, abusing substances, engaging in unsafe sex, or driving recklessly. Engaging in one or more of these impulsive behaviors is often the reason for admission to a hospital.

Treatment

Treatment for people with this disorder involves long-term psychotherapy, such as individual counseling and group or family therapy. The purpose of psychotherapy is to help the participants identify problem areas and work to change behavior and attitudes or modify feelings. The American Psychiatric Association recommends dialectical behavior therapy (DBT) for patients with BPD. This therapy includes individual counseling, telephone support, and skills training and has been shown to reduce self destructive and impulsive episodes, anxiety, and hospitalization. In addition, DBT could also be used to help the family members of patients. Patients with personality disorders can also benefit from milieu therapy. Milieu therapy uses the structured environment of a hospital or group home setting to help patients participate as active members of the milieu community and practice social behaviors. Medications are not indicated for personality disorders, although they are sometimes prescribed when there is a concurrent mood disorder.

❖ NURSING MANAGEMENT

■ Assessment (Data Collection)

You need to collect information about how the individual views himself and others. Obtain a history of former relationships and identify how the individual typically expresses feelings. It is important not to make

Box 49-4	Guide for Assessing Patients with Personality Disorders

Observe and assess for the following:
- Low self-esteem
- Constant seeking of praise and admiration
- Self-centeredness
- Extreme envy of others
- Anger and possible rage when others do not share the same point of view
- Acting without thinking; impulsivity
- Consistent poor judgment in making decisions
- Unreliability
- Evidence of self-destructive behavior
- Treatment of others as objects, not people
- Expression of a need to control others
- Excessive use of manipulation to get needs met

a hasty judgment and label a person with a personality disorder. For example, adolescents may impulsively act out with substances and have identity problems, but these traits often disappear with maturity. In addition, when a patient is labeled as "borderline," nurses may view the patient as "hopeless." Box 49-4 lists examples of behaviors nurses might observe when assessing a personality disorder.

■ Nursing Diagnosis

Typical nursing diagnoses for BPD may include:
- Social isolation related to immature and manipulative behavior
- Chronic low self-esteem related to childhood abuse and neglect
- Ineffective coping related to controlling emotional state outbursts
- Anxiety related to perceived threats of abandonment
- Risk for self-mutilation related to feelings of guilt and rejection

■ Planning

Sample outcomes for the nursing diagnoses above include:
- Patient will discuss one example of how his behavior alienates others by the end of the week.
- Patient will share two things that he likes about himself in today's group meeting.
- Patient will identify three methods to cope with intense emotions (e.g., anger at staff or significant others) within 1 week.
- Patient will identify situations that provoke feelings of abandonment (e.g., favorite nurse is on vacation) and state two methods to reduce accompanying anxiety during this shift.
- Patient will substitute a safe behavior (e.g., talking to nurse, counting to 100) for self-mutilating behavior when experiencing feelings of guilt or rejection during hospitalization.

Planning for the care of a patient with BPD requires involvement of the entire team to define goals and to avoid the patient's inevitable attempts at staff manipulation. If possible, some staff debriefing time will help everyone to maintain a professional and optimistic focus when working with patients who have this disorder.

 Assignment Considerations

Interpersonal Skills

When planning care for your patients, incorporate the strengths and interpersonal skills of your team members and make assignments appropriately. For example, your patient is a 23-year-old woman who needs an escort to attend a group therapy class outside of the unit. She is known for her attempts to manipulate male staff members; therefore assign a mature female nursing assistant who is familiar with the patient's manipulative behavior.

■ Implementation

For individuals with BPD, setting limits is a priority intervention. Individuals must be taught healthy and nonmanipulative ways to have their needs met. To work with patients who have BPD, the staff needs to maintain good boundaries without being controlling, rigid, and inflexible. Patients with this disorder often ask you to "bend the rules" or grant special privileges. **The staff needs to consistently set limits with caring and empathy, offer a rationale, and decline negotiation.** If the patient views the limit setting as punitive, the behavior is certain to recur at a later time. This does not mean that the patient will always gladly accept the limit setting and be grateful for your concern. It does mean that you are assisting the patient in developing some internal sense of boundaries and subsequent changes in behavior.

It is also necessary to maintain a safe environment for patients with BPD because they can be impulsive and do not have internal control. It may be necessary to initiate suicide precautions or help the patient who is self-mutilating to stop this behavior. See Chapter 46 for information on suicide precautions.

Patients with personality disorders have an ability to "get under the skin" of caregivers. If you note a particularly intense reaction to a patient (excessive sympathy, empathy, anger, or frustration), it is important to talk about these feelings with a more experienced nurse or a peer whom you trust. Identify and express the feelings that the patient's behavior evokes in you. Your awareness of your own feelings will help you to modify your reactions and focus on the therapeutic aspects of your relationship with the patient. Evidence suggests that the strength of the therapeutic alliance is related to overall outcomes of treatment (Lamont & Brunero, 2009). In addition, the nurse's skills and attitudes are just as important as any prescribed medical intervention (Swift, 2009).

■ Evaluation

Achievement of long-term outcomes is demonstrated by new coping strategies for handling stressors, verbalizing anger without acting out, increasing independent decision making, and decreasing manipulative behaviors to have needs met. It is expected that in times of stress, the patient will revert to previously learned behaviors. When the stress has passed, you should encourage the patient to continue implementing new behaviors.

COMMUNITY CARE

At one time individuals with thought disorders were hospitalized indefinitely. With the introduction of antipsychotic medications, hospitalization is reserved for medication stabilization; then patients are released to a less restrictive type of care. In fact, community mental health teams are shown to increase patients' acceptance of treatment and reduce the need for hospitalization (Malone et al., 2009).

 Elder Care Points

Although elderly schizophrenics are few in number, they can present unique challenges for nurses who work in long-term care. Because of the negative symptoms of social withdrawal, apathy, and sometimes paranoia, schizophrenic elders are not as likely to seek out nurses for help. They may ignore physical problems and often will not seek help for pain associated with physical disabilities.

 Safety Alert

Be Alert for Suicidal Ideations

Approximately 50% of patients who have schizophrenia think about suicide sometime during their lifetime. Community health nurses are in a position to make regular contact with these patients; assess for suicide even if the patient does not raise the issue; clearly communicate the intention to see the patient again; and help the patient to make a crisis response plan that includes hospitalization as needed (Meerwijk et al., 2010) (see Chapter 46).

Patients with personality disorders are not hospitalized unless they present an imminent danger to themselves via self-mutilation or suicidal gestures. Again, nurses come into contact with personality disorders in a variety of settings outside a psychiatric hospital. Setting limits and appropriate boundaries continues to be an effective intervention, regardless of the setting.

Patients with chronic mental illness are at high risk for social problems and may have limited encounters with health care professionals. For example, patients with schizophrenia are at a high risk for homelessness, and patients with personality disorders, particular antisocial personality disorder, are more likely to be incarcerated. In accordance with *Healthy People 2020* goals, a greater percentage of people who are homeless and those who are in jail need mental health screening and access to treatment.

Get Ready for the NCLEX® Examination!

Key Points

- Thought disorders are characterized by disorganized thoughts and behavior and hallucinations. Mood and interpersonal relationships are altered.
- Schizophrenia is the most commonly diagnosed thought disorder and usually develops in late adolescence or the early 20s.
- The positive symptoms of schizophrenia (hallucinations, delusions, and disordered thinking) can be treated with antipsychotic medications.
- The negative symptoms of schizophrenia (apathy, social isolation, psychomotor retardation, blunted affect, poverty of thoughts, and lack of motivation) are responsive to some of the newer atypical medications but are more difficult to treat. Long-term social skills training and ongoing family and community support are essential.
- Elders who are taking antipsychotics are at a greater risk for developing extrapyramidal symptoms, tardive dyskinesia, and neuroleptic malignant syndrome. Beginning doses should be one half to one third of the normal adult dose.

- General nursing management includes establishing trust and rapport, encouraging social skills, administering medications and monitoring effects, and educating the patient and family about the illness and the therapeutic regimen.
- Personality disorders are characterized by enduring traits. The four hallmarks of personality disorders are inflexible and maladaptive response to life events, serious difficulty in personal and work relationships, a tendency to evoke interpersonal conflict, and a tendency to evoke a negative empathic response from others.
- Borderline personality disorder is the most prevalent personality disorder.
- For a patient with a personality disorder, assess the patient's view of self and others, expression of feelings, and behaviors that are interfering with routine life and relationships.
- General nursing management of patients with personality disorders includes building trust, setting limits, teaching coping skills, preventing self-harm, and encouraging insight into behavior.

Additional Learning Resources

 SG Go to your Study Guide for additional learning activities to help you master this chapter content.

evolve Go to your Evolve website (http://evolve.elsevier.com/deWit/medsurg) for the following FREE learning resources:
- Animations, audio, and video
- Answers and rationales for questions and activities
- Concept Map Creator
- Glossary with pronunciations in English and Spanish
- Interactive Review Questions and Exercises and more!

🖱 Online Resources
- National Institute of Mental Health, www.nimh.nih.gov/health/topics/schizophrenia/index.shtml
- Mayo Clinic, www.mayoclinic.com/health/borderline-personality-disorder/DS00442
- National Alliance on Mental Illness, www.nami.org

Review Questions for the NCLEX® Examination

1. An elderly male patient on antipsychotic medications develops a flat affect with drooling and a shuffling gait. He has slowed movements, tremors, motor restlessness, apprehension, and irritability. The nurse would obtain an order for which medication?
   1. Benztropine (Cogentin)
   2. Haloperidol (Haldol)
   3. Chlorpromazine (Thorazine)
   4. Perphenazine (Trilafon)

2. The nurse is administering medication to a familiar patient, who has been on the unit for several weeks. When asked to state his name, the patient replies, "I am Jesus Christ, the son of God." What is the best nursing action?
   1. Give the medication, because the nurse knows he is confused.
   2. Document that the patient cannot state his name and hold the medication.
   3. Hold the medication until the family can bring in a picture identification.
   4. Have a second nurse verify his identity and document accordingly.

3. The nurse discusses the effects of a patient's antipsychotic medication. Which patient statement indicates a need for further teaching?
   1. "The medication helps me to think more logically."
   2. "The medication makes my mouth dry."
   3. "The medication improves my mood."
   4. "The medication helps to stop the voices."

4. A patient reports that he has been taking thioridazine (Mellaril) for more than 12 months. Which symptom is the cause for greatest concern?
   1. Muscle rigidity
   2. Tongue protrusion
   3. Photophobia
   4. Motor restlessness

5. When talking with a patient who is having active hallucinations, what is the priority action?
   1. Assess the content and themes of hallucinations.
   2. Give an antipsychotic medication.
   3. Take the patient to a secluded area.
   4. Set boundaries and explain rationale.

6. The patient is suspicious and believes that he is surrounded by terrorists. He tells the nurse, "They put anthrax in the food and there is a bomb in the bathroom." What is the most therapeutic response?
   1. "Who do you think is doing all these things?"
   2. "Let's go together and check the bathroom."
   3. "Tell me why you believe these things are happening."
   4. "I believe that the hospital is a safe place."

7. A patient is readmitted for an acute psychotic episode. He appears to be having command hallucinations. What is the priority nursing diagnosis?
   1. Disturbed sensory perception
   2. Risk for self- or other-directed violence
   3. Anxiety
   4. Ineffective coping

8. A nursing student is caring for a patient with a personality disorder. Which statement by the student indicates a need for additional training and education on setting boundaries?
   1. "I can spend 20 minutes talking with you and then I have to pass medications."
   2. "I understand that you are bored, but you have to complete the task."
   3. "If you promise not to cause trouble, I'll give you the magazine."
   4. "When someone is speaking in group, it is polite to listen while they speak."

9. A patient demonstrates negative symptoms of apathy, social isolation, and lack of motivation. To establish trust, what should the nurse do? *(Select all that apply.)*
   1. Offer self and be available.
   2. Reorient to person, place, and time.
   3. Keep all promises.
   4. Invite the patient to join groups.
   5. Leave the door open for future interactions.
   6. Encourage independence in ADLs.

10. A patient is becoming progressively louder and more aggressive about getting a personal item (belt) that was taken from him for safety precautions. What intervention(s) should the nurse use? *(Select all that apply.)*
    1. Continuously assess for pacing, fidgeting, and increase in verbalizations.
    2. Maintain a calm, self-assured attitude, even if frightened.
    3. Listen and state, "I care and want to help."
    4. Move in close to the patient to reassure him.
    5. Give the patient the belt and set strict limits on his behavior.
    6. Stand to the side or sideways to present a smaller target.
    7. Explain the hospital policy and offer him a copy.

Critical Thinking Activities

Scenario A
You are caring for Mrs. Leiber, a 65-year-old who has a fixed delusional system with many religious overtones. You notice that she is pacing and becoming increasingly agitated. She begins to yell in a loud voice about God and salvation and not being saved.

1. How might you approach Mrs. Leiber and assist her to de-escalate?

2. What behaviors would cause you to consider physically restraining Mrs. Leiber?

Scenario B
Mr. John Hammer, 42 years old, was recently discharged from a psychiatric facility after an extended stay. He comes to the clinic for a renewal of his antipsychotic medications, accompanied by his elderly father, who reports that his son is noncompliant with medications and has limited social interaction.

1. What nursing interventions could increase Mr. Hammer's compliance with therapy?

2. What type of community referrals would be appropriate for this patient and his family?

Scenario C
A 32-year-old patient, Betsy Johnston, arrives at the clinic with a superficial scratch on the wrist. She begins to cry, "You are the best nurse here. You're always so kind and understanding. Would you call my boyfriend and tell him that I am here? I cut myself because we just broke up." You know Ms. Johnston because she has been in the clinic many times with similar minor injuries. In the past, she has been manipulative and verbally abusive toward the staff.

1. What behaviors suggest that Ms. Johnston may have a personality disorder?

2. How would you respond to her request to call the boyfriend?

Scenario D
Mr. Mueller is admitted to the psychiatric unit for chronic schizophrenia. It is very difficult to understand Mr. Mueller, because he has thought disorders and manifests word salad, neologisms, and loose associations. He has not demonstrated any aggressive behaviors toward anyone, but he is unable to sustain interaction for more than a few seconds at a time.

1. What interventions could be used for the nursing diagnosis of Impaired verbal communication related to cognitive impairment?

2. Write a communication goal that would be appropriate for Mr. Mueller.

3. Identify an activity that would be appropriate for this patient.

Most Common Laboratory Test Values

Table A-1   Reference Intervals for Hematology

TEST	CONVENTIONAL UNITS	SI UNITS
Acid hemolysis (Ham test)	No hemolysis	No hemolysis
Alkaline phosphatase, leukocyte	Total score, 14-100	Total score, 14-100
Cell counts		
Erythrocytes		
Males	4.6-6.2 million/mm^3	4.6-6.2 × 10^{12}/L
Females	4.2-5.4 million/mm^3	4.2-5.4 × 10^{12}/L
Children (varies with age)	4.5-5.1 million/mm^3	4.5-5.1 × 10^{12}/L
Leukocytes, total	4500-11,000/mm^3	4.5-1.0 × 10^9/L
Leukocytes, differential counts*		
Myelocytes	0%	0/L
Band neutrophils	3%-5%	150-400 × 10^6/L
Segmented neutrophils	54%-62%	3000-5800 × 10^6/L
Lymphocytes	25%-33%	1500-3000 × 10^6/L
Monocytes	3%-7%	300-500 × 10^6/L
Eosinophils	1%-3%	50-250 × 10^6/L
Basophils	0%-1%	15-50 × 10^6/L
Platelets	150,000-400,000/mm^3	150-400 × 10^9/L
Reticulocytes	25,000-5,000/mm^3 (0.5%-1.5% of erythrocytes)	25-75 × 10^9/L
Coagulation tests		
Bleeding time (template)	2.75-8.00 min	2.75-8.00 min
Coagulation time (glass tube)	5-15 min	5-15 min
D-Dimer	<0.5 mcg/mL	<0.5 mg/L
Factor VIII and other coagulation factors	50%-150% of normal	0.5-1.5 of normal
Fibrin split products (Thrombo-Welco test)	<10 mcg/mL	<10 mg/L
Fibrinogen	200-400 mg/dL	2.0-4.0 g/L
Partial thromboplastin time, activated (aPTT)	20-25 sec	20-35 sec
Prothrombin time (PT)	12.0-14.0 sec	12.0-14.0 sec
Coombs' test		
Direct	Negative	Negative
Indirect	Negative	Negative
Corpuscular values of erythrocytes		
Mean corpuscular hemoglobin (MCH)	26-34 pg/cell	26-34 pg/cell
Mean corpuscular volume (MCV)	80-96 μm^3	80-96 fL
Mean corpuscular hemoglobin concentration (MCHC)	32-36 g/dL	320-360 g/L
Haptoglobin	20-165 mg/dL	0.20-1.65 g/L
Hematocrit		
Males	40-54 mL/dL	0.40-0.54 g/L
Females	37-47 mL/dL	0.37-0.47 g/L
Newborns	49-54 mL/dL	0.49-0.54 g/L
Children (varies with age)	35-49 mL/dL	0.35-0.49 g/L
Hemoglobin		
Males	13.0-18.0 g/dL	8.1-11.2 mmol/L
Females	12.0-16.0 g/dL	7.4-9.9 mmol/L
Newborns	16.5-19.5 g/dL	10.2-12.1 mmol/L
Children (varies with age)	11.2-16.5 g/dL	7.0-10.2 mmol/L

Continued

Table A-1 Reference Intervals for Hematology—cont'd

TEST	CONVENTIONAL UNITS	SI UNITS
Hemoglobin, fetal	<1.0% of total	<0.01 of total
Hemoglobin A1C	3%-5% of total	0.03-0.05 of total
Hemoglobin A2	1.5%-3.0% of total	0.015-0.03 of total
Hemoglobin, plasma	0.0-5.0 mg/dL	0.0-3.2 µmol/L
Methemoglobin	30-130 mg/dL	19-80 µmol/L
Erythrocyte sedimentation rate (ESR) Wintrobe • Males • Females Westergren • Males • Females	 0-5 mm/hr 0-15 mm/hr 0-15 mm/hr 0-20 mm/hr	 0-5 mm/hr 0-15 mm/hr 0-15 mm/hr 0-20 mm/hr

From McCloskey, L.J. (2010). Reference intervals for interpretation of laboratory test values. In Bope, E.T., Rakel, R.E. & Kellerman, R., *Conn's Current Therapy 2010*. Philadelphia: Saunders.
*Conventional units are percentages; SI units are absolute cell counts.

Table A-2 Reference Intervals* for Clinical Chemistry (Blood, Serum, and Plasma)

ANALYTE	CONVENTIONAL UNITS	SI UNITS
Acetoacetate plus acetone Qualitative Quantitative	 Negative 0.3-2.0 mg/dL	 Negative 30-200 µmol/L
Acid phosphatase, serum (thymolphthalein monophosphate substrate)	0.1-0.6 U/L	0.1-0.6 U/L
ACTH (see Corticotropin)		
Alanine aminotransferase (ALT), serum (SGPT)	1-45 U/L	1-45 U/L
Albumin, serum	3.3-5.2 g/dL	33-52 g/L
Aldolase, serum	0.0-7.0 U/L	0.0-7.0 U/L
Aldosterone, plasma Standing Recumbent	 5-30 ng/dL 3-10 ng/dL	 140-830 pmol/L 80-275 pmol/L
Alkaline, phosphatase (ALP), serum Adult Adolescent Child	 35-150 U/L 100-500 U/L 100-350 U/L	 35-150 U/L 100-500 U/L 100-350 U/L
Ammonia nitrogen, plasma	10-50 µmol/L	10-50 µmol/L
Amylase, serum	25-125 U/L	25-125 U/L
Anion gap, serum calculated	8-16 mEq/L	8-16 mmol/L
Ascorbic acid, blood	0.4-1.5 mg/dL	23-85 µmol/L
Aspartate aminotransferase (AST), serum (SGOT)	1-36 U/L	1-36 U/L
Base excess, arterial blood, calculated	0 ± 2 mEq/L	0 ± 2 mmol/L
Bicarbonate Venous plasma Arterial blood	 23-29 mEq/L 21-27 mEq/L	 23-29 mmol/L 21-27 mmol/L
Bile acids, serum	0.3-3.0 mg/dL	0.8-7.6 mmol/L
Bilirubin, serum Conjugated Total	 0.1-0.4 mg/dL 0.3-1.1 mg/dL	 1.7-6.8 µmol/L 5.1-19.0 µmol/L
Calcium, serum	8.4-10.6 mg/dL	2.10-2.65 mmol/L
Calcium, ionized, serum	4.25-5.25 mg/dL	1.05-1.30 mmol/L
Carbon dioxide, total, serum or plasma	24-31 mEq/L	24-31 mmol/L
Carbon dioxide tension (Pco_2), blood	35-45 mm Hg	35-45 mm Hg

*Reference values may vary, depending on the method and sample source used.

Table A-2 | Reference Intervals for Clinical Chemistry (Blood, Serum, and Plasma)—cont'd

ANALYTE	CONVENTIONAL UNITS	SI UNITS
β-Carotene, serum	60-260 mcg/dL	1.1-8.6 µmol/L
Ceruloplasmin, serum	23-44 mg/dL	230-440 mg/L
Chloride, serum or plasma	96-106 mEq/L	96-106 mmol/L
Cholesterol, serum or EDTA plasma 　Desirable range 　Low-density lipoprotein (LDL) cholesterol 　High-density lipoprotein (HDL) cholesterol	 <200 mg/dL 60-180 mg/dL 30-80 mg/dL	 <5.20 mmol/L 1.55-4.65 mmol/L 0.80-2.05 mmol/L
Copper	70-140 mcg/dL	11-22 µmol/L
Corticotropin (ACTH), plasma, 8 AM	10-80 pg/mL	2-18 pmol/L
Cortisol, plasma 　8 A.M. 　4 P.M. 　10 P.M.	 6-23 mcg/dL 3-15 mcg/dL <50% of 8 AM value	 170-630 µmol/L 80-410 µmol/L <50% of 8 AM value
Creatine, serum 　Males 　Females	 0.2-0.5 mg/dL 0.3-0.9 mg/dL	 15-40 µmol/L 25-70 µmol/L
Creatine kinase (CK), serum 　Males 　Females	 55-170 U/L 30-135 U/L	 55-170 U/L 30-135 U/L
Creatinine kinase MB isoenzyme, serum	<5% of total CK activity <5% of ng/mL by 　immunoassay	<5% of total CK activity <5% of ng/mL by 　immunoassay
Creatinine, serum	0.6-1.2 mg/dL	50-110 µmol/L
Estradiol-17β, adult 　Males 　Females 　• Follicular 　• Ovulatory 　• Luteal	 10-65 pg/mL 30-100 pg/mL 200-400 pg/mL 50-140 pg/mL	 35-240 pmol/L 110-370 pmol/L 730-1470 pmol/L 180-510 pmol/L
Ferritin, serum	20-200 ng/mL	20-200 mcg/L
Fibrinogen, plasma	200-400 mg/dL	2.0-4.0 g/L
Folate, serum 　Erythrocytes	3-18 ng/mL 145-540 ng/mL	6.8-4.1 nmol/L 330-120 nmol/L
Follicle-stimulating hormone (FSH), plasma 　Males 　Females, premenopausal 　Females, postmenopausal	 4-25 mU/mL 4-30 mU/mL 40-250 mU/mL	 4-25 U/L 4-30 U/L 40-250 U/L
Gastrin, fasting, serum	0-100 pg/mL	0-100 mg/L
Glucose, fasting, plasma or serum	70-100 mg/dL	3.9-5.55 nmol/L
γ-Glutamyltransferase (GGT), serum	5-40 U/L	5-40 U/L
Growth hormone (hGH), plasma, adult, fasting	0-6 ng/mL	0-6 mcg/L
Haptoglobin, serum	20-165 mg/dL	0.20-1.65 g/L
β-Hydroxybutyrate	0.3-2.8 mg/dL	20-280 µmol/L
Immunoglobulins, serum (see Table A-8, Reference Intervals for Tests of Immunologic Function)		
Iron, serum	75-175 mcg/dL	13-31 µmol/L
Iron-binding capacity, serum 　Total 　Saturation	 250-410 mcg/dL 20%-55%	 45-73 µmol/L 0.20-0.55
Lactate 　Venous whole blood 　Arterial whole blood	 5.0-20.0 mg/dL 5.0-15.0 mg/dL	 0.6-2.2 mmol/L 0.6-1.7 mmol/L
Lactate dehydrogenase (LD), serum	110-220 U/L	110-220 U/L
Lipase, serum	10-140 U/L	10-140 U/L

Continued

Table A-2   Reference Intervals for Clinical Chemistry (Blood, Serum, and Plasma)—cont'd

ANALYTE	CONVENTIONAL UNITS	SI UNITS
Lutropin (LH), serum		
Males	1-9 U/L	1-9 U/L
Females		
• Follicular phase	2-10 U/L	2-10 U/L
• Midcycle peak	15-65 U/L	15-65 U/L
• Luteal phase	1-12 U/L	1-12 U/L
• Postmenopausal	12-65 U/L	12-65 U/L
Magnesium, serum	1.3-2.1 mg/dL	0.65-1.05 mmol/L
Osmolality	275-295 mOsm/kg water	275-295 mOsm/kg water
Oxygen, blood, arterial, room air		
Partial pressure (PaO$_2$)	80-100 mm Hg	80-100 mm Hg
Saturation (SaO$_2$)	95%-98%	95%-98%
pH, arterial blood	7.35-7.45	7.35-7.45
Phosphate, inorganic, serum		
Adult	3.0-4.5 mg/dL	1.0-1.5 mmol/L
Child	4.0-7.0 mg/dL	1.3-2.3 mmol/L
Potassium		
Serum	3.5-5.0 mEq/L	3.5-5.0 mmol/L
Plasma	3.5-4.5 mEq/L	3.5-4.5 mmol/L
Progesterone, serum, adult		
Males	0.0-0.4 ng/mL	0.0-1.3 mmol/L
Females		
• Follicular phase	0.1-1.5 ng/mL	0.3-4.8 mmol/L
• Luteal phase	2.5-28.0 ng/mL	8.0-89.0 mmol/L
Prolactin, serum		
Males	1.0-15.0 ng/mL	1.0-15.0 mcg/L
Females	1.0-20.0 ng/mL	1.0-20.0 mcg/L
Protein, serum, electrophoresis		
Total	6.0-8.0 g/dL	60-80 g/L
Albumin	3.5-5.5 g/dL	35-55 g/L
Globulins		
• α_1	0.2-0.4 g/dL	2.0-4.0 g/L
• α_2	0.5-0.9 g/dL	5.0-9.0 g/L
• β	0.6-1.1 g/dL	6.0-11.0 g/L
• γ	0.7-1.7 g/dL	7.0-17.0 g/L
Pyruvate, blood	0.3-0.9 mg/dL	0.03-0.10 mmol/L
Rheumatoid factor	0.0-30.0 IU/mL	0.0-30.0 kIU/L
Sodium, serum or plasma	135-145 mEq/L	135-145 mmol/L
Testosterone, plasma		
Males, adult	300-1200 ng/dL	10.4-41.6 nmol/L
Females, adult	20-75 ng/dL	0.7-2.6 nmol/L
Pregnant females	40-200 ng/dL	1.4-6.9 nmol/L
Thyroglobulin	3-42 ng/mL	3-42 mcg/L
Thyrotropin (hTSH), serum	0.4-4.8 μIU/mL	0.4-4.8 mIU/L
Thyrotropin-releasing hormone (TRH)	5-60 pg/mL	5-60 ng/L
Thyroxine (FT$_4$), free, serum	0.9-2.1 ng/dL	12-27 pmol/L
Thyroxine (T$_4$), serum	4.5-12.0 mcg/mL	58-154 nmol/L
Thyroxine-binding globulin (TBG)	15.0-34.0 mcg/mL	15.0-34.0 mg/L
Transferrin	250-430 mg/dL	2.5-4.3 g/L
Triglycerides, serum, after 12-hr fast	40-150 mg/dL	0.4-1.5 g/L
Triiodothyronine (T$_3$), serum	70-190 ng/dL	1.1-2.9 nmol/L
Triiodothyronine uptake, resin (T$_3$RU)	25%-38%	0.25-0.38
Troponin I	0.05-0.50 ng/mL	0.05-0.50 ng/mL

Table A-2   Reference Intervals for Clinical Chemistry (Blood, Serum, and Plasma)—cont'd

ANALYTE	CONVENTIONAL UNITS	SI UNITS
Urate		
Males	2.5-8.0 mg/dL	150-480 µmol/L
Females	2.2-7.0 mg/dL	130-420 µmol/L
Urea, serum or plasma	24-49 mg/dL	4.0-8.2 nmol/L
Urea, nitrogen, serum or plasma	11-23 mg/dL	8.0-16.4 nmol/L
Viscosity, serum	1.1-1.8 × water	1.1-1.8 × water
Vitamin A, serum	20-80 mcg/dL	0.70-2.80 µmol/L
Vitamin B_{12}, serum	180-900 pg/mL	133-664 pmol/L

Table A-3   Reference Intervals* for Therapeutic Drug Monitoring (Serum or Plasma)

ANALYTE	THERAPEUTIC RANGE	TOXIC CONCENTRATIONS	PROPRIETARY NAME(S)
Analgesics			
Acetaminophen	10-40 mcg/mL	>150 mcg/mL	Tylenol, Datril
Salicylate	100-250 mcg/mL	>300 mcg/mL	Aspirin, Bufferin
Antibiotics			
Amikacin	20-30 mcg/mL	Peak >35 mcg/mL Trough >10 mcg/mL	Amkin
Gentamicin	5-10 mcg/mL	Peak >10 mcg/mL Trough >2 mcg/mL	Garamycin
Tobramycin	5-10 mcg/mL	Peak >10 mcg/mL Trough >2 mcg/mL	Nebcin
Vancomycin	5-35 mcg/mL	Peak >40 mcg/mL Trough >10 mcg/mL	Vancocin
Anticonvulsants			
Carbamazepine	5-12 mcg/mL	>15 mcg/mL	Tegretol
Ethosuximide	40-100 mcg/mL	>250 mcg/mL	Zarontin
Phenobarbital	15-40 mcg/mL	40-100 ng/mL (varies widely)	Luminal
Phenytoin	10-20 mcg/mL	>20 mcg/mL	Dilantin
Primidone	5-12 mcg/mL	>15 mcg/mL	Mysoline
Valproic acid	50-100 mcg/mL	>100 mcg/mL	Depakene
Antineoplastics and Immunosuppressives			
Cyclosporine	100-300 ng/mL	>400 ng/mL	Sandimmune
Methotrexate, high-dose, 48 hr	Variable	>1 µmol/L, 48 hr after dose	
Tacrolimus (FK-506), whole blood	3-20 mcg/L	>15 mcg/L	Prograf
Bronchodilators and Respiratory Stimulants			
Caffeine	3-15 ng/mL	>30 ng/mL	Elixophyllin
Theophylline (aminophylline)	10-20 mcg/mL	>30 mcg/mL	Quibron
Cardiovascular Drugs			
Amiodarone (obtain specimen more than 8 hr after last dose)	1.0-2.0 mcg/mL	>2.0 mcg/mL	Cordarone
Digoxin (obtain specimen more than 6 hr after last dose)	0.8-2.0 ng/mL	>2.4 ng/mL	Lanoxin
Disopyramide	2-5 mcg/mL	>7 mcg/mL	Norpace
Flecainide	0.2-1.0 mcg/mL	>1 mcg/mL	Tambocor

*Values may vary depending on the method and sample collection device used. Always consult the reference values provided by the laboratory performing the analysis.

Continued

Table A-3 Reference Intervals for Therapeutic Drug Monitoring (Serum or Plasma)—cont'd

ANALYTE	THERAPEUTIC RANGE	TOXIC CONCENTRATIONS	PROPRIETARY NAME(S)
Lidocaine	1.5-5.0 mcg/mL	>6 mcg/mL	Xylocaine
Mexiletine	0.7-2.0 mcg/mL	>2 mcg/mL	Mexitil
Procainamide	4-10 mcg/mL	>12 mcg/mL	Pronestyl
Procainamide plus NAPA (N-acetyl procainamide)	8-30 mcg/mL	>30 mcg/mL	
Propranolol	50-100 ng/mL	Variable	Inderal
Quinidine	2-5 mcg/mL	>6 mcg/mL	Cardioquin, Quinaglute
Tocainide	4-10 ng/mL	>10 ng/mL	Tonocard
Psychopharmacologic Drugs			
Amitriptyline	120-150 ng/mL	>500 ng/mL	Elavil, Triavil
Bupropion	25-100 ng/mL	Not applicable	Wellbutrin
Desipramine	150-300 ng/mL	>500 ng/mL	Norpramin
Imipramine	125-250 ng/mL	>400 ng/mL	Tofranil
Lithium (obtain specimen 12 hr after last dose)	0.6-1.5 mEq/L	>1.5 mEq/L	Lithobid
Nortriptyline	50-150 ng/mL	>500 ng/mL	Aventyl, Pamelor

Table A-4 Reference Intervals* for Clinical Chemistry (Urine)

ANALYTE	CONVENTIONAL UNITS	SI UNITS
Acetone and acetoacetate, qualitative	Negative	Negative
Albumin		
Qualitative	Negative	Negative
Quantitative	10-100 mg/24 hr	0.15-1.5 µmol/day
Aldosterone	3-20 mcg/24 hr	8.3-55 nmol/day
δ-Aminolevulinic acid (δ-ALA)	1.3-7.0 mg/24 hr	10-53 µmol/day
Amylase	<17 U/hr	<17 U/hr
Amylase/creatinine clearance ratio	0.01-0.04	0.01-0.04
Bilirubin, qualitative	Negative	Negative
Calcium (regular diet)	<250 mg/24 hr	<6.3 nmol/day
Catecholamines		
Epinephrine	<10 mcg/24 hr	<55 nmol/day
Norepinephrine	<100 mcg/24 hr	<590 nmol/day
Total free catecholamines	4-126 mcg/24 hr	24-745 nmol/day
Total metanephrines	0.1-1.6 mg/24 hr	0.5-8.1 µmol/day
Chloride (varies with intake)	110-250 mEq/24 hr	110-250 mmol/day
Copper	0-50 mcg/24 hr	0.0-0.80 µmol/day
Cortisol, free	10-100 mcg/24 hr	27.6-276 nmol/day
Creatine		
Males	0-40 mg/24 hr	0.0-0.30 mmol/day
Females	0-80 mg/24 hr	0.0-0.60 mmol/day
Creatinine	15-25 mg/kg/24 hr	0.13-0.22 mmol/kg/day
Creatinine clearance (endogenous)		
Males	110-150 mL/min/1.73 m^2	110-150 mL/min/1.73 m^2
Females	105-132 mL/min/1.73 m^2	105-132 mL/min/1.73 m^2
Cystine or cysteine	Negative	Negative
Dehydroepiandrosterone		
Males	0.2-2.0 mg/24 hr	0.7-6.9 µmol/day
Females	0.2-1.8 mg/24 hr	0.7-6.2 µmol/day

*Values may vary, depending on the method used.

Table **A-4** Reference Intervals for Clinical Chemistry (Urine)—cont'd

ANALYTE	CONVENTIONAL UNITS	SI UNITS
Estrogens, total		
Males	4-25 mcg/24 hr	14-90 nmol/day
Females	5-100 mcg/24 hr	18-360 nmol/day
Glucose (as reducing substance)	<250 mg/24 hr	<250 mg/day
Hemoglobin and myoglobin, qualitative	Negative	Negative
Hemogentisic acid, qualitative	Negative	Negative
17-Hydroxycorticosteroids		
Males	3-9 mg/24 hr	8.3–25 µmol/day
Females	2-8 mg/24 hr	5.5–22 µmol/day
5-Hydroxyindoleacetic acid		
Qualitative	Negative	Negative
Quantitative	2-6 mg/24 hr	10-31 µmol/day
17-Ketogenic steroids		
Males	5-23 mg/24 hr	17-80 µmol/day
Females	3-15 mg/24 hr	10-52 µmol/day
17-Ketosteroids		
Males	8-22 mg/24 hr	28-76 µmol/day
Females	6-15 mg/24 hr	21-52 µmol/day
Magnesium	6-10 mEq/24 hr	3-5 mmol/day
Metanephrines	0.05-12.00 ng/mg creatinine	0.03-0.70 mmol/mmol creatinine
Osmolality	38-1400 mOsm/kg water	38-1400 mOsm/kg water
pH	4.6-8.0	4.6-8.0
Phenylpyruvic acid, qualitative	Negative	Negative
Phosphate	0.4-1.3 g/24 hr	13-42 mmol/day
Porphobilinogen		
Qualitative	Negative	Negative
Quantitative	<2 mg/24 hr	<9 µmol/day
Porphyrins		
Coproporphyrin	50-250 mcg/24 hr	77-380 nmol/day
Uroporphyrin	10-30 mcg/24 hr	12-36 nmol/day
Potassium	25-125 mEq/24 hr	25-125 mmol/day
Pregnanediol		
Males	0.0-1.9 mg/24 hr	0.0-6.0 µmol/day
Females		
• Proliferative phase	0.0-2.6 mg/24 hr	0.0-8.0 µmol/day
• Luteal phase	2.6-10.6 mg/24 hr	8-33 µmol/day
• Postmenopausal	0.2-1.0 mg/24 hr	0.6-3.1 µmol/day
Pregnanetriol	0.0-2.5 mg/24 hr	0.0-7.4 µmol/day
Protein, total		
Qualitative	Negative	Negative
Quantitative	10-150 mg/24 hr	10-150 mg/day
Protein/creatinine ratio	<0.2	<0.2
Sodium (regular diet)	60-260 mEq/24 hr	60-260 mmol/day
Specific gravity		
Random specimen	1.003-1.030	1.003-1.030
24-hr collection	1.015-1.025	1.015-1.025
Urate (regular diet)	250-750 mg/24 hr	1.5-4.4 mmol/day
Urobilinogen	0.5-4.0 mg/24 hr	0.6-6.8 µmol/day
Vanillylmandelic acid (VMA)	1.0-8.0 mg/24 hr	5-40 µmol/day

Table A-5   Reference Intervals for Toxic Substances

ANALYTE	CONVENTIONAL UNITS	SI UNITS
Arsenic, urine	<130 mcg/24 hr	<1.7 µmol/day
Bromides, serum, inorganic Toxic symptoms	<100 mg/dL 140-1000 mg/dL	<10 mmol/L 14-100 mmol/L

Carboxyhemoglobin, blood
    Urban environment
    Smokers
	Saturation, percent
	<5%
	<12%
		
		<0.05
		<0.12

Symptoms
    Headache
    Nausea and vomiting
    Potentially lethal
	
	>15%
	>25%
	>50%
		
		>0.15
		>0.25
		>0.50

Ethanol, blood
 	
    Intoxication
 	
    Marked intoxication
 	
    Alcoholic stupor
 	
    Coma
	<0.05 mg/dL
	<0.005%
	>100 mg/dL
	>0.1%
	300-400 mg/dL
	0.3%-0.4%
	400-500 mg/dL
	0.4%-0.5%
	>500 mg/dL
	>0.5%
		<1.0 mmol/L
		
		>22 mmol/L
		
		65-87 mmol/L
		
		87-109 mmol/L
		
		>109 mmol/L

Lead, blood
    Adults
    Children
	
	<20 mcg/dL
	<10 mcg/dL
		
		<1.0 µmol/L
		<0.5 µmol/L

Lead, urine	<80 mcg/24 hr	<0.4 µmol/day
Mercury, urine	<10 mcg/24 hr	<150 nmol/day

Table A-6   Reference Intervals for Tests Performed on Cerebrospinal Fluid

TEST	CONVENTIONAL UNITS	SI UNITS
Cells	<5 mm^3; all mononuclear	<5 × 10^6/L, all mononuclear
Protein electrophoresis	Albumin predominant	Albumin predominant
Glucose	50-75 mg/dL (20 mg/dL less than in serum)	2.8-4.2 mmol/L (1.1 mmol/L less than in serum)

IgG
    Children <14 yr
    Adults
	
	<8% of total protein
	<14% of total protein
		
		<0.08 of total protein
		<0.14 of total protein

IgG index	0.3-0.6	0.3-0.6
Oligoclonal banding on electrophoresis	Absent	Absent
Pressure, opening	70-180 mm H$_2$O	70-180 mm H$_2$O
Protein, total	15-45 mg/dL	150-450 mg/L

Table A-7   Reference Intervals for Tests of Gastrointestinal Function

TEST	CONVENTIONAL UNITS
Bentiromide	6-hr urinary arylamine excretion >57% excludes pancreatic insufficiency
β-Carotene, serum	60-250 ng/dL

Fecal fat estimation
    Qualitative
    Quantitative
	
	No fat globules seen by high-power microscope
	<6 g/24 hr (>95% coefficient of fat absorption)

Gastric acid output
    Basal
    • Males
    • Females
	
	0.0-10.5 mmol/hr
	0.0-5.6 mmol/hr

Table A-7 | Reference Intervals for Tests of Gastrointestinal Function—cont'd

TEST	CONVENTIONAL UNITS
Gastric acid output—Cont'd	
Maximum (after histamine or pentagastrin)	
• Males	9.0-48.0 mmol/hr
• Females	6.0-31.0 mmol/hr
Ratio: basal/maximum	
• Males	0.0-0.31
• Females	0.0-0.29
Secretin test, pancreatic fluid	
Volume	>1.8 mL/kg/hr
Bicarbonate	>80 mEq/L
D-Xylose absorption test, urine	>20% of ingested dose excreted in 5 hr

Table A-8 | Reference Intervals for Tests of Immunologic Function

TEST	CONVENTIONAL UNITS	SI UNITS
Complement, serum		
C3	85-175 mg/dL	0.85-1.75 g/L
C4	15-45 mg/dL	150-450 mg/L
Total hemolytic (CH$_{50}$)	150-250 U/mL	150-250 U/mL
Immunoglobulins, serum, adult		
IgG	640-1350 mg/dL	6.4-13.5 g/L
IgA	70-310 mg/dL	0.70-3.1 g/L
IgM	90-350 mg/dL	0.90-3.5 g/L
IgD	0.0-6.0 mg/dL	0.0-60 mg/L
IgE	0.0-430 ng/dL	0.0-430 mg/L
Autoantibodies, serum, adult		
Antinuclear antibody	<1:40	
Anti-dsDNA antibody	0-40 IU	0-40 IU/mL
Anti-CCP	0-19 units	
Rheumatoid factor	0-30 mg/dL	

Table A-9 | Lymphocyte Subsets, Whole Blood, Heparinized

ANTIGEN(S) EXPRESSED	CELL TYPE	PERCENTAGE (%)	ABSOLUTE CELL COUNT
CD3	Total T cells	56-77	860-1880
CD19	Total B cells	7-17	140-370
CD3 and CD4	Helper-inducer cells	32-54	550-1190
CD3 and CD8	Suppressor-cytotoxic cells	24-37	430-1060
CD3 and DR	Activated T cells	5-14	70-310
CD2	E rosette T cells	73-87	1040-2160
CD16 and CD56	Natural killer (NK) cells	8-22	130-500
Helper/suppressor ratio: 0.8-1.8			

Table A-10 | Reference Values for Semen Analysis

TEST	CONVENTIONAL UNITS	SI UNITS
Volume	2-5 mL	2-5 mL
Liquefaction	Complete in 15 min	Complete in 15 min
pH	7.2-8.0	7.2-8.0
Leukocytes	Occasional or absent	Occasional or absent
Spermatozoa		
Count	$60\text{-}150 \times 10^6$ mL	$60\text{-}150 \times 10^6$ mL
Motility	>80% motile	>0.80 motile
Morphology	80%-90% normal forms	>0.80-0.90 normal forms
Fructose	>150 mg/dL	>8.33 mmol/L

Assume that every person is potentially infected or colonized with an organism that could be transmitted in the health care setting and apply the following infection control practices during the delivery of health care. *Category 1B/1 C*

A. HAND HYGIENE

1. During the delivery of health care, avoid unnecessary touching of surfaces in close proximity to the patient to prevent (1) contamination of clean hands from environmental surfaces and (2) transmission of pathogens from contaminated hands to surfaces.
2. When your hands are visibly dirty, contaminated with proteinaceous material, or visibly soiled with blood or body fluids, wash your hands with either a non-antimicrobial soap and water or an antimicrobial soap and water. *Category 1A*
3. If your hands are not visibly soiled, or after removing visible material with non-antimicrobial soap and water, decontaminate your hands. The preferred method of hand decontamination is with an alcohol-based hand rub. Alternatively, hands may be washed with an antimicrobial soap and water. Frequent use of alcohol-based hand rub immediately following handwashing with non-antimicrobial soap may increase the frequency of dermatitis. *Category 1B*
   Perform hand hygiene:
   • Before having direct contact with patients
   • After contact with blood, body fluids or excretions, mucous membranes, nonintact skin, or wound dressings
   • After contact with a patient's intact skin (e.g., when taking a pulse or blood pressure or lifting a patient)
   • If your hands will be moving from a contaminated body site to a clean body site during patient care
   • After contact with inanimate objects (including medical equipment) in the immediate vicinity of the patient
   • After removing gloves

4. Wash your hands with non-antimicrobial soap and water or with antimicrobial soap and water if contact with spores (e.g., *Clostridium difficile* or *Bacillus anthracis*) is likely to have occurred. The physical action of washing and rinsing your hands under such circumstances is recommended because alcohols, chlorhexidine, iodophors, and other antiseptic agents have poor activity against spores. *Category II*
5. Do not wear artificial fingernails or extenders if duties include direct contact with patients who are at high risk for infection and associated adverse outcomes (e.g., those in intensive care units [ICUs] or operating rooms). *Category 1A*
   • Develop an organizational policy on the wearing of nonnatural nails by health care personnel who have direct contact with patients outside of the groups specified above.

B. PERSONAL PROTECTIVE EQUIPMENT (PPE)

Observe the following principles of use:
   • Wear PPE when the nature of anticipated patient interaction indicates that contact with blood or body fluids may occur. *Category 1B/1 C*
   • Prevent contamination of clothing and skin during the process of removing PPE. *Category II*
   • Before leaving the patient's room or cubicle, remove and discard PPE. *Category 1B/1 C*

GLOVES

Wear gloves when it can be reasonably anticipated that contact with blood or other potentially infectious materials, mucous membranes, nonintact skin, or potentially contaminated intact skin (e.g., of a patient incontinent of stool or urine) could occur. Wear gloves with fit and durability appropriate to the task. Wear disposable medical examination gloves for providing direct patient care. Wear disposable medical examination gloves or reusable utility gloves for cleaning the environment or medical equipment. Remove gloves after contact with a patient and/or the surrounding environment (including medical equipment) using proper technique to prevent hand contamination. Do not wear the same pair of gloves for the care of more than one patient. Do not wash gloves for the purpose of reuse since this practice has been associated with transmission of pathogens. Change gloves during patient care if your hands will move from a contaminated body site (e.g., perineal area) to a clean body site (e.g., face).

---

*Sections pertinent to adult health care nursing extracted from Siegel, J.D., Rhinehart, E., Jackson, M., et al. (2007). *Guideline for Isolation Precautions: Preventing Transmission of Infectious Agents in Healthcare Settings 2007*. Atlanta: Centers for Disease Control and Prevention.

GOWNS

Wear a gown that is appropriate to the task to protect skin and prevent soiling or contamination of clothing during procedures and patient care activities when contact with blood, body fluids, secretions, or excretions is anticipated. Wear a gown for direct patient contact if the patient has uncontained secretions or excretions. Remove gown and perform hand hygiene before leaving the patient's environment. Do not reuse gowns, even for repeated contacts with the same patient. Routine donning of gowns on entrance into a high-risk unit (e.g., ICU, neonatal ICU [NICU]) is not indicated.

MOUTH, NOSE, AND EYE PROTECTION

Use PPE to protect the mucous membranes of your eyes, nose, and mouth during procedures and patient care activities that are likely to generate splashes or sprays of blood, body fluids, secretions, and excretions. Select masks, goggles, face shields, and combinations of each according to the need anticipated by the task performed. During aerosol-generating procedures (e.g., bronchoscopy, suctioning of the respiratory tract [if not using in-line suction catheters], endotracheal intubation) in patients who are not suspected of being infected with an agent for which respiratory protection is otherwise recommended (e.g., *Mycobacterium tuberculosis*, SARS, or hemorrhagic fever viruses), wear one of the following: a face shield that fully covers the front and sides of the face, a mask with attached shield, or a mask and goggles (in addition to gloves and gown).

PATIENT CARE EQUIPMENT AND INSTRUMENTS/DEVICES

Establish policies and procedures for containing, transporting, and handling patient care equipment and instruments/devices that may be contaminated with blood or body fluids. Remove organic material from critical and semicritical instruments/devices, using recommended cleaning agents before high-level disinfection and sterilization to enable effective disinfection and sterilization processes. Wear PPE (e.g., gloves, gown), according to the level of anticipated contamination when handling patient care equipment and instruments/devices that are visibly soiled or may have been in contact with blood or body fluids.

CARE OF THE ENVIRONMENT

Establish policies and procedures for routine and targeted cleaning of environmental surfaces as indicated by the level of patient contact and degree of soiling. Clean and disinfect surfaces that are likely to be contaminated with pathogens, including those that are in close proximity to the patient (e.g., bed rails, overbed tables) and frequently touched surfaces in the patient care environment (i.e., door knobs, surfaces in and surrounding toilets in patients' rooms) on a more frequent schedule compared to that for other surfaces (e.g., horizontal surfaces in waiting rooms). Use Environmental Protection Agency (EPA)–registered disinfectants that have microbiocidal (i.e., killing) activity against the pathogens most likely to contaminate the patient care environment. Use in accordance with manufacturer's instructions. Review the efficacy of in-use disinfectants when evidence of continuing transmission of an infectious agent (e.g., rotavirus, *C. difficile,* norovirus) may indicate resistance to the in-use product and change to a more effective disinfectant as indicated.

TEXTILES AND LAUNDRY

Handle used textiles and fabrics with minimum agitation to avoid contamination of air, surfaces, and persons. If laundry chutes are used, ensure that they are properly designed, maintained, and used in a manner to minimize dispersion of aerosols from contaminated laundry.

SAFE INJECTION PRACTICES

The following recommendations apply to the use of needles, cannulas that replace needles, and, where applicable, intravenous delivery systems. Use aseptic technique to avoid contamination of sterile injection equipment. Do not administer medications from a syringe to multiple patients even if the needle or cannula of the syringe is changed. Needles, cannulas, and syringes are sterile, single-use items; they should not be reused for another patient nor to access a medication or solution that might be used for a subsequent patient. Use fluid infusion and administration sets (i.e., intravenous bags, tubing, and connectors) for one patient only and dispose of appropriately after use. Consider a syringe or needle/cannula contaminated once it has been used to enter or connect to a patient's intravenous infusion bag or administration set. Use single-dose vials for parenteral medications whenever possible. Do not administer medications from single-dose vials or ampules to multiple patients or combine leftover contents for later use. If multidose vials must be used, both the needle or cannula and syringe used to access the multidose vial must be sterile. Do not keep multidose vials in the immediate patient treatment area, and store them in accordance with the manufacturer's recommendations; discard if sterility is compromised or questionable. Do not use bags or bottles of intravenous solution as a common source of supply for multiple patients.

Infection control practices for special lumbar puncture procedures: wear a surgical mask when placing a catheter or injecting material into the spinal canal or subdural space (i.e., during myelograms, lumbar puncture, and spinal or epidural anesthesia).

WORKER SAFETY

Adhere to federal and state requirements for protection of health care personnel from exposure to bloodborne pathogens.

Standard Steps for All Nursing Procedures

AT THE BEGINNING OF THE PROCEDURE

STEP A: PERFORM TASK ACCORDING TO PROTOCOL

- Mentally review the steps of the task beforehand. If you are uncertain how to do a task, ask your team leader, resource nurse, instructor, or charge nurse.
- Plan for efficiency of time and effort while delivering safe care.

STEP B: CHECK ORDERS, COLLECT EQUIPMENT AND SUPPLIES, AND PERFORM HAND HYGIENE

- Verify that the procedure is to be done for the patient.
- Check the agency's policies and procedures manual for the accepted method of performing the procedure.
- Process equipment and supply charges.
- Take all equipment and supplies to the patient's room.

STEP C: IDENTIFY AND PREPARE PATIENT

- Greet the patient, introduce yourself, and check the patient's identification band. Use two identifiers during the identification process.
- Explain what you are going to do in terms the patient can understand.
- Elicit questions and answer clearly.
- Provide necessary teaching related to the procedure to be performed.

STEP D: PROVIDE PRIVACY, INSTITUTE SAFETY PRECAUTIONS, ARRANGE SUPPLIES AND EQUIPMENT

- Close the door or curtains and drape the patient before beginning the procedure or discussing information the person might want kept confidential.
- Check equipment for breaks or wear and for safety.
- Set up the equipment and supplies in an orderly, methodical fashion.
- Raise the bed to an appropriate working height.
- Raise the side rail before turning the patient and be certain that the wheels are locked.
- Perform hand hygiene to prevent contaminating the patient with organisms from the chart, the nurses' station, and the supply room.

DURING THE PROCEDURE

STEP E: USE STANDARD PRECAUTIONS AND ASEPTIC TECHNIQUE AS APPROPRIATE

- Protect yourself from blood and body fluids by wearing gloves.
- If there is a danger of splashing blood or body fluids, wear protective glasses or goggles and an impermeable cover gown or apron.
- Be very careful with sharp instruments and needles so as not to nick your skin. (See Appendix B, Standard Precautions.)

AT THE END OF THE PROCEDURE

STEP X: REMOVE GLOVES AND OTHER PROTECTIVE EQUIPMENT

- After making certain the patient is clean and dry, dispose of used supplies, remove goggles and other protective equipment, and discard or store appropriately.
- To remove gloves without contaminating yourself, begin by pulling one glove off without touching your skin; hold the removed glove in the palm of the remaining gloved hand and then reach to the inside of the other glove and roll it down the hand.
- Dispose of the gloves in the trash.
- Perform hand hygiene immediately.

STEP Y: RESTORE UNIT

- Collect the used equipment; dispose of, clean, or store items in the proper places.
- Make the person comfortable, tidy the bed and unit, place the call light and personal items within reach, and provide for safety by lowering the bed.
- Remove used equipment.
- Place soiled linens in a soiled-linen hamper.
- Clean reusable items and return them to the storage or processing area (central supply). Discontinue use of the equipment on the computer so no further charges will be made.
- Remove unsightly, odorous, or potentially infectious trash from the room.
- Inquire if anything else is needed.
- Perform hand hygiene before leaving the room.

STEP Z: RECORD AND REPORT PROCEDURE

- Document assessment findings and the details of the procedure performed, or care given, in the chart. Include any problems encountered and the patient's response to the care or treatment. The recording should be accurate, specific, concise, and appropriate and should include the specific time the procedure was performed and how it was done.
- Report abnormalities encountered to the charge nurse or physician.

CHAPTER 1
1. 1
2. 4
3. 3
4. 3
5. 1
6. 3
7. 4
8. 2
9. 1, 2
10. 2, 3

CHAPTER 2
1. 3
2. 2
3. 3
4. 2
5. 4
6. 3
7. 1, 3
8. 2, 3, 4, 5
9. 1, 2, 4, 5
10. 1, 3, 4, 5

CHAPTER 3
1. 3
2. 2
3. 1
4. 4
5. 3
6. 1
7. 2
8. 1, 2, 3
9. 1, 2, 5
10. 1, 3

CHAPTER 4
1. 2
2. 2
3. 1
4. 3
5. 2
6. 1
7. 3
8. 1, 4, 5
9. 1, 3, 5
10. 1, 2, 3

CHAPTER 5
1. 3
2. 4
3. 4
4. 1
5. 2

6. 1
7. 2
8. 2
9. 1, 4, 5
10. 1, 2, 3, 5

CHAPTER 6
1. 1
2. 2
3. 4
4. 4
5. 2
6. 2
7. 4
8. 2
9. 3
10. 2, 3, 4

CHAPTER 7
1. 4
2. 2
3. 3
4. 4
5. 2
6. 2
7. 1
8. 2
9. 1
10. 1, 2, 3, 4

CHAPTER 8
1. 1
2. 4
3. 4
4. 2
5. 3
6. 2
7. 3
8. 3
9. 1, 3, 4
10. 1, 3, 5

CHAPTER 9
1. 1
2. 4
3. 4
4. 4
5. 3
6. 3
7. 1
8. 1
9. 1, 3, 4
10. 2, 3, 4

CHAPTER 10
1. 2
2. 1
3. 1
4. 2
5. 2
6. 4
7. 2
8. 1
9. 1
10. 2

CHAPTER 11
1. 3
2. 1
3. 3
4. 4
5. 1
6. 1
7. 4
8. 1
9. 1, 2
10. 1, 2, 3

CHAPTER 12
1. 3
2. 3
3. 1
4. 3
5. 2
6. 1
7. 2, 3, 4
8. 1, 2, 3, 4
9. 1, 4, 5
10. 1, 2, 3, 4

CHAPTER 13
1. 3
2. 4
3. 2
4. 4
5. 3
6. 2
7. 2
8. 2
9. 3
10. 1, 3, 5

CHAPTER 14
1. 3
2. 2
3. 1, 2, 5
4. 2
5. 2, 3, 4, 5, 6

6. 1, 4, 5
7. 2
8. 2
9. 2
10. 4

CHAPTER 15
1. 4
2. 2
3. 3
4. 2
5. 2
6. 1
7. 2
8. 4
9. 2, 3, 5
10. 1, 3, 5

CHAPTER 16
1. 3
2. 2, 5
3. 1
4. 4
5. 1
6. 2
7. 1
8. 2, 4
9. 2
10. 3, 4, 1, 2

CHAPTER 17
1. 1
2. 2, 3, 5
3. 3
4. 2
5. 4
6. 1, 3, 4, 6
7. 3
8. 2
9. 2-5 weeks
10. 1, 3, 5, 6

CHAPTER 18
1. 2, 4, 5
2. 3
3. 0.6
4. 1
5. 2
6. 1
7. 3
8. 2, 4, 5
9. 2
10. 2, 3, 4

CHAPTER 19
1. 4
2. 1, 2, 3, 4, 6
3. 3
4. 2
5. 4
6. 2
7. 1
8. 1
9. 2
10. 1, 3, 4, 5, 6

CHAPTER 20
1. 3, 4
2. 2
3. 1
4. 2
5. 2
6. 4
7. 2
8. 3
9. 3
10. 3

CHAPTER 21
1. 1, 2, 3
2. 2
3. 3
4. 1
5. 1, 2, 4, 5
6. 1
7. 4
8. 3
9. 1, 2, 5
10. 4

CHAPTER 22
1. 2
2. 2
3. 2
4. 1
5. 3
6. 2
7. 3
8. 1
9. 2
10. 2, 4, 5

CHAPTER 23
1. 3
2. 1, 3, 4
3. 1
4. 2
5. 2

6. Cushing's triad
7. 3
8. 2, 3, 4
9. 3
10. 1

CHAPTER 24
1. 3
2. 1, 2, 3, 4
3. 4
4. Arteriovenous malformation
5. 1, 2, 3, 5
6. 1
7. 2
8. 1, 2, 3
9. 3
10. 2

CHAPTER 25
1. 3
2. 1, 3, 4
3. 1
4. 4
5. Cholinergic crisis
6. 2
7. 1
8. 3
9. 3
10. 3, 4

CHAPTER 26
1. 4
2. 2
3. 1, 3, 5
4. 2
5. 4
6. 4
7. 3
8. 2
9. 2
10. 1, 4, 5

CHAPTER 27
1. 2
2. 2
3. 4
4. 3
5. Retinopathy
6. 1, 2, and 5
7. 1
8. 2
9. 2
10. 1, 3, 4

CHAPTER 28
1. 3
2. 3
3. 2
4. 2
5. 3
6. 3
7. 4
8. 1, 2, 3
9. 1, 2, 3
10. 20.83 or 21 gtt/min

CHAPTER 29
1. 4
2. 3
3. 1, 2, 3, 4
4. 1
5. 2
6. 3
7. 3
8. 2
9. 3, 6
10. 1000 mL/hr

CHAPTER 30
1. 2
2. 2
3. 3
4. 2
5. 4
6. 4
7. 3
8. 4
9. 1, 3, 5
10. 2, 3, 4

CHAPTER 31
1. 3
2. 3
3. 1
4. 2
5. 2
6. 3
7. 3
8. 2
9. 4
10. 1, 2, 4

CHAPTER 32
1. 2
2. 1, 4, 5
3. 2
4. 4
5. 2
6. 2
7. 3
8. 2
9. 3
10. 2

CHAPTER 33
1. 3
2. 2
3. 1
4. 2
5. 4
6. 3
7. 3
8. 3
9. 2
10. 1, 3, 4

CHAPTER 34
1. 1
2. 3
3. 3
4. 2
5. 3

6. 4
7. 2
8. 2, 3
9. 1, 2, 5
10. creatinine

CHAPTER 35
1. 1
2. 1
3. 2
4. 2
5. 3, 5, 1, 2, 4
6. 3
7. 1, 3, 4, 5
8. 1, 3, 4, 5
9. 2
10. 4

CHAPTER 36
1. 4
2. 2
3. 1
4. 2
5. 2
6. 1
7. 2
8. 2
9. 3
10. 1, 2, 4, 5

CHAPTER 37
1. 2
2. 1
3. 2
4. 1, 4
5. 1, 3, 4, 5
6. 2
7. 2
8. 1
9. 1, 2, 4, 5
10. 1

CHAPTER 38
1. 3
2. 1, 3, 7
3. 1, 2, 4, 5
4. 3
5. 4
6. 4
7. 2
8. 2
9. 1
10. 2

CHAPTER 39
1. 2
2. 2
3. 3
4. 4
5. 2
6. 2
7. 1
8. 1, 3, 4, 5
9. 3, 4
10. 2, 4, 5

CHAPTER 40
1. 2
2. 3
3. 2
4. 2
5. 2
6. 2
7. 2
8. 1, 2, 5
9. 1, 2, 4
10. Peyronie's disease

CHAPTER 41
1. 1
2. 2
3. 1
4. 2
5. 1
6. 1, 2, 4
7. 2, 3, 4
8. 1, 2, 5
9. 1, 2, 4
10. Ophthalmia neonatorum

CHAPTER 42
1. 2, 4, 5
2. 1
3. 2
4. 2
5. 3
6. 1
7. 3
8. 4
9. 1, 5
10. 1, 2, 3, 4, 5

CHAPTER 43
1. 1, 2, 4, 5
2. 1, 2, 3, 5
3. 3
4. 4
5. 1, 2, 3, 5
6. 1
7. 4
8. 2
9. 3, 4
10. 4, 3, 2, 1

CHAPTER 44
1. 4
2. 4
3. 3
4. 2
5. 3
6. 1
7. 4
8. 2
9. 1, 3, 4
10. 250 drops/min

CHAPTER 45
1. 1
2. 3
3. 4
4. 2

5. 1, 3, 4, 6
6. 4
7. 4
8. 4
9. 2
10. 3

CHAPTER 46
1. 3
2. 3
3. 4
4. 2
5. 2
6. 3, 4, 5, 7
7. 2
8. 1, 2, 5, 7
9. 1
10. 1

CHAPTER 47
1. 2
2. 2
3. 4
4. 2
5. 1
6. 2
7. 2
8. 1, 2, 3, 6
9. 3
10. 3

CHAPTER 48
1. 4
2. 3
3. 4
4. 3
5. 2
6. 1, 2, 6
7. 1
8. 2
9. 3
10. 1

CHAPTER 49
1. 1
2. 4
3. 3
4. 1
5. 1
6. 4
7. 2
8. 3
9. 1, 3, 4, 5
10. 1, 2, 3, 6

These standards and competencies are intended to better define the range of capabilities, responsibilities, rights, and relationship to other health care providers for scope and content of practical/vocational nursing education programs. The guidelines will assist:

- Educators in development, implementation, and evaluation of practical/vocational nursing curricula.
- Students in understanding expectations of their competencies on completion of the educational program.
- Prospective employers in appropriate utilization of the practical/vocational nurse.
- Consumers in understanding the scope of practice and level of responsibility of the practical/ vocational nurse.

A. PROFESSIONAL BEHAVIORS

Professional behaviors, within the scope of nursing practice for a practical/vocational nurse, are characterized by adherence to standards of care, accountability for one's own actions and behaviors, and use of legal and ethical principles in nursing practice. Professionalism includes a commitment to nursing and a concern for others demonstrated by an attitude of caring. Professionalism also involves participation in life-long self-development activities to enhance and maintain current knowledge and skills for continuing competency in the practice of nursing for the LP/VN, as well as individual, group, community, and societal endeavors to improve health care.

Upon completion of the practical/vocational nursing program the graduate will display the following program outcome:

- Demonstrate professional behaviors of accountability and professionalism according to the legal and ethical standards for a competent licensed practical/vocational nurse.

Competencies which demonstrate this outcome has been attained:

1. Comply with the ethical, legal, and regulatory frameworks of nursing and the scope of practice as outlined in the LP/VN nurse practice act of the specific state in which licensed.
2. Utilize educational opportunities for life-long learning and maintenance of competence.
3. Identify personal capabilities and consider career mobility options.
4. Identify own LP/VN strengths and limitations for the purpose of improving nursing performance.
5. Demonstrate accountability for nursing care provided by self and/or directed to others.
6. Function as an advocate for the health care consumer, maintaining confidentiality as required.
7. Identify the impact of economic, political, social, cultural, spiritual, and demographic forces on the role of the licensed practical/vocational nurse in the delivery of health care.
8. Serve as a positive role model within health care settings and the community.
9. Participate as a member of a practical/vocational nursing organization.

B. COMMUNICATION

Communication is defined as the process by which information is exchanged between individuals verbally, non-verbally, and/or in writing or through information technology. Communication abilities are integral and essential to the nursing process. Those who are included in the nursing process are the licensed practical/vocational nurse and other members of the nursing and health care team, client, and significant support person(s). Effective communication demonstrates caring, compassion, and cultural awareness, and is directed toward promoting positive outcomes and establishing a trusting relationship.

Upon completion of the practical/vocational nursing program the graduate will display the following program outcome:

- Effectively communicate with patients, significant support person(s), and members of the interdisciplinary health care team incorporating interpersonal and therapeutic communication skills.

Competencies which demonstrate this outcome has been attained:

1. Utilize effective communication skills when interacting with clients, significant others, and members of the interdisciplinary health team.

2. Communicate relevant, accurate, and complete information.
3. Report to appropriate health care personnel and document assessments, interventions, and progress or impediments toward achieving client outcomes.
4. Maintain organizational and client confidentiality.
5. Utilize information technology in support and communicate the planning and provision of client care.
6. Utilize appropriate channels of communication.

C. ASSESSMENT*

Assessment is the collection and processing of relevant data for the purposes of appraising the client's health status. Assessment provides a holistic view of the client which includes physical, developmental, emotional, psychosocial, cultural, spiritual, and functional status. Assessment involves the collection of information from multiple sources to provide the foundation for nursing care. Initial assessment provides the baseline for future comparisons in order to individualize client care. Ongoing assessment is required to meet the client's changing needs.

Upon completion of the practical/vocational nursing program the graduate will display the following program outcome:

- Collect holistic assessment data from multiple sources, communicate the data to appropriate health care providers, and evaluate client responses to interventions.

Competencies which demonstrate this outcome has been attained:

1. Assess data related to basic physical, developmental, spiritual, cultural, functional, and psychosocial needs of the client.
2. Collect data within established protocols and guidelines from various sources, including client interviews.
3. Assess data related to the client's health status, identify impediments to client progress and evaluate response to interventions.
4. Document data collection, assessment, and communicate findings to appropriate member(s) of the health care team.

D. PLANNING

Planning encompasses the collection of health status information, the use of multiple methods to access information, and the analysis and integration of knowledge and information to formulate nursing care plans and care actions. The nursing care plan provides

*As approved and adopted by NAPNES Board of Directors May 5, 2007.

direction for individualized care, and assures the delivery of accurate, safe care through a definitive pathway that promotes the client's and support person(s)'s progress toward positive outcomes.

Upon completion of the practical/vocational nursing program the graduate will display the following program outcome:

- Collaborate with the registered nurse or other members of the health care team to organize and incorporate assessment data to plan/revise patient care and actions based on established nursing diagnoses, nursing protocols, and assessment and evaluation data.

Competencies which demonstrate this outcome has been attained:

1. Utilize knowledge of normal values to identify deviation in health status to plan care.
2. Contribute to formulation of a nursing care plan for clients with non-complex conditions and in a stable state, in consultation with the registered nurse and as appropriate in collaboration with the client or support person(s) as well as members of the interdisciplinary health care team using established nursing diagnoses and nursing protocols.
3. Prioritize nursing care needs of clients.
4. Assist in the review and revision of nursing care plans with the registered nurse to meet the changing needs of clients.
5. Modify client care as indicated by the evaluation of stated outcomes.
6. Provide information to client about aspects of the care plan within the LP/VN scope of practice.
7. Refer client as appropriate to other members of the health care team about care outside the scope of practice of the LP/VN.

E. CARING INTERVENTIONS

Caring interventions are those nursing behaviors and actions that assist clients and significant others in meeting their needs and the identified outcomes of the plan of care. These interventions are based on knowledge of the natural sciences, behavioral sciences, and past nursing experiences. Caring is the "being with" and "doing for" that assists clients to achieve the desired outcomes. Caring behaviors are nurturing, protective, compassionate, and person-centered. Caring creates an environment of hope and trust where client choices related to cultural, religious, and spiritual values, beliefs, and lifestyles are respected.

Upon completion of the practical/vocational nursing program the graduate will display the following program outcome:

- Demonstrate a caring and empathic approach to the safe, therapeutic, and individualized care of each client.

Competencies which demonstrate this outcome has been attained:

1. Provide and promote the client's dignity.
2. Identify and honor the emotional, cultural, religious, and spiritual influences on the client's behalf.
3. Demonstrate caring behaviors toward the client and significant support person(s).
4. Provide competent, safe, therapeutic, and individualized nursing care in a variety of settings.
5. Provide a safe physical and psychosocial environment for the client and significant other(s).
6. Implement the prescribed care regimen within the legal, ethical, and regulatory framework of practical/vocational nursing practice.
7. Assist the client and significant support person(s) to cope with and adapt to stressful events and changes in health status.
8. Assist the client and significant other(s) to achieve optimum comfort and functioning.
9. Instruct client regarding individualized health needs in keeping with the licensed practical/vocational nurse's knowledge, competence, and scope of practice.
10. Recognize client's right to access information and refer requests to appropriate person(s).
11. Act in an advocacy role to protect client rights.

F. MANAGING

Managing care is the effective use of human, physical, financial, and technological resources to achieve the client identified outcomes while supporting organizational outcomes. The LP/VN manages care through the processes of planning, organizing, and directing.

Upon completion of the practical/vocational nursing program, the graduate will display the following program outcome:

• Implement patient care, at the direction of a registered nurse, licensed physician, or dentist through performance of nursing interventions or directing aspects of care, as appropriate, to unlicensed assistive personnel (UAP).

Competencies which demonstrate this outcome has been attained:

1. Assist in the coordination and implementation of an individualized plan of care for clients and significant support person(s).
2. Direct aspects of client care to qualified UAPs commensurate with abilities and level of preparation and consistent with the state's legal and regulatory framework for the scope of practice for the LP/VN.
3. Supervise and evaluate the activities of UAPs and other personnel as appropriate within the state's legal and regulatory framework for the scope of practice for the LP/VN as well as facility policy.
4. Maintain accountability for outcomes of care directed to qualified UAPs.
5. Organize nursing activities in a meaningful and cost-effective manner when providing nursing care for individuals or groups.
6. Assist the client and significant support person(s) to access available resources and services.
7. Demonstrate competence with current technologies.
8. Function within the defined scope of practice for the LP/VN in the health care delivery system at the direction of a registered nurse, licensed physician, or dentist.

NFLPN Nursing Practice Standards for the Licensed Practical/Vocational Nurse*

Nursing Practice Standards is one of the ways that NFLPN meets the objective of its bylaws to address principles and ethics and also to meet another Article II objective, "To interpret the standards of practical (vocational) nursing."

In recent years, LPNs and LVNs have practiced in a changing environment. As LPNs and LVNs practice in expanding roles in the health care system, *Nursing Practice Standards* is essential reading for LPNs, LVNs, PN, and VN students and their educators, and all who practice with LPNs and LVNs.

NURSING PRACTICE STANDARDS FOR THE LICENSED PRACTICAL/ VOCATIONAL NURSE

PREFACE

The Standards were developed and adopted by NFLPN to provide a basic model whereby the quality of health service and nursing service and nursing care given by LP/VNs may be measured and evaluated.

These nursing practice standards are applicable in any practice setting. The degree to which individual standards are applied will vary according to the individual needs of the patient, the type of health care agency or services, and the community resources.

The scope of licensed practical nursing has extended into specialized nursing services. Therefore specialized fields of nursing are included in this document.

THE CODE FOR LICENSED PRACTICAL/ VOCATIONAL NURSES

The Code, adopted by NFLPN in 1961 and revised in 1979, provides a motivation for establishing, maintaining, and elevating professional standards. Each LP/VN, upon entering the profession, inherits the responsibility to adhere to the standards of ethical practice and conduct as set forth in this Code.

1. Know the scope of maximum utilization of the LP/VN as specified by the nurse practice act and function within this scope.
2. Safeguard the confidential information acquired from any source about the patient.

---

*From National Federation of Licensed Practical Nurses, Inc.

3. Provide health care to all patients regardless of race, creed, cultural background, disease, or lifestyle.
4. Uphold the highest standards in personal appearance, language, dress, and demeanor.
5. Stay informed about issues affecting the practice of nursing and delivery of health care and, when appropriate, participate in government and policy decisions.
6. Accept the responsibility for safe nursing by keeping oneself mentally and physically fit and educationally prepared to practice.
7. Accept responsibility for membership in NFLPN and participate in its efforts to maintain the established standards of nursing practice and employment policies that lead to quality patient care.

INTRODUCTORY STATEMENT

DEFINITION

Practical/Vocational nursing means the performance for compensation of authorized acts of nursing that utilize specialized knowledge and skills and that meet the health needs of people in a variety of settings under the direction of qualified health professionals.

SCOPE

Licensed Practical/Vocational nurses represent the established entry into the nursing profession and include specialized fields of nursing practice.

Opportunities exist for practicing in a milieu where different professions unite their particular skills in a team effort: to preserve or improve an individual patient's functioning and to protect health and safety of patients.

Opportunities also exist for career advancement within the profession through academic education and for lateral expansion of knowledge and expertise through both academic/continuing education and certification.

STANDARDS

EDUCATION

The Licensed Practical/Vocational Nurse
1. Shall complete a formal education program in practical nursing approved by the appropriate nursing authority in a state.

2. Shall successfully pass the National Council Licensure Examination for Practical Nurses.
3. Shall participate in initial orientation within the employing institution.

LEGAL/ETHICAL STATUS

The Licensed Practical/Vocational Nurse

1. Shall hold a current license to practice nursing as an LP/VN in accordance with the law of the state wherein employed.
2. Shall know the scope of nursing practice authorized by the nurse practice act in the state wherein employed.
3. Shall have a personal commitment to fulfill the legal responsibilities inherent in good nursing practice.
4. Shall take responsible actions in situations wherein there is unprofessional conduct by a peer or other health care provider.
5. Shall recognize and have a commitment to meet the ethical and moral obligations of the practice of nursing.
6. Shall not accept or perform professional responsibilities that the individual knows he or she is not competent to perform.

PRACTICE

The Licensed Practical/Vocational Nurse

1. Shall accept assigned responsibilities as an accountable member of the health care team.
2. Shall function within the limits of educational preparation and experience as related to the assigned duties.
3. Shall function with other members of the health care team in promoting and maintaining health, preventing disease and disability, caring for and rehabilitating individuals who are experiencing an altered health state, and contributing to the ultimate quality of life until death.
4. Shall know and utilize the nursing process in planning, implementing, and evaluating health services and nursing care for the individual patient or group.
   a. Planning: The planning of nursing includes:
      (1) Assessment/data collection of health status of the individual patient, the family, and community groups
      (2) Reporting information gained from assessment/data collection
      (3) The identification of health goals.
   b. Implementation: The plan for nursing care is put into practice to achieve the stated goals and includes:
      (1) Observing, recording, and reporting significant changes that require intervention or different goals
      (2) Applying nursing knowledge and skills to promote and maintain health, to prevent disease and disability and to optimize functional capabilities of an individual patient

      (3) Assisting the patient and family with activities of daily living and encouraging self-care as appropriate
      (4) Carrying out therapeutic regimens and protocols prescribed by personnel pursuant to authorized state law
   c. Evaluations: The plan for nursing care and its implementations are evaluated to measure the progress toward the stated goals and will include appropriate person and/or groups to determine:
      (1) The relevancy of current goals in relation to the progress of the individual patient
      (2) The involvement of the recipients of care in the evaluation process
      (3) The quality of the nursing action in the implementation of the plan
      (4) A re-ordering of priorities or new goal setting in the care plan
5. Shall participate in peer review and other evaluation processes.
6. Shall participate in the development of policies concerning the health and nursing needs of society and in the roles and functions of the LP/VN.

CONTINUING EDUCATION

The Licensed Practical/Vocational Nurse

1. Shall be responsible for maintaining the highest possible level of professional competence at all times.
2. Shall periodically reassess career goals and select continuing education activities that will help achieve these goals.
3. Shall take advantage of continuing education and certification opportunities that will lead to personal growth and professional development.
4. Shall seek and participate in continued education activities that are approved for credit by appropriate organizations, such as the NFLPN.

SPECIALIZED NURSING PRACTICE

The Licensed Practical/Vocational Nurse

1. Shall have had at least 1 year's experience in nursing at the staff level.
2. Shall present personal qualifications that are indicative of potential abilities for practice in the chosen specialized nursing area.
3. Shall present evidence of completion of a program or course that is approved by an appropriate agency to provide the knowledge and skills necessary for effective nursing services in the specialized field.
4. Shall meet all of the standards of practice as set forth in this document.

GLOSSARY

authorized (acts of nursing) Those nursing activities made legal through state nurse practice acts.
career advancement A change of career goal.

lateral expansion of knowledge An extension of the basic core of information learned in the school of practical nursing.

LPN/LVN A combined abbreviation for licensed practical nurse and licensed vocational nurse. LVN is the title used in California and Texas for the nurses who are called LPNs in other states.

milieu One's environment and surroundings.

peer review A formal evaluation of performance on the job by other LPN/LVNs.

protocols Courses of treatment that include specific steps to be performed in a stated order.

special nursing practice A restricted field of nursing in which a person is particularly skilled and has specific knowledge.

therapeutic regimens Regulated plans designed to bring about effective treatment of disease.

American Hospital Association: The Patient Care Partnership—Understanding Expectations, Rights, and Responsibilities*

When you need hospital care, your physician and the nurses and other professionals at our hospital are committed to working with you and your family to meet your health care needs. Our dedicated physicians and staff serve the community in all its ethnic, religious, and economic diversity. Our goal is for you and your family to have the same care and attention we would want for our families and ourselves.

The sections explain some of the basics about how you can expect to be treated during your hospital stay. They also cover what we will need from you to care for you better. If you have questions at any time, please ask them. Unasked or unanswered questions can add to the stress of being in the hospital. Your comfort and confidence in your care are very important to us.

WHAT TO EXPECT DURING YOUR HOSPITAL STAY

HIGH-QUALITY HOSPITAL CARE

Our first priority is to provide you the care you need, when you need it, with skill, compassion, and respect. Tell your caregivers if you have concerns about your care or if you have pain. You have the right to know the identity of physicians, nurses, and others involved in your care, and you have the right to know when they are students, residents, or other trainees.

A CLEAN AND SAFE ENVIRONMENT

Our hospital works hard to keep you safe. We use special policies and procedures to avoid mistakes in your care and keep you free from abuse or neglect. If anything unexpected and significant happens during your hospital stay, you will be told what happened, and any resulting changes in your care will be discussed with you.

INVOLVEMENT IN YOUR CARE

You and your physician often make decisions about your care before you go to the hospital. Other times, especially in emergencies, those decisions are made during your hospital stay. When decision making takes place, it should include:

Discussing Your Medical Condition and Information about Medically Appropriate Treatment Choices

To make informed decisions with your physician, you need to understand:

- The benefits and risks of each treatment
- Whether your treatment is experimental or part of a research study
- What you can reasonably expect from your treatment and any long-term effects it might have on your quality of life
- What you and your family will need to do after you leave the hospital
- The financial consequences of using uncovered services or out-of-network providers

Please tell your caregivers if you need more information about treatment choices.

Discussing Your Treatment Plan

When you enter the hospital, you sign a general consent to treatment. In some cases, such as surgery or experimental treatment, you may be asked to confirm in writing that you understand what is planned and agree to it. This process protects your right to consent to or refuse a treatment. Your physician will explain the medical consequences of refusing recommended treatment. It also protects your right to decide if you want to participate in a research study.

Getting Information from You

Your caregivers need complete and correct information about your health and coverage so that they can make good decisions about your care. That includes:

- Past illnesses, surgeries, or hospital stays
- Past allergic reactions
- Any medicines or dietary supplements (such as vitamins and herbs) that you are taking
- Any network or admission requirements under your health plan

Understanding Your Health Care Goals and Values

You may have health care goals and values or spiritual beliefs that are important to your well-being. They will be taken into account as much as possible throughout your hospital stay. Make sure your physician, your family, and your care team know your wishes.

Understanding Who Should Make Decisions When You Cannot

If you have signed a health care power of attorney stating who should speak for you if you become unable to make health care decisions for yourself, or a "living will" or "advance directive" that states your wishes about end-of-life care, give copies to your physician, your family, and your care team. If you or your family need help making difficult decisions, counselors, chaplains, and others are available to help.

PROTECTING YOUR PRIVACY

We respect the confidentiality of your relationship with your physician and other caregivers, and the sensitive information about your health and health care that are part of that relationship. State and federal laws and hospital operating policies protect the privacy of your medical information. You will receive a Notice of Privacy Practices that describes the ways that we use, disclose, and safeguard patient information and that explains how you can obtain a copy of information from our records about your care.

PREPARING YOU AND YOUR FAMILY FOR WHEN YOU LEAVE THE HOSPITAL

Your physician works with hospital staff and professionals in your community. You and your family also play an important role in your care. The success of your treatment often depends on your efforts to follow medication, diet, and therapy plans. Your family may need to help care for you at home.

You can expect us to help you identify sources of follow-up care and to let you know if our hospital has a financial interest in any referrals. As long as you agree that we can share information about your care with them, we will coordinate our activities with your caregivers outside the hospital. You can also expect to receive information and, when possible, training about the self-care you will need when you go home.

HELP WITH YOUR BILL AND FILING INSURANCE CLAIMS

Our staff will file claims for you with health care insurers or other programs such as Medicare and Medicaid. They also will help your physician with needed documentation. Hospital bills and insurance coverage are often confusing. If you have questions about your bill, contact our business office. If you need help understanding your insurance coverage or health care plan, start with your insurance company or health benefits manager. If you do not have health care coverage, we will try to help you and your family find financial help or make other arrangements. We need your help with collecting needed information and other requirements to obtain coverage or assistance.

Reader References

GENERAL RESOURCES

Ackley, B. J., Ladwig, G. B., Swan, B. A., & Tucker, S. J. (2008). *Evidence-Based Nursing Care Guidelines: Medical Surgical Interventions*. St. Louis: Mosby.

Ackley, B. J., & Ladwig, G. B. (2011). *Nursing Diagnosis Handbook: An Evidence-Based Guide to Planning Care* (9th ed.). St. Louis: Mosby.

Alfaro-Lefevre, R. (2009). *Critical Thinking and Clinical Judgment: A Practical Approach to Outcome-Focused Thinking* (4th ed.). St. Louis: Elsevier.

Agency for Health Care Policy and Research. (1994). *Pressure Ulcer Treatment*. Rockville, MD: U.S. Department of Health and Human Services, Public Health Service.

American Cancer Society. (2011). *Cancer Facts and Figures, 2011*. Atlanta: American Cancer Society.

American Cancer Society. (2011). *Colorectal Cancer Facts and Figures*. Atlanta: American Cancer Society.

American Heart Association. (2010). *Handbook of Emergency Cardiovascular Care*. Dallas: American Heart Association.

American Heart Association, (Eds.), (2011). *Heart Disease and Stroke Statistical Update–2011 Update*. Dallas: American Heart Association.

American Pain Society. (2008). *Principles of Analgesic Use in the Treatment of Acute Pain and Cancer Pain* (6th ed.). Glenview, IL: American Pain Society.

American Psychiatric Association. (2000). *Diagnostic and Statistical Manual of Mental Disorders* (4th ed.). Text Revision. Washington, DC: American Psychiatric Association.

Applegate, E. (2011). *The Anatomy and Physiology Learning System* (4th ed.). Philadelphia: Elsevier Saunders.

Beers, M., & Berkow, R. (Eds.). (2005). *The Merck manual of diagnosis and therapy online*. Retrieved from www.merckmanuals.com/professional/index.html.

Bioterrorism Institute, Ltd. (2005). *Bioterrorism Basics for Nurses CE Program*. Columbus, OH: Bioterrorism Institute.

Black, J. M., & Hawks, J. H. (2009). *Medical-Surgical Nursing: Clinical Management for Positive Outcomes* (8th ed.). Philadelphia: Elsevier Saunders.

Carpenito-Moyet, L. J. (2008). *Nursing Diagnosis: Application to Clinical Practice* (12th ed.). Philadelphia: Lippincott Williams & Wilkins.

Centers for Disease Control and Prevention. (1998). Update: Universal precautions for prevention of transmission of human immunodeficiency virus, hepatitis B virus, and other blood-borne pathogens in health-care settings. *MMWR Morbidity and Mortality Weekly Report, 377*.

Centers for Disease Control and Prevention. (2007). *Recommendations for isolation precautions in hospitals*. Retrieved from www.cdc.gov/hicpac/pdf/isolation/isolation2007.pdf.

Centers for Disease Control and Prevention. (2008). Revised classification system for HIV infection and expanded surveillance case definition for AIDS among adolescents and adults. *MMWR Morbidity and Mortality Weekly Report, 57*(RR-10).

Centers for Disease Control and Prevention, National Center for Injury Prevention and Control. (2009). *10 Leading causes of death*. United States. Retrieved from www.cdc.gov/nchs/fastats/lcod.htm.

Christensen, B., & Kockrow, E. (2011). *Adult Health Nursing* (6th ed.). St. Louis: Mosby.

Christensen, B., & Kockrow, E. (2011). *Foundations of Nursing* (6th ed.). St. Louis: Mosby.

Corbett, J. V. (2008). *Laboratory Tests and Diagnostic Procedures with Nursing Diagnosis* (7th ed.). Upper Saddle River, NJ: Prentice Hall.

deWit, S. C. (2009). *Fundamental Concepts and Skills for Nursing* (3rd ed.). Philadelphia: Elsevier Saunders.

Dorland, I., & Newman, W. A. (2011). *Dorland's Illustrated Medical Dictionary* (32th ed.). Philadelphia: Saunders.

Ebersole, P., Hess, P., Touhy, T., et al. (2008). *Toward Healthy Aging: Human Needs and Human Response* (7th ed.). St. Louis: Mosby.

Ebersole, P., Hess, P., Touhy, T., et al. (2010). *Gerontological Nursing and Healthy Aging* (3rd ed.). St. Louis: Mosby.

Ellsworth, A. J., Witt, D. M., Dugdale, D. C., et al. (2004). *Mosby's Medical Drug Reference*. St. Louis: Mosby.

Emergency Nurses Association. (2009). *Sheehy's Emergency Nursing: Principles & Practice* (5th ed.). St. Louis: Mosby.

Fischbach, F., & Dunning, M. B. (2011). *A Manual of Laboratory and Diagnostic Tests* (8th ed.). Philadelphia: Lippincott Williams & Wilkins.

Fontaine, K. L. (2009). *Complementary and Alternative Therapies for Nursing Practice* (3rd ed.). Upper Saddle River, NJ: Prentice Hall.

Fortinash, K., & Holoday-Worret, P. (2007). *Psychiatric Nursing Care Plans* (5th ed.). St. Louis: Mosby.

Giger, J. N., & Davidhizar, R. E. (2008). *Transcultural Nursing: Assessment & Interventions* (5th ed.). St Louis: Mosby.

Goldman, L., Bennet, J., & Ausiello, D. (Eds.). (2004). *Cecil Textbook of Medicine* (22nd ed.). Philadelphia: Saunders.

Gould, B. E., & Dyer, R. M. (2011). *Pathophysiology for the Health Professions* (4th ed.). Philadelphia: Saunders.

Guyton, A. C., & Hall, J. E. (2011). *Textbook of Medical Physiology* (12th ed.). Philadelphia: Elsevier Saunders.

Haugen, N., & Galura, S. (2011). *Ulrich & Canale's Nursing Care Planning Guides: Prioritization, Delegation, and Critical Thinking*. St. Louis: Saunders.

Herlihy, B., & Maebius, N. K. (2010). *The Human Body in Health and Illness* (4th ed.). St. Louis: Saunders.

Hill, S., & Howlett, H. (2009). *Success in Practical/Vocational Nursing: From Student to Learner* (6th ed.). Philadelphia: Elsevier Saunders.

Hodgson, B. B., & Kizior, R. J. (2012). *Saunders Nursing Drug Handbook 2012*. Philadelphia: Saunders.

Huether, S. E., & McCance, K. L. (2008). *Understanding Pathophysiology* (4th ed.). St. Louis: Mosby.

Ignatavicius, D. D., & Workman, M. L. (2010). *Medical-Surgical Nursing: Critical Thinking for Collaborative Care* (6th ed.). Philadelphia: Elsevier Saunders.

Jarvis, C. (2008). *Physical Examination & Health Assessment* (5th ed.). Philadelphia: Saunders.

Joint Commission on Accreditation of Healthcare Organizations. (2003). *Universal Protocol for Preventing Wrong Site, Wrong Procedure, Wrong Person Surgery*. Chicago: The Joint Commission.

Joint National Committee on Prevention, Detection, Evaluation, and Treatment of High Blood Pressure. (2003). *The Seventh Report of the Joint National Committee on prevention, detection, evaluation and treatment of high blood pressure*. Available at www.nhlbi.nih/gov/guidelines/hypertension.

Kee, J. L., Hayes, E. R., & McCuistion, L. E. (2009). *Pharmacology: A Nursing Process Approach* (6th ed.). Philadelphia: Saunders.

Kee, L. L. (2009). *Laboratory & Diagnostic Tests with Nursing Implications* (8th ed.). Upper Saddle River, NJ: Pearson Prentice Hall.

Kübler-Ross, E. (1969). *On Death and Dying*. New York: Macmillan.

Kumar, V., Abbas, A. K., & Fausto, N. (Eds.). (2010). *Robbins and Cotran Pathologic Basis of Disease* (8th ed.). Philadelphia: Saunders.

Lantus Prescribing Information. Retrieved from http://products.sanofi-aventis.us/lantus/lantus.html.

Lehne, R. A. (2010). *Pharmacology for Nursing Care* (7th ed.). Philadelphia: Saunders.

Lewis, S. L., Heitkemper, M. M., Dirksen, S. R., et al. (2010). *Medical-Surgical Nursing: Assessment and Management of Clinical Problems* (8th ed.). St. Louis: Mosby.

Linton, A., & Lach, H. (2007). *Matteson & McConnell's Gerontological Nursing: Concepts and Practice* (3rd ed.). St. Louis: Mosby.

Linton, A., Matteson, M., & Maebius, N. (2011). *Introduction to Medical-Surgical Nursing* (5th ed.). Philadelphia: Saunders.

Lowdermilk, D. L., & Perry, S. E. (2001). *Maternity and Women's Health Care* (9th ed.). St. Louis: Mosby.

Mahan, K., & Escott-Stump, S. (2008). *Krause's Food, Nutrition, & Diet Therapy* (12th ed.). Philadelphia: Saunders.

Mandell, G. L., Bennett, J. E., & Dolin, R. (2005). *Mandell, Douglas, and Bennett's Principles and Practice of Infectious Disease* (6th ed.). Philadelphia: Elsevier Saunders.

Meiner, S. (2010). *Gerontologic Nursing* (4th ed.). St. Louis: Mosby.

Micozzi, M. S. (2011). *Fundamentals of Complementary and Integrative Medicine* (4th ed.). Philadelphia: Saunders.

National Cancer Institute. (2011). *Cancer trials information*. Retrieved from www.cancer.gov/clinicaltrials.

National Pressure Ulcer Advisory Panel. (2006b). *PUSH tool 3.0*. Retrieved from http://222.npuap.org/positn5.html.

National Stroke Association. (2011). *Stroke prevention*. Retrieved from www.stroke.org/site/PageServer?pagename=prevent.

Office of Disease Prevention and Health Promotion. (2011). *Healthy People 2020*. Rockville, MD: U.S. Department of Health and Human Services.

O'Toole, M. (Ed.). (2005). *Miller-Keane Encyclopedia and Dictionary of Medicine, Nursing, and Allied Health* (7th ed.). Philadelphia: Saunders.

Pagana, K. D., & Pagana, T. J. (2010). *Mosby's Diagnostic and Laboratory Test Reference* (10th ed.). St. Louis: Elsevier Mosby.

Peckenpaugh, N. J. (2010). *Nutrition Essentials and Diet Therapy* (11th ed.). St. Louis: Mosby.

Perry, A. G., & Potter, P. A. (2010). *Clinical Nursing Skills & Techniques* (7th ed.). St. Louis: Mosby.

Perry, A. G., Potter, P. A., & Elkin, M. K. (2012). *Nursing Interventions & Clinical Skills* (5th ed.). St. Louis: Mosby.

Preusser, B. A. (2009). *Winningham & Preusser's Critical Thinking Cases in Nursing: Medical-Surgical Pediatric, Maternity, and Psychiatric Case Studies* (4rd ed.). St. Louis: Mosby.

Purnell, L. D., & Paulanka, B. J. (2008). *Transcultural Health Care: A Culturally Competent Approach* (3rd ed.). Philadelphia: Davis.

Roth, J. J., & Hughes, W. B. (2004). *The Essential Burn Unit Handbook*. St. Louis: Quality Medical Publishing.

Rothrock, J. C. (2010). *Alexander's Care of the Patient in Surgery* (14th ed.). St. Louis: Mosby.

Schlenker, E. D., & Roth, S. L. (2010). *Williams' Essentials of Nutrition and Diet Therapy*. (10th ed.). St. Louis: Mosby.

Skidmore-Roth, L. (2010). *Mosby's Handbook of Herbs & Natural Supplements* (4th ed.). St. Louis: Mosby.

Skidmore-Roth, L. (2011). *Mosby's Nursing Drug Reference*. St. Louis: Elsevier Mosby.

Smeltzer, S. C., Bare, B. G., Hinkle, J. L., et al. (2010). *Brunner & Suddarth's Textbook of Medical-Surgical Nursing* (12th ed.). Philadelphia: Lippincott Williams & Wilkins.

Snyder, M., & Lindquist, R. (2006). *Complementary/Alternative Therapies in Nursing* (5th ed.). New York: Springer.

Stanhope, M., & Lancaster, J. (Eds.), (2008). *Public Health Nursing: Population-Centered Health Care in the Community* (7th ed.). St Louis: Mosby.

Stuart, G. W., & Laraia, M. T. (2009). *Principles and Practice of Psychiatric Nursing* (9th ed.). St. Louis: Elsevier Mosby.

Thibodeau, G. A., & Patton, K. T. (2010). *The Human Body in Health & Disease* (5th ed.). St. Louis: Elsevier Mosby.

U.S. Department of Health and Human Services. (2002). *Disasters and emergencies*. Retrieved from www.usa.gov/Citizen/Topics/PublicSafety/Disasters.shtml.

U.S. Department of Health and Human Services, Centers for Disease Control and Prevention. (2011). *National diabetes fact sheet: General information and national estimates on diabetes in the United States*. Atlanta: USDHHS. Retrieved from www.cdc.gov/diabetes/pubs/factsheet11.htm.

U.S. Department of Health and Human Services, National Center for Health Statistics. (2011). *Health*. United States. Retrieved from www.cdc.gov/nchs/hus.htm.

Varcarolis, E. M. (2011). *Manual of Psychiatric Nursing Care Plans* (3rd ed.). Philadelphia: Saunders.

Varcarolis, E. M., & Halter, M. J. (2009). *Foundations of Psychiatric Mental Health Nursing: A Clinical Approach* (6th ed.). Philadelphia: Saunders.

Weber, J., & Kelley, J. (2009). *Health Assessment in Nursing* (4th ed.). Philadelphia: Lippincott Williams & Wilkins.

Wold, G. H. (2011). *Basic Geriatric Nursing* (5th ed). St. Louis: Mosby.

Zerwekh, J., & Claborn, J. (2010). *Illustrated Study Guide for the NCLEX-PN* (7th ed.). St. Louis: Mosby.

CHAPTER 1

National Council of State Boards of Nursing. (1995). *Delegation: Concepts and Decision-Making Process*. Chicago: National Council Position Paper.

National Council of State Boards of Nursing. (2005). *Working with others: A position paper*. Chicago: National Council of State Boards of Nursing. Retrieved from www.ncsbn.org.

CHAPTER 2

Institute for Healthcare Improvement. (2009). *What is a bundle?* Retrieved from www.ihi.org/ihi//Topics/Critical.

Joint Commission. (2010). *National patient safety goals*. Retrieved from www.jointcommission.org/NR/rdonlyres/1F0FC18B-8974-4852-A5FA-2EA4E191968B/0/NPSGChapterOutline_FINAL_CAH_2010.pdf.

Spector, N. (2005). *Practical nurse scope of practice [White paper]*. Chicago: National Council of State Boards of Nursing. Retrieved from www.ncsbn.org.

CHAPTER 3

Centers for Disease Control and Prevention. (2002). *Guidelines for the prevention of intravascular catheter-related infections*. Retrieved from www.cdc.gov/mmwr/preview/mmwrhtml/rr5110a1.htm.

Institute for Healthcare Improvement. (2010). *Intervention—central line bundle*. Retrieved from www.IHI/Programs/campaign/CentralLineInfection.htm.

CHAPTER 4

Bratzler, D. W. (2009). *The surgical infection prevention and surgical care improvement projects: National initiative to improve surgical care*. Retrieved from http:acute.hshg.com/scip_ipg/scip_spreadtoolkit/B_Bratzler_scip-webex.ppt.

Evans, S. (Ed.). (2007). Perfect harmony: Music therapy eases anxiety and pain in the perioperative setting. *ADVANCE for Nurses, 4*(2), 25–26.

Farmer, S. L., Wren, M. N., Towler, S. C., et al. (2002). The theory and practice of bloodless surgery. *Transfusion and Apheresis Society Journal, 27*(1), 29–43.

Griffin, F. A. (2005). Best-practice protocols: Preventing surgical site infection. *Nursing Management, 36*(11), 20–26.

Joint Commission. (2009). *Universal protocol.* Retrieved from www.jointcommission.org/PatientSafety/UniversalProtocol.

Maltby, J. R. (2000). *Update in anesthesiology, 12*(2), 1–2. Retrieved from www.nda.ox.ac.uk/sfsa/html/u12/u1202_01.htm.

Melling, A. C., Ali, B., Scott, E. M., & Leaper, D. J. (2002). Effects of preoperative warming on the incidence of wound infection after clean surgery: A randomized controlled trial. *Lancet, 359* (9304), 445–446.

Tonnesen, P. R., Nielsen, J. B., Lauritzen, J. B., & Moller, A. M. (2009). Smoking and alcohol intervention before surgery: Evidence for best practice. *British Journal of Anaesthesia, 102*(3), 297–306.

CHAPTER 5

Barclay, L. (2006). *Gum chewing may speed recovery from postoperative ileus.* Retrieved from www.medscape.com/viearticle/524084?src=mp.

Hommertzheim, R., & Steinke, E. E. (2006). Malignant hyperthermia: The perioperative nurse's role. *AORN, 83*(1), 149–164.

Joint Commission. (2008). *Specifications manual for national hospital inpatient quality measures, version 3.0c.* Retrieved from www.jointcommission.org/PerformanceMeasurement/PerformanceMeasurement/Current+NHQM+Manual.htm.

Weinstein, R. A. *Highlights from the 12th SHEA: Back to basics: Safeguarding the operating room and the surgical patient.* Retrieved from www.medscape.com/viewarticle/438961_4.

Winslow, E. H., & Brosz, D. L. (2008). Graduated compression stockings in hospitalized postoperative patients: Correctness of usage and size. *American Journal of Nursing, 108*(9), 40–50.

CHAPTER 6

Centers for Disease Control and Prevention. (2002). Guidelines for the prevention of intravascular catheter-related infections. *MMWR Morbidity and Mortality Weekly Report Recommended Reports, 51*(RR-10), 1–26.

Centers for Disease Control and Prevention. (2010). *Prion diseases.* Retrieved from www.cdc.gov/ncidod/dvrd/prions.

Institute for Healthcare Improvement. (2011). *Implement the central line bundle.* Retrieved from www.ihi.org/IHI/topics/criticalcare/intensivecare/changes/implementthecentrallinebundle.htm.

Joint Commission. (2010). Available at www.thejoint commission.org.

CHAPTER 7

Doheny, K. (2010). *Acupuncture may east chronic back pain.* WebMD. Retrieved from www.webmd.com/back-pain/news/2009051/acupuncture-may-ease-chronic-back-pain.

Titler, M., Herrk.Schilling, M., et al. (2003). Acute pain treatment for older adults hospitalized with hip fracture: Current nursing practices and perceived barriers. *Applied Nursing Research, 16*(4), 211–227.

Yuan, J., Purepong, N., Kerr, D. P., et al. (2008). Effectiveness of acupuncture for low back pain: A systematic review. *Spine, 33* (23), E887–E900.

CHAPTER 8

American Cancer Society. (2000). *American Cancer Society's Guide to Complementary and Alternative Cancer Methods.* Atlanta: American Cancer Society.

American Cancer Society. (2009, November). *American Cancer Society responds to changes to USPSTF mammography guidelines.* Press release. Atlanta. Retrieved from www.cancer.org/docroot/MED/content/MED_2_1x_American_Cancer_Society_Responds_to_Changes_to_USPSTF_Mammography_Guidelines.asp.

American Cancer Society. (2010). *Cancer Facts and Figures, 2010.* Atlanta: American Cancer Society, Inc.

Evans, R. C., & Rossner, A. L. (2005). Alternatives in cancer pain treatment: The application of chiropractic care. *Seminars in Oncology Nursing, 21*(3), 184–189.

Futreal, P. A., Lachlan, C., Marshall, M., et al. (2004). A census of human cancer genes. *Nature Reviews Cancer, 4,* 177–183. doi:10.1038/nrc1299.

King, K., & Klawitter, B. (2007). *Nutrition Therapy: Advanced Counseling Skills.* Baltimore, MD: Lippincott Williams & Wilkins.

Kornmehl, C. L. (2007). *The value of exercise during radiation therapy for breast and prostate cancer.* Retrieved from www.articlealley.com/article_134929_23.html.

M.D. Anderson Cancer Center. (2009). *About complementary/integrative medicine.* Retrieved from www.mdanderson.org/education-and-research/resources-for-professionals/clinical-tools-and-resources/cimer/about-complementary-integrative-medicine/index.html.

Meier, D. E., Isaacs, S. L., & Hughes, R. (2010). *Palliative care: Transforming the care of serious illness.* San Francisco, CA: Jossey-Bass.

National Cancer Institute. (2010). *Tamoxifen.* Retrieved from www.cancer.gov/cancertopics/factsheet/Therapy/tamoxifen.

National Comprehensive Cancer Network (NCCN). (2009). *Clinical practice guidelines in oncology.* Retrieved from www.nccn.org/index.asp.

Shelton, B. K. (2003). Evidence-based care for the neutropenic patient with leukemia. *Seminars in Oncology Nursing, 19*(2), 133–141.

Smith, J. J., Tully, P., & Padberg, R. M. (2005). Chemoprevention: A primary cancer prevention strategy. *Seminars in Oncology Nursing, 21*(4), 243–251.

Steinhauser, K. E., Christakis, N. A., Clipp, E. C., et al. (2007). Factors considered important at the end of life by patients, family, physicians, and other care providers. *JAMA, 284*(19), 2476–2482.

Tabar, P., Yen, F., Vitak, B., et al. (2003). Mammography service screening and mortality in breast cancer patients: 20-year follow-up before and after introduction of screening. *Lancet, 361*(9367), 1405–1410.

CHAPTER 9

Joint Commission. (2010). *National patient safety goals: Long-term care.* Retrieved from www.jointcommission.org/GeneralPublic/NPSG/10_npsgs.htm.

CHAPTER 10

Advisory Committee on Immunization Practices, 2010. (January 14, 2011). Updated recommendations for use of tetanus toxoid, reduced diphtheria toxoid and acellular pertussis vaccine (Tdap). *MMWR Morbidity and Mortality Weekly Report.*

Centers for Disease Control and Prevention. (2011). *Vaccines and immunization schedules.* Retrieved from www.cdc.gov/vaccines/recs/schedules/default.htm.

Dyer, R., & Gould, B. (2010). *Pathophysiology for the Health Professions* (4th ed.). Philadelphia: Elsevier Sciences.

CHAPTER 11

AETC National Resource Center. (2009). *HIV Classification: CDC and WHO Staging Systems.* www.aidsetc.org/aidsetc?page=cm-105_disease#b-4.

American Academy of HIV Medicine. (2007). *AAHIVM Fundamentals of HIV Medicine for the HIV Specialist.* Chicago: American Academy of HIV Medicine and Medical Education Collaborative, Inc.

American Cancer Society. (2009). *What are the key statistics about Kaposi sarcoma?* Retrieved from www.cancer.org/Cancer/KaposiSarcoma/DetailedGuide/kaposi-sarcoma-what-is-key-statistics.

Anish, P., Mahajan, A. P., Stemple, L., et al. (2009). Consistency of state statutes with the Centers for Disease Control and Prevention HIV testing recommendations for health care settings. *Annals of Internal Medicine, 150*(4), 263–269.

Centers for Disease Control and Prevention. (2006). *Revised recommendations for HIV testing of adults, adolescents, and pregnant women in health-care settings.* Retrieved from www.cdc.gov/mmwr/preview/mmwrhtml/rr5514a1.htm.

Centers for Disease Control and Prevention. (2009a). *HIV/AIDS Surveillance Report, 2007* (Vol. 19). Atlanta: U.S. Department of Health and Human Services.

Centers for Disease Control and Prevention. (2009b). *HIV/AIDS surveillance by race/ethnicity (through 2007).* Retrieved from www.cdc.gov/hiv/topics/surveillance/resources/slides/race-ethnicity/index.htm.

Centers for Disease Control and Prevention. (2010). *How is HIV passed from one person to another?* Retrieved from www.cdc.gov/hiv/resources/qa/transmission.htm.

Highleyman, L. (2009). *Non-Hodgkin lymphoma mortality remains high for people with HIV, but antiretroviral therapy reduces risk.* Retrieved from www.hivandhepatitis.com/2009icr/croi/docs/040309_a.html.

Lehman, E., Huy, J., Levy, E., et al. (2010). Bloodborne pathogen risk reduction activities in the body piercing and tattooing industry. *American Journal of Infection Control, 38*(2), 130–138.

National Center for Health Statistics. (2009). *National Vital Statistics Reports (NVSR), Deaths: Final Data for 2006* (Vol. 57, No. 14). Washington, D.C.: U.S. Census Bureau.

National Institute on Aging. (2009). Today's research on aging. *Population Reference Bureau, 18*, 1–7.

Ponce, C. A., Gallo, M., Bustamante, R., & Vargas, S. L. (2010). Pneumocystis colonization is highly prevalent in the autopsied lungs of the general population. *Clinical Infectious Diseases, 50*(3), 347–353.

Romanelli, F., & Matheny, S. (2009). HIV infection: The role of primary care. *American Family Physician, 80*(9), 946–952.

Stringer, J. R., Beard, C. B., Miller, R. F., & Wakefield, A. E. (2002). A new name (*Pneumocystis jiroveci*) for Pneumocystis from humans. *Emerging Infectious Diseases, 8*(9), 891–896.

CHAPTER 12

Altekruse, S. F., Kosary, C. L., Krapcho, M., et al. (2009). *SEER Cancer Statistics Review, 1975-2007.* Bethesda, MD: National Cancer Institute.

American Cancer Society. (2009). *Cancer Facts and Figures 2009.* Atlanta: American Cancer Society.

Bernatsky, S., Boivin, J. F., Joseph, L., et al. (2006). Mortality in systemic lupus erythematosus. *Arthritis and Rheumatism, 54*, 2550–2557.

Dores, G., Coté, T., & Lois, B. T. (2009). New malignancies following Hodgkin lymphoma, non-Hodgkin lymphoma and myeloma. In *SEER Cancer Statistics Review, 1975-2007.* Bethesda, MD: National Cancer Institute.

Grammatikos, A. P. (2008). The genetic and environmental basis of atopic diseases. *Annals of Medicine, 40*(7), 482–495.

Jemal, A., Murray, T., Ward, E., et al. (2005). Cancer statistics, 2005. *CA: A Cancer Journal for Clinicians, 55*(1), 10–30.

National Cancer Institute. (2011). *SEER stat fact sheets: Non-Hodgkin lymphoma.* http://seer.cancer.gov/statfacts/html/nhl.html# survival.

Wolfe, F., Smythe, H., Yunus, M., et al. (1990). The American College of Rheumatology 1990 criteria for the classification of fibromyalgia: Report of the Multicenter Criteria Committee. *Arthritis and Rheumatism, 33*, 160–172.

CHAPTER 13

Agency for Healthcare Research and Quality. (2008). *Helping smokers quit.* Retrieved from www.ahrq.gov/clinic/tobacco/clinhlpsmksqt.htm.

American Cancer Society. (2010). *What are the risk factors for laryngeal and hypolaryngeal cancers?* Retrieved from www.ahrq.gov/clinic/tobacco/clinhlpsmksqt.htm.

Centers for Disease Control and Prevention. (2009a). *Quanti-FERON®-TB gold test.* Retrieved from www.cdc.gov/tb/publications/factsheets/testing/QFT.htm.

Centers for Disease Control and Prevention. (2009b). Updated guidelines for the use of nucleic acid amplification tests in the diagnosis of tuberculosis. *MMWR Morbidity and Mortality Weekly Report, 58*(01), 7–10. Retrieved from www.cdc.gov/mmwr/preview/mmwrhtml/mm5801a3.htm.

Moore, D. A. (2007). Future prospects for the MODS assay in multidrug-resistant tuberculosis diagnosis. *Future Medicine, 2*(2), 97–101.

CHAPTER 14

American Cancer Society. (2009). *Overview: Laryngeal and hypopharyngeal cancer.* Retrieved from www.cancer.org/acs/groups/cid/documents/webcontent/003216-pdf.

American Heart Association. (2009). *Heimlich maneuver.* Retrieved from www.americanheart.org/presenter.jhtml?identifier=4605.

Centers for Disease Control and Prevention. (2009). *Antibiotic resistance questions and answers.* Retrieved from www.cdc.gov/getsmart/antibiotic-use/anitbiotic-resistance-faqs.html#h.

Charra, B., Hachimi, A., Benslama, A., & Motaouakki, S. (2009). Tracheotomy versus prolonged intubation in medical intensive care unit patients. *SIGNA VITAE, 4*(1), 21–23.

Mayo Clinic. (2009). *Tonsillitis: Treatment and drugs.* Retrieved from www.mayoclinic.com/health/tonsillitis/DS00273/DSECTION=treatments-and-drugs.

National Reye's Syndrome Foundation. (2009). *What is the role of aspirin?* Retrieved from www.reyessyndrome.org.

Prasad, A. S., Beck, F. W. J., Bao, B., et al. (2008). Duration and severity of symptoms and levels of plasma interleukin-1 receptor antagonist, soluble tumor necrosis factor receptor, and adhesion molecules in patients with common cold treated with zinc acetate. *Journal of Infectious Diseases, 197*(15), 795–802.

CHAPTER 15

American Cancer Society. (2010). *Lung cancer fact sheet.* Retrieved from www.cancer.org/downloads/PRO/LungCancer.pdf.

American Lung Association. (2010a). *Pneumonia fact sheet.* Retrieved from www.lungusa.org/lung-disease/influenza/in-depth-resources/pneumonia-fact-sheet.html.

American Lung Association. (2010b). *Chronic obstructive pulmonary disease fact sheet.* Retrieved from www.lungusa.org/lung-disease/copd/resources/facts-figures/COPD-Fact-Sheet.html.

American Lung Association. (2010c). *Lung cancer breakthrough.* Retrieved from www.lungusa.org/about-us/our-impact/top-stories/lung-cancer-breakthrough.html.

Atkinson, M. (2010). *Pneumonia. Evidence-based nursing monographs.* Retrieved from www.nursingconsult.com.ezproxy.lib.utexas.edu/das/ebnm/view/199287821-2?DOCID=191486&sid=992458256&summaryresults=true&SEQNO=1.

Bloomfield, R., Noble, D. W., & Webster, N. R. (2009). Prone position for acute respiratory failure in adults (Protocol). *Cochrane Database of Systematic Reviews, 2009*(4). CD008095. doi:10.1002/14651858.CD008095.

Centers for Disease Control and Prevention. (2009). Recommended adult immunization schedule-United States, 2009. *MMWR Morbidity and Mortality Weekly Report, 57*(53), Q1–Q4. Retrieved from www.cdc.gov/mmwr/PDF/wk/mm5753-Immunization.pdf.

Centers for Disease Control and Prevention. (2010). *West Nile virus.* Retrieved from www.cdc.gov/ncidod/dvbid/westnile/qa/transmission.htm.

Clin-eguide. (2005). *Barberry.* Retrieved from http://clineguide.ovid.com.

Collins, T., & Lipke, G. (2009). Reducing VAP in your hospital. *Journal for Respiratory Care Practitioners, 22*(5), 34–36.

Eisenstadt, E. S. (2010). Dysphagia and aspiration pneumonia in older adults. *Journal of the American Academy of Nurse Practitioners, 22,* 17–22.

Gadek, J. E., DeMichele, S. J., Karlstad, M. D., et al. (1999). Effect of enteral feeding with eicosapentaenoic acid, gamma-linolenic acid, and antioxidants in patients with acute respiratory distress syndrome. Enteral nutrition in ARDS study group. *Critical Care Medicine, 27*(8), 1409–1420.

Glastonbury, S. (2009). Herbal medicine: Role in the management of chronic obstructive pulmonary disease (COPD). *Australian Journal of Medical Herbalism, 21*(1), 3–8.

Horowitz, M. A. (2010). *Initiative for vaccine research: rBCG30.* World Health Organization. Retrieved from www.who.int/vaccine_research/diseases/tb/vaccine_development/rbcg30/en/index.html.

Institute for Clinical Symptoms Improvement. (2009). *Health care order set: Prevention of ventilator-associated pneumonia* (4th ed). Retrieved from www.icsi.org.

Institute for Clinical Symptoms Improvement. (2010). *Health care guideline: Venous thromboembolism diagnosis and treatment* (10th ed). Retrieved from www.icsi.org.

Joint Commission. (2010). *A comprehensive review of development and testing for national implementation of hospital core measures.* Retrieved from www.jointcommission.org.

Manning, P., Gibson, P. G., & Lasserson, T. J. (2008). Ciclesonide versus placebo for chronic asthma in adults and children. *Cochrane Database of Systematic Reviews, 2008*(2), CD006217. doi:10.1002/14651858.CD006217.pub2.

Mayo Clinic Staff. (2009). *Tuberculosis: Treatments and drugs.* Retrieved from www.mayoclinic.com/health/tuberculosis/DS00372/DSECTION=treatments-and-drugs.

Mayo Clinic. (2010). *Video-assisted thoracoscopic surgery (VATS).* Retrieved from www.mayoclinic.org/video-assisted-thoracic-surgery.

Menzies, D., Long, R., Trajman, A., et al. (2008). Adverse events with 4 months of rifampin therapy or 9 months of isoniazid therapy for latent tuberculosis infection. *Annals of Internal Medicine, 19*(10), 689–697.

Mesothelioma Research Foundation. (2010). *Mesothelioma causes.* Retrieved from www.mesorfa.org/about-meso/causes.php.

National Cancer Institute. (2010). *Diet may protect against gene changes in smokers.* Retrieved from www.cancer.gov/newscenter/pressreleases/Dietaryfactorslungcancer.

National Human Genome Research Institute. (2009). *Learning about cystic fibrosis.* Retrieved from www.genome.gov/pfv.cfm?pageID.

National Institute of Allergy and Infectious Diseases. (2009). *Tuberculosis.* Retrieved from www.niaid.nih.gov/topics/tuberculosis/research/pages/niaidlabs.aspx.

Rascon-Aguilar, I. E., Pamer, M., Wludyka, P., et al. (2006). Role of gastroesophageal reflux symptoms in exacerbations of COPD. *Chest, 130*(4), 1096–1101.

Restrepo, M., Mortensen, E. M., & Anzueto, A. (2010). Common medications that increase the risk for developing community-acquired pneumonia. *Current Opinion in Infectious Diseases, 23*(2), 145–151.

Taccone, P., Pesenti, A., Latini, R., et al. (2009). Prone positioning in patients with moderate and severe acute respiratory distress syndrome: A randomized controlled trial. *JAMA, 302*(18), 1977–1984.

Talat, N., Perry, S., & Parsonnet, J. (2010). Vitamin D deficiency and tuberculosis progression. *Emerging Infectious Diseases,* May [Epub ahead of print], 1–7.

Tolentino-Delos Reyes, A. F., Ruppert, S. D., & Shiao, S. Y. P. K. (2007). Evidence-based practice: Use of the ventilator bundle to prevent ventilator-associated pneumonia. *American Journal of Critical Care, 16*(1), 20–27.

Troosters, T., Gosselink, R., Janssens, W., et al. (2010). Exercise training and pulmonary rehabilitation: New insights and remaining challenges. *European Respiratory Review, 19,* 24–29.

World Health Organization. (2010). *Cumulative number of confirmed human cases of avian influenza A/(H5N1) reported to WHO.* Retrieved from www.who.int/csr/disease/avian_influenza/country/cases_table_2010_04_21/en/index.html.

Zakay-Rones, A., Thom, E., Wollan, T., et al. (2004). Randomized study of the efficacy and safety of oral elderberry extract in the treatment of influenza A and B virus infections. *Journal of International Medical Research, 32*(2), 132–140.

CHAPTER 16

Agnihotri, P., Telfer, M., Butt, Z., et al. (2007). Chronic anemia and fatigue in elderly patients: Results of a randomized, double-blind, placebo-controlled, crossover exploratory study with epoetin alfa. *Journal of the American Geriatric Society, 55*(10), 1557–1565.

CHAPTER 17

Agnihotri, P., Telfer, M., Butt, Z., et al. (2007). Chronic anemia and fatigue in elderly patients: Results of a randomized, double-blink, placebo-controlled, crossover exploratory study with epoetin alfa. *Journal American Geriatric Society, 55*(10), 1557–1565.

Becker, J. U., & Wira, C. R. (2009). *Disseminated intravascular coagulation.* Retrieved from http://emedicine.medscape.com/article/779097-overview.

Bennett, D. R. (2006). Pain management for sickle cell disease in children and adults. *Cochrane Reviews.* Retrieved from www.2.cochrane.org/reviews/en/ab003350.html.

Besa, E., & Woermann, U. (2009). *Chronic myelogenous leukemia.* Retrieved from http:emedicine.medscape.com/article/199425-overview.

Bizumukama, L., Ferster, A., Gulbis, B., et al. (2009). In vitro inhibitory effects of disodium cromoglycate on ionic transports involved in sickle cell dehydration. *Pharmacology, 2009*(83), 318–322.

Brawley, O. W., Cornelius, L. J., Edwards, L. R., et al. (2008). National Institutes of Health consensus development conference statement: Hydroxyurea treatment for sickle cell disease. *Annals of Internal Medicine, 148*(12), 148–150.

British Columbia Ministry of Health. (2006). *Investigation & Management of B12 and Folate Deficiency.* Victoria, BC: Guidelines & Protocols Advisory Committee.

DeRanieri, J. T. (2008). *Evidence-based nursing monographs: Leukemia.* Retrieved from www.nursingconsult.com/das/news/body/2/ebnm/0193303/.html?nid=193303.

Gentili, A. (2009). *Folic acid deficiency.* Retrieved from http://emedicine.medscape.com/article/200184-overview.

National Cancer Institute. (2008). *Bone marrow transplantation and peripheral blood stem cell transplantation.* Retrieved from www.cancer.gov/cancertopics/factsheet/therapy/bone-marrow-transplant.

National Cancer Institute. (2010). *Leukemia.* Retrieved from www.cancer.gov/cancertopics/type/leukemia.

Nichols, W. L., Hultin, M. B., James, A. H., et al. (2008). Haemophilia. *Haemophilia, 14*(2), 171–232.

Platt, A., & Beasley, J. (2007). How much do you know about sickle-cell disease? *LPN, 3*(4), 32–37.

Singh, N. K., & Gangappa, M. (2007). Acute immune thrombocytopenia associated with hepatitis E in an adult. *American Journal of Hematology.* Retrieved from http://onlinelibrary.wiley.com/doi/10.1002/ajh.20960/abstract.

CHAPTER 18

American Heart Association. (2009). *Cardiovascular disease statistics.* Retrieved from www.americanheart.org/presenter.jhtml?identifier=4478.

Brooks, L. (2007). *New guidelines for treatment of hypertension in the prevention and management of ischemic heart disease*. Retrieved from www.medscape.com/viewarticle/448277.

Felker, G. M., Cuculich, P. S., & Gheorghiade, M. (2006). The Valsalva maneuver: A bedside "biomarker" for heart failure. *American Journal of Medicine, 119*(2), 117–122.

Gami, A. S., Witt, B. J., Howard, D. E., et al. (2007). Metabolic syndrome and risk of incident cardiovascular events and death. *American College of Cardiology, 49*(4), 403–414.

Halford, S. (2003). Diamorphone or morphine for ischaemic cardiac chest pain. In *Best Bets Best Evidence Topics*. Retrieved from www.bestbets.org/bets/bet/php?id=351.

Hlatky, M. A., Boothroyd, D., Vittinghoff, E., et al. (2002). Lessons learned from the Women's Initiative Study. *Southern Medical Journal, 97*, 116–120.

National Heart Lung and Blood Institute. (2002). *Primary prevention of hypertension: A clinical public health advisory*. National Heart Lung and Blood Institute Education Program.

National Institute on Drug Abuse. (2009). *Cocaine*. Retrieved from www.nida.nih.gov/DrugPages/Cocaine.html.

Qaseem, A., Vijan, S., Snow, V., et al. (2007). Glycemic control and type 2 diabetes mellitus: The optimal hemoglobin A1c targets. A guidance statement from the American College of Physicians. *Annals of Internal Medicine, 147*(6), 417–422.

CHAPTER 19

Agency for Healthcare Research and Quality, Segal, J. B., Eng, J., Jenckes, M. W., et al. (2003, March). *Diagnosis and Treatment of Deep Venous Thrombosis and Pulmonary Embolism*. Evidence Report/Technology Assessment Number 68. AHRQ Publication No. 03-E016 Rockville, MD: Agency for Healthcare Research and Quality.

Anderson, F. A., & Audet, A. M. (2011). *Best practices: Preventing deep vein thrombosis and pulmonary embolism*. University of Massachusetts Medical School Center for Outcomes Research. Retrieved from www.outcomes-umassmed.org/dvt/best_practice.

Bartley, M. (2006). Preventing venous embolism. *Nursing2006, 36*(1), 64cc1–64cc4.

Flack, J. M., Sica, D. A., Bakris, G., et al. (2010). Management of high blood pressure in blacks. *Hypertension, 2010*(56), 780.

Johnson, S. (2006). Exercise and peripheral arterial disease. *Annals of Internal Medicine, 144*(9), 699–700.

Kakkos, S. K., Daskalopoulou, S. S., Daskalopoulos, M. E., et al. (2006). Review on the value of graduated elastic compression stockings after deep vein thrombosis. *Thrombosis and Haemostasis, 90*(4), 441–445.

Kartikeyan, G., & Eikelboom, J. W. (2009). Treatment of intermittent claudication. *British Medical Journal*, (338), b46.

Lew, W. K., & Weaver, F. A. (2010). *Varicose veins*. Retrieved from http://emedicine.medscape.com/article/462579.

Research Activities (Eds.). (2006). Management of chest pain in patients with hypertension differs in men, women, and ethnic groups. *Research Activities*, Jan(305), 5–6.

Schreiber, D. (2010). *Deep venous thrombosis and thrombophlebitis: Treatment and medication*. Retrieved from http://emedicine.medscape.com/article/758140-treatment.

Singh, N., O'Donnell, S. D., Gillespie, D. L., & Goff, J. M. (2009). *Atherosclerotic disease of the carotid artery*. Retrieved from http://emedicine.medscape.com/article/463147-overview.

Torpy, J. M., Burke, A. E., & Glass, R. M. (2008). Thrombophlebitis. *JAMA, 300*(14), 1718–1720.

Van Wicklin, S. A., Ward, K. S., & Cantrell, S. W. (2006). Implementing a research utilization plan for prevention of deep vein thrombosis. *AORN Journal, 83*(6), Retrieved from www.nursingconsult.com/das/article/body/169669796-2/jorg=journal&source=MI&s.

Vazquez, S. R., & Kahn, S. R. (2010). Postthrombotic syndrome. *Circulation, 121*, e217–e219.

Weiss, R., & Feied, C. F. (2009). *Venous insufficiency*. Retrieved from http://emedicine.medscape.com/article/1085412-overview.

Widdon, L. L. (2007). Saphenous vein ablation: Radiofrequency and laser. *Baylor Medical Center Proceedings, 20*(2), 136–139.

Wound, Ostomy & Continence Nurses Society. (2011). *Clinical fact sheet: Venous insufficiency (stasis)*. Retrieved from www.wocn.org.

Zolli, A. (2004). Foot ulceration due to arterial insufficiency: Role of cilostazol. *Journal of Wound Care, 13*(2), 45–47.

CHAPTER 20

American Dietetic Association. (2006). Scientific statements and recommendations on dietary fat intake. *Journal of the American Dietetic Association, 106*(11), 1896–1906.

Carroll, P. (2008). *Heart failure*. Retrieved from www.nursingconsult.com/das/news/body/2/ebnm/0/195200/1.html?nid=195200&d.

Coviello, J. (2009). Heart failure: An update. *Home Healthcare Nurse, 27*(6), 354–362.

Heart Center Online. (2007). *Herbal extract shows some benefit for heart failure*. Retrieved from http://heart.health.ivillage.com/newsStories/newsprintfriendly.cfm?newsid=85751.

Heart Failure Society of America. (2009). *Diet and nutrition: Recommendations*. Retrieved from www.heartfailureguideline.org/index.cfm?id=47&s=1.

Jessup, M., Abraham, W. T., Casey, D. E., et al. (2009). *2009 Focused update: ACCF/AHA guidelines for the diagnosis and management of heart failure in adults*. Retrieved from http://circ.ahajournals.org/cgi/content/extract/119/14/1977.

Joint Commission. (2009). *Specifications manual for national quality measures*. Retrieved from www.jointcommission.org/PerformanceMeasurement/PerformanceMeasurement/Current+NHQM+Manual.htm.

Kutzieb, T. P., & Reiner, A. S. (2006). *Heart failure management*. Retrieved from www.patient.co.uk/doctor/Heart-Faiure-Management.htm.

MayoClinic.com. (2006). *Heart failure*. Retrieved from www.mayoclinic.com/health/heartfailure/DS00061/DSECTION.

Repasky, T. M., & Pfeil, C. (2005). Experienced critical care nurse-led rapid response team rescues patients on in-patient units. *Journal of Emergency Nursing, 31*(94), 376–379.

Yu, D. S., Thompson, D. R., & Lee, D. T. (2006). Disease management programs for older people with heart failure: Crucial characteristics which improve post-discharge outcomes. *European Heart Journal, 27*(5), 596–612.

Zipes, D. P., Camm, A. J., Borggrefe, M., et al. (2006). ACC/AHA/ESC guidelines for management of patients with ventricular arrhythmias and the prevention of sudden cardiac death—executive summary. *European Heart Journal, 27*(10), 2099–2140.

CHAPTER 21

American College of Cardiology/American Heart Association. (2004). *ACC/AHA guidelines for the management of patients with ST-elevation myocardial infarction—Executive summary*. Retrieved from www.acc.org/qualityandscience/clinical/guidelines/stemi/Guideline1/PrehospitalIssues.htm.

American Heart Association. (2009a). *American Heart Association diet*. Retrieved from http://diet.lovetoknow.com/wiki/American_Heart_Association_Diet.

American Heart Association. (2009b). *Heart transplants: Statistics*. Retrieved from www.americanheart.org/presenter/jhtml?identifier=4588.

American Heart Association. (2010). *Aspirin in heart attack and stroke prevention*. Retrieved from www.americanheart.org/presenter.ajhtml?identifier_4456.

Bird, M. W., Woods, A. G., & Warren, N. A. (2009). Factors influencing treatment delays for acute myocardial infarction. *Critical Care Nursing Quarterly, 32*(1), 19–23.

Boden, W., O'Rourke, R., Teo, K., et al. (2007). Optimal medical therapy with or without PCI for stable coronary disease. *New England Journal of Medicine, 356*(15), 1503–1516.

Brown, J. (2011). *Minimally invasive direct coronary artery bypass MID-CAB.* Retrieved from http://biomed.brown.edu/Courses/BI108/BI108_2000Groups/Heart_Surgery/MIDCAB.htm.

Cochrane Library. (2010). *Oxygen therapy for acute myocardial infarction.* Retrieved from www.cochranejournalclub.com/oxygen-therapy-for-acute-myocardial-infarction-clinical.

Hayes, S. N., Johnson, P. A., Pina, I. L., et al. (2009). *All about Eve: Unique aspects of CVD in women.* Retrieved from http://cme.medscape.com/viewarticle/704684_print.

Jolliffe, J. A., Rees, K., Taylor, R. S., et al. (2005). Exercise-based rehabilitation for coronary heart disease. *Cochrane Database of Systematic Reviews, 4.* Cochrane Heart Group.

Juurlink, D. N., Gomes, T., Ko, D. T., et al. (2009). *A population-based study of the drug interaction between proton pump inhibitors and clopidogrel.* Retrieved from www.cmaj.ca.

Maryland Heart Center. (2009). *Heart transplantation.* Retrieved from www.umm.edu/heart/elig_crit.htm.

Nursing2009 (Eds.). (2009). Proton pump inhibitors neutralize clopidogrel. *Nursing2009, 39*(4), 2.

Patient.co.uk. (2011). *Cardiac rehabilitation.* Retrieved from www.patient.co.uk/doctor/Cardiac-Rehabilitation.htm.

Plomondon, M. E. (2003). Factors influencing risk-adjusted patient satisfaction after coronary artery bypass graft. *American Journal of Cardiology, 92*(2), 206–208.

Rivera-Bou, W. L. & Brown, D. F. M. (2010). *Thrombolytic therapy for acute myocardial infarction.* Retrieved from http://emedicine.medscape.com/article/811234-overview.

Rosenfeld, A. (2005). Understanding treatment-seeking delay in women with acute myocardial infarction: Description of decision-making patterns. *Journal of Critical Care, 14*(4), 285–293.

Skinner, J. S. & Cooper, A. (2011). *PTCA with or without stenting versus medical treatment alone. Clinical evidence.* Retrieved from http://clinicalevidence.bmj.com/ceweb/conditions/cvd/0206/0206_117.jsp.

CHAPTER 22

Murthy, T. (2009). A new score to validate coma in emergency department—FOUR score. *Indian Journal of Neurotrauma, 6*(1), 59–62.

Paik, N. J. (2008). *Dysphagia.* Retrieved from http://emedicine.medscape.com/article/324096-overview.

Rackley, R., Vasavada, S. P., & Ingber, M. S. (2009). *Neurogenic bladder.* Retrieved from http://emedicine.medscape.com/article/453539-overview.

Royal-Evans, C., & Marcus, R. (2004). *A survey of the use of evidence-based practice in treatment of aphasia.* Presented at the Clinical Aphasiology Conference, Park City, UT, May 2004.

CHAPTER 23

Agency for Healthcare Research and Quality. (2007). *Acute management of autonomic dysreflexia: Individuals with spinal cord injury presenting to healthcare facilities.* Retrieved from www.guideline.gov/summary/summary.aspx?doc_id&2190?nbr.

American Association of Neuroscience Nurses. (2007). *Guide to the Care of the Patient with Intracranial Pressure Monitoring.* Glenview, IL: American Association of Neuroscience Nurses.

American Pain Society. (2010). *A new look at heat treatment for pain disorders,* part 2. Retrieved from www.ampainsoc.org/pub/bulletin/win05/inno1.htm.

Dawodu, S. T. (2009). *Traumatic brain injury (TBI)—Definition, epidemiology, pathophysiology.* Available at http://emedicine.medscape.com/article/326510-overview.

Garde, A. (2009). Experiences with dexamethasone treatment of intracranial pressure caused by brain tumors. *Acta Neurologica Scandinavica, 41*(S13), 439–444.

Hartl, R., Gerber, L. M., Ni, Q., & Ghajar, J. (2008). Effect of early nutrition on deaths due to severe traumatic brain injury. *Journal of Neurosurgery, 109*(7), 50–56.

National Guideline Clearing House. (2009). *Nursing management of adults with severe traumatic brain injury.* Retrieved from www.guideline.gov/content.aspx?id=13576.

National Spinal Cord Injury Association. (2009). *Autonomic dysreflexia.* Retrieved from www.spinalcord.org/news.php?dep=17&page=94&list=aa78.

National Spinal Cord Injury Statistical Center. (2009). *Facts and figures at a glance 2009.* Retrieved from www.nscisc.uab.edu/public_content/facts_figures_2009.aspx.

Neiman, R. (2008). *Israeli device helps paraplegics stand tall.* Retrieved from www.israel21c.org/health/israeli-device-helps-paraplegics-stand-tall.

Patel, R. K., & Slipman, C. W. (2009). *Lumbar degenerative disk disease: Treatment and medication.* Retrieved from http://emedicine.medscape.com/article/309767-treatment.

Perina, D. G. (2009). *Back pain, mechanical.* Retrieved from http://emedicine.medscape.com/article/822462-overview.

Rehabilitation Institute of Chicago. (2009). *New study improves walking in patients with spinal cord injury.* Retrieved from www.ric.org/aboutus/mediacenter/press/2009/spinalcordinjury.aspx.

Schreiber, D. (2009). Spinal cord injuries. From Olson, D. A. (2009). *Head injury: Treatment and medication.* Retrieved from http://emedicine.medscape.com/article/793582-overview.

CHAPTER 24

Agarwal, P., & Berman, S. A. (2011). *Neurologic effects of cocaine.* Retrieved from http://emedicine.medscape.com/article/1174408-overview.

Agency for Healthcare Research and Quality. (2009). *Acute stroke: Evaluation and treatment.* Retrieved from www.ahrq.gov/clinic/epcsums/acstrokesum.htm.

American Heart Association. (2009). *Stroke statistics.* Retrieved from www.americanheart.org/presenter.jhtml?identifier=4725.

Carroll, E., & Berbadis, S. R. (2009). *Complex partial seizures.* Retrieved from http://emedicine.medscape.com/article/1183962-overview.

Chawla, J. (2009). *Migraine headache: Treatment and medication.* Retrieved from http://emedicine.medscape.com/article/1142556-treatment.

Dugdale, D. C., & Hoch, D. B. (2009). *Subarachnoid hemorrhage.* MedlinePlus. Retrieved from www.nlm.nih.gov/medlineplus/ency/article/000701.htm.

Emedicine Health (Eds.). (2010). *Alternative and complementary approaches to migraine.* Retrieved from www.emedicinehealth.com/alternative_and_complementary-approaches_to_migraine.

Epilepsy Action (Ed.). (2010). *Status epilepticus.* Retrieved from www.epilepsy.org.uk/info/status.html.

Food and Drug Administration. (2009). *Metoclopramide-containing drugs.* Retrieved from www.fda.gov/Safety/MedWatch/SafetyInformation/SafetyAlertsforHumanMedical Professionals.

Frieden, J. (2010). *FDA okays Botox to prevent migraines.* MedPage Today. Retrieved from www.medpagetoday.com/tbprint.cfm?tbid-22781.

Gever, J. (2009). *AAPM: Intractable migraines improved by nerve stimulation.* Retrieved from www.medpagetoday.com/MeetingCoverage/AAPM/12721.

Goldstein, J. N. (2009). *Transient ischemic attack*. Retrieved from http://emedicine.medscape.com/article/794281-overview.

Goldstein, J. N., & Kukami, R. (2011). *Transient ischemic attack*. Retrieved from http://emedicine.medscape.com/article/1910519-overview.

Gutierrez, D. (2008). *Music therapy helps patients recover brain function following stroke*. Retrieved from www.naturalnews.com/z024455.html.

Jauch, E. C., & Lutsep, H. L. (2011). *Acute management of stroke*. Retrieved from http://emedicine.medscape.com/article/1159752-overview.

Ko, D. Y., & Sahai-Srivastava, S. (2009). *Generalized tonic-clonic seizures*. Retrieved from http://emedicine.medscape.com/article/1184608-overview.

Lutsep, H. I. (2009). *Mechanical thrombolysis in acute stroke*. Retrieved from http://emedicine.medscape.com/article/1163240-overview.

Monnell, K., Zachariah, S. B., & Khoromi, S. (2009). *Bell palsy*. Retrieved from http://emedicine.medscape.com/article/1146903-overview.

Razonabie, R. R., & Keating, M. R. (2009). *Meningitis*. Retrieved from http://emedicine.medscape.com/article/232915-overview.

Registered Nurses Association of Ontario. (2010). *Stroke assessment across the continuum of care: Practice recommendations*. Retrieved from www.rnao.org/Page.asp?PageID=924&ContentID=820.

Saver, C. (2007). *Cerebrovascular accident (CVA)*. Retrieved from www.nursingconsult.com/das/news/body/2/ebnm/0/189174/1.html.

Scottish Intercollegiate Guidelines Network. (2005). *Diagnosis and management of epilepsy in adults*. Retrieved from www.sign.ac.uk/guidelines/fulltext/70/index.html.

Stroke Center. (2010). *Stroke statistics*. Retrieved from www.strokecenter.org/patients/stats.htm.

Vavazos, J. E., & Berman, S. A. (2009). *Status epilepticus*. Retrieved from http://emedicine.medscape.com/article/1164462-overview.

Vega, C. (2007). *Stimulant abuse may increase stroke among young adults*. CME/CE presentation. Retrieved from www.medscape.com/viewarticle/555229.

Walker, E. P. (2011). *FDA approves wearable device for glioblastoma*. Retrieved from www.medpagetoday.com/Hematology/Oncology/BrainCancer/25958?utm.

Wright, C. B., Moon, Y., Paik, M. C., et al. (2009). Inflammatory biomarkers of vascular risk as correlates of leukoariosis. *Stroke, 2009*(40), 3466.

CHAPTER 25

Armon, C. (2010). *Amyotrophic lateral sclerosis*. Retrieved from http://emedicine.medscape.com/article/1170097-overview.

Centers for Disease Control and Prevention. (2006). *Vaccines and immunizations*. Retrieved from www.cdc.gov/vaccines/vac-gen/side-effects.htm.

Davids, H. R., Oleszek, J. L., & Cha-Kim, A. (2009). *Guillain-Barré syndrome*. Retrieved from http://emedicine.medcscape.com/article/315632-overview.

Multiple Sclerosis Association of America. (2007). *Introduction: Multiple sclerosis*. Retrieved from www.msaa.com/publications/cooling/contnts.htm.

National Institute of Neurological Diseases and Stroke. (2007). *NINCS deep brain stimulation for Parkinson's disease*. Retrieved from www.ninds.nih.gov/disorders/deep_brain_stimulation/deep_brain_stimulation.htm.

Shah, A. K. (2009). *Myasthenia gravis*. Retrieved from http://emedicine.medscape.com/article/1171206-overview.

Susman, E. (2010). *Stem cell implant to the brain helps improve Parkinson's symptoms*. Presented at SIR. Retrieved from www.docguide.com/news/content.nsf/NewsPrint/85257102 0057CCF6852574160051.

Roberts, A., & Harper-Bennie, J. (2010). *Multiple sclerosis and cooling*. Retrieved from www.msassociation.org/publications/cooling/#cooling.

WebMD (Ed.). (2010). *Multiple sclerosis exercise*. Retrieved from www.webmd.com/multiple-sclerosis/guide/multiple-sclerosis-exercise.

WebMD (Ed.). (2010). *Pallidotomy (posteroventral pallidotomy) for Parkinson's disease*. Retrieved from www.webmd.com/parkinsons-disease/palliodotomy-posteroventral-pallidotomy-for-parkinson's-disease.

CHAPTER 26

Bankhead, C. (2009). *Drug delivery via contact lenses passes early test*. Retrieved from www.medpagetoday.com/tbprint.cfm?tbid=15205.

Braille Institute of America. (2010). *Facts about sight loss and definitions of blindness*. Retrieved from www.brailleinstitute.org/facts_abou_sight_loss.

Eyecareamerica. (2010). *Recommended intervals for regular eye exams*. Retrieved from www.eyecareamerica.org/eyecare/treatment/eye-exams.cfm.

Healthy Hearing. (2010). *Hearing aids: Early use prevents auditory atrophy*. Retrieved from www.healthyhearing.com/content/news/Hearing-aids/Other/47578-hearing-aid.

Linus Pauling Institute. (2010). *Carotenoids*. Retrieved from http://lpi.oregonstate.edu/infocenter/phytochemicals/carotenoids.

National Eye Institute. (2010). *U. S. Latinos have high rates of developing vision loss and certain eye conditions*. Retrieved from www.nei.nih.gov/news/pressreleases/050110.asp.

National Institute on Deafness and Other Communication Disorders (NIDCD). (2010a). *Quick statistics*. Retrieved from www.nidcd.nih.gov/health/statistics/quick.htm.

National Institute on Deafness and Other Communication Disorders (NIDCD). (2010b). *Wise ears! Tips: Hearing matters—protect it*. Retrieved from www.nidcd.nih.gov/health/wise/tips.asp.

Ross, M., & Ross, M. (2005). *Rehabilitation engineering research center on hearing enhancement: Evidence-based audiology*. Retrieved from www.hearingresearch.org/Dr.Ross/Evidence-based_Audiology.htm.

CHAPTER 27

Bell, J. A. (2008). *Glaucoma, primary open angle*. Retrieved from http://emedicine.medscape.com/article/126147-overview.

Comer, G. M., Ciulla, T., & Criswell, M. H. (2008). *ARMD, exudative*. Retrieved from http://emedicine.medscape.com/article/1226030-overview.

Gates, G., Verrall, A., Green, J. D., et al. (2006). Meniett clinical trial: Long-term follow-up. *Archives of Otolaryngology—Head and Neck Surgery, 132*(12), 1311–1316.

Harvard Eye Associates. (2010). *CrystaLens, ReZoom and ReSTOR Lens Implants*. Retrieved from www.harvardeye.com/cataract/lens-implants.html.

Mayer, J. (2010). Age-related macular degeneration and antioxidant vitamins: Recent findings. *Clinical Nutrition and Metabolism Care, 13*(1), 28–33.

National Guideline Clearinghouse. (2008). *Age-related macular degeneration*. Retrieved from www.guideline.gov/summary/summary.aspx?view_id=1&doc_id=14275.

Science News (Ed.). (2010). *Fish oil may help protect against retinal degenerative diseases*. Retrieved from www.sciencedaily.com/releases/2006/04/060505234728.htm.

WebMD (Ed.). (2010). *Eye health center: Tonometry*. Retrieved from www.webmd.com/eye-health/tonometry.

Zapanta, P. E., & Van Dusen, R. (2009). *Vestibular rehabilitation*. Retrieved from http://emedicine.medscape.com/article/883878-overview.

CHAPTER 28

American Cancer Society. (2010). *American Cancer Society guidelines for the early detection of cancer.* Retrieved from www.cancer.org/docroot/PED/content/PED_2_3X_ACS_Cancer_Detection_Guidelines_36.asp?sitearea=PED.

Clin-eguide. (2009). *Evidence-based guideline: Cholelithiasis: Prevention.* Retrieved from http://clineguide.ovid.com.

Clin-eguide. (2010). *Guideline: Cirrhosis.* Retrieved from http://clineguide.ovid.com.

Kullberg, E., Forsell, M., Wedel, P., et al. (2009). Dental hygiene education for nursing staff. *Geriatric Nursing, 30*(5), 329–333.

Mehta, G., & Rothstein, K. D. (2009). Health maintenance issues in cirrhosis. *Medical Clinics of North America, 93*(4), 901–915.

National Digestive Diseases Information Clearinghouse. (2007). *Gallstones.* Retrieved from http://digestive.niddk.nih.gov/ddiseases/pubs/gallstones.

Pinto, S. (2008). *Evidence-Based Care Sheet: Hydration: Maintaining Oral Hydration in Older Adults.* Glendale, CA: Cinahl Information Systems.

Yantis, M. A. (2009). Probiotics can thwart antibiotic-associated diarrhea. *Nursing2009, 39*(3), 58.

CHAPTER 29

American Cancer Society. (2009a). *Esophageal cancer.* Retrieved from www.cancer.org/downloads/PRO/EsophagealCancer.pdf.

American Cancer Society. (2009b). *What's new in stomach cancer research and treatment?* Retrieved from www.cancer.org/Cancer/StomachCancer/DetailedGuide/stomach-cancer-new-research.

American Cancer Society. (2010). *Oral cancer.* Retrieved from www.cancer.org/downloads/PRO/OralCancer.pdf.

Clin-eguide. (2009). *Guideline: Peptic ulcer.* Retrieved from http://clineguide.ovid.com.

Dugdale, D. (2009). *Medical encyclopedia: Mouth sores.* Retrieved from www.nlm.nih.gov/medlineplus/ency/article/003059.htm.

Fisichella, P. M. A., & Patti, M. (2009). *Gastroesophageal reflux disease.* Retrieved from http://emedicine.medscape.com/article/176595-overview.

Mayo Clinic Health Letter. (2010). Barrett's esophagus. *Mayo Clinic Health Letter, 28*(4), 1–3.

National Cancer Institute. (2009). *Stomach (gastric) cancer.* Retrieved from www.cancer.gov/cancerinfo/types/stomach.

National Clearinghouse Guidelines. (2009). *American Association of Clinical Endocrinologists, The Obesity Society, and American Society for Metabolic and Bariatric Surgery medical guidelines for clinical practice for the perioperative nutritional, metabolic, and nonsurgical support of the bariatric surgery patient.* Retrieved from www.ngc.gov/summary/summary.aspx?ss=15&doc_id=13022&nbr=006716&string=%22BARIATRIC+SURGERY%22.

Nazario, B. (2009). *Heartburn and asthma.* Retrieved from www.webmd.com/asthma/guide/heartburn-asthma.

Nazarko, L. (2010). Recognizing and managing dysphagia. *Nursing and Residential Care, 12*(3), 133–138.

Neafsey, P. J. (2004). Double trouble: Acetaminophen increases the risk of upper GI complications for people taking NSAIDs. *Home Healthcare Nurse, 22*, 641–642.

Patel, J. A., Patel, N. A., Piper, G. L., et al. (2009). Perioperative management of cholelithiasis in patients presenting for laparoscopic Roux-en-Y gastric bypass: Have we reached a consensus? *American Surgeon, 75*(6), 470–476.

Pinto, S., & Schub, T. (2009). *Evidence-Based Care Sheet: Gastroesophageal Reflux Disease.* Glendale, Calif.: Cinahl Information Systems.

Sreedharan, A., Harris, K., Crelin, A., et al. (2009). Interventions for dysphagia in oesophageal cancer. *Cochrane Database of Systematic Reviews, 2009*(4), CD005048. doi:10.1002/14651858.CD005048.pub2.

Weight-Control Information Network. (2010). *Statistics related to overweight and obesity.* Retrieved from www.win.niddk.nih.gov/statistics/index.htm#overweight.

CHAPTER 30

American Cancer Society. (2010a). *Colorectal cancer.* Retrieved from www.cancer.org.

American Cancer Society. (2010b). *American Cancer Society guidelines for the early detection of cancer.* Retrieved from www.cancer.org/Healthy/FindCancerEarly/CancerScreening Guidelines/american-cancer-society-guidelines-for-the-early-detection-of-cancer.

Beach, P. (2008). *Ulcerative colitis. Mosby's Nursing Consult: Evidence-based nursing monographs.* Retrieved from www.nursingconsult.com.ezproxy.lib.utexas.edu/das/ebnm/view/165337129-2?DOCID=199100&sid=903621103&SEQNO=8.

Black, P. (2009). Cultural and religious beliefs in stoma care nursing. *British Journal of Nursing, 18*(13), 790–793.

Burch, J. (2009). An update on available stoma appliances in the community. *British Journal of Nursing, 14*(4), 146–150.

Carroll, P. (2009). *Diverticular disease: Diverticulosis and diverticulitis. Mosby's Nursing Consult: Evidence-Based nursing monographs.* Retrieved from www.nursingconsult.com.ezproxy.lib.utexas.edu/das/ebnm/view/165337129-2?DOCIDs.=204098&sid=903621103&SEQNO=6.

Clin-eguide. (2008). *Guideline: Appendicitis.* Retrieved from http://clineguide.ovid.com.

Evans, N. P., Misyak, S. A., Schmelz, E. M., et al. (2010). Conjugated linoleic acid ameliorates inflammation-induced colorectal cancer in mice through activation of PPAR1-3. *Journal of Nutrition, 140*(3), 515–521.

Harvard Women's Health Watch. (2009). *Experts revise guidelines for irritable bowel syndrome.* Retrieved from www.health.harvard.edu/fhg/updates/experts-revise-guidelines-for-irritable-bowel-syndrome.shtml.

Hocevar, B. J., Robinson, B., & Gray, M. (2010). Does chewing gum shorten the duration of postoperative ileus in patients undergoing abdominal surgery and creation of a stoma? *Journal of Wound Ostomy and Continence Nursing, 37*(2), 140–146.

Mayo Clinic. (2009). *Colon cancer: Risk factors.* Retrieved from www.mayoclinic.com/health/colon-cancer/DS00035/DSECTION=risk-factors.

Tocco, S. (2009). *Crohn disease. Mosby's Nursing Consult: Evidence-Based nursing monographs.* Retrieved from www.nursingconsult.com.ezproxy.lib.utexas.edu/das/body/165337129-2/ebn.

Wilkes, G. (2008). *What's new in cancer: Update for the practicing nurse. Mosby's Nursing Consult: Clinical Updates.* Retrieved from www.nursingconsult.com.ezproxy.lib.utexas.edu/das/stat/view/195364177-2/cup?nid=198216&sid=983845367&summaryresults=true&SEQNO=1.

CHAPTER 31

Allegretti, P. (2009). *Cirrhosis. Clin-eguide 5-minute clinical suite.* Retrieved from http://clineguide.ovid.com.

American Cancer Society. (2010). *Overview: Pancreatic cancer.* Retrieved from www.cancer.org/acs/groups/cid/documents/webcontent/003071-pdf.

Carroll, P. (2009). *Pancreatitis. Mosby's Nursing Consult: Evidence-Based nursing monographs.* Retrieved from www.nursingconsult.com.ezproxy.lib.utexas.edu/das/stat/view/16533 7129-2/ebnm?nid=212402.

Centers for Disease Control and Prevention. (2010). *Chronic liver disease or cirrhosis.* Retrieved from www.cdc.gov/nchs/fastats/liverdis.htm.

Degli-Esposti, S. D. (2010). *Hepatitis C.* Retrieved from http://clineguide.ovid.com.

Dentinger, C. M. (2009). Hepatitis A: An update. *American Journal of Nursing, 109*(8), 29–32.

Heron, M. (2010). Deaths: Leading causes for 2006. *National Vital Statistics Reports, 58*(14), 1–100.

Laino, C. (2009). *New drug may treat pancreatic cancer.* Retrieved from www.webmd.com/cancer/pancrea tic-cancer/news/20090924/new-drug-may-treat-pancreatic- cancer.

Litchenfeld, L. (2007). *Healthy gums may prevent pancreatic cancer, new drug could treat it.* abcNews/Health. Retrieved from http://abcnews.go.com/Health/CancerPrevention AndTreatment/story?id=2800201&page=1.

McCready, R. (2009). The use of the Molecular Adsorbent Recirculating System (MARS)™ albumin dialysis for the treatment of liver failure: A nursing perspective. *Canadian Association of Critical Care Nurses, 20*(3), 18–22.

Mehta, G., & Rothstein, K. D. (2009). Health maintenance issues in cirrhosis. *Medical Clinics of North America, 93*(4), 901–915.

Morbidity and Mortality Weekly Report Quick Guide. (2010). Recommended adult immunization schedule—United States, 2010. *MMWR Morbidity and Mortality Weekly Report, 59*(1), 1–4.

Mosby's Nursing Consult. (2008). *FDA approves Viread for the treatment of chronic hepatitis B. Drug Information.* Retrieved from www.nursingconsult.com.ezproxy.lib.utexas.edu/das/stat/view/200054724-2/drug?nid=198413&sid=994636272&summaryresults=true&SEQNO=2.

National Cancer Institute Cancer Bulletin. (2007). *Sorafenib for advanced liver cancer increases survival.* Retrieved from www.cancer.gov/clinicaltrials/results/sorafenib-liver0607.

National Digestive Diseases Information Clearinghouse. (2007). *Gallstones.* Retrieved from http://digestive.niddk.nih.gov/ddiseases/pubs/gallstones/index.htm#6.

NIH News Release. (2010). *NIH study offers hope to patients with nonalcoholic steatohepatitis.* Retrieved from www.nih.gov/news/health/apr2010/niddk-28.htm.

ScienceDaily. (2009). *New drug achieves pancreatic cancer tumor remission and prevents recurrence, study suggests.* Retrieved from www.sciencedaily.com/releases/2009/04/090419170025.htm.

Thomas, B. R. (2009). Cholecystectomy: Take a look at two options. *Nursing2009, 39*(2), 36–39.

CHAPTER 32

American Association of Orthopedic Surgeons. *Smoking and musculoskeletal health.* (2010). Retrieved from http://orthoinfo.aaos.org/topic.cfm?topic=A00192.

Brockenbrough, G. (2009). Steroid use may be linked to risk for some musculoskeletal diseases in pro athletes. *Orthopedics Today, 29*(10), 53.

Cameron, I. D., Murray, G. R., Gillespie, L. D., et al. (2010). Interventions for preventing falls in older people in nursing care facilities and hospitals. *Cochrane Database of Systematic Reviews, 2010*(6). Retrieved from www2.cochrane.org/reviews/en/ab005465.html.

Chandran, V. (2010). Genetics of psoriasis and psoriatic arthritis. *Indian Journal of Dermatology, 55*(2), 151–156.

Habif, T. (2009). *Clinical Dermatology* (5th ed.). St Louis: Mosby.

Kalro, B. (2009). Vitamin D and the skeleton. *Alternative Therapies in Women's Health, 11*(4), 25–32.

Phillips, F. (2009). Maintaining healthy bones. *Practice Nurse, 37*(8), 14–18.

Rutledge, D., & Schub, T. (2010). *Evidence-based care sheet: Fall prevention in hospitalized patients.* Glendale, CA: Cinahl Information Systems.

Yeom, H. A., Keller, C., & Fleury, J. (2009). Interventions for promoting mobility in community-dwelling older adults. *Journal of the American Academy of Nurse Practitioners, 21,* 95–100.

CHAPTER 33

Amanatullah, D. F., Cheung, Y., & Di Cesare, P. E. (2010). Hip resurfacing arthroplasty: A review of the evidence for surgical technique, outcome, and complications. *Orthopedic Clinics of North America, 41*(2), 263–272.

Anderson, O. (2010). Ask the experts. *Alive: Canadian Journal of Health and Nutrition,* Apr (330), 61.

Ault, A. (2010). *FDA warns on fracture risks with PPIs. Mosby's Nursing Consult: Drug information: Drug news.* Retrieved from www.nursingconsult.com.ezproxy.lib.utexas.edu/das/pharm/view/203808219-4.

Bakody, E. (2009). Orthopaedic plaster casting: Nurse and patient education. *Nursing Standard, 23*(51), 49–56.

Blakley, T. (2009). Medicinal herbs for muscles and joints. *Massage Magazine, 156,* 92.

Bliuc, D., Nguyen, N. D., Milch, V. E., et al. (2009). Mortality risk associated with low-trauma osteoporotic fracture and subsequent fracture in men and women. *JAMA, 301*(5), 513–521.

Brown, D. A. (2009). Osteoporosis—not just for women. *American Nurse Today, 4*(3), 10–12.

Callahan, L. F., Wiley-Exley, E. K., & Mielenz, T. J. (2009). Use of complementary and alternative medicine among patients with arthritis. *Preventing Chronic Disease, 6*(2), A44.

Chustecka, Z. (2010). *Denosumab "promising" in treatment of giant cell tumor of bone.* Medscape Medical News. Retrieved from www.medscape.com/viewarticle/716889.

Clin-eguide. (2007). *Spinal surgery: Kyphoplasty.* Retrieved from http://clineguide.ovid.com.

Cluett, J. (2010). *ACI—Autologous chondrocyte implantation: What is autologous chondrocyte implantation (ACI)?* Retrieved from http://orthopedics.about.com/od/hipknee/a/aci.htm.

Kalro, B. (2009). Vitamin D and the skeleton. *Alternative Therapies in Women's Health, 11*(4), 25–32.

Kern, U., Alkemper, B., & Kohl, M. (2006). Management of phantom pain with a textile, electromagnetically-acting stump liner: A randomized, double-blind, crossover study. *Journal of Pain Symptom Management, 32*(4), 352–360.

Lowes, R. (2010). *FDA says no "clear connection" between bisphosphonate use and femur fracture risk.* Retrieved from www.medscape.com/viewarticle/718352?sssdmh=dm1.600751&src=nldne&uac=139100FR.

Lucas, B. (2009). Osteoarthritis: Management and treatments. *Nurse Prescribing, 7*(1), 7–12.

Manheimer, E., Cheng, K., Linde, K., et al. (2004). Acupuncture for peripheral joint osteoarthritis. *Cochrane Reviews,* (6). Retrieved from www2.cochrane.org/reviews/en/ab001977.html.

Napoli, M. (2009). The marketing of osteoporosis. *American Journal of Nursing, 109*(4), 58–61.

National Cancer Institute. (2009). *Zoledronate in preventing osteoporosis and bone fractures in patients with locally advanced nonmetastatic prostate cancer undergoing radiation therapy and hormone therapy.* Retrieved from http://clinicaltrials.gov/ct/show/NCT00329797?order=2.

National Guideline Clearinghouse. (2009). *Skeletal pin site care.* Retrieved from www.guideline.gov/summary/summary.aspx?ss=15&doc_id=7420&nbr=004379&string=nursing.

Neal-Boylan, L. (2009). Update on rheumatology: Part 1. *Home Healthcare Nurse, 27*(5), 286–298.

Qaseem, A., Snow, V., Shekeel, P., et al. (2008). Pharmacologic treatment of low bone density or osteoporosis to prevent fractures: A clinical practice guideline from the American College of Physicians. *Annals of Internal Medicine, 149*(6), 404–411.

Santy, J., Vincent, M., & Duffield, B. (2009). The principles of caring for patients with Ilizarov external fixation. *Nursing Standard, 23*(26), 50–55.

Scannell, B. P. (2010). Skeletal traction versus external fixation in the initial temporization of femoral shaft fractures in severely injured patients. *Journal of Trauma—Injury, Infection, and Critical Care, 68*(3), 633–638.

Shimoda, H., Shan, S., & Tanaka, J. (2010). Anti-inflammatory properties of red ginger (*Zingiber officinale* var. *Rubra*) extract and suppression of nitric oxide production by its constituents. *Journal of Medicinal Food, 13*(1), 156–162.

Wehmer, M. A. (2009). *Amputation: Helping patients successfully recover from surgery. Mosby's Nursing Consult: Clinical updates.* Retrieved from www.nursingconsult.com.ezproxy.lib.utexas.edu/das/stat/view/206669901-2/cup?nid=206424&sid=1016071912&summaryresults=true& SEQNO=1.

Wright, E. (2009). Neurovascular impairment and compartment. *Paediatric Nursing, 21*(3), 25–29.

CHAPTER 34

Albo, M. E., Richter, H. E., Brubaker, L., et al. (2007). Burch colposuspension versus fascial sling to reduce urinary stress incontinence. *New England Journal of Medicine, 356*(21), 2143–2155.

Chettle, C. C. (2008). Nurses critical as reimbursement dries up for catheter associated UTIs. *Nursing Spectrum, 21*(16), 26–31.

Dowling-Castronovo, A., & Specht, J. K. (2009). Assessment of transient urinary incontinence in older adults. *American Journal of Nursing, 109*(2), 62–72.

Geriatric Medicine. (2009). Urinary incontinence in older people. *Nursing Older People, Supplement,* 1–22.

Gould, C., Umscheid, C. A., Agarwal, R. K., et al. (2009). *Guideline for Prevention of Catheter-Associated Urinary Tract Infections.* Healthcare Infection Control Practices Advisory Committee. Atlanta: Division of Healthcare Quality Promotion Centers for Disease Control and Prevention.

Katz, A. (2009). When worlds collide: Urinary incontinence and female sexuality. *American Journal of Nursing, 109*(3), 59–63.

National Kidney Foundation. (2010). *Is cystatin C a more accurate filtration marker than creatinine?* Retrieved from www.kidney.org/professionals/KLS/gfr.cfm#24.

Pavlovich-Danis, S. J. (2009). Going…going…gone—Understanding overactive bladder. *Nursing Spectrum,* Winter 2009 CE catalogue, 32–38. Retrieved from www.nurse.com.

CHAPTER 35

American Cancer Society. (2009). *Overview of bladder cancer.* Retrieved from www.cancer.org/docroot/CRI/CRI_2_1x.asp?rnav=criov&dt=44.

Clin-eguide. (2009). *Treatments: Continuous renal replacement therapy.* Retrieved from http://clineguide.ovid.com.

Clin-eguide. (2010). *Zortress approved to prevent organ rejection in adult kidney transplant recipients.* Facts and Comparisons ®eAnswers. Retrieved from http://clineguide.factsandcomparisons.com.ezproxy.lib.utexas.edu/News/NewsArticle.aspx?id=8762.

Dirkes, S., & Hodge, K. (2008, February). Continuous renal replacement therapy in the adult intensive care unit: History and current trends. *Critical Care Nurse, Supplement,* 8–27.

Emergency Nurses' Association. (2010). *Sheehy's Emergency Nursing* (6th ed.). St. Louis: Mosby.

Finkielstein, V. A., & Goldfarb, D. S. (2006). Strategies for preventing calcium oxalate stones. *Canadian Medical Association Journal, 174*(10), 1407–1410.

Guay, D. (2009). Cranberry and urinary tract infections [Review]. *Drugs, 69*(7), 775–807.

Napoli, D. (2010). *Benazepril/amlodipine may slow chronic kidney disease progression. Mosby's Nursing Consult: Drug information.* Retrieved from www.nursingconsult.com.ezproxylib.utexas.edu/das/pharm/view/203971097-2.

Pizzorno, J. E., Murray, M. T., & Joiner-Bey, H. (2008). *The Clinician's Handbook of Natural Medicine* (2nd ed.). Edinburgh: Churchill Livingstone.

Swearingen, P. L. (2007). *Manual of Medical-Surgical Nursing Care* (6th ed.). St. Louis: Mosby.

United Ostomy Association. (2010). *Discussion board: Indiana pouch.* Retrieved from www.uoaa.org.

CHAPTER 36

American Diabetes Association. (2009). Standards of medical care in diabetes. *Diabetes Care, 32*(Suppl. 1), S13–S61.

CHAPTER 37

Brown, S. R., Lee, S., Brown, T. A., et al. (2010). Effect of race on thyroid cancer care in an equal access healthcare system. *American Journal of Surgery, 199*(5), 685–689.

Clin-eguide. (2009). *Adrenal hypofunction. Diseases and conditions.* Retrieved from http://clineguide.ovid.com.

Cook, L. K. (2009). Pheochromocytoma. *American Journal of Nursing, 109*(2), 50–53.

Ferri, F. (2010). *Ferri's Clinical Advisor* (1st ed.). St. Louis: Mosby.

Holcomb, S. S. (2009). Thyroid storm. *Nursing2009, 39*(11), 72.

Khatta, M. (2011). Arrival of vandetanib. *Advance for Nurses, 13*(6), 46.

Osterwell, N. (2009). *Propylthiouracil linked with risk for serious liver damage, death.* Retrieved from www.medscape.com/viewarticle/703851.

CHAPTER 38

American Diabetes Association. (2009). Standards of medical care in diabetes. *Diabetes Care, 32*(Suppl. 1), S13–S61.

American Dietetic Association. (2009). *ADA diabetes type 1 and 2 evidence-based nutrition practice guideline for adults.* ADA Evidenced Analysis Library. Retrieved from www.adaevidencelibrary.com.

Bonham, P. A. (2007). Healing the wounds: Assessing and managing diabetic neuropathy to avoid amputation. *ADVANCE for Nurses, 4*(4), 30–32.

Centers for Disease Control and Prevention. (2010). *National diabetes fact sheet, 2010.* Retrieved from www.cdc.gov/nchs/fastats/diabetes.htm.

Finfer, S., & Delaney, A. (2008). Tight glycemic control in adults. *JAMA, 300*(8), 963–965.

Kapustin, J. (2008). Latent autoimmune diabetes in adults. *Journal of Nurse Practitioners, 4*(9), 681–687.

Lee, F. T. H. (2009). Advances in diabetes therapy in the elderly. *Journal of Pharmacy Practice and Research, 39*(1), 63–66.

Luger, S., & Chabanuk, A. J. (2009). Management of type 2 diabetes. *Home Healthcare Nurse, 27*(2), 92–101.

Medtronic Minimed. (2010). *Introducing the Guardian® Real-Time Continuous Glucose Monitoring System.* Retrieved from www.minimed.com/products/guardian/.

Miller, D. K. (2009). Are you ready to care for a patient with an insulin pump? *Nursing2009, 39*(10), 57–60.

Moquin, B., Blackman, M. R., Mitty, E., et al. (2009). Complementary and alternative medicine (CAM). *Geriatric Nursing, 30*(3), 196–203.

National Institutes of Health NIH News. (2010). *Computers analyze environmental factors in diabetes.* Retrieved from www.nih.gov/news/health/may2010/nigms-20.htm.

Ruggenenti, P., Remuzzi, A., & Remuzzi, G. (2008). Decision time for pancreatic islet-cell transplantation. *Lancet, 371* (9616), 883–884.

Sun, Q., Spiegelman, D., van Dam, R. M., et al. (2010). White rice, brown rice, and risk of type 2 diabetes in U.S. men and women. *Archives of Internal Medicine, 170*(11), 961–969.

CHAPTER 39

American College of Obstetricians and Gynecologists. (2008). *Premenstrual syndrome practice bulletin #15.* Washington, D.C.: American College of Obstetricians and Gynecologists. Retrieved from www.nccam.nih.gov.

American College of Obstetricians and Gynecologists. (2009a). Emergency contraception: Professional update. *Contemporary OB/GYN, 54*(9), 14.

American College of Obstetricians and Gynecologists. (2009b). Committee Opinion #444: Choosing the route of hysterectomy for benign disease. *Journal of Obstetrics, Gynecology, and Neonatal Nursing, 114*(5), 1156–1158.

American College of Obstetricians and Gynecologists. (2009c, December). Committee on Practice Bulletins, Practice Bulletin #109: Cervical cytology screening. *Journal of Obstetrics, Gynecology, and Neonatal Nursing.* Retrieved from www.acog.org/publications/educational_bulletins/pb109.cfm.

Akl, M., & Magrina, J. (2009). Will robots transform gynecologic surgery? *Contemporary OB/GYN, 54*(9), 26–33.

Bachman, G. (2009). Efficacy and safety of low dose regimes of conjugated estrogen creams administered vaginally. *Menopause, 16*, 735.

BFAR Information and Support. (Breastfeeding after Breast and Nipple Surgeries). (2011). *Is it possible to breastfeed after breast reduction surgery?* Retrieved from http://bfar.org/possible-reduction.shtml.

Breslin, E. T., & Lucas, V. A. (2003). *Women's Health Nursing: Toward Evidence-Based Practice.* Philadelphia: Saunders.

Cass, I., & Karlan, B. (2003). Neoplasms of the ovary and fallopian tube. In J. Scott, R. Gibbs, B. Karlan & A. Haney (Eds.), *Danforth's Obstetrics and Gynecology* (9th ed.). Philadelphia: Lippincott Williams & Wilkins.

Clinical Insights. (2010). *Contemporary OB/GYN, 55*(1), 14.

Cummings, S. (2009). Denosumab for prevention of fractures in postmenopausal women with osteoporosis. *New England Journal of Medicine, 361*, 756.

Fontenot, H., & Harris, A. (2008). Latest advances in hormonal contraception. *Journal of Obstetrics, Gynecology, and Neonatal Nursing, 37*(5), 369–374.

Food and Drug Administration. (2010). FDA approves Lysteda to treat heavy menstrual bleeding. *Contemporary OB/GYN, 54*(12), 12.

Fu, M., Ridner, S., & Armer, J. (2009). Post breast cancer lymphedema. *American Journal of Nursing, 109*(7), 48–53.

Holtorf, K. (2009). The bioidentical hormone debate: Are bioidentical hormones (estriadol, estriol, and progesterone) safer or more efficacious than commonly used synthetic versions in hormone replacement therapy? *Postgraduate Medicine, 121*(1), 73–85.

Horbach, N., Lee, T., Levy, B., et al. (2006, May). Laparoscopic supercervical hysterectomy. *Contemporary OB/GYN,* Special Addendum.

Htay, T. T. (2011). *Premenstrual dysphoric disorder.* Retrieved from http://emedicine.medscape.com/article/293257-overview.

James, A. (2009). Von Willebrand disease and other bleeding disorders in women. *American Journal of Obstetrics and Gynecology, 4*(201), 12.

Kaunitz, A. (2005). Beyond the pill. *Journal of Obstetrics and Gynecology, 192*, 998–1004.

Kelland, K. (2011). *Cancer study backs Roche's Herceptin with chemo.* Retrieved from http://reuters.com/assets/print?aid= USLDE 60R0AF20100129,8/16/2011.

Kerlikowski, K. (2009). Evidence-Based breast cancer prevention: The importance of individual risk. *Annals of Internal Medicine, 151*, 750.

Klisc, K., & Kaplan, C. (2009). HPV prevention update. *ADVANCE for Nurse-Practitioners, 17*(11), 28–29.

Morch, L. (2009). Hormone therapy and ovarian cancer. *JAMA, 15*(302), 398.

National Cancer Institute. (2011). *Ovarian cancer prevention.* Retrieved from www.cancer.gov/cncertopics/pdq/prevention/ovarian/Patient/page3.

National Center for Complementary and Alternative Medicine. (2011). *Menopausal symptoms and CAM.* Retrieved from http://nccam.nih.gov/health/menopause/menopause symptoms.htm.

Olson, A., Link, J., Waisman, J., et al. (2009, August). Breast cancer patients unknowingly dose themselves with estrogen by using topical moisturizers. *Journal of Clinical Oncology,* (23), 1225.

Prentice, R. (2009). Benefits and risks of postmenopausal hormone therapy when initiated soon after menopause. *American Journal of Epidemiology, 1*(170), 12.

Samra-Latif, O. M. (2011). *Contraception.* Retrieved from http://emedicine.medscape.com/article/24807-overview.

Stenchever, M. A. (2004). Physiology of micturition, diagnosis of voiding dysfunctions and incontinence, surgical and non-surgical management. In M. A. Stenchever, et al. (Eds.), *Comprehensive Gynecology* (5th ed.). St. Louis: Mosby.

Stewart, E. A., Rabinovici, J., Tempany, C. M., et al. (2006). Clinical outcomes of focused ultrasound surgery for the treatment of uterine fibroids. *Fertility and Sterility, 85*, 22–29.

Weil, E. (2009). The debate over bioidentical hormones. *Nurse Practice, 17*(9), 37–40.

CHAPTER 40

American Cancer Society. (2009). *What are the key statistics about testicular cancer?* Retrieved from www.cancer.org/docroot/cri/content/cri_2_4_1x_what_are_the_key_statistics_for_testicular_cancer_41.asp.

American Urological Association (AUA) *Guidelines on management of BPH: Diagnosis and treatment recommendations.* Retrieved from www.AUAnet.org/guidelines/main_reports/BPH_management/chapt_1_appendix.pdf.

Barnett, S., Kramer, K., Hagerty, S., et al. (2009). Use of 5 a-reductase inhibitors for prostate cancer chemoprophylaxis: American Society of Clinical Oncology and American Urological Association clinical practice guidelines 2008. *Journal of Clinical Urology, 181*, 1642–1657.

DeFleurian, G. (2009). Occupational exposures obtained by questionnaires in clinical practice and their association with semen quality. *Journal of Andrology, 30*, 566.

Hussar, D. (2010). New drugs 2010. *Nursing2010, 40*(2), 39.

Horvath, A., Korde, L., Greene, M., et al. (2009). *Functional phosphodiesferase 11A mutations may modify the risk of familial testicular germ cell tumors human cancer research.* Retrieved from www.NIH.GOV/news/health/june2009/NICHd-29.

Jackson, G., Rosen, R., Kloner, R., & Kostis, J. (2006). The Second Princeton Consensus on Sexual Dysfunction and Cardiac Risk: New guidelines for sexual medicine. *Journal of Sexual Medicine, 3*(1), 28–36.

Mulcathy, N. (2010). *The Progensa urine test detects prostate cancer cells.* The 2010 CUCA Symposium. Abstract #5. Presented March 5, 2010, at the Genito-Urinary Cancer Symposium. Retrieved from www.medpagetoday.com/MeetingCoverage/ASCOGU/18855.

Smith, M. (2009). Denosumab in men receiving androgen deprivation therapy for prostate cancer. *New England Journal of Medicine, 361,* 745.

U.S. Preventive Services Task Force. (2008). Screening for prostate cancer in the United States: Recommendation statement. *Annals of Internal Medicine, 1149*(3), 185–191.

Wold, G. (2008). *Basic Geriatric Nursing* (4th ed.). Philadelphia: Mosby.

CHAPTER 41

Centers for Disease Control and Prevention. (2007). *Sexually transmitted diseases in the U.S. 2006. National surveillance data for chlamydia, gonorrhea and syphilis.* Retrieved from www.cdc.gov.

Klisz, C., & Kaplan, C. (2009). HPV update. *ADVANCE for Nurse-Practitioners, 17*(11), 28–29.

Kurtyka, D. (2010). HIV infection 2010: From terminal disease to chronic infection. *ADVANCE for Nurse-Practitioners, 18*(1), 33–39.

Lennox, J. (2009). Safety and efficacy of raltegravir versus afarirenz-based combination therapy in treatment of new patients with HIV-1 infection. *Lancet, 374*(9), 796.

Munoz, N. (2009). Safety, immunogenicity and efficacy of quadravalent HPV types 6, 11, 16, 18 in women aged 24-45 years. *Lancet, 373*(6), 1949.

Swan, A. (2009). Acute HIV infections in primary care. *ADVANCE for Nurse-Practitioners, 17*(9), 49–54.

Wold, G. (2008). *Basic Geriatric Nursing* (4th ed.). Philadelphia: Mosby.

CHAPTER 42

American Academy of Dermatology. (2010). *Facts about sunscreens.* Retrieved from www.aad.org/media/background/factsheets/fact_sunscreen.htm.

Ayello, E. A., & Sibbald, R. G. (2008). Preventing pressure ulcers and skin tears. In E. Capezuti, D. Zwicker & M. Mezey et al. (Eds.), *Evidence-Based Geriatric Nursing Protocols for Best Practice.* (3rd ed.). New York: Springer.

Bolhuis, J. (2008). Evidence-Based skin tear protocol. *Long-Term Living: For the Continuing Care Professional, 57*(6), 48–52.

D'Avanzo, C. (2008). *Pocket Guide to Cultural Health Assessment* (4th ed.). St. Louis: Mosby.

Fleck, C. A., & Kesselman, P. (2009). What's new in wound care products. *Podiatry Management, 28*(6), 159–168.

Fox, R. (2009). Psychodermatology: A new approach to protect the skin. *Life Extension, 15*(7), 67–73.

Johnson, D., Lineweaver, L., & Maze, L. M. (2009). Patients' bath basins as potential sources of infection: A multicenter sampling study. *American Journal of Critical Care, 18*(1), 31–38.

Kalro, B. (2009). Vitamin D and the skeleton. *Alternative Therapies in Women's Health, 11*(4), 25–32.

Miner, K., Katz, M., & Razor, B. (2009). Skin tear prevention and management. *Nevada RNFormation, 18*(4), 14.

Strayer, D. A., & Schub, T. (2009). *Melanoma: Risk factors and prevention. Evidence-based care sheet.* Glendale, CA: Cinahl Information Systems.

CHAPTER 43

American Burn Association. (2007). *Burn incident fact sheet.* Retrieved from www.ameriburn.org/resources_factsheet.php.

American Burn Association White Paper. (2009). *Surgical Management of the Burn Wound and Use of Skin Substitutes.* Chicago: American Burn Association.

American Burn Association. (2011). *Burn incidence and treatment in the United States: 2011 fact sheet.* Retrieved from www.ameriburn.org/resources_factsheet.php.

American Cancer Society. (2011a). *Melanoma skin cancer: What are the key statistics.* Retrieved from www.cancer.org/Cancer/SkinCancer-Melanoma/DetailedGuide/melanoma-skin-cancer-key-statistics.

American Cancer Society. (2011b). *Treating skin cancer—Melanoma.* Retrieved from www.cancer.org/Cancer/SkinCancer-Melanoma/DetailedGuide/melanoma-skin-cancer-treating-immunotherapy.

Arnstein, P. (2010). What's the best way to cool my patient's burn pain? *Nursing2010, 40*(3), 61–62.

Brimhall, A. K., King, L. N., Licciardone, J. C., et al. (2008). Safety and efficacy of alefacept, efalizumab, etanercept and infliximab in treating moderate to severe plaque psoriasis: a meta-analysis of randomized controlled trials. *British Journal of Dermatology, 159*(2), 274–285.

Centers for Disease Control and Prevention. (2011). *Shingles disease—Questions and answers (herpes zoster).* Retrieved from www.cdc.gov/vaccines/vpd-vac/shingles/dis-faqs.htm.

Chan, M. M., & Chan, G. M. (2009). Nutritional therapy for burns in children and adults. *Nutrition, 25*(3), 261–269.

Combest, W. L. (2007). *Tea tree.* Retrieved from www.uspharmacist.com.

Connor-Ballard, P. A. (2009a). Understanding and managing burn pain: Part 1. *American Journal of Nursing, 109*(4), 48–54.

Connor-Ballard, P. A. (2009b). Understanding and managing burn pain: Part 2. *American Journal of Nursing, 109*(5), 56–63.

Crowe, T., & Brockbank, C. (2009). Nutrition therapy in the prevention and treatment of pressure ulcers. *Wound Practice and Research, 17*(2), 90–98.

Demling, R. H., & De Santi, L. (2004). *Managing the burn wound.* Burnsurgery.org. Retrieved from www.burnsurgery.org.

Drugs.com. (2010). *FDA approves Veltin.* Retrieved from www.drugs.com/newdrugs/stiefel-gsk-receives-fda-approval-veltin-clindamycin-phosphate-tretinoin-gel-1-2-0-025-2220.html.

Farage, M. A., Miller, K. W., Berardesca, E., et al. (2009). Clinical implications of aging skin. *American Journal of Clinical Dermatology, 10*(2), 73–86.

Fleck, C. A., & Kesselman, P. (2009). What's new in wound care products. *Podiatry Management, 28*(6), 159–168.

Gestring, M. (2011). *Negative pressure wound therapy.* Retrieved from www.uptodate.com/contents/negativ-pressure-wound-care.

Hansen, D. S., Langemo, D., Anderson, J., et al. (2009). Can pressure mapping prevent ulcers? *Nursing2009, 39*(6), 50–51.

Hartner, K. (2007). In your own skin. *ADVANCE for Nurses, 5*(20), 33–34.

Hilton, L. (2009). Healing stubborn wounds. *Dermatology Times, 30*(3), 44.

Houghton, P. E., Campbell, K. E., Fraser, C. H., et al. (2010). Electrical stimulation therapy increases rate of healing of pressure ulcers in community-dwelling people with spinal cord injury. *Archives of Physical Medicine and Rehabilitation, 91*(5), 669–678.

Hudak, S., Sharkey, S., Engleman, M., et al. (2008). Pressure ulcer plan is working. *Provider, 34*(5), 34–39.

Kimball, A. B., Guerin, A., Latremouille-Viau, D., et al. (2010). Coronary heart disease and stroke risk in patients with psoriasis: Retrospective analysis. *American Journal of Medicine, 123*(4), 350–357.

Klein, J. M. (2009). The psychiatric nurse in the burn unit. *Perspectives in Psychiatric Care, 45*(1), 71–73.

Klein, J. M., & Hoffman, C. A. (2010). Relaxation and visual imagery techniques: Do they work? Can they really help burn patients? *MEDSURG Nursing, 19*(3), 169–175.

Meier, F., Guenova, E., Clasen, S., et al. (2009). Significant response after treatment with the mTOR inhibitor sirolimus in combination with carboplatin and paclitaxel in metastatic melanoma patients. *Journal of the American Academy of Dermatology, 60*(5), 863–868.

Meinking, T. L., Villar, M. E., Vicaria, M., et al. (2010). The clinical trials supporting benzyl alcohol lotion 5% (Ulesfia™): A safe and effective topical treatment for head lice (pediculosis humanus capitis). *Pediatric Dermatology, 27,* 19–24.

Murphy, P., Colwell, C., Pineda, G., et al. (2009). Burning issues. *EMS Magazine, 38*(10), 83–90.

National Institutes of Health. (2007). *Tai Chi boosts immunity to shingles virus in older adults, NIH-sponsored study reports.* NIH News Press. Retrieved from http://nccam.nih.gov.

Riley, M. M. S. (2008). *Shingles (herpes zoster). Mosby's Nursing Consult: Evidence-based monographs.* Retrieved from www.nursingconsult.com.ezproxy.lib.utexas.edu/das/ebnm/view/165337129-2?DOCID=194108& sid=903621103&SEQNO=10.

Strayer, D. A., & Schub, T. (2009). *Melanoma: Risk factors and prevention. Evidence-Based care sheet.* Glendale, CA: Cinahl Information Systems.

van Rijswijk, L., & Lyder, C. (2008). Pressure ulcers: Were they there on admission? *American Journal of Nursing, 108*(11), 27–28.

Wahl, W. L., Arbabi, S., Zalewski, C., et al. (2010). Intensive care unit core measures improve infectious complications in burn patients. *Journal of Burn Care and Research, 31*(1), 190–195.

Wendling, P. (2009). *Targeted therapy PLX4032 takes center stage in metastatic melanoma. Mosby's Nursing Consult: News.* Retrieved from www.nursingconsult.com.ezproxy.lib.utexas.edu/das/stat/view/219111858-2/mnfp?date=week&nid=212554&sid=1055176832& SEQNO=23.

Yarnell, E., Abascal, K., & Rountree, R. (2009). Herbs for herpes simplex infections. *Alternative and Complementary Therapies, 15*(2), 69–73.

CHAPTER 44

Ahmad, Z. (2009). The very real threat of bioterrorism: Are we prepared? *Internet of Journal of Rescue and Disaster Medicine, 8*(1).

American Red Cross. (2010). *Prepare your home and family.* Retrieved from http://www.redcross.org/portal/site/en/menuitem.d8aaecf214c576bf971e4cfe43181aa0/?vgnextoid=72c51a53f1c37110VgnVCM1000003481a10aRCRD.

Barishansky, R. M., & Langan, J. (2009). Surge capacity. *EMS, 38*(4), 36–40.

Bhardwaj, P., Srivastava, J., & Karan, J. (2009). Bioterrorism: An imminent public health threat. *Internet Journal of Epidemiology.* Retrieved from www.ispub.com/journal/the_internet_journal_of_epidemiology/volume_7_number_1_24/article_printable/bioterrorism-an-imminent-public-health-threat.html.

Brinker, A., Prior, K., & Schumacher, J. (2009). Personal protection during resuscitation of casualties contaminated with chemical or biological warfare agents—A survey of medical first receivers. *Prehospital and Disaster Medicine, 24*(6), 525–528.

Centers for Disease Control and Prevention. (2010). *Bioterrorism agents/disease.* Retrieved from http://emergency.cdc.gov/agent/agentlist-category.asp.

Centers for Disease Control and Prevention. (2011a). *Outbreak postings.* Retrieved from www.cdc.gov/ncidod/dvrd/spb/outbreaks/index.htm.

Centers for Disease Control and Prevention. (2011b). *What you need to know when the power goes out unexpectedly.* Retrieved from www.bt.cdc.gov/disasters/poweroutage/needtoknow.asp.

Chappell, J. R., & Bridges, D. (2009). Prepared or unprepared for pandemic flu? *Journal of Christian Nursing, 26*(2), 80–85.

Couig, M. P., Martinelli, A., & Lavin, R. P. (2005). The National Response Plan: Health and Human Services takes the lead for emergency support function. *Disaster Management & Response, 3*(2), 34–40.

Crisis Management Consultants. (2010). *Developing and managing a human service disaster response team in your community.* Retrieved from www.crisisinc.com/disaster-psychology.

Donnellan, M. E. (2009). *Are we ready? RT for decision makers.* Retrieved from www.rtmagazine.com/issues/articles/2010-04_05.asp.

Drill, H. (2009). If disaster strikes. *Practical Nurse, 63*(6), 22–25.

Emergency Nurses Association (ENA). (2010). *Sheehy's Emergency Nursing: Principles and Practice* (6th ed.). St. Louis: Mosby.

Federal Emergency Management Agency (FEMA). (2010). *Emergency water storage and purification guidelines.* Retrieved from http://www.prepareandsurvive.info/documents/WaterPurificationandStorage.pdf.

Federal Emergency Management Agency (FEMA). (2011). *After a chemical attack.* Retrieved from www/fema.gov/hazard/terrorism/chem/chem_after.shtm.

Grimes, D. E., & Mendias, E. P. (2010). Nurses' intentions to respond to bioterrorism and other infectious disease emergencies. *Nursing Outlook, 58*(1), 10–16.

Kelen, I., McCarthy, M. L., Kraus, C. K., et al. (2009). Creation of surge capacity by early discharge of hospitalized patients at low risk for untoward events. *Disaster Medicine and Public Health Preparedness, 3*(2 Suppl.), S10–S16.

Legg, T. J. (2009). Nursing in disaster situations: Are you prepared to answer the call? *Pennsylvania Nurse, 64*(2), 4–7.

Mosby's Nursing Consult. (2010). *Biological terrorism agents. Patient teaching handouts.* Retrieved from www.nursingconsult.com.

Minnesota Department of Health (MDH). (2008). *MDH Chemical Terrorism Poster.* Retrieved from http://www.health.state.mn.us/divs/phl/labep/posters.html.

Peterman, S. (2010). *Preparing for disaster: How will you respond? Mosby's Nursing Consult: Clinical updates.* Retrieved from www.nursingconsult.com.ezproxy.lib.utexas.edu/das/stat/view/194941733-4/cup.

Peterson, C. A. (2006). Be safe, be prepared: Emergency system for advanced registration of volunteer health professionals in disaster response. *Online Journal of Issues in Nursing.* Retrieved from www.nursingworld.org/MainMenuCategories/ANA Marketplace/ANAPeriodicals/OJIN/TableofContents/Volume112006/No3Sept06/tpc31_216083.aspx.

Powers, R. (2009). Evidence-based ED disaster planning. *Journal of Emergency Nursing, 35*(3), 218–223.

Radiation Emergency Medical Management. (2010a). *Countermeasure for treatment. Managing internal contamination.* Retrieved from www.remm.nlm.gov/int_contamination.htm#blocking agents.

Radiation Emergency Medical Management. (2010b). *Protecting responding personnel.* Retrieved from www.remm.nlm.gov/ext_contamination.htm#personnel.

Rebmann, T. (2009). Assessing hospital emergency management plans: A guide for infection preventionists. *American Journal of Infection Control, 37*(9), 708–714.

Science & Technology Review. (Eds.). (2010). *Responding to a terrorist attack involving chemical warfare agents.* Retrieved from https//str.llnl.gov/Mar10/koester.html.

Stoppler, M. C. (2007). *Medical triage: Code tags and triage terminology.* Medicinenet.com. Retrieved June, 22, 2011 from http://www.medicinenet.com/script/main/art.asp?articlekey=79529.

Todd, R. (2006). Infection control and hurricane Katrina. *American Journal of Nursing, 106*(3), 29–31.

Twedell, D. (2009). Duty to care. *Journal of Continuing Education in Nursing, 40*(2), 53–54.

CHAPTER 45

American Heart Association. (2010). 2010 American Heart Association guidelines for cardiopulmonary resuscitation and emergency cardiovascular care science. *Circulation, 122,* S640–S656.

Brege, D. J. (2009). Recognizing and treating heatstroke. *Nursing Made Incredibly Easy! 7*(4), 13–18.

Camacho, M. (2009). Ingested poisons in adults. *Nursing Made Incredibly Easy! 7*(3), 23–25.

Champion, J. D. (2009). *Recognizing and preventing elder abuse.* Retrieved from www.nursingconsult.com.ezproxy.lib.utexas.edu/das/stat/view/165337129-2/cup.

Edlich, R. F. (2010). *Cold injuries.* http://emedicine.medscape.com/article/1278523-overview#aw2aab6b6.

Ferri, F. F. (2011). *Ferri's Clinical Advisor 2011.* St. Louis: Mosby.

Glow, S. D. (2009). *Caring for patients with sepsis according to the guidelines. Mosby's Nursing Consult: Clinical updates.* Retrieved from www.nursingconsult.com/das/stat/view/223886186-6/cup?nid=207446&sid=1073293776&SEQNO=1.

Habif, T. P. (2010). *Clinical Dermatology* (5th ed.). St. Louis: Mosby.

Harding, A. D. (2010). Poison control in the emergency department. *Journal of Emergency Nursing, 36*(3), 242–244.

Harvard Women's Health Watch. (2009). Recognizing and avoiding tick-borne illness. *Harvard Women's Health Watch, 16*(10), 4–6.

Hussey, L. (2010). *Emergency nursing care of patients with abdominal trauma. Clinical Updates.* Retrieved from www.nursingconsult.com/das/stat/view/223886186-2/cup?nid=196357&sid=1073256366&SEQNO=1.

Hyett, J. M. (2009). How to respond when lightning strikes. *Nursing2009, 39*(7), 32–35.

March, P. D., & Grose, S. (2010). *Patient Assault.* Glendale, CA: Cinahl Information Systems.

National Oceanic and Atmospheric Administration. (2009). *Heat wave.* Washington D. C: U.S. Department of Commerce.

National Safety Council. (2010). *Summary from injury facts, 2010 edition.* Retrieved from www.nsc.org/news_resources/injury_and_death_statistics/Documents/Summary_2010_Ed.pdf.

Olive, P. (2007). Care for emergency department patients who have experienced domestic violence: A review of the evidence base. *Journal of Clinical Nursing, 16*(9), 1736–1748.

Olshaker, J. S. (2009). Managing emergency department overcrowding. *Emergency Medical Clinics of North America, 27*(4), 593–603.

Pines, J. M., Pollack, C. V., Diercks, D. B., et al. (2009). The association between emergency department crowding and adverse cardiovascular outcomes in patients with chest pain. *Academic Emergency Medicine, 16*(7), 617–625.

Pinto, S., & Grose, S. (2010). *Intimate Partner Violence: Psychological Aspects.* Glendale, CA: Cinahl Information Systems.

Schaeffer, S., & Badillo, R. B. (2009). Poison control therapy. *American Journal of Nursing, 109*(12), 42–45.

Schub, E. (2010). *Sepsis and Septic Shock.* Glendale, CA: Cinahl Informations Systems.

Schub, T., & Grose, S. (2010). *Elder Abuse.* Glendale, CA: Cinahl Informations Systems.

Schub, T., & Jaffe, S. E. (2010). *Intimate Partner Violence: Physical Abuse.* Glendale, CA: Cinahl Informations Systems.

Strickler, J. (2007). *Hypovolemic shock. Mosby's Nursing Consult: Evidence-Based Nursing Monographs.* Retrieved from www.nursingconsult.com/das/stat/view/223886186-2/ebnm?fromglu=true&nid=189178.

Tocco, S. (2009). *Neurogenic shock. Mosby's Nursing Consult: Evidence-Based Nursing Monographs.* Retrieved from www.nursingconsult.com/das/stat/view/223886186-2/ebnm?fromglu=true&nid=207656.

Venema, A. M., Groothoff, J. W., & Bierens, J. (2010). The role of the bystander during rescue and resuscitation of drowning victims. *Resuscitation, 81*(4), 434–439.

Wendling, P. (2010). *Study: Uninsured were more likely to die after trauma. Mosby's Nursing Consult: Nursing News.* Retrieved from www.nursingconsult.com.ezproxy.lib.utexas.edu/das/stat/view/214656874-4/mnfp?date=week&nid=216983&sid=1039126648&SEQNO=26.

Wilmot, L. A. (2010). Shock: Early recognition and management. *Journal of Emergency Nursing, 36*(2), 134–139.

CHAPTER 46

Costell, S. (2003). Evidence-based treatment of mood disorders. *Nursing Clinics of North America, 38,* 21–33.

Diazgranados, N., Ibrahim, L., Brutsche, N. E., et al. (2010). A randomized add-on trial of an N-methyl-d-aspartate antagonist in treatment-resistant bipolar depression. *Archives of General Psychiatry, 67*(8), 793–802.

Harvard Medical School. (2009). Manipulating memory to overcome fear. *Harvard Mental Health Letter, 26*(1), 4–5.

Helwick, C. (2010). *Virtual reality exposure enhances treatment of PTSD.* Retrieved from www.medscape.com/viewarticle/722512.

Kavanaugh, A., & McLoughlin, D. M. (2009). Electroconvulsive therapy and nursing care. *British Journal of Nursing, 18*(22), 1370–1377.

Lyons, D. L., Grimley, S. M., & Sydnor, L. (2009). Delirium and dementia: Double trouble. *LPN2009, 5*(2), 38–45.

Maratos, A., Gold, C., Wang, X., et al. (2008). Music therapy for depression. *Cochrane Database of Systematic Reviews, 2010*(7).

National Institute of Mental Health. (2009). *Brain stimulation therapies.* Retrieved from www.nimh.nih.gov/health/topics/brain-stimulation-therapies/brain-stimulation-therapies.shtml.

Peden, A. R., Rayens, M. K., Hall, L. A., et al. (2005). Testing an intervention to reduce negative thinking, depressive symptoms and chronic stressors in low-income single mothers. *Journal of Nursing Scholarship, 37*(3), 268–274.

Phillips, L. L., Paukert, A. L., Stanley, M. A., et al. (2009). Incorporating religion and spirituality to improve care for anxiety and depression in older adults. *Geriatrics, 64*(8), 15–18.

SAMHSA's National Registry of Evidence-based Programs. (2007). *Network therapy.* Retrieved from www.nrepp.samhsa.gov/ViewIntervention.aspx?id=90.

Sherman, F. T. (2009). Life-saving treatment for depression in elderly. *Geriatrics, 64*(4), 8–12.

Smith, M., & Brighton, V. (2009). Detection and assessment of late-life anxiety. *Journal of Gerontological Nursing, 35*(7), 9–14.

Westgard, E. (2009). Coming home with posttraumatic stress disorder. *American Journal of Nursing, 109*(5), 11.

Wilson, D. (2009). Anxiety and depression: It all starts with stress. *Integrative Medicine, 8*(3), 42–45.

CHAPTER 47

Agency for Healthcare Research and Quality (AHRQ). (2009). *Counseling and interventions to prevent tobacco use and tobacco-caused disease in adults and pregnant women reaffirmation recommendation statement.* Retrieved from www.ahrq.gov/clinic/uspstf09/tobacco/tobaccors2.htm.

Back, S. E., Payne, R. L., Simpson, A. N., et al. (2010). Gender and prescription opioids: Findings from the National Survey on Drug Use and Health. *Addictive Behaviors, 35*(11), 1001–1007.

Bates, B. (2009). *Personality disorders elevate risk of substance abuse. Mosby's Nursing Consult: Nursing News.* Retrieved from www.nursingconsult.com.ezproxy.lib.utexas.edu/das/stat/view/214656874-4/mnfp?date=week&nid=214774&sid=1039126648&SEQNO=41.

Boschert, S. (2010). *Zero tolerance links addiction programs for physicians, convicts. Mosby's Nursing Consult: Nursing News.* Retrieved from www.nursingconsult.com.ezproxy.lib.utexas.edu/das/stat/view/214656874-4/mnfp?date=week&nid=218695&sid=1039126648&SEQNO=16.

Calhoun, P. S., McDonald, S. D., Guerra, V. S., et al. (2010). Clinical utility of the primary care–PTSD screen among U.S. veterans who served since September 11, 2001. *Psychiatry Research, 178*(2), 330–335.

Clark, J. (2008). The danger next door: Methamphetamine. *RN, 71*(5), 22–26.

Cleary, M., Hunt, G. E., Matheson, S., et al. (2009). Psychosocial treatments for people with co-occurring severe mental illness and substance misuse: Systematic review. *Journal of Advanced Nursing, 65*(2), 238–258.

Clin-eguide. (2009a). *Guideline: Alcohol withdrawal.* Retrieved from http://clineguide.ovid.com.

Clin-eguide. (2009b). *Guideline: Substance abuse.* Retrieved from http://clineguide.ovid.com.

Cohen, J. (2011). *Alcohol intoxication.* Retrieved from www.emedicinehealth.com/alcohol_intoxication/article_em.htm.

Copp, M. A. (2009). Drug addiction. *RN, 72*(4), 40–44.

DuPont, R. L., McLellan, A. T., White, W. L., et al. (2009). Setting the standard for recovery: Physicians' health programs. *Journal of Substance Abuse Treatment, 36*(2), 159–171.

Durkin, A., & O'Connor, L. G. (2009). Preventing unsafe alcohol consumption on the 21st birthday. *Journal of Psychosocial Nursing, 47*(5), 29–33.

Fals-Stewart, W., & Lam, W. K. (2010). Computer-assisted cognitive rehabilitation for the treatment of patients with substance use disorders: A randomized clinical trial. *Experimental Clinical Psychopharmacology, 18*(1), 87–98.

Glaucoma Research Foundation. (2011). *Medical marijuana.* Retrieved from www.glaucoma.org/treatment/medical-marijuana.php.

Martell, B. A., Orson, F. M., Poling, J., et al. (2009). Cocaine vaccine for the treatment of cocaine dependence in methadone-maintained patients. *Archives of General Psychiatry, 66*(10), 1116–1123.

Matthews, R. (2009). *Target treatment for elders' alcohol and substance abuse. Mosby's Nursing Consult: Nursing News.* Retrieved from www.nursingconsult.com.ezproxy.lib.utexas.edu/das/stat/view/214656874-4/mnfp?date=week&nid=214733&sid=1039126648 &SEQNO=42.

McCabe, S. E., Bostwick, W. B., Hughes, T. L., et al. (2010). The relationship between discrimination and substance use disorders among lesbian, gay, and bisexual adults in the United States. *American Journal of Public Health, 100*(10), 1946–1952.

McQueen, J., Howe, T. E., & Mains, D. (2009). Brief interventions for heavy alcohol users admitted to general hospital wards. *Cochrane Database of Systematic Reviews, 2009*(3) CD005191. doi:10.1002/14651858.CD005191.pub2. Retrieved from www2.cochrane.org/reviews/en/ab005191.html.

Morbidity and Mortality Weekly Report. (2010). Emergency department visits involving nonmedical use of selected prescription drugs—United States, 2004–2008. *Morbidity and Mortality Weekly Report (MMWR), 59*(23), 705–709.

Pinto, S., & Schub, T. (2009). *Substance Abuse in Healthcare Professionals. Evidence-Based Care Sheet.* Glendale, CA: Cinahl Information Systems.

Pinto, S., & Walsh, K. (2008). *Substance Abuse in Older Adults. Evidence-Based Care Sheet.* Glendale, CA: Cinahl Information Systems.

SAMHSA's National Registry of Evidence-based Programs. (2007). *Network therapy.* Retrieved from www.nrepp.samhsa.gov/ViewIntervention.aspx?id=90.

Stevenson, J. S., & Masters, J. A. (2005). Predictors of alcohol misuse and abuse in older women. *Journal of Nursing Scholarship, 37*(4), 329–335.

Tan, W. C., Lo, D., Jong, A., et al. (2009). Marijuana and chronic obstructive lung disease: A population based study. *Canadian Medical Association Journal, 180*(8), 814–820.

Thomas, C. P., Reif, S., Haq, S., et al. (2008). Use of buprenorphine for addiction treatment: Perspectives of addiction specialists and general psychiatrists. *Psychiatric Services, 59*(8), 909–916.

Tierney, J. A. (2009). Identification and treatment of alcohol abuse, dependence, and withdrawal. *ISNA Bulletin, 35*(2), 10–14.

Wells, G. M. (2010). The effect of religiosity and campus alcohol culture on collegiate alcohol consumption. *Journal of American College Health, 58*(4), 295–304.

Yalom, I. D., & Leszcz, M. (2005). *The Theory and Practice of Group Psychotherapy* (5th ed.). New York: Basic Books.

Zarling, K. K. (2007). Tobacco cessation assistance. In B. J. Ackley et al. (Eds.), *Evidence-Based Nursing Care Guidelines: Medical-Surgical Interventions.* St. Louis: Mosby.

CHAPTER 48

Alzheimer's Association. (2011). *Alzheimer's disease facts and figures.* Retrieved from www.alz.org/documents_custom/2011_Facts_Figures_Fact_Sheet.pdf; www.alz.org/national/documents/checklist_10signs.pdf.

Alzheimer's Association International Conference on Alzheimer's Disease. (2010). *Four new research studies describe experimental immunotherapies for Alzheimer's.* Retrieved from www.alz.org/icad/2010_release_four_071310_1230pm.asp.

Ancoli-Israel, S., Palmer, B. W., Cooke, J. R., et al. (2008). Cognitive effects of treating obstructive sleep apnea in Alzheimer's disease: A randomized controlled study. *Journal of American Geriatric Society, 56*(11), 2076–2081.

Bassil, N., & Grossberg, G. T. (2009a). Evidence-based approaches to preventing Alzheimer's disease: Part 1. *Primary Psychiatry, 16*(6), 29–35.

Bassil, N., & Grossberg, G. T. (2009b). Evidence-based approaches to preventing Alzheimer's disease: Part 2. *Primary Psychiatry, 16*(7), 33–38.

Bennett, P. L. (2009). Alzheimer's disease: Seeing the signs early. *Journal of the American Academy of Nurse Practitioners, 21,* 588–595.

Buettner, L. L., Lundegren, H., Lago, D., et al. (1996). Therapeutic recreation as an intervention for persons with dementia and agitation: An efficacy study. *American Journal of Alzheimer's Disease and Other Dementias, 11*(5), 4–12.

Coakley, A. B., & Mahoney, E. K. (2009). Creating a therapeutic and healing environment with a pet therapy program. *Complementary Therapies in Clinical Practice, 15*(3), 141–146.

Drugs.com. (2010). *Zyprexa.* Retrieved from www.drugs.com/pdr/zyprexa.html.

Folstein, M. F., Folstein, S. E., & McHugh, P. R. (1975). A practical method of grading the cognitive state of patients for the clinician. *Journal of Psychiatric Research, 12*(3), 189–198.

Freysteinson, W. M. (2009). Therapeutic mirror interventions. *Journal of Holistic Nursing, 27*(4), 241–252.

Grossberg, G. T., Christensen, D. D., Griffith, P. A., et al. (2010). The art of sharing the diagnosis and management of Alzheimer's disease with patients and caregivers: Recommendations of an expert consensus panel. *Primary Care Companion Journal of Clinical Psychiatry, 12*(1) PCC.09cs00833.

Kalapatapu, R. K., & Neugroschi, J. A. (2009). Update on neuropsychiatric symptoms of dementia: Evaluation and management. *Geriatrics, 64*(4), 20–26.

Lyons, D. L., Grimley, S. M., & Sydnor, L. (2009). Delirium & dementia: Double trouble. *LPN, 5*(2), 38–45.

Manepalli, J., Desai, A., & Sharma, P. (2009). Psychosocial-environmental treatments for Alzheimer's disease. *Primary Psychiatry, 16*(6), 39–46.

McEvoy, P. (2004). Using process mapping to improve nursing practice and patient care. *Professional Nurse, 19*(9), 508–511.

McGuinness, B., Wilson, D., Todd, S., & Passmore, P. (2009). Effective use of drugs in Alzheimer's disease. *Practice Nursing, 20*(6), Supplement, S11–S14.

Nadler-Moodie, M. (2009). Clinical practice guideline. 1-Hour face-to face assessment of a patient in a mechanical restraint. *Journal of Psychosocial Nursing, 47*(6), 37–43.

Nazarko, L. (2009). Dementia care: The use and abuse of antipsychotic drugs. *Nursing and Residential Care, 11*(3), 138–142.

Nguyen, M. (2009). Nurse's assessment of caregiver burden. *MEDSURG Nursing, 18*(3), 147–151.

Qaseem, A., Snow, V., Cross, J. T., Jr, et al.; American College of Physicians/American Academy of Family Physicians Panel on Dementia. (2008). Current pharmacologic treatment of dementia: A clinical practice guideline from the American College of Physicians and the American Academy of Family Physicians. *Annals of Internal Medicine, 148*(5), 370–378.

Rohl, C. (2006). Hussey, L. (2011, updated). *Tailoring nursing care to the special needs of Alzheimer's patients. Mosby's Nursing Consult: Clinical updates.* Retrieved from www.nursing consult.com/nursing/clinical-updates/full-text?clinical_ update_id=200542.

Rutledge, D. N., & March, P. D. (2008). *Restraint and seclusion: Minimizing use in psychiatric facilities.* Glendale, CA: Cinahl Information Systems.

Sullivan, M. G. (2010). *Updated Alzheimer's diagnostic criteria may identify disease earlier. Mosby's Nursing Consult: Nursing News.* Retrieved from www.nursingconsult.com.ezproxy.lib. utexas.edu/das/stat/view/215920407-2/mnfp?date=week& nid= 220139&sid=1042722311&SEQNO=1.

CHAPTER 49

American Psychiatric Association. (2004). *Practice Guideline for the Treatment of Patients with Schizophrenia* (2nd ed.). Arlington, VA: American Psychiatric Association.

American Psychiatric Association. (2007). *Diagnostic and Statistical Manual of Mental Disorders* (4th ed). Text Revision. Washington, D.C.: American Psychiatric Association.

Amminger, G. P., Schafer, M. R., Papageorgiou, K., et al. (2010). Long-chain omega-3 fatty acids for indicated prevention of psychotic disorders: A randomized, placebo-controlled trial. *Archives of General Psychiatry, 67*, 146–154.

Bryan, C. A., Mistovich, J. J., Krost, W. S., et al. (2009). In two minds? EMS care of the schizophrenic patient. *EMS, 38*(12), 63–71.

Calandra, J. (2009). Schizophrenia: What do we really know? *Nursing Spectrum, 22*(8), 22–25.

Drugs.com. (2010). *Abilify (aripiprazole) food and lifestyle interactions.* Retrieved from www.drugs.com/food-interactions/ aripiprazole,abilify.html.

Hoban, S. (2010). Caring for a patient with schizophrenia in a med-surg unit. *Nursing2010, 40*(1), 44–48.

Lamont, S., & Brunero, S. (2009). Personality disorder prevalence and treatment outcomes: A literature review. *Mental Health Nursing, 30*(10), 631–637.

Malone, D., Marriott, G., Newton-Howes, S., et al. (2009). Community mental health teams for people with severe mental illnesses and disordered personality. *Schizophrenia Bulletin, 35*(1), 13–14.

Matheson, S. L., Green, M. J., Loo, C., et al. (2010). Quality assessment and comparison of evidence for electroconvulsive therapy and repetitive transcranial magnetic stimulation for schizophrenia: A systematic meta-review. *Schizophrenia Research, 118*(1–3), 201–210.

Meerwijk, E. L., van Meijel, B., van den Bout, J., et al. (2010). Development and evaluation of a guideline for nursing care of suicidal patients with schizophrenia. *Perspectives in Psychiatric Care, 46*(1), 65–73.

National Institute of Mental Health. (2007). *NREPP SAMHSA's national registry of evidence-based programs.* Retrieved from www.nrepp.samhsa.gov/ViewIntervention.aspx? id=92Functional Adaptation Skills Training (FAST).

National Institute of Mental Health. (2010). *The numbers count: Mental disorders in America.* Retrieved from www.nimh.nih. gov/health/publications/the-numbers-count-mental-disorders-in-america/index.shtml#Schizophrenia.

Roberson, C. (2009). Schizophrenia. *Alabama Nurse, 36*(2), 6–8.

Starr, D. L. (2004). Understanding those who self-mutilate. *Journal of Psychosocial Nursing, 42*(6), 33–40.

Swift, E. (2009). The efficacy of treatments for borderline personality disorder. *Mental Health Practice, 13*(4), 30–33.

Illustration Credits

CHAPTER 2

2-1, 2-2, 2-3 from deWit, S.C. (2005). *Fundamental Concepts and Skills for Nursing* (3rd ed.). Philadelphia: Saunders.

CHAPTER 3

3-2 from Gould, B.E. (2011). *Pathophysiology for Health Professions* (4th ed.). Philadelphia: Saunders. **3-3** from Jarvis, C. (2004). *Physical Examination and Health Assessment* (4th ed.). Philadelphia: Saunders. **3-5, 3-6** from Ignatavicius, D.D., & Workman, M.L. (2010). *Medical-Surgical Nursing: Critical Thinking for Collaborative Care* (6th ed.). Philadelphia: Saunders. **3-7, 3-8** from deWit, S.C. (2005). *Fundamental Concepts and Skills for Nursing* (2nd ed.). Philadelphia: Saunders. **3-9A** from Lewis, S.L., Heitkemper, M.M., Dirksen, S.R., et al. (2007). *Medical-Surgical Nursing: Assessment and Management of Clinical Problems* (7th ed.) St. Louis: Mosby. **3-9B** from Elkin, M.K., Perry, A.G., & Potter, A.G. (2004). *Nursing Interventions and Clinical Skills* (3rd ed.). St. Louis: Mosby.

CHAPTER 4

4-1 from deWit, S.C. (2009). *Fundamental Concepts and Skills for Nursing* (3rd ed.). **4-3** courtesy Southwest Washington Medical Center, Vancouver, WA.

CHAPTER 5

5-1, 5-5A-B, 5-6 from deWit, S.C. (2005). *Fundamental Concepts and Skills for Nursing* (3rd ed.). Philadelphia: Saunders. **5-2** from Black, J.M., & Hawks, J.H. (2005). *Medical-Surgical Nursing: Clinical Management for Positive Outcomes* (7th ed.). Philadelphia: Saunders.

CHAPTER 6

6-1 redrawn from Sattar, S.A., & Springthorpe, V.S. (2004), in Rutala, W.A. (Ed.), *Disinfection, Sterilization and Antisepsis.* Washington, DC: Association for Professionals in Infection Control and Epidemiology, Inc., (APIC). **6-2** from Applegate, E. (2006). *The Anatomy and Physiology Learning System* (3rd ed.) Philadelphia: Saunders. **6-3** from deWit, S.C. (2009). *Fundamental Concepts and Skills for Nursing* (3rd ed.). Philadelphia: Saunders.

CHAPTER 7

7-1 from deWit, S.C. (2009). *Fundamental Concepts and Skills for Nursing* (3rd ed.). Philadelphia: Saunders. **7-2** from Lewis, S.L., Heitkemper, M.M., Dirksen, S.R., et al. (2011). *Medical-Surgical Nursing: Assessment and Management of Clinical Problems* (8th ed.). St. Louis: Mosby. **7-3** from Hockenberry, M.J., Wilson, D., & Winkelstein, M. (2009). *Wong's Essentials of Pediatric Nursing* (8th ed.). St. Louis: Mosby. **7-4** copyright 2002, reprinted with permission from The Regents of the University of Michigan. **7-5** from Monahan, F.D., Neighbors, M., Sands, J.K.,

et al (2007). *Medical-Surgical Nursing: Health and Illness Perspective* (8th ed.). St. Louis: Mosby. **7-6** from Lewis, S.L., Heitkemper, M.M., Dirksen, S.R., et al. (2007). *Medical-Surgical Nursing: Assessment and Management of Clinical Problems* (7th ed.) St. Louis: Mosby.

CHAPTER 8

8-1 from American Cancer Society. *Cancer Facts & Figures 2010.* Atlanta: American Cancer Society. **8-2** from Huether, S.E., & McCance, K.L. (2004). *Understanding Pathophysiology* (3rd ed.). St. Louis: Mosby. **8-3** from Monahan, F.D., Neighbors, M., Sands, J.K., et al (2007). *Medical-Surgical Nursing: Health and Illness Perspective* (8th ed.). St. Louis: Mosby. **8-4** courtesy Cyberknife Center, Southwestern Washington Medical Center, Vancouver, WA. **8-7** from deWit, S.C. (2009). *Fundamental Concepts & Skills for Nursing* (3rd ed.). Philadelphia: Saunders.

CHAPTER 9

9-5 from Katz S, Down TD, Cash HR, et al. (1970). Progress in the development of the Index of ADL. *Gerontologist*, 10:20-30. Copyright The Gerontologist Society of America. Reproduced with permission of the publisher.

CHAPTER 10

10-3 from Huether, S.E., & McCance, K.L. (2004). *Understanding Pathophysiology* (3rd ed.). St. Louis: Mosby. **10-6** from Herlihy, B., & Maebius, N.K. (2007). *The Human Body in Health and Illness* (3rd ed.). Philadelphia: Saunders. **10-7** from Applegate, E. (2000). *The Anatomy and Physiology Learning System* (2nd ed.). Philadelphia: Saunders.

CHAPTER 11

11-1 from Black, J.M., & Hawks, J.H. (2009). *Medical-Surgical Nursing: Clinical Management for Positive Outcomes* (8th ed.). Philadelphia: Saunders. **11-2** from Gould, B.E. (2002). *Pathophysiology for Health Professions* (2nd ed.). Philadelphia: Saunders.

CHAPTER 12

12-2 from Gould, B.E. (2002). *Pathophysiology for Health Professions* (2nd ed.). Philadelphia: Saunders. **12-3** from Ignatavicius, D.D., & Workman, M.L. (2010). *Medical Surgical Nursing: Critical Thinking for Collaborative Care* (6th ed.) Philadelphia: Saunders. **12-4** from Lewis, S.L., Heitkemper, M.M., Dirksen, S.R., et al. (2011). *Medical-Surgical Nursing: Assessment and Management of Clinical Problems* (8th ed.) St. Louis: Mosby. **12-5** from Black, J.M., & Hawks, J.H. (2009). *Medical-Surgical Nursing: Clinical Management for Positive Outcomes* (8th ed.). Philadelphia: Saunders. **12-6** from Lewis, S.L., Heitkemper,

M.M., Dirksen, S.R., et al. (2007). *Medical-Surgical Nursing: Assessment and Management of Clinical Problems* (7th ed.) St. Louis: Mosby. **12-7** From Freundlich, B., & Leventhal, L. (1997). Diffuse pain syndromes. In J.H. Klippel (Ed.), *Primer on the Rheumatic Diseases* (11th ed.). Atlanta: Arthritis Foundation.

CHAPTER 13

13-5 from Dorland (2003). *Dorland's Illustrated Medical Dictionary* (30th ed.). Philadelphia: Saunders. **13-12** from deWit, S.C. (2009). *Fundamental Concepts and Skills for Nursing* (3rd ed.). Philadelphia: Saunders.

CHAPTER 14

14-2 from Lewis, S.L., Heitkemper, M.M., Dirksen, S.R., et al. (2011). *Medical-Surgical Nursing: Assessment and Management of Clinical Problems* (8th ed.) St. Louis: Mosby. **14-3, 14-4, 14-5** from deWit, S.C. (2005). *Fundamental Concepts and Skills for Nursing* (2nd ed.). Philadelphia: Saunders. **14-7** from Black, J.M., & Hawks, J.H. (2009). *Medical-Surgical Nursing: Clinical Management for Positive Outcomes* (8th ed.). Philadelphia: Saunders. **14-8** from Lewis, S.L., Heitkemper, M.M., Dirksen, S.R., et al. (2007). *Medical-Surgical Nursing: Assessment and Management of Clinical Problems* (7th ed.) St. Louis: Mosby. **14-9** courtesy Passey-Muir, Inc., Irvine, CA.

CHAPTER 15

15-6 from Harkreader, H., & Hogan, M.A. (2004). *Fundamentals of Nursing: Caring and Clinical Judgment* (2nd ed.). Philadelphia: Saunders. **15-7, 15-8** from deWit, S.C. (2009). *Fundamental Concepts and Skills for Nursing* (3rd ed.). Philadelphia: Saunders.

CHAPTER 16

16-1 from Thibodeau, G.A., & Patton, K.T. (2010). *The Human Body in Health and Disease* (5th ed.). St. Louis: Mosby. **16-2** from Applegate, E. (2006). *The Anatomy and Physiology Learning System* (3rd ed.) Philadelphia: Saunders.

CHAPTER 17

17-2 Ignatavicius, D.D., & Workman, M.L. (2010). *Medical-Surgical Nursing: Critical Thinking for Collaborative Care* (6th ed.). Philadelphia: Saunders. **17-3** from Lewis, S.L., Heitkemper, M.M., Dirksen, S.R., et al. (2011). *Medical-Surgical Nursing: Assessment and Management of Clinical Problems* (8th ed.) St. Louis: Mosby. **17-4, 17-5** from Lewis, S.L., Heitkemper, M.M., Dirksen, S.R., et al. (2007). *Medical-Surgical Nursing: Assessment and Management of Clinical Problems* (7th ed.) St. Louis: Mosby.

CHAPTER 18

18-1, 18-3, 18-9 from Lewis, S.L., Heitkemper, M.M., Dirksen, S.R., et al. (2007). *Medical-Surgical Nursing: Assessment and Management of Clinical Problems* (7th ed.) St. Louis: Mosby. **18-2** from Lewis, S.L., Heitkemper, M.M., Dirksen, S.R., et al. (2011). *Medical-Surgical Nursing: Assessment and Management of Clinical Problems* (8th ed.) St. Louis: Mosby. **18-6** from Huether, S.E., & McCance, K.L. (2004). *Understanding Pathophysiology* (3rd ed.). St. Louis: Mosby. **18-11** from Jarvis, C. (2004). *Physical Examination and Health Assessment* (4th ed.). Philadelphia: Saunders.

CHAPTER 19

19-1, 19-3 from *Mosby's Dictionary of Medicine, Nursing, and Health Professions* (8th ed.). (2009). St. Louis: Mosby. **19-2** from Black, J.M., & Hawks, J.H. (2009). *Medical-Surgical Nursing: Clinical Management for Positive Outcomes* (8th ed.). Philadelphia: Saunders. **19-4** courtesy Cameron Bangs, M.D. **19-5** from Monahan, F.D., Neighbors, M., Sands, J.K., et al (2007). *Medical-Surgical Nursing: Health and Illness Perspective* (8th ed.). St. Louis: Mosby. **19-6, 19-7** from Kamal, A., & Brockelhurst, J.C. (1991). *Color Atlas of Geriatric Medicine* (2nd ed.). St. Louis: Mosby. **19-8** from Thibodeau, G.A., & Patton, K.T. (2010). *The Human Body in Health and Disease* (5th ed.). St. Louis: Mosby. **19-9** from Swartz, M. (2009). *Textbook of Physical Diagnosis: History and Examination* (6th ed.). Philadelphia: Saunders. **19-10** from Black, J.M., & Hawks, J.H. (2005). *Medical-Surgical Nursing: Clinical Management for Positive Outcomes* (7th ed.). Philadelphia: Saunders.

CHAPTER 20

20-1 from Bloom, A., Watkins, P.H., & Ireland, J. (1992). *Color Atlas of Diabetes* (2nd ed.). St. Louis: Mosby. **20-2** courtesy Thoratec, Pleasanton, CA. **20-3** courtesy Datascope Corp., Montvale, NJ. **20-4, 20-5, 20-6** from Aehlert, B. (2002). *EKGs Made Easy* (2nd ed.). St. Louis: Mosby. **20-7** from Lewis, S.L., Heitkemper, M.M., Dirksen, S.R., et al. (2011). *Medical-Surgical Nursing: Assessment and Management of Clinical Problems* (8th ed.) St. Louis: Mosby. **20-8** from Kumar, V., Abbas, A., & Fausto, N. (2005). *Robbins & Cotran's Pathologic Basis of Disease* (7th ed.). Philadelphia: Saunders. **20-9** from Gould, B.E. (2002). *Pathophysiology for Health Professions* (2nd ed.). Philadelphia: Saunders.

CHAPTER 21

21-1 from Lewis, S.L., Heitkemper, M.M., Dirksen, S.R., et al. (2007). *Medical-Surgical Nursing: Assessment and Management of Clinical Problems* (7th ed.) St. Louis: Mosby. **21-2** from Chabner, D.A. (2001). *The Language of Medicine* (6th ed.). Philadelphia: Saunders. **21-4** from Lewis, S.L., Heitkemper, M.M., Dirksen, S.R., et al. (2011). *Medical-Surgical Nursing: Assessment and Management of Clinical Problems* (8th ed.) St. Louis: Mosby.

CHAPTER 22

22-1 from Applegate, E. (2000). *The Anatomy and Physiology Learning System* (2nd ed.). Philadelphia: Saunders. **22-4** from Ignatavicius, D.D., & Workman, M.L. (2010). *Medical-Surgical Nursing: Critical Thinking for Collaborative Care* (6th ed.). Philadelphia: Saunders. **22-8** from deWit, S.C. (2005). *Fundamental Concepts and Skills for Nursing* (2nd ed.). Philadelphia: Saunders. **22-9** from Jarvis, C. (2004). *Physical Examination and Health Assessment* (4th ed.). Philadelphia: Saunders.

CHAPTER 23

23-2 from Black, J.M., & Hawks, J.H. (2005). *Medical-Surgical Nursing: Clinical Management for Positive Outcomes* (7th ed.). Philadelphia: Saunders. **23-3** from Bingham, B.J.B., Hawke, M., & Kwok, P. (1992). *Clinical Atlas of Otolaryngology.* St. Louis: Mosby. **23-5** from Chipps, E., Clanin, N., & Campbell, V. (1992). *Neurologic Disorders.* St. Louis: Mosby. **23-7, 23-14** from Lewis, S.L., Heitkemper, M.M., Dirksen, S.R., et al. (2007). *Medical-Surgical Nursing: Assessment and Management of Clinical*

Problems (7th ed.) St. Louis: Mosby. **23-8** from Thibodeau, G. A., & Patton, K.T. (2010). *The Human Body in Health and Disease* (5th ed.). St. Louis: Mosby. **23-9** from Ignatavicius, D.D. & Workman, M.L. (2010). *Medical-Surgical Nursing: Critical Thinking for Collaborative Care* (6th ed.). Philadelphia: Saunders. **23-10** courtesy Michael S. Clement, M.D., Mesa, AZ. **23-11** courtesy Acromed Corp., Cleveland, OH. **23-12** courtesy Kinetic Concepts, Inc., San Antonio, TX. **23-13** from deWit, S.C. (2009). *Fundamental Concepts and Skills for Nursing* (3rd ed.). Philadelphia: Saunders.

CHAPTER 24

24-3 from Cotran, R.S., Kumar, V., & Collins, T. (1999). *Robbins Pathologic Basis for Disease* (6th ed.). Philadelphia: Saunders. **24-5** from Black, J.M., & Hawks, J.H. (2005). *Medical-Surgical Nursing: Clinical Management for Positive Outcomes* (7th ed.). Philadelphia: Saunders.

CHAPTER 25

25-1, 25-4 from Lewis, S.L., Heitkemper, M.M., Dirksen, S.R., et al. (2011). *Medical-Surgical Nursing: Assessment and Management of Clinical Problems* (8th ed.) St. Louis: Mosby. **25-3** from Perkin, D.G. (2002). *Mosby's Color Atlas and Text of Neurology.* St. Louis: Mosby. **25-5** from Stevens, A., & Lowe, J. (2000). *Pathology: Illustrated Review in Color* (2nd ed.). London: Mosby. **25-6** courtesy Heather Boyd-Monk and Wills Eye Hospital, Philadelphia. PA.

CHAPTER 26

26-3 from Swartz, M. (2009). *Textbook of Physical Diagnosis: History and Examination* (6th ed.). Philadelphia: Saunders. **26-4, 26-8** from Albert, D.M., & Jakobiec, F.A. (1994). *Principles and Practice of Ophthalmology* (vol. 3). Philadelphia: Saunders. **26-6, 26-11** from Ignatavicius, D.D., & Workman, M.L. (2006). *Medical-Surgical Nursing: Critical Thinking for Collaborative Care* (5th ed.). Philadelphia: Saunders. **26-10** from Jarvis, C. (2004). *Physical Examination and Health Assessment* (4th ed.). Philadelphia: Saunders. **26-13** from Black, J.M., & Hawks, J.H. (2005). *Medical-Surgical Nursing: Clinical Management for Positive Outcomes* (7th ed.). Philadelphia: Saunders.

CHAPTER 27

27-3, 27-5 courtesy Ophthalmic Photography at the University of Michigan, W.K. Kellogg Eye Center, Ann Arbor, MI. **27-6** from Lehne, R.A. (2004). *Pharmacology for Nursing Care* (5th ed.). Philadelphia: Saunders. **27-7, 27-8** from Phipps, W.F., Monahan, F.D., Sands, J.K., et al. (2003). *Medical-Surgical Nursing: Health and Illness Perspective* (7th ed.). St. Louis: Mosby. **27-10** courtesy Macula Foundation, Inc., New York.

CHAPTER 28

28-5 from deWit, S.C. (2005). *Fundamental Concepts and Skills for Nursing* (2nd ed.). Philadelphia: Saunders.

CHAPTER 29

29-6 from Lewis, S.L., Heitkemper, M.M., Dirksen, S.R., et al. (2007). *Medical-Surgical Nursing: Assessment and Management of Clinical Problems* (7th ed.) St. Louis: Mosby.

CHAPTER 30

30-1 from Swartz, M. (2002). *Textbook of Physical Diagnosis: History and Examination* (4th ed.). Philadelphia: Saunders. **30-7, 30-7, 30-8** from deWit, S.C. (2005). *Fundamental Concepts and Skills for Nursing* (2nd ed.). Philadelphia: Saunders.

CHAPTER 31

31-1 from Ignatavicius, D.D., & Workman, M.L. (2006). *Medical-Surgical Nursing: Critical Thinking for Collaborative Care* (5th ed.). Philadelphia: Saunders. **31-3** from Lewis, S.L., Heitkemper, M.M., Dirksen, S.R., et al. (2007). *Medical-Surgical Nursing: Assessment and Management of Clinical Problems* (7th ed.) St. Louis: Mosby.

CHAPTER 32

32-3 from Mourad, L.A. (1991). *Orthopedic Disorders.* St. Louis: Mosby. **32-6** courtesy Hill-Rom Company, Batesville, IN.

CHAPTER 33

33-2, 33-8 from Black, J.M., & Hawks, J.H. (2005). *Medical-Surgical Nursing: Clinical Management for Positive Outcomes* (7th ed.). Philadelphia: Saunders. **33-5** from Roberts, J.R., & Hedges, J.R. (2009). *Clinical Procedures in Emergency Medicine* (5th ed.). Philadelphia: Saunders. **33-7** from Townsend, C. M., Beauchamp, R.D., Evers, B.M., et al. (2007). *Sabiston Textbook of Surgery* (18 ed.). **33-10** from Ignatavicius, D.D., & Workman, M.L. (2006). *Medical-Surgical Nursing: Critical Thinking for Collaborative Care* (5th ed.). Philadelphia: Saunders. **33-11** courtesy Otto Bock HealthCare, Minneapolis, MN.

CHAPTER 34

34-1 from Ignatavicius, D.D., & Workman, M.L. (2006). *Medical-Surgical Nursing: Critical Thinking for Collaborative Care* (5th ed.). Philadelphia: Saunders. **34-2** from Lewis, S.L., Heitkemper, M.M., Dirksen, S.R., et al. (2011). *Medical-Surgical Nursing: Assessment and Management of Clinical Problems* (8th ed.) St. Louis: Mosby. **34-3,** from Ignatavicius, D.D., & Workman, M.L. (2010). *Medical Surgical Nursing: Critical Thinking for Collaborative Care* (5th ed.). Philadelphia: Saunders. **34-4** from Pagana, K.D., & Pagana, T.J. (2005). *Mosby's Diagnostic and Laboratory Test Reference* (7th ed.). St. Louis: Mosby.

CHAPTER 35

35-1, from Lewis, S.L., Heitkemper, M.M., Dirksen, S.R., et al. (2011). *Medical-Surgical Nursing: Assessment and Management of Clinical Problems* (8th ed.) St. Louis: Mosby. **35-2** from Ignatavicius, D.D., & Workman, M.L. (2010). *Medical-Surgical Nursing: Critical Thinking for Collaborative Care* (6th ed.). Philadelphia: Saunders. **35-3** from Lewis, S.L., Heitkemper, M.M., Dirksen, S.R., et al. (2007). *Medical-Surgical Nursing: Assessment and Management of Clinical Problems* (7th ed.) St. Louis: Mosby. **35-4, 35-7** from Black, J.M., & Hawks, J.H. (2005). *Medical-Surgical Nursing: Clinical Management for Positive Outcomes* (7th ed.). Philadelphia: Saunders. **35-5, 35-6** from Ignatavicius, D.D., & Workman, M.L. (2006). *Medical-Surgical Nursing: Critical Thinking for Collaborative Care* (5th ed.). Philadelphia: Saunders. **35-8** From

Glossary

A

abduction Movement away from the midline of the body.

ablation The removal of a part, as by incision; eradication.

ablation therapy A treatment for hyperthyroidism using radioactive iodine (^{131}I).

abrasion A wound caused by rubbing or scraping the skin or mucous membrane.

absorption The passage of liquids or other substances through a body surface and into its tissues and fluids, as in absorption of the end products of digestion into the intestinal villi.

abuse Misuse; excessive or improper use.

acceptance Admission of reality, as in the reality of death; the final stage in the process of dealing with dying and death.

accommodation Adjustment, especially of the ocular lens for seeing objects at varying distances.

achlorhydria The absence of hydrochloric acid from maximally stimulated gastric secretions.

acid A substance that yields hydrogen ions in solution.

acid-base balance A normal condition in which the narrow range of normal pH and the normal ratio of carbonic acid to bicarbonate ions are maintained.

acidosis A condition in which the pH of body fluids is below normal range because of either a loss of base bicarbonate or an accumulation of acid.

acquired Occurring from factors outside the organism, as in response to the environment.

acquired immunity Immunity involving the functioning of the immune system acquired by natural infection or vaccination (active immunity), or transfer of antibody from an immune donor (passive immunity).

acquired immunodeficiency syndrome (AIDS) A group of symptoms believed to be caused by a virus (HIV) that infects and destroys T lymphocytes.

acromegaly A chronic disease of adults caused by hypersecretion of the pituitary growth hormone and characterized by enlargement of many parts of the skeleton.

active immunity Immunity acquired by producing one's own antibody.

active transport Movement of substances from an area of lower concentration to an area of higher concentration.

acuity The degree of seriousness of illness or injury.

acupressure The application of digital pressure on a part of the body to relieve pain or produce anesthesia.

acupuncture A technique for treating certain painful conditions and for producing regional anesthesia by passing long, thin needles through the skin to specific points.

acute myocardial infarction Ischemic necrosis of an area of the heart muscle resulting from sudden occlusion of blood flow through one or more branches of the coronary arteries.

acute pain Sharp, severe pain.

addiction A psychological craving for alcohol or drugs with the presence of withdrawal symptoms if the substance cannot be obtained.

Addisonian crisis Sudden insufficiencies of the mineralocorticoids and the glucocorticoids that can lead to shock.

adduction Movement toward the midline of the body.

adenohypophysis The anterior lobe of the pituitary gland.

adhesion A fibrous band that binds together two parts that are normally separated; often occurs after surgery in the abdomen.

adjuvant That which assists, such as a drug added to a prescription that enhances the action of the principal ingredient.

adrenergic Having action that mimics that of the sympathetic nervous system.

adrenocortical Indicating the cortex of the adrenal gland.

adrenocorticotropic hormone (ACTH) A "tropic" hormone of the anterior pituitary gland. This hormone acts on the adrenal cortex.

adulthood A stage of life at which the individual has reached biologic maturity, usually at age 20 in humans.

advance directive A document prepared while an individual is alive and competent containing information for future health care.

adventitious Acquired; arising sporadically.

aerobe A microorganism that requires oxygen for survival.

aerobic Requiring oxygen to live.

aerosol A suspension of a drug or other substance that is dispensed in a cloud or mist.

affect The external expression; mood.

ageism Prejudice against aging and elderly people.

agent A party authorized to act on behalf of another.

agglutination One type of antigen-antibody reaction in which a solid antigen clumps together with a soluble antibody.

agnosia The loss of the power to recognize the significance of sensory stimuli.

agranulocytosis A condition of deficiency, or absolute lack, of granulocytic white blood cells.

airway The passage by which air enters and leaves the lungs; also, a device used to secure unobstructed respiration.

akathisia A condition of motor restlessness; a common extrapyramidal side effect of neuroleptic drugs.

albumin, serum A plasma protein formed principally in the liver and constituting about 60% of the protein concentration in the plasma.

aldosterone A mineralocorticoid steroid hormone produced by the adrenal cortex. Works in the renal tubules to retain sodium and conserve water by reabsorption; increases urinary potassium excretion.

alkalosis A condition in which the pH of body fluids is above normal because of either a loss of acid or an accumulation of base bicarbonate.

allergen(s) Any substance capable of triggering an exaggerated immune response.

allergy (allergies) An abnormal and individual hypersensitivity to a particular allergen; acquired by exposure to the allergen and manifested after reexposure.

alleviate To relieve; to make easier to bear.

alliance An agreement to cooperate made between a free-standing independent facility and a hospital.

allogeneic Having a different genetic constitution but belonging to the same species.

allograft Transplant tissue obtained from the same species.

alogia A psychiatric term meaning poverty of thoughts.

alopecia Baldness or loss of hair.

Alzheimer's disease (AD) The most common degenerative disease of the brain, with no known cause or cure. The disease causes loss of neurons in the frontal and temporal lobes and affects people over the age of 65, but can also strike younger people.

amenorrhea The absence of menstruation.

anabolic Constructive in nature; the opposite of catabolic.

anabolism The building up of the body substance; the constructive phase of metabolism.

anaerobe An organism that lives in an oxygen-free environment.

anaerobic Able to live in an oxygen-free environment.

analgesia The absence of normal sense of pain.

analgesic(s) A pain reliever.

anaphylaxis An unusual or exaggerated allergic reaction.

anasarca Generalized massive edema resulting from severe depletion of albumin.

anastomosis A communication between two tubular organs; also surgical, traumatic, or pathologic formation of a connection between two normally distinct structures.

androgen(s) Any steroid hormone that promotes male characteristics.

anemia(s) A condition in which there are too few functioning red blood cells to meet the oxygen needs of tissues.

anesthesia The loss of feeling or sensation.

aneurysm A sac formed by localized dilation of the wall of a blood vessel or the heart.

anger A feeling of hostility and bitterness against a situation or person; the second stage in acceptance of death.

angina pectoris Exertional chest pain caused by ischemia of the heart muscle and increased demand for oxygen.

angioedema A vascular reaction representing localized edema caused by dilation and characterized by development of giant wheals.

angiography Radiographic studies of the arteries, veins, or lymph vessels of the body.

animate Alive.

anion A negatively charged atomic particle.

ankylosis Abnormal immobility and consolidation and obliteration of a joint.

anorexia A lack or loss of appetite for food.

anorexia nervosa An eating disorder in which there is an aberration of eating patterns, severe weight loss, and malnutrition.

anosmia The absence of the sense of smell; also called *anosphresia* and *olfactory anesthesia.*

anovulation Failure of the ovary to produce or release mature eggs.

antibiotic An agent that is capable of either killing or inhibiting the growth of microorganisms.

antibody (antibodies) An immunoglobulin molecule that is capable of adhering to and interacting only with the antigen that induced its synthesis.

anticoagulants Substances that suppress, delay, or nullify the coagulation of blood.

antidiuretic hormone A hormone that decreases the production of urine by increasing the reabsorption of water by the renal tubules. It is secreted by the hypothalamus and stored in the posterior lobe of the pituitary gland.

antidysrhythmic agents Substances that help return the heart rate and rhythm to more normal values and restore the origin of the heart's electrical activity to its natural pacemaker.

antiemetic An agent that prevents or relieves nausea and vomiting.

antifungal(s) An agent that is destructive to or inhibitive of the growth of fungi.

antigen(s) Any substance that can produce an antagonist.

antigen-antibody reaction An immune response that occurs when an antibody comes into contact with the specific antigen for which it was formed. In a transfusion reaction, the response is a clumping together, or agglutination, of the red blood cells carrying the antigens.

antihistamine An agent that counteracts the effects of histamine; used to relieve the symptoms of an allergic reaction.

antihypertensive A medication to prevent or control high blood pressure.

antimicrobial agent A substance capable of either killing or suppressing the multiplication and growth of micro-organisms.

antineoplastic agent A substance that inhibits the maturation and proliferation of malignant cells.

antiseptic(s) Any substance that inhibits the growth of bacteria outside the body; in contrast, a germicide kills the bacteria outright.

antitoxin A specific kind of antibody produced in response to the presence of a toxin.

antitussive An agent that inhibits the cough reflex in the cough center in the brain.

antivenin A substance used to neutralize the venom of a poisonous animal.

anuria Diminished or absent production of urine by the kidney.

apathetic thyrotoxicosis Milder hyperthyroidism signs and symptoms seen in the elderly patient compared with symptoms seen in the typical adult patient.

aphakic eye An eye without a lens, as after a cataract extraction.

aphasia A defect in or loss of the power of expression by speech, writing, or signs or in the comprehension of spoken or written language.

aphonia The loss of the voice.

apical Pertaining to the apex of a structure; particularly the heart.

aplastic Having deficient or arrested development.

aplastic anemia Deficient red cell production due to a bone marrow disorder.

apnea Temporary cessation of breathing.

apraxia The loss or impairment of acquired motor skills.

arrhythmia (also dysrhythmia) Variation from the normal rhythm, especially of the heartbeat.

arteriosclerosis A group of diseases characterized by thickening and loss of elasticity of the arterial walls.

arthritis Inflammation of a joint.

arthrocentesis The surgical puncture of a joint cavity for aspiration of synovial fluid.

arthroplasty Surgery of a joint to increase mobility or decrease pain.

arthroscopy Endoscopic examination of the interior of a joint.

ascites The accumulation of edematous fluid within the peritoneal cavity.

asepsis, medical The destruction and containment of infectious agents after they leave the body of a patient with an infectious disease.

assessment, nursing Data-gathering activities for the purpose of collecting a complete, relevant database from which a nursing diagnosis can be made.

asterixis A motor disturbance marked by intermittent lapse of an assumed posture; a characteristic of hepatic coma. Also called "flapping tremor."

asthma A condition marked by recurrent attacks of paroxysmal dyspnea, with wheezing due to spasmodic contraction of the bronchi.

astigmatism An error of refraction in which light rays are not sharply focused on the retina because of abnormal curvature of the cornea or lens.

ataxia Uncoordinated motor movements.

atelectasis The collapsed or airless state of the lung.

atherosclerosis A disease process in which fibrinous plaques are laid down on the inner walls of the arteries, thus narrowing the lumens of the vessels and predisposing them to the development of intravascular clots.

atopy The tendency to develop allergies.

atrial fibrillation Rapid, irregular, and ineffective contractions of the atria.

atrial natriuretic peptide A hormone involved in the regulation of renal and cardiovascular homeostasis. It is produced in the atrium and helps to normalize blood pressure and volume.

atrophy Wasting, or a decrease in size, from lack of use.

atypical antipsychotics Newer medications used for treating schizophrenia with fewer side effects.

audiometry The measurement of sound perception.

audit An official examination of the record of all aspects of patient care.

aura A peculiar sensation preceding the appearance of more definite symptoms, especially a sensation, that occurs immediately before an epileptic seizure.

aural Pertaining to the ear.

auscultation Listening for sounds produced within the body, usually with a stethoscope.

autograft A graft transferred from one part of a patient's body to another.

autoimmune A defective cellular immune response in which antibodies are produced against normal parts of the person's body.

autoimmune disease A disease caused by the body's failure to recognize its own cells, thus rejecting them as it would a foreign substance.

autoimmune thyroiditis (Hashimoto's thyroiditis) Body produces antibodies against the thyroid, which in turn destroy the gland.

autoinoculation Inoculation with microorganisms from one's own body.

autologous Indicating something that has its origin within an individual, as in transfusion with one's own blood.

automated external defibrillator (AED) A defibrillator found in many public places used to treat cardiac arrest.

automatisms Repetitive, automatic actions such as lip smacking.

autonomic dysreflexia Hyperreflexia, an uninhibited and exaggerated reflex response of the autonomic nervous system to some type of stimulation.

avolition A lack of motivation.

avulsion The tearing away of part or all of an organ or structure.

axon The projection, or process, of a neuron that transmits impulses away from the cell body.

azotemia Retention in the blood of urea, creatinine, and other nitrogenous protein metabolites that are normally eliminated in the urine.

B

Babinski's reflex A reflex action elicited by stimulating the sole of the foot and characterized by dorsiflexion of the great toe and flaring of the smaller toes. A positive Babinski reflex indicates an abnormality in the motor control pathways of the nervous system.

bacteria Microscopically small organisms belonging to the plant kingdom, some of which are capable of producing disease in humans.

bacterial vaginosis A bacterial disease of the vagina.

bactericidal Able to kill bacteria.

bacteriophage A virus that destroys bacteria by lysis. The virus is usually of a type specific for the particular kind of bacteria it attacks.

bacteriostatic Able to slow duplication of bacteria.

bargaining An attempt to make an arrangement whereby one gives something in order to gain something in return; the third stage in acceptance of death.

bariatrics The field of medicine that focuses on the treatment and control of obesity and diseases associated with obesity.

base A substance that combines with acids to form salts.

basal insulin Amount of insulin that would normally be produced by the pancreas.

basement membrane The noncellular layer that secures the overlying epithelium to the underlying tissue.

behavior The manner in which one conducts oneself in response to social stimuli, an inner need, or a combination of the two.

belief A currently held idea or value derived from culture and experience.

benign Not very harmful; nonmalignant.

benign pituitary adenoma A benign tumor of the pituitary gland that secretes growth hormone (GH), leading to continued growth. It can also antagonize the effect of the hormone insulin, resulting in increased blood glucose.

bereaved Experiencing the reaction of grief and sadness on learning of the loss of a loved one.

biliary Pertaining to bile, the bile ducts, or the gallbladder.

biliary colic Acute pain resulting from obstruction of a bile duct, usually caused by cholelithiasis.

binder A broad bandage most commonly used as an encircling support of the abdomen or chest.

biofeedback A training program designed to develop one's ability to control the autonomic (involuntary) nervous system.

biologic dressing Materials obtained from a patient's intact skin, cadavers, or animals that is used to treat burn victims.

biologic response modifier (BRM) An agent that manipulates the immune system in hopes of controlling or curing a malignancy.

biomedicine Biologic medicine; focuses on the biologic aspects of medicine.

biopsy Removal of living cells for the purpose of examining them microscopically.

biosynthetic A biologic substance created by chemical processes. A term used for artificial skin that can be used as a temporary measure for grafting in burn victims.

bioterrorism An attack that involves the deliberate release of microorganisms or toxins derived from living organisms that cause disease or death to humans, animals, or plants on which we depend for food.

bipolar disorder A mood disorder in which manic and depressive episodes occur.

bisexual An individual who is sexually attracted to others of either sex.

bivalve Split through all layers of the material.

bladder, cord A dysfunction of the urinary bladder caused by damage to the spinal cord.

bladder, neurogenic A dysfunction of the urinary bladder caused by a lesion of the central or peripheral nervous system and characterized by lack of awareness of the need to void.

blepharitis An infection of the glands and lash follicles along the margin of the eyelid.

blood gases, arterial (ABGs) The partial pressure exerted by oxygen and carbon dioxide in the arterial blood. ABGs reflect the ability of the lungs to exchange these gases, the effectiveness of the kidneys to retain and eliminate bicarbonate, and the efficiency of the heart as a pump.

B-lymphocyte A sensitized lymphocyte that is responsible for antibody formation and the development of humoral immunity.

bolus dose A dose of short- or rapid-acting insulin that is used to manage elevations in blood glucose and bring the next blood glucose measurement into range.

borborygmi Gurgling, splashing sounds normally heard over the large intestine; rumbling in the bowels.

borderline personality disorder A mental disorder defined by the DSM-IV as "a pattern of instability in interpersonal relationships, self-image and affect, and marked impulsivity."

botulism Food poisoning caused by a neurotoxin produced by *Clostridium botulinum*, sometimes found in improperly canned or preserved foods.

bradycardia An abnormally slow heart rate, usually less than 60 beats per minute.

bradykinesia Slow movement; a symptom seen with Parkinson's disease.

bradypnea Abnormally slow breathing.

bronchiectasis Chronic dilation of the bronchi marked by fetid breath and paroxysmal coughing, with the expectoration of mucopurulent matter.

bronchodilator A drug that acts directly on the smooth muscles of the bronchi to relax them and relieve bronchospasm.

bronchogram A radiograph of the bronchial tree using a radiopaque substance that is introduced into the trachea.

bronchoscopy Insertion of an endoscope for diagnosis and treatment of disorders of the bronchi.

bruit An abnormal sound of venous or arterial origin heard on auscultation.

bulimia nervosa A mental disorder occurring predominantly in females characterized by episodes of binge eating that continue until terminated by abdominal pain, sleep, or self-induced vomiting.

bulla (bullae) A blister; a round, fluid-filled lesion of the skin, usually more than 5 mm in diameter.

burns, full-thickness Burns in which all of the epithelializing elements of the skin and those tissues lining the sweat glands, hair follicles, and sebaceous glands are destroyed.

burns, partial-thickness Burns in which the epithelializing elements remain intact.

C

cachexia A profound state of general ill health and malnutrition.

calculus (calculi) An abnormal concretion, usually of mineral salts, occurring mainly in hollow organs or their passages (e.g., renal calculus, or kidney stone).

callus A thickened area of the epidermis caused by pressure or friction.

caloric testing Testing to check the oculovestibular reflex. A patient's eye movements are observed while the external ear canal is irrigated with cold water. Absence of eye movement indicates a brainstem lesion.

candidiasis An infection with a fungus of the genus *Candida*, especially *C. albicans*. It is usually a superficial infection of the moist cutaneous areas of the body, although it becomes more severe in immunocompromised patients.

capitation A payment method wherein the health care provider is paid a monthly contracted rate for each member patient assigned regardless of the type or number of services provided.

capnography Measurement of inhaled and exhaled carbon dioxide as recorded on a capnogram.

caput medusa Dilated cutaneous veins around the umbilicus in patients suffering from cirrhosis of the liver.

carbuncles A collection of infected hair follicles. Most often occur on the back of the neck, the upper back, and the lateral thighs.

carcinogen Any substance or agent that produces or increases the risk of developing cancer in humans or lower animals.

carcinoma(s) A malignant growth made up of epithelial cells.

cardiac glycosides A group of compounds containing a carbohydrate molecule (e.g., digitalis) that affect the contractile force of the heart muscle.

cardiac tamponade Compression of the heart caused by collection of fluid in the pericardial sac.

cardiogenic shock A shock state caused by pump failure of the heart.

cardiomyopathy Disease of the myocardium, especially due to primary disease of the heart muscle.

cardiomyoplasty A procedure wherein the latissimus dorsi muscle is detached from its natural position, brought around to the front of the body and wrapped around the heart. A pacemaker, connected to the heart and back muscle, helps boost the heart's pumping action.

cardiopulmonary resuscitation The reestablishment of heart and lung action after they have suddenly stopped.

cardiotonic(s) An agent having the effect of strengthening contractions of the heart muscle.

cardioversion A mild electrical shock delivered to the heart at a specific time in the cardiac cycle to interrupt the abnormal rhythm and begin a new, normal rhythm of electrical impulse and contraction.

carpopedal spasm A spasm of the hand, thumbs, foot, or toes that accompanies tetany.

carriers People who harbor infectious organisms within their bodies without manifesting any outward symptoms of the infection.

cartilage A type of connective tissue in which fibers and cells are embedded in a semisolid gel material.

catabolic Destructive in nature; the opposite of anabolic.

catabolism The phase of metabolism in which larger molecules are broken down and energy is released; the destructive phase of metabolism.

cataract(s) An opacity of the lens of the eye.

catecholamines One of a group of biogenic amines having a sympathomimetic action; examples are dopamine, norepinephrine, and epinephrine.

category-specific precautions A system of precautionary measures organized according to types of diseases (e.g., respiratory or enteric) and employed to prevent the spread of disease.

cations Positively charged atomic particles.

cauterize To burn with a cautery, or to apply one.

CD lymphocyte A type of lymphocyte that is the master regulator of the human immune system. It is the primary site of replication for HIV.

cell(s) The basic structural unit of living organisms.

cell-mediated immunity Immunity resulting from activation of sensitized lymphocytes.

cellulitis Inflammation of cellular or connective tissue.

central hearing loss Impaired perception of sound caused by pathology above the junction of the eighth cranial nerve and the brainstem (in the brain).

cerumen Earwax.

chalazion An infection of the meibomian gland of the eye; an internal stye.

chancre A primary syphilis skin lesion that begins as a papule and develops into a red, bloodless, painless ulcer with a scooped-out appearance.

chemonucleolysis Treatment of a herniated intervertebral disk by dissolution of a portion of the nucleus pulposus by injection of a chemolytic agent.

chemotherapy Use of chemicals, especially drugs, in the treatment of such diseases as cancer, infection, and some mental illnesses.

cholecystectomy The removal of the gallbladder.

cholecystitis An inflammation of the gallbladder.

choledocholithiasis The condition in which gallstones lodge in the common bile duct.

cholelithiasis The presence of stones within the gallbladder or biliary tract.

cholinergic An agent that produces the effect of acetylcholine.

chorea Involuntary muscle twitching.

chronic pain Pain of long duration showing little change or slowly progressive pain.

chronologic Occurring in a natural time sequence.

Chvostek sign Low calcium level manifests as muscle irritability when the facial nerve is gently tapped.

chyme The mixture of partly digested food and digestive secretions found in the stomach and small intestine during digestion of a meal.

cirrhosis A liver disease characterized by diffuse interlacing bands of fibrous tissue dividing the hepatic parenchyma into micronodular or macronodular areas.

cirrhosis of the liver A condition characterized by destruction of normal hepatic structures and their replacement with necrotic tissue and scarring.

claudication, intermittent A syndrome characterized by intensification of limb pain as exercise is increased; related to occlusion of arteries in the legs.

climacteric Endocrine, somatic, and psychic changes occurring at the end of the female reproductive period (menopause); also, normal diminution of testicular activity in the male.

clinical pathway A tool used to track patient progress along a set path in a managed care system.

clonic Alternating contraction and relaxation of muscles.

clonus Abnormal neuromuscular activity, characterized by rapidly alternating involuntary contraction and relaxation of skeletal muscle; occurs with epileptic seizure.

coarctation Narrowing (of the aorta).

code of ethics A set of rules governing one's conduct.

co-dependency A behavior pattern in which a family member or friend of a substance abuser attempts to control the behavior of the dependent person.

cognition The mental processes of perception, memory, judgment, and reasoning.

co-insurance Insurance in which both the insurer and the patient pay the medical bill.

coitus Sexual intercourse.

colectomy The removal of part of the colon.

colic A spasm causing pain; may be biliary, renal, intestinal, or uterine.

collaboration The act of working or cooperating with another.

collaborator One who works cooperatively with another.

collagen A fibrous protein found in skin, bone, cartilage, and ligaments.

colonization The process in which a group of organisms, especially bacteria, live together and multiply.

colostomy (colostomies) The surgical creation of an opening in the colon to allow fecal material to pass outside.

colporrhaphy The operation of suturing the vagina.

colposcopy The visual examination of the vagina and cervix with a specially designed endoscope that allows the detection of malignant growths in their early stages.

comedo (comedones) A plug of keratin and sebum in an enlarged pore; a blackhead.

communicable disease A disease that may be transmitted directly or indirectly from one individual to another.

compartment syndrome External or internal pressure that seriously restricts circulation to the area.

complement system A complex series of enzymatic proteins that interact to combine with the antigen-antibody complex, producing lysis of intact antigen cells.

complement system of proteins A series of protective proteins that are activated in the inflammatory response.

complementary and alternative medicine (CAM) Types of treatments for medical disorders that do not rely on traditional medicine, but frequently are combined with traditional medical treatment for a disorder.

complete blood count (CBC) The number of each kind of cell in a sample of blood.

compliance An expression of the ability of lung tissue to distend when filled with air.

computed tomography (CT) scan A computer-aided technique in which small sections of tissue within an organ can be visualized by radiograph.

concept(s) An idea, thought, or notion derived from experiences and information acquired from one's external environment.

concussion A term used to describe a closed head injury in which the brain is compressed by a portion of the skull at the time of the blow and temporary ischemia of the brain tissue results.

conductive hearing loss Impaired perception of sound caused by a dysfunction of either the external or the middle ear.

confabulation A behavioral reaction to memory loss in which the patient fills in memory gaps with made-up facts and experiences.

confusion The state of not being aware of or oriented to time, place, or self.

congenital Present at birth.

congestive heart failure The exhaustion of the heart muscle and a resultant engorgement of the heart's chambers and the blood vessels. Eventually, sluggish blood flow leads to retention of fluid and edema in the lungs and elsewhere in the body.

conjugate Working in union; equally coupled.

conjunctivitis An inflammation of the membrane covering the eyeball and lining the eyelids.

consciousness Responsiveness of the mind to impressions made by the senses.

contactant A substance that produces an allergic or sensitivity response when in direct contact with the skin.

contamination The presence of a noxious agent, such as bacteria or radiation, in a place where it is not wanted.

contracture An adaptive shortening of skeletal muscle tissue that is not subjected to normal stretching and contraction.

contralateral On or affecting the opposite side of the body.

contusion A bruise; an injury of a part without a break in the skin.

conventional antipsychotics Neuroleptics used to treat the positive symptoms of schizophrenia. Cause serious and unpleasant side effects and are becoming less commonly prescribed.

convulsion A state of involuntary muscle contractions and relaxations.

copayment The amount a member of an HMO has to pay for each visit to the health care provider.

COPD Chronic obstructive pulmonary disease.

coronary artery bypass graft (CABG) Surgery in which a blood vessel is grafted onto the coronary artery to improve blood flow.

coronary insufficiency Decreased or insufficient blood flow in the coronary arteries.

coronary occlusion The closing off of a coronary artery and interruption of its blood flow.

cor pulmonale Heart disease characterized by hypertrophy of the right ventricle due to pulmonary hypertension.

corrosive Containing a destructive agent that produces disintegration or wearing away.

cost containment The need to hold costs to within fixed limits.

counterregulatory hormones Growth hormone, glucagons, and epinephrine that are released during the night that cause an increase in blood glucose. They act "counter" to insulin.

coup-contrecoup injury An injury that occurs when the head is moving rapidly and hits a stationary object. The contents within the cranium hit the inside of the skull (coup) and then bounce back and hit the opposite side, causing a second injury (contrecoup).

crackles An abnormal respiratory sound heard on auscultation during inspiration; can be a bubbling noise or a popping sound. Crackles do not clear with coughing.

creatinine A nonprotein substance that is formed in muscle in relatively small and constant amounts, passes into the bloodstream, and is eliminated by the kidneys. Urine creatinine levels are diminished when glomerular filtration is impaired.

Credé technique Exerting downward pressure with the open hand over the suprapubic area to facilitate emptying of the urinary bladder.

cremasteric reflex The retraction of the testicles when the inner thigh is stroked. This reflex is absent with testicular torsion.

crepitation A sound like that of hair rubbed between the fingers; occurs when bone fragments rub together.

cretinism A congenital condition due to lack of thyroid secretion, characterized by arrested physical and mental development, dystrophy of the bones and soft parts, and lowered basal metabolism.

criterion A standard for judging a condition or establishing a diagnosis.

critical thinking Purposeful, considered, organized cognitive processing used to examine a problem or situation or evaluate the thinking of others.

crust An outer layer of solid matter formed by dried exudate or secretion.

cryoprecipitate Any precipitate that forms as a result of cooling.

cryosurgery The destruction of tissue by application of extreme cold, as in removal of cataracts.

cryotherapy The therapeutic use of cold or freezing.

cryptorchidism (cryptorchism) The failure of one or both of the testes to descend into the scrotum during fetal life.

culdoscopy The direct inspection of the female viscera through an endoscope introduced into the pelvic cavity through the posterior vaginal fornix.

culture The propagation of microorganisms or living tissue cells in media conducive to their growth.

curettage Cleansing of a surface of an organ with a spoon-shaped instrument (curet).

Curling's ulcer A type of ulcer caused by decreased perfusion to other organs, which causes changes in the gastric mucosa.

cyanosis A bluish tinge to the skin caused by lack of oxygen and accumulation of carbon dioxide in the blood.

cystitis An inflammation of the urinary bladder.

cystocele A protrusion or herniation of the bladder through the wall of the vagina.

cystogram A radiograph of the urinary bladder using a contrast medium.

cystoscopy Endoscopic examination of the interior of the bladder.

cytokine A low-molecular-weight protein secreted by various cell types and involved in cell-to-cell communication. It coordinates antibody and T cell immune interactions and augments immune reactivity.

cytology The study of cells, their origin, structure, function, and pathology.

cytotoxic Destructive to cells.

D

dactylitis An inflammation of a finger or toe.

database A collection of facts and figures for analysis from which conclusions may be drawn.

data collection The systematic collection of physical and psychosocial data for a patient who is having a problem. Part of assessment within the nursing process.

dawn phenomenon A condition sometimes encountered in type 1 diabetes characterized by increased blood glucose in the morning caused by release of hormones during the night.

deaf Partially or completely lacking the sense of hearing.

death(s) The cessation of all physical and chemical processes that invariably occurs in all living organisms. *See also* Dying.

débride Peel away dead tissue.

débridement The removal of all foreign material and dead tissues from or adjacent to a traumatic or infected lesion until healthy tissue is exposed.

debriefing Questioning of personnel involved and obtaining knowledge about function and problems that occurred (during a disaster).

decerebrate posturing Extensor posturing; the arms are stiffly extended and held close to the body and the wrists are flexed outward. Indicates damage to the midbrain or brainstem.

decontamination The freeing of a person or an object of some contaminating substance such as radioactive material.

decorticate posturing Flexor posturing; extension of the legs and internal rotation and adduction of the arms with the elbows bent upward. Indicates damage to the cortex.

decubitus ulcer(s) A breakdown in the skin and underlying tissues caused by long-standing pressure, ischemia, and damage to the underlying tissue.

deductible The yearly amount an insured person must spend out-of-pocket before a medical insurance plan begins to pay its share.

defecate To evacuate the bowels; to have a bowel movement.

defibrillation Stopping fibrillation of the heart with electrical current.

dehiscence The separation of all layers of a surgical wound.

dehydration Excessive loss of water from tissues of the body.

delegate To authorize and send another as one's representative (to carry out a task).

delegation Allocation of patient care activities to team members.

delirium An altered state of consciousness that is usually acute and of short duration.

delusion A false, fixed belief that cannot be changed with rational explanation.

dementia A broad impairment of intellectual function that usually is progressive.

demyelination Destruction of the myelin sheath of nerve tissue.

demyelinization Demyelination.

dendrite Any of the thread-like extensions of the cytoplasm of a neuron.

denial A defense mechanism in which the existence of intolerable conditions is unconsciously rejected; the first stage in the acceptance of death.

denuded When the protective layer or covering is removed through surgery, trauma, or pathologic change.

deoxyribonucleic acid (DNA) The primary genetic material of all cellular organisms.

dependency The state of reliance on a substance; implies that there are physical and psychological symptoms of addiction. Term used to describe substance use disorder.

dependent (nursing action) Requiring an order from a health care provider.

dependent rubor The dusky-red color dangling feet soon take on after elevating the feet and legs above the heart for 1 to 2 minutes. This indicates arterial insufficiency.

depression A morbid sadness, dejection, or melancholy; a stage in the acceptance of death.

depression (of immune function) The decreased ability of the immune system to function normally.

dermabrasion Planing of the skin done by mechanical means to smooth the skin and remove scars.

dermatitis An inflammation of the skin.

dermatology The medical specialty concerned with diagnosing and treating skin disorders.

dermatome A nerve tract.

dermatophytosis Any superficial fungal infection caused by a dermatophyte and involving the stratum corneum of the skin, hair, and nails.

detoxification The process of ridding the body of a drug without causing harmful ill effects.

developmental task(s) A task that should be completed during a specific life period to ensure continuing psychosocial growth and maturity.

deviation Departure from normal.

diabetes insipidus (DI) Occurs as a result of decreased production of the antidiuretic hormone (ADH) and is characterized by the production of copious amounts of dilute urine.

diabetic nephropathy Kidney disease secondary to high blood glucose level.

diabetic neuropathy A disorder of the peripheral nerves that is associated with diabetes mellitus and is characterized by sexual impotence in the male, neurogenic bladder, and pain or loss of feeling in the lower extremities.

diabetogenic Causing diabetes.

diagnosis, nursing A concise statement of a patient's actual or potential health problems that nurses, because of their education and experience, are able and licensed to treat.

diagnosis-related groups (DRGs) The classifications used to determine Medicare payments for patient care based on medical diagnoses.

dialysis The diffusion of solute molecules through a semipermeable membrane, the molecules passing from the more concentrated solution to the less concentrated one.

dialysis, peritoneal The use of the peritoneum as a dialyzing membrane to remove waste products that have accumulated in the body as a result of renal failure.

diaphoresis Excessive perspiration.

diastole The phase of the cardiac cycle in which the heart muscle relaxes between contractions; during this phase the two ventricles are dilated by blood flowing through them. Diastolic blood pressure is recorded as the bottom number in the pressure measurement.

diastolic blood pressure Arterial pressure during diastole.

diffusion The spontaneous mixing of the molecules or ions of two or more substances; the result of random thermal motion.

digital Pertaining to or resembling a finger or toe.

digitalization The initial administration of digitalis to build up a therapeutic blood level of the drug.

diplopia Double vision; seeing two images.

disability Difficulty in performing certain tasks because of impairment.

disaster A natural or human-caused (bioterrorism or nuclear) event that overwhelms the community's existing emergency resources.

disease One possible outcome due to an infection.

disease-specific precautions A system of precautionary measures organized according to the specific infectious disease presented by the patient.

disinfectant(s) An agent that destroys infection-producing organisms.

dislocation Stretching or tearing of ligaments around a joint with complete displacement of a bone.

disseminated Widespread.

disseminated intravascular coagulation (DIC) A disorder characterized by reduction in the elements involved in blood coagulation due to their utilization in widespread blood clotting within the vessels; the activation of the clotting mechanism may arise from any of a number of disorders.

distal In a position farthest from the point of reference.

distraction Diversion of attention from present experience (i.e., pain).

diuresis The excretion of excess fluid in the urine.

diuretic(s) An agent that promotes secretion of urine.

diurnal Happening during daylight hours.

diverticulitis The inflammation of the diverticula.

diverticulosis The presence of diverticula, in the absence of diverticulitis.

diverticulum (diverticula) A small blind pouch resulting from a protrusion of the mucosa of a hollow organ through weakened areas in the organ's muscle wall.

documentation The recording of significant information on a patient's chart.

dowager's hump An abnormal backward curve of the cervical spine that is the result of osteoporosis and/or Cushing syndrome.

Down syndrome A congenital disorder characterized by physical malformations and some degree of mental retardation; also called *trisomy 21 syndrome* because there is a defect in chromosome 21.

DRGs *See* Diagnosis-related groups.

drusen Yellow exudates found beneath the retinal pigment epithelium, representing extracellular debris.

dual diagnosis The diagnosis of a patient with a substance abuse problem and a mental health disorder.

dumping syndrome A group of symptoms caused by too-rapid passage of food through the upper gastrointestinal tract.

dying A stage of life; a process that, from a medical point of view, begins when a person has a disease that is untreatable and inevitably ends in death; or the final stages of a fatal disease. *See also* Death(s).

dynamic Having vital force or inherent power.

dysarthria Slurring or indistinct speech articulation; difficulty speaking.

dyscrasia An imbalance of formed elements, as in blood dyscrasia.

dysfunctional uterine bleeding Uterine bleeding at times other than during normal menstruation.

dysmenorrhea Painful or difficult menstruation.

dyspareunia Difficult or painful coitus in women.

dyspepsia Impairment of the power or function of digestion; usually applied to epigastric discomfort following meals.

dysphagia Difficulty in swallowing.

dysphasia Difficulty speaking; usually caused by a brain lesion.

dyspnea Labored or difficult breathing.

dysrhythmia A variation from the normal rhythm, especially of the heartbeat.

dysthymia A disturbance in mood that may manifest in either depression or elation.

dystonic reactions Acute contractures of the tongue, face, neck, and back.

dysuria Painful urination.

E

eccentric Departing from conventional custom or practice; differing conspicuously in behavior, appearance, or opinions.

ecchymosis (ecchymoses) An irregularly shaped, blue-black skin discoloration caused by bleeding beneath the skin.

ECG (also EKG) *See* Electrocardiogram.

ectopic Located away from normal position, as in ectopic pregnancy.

ectropion An outward turning of the eyelid.

edema An accumulation of fluid surrounding the cell.

edematous Pertaining to, or affected with, edema (abnormal fluid in the tissue).

EEG *See* Electroencephalogram.

effleurage A massage technique with long, light or firm strokes over the spine and back. May be circular strokes done with the fingertips.

effluent A discharge or outflow (i.e., the contents flowing out of an ileostomy or colostomy).

effusion An escape of fluid into a part or tissue, as an exudation or transudation.

ejaculation Ejection of the seminal fluid from the male urethra.

elastance The extent to which the lungs are able to return to their original position after being barely distended.

electrocardiogram The record produced by amplification of the electrical impulses normally generated by the heart.

electroconvulsive therapy (ECT) The oldest form of brain stimulation therapy used for severe depression. Considered after several unsuccessful regimens of medication. Consists of electric shock to the brain via electrodes applied to the temples. This shock artificially induces a grand mal seizure lasting 30 to 90 seconds.

electroencephalogram A recording of changes in electric potentials in various areas of the brain.

electrolyte(s) A chemical substance that, when dissolved in water, dissociates into ions and thus is capable of conducting an electric current.

electromyography The recording and study of intrinsic electrical properties of skeletal muscle; useful in diagnosing neuromuscular disorders.

elimination Discharge from the body of indigestible materials and waste products of metabolism.

embolism A sudden obstruction of arterial blood flow by a blood clot or a mass that has been brought to the site in the bloodstream.

embolus A clot or plug of material (usually from a thrombus) carried by blood flow that lodges in a vessel and obstructs blood flow.

emesis Substance produced by vomiting.

empathy The ability to recognize and share the emotions and states of mind of another; understanding another's behavior.

emphysema A chronic pulmonary disease characterized by increase beyond normal in the size of air spaces distal to the terminal bronchiole with destructive changes in their walls.

empyema The presence of infected and purulent exudate within the pleural cavity.

enabling Doing something for a substance-dependent person that keeps the person from facing consequences. Term used with substance abuse.

encapsulated Surrounded by a fibrous capsule.

encephalopathy Any dysfunction of the brain.

endarterectomy The surgical removal of thickened atheromatous areas of the innermost layer of an artery.

endemic Present in a community at all times.

endocarditis An inflammation of the membrane lining the cavities of the heart and of the connective tissue bed on which it lies.

endocrine Secreting internally; refers to glandular function.

endogenous Coming from within.

endometriosis The presence of endometrial tissue in locations outside the uterus.

endorphin(s) Any of a group of opiate-like peptides naturally produced by the body.

endoscopy Examination with an endoscope that allows for direct visual inspection of the interior of hollow organs and body cavities.

endotoxin(s) A heat-stable toxin that is present in the intact bacterial cell wall, is pyrogenic, and is capable of increasing capillary permeability.

endotracheal intubation Airway management with a catheter or tube inserted through the mouth or nose into the trachea.

engraftment Successful establishment of the graft in bone marrow transplantation.

enteral feeding Feeding a patient by means of a tube passed into the stomach from the nasal passage.

enterocele A hernia containing intestines.

enterostomal Related to an abdominal stoma, or artificial opening of the intestine onto the surface of the body.

entropion Inversion of the eyelid margin.

enucleation Removal of an organ or other mass intact (e.g., the eyeball from the orbit).

environment All the physical and psychological factors that influence or affect the life or survival of an individual.

enzyme Any protein that acts as a catalyst, increasing the rate at which chemical reaction occurs.

epidemic(s) A disease that simultaneously attacks many people in a geographic area, is widely diffused, and spreads rapidly.

epidermophytosis A fungal infection that most often affects the feet, especially between the toes; also called *athlete's foot* or *dermophytosis*.

epididymis A small oblong body resting on and beside the posterior surface of the testes that constitutes the first part of the excretory duct of each testis.

epidural Situated on or outside the dura mater.

epidural hematoma A hematoma caused by rapid leakage of blood from the middle meningeal artery, which quickly elevates intracranial pressure.

epigastric Pertaining to the region over the pit of the stomach.

epilepsy A group of neurologic disorders characterized by recurrent episodes of convulsive seizures, sensory disturbances, abnormal behaviors, loss of consciousness, or all of these.

epistaxis Nosebleed.

equilibrium Balance.

erection The state of swelling, hardness, and stiffness observed in the penis of the male and to a lesser extent in the clitoris of the female.

erythema Redness of the skin.

erythrasma A chronic bacterial infection of the major skinfolds, marked by red or brownish patches on the skin.

erythrocyte sedimentation rate The rate at which red blood cells settle out of unclotted blood in 1 hour.

erythropoiesis Formation of red blood cells, or erythrocytes.

eschar A castoff of dead tissue, as from a burn, corrosive application, or gangrene.

escharotomy Surgical incision of a constricting eschar in a burn victim to permit the cut edges to separate and restore blood flow to unburned tissue.

esophageal varices Varicosities of branches of the azygous vein that connects with the portal vein in the lower esophagus; related to portal hypertension and cirrhosis of the liver.

estrogens The female sex hormones, including estradiol, estriol, and estrone.

etiology Study of the cause of disease; origin.

euthanasia An easy or painless death; active euthanasia, or mercy killing, is the deliberate ending of the life of a person who is incurably and terminally ill; passive euthanasia is the withholding of "heroic" measures and allowing the person to die.

euthymia A normal mood or feeling state.

evaluation, of outcome Appraisal of the patient's progress toward achievement of the goals and objectives stated in the nursing care plan.

evaluation, of process Appraisal of nursing activities and what has been done to assess, plan, and implement nursing care.

evaluation, of structure Appraisal of the physical facilities, equipment, staffing, and other characteristics of an agency that affect the quality of nursing care.

evisceration (1) extrusion of internal organs; (2) removal of the contents of the eyeball, leaving the sclera intact.

excess An amount beyond what is usual or necessary.

excoriation Any superficial loss of substance, such as that produced by scratching the skin.

excursion Range of movement (of the lungs).

exercises, isometric Active exercises performed against stable resistance, without change in the length of the muscle.

exfoliate To separate or peel off in scales, layers, or flakes.

exocrine Secreting externally via a duct.

exogenous Coming from outside.

exophthalmos Abnormal protrusion of the eyeball.

exotoxin A potent toxin formed and excreted by the bacterial cell.

Expanded Precautions Use of Standard Precaution techniques with additional protective actions specific to the organism and location involved.

expected outcomes Results expected to be achieved by the patient from health care provided and personal contributions.

expectorate To spit out saliva or cough up materials from the air passageways leading to the lungs.

extension A movement that brings a limb into or toward a straight position by increasing the angle between the bones forming a joint; opposite of flexion.

extracellular Outside of the cell.

extracellular fluids Body fluids outside the cell walls that constitute the environment of each cell.

extracorporeal Outside the body.

exudate Fluid that contains dead cells, serum, phagocytes, bacteria, or pus.

F

fasiotomy Linear incisions in the fascia down the extremity.

fecal impaction The accumulation of putty-like or hardened feces in the rectum or sigmoid colon.

feedback The process of providing a system with information about its output.

feedback, negative A corrective action in which a system is informed that its output is not satisfactory and a change is needed.

feedback, positive Information that tells a system its output is satisfactory.

fee-for-service Fee paid for services provided; a type of medical practice.

fetor hepaticus Foul-smelling breath associated with severe liver disease.

fibroid A thickened vascular mass in the uterus.

fibroma A fibrous, encapsulated connective tissue tumor.

fibrosis Fibrous tissue formation.

filtration Passage of a gas or liquid through a filter to separate out unwanted matter.

fistula(s) Any abnormal, tubelike passage within the body between two internal organs or leading from an internal organ to the body surface.

flaccid Limp, weak, or relaxed.

flatus Gas in the digestive tract.

flexion A movement that brings a limb into or toward a bent position by decreasing the angle between the bones forming a joint; opposite of extension.

flight of ideas Going from topic to topic in conversation with little or no connection.

flora Plant life, as distinguished from animal life.

fluid(s) The water and substances dissolved in it that form the internal environment.

fluid balance Equilibrium between the amount of fluid taken into the body and that lost through urine, feces, the lungs, skin, and possibly vomiting and fistulas.

fluid deficit(s) A fluid imbalance in which there is not enough fluid in one or more of the body's fluid compartments as a result of either inadequate intake or excessive loss.

fluid excess A fluid imbalance in which too much fluid accumulates in one or more of the body's fluid compartments as a result of either excessive intake or inadequate loss. *See also* Edema.

fluids, transcellular Body fluids that pass through cellular structures and eventually are eliminated from the body.

follicular pharyngitis An inflammation of the pharynx accompanied by purulent infection.

fracture(s) Interruption in the continuity of a bone.

friction rub A high-pitched, scratchy sound heard with the diaphragm of the stethoscope placed at the lower left sternal border of the chest; a symptom of pericarditis.

fructosamine assay A test that may be used to monitor control of glucose over a period of 2 to 3 weeks.

fulguration Destruction by electric cautery.

functional disorder A disorder that affects the function but not the structure of the body or body part.

fungus (fungi) A member of a group of organisms (mushrooms, yeasts, molds, etc.) that thrive in a warm, moist climate. Can cause infections that are difficult to eradicate because fungi tend to reproduce by means of spores that are resistant to ordinary disinfectants and antiseptics.

furuncles Inflammations of hair follicles. Also called *boils*.

G

galactosemia A genetic disorder in which there is a lack of the enzyme necessary for proper metabolism of galactose.

gangrene A necrosis, or death, of tissue, usually caused by deficient or absent blood supply.

gastritis An inflammation of the mucous membrane lining the stomach.

gastrojejunostomy The surgical creation of an anastomosis between the stomach and jejunum.

gastroparesis Delayed gastric emptying.

gastrostomy The surgical creation of an opening into the stomach to administer food and liquids.

gate control theory The proposal that synapses in the dorsal horn of the spinal cord act as gates and that pain signals compete with signals of other kinds of stimuli for passage through the gate and transmission to the brain.

gene One of the self-reproducing biologic units of heredity that make up segments of the DNA molecule that controls cellular reproduction and function.

generalized anxiety disorder A persistent, unrealistic, or excessive worry about two or more life circumstances.

genital Pertaining to the genitals (reproductive organs).

geriatrics The medical treatment of diseases commonly associated with aging and elderly persons.

gerontology The study of the problems of aging in all its aspects.

gigantism Excessive size. Seen in children with excessive secretion of growth hormone.

gingivitis An inflammation of the gingivae.

glaucoma A group of diseases of the eye, characterized by increased intraocular pressure, that can produce blindness if not managed successfully.

global amnesia Irretrievable total loss of memory.

globulin(s) A general term for proteins; separated into five fractions by serum protein electrophoresis and classified in order of decreasing electrophoretic mobility. The fractions are alpha$_1$, alpha$_2$, beta$_1$, beta$_2$, and gamma globulins.

glucagon(s) A polypeptide hormone secreted by the alpha cells of the islets of Langerhans.

glucocorticoid Any hormone released from the adrenal cortex that increases glucogenesis and thus raises the level of liver glycogen and blood glucose.

glucogenesis The formation of glucose from glycogen.

glucometer Blood glucose–monitoring machine.

glucose intolerance The inability to properly metabolize glucose.

glucose tolerance test A test to detect abnormal glucose metabolism; assists in diagnosis of diabetes mellitus.

glycemic Referring to the amount of glucose present in a substance.

glycemic control Control of glucose in the blood.

glycosuria Glucose in the urine.

glycosylated hemoglobin (Hb A$_{1c}$; A1C) Hemoglobin with glucose attached to it; periodic measurements of hemoglobin A$_{1c}$ can help determine a diabetic patient's average blood glucose level over a period of 3 to 4 months.

goal(s) A broad statement describing what is to be accomplished over a specified period.

goiter An enlargement of the thyroid gland.

gonads Gamete-producing glands; the ovaries and testicles.

goniometry The measurement of range of motion in a joint.

graft An implant or transplant of tissue or an organ.

gram negative Having the pink color of the counterstain used in Gram's method of staining microorganisms.

gram positive Retaining the violet color of the stain used in Gram's method of staining microorganisms.

granulocyte A leukocyte containing abundant granules in its cytoplasm; granulocytes include neutrophils, eosinophils, and basophils.

gynecomastia The development of abnormally large mammary glands in the male.

H

hallucination A sensory perception (touching, tasting, feeling, hearing, seeing) that occurs without external stimulation.

hand hygiene The primary intervention any health care provider can use to control the spread of infection; performed with soap and water, if the hands are visibly soiled, or with an alcohol-based hand-sanitizing solution.

handicap A social disadvantage that exists because of a disability.

"Hands-Only CPR" Intended only for lay rescuers and only chest compressions are delivered; rescue breathing or mouth-to-mouth resuscitation are not included.

Haversian system A canal system that runs through the bones and contains the blood and lymph vessels.

health The ability to function well physically and mentally and to express the full range of one's potential.

health care–associated infection Formerly known as a *nosocomial* infection. Can occur when a patient is cared for in any kind of health care setting.

health care–associated pneumonia (HCAP) Pneumonia that develops due to conditions related to being in a health care facility or receiving health care.

health maintenance organization (HMO) A type of group health care practice that provides basic and supplemental health maintenance and treatment services to enrollees who prepay a fixed periodic fee that is set without regard to the amount or kind of services received.

Healthy People 2020 A federal government mandate with goals for improving the health of the American people, with particular attention to health concerns of people in minority groups.

hearing loss Impaired perception of sound.

heat exhaustion A disorder resulting from overexposure to heat or to the sun; also called *heat prostration*. It is caused by excessive perspiration and loss of body water and salt.

heatstroke A life-threatening condition resulting from prolonged exposure to environmental heat; also called *sunstroke*.

Helicobacter pylori A species of gram-negative, microaerophilic bacteria of the family Spirillaceae that causes gastritis and pyloric ulcers in humans.

helping relationship A relationship in which at least one of the parties intends to promote growth, development, maturity, improved functioning, and improved coping in the life of the other.

hemarthrosis A collection of blood in the joint space.

hematemesis Vomiting of blood.

hematocrit The volume percentage of red blood cells in whole blood.

hematoma(s) A localized collection of blood, usually clotted, that has leaked from adjacent blood vessels into an organ, space, or tissue.

hematuria Blood in the urine.

hemianopsia Blindness for half the field of vision in one or both eyes.

hemicolectomy Removal of part of the colon.

hemiparesis Weakness affecting only one side of the body.

hemiparesthesia Abnormal sensation on one side of the body.

hemiplegia Paralysis of one half, or one side, of the body.

hemodialysis The removal of nitrogenous wastes from the blood by circulating arterial blood through a dialysate and returning it to the venous circulation.

hemodynamics The study of the movements of blood and the pressures being exerted in the blood vessels and the chambers of the heart.

hemoglobin The protein found in red blood cells that transports molecular oxygen in the blood; oxygenated hemoglobin (oxyhemoglobin) is bright red; unoxygenated hemoglobin is darker.

hemoglobinuria The presence of free hemoglobin in the urine.

hemolysis The rupture of red blood cells with release of hemoglobin into the plasma.

hemolytic Pertaining to the breakdown of red blood cells.

hemophilia An inherited disorder in which there is deficiency of one or more specific clotting factors in the blood.

hemoptysis Coughing and spitting of blood that can originate in the lungs, larynx, or trachea.

hemorrhoid A varicosity of a vein of the rectum. It may be internal (inside the sphincter muscles of the anus) or external (outside the sphincter muscles).

hemorrhoidectomy The removal of hemorrhoids.

hemothorax A collection of blood in the pleural cavity.

hepatic encephalopathy Degenerative changes in the brain associated with liver failure.

hepatitis An inflammation of the liver.

hernia The protrusion or projection of an organ or a part of an organ through the wall of the cavity that normally contains it.

hernioplasty The repair of a hernia.

herniorrhaphy The surgical repair of a hernia.

herpesvirus Any of a large group of DNA viruses found in many animal species. Type 1 herpes simplex virus (HSV) produces lesions that are primarily nongenital. Type 2 HSV lesions most often are genital.

heterosexual A person who is sexually attracted to people of the opposite sex.

hiatal hernia Protrusion of a portion of the stomach through the opening in the diaphragm through which the esophagus passes.

hierarchy The arrangement of objects, elements, or values in a graduated series.

hirsutism The excessive growth of hair on the body.

HIV The causative agent for AIDS; *see* Human immuno-deficiency virus.

HLA Human leukocyte antigen.

HMO *See* Health maintenance organization.

holism The belief that each person is a unified whole.

holistic health care Attention to the mental, social, spiritual, and physical aspects of health and illness.

Homans' sign Pain on passive dorsiflexion of the foot; a sign of thrombosis of deep calf veins.

homeopathy A practice based on the theory that a substance that produces symptoms of a disease when given in large doses to a healthy individual will cure the same symptoms when administered in small amounts.

homeostasis A tendency of biologic systems to maintain stability in the internal environment while continually adjusting to changes necessary for survival.

homonymous hemianopia Blindness or defective vision in the right or left halves of the visual fields of both eyes.

homosexual A person who is sexually attracted to people of the same sex.

homozygous Having inherited a genetic trait from both parents.

hordeolum An external stye.

hormone A chemical produced by the cells of the body and transported by the bloodstream to target cells and organs on which it has a regulatory effect.

hospice A program that provides a continuum of home and inpatient care for terminally ill individuals and their families.

hospital-acquired pneumonia (HAP) Pneumonia symptoms that occur more than 48 hours after admission.

host An organism in which another parasitic organism is nourished and harbored.

human immunodeficiency virus (HIV) A retrovirus that integrates itself into the genetic material of the cell it infects, changing the DNA of the host cell.

human needs Basic needs for survival and personal growth shared by all humans.

human needs theory The proposal that basic human needs act as stimuli to human behavior; Maslow postulated five levels of human needs: physiologic, safety and security, love and belonging, esteem, and self-actualization.

humoral Pertaining to body fluids or substances contained in them.

humoral immunity Antibody-mediated immunity, the result of B-cell action and the production of antibodies.

hydrocephalus Increased cerebrospinal fluid in the ventricles of the brain.

hydronephrosis Distention of the renal pelvis and calices with urine that cannot flow through obstructed ureters.

hydrostatic pressure The pressure or force due to the presence of a fluid.

hyperalimentation Total parenteral nutrition.

hypercalcemia An excessive amount of calcium in the blood (i.e., more than 5.5 mEq/L or 11 mg/dL).

hypercapnia An excessive amount of carbon dioxide in the blood.

hyperchloremia An excessive amount of chloride in the blood.

hyperesthesia Abnormal sensitivity to stimuli.

hyperglycemia An above-normal level of blood sugar, as in diabetes.

hyperkalemia An excessive amount of potassium in the blood.

hyperlipidemia An excessive amount of lipids in the blood.

hypermagnesemia An excessive amount of magnesium in blood plasma.

hypernatremia An excessive amount of sodium in the blood.

hyperopia A visual defect in which parallel light rays reaching the eye focus behind the retina; farsightedness.

hyperphosphatemia An excessive amount of phosphates in the blood.

hyperplasia An increase in the number of cells of an organ; extra cell growth.

hyperpyrexia An extremely elevated temperature.

hypersecretion Oversecretion.

hypersensitivity An exaggerated immune response to an agent perceived by the body to be foreign. *See also* Allergy (allergies).

hypersomnia Sleeping for long periods.

hypertension Persistently high blood pressure; in adults, a systolic pressure equal to or greater than 140 mm Hg and a diastolic pressure equal to or greater than 90 mm Hg.

hyperthermia Unusually high fever.

hypertonic Of greater concentration.

hypertonic solution A solution in which the osmotic pressure (concentration) is greater than that of body fluids.

hypertrophy An increase in size of a structure or organ.

hyperuricemia An excessive amount of uric acid in the urine.

hyperventilation An abnormal breathing pattern in which an above-normal amount of air is inhaled into the lungs.

hypervolemia An abnormal increase in the volume of circulating blood.

hypesthesia A dysesthesia consisting of abnormally decreased sensitivity, particularly to touch. Also called *hypoesthesia*.

hypnosis A subconscious condition, usually artificially induced, in which there is a response to suggestions and commands made by the hypnotist.

hypoalbuminemia An abnormally low level of albumin in the blood.

hypocalcemia An abnormally low level of calcium in the blood (i.e., less than 4.5 mEq/L or 8.5 mg/dL).

hypocapnia An abnormally low level of carbon dioxide in the blood, resulting from hyperventilation.

hypochloremia An abnormally low level of chloride in the blood.

hypochromic Pertaining to a condition of the blood in which the red blood cells have a reduced hemoglobin content.

hypodermoclysis Injection of fluid into subcutaneous tissue via continuous infusion.

hypoesthesia *See* Hypesthesia.

hypogammaglobulinemia An immune deficiency characterized by abnormally low levels of generally all classes of serum gamma globulins with increased susceptibility to infectious diseases.

hypoglycemia An abnormally low level of blood sugar.

hypoglycemic agents Agents that lower the blood sugar level (i.e., oral medications that are used to treat some forms of diabetes mellitus).

hypokalemia An abnormally low level of potassium in the blood.

hypomagnesemia An abnormally low level of magnesium in the blood plasma.

hypomania Inflated or irritable mood for at least 4 days.

hyponatremia An abnormally low level of sodium in the blood.

hypophosphatemia An abnormally low level of phosphates in the blood.

hypophysectomy Excision of the hypophysis cerebri.

hyposecretion Undersecretion.

hyposensitization A treatment used in managing hypersensitivity to a known allergen; the program involves regular injections of minute quantities of selected antigens over an extended period.

hypothalamus That portion of the diencephalon that lies beneath the thalamus at the base of the cerebrum; it activates, controls, and integrates many of the body's vital functions (e.g., regulation of metabolism, volume of body fluids, electrolyte content, and release of hormones).

hypothermia A serious loss of body heat caused by prolonged exposure to cold.

hypothyroidism Deficient activity of the thyroid gland.

hypotonic Of lesser concentration.

hypotonic solution One in which the osmotic pressure (concentration) is less than that of body fluids.

hypotonic state Pertaining to abnormally decreased muscular tone or tension.

hypoventilation An abnormal breathing pattern in which insufficient amounts of air are inhaled into the lungs.

hypovolemia Diminished blood volume.

hypoxemia Insufficient oxygenation of the blood.

hypoxia Deficiency of oxygen.

hysterectomy Surgical removal of the uterus.

I

iatrogenic Caused by medical treatment or diagnostic procedure.

iatrogenic disorder An adverse condition induced by effects of treatment by a physician or surgeon.

icterus Bile pigmentation of the tissues, membranes, and secretions.

idiopathic Of unknown cause.

idiosyncrasy A special characteristic by which a person differs from others.

ileal conduit A surgically created passageway that uses a portion of the ileum to direct the flow of urine from the ureters to the outside of the body.

ileostomy (ileostomies) An artificial opening in the ileum, created surgically, to drain fecal material from the small intestine.

ileus Intestinal obstruction, especially failure of peristalsis.

illusion A misperception of an actual sensory perception; misinterpretation of reality.

imagery Imagination; the calling up of mental pictures or events.

immune deficiency A lack of immune bodies and resultant impairment of the immune response to foreign agents.

immunity Resistance to a specific disease.

immunity, active Immunity acquired by producing one's own antibody.

immunity, passive Immunity acquired from a source other than one's own body, such as by transfer of antibody or lymphocytes from an immune donor.

immunization The process of rendering an individual immune by passive immunity or of becoming immune by active immunity.

immunocompetence The capacity to develop an immune response after exposure to antigen.

immunoglobulin(s) A protein of animal origin with known antibody activity and a major component of humoral immunity. *See also* Antibody (antibodies).

immunoscintigraphy A radioactive scan of the immune structures.

immunosuppression The deliberate inhibition of antibody formation; used in transplantation to prevent rejection of the donor organ.

immunotherapy Development of passive immunity in a person by administration of preformed antibody; also, the administration of immunopotentiators and immunocompetent lymphoid tissue for cancer treatment.

impairment Dysfunction of a specific organ or body system.

impetigo An infection of the skin, usually by streptococci or staphylococci.

implementation A deliberate action performed to achieve a goal; carrying out of nursing interventions.

impotence Inability of the male to achieve or maintain an erection.

impulsive Acting in response to an impulse because the action brings emotional release or pleasure even though the action may be harmful to oneself or socially unacceptable.

inanimate Not alive; dull, lifeless.

incidence The rate at which certain events occur.

incontinence An alteration in the control of bowel or urinary elimination, or both.

incubation The interval between exposure to infection and the appearance of the first symptom.

index of suspicion Keen observation to detect problems that are not initially obvious, but suspected because of history or circumstances that underlie the patient's decision to seek care.

induration An abnormally hard spot or place.

infarct A localized area of necrosis produced by ischemia caused by obstructed arterial supply or inadequate venous drainage.

infarction Occurrence of a localized area of dead tissue produced by inadequate blood flow.

infection The invasion and multiplication of pathogenic microorganisms in body tissue.

inference A deduction or conclusion.

infertility The condition of inability to produce offspring.

inflammation An immediate cellular response to any kind of injury to the cells and tissues.

ingestants Any substances taken orally, such as food or drink.

ingestion The taking of any substance, such as food, drugs, water, or chemicals, by mouth or through the digestive system.

inhalants Medication or compounds suitable for inhaling.

initial The beginning of a thing or process; the first.

injectables Fluids capable of being injected.

innate Belonging to the essential nature of something; existing in or belonging at birth.

innate immunity A person's natural (inborn) immunity to certain diseases.

inotropic Pertaining to the force or energy of muscular contractions, particularly of the heart.

insensible Unconscious; without feeling or consciousness.

inspection The process of visual examination.

insomnia A sleep disorder; an inability to sleep.

insufficiency The condition of being inadequate for a given purpose.

insulin A naturally occurring hormone secreted by the beta cells of the islets of Langerhans in the pancreas in response to increased levels of glucose in the blood.

insulin-dependent diabetes mellitus Type 1 diabetes; a form of the disease that requires replacement of endogenous insulin with regular injections of exogenous insulin.

insulin resistance A situation where insulin interaction with glucose becomes less efficient and fat metabolism is abnormal.

intention tremor A tremor that occurs on attempt at voluntary movement.

interdisciplinary (collaborative) care plan A care plan composed through collaboration of all of the health care team members caring for a patient.

intermittent claudication Cramping pain in the muscles of the lower extremities brought on by exercise and relieved by rest. A common symptom of arterial insufficiency; pain usually occurs in the calves of the legs, but can also affect the muscles of the thighs and buttocks.

interstitial Placed or lying between.

interstitial fluids Body fluids that are located in the tissue spaces around the cells. *See also* Edema.

intervention Nursing activities performed by the nurse to meet the specified goals of a nursing care plan.

intracellular Within cells.

intracellular fluids Body fluids that are within cell walls.

intractable pain Hard-to-manage pain; pain not relieved by ordinary methods.

intraocular Within the eye.

intrathecal Injected into the subarachnoid space of the spinal cord via lumbar puncture.

intrathoracic Within the thoracic cavity.

intravascular fluids Body fluids within the blood vessels; they are composed of plasma and the substances it transports.

intravenous therapy The administration of fluids through a vein.

intussusception Telescoping of one part of the bowel into another.

inuria Abnormal presence of protein in the urine.

ions Atoms or groups of atoms that have an electric charge through the gain or loss of an electron.

ipsilateral On or affecting the same side of the body.

iridectomy Excision of part of the iris.

ischemia A deficiency of blood supply to a part as a result of functional constriction of a blood vessel or of actual obstruction, as by a clot.

Islets of Langerhans Pancreatic cells. Beta cells, which secrete insulin, are found in these cells.

isolation technique Special precautionary procedures used to set apart a patient with a communicable disease; the purpose is to prevent the spread of infectious agents from the patient to others.

isometric Having equal dimensions; maintaining the same length.

isometric exercises Exercises that involve generating tension between two opposing sets of muscles.

isotonic Of equal solute concentration.

isotonic contraction A contraction that occurs when tension is developed in a muscle.

isotonic solution A solution in which the osmotic pressure is the same as that of intracellular fluid (e.g., normal saline [0.9% concentration]).

isotope One of a series of chemical elements that have nearly identical chemical properties but differ in their atomic weight and electric charge. Many isotopes are radioactive.

J

jaundice A yellowing of the skin and mucous membranes that reflects excessively high blood levels of bilirubin (bile pigment).

K

keloid Excessive, abnormal scar formation in the skin following trauma or surgical incision.

keratitis An inflammation of the cornea.

keratosis (keratoses) Any horny growth, such as a wart or callosity; usually either actinic keratosis or a seborrheic keratosis.

ketoacidosis The accumulation of ketone bodies in the blood because of incomplete metabolism of fats, resulting in metabolic acidosis.

ketonuria The presence of acetone bodies in the urine.

ketosis The accumulation in the body of the ketone bodies: acetone, beta-hydroxybutyric acid, and acetoacetic acid.

kinetic motion The motion of material bodies and the forces and energy associated with it.

Korsakoff's syndrome Substance-induced persisting dementia.

Kupffer's cells Large, highly phagocytic cells in the liver; they form part of the reticuloendothelial system.

kyphosis An abnormally increased curvature of the thoracic spine, which gives a "hunchback" appearance.

L

labile Unsteady, not fixed; easily disarranged.

labyrinthitis An inflammation of the internal ear, including the vestibule, cochlea, and semicircular canal.

laparoscopy The examination of the peritoneal cavity with a fiberoptic instrument inserted through a small abdominal incision.

laryngectomy The partial or total removal of the larynx by surgical excision; the person who has had a laryngectomy is called a *laryngectomee.*

laryngitis An inflammation of the larynx.

laryngoscopy Direct or indirect visual examination of the larynx.

laser Stands for *light amplification by stimulated emission of radiation;* converts light wavelengths into one small, intense, unified beam of single-wavelength radiation; used for diagnosis and surgery.

latent Not obvious; hidden.

latent TB infection (LTBI) Terminology for an infection with *Mycobacterium tuberculosis* but no current active disease.

lesion A circumscribed area of pathologically altered tissue.

leukapheresis A process by which blood is withdrawn from a vein, white blood cells are removed, and the remaining blood is reinfused in the patient.

leukemia A malignant disease of the blood-forming organs, marked by abnormal proliferation and development of leukocytes and their precursors in the blood and bone marrow.

leukocyte A colorless blood cell whose chief function is to protect the body against pathogenic microorganisms.

leukocytosis An increase in the number of white blood cells, or leukocytes, in the blood.

leukopenia A reduction in the number of leukocytes in the blood to 5000 or less.

leukoplakia Patches of thickened, white tissue on mucous membrane; considered a precursor to cancer.

leukotrienes A class of biologically active compounds that occur naturally in leukocytes and produce allergic and inflammatory reactions similar to those of histamine.

level of consciousness (LOC) A standardized system to describe the state of consciousness (i.e., alert wakefulness, drowsiness, stupor, or coma).

Lhermitte's sign An electric shock–like sensation felt along the spine when the neck is flexed.

libido The conscious or unconscious sexual drive.

lifestyle habits Entrenched practices related to work, recreation, diet, exercise, and other activities of daily living.

ligament Connective tissue that joins the bones of a joint together.

ligate To tie or bind.

lipodystrophy A disturbance of or defect in fat metabolism.

lipoma A fatty tumor.

lipoprotein Any of the macromolecular complexes that are transported in the blood.

lithiasis The formation of stones.

lithotripsy The crushing of a calculus in the kidney, bladder, urethra, or gallbladder.

loose associations Disordered thinking with little connection between thoughts.

lordosis An abnormal forward curvature of the spine.

lozenge(s) A medicated tablet or disk.

lucid Clear, especially applied to clarity of the mind.

lymphadenitis An inflammation of the lymph nodes.

lymphadenopathy A disease of the lymph nodes, often producing enlargement.

lymphangiography Radiography of lymphatic vessels after injection of a contrast medium.

lymphangitis An inflammation of the lymph vessels.

lymphatic system An accessory system by which fluids can flow from tissue spaces into the blood.

lymphedema The swelling of tissues drained by the lymphatic system.

lymph nodes Small bundles of lymphatic tissue containing lymphocytes, the functions of which are filtration and phagocytosis.

lymphocyte A mononuclear, nongranulous leukocyte that is chiefly a product of lymphoid tissue and is important in the development of immunity.

lymphocyte, sensitized A nongranular lymphocyte that has been processed either by the thymus (T lymphocyte) or an unknown processing area (B lymphocyte) and is responsible for either cellular or humoral immunity.

lymphocyte-transforming factor A protein mediator that causes transformation and clonal expansion of nonsensitized lymphocytes that produce a toxin destructive to antigen.

lymphoma Any neoplastic disorder of lymphoid tissue.

lyse To produce decomposition; to destroy.

lysis The gradual decline of a fever or disease; the opposite of crisis.

M

macrophage(s) A large, mononuclear phagocyte derived from monocytes; macrophages are components of the reticuloendothelial system.

macrophage-activating factor A mediator released by sensitized lymphocytes on contact with an antigen, the function of which is to induce in macrophages an increased content of lysosomal enzymes, more aggressive phagocytosis, and increased mitosis.

macrophage chemotaxis factor A protein mediator released by sensitized lymphocytes on contact with antigen, the function of which is to attract macrophages to the antigen site.

macule (macula) A discolored spot on the skin that is not raised above the surface.

major depressive disorder A mental disorder in which at least five symptoms characteristic of depression have been present for at least 2 weeks. Some of these symptoms include an overwhelming feeling of sadness, inability to feel pleasure or interest in daily activities, weight gain or loss not attributed to dieting, sleep disturbances, fatigue, difficulty concentrating, and suicidal thoughts.

malignancy *See* Carcinoma.

malignant Becoming progressively worse; resisting treatment and resulting in death; having the properties of anaplasia, invasiveness, and metastasis.

mammography The x-ray examination of the soft tissues of the breast.

mammoplasty Plastic surgery of the breast.

managed care Organization of health care delivery that coordinates care delivery by various health team members in a timely, cost-effective manner.

mania An elevation in mood characterized by feelings of elation, excitement, or extreme irritability.

mass casualties Casualties in such numbers that the normal health care system has difficulty providing adequate care.

mastication Chewing.

mean, mathematical An average (e.g., mean corpuscular hemoglobin concentration, which is the concentration of hemoglobin in the average erythrocyte).

measurable The ability to be expressed numerically, or to be described as to the extent or quantity (of a substance, energy, or time).

mechanism of injury Refers to how the injury occurred.

mediastinum The mass of tissues and organs separating the sternum in front and the vertebral column behind.

mediate To accomplish by indirect means; to act between two parties or sides.

Medicaid A federally funded state-operated program that provides medical assistance to eligible people with low incomes.

Medicare A federally funded national health insurance program in the United States for people over 65 years old.

medical nutrition therapy A registered dietician (RD) or a certified diabetes educator (CDE) performs an in-depth assessment of type of diabetes, height-to-weight ratio, usual dietary intake, food preferences, exercise level, and daily schedule. A range of interventions are considered when designing a plan that is individualized for the patient.

meditation The act of contemplative thinking.

melanoma A malignant, darkly pigmented mole or tumor of the skin.

melena Black, tarry stools.

menarche The onset of menstruation.

Ménière's disease A group of symptoms produced by an increase in fluid in the labyrinthine spaces with swelling and congestion of the mucosa of the cochlea.

menopause The span of time during which the menstrual cycle wanes and gradually stops; *see* Climacteric.

menorrhagia Excessive menstruation.

menses The onset of the menstrual cycle.

menstruation The shedding of the uterine lining.

mentate To think.

MET Acronym for "metabolic equivalent of task," a measure of heat production by the body. This term is used with cardiac rehabilitation patients.

metabolic acidosis A condition in which the pH of body fluids is below 7.4 because of either an excessive production of carbonic acid through the oxidation of fats, or a loss of bicarbonate.

metabolic alkalosis A condition in which the pH of body fluids is above 7.4 because of either an excessive loss of acid, an above-normal intake or retention of base, or a low level of potassium in the blood.

metabolism The sum of the physical and chemical processes by which living tissue is formed and maintained and by which large molecules are disassembled to provide energy.

metastasis The movement of disease from one organ or body part to a distant location; for example, the migration of microorganisms and of malignant cells.

metrorrhagia Uterine bleeding occurring at irregular intervals and sometimes for prolonged periods.

microalbuminuria Presence of albumin in the urine, which is suggestive of *early* kidney disease.

microcytic Pertaining to a smaller-than-normal cell.

micron A unit of linear measure; equal to 0.001 mm.

micturition The voiding of urine.

milieu therapy Therapy in a structured environment of a hospital or group home setting to help patients participate as active members of the milieu community and practice social behaviors.

milliequivalent One-thousandth of a chemical equivalent, expressed as mEq; the concentration of electrolytes in a certain volume of solution is usually expressed as milliequivalents per liter (mEq/L).

mineralocorticoids A group of hormones elaborated by the adrenal cortex that have an effect on sodium, chloride, and potassium levels in extracellular fluid.

miotic A drug that constricts the pupil.

mitosis A type of cell division of somatic cells in which each daughter cell contains the same number of chromosomes as the parent cell. It is the process by which the body grows and by which somatic cells are replaced.

mittelschmerz A sharp pain in the right or left lower quadrant, sometimes felt at midcycle around the time of ovulation.

modulation The fourth of four phases associated with nociceptive pain wherein the brain sends signals back down the spinal cord by release of neurotransmitters.

monocytes Mononuclear phagocytic leukocytes.

monoparesis Weakness in one limb.

monoplegia Paralysis of one limb.

morphologic Related to the science of structures and forms without regard to function.

mucolytic Dissolving or destroying mucus.

mucorrhea The free discharge of mucus.

mucositis An inflammation of a mucous membrane.

multidrug-resistant organism (MDRO) A pathogen that has mutated due to inadequate dosages or delays in administration of antimicrobial medication and is now resistant to many medications.

multisystem organ dysfunction syndrome (MODS) A syndrome in which there is concurrent dysfunction of several organs.

muscle tone The readiness of a muscle to contract and relax normally.

mutation An unusual change in a gene occurring spontaneously or by induction. Mutation can occur in pathogenic organisms.

mycosis (mycoses) Any disease caused by a fungus.

mydriatic Dilating the pupil.

myocardial infarction (MI) Necrosis of the myocardium as a result of interruption of the blood supply to the area.

myocarditis An inflammation of the heart muscle.

myomectomy Surgical removal of a tumor from the uterine wall, accomplished by use of an endoscope.

myopia The error of refraction in which parallel light rays focus in front of the retina; nearsightedness.

myringotomy An incision into the eardrum.

myxedema A condition in the adult in which there are low thyroid levels.

N

nebulizer An atomizer; a device for delivering drugs or water to the respiratory tract by forcing air or oxygen through a solution.

necrosis The changes that occur as a result of death of cells; caused by enzymatic degradation.

necrotic Pertaining to death of a portion of tissue.

negative feedback In the endocrine system, if the hormonal need of a target tissue is being satisfied, production or secretion of the hormone will be inhibited.

negative symptoms One of the two divisions of signs and symptoms of schizophrenia; include apathy, social isolation, psychomotor retardation, and lack of motivation.

neologism(s) In psychiatry, a new word whose meaning may be known only to the person using it and may be related to his or her conflicts.

neoplasm A tumor; any new and abnormal growth.

nephron The structural and functional unit of the kidney, which consists of the renal corpuscle, the proximal convoluted tubule, limbs of the loop of Henle, the distal convoluted tubule, and the collecting tubule; thus each nephron is able to form urine independently.

nephrosclerosis Atherosclerotic disease of the small renal arteries related to hypertension and eventual destruction of renal cells.

nephrostomy Formation of an artificial fistula into the renal pelvis of the kidney.

nephrostomy tubes Tubes inserted to drain the renal pelvis.

networking Meeting people, exchanging phone numbers, expressing interest in other people and what they are doing, and establishing a business relationship that might be mutually beneficial.

neuroglycopenia A shortage of glucose in the brain.

neuron Any of the conducting cells of the nervous system; consists of a cell body containing the nucleus and cytoplasm and the axon and dendrites.

neuropathic pain Pain associated with a dysfunction of the nervous system; specifically, an abnormality in the processing of sensations.

neuropathy Any disease of the nerves.

neutropenia An abnormal decrease in the number of neutrophils in the blood.

neutrophilia An increase in the number of neutrophils in the blood.

neutrophils Granular leukocytes; also called *polymorphonuclear leukocytes.*

nociceptive pain Pain associated with pain stimuli from either somatic or visceral structures.

nocturia Excessive urination during the night.

nodules Small masses of tissue that can be detected by touch.

noncommunicable Cannot be carried from one person to another.

non–insulin-dependent diabetes mellitus Type 2 diabetes; a form of diabetes in which levels of endogenous insulin are adequate and control can be managed by diet and exercise and perhaps by an oral hypoglycemic agent.

nonjudgmental Avoiding judgment based on one's personal standards.

normal flora Flora most often found on or in body systems that have some form of contact with the outside environment. This flora prevents most harmful microorganisms from colonizing the body.

normo- A combining form indicating normal or usual.

North American Nursing Diagnosis Association–International (NANDA-I) An organization that formulates and validates nursing diagnoses.

nosocomial Pertaining to or originating in a hospital.

nuchal rigidity Stiffness and pain in the neck from inflammation of the meninges.

nurse practice act A legal statute describing the parameters of nursing practice.

nursing The diagnosis and treatment of human responses to actual or potential health problems. *See also* Nursing process.

nursing care plans Written plans of care that serve to communicate to the nursing staff and others the specific nursing diagnoses and prescribed nursing orders for directing and evaluating the effectiveness of the care given.

nursing diagnosis A statement of a health problem or of a potential problem in the patient's health status that a nurse is licensed and competent to treat.

nursing interventions Acts by nurses that implement the nursing care plan.

nursing process A goal-directed series of activities whereby the practice of nursing accomplishes its goal of alleviating, minimizing, or preventing real or potential health problems.

nystagmus Involuntary, rapid rhythmic movement of the eyeball.

O

objective data Information obtained through the senses or measured by instruments.

objectives Well-defined steps toward the accomplishment of a goal; they should be realistic, be stated in measurable terms, and include the conditions under which they will be accomplished.

observation The act of watching carefully and attentively.

obsessive Having ideas, thoughts, or impulses that are persistent to an excessive degree.

obsessive-compulsive disorder A mental disorder characterized by recurrent or intrusive thoughts and rituals that can become overwhelming to the point of interfering with normal life.

obturator A device that is placed into a large-bore cannula during insertion to prevent potential blockage by tissues.

occult Obscure; concealed; hidden.

occult blood Hidden blood.

oculogyric crisis A side effect of antipsychotic medication characterized by uncontrolled rolling back of the eyes.

olfaction The act of smelling.

oligomenorrhea Decreased menstruation. Usually refers to menstrual periods that occur at an interval of 45 days or longer.

oliguria A diminished amount of urine formation.

oncogene A gene in a virus that has the ability to induce a cell to become malignant.

oncology The study of tumors.

onychomycosis A fungal infection of the fingernail or toenail.

oophoritis An inflammation of an ovary; ovaritis.

open access plan An insurance plan in which the patient can see any health care provider.

ophthalmologist A physician who specializes in treating eye disorders.

ophthalmoscope An instrument for examining the eye. The direct ophthalmoscope is used to inspect the back portion of the interior of the eyeball; the indirect ophthalmoscope permits stereoscopic inspection of the interior of the eye.

opportunistic infections (OIs) Infections that develop in an individual with a depressed immune system from organisms commonly found in the environment that are usually harmless.

opportunistic pathogen A fungus or bacterium, usually harmless, that causes infection in a person with a depressed immune system.

optic chiasm The part of the hypothalamus formed by the decussation, or crossing, of the fibers of the optic nerve from the medial half of each retina.

optician A specialist in the making of optical apparatus (e.g., eyeglasses).

optometrist A professional person trained to examine the eyes and prescribe eyeglasses or contact lenses to correct irregularities of vision.

orchiectomy The excision of one or both testes.

orchitis An inflammation of the testes.

orthopedic Referring to the correction of deformities of the musculoskeletal system.

orthopnea The ability to breathe easily only in the upright position.

orthopneic position Sitting up in bed with two or three pillows behind the back.

orthostatic hypotension A fall in blood pressure that occurs when standing up from a sitting or lying position or when standing in a fixed position; it is characterized by dizziness, syncope, and blurred vision.

oscilloscope An instrument that makes visible on a screen the nature of an electrical current.

osmolality The osmotic pressure of a solution, expressed in osmoles or milliosmoles (mOsm) per kilogram of water.

osmosis The passage of solvent from a solution of lesser concentration to one of greater concentration through a selectively permeable membrane.

osmotic pressure Pressure that develops when two solutions of different concentrations are separated by a semipermeable membrane.

ossification Formation of or conversion into bone or a bony substance.

osteomyelitis A bacterial infection of the bone.

osteoporosis A porous condition of bone due to demineralization associated with aging.

otalgia Pain in the ear.

OTC Over the counter; available without a prescription.

otitis media An inflammation of the middle ear.

otorrhea An inflammation of the ear with purulent discharge.

otoscope An instrument for examining the ear canal and eardrum.

outcome The result of an action.

ovulation The periodic ripening and rupture of the mature graafian follicle and the discharge of the ovum from the cortex of the ovary.

oxidation The process by which a substance combines with oxygen.

P

pacemaker A mechanical device that provides electrical stimulation when an anatomic pacemaker fails; a cardiac pacemaker provides electrical stimulation when there is heart block.

pain A feeling of distress or suffering caused by stimulation of specialized nerve cells; considered to occur whenever a person says it is present.

pain threshold The point at which pain is perceived.

pain tolerance The length of time or intensity at which a person will endure pain before outwardly responding to it.

palliative Designed to relieve symptoms when a disease cannot be cured.

palliative care Comfort care.

palliative surgery Surgery performed to make a patient more comfortable.

palmar erythema A persistent redness of the palms, which may be seen in liver disease.

palpation A physical examination technique in which the texture, size, consistency, and location of body parts are felt with the hands.

palpitation A rapid, violent, or throbbing pulsation, as an abnormally rapid throbbing or fluttering of the heart.

pancreatitis An inflamed condition of the pancreas.

pandemic An international outbreak of disease.

panhysterectomy The surgical removal of the entire uterus.

papule A small, round, solid, elevated lesion of the skin.

paracentesis The surgical puncture of a cavity to aspirate fluid.

paradoxical respirations Respirations in which, on inhalation, the traumatized portion of the chest wall moves inward rather than outward.

paralytic ileus The absence of peristalsis; paralysis of the intestines.

paranoia A mental disorder in which a person exhibits delusions of persecution or of grandeur or a combination of both.

paraplegia Paralysis of the lower extremities.

parathormone A hormone produced and secreted by the parathyroid gland.

parenteral Administered by a route other than the digestive tract.

paresthesia A feeling of tingling or numbness.

passive immunity Immunity acquired by transfer of antibody or lymphocytes from an immune donor.

patent Wide open.

pathogen A microorganism or substance capable of producing a disease.

pathologic Caused by a disease.

patient advocate A person who will advocate on the patient's behalf with the hospital, insurance company, or health care personnel.

PCA Patient-controlled analgesia.

pediculosis An infestation with lice.

pelvic inflammatory disease Any inflammation in the pelvis that occurs outside the uterus, uterine tubes, and ovaries.

peptic ulcer The loss of tissue lining the esophagus, stomach, or duodenum.

perception The recognition and interpretation of sensory stimuli that serve as a basis for comprehending, learning, and knowing or for motivating a particular action or reaction. Also, the third of four phases associated with nociceptive pain, during which impulses reach the brain and pain is recognized.

percussion The physical examination technique of tapping the body surface with the fingertips or fist to evaluate the size, borders, and consistency of some of the internal organs or to detect the presence of fluid in a body cavity.

percutaneous Through the skin.

perforation A hole or break in the retaining walls or membranes of an organ, as in perforated ulcer and perforated eardrum.

perfusion Supplying tissues and organs with nutrients and oxygen by blood flow through the arteries.

pericardial effusion A collection of serous or purulent exudate in the pericardial cavity.

pericardiocentesis The surgical puncture of the pericardial cavity for aspiration of fluid.

pericardiotomy The surgical incision of the pericardium.

pericarditis An inflammation of the sac that encloses the heart and the roots of the great vessels.

periodontal Located around a tooth.

perioperative Pertaining to the period extending from the time of hospitalization for surgery to the time of discharge.

periorbital Surrounding the socket of the eye.

peristomal Pertaining to the area around a stoma.

peripheral Pertaining to the area outside the central region or structure.

peristalsis Involuntary wavelike contraction of organs with both longitudinal and circular muscle fibers that passes along the organ and propels its contents, as in peristalsis of the digestive tract.

peritonitis An inflammation of the serous sac that lines the abdominal cavity and encloses the abdominal organs.

permeable Permitting passage of a substance.

personality disorder A mental disorder characterized by inflexible and maladaptive responses to life events, serious difficulty in personal and work relationships, a tendency to evoke interpersonal conflict, and a tendency to evoke a negative empathic response from others.

personal protective equipment (PPE) Equipment that forms some type of barrier to protect a person from exposure to blood-borne pathogens, body fluids, or other potentially infectious materials (e.g., gloves, covering gowns, and face masks).

pessary A hard rubber ring inserted in the vagina to help keep the abdominal organs in place.

petechiae Very small, nonraised, round, purplish spots, caused by intradermal or submucosal bleeding, that later turn blue or yellow.

pH The concentration of hydrogen (H) in a solution; the higher the concentration of hydrogen ions, the lower the pH of the solution.

phacoemulsification A technique of cataract extraction in which high-frequency vibrations are used to fragment the lens.

phagocytosis The engulfing of microorganisms and other foreign matter by phagocytes.

phantom pain A sensation of discomfort occurring where an extremity has been amputated.

pharyngitis An inflammation or infection of the pharynx that usually produces a sore throat.

phenylketonuria A genetic disorder in which there is a defect in the metabolism of phenylalanine resulting in the presence of this amino acid in the urine.

phlebitis An inflammation of a vein.

phlebotomy The surgical opening of a vein to draw blood, often done with a needle.

phobic disorder Excessive fear of a situation or object.

photocoagulation The alteration of proteins in tissue by the use of light energy in the form of ordinary light rays or a laser beam.

photodynamic therapy A type of chemotherapy in which the action of the drug is enhanced by exposure to light.

photophobia Difficulty tolerating light.

pilonidal Pertaining to, characterized by, or having a tuft of hairs.

pilonidal sinus A lesion located at the cleft of the buttocks in the sacrococcygeal region; also called *pilonidal cyst.*

placebo(s) A supposedly inactive substance or procedure that can have either positive or negative effects on the relief of symptoms and that is usually given under the guise of effective treatment or in clinical trials of new drugs.

planning A phase of the nursing process in which a plan is developed with the patient, family, or significant other to provide a blueprint for nursing intervention to achieve specified goals. *See also* Nursing care plans.

plaque A patch or flat area.

plasma The liquid portion of blood in which formed elements are suspended; it contains plasma proteins, inorganic salts, nutrients, gases, wastes from the cells, and various hormones and enzymes.

plasma cell A spherical or ellipsoidal cell involved in the synthesis, storage, and release of antibody.

plasmapheresis The separation of the cells and components of the blood.

platelets The smallest formed elements in the blood; important in coagulation and blood clotting.

plethora A general term denoting a red, florid complexion or an excess of blood.

pleurisy An inflammation of the pleura.

Pneumocystis jiroveci An opportunistic pathogen producing infection of the lung associated with acquired immunodeficiency syndrome (AIDS); formerly *Pneumocystis carinii.*

pneumonectomy The excision of lung tissue, especially of an entire lung.

pneumonia An inflammation of the lungs with consolidation.

pneumothorax The accumulation of air or gas in the pleural cavity, resulting in collapse of the lung on the affected side.

point-of-service (POS) option An option offered by some managed care plans in which a member pays an extra fee to see a desired physician outside of the care plan.

polyarteritis Multiple sites of inflammatory and destructive lesions in the arterial system.

polycystic ovarian syndrome An endocrine disturbance characterized by anovulation, amenorrhea, hirsutism, and infertility.

polycythemia An elevation in the total number of blood cells.

polydipsia Excessive thirst that results in drinking large quantities of water.

polymorphonuclear leukocytes The fully developed cells of the granulocyte series, especially neutrophils the nuclei of which contain three or more lobes.

polyphagia Increased hunger.

polyuria The production of an excessive amount of urine.

positive symptoms One of the two divisions of signs and symptoms seen with schizophrenia; includes hallucinations, delusions, and disordered thinking.

postictal state The condition of a person right after a seizure.

post-traumatic stress disorder A mental disorder characterized by recurrent symptoms of anxiety that some individuals may experience after encountering an extreme, life-threatening event. Nightmares or flashbacks may be part of the symptoms.

PPO *See* Preferred provider organization.

precancerous Term used to refer to a growth that is not yet, but probably will become, cancerous.

precipitate A deposit separated from a suspension or solution by precipitation; the reaction of a reagent that causes the deposit to fall to the bottom or float near the top.

preferred provider organization (PPO) An organization of physicians, hospitals, and pharmacists whose members discount their services to subscriber patients.

premenstrual syndrome A group of symptoms experienced by some women for several days before the onset of the menstrual period.

prepuce The foreskin or fold of skin over the glans penis in the male.

presbycusis Impairment of hearing in old age.

presbyopia Farsightedness that occurs normally with aging.

pressor A substance that causes a rise in blood pressure. Norepinephrine is an example of a "pressor" hormone. Norepinephrine maintains blood pressure.

pressure ulcer A sore caused by pressure from a splint or other appliance or from the body itself when it has remained immobile in bed for extended periods.

preventive Hindering the occurrence of something, especially disease.

priapism A prolonged penile erection resulting in a large, hard, and painful penis unrelated to sexual desire or activity.

primary union The joining of two edges of a wound that are close together, resulting in a thin scar after healing; also called *healing by first intention.*

priority Preference established on the basis of emergency or need.

priority setting Setting the sequence of actions according to importance or priority.

problem-oriented medical record (POMR) A system of documentation in which the information is arranged according to specific problems presented by the patient at the time of seeking health care. The four components are database, problem list, initial plan, and follow-up. *See also* Progress notes.

process A series of actions that move from one point to another on the way to completing a goal.

prodromal stage The early or very beginning stage of an illness.

prodrome An early sign of a developing condition or disease.

prognosis The predicted outcome of the course of a disease.

progress notes Entries in the medical record describing what has been done in the care of the patient and his or her response to the intervention.

prolapse The falling down or displacement of a part or all of an organ, as in prolapse of a stoma and prolapse of the uterus.

promoter(s) A type of epigenetic carcinogen that promotes neoplastic growth only after initiation by another substance; a co-carcinogen.

prophylactic Something done or used to prevent infection or disease.

prospective payment system A payment system for reimbursing hospitals for inpatient health care services in which a predetermined rate is set for treatment of specific illnesses.

prostaglandins A group of naturally occurring fatty acids that stimulate contraction of the uterine and other smooth-muscle tissue.

prostate-specific antigen (PSA) A protein produced by the prostate that is present in elevated levels in patients with cancer or other diseases of the prostate.

prosthesis An artificial substitute for a missing part, such as an eye, limb, or tooth, used for functional or cosmetic reasons, or both.

protease inhibitor A drug that works at the last stage of viral reproduction.

protective isolation Special precautionary procedures to minimize exposure to infectious agents in a patient who has an immune deficiency or who is otherwise susceptible to infection.

proteinuria An excess of serum proteins in the urine.

protocol The plan for a course of medical treatment.

Protozoa A phylum comprising the unicellular organisms; most are free-living, but some lead commensalistic, mutualistic, or parasitic existences.

provider Someone or an agency that provides health care services.

proximal Closest to a point of reference.

pruritus Itching.

pseudocyst An abnormal or dilated cavity resembling a true cyst but not lined with epithelium. Also called *adventitious cyst* or *false cyst.*

psychoactive substances Mind-altering agents capable of changing or altering a person's mood, behavior, cognition, arousal level, level of consciousness, and perceptions.

psychomotor retardation A slowing of speech, movement, and thought process often seen in the depressed patient.

psychotic features Hallucinations, delusions, and grossly disorganized behavior.

ptomaines Toxic substances produced by the action of putrefactive bacteria on proteins and amino acids.

ptosis The dropping of an organ below its usual position, for example, lowering of the eyelid so that it partially or completely covers the cornea.

pulmonary edema A diffuse accumulation of fluid in the tissues and air spaces of the lung.

pulmonary embolus A mass of clotted blood or other formed element in the lung.

pulse deficit The difference between the radial and apical pulse rates.

pulsus paradoxus A drop in systolic blood pressure of greater than 10 mm Hg on inspiration.

purpura Purplish areas caused by bleeding into the skin or mucous membranes.

purulence The condition of producing or discharging pus.

purulent Full of pus.

pus A liquid product of inflammation composed of albuminous substances, a thin fluid, and leukocytes; generally yellow.

pustule A small, round, pus-filled lesion of the skin.

pyelogram A radiograph of the kidney and ureters after injection of a contrast medium that may be administered intravenously (IV pyelogram) or by way of the ureters (retrograde pyelogram).

pyelonephritis An inflammation of the kidney and renal pelvis.

pyrogen Any agent that causes fever.

pyuria Pus in the urine.

Q

quadriplegia Paralysis of all four extremities.

quadriplegic A person with paralysis of all four limbs.

R

rad Radiation absorbed dose; the unit used for measuring doses of radiation.

radiation therapy The use of radiant energy from radioactive materials or high-voltage x rays to treat disease.

radioimmunoassay A laboratory method for measuring minute quantities of specific antibodies or any antigen, such as a hormone or drug, against which antibodies have been produced.

radionuclide A radioactive substance given to the patient before radiography or scanning.

radiopaque Not penetrable by x rays; appears white on radiograph.

rales Abnormal respiratory sounds heard on auscultation with a stethoscope indicating some pathologic condition.

range of motion The extent, measured in degrees of a circle, through which a joint can be extended and flexed.

rationalization A defense mechanism in which a patient finds logical reasons (justification) for his or her behavior while ignoring the real reasons.

realistic Attainable, based on the patient's condition and desire.

rectocele A protrusion of the rectum and posterior vaginal wall into the vagina.

recurrent Returning at intervals.

referred pain Pain felt in a part away from its point of origin.

reflex (reflexes) The sum of any particular autonomic (automatic) response mediated by the nervous system and not requiring conscious movement.

refraction The determination of refractive errors (inability to focus light rays on the retina) and their correction with eyeglasses.

regeneration The natural renewal of a structure.

regimen A prescribed scheme of diet, exercise, or activity to achieve certain ends.

rehabilitation The processes of treatment and education that help the disabled individual attain maximum function, a sense of well-being, and a personally satisfying level of independence.

remittent Having alternating periods of abating and returning, such as a fever that comes and goes.

replicate To duplicate, reproduce, or copy.

replication The process of duplicating or reproducing.

reservoir A passive host or carrier that harbors pathogenic organisms without harm to itself and is a source from which others can be infected.

residual urine Urine that remains in the bladder immediately after urination.

resorption Taking in or absorbing again.

respiration The taking in of oxygen, its utilization in the tissues, and the giving off of carbon dioxide.

respiratory acidosis A condition in which the pH of body fluids is below 7.4 because of failure of the lungs to remove sufficient amounts of carbon dioxide.

respiratory alkalosis A condition in which the pH of body fluids is above 7.4 because of excessive removal of carbon dioxide by the lungs, as in hyperventilation.

resuscitation Revival after apparent death.

reticuloendothelial system A network of cells and tissues found throughout the body, especially in the blood, connective tissue, spleen, liver, lungs, bone marrow, and lymph vessels; these cells play a role in blood cell formation and destruction and in inflammation and immunity.

retinopathy A pathologic condition of the retina associated with diabetes mellitus.

retrograde Moving backward; degenerating from a better to a worse state.

retrospective Dealing with the past.

retrospective payment system Medicare payment based on actual costs submitted to government; used before 1983.

retrovirus A type of virus that contains RNA.

reverse transcriptase An enzyme that is present in retroviruses.

rhinitis An inflammation of the mucous membrane of the nose.

rhinoplasty A plastic surgical operation on the nose, either reconstructive, restorative, or cosmetic.

rhonchi Coarse rattling sounds in the bronchial tubes caused by a partial obstruction.

Rickettsia A genus of small, rod-shaped to round microorganisms found in tissue cells of lice, fleas, ticks, and mites and transmitted to humans by their bites.

rigor mortis The stiffness that occurs in dead bodies.

robotics The science of designing mechanical, computerized instruments for procedures.

Roux-en-Y Any Y-shaped anastomosis in which the small intestine is included.

rubor A dusky-red color seen in patients with arterial insufficiency.

rugae Ridges or folds on a mucous membrane.

S

safer sex Any sexual practice that is performed with the use of a barrier to prevent the exchange of body fluids.

salpingitis An inflammation of a uterine tube.

sarcoidosis A chronic, progressive, systemic granulomatous reticulosis of unknown etiology, involving almost any organ or tissue.

sarcoma A tumor, often highly malignant, composed of cells derived from connective tissue.

scabies An infestation with the mange mite.

scaling The shedding of small, thin, dry layers of skin.

scarring The replacement of damaged tissue with fibrous tissue.

schizophrenia A mental illness that causes unusual, bizarre behavior (hallucinations and delusions).

scleropathy The injection of a solution that causes the vessel to dry up and disintegrate.

scoliosis Lateral curvature of the spine.

scotoma An area of lost vision in the visual field.

sebaceous Containing or pertaining to sebum, an oily, fatty matter secreted by the sebaceous glands.

secondary union The healing of a wound in which the edges are far apart and cannot be brought together; the wound fills with granulation tissue and heals from the edges inward.

sedative(s) An agent that calms nervousness, irritability, and excitement.

seizure(s) An attack of uncontrollable muscular contractions; a convulsion.

self-care The process whereby one initiates and carries out certain health practices to maintain life, health, and personal well-being.

semen A thick, opalescent, viscid secretion discharged from the urethra of the male at the climax of sexual excitement (orgasm).

seminal Concerning the semen or seed.

senile lentigines Areas where melanocytes increase in production, producing brown age spots.

senile purpura Dark purplish red ecchymoses occurring on the forearms and backs of the hands in the elderly.

sensitivity reaction An exaggerated response to agents perceived by the body as foreign.

sensorineural hearing loss Impaired perception of sound caused by a dysfunction in the inner ear or the eighth cranial nerve.

sensory loss Impairment of acuity of sight, hearing, taste, touch, and smell.

sentinel infections Infections that may indicate an underlying immunosuppression.

sentinel node biopsy A biopsy of lymph nodes that receive drainage from the anatomic area of a breast cancer to determine spread of the disease.

sepsis Infection, contamination (refers to infection in the blood).

septicemia Invasion of the bloodstream by infective microorganisms.

sequelae An abnormal condition that follows and is the result of a disease.

seroconversion The point at which antibodies to specific antigens are detectable in the blood.

seroma A collection of serum forming a tumor-like mass.

serosanguineous Containing both serum and blood.

serum (sera) The clear, liquid portion of blood that does not contain fibrinogen or blood cells. Immune serum is blood serum from the bodies of people or animals that have produced antibody; inoculation with such serum produces passive immunity.

serum sickness A hypersensitivity reaction to a foreign serum or other antigen.

sexually transmitted infection An infection that is transmitted by sexual intercourse.

shearing action Superficial layers of tissue are pulled and stretched across deeper layers of tissue.

shedding Losing or casting off by a natural process.

Sheehan syndrome A rare but serious postpartum complication that involves infarction of the pituitary gland secondary to postpartum hemorrhage.

shock Acute peripheral circulatory failure due to derangement of circulatory control or loss of circulating fluid.

shunting Physiologically bypassing, as when blood flows past the alveoli but the membrane is thickened and gases cannot cross into or out of the blood.

sickle cell disease All those genetic disorders in which sickle hemoglobin is found in the red cells.

slit lamp An instrument for examining the surface of the eye through a biomicroscopic lens.

smear A specimen for microscopic and cytologic study; the material is spread thinly and evenly across a slide with a swab or loop.

SOAP Acronym for *Subjective* and *Objective* data, *Assessment*, and *Planning*.

solute The substance that is dissolved in a solution.

Somogyi effect A rebound phenomenon due to overtreatment with insulin.

source-oriented record keeping A system of documentation in which information is arranged according to the person, department, or other source of information.

specific gravity The weight of a substance compared with the weight of an equal amount of another substance taken as a standard; for liquids, the standard usually is water (specific gravity of 1).

spermatozoa The mature male sex or germ cells formed within the seminiferous tubules of the testes.

spider angioma A form of telangiectasis with a central elevated red dot the size of a pinhead from which small blood vessels radiate; often occurs with liver disease.

spirochete Any organism that is a member of the order Spirochaetales.

spirometer An instrument for measuring air taken into and expelled from the lungs.

splenomegaly Enlargement of the spleen.

splitting A personality trait that involves initial idealization of a caregiver or friend, followed by a devaluing of that same person.

spores Reproductive cells, usually unicellular, produced by plants and some protozoa.

sprain The wrenching or twisting of a joint with partial or complete tearing of the ligaments.

sputum A substance expelled by coughing or clearing the throat.

Standard Precautions Precautions designed to prevent the transmission of microorganisms from one patient to another as well as to protect the health care worker from unnecessary exposure to infection.

stapedectomy The surgical removal of the stirrup of the middle ear and its replacement with a prosthetic device.

stasis Standing still; stagnation; usually refers to fluid.

status epilepticus A grave condition in which there is a rapid, unrelenting series of convulsive seizures without intervening periods of consciousness and with absence of respiration. Irreversible brain damage may occur if seizures are not controlled.

steatorrhea Stool that is bulky, frothy, and foul smelling and usually floats in the toilet.

stem cells Generalized mother cells, the descendants of which specialize, often in different functions; an example is an undifferentiated mesenchymal cell that is the progenitor of the blood and fixed-tissue cells of the bone marrow.

stenosis The narrowing or contraction of a passageway or opening.

stent A tubular device to give support to the interior of a vessel or tube, preventing its collapse.

stereotaxis A method of precisely locating areas in the brain.

stereotype(s) A simplification used to describe all members of a specific group without exception.

sterilization, microbe The process of rendering an article free of microorganisms and their pathogenic products.

Steri-Strips Small, reinforced, adhesive strips placed over a healing incision to hold it together after sutures are removed.

STI Sexually transmitted infection.

stoma(s) A mouth-like opening, especially one that is created surgically for the elimination of urine or fecal material.

stomatitis A generalized inflammation of the oral mucosa.

strabismus A deviation of the eye that cannot be controlled voluntarily.

strain The pulling or tearing of either muscle or tendon, or both.

stress incontinence The loss of urine during a sneeze of cough.

stridor A harsh, high-pitched respiratory sound such as the inspiratory sound often heard in acute laryngeal obstruction.

stromal cells Connective tissue cells of the supporting tissue or matrix of an organ.

stye An infected swelling near the margin of the eyelid.

subcutaneous Beneath or to be introduced beneath the skin.

subcutaneous emphysema Interstial emphysema characterized by the presence of air in the subcutaneous tissue, usually caused by intrathoracic injury.

subdural hematoma The accumulation of blood in the subdural space.

subjective data Data that the patient provides about a symptom that cannot be seen, felt, or heard by an examiner (e.g., pain).

subluxation A partial or incomplete dislocation of a bone from its place in a joint.

substance use disorder A problem with alcoholism or drug abuse.

subsystem A system within a larger system.

"sucking" chest wound A wound in which the pleural cavity has been penetrated, allowing air and gas to enter the cavity and produce pneumothorax.

suicidal gestures Things done or said that indicate a patient is contemplating committing suicide.

sundowning The phenomenon of becoming confused and disoriented at night, although oriented during the day.

suppression Inhibition, such as interfering with immune response.

suprasystem A highly complex system.

surge capacity The maximum services that a facility can offer when every resource is mobilized.

susceptible Being predisposed or sensitive to the effects of an infectious disease, allergen, or other pathogenic agent; lacking immunity or resistance.

sympathectomy A surgical excision or interruption in some portion of the sympathetic nerve pathways.

syncope Fainting.

syndrome A combination of signs and symptoms associated with a pathologic process or disease.

syndrome of inappropriate antidiuretic hormone (SIADH) Excessive amounts of ADH are produced, resulting in fluid retention.

synovial fluid The transparent viscid fluid found in joint cavities, bursae, and tendon sheaths.

synthesis The process or processes involved in the formation of a complex substance from simpler elements or compounds; opposite of decomposition.

synthesize To put together (data) into a logical whole.

system An organized whole composed of interacting parts.

systemic inflammatory response syndrome (SIRS) A condition in which the body's inflammatory response feedback mechanism fails, causing signs and symptoms (tachycardia, tachypnea, hypotension, oliguria, and fever) without a documented source of infection.

systole The phase of the cardiac cycle in which the ventricles contract and force blood into the aorta and pulmonary arteries; the systolic pressure is recorded as the top number in a blood pressure reading.

systolic blood pressure Arterial pressure during systole.

T

tachycardia An abnormally rapid heart rate, usually over 100 beats per minute.

tachypnea Abnormal rapidity of respiration.

tamponade The stoppage of blood flow to an organ or part of the body by pressure.

tardive dyskinesia A common extrapyramidal side effect seen with antipsychotics; patients may exhibit lip-smacking, tongue protrusion, blinking, sucking, chewing, and lateral jaw movements.

target cells/tissues Cells and tissues that are affected by a specific hormone.

tendons Connective tissue that connects the muscles to the bones.

TENS Transcutaneous Electrical Nerve Stimulation.

tertiary Third in order or stage.

testis The male gonad. One of two reproductive glands located in the scrotum that produce the male reproductive cells and the male hormone, testosterone.

tetany The continuous tonic spasm of a muscle; associated with calcium deficit, vitamin D deficiency, and alkalosis.

tetraplegia Another term for quadriplegia (paralysis of all four extremities).

thalamus Either of two large structures composed of gray matter and situated at the base of the cerebrum that act as a relay station for impulses traveling from the spinal cord and brainstem to the cerebral cortex.

thanatologist One who studies death.

thanatology The medicolegal study of the dying process and death.

theory (theories) A belief, policy, or principle proposed or followed as the basis of action.

therapeutic Having medicinal or healing properties.

therapeutic alliance Relationship between the patient and nurse established for the purpose of helping the patient to build trust and achieve therapeutic goals.

thermal Pertaining to heat.

thoracentesis The surgical puncture and drainage of the thoracic cavity.

thoracotomy The surgical incision of the wall of the chest.

thought disorder A mental disorder characterized by disorganized thought, behavior, and hallucinations. Mood and interpersonal relationships are altered.

thrombectomy The excision of a clot.

thrombocytopenia A decreased number of platelets.

thrombocytopenic purpura A bleeding disorder characterized by a marked decrease in the number of platelets, resulting in multiple bruises, petechiae, and hemorrhage into the tissues.

thrombolytic Dissolving or splitting up a thrombus.

thrombophlebitis An inflammation of a vein related to formation of a blood clot within the vessel.

thrombosis The formation, development, or presence of a blood clot within a blood vessel.

thrombus A blood clot that obstructs a blood vessel or a cavity of the heart.

thymus An endocrine gland that lies in the upper chest beneath the sternum and that, during fetal life, sensitizes certain stem cells that eventually become T lymphocytes.

thyrocalcitonin A hormone secreted by the thyroid gland.

thyroid crisis A sudden increase in the output of thyroxine and resultant extreme elevation of all body processes.

thyroid panel A group of tests performed to evaluate thyroid function.

thyroid storm *See* Thyroid crisis.

thyrotoxicosis A toxic condition due to hyperactivity of the thyroid gland.

thyroxine (T$_4$) A hormone secreted by the thyroid gland.

time-referenced Measured by an educated guess as to how long it will take to attain the outcome.

tinea Ringworm; a name applied to many different kinds of fungal infections of the skin. The specific type usually is designated by a modifying term (e.g., tinea capitis, or ringworm of the scalp).

tinea pedis A fungal infection of the foot; also called *athlete's foot*.

tinnitus A ringing, buzzing, or other continuous noise in the ear.

T lymphocytes White cells destined to provide cellular immunity that have passed through the thymus and migrated to the lymph nodes.

tolerance Increased resistance to a drug or substance that occurs when there is a need for increased amounts of substances to achieve the desired effect. Term used with substance use disorder.

tonic A state of rigid contraction of the muscles.

tonometer An instrument for measuring tension or pressure, especially intraocular pressure.

tophus (tophi) A deposit of sodium biurate in tissues near a joint, in the ear, or in bone, as occurs in gout.

topical Pertaining to the surface of a part of the body, as in topical medications applied to an area of the skin.

torsion The act of twisting or condition of being twisted.

total parenteral nutrition Intravenous feeding to provide all nutritional needs over time.

tourniquet A device for compressing an artery or vein; its use as an emergency measure to relieve hemorrhage is generally recommended only if the victim's life is threatened and other measures fail to stop massive blood loss.

toxin A poisonous substance.

tracheostomy A surgical incision into the trachea to insert a tube through which the patient can breathe.

traction The exertion of a pulling force, as that applied to a fractured bone or dislocated joint, to maintain proper positioning.

tranquilizers A group of agents that provide calm and relief from anxiety.

transcellular Between cells, but within an epithelial membrane.

transcellular fluid Secretions and excretions that move through cell membranes and eventually leave the body.

transduction The first of four phases associated with nociceptive pain. Tissue damage stimulates the nociceptors and initiates pain sensation.

transfer factor A factor occurring in sensitized lymphocytes that recruits additional lymphocytes and transfers to them the ability to confer cell-mediated immunity.

transformation A change to another form.

transfusion The administration of whole blood or blood components directly into the bloodstream.

transmission The second of four phases associated with nociceptive pain. Involves movement of sensation to the spinal cord.

triage The classification of casualties in an emergency room or location of a disaster by the gravity of the injury, urgency of treatment, and place for treatment.

triiodothyronine (T$_3$) A hormone secreted by the thyroid gland.

Trousseau sign Low calcium level manifested as a carpal spasm elicited by inflating a blood pressure cuff above the systolic blood pressure.

tuberculin test An evaluation of sensitivity to the tubercle bacillus; the most common method is intradermal injection of a purified protein derivative of tuberculin (the Mantoux test); a positive reaction indicates the need for further diagnostic procedures.

tuberculosis Any of the infectious diseases caused by species of *Mycobacterium* and characterized by the formation of tubercles and caseous necrosis in the tissues.

tumor marker A blood test to detect biochemical substances synthesized and released into the bloodstream by tumor cells; used mainly to confirm a diagnosis of cancer or response to cancer therapy.

tumor-node-metastasis (TNM) staging system A system for classifying cancers according to the extent to which the malignancy has spread.

turgor The normal tension of a cell; swelling, distention.

tympanoplasty An operative procedure on the eardrum or ossicles of the middle ear to restore or improve hearing in patients with a conductive hearing loss.

U

ultrasonography An imaging technique in which deep anatomic structures are recorded by depicting the echoes of ultrasonic waves that have been directed into the tissues; the echoes (reflections) returning from the structures are converted into electrical impulses that are displayed on a screen, thus presenting a "picture" of the tissues being examined.

unlicensed assistive personnel (UAP) Nursing assistants, technicians, unit secretaries, and aides who do not hold a professional license to perform some aspects of health care delivery and are hired to perform specific repetitive tasks.

urea nitrogen A major protein metabolite that is not recycled by the body but is excreted in the urine; blood urea nitrogen levels indicate the ability of the kidney to filter and excrete waste products.

uremia Retention in the blood of urea, creatinine, and other nitrogenous wastes normally eliminated in the urine; more correctly called *azotemia*.

ureterostomy (ureterostomies) Surgical creation of a stoma to divert urine to the outside.

urinalysis Analysis of a sample of urine, most often done to detect protein, glucose, acetone, blood, pus, and casts.

uroflowmetry Pressure flow studies of the bladder.

urticaria Hives.

V

vaccination The injection of a vaccine into the body to produce immunity to a specific disease.

vaccines Suspensions of attenuated or killed microorganisms administered by injection to provide active immunity to infectious disease.

vagotomy The interruption of impulses carried by the vagus nerve or nerves; may be done to reduce the production of gastric secretions and to inhibit gastric motility, as part of the treatment for peptic ulcer.

Valsalva maneuver An increase of thoracic pressure by forcible exhalation against the closed glottis, as in straining at stool.

value A personal belief about the worth of something that is cherished or held dear.

valvuloplasty A procedure in which a balloon catheter is threaded via the circulatory system through the heart and into the valve. The balloon is inflated to break open a stenosed valve.

varices Twisted and swollen veins.

varicose veins Enlarged and tortuous veins in which the distorted shape is the result of accumulations of pooled blood.

vascular dementia A broad term used to describe any type of dementia caused by vessel disease.

vascular disorders An abnormal functioning of blood vessels, either arterial or venous. Peripheral arterial disorders are most commonly caused by atherosclerosis. Peripheral venous problems are caused by defective valvular function.

vasectomy Excision of the vas (ductus) deferens, or a portion of it; bilateral vasectomy results in sterility.

vasoactive Tending to cause vasodilation or vasoconstriction.

vector(s) A carrier, usually one that transmits disease.

venereal Pertaining to or resulting from sexual intercourse.

ventilation The movement of air from the external environment to the gas exchange units of the lung.

ventilator associated pneumonia (VAP) Pneumonia that occurs 48 to 72 hours after endotracheal intubation.

vertigo A sensation of movement of one's self or of one's surroundings.

vesicant Blistering; causing or forming blisters.

vesicle A small sac containing a serous liquid; a small blister.

vesicostomy The formation of an opening into the urinary bladder.

viable Capable of living.

virulence The degree of ability of an organism to cause disease.

viscera The internal organs contained within a cavity.

viscous Sticky, gummy, gelatinous; thicker than usual.

vitrectomy The removal of the contents of the vitreous chamber, and replacing them with a sterile physiologic saline solution.

volvulus A twisting of the bowel upon itself, causing obstruction.

vulvectomy The excision of the vulva.

W

wart An epidermal growth of viral origin.

Wernicke's encephalopathy Damage to brain cells caused by chronic alcohol abuse.

wheal A localized area of edema on the body surface.

wheeze A form of rhonchus characterized by a high-pitched or low-pitched musical quality caused by airflow through a narrowed airway.

withdrawal Symptoms that are the opposite of the symptoms caused by the ingestion of chemicals or drugs.

word salad A meaningless mixture of words and phrases characteristic of advanced schizophrenia.

X

xanthelasma A planar xanthoma involving the eyelid(s).

xanthoma A lipid deposit in the skin.

xenograft A surgical graft of tissue from an individual of one species to an individual of a different species.

xerostomia The lack of saliva; dry mouth.

Y

yeast A term for fungi that reproduce by budding.

Z

zygomatic Pertaining to the zygomatic bone.

Index

Note: Page numbers followed by *b* indicate boxes, *f* indicate figures and *t* indicate tables.

A

A1c test, 827, 828*t*
AAA; *See* Abdominal aortic aneurysm
Abdomen
  assessment in blood disorders, 339–340
  distention in peritonitis, 673
  nursing care plan for wound of, 117*b*
  quadrants of, 21*f*, 632*f*
  secondary survey of, 1023*b*
  trauma to, 1025–1026
Abdominal aortic aneurysm, 411
Abdominal breathing, 322*b*
Abdominal hernia, 663–664, 664*f*
Abdominal pain
  in appendicitis, 672
  in bowel ischemia, 670
  in chronic pancreatitis, 710
  in diverticulitis, 668
  in gastroenteritis, 649
  in irritable bowel syndrome, 665
  in liver cancer, 708
  peppermint oil for, 665*b*
  in peritonitis, 673
Abdominal thrusts, 281–282, 282*f*
Abdominal tone, 625*b*
Abdominoperineal resection, 675
Abducens nerve, 475*t*
Abduction contracture, 756
Abilify; *See* Aripiprazole
Ablation therapy in hyperthyroidism, 840
Abnormal uterine bleeding, 904–905, 905*b*
Abrasion, corneal, 577*t*
Abscess
  anorectal, 686–687
  brain, 544–545
  pancreatic, 709
Absence seizure, 524
Absorption, 623
Abstinence as contraception, 884*t*
Abuse, 1066*b*
  child, 1041
  domestic, 1041–1042, 1041*b*
  elder, 1042
Acamprosate calcium, 1069, 1069*t*
Acarbose, 862*t*
Acceleration-deceleration injury, 501, 501*f*
Accessory organs of gastrointestinal system, 621–622
Accidental amputation, 758*b*
Accidental poisoning, 1028–1029, 1029*b*
Accolate; *See* Zafirlukast
Accommodation, 488, 594, 595*f*
Accupril; *See* Quinapril
Accutane; *See* Isotretinoin
Acebutolol, 438*t*
Acetaminophen
  for cancer pain, 170*t*
  overdose of, 136*b*, 745*b*
  therapeutic drug monitoring reference intervals for, 1123*t*
Acetazolamide, 602*t*
Acetylcholine, 477*t*, 1103
  myasthenia gravis and, 563
  in Parkinson's disease, 551, 552*f*

Acetylcysteine, 308*t*
Achilles tendon reflex, 480
Achilles tendon rupture, 736
Achlorhydria, 657
Acid, 45*b*
Acid-base imbalances, 47–50, 47*t*, 50*f*
  arterial blood gas analysis for, 47–48
  data collection for, 57*b*
  home care in, 50
  metabolic acidosis in, 48
  metabolic alkalosis in, 49–50
  respiratory acidosis in, 48
  respiratory alkalosis in, 48–49
Acid-base system, 45–46, 45*b*, 46*f*
Acidosis, 41, 45*b*, 50*f*
Acinar cell, 621*f*
Aciphex; *See* Rabeprazole
Acne, 967–969
Acne rosacea, 967
Acne vulgaris, 967
Acoustic nerve, 475*t*
Acoustic neuroma, 614
Acquired hemophilia, 361
Acquired immunity, 104, 104*b*
Acquired immunodeficiency syndrome, 215–231, 942*t*
  blood-borne pathogen exposure and health care workers, 230–231
  community education and care in, 229–230
  confidentiality and disclosure issues in, 230, 230*b*
  data collection in, 225–231, 225*t*, 226*b*
  diagnosis of, 219, 219*b*, 220*b*, 220*t*
  improving food intake in, 229*b*
  major nursing goals for, 228*b*
  management of, 220–221, 222*t*
  neurologic complications in, 225
  nurse with, 230*b*
  nursing diagnoses in, 226, 227*t*
  occupational exposure to human immunodeficiency virus and, 230*b*
  opportunistic infections in, 221–224
    candidiasis in, 224
    coccidiomycosis in, 223–224
    cryptococcosis in, 223–224
    cryptosporidiosis in, 224
    cytomegalovirus in, 222–223
    hepatitis in, 223
    herpes simplex virus in, 221–223
    histoplasmosis in, 223
    Kaposi sarcoma in, 225, 225*f*
    lymphomas in, 225
    Mycobacterium avium complex in, 223
    Pneumocystis jiroveci in, 224
    toxoplasmosis in, 224, 224*b*
    tuberculosis in, 223
    varicella-zoster virus in, 221–222, 222*b*
  pathophysiology of, 216*f*, 217, 217*t*
  patient teaching in, 228*b*
  risk in over-50 population, 229
  signs and symptoms of, 219
  transmission of, 217–218, 217*b*
  wasting syndrome in, 229

Acquired immunodeficiency syndrome (*Continued*)
  WHO classification for staging of, 221*b*
Acromegaly, 834, 834*f*
ACTH; *See* Adrenocorticotropic hormone
Actidil; *See* Triprolidine
Actinic keratoses, 975
Activated partial thromboplastin time, 337*t*, 626*t*
Active immunity, 203
Active transport, 33, 33*f*
Activities of daily living
  chronic illness and, 186–187
Activity
  intolerance in blood disorders, 340
  postoperative, 88
Actos; *See* Pioglitazone
Acupressure
  for back pain, 518*b*
  as method of pain management, 139–140
Acupuncture
  for back pain, 518*b*
  for diabetic neuropathy, 876*b*
  as method of pain management, 139–140
Acute adrenal insufficiency, 848–852
Acute bacterial prostatitis, 932
Acute blood loss, 347*t*
Acute bronchitis, 293–294
Acute cholecystitis, 691*t*
Acute coronary syndrome, 452, 455–461
Acute dystonia, 1106*f*
Acute gastritis, 650
Acute glomerulonephritis, 789
Acute hemolytic reaction, 365*t*
Acute hypoparathyroidism with tetany, 846
Acute liver failure, 701
Acute lymphocytic leukemia, 355
Acute myelogenous leukemia, 355
Acute otitis media, 612
Acute pain, 127, 127*t*, 128*f*
Acute pancreatitis, 708–710, 709*f*
Acute pulmonary edema, 431
Acute radiation syndrome, 1010*t*
Acute renal failure, 794, 798–801, 799*f*
Acute respiratory distress syndrome, 314, 314*b*
Acute tonsillitis, 281
Acute transfusion reactions, 365*t*
Acute tubular necrosis, 799–800
Acute viral rhinitis, 277–279, 278*t*, 279*b*
Addiction, 1066*b*
Addisonian crisis, 848–852
Addison's disease, 244*t*, 847–848, 848*b*, 849*b*
Adefovir dipivoxil, 696*t*
Adenocard; *See* Adenosine
Adenohypophysis, 823
Adenoids, 196
Adenosine, 438*t*
Adenosine stress test, 378*t*
ADH; *See* Antidiuretic hormone
Adhesion, intestinal obstruction and, 623
Adipose tissue, 953*f*

Adjuvant medications for pain management, 126
Admission form review, 19
Adrenal cortex, 819*t*
Adrenal corticosteroids, 821
Adrenal disorders, 847–853
  acute adrenal insufficiency in, 848–852
  Addison's disease in, 847–848, 848*b*, 849*b*
  corticosteroids for, 853*b*
  Cushing syndrome in, 852–853, 852*f*
  pheochromocytoma in, 847
Adrenal gland, 476*t*, 818, 824*f*
Adrenal hormones, 821, 821*f*, 822*f*
Adrenal medulla, 819*t*
Adrenergic action vasoconstrictors, 514*t*
Adrenergic inhibitors, 402*t*
Adrenocortical insufficiency, 847–848, 848*b*
Adrenocorticotropic hormone, 819*t*, 823, 824*b*
  Addisonian crisis and, 848
  Addison's disease and, 847
  Cushing syndrome and, 852–853, 852*f*
  pituitary hypofunction and, 835*t*
Adrenocorticotropic hormone stimulation test, 824*b*
Adult respiratory distress syndrome, 314
Adventitious lung sounds, 264
Advocate, 3
AED; *See* Automated external defibrillator
Aerobid; *See* Flunisolide
Aerolate; *See* Aminophylline
Aerosols, 320
Affect, 1052
Afinitor; *See* Everolimus
Age
  skin disorder prevention and, 955
  surgical risk factors and, 67*t*
Age-related macular degeneration, 608
Age spots, 954, 954*f*
Agent in infection, 100, 102*b*
Agglutination, 941
Aggressive patient, 1113*b*
Aging-related changes
  in cardiovascular system, 375
  of ear, 580
  in endocrine system, 822
  of eye, 570–571, 570*f*, 571*f*
  in female reproductive system, 882
  in gastrointestinal system, 621, 623
  in hematologic system, 334
  in immune and lymphatic systems, 197–198
  in integumentary system, 953–954, 954*f*
  in male reproductive system, 920, 920*b*
  in musculoskeletal system, 718
  in natural defense mechanisms, 106*t*
  in neurologic system, 478
  in respiratory system, 260
  in urinary system, 766
Agitation
  complementary and alternative medicine for, 1094*b*
  in manic patient, 1051
Agranulocyte, 207*t*, 333, 333*f*
Agranulocytosis, 334–335
  clozapine-induced, 1106*b*
AICD; *See* Automatic implantable cardioverter-defibrillator
AIDS; *See* Acquired immunodeficiency syndrome
AIDS dementia, 225
AIDS dementia complex, 1093
Airborne precautions, 106*t*
Airflow after laryngectomy, 284*f*
Airway
  burn injury of, 984
  ineffective clearance of, 271–272

Airway (*Continued*)
  obstruction of, 281–282, 282*f*, 284*f*
    choking emergency in, 1032
    in unconscious person, 1022
  postoperative assessment of, 83*b*
  primary survey and, 1023*b*
  trauma and, 1022–1023, 1024*f*
Akathisia, 1105, 1106*f*, 1107*t*
Akineton; *See* Biperiden
Al-Anon, 1078–1081
Alanine aminotransferase, 626*t*
  in acute viral hepatitis, 696*t*
  in gallstones, 692
Alateen, 1078–1081
Albumin, 331, 626*t*
Albumin dialysis, 703
Albuterol, 308*t*
Alcaine; *See* Proparacaine
Alcohol use, 1068, 1068*b*
  age-related macular degeneration and, 608*b*
  cancer and, 150
  characteristics of alcohol and, 1072*t*
  chronic pancreatitis and, 710
  drugs for acute alcohol withdrawal, 1069*t*
  focused assessment in, 1076*b*
  hypertension and, 385
  immune response and, 203
  moderation in, 395*b*
  oral cancer and, 644
  peptic ulcer and, 650
  religion and, 1068*b*
  as surgical risk factor, 67*t*
  twelve-step program for, 1071, 1071*b*
Alcoholics Anonymous, 1071, 1071*b*
Alcoholism, 1068
Aldactone; *See* Spironolactone
Aldolase, 720*t*
Aldomet; *See* Methyldopa
Aldosterone, 32, 766*t*, 819*t*, 821, 822*f*, 824*b*
Alendronate, 892
Aliskiren, 402*t*
Alkaline phosphatase, 626*t*, 696*t*, 720*t*
Alkalosis, 44–45, 45*b*, 50*f*
Alkylamines, 239*t*
Alkylating agents, 163*t*
ALL; *See* Acute lymphocytic leukemia
Allegra; *See* Fexofenadine
Allergen
  identification of, 237, 237*t*
  non-IgE dependent, 241
Allergic rhinitis, 277, 278*t*
Allergy, 236–239
  blood transfusion-related, 365*t*
  desensitization for, 238–239
  diagnostic tests for, 237–238
  drug, 238, 863*b*
  drug therapy for, 238, 239*t*
  etiology and pathophysiology of, 236–237, 236*f*
  food, 238
  identification of allergens in, 237, 237*t*
  latex, 238
  signs and symptoms of, 237
Allodynia, 254
Allogenic bone marrow transplantation, 364
Allograft for burn injury, 986–987
Allopurinol, 755
Alogia, 1104
ALP; *See* Alkaline phosphatase
Alpha-antitrypsin, 302
Alpha blockers
  for benign prostatic hyperplasia, 927
  for vascular disorders, 402*t*

Alpha globulins, 331
Alpha-glucosidase inhibitors, 862*t*
Alpha-reductase inhibitors, 927
Alprazolam, 1049*t*
ALS; *See* Amyotrophic lateral sclerosis
ALT; *See* Alanine aminotransferase
Alteplase, 531*t*
Alveolar membrane, 258, 258*f*
Alveolus, 259
Alvesco; *See* Ciclesonide
Alvimopan, 675
Alzheimer's disease, 559, 1087–1088
  cultural considerations in, 1093*b*
  diagnosis of, 1088
  etiology and pathophysiology of, 1087
  nursing care plan for, 1090*b*
  nursing diagnosis and planning in, 1089–1092, 1095
  signs and symptoms of, 1087–1088, 1087*b*
  treatment of, 1088, 1089*f*
  warning signs of, 1089*b*
Amantadine, 554*t*, 1074–1075
Amaryl; *See* Glimepiride
Ambulation with assistive devices, 730–731, 730*b*, 731*b*
AMD; *See* Age-related macular degeneration
Amenorrhea, 904
American Sign Language, 590
Amiloride, 696*t*
Amino acids, 335*b*
Aminoglycosides, 786*t*
Aminophylline, 308*t*
Aminosalicylic acid, 671–672
Amiodarone, 438*t*, 1123*t*
Amitiza; *See* Lubiprostone
Amitriptyline, 1056*t*, 1123*t*
AML; *See* Acute myelogenous leukemia
Ammonia tests for gastrointestinal disorders, 626*t*
Amoxicillin, 647*t*
Amoxil; *See* Amoxicillin
Amphetamines, 1072*t*, 1074
Amputation, 758–760, 758*b*, 759*f*, 760*b*, 760*f*
  diabetes-related, 875–876
Amsler grid, 574*t*, 609, 609*f*
Amyotrophic lateral sclerosis, 559
Anabolism, 623
Anafranil; *See* Clomipramine
Analgesics, 134–136, 135*t*
  for cancer pain, 170*t*
  cautions in taking of, 546*b*
  nursing responsibilities in administration of, 137, 137*b*
  side effects and complications of, 137–138
  therapeutic drug monitoring reference intervals for, 1123*t*
Analysis in nursing process, 24–25
Anaphylactic shock, 241–243, 241*b*, 242*f*, 1036–1037
  blood transfusion-related, 365*t*
Anaphylaxis, 236, 241–243, 241*b*, 242*f*
  in insect bites and stings, 1031
  postoperative, 93
Anasarca, 226
Anastomosis
  in colorectal cancer, 675
  in gastric resection, 656
Ancef; *See* Cefazolin
Androgens, 819*t*, 919
Anemia, 346–349
  aplastic, 352, 352*f*
  data collection in, 349–351, 351*b*, 351*f*
  diagnosis of, 337*t*, 348
  etiology of, 346–347, 347*t*
  in leukemia, 355*t*, 359

Anemia (*Continued*)
  pathophysiology of, 347, 347*f*, 348*f*
  signs and symptoms of, 348, 348*t*
  treatment of, 349, 349*t*
  types of, 353*t*
Anesthesia, 75–76, 77*t*
  general, 76
  local, 76
  procedural sedation, 76
  regional, 76
Aneurysm, 411–412
  abdominal aortic, 411
  cerebral, 533–534
  rupture of, 411
Aneurysm repair, 534*f*
Angel dust, 1076
Angina pectoris, 453–455, 455*f*, 456*b*
Angioedema, 241, 1036
Angiogram, 378*t*
Angiotensin converting enzyme, 400
Angiotensin converting enzyme inhibitors
  for chronic renal failure, 804*t*
  for heart failure, 429, 429*t*
  for vascular disorders, 402*t*
Angiotensin I, 374, 374*f*, 400, 400*f*
Angiotensin II, 374, 374*f*, 400, 400*f*
Angiotensin-receptor blockers, 429*t*
Angiotensinogen, 400, 400*f*
Angle-closure glaucoma, 605
Angry patient, 1113*b*
Anhedonia, 1104
Animal bite, 1030
Anion, 40
Anion imbalances, 45
Ankle-brachial index, 384
Ankylosis, 728
Anorectal disorders, 685–687
  abscess and fistula in, 686–687
  hemorrhoids in, 684*f*, 685–686
  pilonidal sinus in, 686
Anorexia, 212
  in cancer, 166–167
  in gastrointestinal system disorders, 633–635
  in hematologic disorders, 343
  in liver cancer, 708
  in pancreatic cancer, 712
Anorexia nervosa, 640, 1060
Anovulation, 905
Antabuse; *See* Disulfiram
Antacids, 647*t*
Anterior chamber, 568, 569*f*
Anterior colporrhaphy, 901*t*, 903–904
Anterior cruciate ligament injury, 735
Anterior fornix, 881*f*
Anterior pituitary, 819*t*
Anterograde amnesia, 1072
Anthrax, 1011–1013, 1011*t*
Anti-rejection medications, 234*t*
Antianxiety medications, 1048, 1071, 1072*t*
Antibacterial agents, 119*t*
Antibiotics, 118, 119*t*, 647*t*
  administration of, 114*t*
  antitumor, 163*t*
  for eye disorders, 602*t*
  for liver disorders, 696*t*
  for pyelonephritis, 788–789
  therapeutic drug monitoring reference intervals for, 1123*t*
  for upper gastrointestinal disorders, 647*t*
Antibody, primary humoral response and, 199–200
Antibody-mediated immunity, 199–200, 200*f*

Anticholinergics
  for chronic obstructive pulmonary disease and asthma, 308*t*
  for eye disorder diagnosis, 602*t*
  for Parkinson's disease, 554*t*
  ulcerative colitis and, 671*b*
Anticholinesterase therapy, 563
Anticipatory guidance for dying cancer patient, 173–174
Anticonvulsants, 524–525, 525*b*
  in pain management, 136
  therapeutic drug monitoring reference intervals for, 1123*t*
Antidepressants, 1056*t*
  in pain management, 136
  triptans and, 545*b*
Antidiarrheals, 37*t*, 636, 666*t*
Antidiuretic hormone, 766*t*, 819*t*
  diabetes insipidus and, 835–836
  in regulation of body fluids, 31
  syndrome of inappropriate secretion of antidiuretic hormone and, 837, 837*f*
Antidysrhythmics, 438*t*
Antiemetics, 37*t*
Antiepileptic drugs, 524–525, 525*b*
Antiflatulants, 666*t*
Antifungals, 118, 119*t*, 602*t*
Antigen-antibody response, 201
Antihelminthic agents, 119*t*
Antihistamines
  for allergic rhinitis and sinusitis, 278*t*
  for allergy, 238, 239*t*
Antihypertensives, 401, 402*t*
  for acute glomerulonephritis, 789
  administration of, 403*b*
  for chronic renal failure, 804*t*
Antiinflammatory drugs, 135*t*
  for allergy, 238, 239*t*
  for chronic obstructive pulmonary disease and asthma, 308*t*
  for dysmenorrhea, 903*t*
  gastrointestinal intolerance and, 748*b*
  for glaucoma, 602*t*
  for gout, 755
  for pain in osteoporosis, 756–757
  peptic ulcer and, 650
  for rheumatoid arthritis, 747–748, 748*t*
Antimetabolites, 163*t*
  for blood disorders, 349*t*
  for liver disorders, 696*t*
Antimicrobial agents, 114*t*, 118, 119*t*
Antimuscarinics, 780*t*
Antineoplastic drugs, 163*t*, 1123*t*
Antinuclear antibodies, 720*t*
Antioxidants, 571*b*
Antiparkinsonian drugs, 554*t*
Antipsychotic drugs, 1095*b*, 1109, 1113
Antiretrovirals, 222*t*, 696*t*
Antisocial personality disorder, 1114*b*
Antispas; *See* Dicyclomine hydrochloride
Antispasmodics, 647*t*, 666*t*
Antithymocyte globulin, 234*t*
Antithyroid antibody titer, 824*b*
Antithyroid drugs, 840, 844*b*
Antitoxin, 200
Antitumor antibiotics, 163*t*
Antitussive agents, 272
Antivirals, 118, 119*t*, 295*b*
  for eye disorders, 602*t*
  for Parkinson's disease, 554*t*
Antrectomy, 656
Anuria, 775*b*, 789
Anus, 620, 621*f*

Anxiety
  behavioral effects of, 1046*f*
  levels of, 1046*t*
Anxiety disorders, 1045–1048, 1046*f*
  complementary and alternative medicine in, 1050*b*
  cultural considerations in, 1049*b*
  diagnosis of, 1047
  elderly patient and, 1049*b*, 1050*b*
  generalized anxiety disorder in, 1046–1047
  history taking in, 1048–1049
  obsessive-compulsive disorder in, 1047
  phobic disorder in, 1047
  post-traumatic stress disorder in, 1047–1048, 1047*b*
  promotion of relaxation in, 1050*b*
  treatment of, 1048, 1048*b*, 1049*t*
Anxiolytics, 1048
  abuse of, 1071
  characteristics of, 1072*t*
Aorta, 374
Aortic dissection, 411
Aortic regurgitation (insufficiency), 445
Aortic stenosis, 445
Aortoiliac bypass, 409
Apathetic thyrotoxicosis, 839
Aphasia, 495–496, 496*b*, 530–532
Aphonia, 262
Apical pulse, 21*f*, 387
Aplastic anemia, 334–335, 352, 352*f*, 353*t*
Apnea, 259, 273, 273*f*
Apneustic breathing, 273, 273*f*, 507*f*
Apo-timol; *See* Timolol
Apocrine sweat gland, 953*f*
Apokyn; *See* Apomorphine
Apolipoprotein E4
  genotyping, 1088
Apomorphine, 554*t*
Appendicitis, 672–673
Appendix, 620
Applanation tonometer, 602*f*
Apraclonidine, 602*t*
Apresoline; *See* Hydralazine
Aprida SoloStar prefilled insulin pen, 864
APTT; *See* Activated partial thromboplastin time
AquaMEPHYTON; *See* Vitamin K
Aqueous humor, 569
Aranesp; *See* Darbepoetin
Arcus senilis, 570, 570*f*
Aricept; *See* Donepezil
Aripiprazole, 1106
Aromatase inhibitors, 912*b*
Aromatherapy, 1097*b*
Arrector pili muscle, 953*f*
Arrhythmia, 435
ART; *See* Assisted reproductive therapy
Artane; *See* Trihexyphenidyl
Arterial blood gas analysis, 47–48
Arterial blood pressure, 374
Arterial disease, 408*t*, 409
Arterial insufficiency, 407–409, 408*t*
Arterial thrombosis, 408
Arterial ulcer, 407–408, 408*f*
Arteries, 373, 373*f*
  autonomic system effects on, 476*t*
  of brain, 529*f*
  of lower extremity, 407*f*
Arteriogram, 378*t*
Arteriosclerosis, 375, 406
  coronary artery disease and, 451
  orthostatic hypotension and, 400*b*
  sensorineural hearing loss and, 581
Arteriovenous access, 805, 806*f*
Arteriovenous fistula, 805, 806*f*

Arteriovenous malformation, 528–530, 530f
Arthritis
    complementary and alternative medicine
        for, 746b
    elderly use of nonsteroidal
        antiinflammatory drugs and, 746b
    evaluation of safety of complementary and
        alternative medicine in, 747b
    Healthy People 2020 goals for, 745b
    osteoarthritis, 745–746, 747t
    psoriatic, 969
    rheumatoid, 244t, 746–750, 747t, 748t
        diet and, 754
        heat and cold applications in,
            754, 754b
        history taking in, 750–753, 753b
        joint replacement for, 749–750, 749f, 750b,
            750f
        nursing care plan for total hip
            replacement in, 751b
        psychosocial care in, 755
        rest and exercise for, 753–754
        surgical intervention and orthopedic
            devices for, 749
Arthrocentesis, 720t
Arthrography, 720t
Arthroplasty, 749
Arthroscopy, 720t
Artificial airway, 282, 282f
Artificial eye, 597–598
Artificial sphincter implant, 780–781
Asbestos exposure, 302
Ascending colostomy, 679, 680f
Ascites, 40–41, 631
    in acute liver failure, 701
    in cirrhosis, 702f
Asmanex; See Mometasone
Aspartate aminotransferase, 626t
    in acute viral hepatitis, 696t
    in gallstones, 692
Aspergillosis, 298
Aspiration pneumonia, 92t
Aspirin
    avoidance in hemophilia, 362b
    for cancer pain, 170t
    for colon polyps, 675b
    peptic ulcer and, 650
    to prevent myocardial infarction, 453b
    for prevention of stroke recurrence, 530, 531t
    Reye syndrome and, 279b
Assessment in nursing process, 17–24
Assignment, 3–4, 4b
Assist-mode ventilation, 325
Assisted reproductive therapy,
    890, 890b
Assistive-adaptive devices, 186t, 187f
Assistive devices for ambulation, 730–731,
    730b, 731b
AST; See Aspartate aminotransferase
Astelin; See Azelastine
Asterixis, 707
Asthma, 305–310
    pathophysiology of, 305f
    patient teaching in, 307b, 310
    peak flowmeter for, 307b
    psychosocial care in, 310
    rehabilitation in, 307–310
    signs and symptoms of, 305–306
    treatment of, 306–307, 306t, 308t
Astigmatism, 594–595
Asymptomatic inflammatory prostatitis, 933
Atarax; See Hydroxyzine
Ataxia
    after stroke, 530–532
    phenytoin-related, 547

Ataxic breathing, 507f
Atelectasis, 84, 92t, 303
Atenolol, 402t, 438t
Atherosclerosis, 374, 406
    coronary artery disease and, 451
    progression of, 452f
Athlete's foot, 972, 973
Ativan; See Lorazepam
Atopic dermatitis, 967
Atopy, 237
Atorvastatin, 454t
Atrial fibrillation, 437–438, 437f
Atrial flutter, 437–438, 437f
Atrial natriuretic peptide, 32
Atrioventricular node, 372
Atromid; See Clofibrate
Atrophic gastritis, 649–650
Atropine, 438t
Atrovent; See Ipratropium
Attitude of nurse, 15
Atypical antidepressants, 1056t
Atypical antipsychotics, 1106
Audiometry, 584t
Auditory brainstem response, 584t
Auditory hallucination, 1103
Auditory meatus, 579
Auditory ossicle, 579, 580f
Augmentation mammoplasty, 912
Aura in seizure, 524
Aural speculum, 582–583
Auscultation
    of bowel sounds, 631–632, 632f
    of heart sounds, 386, 386f
    use in data collection, 20–21, 21f
Autoantibody, 197t
Autograft for burn injury, 986–987, 988f
Autoimmune diseases, 198–199, 243
    diagnosis of, 234–235, 234b,
        243–245
    gastrointestinal effects of, 623
    signs and symptoms of, 243, 244t
    systemic lupus erythematosus in, 245–248,
        246f, 247t, 248b
    treatment and nursing management
        of, 245
Autoimmune hemolytic anemia, 244t
Autoimmune hepatitis, 244t
Autoimmune thyroiditis, 845
Autoimmunity, 202
Autoinoculation of virus, 970
Autologous blood transfusion, 64, 362
Autologous bone marrow transplantation,
    364
Automated external defibrillator, 1033
Automatic implantable cardioverter-
    defibrillator, 442
Automatisms, 524
Autonomic dysreflexia, 514–515
Autonomic nervous system, 476t, 490
Avandia; See Rosiglitazone
Avelox; See Moxifloxacin
Avian flu, 294b
Avoidant personality disorder, 1114b
Avolition, 1104
Axid; See Nizatidine
Axon, 1102–1103, 1103f
Azatadine, 239t
Azathioprine, 808
Azelaic acid, 968
Azelastine, 239t
Azelastine nasal, 278t
Azilect; See Rasagiline
Azmacort; See Triamcinolone
Azotemia, 802, 927
Azulfidine; See Sulfasalazine

B
B lymphocyte, 199
Babinski's reflex, 480, 485f
Bacillary dysentery, 1004t
Bacille Calmette-Guérin, 204–205
Bacillus anthracis, 1011t
Back pain, 517–520, 517f
    in osteoporosis, 756–757
Back stretching exercises, 729b
Baclofen, 514t
Bacteremia, 113t
Bacteria, 101–102
Bacterial infection
    in acquired immunodeficiency syndrome,
        223
    cutaneous, 970
    in meningitis, 541–543, 542f, 1004t
    in pharyngitis, 281
    sexually-transmitted, 940b
    in tonsillitis, 281
    upper respiratory, 279
Bacterial vaginosis, 907t, 939
Bacteriologic tests, 116
Bactrim; See Trimethoprim-sulfamethoxazole
Baird Body Image Assessment Tool, 190
Balance, 479
    dizziness and vertigo and, 589
    Romberg test for, 585
Balanced suspension, 740, 740f
Balloon tracheostomy tube, 286
Bandaging of stump, 759, 759f, 760b
Banzel; See Rufinamide
Baraclude; See Entecavir
Barber's itch, 972
Barbiturates
    abuse of, 1071
    characteristics of, 1072t
    for increased intracranial pressure, 508
Bariatric surgery, 641–642, 642f
Barium enema, 626t
Barotrauma, mechanical ventilation-related,
    327t
Barrel chest, 262–263, 264f
Barrett's esophagus, 645
Basal body temperature as contraception, 884t
Basal cell carcinoma, 967, 975, 975f
Basal cell layer of skin, 953f
Basal insulin, 863–864
Basal metabolism, 476t
Base, 45b
Basiliximab, 234t
Basophil, 197t, 207t
Bathing
    giving medicated bath, 962
    observation while, 960b
Battle's sign, 501–502, 502f
Beclomethasone, 278t, 308t
Beclovent; See Beclomethasone
Bee sting, 1031
Beginning-of-shift assessment, 21b
Behavior
    in Alzheimer's disease, 1087b
    difficult, 9
    grief and mourning response and,
        513, 513t
    substance abuse and, 1066f
Behavioral Pain Scale, 129–130, 130f
Behavioral therapy, 1048
    for substance abuse, 1069–1071
Bell's palsy, 548
Below-the-knee amputation, 759f
Benadryl; See Diphenhydramine
Benazepril, 402t
Bence Jones protein test, 337t
Benign disorders of breast, 908–909

Benign neoplasm, 145
Benign pituitary adenoma, 834
Benign prostatic hyperplasia, 927–931, 927f
Bentyl; See Dicyclomine hydrochloride
Benzodiazepines, 1048, 1048b, 1049t
    abuse of, 1071
    for acute alcohol withdrawal, 1069, 1069t
Benztropine, 554t
Beta-adrenergic blockers, 402t
    for dysrhythmias, 438t
    for glaucoma, 602t
    for heart failure, 429, 429t
Beta globulins, 331
Betapace; See Isotalol
Bethanechol, 780t
Bi-leaflet mechanical valve, 446f
Biaxin; See Clarithromycin
Bicarbonate, 48
    in acid-base balance, 47
    normal ranges and functions of, 41t
Bicarbonate-carbonic acid buffer system, 46, 46f
Biceps reflex, 480
Biguanides, 862t
Bile acid sequestrants, 454t
Bilevel positive airway pressure, 326
Biliary cirrhosis, 701
Biliary colic, 691, 696
Bilirubin, 696t
Billings method of contraception, 884t
Billroth I and II procedures, 656, 656f
Binder method of pain management, 139
Biobrane, 986–987
Biofeedback
    as method of pain management, 139
    for pelvic floor strengthening, 903b
    in seizure disorders, 525
    in tinnitus, 589
Bioidentical hormones, 891
Biologic agents in bioterrorism, 1011–1015
Biologic disaster, 1010–1015, 1013f, 1014f
Biologic dressings for burn injury, 986–987
Biologic response modifiers, 165, 349t, 358
Biologic therapy for rheumatoid arthritis, 748t
Biomarkers in Alzheimer's disease, 1088
Biomedicine, 10
Biopsy
    in cancer detection, 153–154
    liver, 626t
    lung, 268
    lymph node, 207t
    in musculoskeletal disorders, 720t
    renal, 768b, 768f, 769t
    for sexually transmitted infections, 941
    skin, 957
Biosynthetic skin, 986–987
Bioterrorism, 1010–1015, 1013f, 1014f
    category A agents in, 1011t
    debriefing in, 1016
    nursing management in, 1016, 1016f
Biot's respiration, 273, 273f
BiPAP; See Bilevel positive airway pressure
Biperiden, 554t
Bipolar disorder, 1049t, 1051–1052, 1051t, 1052b
Bisacodyl, 666t
Bismuth salts, 37t, 38
Bismuth subsalicylate, 666t
Bisoprolol, 402t
Bisphosphonates
    for osteoporosis, 756b, 757b
    for prostate cancer, 935t
Bites and stings, 1030–1032
Bivalved cast, 742
Biventricular pacemaker, 430
Bivona Fome-Cuf tracheostomy tube, 285f

Black widow spider, 1031
Blackhead, 967–968
Blackout, alcohol use and, 1068
Bladder, 764, 919f
    autonomic system effects on, 476t
    cancer of, 152t, 795–798, 796f
    cystitis and, 785–788
    functions of, 765–766
    pain in, 774–775
    patient teaching in health of, 767b
    trauma to, 794–795
Bladder scan, 769t
Bladder training, 493–494, 782b
Blakemore-Sengstaken tube, 707, 707f
Blastomycosis, 298
Bleeding
    abnormal uterine, 904–905, 905b
    after cerebral aneurysm repair, 534
    after kidney surgery, 791
    breakthrough, 904
    cancer treatment-related, 169b
    in disseminated intravascular coagulation, 362
    gastrointestinal
        mechanical ventilation-related, 327t
        in peptic ulcer, 651, 653b
    in hematologic disorders, 343, 343b, 343f
    intracerebral, 541
    low platelet count and, 360b
    postoperative, 92t, 93
    pressure points for, 343f
    primary survey and, 1023b
    rectal
        in colorectal cancer, 675
        in diverticulitis, 668
        in inflammatory bowel disease, 671
    techniques to control, 343b
    trauma-related, 1023–1024
Bleeding time, 337t
Blepharitis, 577t
Blindness, 571
    diabetes-related, 874–875
Bloating in irritable bowel syndrome, 665
Blood
    autonomic system effects on, 476t
    components of, 331, 335
    effects of aging on, 334
    functions of, 331
    maturation of cells in, 195, 196f
    oozing of, 342b
    production of, 332, 333f
    red blood cells in, 332
    in urine, 773
    viscosity of, 374
    white blood cells in, 332–333
Blood agents in chemical disaster, 1007t
Blood-borne pathogen exposure, 230–231
Blood disorders, 346–367
    anemia in, 346–349
        aplastic, 352, 352f
        data collection in, 349–351, 351b, 351f
        diagnosis of, 348
        etiology of, 346–347, 347t
        nutrition considerations in, 348b
        pathophysiology of, 347, 347f, 348f
        signs and symptoms of, 348, 348t
        treatment of, 349, 349t
        types of, 353t
    bone marrow and stem cell transplantation in, 364–366
    causes of, 334–335, 334b, 335b
    common problems related to, 343–344
        anorexia in, 343
        bone marrow failure in, 344
        excessive bleeding in, 343, 343b, 343f

Blood disorders (Continued)
        fatigue in, 343
        infection in, 343–344
        pain in, 343
    community care in, 367
    data collection for, 336–340, 339b
    diagnostic tests and procedures in, 336, 337t
    disseminated intravascular coagulation in, 362
    hemophilia in, 361–362, 361f
    home care in, 342b
    leukemia in, 355–359
        etiology of, 355, 355t
        nursing care plan for, 357b
        signs and symptoms of, 355–356
        treatment of, 356–357, 356b
    multiple myeloma in, 360–361
    nursing diagnoses in, 340–341, 341t
    physical assessment in, 339–340
    polycythemia vera in, 354–355
    prevention of, 335–336, 336b
    sickle cell disease in, 353–354, 353f, 354f
    therapies for, 362–367
        biologic response modifiers in, 358
        iron therapy in, 366–367
        leukapheresis in, 364
        oxygen therapy in, 366
        splenectomy in, 367
        transfusions in, 362–364
        vitamin B_{12} therapy in, 367
    thrombocytopenia in, 359–360, 359f
Blood drawing from central line, 56
Blood flow, 372f
Blood glucose, 23
    hemoglobin A_{1c} level and, 829t
    insulin and, 824f
Blood glucose monitor, 867, 867f
Blood loss, 347t, 1035t
Blood pressure, 374, 374f
    classification of, 399t
    hypertension and, 398–404
        in acute glomerulonephritis, 789
        antihypertensive therapy for, 401, 402t, 403b
        blood pressure classification and, 399t
        in cardiovascular disorders, 375
        complementary and alternative medicine for, 405b
        complications of, 401, 406b
        cultural considerations in, 400b
        decreasing dietary sodium and, 405b
        end-stage kidney disease and, 766–767
        etiology of, 398–400
        heart failure and, 426–427
        hypertensive crisis and, 401–404
        monitoring of, 406b
        pathophysiology of, 400, 400f
        retinopathy and, 608
        risk factors for, 399t
        signs and symptoms of, 400–401
    measurement of, 387
    sodium and, 448
Blood products, 363t, 364b
    checking during emergency situation, 1035b
    HIV exposure and, 218
Blood tests, 207t, 1120t
Blood transfusion, 362–364
    autologous, 64
    blood products used in, 363t
    consent for, 362b
    HIV exposure and, 218
    Jehovah's Witness patient and, 64b
    reaction to, 364, 364b, 365t

Blood urea nitrogen, 767, 767b, 769t
Blood vessels, 373–374, 373f
  autonomic system effects on, 476t
  kidney health and, 767b
Blood volume, 374
Bloodless surgery, 64
Blunt chest trauma, 446–447
Blunt trauma, 1025–1026
BMI; See Body mass index
BNP; See Brain natriuretic peptide
Body defenses, 103–108, 104b, 106t
Body fluids, 31–33, 31f, 31t, 32b
Body louse, 974
Body mass index, 641
Body piercings, HIV exposure and, 218
Boil, 970
Bolus dose in insulin therapy, 863–864
Bone(s), 716, 717f
  fracture of, 736–742
    braces and splints for, 739–740, 739f
    casts for, 739, 739f, 744–745
    complications of, 741–742, 742f
    etiology and pathophysiology of, 736–737
    external fixation for, 738–739, 739f
    initial assessment in, 742–743
    internal fixation for, 738, 738f
    nasal, 282–283
    osteoporotic, 756b
    physical assessment of neurovascular status in, 743b
    proton pump inhibitors and, 737b
    reduction, surgery, and stabilization in, 738
    signs and symptoms of, 737
    traction for, 740, 740f, 744b
    types of, 737b, 737f
  functions of, 717
  nutrition for growth and density of, 719b, 756b
  Paget disease of, 757
  sickle cell disease and, 354f
  terms related to bone markings, 718t
  of thorax, 259
Bone marrow, 195, 196f, 197t
  as body defense, 105
  cancer treatment-related suppression of, 168–169
  effects of aging on, 334
  failure in hematologic disorders, 344
Bone marrow aspiration and biopsy, 337t
Bone marrow donation, 366, 366b
Bone marrow transplantation, 165
  in blood disorders, 364–366
  for sickle cell disease, 354
Bone scan, 720t
Bone tumor, 757–758
Bony pelvis, 881
Borderline personality disorder, 1114b
Bortezomib, 657–658
Botulism, 1011t, 1013, 1029
Bowel incontinence, 637
Bowel ischemia, 670
Bowel prep, 631b
Bowel sounds, 21f, 631–632, 632f
Bowel training program, 494–495
Bowman's capsule, 764, 765f
BPH; See Benign prostatic hyperplasia
Brace for fracture, 739–740, 739f
Brachial artery pressure point, 343f
Brachial pulse, 387f
Brachioradialis reflex, 480
Brachytherapy, 159
  for breast cancer, 912f
  for prostate cancer, 935t

Braden scale, 979f
Bradycardia, 435
Bradykinesia, 552, 552f
Bradypnea, 262, 273f
Brain, 472, 473f, 473t, 474f
  abscess of, 544–545
  contusion of, 501
  exercise for, 1087b
  major arteries of, 529f
  sickle cell disease and, 354f
  tumor of, 171t, 539–541, 540f, 540t, 541f
Brain attack, 528–534
  after carotid endarterectomy, 413b
  cerebral aneurysm and arteriovenous malformation in, 528–530, 530f
  complications of, 534, 535f
  diagnosis of, 532, 532f
  dysphagia in, 539b
  etiology of, 528
  nursing care plan for, 536b
  pathophysiology of, 528–530, 529f
  prevention of, 530
  rehabilitation in, 538–539
  risk factors for, 528b
  signs and symptoms of, 530–532, 530b, 531f
  surgery for obstruction in, 533–534, 534f
  treatment of, 531t, 532–534
Brain disorders, 523–548
  bacterial meningitis in, 541–543, 542f
  Bell's palsy in, 548
  brain abscess in, 544–545
  brain tumor in, 539–541, 540f, 540t, 541f
  encephalitis in, 544
  headache in, 545–546, 546b
  seizure disorders and epilepsy in, 523–526, 525b
  stroke in, 528–534
    cerebral aneurysm and arteriovenous malformation in, 528–530, 530f
    complications of, 534, 535f
    diagnosis of, 532, 532f
    dysphagia in, 539b
    etiology of, 528
    nursing care plan for, 536b
    pathophysiology of, 528–530, 529f
    prevention of, 530
    rehabilitation in, 538–539
    risk factors for, 528b
    signs and symptoms of, 530–532, 530b, 531f
    surgery for obstruction in, 533–534, 534f
    treatment of, 531t, 532–534
  transient ischemic attack in, 527–528
  trigeminal neuralgia in, 546–547, 547f
  viral meningitis in, 543
Brain natriuretic peptide, 378t
Brain scan, 481t
Brainstem, 472, 473f, 473t
BRCA1 and BRCA2 genes, 910
Breakthrough bleeding, 904
Breast, 882, 883
  fibroadenoma of, 908
  fibrocystic changes of, 908
  intraductal papilloma of, 908–909
  magnetic resonance imaging of, 895t
  ultrasonography of, 895t
Breast biopsy, 895t
Breast cancer, 909–915
  breast reconstructive surgery for, 912, 913f
  early detection of, 153b
  etiology and pathophysiology of, 909–910
  legal and ethical considerations in, 910b
  metastasis of, 171t
  nursing care plan for breast lumpectomy and, 911b

Breast cancer (Continued)
  postmastectomy exercises and, 914f
  prevention of, 910
  risk factors for, 152t, 909b
  signs and symptoms of, 910
  stages of, 909t
  treatment of, 910–912, 912f
Breast reconstructive surgery, 912, 913f
Breast self-examination, 892–893, 893f
Breathing, primary survey and, 1023b
Breathing exercises, 322–323, 322b
Breathing patterns
  in coma, 507f
  ineffective, 272–273, 272f, 273f
  in neurologic disorders, 492
Breathlessness, 272
Bretylium, 438t
Bretylol; See Bretylium
Brevibloc; See Esmolol
Bricker's conduit, 796f, 797
Briggs adapter, 323t
Brimonidine, 602t
Broad spectrum antibacterials, 118
Bromocriptine mesylate, 554t, 862t
Brompheniramine, 239t, 278t
Bronchial breath sounds, 264t
Bronchiectasis, 301–302
Bronchiole, 258, 258f
Bronchitis
  acute, 293–294
  chronic, 303, 304t
Bronchodilators, 317
  administration of, 321b
  for asthma, 307, 308t
  therapeutic drug monitoring reference intervals for, 1123t
Bronchoscopy, 265t
Bronchovesicular breath sounds, 264t
Bronchus, 258, 258f
Brown recluse spider, 1031
Brown rice, 856b
Brudzinski's sign, 542, 542f
Bruising
  cancer treatment-related, 169b
  in thrombocytopenia, 359f
Bruit, 387, 806
  carotid, 413
BSE; See Breast self-examination
Bucca swab, 136
Buccal mucosa, 136
Buck's extension traction, 740, 740f
Budesonide, 278t, 308t
Buerger's disease, 413
Buffer pairs, 46
Bulbourethral gland, 919
Bulimia nervosa, 640, 1060
Bulk-forming laxative, 666t
Bullous pemphigoid, 244t
Bumetanide, 402t
Bumex; See Bumetanide
BUN; See Blood urea nitrogen
Bundles concept of Institute for Healthcare Improvement, 16
Bunion, 736
Buprenorphine, 1069t, 1073
Bupropion, 1056t, 1069t, 1123t
Burkitt's lymphoma, 149
Burn, 981–989, 1031–1032
  chemical, 1032
  classification of, 982f, 983f, 984t
  complications of, 988
  debridement for, 986
  electrical, 981, 1031–1032, 1032f
  emergency treatment of, 983–984, 984b

Burn (Continued)
  escharotomy for, 986, 987f
  etiology and pathophysiology of, 981–982
  fluid resuscitation and prevention of shock in, 985, 985b
  grafting for, 986–988, 988f
  infection prevention in, 985–986, 992
  itching in, 993
  nursing care plan for, 990b
  nutritional support in, 993
  pain management in, 985, 989–992, 992b
  patient-family education in, 993
  psychosocial support in, 993
  rehabilitation for, 988–989, 989f
  respiratory support in, 984–985
  signs and symptoms of, 982
  topical medications for, 987t
  wound treatment in, 986–988
Bursa, 716
Bursitis, 736
BuSpar; See Buspirone
Buspirone, 1048, 1049t
Butterfly rash, 246f
Byetta; See Exenatide

C
C-A-B cardiopulmonary resuscitation guidelines, 1032–1033
C-peptide, 828t
C-reactive protein, 207t, 378t
CABG; See Coronary artery bypass graft
CAD; See Coronary artery disease
Caffeine
  hypertension and, 405
  therapeutic drug monitoring reference intervals for, 1123t
CAGE questionnaire, 1076–1077
Calan; See Verapamil
Calcaneus, Achilles tendon rupture and, 736
Calcitonin, 819t, 824b
Calcitriol, 766t, 804t
Calcium
  blood measurement of, 720t
  imbalances of, 42t, 44–45, 45f
  intake for immobilized patient, 743b
  normal ranges and functions of, 41t
  supplementation of
    for bone growth and density, 719b
    for chronic renal failure, 804t
    for colon polyps, 675b
    for osteoporosis, 756
Calcium channel blockers
  for dysrhythmias, 438t
  for heart failure, 429t
  for vascular disorders, 402t
Calcium oxalate stones, 792t
Calcium phosphate stones, 792t
Calculi
  bladder training program and, 494
  renal, 791–794, 792f, 792t
Calendar method of contraception, 884t
Calf, fascial compartments of, 742f
Caloric test, 480–485, 584t, 613–614
CAM; See Complementary and alternative medicine
Camphorated opium tincture, 37t
Campral; See Acamprosate calcium
Camptosar; See Irinotecan
Cancer, 144–174; See also specific cancer
  biologic response modifiers for, 165
  bone marrow and stem cell transplantation for, 165
  causes of, 147–149, 147t
    chemical carcinogens in, 148
    chronic irritation in, 148

Cancer (Continued)
    genetic predisposition in, 149
    promotors in, 148
    radiation in, 148–149
    radon gas in, 149
    viruses in, 149
  chemotherapy for, 161–164, 163t, 164f, 164t
  classification of, 146
  complementary and integrative medicine in, 166
  contributing factors in, 149–150
  data collection in, 155
  detection of, 151–155, 151b, 153b
    biopsy in, 153–154
    endoscopy in, 154
    laboratory tests in, 154–155, 155b
    radiologic studies in, 154
  dying patient and, 172–174, 172b, 173t
    anticipatory guidance and, 173–174
    end-stage symptom management and, 174
    palliative care for, 172–174
    terminal hydration and, 174
  evaluating effectiveness of medical treatment for, 166
  gene therapy for, 165
  hormone therapy for, 164–165
  impact of, 144–145, 145f
  metastasis of, 146–147, 147f
  nursing care plan for, 156b
  nursing diagnoses in, 155, 155b
  oncologic emergencies and, 171–172
  physiology of, 145–146, 146f
  prevention of, 150–151, 151b
  radiation therapy for, 159–161
    external, 159–160, 159f, 160b
    internal, 160–161, 161b, 162f
    radiation dosimeter badge and, 162f
    side effects of, 162t
  risk factors for, 152t
  surgery for, 158–159
  treatment problems in, 166–172
    alopecia in, 169
    anorexia, mucositis, and weight loss in, 166–167
    bleeding and bruising with low platelet count in, 169b
    constipation in, 167
    cystitis in, 167–168
    fatigue in, 169
    fear and ineffective coping and, 171
    hyperuricemia in, 169
    immunosuppression, bone marrow suppression, and infection in, 168–169
    metastatic disease and, 170–171, 171t
    nausea, vomiting, and diarrhea in, 167
    pain in, 169–170, 170t
    patient education in, 168b
Candidiasis, 972
  in acquired immunodeficiency syndrome, 224
  sexually transmitted, 939
Canker sore, 643b
Cannabis, 1072t, 1075–1076
Capastat; See Capreomycin
CAPD; See Continuous ambulatory peritoneal dialysis
Capecitabine, 675
Capillary, 373
Capillary refill test, 388
Capitation, 4–5
Capnography, 76
Capoten; See Captopril

Capreomycin, 300t
Captopril, 402t
Caput medusa, 701
Carafate; See Sucralfate
Carbamazepine
  for seizures, 525b
  therapeutic drug monitoring reference intervals for, 1123t
Carbenicillin, 786t
Carbex; See Selegiline
Carbinoxamine, 239t
Carbohydrate counting, 865b, 865t
Carbon dioxide, 259, 260
Carbon monoxide poisoning, 1030
Carbonic acid, 47
Carbonic anhydrase inhibitors, 602t
Carbuncle, 970
Carcinogen, 147, 147t
  avoiding and limiting exposure to, 151b
  chemical, 148
  physical, 148–149
Carcinoma, 146
Cardene; See Nicarpidine
Cardiac catheterization, 378t, 459
Cardiac cirrhosis, 701
Cardiac conduction disorders; See Dysrhythmias
Cardiac conduction system, 372, 373f, 435f
Cardiac cycle, 373
Cardiac disorders; See Heart disease
Cardiac monitoring, 384
Cardiac output, 373
  mechanical ventilation-related impairment of, 327t
Cardiac pacemaker, 440–441, 441b, 441f
Cardiac resynchronization therapy, 430
Cardiac sphincter, 620
Cardiac surgery, 464–469
  community care in, 469
  coronary artery bypass graft in, 465–466, 465f
  heart transplantation in, 466
  nursing care plan for, 467b
  open heart surgery in, 464–465
  percutaneous transluminal coronary angioplasty in, 464, 464f
  postoperative care in, 469
  preoperative care in, 466–468
  transmyocardial laser revascularization in, 464
Cardiac tamponade
  in cancer, 171
  in multiple trauma, 1026
  in penetrating chest trauma, 446–447
  in pericarditis, 443
Cardiac trauma, 446–447
Cardiac treadmill stress test, 377f, 378t
Cardiac valve, 371
Cardiac valve disorders, 444–446, 446f
Cardinal positions of eye movement, 487f
Cardiogenic shock, 461–464, 461t, 1035–1036, 1035f
Cardiomyopathy, 385, 444, 444b
Cardiopulmonary resuscitation, 1032–1033, 1034t
Cardiovascular disease, 375–384
  causes of, 375–376
  common problems in, 393–395
    altered tissue perfusion in, 394–395
    edema in, 393–394
    fatigue and dyspnea in, 385b, 393
    impaired tissue integrity in, 395
    pain in, 394
  diabetes mellitus and, 875

Cardiovascular disease (*Continued*)
  diagnostic tests and procedures in, 377–384, 377f, 378t, 384f
  history taking in, 384–385, 385b
  metabolic syndrome and, 377b
  nursing diagnoses in, 388–392, 389t
  physical assessment in, 385–388, 386b, 386f, 386t
    blood pressure and, 387
    bruits and, 387
    pulses in, 387, 387b, 387f
    skin and, 388
  prevention of, 376–377
  risk factors for, 377t
  as surgical risk factor, 67t
  warning signs of heart attack, 376b
  women and, 375, 375b
Cardiovascular system, 371–395
  blood pressure and, 374, 374f
  blood vessels of, 373–374, 373f
  changes with aging, 375
  chronic renal failure and, 803f
  cirrhosis and, 703f
  heart in, 371–372, 372f
    cardiac cycle and, 373
    conduction system of, 372, 373f
    ejection fraction and, 373
    physical examination of, 386b
    severe anemia and, 348t
Cardioversion, 440
Cardizem; *See* Diltiazem
Cardura; *See* Doxazosin
Caregiver stress, 193b, 1098
Carnitine, 409b, 699
Carotid artery pressure point, 343f
Carotid bruit, 413
Carotid duplex Doppler studies, 378t, 481t
Carotid endarterectomy, 413b
Carotid pulse, 387f
Carpal bones, 717f
Carpal tunnel syndrome, 736
Carpentier-Edwards aortic pericardial valve, 446f
Carpopedal spasm, 44
Cartilage, 716
Carvedilol, 402t, 438t
Cascara sagrada, 666t
Cast, 739, 739f, 742, 744–745
Castor oil, 666t
Cat bite, 1030
Catabolism, 623
Catapres; *See* Clonidine
Cataract, 572, 598–600, 598f, 599b
Catatonic schizophrenia, 1105t
Catechol *O*-methyltransferase inhibitors, 554t
Catheter
  central venous
    care of, 56–57, 56f
    flushing of, 55–56, 55b
    placement in subclavian vein, 56f
  Foley, 794t, 985
  intraventricular, 507
  peripheral nerve, 136
  peripherally inserted central, 56, 56f, 660
  sleeved, 294
  suprapubic, 794t
  Swan-Ganz, 378t
  Tenckhoff, 806–807, 807f
  transtracheal, 323t
  urinary, 776–777, 776b, 776f, 794t
Catheter embolus in intravenous therapy, 54t
Cation, 40
CAVH; *See* Continuous arteriovenous hemofiltration

CAVHD; *See* Continuous arteriovenous hemodialysis
CBC; *See* Complete blood count
Cefazolin, 786t
Cefepime, 786t
Cefixime, 786t
Ceftazidime, 786t
Celexa; *See* Citalopram
Celiac disease, 244t, 673–674
Cell-mediated immunity, 201
Cellulitis, 388, 408f, 970
Central acting agents, 402t
Central hearing loss, 589
Central nervous system, 472, 473f; *See also* Neurologic system
  in control of respiration, 259
  peripheral nervous system interaction with, 474–475, 475f
Central nervous system depressants abuse, 1071–1073, 1072b, 1072t
Central nervous system stimulants abuse, 1072t, 1074–1075, 1074f
Central neurogenic hyperventilation, 507f
Central venous catheter
  care of, 56–57, 56f
  flushing of, 55–56, 55b
  placement in subclavian vein, 56f
Cephalosporins, 786t
Cephulac; *See* Lactulose
Cerebellar tumor, 541
Cerebellum, 473f, 473t
Cerebral aneurysm, 528–530, 530f, 533–534
Cerebral angiography, 481t
Cerebral perfusion pressure, 507
Cerebrospinal fluid, 475, 477f
Cerebrospinal fluid analysis and culture, 481t, 1126t
Cerebrovascular accident, 528–534
  after carotid endarterectomy, 413b
  cerebral aneurysm and arteriovenous malformation in, 528–530, 530f
  complications of, 534, 535f
  diagnosis of, 532, 532f
  dysphagia in, 539b
  etiology of, 528
  nursing care plan for, 536b
  pathophysiology of, 528–530, 529f
  prevention of, 530
  rehabilitation in, 538–539
  risk factors for, 528b
  signs and symptoms of, 530–532, 530b, 531f
  surgery for obstruction in, 533–534, 534f
  treatment of, 531t, 532–534
Cerebrum, 473f, 473t, 474f
Cerebyx; *See* Fosphenytoin
Certolizumab pegol, 672
Cerumen, 579, 580
  impacted, 612
Ceruminous gland, 952
Cervical cancer, 907
  early detection of, 153b
  risk factors for, 152t
Cervical cap contraception, 884t
Cervical traction, 740
Cervical vertebrae, 510f, 717f
Cervix, 881f
  inflammation of, 906
Cetirizine, 239t, 278t
Cetuximab, 675
Chain of infection, 108, 108b, 108f
Chalazion, 577t
Chambers of heart, 371
Chantix; *See* Varenicline
Charge nurse, 3–4, 4b

Chart review, 22
Charting, 16, 16b, 26
Chemical barriers to infection, 103–104
Chemical burn, 597, 981–982, 1032
Chemical carcinogen, 148
Chemical disaster, 1006–1009, 1007t, 1008b
Chemical predictor test of contraception, 884t
Chemical stress test, 378t
Chemoreceptor, 259
Chemotactic factors, 197t
Chemotherapeutic agents, 136, 163t
Chemotherapy, 161–164, 163t, 164f
  for bone tumor, 758
  for brain tumor, 540, 540f
  for breast cancer, 911–912
  for colorectal cancer, 675
  elderly and, 935b
  for gastric cancer, 657–658
  for Hodgkin's lymphoma, 250
  for leukemia, 356, 356b
  for liver cancer, 708
  for multiple myeloma, 360
  for prostate cancer, 935t
  for skin cancer, 976
  toxic effects of, 164t
Chest
  injuries of, 312–313, 446–447, 1024–1025
  secondary survey of, 1023b
Chest compressions, airway, breathing guidelines, 1032–1033
Chest pain, 453–455, 455f, 456b
  in cardiovascular disease, 385–386, 386t
  in myocardial infarction, 458
Chest physiotherapy, 321
Chest radiography, 265t, 378t
Chest tube, 316–317, 316f
Chewing gum postoperatively, 682b
Cheyne-Stokes respiration, 273, 273f, 507f
Chickenpox, 222b, 971, 1013–1014, 1014f
Child abuse, 1041
Chlamydia spp., 103
Chlamydia trachomatis, 942t
  in epididymitis, 932
  nursing care plan for, 949b
  in pelvic inflammatory disease, 939
Chlor-Trimeton; *See* Chlorpheniramine
Chlordiazepoxide, 1049t, 1069t
Chloride
  imbalances of, 45
  normal ranges and functions of, 41t
Chlorine agents in chemical disaster, 1007t
Chlorpheniramine, 239t, 278t
Choking, 282f, 1032
Choking agents, 1007t
Cholangiocarcinoma, 708
Cholecystectomy, 692
Cholecystitis, 691, 691t
Choledocholithiasis, 690, 691f
Cholelithiasis, 690–694, 691f, 691t
  ethnic predisposition to, 690b
  patient teaching in, 692b
  postcholecystectomy diet and, 692b
  postoperative care in, 693–694, 693b, 693f
Cholera, 1004t
Cholescintigraphy, 692
Cholesterol
  lowering in diet, 453b
  vertical auto profile of, 378t
Cholesterol absorption inhibitor, 454t
Cholestyramine, 454t
Cholinergic agents, 602t
Cholinergic crisis, 564b
Cholinesterase inhibitors, 602t
Chondroitin, 746b
Chondroma, 757

Chorea, 562
Choroid, 568, 569f
Christmas disease, 361
Chronic airflow limitation, 302
Chronic bacterial prostatitis, 933
Chronic bronchitis, 303, 304t
Chronic cholecystitis, 691t
Chronic gastritis, 650
Chronic glomerulonephritis, 789–790
Chronic illness, 177–193
  documentation in long-term care and, 187
  fall prevention in, 183–184, 183b, 184b
  family caregiver and, 192–193, 193b
  home care in, 191–193, 191f
  maintaining function in, 187
  management of confusion and
      disorientation in, 185–186, 186f
  medication assessment in, 184b
  nursing care plan for immobilized patient,
      180b
  prevention of immobility in, 178–179, 178b,
      179t
  promotion of independence in, 186–187,
      186t, 187f
  rehabilitation care in, 179–189, 191f
    data collection in, 189–190, 189b, 190b
    nursing diagnoses in, 190, 191b
    rehabilitation programs and, 187–188
    rehabilitation team and, 188–189, 189f
  safe environment and, 183, 183b
  security devices and, 184–185, 184b, 185b
Chronic irritation, cancer and, 148
Chronic lymphocytic leukemia, 355
Chronic myelogenous leukemia, 355
Chronic obstructive pulmonary disease,
    262–263, 287t, 290–292
  chronic bronchitis in, 303
  complementary and alternative medicine
      for, 304b
  complications of, 304–305
  drug therapy for, 308t
  emphysema in, 303, 303f
  nutritional suggestions for, 304b
  patient teaching in, 307b
  smoking cessation and, 307–310
Chronic pain, 126f, 127, 128, 495
Chronic pancreatitis, 710
Chronic renal failure, 801–808
  diabetes mellitus and, 802b
  diagnosis of, 802–803
  dietary restrictions in, 810t
  drug therapy for, 804t
  hemodialysis for, 805–806, 805f, 806f, 811b
  kidney transplantation for, 808, 808b, 808f
  nursing care plan for, 812b
  nursing management of, 808–811,
      810f, 810t
  pathophysiology of, 802
  peritoneal dialysis for, 806–808, 807f
  renal stenosis and, 791
  signs and symptoms of, 802, 803f
Chronic venous insufficiency, 388, 420–421,
    421f
Chvostek's sign, 44, 45f, 845–846
Chyme, 621
Ciclesonide, 278t, 308t
Cigarette smoking; See Smoking
Cilia, 257
Ciliary body, 568, 569f
CIM; See Complementary and integrative
    medicine
Cimetidine, 647t
Cimzia; See Certolizumab pegol
Cinnamon, 304b
Ciprofloxacin, 786t, 788–789

Circulating nurse, 75, 75b, 76b
Circulation
  postoperative, 83b, 85, 85f
  primary survey and, 1023b
Circulatory overload
  blood transfusion-related, 365t
  intravenous therapy-related, 54t
Cirrhosis, 701–703, 702f, 703f, 704b, 707f, 1068
Citalopram, 1056t
Citracel; See Methylcellulose
CK; See Creatine kinase
Clarinex; See Desloratadine
Clarithromycin
  for peptic ulcer, 652
  for upper gastrointestinal disorders, 647t
Claritin; See Loratadine
Classic hemophilia, 361
Clavicle, 717f
Cleansing
  of burn injury, 986
  of pressure ulcer, 981
Clemastine, 239t, 278t
Climacteric, 882
Clinical chemistry reference intervals, 1120t
Clinical judgment, 14–16
Clinical standards, 2, 17–27
Clistin; See Carbinoxamine
Clitoris, 881, 881f
CLL; See Chronic lymphocytic leukemia
Clofibrate, 454t
Clomipramine, 1056t
Clonazepam, 525b
Clonidine, 402t
Clonus, 480
Closed drainage system, 316–317, 316f
Closed dressing, 963
Closed fracture, 737b
Closed reduction, 738
Clostridium botulinum, 1011t, 1013
Clostridium perfringens, 1029
Clozapine, 1106b
Clozaril; See Clozapine
Clubbing of fingers, 263f
Cluster breathing, 507f
Cluster headache, 546
CMG; See Cystometrography
CML; See Chronic myelogenous leukemia
CMV; See Cytomegalovirus
Co-dependency, 1067–1068
Co-insurance, 4
Coagulation tests, 337t, 1119t
Coarctation, 375
Coarse crackles, 263–264
Cobalamin, 335b
Cocaine, 528b, 1074, 1074f
  characteristics of, 1072t
  heart disease and, 376–377
Coccidiomycosis, 223–224, 298
Coccyx, 510f, 717f
Cochlea, 580, 580f
Cochlear implant, 590–591, 591f
Cochlear nerve, 580f
Codeine, 170t
Cogentin; See Benztropine
Cognex; See Tacrine
Cognition, 1085, 1094
Cognitive-behavioral therapy, 1048, 1106–1108
Cognitive disorders, 1085–1099
  AIDS dementia complex in, 1093
  Alzheimer's disease in, 1087–1088
    diagnosis of, 1088
    etiology and pathophysiology of, 1087
    nursing care plan for, 1090b
    nursing diagnosis and planning in,
        1089–1092, 1095

Cognitive disorders (Continued)
    signs and symptoms of, 1087–1088, 1087b
    treatment of, 1088, 1089t
    warning signs of, 1089b
  antipsychotic drugs for, 1095b
  community care in, 1099
  data collection in, 1093–1094, 1094b
  delirium in, 1085–1086
  dementia in, 1086–1087, 1086b
  family assessment in, 1098, 1099b
  guidelines for reality orientation in, 1096b
  substance-induced delirium in, 1086
  use of restraints in, 1096, 1096b, 1097b
  vascular dementia in, 1093
Coin rubbing, 958b
Colace; See Docusate sodium
Colchicine, 755
Cold light inspection, 957
Cold sore, 970b
Cold therapy
  for pain management, 138
  patient teaching in, 754b
  to relieve pain in appendicitis, 673b
  in rheumatoid arthritis, 754, 754b
Colectomy, 675
Colesevelam, 454t
Colestid; See Colestipol
Colestipol, 454t
Collaborative care, 2–3
Collaborative care plan, 27
Colon, 620
  conjugated linoleic acid and, 674b
  normal flora of, 101t
Colon conduit, 796f
Colonoscopy, 626t
Colony-stimulating factor, 364
Color
  of exudate, 981t
  of hair, 953
  of urine, 774t
Color pain scale, 129
Color vision test, 574t
Colorectal cancer, 674–679
  cultural considerations in, 674b
  diagnosis of, 675
  early detection of, 153b
  etiology of, 674
  foods contributing to, 623b
  metastasis of, 171t
  nursing care plan for, 676b
  pathophysiology of, 674–675
  risk factors for, 152t
  signs and symptoms of, 675
  treatment of, 675
Colostomy, 679–680, 679f, 685f
  in colorectal cancer, 675
  irrigation of, 683
Colporrhaphy, 901t, 903–904
Colposcopy, 895t
Coma, myxedema, 845
Combative patient, 1040–1041, 1041b
Combination insulin preparations, 863t
Combivent; See Ipratropium and albuterol
Comedos, 967
Comfort care, 172
Command hallucination, 1108
Comminuted fracture, 737b, 737f
Commissurotomy, 446
Common cold, 277–279, 278t, 279b
Communicable diseases with epidemic
    potential, 1004t
Communication, 2
  after laryngectomy, 289, 289f
  critical thinking and, 16, 16b
  with hearing-impaired person, 575, 587b

Communication (*Continued*)
  in history taking in sexually transmitted
    infections, 941*b*
  staff, 26–27
  standards of practice and, 1134–1135
Community care
  in acquired immunodeficiency syndrome,
    229–230
  in blood disorders, 367
  in cognitive disorders, 1099
  in diabetes mellitus, 877
  in ear disorders, 591, 617
  in endocrine disorders, 831, 853
  in eye disorders, 579, 611–612
  in female reproductive system
    disorders, 915
  in fluid imbalances, 59
  in gastrointestinal disorders, 687
  in heart disease, 448, 469
  infection prevention and control and,
    120–121
  in integumentary disorders, 994
  in lower respiratory system disorders, 327
  in male reproductive disorders, 935–936
  in musculoskeletal disorders, 760–761
  in neurologic disorders, 565
  pain management and, 140–141
  postoperative, 97
  in psychological disorders, 1062
  in sexually transmitted infections, 950
  in substance abuse, 1081–1082
  in upper respiratory system disorders,
    289–290
  in urinary system disorders, 811–812
Community preparedness in disaster,
  999–1000
Compartment syndrome, 741–742
Compassion, 9
Compazine; *See* Prochlorperazine maleate
Compensatory hypertrophy, 790
Competence, 8
Complement assay, 207*t*
Complement system of proteins, 197*t*,
  198, 202
Complementary and alternative
    medicine, 10
  for acquired immunodeficiency syndrome,
    221*b*
  acupuncture for neuropathy in, 876*b*
  for acute respiratory distress syndrome,
    314*b*
  for age-related macular degeneration, 608*b*
  for anxiety, 1050*b*
  aromatherapy in, 1097*b*
  for burn injury, 992*b*, 993*b*
  for calming agitated patient, 1094*b*
  L-carnitine in, 409*b*
  for cold sores, 970*b*
  for colon polyps, 675*b*
  for depression, 1055*b*
  for dysmenorrhea, 902
  for emphysema, 304*b*
  for erectile dysfunction, 925*t*
  evaluation of safety of, 747*b*
  for fibrocystic breast changes, 908*b*
  for healthy bladder, 795*b*
  for heart failure and coronary artery
    disease, 431*b*
  for hepatitis, 699*b*, 701*b*
  herbals and supplements in, 65*b*
  for hypercholesterolemia, 453*b*
  for hypertension, 405*b*
  for infectious diarrhea, 636*b*
  for infertility, 889*b*
  for influenza, 295*b*

Complementary and alternative
    medicine (*Continued*)
  massage in, 1097*b*
  for menopause, 891–892, 891*b*
  music therapy in, 1110*b*
  for nail fungus, 972*b*
  for nausea, 635*b*
  omega-3 fatty acids and, 1103*b*
  for osteoarthritis, 746*b*
  for pain, 140*b*, 1073*b*
    abdominal, 665*b*
    back, 518*b*
    headache, 546*b*
  for pancreatic health, 710*b*
  for Parkinson's disease, 553*b*
  for pelvic floor strength, 903*b*
  pet therapy in, 1088*b*
  for pneumonia, 297*b*
  postoperative chewing of gum and,
    682*b*
  for preventing nausea, 35*b*
  for promoting good liver function, 699*b*
  to reduce urine odor, 798*b*
  sedative effects of herbs and, 1087*b*
  for shingles, 972*b*
  for sore muscles, 735*b*
  for stomatitis, 643*b*
  for stopping hiccoughs, 88*b*
  tai chi in, 719*b*
  transvaginal electrical stimulation in, 780*b*
  for tuberculosis, 299*b*
  for ultraviolet radiation protection, 955*b*
  for upper respiratory infection, 279*b*
  using mirrors to stimulate responses, 1098*b*
  for varicose veins, 419*b*
  for vitamin C for cystitis, 788*b*
  vitamin E and nonalcoholic steatohepatitis
    and, 701*b*
Complementary and integrative medicine in
  cancer, 166
Complete blood count, 207*t*, 337*t*
Complete fracture, 737*b*
Complete heart block, 437*f*, 438
Compliance, 259
Compound fracture, 737*b*, 737*f*
Compulsive act, 1047
Computed tomography
  in cancer, 154
  in cardiovascular disease, 378*t*
  in gallstones, 692
  in gastrointestinal disorders, 626*t*
  in musculoskeletal disorders, 720*t*
  in neurologic disorders, 481*t*
  in respiratory disorders, 265*t*
  in urologic disorders, 769*t*
Computer-assisted cognitive rehabilitation,
  1074–1075
Comtan; *See* Entacapone
Concussion, 500
Condom, 884*t*, 888*f*
Conduction system of heart, 372, 373*f*
Conductive hearing loss, 581, 581*b*
Conduits, 796*f*
Condyle, 718*t*
Condylomata acuminata, 942*t*
Cones, 569
Confabulation, 1071, 1086–1087
Confidentiality, acquired immunodeficiency
  syndrome and, 230, 230*b*
Confrontation test, 574*t*
Confusion
  in cystitis, 786*b*
  in encephalitis, 544
  management in chronic illness, 185–186, 186*f*
  in neurologic disorders, 495

Congenital cataracts, 598
Conical excision, 901*t*
Conization, 901*t*
Conjugated linoleic acid, 674*b*
Conjunctiva, 569, 569*f*
Conjunctivitis, 577*t*
Conscious sedation, 76, 77*t*
Consensual reflex of pupil, 488
Consent
  for surgery, 68–70, 68*b*
  for transfusion, 362*b*
Consolidation therapy, 356
Constipation
  cancer treatment-related, 167
  in colon diverticula, 668
  in colorectal cancer, 675
  in gastrointestinal system disorders, 636
  in irritable bowel syndrome, 665
  narcotic-induced, 137*b*
Contact dermatitis, 966–967
Contact dissolution therapy for gallstones,
  692–693
Contact isolation requirements, 967*b*
Contact laxatives, 666*t*
Contact precautions, 106*t*
Contactant allergens, 237*t*
Continuous ambulatory peritoneal dialysis,
  807
Continuous arteriovenous hemodialysis,
  800–801
Continuous arteriovenous hemofiltration,
  800–801
Continuous bladder irrigation, 928–929, 930*f*
Continuous cycling peritoneal dialysis,
  807
Continuous hemofiltration, 800–801
Continuous passive motion of joint, 729, 729*f*
Continuous positive airway pressure, 326
Continuous renal replacement therapies,
  800–801
Continuous venovenous hemofiltration,
  800–801
Contraception
  female, 883–890, 888*f*
  male, 920–921
  methods of, 884*t*
  sexually transmitted infections and, 939*b*
Contracture, 727–728, 728*f*
  abduction, 756
  after burn injury, 988
Contralateral, term, 502
Contrast dye, 459*b*
Controlled-mode ventilation, 325
Contusion
  brain, 501
  myocardial, 446–447
Conventional antipsychotics, 1105
Coordination, 479
  in multiple sclerosis, 558
Copayment, 4
COPD; *See* Chronic obstructive pulmonary
  disease
Coping
  in cancer, 171
  in infection, 118–120
  in irritable bowel syndrome, 665
  in neurologic disorders, 497
  spiritual beliefs and, 1049*b*
Copperhead snake, 1030
Cor pulmonale, 304–305
Coral snake, 1030
Cordarone; *See* Amiodarone
Coreg; *See* Carvedilol
Corgard; *See* Nadolol
Corium, 952

Cornea, 568, 569f
Corneal abrasion, 577t
Corneal staining, 574t
Corneal transplantation, 596–597, 596f
Corneal ulcer, 577t, 596
Coronary angiography, 378t
Coronary arteries, 372, 372f
Coronary artery bypass graft, 465–466, 465f
Coronary artery disease, 451–464
    complementary and alternative medicine for, 431b
    diagnosis of, 452
    etiology of, 451
    heart failure in, 426–427
    hypertension and, 401
    menopause and, 891
    nutrition considerations in, 453b
    pathophysiology of, 452, 452f
    signs and symptoms of, 452, 452b
    treatment of, 452–453, 454t
Coronary artery stent, 464f
Coronary insufficiency, 452
Coronary occlusion, 458f
Coronary ultrasound, 378t
Correction dose in insulin therapy, 863–864
Corticosteroids
    for adrenal disorders, 853b
    for chronic obstructive pulmonary disease, 317
    for Crohn's disease, 671–672
    for glaucoma, 602t
    for head and spinal cord injury, 514t
    for rheumatoid arthritis, 747–748, 748t
Cortisol, 766t, 819t, 821, 822f, 824b
Cortisone, 852
Corvert; See Ibutilide
Cosmetic surgery, 63t
Cost containment, 6, 7b
Cottonmouth snake, 1030
Cough etiquette, 110–111, 112f
Coughing
    in acute respiratory distress syndrome, 314
    after transsphenoidal hypophysectomy, 835b
    ineffective airway clearance and, 271
    preoperative instructions in, 71–72, 71b, 71f
Coumadin; See Warfarin
Coup-contrecoup injury, 501, 501f
Cowper's gland, 919
CPAP; See Continuous positive airway pressure
CPK; See Creatine phosphokinase
CPR; See Cardiopulmonary resuscitation
Crab lice, 974
Crack cocaine, 1074, 1074f
Crackles, 263–264
Cranberry juice, 533b
Cranial nerve disorders, 546–547
    Bell's palsy in, 548
    trigeminal neuralgia in, 546–547, 547f
Cranial nerves, 472, 475t, 479, 480t
Craniotomy, 541
Creatine kinase, 720t
Creatine kinase-MB, 378t, 459t
Creatine phosphokinase, 378t, 459t, 720t
Creatinine, 765
Creatinine clearance, 767, 769t, 802–803
Cremasteric reflex, 926
Crepitation, 283, 718
Crestor; See Rosuvastatin
Critical incident stress debriefing, 1016

Critical thinking, 14–27
    attitude and, 15
    clinical judgment and, 14–16
    communication skills and, 16, 16b
    Institute for Healthcare Improvement bundles and, 16
    interdisciplinary care plan and, 27
    Joint Commission National Patient Safety Goals and, 16–17, 17b
    Joint Commission National Quality Core Measures and, 17, 17b
    nursing process and, 16–17
        analysis and nursing diagnosis in, 24–25
        assessment in, 17–24
        care plan for imbalanced nutrition and, 18b
        evaluation in, 27
        implementation in, 26–27
        integration of, 16, 17–27
        phases of, 15b
        planning in, 26
Crohn's disease, 244t, 670–672, 670t, 671f
Cromolyn sodium, 278t, 308t
CRRTs; See Continuous renal replacement therapies
CRT; See Cardiac resynchronization therapy
Crutches, 730, 730b, 731b
Crutchfield tongs, 512f
Cryoprecipitate, 363t
Cryosurgery
    in intracapsular cataract extraction, 598–600
    in prostate cancer, 935t
Cryotherapy
    for esophageal cancer, 645
    for hemorrhoids, 686
    for liver cancer, 708
Cryothermia, 77t
Cryptococcosis, 223–224, 298
Cryptosporidiosis, 224
Cuffed tracheostomy tube, 286
Cullen's sign, 1025–1026
Cultural assessment, 7b, 65b
Cultural considerations
    in acquired immunodeficiency syndrome, 218b
    in alcohol use, 1068b
    in Alzheimer's disease, 1093b
    in anxiety disorders, 1049b
    in bone marrow donations, 366b
    in cancer, 149b
    in coin rubbing, 958b
    in colorectal cancer, 674b
    in contraception choices, 939b
    in coronary artery disease, 451b
    in cultural preferences, 10b
    in diabetes mellitus, 857b
    in diet variations, 405b
    in drug metabolism, 72b
    in dyspnea, 385b
    ethnic considerations for pneumococcal vaccine, 296b
    in ethnic predisposition to gallstones, 690b
    in eye contact, 1110b
    in eye disease, 572b
    in female reproductive system disorders, 894b
    in fertility, 889b
    financial burden and, 66b
    in gallstone risk, 624b
    in gastric cancer, 657b
    in genetic hematologic tendencies, 334b
    in hepatitis B, 694b
    hot and cold foods and, 118b

Cultural considerations (Continued)
    in hypertension, 400b
    in Jehovah's Witness and blood transfusions, 64b
    in lactose intolerance, 674b
    in language barriers in psychiatric patient, 1109b
    in liver-related deaths, 701b
    media effects on sexually transmitted infections and, 939b
    in ostomy care, 683b
    in pain perception and treatment, 131b
    in pancreatic cancer, 710b
    in penile cancer, 933b
    in performing wound care, 94b
    in post-traumatic stress disorder, 1047b
    in retinal detachment, 605b
    in smoking, 1075b
    in stroke, 528b
    in thyroid cancer, 845b
    in tuberculosis, 298b
    in type 2 diabetes mellitus, 857b
    uninsured trauma patient and, 1026b
    in women's health, 894b
Cultural needs of patient, 9–10, 10b
Cultural preferences, 10b
Culture and sensitivity, 207t
    cerebrospinal fluid, 481t
    for sexually transmitted infections, 941
    in skin disorders, 957
    synovial fluid, 720t
    in tuberculosis, 299
Curative surgery, 63t
Curling's ulcer, 982, 988
Cushing syndrome, 852–853, 852f
Cutaneous anthrax, 1011t
Cutaneous disorders; See Skin disorders
Cutaneous ureterostomy and vesicotomy, 796–797, 796f
CVA; See Cerebrovascular accident
Cyanide, 1007t
Cyanosis, 262
Cyberknife procedure, 540
Cyclocryotherapy, 604
Cycloplegics, 602t
Cycloserine, 300t
Cycloset; See Bromocriptine mesylate
Cyclosporine
    for kidney transplantation, 808
    therapeutic drug monitoring reference intervals for, 1123t
Cymbalta; See Duloxetine
Cyst, pilonidal, 686
Cystatin C, 767
Cystic fibrosis, 301–302
Cystine stones, 792t
Cystitis, 785–788, 786b
    cancer treatment-related, 167–168
    vitamin C for, 788b
Cystocele, 903
Cystogram, 769t
Cystometrography, 769t
Cystoscopy, 769t, 922t
Cytokines, 197t, 199–200
Cytology, 151
Cytomegalovirus, 222–223
Cytotec; See Misoprostol
Cytotoxic T cell, 197t

D

d-Dimer test, 265t, 337t
Daclizumab, 234t
Daily focused assessment, 22
Dakin's solution, 987t
Darbepoetin, 804t

Daricon; *See* Oxyphencyclamine hydrochloride
Data collection, 17–24
 auscultation in, 20–21, 21*f*
 chart review in, 22
 diagnostic tests in, 23–24
 inspection and observation in, 20
 interview and, 19–20, 19*b*, 20*b*
 olfaction in, 20
 palpation in, 20
 percussion in, 22
 physical assessment and, 20
 practical daily focused assessment in, 22
 preoperative, 64–67, 65*b*
 prioritizing in, 22–23
Dawn phenomenon, 874
Death
 psychological process of, 172
 spiritual beliefs and practices regarding, 173*t*
Death rattle, 174
Debridement
 of burn injury, 986
 of pressure ulcer, 980–981
Debriefing in bioterrorism, 1016
Decerebrate posturing, 487, 487*f*
Decongestants
 for allergic rhinitis and sinusitis, 278*t*, 279
 for allergy, 239*t*
Decontamination
 chemical agents and, 1007*t*
 in nuclear disaster, 1009
 removal and disposal of contaminated clothing, 1009*b*
Decorticate posturing, 487, 487*f*
Deductible, 4
Deep brain stimulation, 554, 1057
Deep breathing, 71–72, 71*b*, 71*f*
Deep full-thickness burn, 984*t*
Deep partial-thickness burn, 984*t*
Deep vein thrombosis, 414, 415–416, 415*f*
 after joint replacement, 750
 nursing care plan for, 417*b*
 in pancreatic cancer, 712*b*
 in spinal cord injury, 515
Defense mechanisms, 1067*t*
Defibrillation, 1023*b*
Deficient fluid volume, 34–38, 34*b*, 34*f*, 36*b*, 37*t*
Degenerative neurologic disorders, 551–565
 Alzheimer's disease in, 559
 amyotrophic lateral sclerosis in, 559
 community care in, 565
 Guillain-Barré syndrome in, 560–561
 Huntington's disease in, 562
 multiple sclerosis in, 557*t*, 558*f*
 myasthenia gravis in, 562–563, 563*f*, 564*b*
 Parkinson's disease in, 551–554
  complications of, 554
  diagnosis of, 552, 552*f*
  etiology of, 551
  nursing care plan for, 555*b*
  pathophysiology of, 551, 552*f*
  patient teaching in, 557*b*
  signs and symptoms of, 552, 552*f*
  surgery for, 554
  treatment of, 553–554, 553*b*, 554*t*
 poliomyelitis and postpolio syndrome in, 562
Dehiscence, 91–93, 92*t*, 93*f*
Dehydration, 34–35, 34*b*, 67*t*
Delayed hypersensitivity, 201
Delayed menstruation contraception, 884*t*
Delegation, 3–4, 4*b*

Delirium, 1085–1086
 end of life care in, 174
 in neurologic disorders, 495
 quick assessment guide for, 1094*b*
 substance-induced, 1086
Delusion, 1085–1086, 1102
Demadex; *See* Torsemide
Dementia, 1086–1087, 1086*b*
 AIDS dementia complex, 1093
 in Alzheimer's disease, 559, 1087–1088
  diagnosis of, 1088
  etiology and pathophysiology of, 1087
  nursing care plan for, 1090*b*
  nursing diagnosis and planning in, 1089–1092, 1095
  signs and symptoms of, 1087–1088, 1087*b*
  treatment of, 1088, 1089*t*
  warning signs of, 1089*b*
 quick assessment guide for, 1094*b*
 using mirrors to stimulate responses in, 1098*b*
 vascular, 1093
Demerol; *See* Meperidine
Demyelination
 in Guillain-Barré syndrome, 560
 in multiple sclerosis, 557, 558*f*
Dendrite, 1102–1103, 1103*f*
Dengue fever, 1004*t*
Denial, 1066–1067, 1067*t*
Denosumab, 890–891
Deoxyribonucleic acid, 145
Depakene; *See* Valproic acid
Depakote; *See* Divalproex
Dependency, 1065–1066, 1066*b*
Dependent edema, 39, 428, 428*f*
Dependent personality disorder, 1114*b*
Depo-Provera, 884*t*
Depressants abuse, 1071–1073, 1072*b*, 1072*t*
Depression, 1055–1057
 after heart surgery, 469
 antidepressants for, 1056*t*
 in bipolar disorder, 1051
 complementary and alternative medicine for, 1055*b*
 suicidal patient and, 1057*b*
Dermabrasion, 968
Dermatitis, 966–967
Dermatome, 221–222, 472, 474*f*
Dermatophytoses, 972
Dermis, 952–953, 953*f*
Descending colostomy, 680, 680*f*
Desensitization therapy, 238–239
Desipramine, 1123*t*
Desloratadine, 239*t*, 278*t*
Desmopressin
 for diabetes insipidus, 837
 for von Willebrand disease, 361
Desvenlafaxine, 1056*t*
Desyrel; *See* Trazodone
Detoxification, 1069
Detrol; *See* Tolterodine
Deviated septum, 279
DEXA; *See* Dual energy x-ray absorptiometry
Dexamethasone, 507
Dexamethasone suppression test, 824*b*
Dexchlorpheniramine, 239*t*
Dexlansoprazole, 647*t*
Dextrose in saline, 52*t*
Dextrose in water, 52*t*
Di-Gel; *See* Simethicone
DiaBeta; *See* Glyburide
Diabetes insipidus, 508–509, 835–837, 836*f*

Diabetes mellitus, 244*t*, 856–877
 chronic pancreatitis and, 710
 chronic renal failure and, 802*b*
 community care in, 877
 cultural considerations in, 857*b*
 diagnostic tests for, 828*t*, 829*t*
 in elderly
  exercise and, 861*b*
  patient teaching and, 873*b*
  weight loss and, 860*b*
 etiology and pathophysiology of, 858
 hypoglycemia in
  hyperglycemia *versus*, 873*b*
  ketoacidosis *versus*, 871*t*
 insulin therapy in, 863–865
  exercise and, 862*b*
  guidelines for subcutaneous injection in, 864*b*
  insulin pump in, 865, 865*f*
  prefilled injection pens for, 864*b*
  preoperative and postoperative management of, 866, 866*b*
  rotation of injection sites in, 864*f*
  types of insulin for, 863*t*
 long-term problems in, 874–876
  cardiovascular disease in, 875
  diabetic neuropathy in, 876, 876*b*
  metabolic syndrome in, 875
  nephropathy in, 875
  peripheral vascular disease in, 875–876
  retinopathy in, 876
 management of, 859–866
  carbohydrate counting in, 865*b*, 865*t*
  data collection in, 867, 867*b*
  diet in, 860
  exercise in, 860–861
  injectable hypoglycemic agents in, 866, 866*b*, 866*t*
  islet cell transplantation in, 866
  oral hypoglycemic agents in, 862–863, 862*t*
  preoperative and postoperative, 866, 866*b*
 nursing care plan for, 868*b*
 nursing diagnoses in, 867–868
 nutrition considerations in
  brown rice and whole grains and, 856*b*
  diet soda and, 875*b*
 patient teaching in, 861*f*, 867*f*, 871–873, 872*f*
  elderly patient and, 873*b*
  foot care and, 875*b*
  home treatment of hypoglycemia and, 861*b*
  sick days and, 872*b*
  travel instructions and, 872*b*
 preoperative and postoperative, 866
 retinopathy in, 608
 short-term problems in, 873–874
  diabetic ketoacidosis in, 873
  hyperglycemic hyperosmolar nonketotic syndrome in, 874
  hypoglycemia in, 874
  rebound hyperglycemia in, 874
 signs, symptoms, and diagnosis of, 858–859
 surgical risk factors in, 67*t*
 types of, 856–858, 857*b*, 857*t*, 858*b*
 venous stasis ulcer in, 421
Diabetic ketoacidosis, 871*t*, 873
Diabetic nephropathy, 802*b*, 860, 875
Diabetic neuropathy, 876, 876*b*
Diabetic retinopathy, 608, 876
Diagnosis-related groups, 5
Diagnostic surgery, 63*t*

Diagnostic tests
for allergies and hypersensitivities, 237–238
for cancer, 153–154, 153b
for cardiovascular disease, 377–384, 377f, 378t, 384f
data collection and, 23–24
for diabetes mellitus, 828t, 829t
for ear disorders, 582–585, 584t
for endocrine disorders, 825–828, 825t, 827f
for eye disorders, 573, 573f, 574t
for female reproductive disorders, 894, 895t
for gastrointestinal system disorders, 625–631, 626t
for hematologic disorders, 336, 337t
for human immunodeficiency virus, 219, 220b, 220t
for immune and lymphatic disorders, 206–209, 207t
for immune disorders, 234–235, 234b
for infection, 116
for integumentary disorders, 957–958
for male reproductive disorders, 921–922, 922t
for musculoskeletal disorders, 719–723, 720t, 723f
for neurologic disorders, 481t, 489, 489f
preoperative, 66, 66b
for respiratory disorders, 264–268, 265t, 268f, 269f
for sexually transmitted infections, 941
for urinary system disorders, 767–768, 768f, 769t
Dialose; See Docusate potassium
Dialysis
albumin, 703
hemodialysis, 800, 805–806, 805f, 806f, 811b
dietary restrictions in, 810t
noncompliance in, 811b
peritoneal, 800, 806–808, 807f, 810t
Diamox; See Acetazolamide
Diaphragm, 259
Diaphragm contraception, 884t, 888f
Diaphragmatic breathing, 322b
Diaphragmatic hernia, 645–646
Diaphysis, 717f
Diarrhea, 38
in bowel ischemia, 670
cancer treatment-related, 167
in colorectal cancer, 675
in diverticulitis, 668
drug therapy for, 37t
in gastroenteritis, 649
in gastrointestinal system disorders, 636–637
in inflammatory bowel disease, 671
in irritable bowel syndrome, 665
Diascopy, 957
Diastolic failure, 428
Diazepam, 1049t, 1069t
DIC; See Disseminated intravascular coagulation
Dicyclomine hydrochloride, 647t, 666t
Diencephalon, 473f, 473t
Diet
adding protein to, 367b
after roux-en-Y gastric bypass, 643
for burn injury patient, 993
cancer and, 150
decreasing sodium in, 405b
diabetes mellitus and, 860
for diverticular disease, 668b
for gallstones, 692, 692b

Diet (Continued)
for gastroesophageal reflux disease, 646–649
guidelines for vomiting, 649b
heart disease and, 447–448, 448b
heart-healthy, 430b
for hemorrhoids, 686
for hyperthyroidism, 840–841
for irritable bowel syndrome, 665
ketogenic, 525
lowering fat and cholesterol in, 453b
memory and, 1087b
ostomy and, 685
for peptic ulcer, 655
renal failure and, 810f, 810t
rheumatoid arthritis and, 754
for skin disorder prevention, 954–955
Differential blood cell count, 333, 337t
Difficult behavior, 9
Diffusion, 32, 33f
Digital pressure points, 343f
Digital rectal examination, 922t, 927
Digitalis
for heart failure, 429t, 430
toxicity of, 447
Digoxin, 430, 438t, 1123t
Dilantin; See Phenytoin
Dilated cardiomyopathy, 444b
Dilation and evacuation, 895t, 901t
Diltiazem, 402t, 438t
Dimetane; See Brompheniramine
Dipentum; See Olsalazine
Diphenhydramine, 239t, 278t, 364
Diphenoxylate atropine, 37t
Diphenoxylate hydrochloride, 666t
Dipivefrin, 602t
Diplopia, 562
Dipyridamole stress test, 378t
Direct-acting vasodilators, 402t
Direct commissurotomy, 446
Direct inguinal hernia, 663–664, 664f
Direct reflex of pupil, 488
Direct renin inhibitors, 402t
Dirty bomb, 1009
Disability, 177
prevention in musculoskeletal disorders, 727–730, 728f, 729b, 729f
primary survey and, 1023b
Disaster, 997
biologic, 1010–1015, 1013f, 1014f
chemical, 1006–1009, 1007t
nuclear, 1009–1010, 1009f, 1010t
psychological responses to, 1001
Disaster Medical Assistance Team, 999
Disaster preparedness and response, 997–1016, 998f
bioterrorism and, 1010–1015, 1013f, 1014f
category A agents in, 1011t
debriefing in, 1016
nursing management in, 1016, 1016f
care of special populations and, 1003
in chemical disaster, 1006–1009, 1007t, 1008b
communicable diseases with epidemic potential and, 1004t
community preparedness and, 999–1000
earthquake and, 999b
hospital preparedness and, 1000–1001
hurricane and, 999b, 1000b
in nuclear disaster, 1009–1010, 1009f, 1010t
nursing management in reconstruction stage, 1006

Disaster preparedness and response (Continued)
nursing roles and responsibilities in, 1002–1003
in pandemic influenza infection, 1015–1016
preparing of disaster supplies and, 998b
psychological responses to disaster and, 1001
tornado and flood and, 999b
triage and, 1001–1006, 1001t, 1002f
water and food safety and, 1003–1006, 1003b, 1006b
wildfire and, 999b
Discharge planning, 94–97, 97b
in prostatectomy, 930, 935b
in total hip replacement, 750b
Disclosure issues in acquired immunodeficiency syndrome, 230, 230b
Disease, 100
Disease-modifying antirheumatic drugs, 747–748, 748t
Disease-producing pathogens, 101–103
Diskectomy, 518–519
Dislocation, 735
Disopyramide, 438t, 1123t
Disorganized schizophrenia, 1105t
Disorientation, 185–186, 186f
Displacement, 1067t
Disposal of sharps, 230b
Disseminated intravascular coagulation, 362
in cancer, 171
in plague, 1013
Distraction as method of pain management, 138–139
Distributive shock, 1036, 1037f
Disulfiram, 1069, 1069t
Ditropan; See Oxybutynin
Diulo; See Metolazone
Diuresis, 836
Diuretics
for acute glomerulonephritis, 789
administration of, 403b
for chronic renal failure, 804t
contraindication in hyperparathyroidism, 847b
for heart failure, 429, 429t
for liver disorders, 696t
for vascular disorders, 402t
Divalproex, 525b
Diverticula, 665–668
Diverticulitis, 668
Diverticulosis, 665
Diving injury, 1019–1020
Dizziness
in ear disorders, 589
in Mèniére's disease, 613–614
DMAT; See Disaster Medical Assistance Team
Dobbhoff tube, 659b
Dobutamine echocardiogram, 378t
Dobutamine stress test, 378t
Documentation
in long-term care, 187
of pressure ulcer, 981
Docusate potassium, 666t
Docusate sodium, 666t
Dofetilide, 438t
Dog bite, 1030
Doll's eye reflex, 480–485
Domestic violence and abuse, 1041–1042, 1041b
Donepezil, 1089t
Dopamine, 477t, 1103
for head and spinal cord injury, 514t
Parkinson's disease and, 551, 552f

Dopamine agonist, 862*t*
Doppler flow studies, 384, 481*t*
Doribax; *See* Doripenem
Doripenem, 786*t*
Dorsalis pedis pulse, 387*f*
Dorzolamide, 602*t*
Double-barreled colostomy, 679, 679*f*
Double-cannula tracheostomy tube, 285
Dowager's hump, 891, 891*f*
Doxazosin, 402*t*
DPP-4 inhibitors, 862*t*
Drain, 90, 90*f*, 91*f*
Drainage in skin disorders, 957*b*
Dressings, 90
　for burn injury, 988
　for pressure ulcer, 981
　for skin disorders, 963
Dressler syndrome, 443–444, 461*t*
DRGs; *See* Diagnosis-related groups
Dristan; *See* Oxymetazoline
Droplet precautions, 106*t*
Drug(s)
　ethnic considerations in metabolism of, 72*b*
　interactions with proton pump inhibitors, 652*b*
Drug abuse, 1065–1082
　alcohol in, 1068, 1068*b*
　central nervous system depressants in, 1071–1073, 1072*b*
　characteristics of abused substances in, 1072*t*
　common terminology in, 1066*b*
　community care in, 1081–1082
　data collection in, 1076–1077, 1076*b*
　defense mechanisms and, 1067*t*
　drug therapy for, 1069*t*
　effects on family and friends, 1067–1068
　elderly and, 1077*b*, 1082*b*
　family interventions in, 1078–1081
　hallucinogens and inhalants in, 1076
　health care worker and, 1081
　hepatitis C and, 694
　marijuana in, 1075–1076
　nicotine in, 1075, 1075*b*
　nursing care plan for, 1079*b*
　nursing diagnoses in, 1077
　one-to-one observation in, 1078*b*
　opiates in, 1073–1074, 1073*b*
　signs and symptoms of, 1066–1067, 1066*f*
　stimulants in, 1074–1075, 1074*f*
　as surgical risk factor, 67*t*
　twelve-step program for, 1071, 1071*b*
Drug allergy, 238
　sulfa, 863*b*
Drug-eluting stent, 464
Drug-induced disorders
　gynecomastia in, 927
　immunosuppression in, 233–234
　parkinsonism in, 1105
　peptic ulcer in, 650
　skin eruption in, 958
Drug therapy
　for allergies, 238, 239*t*
　for anxiety, 1049*t*
　aspirin cautions and, 279*b*
　aspirin precautions in hemophilia, 362*b*
　for blood disorders, 349*t*
　for burn injury, 987*t*
　cautions in taking analgesics, 546*b*
　for chronic obstructive pulmonary disease, 308*t*
　for chronic obstructive pulmonary disease and asthma, 317–320, 321*b*
　for chronic renal failure, 804*t*

Drug therapy (*Continued*)
　for cognitive disorders, 1089*t*
　color of urine and, 774*t*
　for dysmenorrhea, 903*t*
　for dysrhythmias, 438*t*
　for erectile dysfunction, 925*t*
　for eye disorders, 602*t*
　for gastric cancer, 657–658
　for gastroesophageal reflux disease, 646–649
　for heart disease, 447
　for heart failure, 429–431, 429*t*
　hepatotoxicity of, 624*b*
　for hypercholesterolemia, 454*t*
　for irritable bowel syndrome, 665
　medication assessment in, 184*b*
　monitoring of drug side effects in, 352*b*
　for osteoporosis, 756*b*
　ototoxic, 582*b*, 583*b*
　for pain, 134–138, 135*t*
　for Parkinson's disease, 553–554, 553*b*, 554*t*
　proton pump inhibitors and cardiac problems, 646*b*
　for rheumatoid arthritis, 747–748, 748*t*
　for schizophrenia, 1105–1108, 1106*f*, 1107*t*
　for seizures, 525*b*
　selegiline cautions in, 553*b*
　for spinal cord injury, 514*t*
　for stroke, 531*t*
　for substance abuse, 1069*t*
　as surgical risk factor, 67*t*
　for upper gastrointestinal system disorders, 647*t*
　for urinary incontinence, 779–780
　for urinary tract infections, 786*t*
　warnings about antiviral medications, 295*b*
Drusen, 609
Dry age-related macular degeneration, 609
Dry eyes, 571*b*
Dry skin, 955*b*
Dry-suction system, 317
Dual diagnosis, 1055
　in substance abuse, 1065–1066
Dual energy x-ray absorptiometry, 720*t*
Dulcolax; *See* Bisacodyl
Duloxetine, 1049*t*, 1056*t*
Dumping syndrome, 642, 657
Duodenal ulcer, 650
DVT; *See* Deep vein thrombosis
Dyazide; *See* Hydrochlorothiazide
Dying patient, 172–174, 172*b*, 173*t*
　anticipatory guidance and, 173–174
　end-stage symptom management and, 174
　palliative care for, 172–174
　terminal hydration and, 174
Dyrenium; *See* Triamterene
Dysarthria, 530–532
Dyscrasias, 334
Dysfunctional uterine bleeding, 904
Dysmenorrhea, 902–903, 903*t*
Dyspareunia, 890
Dysphagia, 493, 643–644
　in Parkinson's disease, 554
　in stroke, 536, 539*b*
Dysphasia, 532
Dyspnea, 259, 272
　in acute respiratory distress syndrome, 314
　in anaphylactic reaction, 241
　in cardiovascular disease, 385*b*, 393
　end of life care in, 174
Dysreflexia, autonomic, 514–515
Dysrhythmias, 435–442

Dysrhythmias (*Continued*)
　after myocardial infarction, 461*t*
　aging and, 375
　atrial flutter and fibrillation in, 437–438, 437*f*
　automatic implantable cardioverter-defibrillator for, 442
　cardiac monitoring of, 384, 384*f*
　cardiac pacemaker for, 440–441, 441*b*, 441*f*
　cardioversion for, 440
　complete heart block in, 438
　drug therapy for, 438*t*
　etiology of, 435
　evaluation of ECG rhythm strip in, 435*b*
　pathophysiology of, 435, 435*f*
　premature ventricular contractions in, 438
　radiofrequency catheter ablation for, 442
　signs and symptoms of, 435–436, 436*f*
　ventricular fibrillation in, 440
　ventricular tachycardia in, 438–440
Dysthymia, 1051
Dystonic reaction, 1105
Dysuria, 775
　in cystitis, 786
　in urethritis, 788
　in vaginal infection, 906

E
Ear, 579–580
　changes with aging, 580
　functions of, 580
　irrigation of, 585*f*
　ototoxic drugs and, 582*b*, 583*b*
　range of sounds audible and hazardous to, 582*t*
　structures of, 579–580, 580*f*
　tuning fork tests and, 583
　visual examination of, 582–583, 583*f*
Ear disorders, 612–615
　acoustic neuroma in, 614
　community care in, 591, 617
　diagnostic tests for, 584*t*
　dizziness and vertigo in, 589
　external otitis in, 612
　hearing loss in, 581–591, 581*b*
　　care of hearing aid for, 587*b*
　　common causes of, 581*b*
　　communication in, 587–588, 587*b*
　　community care in, 591
　　coping with, 581*b*
　　rehabilitation in, 590–591, 590*f*, 591*f*
　impacted cerumen and foreign bodies in, 612
　instillation of ear medications in, 587, 587*f*, 588*b*
　labyrinthitis in, 613
　Mèniére's disease in, 613–614
　nursing diagnoses for, 586*t*
　otitis media in, 612–613
　otosclerosis and hearing loss in, 614–615
　tinnitus in, 589–590
Ear surgery, 615–617
　home care after, 617*b*
　nursing care plan for tympanoplasty in, 615*b*
　postoperative care in, 617, 617*f*
　preoperative care in, 615–617
Earthquake, 999*b*
Earwax, 579
　impacted, 612
Eating disorders, 640–642, 1060–1061
　anorexia nervosa in, 640, 1060
　bulimia nervosa in, 640, 1060
Ebola virus, 1011*t*, 1014–1015

Ecchymosis
  cancer treatment-related, 169b
  in thrombocytopenia, 359f
Eccrine sweat gland, 953f
ECG; See Electrocardiography
Echocardiography, 378t
ECT; See Electroconvulsive therapy
Ectropion, 571, 571f, 576t
Edema, 39–40
  in cardiovascular disease, 393–394
  in deep vein thrombosis, 415
  laryngeal, 281–282
  pulmonary, 431
Edrophonium test, 563
Educational competencies, 1134–1136
Effexor; See Venlafaxine
Effleurage, 902
EGD; See Esophagogastroduodenoscopy
Ejaculation, 919
Ejaculation disorders, 924
Ejaculatory duct, 919f
Ejection fraction, 373
  in diastolic failure, 428
Elastance, 260b
Elastase, 302
Elavil; See Amitriptyline
Eldepryl; See Selegiline
Elder abuse, 1042
Elderly
  actinic keratoses in, 975b
  aging-related changes in testosterone, 920b
  anemia in, 347b
  antipsychotic medications and, 1106b
  anxiety disorders in, 1049b, 1050b
  aortic stenosis in, 445b
  arthritis in, 746b, 749b
  blood pressure measurement in, 388b
  blood transfusion in, 363b
  brown recluse spider bite and, 1031b
  bruising in, 339b
  cancer in, 151b
  cerumen impaction in, 612b
  chemotherapy and, 356b, 935b
  cold tolerance and, 410b
  constipation in, 636b
  coronary blood flow in, 452b
  crutches and, 731b
  decreased immune function in, 359b
  dehydration in, 58b, 414b
  dementia in, 1086b
  depression in, 633b, 1055b
  diabetes mellitus in
    exercise and, 861b
    patient teaching and, 873b
    weight loss and, 860b
  drug-induced disorders in
    constipation in, 137b
    emotional distress in, 1050b
    hepatitis in, 699b
  drug tolerance and, 137b
  dry eyes in, 571b
  dry skin in, 955b
  dysrhythmias in, 440b
  erectile dysfunction in, 924b
  exposure to colds and coughs, 261b
  eye surgery in, 597b
  fall precautions for, 724b
  fasting and, 631b
  female reproductive system disorders in, 915b
  fluid and electrolyte shifts in, 87b
  fracture in, 737b, 741b
  gallstones in, 692b
  hair loss in, 408b
  heart failure in, 426b, 432b, 434b, 437f

Elderly (Continued)
  heart murmur in, 386b, 443b
  heat application and, 138b
  Helicobacter pylori and, 650b
  hepatitis in, 694b
  high-risk medications and, 138b
  human immunodeficiency virus infection in, 229, 229b
  hyperthyroidism in, 839b
  hypothermia in, 1027b
  hypothyroidism in, 844b
  hypoventilation and, 84b
  immobility and, 178b
  immune function of, 203b, 235b
  impaired swallowing in, 644b
  infection detection in, 116b
  interview of, 19b
  intestinal obstruction in, 669b
  intravenous therapy and, 54b
  iron supplementation and, 351b
  medication assessment in, 632b
  menopause and, 890b
  musculoskeletal disorders in, 724b, 731b
  myocardial infarction in, 459b
  obesity in, 641b
  oliguria in, 800b
  onychomycosis in, 972–973, 973f
  oral rehydration for, 635b
  orthostatic hypotension in, 400b
  osteoporosis in, 755b, 756b
  ostomy care and, 682b
  ototoxicity of analgesic medications and, 582b
  pacemaker and, 441b
  pain in, 84b, 134t
    back, 518b
    chronic, 128b
    pain scales for, 130b
    perception of, 127b
    reporting of, 129b
  Pap smear and, 894b
  patient teaching and, 915b
  peptic ulcer in, 651b
  pernicious anemia in, 340b
  pneumococcal vaccine and, 274b
  pneumonia and influenza in, 298b
  poor nutrition in, 336b
  positioning of, 86b
  preoperative depression in, 66b
  preoperative medications and, 74b, 76b
  preoperative teaching and, 68b, 70b
  protein intake and, 104b
  pulmonary hygiene and, 321b
  rehabilitation and, 188b
  rehydration and, 38b
  renal failure in, 768b
  schizophrenia in, 1116b
  sexual activity and, 923b
  shingles in, 971b
  shock in, 1033b
  skin tears in, 956b
  skin turgor in, 960b
  smoking and alcohol intake history of, 262b
  spiritual beliefs and coping of, 1049b
  substance abuse in, 1077b, 1082b
    alcohol in, 1068b
    benzodiazepines in, 1072b
  substance-induced delirium in, 1086b
  surgical complications in, 64b
  taste and smell sensation changes in, 633b
  toileting and, 781b
  upper respiratory infections and, 279b
  urinary system disorders in, 768b

Elderly (Continued)
  urinary tract infection in, 786b
  vaginal bleeding in, 905b
  varicose veins in, 419b
  wound healing in, 89b
Elderspeak, 1098b
Elective surgery, 63t
Electric shock, 1031–1032, 1032f
Electrical burn, 981
Electrocardiography, 378t, 435b
Electroconvulsive therapy, 1057, 1106
Electroencephalography, 481t, 503f
Electrolyte(s), 40–45, 41t, 42t
Electrolyte imbalances, 40–45, 41t, 42t
  calcium and, 44–45, 45f
  cardiac dysrhythmias and, 434
  chloride and phosphate and, 45
  data collection for, 57b
  in hemodialysis, 805
  magnesium and, 45
  potassium and, 44
  sodium and, 40–43
Electromyography, 481t, 720t, 769t
Electronic artificial larynx, 289, 290f
Electronic health record, 26
Electronic speech aid, 289
Electronystagmography, 584t
Electrophysiology studies, 378t
Electroretinography, 574t
Elimination
  postoperative, 86–87
  preoperative, 70
Eloxatin; See Oxaliplatin
Embolism
  in cerebrovascular accident, 528
  fat, 741
  postoperative prevention of, 85b, 88
  pulmonary, 311–312
Embolization therapy in pancreatic cancer, 712
Embolus, 406
Emergency care, 1021–1026
  in burn injury, 983–984, 984b
  in electric shock, 1031–1032, 1032f
Emergency contraception, 884t, 887–888
Emergency preparedness plan, 1000
Emergent surgery, 63t
EMG; See Electromyography
Emotional impact of infertility, 889b
Emotional shock, 1001
Empathy, 7–8
Emphysema, 303, 303f, 304t
  subcutaneous, 315–316
Employment opportunities in medical-surgical nursing, 3, 3b
Empyema, 298
Enabling in substance abuse, 1067
Enalapril, 402t, 804t
Encapsulated neoplasm, 145
Encephalitis, 544
Encephalopathy
  in cirrhosis, 703, 707
  Wernicke's, 1071
End colostomy, 679
End-of-life care
  pain management in, 138b
  symptom management in, 174
End-stage renal disease, 798
Endocarditis, 376, 442–443, 443f
Endocardium, 371
Endocrine disorders, 823–828
  adrenal, 847–853
    acute adrenal insufficiency in, 848–852
    Addison's disease in, 847–848, 848b, 849b

Endocrine disorders (*Continued*)
   corticosteroids for, 853*b*
   Cushing syndrome in, 852–853, 852*f*
   pheochromocytoma in, 847
causes of, 823–824
community care in, 831, 853
diabetes mellitus in, 244*t*, 856–877
   brown rice and whole grains and, 856*b*
   carbohydrate counting in, 865*b*, 865*t*
   cardiovascular disease and, 875
   chronic pancreatitis and, 710
   chronic renal failure and, 802*b*
   community care in, 877
   cultural considerations in, 857*b*
   data collection in, 867, 867*b*
   diabetic ketoacidosis in, 873
   diabetic neuropathy and, 876, 876*b*
   diagnostic tests for, 828*t*, 829*t*
   diet in, 860
   diet soda and, 875*b*
   in elderly, 861*b*
   etiology and pathophysiology of, 858
   exercise in, 860–861
   foot care and, 875*b*
   hyperglycemic hyperosmolar nonketotic
      syndrome in, 874
   hypoglycemia in, 861*b*, 871*t*, 873*b*, 874
   injectable hypoglycemic agents in, 866,
      866*b*, 866*t*
   insulin therapy in, 863–865;
      See also Insulin therapy
   islet cell transplantation in, 866
   metabolic syndrome and, 875
   nephropathy and, 875
   nursing care plan for, 868*b*
   nursing diagnoses for, 867–868
   oral hypoglycemic agents in, 862–863,
      862*t*
   patient teaching in, 861*f*, 867*f*, 871–873,
      872*f*
   peripheral vascular disease and, 875–876
   preoperative and postoperative
      management in, 866, 866*b*
   rebound hyperglycemia in, 874
   retinopathy and, 608, 876
   sick days and, 872*b*
   signs, symptoms, and diagnosis of,
      858–859
   surgical risk factors in, 67*t*
   travel instructions and, 872*b*
   types of, 856–858, 857*b*, 857*t*, 858*b*
   venous stasis ulcer in, 421
diagnostic tests and procedures in, 825–828,
   825*t*, 827*f*, 828*t*, 829*t*
history taking in, 829, 829*b*
nursing diagnoses for, 829, 829*t*
parathyroid, 845–847, 846*t*
   hyperparathyroidism in, 846–847, 846*b*
   hypoparathyroidism in, 845–846
pituitary, 833–838
   diabetes insipidus in, 835–837, 836*f*
   hypofunction in, 835, 835*f*
   syndrome of inappropriate secretion of
      antidiuretic hormone in, 837–838,
      837*f*
   tumors in, 833–835, 834*f*
prevention of, 824, 824*b*
thyroid
   goiter in, 838–839, 839*f*
   hyperthyroidism in, 839–840,
      840*f*, 841*b*
   hypothyroidism in, 844–845, 844*b*
   myxedema coma in, 845
   thyroid cancer in, 845
   thyroid storm in, 843, 843*b*, 844*b*

Endocrine disorders (*Continued*)
   thyroidectomy in, 840–844
   thyroiditis in, 845
Endocrine pancreas, 821
Endocrine system, 818–831
   adrenal hormones in, 821, 821*f*, 822*f*
   chronic renal failure and, 803*f*
   effects of aging on, 822
   functions of, 819, 819*t*
   organs and structures of, 818, 819*t*, 824*f*
   pancreatic hormones in, 821–822,
      823*f*, 824*f*
   parathyroid glands in, 821
   pituitary hormones in, 819, 820*f*
   thyroid hormones in, 819–821
Endolymph, 580
Endometrial biopsy, 895*t*
Endometrial cancer, 152*t*
Endometriosis, 906
Endorphins, 125, 477*t*
Endoscopic retrograde
   cholangiopancreatography, 626*t*, 692
Endoscopy
   in cancer detection, 154
   in gastric cancer, 657
   in gastrointestinal disorders, 626*t*
   in peptic ulcer, 651
   in urologic disorders, 769*t*
Endotracheal intubation, 284–286, 285*f*
Endotracheal suctioning, 293, 293*f*, 294*f*
Endotracheal tube, 282*f*
Energy expenditure in metabolic equivalents,
   463, 463*t*
ENG; *See* Electronystagmography
Enkephalins, 477*t*
Entacapone, 554*t*
Entecavir, 696*t*
Enteral nutrition, 658–659, 659*b*, 659*f*, 660*b*
   for burn patient, 993
Entereg; *See* Alvimopan
Enterocele, 903
Enterotoxigenic coli, 1029
Entropion, 576*t*
Enucleation, 597–598
Environment
   cancer and, 150–151
   protective, 110
   safety in chronic illness and, 183, 183*b*
   skin disorder prevention and, 955
   spread of infection and, 101*f*, 102*b*
   standard precautions and, 1129
Enzyme-linked immunosorbent assay, 219,
   219*b*
Eosinophil, 197*t*, 207*t*
Epicardium, 371
Epicondyle, 718*t*
Epidermis, 952–953, 953*f*
Epididymis, 918, 919*f*, 926*f*
Epididymitis, 926*f*, 932
Epidural analgesic, 124
Epidural anesthesia, 77*t*
Epidural hematoma, 501, 501*f*
Epidural infusion, 56
Epigastric pain
   in pancreatic cancer, 712
   in peptic ulcer, 651
Epiglottis, 257, 258, 258*f*
Epilepsy, 523–526, 525*b*
Epinephrine, 477*t*, 819*t*, 821, 821*f*
Epiphysis, 717*f*
Epistaxis, 280, 280*f*
Epivir; *See* Lamivudine
Epoetin alfa, 349*t*, 804*t*
Epogen; *See* Epoetin alfa
Epstein-Barr virus, 149

Equipment, standard precautions and,
   1128–1129
Erbitux; *See* Cetuximab
ERCP; *See* Endoscopic retrograde
   cholangiopancreatography
Erectile dysfunction, 923–924, 924*b*, 924*f*, 925*t*
Erection, 919
Errors of refraction, 594–595, 595*f*
Erythema, 245
Erythrasma, 957
Erythrocyte, 332, 333*f*, 1119*t*
Erythrocyte count, 337*t*
Erythrocyte sedimentation rate, 337*t*
Erythropoiesis, 332, 333*f*, 335*b*
Erythropoietin, 347–348, 766*t*
Eschar, 980–981
Escharotomy, 986, 987*f*
Escitalopram, 1056*t*
Esidrix; *See* Hydrochlorothiazide
Esmolol, 438*t*
Esomeprazole, 647*t*
Esophageal cancer, 645
Esophageal diverticula, 668
Esophageal varices, 704–707
Esophagectomy, 645
Esophagogastroduodenoscopy, 626*t*
   in esophageal cancer, 645
   in gastroesophageal reflux disease, 646
Esophagus, 620, 621*f*
ESR; *See* Erythrocyte sedimentation rate
Essential oils, 1050*b*
Estradiol valerate and dienogest, 883–887
Estrogen, 819*t*
   in aromatase inhibitors, 912
   in hormone replacement therapy, 891
   menopause and, 890*b*
ESWL; *See* Extracorporeal shockwave
   lithotripsy
Ethambutol, 300*t*
Ethanolamines, 239*t*
Ethical considerations
   in breast cancer, 910*b*
   in confidentiality and HIV, 230*b*
   in consent for blood administration,
      362*b*
   in documentation of patient teaching, 505*b*
   in documentation of skin lesions, 960*b*
   in giving surgical consent, 68*b*
   in immunizations, 204*b*
   in intravenous therapy, 51*b*
   in liver transplantation, 707*b*
   in morning-after pill, 888*b*
   in narcotic pain control at end of life, 138*b*
   in noncompliance with tuberculosis
      medication, 299*b*
   in nurse use of tobacco, 1075*b*
   in protected health information, 22*b*
   in rights of psychiatric patients, 1108*b*
   in substance abuse among health care
      workers, 1067*b*
   suicidal patient and, 1059*b*
   in testing for BRCA1 and BRCA2 genes,
      910*b*
   in urinary catheterization, 776*b*
   in use of restraints, 184*b*, 1096*b*
   when nurse is HIV positive, 230*b*
Ethionamide, 300*t*
Ethmoid sinus, 258*f*
Ethmozine; *See* Monricizine
Ethosuximide, 525*b*, 1123*t*
Ethylenediamine, 239*t*
Eupnea, 273*f*
Eustachian tube, 579, 580*f*
Evacuation after ostomy, 682–683
Evaluation in nursing process, 27

Everolimus, 798
Evisceration, 91–93, 92*t*, 93*f*
Evoked potential studies, 481*t*
Evoked-response audiometry, 584*t*
Ex-Lax; *See* Phenolphthalein
Excess adrenocorticotropic hormone, 852–853, 852*f*
Excess fluid volume, 38–40, 40*f*
Excisional biopsy, 957
Exelon; *See* Rivastigmine
Exenatide, 866*t*
Exercise
  after roux-en-Y gastric bypass, 643
  for arterial occlusive disease, 409
  for brain, 1087*b*
  in cardiovascular disease, 395
  diabetes mellitus and, 860–861
    elderly person with, 861*b*
    insulin therapy and, 862*b*
  Kegel, 780*b*
  postmastectomy, 914*f*
  quadriceps and gluteal muscle, 729*b*
  range of motion, 728–729
  to reduce gas and bloating, 635*b*
  in rheumatoid arthritis, 753–754
  for varicose veins, 420
Exercise stress test, 377*f*, 378*t*
Exertional angina, 455
Exocrine pancreas, 821
Exophthalmos, 576, 595–596, 839, 840*f*
Expanded precautions, 106*t*, 109
Expected outcomes, 26
Expectorate, 257
Expiration, 259
Expiratory reserve volume, 269*f*
Exposure, primary survey and, 1023*b*
Expressive aphasia, 495
Extended care
  pain management and, 140
  in upper respiratory system disorders, 290
Extensor posturing, 487, 487*f*
External beam radiation, 935*t*
External fixation of fracture, 738–739, 739*f*
External hemorrhoids, 684*f*, 685
External mammary artery pressure point, 343*f*
External otitis, 612
External radiation therapy, 159–160, 159*f*, 160*b*, 162*t*
External urethral sphincter, 765
Extracapsular cataract extraction, 598
Extracellular fluid, 31–32, 31*f*
Extracorporeal circulation, 464–465
Extracorporeal shockwave lithotripsy, 793
Extraocular muscle function test, 574*t*
Extrapulmonary tuberculosis, 301
Extrapyramidal side effects of antipsychotics, 1105, 1107*t*
Extravasation in intravenous therapy, 54*t*
Exudate, 105
  color of, 981*t*
  sampling of, 957
Eye, 568–571
  autonomic system effects on, 476*t*
  basic care of, 571–572
  changes with aging, 570–571, 570*f*, 571*f*
  chronic renal failure and, 803*f*
  diabetic retinopathy and, 876
  functions of, 569, 570*f*
  hyperthyroidism and, 839, 840*f*
  inability to close, 493
  muscles of, 570*t*
  normal flora of, 101*t*
  personal protective equipment for, 1129
  prevention of injury to, 572
  severe anemia and, 348*t*

Eye (*Continued*)
  sickle cell disease and, 354*f*
  structures of, 568–569, 569*f*
Eye contact, 1110*b*
Eye disorders, 571, 594–610
  abnormalities of lid position in, 576*t*
  application of eye patch in, 607*b*
  cataract in, 598–600, 598*f*, 599*b*
  community care in, 579, 611–612
  corneal transplantation in, 596–597, 596*f*
  corneal ulcer in, 596
  cultural considerations in, 572*b*
  danger signals of eye disease and, 572*b*
  diagnostic tests for, 573, 573*f*, 574*t*
  drug therapy for, 602*t*
  errors of refraction in, 594–595, 595*f*
  eye trauma in, 597–598, 597*f*
  glaucoma in, 600–601
    danger signals of, 602*b*
    etiology of, 600–601
    narrow-angle, 605
    nursing management of, 604–605, 604*f*
    open-angle, 602–605, 602*f*
    pathophysiology of, 601, 601*f*
    patient teaching in, 605*b*
  history taking in, 573–576
  home care after retinal surgery, 607*b*
  instillation of eyedrops and eye ointment in, 578*b*
  keratitis in, 595–596
  macular degeneration in, 608–610, 609*f*
  physical examination in, 573*f*, 576
  postoperative care in, 611, 611*f*
  preoperative care in, 610
  prevention of visual loss and, 572, 573*f*
  retinal detachment in, 605–607, 606*f*
  retinopathy in, 608
  signs and symptoms of, 577*t*
  uveitis in, 595
  xanthelasma in, 577*f*
Eye movement positions, 487*f*
Eye ointment, 578*b*, 597, 597*f*
Eye patch, 607*b*, 611, 611*f*
Eye surgery, 610–611
  for cataracts, 598–600, 599*b*
  in elderly, 597*b*
  patient teaching in, 600*b*
  postoperative care in, 611
  preoperative care in, 610
Eyeball, 568, 569*f*
Eyedrops instillation, 578*b*, 611, 611*f*
Eyelashes, 569
Eyelid, 569, 576*t*
Ezetimibe, 454*t*

F

Face, secondary survey of, 1023*b*
Face shield, 111*f*
Facet, 718*t*
Facial nerve, 475*t*, 580*f*
Fainting, 387–388
Fallopian tube, 881, 881*f*
Falls
  during bathing, 962*b*
  disorders and problems increasing risk of, 183*b*
  impaired vision and, 610*b*
  orthostatic hypotension and, 401*b*
  in Parkinson's disease, 555–557
  precautions for, 724*b*
  risk assessment for, 184*b*
  vitamin D association with decreased risk for, 724*b*

Family
  effects of substance abuse on, 1067–1068
  preoperative instructions to, 72
Family caregiver, 192–193, 193*b*
Family coping
  in cognitive disorders, 1098, 1099*b*
  in neurologic disorders, 497
  in substance abuse, 1078–1081
Famotidine, 647*t*
Farsightedness, 594, 595*f*
Fascia, 716
Fasciotomy, 742
FAST; *See* Focused abdominal sonography for trauma
Fasting, elderly and, 631*b*
Fasting blood glucose, 828*t*
Fat(s), lowering in diet, 453*b*
Fat embolism, 741
Fatigue
  in anemia, 348
  cancer treatment-related, 169
  in cardiovascular disease, 393
  in diabetes insipidus, 836
  in diabetes mellitus, 859
  in hematologic disorders, 343
  in multiple sclerosis, 558
  in respiratory disorders, 274
  in urinary disorders, 775–776
Fear
  of cancer, 171
  of dying, 172, 172*b*
  of surgery, 67*t*
Fecal analysis, 626*t*
Fecal immunochemical test, 151, 625–631
Fecal occult blood test, 151, 625–631
Federal Emergency Management Agency, 999
Fee-for service, 4
Feeding tube, 658–659, 659*b*, 659*f*, 660*b*
  for burn patient, 993
Feen-a-Mint; *See* Phenolphthalein
Felbamate, 525*b*
Felbatol; *See* Felbamate
FEMA; *See* Federal Emergency Management Agency
Female condom, 884*t*
Female reproductive disorders, 880–915
  abnormal uterine bleeding in, 904–905, 905*b*
  bacterial vaginosis in, 939
  breast cancer in, 909–915
    breast reconstructive surgery for, 912, 913*f*
    etiology and pathophysiology of, 909–910
    legal and ethical considerations in, 910*b*
    nursing care plan for breast lumpectomy and, 911*b*
    postmastectomy exercises and, 914*f*
    prevention of, 910
    risk factors for, 909*b*
    signs and symptoms of, 910
    stages of, 909*t*
    treatment of, 910–912, 912*f*
  candidiasis in, 939
  cervical cancer in, 907
  community care in, 915
  cultural considerations in, 894*b*
  diagnostic tests for, 888*f*, 894, 897*b*
  dysfunctional uterine bleeding in, 904
  dysmenorrhea in, 902–903, 903*t*
  endometriosis in, 906
  fibroadenoma in, 908
  fibrocystic breast changes in, 908, 908*b*
  gynecologic surgical procedures in, 901*t*
  history taking in, 894, 897*b*
  home care in, 915
  infertility and, 888–890, 889*b*, 890*b*

Female reproductive disorders (*Continued*)
 intraductal papilloma in, 908–909
 leiomyoma in, 905
 lower genital tract inflammations in, 906, 907*t*
 nursing care plan for hysterectomy and, 898*b*
 older adult and, 915*b*
 ovarian cancer in, 908, 908*b*
 pelvic inflammatory disease in, 939
 pelvic relaxation syndrome in, 903–904
 polycystic ovarian syndrome in, 904
 premenstrual dysphoric disorder in, 902
 premenstrual syndrome in, 902
 toxic shock syndrome in, 906–907
 uterine cancer in, 907–908
 vulvar cancer in, 907
Female reproductive system, 881–894
 accessory organs of, 882
 aging-related changes in, 882
 breast and, 883
 contraception and fertility and, 883–890, 884*t*, 888*f*
 external structures of, 881
 fetal sexual development and, 882
 health promotion and disease prevention and, 892–894
  diagnostic tests and, 888*f*, 894, 897*b*
  health screening and assessments in, 892–894, 893*f*
 infertility and, 888–890, 889*b*, 890*b*
 internal structures of, 881, 881*f*
 maturation of, 882
 menopause and, 882, 889*b*, 890–892, 890*b*, 891*f*, 892*b*
 menstruation and, 883
 phases of reproductive cycle and, 882, 882*b*
Femoral artery pressure point, 343*f*
Femoral hernia, 664*f*
Femoral pulse, 387*f*
Femoropopliteal bypass graft, 409, 410*f*
Fenestrated tracheostomy tube, 285, 285*f*
Fenofibrate, 454*t*
Fentanyl
 for cancer pain, 170*t*
 transdermal patch, 136*b*
Feraheme; *See* Ferumoxytol
Ferrous sulfate, 804*t*
Fertility
 contraception and, 883–890
 cultural considerations in, 889*b*
Ferumoxytol, 804*t*
Festerdine, 779–780, 780*t*
Fetal sexual development, 882
FEV₁; *See* Forced expiratory volume in 1 second
Fever, 209–211
 in bacterial meningitis, 542
 blood transfusion-related, 365*t*
 in diverticulitis, 668
 in gallbladder disorders, 691*t*
 in inflammatory bowel disease, 671
 as mechanism to prevent infection, 104
 during thyroid storm, 844*b*
Fever blister, 643
Fexofenadine, 239*t*, 278*t*
Fiberoptic bronchoscopy, 269*f*
Fibric acid derivatives, 454*t*
Fibrillation
 atrial, 437–438, 437*f*
 ventricular, 437*f*, 440
Fibrin, 333
Fibrinogen, 331
Fibroadenoma, 908

Fibroblast, 952
Fibrocystic breast changes, 908, 908*b*
Fibroids, 905
Fibroma, 757
Fibromyalgia, 253–254, 254*b*, 254*f*
Fibula, 717*f*
Fight-or-flight reaction, 1103
Filgrastim, 349*t*
Filtration, 33, 33*f*
Fine crackles, 263–264
Fine-needle aspiration of thyroid, 845
Finger, clubbing of, 263*f*
Fingernails
 fungal infection of, 972–973, 972*b*, 973*f*
 iron deficiency anemia and, 351*f*
Fire ant bite, 1031
Fire safety, 999*b*
First aid, 1020–1021, 1021*t*
 in burn injury, 983–984, 984*b*
First-degree heart block, 436
Fissure, 718*t*
Fistula
 anorectal, 686–687
 arteriovenous, 805, 806*f*
Fistulectomy, 901*t*
FIT; *See* Fecal immunochemical test
FLACC pain scale, 129–130, 130*f*
Flaccid paralysis
 in encephalitis, 544
 positioning in, 729
Flagyl; *See* Metronidazole
Flail chest, 1024
Flamazine; *See* Silver sulfadiazine
Flank pain, 775
Flashback in LSD use, 1076
Flatus, 635
Flecainide, 438*t*, 1123*t*
Fletcher's Castoria; *See* Senna
Flexible sigmoidoscopy, 626*t*
Flexion contracture of knee and hip, 728, 728*f*
Flexor posturing, 487, 487*f*
Flight of ideas, 1051
Flomax; *See* Tamsulosin
Flonase; *See* Fluticasone
Flood, 999*b*
Flovent; *See* Fluticasone
Floxuridine, 708
Fluid deprivation test, 824*b*
Fluid imbalances, 33–40
 in acute renal failure, 801
 community care and, 59
 data collection for, 57*b*
 home care in, 40
 postoperative, 92*t*
 in respiratory disorders, 274
 volume deficit in, 34–38, 34*b*, 34*f*, 36*b*, 37*t*
 volume excess in, 38–40, 40*f*
Fluid intake
 immobilized patient and, 743*b*
 in kidney stones, 793
 preoperative, 70
 renal health and, 767
Fluid overload
 in cardiovascular disease, 393–394
 in hemodialysis, 805
Fluid restriction
 in renal failure, 810*t*
 in syndrome of inappropriate secretion of antidiuretic hormone, 838
Fluid resuscitation
 in burn, 985, 985*b*
 in hyperglycemic hyperosmolar nonketotic syndrome, 874
Fluid retention, mechanical ventilation-related, 327*t*

FluidAir bed, 728*f*, 730
Fluids and electrolytes, 30–59
 acid-base imbalances and, 47–50, 47*t*, 50*f*
  arterial blood gas analysis for, 47–48
  home care in, 50
  metabolic acidosis in, 48
  metabolic alkalosis in, 49–50
  respiratory acidosis in, 48
  respiratory alkalosis in, 48–49
 acid-base system and, 45–46, 45*b*, 46*f*
 distribution and regulation of body fluids, 31–33, 31*f*, 31*t*, 32*b*, 33*f*
 electrolyte imbalances and, 40–45, 41*t*, 42*t*
  calcium and, 44–45, 45*f*
  chloride and phosphate and, 45
  magnesium and, 45
  potassium and, 44
  sodium and, 40–43
 fluid imbalances and, 33–40
  community care and, 59
  deficient fluid volume in, 34–38, 34*b*, 34*f*, 36*b*, 37*t*
  excess fluid volume in, 38–40, 40*f*
  home care in, 40
 intravenous fluid therapy and, 50–57
  administration of, 51–53, 53*b*
  calculation and regulation of flow rate in, 53–57
  central line care in, 56–57, 56*f*
  complications of, 54*t*
  flushing PRN locks or central IV lines in, 55–56
  home care and, 59*b*
  intravenous solutions for, 52*t*
  partial or total parenteral nutrition and, 56–57, 57*b*
  troubleshooting intravenous flow in, 55*t*
 movement of, 32–33
 nursing management of, 58–59
 osmolality and, 40
 postoperative assessment of, 83*b*
 postoperative maintenance of, 86–87
 restrictions in renal failure, 810*t*
Fluke, 103
Flunisolide, 278*t*, 308*t*
Fluorescein, 602*t*
Fluorescein angiography, 574*t*
Fluoroquinolones, 786*t*
5-Fluorouracil
 for colorectal cancer, 675
 for liver cancer, 708
 for liver disorders, 696*t*
 for pancreatic cancer, 712
Fluoxetine, 1056*t*, 1074–1075
Flushing PRN locks, 55–56, 55*b*
Fluticasone, 278*t*, 308*t*
Flutter valve, 317
Fluvastatin, 454*t*
Foam-cuffed tracheostomy tube, 286
FOBT; *See* Fecal occult blood test
Focused abdominal sonography for trauma, 1026
Focused assessment, 22
Foley catheter, 794*t*
 for burn victim, 985
Folic acid
 for chronic renal failure, 804*t*
 for colon polyps, 675*b*
 foods high in, 348*b*
 needed for erythropoiesis, 335*b*
Follicle-stimulating hormone, 819*t*
 ovarian cycle and, 882
 pituitary hypofunction and, 835*t*
 in sperm production, 919
Follicle-stimulating hormone study, 922*t*

Follicular pharyngitis, 280
Food(s)
  contributing to colon cancer, 623b
  cultural considerations and, 118b
  gas-forming, 665
  intake in acquired immunodeficiency
    syndrome, 229b
  iron and folic acid in, 348b
  preoperative intake of, 70
  safe handling of, 1029b
  safety in disaster, 1003–1006, 1006b
  sodium in, 41b
  for thickening stool, 636b
  triggers of migraine headache, 545b
  vitamin C in, 89b
Food allergy, 238
Food diary, 665b
Food poisoning, 1029–1030, 1029b
Foot
  Achilles tendon rupture and, 736
  care in diabetes mellitus, 875b
  exercises of, 71b, 71f
Footdrop, 728, 728f
Foradil; See Formoterol
Foramen, 718t
Forced exhalation coughing, 71b
Forced expiratory volume in 1 second, 268,
    269f
Forced vital capacity, 268, 269f
Forearm, fascial compartments of, 742f
Foreign body
  in ear, 612
  in eye, 597, 597f
ForeseeHome Monitor, 610
Formoterol, 308t
Fortaz; See Ceftazidime
Fosamax; See Alendronate
Fosfomycin tromethamine, 786t
Fosinopril, 402t
Fosphenytoin, 525b
Fossa, 718t
Four-point crutch gait, 730b
FOUR score, 486
Fovea, 718t
Fovea centralis, 569
Fracture, 736–742
  braces and splints for, 739–740, 739f
  casts for, 739, 739f, 744–745
  complications of, 741–742, 742f
  etiology and pathophysiology of, 736–737
  external fixation for, 738–739, 739f
  initial assessment in, 742–743
  internal fixation for, 738, 738f
  nasal, 282–283
  osteoporotic, 756b
  physical assessment of neurovascular
    status in, 743b
  proton pump inhibitors and, 737b
  reduction, surgery, and stabilization in, 738
  of ribs, 1024
  signs and symptoms of, 737
  traction for, 740, 740f, 744b
  types of, 737b, 737f
FRAMES acronym, 1069–1071
Francisella tularensis, 1011t, 1014
FRC; See Functional residual capacity
Frequency, 775b
  in urethritis, 788
Fresh frozen plasma, 363t
Friction rub, 443
Frontal sinus, 258f
Frostbite, 1027–1028, 1028b
Fructosamine assay, 827, 828t
FSH; See Follicle-stimulating hormone
FTA-ABS blood test, 584t

Full Outline of UnResponsiveness score, 486
Full-thickness burn, 982–983, 983f, 984t
Functional assessment in rehabilitation,
    189–190, 189b
Functional incontinence, 777
Functional residual capacity, 268, 269f
Fungal infection
  in acquired immunodeficiency syndrome,
    223–224
  cutaneous, 972–973, 972b, 973b, 973f
  respiratory, 298
Fungi, 103
Furadantin; See Nitrofurantoin
Furosemide, 402t
  for chronic renal failure, 804t
  for liver disorders, 696t
Furuncle, 970
FVC; See Forced vital capacity

G
Gabapentin, 525b
Gabitril; See Tiagabine
GAD; See Generalized anxiety disorder
Galantamine, 1089t
Gallbladder, 621, 621f
  autonomic system effects on, 476t
  disorders of, 623–624, 625
  functions of, 622–623
  sickle cell disease and, 354f
Gallium scan, 720t
Gallstones, 623, 690–694, 691f, 691t
  cultural considerations in, 624b
  ethnic predisposition to, 690b
  patient teaching in, 692b
  postcholecystectomy diet and, 692b
  postoperative care in, 693–694, 693b, 693f
Gamma-aminobutyric acid, 477t
Gamma globulins, 331
Gamma-glutamyl transpeptidase, 626t, 696t
Gamma knife procedure, 540
Gangrene
  in cardiovascular disease, 388
  diabetes-related, 875–876
  in thromboangiitis obliterans, 413
  of toes, 408f
Gantanol; See Sulfamethoxazole
Gantrisin; See Sulfisoxazole
Garamycin; See Gentamicin
Garlic, 205b
Gas exchange, 259–260
Gas-forming foods, 665
Gastric analysis, 626t, 651–652
Gastric bypass, 642, 642f
Gastric cancer, 657–658, 657b
Gastric distention
  after intrathoracic surgery, 316
  mechanical ventilation-related, 327t
Gastric resection, 656
Gastritis, 649–650
Gastrocolic reflex, 621
Gastroenteritis, 649
Gastroesophageal reflux disease, 646–649,
    646b
  Barrett's esophagus and, 645
  in chronic obstructive pulmonary disease,
    305
  male sexual dysfunction and, 923
  Nissen fundoplication surgery for, 649f
Gastroesophageal sphincter, 620
Gastrointestinal anthrax, 1011t
Gastrointestinal bleeding
  mechanical ventilation-related, 327t
  in peptic ulcer, 651, 653b
Gastrointestinal decompression, 658, 658b,
    669, 669f

Gastrointestinal function
  chronic renal failure and, 803f
  cirrhosis and, 703f
  effects of aging on, 621, 623
  postoperative assessment of, 83b
  postoperative promotion of, 87
  reference intervals for tests of, 1126t
  severe anemia and, 348t
Gastrointestinal scintigraphy, 626t
Gastrointestinal system, 620–637
  accessory organs of, 621–622
  functions of, 620–621, 622f
  organs and structures of, 620,
    621f, 622f
Gastrointestinal system disorders
  anorectal, 685–687
    abscess and fistula in, 686–687
    hemorrhoids in, 684f, 685–686
    pilonidal sinus in, 686
  anorexia nervosa in, 640
  bulimia nervosa in, 640
  causes of, 623–624, 624b
  cholelithiasis and cholecystitis in, 690–694,
    691f, 691t
    ethnic predisposition to, 690b
    patient teaching in, 692b
    postcholecystectomy diet and, 692b
    postoperative care in, 693–694,
      693b, 693f
  common problems related to, 633–637
    accumulation of flatus in, 635
    anorexia in, 633–635
    bowel incontinence in, 637
    constipation in, 636
    diarrhea in, 636–637
    nausea and vomiting in, 635
  community care in, 687
  data collection in, 631–632, 631b
  diagnostic tests for, 625–631, 626t
  drug therapy for, 666t
  hepatic, 694–698
    causes of, 624
    cirrhosis in, 701–703, 702f, 703f, 704b,
      707f
    deaths in, 701b
    drug therapy for, 696t
    hepatitis in, 694–698; See also Hepatitis
    liver cancer in, 149, 708
    liver transplantation for, 707, 707b
    prevention of, 625
    as surgical risk factor, 67t
  lower, 663–687
    abdominal and inguinal hernias in,
      663–664, 664f
    appendicitis in, 672–673
    bowel ischemia in, 670
    colorectal cancer in, 674–679;
      See also Colorectal cancer
    diverticula in, 665–668
    inflammatory bowel disease in, 670–672,
      670t, 671f
    intestinal obstruction in, 668–670, 669b,
      669f
    irritable bowel syndrome in, 664–665,
      665b
    malabsorption in, 673–674
    ostomy surgery and care in, 679–681;
      See also Ostomy
    peritonitis in, 673
  nursing diagnoses for, 633, 634t
  obesity in, 640–642; See also Obesity
  pancreatic, 708–713
    acute pancreatitis in, 708–710,
      709f
    chronic pancreatitis in, 710

Gastrointestinal system disorders (*Continued*)
  physical assessment in, 632*b*, 632*f*
  prevention of, 624–625
  upper, 640–660
    dietary guidelines for vomiting in, 649*b*
    drug therapy for, 647*t*
    dysphagia in, 643–644
    enteral nutrition for, 658–659, 659*b*, 659*f*, 660*b*
    esophageal cancer in, 645
    gastric cancer in, 657–658, 657*b*
    gastritis in, 649–650
    gastroenteritis in, 649
    gastroesophageal reflux disease in, 646–649, 646*b*, 649*f*
    gastrointestinal decompression for, 658, 658*b*
    hiatal hernia in, 645–646
    oral cancer in, 644
    peptic ulcer in, 650–652; *See also* Peptic ulcer
    stomatitis in, 643
    total parenteral nutrition for, 660, 660*b*
Gastroparesis, 876
Gastrostomy, 659, 659*f*, 660*b*
Gate control theory of pain, 124, 125*f*
Gel application, 963*b*
Gemcitabine, 712
Gemfibrozil, 454*t*
Gene therapy in cancer, 165
General anesthesia, 76, 77*t*
Generalized anxiety disorder, 1046–1047
Generalized edema, 39
Generalized seizure, 524
Genetic predisposition for cancer, 149
Genital herpes, 942*t*
Genital infection, 906, 907*t*
Genitourinary system
  secondary survey of, 1023*b*
Gentamicin, 786*t*
  for burn injury, 987*t*
  for plague, 1013
  therapeutic drug monitoring reference intervals for, 1123*t*
Geocillin; *See* Carbenicillin
GERD; *See* Gastroesophageal reflux disease
Gestational diabetes, 857*t*, 858
GGT; *See* Gamma-glutamyl transpeptidase
Giant cell arteritis, 244*t*
Gigantism, 834
Ginger, 304*b*, 635*b*
Ginger tea, 35
Gingivitis, 339
Glands
  autonomic system effects on, 476*t*
  cutaneous, 952
Glasgow Coma Scale, 486, 486*t*
Glaucoma, 600–601
  danger signals of, 602*b*
  etiology of, 600–601
  narrow-angle, 605
  nursing management of, 604–605, 604*f*
  open-angle, 602–605, 602*f*
  pathophysiology of, 601, 601*f*
  patient teaching in, 605*b*
Glimepiride, 862*t*
Glipizide, 862*t*
Global amnesia, 1097–1098
Global aphasia, 495
Glomerular filtration rate, 765

Glomerulonephritis, 766
  acute, 789
  chronic, 789–790
  chronic renal failure and, 801–802
Glossectomy, 644
Glossopharyngeal nerve, 475*t*
Gloves, 111*f*, 1128
Glucagon, 819*t*, 823*f*
Glucocorticoids, 819*t*, 821, 822*f*
  peptic ulcer and, 650
Glucometer, 867, 867*f*
Glucophage; *See* Metformin
Glucosamine, 746*b*
Glucose, 23
Glucose intolerance, 834
Glucose tolerance test, 827, 828*t*
Glucotrol; *See* Glipizide
Glutathione, 699
Gluteal setting, 729*b*
Glyburide, 862*t*
Glycemic control, 859
Glycosuria, 859
Glycosylated hemoglobin test, 827
Glyset; *See* Miglitol
Goal setting in addiction therapy, 1077
Goals, expected outcomes and, 26
Goggles, 111*f*
Goiter, 824*b*, 838–839, 839*f*
Gonadotropin-releasing hormone, 919
Gonads, 918
Goniometry, 719, 723*f*
Gonorrhea, 942*t*
Good Samaritan laws, 1020–1021, 1021*t*
Goodpasture's syndrome, 244*t*
Gout, 755
Government-sponsored health insurance, 5–6
Gown, 111*f*, 1129
Grafting in burn, 986–988, 988*f*
Gram negative stain, 941
Gram positive stain, 941
Granulocyte, 332, 333*f*
Granulocyte colony-stimulating factor, 364
Granulocyte-macrophage colony-stimulating factor, 364
Granuloma, 670–671
Grapeseed extract, 405*b*
Graves' disease, 244*t*, 839, 840*f*
Great toe bunion, 736
Greenstick fracture, 737*b*, 737*f*
Grey-Turner's sign, 1025–1026
Grief, 513, 513*t*
Grieving, 172, 172*b*
Group health insurance, 5
Group therapy, 1048
  for substance abuse, 1069–1071
Growth hormone, pituitary hypofunction and, 835*t*
Guanabenz, 402*t*
Guanarito virus, 1014–1015
Guanethidine, 402*t*
Guided imagery, 139
Guillain-Barré syndrome, 244*t*, 560–561
  pancreatic health and, 710*b*
Gums, pancreatic health and, 710*b*
Gynecologic history, 897*b*
Gynecologic surgery, 901*t*, 906
Gynecologic tests, 895*t*
Gynecomastia, 927

H
H1N1 influenza, 294*b*
Haemophilus influenzae type B otitis media, 612
HAI; *See* Health care-associated infection
Hair, 952, 953*f*
Hair loss, cancer treatment-related, 169

Hallucination, 1085–1086
  auditory, 1103
  command, 1108
Hallucinogens, 1072*t*, 1076
Hallux valgus, 736
Halo sign, 502, 502*f*
Halo traction, 512*f*
Haloperidol, 1086*b*
Hand, fascial compartments of, 742*f*
Hand hygiene, 108–109, 1128
Handicap, 177
Hands-only cardiopulmonary resuscitation, 1032–1033
Hartmann's solution, 52*t*
Harvester ant bite, 1031
Hashimoto's thyroiditis, 244*t*, 845
Haversian system, 716
Hawthorne, 431*b*
Head, secondary survey of, 1023*b*
Head halter traction, 740*f*
Head injury, 500–508
  diagnosis of, 502, 503*f*
  drug therapy for, 514*t*
  etiology of, 500
  increased intracranial pressure in, 506–508
    complications of, 508
    etiology and pathophysiology of, 506, 506*f*
    signs and symptoms of, 506–507, 507*f*
    treatment of, 507–508, 508*b*
  levels of consciousness and, 502*b*
  nursing care plan for, 504*b*
  pathophysiology of, 500–501, 501*f*
  patient teaching in, 505*b*
  signs and symptoms of, 501–502, 502*b*, 502*f*
  surgery for, 503
Head lice, 973–974, 974*f*
Headache, 542, 545–546, 546*b*
Health care-associated infection
  cost of, 112–113
  medical and surgical asepsis and, 115
  nursing interventions in, 110, 113*t*
  risk factors for, 113*t*
  sepsis and septic shock in, 115
  surveillance and reporting in, 114–115
Health care-associated pneumonia, 296–297
Health care financing, 4–6
Health care goals, 6–10
Health care team collaboration, 2–3
Health care worker
  blood-borne pathogen exposure and, 230–231
  with HIV infection, 230*b*
  safety in psychiatric unit, 1104*b*
  safety through standard precautions, 1129
  substance abuse and, 1081
Health history, preoperative, 65*b*
Health insurance, 4–6, 5*b*, 6*b*
Health Insurance Portability and Accountability Act, 22*b*
Health maintenance organization, 5
Health promotion
  in arthritis, 745*b*
  in aspirin to prevent myocardial infarction, 453*b*
  in assessment and management of hypertension, 406*b*
  in avoiding hepatitis, 625*b*
  in bladder health, 767*b*
  in cataract prevention, 598*b*
  in colon cancer preventive measures, 674*b*
  in danger signals of glaucoma, 572*b*, 602*b*
  in dangers of cocaine and methamphetamine, 528*b*

Health promotion (*Continued*)
in dangers of toxic agents, 352*b*
in diet and memory, 1087*b*
in drinking in moderation, 395*b*
in drinks and substances to avoid in bladder control, 782*b*
in effects of smoking, 148*b*
in exercise for brain, 1087*b*
in goiter prevention, 824*b*
Healthy People 2020 and, 6–7, 7*b*
in heart-healthy lifestyle recommendations, 448*b*
in hepatitis B, 698*b*
in hypersensitivity reactions, 240*b*
in insulin and exercise, 862*b*
in maintaining abdominal tone, 625*b*
in maintaining healthy immune system, 203*b*
in meningitis immunization, 542*b*
in poison prevention, 1029*b*
in preparing disaster supplies, 998*b*
in preparing safe water, 1003*b*
in preventing blood disorders, 336*b*
in preventing cardiovascular disease in women, 375*b*
in preventing infections at home, 121*b*
in preventing sexually transmitted infections, 950*b*
in preventing spread of herpes virus, 970*b*
in preventing toxoplasmosis, 224*b*
in protecting nervous system, 479*b*
in protection against mosquitoes and ticks, 544*b*
in protection from influenza, 295*b*
in risk factors for stroke, 528*b*
in safe food handling, 1029*b*
in safe sexual practices, 218*b*
in signs of possible throat cancer, 283*b*
in smoking
   age-related macular degeneration and, 608*b*
   musculoskeletal health and, 719*b*
   tobacco cessation and, 261*b*, 712*b*
in stretching for upper back, 729*b*
in sun exposure precautions, 955*b*
in symptoms of ovarian cancer, 908*b*
in testicular self-evaluation, 921*b*, 921*f*, 933*b*
in using CAM therapies for menopause, 891*b*
in warning signs of cancer, 151*b*
in warning signs of heart attack, 376*b*
in women's health care, 892–894
   diagnostic tests and, 888*f*, 894, 897*b*
   health screening and assessments in, 892–894, 893*f*
Hearing aid, 587*b*, 588–589, 590, 590*f*
Hearing-assistive devices, 591
Hearing impairment, 588–589
Hearing loss, 585–591
common causes of, 581*b*
communication in, 587–588, 587*b*
community care in, 591
coping with, 581*b*
in labyrinthitis, 613
in Mèniére's disease, 613–614
in otosclerosis, 614–615
rehabilitation in, 590–591, 590*f*, 591*f*
Heart, 371–372, 372*f*
aging-related changes in, 375
autonomic system effects on, 476*t*
cardiac cycle and, 373
conduction system of, 372, 373*f*
ejection fraction and, 373
sickle cell disease and, 354*f*
Heart attack, 455–461

Heart attack (*Continued*)
aspirin in prevention of, 453*b*
cardiogenic shock in, 1035
complications after, 461*t*
diabetes-related, 875
diagnosis of, 459, 459*t*
emotional and behavioral responses to, 462*b*
etiology and pathophysiology of, 458, 458*f*
Joint Commission Core Measures for, 460*b*
patient teaching in, 463*b*
rehabilitation in, 462–464, 463*t*
signs and symptoms of, 458–459
treatment of, 459–460, 460*b*
warning signs of, 376*b*
Heart block, 436, 438
Heart disease, 426–448
angina pectoris in, 453–455, 455*f*, 456*b*
cardiac trauma in, 446–447
cardiogenic shock in, 461–464
cardiomyopathy in, 444, 444*b*
causes of, 375–376
common problems in, 393–395
   altered tissue perfusion in, 394–395
   edema in, 393–394
   fatigue and dyspnea in, 385*b*, 393
   impaired tissue integrity in, 395
   pain in, 394
community care in, 448
coronary artery disease in, 451–464
   complementary and alternative medicine for, 431*b*
   diagnosis of, 452
   etiology of, 451
   heart failure in, 426–427
   hypertension and, 401
   nutrition considerations in, 453*b*
   pathophysiology of, 452, 452*f*
   signs and symptoms of, 452, 452*b*
   treatment of, 452–453, 454*t*
diagnostic tests and procedures in, 377–384, 377*f*, 378*t*, 384*f*
dietary control in, 447–448, 448*b*
drug therapy for, 447
dysrhythmias in, 435–442
   atrial flutter and fibrillation in, 437–438, 437*f*
   automatic implantable cardioverter-defibrillator for, 442
   cardiac pacemaker for, 440–441, 441*b*, 441*f*
   cardioversion for, 440
   complete heart block in, 438
   drug therapy for, 438*t*
   etiology of, 435
   evaluation of ECG rhythm strip in, 435*b*
   pathophysiology of, 435, 435*f*
   premature ventricular contractions in, 438
   radiofrequency catheter ablation for, 442
   signs and symptoms of, 435–436, 436*f*
   ventricular fibrillation in, 440
   ventricular tachycardia in, 438–440
heart failure in, 426–431
   acute pulmonary edema and, 431
   classification of, 427*t*
   drug therapy for, 429–431, 429*t*
   etiology of, 426–427, 427*f*
   Joint Commission core measures for, 434*b*
   left-sided, 428*t*, 431–432
   nursing care plan for, 432*b*
   nutrition considerations in, 430*b*
   pathophysiology of, 427–428, 427*b*

Heart disease (*Continued*)
   right-sided, 428*t*, 432
   signs and symptoms of, 428–429, 428*f*
   treatment of, 430–431, 430*f*, 431*f*
   warfarin for, 434*b*
history taking in, 384–385, 385*b*
infective endocarditis in, 442–443, 443*f*
metabolic syndrome and, 377*b*
myocardial infarction in, 455–461
   aspirin to prevent, 453*b*
   complications after, 461*t*
   diagnosis of, 459, 459*t*
   emotional and behavioral responses to, 462*b*
   etiology and pathophysiology of, 458, 458*f*
   rehabilitation in, 462–464, 463*t*
   signs and symptoms of, 458–459
   treatment of, 459–460, 460*b*
   warning signs of, 376*b*
nursing diagnoses in, 388–392, 389*t*
oxygen therapy in, 447
pericarditis in, 443–444, 443*f*
physical assessment in, 385–388, 386*b*, 386*f*, 386*t*
   blood pressure and, 387
   bruits and, 387
   pulses in, 387, 387*b*, 387*f*
   skin and, 388
prevention of, 376–377
risk factors for, 377*t*
as surgical risk factor, 67*t*
valvular, 444–446
   aortic regurgitation in, 445
   aortic stenosis in, 445
   medical treatment for, 445–446
   mitral regurgitation in, 445
   mitral stenosis in, 445
   valve replacement surgery for, 446, 446*f*
warning signs of heart attack, 376*b*
women and, 375, 375*b*
Heart failure, 375–376, 426–431
acute pulmonary edema and, 431
after myocardial infarction, 461*t*
classification of, 427*t*
complementary and alternative medicine for, 431*b*
drug therapy for, 429–431, 429*t*
etiology of, 426–427, 427*f*
Joint Commission core measures for, 434*b*
left-sided, 428*t*, 431–432
nursing care plan for, 432*b*
nutrition considerations in, 430*b*
pathophysiology of, 427–428, 427*b*
right-sided, 428*t*, 432
signs and symptoms of, 428–429, 428*f*
treatment of, 430–431, 430*f*, 431*f*
warfarin for, 434*b*
Heart transplantation, 431, 466
Heartburn, 646
Heat application
as method of pain management, 138
patient safety in, 754*b*
patient teaching in, 754*b*
in rheumatoid arthritis, 754
Heatstroke, 1026–1027
Heimlich valve, 317
Helicobacter pylori
in gastric cancer, 657
in gastritis, 649
in peptic ulcer, 650
Helicobacter pylori antibody test, 626*t*
Helminths, 103
Hemarthrosis, 340, 361, 361*f*

Hematemesis
  in esophageal varices, 704
  in peptic ulcer, 651
Hematocrit, 23, 336
  normal values of, 207t
  reference intervals for, 1119t
Hematologic disorders, 346–367
  anemia in, 346–349
    aplastic, 352, 352f
    data collection in, 349–351, 351b, 351f
    diagnosis of, 348
    etiology of, 346–347, 347t
    nutrition considerations in, 348b
    pathophysiology of, 347, 347f, 348f
    signs and symptoms of, 348, 348t
    treatment of, 349, 349t
    types of, 353t
  bone marrow and stem cell transplantation
    in, 364–366
  causes of, 334–335, 334b, 335b
  common problems related to, 343–344
    anorexia in, 343
    bone marrow failure in, 344
    excessive bleeding in, 343, 343b, 343f
    fatigue in, 343
    infection in, 343–344
    pain in, 343
  community care in, 367
  data collection for, 336–340, 339b
  diagnostic tests and procedures in,
    336, 337t
  disseminated intravascular coagulation in,
    362
  hemophilia in, 361–362, 361f
  home care in, 342b
  leukemia in, 355–359
    etiology of, 355, 355t
    nursing care plan for, 357b
    signs and symptoms of,
      355–356
    treatment of, 356–357, 356b
  multiple myeloma in, 360–361
  nursing diagnoses in, 340–341, 341t
  physical assessment in, 339–340
  polycythemia vera in, 354–355
  prevention of, 335–336, 336b
  sickle cell disease in, 353–354, 353f, 354f
  therapies for, 362–367
    biologic response modifiers in, 358
    iron therapy in, 366–367
    leukapheresis in, 364
    oxygen therapy in, 366
    splenectomy in, 367
    transfusions in, 362–364
    vitamin B$_{12}$ therapy in, 367
  thrombocytopenia in, 359–360, 359f
Hematologic system, 331–344
  changes with aging, 334
  chronic renal failure and, 803f
  cirrhosis and, 703f
  components of blood and, 331, 335
  functions of blood and, 331
  lymphatic system interaction with vascular
    system and, 334
  nutrients needed for erythropoiesis and,
    335b
  plasma proteins and, 331
  platelets and, 333–334
  production of blood cells and, 332, 333f
  red blood cells and, 332
  white blood cells and, 332–333
Hematology, 334, 1119t
Hematoma, 89, 146
Hematuria, 773
Hemicolectomy, 675

Hemiglossectomy, 644
Hemiparesis, 492, 530–532
Hemiplegia, 492, 530–532
Hemochromatosis, 708
Hemodialysis, 800, 805–806, 805f, 806f, 811b
  dietary restrictions in, 810t
  noncompliance in, 811b
Hemodynamic monitoring, 378t
Hemoglobin, 23
  normal values of, 207t
  reference intervals for, 1119t
Hemoglobin A1C test, 24
Hemoglobin A1c test, 827, 828t
Hemoglobin electrophoresis, 337t
Hemolysis, 334, 347
Hemolytic anemia, 347, 349
Hemolytic jaundice, 701–702
Hemophilia, 361–362, 361f
Hemoptysis
  in plague, 1013
  in tuberculosis, 298–299
Hemorrhage
  abnormal uterine, 904–905, 905b
  after cerebral aneurysm repair, 534
  after kidney surgery, 791
  breakthrough, 904
  cancer treatment-related, 169b
  in disseminated intravascular coagulation,
    362
  gastrointestinal
    mechanical ventilation-related, 327t
    in peptic ulcer, 651, 653b
  in hematologic disorders, 343, 343b, 343f
  intracerebral, 541
  low platelet count and, 360b
  postoperative, 92t, 93
  pressure points for, 343f
  primary survey and, 1023b
  rectal
    in colorectal cancer, 675
    in diverticulitis, 668
    in inflammatory bowel disease, 671
  subarachnoid, 530
  techniques to control, 343b
  trauma-related, 1023–1024
Hemorrhagic fever, 1011t
Hemorrhoidectomy, 686
Hemorrhoids, 684f, 685–686
Hemothorax, 313, 313f, 1025
Hemovac drainage system, 90, 90f
Heparin-induced thrombocytopenia, 416
Hepatic disorders, 694–698
  causes of, 624
  cirrhosis in, 701–703, 702f, 703f, 704b, 707f
  deaths in, 701b
  drug therapy for, 696t
  hepatitis in, 694–698
  liver cancer in, 149, 708
  liver transplantation for, 707, 707b
  prevention of, 625
  as surgical risk factor, 67t
Hepatitis
  in acquired immunodeficiency syndrome,
    223
  avoiding contraction of, 625b
  complementary and alternative medicine
    for, 699b, 701b
  complications of, 701
  diagnosis of, 695–696, 696t
  epidemic potential in natural disaster, 1004t
  etiology and pathophysiology of, 694
  focused assessment in, 698b
  home care considerations in, 699b
  liver cancer risk and, 149
  prevention of, 699–701

Hepatitis (*Continued*)
  signs and symptoms of, 694–695, 695t
  treatment of, 696–698, 696t
Hepatitis A virus, 694, 695t, 699b
Hepatitis B virus, 694, 695t
  among Asian Americans, 694b
  community care in, 713
  health promotion goals for, 698b
  home care considerations in, 699b
  liver cancer and, 149
  sexually transmitted, 942t
Hepatitis C virus, 694, 695t
  home care considerations in, 699b
  intravenous drug use and, 694
  risk in hemodialysis, 805
  transmission of, 699b
Hepatitis D virus, 694, 695t
Hepatitis E virus, 694, 695t
Hepatobiliary scintigraphy, 626t
Hepatoiminodiacetic acid scan, 626t, 692
Hepatoma, 708
Hepatotoxicity of antipsychotics, 1105–1106
Hepsera; *See* Adefovir dipivoxil
Herbal supplements, 65b
  for benign prostatic hyperplasia, 928
  for infertility, 889b
  sedative effects of, 1087b
Hernia, 669f
  hiatal, 645–646
  inguinal, 663–664, 664f
Herniated disk, 517–520, 517f
Hernioplasty, 664
Herniorrhaphy, 664
Heroin, 1073
Herpes simplex virus, 970–971, 970b, 970f
  in acquired immunodeficiency syndrome,
    221–223
  in Bell's palsy, 548
Herpes zoster, 971–972, 971b, 971f, 972b
Hesitancy, 775b
Heterotopic ossification, 515
Hiatal hernia, 645–646, 649f
Hiccoughs, 88b
HIDA scan, 692
High-fiber diet
  for diverticular disease, 668b
  for hemorrhoids, 686
  for immobilized patient, 743b
  for irritable bowel syndrome, 665
High-frequency jet ventilation, 325
High-intensity focused ultrasound, 929t
Highway safety, 1019
Hip
  flexion contracture of, 728, 728f
  total replacement of, 749–750, 749f, 750f, 751b
Hip abductor wedge, 750b, 750f
HIPAA; *See* Health Insurance Portability and
    Accountability Act
Hirsutism
  in Cushing syndrome, 852
  in polycystic ovarian syndrome, 904
Histamine, 197t
Histamine$_2$ receptor antagonists, 646, 647t
Histoplasmosis, 223, 298
Histrionic personality disorder, 1114b
HIT; *See* Heparin-induced thrombocytopenia
HIV; *See* Human immunodeficiency virus
HIV encephalopathy, 225
HMG-CoA reductase inhibitors, 454t
HMO; *See* Health maintenance organization
Hoarseness, 262
Hodgkin's lymphoma, 249–250, 251f, 252f
Holistic assessment, 7b
Holistic care, 7–10, 7b
Holter monitor, 378t

Home care
  in acid-base imbalances, 50
  after ear surgery, 617b
  after retinal surgery, 607b
  in chronic illness, 191–193, 191f
  in dehiscence or evisceration, 93b
  evaluation of treatment in, 342b
  in female reproductive system disorders, 915
  in fluid imbalances, 40
  in hepatitis, 699b
  in hypoglycemia, 861b
  infection prevention and control and, 121, 121b
  in intravenous fluid therapy, 59b
  maintaining medication record in, 134b
  in musculoskeletal disorders, 760
  pain management and, 141
  postoperative instructions and, 97b
  of tracheostomy, 286b
  in upper respiratory system disorders, 290
Home safety, 1019, 1020b
Homeostasis, 198
Homocysteine, 378t
Homograft for burn injury, 986–987
Homonymous hemianopsia, 532, 532f
Honeymoon cystitis, 785
Hookworm, 103
Hordeolum, 577t
Hormone(s), 819t, 822
  adrenal, 821, 821f, 822f
  effects of aging on, 822
  in inflammatory response, 108
  for osteoporosis, 756b
  pancreatic, 821–822, 823f, 824f
  pituitary, 819, 820f
  in renal function, 766t
  thyroid, 819–821
Hormone replacement therapy, 891–892
Hormone therapy
  for cancer, 163t, 164–165
  for prostate cancer, 935t
Hornet sting, 1031
Horny cell layer of skin, 953f
Hospital-acquired infection, 89–90
Hospital-acquired pneumonia, 296–297
Hospital preparedness in disaster, 1000–1001
Host in infection, 100, 102b
Hostile patient, 1113b
Hot and cold foods, 118b
HPV; See Human papillomavirus
Human bite, 1030
Human immunodeficiency virus, 942t;
    See also Acquired immunodeficiency
    syndrome
  exposure to, 217–218, 217b
  life cycle of, 216f, 217t
Human immunodeficiency virus testing, 219, 220b, 220t
Human papillomavirus, 942t
  oral cancer and, 644
  prevention of, 940
Humerus, 717f
Humidification, 320–321
Huntington's disease, 562
Hurricane, 999b, 1000b
Hydralazine, 402t
Hydrea; See Hydroxyurea
Hydrocele, 925–926, 926f
Hydrocephalus
  in bacterial meningitis, 542
  brain tumor-related, 541
  increased intracranial pressure-related, 508
  subarachnoid hemorrhage and, 534
Hydrochlorothiazide, 402t

Hydrocodone, 170t
Hydrocortisone, 821, 822f
HydroDIURIL; See Hydrochlorothiazide
Hydromorphone, 170t
Hydronephritis, 790–791
Hydronephrosis, 927
Hydrostatic pressure, 33
Hydroureter, 927
17-Hydroxycorticosteroids, 824b
Hydroxyurea, 349t, 354
Hydroxyzine, 37t
Hyoscyamine, 666t
Hyperalgesia in fibromyalgia, 254
Hyperbaric oxygen, 409
Hypercalcemia, 42t, 45
  in cancer, 171
  in multiple myeloma, 360
Hypercapnia, 272–273, 314–315
Hypercarbia, 314–315
Hyperchloremia, 45
Hypercholesterolemia, 454t
Hyperesthesia in Guillain-Barré syndrome, 560
Hyperglycemia
  in diabetes mellitus, 859
  hypoglycemia versus, 873b
  rebound, 874
  visual loss and, 573
Hyperglycemic hyperosmolar nonketotic syndrome, 874
Hyperkalemia, 42t, 44, 982
Hyperlipidemia, 452
Hypermagnesemia, 42t, 45
Hypernatremia, 41–43, 42t
Hyperopia, 594, 595f
Hyperparathyroidism, 846–847, 846b, 846t
Hyperphosphatemia, 42t, 45
Hyperpigmentation, 967
Hyperpyrexia, 209–211
Hyperreflexia, 514–515
Hypersecretion, 823–824
Hypersensitivity, 236–239
  desensitization for, 238–239
  diagnostic tests for, 237–238
  drug therapy for, 238, 239t
  to drugs, 238
  etiology and pathophysiology of, 236–237, 236f
  to foods, 238
  identification of allergens in, 237, 237t
  to latex, 238
  nursing goals for, 240b
  signs and symptoms of, 237
  substances causing, 241b
Hypersomnia, 1052
Hypertension, 398–404
  in acute glomerulonephritis, 789
  antihypertensive therapy for, 401, 402t, 403b
  blood pressure classification and, 399t
  in cardiovascular disorders, 375
  complementary and alternative medicine for, 405b
  complications of, 401, 406b
  cultural considerations in, 400b
  decreasing dietary sodium and, 405b
  end-stage kidney disease and, 766–767
  etiology of, 398–400
  heart failure and, 426–427
  hypertensive crisis and, 401–404
  monitoring of, 406b
  pathophysiology of, 400, 400f
  retinopathy and, 608
  risk factors for, 399t
  signs and symptoms of, 400–401

Hypertensive crisis, 401–404
Hypertensive urgency, 401–404
Hyperthermia, 209–211
Hyperthyroidism, 839–840, 840f, 841b
Hypertonic saline test, 824b
Hypertonic solution, 32–33, 51
Hypertrophic cardiomyopathy, 444b
Hyperuricemia, cancer treatment-related, 169
Hyperventilation, 47
Hypervolemia, 39
Hypnosis, 77t, 139
Hypocalcemia, 42t, 44
Hypocapnia, 273
Hypochloremia, 45
Hypodermoclysis, 56
Hypofunction of pituitary gland, 835, 835t
Hypoglossal nerve, 475t
Hypoglycemia, 23, 874, 876–877, 1026
  complications in, 876
  diagnosis and treatment of, 876
  in elderly, 860b, 861b
  etiology and pathophysiology of, 876
  home treatment of, 861b
  hyperglycemia versus, 873b
  insulin infusion and, 866b
  ketoacidosis versus, 871t
  signs and symptoms of, 876
Hypoglycemic agents
  injectable, 866, 866b, 866t
  oral, 862–863, 862t
Hypokalemia, 42t, 44, 394b
Hypomagnesemia, 42t, 45
Hypomania, 1051
Hyponatremia, 40–41, 42t
  in burn injury, 982
  in syndrome of inappropriate secretion of antidiuretic hormone, 838
Hypoparathyroidism, 845–846, 846t
Hypophosphatemia, 42t, 45
Hypophysectomy, 834, 834f, 835b
Hyposecretion, 823–824
Hypostatic pneumonia, 84, 92t
Hypothalamus, 473f, 473t, 819t, 919
Hypothermia, 1027, 1027b
Hypothyroidism, 844–845, 844b
  ablation therapy-related, 840
  self-care management of, 844b
Hypotonic solution, 32–33, 51
Hypoventilation, 47
Hypovolemia, 39, 346, 1033–1035
Hypovolemic shock, 1033–1035, 1035t, 1036f
  in multiple trauma, 1026
  in peptic ulcer-related gastrointestinal bleeding, 651
  postoperative, 93
Hypoxemia, 48–49
Hypoxemic respiratory failure, 314
Hypoxia, 260b, 274
Hysterectomy, 901t, 903–904
  nursing care plan for, 898b
  for uterine fibroids, 905
Hysteroscopic endometrial ablation, 905
Hysteroscopy, 895t, 905
Hytrin; See Terazosin

I
IABP; See Intraaortic balloon pump
Iatrogenic, term, 203
IBD; See Inflammatory bowel disease
IBS; See Irritable bowel syndrome
Ibuprofen
  for cancer pain, 170t
  for dysmenorrhea, 903t
Ibutilide, 438t
Icterus, 701–702

Ideas of reference, 1104
Identification as defense mechanism, 1067*t*
Ileal conduit, 796*f*, 797
Ileal reservoir, 796*f*, 797
Ileoanal reservoir, 681*f*
Ileocecal valve, 620
Ileostomy, 680–681, 680*f*, 685*b*
Ilium, 717*f*
Illusion, 1085–1086, 1104
Imaging studies
    of breast, 895*t*
    in cancer, 154
    in cardiovascular disease, 378*t*
    in ear disorders, 584*t*
    in gallstones, 692
    in gastrointestinal disorders, 626*t*
    in head injury, 503*f*
    in immune and lymphatic disorders,
        206–209
    in musculoskeletal disorders, 720*t*
    in neurologic disorders, 481*t*
    in respiratory disorders, 265*t*
    in stroke, 529*f*
    in tuberculosis, 299
    in urinary disorders, 767–768, 769*t*
Imbalanced nutrition, 18*b*
Imipramine, 1056*t*, 1123*t*
Immediate hypersensitivity, 236, 236*f*
Immediate preoperative care, 72–74
Immobility, 724
    in Guillain-Barré syndrome, 562
    in neurologic disorders, 492
    nursing care plan for, 180*b*
    prevention of, 178–179, 178*b*, 179*t*
Immobilization in spinal cord injury, 512,
        512*f*, 513*f*
Immune deficiency, 198–199
    in acquired immunodeficiency syndrome;
        See Acquired immunodeficiency
        syndrome
    diagnosis and treatment in, 234–235, 234*b*
    prevention of infection in, 235*b*
Immune disorders, 233–254
    allergy in, 236–239
        desensitization for, 238–239
        diagnostic tests for, 237–238
        drug therapy for, 238, 239*t*
        to drugs, 238
        etiology and pathophysiology of,
            236–237, 236*f*
        to foods, 238
        identification of allergens in, 237, 237*t*
        to latex, 238
        signs and symptoms of, 237
    anaphylactic shock in, 241–243, 241*b*, 242*f*
    autoimmune, 243
        diagnosis of, 234–235, 234*b*,
            243–245
        signs and symptoms of, 243,
            244*t*
        systemic lupus erythematosus in,
            245–248, 246*f*, 247*t*, 248*b*
        treatment and nursing management of,
            245
    data collection in, 205–209, 206*b*
    diagnostic tests for, 206–209, 207*t*
    nursing diagnoses for, 210*t*
    prevention of, 204–205, 204*b*, 204*f*
Immune function reference intervals, 1127*t*
Immune system, 195–212
    effects of aging on, 197–198
    fever and, 209–211
    functions of, 196–197, 197*t*
    immunosuppression and, 212
    maturation of blood cells and, 196*f*

Immune system (*Continued*)
    nutrition and, 212
    organs and structures of, 195–198,
        196*f*, 197*t*
    protective mechanisms of, 198–203
        immune response in, 198–203, 200*f*, 201*t*,
            202*f*
        immunity against disease and, 202–203,
            202*f*
        inflammatory response in, 198, 199*f*
        types of immunity in, 199–202
Immune thrombocytopenic purpura, 359
Immunity
    compromised, 228*b*
    tuberculosis and, 301
    types of, 199–202, 202*f*
Immunization, 204–205
Immunocompetence, 215
Immunoglobulins, 207*t*
Immunomodulators, 308*t*, 696*t*
Immunoscintigraphy, 206–209
Immunosuppression, 212
    cancer treatment-related, 168–169
Immunosuppressives
    ideal actions of, 234*b*
    for kidney transplantation, 808
    for pain management, 136
    therapeutic drug monitoring reference
        intervals for, 1123*t*
Immunotherapy, 165
Imodium; *See* Loperamide
Impacted cerumen, 612
Impairment, 177
Impedance plethysmography, 378*t*
Imperforate hymen, 904
Implanted infusion port, 163, 164*f*
Implementation in nursing process, 26–27
Impotence, 923–924
Impulsivity in borderline personality
    disorder, 1114
Imuran; *See* Azathioprine
IMV; *See* Intermittent mandatory ventilation
In vitro fertilization, 890*b*
Incarcerated hernia, 663–664
Incentive spirometer, 71*b*
Incomplete fracture, 737*b*
Incontinence
    after stroke, 532
    in neurologic disorders, 493–495
Increased intracranial pressure, 506–508
    in brain tumor, 539
    complications of, 508
    etiology and pathophysiology of,
        506, 506*f*
    nursing care plan for, 504*b*
    signs and symptoms of, 506–507, 507*f*
    treatment of, 507–508, 508*b*
Incretin mimetics, 866, 866*t*
Incus, 579, 580*f*
Indapamide, 402*t*
Independence promotion in chronic illness,
    186–187, 186*t*, 187*f*
Inderal; *See* Propranolol
Index of suspicion, 1022
Indiana pouch, 797
Indirect inguinal hernia, 663–664, 664*f*
Ineffective airway clearance, 271
Ineffective breathing patterns, 272–273, 272*f*
Infarct, 435
Infarction, 458
Infection, 100–103
    body defense against, 103–108, 104*b*,
        106*t*
    cancer treatment-related, 168–169
    chain of, 108, 108*b*, 108*f*

Infection (*Continued*)
    cutaneous, 966–970
        acne in, 967–969
        contact isolation requirements in, 967*b*
        dermatitis in, 966–967
        fungal, 972–973, 972*b*, 973*f*
        herpes simplex in, 970–971, 970*b*, 970*f*
        herpes zoster in, 971–972, 971*b*,
            971*f*, 972*b*
        in intravenous therapy, 54*t*
        psoriasis in, 969, 969*f*
        Stevens-Johnson syndrome in, 969–970
    diagnostic tests for, 116
    disease-producing pathogens and, 101–103
    factors influencing, 101, 102*b*
    at fracture site, 741
    fungal
        in acquired immunodeficiency
            syndrome, 223–224
        cutaneous, 972–973, 972*b*, 973*b*, 973*f*
        recurrent, 973*b*
        respiratory, 298
    health care-associated
        cost of, 112–113
        medical and surgical asepsis and, 115
        nursing interventions in, 110, 113*t*
        risk factors for, 113*t*
        sepsis and septic shock in, 115
        surveillance and reporting in, 114–115
    hospital-acquired, 89–90
    immune response and, 108
    inflammatory response and, 105–107, 107*f*
    intravenous therapy-related, 54*t*
    mechanical ventilation-related, 327*t*
    normal flora and, 105
    parasitic
        in acquired immunodeficiency
            syndrome, 224
        in pediculosis and scabies, 973–974, 974*f*
    postoperative prevention of, 86
    respiratory tract, 294, 300*t*
        otitis media and, 612
        prevention of, 113*t*
        risk for, 261*b*, 273–274
    risk for
        in hematologic disorders, 343–344
        in leukemia, 355*t*
        in spinal cord injury, 515
    risk in diabetes mellitus, 859
    sexually transmitted, 938–950, 942*t*
        bacterial vaginosis in, 939
        candidiasis in, 939
        chlamydial infection in, 949*b*
        community care in, 950
        contraception choices and, 939*b*
        diagnostic tests for, 941
        history taking in, 941–948, 941*b*, 948*b*
        human papillomavirus in, 940
        lesions in, 940, 940*b*
        media effects on, 939*b*
        pelvic inflammatory disease in, 939
        prevention of, 948–950, 950*b*
        reporting of, 940
        risk factors for, 939–940
        transmission of, 940–941
    susceptibility to, 110*t*
    urinary tract
        cystitis in, 785–788
        drug therapy for, 786*t*
        in elderly, 786*b*
        postoperative, 92*t*
        prevention of, 113*t*, 788*b*
        pyelonephritis in, 788–789
        urethritis in, 788
    wound, 91, 92*t*

Infection prevention and control, 108–111
in abdominal wound, 117*b*
after tracheostomy, 286
antimicrobial agents for, 114*t*, 118, 119*t*
in burn, 985–986, 992
during cancer treatment, 168*b*
community care and, 120–121
cultural considerations in, 118*b*
data collection in, 115–116
expanded precautions in, 106*t*, 109
hand hygiene in, 108–109
health care-associated infections and
cost of, 112–113
medical and surgical asepsis and, 115
nursing interventions against, 110, 113*t*
risk factors for, 113*t*
sepsis and septic shock in, 115
surveillance and reporting in,
114–115
home care and, 121, 121*b*
in home of HIV positive person, 228*b*
in immune disorders, 235*b*
in immunodeficient patient, 235*b*
long-term care and, 121
patient teaching in, 109–110, 120*b*
personal protective equipment in, 109–110,
111*f*
protective environment in, 110
respiratory hygiene and cough etiquette in,
110–111, 112*f*
standard precautions in, 109, 109*b*
in tuberculosis, 301
Infective endocarditis, 442–443, 443*f*
Inferior vena cava, 374
Infertility, 888–890, 889*b*, 890*b*
complementary and alternative medicine
for, 889*b*
emotional impact of, 889*b*
female, 888–890
male, 924–925
Infiltration in intravenous therapy, 54*t*
Inflammation, 105–107, 107*f*
in burn injury, 982
in bursitis, 736
in cholecystitis, 691
in cirrhosis, 702*b*
in epididymitis, 932
in gastritis, 649–650
in orchitis, 932
in peritonitis, 673
in prostatitis, 932–933
Inflammatory bowel disease, 670–672, 670*t*,
671*f*
Inflammatory heart disease, 442–444
cardiomyopathy in, 385, 444, 444*b*
infective endocarditis in, 442–443, 443*f*
pericarditis in, 376, 443–444, 443*f*
Inflammatory infections of skin, 966–970
acne in, 967–969
contact isolation requirements in, 967*b*
dermatitis in, 966–967
psoriasis in, 969, 969*f*
Stevens-Johnson syndrome in, 969–970
Inflammatory musculoskeletal disorders,
745–750
Lyme disease in, 745
osteoarthritis in, 745–746, 746*b*, 747*t*
Inflammatory urinary disorders, 785–790
acute glomerulonephritis in, 789
chronic glomerulonephritis in, 789–790
cystitis in, 785–788
nephrotic syndrome in, 790
pyelonephritis in, 788–789
urethritis in, 788
Infliximab, 666*t*, 672

Influenza, 294–295, 294*b*, 295*b*
pandemic, 1015–1016
Influenza vaccine, 261
Infratentorial brain tumor, 539–540
Ingestant allergens, 237*t*
Inguinal hernia, 663–664, 664*f*
Inhalant allergens, 237*t*
Inhalants abuse, 1076
Inhalation anesthesia, 77*t*
Inhalational anthrax, 1011*t*
Inhaled poisons, 1030
Injectable allergens, 237*t*
Injectable contraceptives, 884*t*
Injectable hypoglycemic agents, 866,
866*b*, 866*t*
Injection practices, 1129
Injury prevention, postoperative, 85–86
Inner ear, 580
labyrinthitis and, 613
Mèniére's disease and, 613
otosclerosis and, 614–615
Inotropic agonists, 429*t*
Inotropin; *see* Dopamine
Insect bites and stings, 1031, 1031*b*
Insensible water loss, 33–34
Inspection, 20
Inspiration, 259
Inspiratory capacity, 269*f*
Inspiratory reserve volume, 269*f*
Instillation
of ear medications, 587, 587*f*, 588*b*
of eyedrops, 578*b*
Institute for Healthcare Improvement
bundles, 16
Instruments, standard precautions and, 1129
Insulin, 819*t*, 822, 823*f*
benign pituitary adenoma effects on, 834
blood glucose and, 824*f*
effects of aging on, 822
Insulin pen injector, 864*b*
Insulin pump, 865, 865*f*
Insulin reaction, 1026
Insulin resistance, 857
Insulin therapy, 863–865
exercise and, 862*b*
guidelines for subcutaneous injection in,
864*b*
insulin pump in, 865, 865*f*
prefilled injection pens for, 864*b*
preoperative and postoperative
management of, 866, 866*b*
rotation of injection sites in, 864*f*
types of insulin for, 863*t*
Insulin-to-carbohydrate ratios, 860, 865*b*
Intake and output
after ostomy, 682
in kidney transplantation, 809–810, 810*f*
measuring of, 777
Intal; *See* Cromolyn sodium
Integumentary disorders, 966–994
application of wet compresses or dressings
in, 963
bacterial infections in, 970
burns in, 981–989
classification of, 982*f*, 983*f*, 984*t*
complications of, 988
debridement for, 986
emergency treatment of, 983–984, 984*b*
escharotomy for, 986, 987*f*
etiology and pathophysiology of,
981–982
fluid resuscitation and prevention of
shock in, 985, 985*b*
grafting for, 986–988, 988*f*
infection prevention in, 985–986, 992

Integumentary disorders (*Continued*)
itching in, 993
nursing care plan for, 990*b*
nutritional support in, 993
pain management in, 985, 989–992, 992*b*
patient-family education in, 993
psychosocial support in, 993
rehabilitation for, 988–989, 989*f*
respiratory support in, 984–985
signs and symptoms of, 982
topical medications for, 987*t*
wound treatment in, 986–988
causes of, 954
community care in, 994
cultural considerations in, 958*b*
diagnostic tests and procedures in, 957–958
in elderly, 960*b*
fungal infections in, 972–973, 972*b*,
973*b*, 973*f*
history taking in, 958
inflammatory infections in, 966–970
acne in, 967–969
contact isolation requirements in, 967*b*
dermatitis in, 966–967
psoriasis in, 969, 969*f*
Stevens-Johnson syndrome in, 969–970
laundry requirements in, 962
medicated baths for, 962
nursing diagnoses for, 960, 961*t*
pediculosis and scabies in, 973–974, 974*f*
physical assessment in, 958–960, 958*f*, 959*b*
pressure ulcers in, 977–981
bony prominence susceptible to skin
breakdown and, 977*f*
Braden scale for, 979*f*
cleansing and dressing of, 981
color of purulent exudate in, 981*t*
debridement of, 980–981
documentation of, 981
risk factors and prevention of, 977–978,
978*b*
signs and symptoms of, 978–980, 980*f*
prevention of, 954–956
self-assessment of skin in, 960*b*
skin cancer in, 974–977, 975*f*,
976*f*, 976*t*
skin drainage or weeping in, 957*b*
skin integrity and, 956–958, 956*b*
tinea pedis in, 973
topical therapy for, 963, 963*b*
types of skin lesions in, 959*t*
viral infections in, 970–972
herpes simplex virus in, 970–971,
970*b*, 970*f*
herpes zoster in, 971–972, 971*b*,
971*f*, 972*b*
Integumentary system, 952–963
changes with aging, 953–954, 954*f*
chronic renal failure and, 803*f*
cirrhosis and, 703*f*
functions of skin and, 953
structure of skin, hair, and nails in,
952, 953*f*
sun exposure precautions and, 955*b*
ultraviolet radiation protection and, 955*b*
Intellectualization, 1067*t*
Interdisciplinary care plan, 27
Interferons, 107, 165
Interleukins, 165
Intermediate acting insulin, 863*t*
Intermittent claudication, 385, 407
Intermittent mandatory ventilation, 325–326
Internal fixation of fracture, 738, 738*f*
Internal hemorrhoids, 684*f*, 685
Internal mammary artery graft, 465*f*

Internal radiation therapy, 160–161, 161*b*, 162*f*, 162*t*
Internal urethral sphincter, 764
Interpersonal therapy, 1048
Intervertebral disk rupture, 517–520, 517*f*
Interview, 19–20, 19*b*, 20*b*
Intestinal gas, 635
Intestinal obstruction, 623, 668–670, 669*b*, 669*f*
  ileostomy-related, 685*b*
Intoxication, 1068–1071
Intraaortic balloon pump, 431, 431*f*
Intracapsular cataract extraction, 598
Intracellular fluid, 31–32, 31*f*
Intracerebral hematoma, 501, 501*f*
Intracerebral hemorrhage, 541
Intracranial pressure elevation, 506–508
  complications of, 508
  etiology and pathophysiology of, 506, 506*f*
  nursing care plan for, 504*b*
  signs and symptoms of, 506–507, 507*f*
  treatment of, 507–508, 508*b*
Intracranial tumor, 539–541, 540*f*, 540*t*, 541*f*
Intractable pain, 136
Intracytoplasmic sperm injection, 890*b*
Intraductal papilloma, 908–909
Intramuscular analgesics, 136
Intraocular pressure test, 574*t*
Intraoperative care, 74
Intrarenal acute renal failure, 799
Intrathecal contrast-enhanced computed tomography, 481*t*
Intrathoracic surgery, 315–317
Intrauterine device, 884*t*, 888
Intravenous analgesics, 136
Intravenous anesthesia, 77*t*
Intravenous feeding, 660
Intravenous fluid therapy, 50–57
  administration of, 51–53, 53*b*
  calculation and regulation of flow rate in, 53–57
  central line care in, 56–57, 56*f*
  complications of, 54*t*
  flushing PRN locks or central IV lines in, 55–56
  home care and, 59*b*
  intravenous solutions for, 52*t*
  partial or total parenteral nutrition and, 56–57, 57*b*
  troubleshooting intravenous flow in, 55*t*
Intravenous pyelogram, 769*t*
Intravenous solutions, 52*t*
Intraventricular catheter, 507
Intussusception, 668, 669*f*
Invasive treatments in pain management, 137
Iodine deficiency in goiter, 839
Ionizing radiation, 159
  leukemia and, 355
Ipratropium, 308*t*
Ipratropium and albuterol, 308*t*
Ipsilateral, term, 502
Irinotecan, 675
Iris, 568, 569*f*
Iron
  for chronic renal failure, 804*t*
  foods high in, 348*b*
  needed for erythropoiesis, 335*b*
Iron deficiency anemia, 347, 353*t*
Iron therapy, 366–367
Irreducible hernia, 663–664
Irrigation
  of ear, 585*f*
  in ostomy care, 682–683
Irritable bowel syndrome, 664–665, 665*b*

Ischemia
  bowel, 670
  in cardiovascular disorders, 375
Ischium, 717*f*
Islet cell transplantation, 866
Islets of Langerhans, 621*f*, 819*t*
Ismelin; *See* Guanethidine
Isocarboxazid, 1056*t*
Isometric exercises, 728–729, 729*b*
Isoniazid, 300*t*
Isoptin; *See* Verapamil
Isotalol, 438*t*
Isotonic solution, 32–33, 50
Isotretinoin, 968
Itching, 958
  burn-related, 993
  in cirrhosis, 701
  in hemorrhoids, 686
  in louse infestation, 974
  in urethritis, 788
  vaginal, 890, 906
IUD; *See* Intrauterine device
IVP; *See* Intravenous pyelogram

J

Jackson-Pratt drain, 90, 90*f*, 91*f*
JAMCO mnemonic, 1093–1094, 1094*b*
Januvia; *See* Sitagliptin
Japanese encephalitis, 1004*t*
Jaundice, 339
  in gallstones, 691, 691*t*
  hemolytic, 701–702
Jaw-thrust maneuver, 81, 82*f*
Jehovah's Witness, blood transfusion and, 64*b*
Jejunostomy, 659–660, 659*b*, 659*f*, 660*b*
Jock itch, 972
Joint, 716
  assessment in blood disorders, 340
  dislocation of, 735
  protection of, 753*b*
  sickle cell disease and, 354*f*
Joint Commission Core Measures, 17, 17*b*
  for heart failure, 434*b*
  for myocardial infarction, 460*b*
Joint contracture, 727–728, 728*f*
Joint replacement, 749–750, 750*b*
  postoperative care in, 749–750, 750*f*
  preoperative care in, 749
  total hip replacement in, 749–750, 749*f*, 750*f*, 751*b*
Junin virus, 1011*t*, 1014–1015

K

Kanamycin, 300*t*
Kantrex; *See* Kanamycin
Kaolin-pectin, 37*t*, 38
Kaolin-pectin combinations, 666*t*
Kaopectate; *See* Kaolin-pectin
Kapidex; *See* Dexlansoprazole
Kaposi sarcoma, 225, 225*f*
Karnofsky Performance Scale, 225*t*
Kayexalate; *See* Sodium polystyrene
Kegel exercises, 780*b*
Keloid, 958, 958*f*
Keppra; *See* Levetiracetam
Keratitis, 571, 577*t*, 595–596
Keratoplasty, 596–597, 596*f*
Keratoses, 958
Kernig's sign, 542, 542*f*
Ketoacidosis, 48, 857
  hypoglycemia *versus*, 871*t*
  monitoring for, 871
Ketogenic diet, 525
Ketone(s), 873
Ketone bodies, 828*t*

Ketoprofen, 170*t*
17-Ketosteroids, 824*b*
Kidney, 764, 765*f*
  acute renal failure and, 794, 798–801
  autonomic system effects on, 476*t*
  cancer of, 798
  chronic renal failure and, 801–808
    diabetes mellitus and, 802*b*
    diagnosis of, 802–803
    drug therapy for, 804*t*
    hemodialysis for, 805–806, 805*f*, 806*f*, 811*b*
    kidney transplantation for, 808, 808*b*, 808*f*
    nursing care plan for, 812*b*
    nursing management of, 808–811, 810*f*, 810*t*
    pathophysiology of, 802
    peritoneal dialysis for, 806–808, 807*f*
    signs and symptoms of, 802, 803*f*
  diabetic nephropathy and, 802*b*, 860, 875
  functions of, 765, 766*t*
  glomerulonephritis and, 766
    acute, 789
    chronic, 789–790
    chronic renal failure and, 801–802
  nephrotic syndrome and, 790
  patient teaching in health of, 767*b*
  potentially nephrotoxic substances and, 767*b*
  pyelonephritis and, 788–789
  sickle cell disease and, 354*f*
  trauma to, 794
Kidney, ureter, bladder study, 769*t*
Kidney stones, 791–794, 792*f*, 792*t*
Kidney transplantation, 808, 808*b*, 808*f*
Kiesselbach's area, 258*f*
Killer T cell, 197*t*, 201
Kinins, 197*t*
Klonopin; *See* Clonazepam
Knee
  anterior cruciate ligament injury of, 735
  below-the-knee amputation, 759*f*
  flexion contracture of, 728, 728*f*
  meniscal injury of, 736
  total replacement of, 750
Knee jerk, 479–480
Kock pouch, 680, 681*f*, 683, 796*f*, 797
Konsyl; *See* Psyllium
Korsakoff's syndrome, 1071
KUB; *See* Kidney, ureter, bladder study
Kübler-Ross stages of dying, 172, 172*b*
Kupffer cell, 105
Kussmaul's respiration, 273, 273*f*
Kyphoplasty, 757
Kyphosis, 259, 718, 724

L

Labetalol, 402*t*
Labia majora, 881, 881*f*
Labia minora, 881, 881*f*
Laboratory tests
  in acute viral hepatitis, 696*t*
  in cancer detection, 154–155, 155*b*
  in cardiovascular disease, 378*t*
  in gastrointestinal disorders, 626*t*
  in immune and lymphatic disorders, 206, 207*t*
  preoperative, 66, 66*b*
  reference values in, 1119–1128
Labyrinthitis, 613
Lacosamide, 525*b*
Lacrimal gland, 569
Lactated Ringer's solution, 52*t*
Lactation, 882

Lactose intolerance, 673–674, 674*b*
Lactulose, 696*t*
Laumennec's cirrhosis, 701
Lamictal; *See* Lamotrigine
Laminectomy, 519
Lamivudine, 696*t*
Lamotrigine, 525*b*
Language barriers, psychiatric patient and, 1109*b*
Lanoxin; *See* Digoxin
Lansoprazole, 647*t*
Lantus SoloStar, 864
Lanugo, 1061
Laparoscopic adjustable gastric banding, 640–660
Laparoscopic cholecystectomy, 692, 692*b*
Laparoscopic radical prostatectomy, 929*t*
Laparoscopic surgical fundoplication, 649, 649*f*
Large intestine, 620, 621*f*, 622*f*
Laryngeal cancer, 283–289
    communication after laryngectomy and, 289, 289*f*
    endotracheal intubation and tracheostomy in, 284–286, 285*f*
    etiology and pathophysiology of, 283
    home care of tracheostomy in, 286*b*
    nursing care plan for laryngectomy, 287*b*
    nursing management of, 286–289
    nutrition considerations in, 289*b*
    rehabilitation in, 289, 290*f*
    signs and symptoms of, 283, 283*b*
    treatment of, 283–286, 284*f*
Laryngeal edema, 281–282
Laryngectomy, 283
    airflow after, 284*f*
    nursing care plan for, 287*b*
    nutrition considerations in, 289*b*
Laryngitis, 262, 280
Laryngoscope, 284, 285*f*
Laryngoscopy, 265*t*
Larynx, 257, 258, 258*f*
Laser cauterization of uterine fibroids, 905
Laser in situ keratomileusis, 595
Laser iridotomy, 605
Laser prostatectomy, 929*t*
Laser surgery in eye disorders, 604, 606
Laser trabeculoplasty, 605
LASIK surgery, 595
Lasix; *See* Furosemide
Lassa virus, 1011*t*, 1014–1015
Latent autoimmune diabetes, 857*t*, 858
Latent TB infection, 298
Latex allergy, 65*b*
Laundry
    requirements in skin disorders, 962
    standard precautions and, 1129
Laxatives, 666*t*
    after eating binge, 640
    for liver disorders, 696*t*
Lea's shield contraception, 884*t*
Left atrium, 371
Left coronary artery, 372, 372*f*
Left-sided brain damage, 535*f*
Left-sided heart failure, 428, 428*t*, 431–432
Left ventricle, 371
Left ventricular assist device, 430, 430*f*
Leg, fascial compartments of, 742*f*
Leg exercises, 71*b*, 71*f*
Legal and ethical considerations
    in breast cancer, 910*b*
    in confidentiality and HIV, 230*b*

Legal and ethical considerations (*Continued*)
    in consent for blood administration, 362*b*
    in documentation of patient teaching, 505*b*
    in documentation of skin lesions, 960*b*
    in giving surgical consent, 68*b*
    in immunizations, 204*b*
    in intravenous therapy, 51*b*
    in liver transplantation, 707*b*
    in morning-after pill, 888*b*
    in narcotic pain control at end of life, 138*b*
    in noncompliance with tuberculosis medication, 299*b*
    in nurse use of tobacco, 1075*b*
    in protected health information, 22*b*
    in rights of psychiatric patients, 1108*b*
    in substance abuse among health care workers, 1067*b*
    suicidal patient and, 1059*b*
    in testing for BRCA1 and BRCA2 genes, 910*b*
    in urinary catheterization, 776*b*
    in use of restraints, 184*b*, 1096*b*
    when nurse is HIV positive, 230*b*
Leiomyoma, 905
Lens, 568, 569*f*
    accommodation and, 594, 595*f*
Lentigo maligna melanoma, 976*t*
Leptospirosis, 1004*t*
Lescol; *See* Fluvastatin
Leucovorin, 675
Leukapheresis, 356, 364
Leukemia, 146, 355–359
    etiology of, 355, 355*t*
    nursing care plan for, 357*b*
    risk factors for, 152*t*
    signs and symptoms of, 355–356
    treatment of, 356–357, 356*b*
Leukocyte, 332, 333*f*
    normal range of, 207*t*
    reference intervals for, 1119*t*
Leukocyte count, 336, 337*t*
Leukocytosis, 105
Leukopenia, 334–335, 1068
Leukoplakia, 644
Leukotriene(s), 197*t*
Leukotriene inhibitor, 308*t*, 320
Leukotriene modifiers, 308*t*
Levalbuterol, 308*t*
Levaquin; *See* Levofloxacin
Level of consciousness
    in head injury, 502*b*
    in neurologic disorders, 486, 486*t*
Levetiracetam, 525*b*
Levodopa, 554*t*
Levodopa-carbidopa, 554*t*
Levofloxacin, 786*t*
Levonorgestel-releasing intrauterine system, 903*t*
Levsin; *See* Hyoscyamine
Lewisite, 1007*t*
Lexapro; *See* Escitalopram
LH; *See* Luteinizing hormone
Libido, 920
Librium; *See* Chlordiazepoxide
Licensed practical/vocational nurse, 1–3
    in home care, 192
    nursing practice standards for, 1137
    role in rehabilitation, 189
Lidocaine
    for dysrhythmias, 438*t*
    therapeutic drug monitoring reference intervals for, 1123*t*
Lifestyle alterations in gastroesophageal reflux disease, 646*b*

Lifting and turning of patient, 727
Ligament, 716
    dislocation and, 735
    sprain of, 734–735
Lightning strike, 1032*b*
Lioresal; *See* Baclofen
Lip-reading, 590
Lipitor; *See* Atorvastatin
Lipoprotein-associated phospholipase, 481*t*
Lisinopril, 402*t*
Lithiasis, 791
Lithium carbonate, 1051–1052, 1051*t*, 1123*t*
Lithotripsy for gallstones, 693
Livaio; *See* Pitavastatin
Liver, 621, 621*f*
    autonomic system effects on, 476*t*
    in body defense against infection, 105
    drugs and substances toxic to, 624*b*
    functions of, 622–623
    sickle cell disease and, 354*f*
Liver biopsy, 626*t*
Liver disorders, 694–698
    cancer in, 149, 708
    causes of, 624
    cirrhosis in, 701–703, 702*f*, 703*f*, 704*b*, 707*f*
    deaths in, 701*b*
    drug therapy for, 696*t*
    hepatitis in, 694–698
        in acquired immunodeficiency syndrome, 223
        avoiding contraction of, 625*b*
        complementary and alternative medicine for, 699*b*, 701*b*
        complications of, 701
        diagnosis of, 695–696, 696*t*
        epidemic potential in natural disaster, 1004*t*
        etiology and pathophysiology of, 694
        focused assessment in, 698*b*
        home care considerations in, 699*b*
        liver cancer risk and, 149
        prevention of, 699–701
        signs and symptoms of, 694–695, 695*t*
        treatment of, 696–698, 696*t*
    liver transplantation for, 707, 707*b*
    prevention of, 625
    propylthiouracil-related, 840*b*
    as surgical risk factor, 67*t*
Liver spots, 954, 954*f*
Local anesthesia, 76, 77*t*
Localized edema, 39
Log roll, 1023*b*
Lomotil; *See* Diphenoxylate atropine
Long-acting beta-adrenergic agonists, 308*t*
Long acting insulin, 863*t*
Long leg cast, 739
Long spine board, 1025*f*
Long-term care
    in chronic illness, 179–187
    infection prevention and control in, 121
    in neurologic disorders, 565
    pain management in, 140
    use of restraints in, 1097
Longitudinal fracture, 737*f*
Loniten; *See* Minoxidil
Loop colostomy, 679, 685*f*
Loop diuretics
    for heart failure, 429*t*
    for liver disorders, 696*t*
    for vascular disorders, 402*t*
Loose associations, 1109
Loperamide, 37*t*, 666*t*
Lopid; *See* Gemfibrozol
Lopressor; *See* Metoprolol
Loratadine, 239*t*, 278*t*

Lorazepam, 1049*t*
    abuse of, 1072
    for acute alcohol withdrawal, 1069*t*
Lotensin; *See* Benazepril
Lotion application, 963*b*
Lou Gehrig's disease, 559–560
Lovastatin, 454*t*
Lovaza, 454*t*
Low back pain, 517–520, 517*f*
Lower extremity ultrasound, 378*t*
Lower extremity veins and arteries, 407*f*
Lower gastrointestinal system disorders,
        663–687
    abdominal and inguinal hernias in,
        663–664, 664*f*
    appendicitis in, 672–673
    bowel ischemia in, 670
    colorectal cancer in, 674–679
        cultural considerations in, 674*b*
        diagnosis of, 675
        early detection of, 153*b*
        etiology of, 674
        foods contributing to, 623*b*
        metastasis of, 171*t*
        nursing care plan for, 676*b*
        pathophysiology of, 674–675
        risk factors for, 152*t*
        signs and symptoms of, 675
        treatment of, 675
    diverticula in, 665–668
    inflammatory bowel disease in, 670–672,
        670*t*, 671*f*
    intestinal obstruction in, 668–670, 669*b*, 669*f*
    irritable bowel syndrome in, 664–665, 665*b*
    malabsorption in, 673–674
    ostomy surgery and care in, 679–681
        changing collection device after,
            681*f*, 684
        colostomy in, 679–680, 679*f*, 685*f*
        cultural considerations in, 683*b*
        evacuation and irrigation after,
            682–683
        ileostomy in, 680–681, 680*f*
        measurement of intake and output
            after, 682
        patient education in, 684–685
        periostomal skin care after, 683–684
        preoperative care in, 681
        psychosocial concerns in, 684
        stoma care in, 682
    peritonitis in, 673
Lower genital tract inflammations,
        906, 907*t*
Lower respiratory system, 258
Lower respiratory system disorders, 293–327
    acute bronchitis in, 293–294
    acute respiratory distress syndrome in,
        314, 314*b*
    antiviral medications and, 295*b*
    asthma in, 305–310
        pathophysiology of, 305*f*
        patient teaching in, 307*b*, 310
        peak flowmeter for, 307*b*
        psychosocial care in, 310
        rehabilitation in, 307–310
        signs and symptoms of, 305–306
        treatment of, 306–307, 306*t*, 308*t*
    atelectasis in, 303
    bronchiectasis in, 301–302
    chest injuries in, 312–313
    chronic obstructive pulmonary disease in,
        303–305, 304*t*
        chronic bronchitis in, 303
        complementary and alternative medicine
            for, 304*b*

Lower respiratory system disorders
        (*Continued*)
        complications of, 304–305
        drug therapy for, 308*t*
        emphysema in, 303, 303*f*
        nutritional suggestions for, 304*b*
        patient teaching in, 307*b*
        smoking cessation and, 307–310
    community care in, 327
    cystic fibrosis in, 301–302
    empyema in, 298
    extrapulmonary tuberculosis in, 301
    fungal infections in, 298
    influenza in, 294–295, 294*b*, 295*b*
    lung cancer in, 310–311
    lung transplantation in, 312
    obstructive pulmonary disorders in,
        302–311
    occupational lung disorders in, 302
    pleural effusion in, 302
    pleurisy in, 302
    pneumonia in, 295–298
        complementary and alternative medicine
            for, 297*b*
        etiology and pathophysiology of,
            295–296
        hypostatic, 84
        postoperative, 86, 92*t*
        signs and symptoms of, 297
    pneumothorax and hemothorax in,
        313, 313*f*
    primary pulmonary hypertension in, 312
    pulmonary edema in, 314
    pulmonary embolism in, 311–312
    pulmonary fibrosis in, 302
    respiratory failure in, 314–315, 315*b*
    restrictive pulmonary disorders in, 302
    sarcoidosis in, 302
    therapeutic measures in, 315–327
        chest tubes in, 316–317, 316*f*
        drug therapy in, 317–320, 321*b*
        humidification in, 320–321
        intrathoracic surgery in, 315–317
        mechanical ventilation in, 325–327, 326*f*,
            327*b*, 327*t*
        oxygen therapy in, 323–325, 323*f*, 323*t*
        pulmonary hygiene in, 321–322, 321*b*,
            322*b*, 322*f*
    tuberculosis in, 298–301, 298*b*, 300*t*
Lozenge, 280
Lozol; *See* Indapamide
LSD; *See* Lysergic acid diethylamide
Lubiprostone, 666*t*
Lucentis; *See* Ranibizumab
Ludiomil; *See* Maprotiline
Lumbar puncture, 481*t*, 489*f*
Lumbar vertebrae, 510*f*, 717*f*
Luminol; *See* Phenobarbital
Lumpectomy, 158–159, 910, 911*b*
Lung
    auscultation of, 263, 263*f*
    autonomic system effects on, 476*t*
    normal lung sounds, 264*t*
    oxygen and carbon dioxide exchange and,
        259–260
    oxygen delivery and, 258, 258*f*
    protection of, 258–259
    sickle cell disease and, 354*f*
Lung biopsy, 268
Lung cancer, 310–311
    metastasis of, 171*t*
    nursing care plan for, 318*b*
    risk factors for, 152*t*
    smoking and, 148*b*
Lung compliance, 260*b*

Lung disorders, 293–327
    acute bronchitis in, 293–294
    acute respiratory distress syndrome in, 314
    asthma in, 305–310
        pathophysiology of, 305*f*
        patient teaching in, 307*b*, 310
        peak flowmeter for, 307*b*
        psychosocial care in, 310
        rehabilitation in, 307–310
        signs and symptoms of, 305–306
        treatment of, 306–307, 306*t*, 308*t*
    atelectasis in, 303
    bronchiectasis in, 301–302
    cancer in, 310–311
        metastasis of, 171*t*
        nursing care plan for, 318*b*
        risk factors for, 152*t*
        smoking and, 148*b*
    chronic obstructive pulmonary disease in,
        303–305, 304*t*
        chronic bronchitis in, 303
        complementary and alternative medicine
            for, 304*b*
        complications of, 304–305
        drug therapy for, 308*t*
        emphysema in, 303, 303*f*
        nutritional suggestions for, 304*b*
        patient teaching in, 307*b*
        smoking cessation and, 307–310
    cystic fibrosis in, 301–302
    interstitial, 302
    lung transplantation for, 312
    obstructive, 302–311
    occupational, 302
    pneumonia in, 295–298
        complementary and alternative medicine
            for, 297*b*
        etiology and pathophysiology of,
            295–296, 296*f*
        hypostatic, 84
        postoperative, 86, 92*t*
        signs and symptoms of, 297
    pulmonary edema in, 314
    pulmonary fibrosis in, 302
    respiratory failure in, 314–315
    restrictive, 302
    sarcoidosis in, 302
    tuberculosis in, 298–301
        drug therapy for, 300*t*
        ethnic occurrence of, 298*b*
        extrapulmonary, 301
        vitamin D in prevention of, 299*b*
Lung exercises, 71–72, 71*b*, 71*f*
Lung function tests, 268, 269*f*
Lung sounds, 21*f*, 264*t*
Lung transplantation, 312
Lung ventilation and perfusion scan, 265*t*
Lutein, 571
Luteinizing hormone, 819*t*
    ovarian cycle and, 882
    pituitary hypofunction and, 835*t*
    in sperm production, 919
Luteinizing hormone study, 922*t*
LVAD; *See* Left ventricular assist device
Lybrel oral contraceptive, 883–887
Lyme disease, 745
Lymph, 195
Lymph node, 195, 196*f*
Lymph node biopsy, 207*t*
Lymph vessels, 195
Lymphadenopathy, 250
Lymphangiogram, 207*t*
Lymphatic disorders, 249
    fibromyalgia in, 253–254, 254*b*, 254*f*
    lymphedema in, 253, 253*b*

Lymphatic disorders (*Continued*)
  lymphoma in, 146, 249–254
    in acquired immunodeficiency
      syndrome, 240
      Hodgkin's, 249–250, 251*f*, 252*f*
      lymphedema in, 253, 253*b*
      non-Hodgkin's, 250–253
Lymphatic system, 195–212
  effects of aging on, 197–198
  functions of, 196–197, 197*t*
  interaction with vascular system, 334
  organs and structures of, 195–196,
    196*f*
  protective mechanisms of, 198–203
Lymphedema, 253, 253*b*
  after breast surgery, 913–915
Lymphocyte, 207*t*, 333, 333*f*
Lymphocyte immune globulin, 234*t*
Lymphoma, 146
  in acquired immunodeficiency syndrome,
    225
  Hodgkin's, 249–250, 251*f*, 252*f*
  lymphedema in, 253, 253*b*
  non-Hodgkin's, 250–253
Lyrica; *See* Pregabalin
Lysergic acid diethylamide, 1072*t*, 1076
Lysine for canker sore, 643*b*
Lysis, 200

M

Machupo virus, 1014–1015
Macrodantin; *See* Nitrofurantoin
Macrophage, 105, 197*t*
Macugen; *See* Pegaptanib sodium
Macula lutea, 569, 569*f*
Macular degeneration, 608–610, 609*f*
Macule, 959*t*
Mafenide acetate, 987*t*
Magnesium
  for dysrhythmias, 438*t*
  imbalances of, 42*t*, 45
  normal ranges and functions of, 41*t*
Magnesium sulfate, 1069*t*
Magnetic resonance angiography, 481*t*
Magnetic resonance arteriography, 378*t*
Magnetic resonance-guided focused
    ultrasound surgery, 905
Magnetic resonance imaging
  of breast, 895*t*
  in cancer, 154
  in cardiovascular disease, 378*t*
  in ear disorders, 584*t*
  in gastrointestinal disorders, 626*t*
  in head injury, 503*f*
  in musculoskeletal disorders, 720*t*
  in stroke, 529*f*
  in urologic disorders, 769*t*
Magnetic resonance spectroscopy, 481*t*
Magnetic seizure therapy, 1057
Magnetoencephalography, 481*t*
Maintenance therapy, 356
Major depressive disorder, 1055–1057
Major surgery, 63*t*
Malabsorption, 673–674
Malaria, 1004*t*
Maldistribution of fluids, 1036, 1037*f*
Male condom, 884*t*, 888*f*
Male reproductive disorders, 918–936
  benign prostatic hyperplasia in, 927–931,
    927*f*
  community care in, 935–936
  diagnostic tests for, 921–922, 922*t*
  ejaculation disorders in, 924
  epididymitis in, 932

Male reproductive disorders (*Continued*)
  erectile dysfunction in, 923–924, 924*b*, 924*f*,
    925*t*
  history taking in, 921, 921*b*
  hydrocele in, 925–926, 926*f*
  infertility in, 924–925
  orchitis in, 932
  penile cancer in, 933, 933*b*
  Peyronie's disease in, 927
  priapism in, 926–927
  prostate cancer in, 934–935, 935*b*, 935*t*
  prostatectomy in, 931*b*, 935*b*
  prostatitis in, 932–933
  surgical interventions in, 929*t*, 930*f*
  testicular cancer in, 933–934, 933*b*
  testicular torsion in, 926
  varicocele in, 926
Male reproductive system, 918–936
  changes with aging, 920, 920*b*
  contraception and, 920–921
  fertility and, 920
  functions of organs in, 919
  health screening and assessments
    and, 921*b*
  sperm production and, 919–920
  structures of, 918–919, 919*f*
Malignant hypertension, 401
Malignant hyperthermia, 92*t*, 93–94
Malignant melanoma, 975–976, 976*t*
Malignant neoplasm, 145
Malleus, 579, 580*f*
Malnutrition, 67*t*
Mammary gland, 882
Mammography, 154, 895*t*
Managed care, 5
Mandibulectomy, 644
Mania, 1051
Manipulative patient, 1113*b*
Mannitol, 514*t*
Mantoux test, 299
Maprotiline, 1056*t*
Marburg virus, 1011*t*, 1014–1015
Marijuana, 1072*t*, 1075–1076
Marplan; *See* Isocarboxazid
Marshall-Marchetti-Krantz procedure,
    780–781
Mask, 111*f*
Masking, 589
Maslow's hierarchy of needs, 25, 25*f*
Mass casualty, 999
Massage
  for back pain, 518*b*
  as method of pain management, 139
  for osteoarthritis, 746*b*
  for reducing agitation in Alzheimer's
    disease, 1097*b*
Mast cell, 197*t*
Mast cell stabilizer, 278*t*
Mastectomy, 69*b*, 95*b*, 158–159, 910
Mastication, 620
Maxair; *See* Pirbuterol
Maxillary sinus, 258*f*
Maxipime; *See* Cefepime
MDI; *See* Metered-dose inhaler
Meal plan, 860
Mean corpuscular hemoglobin, 207*t*
Mean corpuscular hemoglobin concentration,
    207*t*
Mean corpuscular volume, 207*t*
Measles, 1004*t*
Meatus, 718*t*
Mechanical barriers to infection, 103
Mechanical Embolus Removal in Cerebral
    Ischemia Retriever, 533
Mechanical suctioning, 272

Mechanical ventilation, 325–327, 326*f*,
    327*b*, 327*t*
Mechanism of injury, 1022
Media effects on sexually transmitted
    infections, 939*b*
Median nerve, carpal tunnel syndrome and,
    736
Mediastinal shift, 1025
Mediastinoscopy, 265*t*
Medicaid, 6, 6*b*
Medical-alert bracelet, 861*f*
Medical asepsis, 115
Medical command physician, 1000
Medical nutrition therapy, 860
Medical-surgical nursing, 1–10
  charge nurse/manager of care in, 3–4, 4*b*
  clinical standards in, 2, 17–27
  cost containment and, 6, 7*b*
  cultural needs of patient and, 9–10, 10*b*
  effective communication in, 2
  employment opportunities in, 3, 3*b*
  goals for health care in, 6–10
  health care team collaboration and, 2–3
  health insurance and, 4–6, 5*b*, 6*b*
  health promotion and, 6–7, 7*b*
  holistic care and, 7–10, 7*b*
  patient advocacy and, 3
  patient education and, 2
  patient safety and, 2
  psychological needs of patient and,
    7–9, 9*b*
  role of licensed practical/vocational nurse
    in, 1–3
  social needs of patient and, 9
  spiritual care and, 10, 11*b*
Medicare, 5–6, 5*b*, 6*b*
Medicated bath, 962
Medication assessment in chronic illness, 184*b*
Meditation, 139
Medulla oblongata, 473*f*, 473*t*
Mefenamic acid, 903*t*
Melanocyte, 952, 953*f*
Melanoma, 146, 974–977, 976*f*, 976*t*
  early detection of, 153*b*
  metastasis of, 171*f*
  risk factors for, 152*t*
Melatonin, 819*t*
Melena, 655
Memantine, 1089*t*
Memory
  cognitive disorders and, 1094
  diet and, 1087*b*
Memory T cell, 197*t*
Menarche, 882
Mèniére's disease, 613–614
Meninges, 475, 477*f*
Meningitis
  bacterial, 541–543, 542*f*
  epidemic potential in natural disaster, 1004*t*
  viral, 543
Meningococcal meningitis, 1004*t*
Meniscal injury, 736
Menopause, 882, 889*b*, 890–892, 890*b*,
    891*f*, 892*b*
Menorrhagia, 904
Menses, 882
Menstrual cycle, 882, 882*b*
Menstrual dysfunction, 902–903
  dysmenorrhea in, 902–903, 903*t*
  premenstrual dysphoric disorder in, 902
  premenstrual syndrome in, 902
Menstruation, 883
Mental changes
  in multiple sclerosis, 558
  in neurologic disorders, 486, 486*t*

Mental health disorders, 1045–1062
  anxiety and anxiety disorders in,
    1045–1048, 1046f
      complementary and alternative medicine
        in, 1050b
      cultural considerations in, 1049b
      diagnosis of, 1047
      elderly patient and, 1049b, 1050b
      generalized anxiety disorder in,
        1046–1047
      history taking in, 1048–1049
      levels of anxiety in, 1046t
      obsessive-compulsive disorder in, 1047
      phobic disorder in, 1047
      post-traumatic stress disorder in,
        1047–1048, 1047b
      promotion of relaxation in, 1050b
      treatment of, 1048, 1048b, 1049t
  community care in, 1062
  eating disorders in, 1060–1061
    anorexia nervosa in, 640, 1060
    bulimia nervosa in, 640, 1060
  mood disorders in, 1051–1052
    antidepressants for, 1056t
    bipolar disorder in, 1049t, 1051–1052,
      1051t, 1052b
    complementary and alternative medicine
      for, 1055b
    major depressive disorder in, 1055–1057
    serotonin syndrome and, 1057b
    suicidal patient and, 1059–1060, 1059b
  personality disorders in, 1113–1114, 1114b
    borderline personality disorder in, 1114
    guide for assessment in, 1115b
  schizophrenia in, 1103–1108
    data collection in, 1108
    diagnosis of, 1104, 1105t
    etiology and pathophysiology of, 1103
    nursing care plan for, 1110b
    nursing diagnoses for, 1108
    signs and symptoms of, 1103–1104,
      1104f
    treatment of, 1105–1108, 1106f
  thought disorders in, 1102–1108
    community care in, 1116
    drug therapy for, 1107t
    interventions for angry, hostile,
      aggressive, manipulative, or
      paranoid patient, 1113b
    neurotransmitters and, 1102–1103, 1103f
    patient rights and, 1108b
Mental status
  assessment in blood disorders, 340
  postoperative assessment of, 83b
  in shock, 1033
Menthol application for pain, 138
Meperidine, 668b
MERCI Retriever; See Mechanical Embolus
  Removal in Cerebral Ischemia Retriever
Meridia; See Sibutramine
Mesalamine, 666t
Meshed autograft, 988f
Mesothelioma, 302
Mestinon; See Pyridostigmine
Metabolic acidosis, 47, 47t, 48, 49f
  in burn injury, 982
Metabolic alkalosis, 47t, 49–50
Metabolic emergencies, 1026
Metabolic equivalents, 393, 463, 463t
Metabolic syndrome, 376, 377b, 875
Metabolism, 623
  chronic renal failure and, 803f
  cirrhosis and, 703f
Metacarpals, 717f
Metamucil; See Psyllium

Metastasis, 145–147, 147f
  treatment problems in, 170–171, 171t
Metatarsals, 717f
Metered-dose inhaler, 320
Metformin, 862t, 863b
Methadone, 170t, 1069t
Methamphetamine, 376–377, 528b,
  1074, 1074f
Methimazole, 840
Methotrexate
  for psoriasis, 969
  therapeutic drug monitoring reference
    intervals for, 1123t
Methylcellulose, 666t
Methyldopa, 402t
Methylphenidate, 1074–1075
Methylprednisolone, 234t, 514t
Methylxanthine derivative, 308t
Metoclopramide, 37t, 647t
Metolazone, 402t
Metoprolol, 402t, 438t
Metronidazole
  for pouchitis, 681
  for upper gastrointestinal disorders,
    647t
Metrorrhagia, 904
Mevacor; See Lovastatin
Mexiletine, 438t, 1123t
Mexitil; See Mexiletine
Microalbuminuria, 773, 875
Microlaryngoscopy, 283
Micronase; See Glyburide
Microorganisms, 101–103
Microscopic tests in skin disorders, 957
Microwave therapy in pancreatic cancer, 712
Micturition, 766
Midamor; See Amiloride
Midbrain, 473f, 473t
Middle ear, 579
  otitis media and, 612–613
Miglitol, 862t
Migraine headache, 545–546, 545b, 546b
Miliary tuberculosis, 301
Milieu therapy, 1114
Military personnel, post-traumatic stress
  disorder and, 1047b
Miller-Abbott tube, 669f, 681
Mineralocorticoids, 819t, 821, 822f
Minerals
  for blood disorders, 349t
  for chronic renal failure, 804t
Mini-Mental State Examination, 1093
Minimum Data Set, 187
Minipill, 884t
Minipress; See Prazosin
Minor surgery, 63t
Minoxidil, 402t
Miotics, 602t
Mirapex; See Pramipexole
Mirtazapine, 1056t
Misoprostol, 647t, 652
Mites, 973–974, 974f
Mitotic inhibitors, 163t
Mitral regurgitation (insufficiency), 445
Mitral stenosis, 443f, 445
Mitral valve
  prolapse of, 445
  vegetations on, 442, 443f
Mitral valve annuloplasty, 446
Mittelschmerz, 883
Mixed incontinence, 777
MMSE; See Mini-Mental State Examination
Mobilization, 728
Mobitz I heart block, 436
Mobitz II heart block, 436

Moderate sedation, 76
Modes of ventilation, 325–326
Modified radical mastectomy, 910
MODS; See Multiple organ dysfunction
  syndrome
Modulation of pain, 126, 126f
Mometasone, 278t, 308t
Moniliasis, 939, 972
Monoamine oxidase inhibitors, 1055, 1056t
  cautions for use of, 553b
  for Parkinson's disease, 554t
Monoclonal antibodies, 165
Monocyte, 197t
  in body defense against infection, 105
  normal range of, 207t
Monopril; See Fosinopril
Monricizine, 438t
Mons pubis, 881
Montelukast, 308t
Monurol; See Fosfomycin tromethamine
Mood disorders, 1051–1052
  antidepressants for, 1056t
  bipolar disorder in, 1049t, 1051–1052, 1051t,
    1052b
  complementary and alternative medicine
    for, 1055b
  major depressive disorder in, 1055–1057
  serotonin syndrome and, 1057b
  suicidal patient and, 1057b
Morbidly obese, 641
Morning-after pill, 887–888, 888b
Morphine, 170t
Mosquito bite, 544b
Motivational interviewing, 1048
Motor dysfunction in multiple sclerosis, 558
Motor vehicle accident, 1019
Motrin; See Ibuprofen
Mourning response, 513, 513t
Mouth, 257, 258f, 620, 621f
  normal flora of, 101t
  personal protective equipment for,
    1129
  stomatitis and, 643
  visual examination of, 264–268
Moxifloxacin, 786t
MRI; See Magnetic resonance imaging
MS; See Multiple sclerosis
Mucolytics, 308t
Mucomyst; See Acetylcysteine
Mucorrhea, 665
Mucositis, cancer treatment-related,
  166–167
Mucous membranes, 257, 258f
  assessment in blood disorders, 339
  of bronchioles, 259
  stomatitis and, 643
Multidrug-resistant organisms, 116
Multiple daily injection regimen in insulin
  therapy, 863–864
Multiple-gated acquisition scan, 378t
Multiple myeloma, 360–361
Multiple organ dysfunction syndrome,
  1038
Multiple sclerosis, 244t, 557t, 558f
Multiple trauma, 1026
Mumps orchitis, 932
Muromonab-CD3, 234t
Muscle(s)
  of eye, 569, 569f, 570t
  functions of, 718
  respiratory, 259
  strain of, 735
Muscle relaxants, 137
Muscle spasm, 513–514
Muscle strength, 719

Muscle tone, 728
Muscle weakness
  in diabetes insipidus, 836
  in diabetes mellitus, 859
Musculoskeletal disorders, 734–761
  Achilles tendon rupture in, 736
  ambulation with assistive devices in, 730–731, 730b, 731b
  amputation in, 758–760, 758b, 759f, 760b, 760f
  anterior cruciate ligament injury in, 735
  bone tumors in, 757–758
  bunion in, 736
  bursitis in, 736
  carpal tunnel syndrome in, 736
  causes of, 718–723
  community care in, 760–761
  diagnostic tests and procedures in, 719–723, 720t, 723f
  dislocation in, 735
  elderly and, 724b, 731b
  fractures in, 736–742
    braces and splints for, 739–740, 739f
    casts for, 739, 739f, 744–745
    complications of, 741–742, 742f
    etiology and pathophysiology of, 736–737
    external fixation for, 738–739, 739f
    initial assessment in, 742–743
    internal fixation for, 738, 738f
    osteoporotic, 756b
    physical assessment of neurovascular status in, 743b
    proton pump inhibitors and, 737b
    reduction, surgery, and stabilization in, 738
    signs and symptoms of, 737
    traction for, 740, 740f, 744b
    types of, 737b, 737f
  gout in, 755
  history taking in, 723–724, 723b
  joint protection in, 753b
  lifting and turning patient and, 727
  Lyme disease in, 745
  meniscal injury in, 736
  nursing diagnoses for, 725t
  osteoarthritis in, 745–746, 746b, 747t
  osteoporosis in, 755–757
    diagnosis of, 756
    elderly and, 755b, 756b
    etiology and pathophysiology of, 755
    nutrition and, 756b
    signs and symptoms of, 755–756
    treatment of, 756–757, 756b, 757b
    vertebral compress fractures in, 757
  Paget's disease of bone in, 757
  patient teaching in, 729b
  physical assessment in, 724, 724b
  positioning in, 729
  prevention of, 719–723
  prevention of disability in, 727–730, 728f, 729b, 729f
  psychosocial care in, 731–732
  rheumatoid arthritis in, 746–750, 747t, 748t
    diet and, 754
    heat and cold applications in, 754, 754b
    history taking in, 750–753, 753b
    joint replacement for, 749–750, 749f, 750b, 750f
    nursing care plan for total hip replacement in, 751b
    psychosocial care in, 755
    rest and exercise for, 753–754
    surgical intervention and orthopedic devices for, 749

Musculoskeletal disorders (Continued)
    rotator cuff tear in, 735
    slings and splints for, 730, 730f
    special beds for, 729–730, 730f
    sprain in, 734–735
    strain in, 735
Musculoskeletal system, 716–732
    changes with aging, 718
    effects of smoking on, 719b
    functions of bones in, 717
    functions of muscles in, 718
    nutrition for bone growth and density, 719b
    severe anemia and, 348t
    structures of, 716–717, 717f, 718t
Music therapy, 1110b
    for depression, 1055b
    as method of pain management, 139
Mustard agents, 1007t
Myambutol; See Ethambutol
Myasthenia gravis, 244t, 562–563, 563f, 564b
Mycifradin; See Neomycin
Mycobacterium avium complex, 223
Mycobacterium tuberculosis, 223
Mycoplasma, 103
Mycoses, 972
Mydriatics, 602t
Myelography, 481t
Myeloid leukemia, 355
Myeloperoxidase antigen, 378t
Mylicon; See Simethicone
Myocardial contusion, 446–447
Myocardial infarction, 455–461
    aspirin in prevention of, 453b
    cardiogenic shock in, 1035
    complications after, 461t
    diabetes-related, 875
    diagnosis of, 459, 459t
    emotional and behavioral responses to, 462b
    etiology and pathophysiology of, 458, 458f
    Joint Commission Core Measures for, 460b
    patient teaching in, 463b
    rehabilitation in, 462–464, 463t
    signs and symptoms of, 458–459
    treatment of, 459–460, 460b
    warning signs of, 376b
Myocarditis, 442
Myocardium, 371
Myoglobin, 378t, 459t
Myomectomy, 905
Myopia, 594, 595f
Myringotomy, 613, 617
Mysoline; See Primidone
Myxedema, 844
Myxedema coma, 845

N
N-acetylcysteine, 699
Nadolol, 438t
Nails, 952, 953f
    fungal infection of, 972–973, 972b, 973f
    iron deficiency anemia and, 351f
Nalmefene, 1069, 1069t
Naloxone, 1069t, 1073
Naltrexone, 1069, 1069t
Namendal; See Memantine
NANDA-I, 24
Naproxen
    for cancer pain, 170t
    for dysmenorrhea, 903t
Narcan; See Naloxone
Narcissistic personality disorders, 1114b

Narcotic analgesics, 135t, 1072t
Narcotic antagonist, 1069t
Narcotic-induced constipation, 137b
Nardil; See Phenelzine
Narrow-angle glaucoma, 601f, 605
Narrow spectrum antibacterials, 118
Nasacort; See Triamcinolone
Nasal artificial airway, 282f
Nasal cannula, 323t
Nasal cavity, 257, 258f
Nasal fracture, 282–283
Nasal packing, 280f
Nasal polyp, 279
Nasal prongs, 323t
Nasal septum, 258f
Nasalcrom; See Cromolyn sodium
Nasalide; See Flunisolide
Nasogastric tube
    in bowel ischemia, 670
    in ostomy surgery, 681
Nasonex; See Mometasone
Natazia; See Estradiol valerate and dienogest
National Multiple Sclerosis Society, 559
National Patient Safety Goals, 16–17, 17b
National Quality Core Measures, 17, 17b
Natural killer lymphocyte, 197t
Nausea, 35–38, 35b
    in appendicitis, 672
    in bowel ischemia, 670
    cancer treatment-related, 167
    in gallbladder disorders, 691t
    in gastrointestinal system disorders, 635
    in Mèniére's disease, 613–614
    in peritonitis, 673
    smells and, 635b
Near vision test, 574t
Nearsightedness, 594, 595f
Nebulizer, 320
Neck
    secondary survey of, 1023b
    trauma to, 1024, 1025f
Necrosis in coronary artery disease, 452
Nedocromil, 308t
Needle bladder neck suspension, 780–781
Nefazodone, 1056t
Negative feedback, 822–823, 838, 838f
Negative-pressure ventilator, 325
Negative symptoms of schizophrenia, 1104, 1104f
Neisseria gonorrhoeae, 932, 939
Neo-Synephrine; See Phenylephrine
Neologisms, 1109
Neomycin, 696t
Neoplasm, 145, 224, 225f
Neostigmine, 563
Neovascularization in retinopathy, 608
Nephrectomy, 790–791
Nephrolithotomy, 793
Nephron, 764, 765f
Nephropathy, diabetic, 875
Nephrosclerosis, 801–802
Nephrostomy tube, 790–791, 791b, 794t
Nephrotic syndrome, 790
Nephrotoxic substances, 767b, 768–773
Nerve agents, 1007t
Nerve block, 77t
Nerve conduction, 475–477
Neteglinide, 862t
Neulasta; See Pegfilgrastim
Neupogen; See Filgrastim
Neuregulin-1, 533
Neuro check, 488–489, 489b
NeuroCybernetic Prosthesis, 525
Neurofiber tangles, 1088

Neurogenic shock, 93, 513, 1037
Neuroglycopenia, 876
Neurolemma, 477
Neuroleptic malignant syndrome, 1105–1106, 1107t
Neurologic complications
　in acquired immunodeficiency syndrome, 225
　in intravenous therapy, 54t
Neurologic disorders
　back pain in, 517–520, 517f
　of brain, 523–548
　　bacterial meningitis in, 541–543, 542f
　　Bell's palsy in, 548
　　brain abscess in, 544–545
　　brain tumor in, 539–541, 540f, 540t, 541f
　　encephalitis in, 544
　　headache in, 545–546, 546b
　　seizure disorders and epilepsy in, 523–526, 525b
　　stroke in, 528–534; See also Stroke
　　transient ischemic attack in, 527–528
　　trigeminal neuralgia in, 546–547, 547f
　　viral meningitis in, 543
　causes of, 478
　classification of, 478b
　common care problems in, 492–497
　　aphasia in, 495–496, 496b
　　confusion in, 495
　　dysphagia in, 493
　　impaired mobility in, 492
　　incontinence in, 493–495
　　ineffective breathing pattern in, 492
　　ineffective family coping in, 497
　　pain in, 495
　　psychosocial concerns in, 497
　　self-care deficit in, 492–493
　　sexual dysfunction in, 496–497
　diagnostic tests for, 481t, 489, 489f
　evaluation of neurologic status in, 479–485, 480t, 485f
　head injury in, 500–508
　　diagnosis of, 502, 503f
　　etiology of, 500
　　levels of consciousness and, 502b
　　nursing care plan for, 504b
　　pathophysiology of, 500–501, 501f
　　patient teaching in, 505b
　　signs and symptoms of, 501–502, 502b, 502f
　　surgery for, 503
　increased intracranial pressure in, 506–508
　　complications of, 508
　　etiology and pathophysiology of, 506, 506f
　　signs and symptoms of, 506–507, 507f
　　treatment of, 507–508, 508b
　mental function and level of consciousness in, 486, 486t
　neurologic and neuromuscular status in, 486–487, 487f
　nursing diagnoses for, 489, 490t
　peripheral and degenerative, 551–565
　　Alzheimer's disease in, 559
　　amyotrophic lateral sclerosis in, 559
　　community care in, 565
　　Guillain-Barré syndrome in, 560–561
　　Huntington's disease in, 562
　　multiple sclerosis in, 557t, 558f
　　myasthenia gravis in, 562–563, 563f, 564b
　　Parkinson's disease in, 551–554; See also Parkinson's disease

Neurologic disorders (Continued)
　　poliomyelitis and postpolio syndrome in, 562
　prevention of, 478–479
　pupillary abnormalities in, 488, 488t
　spinal cord injury in, 509–515
　　autonomic dysreflexia in, 514–515
　　deep venous thrombosis in, 515
　　drug therapy for, 514t
　　etiology of, 509, 510f
　　heterotopic ossification in, 515
　　immobilization and surgery in, 512, 512f, 513f
　　infection risk in, 515
　　muscle spasms in, 513–514
　　nursing planning in, 516–517, 516f
　　orthostatic hypotension in, 515
　　pathophysiology of, 509, 511f
　　psychological care in, 512, 513t
　　rehabilitation in, 517
　　renal complications in, 515
　　respiratory management in, 512
　　sexual concerns in, 513
　　signs and symptoms of, 509–510, 511t
　　skin breakdown in, 515
　　spinal shock and neurogenic shock in, 513
　　treatment of, 510–513
　　urinary management in, 512
Neurologic incontinence, 777
Neurologic status
　evaluation of, 479–485, 480t, 485f
　secondary survey of, 1023b
Neurologic system, 472–497
　age-related changes in, 478
　autonomic effects on organs of body, 476t
　chronic renal failure and, 803f
　cirrhosis and, 703f
　cranial nerves in, 475t
　diabetic neuropathy and, 876, 876b
　nerve conduction and, 475–477
　neurotransmitters and, 476, 477t
　organization of, 472–474, 473f, 473t, 474f
　peripheral nervous system and central nervous system interaction and, 474–475, 475f
　protection of, 475, 477f, 479b
　severe anemia and, 348t
Neuroma, acoustic, 614
Neuromuscular blocking agents, 514t
Neuromuscular electrical stimulation, 644
Neuromuscular function testing, 479, 481t
Neuromuscular status in neurologic disorders, 486–487, 487f
Neuron, 472, 473f
Neurontin; See Gabapentin
Neuropathic pain, 125t, 126
Neuropathy, diabetic, 876, 876b
Neurotransmitters, 476, 477t, 1102–1103, 1103f
Neurovascular status in fracture, 743b
Neutropenia, 212
Neutrophil, 197t, 207t
Newborn, pain in, 134t
Nexavar; See Sorafenib
Nexium; See Esomeprazole
NHL; See Non-Hodgkin's lymphoma
Niacin, 454t
Nicarpidine, 402t
Nicobid; See Niacin
Nicorette, 1069t
Nicotine, 1075, 1075b
Nicotine patch, 1069t
Nicotine replacement therapy, 1075
Nicotine transdermal, 1069t

Nicotinex; See Niacin
Nicotinic acid, 454t
Nicotrol, 1069t
Nifedipine, 402t
Nimodipine, 531t
Nissen fundoplication surgery, 649f
Nitrates
　as food preservatives, 623
　for heart failure, 429t
Nitrites, 623
Nitrofurantoin, 786t
Nizatidine, 647t
NMES; See Neuromuscular electrical stimulation
Nociceptive pain, 125–126, 125t, 126f
Nocturia, 766, 775b, 836
Nocturnal confusion, 186
Nocturnal intermittent dialysis, 807
Nodular malignant melanoma, 976t
Noise-induced hearing impairment, 582
Nolvadex; See Tamoxifen
Non-Hodgkin's lymphoma, 250–253
Non-IgE dependent allergens, 241
Non-narcotic analgesics, 135t
Non-rebreather mask, 323t
Non-small cell lung cancer, 311
Non-ST segment elevation myocardial infarction, 455–458
Nonalcoholic steatohepatitis, 701b
Nonbacterial prostatitis/chronic pelvic pain syndrome, 933
Nongonococcal urethritis, 932
Noninvasive positive ventilation, 326
Nonnucleoside reverse transcriptase inhibitors, 222t
Nonpharmacologic approaches to pain management, 138–140, 140f, 170
Nonproductive cough, 262
Nonspecific urethritis, 788
Nonsteroidal antiinflammatory drugs, 135t
　for dysmenorrhea, 903t
　gastrointestinal intolerance and, 748b
　for glaucoma, 602t
　for gout, 755
　for pain in osteoporosis, 756–757
　peptic ulcer and, 650
　for rheumatoid arthritis, 747–748, 748t
Nonsulfonylurea insulin glinides, 862t
Nonunion, 741
Norepinephrine, 477t, 819t, 821, 1103
Normal flora, 100, 101t, 105
Normal sinus rhythm, 436f
Normodyne; See Labetalol
Norpace; See Disopyramide
North American Nursing Diagnosis Association International, 24
Nortriptyline, 1123t
Norwalk virus, 649
Nose, 257, 258f
　epistaxis and, 280, 280f
　fracture of, 282–283
　normal flora of, 101t
　personal protective equipment for, 1129
　rhinitis and, 277–279, 278t, 279b
　visual examination of, 264–268
Nosebleed, 280, 280f
Nosocomial infection; See Health care-associated infection
Novo-Niacin; See Nicotinic acid
NSAIDs; See Nonsteroidal antiinflammatory drugs
Nuchal rigidity
　in bacterial meningitis, 542
　in encephalitis, 544
　in head injury, 501–502

Nuclear disaster, 1009–1010, 1009f, 1010t
Nuclear imaging, 378t, 626t
Nucleoside reverse transcriptase inhibitors, 222t
Nucleotide reverse transcriptase inhibitors, 222t
Numbered pain scale, 129
Nurse practice act, 1–2
Nursing care plan
    for abdominal wound, 117b
    for adrenocortical insufficiency, 849b
    for Alzheimer's disease, 1090b
    for angina, 456b
    for bipolar disorder, 1053b
    for breast lumpectomy, 911b
    for burn victim, 990b
    for cancer, 156b
    for cardiac surgery patient, 467b
    for cataract extraction, 599b
    for Chlamydia trachomatis, 949b
    for chronic renal failure, 812b
    for cirrhosis, 704b
    for colorectal cancer, 676b
    for deep vein thrombosis, 417b
    for deficient fluid volume, 36b
    for diabetes mellitus, 868b
    for head injury and increased intracranial
        pressure, 504b
    for heart failure, 432b
    for hyperthyroidism, 841b
    for hysterectomy, 898b
    for imbalanced nutrition, 18b
    for immobilized patient, 180b
    for laryngectomy, 287b
    for leukemia, 357b
    for lumpectomy, 911b
    for lung cancer, 318b
    for Parkinson's disease, 555b
    for patient with pain, 133b
    for peptic ulcer, 653b
    for prostatectomy, 931b
    for schizophrenia, 1110b
    for shock, 1039b
    for simple mastectomy, 69b, 95b
    for stroke, 536b
    for substance abuse, 1079b
    for systemic lupus erythematosus, 248b
    for total hip replacement, 751b
    for tympanoplasty, 615b
Nursing diagnoses, 24–25
    for acquired immunodeficiency syndrome,
        226, 227t
    for Alzheimer's disease, 1089–1092, 1095
    for borderline personality disorder, 1114
    for cancer, 155, 155b
    for cardiovascular disease, 388–392, 389t
    for diabetes mellitus, 867–868
    for ear disorders, 586t
    for endocrine disorders, 829, 829t
    for gastrointestinal system disorders, 633,
        634t
    for hematologic disorders, 340–341, 341t
    for hypertension, 404–405
    for immune and lymphatic disorders,
        210t
    for musculoskeletal disorders, 725t
    for neurologic disorders, 489, 490t
    for rehabilitation, 190, 191b
    for respiratory disorders, 270t
    for schizophrenia, 1108
    for skin disorders, 960, 961t
    for substance abuse, 1077
    for urinary incontinence, 778t
Nursing interventions, 26
Nursing practice standards, 1137–1140

Nursing process, 15b, 16–17
    analysis and nursing diagnosis in, 24–25
    assessment and data collection in, 17–24
    evaluation in, 27
    implementation in, 26–27
    integration of, 16, 17–27
    planning in, 26
Nutrients needed for erythropoiesis, 335b
Nutrition
    in acquired immunodeficiency syndrome,
        229b
    adding protein to diet, 367b
    after brain injury, 509
    after laryngectomy, 289b
    for bone growth and density, 719b, 756b
    brown rice and whole grains and, 856b
    building red blood cells and, 335b
    cancer prevention and, 150, 150b
    chronic obstructive pulmonary disease
        and, 304b
    colon and conjugated linoleic acid and, 674b
    coronary artery disease and, 453b
    decreasing sodium in diet, 405b
    diet soda and, 875b
    diverticular disease and, 668b
    dysphagia and, 539b
    fat and cholesterol in diet and, 453b
    food triggers of migraine headache, 545b
    foods that thicken stool, 636b
    gallstones and, 692, 692b
    gastric cancer and, 657b
    heart-healthy diet and, 430b
    for immobile musculoskeletal patient, 743b
    immune system and, 212
    iron and folic acid rich foods, 348b
    lung cancer and, 311b
    menopause and, 892b
    phosphorus rich foods, 846b
    potassium rich foods, 44b
    in prevention of infection, 104
    in promoting relaxation, 1050b
    respiratory disorders and, 274
    sodium rich foods, 41b
    vitamin C and protein rich foods, 89b
    vitamin D association with decreased risk
        for falls, 724b
    vitamins and antioxidants beneficial to
        vision, 571b
Nutritional anemia, 347
Nutritional deficiency in malabsorption,
    673–674
Nutritional support in burn injury, 993
Nystagmus, 487
    in labyrinthitis, 613
    testing for, 583–585
Nystatin, 987t

O
Oatmeal bath, 962b
Obesity, 640–642
    bariatric surgery for, 641–642, 642f
    cancer and, 150
    cardiovascular disease and, 376
    development of diabetes mellitus and, 858
    diagnosis of, 641
    etiology and pathophysiology of, 641
    signs and symptoms of, 641
    as surgical risk factor, 67t
    treatment of, 641–642
Objective data, 18
Oblique fracture, 737f
Observation, 20
    in substance abuse therapy, 1078b
    while bathing, 960b
Obsession, 1047

Obsessive-compulsive disorder, 1047
Obsessive-compulsive personality disorder,
    1114b
Obstruction
    airway, 281–282, 282f, 284f
        choking emergency in, 1032
        in unconscious person, 1022
    intestinal, 623, 668–670, 669b, 669f
        ileostomy-related, 685b
    urinary tract, 790–794
        hydronephrosis in, 790–791
        kidney stones in, 791–794, 792f, 792t
        renal stenosis in, 791
Obstructive pulmonary disorders, 261,
    302–311
Obstructive shock, 1036
Obstructive sleep apnea, 282
Obturator of tracheostomy tube, 285
Occipital nerve stimulation, 545–546
Occlusive dressing, 1025
Occult blood, 151
Occupational exposure to human
    immunodeficiency virus,
    230b
Occupational lung disorders, 302
Ocular myasthenia, 562–563
Ocular trauma, 597–598, 597f
Oculocephalic reflex, 480–485
Oculogyric crisis, 1105
Oculomotor nerve, 475t
Oculovestibular reflex, 480–485
Odor of urine, 773
Odors, nausea and, 635b
Ointment application, 963b
Olepto; See Trazodone
Olfaction use in data collection, 20
Olfactory nerve, 475t
Oligomenorrhea, 904
Oliguria, 775b
    in acute glomerulonephritis, 789
    elderly and, 800b
Olsalazine, 666t, 671–672
Omalizumab, 308t
Omega-3 fatty acids, 1103b
Omeprazole, 647t
Omeprazole and sodium
    bicarbonate, 647t
Ommaya reservoir, 540, 540f
Omnaris; See Ciclesonide
Oncogenesis, 147
Oncologic emergency, 171–172
Ondansetron, 37t, 1074–1075
One-way tracheostomy valve box,
    285–286
Onglyza; See Saxagliptin
Onychomycosis, 972–973, 973f
Oocyte, 881
Oophorectomy, 901t
Oophoritis, 939
Open-angle glaucoma, 601f, 602–605, 602f
Open dressing, 963
Open fracture, 737b, 742b
Open heart surgery, 464–465
Open prostatectomy, 929t
Open reduction, 738
Open reduction and internal fixation, 738
Operating room, 75
Ophthalmoscopy, 574t
Opioids, 135t
    abuse of, 1069t, 1073–1074, 1073b
    for cancer pain, 170t
    characteristics of, 1072t
    for pancreatic cancer, 712
    ulcerative colitis and, 671b
Opium tincture, 666t

Opportunistic infections, 217, 221–224, 972
    candidiasis in, 224
    coccidiomycosis in, 223–224
    cryptococcosis in, 223–224
    cryptosporidiosis in, 224
    cytomegalovirus in, 222–223
    hepatitis in, 223
    herpes simplex virus in, 221–223
    histoplasmosis in, 223
    Kaposi sarcoma in, 225, 225f
    lymphomas in, 225
    Mycobacterium avium complex in, 223
    Pneumocystis jiroveci in, 224
    toxoplasmosis in, 224, 224b
    tuberculosis in, 223
    varicella-zoster virus in, 221–222, 222b
Optic disc, 568, 569f
Optic nerve, 475t, 568, 569f, 570f
Optical coherence tomography, 574t
Optimine; See Azatadine
Oral analgesics, 136
Oral cancer, 644
    early detection of, 153b
    risk factors for, 152t
Oral contraceptives, 883–887, 884t,
    888f, 903t
Oral hypoglycemic agents, 862–863, 862t
Oral rehydration, elderly patient
    and, 635b
Orchiectomy, 933
Orchitis, 932
ORIF; See Open reduction and internal
    fixation
Orlistat, 641
Oropharyngeal artificial airway, 282f
Orthopedic, term, 719
Orthopedic devices, 749
Orthopnea, 272
Orthopneic position, 272f
Orthoses, 749
Orthostatic hypotension, 183–184
    antihypertensive therapy-related, 401
    arteriosclerosis and, 400b
    in spinal cord injury, 515
Orthotic bladder substitute, 797
Osmolality, 40
Osmoreceptor, 31
Osmosis, 32–33, 33f
Osmotic diuretics, 514t
Ossification, 718
Osteoarthritis, 745–746, 746b, 747t
Osteogenesis, 741
Osteoma, 757
Osteomyelitis, fracture-related, 741
Osteopenia, 755
Osteoporosis, 755–757
    diagnosis of, 756
    elderly and, 755b, 756b
    etiology and pathophysiology of, 755
    fracture in, 736–737
    menopause and, 890–891, 890b
    in multiple myeloma, 360
    nutrition and, 756b
    signs and symptoms of, 755–756
    treatment of, 756–757, 756b, 757b
    vertebral compress fracture in, 757
Osteotomy, 749
Ostomy surgery, 679–681
    changing collection device after,
        681f, 684
    colostomy in, 679–680, 679f, 685f
    cultural considerations in, 683b
    evacuation and irrigation after,
        682–683
    ileostomy in, 680–681, 680f

Ostomy surgery (Continued)
    measurement of intake and output after,
        682
    patient education in, 684–685
    periostomal skin care after,
        683–684
    preoperative care in, 681
    psychosocial concerns in, 684
    stoma care in, 682
Otitis media, 612–613
Otorrhea, 585
Otosclerosis, 614–615
Otoscope, 582–583, 583f
Ototoxic drugs, 582b, 583b
Oval window, 580
Ovarian cancer, 152t, 908, 908b
Ovarian cycle, 882
Ovarian cycle syndrome, 902
Ovary, 818, 819t, 824f, 881, 881f
Over-the-counter drugs, 767b
Overdose
    of acetaminophen, 136b
    using transdermal fentanyl, 136b
Overflow incontinence, 777
Overhydration, 34b
Ovulation method of contraception, 884t
Ovum, 881
Oxaliplatin, 675
Oxazepam, 1049t
    abuse of, 1072
    for acute alcohol withdrawal, 1069t
Oxcarbazepine, 525b
Oximetry, 265t
Oxybutynin, 779–780, 780t
Oxycodone, 170t
Oxygen, respiration and, 259
Oxygen and carbon dioxide exchange,
    259–260
Oxygen delivery, 258, 258f
Oxygen delivery devices, 323f, 323t
Oxygen saturation, 48
Oxygen therapy, 323–325, 323f, 323t
    in blood disorders, 366
    in heart disease, 447
Oxygen toxicity, mechanical ventilation-
    related, 327t
Oxyhemoglobin, 260
Oxymetazoline, 239t, 278t
Oxyphencyclamine hydrochloride, 666t
Oxytocin, 819t

P
Pacemaker, 440–441, 441b, 441f
Packed red blood cells, 363t
PACU; See Postanesthesia care unit
Paget's disease of bone, 757
Pain, 124–141
    acute, 127, 127t, 128f
    in appendicitis, 672
    in bowel ischemia, 670
    cancer treatment-related, 169–170, 170t
    chest, 453–455, 455f, 456b
        in cardiovascular disease, 385–386, 386t,
            394
        in myocardial infarction, 458
    in cholecystitis, 691
    chronic, 126f, 128
    in chronic pancreatitis, 710
    in compartment syndrome, 742
    complementary and alternative medicine
        for, 1073b
    cultural beliefs affecting pain perception
        and treatment, 131b
    data collection in, 128–131, 129b, 129f, 130f
    in dislocation, 735

Pain (Continued)
    in diverticulitis, 668
    false perceptions of, 134t
    in gastroenteritis, 649
    in Guillain-Barré syndrome, 560
    headache, 545–546, 546b
    in hematologic disorders, 343
    in hemorrhoids, 686
    in hydronephrosis, 790
    in irritable bowel syndrome, 665
    in liver cancer, 708
    in neurologic disorders, 495
    neuropathic, 126
    nociceptive, 125–126, 126f
    patient description of, 130–131, 130t
    in peptic ulcer, 651
    perception of, 126–127
    in peritonitis, 673
    physiologic sources of, 125t
    pleurisy, 302
    postoperative assessment of, 83b
    referred, 130–131, 132f
    in stomatitis, 643
    theories of, 124–125, 125f
    in trigeminal neuralgia, 547
    types and causes of, 128f
    in urinary disorders, 774–775
Pain management, 8–9, 134–140, 135f
    analgesics in, 134–136, 135t
    in burn injury, 985, 989–992, 992b
    community care and, 140–141
    at end of life, 138b, 174
    extended care and, 140
    home care and, 141
    nonpharmacologic approaches in, 138–140,
        140f
    nursing care plan for, 133b
    nursing responsibilities in, 137, 137b
    patient education in, 133b
    postoperative, 87–88
    preoperative, 70
    side effects and complications of pain
        medications, 137–138
Pain rating scales, 129–130, 129f, 130f
Pain threshold, 127
Pain tolerance, 127
Palliative care, 172–174
Palliative surgery, 63t
Palmar erythema, 701
Palpation
    abdominal, 632
    use in data collection, 20
Palpitations, 394, 435
Pamate; See Tranylcypromine
Pancreas, 621f, 622, 818, 819t, 824f
    diabetes mellitus and, 856
    disorders of, 708–713
        acute pancreatitis in, 708–710,
            709f
        cancer in, 152t, 710–713
        causes of, 624
        chronic pancreatitis in, 710
        prevention of, 625
    functions of, 622–623
Pancreatic duct, 621f, 622
Pancreatic hormones, 821–822, 823f, 824f
Pancreatitis
    acute, 708–710, 709f
    chronic, 710
Pancuronium, 514t
Pandemic influenza infection, 1015–1016
Panhysterectomy, 901t, 908
Panitumumab, 675
Pantoprazole, 647t
Pap smear, 894b, 895t

Papillary muscle dysfunction after myocardial infarction, 461t
Papilledema, 506
Papule, 959t
Para-aminobenzoic acid, 300t
Paracentesis, 702–703
Parallel talk, 496
Paralytic ileus, 87, 92t
    after intrathoracic surgery, 316
    intestinal obstruction and, 668–669
    in peritonitis, 673
Paranasal sinuses, 257, 258f
Paranoid patient, 1113b
Paranoid personality disorder, 1114b
Paranoid schizophrenia, 1105t
Paraplegia, 510
Parasitic infection
    in acquired immunodeficiency syndrome, 224
    in pediculosis and scabies, 973–974, 974f
Parasympathetic nervous system, 474
Parathormone, 819t, 821
Parathyroid disorders, 845–847, 846t
    hyperparathyroidism in, 846–847, 846b
    hypoparathyroidism in, 845–846
Parathyroid gland, 818, 819t, 821, 824f
Parathyroid hormone, 766t, 819t, 821
Paregoric; See Opium tincture
Parkinson's disease, 551–554
    complications of, 554
    diagnosis of, 552, 552f
    etiology of, 551
    nursing care plan for, 555b
    pathophysiology of, 551, 552f
    patient teaching in, 557b
    signs and symptoms of, 552, 552f
    surgery for, 554
    treatment of, 553–554, 553b, 554t
Parkland formula, 985
Parlodel; See Bromocriptine mesylate
Parotid gland, 621f
Partial parenteral nutrition, 56–57, 57b
Partial pressure of carbon dioxide, 47
Partial pressure of oxygen, 47
Partial rebreathing mask, 323t
Partial seizure, 524
Partial-thickness burn, 982–983, 983f, 984t
Partial thromboplastin time, 626t
Passive immunity, 202
Passive transport, 32–33
Passy-Muir speaking tracheostomy valve, 289, 289f
Patch test, 237–238
Patella, 717f
Patellar reflex, 480
Patent airway
    postoperative, 84
    tracheostomy and, 286
Pathogens, 101–103
Pathologic fracture, 737f
Patient advocacy, 3
Patient care equipment, standard precautions and, 1129
Patient care partnership, 1140–1142
Patient-controlled analgesia, 136
Patient-endorsed intake, 174
Patient positioning
    bony prominences susceptible to skin breakdown and, 977f
    in musculoskeletal disorders, 729
    to prevent abduction contracture, 756
Patient rights, 1108b
Patient safety, 2
    abdominal pain in appendicitis and, 673b
    acetaminophen overdose and, 745b

Patient safety (Continued)
    bisphosphonates and, 757b
    blood products and, 364b
    in chronic illness, 183, 183b
    contrast dye and, 459b
    in crutches, 731b
    fentanyl patch and, 136b
    in flushing intravenous catheter, 55b
    herpes zoster transmission and, 971b
    in hip abductor wedge, 750b
    in infection prevention in immunodeficient patient, 235b
    in infective endocarditis, 443b
    in intravenous line connection, 51b
    intravenous potassium and, 44b
    in intravenous therapy, 51b, 53b, 55b
    in isometric exercises, 729b
    latex allergy and, 65b
    in liver inflammation, 702b
    low platelet count and, 360b
    marking of surgical site and, 596b
    neurologic changes and, 488b
    in open fracture, 742b
    ototoxic drugs and, 582b
    patient with allergies and, 238b
    postoperative, 85–86
    preventing acetaminophen overdose, 136b
    preventing falls and, 72b, 962b
    in preventing ventilator-acquired pneumonia, 327b
    prevention of embolus, 85b
    prevention of falls from impaired vision, 610b
    prolonged vomiting and, 35b
    in proton pump inhibitors, 464b
    proton pump inhibitors and fracture risk, 737b
    recognition and response to changes in patient condition, 315b
    security devices and, 184–185, 184b, 185b
    sharps disposal and, 230b
    signs of hypokalemia and, 394b
    skin drainage or weeping and, 957b
    in spinal injury, 511b
    during thyroid storm, 844b
    in total parenteral nutrition, 57b
    transfusion reaction and, 364b
    in transmission of hepatitis C, 699b
    in triptans and antidepressant use, 545b
    in varicella transmission, 222b
    verification before surgery, 74b
    in warfarin interaction with cranberry juice, 533b
Patient self-esteem, 8
Patient teaching, 2
    in abdominal and diaphragmatic breathing, 322b
    in accidental amputation care, 758b
    in acquired immunodeficiency syndrome, 228b
    in Addison's disease, 848b
    in angina, 458b
    in antipsychotic medications, 1109b
    in asthma, 310
    in avoiding and limiting exposure to carcinogens, 151b
    in cancer treatment problems, 168b, 169b
    in chronic respiratory disease, 307b
    in compromised immunity, 228b
    in diabetes mellitus, 861f, 867f, 871–873, 872f
        elderly patient and, 873b
        foot care and, 875b
        home treatment of hypoglycemia and, 861b

Patient teaching (Continued)
    sick days and, 872b
        subcutaneous insulin injection and, 864b
        travel instructions and, 872b
    in discharge instructions
        for prostatectomy, 935b
        for same-day surgery patient, 97b
    in epilepsy, 527, 527b
    in exercise to reduce gas and bloating, 635b
    in eye surgery, 600b
    in foods contributing to colon cancer, 623b
    in gastroesophageal reflux disease, 646b
    in glaucoma, 605b
    in head injury, 505b
    in heat and cold applications, 754b
    in home care intravenous therapy, 59b
    in home care of tracheostomy, 286b
    in hurricane preparation, 1000b
    in hypertension, 406b
    in infection prevention and control, 109–110, 120b
    in joint protection, 753b
    in Kegel exercises, 780b
    in kidney health and healthy blood vessels, 767b
    in laparoscopic cholecystectomy, 692b
    in low back pain or spinal surgery, 520b
    in lung exercises, 71b
    in lymphedema, 253b
    in musculoskeletal disorders, 729b
    in myasthenia gravis, 564b
    in oatmeal bath, 962b
    older adult and, 915b
    in ostomy care, 684–685, 685b
    in over-the-counter drugs, 767b
    in pacemaker, 441b
    in pain management, 133b
    in Parkinson's disease, 557b
    in postoperative foot and leg exercises, 71b, 71f
    preoperative, 66–67, 67b
    in preventing falls from orthostatic hypotension, 401b
    in pursed-lip breathing, 321b
    in quadriceps and gluteal muscle exercises, 729b
    in recovery from myocardial infarction, 463b
    in recurrent fungal infections, 973b
    in removal and disposal of contaminated clothing, 1009b
    in self-assessment of skin, 960b
    in self-care management of hypothyroidism, 844b
    in skin care during radiation treatment, 160b
    in sodium-restricted diet, 789b
    in T-tube care, 693b
    in total hip replacement, 750b
    in urinary tract infection prevention, 788b
    in urinary urgency, 774b
    in using peak flowmeter, 307b
    in warfarin, 434b
    in warning signs of stroke, 530b
Patient unit preparation, 74, 74f
Pavulon; See Pancuronium
Payne-Martin classification of skin tears, 956
PCA; See Patient-controlled analgesia
PCP; See Phencyclidine hydrochloride
Peak flowmeter, 268, 269f
Pearson attachment, 740
Pedal edema, 39–40, 40f
Pedal pulse, 387
Pediculosis, 973–974, 974f
PEEP; See Positive end-expiratory pressure

PEG; *See* Percutaneous endoscopic gastrostomy
Pegfilgrastim, 349*t*
Peginterferon alfa-2b, 696*t*
Pelvic examination, 894, 895*t*, 897*b*
Pelvic floor, 881
Pelvic inflammatory disease, 939
Pelvic relaxation syndrome, 903–904
Pelvic rock exercise, 902
Pelvic traction, 740, 740*f*
Pelvic ultrasonography, 895*t*
Penetrating trauma
    abdominal, 1025
    chest, 446–447
Penicillins, 786*t*
Penile implant, 924, 924*f*
Penis, 919, 919*f*
    autonomic system effects on, 476*t*
    cancer of, 933, 933*b*
    Peyronie's disease and, 927
    priapism and, 926–927
    sickle cell disease and, 354*f*
Penrose drain, 90*f*
Pepcid; *See* Famotidine
Peppermint oil, 665*b*
Peptic ulcer, 650–652
    in chronic obstructive pulmonary disease, 305
    complications of, 655
    diagnosis of, 651–652
    etiology of, 650
    focused assessment for, 652*b*
    nursing care plan for, 653*b*
    pathophysiology of, 650–651, 651*f*
    signs and symptoms of, 651
    surgical treatment of, 655–657, 656*f*
    treatment of, 652
Pepto-Bismol; *See* Bismuth subsalicylate
Perception of pain, 126–127, 126*f*
Percussion
    abdominal, 632
    use in data collection, 22
Percutaneous endoscopic gastrostomy, 659, 659*f*, 660*b*
Percutaneous laser diskectomy, 519
Percutaneous transluminal angioplasty, 409
Percutaneous transluminal coronary angioplasty, 464, 464*f*
Pereyra procedure, 780–781
Perforation in peptic ulcer disease, 655
Perfusion, 260, 260*b*
    cardiovascular disease and, 394–395
    shock and, 1033
Pergolide, 554*t*
Pericardial effusion
    in cancer, 171
    in pericarditis, 443, 443*f*
Pericardial space, 371
Pericardial tamponade, 1036
Pericardiocentesis, 444
Pericardiotomy, 444
Pericarditis, 376, 443–444, 443*f*
    after myocardial infarction, 461*t*
    methamphetamine-related, 1074
Pericardium, 371
Perineal prostatectomy, 929*t*, 930*f*
Perineum, 881
Perioperative nursing, 64
Peripheral arterial disease, 407–409, 408*t*
Peripheral nerve catheter, 136
Peripheral nerve disorders
    Alzheimer's disease in, 559
    amyotrophic lateral sclerosis in, 559
    community care in, 565
    Guillain-Barré syndrome in, 560–561

Peripheral nerve disorders (*Continued*)
    Huntington's disease in, 562
    multiple sclerosis in, 557*t*, 558*f*
    myasthenia gravis in, 562–563, 563*f*, 564*b*
    Parkinson's disease in, 551–554
        complications of, 554
        diagnosis of, 552, 552*f*
        etiology of, 551
        nursing care plan for, 555*b*
        pathophysiology of, 551, 552*f*
        patient teaching in, 557*b*
        signs and symptoms of, 552, 552*f*
        surgery for, 554
        treatment of, 553–554, 553*b*, 554*t*
    poliomyelitis and postpolio syndrome in, 562
Peripheral nervous system, 472, 474–475, 475*f*
Peripheral neuropathy
    in AIDS dementia complex, 1093
    in chronic renal failure, 803*f*
Peripheral vascular disease, 406–409
    aneurysm in, 411–412
    Buerger's disease in, 413
    carotid occlusion in, 413
    chronic venous insufficiency in, 420–421, 421*f*
    community care in, 423
    data collection for, 422*b*
    diabetes mellitus and, 875–876
    nursing diagnoses for, 389
    peripheral arterial disease in, 407–409, 408*t*
    Raynaud's disease and phenomenon in, 413–414, 414*f*
    superficial thrombophlebitis in, 415
    as surgical risk factor, 67*t*
    varicose veins in, 416–420, 420*f*
    venous stasis ulcers in, 420–421, 421*f*
    venous thrombosis in, 414–415
Peripheral vascular system, 407*f*
Peripherally acting adrenergic blockers, 402*t*
Peripherally inserted central catheter, 56, 56*f*, 660
Peristalsis, 623
Peritoneal dialysis, 800, 806–808, 807*f*, 810*t*
Peritoneum, 620
Peritonitis, 668, 673, 939
Permanent contraception, 920–921
Permax; *See* Pergolide
Pernicious anemia, 244*t*, 347, 348*f*, 349, 353*t*, 367
Personal protective equipment, 109–110, 111*f*, 1023*b*, 1128–1129
Personality disorders, 1113–1114, 1114*b*
    borderline personality disorder in, 1114
    guide for assessment in, 1115*b*
Pesticide, development of diabetes mellitus and, 858
PET; *See* Positron emission tomography
Pet therapy, 1088*b*
Petechiae, 339
Petit mal seizure, 524
Peyronie's disease, 927
pH, 45*b*, 47
Phacoemulsification, 598–600
Phagocytosis, 102, 105, 332
Phalanges, 717*f*
Phantom pain, 126, 758
Pharmacologic manipulation of neurotransmitters, 1074–1075
Pharyngitis, 280–281
Pharynx, 257, 258*f*, 620, 621*f*
Phazyme; *See* Simethicone
Phenazopyridine, 786*t*
Phencyclidine hydrochloride, 1072*t*, 1076

Phenelzine, 1056*t*
Phenergan; *See* Promethazine
Phenobarbital, 525*b*, 1123*t*
Phenolphthalein, 666*t*
Phenothiazine, 239*t*
Phenylephrine, 239*t*, 278*t*, 602*t*
Phenylpropanolamine, 239*t*
Phenytoin
    after stroke, 531*t*
    ataxia and, 547
    for dysrhythmias, 438*t*
    intravenous, 526
    for seizure, 525*b*
    for substance abuse-related seizure, 1069, 1069*t*
    therapeutic drug monitoring reference intervals for, 1123*t*
Pheochromocytoma, 847
Philadelphia collar, 1025*f*
Phlebitis, 54*t*
Phobic disorder, 1047
Phosgene, 1007*t*
Phosphate
    blood measurement of, 720*t*
    imbalances of, 42*t*, 45
    normal ranges and functions of, 41*t*
Phosphodiesterase inhibitors, 429*t*
Phosphorus
    blood measurement of, 720*t*
    for bone growth and density, 719*b*
    foods high in, 846*b*
    restrictions in renal failure, 810*t*
Photocoagulation in hemorrhoids, 686
Photodynamic therapy
    for age-related macular degeneration, 609–610
    for bladder cancer, 795
    for esophageal cancer, 645
Photophobia, 576, 598
Photorefractive keratectomy, 595
Physical assessment, 20
Physical carcinogens, 148–149
Physical dependence, 1066*b*
Physical symptoms of substance abuse, 1066*f*
Physiologic stress ulcer, 650
Phytoestrogens, 892*b*
PICC; *See* Peripherally inserted central catheter
PID; *See* Pelvic inflammatory disease
Pieces of Pain Scale, 129
Pilocarpine, 602–604
Pilonidal sinus, 686
Pineal gland, 818, 819*t*, 824*f*
Pinna, 579, 580*f*
Pioglitazone, 862*t*
Pipe smoking, 1075
Piperacillin tazobactam, 786*t*
Piperidine, 239*t*
Pirbuterol, 308*t*
Piroxicam, 170*t*
Pit viper, 1030
Pitavastatin, 454*t*
Pitressin; *See* Vasopressin
Pitting edema, 39, 428, 428*f*
Pituitary, 818, 824*f*
Pituitary disorders, 833–838
    diabetes insipidus in, 835–837, 836*f*
    hypofunction in, 835, 835*t*
    syndrome of inappropriate secretion of antidiuretic hormone in, 837–838, 837*f*
    tumors in, 833–835, 834*f*
Pituitary hormones, 819, 820*f*, 825*t*
Placebo, 134*t*
Plague, 1011*t*, 1013

Planning in nursing process, 26
Plaque, 959*t*
Plasma, 331
Plasma cell, 197*t*, 360
Plasma proteins, 331
Plasmapheresis, 789
Platelet, 207*t*, 333–334
Platelet count, 23
  prevention of bleeding and bruising in low count, 169*b*
  in thrombocytopenia, 359
Platelet transfusion, 363*t*
Pleura, 258
Pleural cavity, 259
Pleural effusion, 302
Pleurisy, 302
Pleurx pleural catheter, 317
PMS; *See* Premenstrual syndrome
Pneumaturia, 773
Pneumococcal vaccine, 296*b*
Pneumocystis jiroveci, 224, 298
Pneumonectomy, 311, 316
Pneumonia, 295–298
  aspiration, 92*t*
  in chronic obstructive pulmonary disease, 305
  complementary and alternative medicine for, 297*b*
  epidemic potential in natural disaster, 1004*t*
  etiology and pathophysiology of, 295–296, 296*f*
  hypostatic, 84
  postoperative, 86, 92*t*
  signs and symptoms of, 297
  ventilator-acquired, 327*b*
Pneumostat, 317
Pneumothorax, 261, 282*f*, 1025
Point of maximal impulse, 372
Poison control center, 1028–1029
Poisoning, 1028–1030
  accidental, 1028–1029, 1029*b*
  food, 1029–1030, 1029*b*
  inhaled poisons and, 1030
Polaramine; *See* Dexchlorpheniramine
Poliomyelitis, 562
Polycystic ovarian syndrome, 904
Polycythemia, 303, 339
Polycythemia vera, 354–355
Polydipsia, 859
Polymyalgia rheumatica, 244*t*
Polymyxin G-bacitracin, 987*t*
Polyp, nasal, 279
Polyphagia, 859
Polypharmacy, 19–20
Polysubstance abuse, 1068
Polyuria, 775*b*, 859
Pons, 473*f*, 473*t*
Pontocaine; *See* Tetracaine
Popliteal pulse, 387, 387*f*
Porcine heterograft, 446*f*
Portal cirrhosis, 701
Portal hypertension, 702*f*
Portal systemic encephalopathy, 707
Positioning
  bony prominences susceptible to skin breakdown and, 977*f*
  in musculoskeletal disorders, 729
  to prevent abduction contracture, 756
Positive end-expiratory pressure, 326
Positive-pressure ventilator, 325
Positive symptoms of schizophrenia, 1103, 1104*f*
Positron emission tomography, 378*t*

Positron emission tomography (*Continued*)
  gynecologic, 895*t*
  in neurologic disorders, 481*t*
Post-thrombotic syndrome, 416
Post-traumatic stress disorder, 1047–1048, 1047*b*
Postanesthesia care unit, 81–83, 82*b*, 82*f*
Postcholecystectomy diet, 692*b*
Posterior chamber, 568, 569*f*
Posterior colporrhaphy, 901*t*, 903–904
Posterior fornix, 881*f*
Posterior pituitary, 819*t*
Posterior tibial pulse, 387*f*
Postictal phase of seizure, 524
Postmastectomy exercises, 914*f*
Postnecrotic cirrhosis, 701
Postoperative care, 81–97
  in amputation, 758–759
  in bariatric surgery, 643
  in breast cancer surgery, 913
  in cardiac surgery, 469
  circulation and tissue perfusion maintenance in, 85, 85*f*
  community care and, 97
  data collection and, 83, 83*b*
  in diabetes mellitus, 866, 866*b*
  discharge planning and, 94–97, 97*b*
  in ear surgery, 617, 617*f*
  in eye surgery, 611, 611*f*
  fluid balance and elimination in, 86–87
  in gallstone surgery, 693–694
  in gastric surgery, 656
  gastrointestinal function promotion in, 87
  in head injury, 503
  home care and, 97*b*
  infection prevention and, 86
  injury prevention and, 85–86
  in intrathoracic surgery, 315–317
  in joint replacement, 749–750, 750*f*
  maintenance of ventilation in, 84
  malignant hyperthermia and, 93–94
  pain management in, 87–88
  postanesthesia care unit and, 81–83, 82*b*, 82*f*
  postoperative complications and, 90–94, 92*t*
  postoperative hemorrhage and shock and, 93
  promotion of psychological adjustment and, 94, 94*b*
  in prostatectomy, 928–931, 930*f*
  in renal trauma, 794
  rest and activity promotion in, 88
  in simple mastectomy, 95*b*
  in thyroidectomy, 841–844
  in tonsillitis, 281
  in urinary diversion, 797–798
  vital signs and, 83*b*
  wound healing promotion in, 89–90
    dehiscence and evisceration and, 91–93, 93*f*
    drains and, 90, 90*f*, 91*f*
    dressings and, 90
    primary intention wound healing and, 89*t*
    removal of sutures and staples in, 90, 91*f*
    wound infection and, 91
Postpolio syndrome, 562
Postrenal acute renal failure, 799
Postural drainage, 321, 322*f*
Postural hypotension, 400*b*
Potassium
  foods high in, 44*b*
  imbalances of, 42*t*, 44

Potassium (*Continued*)
  normal ranges and functions of, 41*t*
  restrictions in renal failure, 810*t*
Potassium iodide, 840
Potassium-sparing diuretics
  for heart failure, 429*t*
  for liver disorders, 696*t*
  for vascular disorders, 402*t*
Pott's disease, 301
Powder application, 963*b*
PPE; *See* Personal protective equipment
PPO; *See* Preferred provider organization
PPS; *See* Prospective payment system
PQRST for pain assessment, 385–386, 386*t*
Practical daily focused assessment, 22
Pramipexole, 554*t*
Pramlinitide, 866*b*, 866*t*
Prandin; *See* Repaglinide
Prazosin, 402*t*
Precose; *See* Acarbose
Prediabetes, 857*t*
Preferred provider organization, 5
Pregabalin, 525*b*
Prehypertension, 399*t*
Premarin, 891
Premature atrial contractions, 436
Premature ejaculation, 924
Premature ventricular contractions, 437*f*, 438
Premenstrual dysphoric disorder, 902
Premenstrual syndrome, 902
Preoperative care, 62–78
  in amputation, 758
  in bariatric surgery, 643
  in breast cancer surgery, 913
  in cardiac surgery, 466–468
  data collection in, 64–67, 65*b*
  deep breathing and coughing instructions in, 71–72, 71*b*, 71*f*
  in diabetes mellitus, 866, 866*b*
  in ear surgery, 615–617
  elimination before surgery and, 70
  in eye surgery, 610
  food and fluids before surgery and, 70
  foot and leg exercises instructions in, 71*b*, 71*f*
  in gallstone surgery, 693
  in gastric surgery, 656
  in head injury, 503
  immediate, 72–74
  in intrathoracic surgery, 315
  in joint replacement, 749
  in nephrectomy and nephrostomy, 791
  pain control and, 70
  patient education in, 66–67, 67*b*
  preoperative checklist for, 73*f*
  preoperative laboratory and diagnostic tests and, 66, 66*b*
  preparation of patient unit and, 74, 74*f*
  in prostatectomy, 928
  in renal trauma, 794
  rest and sedation and, 70
  skin preparation for surgery and, 70
  in thyroidectomy, 841
  in tonsillitis, 281
  tubes and equipment in, 70
Preoperative checklist, 73*f*
Prepuce, 919*f*
Prepyloric ulcer, 650
Prerenal acute renal failure, 799
Presbycusis, 589
Presbyopia, 570, 594
Pressor, 821
Pressure dressing for burn injury, 988, 989*f*

Pressure mapping, 980
Pressure points, 343f
Pressure support ventilation, 326
Pressure ulcer, 977–981
    bony prominence susceptible to skin
        breakdown and, 977f
    Braden scale for, 979f
    cleansing and dressing of, 981
    color of purulent exudate in, 981t
    debridement of, 980–981
    documentation of, 981
    risk factors and prevention of, 977–978,
        978b
    signs and symptoms of, 978–980, 980f
Pressured speech, 1051
Prevacid; See Lansoprazole
Priapism, 924, 926–927
Prilosec; See Omeprazole
Primary amenorrhea, 904
Primary biliary sclerosis, 244t
Primary dysmenorrhea, 902
Primary humoral response, 199–201,
    200f, 204f
Primary hypertension, 399
Primary hyperthyroidism, 839
Primary infertility, 889
Primary intention wound healing, 89t
Primary prevention, 892
Primary pulmonary hypertension, 312
Primary sclerosing cholangitis, 244t
Primary survey, 1023b
Primidone
    for seizures, 525b
    therapeutic drug monitoring reference
        intervals for, 1123t
Prinivil; See Lisinopril
Prion, 103
Prioritizing in data collection, 22–23
Priority setting, 25
Pristiq; See Desvenlafaxine
Pro-Banthine; See Propantheline bromide
Probiotics, 636b
Procainamide, 438t, 1123t
Procan; See Procainamide
Procardia; See Nifedipine
Procedural sedation anesthesia, 76, 77t
Prochlorperazine maleate, 37t
Procrit; See Epoetin alfa
Prodromal stage in hepatitis, 699
Prodrome, 221
Productive cough, 262
Professional behaviors, 1134
Progesterone, 819t
Prograf; See Tacrolimus
Prolactin, 819t, 922t
Prolapse
    of female organs, 882
    mitral valve, 445
Prolia; See Denosumab
Promethazine, 37t, 239t
Prometrium, 891
Promotors of cancer, 148
Pronestyl; See Procainamide
Propafenone, 438t
Propantheline bromide, 647t, 666t
Proparacaine, 602t
Propine; See Dipivefrin
Propoxyphene, 170t
Propranolol, 402t
    for cocaine addiction, 1074–1075
    for dysrhythmias, 438t
    therapeutic drug monitoring reference
        intervals for, 1123t
Propylthiouracil, 840, 840b
Prospective payment system, 5

Prostaglandin analogs, 602t
Prostaglandins, 197t
Prostate, 919, 919f
    benign prostatic hyperplasia and, 927–931,
        927f
    infection of, 932–933
Prostate cancer, 934–935, 935b, 935t
    early detection of, 153b
    metastasis of, 171t
    risk factors for, 152t
Prostate-specific antigen, 154, 155b, 922, 922t,
    934
Prostate tissue analysis, 922t
Prostatectomy, 929t, 931b, 935b
    discharge instructions for, 935b
    nursing care plan for, 931b
Prostatitis, 932–933
Prostatodynia, 933
Prosthesis
    patient teaching in care of, 760b
    preoperative assessment of, 65
Prostigmin; See Neostigmine
Protease inhibitors, 222t
Protected health information, 22b
Protective environment, 110
Protective gear, 1023b
Protein
    adding to diet, 367b
    foods high in, 89b
    intake for immobilized patient, 743b
    restrictions in renal failure,
        810f, 810t
    tests for gastrointestinal disorders and, 626t
Proteinuria, 773
Prothrombin time, 337t
    in acute viral hepatitis, 696t
    in gastrointestinal disorders, 626t
Proton pump inhibitors, 464b, 647t
    drug interactions with, 652b
    fractures and, 737b
    for hiatal hernia, 646
    risk for cardiac problems and, 646b
Protonix; See Pantoprazole
Protozoa, 102
Proventil; See Albuterol
Provider, 4
Prozac; See Fluoxetine
Pruritus
    burn-related, 993
    in cirrhosis, 701
    in hemorrhoids, 686
    in louse infestation, 974
    in urethritis, 788
    vaginal, 890, 906
Pseudo-parkinsonism, 1105, 1106f, 1107t
Pseudocyst, pancreatic, 709
Pseudoephedrine, 239t, 278t
Psoriasis, 969, 969f
Psoriatic arthritis, 969
Psychoactive substances, 1065–1066
Psychodynamic therapy, 1048
Psychological adjustment after surgery,
    94, 94b
Psychological assessment, 7b, 65b
Psychological dependence, 1066b
Psychological disorders, 1045–1062
    anxiety and anxiety disorders in,
        1045–1048, 1046f
    complementary and alternative medicine
        in, 1050b
    cultural considerations in, 1049b
    diagnosis of, 1047
    elderly patient and, 1049b, 1050b
    generalized anxiety disorder in,
        1046–1047

Psychological disorders (Continued)
    history taking in, 1048–1049
    levels of anxiety in, 1046t
    obsessive-compulsive disorder in, 1047
    phobic disorder in, 1047
    post-traumatic stress disorder in,
        1047–1048, 1047b
    promotion of relaxation in, 1050b
    treatment of, 1048, 1048b, 1049t
community care in, 1062
eating disorders in, 1060–1061
    anorexia nervosa in, 640, 1060
    bulimia nervosa in, 640, 1060
mood disorders in, 1051–1052
    antidepressants for, 1056t
    bipolar disorder in, 1049t, 1051–1052,
        1051t, 1052b
    complementary and alternative medicine
        for, 1055b
    major depressive disorder in, 1055–1057
    serotonin syndrome and, 1057b
    suicidal patient and, 1059–1060, 1059b
personality disorders in, 1113–1114, 1114b
    borderline personality disorder in, 1114
    guide for assessment in, 1115b
schizophrenia in, 1103–1108
    data collection in, 1108
    diagnosis of, 1104, 1105t
    etiology and pathophysiology of, 1103
    nursing care plan for, 1110b
    nursing diagnoses for, 1108
    signs and symptoms of, 1103–1104,
        1104f
    treatment of, 1105–1108, 1106f
thought disorders in, 1102–1108
    community care in, 1116
    drug therapy for, 1107t
    interventions for angry, hostile,
        aggressive, manipulative, or
        paranoid patient, 1113b
    neurotransmitters and, 1102–1103, 1103f
    patient rights and, 1108b
Psychological needs of patient, 7–9, 9b
Psychological responses to disaster, 1001
Psychosocial care
    in acquired immunodeficiency syndrome,
        226
    in asthma, 310
    in burn injury, 993
    in multiple myeloma, 360–361
    in musculoskeletal disorders, 731–732
    in neurologic disorders, 497
    in ostomy, 684
    in rheumatoid arthritis, 755
    in spinal cord injury, 512, 513t
    in urinary diversion, 798
Psychotherapeutic interventions, 1048b
Psychotherapy, 1114
Psychotic features, 1102
Psyllium, 666t
PT; See Prothrombin time
PTA; See Percutaneous transluminal
    angioplasty
PTH; See Parathyroid hormone
Ptosis, 571, 576t
    in cluster headache, 546
    in myasthenia gravis, 562, 563f
PTSD; See Post-traumatic stress disorder
PTT; See Partial thromboplastin time
PTU; See Propylthiouracil
Puberty, female, 882
Pubic lice, 973–974, 974f
Pubis, 717f
Public information officer, 1000–1001
Pudendum, 881

Pulmicort; *See* Budesonide
Pulmonary agents in chemical disaster, 1007*t*
Pulmonary angiography, 265*t*
Pulmonary disorders; *See* Respiratory disorders
Pulmonary edema, 314, 431
Pulmonary embolism, 92*t*, 311–312
Pulmonary fibrosis, 302
Pulmonary function tests, 265*t*, 268, 268*f*, 269*f*
Pulmonary hygiene, 260*b*, 285*f*
Pulmonary system; *See* Respiratory system
Pulmonary vascular disorders, 304–305
    primary pulmonary hypertension in, 312
    pulmonary embolism in, 311–312
Pulse deficit, 385–386
Pulse measurement, 387, 387*b*, 387*f*
Pulse pressure, 374
Pulsus paradoxus, 443–444
Pumpkin seeds, 928
Punch biopsy, 957
Pupil, 476*t*
Pupil gauge, 487*f*
Pupillary abnormalities, 488, 488*t*
Pupillary reactions, 487–488
Purified protein derivative tuberculin, 299
Purpura, 359
Pursed-lip breathing, 321*b*, 322–323
Purulent exudate, 981, 981*t*
Pus, wound healing and, 89
Pustule, 959*t*
Pyelonephritis, 788–789
Pyloric sphincter, 620, 622*f*
Pyloroplasty with truncal or proximal gastric vagotomy, 656
Pyrazinamide, 300*t*
Pyridium; *See* Phenazopyridine
Pyridostigmine, 563

Q

Quadrants of abdomen, 21*f*
Quadriceps setting, 729*b*
Quadriplegia, 492, 509
QuantiFERON-TB Gold test, 299
Questran; *See* Cholestyramine
Quinapril, 402*t*
Quinidine, 438*t*, 1123*t*

R

RA; *See* Rheumatoid arthritis
Rabeprazole, 647*t*
Radial keratotomy, 595
Radial pulse, 387*f*
Radiation
    as cause of cancer, 148–149
    exposure in nuclear disaster, 1009, 1009*f*, 1010*t*
    sun exposure precautions and, 955*b*
Radiation dosimeter badge, 162*f*
Radiation skin injury, 982
Radiation therapy, 159–161
    for bone tumor, 758
    for breast cancer, 911–912
    for colorectal cancer, 675
    elderly and, 935*b*
    external, 159–160, 159*f*
    internal, 160–161, 161*b*, 162*f*
    for liver cancer, 708
    for prostate cancer, 935*t*
    for skin cancer, 976
    skin care during, 160*b*
Radical hysterectomy, 901*t*
Radical mastectomy, 910
Radical pancreaticoduodenectomy, 712
Radical prostatectomy, 935*t*

Radical surgery, 63*t*
Radioactive iodine uptake, 824*b*
Radiofrequency catheter ablation
    for esophageal cancer, 645
    for liver cancer, 708
    for pancreatic cancer, 712
    for tachydysrhythmias, 442
Radiography in musculoskeletal disorders, 720*t*
Radioimmunotherapy, 708
Radiologic studies
    in cancer, 154
    in cardiovascular disease, 378*t*
    in gallstones, 692
    in gastrointestinal disorders, 626*t*
    in neurologic disorders, 481*t*
    in respiratory disorders, 265*t*
    in tuberculosis, 299
    in urinary disorders, 767–768, 769*t*
Radionuclide renal scan, 769*t*
Radionuclide studies, 154, 481*t*
Radius, 717*f*
Radon gas, 149
Range of motion exercises, 728–729
Range of motion testing, 719
Ranibizumab, 610
Ranitidine, 647*t*
Rapamycin, 234*t*
Rapid acting insulin, 863*t*
Rapid strep test, 268
Rasagiline, 554*t*
Rash in systemic lupus erythematosus, 246*f*
RAST, 237
Rate of flow in intravenous therapy, 53–57, 55*t*
Rationalization, 1066–1067, 1067*t*
Rattlesnake, 1030
Raynaud's disease, 244*t*, 413–414, 414*f*
Raynaud's phenomenon, 244*t*, 413–414
Razadyne; *See* Galantamine
Reaction formation as defense mechanism, 1067*t*
Reality orientation, 1096*b*
Rebetol; *See* Ribavirin
Rebound hyperglycemia, 874
Receptive aphasia, 495
Reconstruction stage in natural disaster, 1006
Reconstructive mammoplasty, 912
Reconstructive surgery of breast, 912, 913*f*
Recovery position, 1020*f*
Rectal bleeding
    in colorectal cancer, 675
    in diverticulitis, 668
    in inflammatory bowel disease, 671
Rectocele, 903
Rectum, 620, 621*f*, 919*f*
Red blood cell, 332, 333*f*
    anemia and, 346–349
        aplastic, 352, 352*f*
        data collection in, 349–351, 351*b*, 351*f*
        diagnosis of, 337*t*, 348
        etiology of, 346–347, 347*t*
        in leukemia, 355*t*, 359
        pathophysiology of, 347, 347*f*, 348*f*
        signs and symptoms of, 348, 348*t*
        treatment of, 349, 349*t*
        types of, 353*t*
    nutrients needed for erythropoiesis, 335*b*
    sickling of, 353*f*
Red blood cell count, 23, 207*t*, 337*t*
Reducible hernia, 663–664
Reduction
    of dislocation, 735
    of fracture, 738
Reduction mammoplasty, 912

Referred pain, 130–131, 132*f*
Reflex(es), 479–485
Reflex arc, 474, 475*f*
Refraction, 569
Refraction errors, 594–595, 595*f*
Refraction test, 574*t*
Regional anesthesia, 76
Reglan; *See* Metoclopramide
Regression, 1067*t*
Regurgitation
    aortic, 445
    mitral, 445
Rehabilitation
    in amputation, 759–760
    in asthma, 307–310
    in burn injury, 988–989, 989*f*
    in chronic illness, 179–189, 191*f*
    data collection in, 189–190, 189*b*, 190*b*
    in hearing loss, 590–591, 590*f*, 591*f*
    in laryngeal cancer, 289, 290*f*
    in myocardial infarction, 462–464, 462*b*, 463*t*
    nursing diagnoses in, 190, 191*b*
    rehabilitation programs in, 187–188
    rehabilitation team in, 188–189, 189*f*
    in spinal cord injury, 517
    in stroke, 538–539
Relaxation
    as method of pain management, 139
    nutrition and, 1050*b*
Religion
    alcohol use and, 1068*b*
    spiritual beliefs and practices regarding death, 173*t*
Remeron; *See* Mirtazapine
Remicade; *See* Infliximab
Remission induction therapy, 356
Renal angiography, 769*t*
Renal biopsy, 768*b*, 768*f*, 769*t*
Renal dialysis, 803–808
Renal failure, 798–801
    acute, 794, 798–801
    chronic, 801–808
        diabetes mellitus and, 802*b*
        diagnosis of, 802–803
        drug therapy for, 804*t*
        hemodialysis for, 805–806, 805*f*, 806*f*, 811*b*
        kidney transplantation for, 808, 808*b*, 808*f*
        nursing care plan for, 812*b*
        nursing management of, 808–811, 810*f*, 810*t*
        pathophysiology of, 802
        peritoneal dialysis for, 806–808, 807*f*
        signs and symptoms of, 802, 803*f*
    dietary restrictions in, 810*f*, 810*t*
    pathophysiology of, 799*f*
Renal staghorn calculus, 791, 792*f*
Renal stenosis, 791
Renal stones, 791–794, 792*f*, 792*t*
Renal system, 764–782
    bladder health and, 767*b*
    changes with aging, 766
    complications in spinal cord injury, 515
    kidney in, 765, 766*t*, 767*b*
    over-the-counter drugs and, 767*b*
    postoperative assessment of, 83*b*
    potentially nephrotoxic substances and, 767*b*
    structures of, 764–765, 765*f*
    terminology related to urine output and flow, 775*b*
    ureter, bladder, and urethra in, 765–766

Renal transplantation, 808, 808b, 808f
Renal ultrasonography, 769t
Renin, 32, 374, 374f, 766t
Renin-angiotensin-aldosterone system, 32, 374f
Repaglinide, 862t
Repetitive transcranial magnetic stimulation, 1057, 1106
Report, 27
Reporting of sexually transmitted infections, 940
Reproductive disorders
  female, 880–915
    abnormal uterine bleeding in, 904–905, 905b
    bacterial vaginosis in, 939
    breast cancer in, 909–915; See also Breast cancer
    candidiasis in, 939
    cervical cancer in, 907
    community care in, 915
    cultural considerations in, 894b
    dysfunctional uterine bleeding in, 904
    dysmenorrhea in, 902–903, 903t
    endometriosis in, 906
    fibroadenoma in, 908
    fibrocystic breast changes in, 908, 908b
    gynecologic surgical procedures in, 901t
    history taking in, 894, 897b
    home care in, 915
    intraductal papilloma in, 908–909
    leiomyoma in, 905
    lower genital tract inflammations in, 906, 907t
    nursing care plan for hysterectomy and, 898b
    older adult and, 915b
    ovarian cancer in, 908, 908b
    pelvic inflammatory disease in, 939
    pelvic relaxation syndrome in, 903–904
    polycystic ovarian syndrome in, 904
    premenstrual dysphoric disorder in, 902
    premenstrual syndrome in, 902
    toxic shock syndrome in, 906–907
    uterine cancer in, 907–908
    vulvar cancer in, 907
  male, 918–936
    benign prostatic hyperplasia in, 927–931, 927f
    community care in, 935–936
    diagnostic tests for, 921–922, 922t
    ejaculation disorders in, 924
    epididymitis in, 932
    erectile dysfunction in, 923–924, 924b, 924f, 925t
    history taking in, 921, 921b
    hydrocele in, 925–926, 926f
    infertility in, 924–925
    orchitis in, 932
    penile cancer in, 933, 933b
    Peyronie's disease in, 927
    priapism in, 926–927
    prostate cancer in, 934–935, 935b, 935t
    prostatectomy in, 931b, 935b
    prostatitis in, 932–933
    surgical interventions in, 929t, 930f
    testicular cancer in, 933–934, 933b
    testicular torsion in, 926
    varicocele in, 926
Reproductive system
  chronic renal failure and, 803f
  cirrhosis and, 703f
  female, 881–894
    accessory organs of, 882

Reproductive system (Continued)
    aging-related changes in, 882
    breast and, 883
    contraception and fertility and, 883–890, 884t, 888f
    external structures of, 881
    fetal sexual development and, 882
    health screening and assessments in, 892–894, 893f
    internal structures of, 881, 881f
    maturation of, 882
    menopause and, 882, 889b, 890–892, 890b, 891f, 892b
    menstruation and, 883
    phases of reproductive cycle and, 882, 882b
  male, 918–936
    changes with aging, 920, 920b
    contraception and, 920–921
    fertility and, 920
    functions of organs in, 919
    health screening and assessments and, 921b
    sperm production and, 919–920
    structures of, 918–919, 919f
Requip; See Ropinirole
Reserpine, 402t
Reservoir, 108, 108b
Residual schizophrenia, 1105t
Residual urine, 766, 775b
Residual volume, 268, 269f
Resistance, 260b
Respiration
  control of, 259
  trauma and, 1022–1023, 1024f
Respirator, 111f
Respiratory acidosis, 47t, 48
Respiratory alkalosis, 47t, 48–49
Respiratory arrest, 281–282, 282f, 284f
Respiratory disorders
  epidemic potential in natural disaster, 1004t
  lower
    acute bronchitis in, 293–294
    acute respiratory distress syndrome in, 314, 314b
    antiviral medications and, 295b
    asthma in, 305–310
    atelectasis in, 303
    bronchiectasis in, 301–302
    chest injuries in, 312–313
    chest tubes for, 316–317, 316f
    chronic bronchitis in, 303
    chronic obstructive pulmonary disease in, 303–305, 304t
    community care in, 327
    cystic fibrosis in, 301–302
    drug therapy for, 317–320, 321b
    emphysema in, 303, 303f
    empyema in, 298
    extrapulmonary tuberculosis in, 301
    fungal infections in, 298
    humidification for, 320–321
    influenza in, 294–295, 294b, 295b
    intrathoracic surgery for, 315–317
    lung cancer in, 310–311
    lung transplantation in, 312
    mechanical ventilation for, 325–327, 326f, 327b, 327t
    obstructive pulmonary disorders in, 302–311
    occupational lung disorders in, 302
    oxygen therapy for, 323–325, 323f, 323t
    pleural effusion in, 302
    pleurisy in, 302
    pneumonia in, 295–298

Respiratory disorders (Continued)
    pneumothorax and hemothorax in, 313, 313f
    primary pulmonary hypertension in, 312
    pulmonary edema in, 314
    pulmonary embolism in, 311–312
    pulmonary fibrosis in, 302
    pulmonary hygiene for, 321–322, 321b, 322b, 322f
    respiratory failure in, 314–315, 315b
    restrictive pulmonary disorders in, 302
    sarcoidosis in, 302
    tuberculosis in, 298–301, 298b, 300t
  prevention of, 261, 261b
  as surgical risk factor, 67t
  upper, 277–290
    airway obstruction and respiratory arrest in, 281–282, 282f, 284f
    community care and, 289–290
    epistaxis in, 280, 280f
    extended care and, 290
    home care and, 290
    laryngeal cancer in, 283–289
    nasal fracture in, 282–283
    obstructive sleep apnea in, 282
    pharyngitis in, 280–281
    sinusitis in, 279–280
    tonsillitis in, 281
    upper respiratory infection and rhinitis in, 277–279, 278t, 279b
Respiratory distress, 306
Respiratory failure, 260b, 273
Respiratory hygiene, 110–111, 112f
Respiratory management
  in burn injury, 984–985
  in spinal cord injury, 512
Respiratory muscles, 259
Respiratory system
  chronic renal failure and, 803f
  role in acid-base balance, 46, 46f
  severe anemia and, 348t
Respiratory tract infection, 294, 300t
  otitis media and, 612
  prevention of, 113t
  risk for, 261b, 273–274
Rest
  postoperative, 88
  preoperative, 70
  in rheumatoid arthritis, 753–754
Restorative program, 183–184
Restorative surgery, 63t
Restraints, 184–185, 184b, 185b
  in cognitive disorders, 1096, 1096b, 1097b
Restrictive cardiomyopathy, 444b
Restrictive pulmonary diseases, 261, 302
Retin-A; See Tretinoin
Retina, 568, 569f
Retinal angiography, 574t
Retinal detachment, 605–607, 606f
Retinoic acid, 968
Retinopathy, diabetic, 608, 876
Retinoscopy, 574t
Retrograde ejaculation, 924, 930
Retrograde pyelogram, 769t
Retropubic prostatectomy, 929t, 930f
Retropubic suspension, 780–781
Retrospective payment system, 5
Retrovirus, 217
Reuptake of neurotransmitters, 1102–1103
Reverse transcriptase, 217
Reversible contraception, 920
Revex; See Nalmefene
ReVia; See Naltrexone
Review of admission forms, 19
Rewarming process, 1028

Reye syndrome, 279b
RFA; See Radiofrequency catheter ablation
Rheumatoid arthritis, 244t, 746–750,
    747t, 748t
    diet and, 754
    heat and cold applications in, 754, 754b
    history taking in, 750–753, 753b
    joint replacement for, 749–750, 749f, 750b,
        750f
    nursing care plan for total hip replacement
        in, 751b
    psychosocial care in, 755
    rest and exercise for, 753–754
    surgical intervention and orthopedic
        devices for, 749
Rheumatoid factor, 720t
Rhinitis, 277–279, 278t, 279b
Rhinocort; See Budesonide
Rhinoplasty, 283
Rhonchi, 263–264
Rhythm method of contraception, 884t
Rhythmol; See Propafenone
Rib, 717f
Rib fracture, 1024
Ribavirin, 696t
RICE acronym, 734–735
Rickettsia, 103
Rifadin; See Rifampin
Rifampin, 300t
Right atrium, 371
Right coronary artery, 372, 372f
Right-sided brain damage, 535f
Right-sided heart failure, 427, 428t, 432
Right ventricle, 371
Rights of psychiatric patient, 1108b
Rigidity in Parkinson's disease, 552, 552f
Ringer's solution, 52t
Ringworm, 972
Rinne test, 583, 584t
Ritalin; See Methylphenidate
Rivastigmine, 1089t
Robotic(s), 62–64
Robotic gynecologic surgery, 906
Rocaltrol; See Calcitriol
Rods, 569
Romberg test, 479, 585
Ropinirole, 554t
Rosiglitazone, 862t
Rosuvastatin, 454t
Rotator cuff tear, 735
RotoRest Delta Advances Kinetic Therapy
    system, 513f, 729–730
Round ligament, 881f
Round window, 580
Roux-en-Y gastric bypass, 642, 642f
Rubor, 388, 407
Rufinamide, 525b
Rugae, scrotal, 919
Rule of nines, 982, 982f
Rupture
    of Achilles tendon, 736
    of aneurysm, 411
    of intervertebral disk, 517–520, 517f
Russell's traction, 740, 740f
RV; See Residual volume
RYGB; See Roux-en-Y gastric bypass

S
Sabia virus, 1014–1015
Sabril; See Vigabatrin
Sacrum, 510f, 717f
Safe injection practices, 1129
Safe sexual practices, 218b
Safety; See Patient safety
Saint John's wort, 1055b

Salem sump tube, 658b
Saline, 52t
Saline nasal spray, 278t
Salmeterol, 308t
Salmonella, 1029
Salpingectomy, 901t
Salpingitis, 939
Samsca; See Tolvaptan
Sanctura; See Trospium
Saphenous vein graft, 465f
Sarcoidosis, 302
Sarcoma, 146
    Kaposi, 225, 225f
Sarcoptes scabiei, 974
Sarin, 1007t
Saw palmetto, 928
Saxagliptin, 862t
Scabies, 973–974, 974f
Scapula, 717f
Scarring after burn injury, 988
Schilling test, 337t
Schizoid personality disorder, 1114b
Schizophrenia, 1103–1108
    community care in, 1116
    data collection in, 1108
    diagnosis of, 1104, 1105t
    in elderly, 1116b
    etiology and pathophysiology of, 1103
    nursing care plan for, 1110b
    nursing diagnoses for, 1108
    signs and symptoms of, 1103–1104, 1104f
    suicidal ideations and, 1116b
    treatment of, 1105–1108, 1106f,
        1107t
Schizotypal personality disorder,
    1114b
Schwann cell, 477
Scintigraphy, 626t
Sclera, 568, 569f
Scleroderma, 244t
Scleropathy, 420
Sclerotherapy in hemorrhoids, 686
Scotoma, 545
Screening
    for prostate cancer, 934
    in women's health care, 892–894
Scrotum, 918, 919f
    masses in, 925–926, 926f
    varicocele and, 926
Scrub person, 75, 75b, 75f, 76b
Sea bands, 35
Seasonale oral contraceptive, 883–887, 884t
Sebaceous gland, 952, 953f
Seborrheic dermatitis, 967
Second-degree heart block, 436
Secondary amenorrhea, 904
Secondary cellular immune response,
    201–202, 204f
Secondary Cushing syndrome, 852
Secondary dysmenorrhea, 902–903
Secondary hypertension, 399
Secondary hyperthyroidism, 839
Secondary infertility, 889
Secondary prevention, 892
Secondary survey, 1023b
Sectral; See Acebutolol
Security devices, 184–185, 184b, 185b
Sedation, preoperative, 70
Sedimentation rate, 336
Segmental mastectomy, 910
Seizure, 523–526, 525b
    after stroke, 534
    in encephalitis, 544
Selective serotonin reuptake inhibitors
    for anxiety, 1048

Selective serotonin reuptake inhibitors
        (Continued)
    for depression, 1055, 1056t
    triptans and, 545b
Selegiline, 553–554, 553b
Self-care
    deficit in neurologic disorders, 492–493
    in management of hypothyroidism, 844b
Self-esteem, 8
Self-mutilating behavior, 1114
Self-talk, 496
Semen, 919
Semen analysis, 922t, 924–925, 1127t
Semicircular canals, 580f
Seminal fluid, 919
Seminal vesicle, 918
Seminiferous tubule, 919
Semipermeable membrane, 32, 33f
Senile lentigines, 954, 954f
Senile purpura, 960
Senna, 666t
Senokot; See Senna
Sensitivity tests, 116
Sensorineural hearing loss, 581, 581b
    in labyrinthitis, 613
    in Mèniére's disease, 613–614
Sensory dysfunction in multiple sclerosis, 558
Sentinel infection in acquired
        immunodeficiency syndrome, 219
Sentinel node biopsy, 910–911
Sepsis, 115, 1037–1038
    blood transfusion-related, 365t
Septic shock, 115, 1037–1038
Septra; See Trimethoprim-sulfamethoxazole
Sequential compression devices, 416
Sequential pneumatic compression device,
    85, 85f
Serax; See Oxazepam
Serevent; See Salmeterol
Seroma, 89
Seromycin; See Cycloserine
Serosanguineous exudate, 981
Serotonin, 477t, 1103
Serotonin syndrome, 1057b
Serous otitis media, 612
Serpaline; See Reserpine
Sertraline, 1056t
Serum albumin, 696t
Serum bilirubin, 626t, 696t
Serum creatinine, 767, 767b, 769t
Serum ferritin, 337t
Serum immunoglobulins, 207t
Serum lipids, 378t
Serum tests
    for diabetes mellitus, 828t
    reference intervals for, 1120t, 1123t
Serum thyroxine, 824b
Serum triiodothyronine, 824b
Severe acute respiratory syndrome, 294b
Sexual dysfunction
    after spinal cord injury, 513
    in neurologic disorders, 496–497
Sexually transmitted infections, 938–950, 942t
    bacterial vaginosis in, 939
    candidiasis in, 939
    chlamydial infection in, 949b
    community care in, 950
    contraception choices and, 939b
    diagnostic tests for, 941
    history taking in, 941–948, 941b, 948b
    human papillomavirus in, 940
    lesions in, 940, 940b
    media effects on, 939b
    pelvic inflammatory disease in, 939
    prevention of, 948–950, 950b

Sexually transmitted infections (*Continued*)
 reporting of, 940
 risk factors for, 939–940
 transmission of, 940–941
Sharps disposal, 230*b*
Shave biopsy, 957
Shearing action, 977
Sheehan syndrome, 835
Shiley and Portex fenestrated tracheostomy
  tube, 285*f*
Shingles, 971, 971*b*, 971*f*, 972*b*
Shock, 1033–1038
 anaphylactic, 241–243, 241*b*, 242*f*,
  1036–1037
 in burn, 985, 985*b*
 cardiogenic, 1035–1036, 1035*f*
 checking blood products in emergency
  situation and, 1035*b*
 distributive, 1036, 1037*f*
 emotional, 1001
 hypovolemic, 1033–1035, 1035*t*,
  1036*f*
 neurogenic, 1037
 nursing care plan for, 1039*b*
 obstructive, 1036
 in peritonitis, 673
 postoperative, 92*t*, 93
 septic, 1037–1038
 signs and symptoms of, 1033, 1034*f*
 spinal, 513
 systemic inflammatory response syndrome
  and, 1038
Shock wave therapy for gallstones, 693
Short-acting beta-adrenergic agonists, 308*t*
Short acting insulin, 863*t*
Short leg cast, 739
Short spine board, 1025*f*
Shoulder, rotator cuff tear of, 735
Shunting, 260*b*
SIADH; *See* Syndrome of inappropriate
  secretion of antidiuretic hormone
Sibutramine, 641
Sick days in diabetes mellitus, 872*b*
Sickle cell anemia, 353*t*
Sickle cell disease, 353–354, 353*f*, 354*f*
Sickle cell trait, 353
Sickledex, 337*t*
Sigmoid colostomy, 680, 680*f*
Sigmoid conduit, 796*f*, 797
Sigmoidostomy, 796*f*
Sign language, 590
Silvadene; *See* Silver sulfadiazine
Silver nitrate, 987*t*
Silver sulfadiazine, 987*t*
Simethicone, 666*t*
Simple face mask, 323*t*
Simple fracture, 737*b*, 737*f*
Simple surgery, 63*t*
SIMV; *See* Synchronized intermittent
  mandatory ventilation
Simvastatin, 454*t*
Sinemet; *See* Levodopa-carbidopa
Single-barreled colostomy, 679
Single-cannula tracheostomy tube, 285
Single photon emission computerized
  tomography
 in neurologic disorders, 481*t*
 in Parkinson's disease, 552, 552*f*
Singulair; *See* Montelukast
Sinoatrial node, 372
Sinus, 257, 258*f*, 718*t*
Sinusitis, 278*t*, 279–280
SIRS; *See* Systemic inflammatory response
  syndrome
Sitagliptin, 862*t*

Sjögren syndrome, 244*t*
Skeletal muscle, 716
 autonomic system effects on, 476*t*
 preventing contractures and, 728
Skeletal muscle relaxants, 514*t*
Skeletal traction, 740
Skeleton, 717*f*
Skin
 assessment of, 958–960, 959*b*
  in blood disorders, 339
  in cardiovascular disease, 388
  postoperative, 83*b*
  for signs of breakdown, 960
 as barrier to infection, 103–105
 bony prominences susceptible to
  breakdown, 977*f*
 breakdown in spinal cord injury, 515
 changes with aging, 953–954, 954*f*
 chronic renal failure and, 803*f*
 cirrhosis and, 703*f*
 dermatomes of, 472, 474*f*
 functions of, 953
 normal flora of, 101*t*
 preparation for surgery, 70
 self-assessment of, 960*b*
 severe anemia and, 348*t*
 sickle cell disease and, 354*f*
 structure of, 952, 953*f*
 sun exposure precautions and, 955*b*
 tearing of, 956–958, 956*b*
 ultraviolet radiation protection and, 955*b*
Skin biopsy, 957
Skin cancer, 974–977, 975*f*, 976*f*
 early detection of, 153*b*
 risk factors for, 152*t*
 types of, 976*t*
Skin care
 after ostomy, 683–684
 integrity of skin and, 956–958, 956*b*
 during radiation therapy, 160, 160*b*
Skin disorders, 966–994
 application of wet compresses or dressings
  in, 963
 bacterial infections in, 970
 causes of, 954
 cultural considerations in, 958*b*
 diagnostic tests and procedures in,
  957–958
 in elderly, 960*b*
 fungal infections in, 972–973, 972*b*,
  973*b*, 973*f*
 history taking in, 958
 inflammatory infections in, 966–970
  acne in, 967–969
  contact isolation requirements in, 967*b*
  dermatitis in, 966–967
  psoriasis in, 969, 969*f*
  Stevens-Johnson syndrome in,
   969–970
 laundry requirements in, 962
 medicated baths for, 962
 nursing diagnoses for, 960, 961*t*
 physical assessment in, 958–960,
  958*f*, 959*b*
 prevention of, 954–956
 self-assessment of skin in, 960*b*
 skin drainage or weeping in, 957*b*
 skin integrity and, 956–958, 956*b*
 topical therapy for, 963, 963*b*
 types of skin lesions in, 959*t*
 viral infections in, 970–972
  herpes simplex virus in, 970–971,
   970*b*, 970*f*
  herpes zoster in, 971–972, 971*b*,
   971*f*, 972*b*

Skin infection, 966–970
 acne in, 967–969
 contact isolation requirements in, 967*b*
 dermatitis in, 966–967
 fungal, 972–973, 972*b*, 973*f*
 herpes simplex in, 970–971, 970*b*, 970*f*
 herpes zoster in, 971–972, 971*b*, 971*f*, 972*b*
 in intravenous therapy, 54*t*
 psoriasis in, 969, 969*f*
 Stevens-Johnson syndrome in, 969–970
Skin lesions, 959*t*
 documentation of, 960*b*
 herpes simplex virus, 970–971, 970*f*
 herpes zoster, 971–972, 971*f*
 reporting of, 977*b*
 in sexually transmitted infections,
  940, 940*b*
 topical therapy for, 963, 963*b*
Skin patch contraception, 884*t*
Skin patch testing, 957
Skin testing, 206
 for allergy, 237–238
 before immunization, 205
 tuberculin, 299
Skin traction, 740
Skin turgor, 34–35, 34*f*
 in elderly, 960*b*
Skull, 717*f*
Skull radiography, 481*t*
SLE; *See* Systemic lupus erythematosus
Sleep as method of pain management, 138
Sleep deprivation in cardiovascular disease, 394
Sleeved catheter in suctioning, 294
Sliding scale in insulin therapy, 864*b*
Sling, 730, 730*f*
Sling procedure for urinary incontinence, 781
Slipped disk, 517–520, 517*f*
Slit-lamp ocular examination, 573*f*, 574*t*
Slo-Bid; *See* Aminophylline
Slo-Niacin; *See* Nicotinic acid
Small intestine, 620, 621*f*, 622*f*
 diverticulitis of, 668
 gastroenteritis and, 649, 649*b*
 normal flora of, 101*t*
Smallpox, 1011*t*, 1013–1014, 1013*f*, 1014*f*
Smear for sexually transmitted infections, 941
Smoking, 1075, 1075*b*
 age-related macular degeneration and, 608*b*
 bladder cancer and, 795
 effects on musculoskeletal system, 719*b*
 esophageal cancer and, 645
 heart disease and, 376–377
 lung cancer and, 148*b*, 295
 oral cancer and, 644
 oxygen therapy and, 325
 pancreatic cancer and, 710–712
 peptic ulcer and, 650
 wound healing and, 89
Smoking cessation, 261*b*, 414*b*, 712*b*
 in Buerger's disease, 413
 in chronic obstructive pulmonary disease,
  321*b*
 in peripheral vascular disease, 411
Snakebite, 1030–1031
Social assessment, 7*b*
Social needs of patient, 9
Sodium
 blood pressure and, 448
 decrease in diet, 405*b*
 foods high in, 41*b*
 imbalances of, 40–43, 42*t*
 normal ranges and functions of, 41*t*
 restrictions in renal failure, 810*t*
Sodium hypochlorite solution, 987*t*
Sodium polystyrene, 804*t*

Sodium-restricted diet, 789
Solifenacin, 779–780, 780t
Solu-Medrol; See Methylprednisolone
Somatic pain, 125, 125t
Somogyi effect, 874
Sonogram, gynecologic, 895t
Sorafenib
    for gastric cancer, 657–658
    for liver cancer, 708
    for renal cancer, 798
Sore throat, 280–281
Specialty beds for musculoskeletal disorders, 729–730, 730f
SPECT; See Single photon emission computerized tomography
Speech
    after stroke, 532
    aphasia and, 495–496, 496b
    production by larynx, 258
Speech reading, 590
Speed shock in intravenous therapy, 54t
Sperm count, 924–925
Sperm production, 919–920
Spermatic cord, 919, 926f
    testicular torsion and, 926
    varicocele and, 926
Spermatocele, 926f
Spermatogenesis, 919
Spermicide, 884t
Sphenoid sinus, 258f
Spica cast, 739
Spider angioma, 701
Spinal accessory nerve, 475t
Spinal anesthesia, 77t
Spinal column divisions, 510f
Spinal cord, 472
Spinal cord compression, 171
Spinal cord injury, 509–515, 1024, 1025f
    autonomic dysreflexia in, 514–515
    deep venous thrombosis in, 515
    drug therapy for, 514t
    etiology of, 509, 510f
    heterotopic ossification in, 515
    immobilization and surgery in, 512, 512f, 513f
    infection risk in, 515
    muscle spasms in, 513–514
    nursing planning in, 516–517, 516f
    orthostatic hypotension in, 515
    pathophysiology of, 509, 511f
    psychological care in, 512, 513t
    rehabilitation in, 517
    renal complications in, 515
    respiratory management in, 512
    sexual concerns in, 513
    signs and symptoms of, 509–510, 511t
    skin breakdown in, 515
    spinal shock and neurogenic shock in, 513
    treatment of, 510–513
    urinary management in, 512
Spinal cord stimulator, 140
Spinal fusion, 519
Spinal immobilization, 1025f
Spinal nerves, 510f
Spinal shock, 513
Spinal surgery, 518–519, 519b, 520b
Spinal tap, 481t
Spine, vertical compression of, 511f
Spine radiography, 481t
Spiral fracture, 737f
Spiritual assessment, 7b, 65b
Spiritual care, 10, 11b
Spironolactone, 402t, 696t
Spleen, 196, 196f
    assessment in blood disorders, 340
    sickle cell disease and, 354f

Spleen sonogram, 207t
Splenectomy, 359–360, 367
Splenomegaly
    in leukemia, 355t
    in polycythemia vera, 354
Splint, 730, 730f, 739–740, 739f
Splitting
    in borderline personality disorder, 1114
    as defense mechanism, 1067t
Sprain, 734–735
Sprue, 673–674
Sputum, 262, 263t
Sputum analysis, 265t, 299
Squamous cell carcinoma, 975, 975f, 976t
SSRIs; See Selective serotonin reuptake inhibitors
ST segment elevation myocardial infarction, 455–458
Stabilization of fracture, 738
Stable angina, 452, 455
Staff communication, 26–27
Staining for sexually transmitted infection, 941
Stamey procedure, 780–781
Standard precautions, 1128–1130, 109, 109b
Standard steps in nursing procedures, 1130–1131
Standards of practice, 1134–1136
Stapedectomy, 614–615
Stapes, 579, 580f
Staphylococcus aureus in toxic shock syndrome, 906–907
Staples, removal of, 90, 91f
Starlix; See Neteglinide
Stasis, 71
Stasis dermatitis, 967
Statins, 454t
Status asthmaticus, 306
Status epilepticus, 524
Steatohepatitis, 701b
Steatorrhea, 674
Stem cell transplantation, 165, 364–366
Stenosis
    aortic, 445
    of left anterior descending coronary artery, 455f
    mitral, 443f, 445
    renal, 791
Stent, 409, 464f
    drug-eluting, 464
Stereotactic neurosurgery, 554
Stereotypes, 10
Sternum, 717f
Stevens-Johnson syndrome, 969–970
Stimulants abuse, 1072t, 1074–1075, 1074f
STIs; See Sexually transmitted infections
Stoma, 283
Stoma care, 682
Stomach, 620, 621f, 622f
    cancer of, 152t, 657–658, 657b
    gastritis and, 649–650
    gastroenteritis and, 649, 649b
Stomatitis, 643
    chemotherapy-related, 359
Stool examination, 625–631, 626t
Strain, 735
Stratum corneum, 952, 953f
Stratum germinativum, 953f
Streptococcus pneumoniae
    in otitis media, 612
    throat culture for, 268
    in tonsillitis, 281
Streptomycin, 300t

Stress
    anxiety and, 1050b
    behavioral effects of, 1046f
    cancer and, 150
    caregiver, 193b
    development of diabetes mellitus and, 858
    hypertension and, 405–406
    peptic ulcer and, 650
Stress echocardiogram, 378t
Stress incontinence, 777, 903
Stretching exercises for back, 729b
Stridor, 49
Stroke, 528–534
    after carotid endarterectomy, 413b
    cerebral aneurysm and arteriovenous malformation in, 528–530, 530f
    complications of, 534, 535f
    diabetes-related, 875
    diagnosis of, 532, 532f
    dysphagia in, 539b
    etiology of, 528
    nursing care plan for, 536b
    pathophysiology of, 528–530, 529f
    prevention of, 530
    rehabilitation in, 538–539
    risk factors for, 528b
    signs and symptoms of, 530–532, 530b, 531f
    surgery for obstruction in, 533–534, 534f
    treatment of, 531t, 532–534
Stroke volume, 373
Stromal cell, 199–200
Struvite stones, 792t
Stump care, 759, 759f, 760b
Stye, 577t
Subarachnoid hemorrhage, 530
Subarachnoid space, 475, 477f
Subclavian artery pressure point, 343f
Subcutaneous analgesics, 136
Subcutaneous emphysema, 315–316
Subcutaneous infusion, 56
Subcutaneous tissue, 952, 953f
Subdural hematoma, 501, 501f
Subjective data, 18
Sublimation, 1067t
Sublingual carbon dioxide level, 265t
Sublingual gland, 621f
Sublingual nitroglycerin, 455
Subluxation, 509, 735
Submandibular gland, 621f
Suboxone; See Buprenorphine
Substance abuse, 1065–1082
    alcohol in, 1068, 1068b
    central nervous system depressants in, 1071–1073, 1072b
    characteristics of abused substances in, 1072t
    common terminology in, 1066b
    community care in, 1081–1082
    data collection in, 1076–1077, 1076b
    defense mechanisms and, 1067t
    drug therapy for, 1069t
    effects on family and friends, 1067–1068
    elderly and, 1077b, 1082b
    family interventions in, 1078–1081
    hallucinogens and inhalants in, 1076
    health care worker and, 1081
    hepatitis C and, 694
    marijuana in, 1075–1076
    nicotine in, 1075, 1075b
    nursing care plan for, 1079b
    nursing diagnoses in, 1077
    one-to-one observation in, 1078b
    opiates in, 1073–1074, 1073b
    signs and symptoms of, 1066–1067, 1066f

Substance abuse (*Continued*)
 stimulants in, 1074–1075, 1074f
 as surgical risk factor, 67t
 twelve-step program for, 1071, 1071b
Substance-induced delirium, 1086
Subtotal gastrectomy, 656
Subtotal parathyroidectomy, 847
Subutex; *See* Buprenorphine
Sucralfate, 647t, 652
Suctioning, 272
 endotracheal and tracheostomy, 293, 293f, 294f
Sudafed; *See* Pseudoephedrine
Suicidal ideations
 in borderline personality disorder, 1114
 in schizophrenia, 1116b
Suicidal patient, 1059–1060, 1059b
Sulfa drug allergy, 863b
Sulfamethoxazole, 786t
Sulfamylon; *See* Mafenide acetate
Sulfasalazine, 666t
Sulfisoxazole, 786t
Sulfonamides, 786t
Sulfonylureas
 allergy to, 863b
 for diabetes mellitus, 862t
Sun exposure precautions, 955b
Sundowning, 186, 1094
Sunitinib
 for gastric cancer, 657–658
 for liver cancer, 708
 for renal cancer, 798
Superficial burn, 984t
Superficial partial-thickness burn, 984t
Superficial spreading melanoma, 976t
Superficial thrombophlebitis, 415
Superior vena cava, 374
Superior vena cava syndrome, 171
Support group for substance abuse, 1073–1074
Suppurative otitis media, 612
Suprapubic catheter, 794t
Suprapubic prostatectomy, 928–929, 929t, 930f
Supratentorial brain tumor, 539–540
Supraventricular tachycardia, 436
Suprax; *See* Cefixime
Surfactant, 259, 260b, 666t
Surfak; *See* Docusate sodium
Surge capacity, 1000
Surgery, 62–78
 anesthesia in, 75–76, 77t
  general, 76
  local, 76
  procedural sedation, 76
  regional, 76
 autologous blood transfusion in, 64
 bariatric, 641–642, 642f
 for benign prostatic hyperplasia, 928, 929t
 bloodless, 64
 for bone tumor, 758
 for brain tumor, 541
 for cancer, 158–159
 cardiac, 464–469
  community care in, 469
  coronary artery bypass graft in, 465–466, 465f
  heart transplantation in, 466
  nursing care plan for, 467b
  open heart surgery in, 464–465
  percutaneous transluminal coronary angioplasty in, 464, 464f
  postoperative care in, 469
  preoperative care in, 466–468

Surgery (*Continued*)
 transmyocardial laser revascularization in, 464
 categories of, 63t
 circulating nurse and scrub person in, 75, 75b, 75f, 76b
 consent for, 68–70, 68b
 data collection before, 64–67, 65b
 deep breathing and coughing instructions before, 71–72, 71b, 71f
 ear, 615–617
  home care after, 617b
  nursing care plan for tympanoplasty in, 615b
  postoperative care in, 617, 617f
  preoperative care in, 615–617
 elimination before, 70
 eye, 610–611
  for cataracts, 598–600, 599b
  in elderly, 597b
  patient teaching in, 600b
  postoperative care in, 611
  preoperative care in, 610
 for female organ prolapse, 903–904
 food and fluids before, 70
 for fracture, 738
 gynecologic, 901t
 for head injury, 503
 immediate preoperative care in, 72–74
 for inflammatory bowel disease, 672
 intraoperative care and, 74
 laparoscopic surgical fundoplication, 649, 649f
 for male urologic disorders, 929t, 930f
 marking of surgical site, 596b
 mastectomy, 69b
 for obstruction in stroke, 533–534, 534f
 for oral cancer, 644
 ostomy, 679–681
  changing collection device after, 681f, 684
  colostomy in, 679–680, 679f, 685f
  cultural considerations in, 683b
  evacuation and irrigation after, 682–683
  ileostomy in, 680–681, 680f
  measurement of intake and output after, 682
  patient education in, 684–685
  periostomal skin care after, 683–684
  preoperative care in, 681
  psychosocial concerns in, 684
  stoma care in, 682
 pain control before, 70
 for pancreatic cancer, 712
 for Parkinson's disease, 554
 patient education before, 66–67, 67b
 for peptic ulcer, 655–657, 656f
 for peritonitis, 673
 postoperative care in; *See* Postoperative care
 potential intraoperative complications in, 77–78
 preoperative care in; *See* Preoperative care
 preoperative checklist for, 73f
 preoperative laboratory and diagnostic tests in, 66, 66b
 preparation of patient unit and, 74, 74f
 rest and sedation before, 70
 for rheumatoid arthritis, 749
 risk of complications in, 66, 67t
 skin preparation for, 70
 for spinal cord injury, 512, 512f, 513f

Surgery (*Continued*)
 surgical holding area and, 75
 surgical suite and, 75
 surgical team and, 74
 teaching postoperative foot and leg exercises before, 71b, 71f
 technical advances in, 62–64
 terminology used in, 64b
 tubes and equipment in, 70
 for urinary incontinence, 780–781
 valve replacement, 446, 446f
Surgical asepsis, 115
Surgical holding area, 75
Surgical suite, 75
Surgical team, 74
Surgically mature stoma, 679
Surrogate mother, 890b
Surveillance and reporting of infection, 114–115
Susceptibility to infection, 110t
Sustained release implant contraception, 884t
Sutent; *See* Sunitinib
Suture removal, 90, 91f
Swallowing
 after laryngectomy, 289b
 dysphagia and, 493, 643–644
Swan-Ganz catheter, 378t
Sweat gland, 476t, 952, 953f
Symlin; *See* Pramlinitide
Symmetrel; *See* Amantadine
Sympathetic nervous system, 474
Sympathomimetics, 602t
Symphysis pubis, 881f
Symptothermal method of contraception, 884t
Synapse, 476
Synaptic cleft, 1102–1103
Synchronized intermittent mandatory ventilation, 325–326
Syncope, 387–388
Syndrome of inappropriate secretion of antidiuretic hormone, 837–838, 837f
Synovectomy, 749
Synovial fluid culture, 720t
Syphilis, 942t
Systemic inflammatory response syndrome, 1037, 1038
Systemic lupus erythematosus, 244t, 245–248
 diagnosis of, 247, 247t
 etiology and pathophysiology of, 246
 nursing care plan for, 248b
 signs and symptoms of, 246–247, 246f
 skin protection in, 247b
Systemic mycoses, 972
Systolic failure, 428

T

T-bar, 323t
T lymphocyte
 in cell-mediated immunity, 201, 202f
 in humoral immunity, 199
t-PA; *See* Tissue plasminogen activator
T-tube drain, 90f, 693, 693b, 693f
Tachycardia, 435
 in anaphylactic reaction, 241
 in anemia, 348
 ventricular, 437f, 438–440
Tachypnea, 273f
 in acute respiratory distress syndrome, 314
 in anemia, 348
 in respiratory distress, 262
Tacrine, 1089t
Tacrolimus
 for kidney transplantation, 808
 therapeutic drug monitoring reference intervals for, 1123t

Tagamet; *See* Cimetidine
Tai Chi, 719*b*, 972*b*
Tambocor; *See* Flecainide
Tamoxifen, 911
Tamponade, 929
Tamsulosin, 780*t*
Tapazole; *See* Methimazole
Tar preparations, 969
Tardive dyskinesia, 1105, 1106*f*, 1107*t*
Target cell, 822
Target tissues, 822
Tarsals, 717*f*
Tasmar; *See* Tolcapone
Tattoo, HIV exposure and, 218
Tavist; *See* Clemastine
Technetium pyrophosphate scan, 378*t*
TEE; *See* Transesophageal echocardiography
Tegretol; *See* Carbamazepine
Tekturna; *See* Aliskiren
Telbivudine, 696*t*
Telecommunication device, 591
Telemetry, 384, 384*f*
Teletherapy, 159
Temazepam, 1072
Temporal arteritis, 244*t*
Temporal artery pressure point, 343*f*
Temporal pulse, 387*f*
Temporary transvenous pacemaker, 440–441, 441*f*
Temsirolimus, 798
Tenckhoff catheter, 806–807, 807*f*
Tender points in fibromyalgia, 254, 254*f*
Tendon, 716
    strain of, 735
Tenofovir, 696–698, 696*t*
Tenormin; *See* Atenolol
TENS; *See* Transcutaneous electrical nerve stimulation
Tensilon test, 563
Tension-free vaginal tape sling procedure, 903–904
Tension headache, 546
Tension pneumothorax, 1025, 1036
Tension release relaxation method, 139
Terazosin, 402*t*
Terminal hydration, 174
Testicular cancer, 153*b*, 926*f*, 933–934, 933*b*
Testicular self-examination, 921*b*, 921*f*, 922*t*, 933*b*
Testicular torsion, 926, 926*f*
Testis, 818, 819*t*, 824*f*, 918, 919*f*, 926*f*
    hydrocele and, 925–926, 926*f*
    orchitis and, 919
Testosterone, 819*t*, 920, 922*t*
Tetanus, 1004*t*
Tetany, 44, 45*f*
    acute hypoparathyroidism with, 846
    in postoperative thyroidectomy patient, 841–843
Tetracaine, 602*t*
Tetracycline, 647*t*
Tetraplegia, 492, 509
Thalamus, 473*f*, 473*t*
Thallium perfusion imaging, 378*t*
Thallium scan, 720*t*
Theo-Dur; *See* Aminophylline
Theophylline, 1123*t*
Therapeutic alliance, 1110
Therapeutic communication, 2, 8
Therapeutic donor insemination, 890*b*
Therapeutic drug monitoring, 1123*t*
Therapeutic immunosuppression, 233–235, 234*b*, 234*t*
Therapeutic nurse-patient relationship, 8–9
Therapeutic suggestion, 139

Therapeutic touch, 9
Thiamine
    for liver disorders, 696*t*
    for substance abuse, 1069*t*, 1071
Thiazide diuretics
    contraindication in hyperparathyroidism, 847*b*
    for heart failure, 429*t*
    for vascular disorders, 402*t*
Thiazolidinediones, 862*t*
Thin prep, 895*t*
Third-degree heart block, 437*f*, 438
Third spacing, 39
Thirst in diabetes insipidus, 836
Thomas splint, 740
Thoracentesis, 265*t*, 302
Thoracic trauma, 1024
Thoracic vertebrae, 510*f*, 717*f*
Thoracotomy, 315
Thought disorders, 1102–1108
    community care in, 1116
    drug therapy for, 1107*t*
    interventions for angry, hostile, aggressive, manipulative, or paranoid patient, 1113*b*
    neurotransmitters and, 1102–1103, 1103*f*
    patient rights and, 1108*b*
    schizophrenia in, 1103–1108
        data collection in, 1108
        diagnosis of, 1104, 1105*f*
        etiology and pathophysiology of, 1103
        nursing care plan for, 1110*b*
        nursing diagnoses for, 1108
        signs and symptoms of, 1103–1104, 1104*f*
        treatment of, 1105–1108, 1106*f*
Three-chamber closed drainage system, 317
Three-point crutch gait, 730*b*
Throat
    normal flora of, 101*t*
    visual examination of, 264–268
Throat cancer, 262, 283–289
    communication after laryngectomy and, 289, 289*f*
    endotracheal intubation and tracheostomy in, 284–286, 285*f*
    etiology and pathophysiology of, 283
    home care of tracheostomy in, 286*b*
    nursing care plan for laryngectomy, 287*b*
    nursing management of, 286–289
    nutrition considerations in, 289*b*
    rehabilitation in, 289, 290*f*
    signs and symptoms of, 283, 283*b*
    treatment of, 283–286, 284*f*
Throat culture, 268, 281
Throat lozenge, 280
Thromboangiitis obliterans, 413
Thrombocyte, 207*t*, 333, 333*f*
Thrombocytopenia, 334–335, 359–360, 359*f*, 1068
Thrombolytic therapy, 416
Thrombophlebitis, 71, 406
    in intravenous therapy, 54*t*
    postoperative, 85, 92*t*
Thrombus, 409
Thrush, 972
Thymosin, 819*t*
Thymus gland, 195, 196*f*, 197*t*, 818, 819*t*, 824*f*
Thyrocalcitonin, 819, 838
Thyroid, 818, 819*t*, 824*f*
    posterior palpation of, 827*f*
Thyroid cancer, 845, 845*b*
Thyroid crisis, 840, 843

Thyroid disorders, 838–845, 838*f*
    cancer in, 845
    goiter in, 838–839, 839*f*
    hyperthyroidism in, 839–840, 840*f*, 841*b*
    hypothyroidism in, 844–845, 844*b*
    myxedema coma in, 845
    thyroid storm in, 843, 843*b*, 844*b*
    thyroidectomy in, 840–844
    thyroiditis in, 845
Thyroid hormones, 819–821
    effects of aging on, 822
    pituitary hypofunction and, 835*t*
    testing of, 825*t*
Thyroid medications, 844*b*
Thyroid-releasing hormone, 838
Thyroid scan, 824*b*
Thyroid-stimulating hormone, 24, 819*t*, 824*b*, 838
Thyroid storm, 843, 843*b*, 844*b*
Thyroidectomy, 840–844, 845
Thyroiditis, 845
Thyrotoxicosis, 843
Thyroxine, 819, 819*t*, 838
TIA; *See* Transient ischemic attack
Tiagabine, 525*b*
Tibia, 717*f*
Tic douloureux, 546–547, 547*f*
Ticarcillin/clavulanic acid, 786*t*
Tick, 544*b*, 1031
Tidal volume, 268, 269*f*
Tikosyn; *See* Dofetilide
Tiladel; *See* Nedocromil
Time-cycled ventilator, 325
Timentin; *See* Ticarcillin/clavulanic acid
Timolol, 402*t*
Tinea barbae, 972
Tinea cruris, 972
Tinea pedis, 972, 973
Tinnitus, 589–590, 613–614
Tissue integrity in cardiovascular disease, 395
Tissue perfusion
    cardiovascular disease and, 394–395
    postoperative, 85, 85*f*
Tissue plasminogen activator, 531*t*, 533
Tissue turgor, 34–35, 34*f*
TLC; *See* Total lung capacity
TNM staging system, 146–147
Tobacco use, 1075, 1075*b*
    age-related macular degeneration and, 608*b*
    bladder cancer and, 795
    effects on musculoskeletal system, 719*b*
    esophageal cancer and, 645
    heart disease and, 376–377
    lung cancer and, 148*b*, 295
    oral cancer and, 644
    oxygen therapy and, 325
    pancreatic cancer and, 710–712
    peptic ulcer and, 650
    wound healing and, 89
Tobramycin, 786*t*, 1123*t*
Tocainamide, 438*t*
Tocainide, 1123*t*
Toe
    bunion of, 736
    gangrene of, 408*f*
Tofranil; *See* Imipramine
Toileting
    establishing schedule of, 781*b*
    immobility and, 724
Tolcapone, 554*t*
Tolerance, 1066–1067, 1066*b*
Tolterodine, 779–780, 780*t*

Tolvaptan, 838
Tomography, 720*t*
Tongue, 621*f*
Tono-Pen, 573*f*
Tonocard; *See* Tocainamide
Tonsil, 196, 196*f*, 257, 258*f*
Tonsillitis, 281
Topamax; *See* Topiramate
Topical analgesics, 136
Topical dye test, 574*t*
Topical therapy
   for burn injury, 987*t*
   for skin disorders, 963, 963*b*
Topiramate, 525*b*
Toprol XL; *See* Metoprolol
Torisel; *See* Temsirolimus
Tornado, 999*b*
Torsemide, 402*t*
Torsion, testicular, 926, 926*f*
Total gastrectomy, 656, 656*f*
Total hip replacement, 749–750, 749*f*,
   750*f*, 751*b*
Total iron-binding capacity, 337*t*
Total knee replacement, 750
Total laryngectomy, 283–284
Total lung capacity, 268, 269*f*
Total mastectomy, 910
Total parenteral nutrition, 56–57, 57*b*,
   660, 660*b*
   in acute pancreatitis, 709
Total serum complement, 207*t*
Total thyroxine, 824*b*
Toviaz; *See* Festerdine
Toxic agents, 352*b*, 1126*t*
Toxic goiter, 839
Toxic shock syndrome, 906–907
Toxin, 200
Toxoplasmosis, 224, 224*b*
TPN; *See* Total parenteral nutrition
Trabeculectomy, 605
Trabeculoplasty, 604
Trachea, 257, 258*f*
Tracheobronchitis, 293
Tracheostomy, 283
   care of, 296, 296*f*, 297*f*
   home care of, 286*b*
   in laryngeal cancer, 284–286, 285*f*
   in oral cancer surgery, 644
   suctioning of, 293, 293*f*, 294*f*
Tracheostomy collar, 323*t*
Tracheostomy tube, 285–286, 285*f*
Traction, 740, 740*f*, 744*b*
Trandate; *See* Labetalol
Transcutaneous electrical nerve stimulation,
   140, 903*b*
Transcutaneous pacemaker, 440–441
Transdermal patch, 136
Transduction of pain, 126, 126*f*
Transesophageal echocardiography,
   378*t*
Transformation of cancer cell, 149
Transfusion, 362–364
   blood products used in, 363*t*
   consent for, 362*b*
   HIV exposure and, 218
Transfusion reaction, 358*t*, 364, 364*b*, 365*t*
Transient ischemic attack, 527–528
Transmission of pain, 126, 126*f*
Transmyocardial laser revascularization, 464
Transplantation
   bone marrow, 165
      in blood disorders, 364–366
      for sickle cell disease, 354
   corneal, 596–597, 596*f*
   heart, 431, 466

Transplantation (*Continued*)
   islet cell, 866
   kidney, 808, 808*b*, 808*f*
   liver, 707
   lung, 312
Transrectal ultrasound, 922*t*
Transsphenoidal surgical approach for
   hypophysectomy, 834*f*
Transtracheal catheter, 323*t*
Transurethral electrovaporization of prostate,
   929*t*
Transurethral incision of prostate, 929*t*
Transurethral microwave thermotherapy,
   929*t*
Transurethral needle ablation, 929*t*
Transurethral photoselective vaporization of
   prostate, 929*t*
Transurethral resection of bladder, 795
Transurethral resection of prostate, 928–929,
   929*t*
Transvaginal electrical stimulation, 780*b*
Transvenous pacemaker, 440–441, 441*f*
Transverse colostomy, 680, 680*f*
Transverse fracture, 737*f*
Tranylcypromine, 1056*t*
Trauma, 1019–1042
   abdominal, 1025–1026
   accidental poisoning and, 1028–1029, 1029*b*
   airway and respiration in, 1022–1023, 1024*f*
   animal bites and, 1030
   bladder, 794–795
   burn, 981–989
      classification of, 982*f*, 983*f*, 984*t*
      complications of, 988
      debridement for, 986
      emergency treatment of, 983–984, 984*b*
      escharotomy for, 986, 987*f*
      etiology and pathophysiology of,
         981–982
      fluid resuscitation and prevention of
         shock in, 985, 985*b*
      grafting for, 986–988, 988*f*
      infection prevention in, 985–986, 992
      itching in, 993
      nursing care plan for, 990*b*
      nutritional support in, 993
      pain management in, 985, 989–992, 992*b*
      patient-family education in, 993
      psychosocial support in, 993
      rehabilitation for, 988–989, 989*f*
      respiratory support in, 984–985
      signs and symptoms of, 982
      topical medications for, 987*t*
      wound treatment in, 986–988
   cardiac, 446–447
   cardiopulmonary resuscitation in,
      1032–1033, 1034*t*
   chemical burns and, 1032
   chest, 1024–1025
   choking emergencies and, 1032
   combative patient and, 1040–1041, 1041*b*
   control of bleeding in, 1023–1024
   domestic violence and abuse and,
      1041–1042, 1041*b*
   electric shock and burns and, 1031–1032,
      1032*f*
   emergency care in, 1021–1026
   to eye, 572
   first aid and Good Samaritan laws,
      1020–1021, 1021*t*
   focused assessment in, 1023*b*
   food poisoning and, 1029–1030, 1029*b*
   frostbite and, 1027–1028, 1028*b*
   head, 500–508
      diagnosis of, 502, 503*f*

Trauma (*Continued*)
      drug therapy for, 514*t*
      etiology of, 500
      increased intracranial pressure in,
         506–508
      levels of consciousness and, 502*b*
      nursing care plan for, 504*b*
      pathophysiology of, 500–501, 501*f*
      patient teaching in, 505*b*
      signs and symptoms of, 501–502,
         502*b*, 502*f*
      surgery for, 503
   heatstroke and, 1026–1027
   highway safety and, 1019
   home safety and, 1019, 1020*b*
   human bites and, 1030
   hypothermia and, 1027, 1027*b*
   inhaled poisons and, 1030
   insect bites and stings and, 1031, 1031*b*
   to kidneys and ureters, 794
   metabolic emergencies and, 1026
   multiple, 1026
   neck and spine, 1024, 1025*f*
   ocular, 597–598, 597*f*
   personal protective equipment and, 1023*b*
   pneumothorax, hemothorax, and tension
      pneumothorax in, 1025
   shock and, 1033–1038
      anaphylactic, 1036–1037
      cardiogenic, 1035–1036, 1035*f*
      checking blood products in emergency
         situation and, 1035*f*
      distributive, 1036, 1037*f*
      hypovolemic, 1033–1035, 1035*t*, 1036*f*
      neurogenic, 1037
      nursing care plan for, 1039*b*
      obstructive, 1036
      septic, 1037–1038
      signs and symptoms of, 1033, 1034*f*
      systemic inflammatory response
         syndrome and, 1038
   snakebite and, 1030–1031
   spinal cord, 509–515
      autonomic dysreflexia in, 514–515
      deep venous thrombosis in, 515
      drug therapy for, 514*t*
      etiology of, 509, 510*f*
      heterotopic ossification in, 515
      immobilization and surgery in, 512, 512*f*,
         513*f*
      infection risk in, 515
      muscle spasms in, 513–514
      nursing planning in, 516–517, 516*f*
      orthostatic hypotension in, 515
      pathophysiology of, 509, 511*f*
      psychological care in, 512, 513*t*
      rehabilitation in, 517
      renal complications in, 515
      respiratory management in, 512
      sexual concerns in, 513
      signs and symptoms of, 509–510, 511*t*
      skin breakdown in, 515
      spinal shock and neurogenic shock in,
         513
      treatment of, 510–513
      urinary management in, 512
   triage in, 1022
   uninsured patient and, 1026*b*
   water safety and, 1019–1020, 1020*f*
Traumatic cataracts, 598
Travel instructions in diabetes mellitus, 872*b*
Trazodone, 1056*t*
Treadmill stress test, 377*f*, 378*t*
Trecator; *See* Ethionamide
Tremor in Parkinson's disease, 552, 552*f*

Tretinoin, 968
Triage, 999, 1022
    disaster preparedness and response and, 1001–1006, 1001t, 1002f
Triage officer, 1000–1001
Triamcinolone, 278t, 308t
Triamterene, 402t, 696t
Triceps reflex, 480
Trichomonas vaginalis, 932
Trichomoniasis, 942t
Tricor; *See* Fenofibrate
Tricyclic antidepressants, 1055, 1056t
Trigeminal nerve, 475t
Trigeminal neuralgia, 546–547, 547f
Trihexyphenidyl, 554t
Triiodothyronine, 819, 819t, 838
Trileptal; *See* Oxcarbazepine
Trimethoprim-sulfamethoxazole, 786t, 788–789
Tripelennamine; *See* Ethylenediamine
Triprolidine, 239t
Triptans, 545b
Trochanter, 718t
Trochlear nerve, 475t
Troponin I, 378t, 459t
Troponin II, 459t
Troponin T, 378t
Trospium, 780t
Trousseau sign, 44, 45f, 845–846
Trovafloxacin, 786t
Trovan; *See* Trovafloxacin
Trusopt; *See* Dorzolamide
Trust, 8
Tubal ligation, 884t
Tube feeding, 658–659, 659b, 659f, 660b
Tubeless gastric analysis, 626t
Tuberculin skin testing, 299
Tuberculosis, 298–301
    in acquired immunodeficiency syndrome, 223
    drug therapy for, 300t
    ethnic occurrence of, 298b
    extrapulmonary, 301
    vitamin D in prevention of, 299b
Tuberosity, 718t
Tubes
    postoperative assessment of, 83b
    in surgery, 70
Tubular necrosis, 766
Tularemia, 1011t, 1014
Tumor
    acoustic neuroma, 614
    brain, 539–541, 540f, 540t, 541f
    classification of, 146
    pheochromocytoma, 847
    pituitary, 833–835, 834f
Tumor lysis syndrome, 171
Tumor markers, 154–155
Tunica adventitia, 374
Tunica intima, 374
Tunica media, 374
Tuning fork tests, 583
Turgor, 34–35, 34f, 960b
Turning
    of patient, 727
    preoperative instructions in, 72
TV; *See* Tidal volume
Twelve-step program for substance abuse, 1071, 1071b
Twenty-four hour urine collection, 768b
Two-hour postprandial blood glucose, 828t
Two-point crutch gait, 730b
Tympanic membrane, 579, 580f
Tympanoplasty, 613
    nursing care plan for, 615b
    in otosclerosis, 615

Type 1 diabetes mellitus, 244t, 857, 857b, 857t
Type 2 diabetes mellitus, 857, 857t
    ethnicity and, 857b
    factors in development of, 858b
    metformin for, 863b
    symptoms of, 857b
Type II second-degree heart block, 436
Typhoid fever, 1004t
Tyzeka; *See* Telbivudine

U
Ulcer
    arterial, 407–408, 408f
    corneal, 577t, 596
    Curling's, 982, 988
    peptic, 650–652
        in chronic obstructive pulmonary disease, 305
        complications of, 655
        diagnosis of, 651–652
        etiology of, 650
        focused assessment for, 652b
        nursing care plan for, 653b
        pathophysiology of, 650–651, 651f
        signs and symptoms of, 651
        surgical treatment of, 655–657, 656f
        treatment of, 652
    pressure, 977–981
        bony prominence susceptible to skin breakdown and, 977f
        Braden scale for, 979f
        cleansing and dressing of, 981
        color of purulent exudate in, 981t
        debridement of, 980–981
        documentation of, 981
        risk factors and prevention of, 977–978, 978b
        signs and symptoms of, 978–980, 980f
    venous stasis, 421–422, 421f
Ulcerative colitis, 670–672, 670t, 671f
Ulna, 717f
Ulnar pulse, 387f
Ultrasonography
    in cardiovascular disease, 378t
    in eye disorders, 574t
    in gastrointestinal disorders, 626t
    gynecologic, 895t
    renal, 769t
Ultrasound arteriography, 481t
Ultraviolet radiation protection, 955b
Umbilical hernia, 664f
Unconscious patient
    airway obstruction in, 1022
    oral care for, 493
Undifferentiated schizophrenia, 1105t
Uni-Dur; *See* Aminophylline
Uninsured patient, trauma and, 1026b
Uniphyl; *See* Aminophylline
Universal signal for choking, 282f
Unlicensed assistive personnel, 3
Unstable angina, 452, 455
Upper gastrointestinal system disorders, 640–660
    dietary guidelines for vomiting in, 649b
    drug therapy for, 647t
    dysphagia in, 643–644
    enteral nutrition for, 658–659, 659b, 659f, 660b
    esophageal cancer in, 645
    gastric cancer in, 657–658, 657b
    gastritis in, 649–650
    gastroenteritis in, 649
    gastroesophageal reflux disease in, 646–649, 646b, 649f

Upper gastrointestinal system disorders (*Continued*)
    gastrointestinal decompression for, 658, 658b
    hiatal hernia in, 645–646
    oral cancer in, 644
    peptic ulcer in, 650–652
    stomatitis in, 643
    total parenteral nutrition for, 660, 660b
Upper GI series, 626t
    in gastric cancer, 657
    in peptic ulcer, 651
Upper respiratory infection, 277–279, 278t, 279b
    otitis media and, 612
Upper respiratory system, 257, 258f
    normal flora of, 101t
Upper respiratory system disorders, 277–290
    airway obstruction and respiratory arrest in, 281–282, 282f, 284f
    community care and, 289–290
    epistaxis in, 280, 280f
    extended care and, 290
    home care and, 290
    laryngeal cancer in, 283–289
        communication after laryngectomy and, 289, 289f
        endotracheal intubation and tracheostomy in, 284–286, 285f
        etiology and pathophysiology of, 283
        home care of tracheostomy in, 286b
        nursing care plan for laryngectomy, 287b
        nursing management of, 286–289
        nutrition considerations in, 289b
        rehabilitation in, 289, 290f
        signs and symptoms of, 283, 283b
        treatment of, 283–286, 284f
    nasal fracture in, 282–283
    obstructive sleep apnea in, 282
    pharyngitis in, 280–281
    sinusitis in, 279–280
    tonsillitis in, 281
    upper respiratory infection and rhinitis in, 277–279, 278t, 279b
Urecholine; *See* Bethanechol
Uremia, 802
Uremic syndrome, 802
Ureter
    functions of, 765–766
    trauma to, 794
Ureteral catheter, 794t
Ureteral stent, 794t
Ureterosigmoidostomy, 796f, 797
Ureterostomy, 796f
Urethra, 764
    female, 881f
    functions of, 765–766
    male, 919, 919f
    urethritis and, 788
Urethral catheter, 794t
Urethral meatus, 881
Urethral pressure study, 769t
Urethral smear, 922t
Urethral sphincter, 764
Urethral stent, 929t
Urethritis, 788
Urge incontinence, 777
Urgency, 774b
Urgent surgery, 63t
Uric acid, 720t, 769t
    chemotherapy-related increase in, 359
    gout and, 755
Uric acid stones, 792t
Urinalysis, 769t
Urinary analgesics, 786t

Urinary antispasmodics, 780*t*
Urinary bladder; *See* Bladder
Urinary catheter, 776–777, 776*b*, 776*f*
Urinary diversion, 795–796, 796*f*
Urinary frequency, 775*b*
  in urethritis, 788
Urinary hesitancy, 775*b*
Urinary ileostomy, 797
Urinary incontinence, 777–782
  aging and, 766
  etiology of, 777
  nursing diagnoses for, 778*t*
  nursing management of, 781–782,
    781*b*, 782*b*
  treatment of, 779–781, 780*b*, 780*t*
Urinary management in spinal cord injury,
    512
Urinary retention, 775*b*, 782
  postoperative, 92*t*
Urinary stasis, 785
  in benign prostatic hyperplasia,
    927
Urinary system, 764–782
  bladder health and, 767*b*
  changes with aging, 766
  complications in spinal cord injury,
    515
  kidney in, 765, 766*t*, 767*b*
  over-the-counter drugs and, 767*b*
  postoperative assessment of, 83*b*
  potentially nephrotoxic substances and,
    767*b*
  structures of, 764–765, 765*f*
  terminology related to urine output and
    flow, 775*b*
  ureter, bladder, and urethra in,
    765–766
Urinary system disorders, 785–812
  acute glomerulonephritis in, 789
  acute renal failure in, 798–801, 799*f*
  bladder cancer in, 795–798, 796*f*
  bladder trauma in, 794–795
  catheters and tubes used in, 794*t*
  causes of, 766–767
  chronic glomerulonephritis in, 789–790
  chronic renal failure in, 801–808
    diabetes mellitus and, 802*b*
    diagnosis of, 802–803
    drug therapy for, 804*t*
    hemodialysis for, 805–806, 805*f*,
      806*f*, 811*b*
    kidney transplantation for, 808,
      808*b*, 808*f*
    nursing care plan for, 812*b*
    nursing management of, 808–811, 810*f*,
      810*t*
    pathophysiology of, 802
    peritoneal dialysis for, 806–808, 807*f*
    signs and symptoms of, 802, 803*f*
  community care in, 811–812
  cystitis in, 785–788
  diagnostic tests and procedures in, 767–768,
    768*f*, 769*t*
  in elderly, 768*b*
  history taking in, 768–773, 773*b*
  hydronephritis in, 790–791
  kidney and ureter trauma in, 794
  kidney cancer in, 798
  measuring intake and output in, 777
  nephrotic syndrome in, 790
  physical assessment in, 773, 774*t*
  prevention of, 767
  pyelonephritis in, 788–789
  renal stenosis in, 791
  renal stones in, 791–794, 792*f*, 792*t*

Urinary system disorders (*Continued*)
  urethritis in, 788
  urinary catheter for, 776–777,
    776*b*, 776*f*
  urinary incontinence in, 777–782
    etiology of, 777
    nursing diagnoses for, 778*t*
    nursing management of, 781–782, 781*b*,
      782*b*
    treatment of, 779–781,
      780*b*, 780*t*
  urinary retention in, 782
  urinary tract infection in
    drug therapy for, 786*t*
    postoperative, 92*t*
    prevention of, 113*t*, 788*b*
Urinary tract infection
  cystitis in, 785–788
  drug therapy for, 786*t*
  in elderly, 786*b*
  postoperative, 92*t*
  prevention of, 113*t*, 788*b*
  pyelonephritis in, 788–789
  urethritis in, 788
Urinary tract obstruction,
    790–794
  hydronephrosis in, 790–791
  kidney stones in, 791–794,
    792*f*, 792*t*
  renal stenosis in, 791
Urinary urgency, 774*b*
Urine, 764
  characteristics of, 773, 774*t*
  reduction of odor of, 798*b*
Urine culture and sensitivity,
    769*t*
Urine osmolality, 769*t*
Urine output
  in acute renal failure, 801
  after burn injury, 985
  measuring of, 777
  postoperative, 86*b*
    in kidney surgery, 792
    in urinary diversion, 797
  in septic shock, 1038
  terminology related to, 775*b*
Urine retention in benign prostatic
    hyperplasia, 927
Urine specimen collection, 777*b*
Urine tests
  for diabetes mellitus, 828*t*
  for endocrine disorders, 824*b*
  reference intervals for, 1124*t*
Urodynamics, 927
Uroflowmetry, 922*t*
Urography, 922*t*
Urologic system; *See* Urinary system
Urticaria, 241
Uterine artery embolization, 905
Uterine cancer, 907–908
  early detection of, 153*b*
  risk factors for, 152*t*
Uterus, 881, 881*f*
  endometriosis and, 906
  fibroids of, 905
  prolapse of, 903
Uveitis, 595

V

Vaccine for human immunodeficiency virus,
    218
Vagal nerve stimulator, 525
Vagina, 881, 881*f*
  inflammation of, 906, 907*t*
  normal flora of, 101*t*

Vaginal discharge, 883
Vaginal ring contraception, 884*t*
Vaginal sponge contraception, 884*t*
Vaginal ultrasonography, 895*t*
Vaginal vestibule, 881
Vaginosis, bacterial, 939
Vagotomy, 656
Vagus nerve, 475*t*
Vagus nerve stimulation, 1057
Valium; *See* Diazepam
Valproic acid, 525*b*, 1123*t*
Valve replacement surgery, 446, 446*f*
Valvular heart disease, 444–446
  aortic regurgitation in, 445
  aortic stenosis in, 445
  medical treatment for, 445–446
  mitral regurgitation in, 445
  mitral stenosis in, 445
  valve replacement surgery for, 446, 446*f*
Vancenase; *See* Beclomethasone
Vanceril; *See* Beclomethasone
Vancomycin, 1123*t*
Varenicline, 1069*t*, 1075
Variant angina, 455
Varicella, 971
Varicella-zoster virus, 221–222, 222*b*
Varicocele, 926, 926*f*
Varicose veins, 416–420, 420*f*
Variola virus, 1011*t*
Vas deferens, 918, 919*f*
Vascular dementia, 1093
Vascular disease, 406–409
  aneurysm in, 411–412
  Buerger's disease in, 413
  carotid occlusion in, 413
  chronic venous insufficiency in,
    420–421, 421*f*
  community care in, 423
  data collection for, 422*b*
  nursing diagnoses for, 389
  peripheral arterial disease in, 407–409, 408*t*
  Raynaud's disease and phenomenon in,
    413–414, 414*f*
  superficial thrombophlebitis in, 415
  as surgical risk factor, 67*t*
  varicose veins in, 416–420, 420*f*
  venous stasis ulcers in, 420–421, 421*f*
  venous thrombosis in, 414–415
Vascular system, 373–374, 373*f*
  changes with aging, 375
  interaction with lymphatic system, 334
Vasectomy, 884*t*, 920–921
Vasoactive substances, 1036
Vasoconstrictors
  for cirrhosis, 707
  for liver disorders, 696*t*
Vasodilators
  for cirrhosis, 707
  for heart failure, 429*t*
  for vascular disorders, 402*t*
Vasopressin, 696*t*
Vasospastic angina, 455
Vasotec; *See* Enalapril
VATS; *See* Video-assisted thoracoscopic
    surgery
VC; *See* Vital capacity
Vectibix; *See* Panitumumab
Vector, 108
Vector-borne diseases, 1004*t*
Vegetations in infective endocarditis, 442
Veins, 373, 373*f*
  of lower extremity, 407*f*
  varicose, 416–420, 420*f*
Velcade; *See* Bortezomib
Veltin Gel, 968

Vena cava filter, 416
Venereal warts, 942*t*
Venlafaxine, 1056*t*
Venogram, 378*t*
Venous disorders, 408*t*, 414–416
  chronic venous insufficiency in,
    420–421, 421*f*
  community care in, 423
  deep vein thrombosis in, 415–416, 415*f*
  superficial thrombophlebitis in, 414–415
  varicose veins in, 416–420, 420*f*
  venous stasis ulcers in, 420–421, 421*f*
  venous thrombosis in, 414–415
Venous spasm in intravenous therapy, 54*t*
Venous stasis ulcer, 421–422, 421*f*
Venous thrombosis, 406
  fracture-related, 741
  postoperative, 85
Ventilation, 260*b*
  postoperative, 84
Ventilation-perfusion scan, 265*t*, 378*t*
Ventilator-acquired pneumonia,
  296–297, 327*b*
Ventolin; *See* Albuterol
Ventricular aneurysm, 461*t*
Ventricular fibrillation, 437*f*, 440
Ventricular tachycardia, 437*f*, 438–440
Ventriculoperitoneal shunt, 541, 541*f*
Venturi mask, 323*t*
Venule, 373
Verapamil, 402*t*, 438*t*
Verelan; *See* Verapamil
Vertebral column, 717*f*
Vertebral fracture, osteoporosis-related, 757
Vertebroplasty, 757
Verteporfin, 609–610
Vertical auto profile, 378*t*
Vertical banded gastroplasty, 640–660
Vertical compression of spine, 511*f*
Vertigo, 589
Vesicants, 163, 1007*t*
Vesicare; *See* Solifenacin
Vesicle, 959*t*
Vesicular breath sounds, 264*t*
Vestibular nerve, 580*f*
Video-assisted thoracoscopic surgery, 315
Vigabatrin, 525*b*
Vimpat; *See* Lacosamide
Viral hemorrhagic fevers, 1014–1015
Viral infection
  in acquired immunodeficiency syndrome,
    221; *See also* Acquired
    immunodeficiency syndrome
  cutaneous, 970–972
    herpes simplex virus in, 970–971,
      970*b*, 970*f*
    herpes zoster in, 971–972, 971*b*,
      971*f*, 972*b*
  in hepatitis
    avoiding contraction of, 625*b*
    complementary and alternative medicine
      for, 699*b*, 701*b*
    complications of, 701
    diagnosis of, 695–696, 696*t*
    etiology and pathophysiology of, 694
    focused assessment in, 698*b*
    home care considerations in, 699*b*
    liver cancer risk and, 149
    prevention of, 699–701
    signs and symptoms of, 694–695, 695*t*
    treatment of, 696–698, 696*t*
  in meningitis, 543
  in rhinitis, 277–279, 278*t*, 279*b*
  sexually transmitted, 940*b*
  type 1 diabetes mellitus and, 858

Viread; *See* Tenofovir
Virtual colonoscopy, 625–631, 626*t*
Virus, 102, 149
Visceral pain, 125, 125*t*
Vistaril; *See* Hydroxyzine
Visual acuity, 574*t*
Visual examination of ear, 582–583, 583*f*
Visual fields test, 574*t*
Visual impairment, 571
  community care in, 579
  diagnostic tests and examinations in, 573,
    573*f*, 574*t*
  falls and, 610*b*
  in glaucoma, 601
  history taking in, 573–576
  nursing interventions for, 578–579,
    579*b*
  physical examination in, 576
  prevention of, 572, 573*f*
  resources for, 611–612
Visual pain scale, 129, 129*f*
Visual pathway, 569, 570*f*
Visudyne; *See* Verteporfin
Vital capacity, 268, 269*f*
Vital signs, postoperative, 83*b*
Vitamin(s)
  beneficial to vision, 571*b*
  for blood disorders, 349*t*
  for chronic renal failure, 804*t*
  for liver disorders, 696*t*
Vitamin B_1
  for liver disorders, 696*t*
  for substance abuse, 1069*t*, 1071
Vitamin B_6
  in erythropoiesis, 335*b*
  for migraine, 546*b*
Vitamin B_{12}, 367
  for chronic renal failure, 804*t*
  deficiency of, 244*t*
  in erythropoiesis, 335*b*
Vitamin C
  for cystitis, 788*b*
  in erythropoiesis, 335*b*
  foods high in, 89*b*
  intake for immobilized patient, 743*b*
  iron and, 366–367
  wound healing and, 89
Vitamin D
  decreased risk for falls and, 724*b*
  intake for immobilized patient, 743*b*
  in prevention of tuberculosis, 299*b*
Vitamin E, 701*b*
Vitamin K, 696*t*
Vitrectomy, 607*b*
Vivitrol; *See* Naltrexone
Voiding, 766
  changes in pattern of, 774
  pain in, 775
Volume-cycled ventilator, 325
Volvulus, 668, 669*f*
Vomiting, 35–38, 35*b*
  in appendicitis, 672
  in bowel ischemia, 670
  cancer treatment-related, 167
  dietary guidelines for, 649*b*
  drug therapy for, 37*t*
  in gallbladder disorders, 691*t*
  in gastroenteritis, 649
  in gastrointestinal system disorders, 635
  in Mèniére's disease,
    613–614
  in pancreatic cancer, 712
  in peritonitis, 673
von Recklinghausen's disease, 846–847, 846*b*,
  846*t*

von Willebrand disease, 361
Vulva, 881
  cancer of, 907
  inflammation of, 906
  self-examination of, 894
Vulvectomy, 901*t*

W
Waist-to-hip ratio, 641
Walking boot, 739–740, 739*f*
Warfarin, 434*b*, 533*b*
Wart, venereal, 942*t*
Washed red blood cells, 363*t*
Wasp sting, 1031
Wasting syndrome in acquired
  immunodeficiency syndrome, 229
Water, sources of and loss of, 31*t*
Water and food safety in disaster, 1003–1006,
  1003*b*, 1006*b*
Water safety, 1019–1020, 1020*f*
Water-seal drainage system, 316*f*
Waterborne communicable diseases, 1004*t*
Weakness
  in diabetes insipidus, 836
  in diabetes mellitus, 859
Weber's test, 583, 584*t*
Wegener's granulomatosis, 244*t*
Weight
  fluid gain or loss and, 35*b*
  obtaining daily, 58*b*
Weight loss
  in cancer, 166–167
  in elderly, 860*b*
  for hypertension, 405
  in inflammatory bowel disease, 671
  in liver cancer, 708
  in pancreatic cancer, 712
  in type 1 diabetes mellitus, 859
Welchol; *See* Colesevelam
Wellbutrin; *See* Bupropion
Wenckebach heart block, 436
Wernicke's encephalopathy, 1071
West Nile virus, 294*b*
Western blot, 219, 219*b*
Wet age-related macular degeneration, 609
Wet compress, 963
Wheal, 241, 957, 959*t*
Wheezing, 263–264
Whipple procedure, 712
Whisper test, 583
White blood cell, 332–333
  leukemia and, 355–359
    etiology of, 355, 355*t*
    nursing care plan for, 357*b*
    risk factors for, 152*t*
    signs and symptoms of,
      355–356
    treatment of, 356–357, 356*b*
White blood cell count, 207*t*
White blood cell transfusion, 363*t*
White noise, 589–590
Whitehead, 967–968
Whole grains, 856*b*
Wildfire, 999*b*
Winter itch, 958
Withdrawal, 1066*b*, 1068–1071
  from benzodiazepines, 1072–1073
  from opiates, 1073
Women's health care; *See also* Female
  reproductive disorders
  breast cancer and, 909–915
    breast reconstructive surgery for, 912,
      913*f*
    early detection of, 153*b*

Women's health care; (*Continued*)
   etiology and pathophysiology of,
     909–910
   legal and ethical considerations in,
     910*b*
   metastasis of, 171*t*
   nursing care plan for breast lumpectomy
     and, 911*b*
   postmastectomy exercises and, 914*f*
   prevention of, 910
   risk factors for, 152*t*, 909*b*
   signs and symptoms of, 910
   stages of, 909*t*
   treatment of, 910–912, 912*f*
  cardiovascular disease and, 375, 375*b*
  cultural considerations in, 894*b*
  diagnostic tests in, 892–893, 895*t*
  health screening and assessments in,
    892–894
Wong Baker FACES Pain Rating Scale,
  129*f*
Wood's light inspection, 957
Word salad, 1109
World Health Organization classification for
  HIV infection and staging, 221*b*
Worms, 103
Wound care
  in burn injury, 986–988
  postoperative assessment in, 83*b*

Wound healing, 89–90
  dehiscence and evisceration and, 91–93, 93*f*
  drains and, 90, 90*f*, 91*f*
  dressings and, 90
  postoperative complications and,
    90–94, 92*t*
  primary intention, 89*t*
  removal of sutures and staples and,
    90, 91*f*
  wound infection and, 91
Wound infection, 91, 92*t*, 113*t*
Wound-related diseases, 1004*t*
Wrist drop, 728, 728*f*
Wrist splint, 730*f*
Wytensin; *See* Guanabenz

X

Xanax; *See* Alprazolam
Xanthelasma, 577*f*
Xeloda; *See* Capecitabine
Xenical; *See* Orlistat
Xenograft for burn injury, 986–987
Xenon computed tomography, 481*t*
Xerography, 720*t*
Xgera; *See* Denosumab
Xolair; *See* Omalizumab
Xopenex; *See* Levalbuterol
Xylocaine; *See* Lidocaine

Y

Yeast infection, 907*t*, 939
Yellow fever, 1004*t*
Yersinia pestis, 1011*t*, 1013
Yoga, 746*b*

Z

Zafirlukast, 308*t*
Zantac; *See* Ranitidine
Zarontin; *See* Ethosuximide
Zaroxolyn; *See* Metolazone
Zeaxanthin, 571
Zebeta; *See* Bisoprolol
Zegerid; *See* Omeprazole and sodium
  bicarbonate
Zetia; *See* Ezetimibe
Zileuton, 308*t*
Zocor; *See* Simvastatin
Zofran; *See* Ondansetron
Zoloft; *See* Sertraline
Zonegran; *See* Zonisamide
Zonisamide, 525*b*
Zosyn; *See* Piperacillin tazobactam
Zyban; *See* Bupropion
Zyflo; *See* Zileuton
Zygote intrafallopian transfer, 890*b*
Zyrtec; *See* Cetirizine

NANDA-I–Approved Nursing Diagnoses, 2012-2014

Domain 1: Health Promotion

Class 1: Health Awareness
Deficient Diversional Activity (00097)
Sedentary Lifestyle (00168)

Class 2: Health Management 153
Deficient Community Health (00215)*
Risk-Prone Health Behavior (00188)†
Ineffective Health Maintenance (00099)
Readiness for Enhanced Immunization Status (00186)
Ineffective Protection (00043)
Ineffective Self-Health Management (00078)
Readiness for Enhanced Self-Health Management (00162)†
Ineffective Family Therapeutic Regimen Management (00080)

Domain 2: Nutrition

Class 1: Ingestion
Insufficient Breast Milk (00216)*
Ineffective Infant Feeding Pattern (00107)
Imbalanced Nutrition: Less Than Body Requirements (00002)
Imbalanced Nutrition: More Than Body Requirements (00001)
Readiness for Enhanced Nutrition (00163)
Risk for Imbalanced Nutrition: More Than Body Requirements (00003)
Impaired Swallowing (00103)

Class 2: Digestion

Class 3: Absorption

Class 4: Metabolism
Risk for Unstable Blood Glucose Level (00179)
Neonatal Jaundice (00194)
Risk for Neonatal Jaundice (00230)*
Risk for Impaired Liver Function (00178)

Class 5: Hydration
Risk for Electrolyte Imbalance (00195)
Readiness for Enhanced Fluid Balance (00160)
Deficient Fluid Volume (00027)
Excess Fluid Volume (00026)
Risk for Deficient Fluid Volume (00028)
Risk for Imbalanced Fluid Volume (00025)

Domain 3: Elimination and Exchange

Class 1: Urinary Function
Functional Urinary Incontinence (00020)
Overflow Urinary Incontinence (00176)
Reflex Urinary Incontinence (00018)
Stress Urinary Incontinence (00017)
Urge Urinary Incontinence (00019)
Risk for Urge Urinary Incontinence (00022)
Impaired Urinary Elimination (00016)
Readiness for Enhanced Urinary Elimination (00166)
Urinary Retention (00023)

Class 2: Gastrointestinal Function
Constipation (00011)
Perceived Constipation (00012)
Risk for Constipation (00015)
Diarrhea (00013)
Dysfunctional Gastrointestinal Motility (00196)
Risk for Dysfunctional Gastrointestinal Motility (00197)
Bowel Incontinence (00014)

Class 3: Integumentary Function

Class 4: Respiratory Function
Impaired Gas Exchange (00030)

Domain 4: Activity/Rest

Class 1: Sleep/Rest
Insomnia (00095)
Sleep Deprivation (00096)
Readiness for Enhanced Sleep (00165)
Disturbed Sleep Pattern (00198)

Class 2: Activity/Exercise
Risk for Disuse Syndrome (00040)
Impaired Bed Mobility (00091)
Impaired Physical Mobility (00085)
Impaired Wheelchair Mobility (00089)
Impaired Transfer Ability (00090)
Impaired Walking (00088)

Class 3: Energy Balance
Disturbed Energy Field (00050)
Fatigue (00093)
Wandering (00154)

Class 4: Cardiovascular/Pulmonary Responses
Activity Intolerance (00092)
Risk for Activity Intolerance (00094)
Ineffective Breathing Pattern (00032)
Decreased Cardiac Output (00029)
Risk for Ineffective Gastrointestinal Perfusion (00202)
Risk for Ineffective Renal Perfusion (00203)
Impaired Spontaneous Ventilation (00033)
Ineffective Peripheral Tissue Perfusion (00204)
Risk for Decreased Cardiac Tissue Perfusion (00200)†
Risk for Ineffective Cerebral Tissue Perfusion (00201)
Risk for Ineffective Peripheral Tissue Perfusion (00228)*
Dysfunctional Ventilatory Weaning Response (00034)

Class 5: Self-Care
Impaired Home Maintenance (00098)
Readiness for Enhanced Self-Care (00182)
Bathing Self-Care Deficit (00108)
Dressing Self-Care Deficit (00109)†
Feeding Self-Care Deficit (00102)
Toileting Self-Care Deficit (00110)
Self-Neglect (00193)†

Domain 5: Perception/Cognition

Class 1: Attention
Unilateral Neglect (00123)

Class 2: Orientation
Impaired Environmental Interpretation Syndrome (00127)

Class 3: Sensation/Perception

Class 4: Cognition
Acute Confusion (00128)
Chronic Confusion (00129)
Risk for Acute Confusion (00173)
Ineffective Impulse Control (00222)*
Deficient Knowledge (00126)
Readiness for Enhanced Knowledge (00161)
Impaired Memory (00131)

Class 5: Communication
Readiness for Enhanced Communication (00157)
Impaired Verbal Communication (00051)

Domain 6: Self-Perception

Class 1: Self-Concept
Hopelessness (00124)
Risk for Compromised Human Dignity (00174)
Risk for Loneliness (00054)
Disturbed Personal Identity (00121)
Risk for Disturbed Personal Identity (00225)*
Readiness for Enhanced Self-Concept (00167)

Class 2: Self-Esteem
Chronic Low Self-Esteem (00119)
Situational Low Self-Esteem (00120)
Risk for Chronic Low Self-Esteem (00224)*
Risk for Situational Low Self-Esteem (00153)

Class 3: Body Image
Disturbed Body Image (00118)

Domain 7: Role Relationships

Class 1: Caregiving Roles
Ineffective Breastfeeding (00104)
Interrupted Breastfeeding (00105)
Readiness for Enhanced Breastfeeding (00106)*
Caregiver Role Strain (00061)
Risk for Caregiver Role Strain (00062)
Impaired Parenting (00056)
Readiness for Enhanced Parenting (00164)
Risk for Impaired Parenting (00057)

Class 2: Family Relationships
Risk for Impaired Attachment (00058)*
Dysfunctional Family Processes (00063)†